Cambridge textbook
of accident and emergency
medicine

Cambridge textbook of accident and emergency medicine

EDITED BY

David Skinner

Accident and Emergency Department,
John Radcliffe Hospital, Oxford, UK

Andrew Swain

Accident and Emergency Department,
General Hospital, Weston-super-Mare, UK

Rodney Peyton

Department of Surgery, South Tyrone Hospital,
Dungannon, Northern Ireland

and

Colin Robertson

Accident and Emergency Department,
Royal Infirmary, Edinburgh, UK

PROJECT CO-ORDINATOR

Fiona Whimster

Bart's City Life Saver, St Bartholomew's Hospital,
London, UK

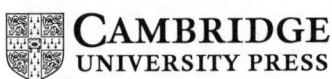

CAMBRIDGE
UNIVERSITY PRESS

PUBLISHED BY THE PRESS SYNDICATE OF THE UNIVERSITY OF CAMBRIDGE
The Pitt Building, Trumpington Street, Cambridge CB2 1RP, United Kingdom

CAMBRIDGE UNIVERSITY PRESS
The Edinburgh Building, Cambridge CB2 2RU, United Kingdom
40 West 20th Street, New York, NY 10011-4211, USA
10 Stamford Road, Oakleigh, Melbourne 3166, Australia

First published in 1997

Printed in the United Kingdom at the University Press, Cambridge

Typeset in Monotype Times New Roman

A catalogue record for this book is available from the British Library

Every effort has been made in preparing this book to provide
accurate and up-to-date information which is in accord with
accepted standards and practice at the time of publication.
Nevertheless,the authors, editors and publisher can make no
warranties that the information contained herein is totally free
from error, not least because clinical standards are constantly
changing through research and regulation. The authors, editors and
publisher therefore disclaim all liability for direct or consequential
damages resulting from the use of material contained in this book.
The reader is strongly advised to pay careful attention to
information provided by the manufacturer of any drugs or
equipment that they plan to use.

  The editors would also like to remind readers of the usage of μg
for micrograms and that particular care should always be taken
when reading and writing dosage figures.

ISBN 0 521 43379 7   hardback

To Juliet

Who has already endured, without complaint, both a major accident and a major emergency.

Contents

List of contributors   ix
Foreword   xiii

PART I GENERAL PRINCIPLES   1

1 The accident and emergency department   3
   D. Skinner, L. Hadfield-Law, M. Deahl,
   A. Copeman and A. Swain

2 Airway management   22
   M.J.A. Parr, J.P. Nolan and P.J.F. Baskett

3 Cardiac arrest and cardiopulmonary resuscitation in adults   62
   C.E. Robertson

4 Cardiopulmonary resuscitation in children   81
   R.M. Bingham

5 Early management of the multiply injured patient   100
   K.I. Maull

6 Shock   118
   I.McA. Ledingham

7 Fluid, electrolyte and acid–base balance   140
   J. Harris, S. Harrod and D. Watson

8 Anaphylaxis   159
   A.G. Bird

9 Coma: initial assessment and management   167
   C. Grange and D. Watson

10 Analgesia and anaesthesia   183
   J.P. Nolan and P.J.F. Baskett

11 Poisoning   206
   J.A. Henry

12 Wound care   235
   J. Heyworth

13 Hospital response to disasters in the UK   257
   M.C. Gavalas and S.A.D. Miles

14 Prehospital care   284
   A: Prehospital care and the ambulance service   284
   M. Ward and M. Willis

B(i): Prehospital cardiac care I: An overview   288
   M. Eisenberg

B(ii): Prehospital cardiac care II: European and American perspectives   298
   R.O. Cummins and J.R. Graves

C(i): Prehospital care of the trauma patient   326
   P.L. Lane

C(ii): Interhospital transport of the trauma patient   340
   P.L. Lane

15 Radiology—emergency imaging   349
   J.G. Murray, J.J. Curtin and G.J. de Lacey

16 Deaths   395
   C. McLauchlan

PART II TRAUMA   409

17 Concepts of trauma management—epidemiology, mechanisms and prevention   411
   P.E. Collicott

18 Head injuries   420
   D. Gentleman, R. Bradford and G. Dunwoody

19 Faciomaxillary and dental emergencies   439
   A: Faciomaxillary and dental trauma   439
   I. Hutchison
   B. Oral and maxillofacial diseases   459
   I. Hutchison

20 Ear, nose and throat emergencies   481
   V.J. Lund and D.J. Howard

21 Ocular trauma and emergencies   498
   R.J. Cooling

22 Trauma to the spine and spinal cord   510
   A. Swain

23 Chest and cardiac trauma   533
   P.A. Driscoll, C.L. Gwinnutt and T.R. Graham

24 Abdominal trauma   558
   B.J. Rowlands

25 Urological trauma 569
R.S. Kirby and S.A.V. Holmes

26 Management of open fractures 581
A.J. Forester and S.P.F. Hughes

27 Hand injury 589
I.W.R. Anderson and A. Sen

28 Upper limb injuries 601
K.M. Willett

29 Paediatric orthopaedics 618
M. Bell

30 Injuries of the lower limb 633
M. Pearse and M. Jackson

31 Injury to the pelvis and proximal femur 648
M. Bircher

32 Sports injuries 659
N. Tubbs

33 Special trauma cases 680
A. Paediatric trauma 680
T.D. Bell and B.L. Enderson
B: Trauma in pregnancy 702
P. Nash
C: Trauma in the elderly 708
G. Hughes
D: Rape, sexual assault and female genital injuries 716
P. Nash

34 Burns and scalds 721
J.M. Ryan

35 Chemical and radiation injuries 733
T. Daynes and A.D. Redmond

36 Electrical and lightning injuries 742
J. Wardrope

37 Near drowning and diving injuries 751
D. Steedman

38 Hypothermia and cold injury 765
E.L. Lloyd

39 Hyperthermia 787
M.T. Ali and J.H. Coakley

40 Ballistic injuries 798
J.W.R. Peyton

41 Rehabilitation of soft tissue injuries 805
N.S.T. Gendi and J. Outhwaite

42 Physiotherapy: the contribution 812
H.R. Trundle

43 Envenomation 822
A.F.T. Brown

PART III MEDICAL, SURGICAL AND
OBSTETRIC EMERGENCIES 837

44 Adult respiratory emergencies 839
K. Jones and F. Morris

45 Cardiovascular emergencies 866
A: Cardiovascular emergencies (excluding arrhythmias) 866
R. Vincent and D.A. Chamberlain
B: Cardiac arrhythmias 897
T.A. Millane and A.J. Camm

46 Vascular emergencies 931
D.C. Mitchell and R.F.M. Wood

47 The acute abdomen 951
B.D. George and R. Campbell

48 Urogenital diseases 969
C.A. Carne and N. Bullock

49 Haematological emergencies, blood products and blood transfusion 978
H.-A. Doughty and M.F. Murphy

50 Acute orthopaedic conditions 1003
H. Ware

51 Inflamed joints and soft tissues 1014
C.B. Colaço and A. Wilson

52 Dermatological emergencies 1029
H.L. Cugnoni and D.W.S. Harris

53 Neurological emergencies 1057
M.K. Sharief and P. Anand

54 The management of psychiatric emergencies 1078
W.D.A. Bruce-Jones and P.D. White

55 Deliberate self-harm and substance misuse 1091
C.V.R. Blacker and B. Charnaud

56 Endocrine emergencies 1102
R. Sheaves and J. Wass

57 Diabetic emergencies 1120
J. Anderson and E. Gale

58 Obstetric emergencies 1137
P. Nash and J. Price

59 Gynaecological emergencies 1148
C. Gilling-Smith, L. Regan and R. Touquet

60 Paediatric emergencies 1173
E.M. Molyneux

61 Management of non-accidental injury 1213
T.F. Beattie

62 Care of the elderly 1220
C. Bowman

63 The febrile patient 1228
A.D. Harries and C. Parry

Index 1251

Contributors

ALI, M.T., Intensive Care Unit, St Bartholomew's Hospital, London, UK

ANAND, P., Department of Neurology, London Hospital Medical College and Royal London Hospital, London, UK

ANDERSON, I.W.R., Department of Accident and Emergency Medicine, Victoria Infirmary, Glasgow, UK

ANDERSON, J., Department of Diabetes and Metabolism, St Bartholomew's Hospital, London, UK

BASKETT, P.J.F., Department of Anaesthesia, Frenchay Hospital, Bristol, UK

BEATTIE, T.F., Accident and Emergency Department, Royal Hospital for Sick Children, Edinburgh, UK

BELL, M., Orthopaedic Department, Royal Hallamshire Hospital, Sheffield, UK

BELL, T.D., Department of Surgery, University of Tennessee Memorial Hospital, Knoxville, Tennessee, USA

BINGHAM, R.M., Department of Anaesthesia, Great Ormond Street Hospital for Sick Children, London, UK

BIRCHER, M., Department of Orthopaedics, St George's Hospital, London, UK

BIRD, A.G., Department of Immunology, Oxford Radcliffe Hospital NHS Trust, Oxford, UK

BLACKER, C.V.R., Department of Psychiatry, Cornwall Healthcare Trust, Royal Cornwall Hospital, Truro, UK

BOWMAN, C., Department of Gerontology, General Hospital, Weston-super-Mare, UK

BRADFORD, R., Department of Neurosurgery, Royal Free Hospital, London, UK

BROWN, A.F.T., Department of Emergency Medicine, Royal Brisbane Hospital, Queensland, Australia

BRUCE-JONES, W.D.A., Bath Mental Health Care Trust, Royal United Hospital, Bath, UK

BULLOCK, N., Departments of Genitourinary Medicine and Urology, Addenbrooke's NHS Trust, Cambridge, UK

CAMM, A.J., Department of Cardiological Sciences, St George's Hospital Medical School, London, UK

CAMPBELL, R., Department of General Surgery, South Tyrone Hospital, Dungannon, Northern Ireland

CARNE, C.A., Departments of Genitourinary Medicine and Urology, Addenbrooke's NHS Trust, Cambridge, UK

CHAMBERLAIN, D.A., Department of Cardiology, Royal Sussex County Hospital, Brighton, UK

CHARNAUD, B., Trengweath Mental Health Unit, Redruth, UK

COAKLEY, J.H., Intensive Care Unit, St Bartholomew's Hospital, London, UK

COLAÇO, C.B., Department of Rheumatology, Central Middlesex Hospital, London, UK

COLLICOTT, P.E., Department of Surgery, University of Nebraska Medical Center, Lincoln, Nebraska, USA

COOLING, R.J., Moorfields Eye Hospital NHS Trust, London, UK

COPEMAN, A., Accident and Emergency Department, Whipps Cross Hospital, London, UK

CUGNONI, H.L., Accident and Emergency Department, Royal Hospitals Trust, London, UK

CUMMINS, R.O., Emergency Medicine Service, University of Washington Medical Center, Seattle, Washington, USA

CURTIN, J.J., Radiology Department, Northwick Park Hospital, Harrow, UK

DAYNES, T., Accident and Emergency Department, North Staffordshire Hospital, Stoke on Trent, UK

DEAHL, M., Department of Psychological Medicine, St Bartholomew's Hospital, London, UK

DE LACEY, G.J., Radiology Department, Northwick Park Hospital, Harrow, UK

DOUGHTY, H.-A., South Thames Blood Transfusion Service, London, UK

DRISCOLL, P.A., Department of Emergency Medicine, Hope Hospital, Salford, UK

DUNWOODY, G., Department of Neurosurgery, Royal Free Hospital, London, UK

EISENBERG, M., Emergency Medicine Service, University of Washington Medical Center, Seattle, Washington, USA

ENDERSON, B.L., Department of Surgery, University of Tennessee Memorial Hospital, Knoxville, Tennessee, USA

FORESTER, A.J., Department of Orthopaedic Surgery, Hammersmith Hospital, London, UK

GALE, E., Department of Diabetes and Metabolism, St Bartholomew's Hospital, London, UK

GAVALAS, M.C., Accident and Emergency Department, University College Hospital, London, UK

GENDI, N.S.T., Rheumatology Department, Basildon Hospital, Basildon, UK

GENTLEMAN, D., Department of Neurosurgery, Dundee Royal Infirmary, Dundee, UK

GEORGE, B.D., Department of General Surgery, John Radcliffe Hospital, Oxford, UK

GILLING-SMITH, C., Department of Obstetrics and Gynaecology, St Mary's Hospital, London, UK

GRAHAM, T.R., Department of Cardiothoracic Surgery, Queen Elizabeth Hospital, Birmingham, UK

GRANGE, C., Department of Anaesthesia and Intensive Care Medicine, St Bartholomew's Hospital, London, UK

GRAVES. J.R., Center for Evaluation of Emergency Medical Services, Seattle-King County Department of Public Health, Seattle, Washington, USA

GWINNUTT, C.L., Department of Anaesthesia, Hope Hospital, Salford, UK

HADFIELD-LAW, L., Accident and Emergency Department, John Radcliffe Hospital, Oxford, UK

HARRIES, A.D., Department of Medicine, Queen Elizabeth Central Hospital, Blantyre, Malawi, Central Africa

HARRIS, D.W.S., Department of Dermatology, The Whittington Hospital NHS Trust, London, UK

HARRIS, J., Department of Anaesthesia, Northwick Park Hospital, Harrow, UK

HARROD, S., Department of Anaesthesia and Intensive Care Medicine, St Bartholomew's Hospital, London, UK

HENRY, J.A., Medical Toxicology Unit, Guy's Hospital, London, UK

HEYWORTH, J., Accident and Emergency Department, Southampton General Hospital, Southampton, UK

HOLMES, S.A.V., Department of Urology, St Mary's Hospital, Portsmouth, UK

HOWARD, D.J., Institute of Laryngology and Otology, London, UK

HUGHES, G., Department of Accident and Emergency Medicine, Bristol Royal Infirmary, Bristol, UK

HUGHES, S.P.F., Department of Orthopaedic Surgery, Hammersmith Hospital, London, UK

HUTCHISON, I., Department of Oral and Maxillofacial Surgery, St Bartholomew's Hospital, London, UK

JACKSON, M., Department of Orthopaedic Surgery, Bristol Royal Infirmary, Bristol, UK

JONES, K., Chest and Heart Unit, Bury General Hospital, Bury, UK

KIRBY, R.S., Department of Urology, St Bartholomew's Hospital, London, UK

LANE, P.L., Trauma Services, Victoria Hospital, London, Ontario, Canada

LEDINGHAM, I.McA., Department of Emergency and Critical Care Medicine, Faculty of Medicine and Health Sciences, United Arab Emirates University, Al-Ain, UAE

LLOYD, E.L., Department of Anaesthesia, Western General Hospital, Edinburgh, UK

LUND, V.J., Institute of Laryngology and Otology, London, UK

MAULL, K.I., Department of Surgery, Stritch School of Medicine, Loyola University, Maywood, Illinois, USA

McLAUCHLAN, C., Accident and Emergency Department, Royal Devon and Exeter Hospital, Exeter, UK

MILES, S.A.D., Accident and Emergency Department, Royal Hospitals' Trust, London, UK

MILLANE, T.A., Adolph Besser Institute of Cardiology, Royal Alexandra Hospital for Children, Sydney, NSW, Australia

MITCHELL, D.C., Department of Vascular Surgery, Southmead Hospital, Bristol, UK

MOLYNEUX, E.M., Accident and Emergency Department, Royal Liverpool Children's Hospital NHS Trust, Liverpool, UK

MORRIS, F., Accident and Emergency Department, Northern General Hospital, Sheffield, UK

MURPHY, M.F., Department of Haematology, St Bartholomew's Hospital, London, UK

MURRAY, J.G., Radiology Department, Northwick Park Hospital, Harrow, UK

NASH, P., Accident and Emergency Department, Neath General Hospital, Neath, UK

NOLAN, J.P., Department of Anaesthesia, Royal United Hospital, Bath, UK

OUTHWAITE, J., The Nuffield Orthopaedic Centre, Oxford, UK

PARR, M.J.A., Department of Anaesthesia, Frenchay Hospital, Bristol, UK

PARRY, C., Wellcome Trust Clinical Research Unit, Centre for Tropical Diseases, Cho Quan Hospital, Ho Chi Minh City, Viet Nam *and* Centre for Tropical Medicine, John Radcliffe Hospital, Oxford, UK

PEARSE, M., Department of Orthopaedic Surgery, Charing Cross Hospital, London, UK

PEYTON, J.W.R., Department of Surgery, South Tyrone Hospital, Dungannon, Northern Ireland

PRICE, J., Obstetrics and Gynaecology Department, Hillingdon Hospital, Uxbridge, UK

REDMOND, A.D., Accident and Emergency Department, North Staffordshire Hospital, Stoke on Trent, UK

REGAN, L., Department of Obstetrics and Gynaecology, St Mary's Hospital, London, UK

ROBERTSON, C.E., Accident and Emergency Department, Royal Infirmary, Edinburgh, UK

ROWLANDS, B.J., Department of Surgery, The Queen's University of Belfast, Belfast, Northern Ireland

RYAN, J.M., The Leonard Cheshire Department of Conflict Recovery, University College Hospital, London, UK

SEN, A., Department of Accident and Emergency Medicine, Victoria Infirmary, Glasgow, UK

SHARIEF, M.K., Department of Neurology, London Hospital Medical College and Royal London Hospital, London, UK

SHEAVES, R., Department of Endocrinology, Jersey General Hospital, Jersey, CI

SKINNER, D., Accident and Emergency Department, John Radcliffe Hospital, Oxford, UK

STEEDMAN, D., Department of Accident and Emergency Medicine, Royal Infirmary, Edinburgh, UK

SWAIN, A., Accident and Emergency Department, General Hospital, Weston-super-Mare, UK

TOUQUET, R., Department of Accident and Emergency Medicine, St Mary's Hospital, London, UK

TRUNDLE, H.R., Trauma Service, John Radcliffe Hospital, Oxford, UK

TUBBS, N., Department of Trauma and Orthopaedic Surgery, University Hospital Birmingham, Birmingham. UK

VINCENT, R., Department of Cardiology, Royal Sussex County Hospital, Brighton, UK

WARD, M., Nuffield Department of Anaesthesia, John Radcliffe Hospital, Oxford, UK

WARDROPE, J., Department of Accident and Emergency Medicine, Northern General Hospital NHS Trust, Sheffield, UK

WARE, H., Department of Orthopaedic Surgery, Chase Farm Hospital, Enfield, Middlesex, UK

WASS, J., Department of Endocrinology, Radcliffe Infirmary, Oxford, UK

WATSON, D., Department of Anaesthesia and Intensive Care Medicine, St Bartholomew's Hospital, London, UK

WHITE, P.D., Department of Psychological Medicine, St Bartholomew's Hospital, London, UK

WILLETT, K. M., Trauma Service, John Radcliffe Hospital, Oxford, UK

WILLIS, M., Norfolk Ambulance NHS Trust, Norwich, UK

WILSON, A., Accident and Emergency Department, The Royal London Hospital, London, UK

WOOD, R.F.M., Department of Surgery, Northern General Hospital, Sheffield, UK

Foreword

"To study the phenomena of disease without books is to sail an uncharted sea, while to study books without patients is not to go to sea at all."

In his lecture entitled 'Books and Men' given at Boston Medical Library in 1901, Sir William Osler further observed that only a maker of books can appreciate the labours of others at their true value. I hope that Osler was wrong on this one occasion because the labours of those involved in the production of this definitive work deserve the appreciation of all who practise in the field of Accident and Emergency Medicine. Our specialty has a very broad canvas, which encompasses aspects of many disciplines and which has been the subject in recent years of several practical pocket-guides for senior house officers, but there is no current British textbook which combines this breadth with such depth of detail and which so comprehensively expounds the theory behind the practice. A substantial reference and referenced text is one of the hallmarks of a clinical discipline and the publication of this book is final recognition of the emergence of the specialty of Accident and Emergency Medicine.

The first 'Casualty' Consultant in the United Kingdom was the late Maurice Ellis, who was appointed to Leeds General Infirmary in 1952 and who was still the only such Consultant when he retired in 1969. He also wrote the first book relevant to his field of work but the *Casualty Officer's Handbook* was mostly related to aspects of trauma, although there was a final chapter on Resuscitation which concluded with the statement that 'a cardiac surgeon, if available, should be urgently summoned to carry out defibrillation'! The year was 1962 and it was a further decade before a pilot scheme of 30 posts confirmed the value of appointing full-time Consultants in charge of Accident and Emergency Departments, The opening chapter of this book briefly summarizes the ensuing growth of the specialty but there were inevitably those who continued to doubt that it should survive and the last of several national enquiries reported as recently as 1980. The previous year, however, Rutherford *et al.* produced their book on *Accident and Emergency Medicine*, which was a more comprehensive work than any previously available and which undoubtedly contributed to the further recognition of the specialty.

Seventeen years elapsed between the publication of the books by Ellis (1962) and by Rutherford *et al.* (1979) and now, after a similar interval of time, we are privileged to receive this *Cambridge Textbook of Accident and Emergency Medicine*, which will surely remain our standard reference for even longer than its predecessors. During these latter seventeen years, Accident and Emergency Medicine has become an established specialty with the emergence of the British Association for Accident & Emergency Medicine and, more recently, of the Faculty of Accident and Emergency Medicine, which has formal links with no less than six Medical Royal Colleges. These links with Royal Colleges of Medicine, Surgery and Anaesthesia recognize that Accident and Emergency Medicine is not an independent specialty but a specialty which is inter-dependent with all other major clinical disciplines. This has been further recognized by the Editors in their choice of contributors, who include not only many of the leading A&E specialists in the United Kingdom but also specialists from other disciplines and from other countries. It is to be hoped that this book will have a similarly diverse readership and it must find a place in every A&E Department and in every hospital library. Those who practise Accident and Emergency Medicine will never be without patients but they will be at risk of sailing Sir William Osler's 'uncharted sea' if they do not seek guidance from this definitive textbook.

Dr David J. Williams FRCP FFAEM — London
President — August 1996
Faculty of Accident and Emergency Medicine

PART I GENERAL PRINCIPLES

1 The accident and emergency department

D. SKINNER[a], L. HADFIELD-LAW[a], M. DEAHL[b], A. COPEMAN[c] and A. SWAIN[d]

[a] Accident and Emergency Department, John Radcliffe Hospital, Oxford, UK
[b] Department of Psychological Medicine, St Bartholomew's Hospital, London, UK
[c] Accident and Emergency Department, Whipps Cross Hospital, London, UK
[d] Accident and Emergency Department, General Hospital, Weston-super-Mare, UK

Chapter plan

Introduction
A&E department design and equipment
A&E department staffing and training
Trauma teams
Cardiac arrest teams
Protection of staff in A&E
Stress and staff support in the A&E department
Patient rights
A&E department management

INTRODUCTION

The accident and emergency (A&E) department is the avenue through which a significant proportion of in-patients enter hospital. As well as being a route for admission, the A&E department will manage approximately 80% of its patients without admission. A thriving, well-resourced, forward-looking and innovative A&E department is key to the success of the hospital.

In the UK, patients with acute injury or illness currently consult either their general practitioner (primary care physician) or their local A&E department. Approximately 11 million people each year seek urgent medical attention in A&E departments in the UK (National Audit Office, 1992a, b). Increasingly, particularly in inner city areas, the A&E department not only provides traditional A&E care but also acts as a primary care resource for a percentage of its population. A&E attendances and admissions continue to increase, year on year (Hobbs, 1995). Most of the increase in emergency admissions is accounted for by acute medical conditions – ischaemic heart disease and respiratory illness (Edwards & Werneke, 1994).

The speciality of 'accident and emergency medicine' has progressed dramatically over the last 30 years, not only by virtue of its recognition as a speciality but also in the level and sophistication of care provided by A&E specialist doctors and nurses.

In 1962 the Platt Report recommended that 'casualty' departments be renamed 'accident and emergency' departments, to emphasize to the public the nature of the service provided, and to discourage casual attenders. Platt also suggested that an orthopaedic surgeon be clinically and managerially responsible for each A&E department.

This arrangement proved unsatisfactory since these orthopaedic surgeons were expected to continue their orthopaedic practice in addition to running the A&E department. In the late 1960s, the new specialty of 'accident and emergency' was created and, in 1972, 32 full-time consultants were appointed to supervise and manage A&E departments. These initial appointments proved to be a success and by January 1992 there were 242 A&E consultants in post in the UK (BAEM, 1992).

The initial 32 A&E consultants were appointed from trainees in other, mainly surgical, specialties but it soon became clear that A&E needed its own training programme. This began in 1976 when senior registrar posts were created and, more recently, career A&E registrar posts have also been established. Further rationalization of the training grades into one higher specialist training grade will occur in 1996 in accordance with the Calman Report. The entry requirement for higher specialist training in A&E at registrar level is one or more of the following: FRCS (fellowship in general surgery of one of the Royal Colleges of Surgeons), MRCP(UK) (membership of the Royal College of Physicians), FRCA (fellowship of the Royal College of Anaesthetists) or FRCSEd(A&E) which is the specialty's own fellowship. The development of the specialty of A&E is far from

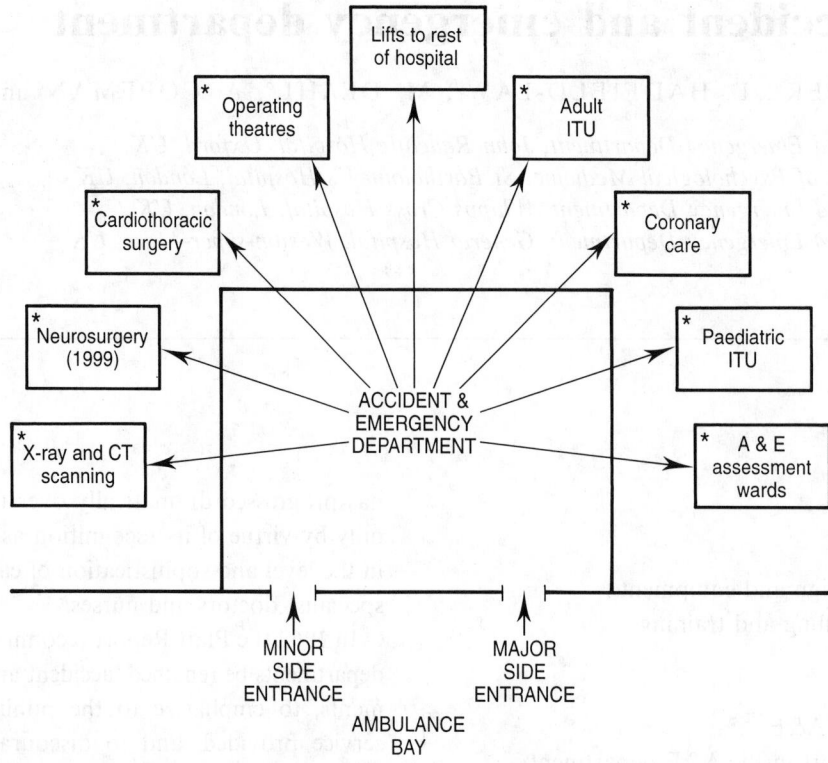

* All on the same level (ground floor) in the hospital as the A & E department

Fig. 1. Relationship of A&E Department to intensive therapy (ITU), coronary care unit (CCU), assessment wards, emergency theatres and X-ray at the John Radcliffe Hospital.

complete with 25% of A&E departments still without an A&E consultant in 1993. Academic departments of A&E are emerging but thus far only three A&E professorial chairs have been established in the UK.

During the time that the specialty has been evolving, the design, sophistication and equipping of A&E departments has developed.

A&E DEPARTMENT DESIGN AND EQUIPMENT

The internal design of an A&E department is crucial to its safe and cost-effective medical, nursing and administrative management. The physical relationship of the A&E department to the rest of the hospital is also critically important for the effective management of patients, particularly those with life-threatening conditions.

Physical relationship of A&E department to the rest of the hospital

Many older style hospitals developed their A&E facility as an offshoot, or extension, of the out-patient department. This area is rarely well sited for the most effective

management of patients. The A&E department should be adjacent, or close, to other critical care areas as well as radiology and CT (computed tomography) scanning. Figure 1 shows the relationship of A&E to the intensive therapy unit, coronary care unit, assessment wards, emergency theatres and X-ray at the John Radcliffe site of the Oxford Radcliffe Hospital. This is an ideal organization of facilities, particularly as they are all sited on level 1 (ground floor), with the ambulance delivery point immediately adjacent. Patients with major injuries are transported directly to the A&E resuscitation room so that, after initial resuscitation, CT scanning can be performed, before transfer to theatre or intensive therapy unit. The proximity of critical care areas is not only beneficial to the patient but also allows cooperation and collaboration between clinicians and nursing staff, both clinically and educationally, which further enhances patient care.

Internal design of the A&E department

Most A&E departments have evolved within existing hospitals and there are relatively few examples of purpose-built facilities. Furthermore, the role of A&E

departments is continually changing. There is therefore no ideal A&E department. In general terms, however, various requirements must be satisfied in order to provide the best service:

1. Easy access for ambulances and the general public.
2. Distinct, ideally separate, access for ambulance and ambulant cases.
3. A close physical relationship between A&E (particularly the resuscitation room) and other critical care areas.
4. A clear distinction between major and minor sides of A&E, arranged so that the nursing and medical staff can move freely between these areas.
5. The resuscitation room must be close to the ambulance entrance. The route from the resuscitation room to CT scanning and other areas should not pass through minor treatment or waiting areas.
6. The trolley and high dependency areas must be arranged so that they can be safely and economically supervised by nursing staff. Nurses must be able to see patients, and vice versa.
7. All patient cubicles must have curtain closure to allow easy egress of staff in the presence of violent patients.
8. Minor cubicles must be easily supervised.
9. The patient waiting area should be welcoming and open-plan, allowing easy surveillance by nursing and security staff.
10. There should be a readily identifiable nursing triage area for the initial assessment of cases on the minor side.
11. There should be a clearly designated reception area affording adequate protection to staff and space for storage of A&E records.
12. There must be fully equipped suture and fracture manipulation theatres.
13. There must be adequate office accommodation for senior medical and nursing staff as well as for a departmental secretary.
14. The department must include a distressed relative/patient interview room with telephone, etc. (see Chapter 16).
15. There must be a rest room for A&E staff.
16. There must be a seminar room for A&E staff teaching and meetings.

A&E equipment

The provision of high-quality equipment is crucially important for the optimal management of A&E patients.

Naturally, the distribution of equipment around the A&E department will depend on the function of each area.

> **Broadly speaking the three areas of most concern are:**
> - The minor side
> - The major side
> - The resuscitation room

The minor side

The equipment required for the cost-effective running of the minor side will be determined by the range of conditions routinely managed. Commonly presenting traumatic conditions, including soft tissue and bony injuries, generate a large workload which can be divided into:

- Assessment, examination, cleansing and closure of wounds (see Chapter 12).
- Assessment and reduction of fractures and dislocations (see Chapters 26–30).

Details of the equipment required for the above will not be discussed here. However, given the large numbers and high turnover of doctors and nurses working in A&E, it is extremely useful to have firm guidelines for suturing techniques, local anaesthetic provision and choice of suture materials. This will ensure a common, high standard of wound care and avoid the use of unnecessarily expensive suture materials. In particular, a standard suture pack should be agreed with the sterile supplies department and minimum standards for sterile technique set within the department. In addition, local policies covering safe practice (e.g. local anaesthesia) will help to avoid disasters which are a constant threat in A&E due to the volume of patients seen and 'round the clock' activity.

Although A&E staff can be expected to deal with a wide variety of fractures and dislocations, reduction techniques and the choice of immobilizing splints should be agreed locally after discussion with orthopaedic colleagues who will usually be responsible for the further care of these patients. Problems can arise, however, with local, regional and general analgesia and anaesthesia techniques (see Chapter 10). Specialist anaesthetic help should be readily sought and available. The days of the single doctor providing both the Bier's block and manipulating the fracture are gladly over. The anaesthetic department should identify an anaesthetic consultant responsible for liaison with the A&E consultant regarding anaesthesia and analgesia in the A&E department.

The major side

The major side of most A&E departments is divided into a series of cubicles. Each cubicle should be large enough to accommodate an A&E trolley leaving adequate space around it for medical and nursing staff and equipment.

Each trolley must have certain basic facilities, including an easily achievable Trendelenberg (head down) position, oxygen cylinder, sucker and other equipment which may be required to sustain or even resuscitate patients being transferred from the A&E department to other hospital areas.

Piped oxygen and suction should be provided to each cubicle which should have a wall-mounted, mains-supplied ophthalmoscope/auroscope. Each cubicle should also have a multidrawer trolley containing, on different trays, the equipment necessary for all procedures likely to be performed in the area (e.g. dressings, catheterization, chest drain insertion, etc.).

Individual A&E departments need to determine which procedures are to be performed in the trolley area, and local policies will clearly dictate the equipment required in each cubicle.

The resuscitation room

Modern A&E departments should be designed with at least three bays in the resuscitation room and these must be equipped to enable all forms of resuscitation, including paediatric, to be performed. Basic equipment in each bay will include: a trolley with head down facility, a trolley-mounted monitor/defibrillator, airway and ventilation equipment and peripheral and central venous cannulation equipment. Several A&E departments have found the provision of an overhead gantry X-ray facility to be extremely valuable for providing high-quality X-rays without disrupting the resuscitation process.

A&E DEPARTMENT STAFFING AND TRAINING

Medical staff

The medical staffing of A&E departments varies widely across the UK. In order to encourage adequate staffing of A&E departments, the British Association for Accident and Emergency Medicine (BAEM) recommended in 1993 staffing levels dependent on patient throughput. They suggested that A&E departments should continue to be consultant-led but should have a full complement of senior house officers (SHOs) together with middle grade medical staff.

Senior house officers

The number of SHOs required is calculated on the assumption that the standard working week is 40 h and it takes into account annual leave and study leave. One SHO working a 40-h week should see 4000 new patients per year and, therefore, for a department seeing 40 000 new patients per year the recommended staffing level would be ten SHOs, if there are no other staff below consultant grade. There is a pro rata reduction of SHOs as their hours increase. The current limit for a UK A&E SHO is 56 hours per week.

Middle and senior grade medical staff

Middle grade staff requirements are calculated, together with SHO numbers, on the basis of the number of doctors required to see a certain workload. A&E consultants are not included in this calculation. Assuming a 40-h week, a department seeing 60 000 new patients per year will require a total staffing level of 15 doctors, including both SHO and middle grade staff. In addition, it is recommended that three full-time consultants would be required for adequate supervision of this number of junior and middle grade staff.

Training grades (registrar and senior registrar)

Registrars and senior registrars are seconded to other specialties during the course of their training and at these times are not available for service work in the A&E department. Approximately 50% of their time is spent on such secondments. In the A&E department they will spend approximately one-third of their time seeing new patients and one-third supervising SHOs and possibly running review clinics. Their contribution to the workload is therefore relatively small.

Although the BAEM issues recommendations concerning appropriate staffing levels, the ratio of senior, middle and junior grades is likely to come under increasing question given the continuing contraction of the junior grades and the implementation of the Calman Report. A change in consultant working practice would seem to be necessary in order to accommodate this reduction in junior doctors and it is certain that significantly larger numbers of consultants will be required in the future.

Nursing staff

Before the emergence of A&E as a specialty, standards of nursing care were, on the whole, minimal and vaguely defined. Nurses assigned to the A&E department were either devoted to their work or, if not, turnover was high. Staffing was scant and correlated to the number of patients seen. Patient registration was completed by nursing staff, as most hospitals could not afford the expense of assigning a clerical officer to the A&E department. Education and training for A&E nurses was derived from work experience. Formal education for the A&E nurse was largely unavailable.

The nature of the A&E workload has changed only slightly over the last few decades. However, standards of patient care, educational sophistication and prehospital management have developed dramatically.

Adequately and specifically trained nursing staff are an essential element in providing quality A&E care. It is no longer acceptable to have any qualified nurse or doctor providing care to patients attending the A&E department.

To ensure recruitment and retention of suitable A&E staff, the senior nurse and A&E consultant should work together. A&E staff should be recruited with a strong emphasis on team work. An effective way of achieving this is by conducting multidisciplinary interviews (Hadfield, 1991).

The A&E service can only be as proficient as those providing that service.

The nurse's role in A&E

Through educational opportunities and the development of A&E as a specialty, the role of the A&E nurse has grown and developed. A specifically trained, committed and energetic A&E nurse can be a mainstay of a well-organized department.

Triage

Triage may be described as a 'process by which a patient is assessed upon arrival, to determine the urgency of their problem, and to designate appropriate health care resources to care for the identified problem' (George, 1976).

In the UK over the last 10–15 years, this role has been assumed by suitably trained and experienced A&E nurses. The process should be carried out in private but with access to other areas of the department (Williams, 1992). Explaining the role of triage and informing patients about waiting times and the system of priority setting, reduces frustration and increases patient satisfaction (Bailey *et al.*, 1987). In addition, a valuable opportunity arises to provide health education whilst the nurse assesses the patient (Rund & Rausch, 1981).

The role of the triage nurse continues to be refined. Particular attention is being paid to this area following the publication of the Patients Charter (Department of Health, 1991) which states that the A&E patient should be seen immediately and the need for treatment assessed.

Expanded nursing practice

The National Audit Office report on A&E services (Murphie & Marsden, 1992) noted the variation in nursing practice between hospitals and the lack of transferability between departments. It seems wasteful, in terms of resources, to allow a nurse to defibrillate and apply plaster of Paris casts in one department, while preventing him/her from doing so in another.

The United Kingdom Central Council's latest guidance ('The Scope of Professional Practice', UKCC, 1992a) emphasizes the nurse's professional accountabilty and places decisions about the boundaries of practice in the hands of the individual practitioner. Its six 'principles' lay down guidelines to help practitioners make those decisions (Carlisle, 1992).

Outdated practices involving the signing, by medical colleagues, of extended role certificates for nurses will no longer be required but will be replaced by a mutual understanding and respect for each others' roles. Clause 4 of the UKCC Code of Conduct, which requires nurses to acknowledge the limits of their competence, underpins the new guidance (UKCC, 1992b). Any functions must lie within those limits and the nurse must be skilled and safe. Hopefully, this will also ensure that patient need is the driving force behind any change in clinical practice.

Skill mix

The search for appropriate skill mix involves a review of the composition of the workforce to establish the best range of skills, using different grades to meet a variety of patient needs. Some consider this initiative merely to be a quest for cost effectiveness (Sheehan, 1993).

Over recent years attention has been drawn to the role of the health care assistant or support workers in A&E. A report commissioned by the Department of Health (University of York, Centre for Health Economics, 1992) suggests that more highly qualified nurses deliver better quality care. It is difficult to justify the use of skill mix to reduce cost if we know that it also reduces quality of care.

Workload versus staffing levels

'The mercurial changes in patient flow and in severity of illness occur hour to hour – day to day – season to season' (Schulmerich, 1984).

The difficulty of matching staffing levels to a constantly fluctuating workload has presented a challenge to managers and clinicians for many years. Traditionally, numbers of staff required were calculated purely on the basis of the number of patients seen per year which, of course, bore no relation to the time and effort consumed by the individual patients. For example, the level of care required by a patient suffering the effects of a hallucinogenic drug far outweighs that required by an individual attending for tetanus immunization following a small cut. This example also supports Vail's theory (1989) that intensity of care does not necessarily relate to seriousness of illness or injury.

In other clinical areas, workload measurements are relatively easy to calculate following patient dependency studies. These place patients in categories according to their care needs, with a view to determining the number of staff and level of skilled care they require.

Problems with devising a similar system for A&E lie with the unpredictable nature of the patients' clinical condition. The range of presenting problems is also wide and varied. Categories based on retrospective studies can be devised but are difficult to validate. Patient turnover is 100% in A&E so such studies can only provide information for staffing averages (Stolley, 1989).

Nevertheless, efforts have been made to determine appropriate A&E nursing staff levels (Buschiazzo, 1984; Kromash, 1984; Butler, 1986; Helmer *et al.*, 1988; Stolley, 1989; Vail, 1989; Connors, 1993).

Other factors should also be considered when matching workload to staffing levels (e.g. geographical layout of the department) (Murphie & Marsden, 1992). The application of set staffing formulae to different hospitals does not seem particularly useful.

Where shortages of staff are evident, working practice, shift arrangements and patterns of patient attendance

should be carefully examined to ensure that the best possible use is made of the resources available. Once evidence is available to show that this has been done, negotiations with A&E service purchasers can begin.

Other staff

In additional to medical and nursing staff, other important groups of personnel are required for the smooth running of an A&E department.

It is essential to have sufficient reception staff to ensure 24 h cover. Most A&E departments are now fully computerized and the reception staff provide an invaluable service in data collection as well as generating medical records after triage.

Radiography staff from the senior grades are usually rostered for A&E work although more junior staff will also work in the A&E department on rotation.

It is essential that physiotherapy is available and some departments now have physiotherapists dedicated to A&E work. They may be based in the A&E department, which is particularly useful as it allows medical and nursing staff to be educated concerning appropriate referrals for physiotherapy.

Portering staff, rostered only to the A&E department, are invaluable. This arrangement encourages teamwork and enables the porters to develop skills specific to A&E work. They often also provide a back-up to security staff when patients become disorderly.

Finally, the smooth running of an A&E department requires an adequate level of support from secretarial and administrative staff.

Medical staff training

Senior house officers

Adequate training of SHOs in the A&E department is essential. Given the diversity of clinical problems it is impossible to totally prepare the new doctor for such a varied workload. For this reason, middle or senior grade staff should always be available to initiate and assist with patient management. At the beginning of each 6-month period the new SHOs should be introduced to the physical organization of the department, and their role within the trauma and cardiac arrest teams must be made clear. Ideally, simulated cardiac and trauma resuscitation scenarios should be organized. It is also desirable that new SHOs should have attended both advanced trauma and cardiac life support courses. Regular teaching sessions, at least once per week, should continue throughout the 6-month post and the department should be staffed by other doctors at these times. Teaching sessions can take on a variety of forms but should include review of interesting X-rays as well as formal case presentations. Tutorials on specific subjects, given by a senior member of A&E staff, should form part of the overall teaching package. Part of the teaching session can also include audit and an invaluable benefit of this regular meeting is the opportunity to discuss individual or collective problems.

Although formal individual performance review may not be essential, SHOs are keen to receive feedback regarding their performance. At the beginning of his/her post, each SHO should ideally be given a 'log book' listing a variety of practical procedures which are likely to be performed during the post. This log should be discussed at the outset and reviewed after 3 months when appropriate adjustments can be made. Formal review should take place near the end of the post when feedback from the SHO is extremely helpful in adjusting teaching and other aspects of junior staff supervision.

Training grades

Guidelines for the training of registrars and senior registrars in A&E are laid down by the Specialist Advisory Committee (SAC, A&E Medicine, Royal College of Physicians). Training posts require approval from the SAC before a position is established, and they are regularly reviewed to ensure that training is satisfactory. One day per week should be allocated for research, and service commitments should not interfere with this.

Communication skills training

Training all staff to be more sensitive to patient needs and to communicate effectively can improve patient outcome and staff morale and reduce risk. One of the first considerations should be why communication is not always effective. Factors may include:

1. Patients who are usually anxious and often dependent.
2. Hospitals frighten lay people.
3. Staff harbour or express hostility to some groups of patients (Shinter & Leddington, 1991).
4. Staff tend only to ask closed questions.
5. Staff frequently interrupt patients.
6. Staff tend not to use 'social cement' with patients (e.g. greetings or introductions) (American Health Consultants Inc., 1989).

Attention can be given to techniques contributing to effective communication, and how these techniques can be taught (Bjorn, 1991).

Data collected by Ward (1990) tentatively suggest that nurses who qualify and then work in A&E may become less welcoming to the patient, more secure in their territory, and less willing to adapt their behaviour to individual patients. Continuing education opportunities covering interpersonal skills are suggested to improve this situation.

TRAUMA TEAMS

All A&E departments should agree with relevant hospital specialties on the form and composition of a trauma team mobilized to manage the multiple injured patient presenting to the A&E department. Driscoll (1992) has shown that survival is enhanced by the use of a well-organized trauma team managing the patient to agreed

---

Responsibilities of members of the trauma team

- Team leader
  - Primary survey
  - Secondary survey
  - Coordinate team effort
  - Overall responsibility for patient while in A&E department
- Anaesthetist
  - Airway control
  - Ventilation
  - Central venous cannulation
  - Fluid balance
- Other doctor
  - All other procedures
  - Chest drain
  - Catheterization
  - Splintage of fractures
  - Removal of clothes, etc.
- Nurses (ideally two)
  - Measure vital signs
  - Record data
  - Removal of clothes
  - Help doctors
  - Attach monitor
- Radiographers
  - Take specific radiographs of cervical spine, chest and pelvis in all patients as soon as possible
  - Coordinate with team
  - Take other radiographs as clinically necessary

Source: *ABC of Major Trauma*, British Medical Journal Publications (1991) Eds Skinner, D., Driscoll, P., Earlam, R.

protocols. Most trauma teams in the UK and North America, as well as elsewhere, manage their patients according to the Advanced Trauma Life Support (ATLS) guidelines produced by the American College of Surgeons Committee on Trauma. Although the ATLS course itself imagines only one doctor and one nurse managing each patient, the system lends itself well to the allocation of tasks to different team members so that a horizontal form of management can take place. The trauma team will comprise both medical and nursing staff with designated, preassigned roles. (For further details on the management of the multiple injured patient refer to Chapter 5.)

CARDIAC ARREST TEAMS

Cardiac arrests in the A&E department are an almost daily occurrence. Depending on staffing levels, the A&E department may be able to provide its own cardiac arrest team for part, or all, of the 24-h period. Clearly it is essential that under these circumstances the team performs to the hospital's Resuscitation Committee guidelines for the management of cardiac arrest. The team will comprise both medical and nursing members and there should be a clearly identified team leader who will not be involved in complex practical procedures but will retain an overview of the entire team's performance. The suggested composition of the cardiac arrest team is shown in Fig 2. (For further details of the management of cardiac arrest, refer to Chapter 3.)

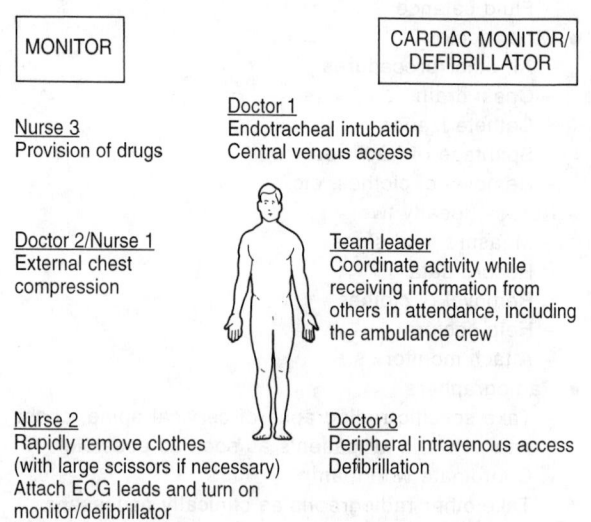

Fig. 2. Roles of the cardiac arrest team. (Courtesy of 'Cardiopulmonary Resuscitation', Skinner D.V. & Vincent, R., Oxford University Press, 1993.)

PROTECTION OF STAFF IN A&E
Infection

A&E staff of all grades are, of necessity, exposed to patients whose infectivity at presentation is unknown. It is essential, therefore, that staff adhere to infection protection guidelines as laid down by the A&E department in consultation with relevant hospitals specialists. All A&E staff should be immunized against hepatitis B and whenever in contact with patient's body fluids, such as blood, urine or faeces, should wear gloves, aprons and goggles. Some departments recommend the use of masks when dealing with multiple injured patients but few have so far adopted this recommendation because of concerns about the resultant inability to relate adequately to the patient. All staff must adhere rigidly to the hospital protocol for needlestick injury.

Violence

A&E staff are particularly at risk of being involved in a violent situation. Risks are increased when patients are physically or mentally ill, under the influence of alcohol or drugs, or simply distressed (Hadfield, 1991).

It is crucial that all staff caring for patients should be familiar with methods of dealing with violence (Mid-Glamorgan Health Authority, 1984). In 1986, a study of 45 A&E departments showed that only 20% reported any training in the handling of violent or aggressive patients (Walsh, 1986).

Preparation for A&E staff should emphasize defusion techniques, as opposed to self-defence training, since the latter can lull individuals into a false sense of security (Power, 1992). Once a situation has erupted, 'flight not fight' is the answer.

Provision of the appropriate training does not relieve A&E department leaders of the managerial responsibility to provide and maintain a safe working environment. Increased awareness of the size and magnitude of the problem of violence has sparked responses from our American colleagues in particular. Ten ways to maintain a safer A&E department are suggested:

1. Improved access, control and visibility of all A&E entrances.
2. Use of metal detectors.
3. Silent alarm systems connected to the security office or local police station.
4. Better waiting area facilities.
5. Designated areas in which to care for psychiatric or potentially violent patients.

6. High-profile police presence in A&E.
7. Careful screening of all A&E staff, to ensure suitability to work in highly stressful situations.
8. Separation of patients with major and minor complaints.
9. Staff debriefing opportunities.
10. Closed circuit televisions to monitor all hospital entrances.

Risk factors associated with violent behaviour in A&E have been noted in a publication of the American College of Emergency Physicians (Gavin, 1988). One department has even recruited German Shepherd dogs to its security force (Eddinger, 1991).

STRESS AND STAFF SUPPORT IN THE A&E DEPARTMENT

Introduction

A&E personnel experience distressing and potentially traumatic events, beyond the realms of 'normal' human experience, on a daily basis. The additional stresses of fatigue, an unpredictable and at times high-intensity workload and rapid turnover of junior and relatively inexperienced staff, all contribute to make the A&E department the most demanding workplace in the hospital.

Serious and sometimes disabling psychological and psychiatric symptoms are well recognized in A&E personnel, rescue workers and members of the emergency services involved in the aftermath of accidents and disaster (McFarlane, 1988). The majority of A&E staff will experience some features of traumatic stress following intense and distressing emergency situations (Hartsough, 1985). Psychological symptoms include fatigue, sadness, dysphoria and poor concentration, heightened arousal and anxiety, guilt, anger and feelings of helplessness, identification with victims and intrusive thoughts which interfere with work. Although many of these symptoms are self-limiting, a number of individuals will go on to develop more serious acute stress reactions, diverse adjustment disorders and post-traumatic stress disorder (PTSD). The prevalence of PTSD may be as high as 30% or more in victims, emergency workers and rescuers alike following serious accidents and disasters (Duckworth, 1986; Cobb & Lindemann, 1943). Serious psychological distress may also occur in 'second-line' support workers such as administrators, control room and reception staff, switchboard operators, hospital ancillary and volunteer workers as well as the families of emergency service personnel.

A variety of individual and situational factors predispose staff to the effects of traumatic stress. Individual vulnerability factors include fatigue and sleep loss, poor physical health, a personal history of psychiatric disorder and a 'neurotic' anxiety-prone personality, as well as a lack of supportive and confiding relationships. Adverse reactions are more likely to occur in staff subject to intense and prolonged exposure to distressing events. Other situational factors which predispose to stress include a lack of adequate training, low morale, working in dangerous conditions, a poor sense of identity and lack of a close-knit cohesive team. Staff who identify with victims, for example those who handle personal effects, are especially vulnerable. Infant deaths, child abuse, victims of sexual assault, mass casualties, body handling and identification are particularly associated with subsequent psychological morbidity (Taylor & Frazer, 1982; Jones, 1985; Deahl et al., 1994) and recognized as stressors that 'can make victims of rescuers' (Ursano & McCarroll, 1990).

Trauma psychology suggests that most victims of severe trauma will endure some distressing symptoms as they assimilate their experience. Psychologists have developed cognitive information-processing models to explain reactions to stressful events (Horowitz, 1974). These predict alternating intrusive symptoms (e.g. nightmares and flashbacks) and avoidance symptoms (e.g. denial and phobic avoidance of situations reminiscent of the trauma). These diminish in intensity with time and form an integral part of the normal stress response. Such symptoms are only considered pathological when they become excessive in frequency, magnitude or duration.

Coping with stressful events

Staff often feel inhibited from openly expressing distress and emotion, fearing criticism from their colleagues and being labelled as 'weak' or 'unprofessional'. Within limits, displaying emotion does not necessarily impair and may even enhance operational efficiency. It may also protect against subsequent psychological morbidity. Humour, particularly black humour, is a well-known and effective coping strategy and common behavioural response amongst A&E staff in times of stress and tragedy. It has important protective effects and should not necessarily be seen as a callous reaction to circumstances. Other staff, conversely, display 'machismo' or the 'stiff upper lip', concealing or suppressing emotions and feelings in order to cope with the demands of stressful situations. Rigid, inflexible thinking and over-intellectualization are also common coping strategies. Although staff who suppress their feelings may appear superficially more 'efficient' and 'in control', there is some evidence to suggest that these coping strategies may actually be associated with a diminished capacity to make decisions and with impaired operational efficiency (Rayner, 1958).

Primary prevention

It is axiomatic that a happy department is a healthy department. Effective leadership and communication lie at the heart of any well-managed organization. The effects of stress are minimized by high morale and effective teamwork, although these may be difficult to cultivate in a department where rapid staff turnover, shift-working, frequent understaffing and the regular use of agency or locum staff militate against the development of good working relationships. The escalating demands of administration and management within the Health Service put increasing pressures on senior medical and nursing staff to leave the 'shop floor' and become less conspicuous to their less experienced juniors. It is vital for senior staff to recognize the importance of setting aside time to spend with their juniors not just in formal meetings and teaching sessions, but informally, 'walking the floor' offering encouragement, support, practical advice and guidance on routine clinical matters. Keeping 'in touch' with the shop floor is not only good for the juniors' morale but enables senior staff to detect problems and troubleshoot at an early stage, allowing an opportunity to intervene before matters get out of hand.

Senior nursing and medical staff should lead by example and allow junior staff the opportunity of seeing and learning from their more experienced colleagues 'getting their hands dirty' in the daily clinical routine. The more accessible and approachable the senior staff make themselves, the more mutual confidence and trust are allowed to develop. Demonstrating a genuine concern for the professional and personal interests and problems of colleagues and juniors alike makes staff feel respected and valued – important factors in promoting morale within the department. This should include practical advice on issues of immediate concern to the junior staff such as careers guidance and counselling.

Communication should always be a two-way process. Regular departmental meetings should be held to brief staff on developments within the hospital that might affect them; information should not be disseminated by rumour and gossip, especially during times of reorganiza-tion and rationalization within the hospital. Regular formal feedback and appraisal of staff performance should be given, including praise where due and criticism framed as constructively as possible. Junior staff should be allowed the opportunity of giving feedback to their more senior colleagues. Communication between departments frequently breaks down and tempers become frayed under stressful working conditions, often at times of maximum fatigue when senior staff are not available to adjudicate. These disputes often concern the appropriateness of patient referrals. The use of treatment protocols and explicit referral policies should be used whenever possible to prevent 'turf wars' breaking out between the junior staff and damaging relations between departments. The role of informal communication should not be underestimated, and social occasions and opportunities to meet outside work can be used as powerful tools to enhance group cohesion and boost team spirit and morale.

Training and regular supervision are both key ingredients in the successful management of a busy department. There is ample evidence to suggest that training enables staff not only to deal more effectively with stressful situations but also helps them cope better emotionally. Regular rehearsal of the hospital's major incident plan is a particular example where training can help protect staff against the emotional impact of events beyond 'normal experience' with which they may well otherwise have difficulty coping. Formal training should not be confined to clinical management problems but should cover other stressful and difficult situations which staff face in their daily routine, such as breaking bad news, dealing with uncooperative, difficult and aggressive patients, as well as recognizing and coping with stress itself. The teaching of systematic treatment protocols such as ALS (Advanced Life Support) and ATLS not only improves clinical performance and the self-confidence of junior staff but teaches important principles of teamwork which can be generalized beyond the resuscitation room and throughout the department. Without doubt, feeling part of a cohesive group and an efficient clinical team is one of the most important protective factors against the effects of stress.

Secondary prevention and intervention following psychological trauma

Staff should always meet as a matter of routine to discuss and reflect upon any serious or major incident that occurs in the department. An 'operational debriefing' enables staff to describe their role as well as their perceptions of what took place and provides a valuable opportunity to learn and improve for the future. It is also important to acknowledge the feelings and emotions that staff take with them from any incident, whether it be an abusive or violent patient, or a distressing clinical situation. This not only helps identify staff in distress, but may itself be therapeutic in minimizing the risk of later, more serious psychological sequelae. This 'emotional' debriefing need not be a formal affair and a 'shoulder to cry on' over a cup of tea may well be as effective as any more formal intervention. No matter how informal, its potential importance cannot be underestimated and it should be a matter of departmental policy that staff do not leave the department following a distressing incident until they have had an opportunity to discuss their feelings.

A variety of counselling and more formal but brief psychotherapeutic techniques have been advocated to help emergency service workers and rescuers exposed to distressing and potentially traumatizing events. Attempts to prevent or minimize morbidity have resulted in calls for the routine provision of early psychological intervention for carers as well as the victims of trauma and the emergence of a 'disaster industry' led by a variety of professional groups, including lay counsellors, psychologists, social workers and psychiatrists who have all sought to establish a role for themselves following traumatic incidents (British Psychological Society, 1990). A recent survey of senior officers of UK emergency services revealed that 72% had some critical incident stress provision within their local service although only 28% felt that sufficient attention was paid to this aspect of staff welfare (Orner et al., 1993). Early interventions are intuitively appealing and a response to perceived need, but whether or not they work is less certain.

Of all the techniques currently available, psychological debriefing (PD) is the most widely advocated preventative intervention at present.

What is psychological debriefing?

Jeffrey Mitchell, an American psychologist, initially described 'critical incident stress debriefing' (CISD) with ambulance personnel in 1983. CISD has been modified and expanded by others including Dyregrov (1989) who coined the term psychological debriefing (PD). It has been used with those directly involved in traumatic events, including hospital staff, emergency service workers and the providers of psychological aftercare.

A PD is a structured intervention designed to promote the emotional processing of traumatic events through the ventilation and normalization of reactions and preparation for possible future experiences. Although initially designed for use in groups, it has also been used with individuals, couples and families. A typical PD takes place 48–72 h after the trauma as a single group meeting lasting approximately 2 h.

Seven stages are passed through during PD. A brief introduction stressing the focus of the intervention and its confidentiality is followed by consideration of the facts of what happened from the varied perspectives of all those attending. The expectations, thoughts and impressions of those involved are then discussed. By this stage of the PD a detailed reconstruction of what happened will have occurred and, at least in theory, led to the open expression of associated emotions including guilt and anger. These are considered in depth and normalized as far as is reasonably possible. Group processes such as universality and peer support are mobilized during group PD which helps with the acceptance of experienced emotions. The emphasis remains on normalization throughout and this is discussed formally towards the end of the PD. In conclusion, the debriefer(s) prepares the participants for future symptoms and reactions, should they occur, and gives guidelines as to when further help should be sought and where it can be found. These points are often reinforced with written information distributed to the participants before they leave.

Through facilitating the ventilation of impressions, reactions and feelings, PD aims to promote emotional processing of the trauma and to reduce and control the frequency and severity of psychological sequelae. Immediacy is thought to enhance the effectiveness of debriefing: the earlier debriefing occurs, the less the opportunity for maladaptive and disruptive cognitive and behavioural patterns to become established (Rachman, 1980).

Does psychological debriefing work?

Research into post-traumatic stress has been hampered by a number of serious methodological difficulties. The unpredictability, setting and chaos of accidents and disaster make research, and in particular controlled studies, extremely difficult to undertake. Many studies are anecdotal and do not employ clear diagnostic criteria or standardized instruments to rate symptoms or outcome (Raphael et al., 1989). Studies frequently fail to specify the content of PD and deal with traumas of varying magnitude in heterogeneous groups of subjects who have had variable exposure to traumatic events. Interpretation of outcome is often problematic and findings are frequently contradictory. Most importantly, a lack of controlled studies makes it difficult to judge the efficacy of any professional intervention given our lack of knowledge of the natural history of post-traumatic stress reactions.

Although numerous anecdotal reports suggest that providing PD does help to reduce subsequent psychological morbidity (Dyregov, 1989; Armstrong *et al.*, 1991; Robinson & Mitchell, 1993), more recent and methodologically more rigorous studies using comparison groups have cast doubt on earlier findings. In general, studies suggest that PD may well reduce symptoms of acute stress following trauma and is appreciated by participants who find it subjectively helpful. Clinical experience suggests that many individuals value the opportunity to express feelings of anger and guilt and derive comfort from the realization that these are a normal emotional response to trauma. Many of the feelings expressed during PD are intensely personal, and disaster workers and victims alike often experience difficulty in confiding in, and tend to be suspicious of, 'outsiders', especially mental health professionals.

At present, there is little evidence to demonstrate that PD has any impact in reducing long-term psychological morbidity such as PTSD. The evidence from methodologically flawed studies suggests that at best PD affords some protection against later sequelae and, at worst, it makes no difference. It is already apparent that individuals receiving PD are not immune to later psychological sequelae. Therefore, whether or not PD is employed following serious traumatic events, formal follow-up to facilitate the identification of individuals who go on to develop serious psychological sequelae is vital.

PD is not without its own risks. Mandatory attendance at a PD has, not surprisingly, been associated with passive participation and resentment (Flannery *et al.*, 1991) and it is widely accepted that debriefers themselves may become 'secondary victims' (Berah *et al.*, 1984; Raphael, 1986; Talbot, 1990). McFarlane (1989) voiced concern that overenthusiasm for primary preventative methods might delay the diagnosis and effective treatment of those who suffer serious psychological sequelae. He argued that 'clear definition of these limitations of the crisis intervention approach and the point at which more formal treatment is required' is needed. His concerns were fuelled by the finding that many emergency workers who developed psychiatric disorders as a result of the Australian bushfires presented late due to other

professionals' fears that labelling on referral to a psychiatrist would occur (McFarlane, 1984).

The current body of knowledge suggests that the presence or absence of other factors – for example a severe acute stress reaction, working under dangerous conditions, 'neurotic' personality traits, a past psychiatric history and an absence of adequate social supports – are likely to affect the psychological outcome of individuals involved in traumatic events more than whether or not they received a debriefing. Indeed, when individuals have an adequate support network and do not have other vulnerability factors, PD may be redundant (Bisson & Deahl, 1994). Some of these individual factors should perhaps receive greater attention when selecting emergency service personnel.

If PD is to be effective, it should be a team responsibility taking place within groups of emergency workers carried out as locally and rapidly as possible. The role of mental health professionals should be directed towards educating these groups rather than trying to deliver a service themselves. If PD or any other professional psychological intervention is to be made available to large numbers of individuals, considerable resources will be required. It is essential, therefore, that the efficacy of PD is properly evaluated. This should give a clearer indication as to whether it should be routinely offered to everyone involved in traumatic events, restricted to 'high-risk' individuals, or abandoned. Who should deliver PD, when, and what form it should take, all remain unanswered questions.

No matter how effective debriefing may be, overenthusiasm for any psychological intervention must not deflect attention from the need to develop those attributes of a department which have been shown to offer individual staff protection against the effects of psychological trauma. In the maelstrom of A&E it is all too easy for staff to overextend themselves both physically and emotionally. A commitment to training, teamwork and proper attention to the promotion and maintenance of morale and welfare of staff must be explicit and given high priority in departmental operational policies in order to avoid unnecessary stress, improve work efficiency and prevent the carers from becoming as ill as those they seek to help.

PATIENT RIGHTS

The majority of those admitted to hospital are apprehensive, even when they have been prepared for admission. It is not surprising, therefore, that A&E patients and their loved ones are often particularly anxious. They will experience the distress of physiological pain and shock, of psychological stress and of social anxiety (Sbaih, 1992).

Results of a study of 200 A&E patients revealed that 98% of the respondents were registered with a general practitioner but 78% had not contacted him/her before attending A&E. Among other reasons, 25% anticipated that they would need an X-ray. Over half (52%) admitted that they did not feel that their problem was an emergency, or were not aware that facilities such as suturing were offered by their general practitioner. Findings such as this strongly suggest a wide gap in patient education (Bellavia & Brown, 1991).

Nguyen-Van-Tam & Baker (1992) investigated 36 patients who had seen their general practitioner before referring themselves to A&E. It is assumed that the general practitioner, having decided not to refer the patient, had already given the appropriate treatment and advice. Such patients often encounter scepticism from A&E staff. However, results show that patients in the group above are just as likely to be admitted as any other group, suggesting that scepticism from staff is unjustified.

Consent and upholding patients' interests

A&E staff still consider the process of informed consent to be a legal obligation. So often the opportunity is missed to make sure that patients' expectations are appropriate. Patients should always be asked to explain the contents of a consent form *before* they sign it. Another safe but time-consuming method is to ask patients to write their own consent form.

A&E staff should consider the following tactics to uphold patients' interests:

1. Do not discharge or turn away patients without being sure that they are not at risk.
2. Make the patients and those accompanying them as comfortable as possible during their stay.
3. Do not hesitate to refer patients to a specialist or other agency unless you are sure that they are not at risk.
4. Always adhere to any hospital or departmental policies or procedures.
5. Make sure that all relevant information is documented.
6. Always act in the best interests of the patient.

A&E DEPARTMENT MANAGEMENT

Changes in the management of A&E services have been amongst the most important developments over recent years. The key to an efficient service is effective leadership. Other important elements include appropriate use of resources (facilities, personnel and equipment) underpinned by strong communication networks and collaboration between individuals both within and outside the department.

The major current problem for many A&E departments is cost containment without compromising the quality of care. The trends and pressures causing these problems are expected to intensify in the foreseeable future.

A separate budget for the A&E service is essential, and standards should be set in accordance with the level of service which can be provided for the funding available.

Effective A&E services also rely on clearly defined roles. Specific job descriptions for each post should reflect its responsibilities and functions.

Leadership, motivation and team building

Many mistakenly believe that managers must learn to motivate staff. Employees actually bring their own motivation but they need their managers to liberate and involve them, to allow them to be accountable and to reach their potential. The leader's role is to help set goals and to facilitate, not to force employees to do as they are told (Hadfield, 1989).

Individual performance review

Ensuring that A&E staff perform well contributes to high-quality patient care. Perhaps one of the most important reasons for staff appraisal is the effect it has on morale. Individual performance review should not be used as a punitive measure; a disciplinary procedure is available for that purpose.

Individual performance review should be used as an opportunity to praise for aspects of the job well done, and to give guidance and help set goals where performance can be improved (Hadfield, 1989).

Financial management

For those who manage an A&E service, one of the most important activities is to respond to the new financial pressures in health care. Service leaders will only be successful in financial management if all members of the A&E team understand this concept (Thurgood, 1993).

Unfortunately, many doctors and nurses have not had the education, training or experience in actively controlling costs and improving efficiency and productivity. To alleviate these difficulties, service leaders must acquire the skills and knowledge to manage the various components of a budget. Once basic concept skills and techniques are learned, effective strategies can be formulated to control costs. These should be underpinned by the fundamental principles of human motivation to ensure success (Blaney & Hobson, 1988).

Following the introduction of resource management, many clinicians have been identified as 'budget holders'. These individuals may be more aptly named 'budget monitors', which would appropriately describe their relationship with senior hospital management teams (Royal College of Nursing Standards of Care Project, 1989).

Risk management

Traditionally, A&E departments have been considered to be high-risk areas. A&E staff are more 'at risk' than other specialities due to violence, stress, litigation and complaints. There are several causes of this vulnerability, which include:

- High turnover of patient population.
- Waiting times.
- Lack of hospital beds for admission.
- Fluctuating workload.
- Delays in transport.
- Broad scope of A&E work.
- More SHOs than any other specialty.
- Limited out-of-hours support from senior A&E staff (except in large centres).
- No previous knowledge of most patients attending.
- Greater proportion of intoxicated, uncooperative, belligerent or violent patients.
- Limited facilities in many departments for observing patients.
- Patients may be reluctant to re-attend even when their condition deteriorates.

Changes in workload in relation to staffing levels in A&E are often the cause of an increase in risk. It is, of course, unrealistic to attempt to plan for every eventuality. Nevertheless, A&E risk management can be achieved through refining department policies and procedures, and improving public relations (American Health Consultants Inc., 1989). Poor patient outcome may be unavoidable, but the department can minimize liability by showing that they did their best (Hadfield, 1989).

A&E patients are usually anxious and have high expectations of the service. Much of the risk associated with such tension can be reduced by approaching patients in a professional and sensitive way. Courtesy must start with the first member of staff to meet the patient.

One of the greatest difficulties A&E patients and staff face is that of long waiting times. Ensuring that someone regularly and sympathetically updates patients and those accompanying them will help to reduce dissatisfaction and unrealistic expectations concerning waiting times. In some departments a full-time volunteer assumes this role.

Staff education concerning communication can be very helpful, the key concept being 'putting patients first'. Training in all aspects of patient care can reduce risk.

Some of the everyday tasks in A&E are important for good patient care and risk reduction. A useful example is clear and comprehensive documentation. The environment can make a major contribution to this. For example, there is often not enough blank space on preprinted forms, and not enough desk space to sit comfortably at to complete records. Once in court, patient records can make or break a hospital's defence. Coroners and civil courts often operate on the theory that 'If it has not been documented, it has not been done'.

To produce satisfactory patient records:

1. Write clearly in black ink (for easy photocopying).
2. Use standard abbreviations.
3. Sign, date and time *every* entry.
4. Be concise and complete.
5. Be truthful and objective, no judgemental comments.
6. Do not leave blank spaces.
7. Delete and initial, do not rub out, 'Tippex' or make illegible.

Medical negligence

A five year study of over 900 hospital negligence claims dealt with by one firm of solicitors showed that 8.5% originated from A&E, which was equal fourth in ranking for frequency, after obstetrics & gynaecology (28%), general surgery (17%) and orthopaedic surgery (15%) (Dr A. L. Gwynne—personal communication). Review of a series of 70 claims involving A&E departments gives some idea of the spectrum of the problem (Table 1). Although responsibility rested with medical staff outside the A&E department in seven cases, A&E staff were considered culpable in 55% of the remainder. In many instances, the source of the problem was multifactorial. For example, admitting hospital teams also provided care or advice which fell below the standard that an A&E department would normally expect in 22% of cases,

Table 1. *Clinical problems encountered in a series of 70 claims of medical negligence in A&E departments*

Problem	Number of patients
Wounds	12
Foreign bodies	6
Hand injuries	11
Fractures/dislocations	10
Spinal injuries	8
Head injuries	4
Acute abdominal problems	4
Major blood vessel rupture	3
Scalds	3
Pneumonia	3
Bones lodged in throat	2
Subarachnoid haemorrhage	1
Heart attack	1
Stroke	1
Drug overdose	1
Resuscitation	1
Pneumothorax	1
Eye injury	1
Drug effect	1
Achilles tendon rupture	1
Alcohol toxicity	1
Childbirth	1

Total number of patients = 70.

and in two instances the care administered by ambulance staff was deficient. A&E mismanagement contributed to six of a total of ten deaths and analysis of three cases was rendered more difficult by evidence that the medical records had been altered after the event. Ten per cent of the claims were considered hypercritical and could not be justified.

The quality of A&E care can be undermined at any stage in the patient's management, from the taking of a history on first presentation to reattendance at a later date. In the series examined, most histories could be defended, but there was sometimes a failure to appreciate the susceptibility of certain patients to illness or injury. The presence of neurological symptoms was disregarded in several cases.

Problems relating to clinical examination most frequently involved inadequate wound exloration (particularly when contamination was likely) and failure to properly assess nerve and tendon function in the hand. Impairment of sensation in the hand warrants direct referral or early review as primary nerve repair produces the best results. The delayed development of boutonnière deformity means that proximal interphalangeal joint injuries should be reviewed urgently if there is a possibility of injury to the extensor expansion. The scaphoid bone must also be routinely examined in all wrist injuries.

Investigations, particularly the requesting and interpretation of X-rays (see Chapter 15), are a potent source of litigation (Touquet et al., 1995). In the cases surveyed, failure to X-ray radio-opaque material lodged in the tissues or the throat was a common feature despite long-established guidance from the medical defence societies on this subject. Further films after surgery sometimes reveal a significant amount of residual debris. The doctor was sometimes misled when the name, date or side of injury marked on the X-rays was not checked. Similarly, the results of pathology tests were not always scrutinized carefully and some tests such as electrocardiographs (ECGs) in patients with chest pain should have been repeated.

The most serious diagnostic failures concerned the misinterpretation of neurological symptoms and signs resulting from brain trauma or incomplete spinal cord injury. In six cases, neurological symptoms were dismissed or attributed erroneously to the effect of drugs or psychiatric disturbance. Some patients with lower limb problems who were examined on a couch were discharged from the A&E department without any assessment of their gait, but could not walk, even with assistance. Others were sent home despite the persistence of severe pain which was subsequently attributed to myocardial infarction, aortic dissection, appendicitis, or similar conditions. A further opinion and hospital admission are justified when pain is severe, even if its cause is not apparent. In many instances, observation on a short-stay ward is helpful as long as the patient is carefully monitored. Unfortunately, this did not happen in two cases and the patients deteriorated irreversibly on the A&E ward. Tried and tested documentation such as Glasgow coma charts should be used when patients are under observation as some local charts do not record important clinical signs.

In most instances, physical procedures undertaken in A&E were beyond reproach but inadequate management of penetrating wounds of knuckle joints and delayed treatment of serious emergencies such as haemorrhage from an aortic aneurysm or testicular torsion were difficult to defend. None of the patients with undiagnosed spinal injury were adequately immobilized.

Referral to admitting teams can be difficult if resident staff are busy or unsupportive. Some problems could have been avoided if the A&E doctor had conveyed an appropriate degree of urgency to the specialist team and not accepted advice over the telephone when the patient should have been seen and reassessed by a more experienced doctor. An even more difficult situation arose if the patient was referred to an inappropriate speciality whose perspective on the case was understandably biased. Referral must not be overplayed but it does represent one of the most important medicolegal safety nets in cases of uncertainty.

As the doctor will not know most A&E attenders and the majority of them will be discharged from the department, it is essential that patients are given appropriate advice and told whom to consult if their symptoms persist or deteriorate. It is very important that this advice is recorded succinctly in the A&E notes but this did not happen in a large number of cases. Some patients feel that they should not return to A&E, even when clinical complications develop and they may, to their detriment, accept a non-urgent appointment from the general practitioner's surgery. When patients did return to A&E, several were unfortunately treated in the same way as they were at their first attendance. It should be assumed that an unscheduled reattendance at the A&E department is a cry for help. If X-rays or other interventions were not thought to be fully justified at the first visit, they should normally be actioned if the patient returns. In several cases, negligence was agreed largely because A&E staff failed to take appropriate action when given a second opportunity. Good communication with general practitioners (normally by letter but sometimes by telephone) helps to ensure a smooth transition of care and allows staff in the community to intervene more effectively if complications develop following the patient's discharge from A&E. Contact with the general practitioner can also bring important information to light.

Damage limitation requires that an attentive history is obtained, followed by a careful but pertinent examination, selection of appropriate investigations and the establishment of a working (rather than final) diagnosis. The diagnosis and treatment, and often their limitations, must be explained to the patient and advice given concerning an appropriate source of further medical care, should this prove necessary. Accurate but concise documentation of these points provides the greatest protection. The use of advice leaflets can help to convey relevant information, reinforce advice, improve efficiency and protect staff against unfair claims.

Whilst a well-structured approach to the assessment and treatment of patients is expected, A&E doctors also have a right to receive as much clinical support as possible. A small departmental reference library and local policy guidelines are invaluable aids for inexperienced doctors.

Ideally, all A&E X-rays should be seen by a radiologist on the next working day when reports should be returned to the A&E department for checking by senior staff. This arrangement can be streamlined further if a system is established which tells the radiologist whether the A&E doctor identifed any abnormality on the film. If the radiologist knows than an important abnormality was missed, a telephone message can be conveyed directly to the A&E department.

The risk of malpractice litigation can also be reduced by timely intervention on the part of the experienced nursing staff who represent an invaluable asset. Senior nurses can keep consultants informed of problems as they arise.

The accepted definition of medical negligence was established in the case of Bolam v Friern Hospital Management Committee (1957) and is often referred to as the Bolam test. This states that a doctor is not guilty of negligence if he or she acted 'in accordance with a practice accepted as proper by a responsible body of medical men skilled in that particular art' – in other words, a common or accepted practice. The Bolam test also refers to the standard being that 'of the ordinary skilled man exercising and professing to have that special skill', which means the A&E doctor of ordinary skill and of the relevant grade. Further reassurance in the Bolam test includes the concept that a doctor 'is not negligent if he is acting in accordance with such a practice, merely because there is a body of opinion who would take a contrary view'. In other words, it would not be negligent to adopt a non-standard technique as long as the treatment would be accepted as proper by a responsible body of medical practitioners. In practice, one needs to ask if the patient received a *reasonable* level of care – a subjective concept. Finally, proof of negligence is based upon it being more likely than not to have occurred (more than a 50% chance), frequently referred to as the balance of probabilities.

A further concept which is important in A&E negligence is the subject of causation. This is assessed by means of the 'but for' principle, meaning that an adverse outcome has to be attributed to the care administered before negligence can be established (e.g. 'but for the treatment given, the complication would not have arisen'). A delayed diagnosis which prolongs discomfort but does not affect the clinical outcome may be the subject of complaint and compensation but is not consistent with medical negligence.

Access to past records is also important. A&E staff can anticipate potential problems by paying particular attention to patients who have been seen recently with the same complaint. If records are not immediately available, difficulties can arise.

The main reasons for legal action against A&E staff are:

- Not communicating with patients which makes them feel like something less than people (American Health Consultants Inc., 1989). Milanesi (in American Health Consultants Inc., 1989) identified the '3 R's' of risk management: recording, reporting and rapport.
- Poor rapport between staff, patients and relatives, which is probably the most frequent cause of communication breakdown. If staff took the time and trouble to concentrate on what is being said to them, and responded appropriately, bad relations could be avoided (Palmer, 1993).

Another factor contributing to communication breakdown is the level of expectation held by patients following treatment in A&E, and what sort of progress they can expect following attendance. Maintaining a strict discharge planning process which incorporates education for all patients, increases their awareness. Policies should include patients in decisions made about their care (e.g. whether or not admission is indicated, or whether regional or local anaesthesia should be considered). Communicating respect for others by involving them in the decision-making process is a valuable technique which costs little.

Saunders (1986) believes that first encounters in all human relationships are crucial. 'If handled well, they can begin the process of strengthening social relationships between interactors and, at the same time, lay the foundation for future productive and mutually beneficial transaction.'

Adequate numbers of motivated, properly educated A&E staff working in a well-equipped and organized department will provide optimum patient care. The availability of such a service to the local community will enhance the public's view of the hospital as a whole.

Bibliography

AMERICAN HEALTH CONSULTANTS INC. (1989). *Reducing Risk in the Emergency Department*. Atlanta: Medical Reports Group.

ARMSTRONG, K., O'CALLAHAN, W. & MARMAR, C.R. (1991). Debriefing Red Cross disaster personnel: the multiple stressor debriefing model. *J. Traum. Stress*, **4**, 581–93.

BAEM. (1992). *The Way Ahead, A&E Services 2001*. London: BAEM.

BAILEY, A., HALLAM, K. & HURST, K. (1987). Nursing practice supplement – triage on trial. *Nursing Times*, **83** (44), 65–6.

BELLAVIA, J. & BROWN, D. (1991). A misuse of resources. *Nursing Times*, **87** (44), 26–9.

BERAH, E.F., JONES, H.J. & VALENT, P. (1984). The experience of a mental health team involved in the early phase of a disaster. *Aust. N.Z. J. Psychiatry*, **18**, 354–8.

BISSON, J.I. & DEAHL, M.P. (1994). Psychological debriefing and prevention of post traumatic stress. *Br. J. Psychiatry*, **165**, 717–20.

BJORN, P.R. (1991). Nurse educator: an approach to the potentially violent patient. *J. Emerg. Nurs.*, **17** (5), 36–9.

BLANEY, D.R. & HOBSON, C.J. (1988). Development financial management skills: an educational approach. *J. Nurs. Admin.*, **18** (6), 13–17.

BOLAM v. FRIERN HOSPITAL MANAGEMENT COMMITTEE (1957). 2 All ER 118, (1957), 1 WLR 582–3.

BRITISH PSYCHOLOGICAL SOCIETY WORKING PARTY (1990). *Psychological Aspects of Disaster*. Leicester: British Psychological Society.

BUSCHIAZZO, L. (1984). Patient classification in an emergency department. *J. Emerg. Nurs.*, **10** (4), 183–4.

BUTLER, W.R. (1986). Emergency department patient classification matrix: development and testing of one tool. *J. Emerg. Nurs.*, **12** (50), 279–85.

CARLISLE, D. (1992). Scope for extensions. *Nursing Times*, **88** (37), 26–8.

COBB, S. & LINDEMANN, E. (1943). Neuropsychiatric observations after the coconut grove fire. *Ann. Surg.*, **117**, 814–24.

CONNORS, A.M. (1993). Patient classification system in a rural emergency department. *Accid. Emerg. Nurs.*, **2**(1), 7–20.

DEAHL, M., GILLAM, A.B., SEARLE, M.M. *et al.* (1994). Psychological sequelae following the Gulf war: factors associated with subsequent morbidity and the effectiveness of psychological debriefing. *Br. J. Psychiatry*, **165**, 60–5.

DEPARTMENT OF HEALTH (1991). *The Patients Charter*. London: HMSO.

DRISCOLL, P.A. (1992). Trauma: today's problems, tomorrow's answers. *Injury*, **23** (3), 151–8.

DUCKWORTH, D.H. (1986). Psychological problems arising from disaster work. *Stress Med.*, **2**, 315–23.

DYREGROV, A. (1989). Caring for helpers in disaster situations: psychological debriefing. *Disaster Manage.*, **2**, 25–30.

EDDINGER, C. (1991). Security dogs in the emergency department: one hospital's solution to the crisis of violence. *J. Emerg. Nurs.*, **17** (5), 23–25A.

EDWARDS, N. & WERNEKE, U. (1994). In the fast lane. *Health Serv. J.*, 104.

FLANNERY, R.B., FULTON, P., TAUSCH, J. *et al.* (1991). A program to help staff cope with psychological sequelae of assaults by patients. *Hosp. Community Psychiatry*, **42**, 935–8.

GAVIN, L.J. ed. (1988). *Emergency Department Violence: Prevention and Management.* Dallas: American College of Emergency Physicians.

GEORGE, J.E. (1976). Emergency nurse triage beware. *Emerg. Leg. Bull.*, Winter.

GOULD, D. (1988). Opportunities for the accident and emergency nurse. *Nursing*, **3** (31), 24–26.

HADFIELD, L.V. (1989). In search of excellence in accident and emergency. *Nursing Standard*, **25** (3), 19.

HADFIELD, L.V. (1991). Violence in the accident and emergency department: differences across the Atlantic. *J. Emerg. Nurs.*, **17** (5), 269–70.

HADFIELD, L.V. (1991). Interviewing together. *Nursing Times*, **87** (38), 13.

HARTSOUGH, P.N. (1985). Emergency organisation role. In *Role Stresses and Support for Emergency Service Workers.* pp. 1–20. Washington: National Institute for Mental Health.

HELMER, F.T., FREITAS, C.A.N. & ONAHA, B. (1988). Determining the required nurse staffing of an emergency department. *J. Emerg. Nurs.*, **14** (6), 352–8.

HOBBS, R. (1995). Rising emergency admissions. *BMJ*, **310**, 207–8.

HOROWITZ, M.J. (1974). Stress response syndromes: character style and dynamic psychotherapy. *Arch. Gen. Psychiatry*, **31**, 768–81.

JONES, D.J. (1985). Secondary disaster victims: the emotional effects of identifying and recovering human remains. *Am. J. Psychiatry*, **142**, 303–7.

KROMASH, E.J. (1984). Patient classification and required nursing time in a paediatric emergency department. *J. Emerg. Nurs.*, **10** (2), 69–73.

McFARLANE, A.C., (1984). The Ash Wednesday bushfires in South Australia: implications for planning for future post-disaster services. *Med. J. Aust.*, **141**, 286–91.

McFARLANE, A.C. (1988). The longitudinal course of post-traumatic morbidity: the range of outcomes and their predictors. *J. Nerv. Ment. Dis.*, **176**, 30–9.

McFARLANE, A.C. (1989). The treatment of post-traumatic stress disorder. *Br. J. Med. Psychol.*, **62**, 81–90.

MID-GLAMORGAN HEALTH AUTHORITY (1984). *Accident and Emergency Department Guidelines and Information Document.* London: Kings Fund.

MITCHELL, J.T. (1983). When disaster strikes ... the critical incident debriefing process. *J. Emerg. Med. Serv.*, **8**, 36–9.

MURPHY, A. & MARSDEN, E. (1992). Accident and emergency departments: value for money. *Nursing Standard*, **7** (7), 6–7.

NATIONAL AUDIT OFFICE (1992a). *NHS Accident and Emergency Departments in Scotland.* London: HMSO.

NATIONAL AUDIT OFFCE (1992b). *NHS Accident and Emergency Departments in England.* London: HMSO.

NGUYEN-VAN-TAM, J.S. & BAKER, D.M. (1992). General practice and accident and emergency care: does the patient know best? *BMJ*, **305**, 157–8.

ORNER, R.J., PAULSON, R., THOMPSON, M. *et al.* (1993). Critical incident stress management services in United Kingdom emergency services. Paper presented at the Second World Congress on Stress, Trauma and Coping in Emergency Service Professions, Baltimore, MD.

PALMER, S. (1993). Conflicting interests? *Nursing Times*, **89** (10), 35.

PLATT REPORT (1962). London: HMSO.

POWER, M. (1992). Scepticism over approach to violence. *Nursing Times*, **88** (33), 9.

RACHMAN, S. (1980). Emotional processing. *Behav. Res. Ther.*, **18**, 51–60.

RAPHAEL, B. (1986). *When Disaster Strikes.* London: Hutchinson.

RAPHAEL, B., LUNDIN, T. & WEISAETH, L. (1989). A research method for the study of psychological and psychiatric aspects of disaster. *Acta Psychiatr. Scand.*, **80** (Suppl. 353).

RAYNER, J.F. (1958). How do nurses behave in disaster? *Nurs. Outlook*, **6**, 572–6.

ROBINSON, R.C. & MITCHELL, J.T. (1993). Evaluation of psychological debriefings. *J. Traum. Stress*, **6**, 367–82.

ROYAL COLLEGE OF NURSING STANDARDS OF CARE PROJECT (1991). *Management in Nursing.* London: RCN.

RUND, D.A. & RAUSCH, T.S. (1981). *Triage.* St. Louis: C.V. Mosby.

SAUNDERS, C. (1986). Opening and closing. In Hargie, O., ed. *A Handbook of Communication Skills.* Kent: Croom Helm.

SBAIH, L. (1992). *Accident and Emergency Nursing: A Nursing Model.* London: Chapman & Hall.

SCHULMERICH, S.C. (1984). Developing a patient classification system for the emergency department. *J. Emerg. Nurs.*, **10** (6), 298–305.

SCHULMERICH, S.C. (1986). Converting patient classification data into staffing requirements for the emergency department. *J. Emerg. Nurs.*, **12** (5), 286–90.

SHEEHAN, A. (1993). Skill mix does not work. *Br. J. Nurs.*, **2** (5), 256.

SHINER, P. & LEDDINGTON, S. (1991). 'Sometimes it makes you frightened to go to hospital ... they treat you like dirt'. *Health Serv. J.*, **101** (7 Nov.), 21–3.

STOLLEY, J. (1989). Establishing reliability and validity of an emergency department patient classification system. *J. Emerg. Nurs.*, **15** (6), 488–94.

TALBOT, A. (1990). The importance of parallel process in debriefing crisis counsellors. *J. Traum. Stress*, **3**, 265–77.

TAYLOR, A.J.W. & FRAZER, A.G. (1982). The stress of post-disaster body handling and victim identification work. *J. Hum. Stress*, **8**, 4–12.

THURGOOD, J. (1993). Definitions and explanations of the new financial vocabulary. *Br. J. Nurs.*, **2** (5), 295–6.

TOUQUET, R., DRISCOLL, P. & NICHOLSON, D. (1995). Teaching in accident and emergency medicine: 10 commandments of accident & emergency radiology. *BMJ*, **310**, 642–5.

UNITED KINGDOM CENTRAL COUNCIL (1992a). *The Scope of Professional Practice*. London: UKCC.

UNITED KINGDOM CENTRAL COUNCIL (1992b). *Code of Professional Conduct*. London: UKCC.

UNIVERSITY OF YORK, CENTRE FOR HEALTH ECONOMICS (1992). *Skill Mix and the Effectiveness of Nursing Care*. University of York.

URSANO, R.J. & McCARROLL, J.E. (1990). The nature of a post-traumatic stressor: handling dead bodies. *J. Nerv. Ment. Dis.*, **178**, 396–8.

VAIL, J.D. (1989). In Lambert, C.E. & Lambert, V.A., ed. *Perspectives in Nursing*. St Louis: C.V. Mosby.

WALSH, M. (1986). Counting the bruises. *Nursing Times*, **82** (80), 62–4.

WARD, R. (1990). Meeting points. *Nursing Times*, **89** (22), 58–60.

WILLIAMS, D.G. (1992). Sorting out triage. *Nursing Times*, **88** (30), 34–6.

Further reading

DYER, C., ed. (1992). *Doctors, Patients and the Law*. Oxford: Blackwell.

TOUQUET, R. & HARRIS, N. (1994). Accident and emergency. In Powers, S. & Harris, N.H., ed. *Medical Negligence*, pp. 435–52. Oxford: Butterworths.

2 Airway management

M.J.A. PARR[a], J.P. NOLAN[b] and P.J.F. BASKETT[c]

[a]Intensive Therapy Unit, Royal North Shore Hospital, St Leonards, NSW, Australia
[b]Department of Anaesthesia, Royal United Hospital, Bath, UK
[c]Department of Anaesthesia, Frenchay Hospital, Bristol, UK

Chapter plan

Introduction
The airway
Ventilation
Management
Ventilation techniques
Monitoring
Pharmacological adjuncts to airway management
Rapid sequence induction of anaesthesia
Inhalational induction of anaesthesia
Summary

INTRODUCTION

The airway is the first priority during resuscitation, and airway management skills are essential for those involved in emergency medicine. In the presence of airway obstruction, hypoxia leading to circulatory arrest can be expected to occur within 4–10 min, with irreversible central nervous system (CNS) damage following quickly. Basic airway management requires relatively simple skills but the clinical scenario is often complex and made more stressful because of lack of time for deliberation. Advanced airway management demands significantly more skill and experience. Effective airway management requires an understanding of functional airway anatomy and physiology, and the skills to assess and intervene rapidly when airway obstruction and ventilatory compromise occur. The basic skill of maintaining an open airway cannot be overemphasized, and should be mastered before attention is directed to advanced airway management techniques.

THE AIRWAY

Anatomy (Fig. 1)

The upper airway extends from the mouth and anterior nares to the inferior larynx.

The nose

The nasal cavity extends from the nostrils to the posterior nares or choanae, where it continues as the nasopharynx. The roof of the nasal cavity contains the olfactory region, lined with olfactory epithelium. The roof lies below the anterior cranial fossa and is formed from the nasal and frontal bones and the cribriform plate of the ethmoid anteriorly and the body of the sphenoid posteriorly. Nasal tubes inserted in the presence of a base of skull fracture may enter the cranial cavity.

The floor of the nasal cavity is formed from the hard palate which is made up of the palatal processes of the maxillae and the horizontal plates of the palatine bones. The soft palate is contiguous with the posterior aspect of the hard palate.

Inside the nose the lateral wall, which is covered in a thick vascular mucous membrane, is formed anteriorly and inferiorly by the nasal surfaces of the maxilla, posteriorly by the perpendicular plate of the palatine bone and superiorly by the ethmoid. The superior and middle conchae or turbinates project into the nasal cavity from their ethmoid attachments; the inferior concha arises from the maxilla and hard palate. The turbinates may be damaged during nasal intubation causing haemorrhage. Below each concha there is a meatus into which the paranasal sinuses open. The nasolacrimal duct opens into the anterior part of the inferior meatus and the eustachian (pharyngotympanic) tube opens just pos-

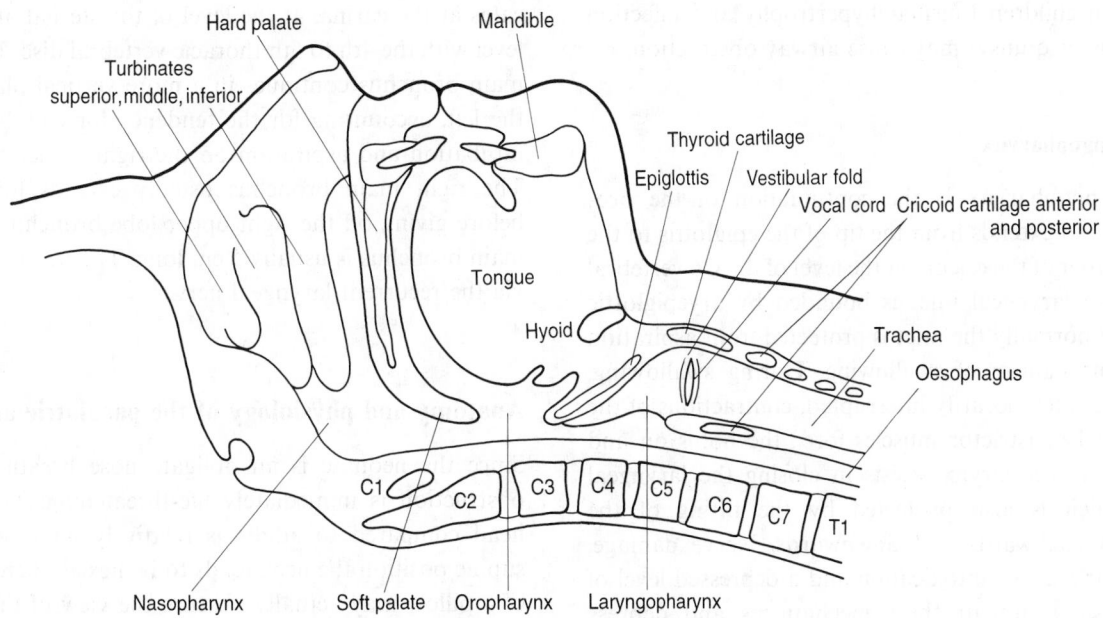

Fig. 1. Sagittal section of the adult upper airway.

terior to the inferior meatus above the level of the soft palate.

The medial wall of the nasal cavity is formed by the nasal septum which in older children and adults is often deviated to one side, making one nostril narrower than the other. The main nasal air passage lies beneath the inferior turbinate; correctly placed nasal tubes following this tract will be directed backwards along the floor of the nose.

The nasal cavity continues as the nasopharynx, lying above and behind the soft palate. The anterior nasopharynx is formed by the soft palate and the posterior boundary is made up of parts of the sphenoid bone, basilar occipital bone and anterior arch of atlas. The lateral walls are made up of the superior constrictor muscle and the pharyngobasilar membrane.

The nasal blood supply arises from the ophthalmic, maxillary and facial arteries. Little's area, on the anterior inferior part of the nasal septum, accounts for 90% of epistaxis and receives a blood supply from the sphenopalatine branch of the maxillary artery and the superior labial branch of the facial artery. Venous drainage is to the pterygoid venous plexus and the facial vein.

The nerve supply of the nasal cavity originates from the olfactory nerve which supplies the olfactory zone; the common sensory supply is from branches of the trigeminal nerve. Beneath the mucous membrane of the upper posterior wall of the nasopharynx there is a collection of lymphoid tissue, the adenoid or naso-

pharyngeal tonsil. In children, adenoids may hypertrophy and obstruct the airway and the pharyngotympanic tube.

The functions of the nasal cavity include providing the respiratory airway, olfactory sensation, humidification, heat exchange, filtering of particulate matter and speech enunciation. Nasal intubation bypasses all these functions, and by impeding the drainage of the paranasal sinuses it can result in sinusitis.

The mouth

The vestibule of the mouth is formed by the lips and cheeks outside, and the teeth and gums inside. The oral cavity is bound by the teeth anteriorly, hard and soft palate above, the tongue below, and the oropharyngeal isthmus behind.

The soft palate contains five muscles: tensor palati, levator palati, palatoglossus, palatopharyngeus, and musculus uvulae. These act in a coordinated manner to close off the mouth from the nasopharynx during speech and swallowing.

The oropharynx

The oropharynx communicates with the oral cavity and the nasopharynx and extends from the soft palate to the tip of the epiglottis. Nodules of lymphoid tissue, the lingual tonsils, extend laterally to join the palatine tonsils. In children tonsillar hypertrophy and infection (tonsillitis or quinsy) may cause airway obstruction.

The laryngopharynx

The laryngopharynx is the continuation of the oropharynx and extends from the tip of the epiglottis to the lower border of the cricoid at the level of the C6 vertebral body. The laryngeal inlet is bounded by aryepiglottic folds and normally the inlet is protected from aspiration by the mechanism of swallowing. During swallowing, breathing is temporarily interrupted, contractions of the pharyngeal constrictor muscles force the bolus on and elevation of the larynx assists in closing the laryngeal inlet, which is also protected by the tilting of the epiglottis backwards and downwards. Nerve damage, nerve blockade, or intoxication and a depressed level of consciousness, impair these mechanisms and depress protective reflexes. In these situations there is a great risk that vomiting or regurgitation will result in pulmonary aspiration.

The larynx

The larynx lies between the laryngopharynx and the trachea and comprises cartilages, membranes and ligaments. The outer wall is made up of thyroid cartilage, cricoid cartilage (the only complete cartilagenous ring of the airway), paired arytenoids, corniculate and cuneiform cartilages, and the cartilage of the epiglottis. The vestibular or quadrate membrane joins the arytenoid and thyroid cartilages and epiglottis; its lower border forms the vestibular fold. The cricothyroid membrane joins the cricoid cartilage to the thyroid cartilage. The free upper border forms the vocal folds (true vocal cords) at the level of the thyroid cartilage notch behind the laryngeal prominence (Adam's apple). When separated, the true vocal cords form the rima glottidis, the narrowest part of the adult airway. The nerve supply to the larynx is from the vagus, via its superior and recurrent laryngeal branches.

The lower airway

The lower airway continues as the trachea and bronchi. The trachea is attached to the cricoid cartilage by the cricotracheal ligament. The adult trachea is 10–12 cm long, with a lumen of 2.5 cm. Sixteen to 20 C-shaped cartilages maintain tracheal patency. The trachea bifur-

cates at the carina, at the level of the sternal angle and level with the 4th to 5th thoracic vertebral disc. The right main bronchus continues in a more vertical plane than the left, accounting for the tendency for endobronchial intubation and aspiration on the right rather than left. The right main bronchus usually extends for 2.5 cm before giving off the right upper lobe bronchus; the left main bronchus is usually 5 cm long. The nerve supply is via the recurrent laryngeal nerve.

Anatomy and physiology of the paediatric airway

Since the neonate is an obligate nose breather, nasal obstruction is immediately life-threatening. The infant head compared to adults is relatively large so in the supine position the neck tends to be flexed; therefore use of a pillow may actually obscure the view of the larynx by increasing flexion. Children have large tongues relative to the size of the oral cavity, and large tonsils and adenoids also increase the risk of upper airway obstruction and may interfere with laryngoscopy. At laryngoscopy, the larynx is more anterior. The epiglottis tends to be a large, U- or V-shaped, floppy structure which may need to be lifted with the laryngoscope blade to obtain a view of the larynx.

The neonatal trachea is narrow (3–4 mm) and short (4–5 cm), increasing the risk of bronchial intubation. Up to the age of 10 years the cricoid cartilage represents the narrowest part of the upper airway. Mucosal ischaemia and trauma at this level is associated with subglottic stenosis. The risk of this is reduced by using uncuffed tracheal tubes. In adults, the narrowest part of the airway is at the vocal cords.

Vagal reflexes are sensitive in children, and instrumentation of the airway in inadequately anaesthetized children can result in laryngospasm, bronchospasm, bradycardia and sinus arrest.

Oxygen consumption is much higher in the child because of the high metabolic rate. This results in a high minute ventilation, manifested as a high respiratory rate. The increased oxygen consumption, coupled with a reduced oxygen reserve, results in rapid arterial oxygen desaturation in the presence of upper airway obstruction or apnoea.

In infants the lung functional residual capacity (FRC) is small and the closing volume of the airways is relatively large. To avoid airway closure in the obtunded or anaesthetized child, continuous positive airway pressure is beneficial.

Airway anatomy and physiology during pregnancy

In pregnancy, capillary engorgement may cause significant swelling of the upper airway and this may be exacerbated by the oedema of pre-eclamptic toxaemia and upper respiratory tract infections. This swelling, together with the weight gain and breast enlargement associated with pregnancy can make intubation more difficult than in the non-pregnant patient.

A reduction in FRC, secondary to elevation of the diaphragm, occurs around term, and 30% of parturients are likely to produce airway closure during normal tidal ventilation. Increased oxygen consumption occurs throughout pregnancy which results in an increased minute ventilation achieved by an increase in tidal volume. The increased oxygen consumption, coupled with a reduced oxygen reserve, results in rapid arterial oxygen desaturation in the presence of upper airway obstruction or apnoea.

Physiological hyperventilation results in a reduced maternal $PaCO_2$ to around 4 kPa (30 mmHg) at term. Excessive hyperventilation produced during artificial ventilation must be avoided because it can result in reduced fetoplacental blood flow and fetal acidosis.

Airway assessment

The urgency of the clinical problem dictates the pace and extent of airway assessment. Airway compromise arises from either direct disease or injury of the airway, or neurological problems. Airway compromise can occur insidiously or suddenly, and the management will depend on the history and the findings on examination.

The history should include the acute event and any premorbid condition of relevance. Airway problems may become apparent only after the history has been taken; for example, the burned patient who has had an inhalational smoke injury may be at risk from delayed airway obstruction. Known airway problems, such as a difficult intubation during a previous anaesthetic, may be revealed during questioning.

Examination involves looking, listening, and feeling to assess the degree of airway obstruction and ventilatory compromise. During this assessment, attention is directed to the rate of ventilation; bradypnoea usually implies CNS depression or injury whilst tachypnoea may indicate upper or lower airway problems. Agitation and cyanosis, which is best detected on the lips or in the mouth, suggest hypoxaemia. The presence of hypertension, tachycardia and vasodilatation in obtunded patients suggests hypercarbia. During partial upper airway obstruction there is a reduction in tidal volume despite increased thoracic and diaphragmatic movement. There may be intercostal recession, supraclavicular retraction, use of accessory muscles and a tracheal tug. Paradoxical chest wall movements may also occur in airway obstruction. Total airway obstruction results in no air movement or breath sounds, though deceptive movements of the chest wall and diaphragm may persist until critical brainstem hypoxia results in respiratory arrest.

The presence of inspiratory or expiratory noise should be assessed. Snoring usually indicates partial obstruction at the pharyngeal level. Stridor, a high-pitched inspiratory noise, is usually associated with partial obstruction at the level of the larynx (inspiratory stridor) or trachea (expiratory stridor).

The quality of speech should be assessed; a hoarse voice implies partial obstruction at laryngeal level, often due to vocal cord dysfunction. Aphonia in a conscious patient is an ominous sign; the patient who is too short of breath to talk is in immediate danger of respiratory decompensation. Wheezing and dyspnoea imply lower airway obstruction. In the unconscious patient, feeling for air movement at the nose and mouth is undertaken at the same time as maintaining the airway .

When assessing the upper airway, a number of easily identified factors may make management difficult. Beards make it more difficult to achieve an air-tight seal during bag and mask ventilation, and a similar problem may be encountered when patients have had their dentures removed. Consequently, there is a case for leaving well-fitting dentures in place. Patients with poor dentition such as loose teeth, protruding upper incisors (buck teeth) or single fangs (peg teeth) are likely to pose problems during intubation.

Mouth opening should be assessed. Adults should be able to produce a 4 cm space (approximately three finger breadths) between upper and lower incisors; inability to do this is associated with difficult laryngoscopy. In the sitting patient, the structures visible on opening the mouth and protruding the tongue can be graded (Fig. 2) (Mallampati et al., 1985; Samsoon & Young, 1987). If the faucial pillars, uvula and soft palate can be seen (grades I and II), laryngoscopy and intubation are unlikely to be difficult. Hypoplastic and receding mandibles normally make laryngoscopy and intubation more difficult. If the distance between the chin and the thyroid notch (thyromental distance) is less than 6.5 cm, visualization of the larynx may be difficult or impossible (Fig. 3).

The range of neck movement must be assessed if

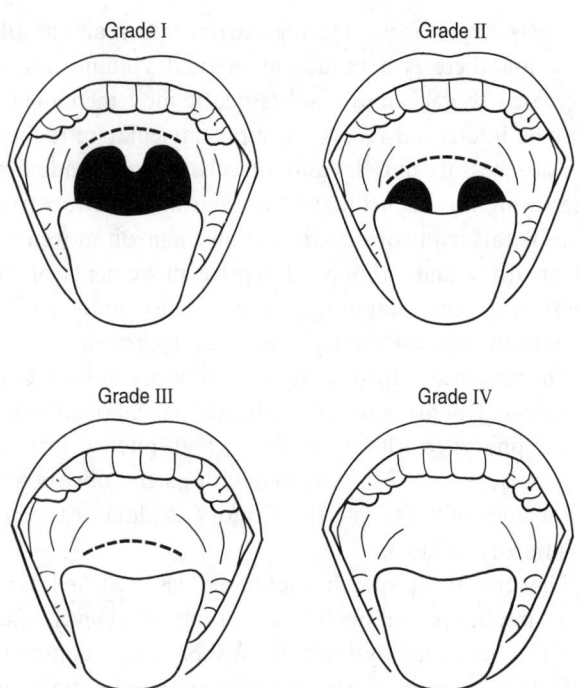

Grade I   Grade II

Grade III   Grade IV

Fig. 2. Structures visible on mouth opening. (Modified from Samsoon & Young, 1987.)

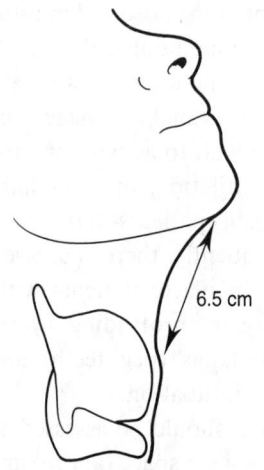

6.5 cm

Fig. 3. The thyromental distance.

possible; patients with short necks have a reduced range of movement. The ideal position for intubation is flexion of the neck (usually on one pillow) and extension at the atlanto-occipital junction, which brings the upper airway into alignment. Pre-existing disease, such as rheumatoid arthritis and ankylosing spondylitis, may severely restrict neck movement. Blunt trauma cases will have reduced head and neck movement because of the need for cervical spine immobilization. Suspicion of a base of skull fracture or the presence of nasal obstruction exclude the nasal route for tracheal intubation.

It is also important to recognize the patient who has potential for delayed airway obstruction, particularly from oedema associated with burns and smoke inhalation, or from trauma that produces an expanding haematoma. Assessment of these patients must include questioning and examination to exclude intraoral and upper airway injuries. The presence or suspicion of such an injury must lower the threshold for electively securing the airway with a tracheal tube. While airway obstruction may not be apparent at the time of presentation, progressive swelling around the airway may produce a hypoxic patient, in whom intubation is impossible and the creation of a surgical airway very difficult.

Airway pathophysiology

A number of conditions are associated with airway complications.

Conditions associated with potential airway problems

- Congenital anatomical abnormalities
- Infection
- Trauma (NB: cervical spine injury)
- Neoplasm
- Foreign body (especially in small children)
- Oedema (trauma, burn, pregnancy, anaphylaxis)
- Rheumatoid arthritis, ankylosing spondylitis
- Poor dentition
- Vocal cord dysfunction
- Obesity

Down's syndrome and achondroplasia are associated with a disproportionately large tongue, Pierre Robin syndrome with micrognathia and Treacher–Collins syndrome with micrognathia and cleft palate. In patients with these syndromes, problems with the airway should be anticipated; recognition is not usually difficult because of marked anatomical abnormalities.

Infections such as epiglottitis, croup and abscesses (dental, submandibular, retropharyngeal, quinsy) pose a major threat to the airway. If there is a risk of sudden upper airway obstruction (e.g.epiglottitis), the patient should be handled only to administer a general anaesthetic (see gas induction of anaesthesia below); direct examination or X-ray are contraindicated until the airway is secured.

Patients with blunt trauma should be assumed to have a cervical spine injury until appropriate X-rays and clinical examination of the cooperative patient have proved otherwise. Cervical spine immobilization, either by manual in-line immobilization or semirigid collar, sand bags and tape, will make laryngoscopy more difficult (Nolan & Wilson, 1993). Trauma patients may have intrinsic or extrinsic airway obstruction. Intrinsic airway obstruction may arise from direct injury with laryngeal disruption or burns, or may result from blood, tissue debris or vomitus. Foreign bodies such as teeth, dentures and missiles may cause obstruction, as may severe maxillary and mandibular fractures. Extrinsic compression by a haematoma or soft tissue swelling may also lead to upper airway obstruction.

Airway obstruction caused by neoplasms is usually insidious, but haemorrhage into a tumour or oedema may result in sudden life-threatening airway obstruction. Foreign body obstruction of the upper airway may be immediately life-threatening and should always be considered in small children presenting with ventilatory distress.

Oedema of the upper airway may be caused by burns, smoke inhalation, angioneurotic oedema or anaphylaxis, and is associated with pregnancy.

Inflammatory diseases such as rheumatoid arthritis, ankylosing spondylitis and scleroderma restrict movement and therefore impair airway manoeuvres. They may also be associated with ventilatory compromise through lung involvement.

Obesity, with tissue swelling and restricted movement, makes airway management more difficult. Obese patients, like parturients and children, have high oxygen consumption and poor oxygen reserves, giving rise to rapid oxygen desaturation when ventilation is impaired.

VENTILATION

Respiratory physiology is complex, requiring intact central and peripheral nervous systems, intact ventilatory mechanics and an adequate oxygen transportation system, which in turn relies on adequate cardiovascular function.

Respiratory control

Central control

Central nervous system (CNS) control of respiration is mediated through respiratory centres in the medulla and pons; these centres receive input from other areas including the reticular activating system. Sleep, sedatives, opioids, general anaesthetics and injury to the respiratory centres result in hypoventilation.

Central causes of hypoventilation

- Unconsciousness
- Opioids
- Sedatives, hypnotics, general anaesthetics
- Marked hypercapnia (carbon dioxide narcosis)
- Post hyperventilation (low $PaCO_2$)
- Brain injury with raised intracranial pressure due to hypoxia, head injury, haemorrhage, thrombosis, infarction or infection

---

The reduction in ventilation may result from a fall in respiratory rate or tidal volume, or a combination of the two.

Ventilation is stimulated by a fall in pH, a rise in carbon dioxide, a fall in O_2 and respiratory stimulant drugs (e.g. doxapram). However, very high levels of carbon dioxide depress ventilation and result in narcosis. Central chemoreceptors in the ventrolateral medulla and peripheral chemoreceptors in the aortic and carotid bodies, respond to changes in carbon dioxide and H^+ concentration.

The normal stimulus to ventilation is the partial pressure of carbon dioxide in arterial blood ($PaCO_2$). In some patients with chronic obstructive pulmonary disease who retain carbon dioxide, this drive has been replaced by a hypoxic drive dependent on low partial pressures of oxygen in arterial blood (PaO_2). If high inspired concentrations of oxygen are given to these patients, hypoventilation with further carbon dioxide retention and decreasing consciousness may occur. However, it is important to remember that hypercarbia kills slowly, hypoxia kills quickly and the need to provide immediate adequate oxygenation is the primary concern. Aim to deliver an inspired oxygen concentration sufficient to provide an adequate PaO_2 without causing a detrimental rise in $PaCO_2$.

Peripheral control

Adequate ventilation also requires intact chest wall and intrapulmonary mechanics. Peripheral causes of impaired ventilation include obstruction to the upper airway, most commonly due to the tongue.

The function of the phrenic and intercostal nerves may be impaired after injury to the spinal cord. Phrenic innervation is via cervical spinal roots C3–5; therefore diaphragmatic function will be maintained with cord lesions below this level. Neuromuscular junction blockade

Peripheral causes of hypoventilation

- Obstructed upper airway (tongue, foreign body, infection, tumour)
- Phrenic and intercostal nerve damage or blockade, spinal cord damage
- Neuromuscular junction blockade (drugs, poisons)
- Inadequate muscle power (injury, pain, pre-existing neuromuscular diseases)
- Failure of chest wall mechanics (flail, muscle injury, kyphoscoliosis)
- Abnormal intrapleural space (pneumothorax, haemothorax)
- Reduced lung compliance (pre-existing pulmonary disease, contusion, collapse)
- Obesity and pregnancy

Table 1. *Normal values for arterial blood gas analysis*

pH	7.34–7.46
PaO_2	12–14.67 kPa (75–100 mmHg)
$PaCO_2$	4.5–6.1 kPa (33–46 mmHg)
Actual bicarbonate	22–26 mmol l^{-1}
Standard bicarbonate	22–26 mmol l^{-1}
Base excess	± 2
Oxygen saturation	96–100%

occurs with neuromuscular blocking drugs and poisoning by organophosphorus compounds. Inadequate respiratory muscle power may result from injury or pre-existing muscle disease. However, pain is a more common cause of restricted deep breathing and coughing. The paradoxical movement of a flail segment of the chest wall may lead to inadequate ventilation of the underlying lung with ventilation/perfusion mismatching. However, underlying pulmonary contusion is a stronger indication for early intubation and ventilation.

Pneumothorax, haemothorax, pleural effusion or empyema will impair pulmonary ventilation. Accumulations of air or fluid in the pleural space cause pulmonary collapse with ventilation/perfusion mismatch and mediastinal shift with reduction in cardiac output, sometimes to the point of cardiac arrest. The pneumothorax may be open to the exterior or closed.

A pneumothorax comes under tension if a valve-like leak in the lung allows gas to escape from the respiratory tract into the pleural space but does not permit its return. A simple closed pneumothorax can be converted to a tension pneumothorax (the commonest life-threatening complication of chest injury and barotrauma) when positive pressure ventilation is used. Haemothorax commonly occurs after blunt or penetrating chest injury and frequently a pneumothorax is also present (haemopneumothorax).

Urgent decompression of the pleural space is required as a life-saving procedure in patients with tension pneumothorax, and early chest drainage is needed for rapidly accumulating blood, air or other foreign material in the pleural space. Temporary decompression of a pneumothorax can be achieved using simple needle thoracostomy. Formal chest tube drainage is required for fluid removal and longer term relief of a pneumothorax (see Chapter 23).

Pulmonary contusion should be suspected in any chest injury and may result in ventilatory failure, ventilation/perfusion mismatch and hypoxaemia, requiring early intubation and ventilation. Reduced lung compliance with impaired ventilation results from direct or indirect pulmonary injury, and will be complicated by any pre-existing pulmonary disease .

Assessment of ventilation

Having ensured an unobstructed airway, ventilation is assessed by looking, listening and feeling. The rate and the degree of chest expansion are assessed, asymmetry of movement is looked for and the presence of subcutaneous emphysema, or a flail segment may be felt. The position of the trachea should be checked and the lung fields are auscultated for breath sounds.

While the minute ventilation (tidal volume × respiratory rate) gives an idea of the adequacy of ventilation, it is necessary to obtain an arterial blood gas sample for analysis. Normal values for arterial blood gas analysis are given in Table 1. Continuous measurement of oxygen saturation of arterial blood by pulse oximetry is a valuable aid to assessment of the adequacy of ventilation, perfusion and oxygenation. End-tidal analysis of carbon dioxide (capnography) gives an estimate of $PaCO_2$ and ventilation; however, in patients with large physiological dead spaces the end-tidal carbon dioxide may not reflect the $PaCO_2$.

Carbon monoxide and cyanide poisoning

Carbon monoxide (CO) has 240 times the affinity of oxygen for haemoglobin. The half-life of carboxyhaemoglobin in a patient breathing 21% oxygen is180–300 min, but this is shortened to 30–80 min by breathing 100% oxygen at 1 atmosphere. It is reduced further to 20–30 min by hyperbaric oxygen (HBO) therapy.

There is evidence to show that HBO therapy (see below) reduces the mortality and morbidity in patients with carbon monoxide poisoning who suffer loss of consciousness. Patients who manifest signs of severe carbon monoxide poisoning with alterations in mental function, cardiovascular dysfunction, pulmonary oedema, or severe acidosis should be considered for HBO regardless of their carboxyhaemoglobin levels. The earlier HBO is initiated the better the outcome. In any event, patients with signs of severe carbon monoxide poisoning should be intubated and ventilated with 100% oxygen.

Oxygen therapy

Oxygen is indicated in any situation where tissue oxygenation is impaired, or to increase the amount of oxygen reserve before any airway procedure. The most efficient method for delivering a high oxygen concentration in the spontaneously breathing patient is to use a tight-fitting mask, with a wide-bore circuit and reservoir bag that is supplied with oxygen at a flow rate greater than the patient's minute ventilation. An alternative method in the spontaneously breathing patient is the use of Venturi devices that deliver set concentrations of oxygen. In the intubated patient with an airtight tracheal tube, delivery of 100% oxygen can be ensured and positive end-expiratory pressure (PEEP) can be used in an attempt to improve oxygenation.

Hyperbaric oxygen therapy

HBO therapy involves a patient breathing 100% oxygen while exposed to chamber pressures above atmospheric. HBO therapy evolved originally as a tool in the management of decompression sickness and arterial gas embolism. To date there are around 12 convincing indications for which HBO has been shown to be beneficial. However, access to HBO is is often limited by lack of an available facility and the dangers of transporting a critically ill patient. In the context of accident and emergency (A&E) medicine, there are a number of conditions for which HBO should be considered:

- Air or gas embolism.
- Carbon monoxide poisoning and smoke inhalation.
- Carbon monoxide poisoning complicated by cyanide poisoning.

- Decompression sickness.
- Gas gangrene.
- Necrotizing soft tissue infections.
- Acute traumatic ischaemia.

Victims of smoke inhalation are frequently exposed to both carbon monoxide and cyanide, which have synergistic toxicity. HBO not only reduces the half-life of carboxyhaemoglobin but also reduces the toxicity of cyanide and augments the antidote treatment (see Chapter 11).

MANAGEMENT

The airway

Airway patency can be established and controlled by basic manual and positional methods (with the aid of adjuncts), or by advanced techniques such as tracheal intubation, cricothyroidotomy and tracheostomy. Although basic airway manoeuvres are vitally important and will often successfully relieve airway obstruction and save lives, continued airway patency and security in the unconscious patient can only be guaranteed by placement of a cuffed tracheal tube.

All A&E doctors should be skilled in the use of basic airway manoeuvres and simple adjuncts. All A&E specialists should be competent in tracheal intubation and cricothyroidotomy.

A comprehensive range of airway procedures is described below.

Basic airway manoeuvres

TECHNIQUES

Chin lift and jaw thrust

The commonest cause of upper airway obstruction in the supine unconscious patient is the tongue falling backwards to occlude the posterior oropharynx . The chin lift (Fig. 4) and jaw thrust (Fig. 5) with head tilt will often relieve this obstruction.

Indication
- Upper airway obstruction.

Contraindication
- None, but caution is required in the presence of suspected cervical spinal injury (avoid head tilt).

Procedure
- The obstruction can usually be overcome by alignment of the head, neck and mandible.
- These manoeuvres lift the base of the tongue off the posterior pharyngeal wall.

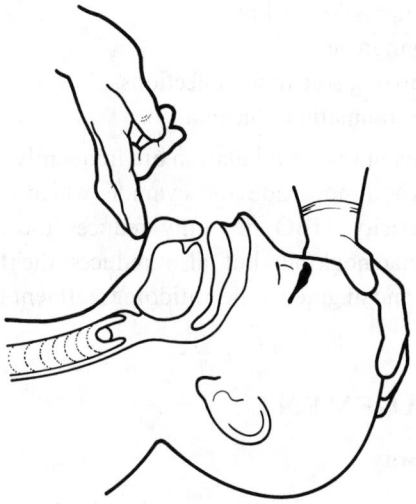

Fig. 4. Head tilt and chin lift.

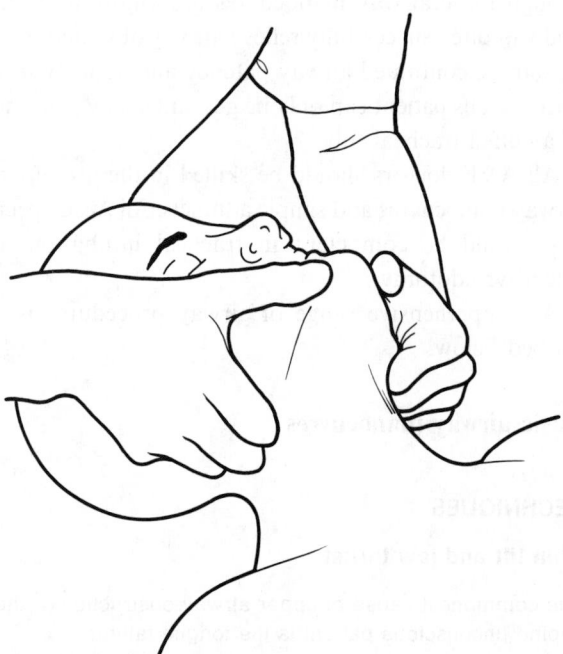

Fig. 5. The jaw thrust.

- The procedure consists of backward tilt of the head, elevation of the tip of the chin (chin lift) and protrusion of the mandible (jaw thrust).
- Cervical spine injury should be suspected in all cases of blunt trauma, particularly those with an altered level of consciousness and those with an injury above the clavicle. The cervical spine cannot be considered cleared until injury is excluded by radiological and clinical examination.

- If a cervical spinal injury is suspected, in-line stabilization of the head and neck should be maintained throughout, thus preventing neck movement.
- An open airway is confirmed by looking, listening and
  feeling for unobstructed air flow.

Potential complications
- Exacerbation of cervical spine injury.

Airway toilet and suctioning

Aspiration of the oropharynx is indicated to remove fluid and debris that is at risk of causing airway obstruction or pulmonary aspiration. Suction apparatus should develop a vacuum of 600 mmHg below atmospheric pressure within 10 sec of being switched on and be able to displace 35 litres of free air min^{-1}. The tonsil sucker (Yankauer) may cause mucosal damage when soft tissues are sucked into the end, and should have several end holes to reduce this risk. (For tracheal suction, refer to the section on intubation.)

The recovery position

This position aids the maintenance of a clear airway and reduces the risk of pulmonary aspiration in the spontaneously breathing, unconscious patient who is not at risk of cervical spine injury. Even a large person can be turned easily by a single small rescuer if the correct technique is used (Fig. 6).

Indication
- Airway maintenance in the unconscious, spontaneously breathing patient.

Relative contraindication
- Suspected spinal injury. If a spinal injury is suspected and turning is required, the patient should be 'log-rolled' into the lateral position. This will require a minimum of four attendants, one of whom maintains manual in-line stabilization of the cervical spine. This will prevent aggravation of spinal injury by rotation or flexion/extension of the spinal column.

Practical procedure
- Kneel beside the supine casualty.
- Ensure the airway is open.
- Place the arm nearest you out at right-angles to his body, elbow bent and palm uppermost.
- Bring the far arm across the chest and place the hand palm down on the shoulder nearest to you with the back of the hand against the cheek.
- Grasp the far leg just above the knee and pull it up, keeping the foot on the ground.
- With the other hand on the far shoulder, pull on the leg to roll the casualty towards you and onto his or her side.
- Adjust the upper leg so that both the hip and knee are bent at right-angles.

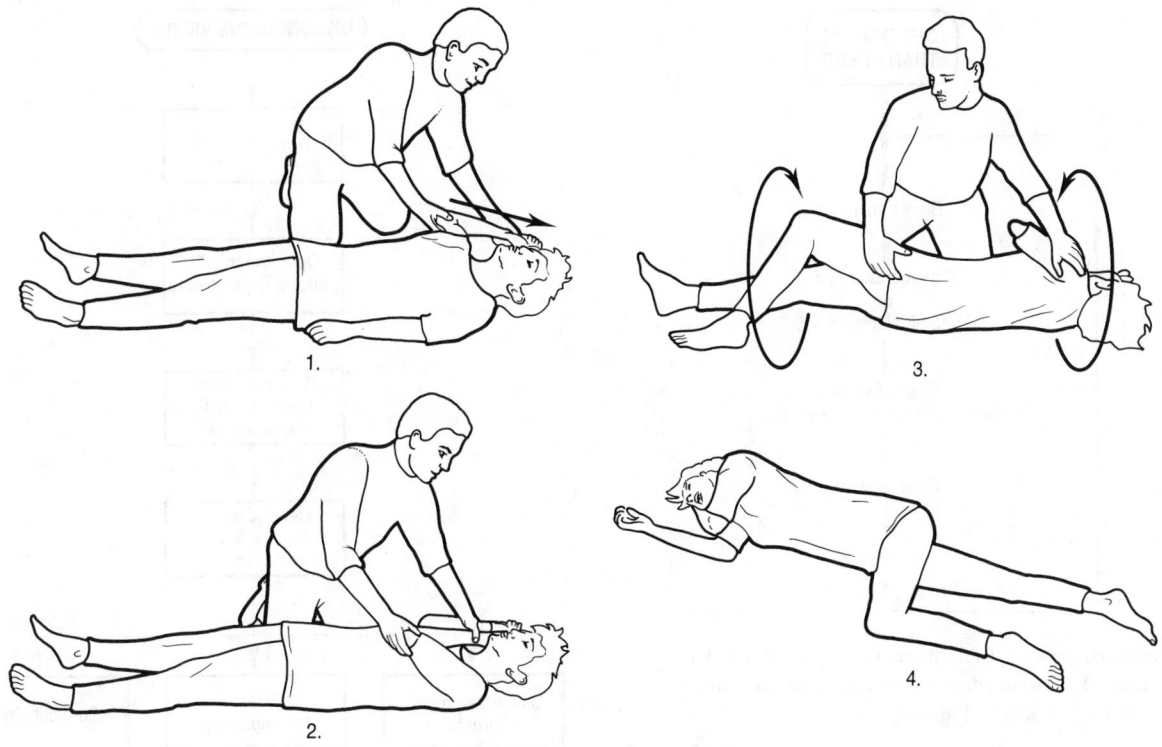

Fig. 6. The recovery position performed by a single rescuer.

- Adjust the hand under the cheek to support the head.
- Check the airway

Potential complications
- Care must be taken not to aggravate injuries to limbs, pelvis or chest, or disturb vascular lines, chest drains, urinary catheters, etc. Pressure injury may occur from an unnoticed item in a pocket or beneath the patient.

Clearance of the upper airway obstructed by solid material

If upper airway obstruction due to a foreign body is witnessed or strongly suspected, manoeuvres should be performed to increase intrathoracic pressure in an attempt to cause expulsion (Figs 7–10).

- *Back blows* should be used in the conscious patient with upper airway obstruction involving solid material and unrelieved by coughing (in the absence of suspected spinal or chest injury). Ideally the patient should be placed in the lateral position with a head down tilt. Alternatively the patient should stand or sit, and lean forward. Children can be placed prone and head down on the rescuer's arm or thigh. A series of five blows are delivered to the middle of the back of the chest, timed to coincide with expiration if possible (Fig. 11).
- *Abdominal thrusts* (Heimlich manoeuvre) may be tried in the conscious patient with upper airway obstruction involving solid material and unrelieved by coughing or

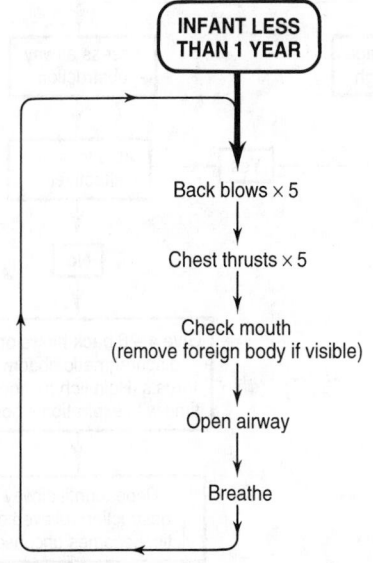

Fig. 7. Paediatric choking. Infant less than 1 year. (From Parr, M.J.A. & Craft, T.M. *Resuscitation: Key Data*, 2nd edn with permission of BIOS Scientific Publishers Ltd..)

back blows. Abdominal thrusts are not recommended in pregnancy, in children less than 1 year old, in patients with suspected spinal, chest or abdominal injury, or extreme obesity. Stand behind the victim wrapping the arms around the patient at the lower margin of the rib

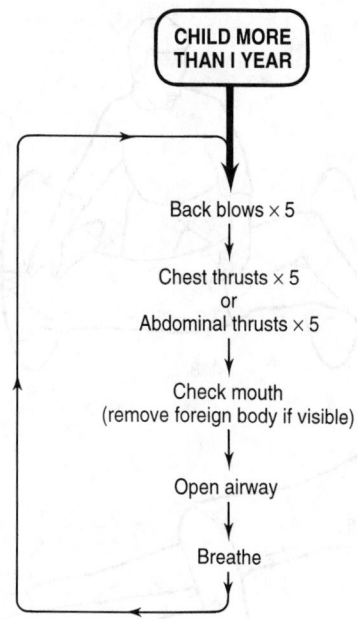

Fig. 8. Paediatric choking. Child more than 1 year. (From Parr, M.J.A. & Craft, T.M. *Resuscitation: Key Data*, 2nd edn with permission of BIOS Scientific Publishers Ltd.)

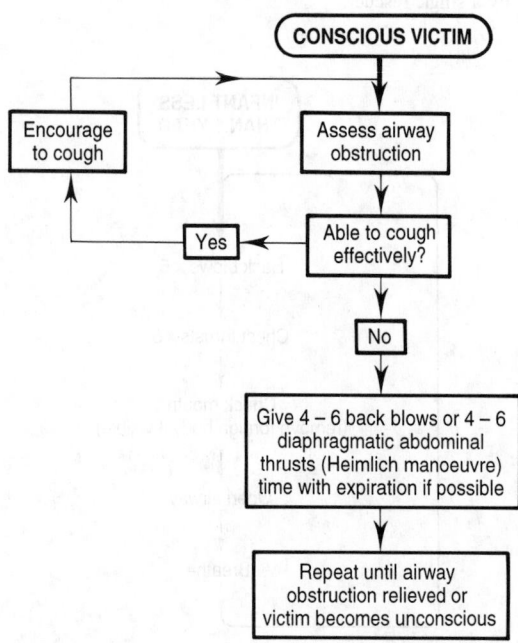

Fig. 9. Adult choking: conscious victim. (From Parr, M.J.A. & Craft, T.M. *Resuscitation: Key Data*, 2nd edn with permission of BIOS Scientific Publishers Ltd.)

cage. Make one hand into a fist, clasp it tightly with the other and give a series of five sharp upward thrusts, timed with expiration if discernible (Fig. 12). If abdominal thrusts do not expel the foreign material be prepared for the patient to lose consciousness and, in

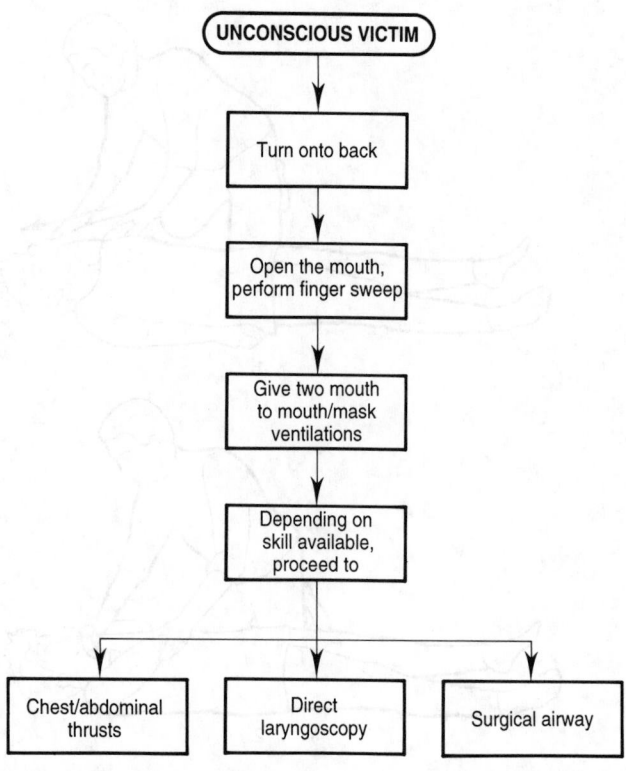

Fig. 10. Adult choking: unconscious victim. (From Parr, M.J.A. & Craft, T.M. *Resuscitation: Key Data*, 2nd edn with permission of BIOS Scientific Publishers Ltd.)

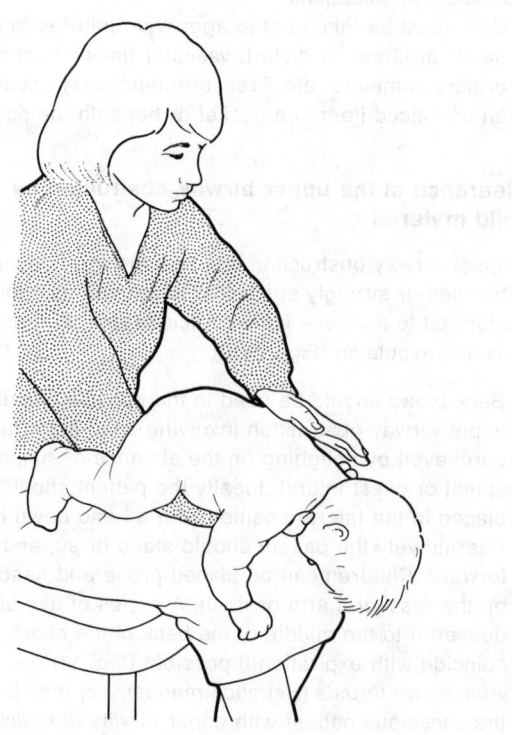

Fig. 11. Performing back blows on small children.

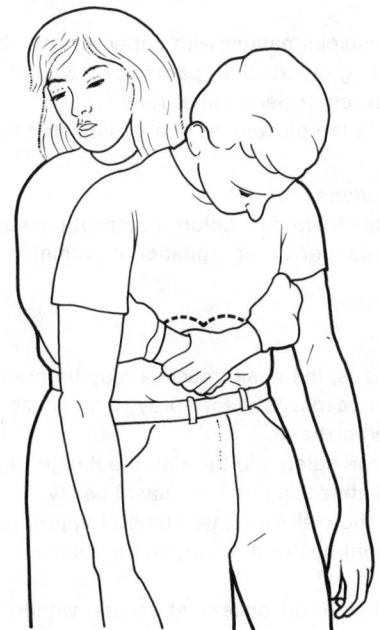

Fig. 12. Abdominal thrusts (Heimlich manoeuvre), standing victim.

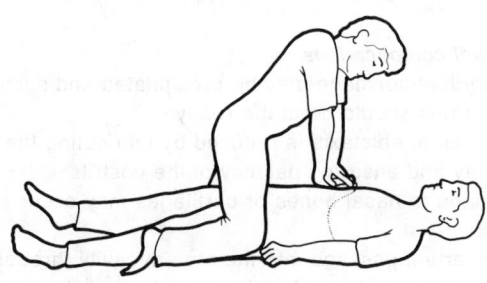

Fig. 13. Abdominal thrusts, supine victim.

adults, attempt to remove the obstruction by finger sweeps. Abdominal thrusts are not recommended in infants because of the risk of visceral injury. If the victim loses consciousness abdominal thrusts may be continued with the victim in the supine position (Fig. 13).

● *Chest thrusts* may be used to replace abdominal thrusts for children. The technique is similar to the chest compressions during cardiopulmonary resuscitation, but they are sharper and more vigorous.

● *Finger sweeps* may be used in the unconscious patient to clear the airway of visible foreign material (gastric contents, blood, false teeth, etc.) that may cause upper airway obstruction. If the material is not visible there are risks of causing deeper impaction of the foreign bodies and of producing soft tissue damage, especially in children.

● *Lateral positioning* with head down tilt is recommended to enhance the removal of fluid foreign material by gravity drainage and suctioning in unconscious patients.

● *Direct laryngoscopy* with suction or forceps removal of debris in an unconscious patient with airway obstruction may be used depending on the skill and experience of the clinician.

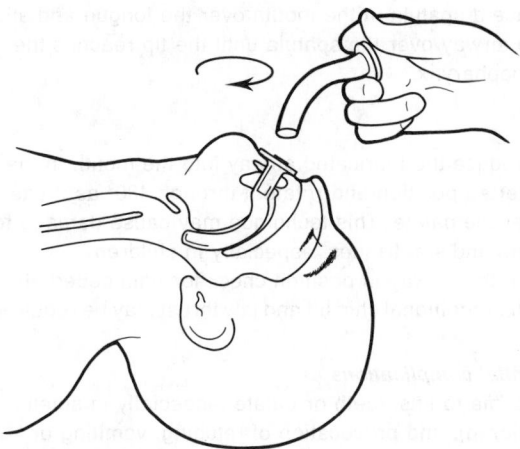

Fig. 14. Insertion of an oropharyngeal (Guedel) airway.

Airway adjuncts

Although a clear airway may be achieved by manual methods in the short term, there are many occasions when airway adjuncts are helpful and necessary. Some will merely retain airway patency; others will also offer some degree of protection against aspiration of foreign material and permit effective artificial ventilation.

TECHNIQUES

The oropharyngeal (Guedel) airway

The oropharyngeal (Guedel) airway prevents backward displacement of the tongue in the unconscious patient and usually provides relief for the rescuer from having to apply prolonged chin lift or jaw thrust. The airway does not protect against aspiration of foreign material. A variety of sizes (000–4) are available. Sizes 2 or 3 are suitable for the average adult (Fig. 14).

Indications

● An oropharyngeal airway is indicated in the unconscious patient with upper airway obstruction or impending obstruction and absent airway reflexes.

● It may also be used to act as a protective bite block when other airways such as a tracheal tube or laryngeal mask airway are in place.

Contraindications

● It is contraindicated in patients with clenched jaws, at-risk dentition, active airway reflexes, active bleeding within the hypopharynx, and those in danger of regurgitation or vomiting of stomach contents.

Procedure

There are two possible techniques for placing an oropharyngeal airway. With the patient in the supine or lateral position, either:

- Place a spatula in the mouth over the tongue and slide the airway over the spatula until the tip reaches the hypopharynx.

  or

- Introduce the lubricated airway into the mouth in the inverted position and rotate it through 180° as it passes over the palate. This technique may cause damage to teeth and soft tissues, especially in children.
- With the airway in position check for unimpeded air entry (additional chin lift and jaw thrust may be required).

Potential complications

- Trauma to lips, teeth or palate (especially in small children), and provocation of retching, vomiting or laryngeal spasm if active reflexes are present. The airway should be removed immediately at the first sign of these events occurring.

The nasopharyngeal airway

The nasopharyngeal airway is passed through the nose so that the tip lies behind the tongue in the laryngopharynx just above the glottis. The specially designed airway is made of soft plastic material and has a collar flange at its proximal end to prevent it disappearing into the nose (Fig. 15). If a purpose-made device is not available, one can be made from a cut-down uncuffed nasotracheal tube of the appropriate size with a large safety pin placed through the proximal end. Nasopharyngeal airways do not protect against aspiration of foreign material. Several sizes are available; a 6.5–7.5 mm airway is suitable for the average adult. They are easier to place than oral airways and are better tolerated by the obtunded patient.

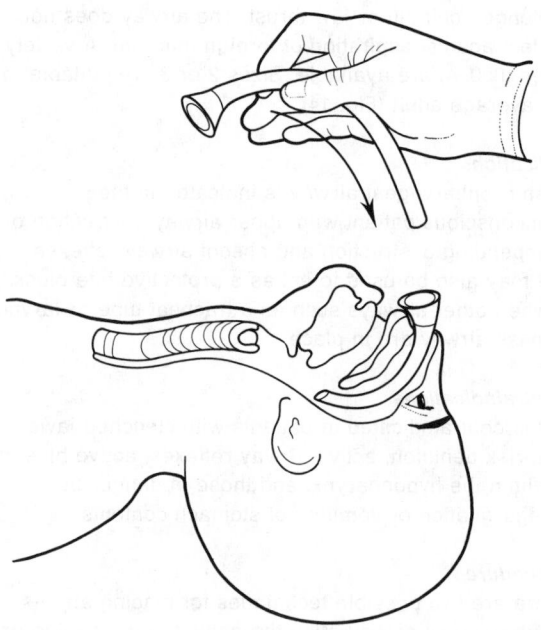

Fig. 15. Insertion of a nasopharyngeal airway.

Indications

- The unconscious patient with upper airway obstruction or impending obstruction, particularly with clenched jaws, seizures or dentition at risk.
- To facilitate the placement of a nasogastric tube.

Contraindications

- Bilateral obstructed or deformed nasal passages.
- Imminent danger of regurgitation or vomiting of stomach contents.

Procedure

- If time allows, the nasal mucosa may be prepared by applying a vasoconstrictor spray to minimize the risk of nasal haemorrhage.
- Pass a large safety pin through the flange to prevent the airway disappearing into the nasal cavity.
- Introduce the well-lubricated tube of appropriate size into the right nostril directing the tip backwards, not upwards.
- If obstruction to advancement occurs, withdraw and try the left nostril. Insert the airway with rotation until the flange impinges on the nostril.
- Check for unimpeded air entry.

Potential complications

- Nasal haemorrhage may be precipitated and suction apparatus should be at the ready.
- The risk of epistaxis is reduced by lubricating the airway and ensuring patency of the nostril.
- Damage to nasal bones or cartilages may occur with force.
- Inadvertent passage into the cranial cavity through a fractured cribriform plate is possible, therefore ensure that the airway is directed backwards not upwards. Use extreme caution in any patient who may have a base of skull fracture.
- Provocation of retching, vomiting or laryngeal spasm are possible although less likely than with the oropharyngeal airway.

Advanced airway manoeuvres

TECHNIQUES

Preoxygenation

Preoxygenation is performed to provide a reservoir of oxygen in the lungs to prevent desaturation during airway procedures. Administration of 100% oxygen in the presence of normal ventilation results in 85–98% nitrogen washout in 2 min, filling the functional residual capacity with oxygen. In normal individuals this reservoir may provide protection from hypoxia for more than 10 min. However, in individuals with pulmonary damage, reduced ventilation, decreased oxygen delivery or increased

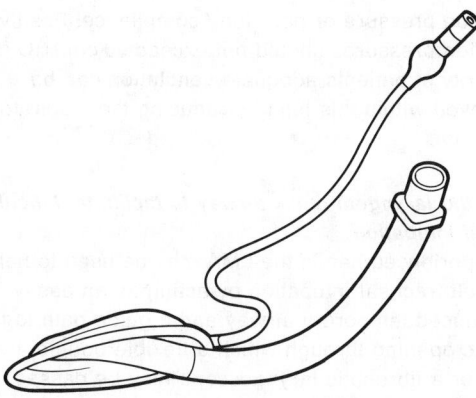

Fig. 16. The laryngeal mask airway.

Table 2. *Laryngeal mask airway sizes and cuff inflation volumes*

Size	Patient	Cuff volume (ml)
1	Neonates/infants up to 6.5 mg	2–4
2	Infants/children 6.5–15 kg	10
2.5	Children 15–30 kg	15
3	Small adults/children 30–50 kg	20
4	Normal and large adults	30
5	Large adults	40

oxygen consumption this safety period may be considerably shorter.

Indications
- Prior to any airway procedure that is likely to interfere with ventilation.

Practical technique
- 100% oxygen should be inhaled at a flow rate greater than the patients minute ventilation for 3 min, via a non-rebreathing circuit with a reservoir bag and a mask with an airtight seal.

The laryngeal mask airway

This airway (LMA) consists of a wide-bore tube with an elliptical inflatable cuff at the distal end which is designed to form a seal around the laryngeal opening, leaving the tube orifice in close proximity to the glottic opening (Fig. 16) (Brain, 1983). The LMA can provide a clear and secure airway without the skill required for laryngoscopy and tracheal intubation (Calder *et al*., 1990). While not guaranteeing protection of the airway in every case, the LMA offers greater security and convenience than most other airways except the tracheal tube. Carefully applied positive pressure ventilation may be provided via the LMA which incorporates a standard connector. The technique can easily be learnt by non-anaesthetists and is easier to perform than intubation or bag and mask ventilation (Pennant & Walker, 1992; Alexander *et al.*, 1993; Martin *et al*, 1993; Anonymous, 1994). The LMA is not intended as a long-term airway in the emergency situation.

The LMA is manufactured in a range of sizes in both standard and reinforced materials suitable for patients ranging from infants to large adults (Table 2).

Indications
- The LMA is indicated for the unconscious patient with absent airway reflexes at risk of airway obstruction who may need artificial ventilation when tracheal intubation is precluded by lack of skill or equipment.
- The LMA has a major role in cases of known or apparently difficult intubation.

Contraindications
- Situations involving high airway inflation pressures (e.g. chronic obstructive pulmonary disease), patients with full stomachs, and those with severe oropharyngeal trauma.

Procedure
- Lubricate the back and sides (but not the aperture) of the completely deflated cuff.
- With the patient in the supine position and the head and neck aligned in the clear airway position, depress the chin to open the mouth.
- Holding the tube like a pen, introduce the LMA into the mouth with the distal aperture facing caudad (Fig. 17).
- Advance the tip, applying it to the surface of the palate until it reaches the posterior pharyngeal wall.

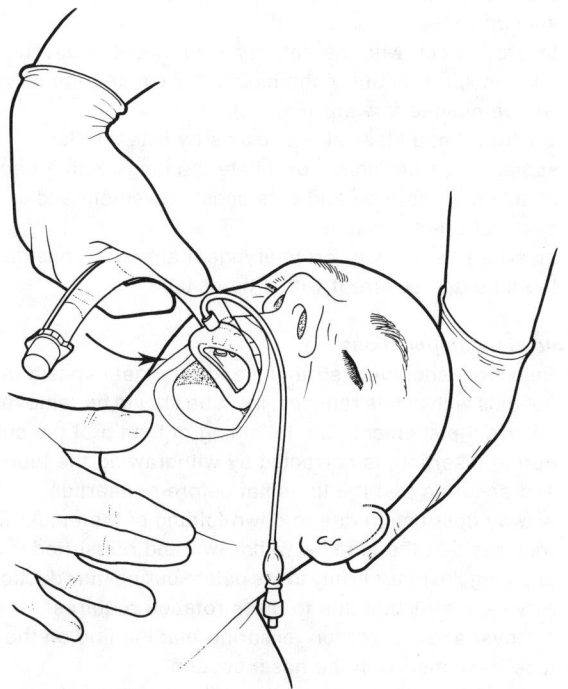

Fig. 17. Technique of inserting the laryngeal mask airway.

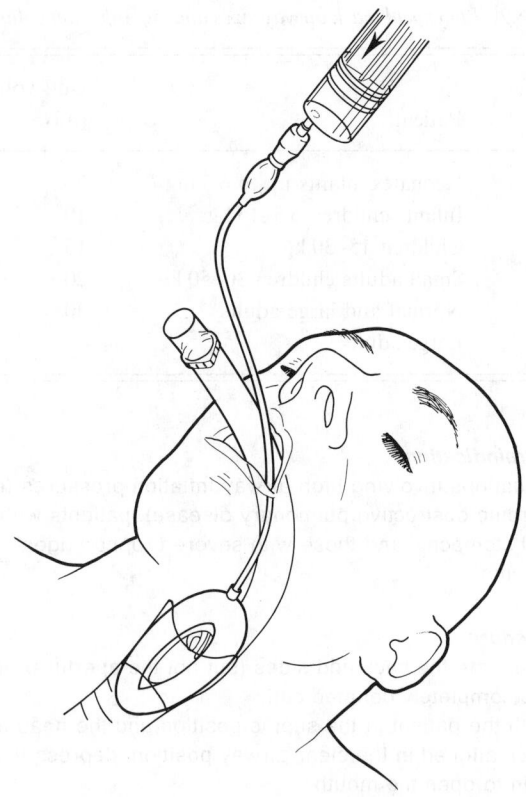

Fig. 18. Technique of inserting the laryngeal mask airway.

- Now move the operating hand to the proximal end of the tube and press the mask into position until resistance is felt as it locates in the back of the laryngopharynx.
- The line on the tube should be aligned with the nasal septum.
- Inflate the cuff with the appropriate amount of air; the tube should rise out of the mouth 1–2 cm and the larynx will be pushed forward (Fig. 18).
- Confirm that a clear airway exists by listening for spontaneous breathing, or inflate the lungs with a bag attached to the tube and note chest movement and bilateral breath sounds.
- Insert a bite block or oropharyngeal airway alongside the tube and secure it with a tie or tape.

Potential complications

- Rejection, coughing, straining and laryngeal spasm in patients with active reflexes; the tube should be removed.
- Incorrect placement, due to folding of the tip of the cuff during insertion, is corrected by withdrawing the tube and ensuring that the tip is flat before reinsertion.
- Airway obstruction due to down folding of the epiglottis, requires that the tube be withdrawn and reinserted, applying the mask firmly to the palate during introduction.
- Airway obstruction due to mask rotation requires removal and reinsertion, ensuring that the line on the tube is aligned with the nasal septum.
- Persistent leakage around the cuff may be due to incorrect sizing, inadequate cuff inflation, excessive lung

inflation pressure or poor lung compliance. Positive inflation pressures should not exceed 20 cm H_2O. In the majority of patients adequate ventilation can be achieved within this limit by reducing the inspiratory flow rate.

Use of the laryngeal mask airway to facilitate difficult tracheal intubation

- In experienced hands the LMA may be used to help with difficult tracheal intubation by acting as an easily introduced temporary airway and a guide path to the glottic opening through which a flexible bougie, tracheal tube or a fibreoptic laryngoscope may be passed (Brain, 1984, 1985; Heath & Allagain, 1991).

The pharyngotracheal lumen airway

The pharyngotracheal lumen airway (PTLA) has been introduced as a substitute for the oesophageal obturator airway which has waned in popularity. This airway consists of two tubes, a longer one with a distal cuff and a shorter one with a large cuff (Fig. 19). Although relatively difficult to introduce, the PTLA does offer security of the airway.

Indications

- The PTLA is indicated for the unconscious patient with absent airway reflexes at risk of airway obstruction who may need artificial ventilation when tracheal intubation is precluded by lack of skill or equipment.

Contraindications

- Severe oropharyngeal trauma.
- Inadequate mouth opening (the device is bulky).

Procedure

- The device is introduced into the mouth blindly and is designed so that the short tube lies just above the glottic opening with the large cuff inflated to obliterate the hypopharynx.
- Normally the longer tube enters the oesophagus and its cuff is inflated to prevent regurgitation of gastric contents and prevent gas entering the stomach.
- Inflation of the short tube ventilates the lungs through the glottic opening.
- If the long tube enters the trachea, ventilation is applied through this route, and the short tube can then act as a guide path for a separate gastric tube to remove stomach contents.

Potential complications

- The cuffs may be damaged by sharp teeth during insertion.
- Further damage to soft tissues may occur in patients with oropharyngeal injuries.
- Massive inflation of the stomach occurs if ventilation is applied to the incorrect tube, so confirmation of correct placement is essential.

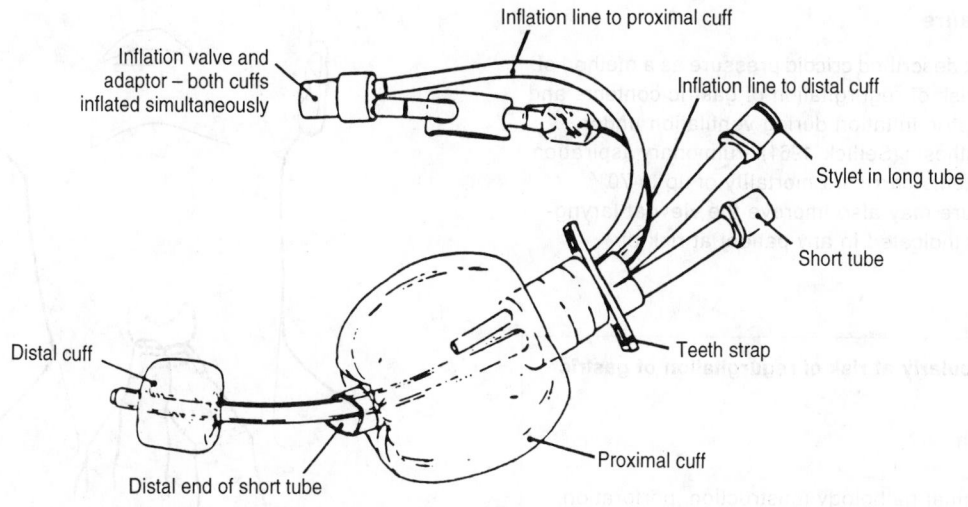

Fig. 19. The pharyngotracheal lumen airway (PTLA).

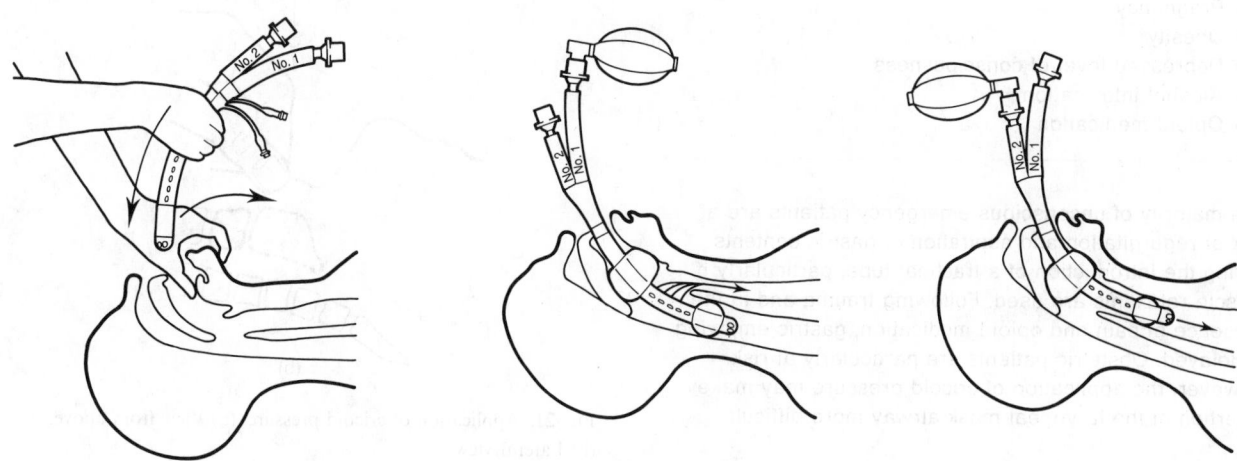

Fig. 20. The Combitube oesophageal/tracheal airway.

The Combitube oesophageal/tracheal airway

The Combitube is a double lumen tube which is designed to ventilate the patient's lungs whether the tube enters the trachea or the oesophagus (Frass *et al.*, 1987). The 'tracheal' channel has an open distal end and the 'oesophageal' channel has a blind end with openings at supraglottic level. There is a small-volume distal cuff and a high-volume (100 ml) cuff designed to occupy the laryngopharynx (Fig. 20).

Indications
- The Combitube is suitable for use in an unconscious patient with absent airway reflexes at risk of airway obstruction who may need artificial ventilation when tracheal intubation is precluded by lack of available skill or equipment.

Contraindications
- As with the PTLA, the Combitube is contraindicated in severe oropharyngeal trauma.

Procedure
- The tube is introduced into the mouth blindly.
- If the tube enters the oesophagus the patient is ventilated via the 'oesophageal' channel through the openings just above the glottic aperture.
- The inflating gas is prevented from passing anywhere else by the distal and hypopharyngeal cuffs.
- If the tube enters the trachea, ventilation should be via the 'tracheal' port, and the hypopharyngeal cuff is redundant.

Potential complications
- The cuffs may be damaged by sharp teeth during insertion.
- Further damage to soft tissues in patients with oropharyngeal injuries may occur.
- Massive inflation of the stomach occurs if ventilation is applied to the incorrect tube, so confirmation of correct placement is essential.

Cricoid pressure

In 1961, Sellick described cricoid pressure as a method of reducing the risk of regurgitation of gastric contents and preventing gastric inflation during ventilation under general anaesthesia (Sellick, 1961). Pulmonary aspiration of gastric contents carries a mortality of up to 70%. Cricoid pressure may also improve the view at laryngoscopy and is indicated in any patient at risk of regurgitation.

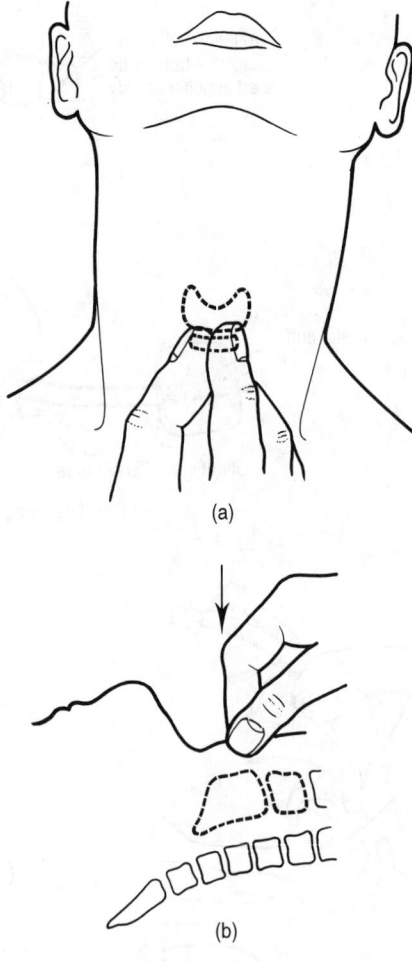

Fig. 21. Application of cricoid pressure. (a) View from above. (b) Lateral view.

Patients particularly at risk of regurgitation of gastric contents

- Full stomach
- Trauma
- Intra-abdominal pathology (obstruction, perforation, paresis)
- Hiatus hernia
- Pregnancy
- Obesity
- Depressed level of consciousness
- Alcohol intoxication
- Opioid medication

The majority of unconscious emergency patients are at risk of regurgitation and aspiration of gastric contents during the introduction of a tracheal tube, particularly if muscle relaxants are used. Following trauma and in the presence of pain and opioid medication, gastric emptying is delayed. Obstetric patients are particularly at risk. However, the application of cricoid pressure may make insertion of the laryngeal mask airway more difficult.

Indications

- To reduce the risk of regurgitation of gastric contents.
- To prevent gastric inflation during positive pressure ventilation via a face mask.

Contraindications

- The conscious patient (properly applied cricoid pressure is painful).

Procedure

Extension of the neck (which is avoided in trauma patients with suspected cervical spine injury) and backward pressure on the cricoid cartilage result in occlusion of the oesophagus against the vertebral body of C5.

- The patient is generally placed in the supine position but can be lying on the left side if circumstances dictate and the intubationist is highly skilled.
- In the conscious patient palpate the cricoid cartilage between the thumb and middle finger with the index finger above (Fig. 21).
- As anaesthesia is induced, apply pressure in a vertical plane.
- A pressure of around 44 N (4 kg) is required, or roughly

the amount of pressure that when applied to the bridge of the nose would feel uncomfortable.

- Apply counter pressure, either with a semirigid cervical collar in trauma patients, or in other patients with the opposite hand placed behind the neck.
- Maintain pressure until the trachea is safely intubated and the cuff inflated.

Potential complications

- If incorrectly applied, cricoid pressure will increase the difficulty of intubation.
- The pressure may need to be adjusted, or very rarely removed, to facilitate intubation.
- Active vomiting against applied cricoid pressure may cause oesophageal or gastric rupture.

Tracheal intubation

Tracheal intubation provides the most reliable, clear and secure airway through which positive pressure ventilation can be applied. The cuff around the distal end of the tube prevents gas leakage during ventilation and guards the

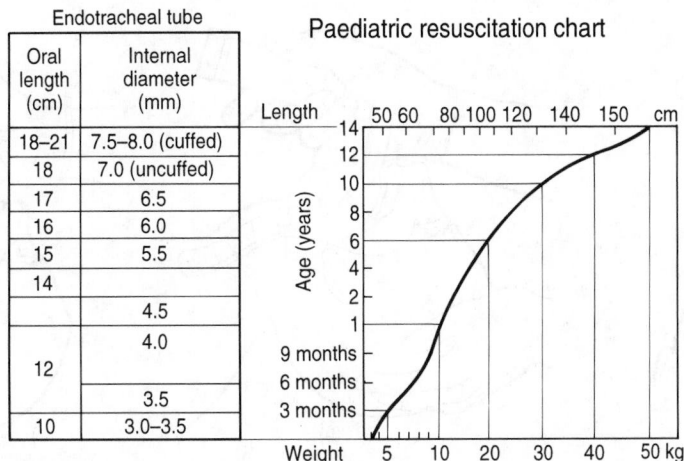

Fig. 22. The Oakley paediatric resuscitation chart. (From *British Medical Journal*, 1 October 1988; **297** by permission of the publisher.)

tracheobronchial tree from aspiration of foreign material. The tube can be passed into the trachea by a variety of means: orally or nasally using direct laryngoscopy to view the passage of the tube through the glottic opening, blind nasally, blind orally with the aid of an Augustine Guide™; orally or nasally using a guiding light wand, with the aid of a fibreoptic laryngoscope, or by using a retrograde cannulation technique.

Tracheal intubation can be performed on patients of any age and a range of tube sizes are available. Tracheal tubes are made longer than is generally needed and usually have to be cut to the appropriate length (see below). All should be fitted with a 15 mm adapter. Conventional tracheal tubes less than 6.5 mm diameter do not have cuffs. Tubes of larger size may be cuffed or uncuffed. For adult anaesthesia and in patients on the intensive therapy unit, cuffed tubes are preferred as they offer protection against aspiration and allow leak-proof positive pressure ventilation.

Methods of assessing the potential difficulty of intubating a patient have been discussed above. It is usually a combination of factors that determines the difficulty of intubation. Unexpected difficulty with intubation can still occur in the absence of any indicators.

Sizing of tubes

The adult trachea will accommodate 7.0–9.0 mm internal diameter (ID) tubes cut to a length of between 21–25 cm (2 cm longer for nasal intubation).Conventionally, in the UK, 8.0 mm ID tubes are used for females and 9.0 mm ID tubes are used for males; American anaesthesiologists tend to intubate the trachea with tubes 1 mm smaller. Tracheal tubes with high-volume, low-pressure cuffs are preferred to those with low-volume, high-pressure cuffs.

In children the correct internal diameter and length can be obtained from charts (Fig. 22) (Oakley *et al.*, 1993), or can be calculated using the following formulae:

Internal diameter (mm) = (Age of child/4) + 4

Length (cm) = (Age of child/2) + 12

[add an additional 1–3 cm for nasal tubes]

Orotracheal intubation using direct laryngoscopy

Unless there are specific contraindications, anaesthetists would normally place a tracheal tube via the oral route, aided by direct laryngoscopy. As long as the necessary skills have been acquired, in the vast majority of circumstances this technique is the quickest and most reliable method for inserting a tracheal tube.

Indications

- Airway obstruction or potential airway obstruction in the unconscious or anaesthetized patient.
- Airway protection in patients at risk of aspiration of foreign material.
- Patients requiring positive pressure ventilation because of actual or impending respiratory failure or for therapeutic reasons such as controlled ventilation for head injury.
- To facilitate PEEP, and high inspired oxygen concentration.
- To gain access to the lower respiratory tract for aspiration of secretions, bronchial lavage, etc.
- To provide a route for delivery of resuscitation drugs.
- Where the airway is at risk during head, neck and airway surgery.

Absolute contraindications

- Absence of available skill and equipment.

Relative contraindications

- Severe maxillofacial trauma with anatomical disruption.
- Inaccessible glottis due to immobility or distorted anatomy from tumour, infection, or massive pharyngeal or laryngeal oedema.

Procedure

- Wherever possible, use a pulse oximeter to monitor the patient's arterial oxygen saturation.

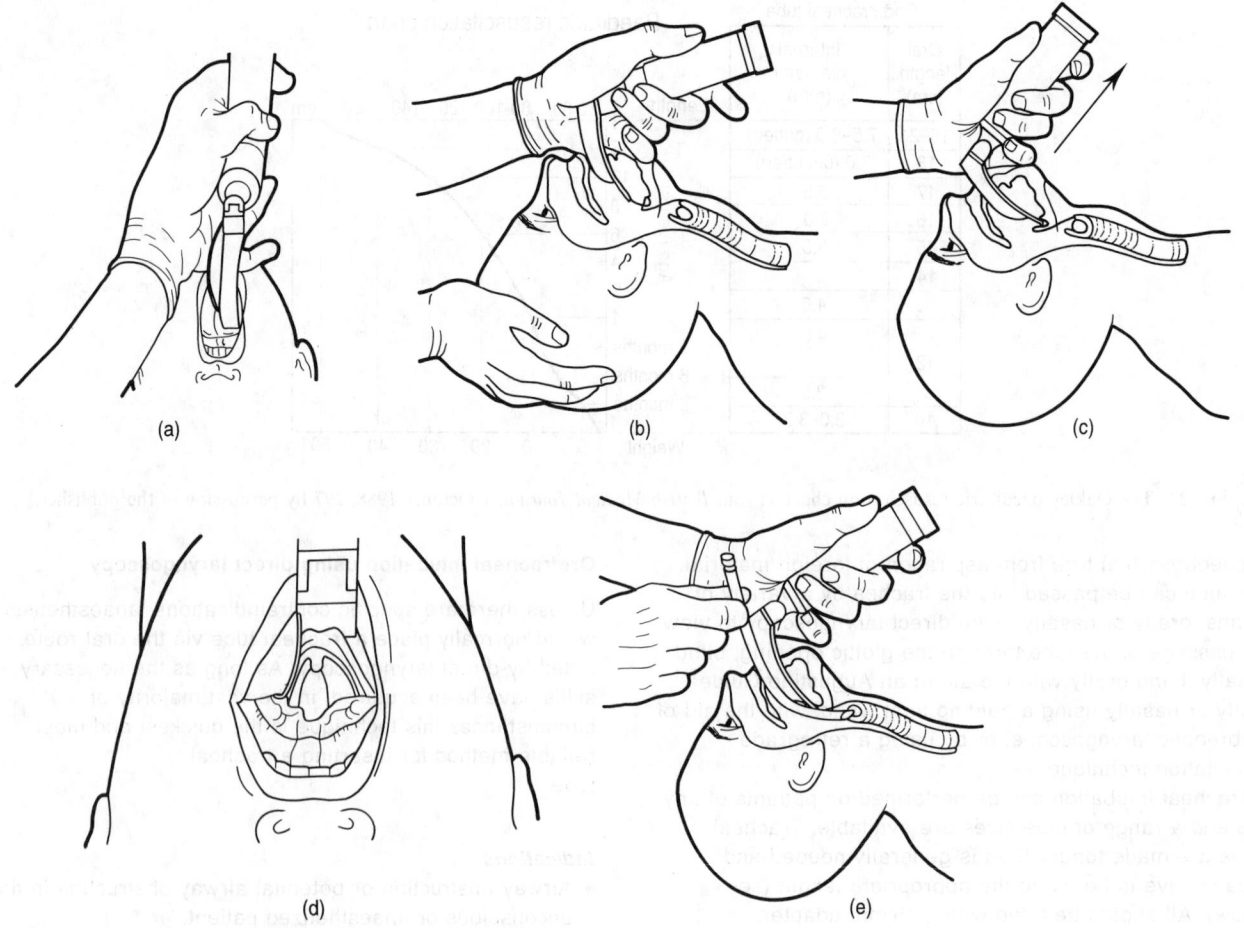

Fig. 23(a–e). Orotracheal intubation.

- Before attempting intubation, briefly ventilate and oxygenate the patient with a bag–valve–mask device (see 'preoxygenation' above).
- Place the patient supine in the clear airway position with one pillow under the head. (Obtaining good views of the larynx at direct laryngoscopy requires that the mouth, oropharynx and larynx are in one plane. Flexion of the neck aligns the larynx and oropharynx, while extension at the atlanto-occipital joint aligns the mouth and oropharynx – "sniffing the morning air" position).
- Using the left hand to hold the laryngoscope handle, insert the laryngoscope blade into the right-hand corner of the mouth ensuring that the lower lip is not caught between the blade and lower teeth.
- Slide the laryngoscope blade towards the posterior pharyngeal wall, aiming for the midline at laryngeal level and displacing the body of the tongue towards the left-hand side of the mouth.
- When the laryngoscope tip reaches the larynx, lift the laryngoscope handle forwards and upwards (towards the junction of the ceiling and the opposite wall) and observe the tip of the laryngoscope blade (Fig. 23).
- If using a curved laryngoscope blade, slide the tip of the blade between the back of the tongue and the base of

the epiglottis (the vallecula), maintaining head tilt by occipital pressure with the right hand. If using a straight laryngoscope blade, place the tip of the blade behind the epiglottis.
- Adjust the tip of blade to improve the view of the cords. Pressure on the cricoid cartilage may improve the view and reduces the possibility of gastric regurgitation.
- Pass the tracheal tube through the right-hand corner of the mouth and between the vocal cords under direct vision. If necessary rotate the tube 90° counter clockwise to ease the passage through the glottic opening.
- If the view is restricted to only the epiglottis or arytenoids, use a gum elastic bougie. The distal end of the bougie should be angled to 45° and if passed directly behind the epiglottis it will usually pass through the vocal cords into the trachea. Tracheal placement of the bougie is confirmed if the bougie is felt to 'click' across the tracheal rings or to be 'held up' in the bronchial tree. Leaving the laryngoscope in the mouth, railroad the tracheal tube over the bougie into the trachea. Keep hold of the tube and withdraw the bougie.
- Once the tube has passed between the vocal cords, it should be advanced so that the cuff lies below the glottis opening.

- Inflate the cuff through the pilot tube until the audible leak associated with positive pressure ventilation ceases. Suspect an incorrectly placed tube in the oesophagus if cuff inflation volumes of more than 10–15 ml are required.
- Confirm correct placement of the tracheal tube (see 'monitoring' below). Check that the tube is in the trachea by observing bilateral chest movement and auscultate breath sounds over both upper lobes in the axillae. Listen over the epigastrium; gurgling sounds suggest oesophageal placement. If an oesophageal detector device is available, connect to the tracheal tube and attempt to aspirate air. Easy aspiration of air and no return of the plunger confirms correct tracheal placement. Difficulty in aspirating air and the generation of a negative pressure suggests oesophageal placement. The detection of carbon dioxide in exhaled air is the gold standard for confirming tracheal intubation and a capnometer should be located permanently in the resuscitation room. However, this technique is unreliable during cardiopulmonary resuscitation, when the end-tidal pCO_2 may be very low or nil.
- Allow 30 sec for the entire procedure of intubation. If the attempt has failed after this time, remove the laryngoscope and tube, and ventilate with oxygen via the bag–valve–mask device for 1–2 min before trying again.
- Secure the tube in place with a tie or tape.

Modifications for children
Because of the anatomical differences (particularly the relatively large and floppy epiglottis) discussed at the beginning of the chapter, most clinicians find a straight-bladed laryngoscope preferable in children below 2 years of age. The straight blade is passed behind the epiglottis (not in front, as is done with the curved blade). The size of tracheal tube is critical as there must be a leak to prevent the possible complication of subglottic stenosis associated with prolonged intubation. In infants and children the narrowest diameter of the airway is at the level of the cricoid ring and not, as in the adult, the space between the vocal cords. Therefore cuffed tubes are not generally used in infants and children under 10 years. A slight leak during positive pressure ventilation is acceptable. Special care must be taken to ensure that bronchial intubation does not occur as the child's trachea is relatively short.

Potential complications
- Trauma to lips, teeth, tongue and structures in the pharynx or larynx.
- Exacerbation of cervical spine injury.
- Failure to intubate.
- Oesophageal intubation. Bronchial intubation.
- Vagal stimulation causing bradycardia may be blocked with anticholinergic medication and must be differentiated from the bradycardia associated with hypoxia.

- Sympathetic stimulation with hypertension and tachyarrhythmias.
- Inducing vomiting, coughing and laryngospasm.
- Aspiration of foreign material (e.g. stomach contents, blood, etc.) during the intubation attempt.
- Kinking of the tracheal tube in the pharynx or mouth.
- Overinflation of the cuff leading to pressure necrosis of the tracheal mucous membrane or ballooning of the cuff to obstruct the lumen of the tube.

Oral intubation aided by the McCoy levering laryngoscope

On many occasions (particularly when attempting to intubate the patient with the head and neck in neutral alignment) laryngoscopy will result in visualization of the epiglottis only. In some of these situations a gentle levering movement of the laryngoscope will improve the view. However, when levering the laryngoscope the upper teeth may inadvertently be used as a fulcrum producing dental damage. Recently, a modification of the standard curved laryngoscope blade, the levering laryngoscope, has been described (McCoy & Mirakur, 1993) (Fig. 24). The levering laryngoscope differs from the standard curved blade as follows:

- The blade has been cut 2.5 cm proximal to the tip and a hinge placed between the two parts.
- A 15.5 cm long lever is attached to the proximal end of the handle.
- The lever is connected to a spring-loaded drum on the proximal end of the blade.
- A connecting shaft links the spring-loaded drum to the hinged tip.

The blade adds 70 g to a standard 100 g blade and can be attached to a standard laryngoscope handle.

Indications
- As for direct oral intubation.
- As an alternative to the gum elastic bougie when the epiglottis only is visualized at laryngoscopy.

Contraindications
- As for direct oral intubation.
- Lack of training and experience with the McCoy blade.

Procedure
- The patient is positioned and laryngoscopy performed as described under direct oral intubation.
- Grasp the laryngoscope handle in the normal manner with the lever lying posterior to the thumb. In this position the blade will be maintained in the usual curved shape.
- Insert the blade tip into the vallecula. Move the thumb from the laryngoscope handle to behind the lever.
- Apply gentle pressure to the handle. Approximately 20° movement of the lever causes the blade tip to elevate 70° upwards, lifting the hyoepiglottic ligament and exposing the larynx.

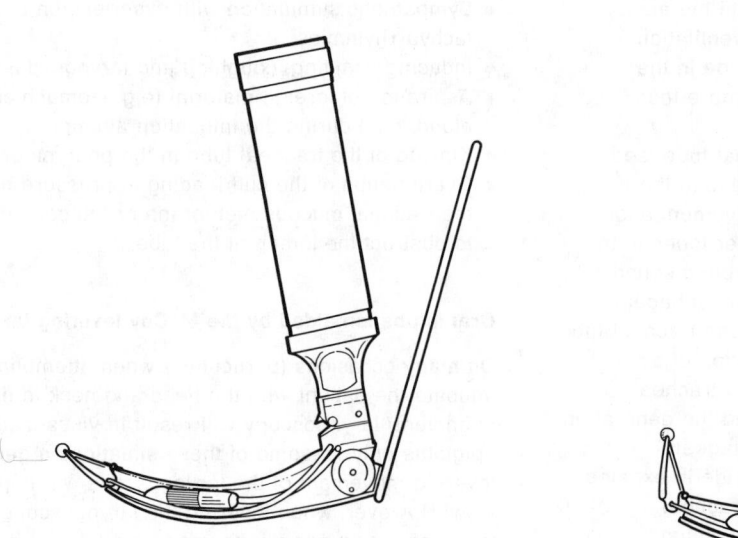
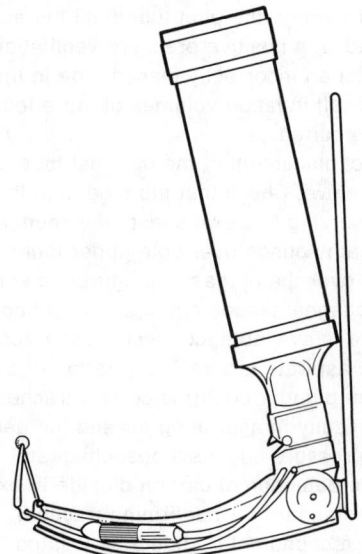

Fig. 24. The McCoy levering laryngoscope.

- Place the tracheal tube in the usual way. Release the lever and withdraw the blade gently from the mouth.
- Check the tube position and secure as described above.

Potential complications

The complications of this technique are similar to those described under direct oral intubation, though the risk of dental damage should, theoretically, be less.

Oral intubation aided by the Bullard laryngoscope

The Bullard intubating laryngoscopes comprise anatomically shaped rigid blades with an attached fibreoptic light source and intubating stylet (Bjoraker, 1990) (Fig. 25). They are designed for indirect oral visualization of the larynx and intubation with virtually no manipulation of the head and neck. The blade can be successfully placed in patients with as little as 6 mm of mouth opening. There are paediatric and adult versions of the Bullard laryngoscope. The adult blade is designed to arch over the tongue and is in a shape that resembles an inverted question mark. The paediatric version has a short L-shaped blade and is recommended for use in patients up to 10 years of age.

Indications

- Oral intubation in patients with limited mouth opening.
- Oral intubation in patients with cervical spine pathology where the head and neck must be kept in neutral alignment.

Contraindications

- Lack of experience with the technique.

Procedure

- Position the patient as for direct oral intubation above.

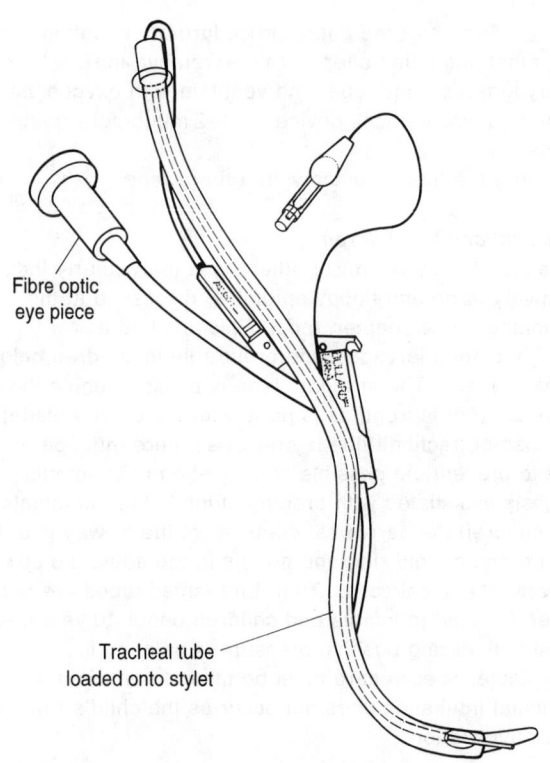

Fibre optic eye piece

Tracheal tube loaded onto stylet

Fig. 25. The Bullard laryngoscope (without handle).

- Load a tracheal tube of appropriate size onto the rigid intubation stylet. The stylet is fastened proximally to the laryngoscope and rides behind the length of the laryngoscope blade.
- Adjust the stylet so that its distal end is within the field of view of the laryngoscope. The stylet protrudes approximately 2 cm from the end of the tracheal tube.

- With the left hand, place the laryngoscope blade, tube and stylet into the pharynx. Aim the stylet tip at the glottic opening.
- Advance the tracheal tube off the stylet and through the vocal cords.
- Check the tube position and secure as described above.

Potential complications.

- Proficient use of the Bullard laryngoscope requires considerable practice.
- The level of skill required for this technique will probably restrict its use to anaesthetists.
- The patient may become hypoxic if the clinician spends too long attempting to intubate the patient with a Bullard laryngoscope.
- The presence of blood or vomit will severely restrict the view.

Digital blind oral intubation

This technique is rarely used but enthusiasts claim that with practice the majority of deeply unconscious patients can be intubated by the digital (or tactile) method. It has been used in the prehospital environment particularly (Stewart, 1984). Its potential advantages include minimal movement of the head and neck, secretions or blood in the airway do not alter the success rate, and it requires minimal equipment.

Indications

- Where intubation is required and the patient is deeply unconscious.
- Lack of experience or equipment for direct oral intubation with the aid of a laryngoscope.

Contraindications

- Any patient who is not deeply unconscious.
- The ability and equipment to perform direct laryngoscopy.

Procedure

- Lubricate the tracheal tube and insert a stylet. The distal end of the stylet should be level with the 'Murphy eye' (the side aperture near the tip of tracheal tubes) of the tracheal tube. Curve the stylet to form a 'J' shape with a gentle hook at the tip.
- Kneel at the side of the patient facing the patient's right shoulder. Hold the tracheal tube in the right hand. Introduce the index and middle fingers of the left hand into the corner of the patient's mouth. Depressing the tongue and opening the mouth, slide the fingers along the tongue until the epiglottis is easily palpated in the midline.
- Pass the tube into the mouth along a path between the two fingers towards the epiglottis. Place the tube behind the epiglottis and with firm, anteriorly directed pressure guide the tube through the glottis.
- Once through the cords, withdraw the stylet and push the tube further into the trachea.

- Check the tube position, inflate the cuff and secure as above.

Potential complications

- The intubator's fingers may be bitten if the patient is not deeply unconscious.
- There may be a higher incidence of laryngeal trauma than with the direct oral technique.

The technique is not as successful as direct oral intubation with a laryngoscope.

Blind oral intubation aided by the lighted stylet

In this method, a lighted stylet (light wand) is passed through the lumen of the tracheal tube so that the light at the end just emerges from the distal end of the tube (Vollmer et al., 1985) (Fig. 26). This technique can be combined with tactile intubation. The principle of the technique is to pass the tube directly through the glottis into the trachea using maximal transillumination to confirm the position of the tube as it is guided from just above the larynx, through the vocal cords and into the trachea.

Indications

- Difficult intubation using direct laryngoscopy.
- Suspected spinal injury where the head and neck must be kept in neutral alignment.

Contraindications

- Lack of experience with the procedure.
- Oropharyngeal injury, inflammation, tumour or airway obstruction due to pharyngeal or laryngeal oedema.

Procedure

- Place the patient supine with the head and neck aligned in the clear airway position.
- Wrap a piece of gauze around the tongue and pull it forward.
- Pass the light wand through the lumen of the tracheal tube so that the lighted end just emerges from the distal end of the tube and bend it to a J shape. The base of the J should be equal in length to the thyromental distance.
- Clip the proximal end of the tube to the wand handle.
- Introduce the tube and wand into the mouth, aiming for the larynx.
- Observe the transillumination anteriorly as the tube passes behind the tongue and into the hypopharynx.
- Advance the tube further. If it passes easily and if the transillumination intensity increases in the midline, it has entered the trachea; if the light intensity diminishes, the tube has entered the oesophagus.
- Transillumination either side of the midline, with difficulty in advancement, indicates incorrect placement in the piriform fossa.

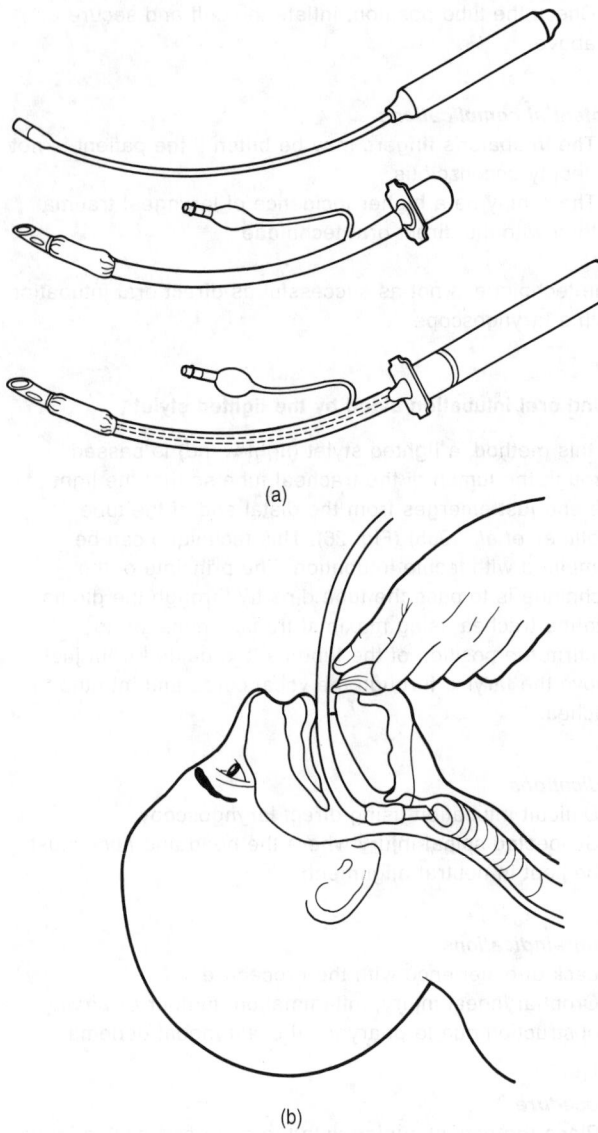

(a)

(b)

Fig. 26(a, b). The light stylet.

Potential complications

- Persistent lodging in the piriform fossa or in front of the epiglottis.
- Damage to pharyngeal or laryngeal structures.

This technique is less successful than oral intubation under direct laryngoscopy. It is likely to be difficult in a brightly lit room or in sunlight.

Blind oral intubation aided by the Augustine Guide

The Augustine Guide™ (Fig. 27) allows oral endotracheal intubation to be performed blindly and without head and neck manipulation (Kovac, 1993). It is a premoulded device designed to fit in a lock and key fashion in the glottis; it

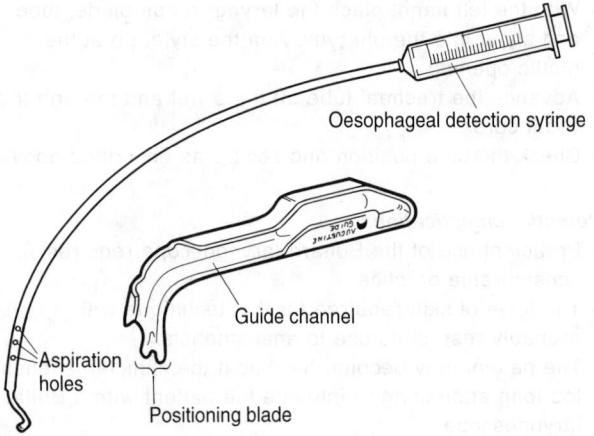

Fig. 27. The Augustine Guide™.

serves as a guide to allow blind insertion of an endotracheal tube. A specially designed stylet (with side aspiration holes at the distal end) is advanced through the Augustine Guide™ channel and the endotracheal tube is then advanced over the stylet into the larynx.

Indications

- Patients with suspected cervical spine fractures who require intubation.

Contraindications

- Wherever possible, it is better to use direct laryngoscopy and oral intubation for urgent advanced airway control.

Procedure

- Place the patient supine with the head and neck in neutral alignment.
- Mount the well-lubricated tracheal tube onto the guiding channel and slide the stylet into the tracheal tube.
- Open the patient's mouth and insert a bite block between the molars on the right.
- Grasp the tip of the tongue with gauze and withdraw the tongue as far as possible.
- Insert the Augustine Guide™, tracheal tube and stylet into the mouth and advance toward the larynx. The distal end of the guide will lock into the glossoepiglottic fold.
- Advance the stylet into the larynx. Attach the 35 ml syringe to the stylet and rapidly aspirate. Free and easy return of air confirms successful placement of the stylet in the trachea. If the stylet enter the oesophagus, aspiration of air is difficult or impossible because the oesophageal walls collapse and occlude the side holes of the stylet.
- On confirming successful entry of the stylet into the trachea, detach the tracheal tube from the guide and advance it over the stylet and into the trachea.

- Remove the stylet and confirm correct location of the tube in the trachea by the standard techniques.

Potential complications

- The Augustine Guide™ may cause injury to the frenulum or to the tongue itself.
- Unrecognized oesophageal intubation is a hazard and correct tube placement must be confirmed with great care.

Blind nasal intubation

The A&E physician who is not experienced in direct laryngoscopy and oral intubation, and who is not familiar with the use of neuromuscular blocking drugs, may prefer the nasotracheal route for intubation. This route is preferred by emergency physicians in the USA and until recently was the technique recommended in the advanced trauma life support manual (American College of Surgeons Committee on Trauma, 1993). Advocates of the nasotracheal technique claim that it results in less movement of the cervical spine in comparison with orotracheal intubation, but the majority of UK anaesthetists would disagree with this (Wood & Lawler, 1992).

Nasotracheal tubes are available with flexible tips which allow the curve of the tube to be varied by traction on a ring pull. This allows the tip of the tube to be adjusted to negotiate the curve from the nose into the hypopharynx and to proceed anteriorly through the glottic opening.

Nasotracheal intubation can also be performed under direct vision by introducing a laryngoscope and using Magill's intubating forceps to guide the distal end of the tracheal tube through the cords. This technique is more difficult than oral intubation and is less likely to be used for emergency airway management in the A&E department. If the operator can perform direct laryngoscopy then it is easier to place an oral tracheal tube.

Indications

- Where the operator is not skilled in direct laryngoscopy and oral intubation.
- A patient with limited mouth opening who requires an tracheal tube.

Contraindications

- Suspected basal skull fracture.
- Nasal obstruction.

Procedure

- Place the patient in a supine position with the head and neck aligned in the clear airway position.
- Introduce the lubricated nasotracheal tube into the right nostril directing it backwards in line with the hard palate. If resistance is encountered, withdraw and try the left nostril.
- Advance the tube through the nasopharynx.
- Occlude the mouth and opposite nostril manually.
- Listen at the proximal end of the tube for breath sounds in the spontaneously breathing patient. Though more

difficult, the technique can also be used in the apnoeic patient.

- Manipulating the larynx and tube, steer the tube so that breath sounds reach maximum intensity and at this point advance the tube during inspiration through the glottic opening into the trachea.
- Auscultate carefully to confirm correct placement in the trachea.

Potential complications

- Bleeding is a common problem.
- Unrecognized oesophageal intubation is a significant risk.
- Coughing, bronchospasm and/or laryngospasm may be provoked.
- Sinusitis is a significant risk with long-term nasal intubation.
- It is possible to push a nasotracheal tube through a fracture in the base of the skull.
- This technique is not as successful as direct laryngoscopy and oral intubation (Dronen et al., 1987).

Retrograde tracheal intubation

Some patients may prove impossible to intubate using the procedures described above. As long as time allows, an alternative method can be to pass a guidewire through the cricothyroid membrane retrogradely (in a cephalad direction) retrieving it in the mouth and railroading the tracheal tube over the guidewire (Fig. 28).

It is generally carried out under local anaesthesia. The procedure is not suitable for the unconscious emergency patient at risk from gastric regurgitation and pulmonary aspiration, when a surgical airway is usually more appropriate.

Fibreoptic intubation techniques

Anaesthetists frequently use fibreoptic intubating bronchoscopes to safely intubate patients with potentially difficult airways. Most of these patients are awake and intubated with the aid of local anaesthesia. If time allows, fibreoptic intubation is probably the method of choice in patients with suspected cervical spine injury. The availability of equipment, experience with the technique, and urgency of intervention limit its efficacy in the emergency situation. Contraindications include upper airway bleeding which makes visualization difficult, nasal obstruction, and any injury which prevents use of the preferred nasal route. It is contraindicated in apnoeic patients.

Tracheal intubation in suspected cervical spine injury

As stated in the section on basic airway manoeuvres, any patient who has sustained significant blunt trauma, particularly above the clavicles, should be assumed to have a cervical spine injury until proven otherwise (American College of Surgeons Committee on Trauma,

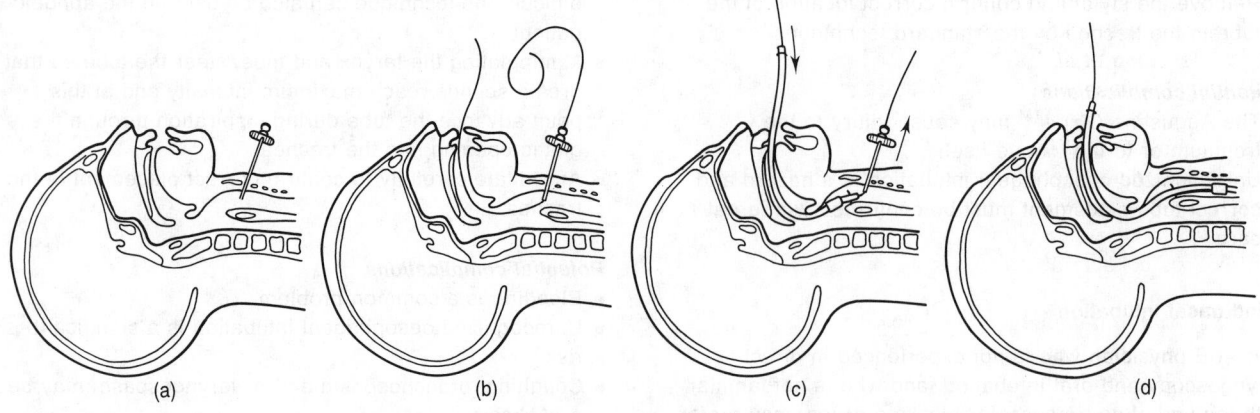

Fig. 28(a–d). Retrograde intubation.

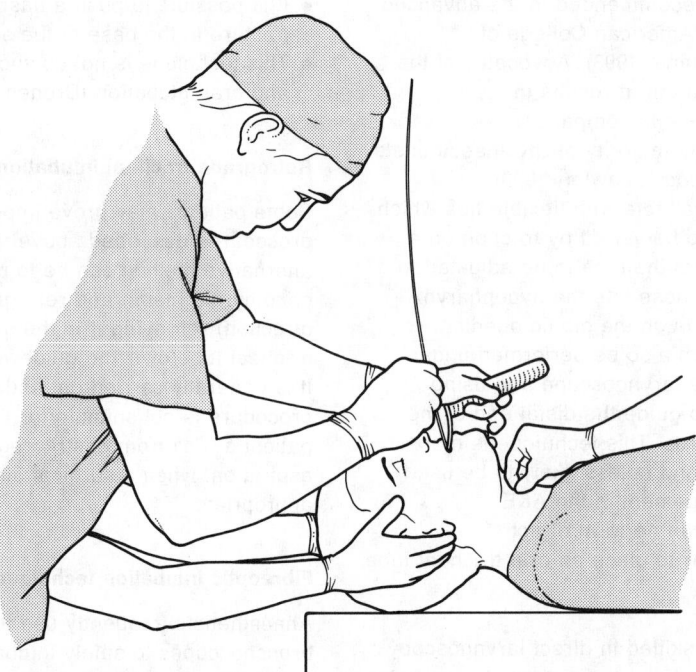

Fig. 29. Manual in-line stabilization of the cervical spine during intubation. Note the use of a gum elastic bougie and cricoid pressure.

1993). In these circumstances, the cervical spine is considered intact only when good-quality radiographs showing the whole of the cervical spine to the C7/T1 junction and a reliable clinical examination are both normal. In a patient with a potential cervical spine injury requiring advanced airway management, the priorities are to secure the airway while preserving neurological function. The best technique for this depends to some extent on the urgency of the situation (Hastings & Marks, 1991) and the skill and experience of the individual clinician. All basic and advanced airway manoeuvres have the potential to produce movement in the unstable cervical spine (Aprahamian *et al.*, 1984; Majernick *et al.*, 1986). It appears that most techniques are relatively safe if performed properly by competent, experienced clinicians.

The majority of cases can be managed by rapid sequence induction of anaesthesia with cricoid pressure, manual in-line stabilization of the head and neck, and orotracheal intubation (Fig. 29). This is the technique that anaesthetists are most familiar with and it has been shown to be safe (Criswell *et al.*, 1994). Manual in-line stabilization must be applied throughout the procedure; in-line *traction* exacerbates some cervical spine injuries and should be avoided (Bivins *et al.*, 1988; Turner, 1989).

Placing the patient's head and neck in neutral alignment will tend to worsen the view at laryngoscopy (Nolan & Wilson, 1993). Intubation is aided greatly by the use of a gum elastic bougie and/or McCoy levering laryngoscope (see above).

Awake, blind nasal intubation (see above) is advocated

by many as the technique of choice for urgent intubation of the patient with a known or suspected cervical spine injury (Meschino *et al.*, 1992). This method is used commonly by those who are not familiar with the use of anaesthetic induction and paralysing agents, laryngoscopy, or oral intubation. However, there are considerable disadvantages to nasal intubation which have been listed previously.

The awake fibreoptic technique is probably the safest but requires considerable experience and is impractical in the emergency situation. The Bullard laryngoscope (see above) allows oral intubation without the need to move the cervical spine, but it utilizes fibreoptics which would be obscured by blood in the airway. Oral or nasal intubation using a lighted stylet would be another option but this technique carries a higher failure rate than intubation under direct vision.

In an emergency and in the event of failure to intubate a patient with suspected cervical spine injury, options include insertion of a laryngeal mask or Combitube to provide a temporary airway, or cricothyroidotomy.

Tracheal intubation in patients with pharyngeal and/or laryngeal oedema

Acute pharyngeal and laryngeal oedema may result from inhalational thermal injury, upper airway infection (including epiglottitis) or anaphylaxis. Airway management in these patients requires great care and intubation should be attempted only by the very experienced. Repeated attempts and inexpert manipulation of the airway will aggravate the oedema and may convert partial into complete airway obstruction. Depending on the exact circumstances, blind intubation techniques (e.g. blind nasal, light wand) and the use of muscle relaxants are frequently contraindicated. The technique of choice is often oral intubation using direct laryngoscopy under deep inhalational general anaesthesia (strongly indicated if acute epiglottitis is suspected; see below), although a rapid sequence induction may also be appropriate in experienced hands. Facilities for cricothyroidotomy must be immediately available.

Tracheal tube suction

Tracheal tube suction is indicated to remove secretions, prevent tube blockage and improve oxygenation. It should be performed with catheters that are less than half the diameter of the tracheal tube, to avoid lung collapse. The catheters should have more than one end hole to reduce the risk of mucosal injury.

Procedure
- Tracheal tube suction should be an aseptic procedure.
- Following preoxygenation with 100% oxygen, an appropriately sized catheter is introduced into the tracheal tube, and intermittent suction applied as it is withdrawn.
- Suction should be limited to less than 10 sec at a time

as prolonged suction attempts will result in oxygen desaturation.

Potential complications
- Introduction of infection.
- Hypoxia from prolonged suctioning.
- Pulmonary collapse and mucosal trauma.
- Arrhythmias and hypotension (vagal effect).

Percutaneous approaches to the airway

Transtracheal intubation may be accomplished directly through the cricothyroid membrane or the upper part of the trachea. The procedure is not without hazard and is reserved for patients in whom translaryngeal intubation is impossible, dangerous or contraindicated.

Percutaneous transtracheal jet ventilation

Lung ventilation may be accomplished using a high-pressure oxygen source delivered through an intratracheal cannula passed through the cricothyroid membrane. The technique may be used in an emergency when other methods for ventilating the lungs are impossible or hazardous. The efficiency and safety of the technique is dependent on unobstructed exhalation and a reliable system for controlling the inspiratory and expiratory times.

Three methods may be used to ventilate the lungs through a transtracheal cannula:

1. A purpose-designed jet injector control system (e.g. the Sanders injector; Fig. 30).
2. Non-compliant narrow-bore tubing connected to a high-pressure oxygen source (60 p.s.i.) (e.g. wall outlet oxygen).
3. An anaesthetic breathing circuit may be attached to the tracheal cannula via a 3 mm tracheal tube connector or via a cuffed tracheal tube plugged into the barrel of a syringe. (A 6.5 mm tube will fit into a 5 ml syringe and an 8.5 mm tube will fit a 10 ml syringe). Ventilation of the lungs using this arrangement is particularly inefficient and much of the effort is dissipated in overcoming the compliance of the system.

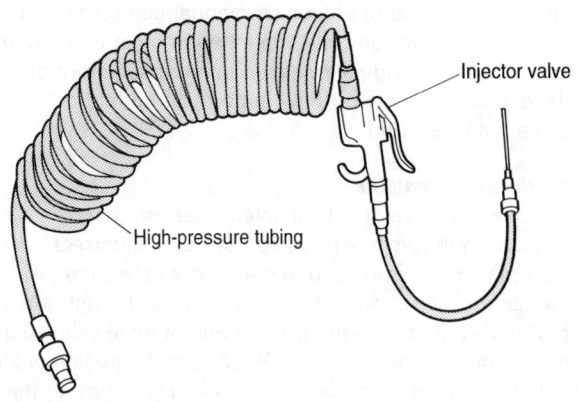

Fig. 30. The Sanders injector.

Wherever possible, the cannula should be connected to a 60 p.s.i. oxygen source, as in (1) or (2) above. Such a system will provide adequate oxygenation for up to 45 min. Jet ventilation through the cricothyroid membrane is relatively inefficient for clearing carbon dioxide from the respiratory tract; hypercapnoea will develop but, in comparison with the effect of severe hypoxia, is less clinically significant.

Indications
- To achieve ventilation in patients with upper airway inspiratory obstruction who cannot be ventilated with a bag–valve–mask device (even with the aid of an oro- or nasopharyngeal airway, a laryngeal mask or other airway), and who cannot be intubated immediately using the translaryngeal route.
- To 'buy time' in patients with upper airway obstruction while more time-consuming methods of translaryngeal intubation, such as the fibreoptic or retrograde techniques, are accomplished.
- In children it is preferred over cricothyroidotomy in the emergency situation because of the risks of laryngeal damage associated with cricothyroidotomy.

Contraindications
- Lower airway obstruction.
- Obstruction to exhalation.
- Laryngeal injury.
- Distorted anatomy of the neck.
- Tracheo-oesophageal fistula.

Procedure
- Unless contraindicated by a potential cervical spine injury, extend the patient's head and neck.
- Insert a 12–14 SWG cannula over needle percutaneously through the cricothyroid membrane into the trachea directing it 30° caudally.
- Confirm correct placement in the trachea by free aspiration of air into a syringe partly filled with sterile water.
- Advance the cannula inferiorly.
- Remove the needle and syringe from the cannula.
- Connect the ventilation apparatus to the cannula.

If using a Sanders injector system, apply intermittent positive pressure to the lungs by manual compression of the injector trigger control. Each inflation must be carefully observed and the trigger released immediately normal chest expansion occurs. Ample time must be left for passive lung deflation.

Potential complications
The procedure is relatively simple to perform but is associated with a major risk of barotrauma.Incorrect needle placement may lead to massive emphysema. An inadequate escape route for exhaled gases through the upper airway, and/or prolonged inflation times, will rapidly cause pulmonary barotrauma. Other complications include needle placement in the oesophagus and puncture of the great vessels in the neck.

Cricothyroidotomy (Fig. 31)

Access to the trachea through the cricothyroid membrane is simpler and less hazardous than tracheostomy and is therefore the preferred method in an emergency, except when there is severe trauma to the larynx.

Indications
The indications for a surgical airway include:

- When intubation has proved impossible.
- Severe anatomical abnormality such as ankylosing spondylitis.
- Cervical spine injury when intubation could prove hazardous.
- Extensive maxillofacial or laryngeal injury.
- Upper airway obstruction which renders intubation impossible (e.g. impacted foreign body, tumour invasion, inflammation and oedema formation).
- When direct access to the trachea is required for aspiration of secretions for an extended period of time and prolonged intubation would be undesirable.
- When prolonged intermittent positive pressure ventilation is required.

Relative contraindications
- Obese bull neck with engorged veins, laryngeal trauma, recent inflammatory conditions of the larynx (tracheostomy is preferred).
- Children who have not yet reached puberty (tracheostomy is preferred except for an emergency short-term airway).

In the two latter conditions there is a danger of subglottic stenosis. The cricothyroidotomy should be replaced by a tracheostomy within 48 h should the indication for a surgical airway remain.

Procedure
- If spinal trauma is excluded, place the patient supine with the head hyperextended on the neck by inserting a sandbag or rolled sheet beneath the shoulders.
- Access will be restricted in patients with cervical spine injury. Some cervical collars permit the procedure to be done through an anterior window in the collar, although this may still be restrictive. If the collar has to be removed to gain access, in-line cervical stabilization must be maintained by an assistant.
- Place the occiput on a soft ring to stabilize the head.
- Tilt the table or trolley 15° head up to reduce venous bleeding.
- Clean and drape the skin over the anterior and lateral aspects of the neck from chin to sternum.
- Identify the cricothyroid membrane by palpation of the dimple just below the thyroid cartilage ('Adam's apple').
- In conscious patients infiltrate the skin and subcutaneous tissue with 1% lignocaine with adrenaline.
- Make a 2–3 cm transverse skin incision over the cricothyroid membrane whilst fixing the larynx with the other hand.

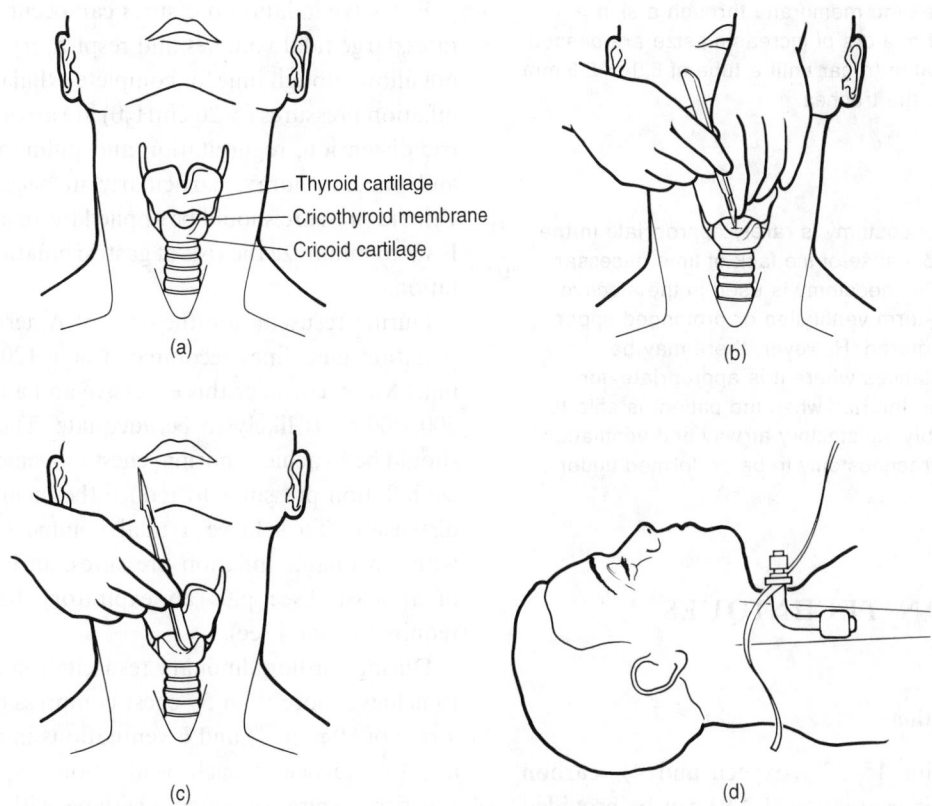

Fig. 31. Cricothyroidotomy.

- Dissect the subcutaneous tissue down to the membrane using artery forceps.
- Incise the membrane transversely, insert the scalpel handle through the incision and rotate it 90° to achieve an airway (artery forceps or tracheal spreader may be used instead of the scalpel handle).
- Insert a lubricated tracheal tube, or 6.0 mm tracheostomy tube, through the incision between the points of a tracheal spreader directing it caudally into the trachea.
- Inflate the cuff through the pilot tube.
- Connect the tracheal or tracheostomy tube to the ventilating apparatus and check for correct placement by observing chest movement and carbon dioxide content of the exhaled air.
- Suture the edges of the skin around the tube.
- Fix the tube in position using tape or sutures.

Potential complications

Complication rates of 8.6–32% have been reported.

- Care should be taken not to pierce the posterior aspect of the airway.
- Bleeding may occur, restricting visual access to the membrane, especially in patients with airway obstruction.
- Tracheal stimulation will make the conscious patient cough and spray blood; universal precautions including a visor are strongly recommended.

- Air embolism may occur in the head up position, particularly in the gasping patient with engorged neck veins.

'Blind' cricothyroidotomy

Purpose-designed cricothyroidotomy sets have been produced which are based on the 'blind stab' principle. Examples include the Portex Minitrach II and the NuTrach. The Portex Minitrach II set includes a scalpel, bougie, 4.0 mm tube and connector and suction catheter. It was originally designed for tracheal access for suction in the intensive care setting but it has also been used to achieve an emergency airway. It may be difficult to locate the stab incision in the membrane with the bougie using this blind technique, especially in the gasping patient whose larynx is moving up and down in relation to the skin. This problem can be minimized by transfixing the skin and membrane by two needles placed laterally to the proposed incision and asking an assistant to hold them so that the original alignment of larynx and skin is maintained. Bleeding may be a hazard in the asphyxiating patient. The 4.0 mm tube provided is too narrow for anything but a very short-term emergency airway. To achieve a better airway the bougie can be reinserted and tracheal tubes of increasing diameter can be introduced until a 6.0 or 6.5 mm tube is accommodated in the trachea.

The NuTrach consists of a patent expandable trocar

system which pierces the membrane through a skin incision. A series of dilators of increasing size are passed through the expandable trocar until a tube of 6.0 or 6.5 mm is accommodated in the trachea.

Tracheostomy

Formal surgical tracheostomy is rarely appropriate in the emergency setting because of the lack of time necessary for the procedure. Tracheostomy is used in the elective situation when long-term ventilation or prolonged upper airway bypass is required. However, there may be emergency circumstances where it is appropriate, for example in laryngeal injuries when the patient is able to maintain a reasonably satisfactory airway and ventilation to allow time for a tracheostomy to be performed under local anaesthesia.

VENTILATION TECHNIQUES

Basic techniques

Expired air ventilation

Expired air contains 15–17% oxygen and 4% carbon dioxide. Expired air ventilation (EAV) can be provided by the direct mouth-to-mouth, mouth-to-nose and mouth to mouth and nose (in infants) methods. The mouth-to-mouth method is recommended for adults by the majority of authorities.

A protective device such as a mask, tube airway or foil may be interposed between the patient and the rescuer to avoid direct contact. Some protective devices have ports to allow for oxygen enrichment of the inspired air. 'Naked' EAV carries with it the advantage that no equipment whatsoever is required and so artificial ventilation can be carried out immediately at any place provided there is a respirable atmosphere. However, there are aesthetic drawbacks to the direct methods and there is also a fear of cross-infection between the patient and rescuer although this is not currently justified by scientific data.

Respiratory rates should equate to normal physiological values related to the patient's age and weight. A rate of $10-12$ breaths/min^{-1} is recommended for adults, 20 min^{-1} for children over 1 year and $25-30$ min^{-1} for infants under 1 year. Tidal volumes should be slightly greater than normal values ranging from 25–50 ml in infants to 500–800 ml in adults. Inspiratory flow rates should mimic normal values of 20–30 litres min^{-1} in adults. Inspiration should take 1.5–2 sec, with twice that time allowed for exhalation.

Excessive inflation pressures can occur with high flow rates, large tidal volumes and respiratory rates which do not allow enough time for complete exhalation. Excessive inflation pressures (>20 cmH$_2$0) are associated with gastric distension, regurgitation and pulmonary aspiration and pneumothorax, particularly in paediatric patients. Cricoid pressure should be applied by an assistant during EAV to minimize the risk of gastric inflation and regurgitation.

During resuscitation the current American Heart Association guidelines recommend 800–1200 ml tidal volume. Many consider this excessive and a tidal volume of 500–700 ml is likely to be adequate. The primary goal should be to achieve normal chest movement and minimize inflation pressures to reduce the incidence of gastric distension. To achieve a tidal volume of 800–1200 ml with reasonable inflation pressures, an inspiratory time of at least 2 sec plus an expiratory time of 2 sec is required (total 4 sec).

During cardiopulmonary resuscitation it is impossible to achieve more than 50 chest compressions (applied at a rate of 80 min^{-1}) and 6 ventilations in a minute using a 5:1 sequence if each ventilation requires 4 sec (in practice, expiration often overlaps with the restart of chest compressions). Is this adequate circulatory support? Reducing the recommended tidal volume to 500–600 ml would reduce the overall time for each ventilation (inspiration and expiration) to, say, 3 sec, allowing time for ten more chest compressions and one more ventilation in each minute. Would this be better? Is there too much emphasis on ventilation in cardiac arrest when carbon dioxide elimination requirement is greatly reduced? Further research is required.

TECHNIQUES

Direct methods of expired air ventilation

Indications
- An apnoeic patient without serious maxillofacial injury in a situation where no equipment is immediately available. Direct expired air ventilation has saved many lives and healthcare professionals faced with an apnoeic patient in a situation without immediate access to equipment should not hesitate to apply it.

Contraindications
- A major maxillofacial injury producing distortion and serious intraoral haemorrhage.
- Obvious mortal injury.
- Patient's expressed wish not to be resuscitated known to the rescuer.

The mouth-to-mouth method

The mouth-to-mouth method is generally recognized by most authorities as the method of choice for providing expired air ventilation.

Procedure

- Place the patient supine with the head and neck aligned in the clear airway position.
- Clear the airway of any foreign material.
- Kneel to one side of the patient's head.
- Pinch the nostrils closed with the finger and thumb of one hand.
- The heel of that hand produces downward pressure on the forehead to maintain head tilt.
- Support the chin with the other hand holding the mouth 1 cm open.
- The rescuer inhales deeply, opens his own mouth widely, seals it over the patient's mouth and blows until the patient's chest rises.
- If inflation is difficult, tilt the head further back, check that the airway is not obstructed by foreign material and try again.
- Once inflation has occurred, the rescuer removes his mouth allowing complete passive exhalation.
- Repeat the process at a rate of 10–12 min^{-1} in adults.
- Unless they interfere, do not remove artificial dental plates as they maintain the normal facial configuration.
- The concentration of inspired oxygen can be increased if oxygen tubing is placed in the rescuer's mouth and a flow rate of 3–5 litres min^{-1} is set.

The mouth-to-nose method

Indications

- The mouth-to-nose method is advocated in patients with major mouth and lip lacerations.
- When the mouth-to-mouth method is ineffective.
- When local cultural preferences dictate that the mouth-to-nose technique is more acceptable.
- In the rescue of victims of immersion.

Contraindication

- Nasal obstruction

Procedure

- The patient and rescuer are placed as for the mouth-to-mouth method.
- Maintain head tilt by downward pressure on the patient's forehead with one hand and seal the patient's lips with the thumb of the other hand which is supporting the chin.
- Inflation of the patient's lungs is provided by the rescuer forming a seal with his lips around the patient's nostrils and blowing until normal inspiratory chest expansion is achieved.
- Assist passive exhalation by opening the patient's mouth in case there is a degree of nasal obstruction.

- Oxygen enrichment may be achieved from oxygen tubing directed into the rescuer's mouth.

The mouth to mouth and nose method

Indications

- This method is used in resuscitation of infants and small children.

Procedure

- The patient and rescuer are positioned as before.
- Place the relatively large infant's head in the neutral rather than the extended position.
- The rescuer applies his mouth over the infant's mouth and nose and blows to achieve normal chest expansion for that child.
- Repeat the process 20–30 times per min.
- Oxygen enrichment may be achieved with oxygen tubing in the rescuer's mouth.

Potential complications

- Only the minimum head extension and neck movement required to achieve a clear airway should be applied in patients with suspected cervical spine injury.
- Ventilation may be inadequate.
- Gastric inflation and regurgitation may occur.

Expired air ventilation using simple protective appliances

Simple inexpensive protective devices are available which are designed to prevent direct contact between patient and rescuer during expired air ventilation. These devices are of three types: the mask, the tube/flange and the foil. They avoid aesthetic concern about direct patient/rescuer contact, especially in the presence of blood, vomit or nasal secretions. They may reduce the possibility of cross-infection. With certain models, oxygen can be added.

The mask type

This device consists of a moulded face mask similar to that used in anaesthesia. Improved models incorporate a unidirectional valve which diverts the patient's expired air away from the rescuer and traps any macroscopic particles emerging from the patient (e.g. Laerdal Pocket Mask; Fig. 32). Mouth-to-mask ventilation is effective and popular with ward nurses as it avoids direct patient contact and unlike bag and mask ventilation it requires no particular strength. The method is particularly suitable for patients with suspected cervical spine injury as the clear airway is provided primarily by jaw thrust and is less dependent on head tilt.

Procedure

- Place the patient supine with the head and neck aligned in the clear airway position.
- Apply the mask to the face to cover the patient's mouth and nose.

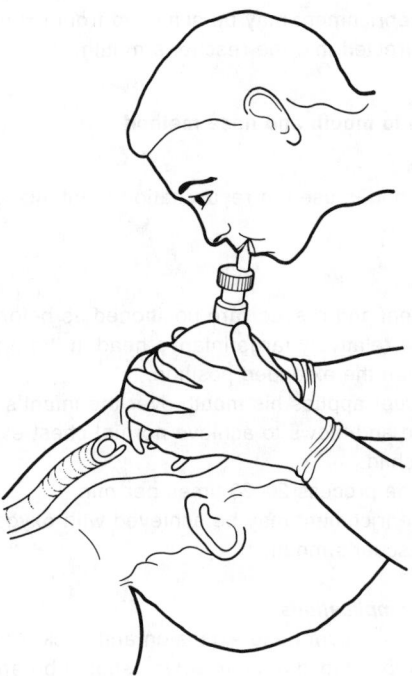

Fig. 32. Expired air ventilation using the mask with non-return valve.

- Using both hands, apply bilateral jaw thrust with the fingers and press the mask tightly onto the face with the outstretched thumbs and thenar eminences.
- The patient's lungs are inflated by blowing into the port of the mask.
- Some adjustment of the mask and hand position may be necessary to prevent leaks at the mask/patient interface.
- If an oxygen nipple is fitted, give oxygen at 8 litres min^{-1} to improve the FiO$_2$ (fraction of inspired oxygen); masks with this fitment are preferred.
- Training is needed to achieve a good technique.

Potential complications
- Inadequate ventilation due to leak.
- Gastric inflation resulting from poor airway alignment.

The foil type

The foil type consist of a small area of plastic film which can be applied to the oronasal region. An orifice with a one-way valve or textile filter is provided to be aligned with the patient's mouth. The resistance to airflow through the valve should not exceed 2 cmH$_2$O. Oxygen enrichment may be provided through tubing from an oxygen source placed under the foil. These devices are inexpensive, compact, lightweight and designed for use by members of the public. Training is important.

Procedure
- Place the patient supine with head and neck aligned in the open airway position.
- Place the foil over the patient's mouth and nose locating the orifice at the mouth.

- Stand or kneel at the side of the patient's head as with the mouth-to-mouth method.
- Apply chin lift with fingers and thumbs to occlude the nostrils and seal the foil to the face.
- Inflate the patient's lungs by blowing over the valve or filtered orifice, as with the mouth-to-mouth method.
- Some adjustment of the hand position may be required to provide an effective seal between the foil and the face.

Potential complications
- On occasion the foil may tear due to contact with the patient's or rescuer's teeth.

The self-inflating bag–valve–mask device

The advantages of the bag–valve–mask device over expired air ventilation are oxygen enrichment and improved hygiene. The device consists of a self-inflating bag, a non-rebreathing valve and a face mask. The unit is capable of inflating the patient's lungs with air or an air/oxygen mixture entrained through an inlet valve. Inflation of the lungs occurs through the patient valve when the bag is compressed and the patient's exhaled air is deviated to the atmosphere during the relaxation and bag re-expansion phase. To a certain extent, upper airway obstruction can be overcome by high upper airway pressures, but this carries an increased risk of gastric insufflation, regurgitation and pulmonary aspiration.

The bag may be used with a face mask or attached to any standard 15 mm connector on a tracheal tube, laryngeal mask, etc. Use of the bag and mask by a single operator requires a particular skill to achieve airway alignment and a seal between the mask and the patient's face with one hand. Many authorities advocate using two rescuers (if available) – one using both hands to align the airway and apply the mask to the face, and one to squeeze the bag (Fig. 33). Rescuers with small hands may find the open palm technique more effective; compressing the bag with an open hand against their chest or thigh.

Oxygen enrichment is best provided using a reservoir

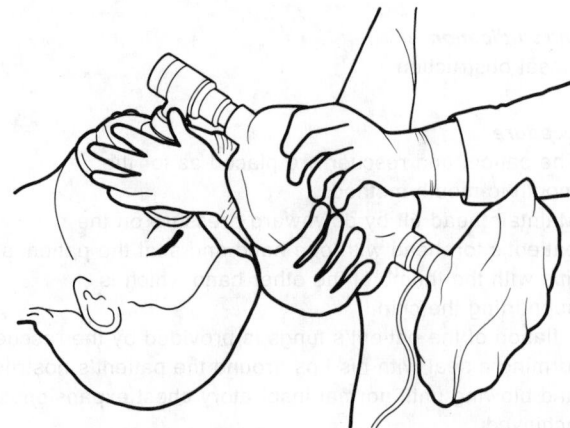

Fig. 33. Two-rescuer technique of ventilation with the bag–valve–mask device.

bag attached to the inflating bag. Inspired oxygen concentrations of 90% are possible with flow rates of 8–10 litres min^{-1} using this system. The addition of oxygen through a nipple directly attached to the inflating bag without a reservoir is much less efficient as the high flow rates necessary to achieve a high FiO$_2$ (15 litres min^{-1}) jam the patient valve in the inspiratory mode.

Indications
- The apnoeic or hypoventilating patient in need of ventilatory support.

Contraindications
- None, except inability to master the technique.

Procedure
- Place the patient supine with the head and neck aligned in the correct airway position.
- Apply the appropriately sized mask firmly to the patient's face using the thumb and forefinger to form a collar around the mask near the port attached to the patient valve.
- The other fingers support the jaw, performing a jaw thrust to maintain a clear airway.
- The air-tight seal is achieved by opposing the thumb and forefinger towards the other fingers.
- Compress the bag with the free hand to inflate the patient's lungs.
- Greater inflation volumes may be achieved using the open palm method and compressing the bag against a part of the operator's anatomy (e.g. thigh or chest).
- PEEP may be applied using a special valve and a filter may be attached to the inlet valve for use when the atmospheric air is contaminated by noxious gases.

Potential complications
- The technique is not easy to acquire and requires continued practice to maintain a patent airway and an airtight seal between the mask and the face throughout.
- The two-man technique reduces the risk of a leak and inadequate tidal volume.
- An inadequate seal results in hypoventilation.
- Poor seals are associated with beards, obesity, abnormal facial anatomy and edentulous patients.
- High inspiratory flow rates or volumes, particularly in the presence of an imperfectly aligned airway, result in gastric inflation and the risk of regurgitation and pulmonary aspiration. Cricoid pressure by an assistant reduces the chances of this occurring.
- The valves should be easy to take apart for cleaning. Incorrect assembly should be impossible.

Advanced techniques

TECHNIQUES

Manually triggered oxygen-powered resuscitators

These devices are powered by a high-pressure (45–60 p.s.i.) oxygen source. Triggering of the inspiratory and expiratory phase is done by manually compressing and releasing a lever or button at the patient valve which is attached to a face mask, tracheal tube or laryngeal mask. Both hands are free to ensure an airtight fit between the mask and the face and control airway alignment. Some models have a triggering device to provide assisted ventilation in time with the patient's own respiratory efforts.

Indications and contraindications
- These are as for the self-inflating bag–valve–mask device.

Procedure when used with a face mask
- The patient is placed supine and the head and neck are aligned in the clear airway position.
- Turn on the oxygen supply.
- Using both hands, the mask is applied over the mouth and nose to form an airtight seal as with mouth-to-mask EAV.
- Inflate the chest by depressing the lever or button trigger on the patient valve. Release the trigger to allow passive exhalation.
- Continue to ensure airway patency on a breath-by-breath basis.

Potential complications
- Lack of direct contact 'feel' during the inspiratory phase may lead to gastric inflation and the risk of regurgitation and pulmonary aspiration in an airway which is less than perfectly controlled.
- The equipment should be designed to restrict the inspiratory flow rates to less than 40 litres min^{-1} and a blow-off valve with audible warning should operate if the inflation pressure reaches 60 cm H$_2$O in adults.

Automatic resuscitators

These devices are small portable ventilators powered by a high-pressure (45–60 p.s.i.) oxygen source. They cycle between inspiration and expiration using a fluid logic arrangement or by electronic control. Cycling should be triggered by volume or time, not pressure. The versatility of control of the inspiratory and expiratory phase varies from model to model. Some models have the facility to ventilate with an air/oxygen mixture and/or a demand valve triggered by the patient's inspiratory efforts. They can be used with a face mask or may be attached to a tracheal tube, laryngeal mask or other sophisticated airway adjunct. Automatic resuscitators provide consistent automatic ventilation at the preset tidal volume, rate and respiratory pattern. Manual methods are, perforce, subject to continual variation. Once the automatic resuscitator is connected to a tracheal tube, the rescuer is free to undertake other tasks (e.g. venous cannulation).

Indications and contraindications
- These are as for the self-inflating bag–valve–mask device.

Procedure when used with a face mask
- Place the patient supine with the head and neck aligned in the clear airway position.
- Turn on the oxygen supply.
- Apply the mask to the mouth and nose to form an airtight seal as with mouth-to-mask ventilation.
- Adjust the controls for tidal volumes and respiratory rate to achieve normal chest expansion at a suitable rate.
- Some models have additional controls to adjust the inspiratory and expiratory times and flow rates and to introduce a triggering mode.
- Adjust the air/oxygen mixture as appropriate (generally 100% oxygen or 60% oxygen).
- Ensure airway patency with each breath.
- As soon as possible connect the device to a tracheal tube or laryngeal mask.

Potential complications
- As with manual triggered devices, there is a loss of feel during inflation with the attendant danger of gastric inflation, regurgitation and aspiration.
- Experience with models which have a low inspiratory flow rate and a blow-off valve with audible warning has shown that the danger of gastric inflation is less than with the self-inflating bag or mouth-to-mask method.

MONITORING

As an absolute minimum, all severely ill patients in the accident department should have their blood pressure, electrocardiograph (ECG), and arterial oxygen saturation (pulse oximeter) monitored. Ideally facilities to monitor end-tidal carbon dioxide and intravascular pressures should also be available.

Blood pressure

The use of an automatic non-invasive blood pressure monitor allows for other simultaneous interventions when staff numbers are limited; some models will also produce a print-out of recordings and save time with documentation. The ability to monitor intra-arterial blood pressure is invaluable during the resuscitation of severely injured patients. All A&E departments should have this facility.

The ECG

The ECG should be continuously monitored during any airway intervention. Some models will also measure ventilation rate from changes in chest wall impedance, although this is often disturbed by artefact interference in the resuscitation setting.

The pulse oximeter

The introduction of pulse oximetry has been a major advance as an adjunct to airway management. The pulse oximeter utilizes the differential absorption of infrared and near-red light by oxy- and deoxyhaemoglobin in pulsatile blood, to provide an estimate of oxygen saturation in arterial blood. The pulse oximeter provides an early visual and auditory warning of arterial oxygen desaturation. Hypothermia and hypotension with peripheral vasoconstriction reduce the chances of getting a reliable signal, and movement artefact may cause interference. Because they are calibrated to read for normal oxyhaemoglobin, the presence of abnormal haemoglobins (e.g. COHb, metHb) renders pulse oximeters inaccurate.

Detection of correct tracheal tube placement

Nothing is more important following intubation than detection of correct placement of the tube in the trachea. Undetected tube placement in the oesophagus will have disastrous consequences and is rightly considered negligent.

A number of methods are available to confirm the presence of the tube in the trachea.

Clinical methods

The following techniques for checking the correct placement of the tracheal tube do not require special equipment:

- Visualize the tube passing between the vocal cords.
- Palpate the tube passing into the larynx.
- Apply positive pressure ventilation and note absence of leak around the cuff, bilateral chest expansion and breath sounds heard in both axillae but not in the epigastric area.

These methods are reliable in the majority of cases.

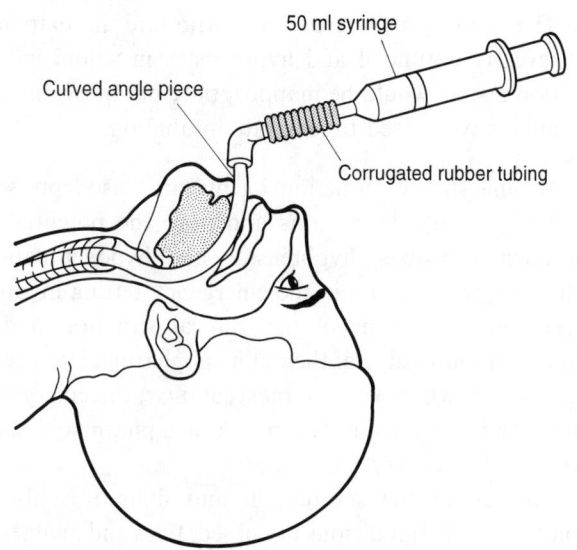

Fig. 34. The Wee oesophageal detector.

The oesophageal detector

The oesophageal detector (Wee, 1988) is a 50 ml syringe or self-inflating bulb applied to the tracheal tube connector (Fig. 34). Aspiration is attempted; free aspiration confirms placement of the tube in the trachea. Resistance to aspiration indicates that the tube is in the oesophagus. This is a very reliable and inexpensive method.

Transillumination

Transillumination involves passing a lighted stylet down the lumen of the tube. Bright transillumination suggests that the tube is in the trachea, while a dull glow suggests that it is in the oesophagus. This method is not completely reliable and depends on observer variation and background lighting.

Carbon dioxide detection

The detection of carbon dioxide from the tube during expiration confirms placement in the trachea. Carbon dioxide can be detected by a capnometer or by a simple inexpensive colorimetric device (e.g. Fenem detector). Carbon dioxide is not produced during cardiac arrest: indeed, measurement of end-tidal carbon dioxide is a useful indication of the efficacy of cardiopulmonary resuscitation and may give some prediction of outcome. Values below 1.3 kPa indicate a poor prognosis and above 2.0 kPa suggest a good outcome.

Table 3. *Techniques for applying local anaesthesia to the airway*

- Nasal mucosa by spray or direct appliction using a cotton pledget
- Mouth and back of pharynx by spray, or gargle
- Posterior tongue by glossopharyngeal nerve block, injection where the tongue opposes the palatoglossal fold
- Superior laryngeal nerve blocks by injection just inferior to the greater cornu of the hyoid cartilage through the neck, or application of local anaesthetic to the piriform fossae at laryngoscopy
- Tracheal anaesthesia by transcricothyroid membrane injection
- Inhalation of nebulized local anaesthetic
- Injecting local anaesthetic down an advancing fibreoptic scope

Visual confirmation of the tracheal tube in the trachea

A fibreoptic laryngoscope is passed through the lumen of the tube. Visualization of the rings of the trachea and the carina confirms correct tube placement. This is the most reliable method.

PHARMACOLOGICAL ADJUNCTS TO AIRWAY MANAGEMENT

Local anaesthesia of the airway

There are numerous techniques for applying local anaesthesia to the airway (Table 3). Lignocaine when applied to mucous membranes will produce anaesthesia in about 1 min which lasts for around 45 min. Concentrations of 2% or 4% are usually used for airway anaesthesia. The maximum dose of lignocaine is 3 mg kg^{-1}.

Cocaine inhibits the reuptake of catecholamines and therefore has vasoconstrictor activity as well as local anaesthetic action. This is a particular advantage when it is used to anaesthetize the nose. Cocaine has a rapid onset of action and surface anaesthesia lasts for around 30–90 min. Concentrations of 4% or 10% are used to a maximum dose of 1.5 mg kg^{-1}.

Attenuating the cardiovascular response to laryngoscopy and intubation

Laryngoscopy and intubation are very powerful stimuli and are frequently associated with hypertension, tachycardia, laryngospasm and bronchospasm, especially in individuals who are inadequately paralysed or not deeply unconscious. This cardiovascular response may be life-threatening to those with critical coronary artery disease, cardiac pathology or those with raised intracranial pressure. Bradycardia, due to vagal stimulation, is also seen during laryngoscopy and intubation, more commonly in children than adults, which is why some advocate administering atropine to children prior to intubation.

A variety of agents have been used in an attempt to reduce the cardiovascular response to laryngoscopy and intubation, including lignocaine, beta-blockade, vasodilators, opioids and general anaesthetic agents. All may have some role but are of limited usefulness in the emergency situation. Therefore airway management in the emergency situation also requires some knowledge of the clinical pharmacology of anaesthetic and vasoactive agents.

Anaesthetic induction agents

Discussion of balanced anaesthesia is beyond the scope of this chapter. However, airway management in the A&E department should not deteriorate into a battle for the airway between patient and clinician. A smooth induction of anaesthesia and paralysis provides optimal conditions for intubation in high-risk patients. The skills necessary to achieve this safely require formal training. Anaesthetic, sedative and analgesic agents are indicated not only for humane reasons, but also to avoid the adverse cardiovascular responses to airway manipulation, particularly laryngoscopy.

Contraindications to the administration of anaesthetic agents include inadequate skill and knowledge on the part of the clinician and assistants, and inadequate resuscitation of the patient. However, in circumstances of profound hypotension and unconsciousness, it may be appropriate to administer a muscle relaxant alone to facilitate tracheal intubation. Whilst remembering that the correct dose of any anaesthetic, sedative or analgesic drug is the titrated dose that is required to produce the desired effect, severely ill or injured patients requiring intubation generally fall into three groups:

1. Patients who are stable or adequately resuscitated, who should receive a standard or reduced dose of induction agent.
2. Patients who are unstable or inadequately resuscitated in whom it is necessary to proceed and who should receive a reduced, titrated dose of induction agent (in this situation factors such as best guess, skill and experience come into play).

3. The third group are those who are in extremis, severely obtunded and hypotensive in whom induction agents would be inappropriate but muscle relaxants may be used to facilitate intubation.

All anaesthetic induction agents are vasodepressors and respiratory depressants and have the potential to produce or worsen hypotension and hypoventilation. Their appropriate use in the emergency setting involves a careful assessment of the clinical situation and a thorough knowledge of their clinical pharmacology. Use agents with which you are most familiar; the emergency situation is not the time to embark on a pharmacological voyage of discovery.

Sedation in the severely ill and injured is also a complex issue. Injudicious use of sedatives and analgesics in the severely ill or injured is likely to result in a severely obtunded patient with cardiovascular compromise, hypoventilation, hypercarbia, hypoxia and depressed protective airway reflexes. Before sedating any patient it is necessary to ask: Why does the patient need sedation? What are the aims of sedation? Will significant clinical signs be obscured by the administration of drugs? It is often safer to opt for general anaesthesia with tracheal intubation, followed by sedation and controlled ventilation. For example, in the case of the combative, intoxicated trauma patient with head and other potentially severe injuries, induction of anaesthesia and intubation will facilitate definitive investigation (e.g. CT (computed tomography) scan) and prevent secondary injury (self-inflicted trauma and secondary brain injury from hypoxia, hypercarbia, hypotension and hypertension).

The anaesthetic agents most commonly used are thiopentone, etomidate, propofol and ketamine. The doses quoted are for anaesthesia in the presence of fluid resuscitation and cardiovascular stability; depending on the clinical circumstances the doses required may be significantly less.

Thiopentone

Thiopentone is a short-acting thiobarbiturate which is contraindicated in porphyria. Following injection of a hypnotic dose, unconsciousness occurs in one arm–brain circulation, the timing of which is dependent on the circulatory status. The hypnosis lasts for 5–10 min. Thiopentone is a potent ventilatory and cardiovascular depressant. The administration of a standard dose to a hypovolaemic patient may cause profound hypotension. Thiopentone has a negative analgesic action. It has a strong alkaline pH and tissue infiltration or intra-arterial injection are likely to lead to serious necrosis. The normal anaesthetic dose is 3–4 mg kg^{-1}.

Etomidate

Etomidate is an imidazole derivative that is also contra-indicated in porphyria. An induction dose of etomidate produces hypnosis in one arm–brain circulation and lasts for 3–12 min. Etomidate is hydrolysed in plasma and liver to inactive metabolites. Of the induction agents available etomidate produces the least cardiovascular depression. It is painful on injection, and induction may be associated with myoclonic jerks. Etomidate also causes adrenocortical suppression and should not be given in repeated dosage or by infusion. The standard induction dose is 0.1–0.3 mg kg^{-1}.

Propofol

Propofol is a phenol derivative. Induction may be associated with pain on injection and some excitatory movement. Like thiopentone it is a potent ventilatory and cardiovascular depressant. Propofol produces a rapid clear-headed recovery and as such is useful as an infusion for sedation and anaesthesia. The standard induction dose is 2–2.5 mg kg^{-1}.

Ketamine

Ketamine is an arylcyclohexylamine related to phencyclidine. It produces a state known as dissociative anaesthesia. Following intravenous injection of 1–2 mg kg^{-1}, hypnosis is delayed longer than one arm–brain circulation and surgical anaesthesia has a duration of 10–15 min. Ketamine has the advantages that it is a powerful analgesic, a good bronchodilator and sympathetic stimulator that may improve cardiac stability. Ketamine may also be give by the intramuscular (IM) route; a dose of 5–10 mg kg^{-1} IM provides surgical anaesthesia for 12–25 min. Disadvantages include an increase in cerebral blood flow, intracranial pressure, cerebral oxygen consumption and muscle tone, and emergence delirium. Ketamine is contraindicated in hypertension and head injury.

Benzodiazepines

Benzodiazepines such as midazolam and diazepam have anxiolytic, hypnotic, relaxant, anticonvulsant and am-nesic actions. They can be given to induce anaesthesia but are more frequently used to provide sedation in combination with an analgesic for intubated patients. Most intubated patients are optimally sedated using a combination of a sedative and an analgesic (see Chapter 10).

Neuromuscular blocking drugs

Indications
- Neuromuscular blocking drugs are used to facilitate intubation and controlled ventilation.

Contraindications
- An absolute contraindication to the uses of neuromuscular blocking agents is inability to control the airway and provide ventilation.

Potential complications
- Administration of neuromuscular blocking agents will impair neurological examination.
- Deprived of protective airway reflexes the patient is at risk of aspiration of gastric contents.
- It is important to remember that when using neuromuscular blockers there is the potential to have patients who are paralysed but aware. This can be avoided by providing adequate sedation and by avoiding repeated or prolonged use of the neuromuscular blockers.

Depolarizing neuromuscular blockers

Suxamethonium

Suxamethonium is the only depolarizing neuromuscular blocker in common use. It is the agent most commonly used to paralyse patients before urgent intubation. Suxamethonium binds to acetylcholine receptors at the neuromuscular junction causing depolarization, manifested as muscle fasciculation. The neuromuscular end-plate then becomes refractory until the suxamethonium is metabolized by plasma cholinesterases. The fasciculations indicate when neuromuscular blockade has occurred; however, occasionally they may not be seen.

Suxamethonium has a rapid onset and short duration of action, generally lasting 3–10 min. Delayed onset is seen in low cardiac output states, and prolonged action ('suxamethonium apnoea') is seen in individuals with abnormal or low levels of plasma cholinesterase.

Adverse effects include dangerous hyperkalaemia that may result in cardiac arrest. This is seen following crush injury, burns and motor neuropathies, including spinal cord injury. The period of greatest risk is from a few days to about 6 months after the injury. It is not a problem immediately after trauma and suxamethonium can safely be used for urgent intubation. Suxamethonium causes transient increases in intraocular, intracranial and intragastric pressure. However, the advantages of speed and safety that it provides for intubation in high-risk groups usually outweigh these disadvantages. With repeated doses, suxamethonium may cause a bradycardia by vagal stimulation and it is a well-recognised trigger for malignant hyperpyrexia. The standard dose is 1 mg kg^{-1} for adults (2 mg kg^{-1} for children).

Non-depolarizing neuromuscular blockers

Pancuronium bromide

Pancuronium is an aminosteroid neuromuscular blocker. It produces neuromuscular blockade lasting around 70 min and a tachycardia by a vagolytic effect. It is considered the long-acting neuromuscular blocker of choice in the high-risk cardiac patient. The standard dose is 0.1 mg kg^{-1}.

Vecuronium bromide

Vecuronium is an aminosteroid with an intermediate duration of action of 20–30 min. It has the least side-effects of the neuromuscular blockers. Cardiovascular stability and lack of histamine release have made it a popular choice for short periods of paralysis. The standard dose of 0.1 mg kg^{-1} will produce paralysis in approximately 2 min.

Rocuronium bromide

Rocuronium is an aminosteroid which is related closely to vecuronium, and has only recently been made available for clinical use. Like vecuronium it has minimal cardiovascular side-effects and has a duration of action of 30 min. Its great advantage is its speed of onset; after a standard intubating dose of 0.6 mg kg^{-1} good to excellent intubating conditions are present in just 1 min.

Atracurium besylate

Atracurium is another intermediate duration neuromuscular blocker lasting 15–35 min. It has the advantage of not relying on liver or renal metabolism; it undergoes spontaneous degradation by Hofmann elimination which is temperature- and pH-dependent. The standard intubation dose is 0.5 mg kg^{-1}.

RAPID SEQUENCE INDUCTION OF ANAESTHESIA

TECHNIQUE

Rapid sequence induction of anaesthesia for emergency tracheal intubation ideally requires four individuals (Fig. 35):

- One applies manual in-line stabilization of the cervical spine.
- One performs preoxygenation and intubation.
- One applies cricoid pressure, and is therefore in an ideal position to perform a cricothyroidotomy, if needed, without abandoning cricoid pressure and the anatomical landmark. A right-handed individual who may be called on to perform a cricothyroidotomy would need to stand on the patient's left side and apply cricoid pressure with the left hand.
- The fourth individual is responsible for administration of anaesthetic and neuromuscular blocking drugs.

While some may consider it a luxury to have four individuals to secure the airway, the speed and safety with which intubation is accomplished justify these numbers.

Indications
- Rapid sequence induction of anaesthesia is performed to minimize the risks of pulmonary aspiration in the presence of a full stomach.

Contraindications
- Inability to control the airway and provide ventilation.
- Lack of skill, equipment or adequate assistance.

Procedure
- As time allows, assess the patient for potential airway problems and cardiovascular stability.
- The procedure requires adequate equipment, drugs and assistance.
- Position the patient supine or in the left lateral position.
- Apply monitors, including pulse oximeter, blood pressure and ECG.
- Venous access is confirmed or established.
- Preoxygenate with high-flow 100% oxygen for as long as is feasible (up to 5 min) while the above are being performed.
- If the patient has a potential cervical spine injury get an assistant to apply manual in-line stabilization of the neck (see above).
- In the unconscious patient, if spontaneous ventilation is

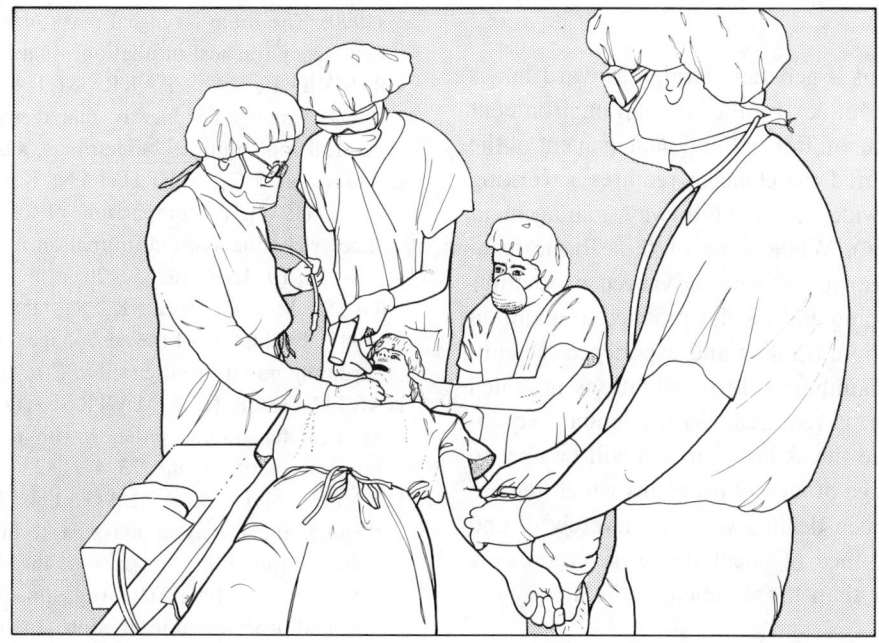

Fig. 35. Rapid sequence induction of anaesthesia for emergency airway control.

inadequate, it is necessary to ventilate the patient with 100% oxygen while cricoid pressure is performed.

- Induction of anaesthesia is accompanied by application of cricoid pressure by an assistant, and immediately followed by suxamethonium 1 mg kg^{-1}.
- If suxamethonium is contraindicated, vecuronium 0.2 mg kg^{-1} or rocuronium 0.6 mg kg^{-1} are alternatives.
- Await the onset of paralysis and intubate the patient.
- If difficulties with intubation are encountered the patient should be oxygenated between attempts.
- Release cricoid pressure only when the tube position is confirmed.
- Secure the tube in place, obtain a chest X-ray at an appropriate moment.

INHALATIONAL INDUCTION OF ANAESTHESIA

In some situations of impending airway obstruction (e.g. epiglottitis) it is inappropriate to administer an intravenous anaesthetic and neuromuscular blocking drug because total airway obstruction with inability to ventilate may follow. In this situation direct examination and investigation of the airway are contraindicated. The patient should be handled only to induce anaesthesia and secure the airway. In experienced anaesthetic hands, an inhalational induction with 100% oxygen and a volatile anaesthetic (most commonly halothane) is often the method of choice. Recognition of imminent airway ob-

struction and the availability of a skilled anaesthetist are needed for safe management of these difficult airway emergencies. Equipment to perform an emergency surgical airway must be immediately available.

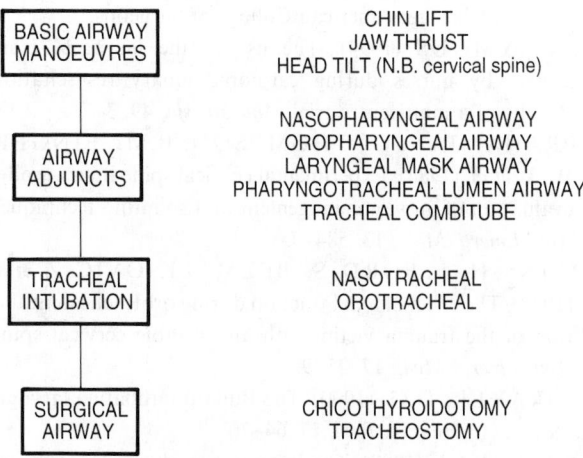

AIRWAY MANAGEMENT

| BASIC AIRWAY MANOEUVRES | CHIN LIFT JAW THRUST HEAD TILT (N.B. cervical spine) |

| AIRWAY ADJUNCTS | NASOPHARYNGEAL AIRWAY OROPHARYNGEAL AIRWAY LARYNGEAL MASK AIRWAY PHARYNGOTRACHEAL LUMEN AIRWAY TRACHEAL COMBITUBE |

| TRACHEAL INTUBATION | NASOTRACHEAL OROTRACHEAL |

| SURGICAL AIRWAY | CRICOTHYROIDOTOMY TRACHEOSTOMY |

Call for help early, anticipate problems and solutions.
Oxygenation should be maintained during all manoeuvres.
The skill and experience of the clinician determine
the nature and extent of intervention.

Consider the merits of:

Awake	versus	Anaesthetized
Spontaneous ventilation	versus	Neuromuscular blockade
Surgical airway	versus	Non-surgical

Fig. 36. Airway management.

SUMMARY

Airway management is generally straightforward but is often made more complex by the stressful environment of the A&E department. For optimal management of the severely ill and injured the clinician requires a working knowledge of a wide range of airway management procedures (Fig. 36). While some of these basic techniques are easily learnt, the more advanced procedures require formal training and regular practice to maintain skill. With appropriate training and experience the clinician will become familiar with the situations in which airway intervention is required. With adequate equipment and assistance the skilled clinician will be able to manage a wide range of airway problems which remain the first priority when dealing with the severely ill and injured. In the absence of adequate oxygenation, any interventions other than those aimed at the airway are redundant.

Bibliography

ALEXANDER, R., HODGSON, P., LOMAX, D. *et al.* (1993). A comparison of the laryngeal mask airway and Guedel airway, bag and facemask for manual ventilation. *Anaesthesia*, **48**, 231–4.

AMERICAN COLLEGE OF SURGEONS COMMITTEE ON TRAUMA (1993). *Advanced Trauma Life Support Program For Physicians: Instructor Manual*. Chicago: American College of Surgeons.

ANONYMOUS (1994). The use of the laryngeal mask airway by nurses during cardiopulmonary resuscitation. Results of a multicentre trial. *Anaesthesia*, **49**, 3–7.

APRAHAMIAN, C., THOMPSON, B.M., FINGER, W.A. *et al.* (1984). Experimental cervical spine injury model: evaluation of airway management and splinting techniques. *Ann. Emerg. Med.*, **13**, 584–7.

BIVINS, H.G., FORD, S., BEZMALINOVIC, Z. *et al.* (1988). The effect of axial traction during orotracheal intubation of the trauma victim with an unstable cervical spine. *Ann. Emerg. Med.*, **17**, 25–9.

BJORAKER, D.G. (1990). The Bullard intubating laryngoscopes. *Anesthesiol. Rev.*, **17**, 64–70.

BRAIN, A.I.J. (1983). The laryngeal mask – a new concept in airway management. *Br. J. Anaesth.*, **55**, 801–5.

BRAIN, A.I.J. (1984). The laryngeal mask airway – a possible new solution to airway problems in the emergency situation. *Arch. Emerg. Med.*, **1**, 229–32.

BRAIN, A.I.J. (1985). Three cases of difficult intubation overcome by the laryngeal mask airway. *Anaesthesia*, **40**, 353–5.

CALDER, I., ORDMAN, A.J., JACKOWSKI, A. *et al.* (1990). The brain laryngeal mask airway. An alternative to emergency tracheal intubation. *Anaesthesia*, **45**, 137–9.

CRISWELL, J.C., PARR, M.J.A. & NOLAN, J.P. (1994). Emergency airway management in patients with cervical spine injuries. *Anaesthesia*, **49**, 900–3.

DRONEN, S.C., MERIGIAN, K.S., HEDGES, K.R. *et al.* (1987). A comparison of blind nasotracheal and succinylcholine assisted intubation in the poisoned patient. *Ann. Emerg. Med.*, **16**, 650–2.

FRASS, M., FRENZER, R., RAUSCHA, R. *et al.* (1987). Evaluation of the oesophageal tracheal combitube in cardiopulmonary resuscitation. *Crit. Care Med.*, **15**, 609–11.

HASTINGS, R.H. & MARKS, J.D. (1991). Airway management for trauma patients with potential cervical spine injuries. *Anesth. Analg.*, **73**, 471–82.

HEATH, M.L. & ALLAGAIN, J. (1991). Intubation through the laryngeal mask: a technique for unexpected difficult intubation. *Anaesthesia*, **46**, 545–8.

KOVAC, A.L. (1993). The Augustine Guide™: a new device for blind orotracheal intubation. *Anesthesiol. Rev.*, **20**, 25–9.

MAJERNICK, T.G., BIENIEK, R., HOUSTON, J.B. *et al.* (1986). Cervical spine movement during orotracheal intubation. *Ann. Emerg. Med.*, **15**, 417–20.

MALLAMPATI, S.R., GATT, S.P., GUGINO, L.D. *et al.* (1985). A clinical sign to predict difficult tracheal intubation: a prospective study. *Can. Anaesth. Soc. J.*, **32**, 429–34.

MARTIN, P.D., CYNA, A.M., HUNTER, W.A.H. *et al.* (1993). Training nursing staff in airway management for resuscitation. *Anaesthesia*, **48**, 133–7.

McCOY, E.P. & MIRAKUR, R.K. (1993). The levering laryngoscope. *Anaesthesia*, **48**, 516–19.

MESCHINO, A., DEVITT, J.H., KOCH, J.P. *et al.* (1992). The safety of awake tracheal intubation in cervical spine injury. *Can. J. Anaesth.*, **39**, 114–17.

NOLAN, J.P. & WILSON, M.E. (1993). Orotracheal intubation in patients with potential cervical spine injuries. An indication for the gum elastic bougie. *Anaesthesia*, **48**, 630–3.

OAKLEY, P.A., PHILLIPS, B., MOLYNEUX, E. *et al.* (1993). Paediatric resuscitation. *Br. Med. J.*, **306**, 1613.

PENNANT, J.H. & WALKER, M.B. (1992). Comparison of the endotracheal tube and laryngeal mask in airway management by paramedical personnel. *Anesth. Anal.*, **74**, 531–4.

SAMSOON, G.L.T. & YOUNG, J.R.B. (1987). Difficult tracheal intubation: a retrospective study. *Anaesthesia*, **42**, 487–90.

SELLICK, B.A. (1961). Cricoid pressure to control regurgitation of stomach contents during induction of anaesthesia. *Lancet*, **ii**, 404–6.

STEWART, R.D. (1984). Tactile orotracheal intubation. *Ann. Emerg. Med.*, **13**, 175–8.

TURNER, L.M. (1989). Cervical spine immobilization with

axial traction: a practice to be discouraged. *J. Emerg. Med.*, **7**, 385–6.

VOLLMER, T.P., STEWART, R.D., PARIS, P.M. *et al.* (1985). Use of a lighted stylet for guided orotracheal intubation in the prehospital setting. *Ann. Emerg. Med.*, **14**, 324–8.

WEE, M.Y.K. (1988). The oesophageal detector device. *Anaesthesia*, **43**, 27–9.

WOOD, P.R. & LAWLER, P.G.P. (1992). Managing the airway in cervical spine injury. A review of the Advanced Trauma Life Support protocol. *Anaesthesia*, **47**, 792–7.

3 Cardiac arrest and cardiopulmonary resuscitation in adults

C.E. ROBERTSON

Accident and Emergency Department, Royal Infirmary, Edinburgh, UK

Chapter plan

The pathophysiology of cardiac arrest
The recognition of cardiac arrest
The pathophysiology of forward blood flow during cardiopulmonary resuscitation
Basic life support
Airway techniques and ventilation
Defibrillation
Drug delivery routes
Drugs used in cardiac arrest
Advanced life support
Open chest cardiopulmonary resuscitation
Post resuscitation care
The cardiac arrest team
Outcome prediction

THE PATHOPHYSIOLOGY OF CARDIAC ARREST

Sudden unexpected cardiac arrest is the commonest cause of death in the developed world. It is estimated that approximately 2500 cardiac arrests occur daily in Europe, 150–200 of these being in the UK. The vast majority of such cases are related to coronary heart disease. In the UK coronary heart disease kills nearly 500 people every day and is the primary cause of premature death for men. The tragedy is that, with appropriate and rapid treatment, the majority of the 60 000 cardiac arrests occurring yearly in the community could be saved.

The marked differences in aetiology between cardiac arrest occurring in children and that occurring in adults are highlighted in Chapter 4. Within the spectrum of adult events, however, the aetiology of cardiac arrest varies. In young adults up to 35 years of age, conditions such as cardiomyopathy, valvular disease and congenital cardiac disorders account for a significant proportion of cases (Safranek *et al.*, 1992). Nevertheless, even in this age group coronary heart disease comprises the largest single aetiology, and in older age groups accounts for over 90% of such events.

For most individuals, the cardiac arrest is entirely unheralded. Although it is assumed that the arrhythmias leading to cardiac arrest occur as a direct consequence of disturbance of the normal electrical activity in ischaemic myocardium, continuous ambulatory electrocardiographic (ECG) monitoring (performed admittedly in individuals with known or suspected heart disease) usually fails to show any ST-T wave changes compatible with ischaemic events. The role of premonitory arrhythmias is unclear in otherwise asymptomatic patients. Recently, the importance of antecedent ventricular arrhythmias such as monomorphic or polymorphic ventricular tachycardia (VT) or torsade de pointes has been highlighted (Bayes de Luna *et al.*, 1989; Tzivoni *et al.*, 1983). These aspects, and the importance of ECG abnormalities such as the long QT syndrome, may be relatively more important in the subgroup of individuals who are subsequently found not to have coronary heart disease.

The vast majority of adult patients experiencing cardiac arrest do so as a consequence of a primary myocardial event. Myocardial ischaemia, which may be reversible or lead to an episode of infarction, is the commonest precipitating event. This may be triggered by fissure and rupturing of an atheromatous plaque with platelet deposition and thrombus formation and propagation, or in some patients due to coronary artery spasm (DeWood *et al.*, 1980; Davies and Thomas, 1984). For ischaemia-related events, fully established transmural myocardial infarcts are associated with the lowest risk of ventricular fibrillation (VF). Evolving or subendocardial infarcts have a higher risk; and the greatest occur in individuals with ischaemic events without actual infarction.

In individuals who survive a cardiac arrest, a number of factors are recognized in the predisposition to further events. These include susceptibility to arrhythmias, poor ventricular function and the presence of an abnormal resting 12-lead ECG. Patients who are not hypertensive, do not smoke, take regular exercise and have a modest alcohol intake also reduce the risk of further arrests. Preventive antiarrhythmic drug therapy is probably of less value than previously thought, and recent large studies have demonstrated adverse effects of antiarrhythmic agents when given prophylactically after established myocardial infarction (Echt *et al.*, 1991; Cardiac Arrhythmia Suppression Trial, 1992). Targeting of specific high-risk groups rather than blunderbuss therapy may prove more efficacious.

Cessation of cardiac activity can occur in one of three ECG modes. In the context of sudden cardiac arrest, VF or pulseless VT is by far the commonest primary arrhythmia to be documented. Ventricular asystole or electromechanical dissociation (EMD) are infrequent primary rhythms, although with the passage of time the ECG traces of VF or EMD will degenerate to produce a complete absence of detectable electrical activity – asystole. It must be acknowledged that our understanding of the natural history of these rhythms is incomplete (Campbell, 1993). Cases of prolonged VF, and even asystole, which have spontaneously reverted to a perfusing rhythm are well documented (Clayton *et al.*, 1993).

Once cardiac arrest has occurred tissue perfusion ceases. The effects of this are most dramatically seen in the brain. Within 10–15 sec of the cessation of cardiac pumping action, loss of consciousness develops because of cerebral hypoxia. Over the next 5 min, neuronal glucose and glycogen stores are progressively depleted and an isoelectric EEG (electroencephalogram) develops (Rossen *et al.*, 1943; Nemoto, 1978; Siesjo, 1992). By the end of this time ATP stores are exhausted. At this stage, even if cardiac output is restored, the cerebral injury is likely to be irrecoverable except in certain special circumstances.

THE RECOGNITION OF CARDIAC ARREST

The diagnosis of cardiac arrest is made on clinical grounds. The cardinal features in the clinical recognition of cardiac arrest are the combination of unconsciousness together with the absence of a major (carotid or femoral) pulse.

It is time-wasting and potentially confusing to look for other associated features. Ineffective 'agonal' respiratory movement may occur for up to several minutes after cardiac arrest. Pupil size or responsiveness to light and the presence or absence of cyanosis or pallor are equally unhelpful. Occasionally, cardiac arrest may present with a grand mal convulsion of short duration.

Once made, the clinical diagnosis of cardiac arrest can be characterized by an ECG trace. Care is required as a number of pitfalls can occur in the interpretation of the ECG monitor trace. In particular, VF can be mimicked by movement artefact (either muscular movement by the patient, or of the leads) and asystole by lead disconnection or an inadequate gain setting. It should also be emphasised that with EMD the clinical picture of cardiac arrest can occur in a patient with an apparently normal ECG trace.

The dictum is: 'When in doubt, treat the patient and not an ECG trace'.

THE PATHOPHYSIOLOGY OF FORWARD BLOOD FLOW DURING CARDIOPULMONARY RESUSCITATION

Because of the inherent difficulties in studying human cardiac arrest, our knowledge of the mechanisms producing forward, or antegrade, blood flow is incomplete (Peters & Ihle, 1990). Extrapolation of data from the animal models commonly used may be inappropriate due to the considerable differences in chest wall configuration and internal anatomy.

The original theory postulated over 30 years ago suggested that during manual closed chest compression the heart was physically 'squeezed' between the sternum anteriorly and the spine posteriorly (Kouwenhoven *et al.*, 1960). During the compression phase the atrioventricular valves would close and prevent retrograde blood flow. At the same time the aortic and pulmonary valves open to allow forward flow. During the relaxation phase the atrioventricular valves open permitting ventricular filling from blood returning via the venae cavae and pulmonary artery, while the aortic and pulmonary valves close to prevent retrograde flow.

In the late 1970s, this 'cardiac' pump theory required re-evaluation when it was observed that patients or experimental animals in cardiac arrest could maintain sufficient antegrade blood flow to remain conscious by

---

Theories of forward blood flow during CPR

Cardiac pump
- Heart compressed between sternum and spine
- Mitral and tricuspid valves close during compression preventing retrograde flow into atria
- Aortic and pulmonary valves open during compression allowing systemic and pulmonary flow
- During relaxation phase mitral/tricuspid valves open permitting ventricular filling, while aortic/pulmonary valves shut preventing retrograde flow

Thoracic pump
- Intrathoracic pressure increased by ventilation and for chest compression
- No valve patency required. Heart acts as a passive conduit
- Forward blood flow occurs due to pressure gradient between intra- and extrathoracic vascular circuits

---

techniques that dramatically increased intrathoracic pressure (Criley *et al.*, 1976; Forney & Ornato, 1980). These techniques included vigorous coughing, positive pressure ventilation or inflation of a pneumatic vest (Halperin *et al.*, 1986; Luce *et al.*, 1983). Clearly, in these patients the cardiac pump theory could not be functioning. Forward blood flow must be produced simply by the increase in intrathoracic pressure. This mechanism of producing forward blood flow has been called the thoracic pump.

For the thoracic pump to function, cerebral perfusion can only occur if a pressure gradient exists between the intra- and extrathoracic circuits when intrathoracic pressure is increased. This has been demonstrated between the carotid arteries and jugular veins. Furthermore, retrograde blood flow must be prevented. Functional valves in the internal jugular and subclavian veins at the thoracic inlet have been shown to prevent transmission of intrathoracic pressure increases as well as retrograde flow to the cerebral venous system (Fisher *et al.*, 1982; Paradis *et al.*, 1981). Meanwhile, the thick-walled carotid arteries, which are relatively resistant to collapse, facilitate antegrade cerebral blood flow (Michael *et al.*, 1984; Yin *et al.*, 1982).

Many studies have been performed to elucidate which of these two theories is operative during CPR in man. The two are not necessarily mutually exclusive. It is possible that at different phases of compression or ventilation, or at different time intervals after cardiac arrest, one or other is operative. For patients undergoing purely intrathoracic pressure increases such as 'cough CPR' the thoracic pump mechanism must be working. However, the balance of evidence now suggests that, when CPR is performed using standard techniques involving chest compression, direct compression of the right and left ventricles actually occurs (Guly *et al.*, 1993; Higano *et al.*, 1990). Further confirmation of this comes from the demonstration of appropriate opening and closure of the atrioventricular, aortic and pulmonary valves by techniques such as transoesophageal echocardiography.

An understanding of the mechanisms involved in forward blood flow is not merely of academic interest. Attempts to maximize the cardiac output achieved during CPR are essential (Robertson & Holmberg, 1992). Even with optimal closed chest compression, cardiac output rarely approaches even a quarter of normal values (Del Guercio *et al.*, 1963; Ditchley *et al.*, 1982). The magnitude of the pressure gradients produced, and the myocardial and cerebral perfusion values obtained, are similarly dismal, irrespective of the means by which antegrade blood flow is produced. The pressure gradients produced during CPR strongly determine the likelihood of restoring spontaneous circulation and maintaining cerebral function (Weil & Noc, 1992). The gradient between aortic diastolic and right atrial pressures (which approximates to the coronary perfusion pressure) is a strong predictor of the success in restoring spontaneous circulation (Niemann *et al.*, 1985). Cerebral perfusion depends upon the gradient between the arterial and venous cerebral circulations during the 'systolic' phase and these levels have also been shown to be important prognostically.

A number of innovative and ingenious techniques have been used to improve myocardial and cerebral perfusion during CPR. Attempts to augment the intrathoracic pressures generated during CPR include the use of an intermittent or continuous compressive force to the abdomen by binding or inflating a garment such as the MAST suit. While some haemodynamic improvements have been noted with these devices, no evidence of improved survival has been demonstrated in large-scale clinical evaluation (Niemann, 1989). Simultaneous chest compression and ventilation has been shown to improve cerebral, but not myocardial, perfusion.

Mechanical devices exist which produce chest compression and ventilation. They have the advantage that they can perform CPR in a preprogrammed compression and ventilation sequence without interruption or tiring. The haemodynamic profiles produced during mechanical CPR are similar to that achieved during optimal manual procedures. Particular complications related to mechanical CPR include an increase in the incidence of sternal fractures as well as their cost, the need for operator familiarity, size and weight considerations (Robertson & Holmberg, 1992). Recently, a new dimension has been added to closed chest cardiac massage techniques. The active compression/ decompression device enables conventional chest compression to be performed but in addition has a suction-cup device that adheres to the anterior chest wall (Cohen *et al.*, 1992a, b). By pulling up vertically this provides active chest expansion in the 'decompression' phase. Early animal and human studies suggest that improved venous return and cardiac filling are produced by this device. This is probably related to the increased negative intrathoracic pressures developed during decompression.

BASIC LIFE SUPPORT

Attempts to reanimate the apparently lifeless are well documented in antiquity, and detailed and entertaining accounts of the historical background to CPR exist (Safar, 1989; Paraskos, 1992).

Basic life support (BLS) is the provision and maintenance of an airway, and the support of ventilation and circulation without the use of any equipment other than simple airway devices or protective shields (BLS Working Party of the European Resuscitation Council, 1992).

All staff involved in patient care, emergency service personnel (ambulance, police, fire, etc.) and all road users requiring to undertake a driving test should be taught BLS. Several European countries include BLS training as part of a graded programme within the school curriculum and this development is to be encouraged.

BLS commences with an assessment of the situation to ensure that neither the rescuer nor the patient are at risk from hazards such as passing traffic, electricity, etc. After confirmation that cardiac arrest is present (i.e. a pulseless and unconscious patient), the rescuer must ensure that help is summoned prior to starting CPR. The airway is then cleared and appropriately positioned (see Chapter 2). Mouth-to-mouth or mouth-to-mask expired air ventilation is given. During mouth-to-mouth ventilation, minimal resistance to breathing should be encountered. To reduce the likelihood of gastric insufflation and

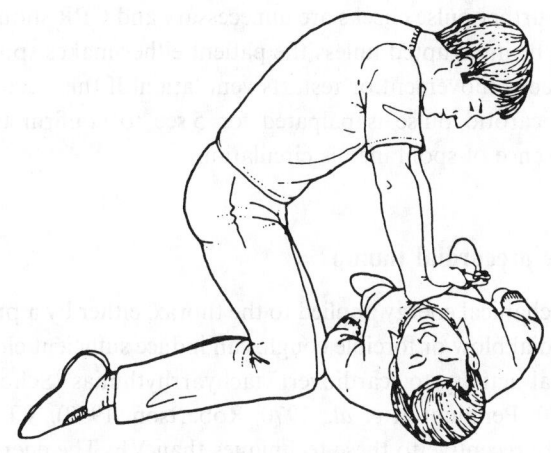

Fig. 1. Chest compression. (Reproduced by permission of the Resuscitation Council (UK).)

distension, with the risk of regurgitation and aspiration, each breath should take about 2 sec (Ruben *et al.*, 1961). The aim is to produce a tidal volume of 800–1200 ml, normally the amount required to produce visible lifting of the chest. The chest should be observed to fall during expiration before the next ventilating breath is given.

Chest compression (Fig. 1) is performed by two-handed pressure over the middle of the lower half of the sternum. Compression should aim to depress the sternum 4–5 cm and be firm, controlled and applied vertically . The duration of the compression and relaxation phases should be equal. The rate of chest compression is approximately 80 min^{-1}. For single-rescuer CPR, a compression/ventilation ratio of 15:2 is recommended. For two-rescuer CPR (Fig. 2) the compression/ventilation ratio is 5:1.

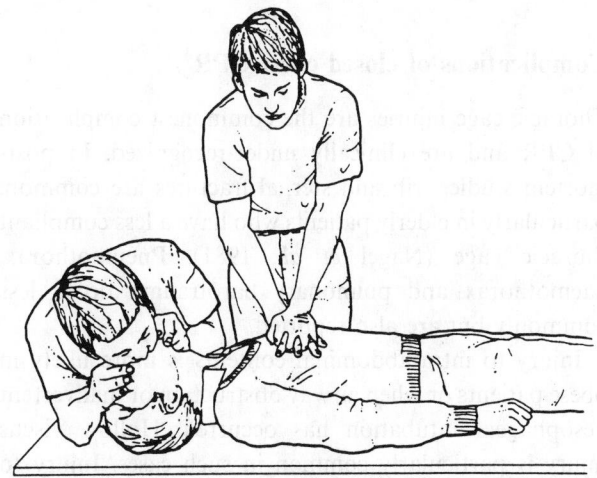

Fig. 2. Two-person cardiopulmonary resuscitation. (Reproduced by permission of the Resuscitation Council (UK).)

Further pulse checks are unnecessary and CPR should not be interrupted unless the patient either makes spontaneous movement or restarts ventilation. If this occurs, the carotid pulse is palpated for 5 sec to confirm the presence of spontaneous circulation.

The precordial thump

Mechanical energy applied to the thorax, either by a precordial blow or forcible cough, can induce sufficient electrical activity to 'cardiovert' tachyarrhythmias (Schott, 1920; Pennington et al., 1970; Robertson, 1992). VT is more receptive to these techniques than VF. The energy required to terminate VT by electrical means may, particularly in the first few seconds of cardiac arrest, be as little as 1–10 J. A precordial blow can generate these levels sufficient to depolarize a critical mass of myocardium and terminate the episode. Conversion rates of 11–40% for VT and 2% for VF have been reported (Caldwell et al., 1985).

For patients in asystole, the electrical stimulus may be sufficient to induce mechanical systole and restart the normal electrical processes involved with resumption of cardiac output.

Physical complications of a precordial thump, such as sternal or rib fractures, myocardial contusion or rupture, do not appear to occur with any greater frequency than following standard chest compression. Concern that a precordial thump may cause VT to deteriorate by producing an acceleration in rate or precipitate VF (Krijne, 1984) is outweighed by the potential for the rapid and successful restoration of a perfusing rhythm in a patient already with the clinical features of cardiac arrest.

Complications of closed chest CPR

Thoracic cage injuries are the commonest complication of CPR and are clinically under-recognized. In post-mortem studies, rib and sternal fractures are common, particularly in elderly patients who have a less compliant thoracic cage (Nagel et al., 1981). Pneumothorax, haemothorax and pulmonary barotrauma occur less commonly but are also reported.

Injury to intra-abdominal contents is more likely in obese patients or when airway obstruction or inadvertent oesophageal intubation has occurred. Hollow viscus injury is particularly common in such cases. Injury to the solid abdominal organs (particularly liver and spleen) is infrequent but when it occurs is associated with a high risk of major haemorrhage (Clark, 1962; Bjork et al., 1980; Power et al., 1984).

AIRWAY TECHNIQUES AND VENTILATION

Tracheal intubation with a cuffed tube is the best method of securing the upper airway and permitting artificial ventilation during cardiac arrest. Prior to intubation, preoxygenation and ventilation can be performed using standard BLS mouth-to-mask or bag–valve–mask techniques. Oropharyngeal (Guedel) or nasopharyngeal airways can be used in association with these techniques to further improve upper airway patency. Bag–valve devices can be used in combination with a face mask or tracheal tube. Single-rescuer use of bag–valve–mask devices is difficult because of the difficulty of maintaining an adequate seal between the mask and face while compressing the bag (Hess & Baran, 1985; Johannigman et al., 1991). Therefore it is recommended that if these devices are used by two rescuers (Jesudian et al., 1985), the first maintains an adequate seal between the mask and the patient's face while the second squeezes the bag.

Tracheal intubation enables the delivery of high concentrations of inspired oxygen, facilitates mechanical ventilation and allows suction of the trachea and lower airway (Carli et al., 1992). The technique and complications are described in Chapter 2. The risks of gastric distension, regurgitation and aspiration, all of which commonly occur during BLS, are minimized by tracheal intubation. Some drugs can also be delivered by the endobronchial route. No longer than 15–30 sec should be allowed for tracheal intubation to be performed.

Following intubation, the position of the tracheal tube is checked. This is performed by direct laryngoscopic examination to confirm that the tube passes directly through the cords. Then auscultate both sides of the chest in the 3rd to 5th interspaces in the midaxillary lines to ensure adequate ventilation. Symmetrical expansion of the chest should also be present. Following tracheal intubation, ventilation using a bag–valve device (with a reservoir to further increase oxygen enrichment) or a mechanical ventilator can then take place. Ventilation is performed with a ventilation/compression frequency of 1:5.

When mechanical ventilation is used, a tidal volume of 10 ml kg^{-1}, a respiratory rate of 12–15 min^{-1} and an inspiratory/expiratory ratio of 1:2 or 1:1.5 is advocated. These values may require to be adjusted according to the physical characteristics of the patient and upon the results of arterial blood gas analysis.

Attempts should be made to maximally increase the inspired oxygen concentration during ventilation. Hypoperfusion during cardiac arrest and CPR leads to tissue hypoxia and this increases in severity with time. Concerns with regard to carbon dioxide retention in patients with obstructive airway disease are invalid in the context of cardiac arrest. Expired air ventilation such as is delivered during BLS provides approximately 16–17% inspired oxygen to the patient. Bag–valve devices attached to an oxygen supply can give FiO_2 (fraction of inspired oxygen) levels of approximately 50%, which can be increased to nearly 90% by the addition of a reservoir to the system. Depending upon the setting chosen, most mechanical ventilators can deliver 100% oxygen.

With good-quality CPR and adequate ventilation using high inspired concentrations of oxygen, PaO_2 and $PaCO_2$ levels can be maintained in or near the normal range for up to 20 min (Steedman & Robertson, 1992). Provided adequate ventilation occurs, and $PaCO_2$ levels are kept near normal, the development of arterial acidaemia due to anaerobic metabolism and lactate production is also significantly delayed.

Capnography with end-tidal carbon dioxide measurement can be used to confirm that tracheal intubation has occurred. Low levels of end-tidal carbon dioxide (below 0.5%) persisting after the first few ventilations suggest malposition of the tracheal tube. Measurement of end-tidal carbon dioxide levels can also be used as an indirect means of assessing cardiac output during CPR (Steedman & Robertson, 1990). End-tidal carbon dioxide levels with normal spontaneous cardiac output are 4–5%. In patients undergoing CPR there is a close relationship between the cardiac output achieved and end-tidal carbon dioxide values (Garnett et al., 1987; Sanders et al., 1985). The return of spontaneous circulation is often heralded by a sudden rise in end-tidal carbon dioxide levels, often above normal values. This is due to a washout phenomenon as the spontaneous return of cardiac output promotes a flush of hypercarbic blood back to the lungs.

The use of alternative devices to protect the airway and permit ventilation are inferior to tracheal intubation (Carli et al., 1992). Devices such as the oesophageal obturator airway, the pharyngotracheal lumen airway and the oesophagotracheal Combitube have been extensively used in North America. Elsewhere, their use is very limited and concerns exist as to their role in inducing oesophageal injury, vomiting and aspiration. Furthermore, the airway is not as well protected and ventilation is not rendered as easily as with a cuffed tracheal tube.

The laryngeal mask (see Chapter 2) has also been recommended for airway management in cardiac arrest but to date limited clinical experience is available regarding its use in this situation (Leach et al., 1993).

In the event of inability to provide an airway by the above means, transtracheal ventilation can be considered. This is particularly indicated if airway obstruction is present and cannot be relieved by other techniques. These techniques are described in Chapter 2.

DEFIBRILLATION

The definitive treatment of VF and pulseless VT is defibrillation (Bossaert & Koster, 1992). During defibrillation, a direct electric current passes across the heart. This depolarizes the myocardium and, if successful, allows the normal myocardial pacemaker cells to restart and control coordinated electrical activity. Only a small proportion of the current administered during external defibrillation actually traverses the myocardium. Parallel electrical pathways through the thoracic cage and lungs can shunt up to 95% of the delivered energy around the myocardium (Lerman & Deal, 1990).

The chance of a defibrillating shock being successful depends on a number of inter-related aspects. These include dynamic variables such as changes in the VF wave form and the vector of the fibrillatory activity at the time the shock is administered, and factors related to transthoracic impedance (Kerber et al., 1981; Sirna et al., 1988).

Mean transthoracic impedance is 70–80 ohms, although this may vary between 15 and 150 ohms. Transthoracic impedance is affected by physical variables such as the body weight and composition of the patient, the electrode

---

Factors affecting transthoracic impedance

- Body weight and composition
- Electrode size
- Electrode pressure
- Phase of ventilation
- Duration of ventricular fibrillation
- Prior shocks
- Metabolic state of myocardium (pH, temperature, ischaemia)
- Antiarrhythmic drugs

---

size, pressure employed and the phase of ventilation. There are also variables such as the duration of VF and the administration of prior shocks – repeated shocks significantly reduce impedance. Thirdly, the defibrillation threshold depends upon the metabolic state of the myocardium, temperature, pH, ischaemia and the presence of antiarrhythmic drugs.

Defibrillation has its own hazards. If the operator is careless, members of the team may be inadvertently shocked. There is a risk of explosion if, prior to defibrillation, nitroglycerin adhesive patches or ointment have not been removed (Wrenn, 1990). Finally, the electrical energy delivered to the patient can itself cause myocardial damage and provoke arrhythmias. Myocardial injury, characterized by mitochondrial dysfunction and free radical generation, has been demonstrated after defibrillation. The magnitude of this insult increases with the energy delivered and the number of shocks used.

For these reasons, the energies selected for the first shock sequence are determined by the balance between the probability of success and the risks of inducing further damage. The first and second shocks are given at 200 J, and further shocks at 360 J. To minimize transthoracic impedence, the optimal electrode pad size is 12– 13 cm and they should be placed firmly (minimum 12 kg pressure) with one paddle below the outer half of the right clavicle and the other over the cardiac apex (V4–5 position). The polarity of the paddles is irrelevant. Conductive gel pads or electrode gel are used to improve contact (Aylward et al., 1985) and the shock should be given during the expiratory phase of ventilation.

Some modern defibrillators can measure transthoracic impedance and automatically deliver a defibrillating shock of the appropriate current. A shock with a current of 30–40 A is thought to be optimal. 'Current-based' defibrillation can prevent the selection and administration of an inappropriately low-energy shock to patients with high transthoracic impedance and vice versa. In the future, this technique may prove to be more efficacious than standard fixed energy shocks (Bossaert & Koster, 1992; Dalzell & Adgey, 1991).

Automatic defibrillators

In the past 5 years, the use of semiautomatic and automatic external defibrillators (AEDs) has become common, particularly for prehospital situations. These machines can detect VF and VT with a high degree of sensitivity and specificity (Dickey et al., 1992). They can then either advise, or automatically give, defibrillating shocks at preselected energy levels.

The prehospital use of AEDs improves the survival of patients with VF and VT by reducing the need for rescuer decision-making and the time taken to deliver the shocks. Most machines have facilities to record and store the events, permitting playback analysis after each resuscitation. AEDs require minimal staff training time. Although the costs of these devices are somewhat higher than for manual devices, their applicability will lead to widespread use in ambulance services, by general practitioners and other members of the emergency services (Cobbe et al., 1991).

DRUG DELIVERY ROUTES

The ideal method of drug administration to a patient in cardiac arrest is one which delivers the drug to the target organ(s), is simple and rapid to perform with minimal expertise and which has minimal complications (Hapnes & Robertson, 1992). At present, no single route has all of these features.

The commonest and simplest method of drug delivery is via a peripheral venous cannula. This requires little expertise and should normally be achieved in under 30 sec. To aid drug delivery from a peripheral line, the limb can be elevated and a fluid flush of 20 ml given. Because circulation times are prolonged during CPR, drug delivery to the heart after peripheral venous administration is delayed (up to 3–5 min) with inadequate drug levels achieved (Hedges et al., 1982; Kuhn et al., 1981). Central venous cannulation allows rapid drug delivery to the right side of the heart but requires considerable expertise and has potentially catastrophic complications.

Potential complications of central venous cannulation during CPR

- Failure to achieve access
- Interruption of CPR
- Pneumothorax
- Haemothorax
- Air embolism
- Local and systemic sepsis
- Catheter embolization
- Arterial puncture
- Thoracic duct puncture (on left)
- Relative contraindication for later thrombolytic therapy

In addition, subclavian vein approaches may require chest compression to be temporarily interrupted while the use of the internal jugular vein may complicate airway management. Some drugs can be delivered via a tracheal tube and then be absorbed via the pulmonary vasculature (Aitkenhead, 1991). If this endobronchial route is used, the drug is administered in two to three times the normal intravenous dose and diluted with normal saline or sterile water to a total volume of 10 ml. After administration ventilation is given to aid dispersal and absorption from the distal airways. Drugs which can be given in this way are adrenaline, atropine and lignocaine. Despite initial enthusiasm, however, drug administration via the endobronchial route during CPR is at best inefficient and in some situations completely ineffective. Adverse effects may occur, and marked persistent decreases in arterial oxygenation have been reported. Adrenaline absorption following endobronchial administration appears to be particularly poor (Quinton et al., 1987). This may be due to local airway factors such as pulmonary oedema and atelectasis in association with the vasoconstrictive actions of adrenaline leading to inhibition of its own absorption.

Theoretically, direct intracardiac drug administration should provide the most rapid drug delivery to the heart (Pedersen et al., 1991). Subxiphoid and left sternal approaches can be used. However the technique requires temporarily stopping chest compression and ventilation and the hazards of pneumothorax, haemothorax, haemopericardium, myocardial injury and coronary artery laceration are considerable (Sabin et al., 1983).

In children, the intraosseous route is a useful technique to allow fluid or drug administration when venous access is impossible. Following delivery to the marrow cavity, drug absorption rapidly occurs via the venous sinusoids which drain directly into the central circulation. Little adult experience is available for this technique.

Human data as to the optimal route for drug administration is scanty and dogmatic statements as to the most applicable route for drug administration in any given clinical situation are difficult. In experienced hands, cannulation of the internal jugular or subclavian veins is likely to give the most rapid and reliable administration of drugs directly into the central circulation. For patients in cardiac arrest, the central veins are usually distended and, with experience, can usually be cannulated rapidly. Peripheral venous cannulation should be considered as the route of choice for inexperienced team members with the endobronchial and intracardiac routes considered as second-line alternatives.

DRUGS USED IN CARDIAC ARREST

Vasopressors

Vasopressors have long been used as adjuncts to improve the success rate in CPR (Crile & Dolley, 1906). Catecholamines, such as adrenaline and noradrenaline, increase aortic diastolic pressure by producing arteriolar vasoconstriction and improve blood delivery to the central circulation by shunting blood back from the skin, skeletal muscle and splanchnic beds (Waller & Robertson, 1991; Paradis & Koscove, 1990). In man, cardiac arrest is associated with the highest endogenous levels of adrenaline and noradrenaline. Levels 300–400 times normal resting values have been recorded (Little et al., 1985). If exogenous catecholamines are given, even greater rises in plasma catecholamine concentrations are produced. At these 'pharmacological' levels, improved myocardial and cerebral perfusion occurs (Michael et al., 1984). Peripheral vasoconstriction is mediated by alpha$_1$-(α_1-) and alpha$_2$-(α_2-)adrenoreceptor stimulation (Lindner & Koster, 1992). In cardiac arrest, the alpha$_2$-receptors play the most significant role in producing vasoconstriction. Hence selective alpha$_1$-agonists such as methoxamine and phenylephrine are less effective than adrenaline and noradrenaline in their haemodynamic actions during cardiac arrest (Brown & Werman, 1990). Myocardial alpha-receptor stimulation also leads to coronary vasoconstriction. Nevertheless, when adrenaline or noradrenaline are given, myocardial blood flow is not reduced because the coronary vessels also have beta-receptors which when stimulated produce vasodilation. Both adrenaline and noradrenaline improve coronary perfusion in a dose-related manner. The effective dose is influenced by the duration of cardiac arrest and the degree of respiratory and metabolic acidosis. In experimental animals, coronary perfusion pressure, myocardial blood flow and restoration of spontaneous output are closely related to the administered dose within the range 0.045–0.2 mg kg^{-1} (Lindner et al., 1991).

Potential disadvantages of catecholamine administration include the development of myocardial contraction band necrosis, increased myocardial oxygen consumption, arterial hypertension, increased incidence of arrhythmias following resuscitation and metabolic effects including hyperglycaemia, hyperlactataemia and increased systemic oxygen demand (Lindner & Koster, 1992).

The optimal dose of adrenaline in cardiac arrest is unclear. The currently recommended intravenous (IV) dose of adrenaline is 1 mg. This is repeated every 2–3 min

(ALS Working Party of the ERC, 1992). When given intravenously, the half-life of adrenaline is very short (minutes) due to rapid metabolism. Recently it has been shown in man that the high endogenous levels of adrenaline which occur during cardiac arrest can be maintained for up to 60 min during good CPR. Animal data show a dose-related effect between catecholamines and their beneficial haemodynamic effects. For these reasons, and because a few human case reports had suggested beneficial outcome, the use of high-dose (5–15 mg) adrenaline and noradrenaline has been advocated (Koscove & Paradis, 1988; Cipolotti et al., 1991). Three large North American multicentre trials have failed to show any benefit from the administration of high-dose adrenaline or noradrenaline in patients with out-of-hospital or in-hospital cardiac arrest (Stiell et al., 1992; Brown et al., 1992; Callahan et al., 1992). Indeed, in a small study, there was no difference in immediate survival or hospital discharge rates for patients randomized to 10 mg, 1 mg of adrenaline, or placebo (Woodhouse et al., 1993).

Antiarrhythmic drugs

While many agents have been shown to have antiarrhythmic properties in patients with cardiac rhythms associated with output, the evidence for their value in cardiac arrest situations is tenuous (Von Planta & Chamberlain, 1992). Many agents have indeed been shown to have proarrhythmic qualities and adversely affect outcome.

There are distinct differences in the use of an antiarrhythmic agent to prevent malignant ventricular arrhythmias and VF and the use of the same drug to facilitate defibrillation. The most commonly used antiarrhythmic agent in the treatment of VT and VF is lignocaine. Lignocaine has relatively little myocardial depressant action and a short half-life (although this is prolonged in the postarrest situation and, by producing hepatic microsomal dysfunction, it actually inhibits its own metabolism). In patients with acute myocardial infarction, lignocaine reduces the incidence of VF, although there is no reduction in mortality (Lie et al., 1974). Experimentally, lignocaine increases the defibrillation threshold and the energy required for successful defibrillation (Dorian et al., 1986). Furthermore, in patients given lignocaine as an adjunct for defibrillation there is a three-fold increase in the incidence of postshock asystole. In VF or pulseless VT, the loading dose of

lignocaine is a bolus of 100 mg IV. Following successful defibrillation a decreasing dose infusion is required to maintain an adequate plasma level. An infusion rate of 3 mg min^{-1} for 3 h followed by 1.5 mg min^{-1} is appropriate but the dose should be reduced in patients with heart failure, the elderly and those with hepatic dysfunction.

Bretylium tosylate is a second-line agent with a variety of actions. It initially causes catecholamine release, followed by subsequent sympathetic blocking actions. It has not been shown to be superior to lignocaine as an aid to defibrillation although there is some evidence to suggest synergy between the two agents.

Other antiarrhythmic drugs advocated for the treatment of VF include procainamide, mexiletine, flecainide, amiodarone and beta-adrenoceptor antagonists. None of these agents has been shown to be more efficacious or to have better haemodynamic effects than lignocaine (Chamberlain, 1991; Waller, 1991). Of the group, amiodarone is probably the most promising but the overwhelming message is that, in the context of established cardiac arrest, antiarrhythmic drug therapy has little, if any, proven beneficial role.

Buffers and alkalizing agents

When cardiac pumping action ceases in cardiac arrest, anaerobic metabolism occurs in tissues producing lactic and other organic acids. This can be detected by the developing acidaemia in arterial or venous samples. With good quality CPR and adequate alveolar ventilation, the development of acidaemia is slow and significant falls in arterial pH do not occur for at least the first 20 min following cardiac arrest (Steedman & Robertson, 1992). The degree to which arterial or venous acidaemia affects myocardial tissue pH levels is less clear. A defined level of acidaemia which requires treatment before the chances of successful outcome are compromised is not known. As an empirical guide, an arterial pH 7.1 ($H^+ > 80$ nmol l^{-1}) may be appropriate for the administration of a buffer (Koster & Carli, 1992). Complex inter-relationships between the development of acidaemia and the activity of endogenous or exogenously administered catecholamines are also important.

The most commonly used buffering agent is sodium bicarbonate. This is usually administered as a hypertonic 8.4% solution which is highly irritant to tissues. When sodium bicarbonate acts as a buffer carbon dioxide is produced. If not removed due to inadequate alveolar ventilation, the resulting severe hypercarbia can lead to a paradoxical intracellular acidosis. This develops because carbon dioxide crosses cell membranes and the blood–brain barrier more rapidly than bicarbonate ions. CSF (cerebrospinal fluid) and myocardial acidosis may therefore be produced following bicarbonate administration (Berenyi et al., 1975) and can depress myocardial contractility (Von Planta et al., 1989). If considered appropriate an intravenous dose of 50 ml of 8.4% sodium bicarbonate (or 1 mmol kg^{-1} body weight) should be given and further doses given following blood gas analysis. Alternative buffer agents such trihydroxymethyl-aminomethane (THAM), Carbicarb (an equimolar combination of sodium bicarbonate and sodium carbonate) and Tribonate (THAM, sodium acetate, sodium bicarbonate and sodium phosphate) may be more efficient and produce less carbon dioxide (Koster & Carli, 1992). However, no clinical studies have confirmed any greater efficacy from their use than sodium bicarbonate. By far the best way to correct acid–base disturbances associated with cardiac arrest is to restore a spontaneous circulation as rapidly as possible.

Calcium and magnesium salts

Ionized calcium is important in normal myocardial contractile function and low levels have been demonstrated in patients with cardiac arrest (Urban et al., 1988). However, calcium ion shifts accompany cerebral ischaemic insults and it is possible that additional calcium administration may adversely affect cerebral function (Dembo, 1981). There is no evidence of any beneficial effect from the administration of calcium salts in patients with asystole or VF (Steuven et al., 1984). For patients with EMD associated with hyperkalaemia or patients taking calcium channel blockers, administration of 10 ml of 10% calcium chloride may be beneficial.

Magnesium is the treatment of choice for polymorphic VT (torsade de pointes) which may present as an arrhythmia associated with cardiac arrest in patients with prolonged QT syndrome. Intracellular magnesium depletion is common in patients on long-term diuretic therapy. Hypomagnesaemia may predispose to malignant ventricular arrhythmias including VF, and magnesium supplementation has been shown to reduce the incidence of arrhythmias by affecting slow sodium channels. The dose of magnesium sulphate is 50 ml of 50% solution infused over 30 min.

Atropine

Atropine has a clear role as a parasympatholytic agent for patients with symptomatic bradyarrhythmias (see Chapter 45b). It is given in a dose of 0.5 mg IV and may be repeated as clinically indicated. Some patients with ventricular asystole have marked increases in vagal tone. Atropine in a single dose of 3 mg IV, to provide complete vagal blockade, is recommended in this situation (Von Planta & Chamberlain, 1992).

ADVANCED LIFE SUPPORT

Figs 3–5 show algorithms for the treatment of VF, Asystole and EMD.

VF algorithm

The treatment of VF and pulseless VT is identical (ALS Working Party of the ERC, 1992). These patients must be defibrillated as rapidly as possible. Only a single precordial thump may precede electrical defibrillation. This takes 2–3 sec and will not delay preparations for defibrillation. If the precordial thump is unsuccessful, then electrical defibrillation must immediately follow. The sequence of energies recommended for the first three defibrillation shocks is 200 J, 200 J and 360 J. With modern defibrillators, these first three shocks can be delivered within 30–45 sec. Provided this is the case, they should not be interrupted by BLS. In situations where the defibrillator is slow to charge or the team is inexperienced in the delivery of defibrillating shocks, one or two sequences of BLS (chest compression:ventilation 5:1) can be administered between shocks. If, after the first three defibrillating shocks, the patient remains in VF attempts should be made to intubate the patient and achieve intravenous access, if these procedures have not already been performed. These interventions must not cause delay in the administration of further defibrillating shocks or the performance of BLS. The leader of the arrest team should allow no longer than 15–30 sec for these procedures to be performed. Adrenaline in a dose of 1 mg IV is administered before further shocks are given but, again, defibrillation should not be delayed merely for drug administration.

A further sequence of shocks, all now at 360 J, is performed. If unsuccessful, the 'loop' is repeated. With each loop, adrenaline is given in a dose of 1 mg every 2–3 min. If the patient remains in VF after three loops

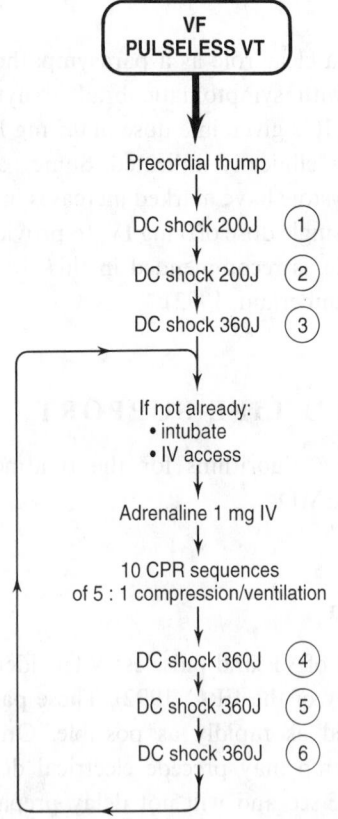

Fig. 3. Algorithm for ventricular fibrillation (VF) or pulseless ventricular tachycardia. (Copyright European Resuscitation Council.)

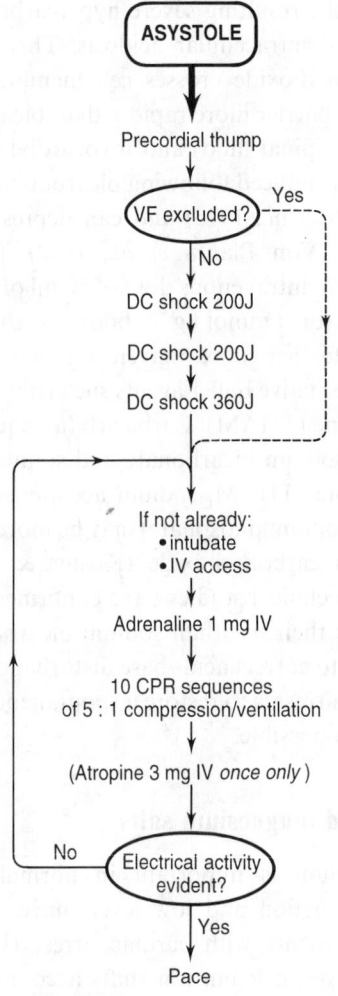

Fig. 4. Algorithm for asystole. (Copyright European Resuscitation Council.)

of the algorithm have been completed, consideration can be made for the administration of an alkalizing agent and/or an antiarrhythmic drug. A dosage of 50 mmol (or 1 mmol kg^{-1} body weight) of sodium bicarbonate is recommended but should ideally be given only in the knowledge of arterial and central venous pH and bicarbonate levels.

The most appropriate antiarrhythmic drug at this stage is probably lignocaine, given as a bolus of 100 mg IV.

For any individual clinical situation, the number of loops performed depends upon the clinical judgement of the team leader and the prospect of successful outcome. Provided it is appropriate to continue resuscitation, however, patients remaining in VF should have continued resuscitation.

Asystole algorithm

The possibility of VF being misdiagnosed as asystole must always be considered. This may occur because of electrical or movement artefact or an inappropriately low-gain setting on the ECG monitor. An unusually directional vector of a VF wave form perpendicular to the sensing electrode can also lead to VF being mistaken for asystole. Since VF is so amenable to treatment and is much more likely to have a successful outcome, the initial defibrillation sequence should be followed if any doubt exists. The sequence of three shocks if given is then followed by tracheal intubation, securing intravenous access and drug administration. Adrenaline 1 mg IV is given to improve myocardial and cerebral perfusion during CPR. A single 3 mg dose of atropine will block excess vagal tone affecting the heart. Recently a role for

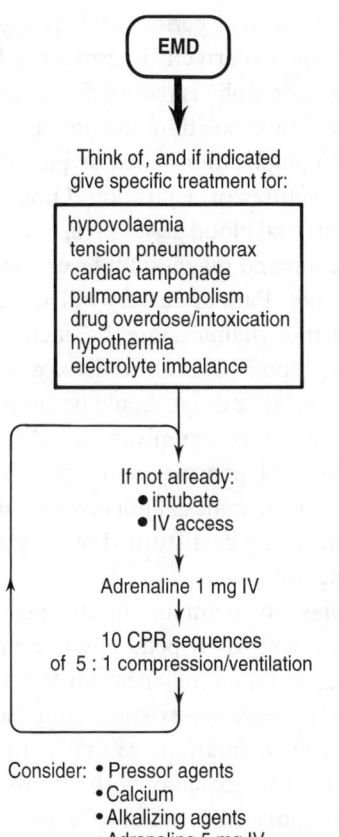

Fig. 5. Algorithm for electromechanical dissociation (EMD). (Copyright European Resuscitation Council.)

aminophylline in bradyasystolic cardiac arrests has been suggested (Viskin *et al.*, 1993).

Electrical pacing can be considered for asystole but only if electrical activity (elicited by the presence of P waves or occasional QRS complexes) has been present. If asystole persists, further loops of the algorithm can be considered, but it must be remembered that the prognosis for asystole, except in certain special situations, is very poor.

Electromechanical dissociation algorithm

It has recently been recognized that situations exist where there are the clinical features of cardiac arrest (i.e. loss of consciousness and absence of a palpable major pulse) but when intra-arterial monitoring is undertaken a pressure wave form can be detected . The term 'pseudo-EMD' has been used for this state (Paradis *et al.*, 1992). In this situation, there is mechanical pumping activity of the heart associated with electrical complexes but the pressures produced are too small to produce a palpable pulse.

In the context of acute myocardial infarction, EMD carries an extremely poor prognosis (Vincent *et al.*, 1981). There are, however, a number of potentially reversible causes of EMD. These include hypovolaemia, tension pneumothorax and pulmonary embolism. If present, specific treatment should be administered for these. Other potentially reversible causes of EMD include hypothermia and drug overdose with agents such as beta-blockers, tricyclic antidepressants or calcium channel blockers. Specific therapy can be targeted for these situations (see Chapter 11). If there is no potentially remediable cause, the standard EMD algorithm should be followed (Fig. 5). Drugs such as pressor agents, calcium salts, alkalizing agents and high-dose adrenaline have been advocated, but there is no objective evidence that these therapies are of specific value.

OPEN CHEST CARDIO-PULMONARY RESUSCITATION

Open chest techniques were routine until the introduction of closed chest compression by Kouwenhoven in 1960. Open chest cardiac massage has been shown experimentally to improve cardiac output, coronary and myocardial perfusion (Weiser *et al.*, 1962; Barnett *et al.*, 1986; DeBehnke *et al.*, 1991) and animal studies have demonstrated significantly higher resuscitation rates.

The technique is neither complex nor time-consuming. The usual emergency department approach is via an incision from the sternum to the mid- or posterior axillary line in the 5th intercostal space. The intercostal muscles and pleura are divided exposing the heart. Incision of the pericardium is not required except in those situations where pericardial tamponade is present. If the pericardium is opened, care should be taken to avoid injury to the phrenic nerve. The heart is then compressed with a two-handed technique or with one hand placed posteriorly and compressing the heart arteriorly against the sternum taking care not to injury the relatively thin-walled atria and right ventricle.

Bleeding from intercostal or the internal mammary vessels is not a problem until a spontaneous circulation is achieved. Following successful restoration of circulation, formal in-theatre closure of the chest with appropriate drainage of the pleural cavities is undertaken.

Early reports of open chest techniques in man were very encouraging but reflected the treatment of patients with markedly different pathophysiological situations from that occurring in sudden cardiac arrest events (Stevenson *et al.*, 1953; Briggs *et al.*, 1956). In the only randomized human trial of open versus closed massage no additional benefit accrued from the open chest technique (Geehr & Auerback, 1985).

At present, despite theoretical advantages and an improved haemodynamic profile, open chest massage cannot be recommended for the routine management of cardiac arrest (Robertson & Holmberg, 1992). In some special situations, however, e.g. pericardial tamponade, patients with recent sternotomy, those undergoing intra-abdominal surgery and patients in whom closed chest CPR is ineffective because of anatomical constraints, an open-chest technique is indicated.

POST RESUSCITATION CARE

General features

In the immediate postresuscitation phase, the aim is to maintain a stable cardiac rhythm and a haemodynamic profile and pulmonary gas exchange as near the patient's normal status as possible (Steen et al., 1992).

Some patients, particularly those with VF who have been rapidly defibrillated, will promptly regain consciousness and have minimal derangement in their haemodynamic parameters. These individuals should have close ECG monitoring, be given high concentrations of oxygen pending arterial blood gas analysis, analgesia for pain and consideration of thrombolysis if evidence of acute myocardial infarction is present on the 12-lead ECG.

The indications for thrombolysis in the context of the postarrest phase include those outlined in Chapter 45A. However, the risks of thrombolysis causing haemorrhage after traumatic CPR must be considered. Greater than 10 min of CPR is commonly considered a contraindication to thrombolytic therapy. CPR for periods less than this should be judged according to the clinical merits and adjudged risks (Tenaglia et al., 1991).

Investigations in the postarrest phase

- 12-lead ECG
- Arterial blood gases
- Chest radiograph
- Urea, creatinine and electrolytes
- Plasma glucose
- (Calcium, magnesium)
- 'Cardiac' enzymes
- Haematocrit

A 12-lead ECG must be performed to recognize infarction or ischaemia and to correctly interpret rhythm abnormalities. Chest radiography is required to assess factors such as the tracheal tube position, the presence of pulmonary oedema and complications such as pneumo- or haemothorax, rib fractures or aspiration. Other investigations will include arterial blood gases, urea, electrolytes, plasma glucose, calcium and magnesium levels, haematocrit and cardiac enzymes. Pain or anxiety will adversely affect the patient's haemodynamic state by increasing catecholamine levels, blood pressure and oxygen demand, and analgesic and sedative drugs should be given appropriately. Drug metabolism is commonly impaired in these patients. The half-lives and pharmacokinetics of drugs such as opioids, benzodiazapines, anticonvulsants and antiarrhythmic drugs may be disturbed because of hepatic and renal dysfunction.

Arrhythmias are common in the postarrest period. Their management will depend upon accurate identification of the arrhythmia, its effect on the haemodynamic status of the patient, pre-existing drug therapy and the therapeutic armamentarium available to the clinician. Electrolyte disturbances may both provoke the development of arrhythmias and lead to refractoriness to therapy. Close attention and appropriate correction of potassium, calcium and magnesium levels is important.

Cerebral protection

Although a proportion of patients will rapidly regain consciousness and remain haemodynamically stable, most (approximately 85%) will not (Thomassen & Wernberg, 1979; Longstreth et al., 1983). For these individuals the full spectrum of intensive care facilities will be required. In particular, attention must be given to correcting or preventing those factors which can adversely affect cerebral viability (Gustafson et al., 1992).

The normal autoregulation processes are deranged following cardiac arrest, and cerebral blood flow is closely related to cerebral perfusion pressure. Therefore both hypotension and hypertension should be avoided (Kagstrom et al., 1983). Measurement of right and left heart filling pressures, cardiac output and oxygen transport variables are usually required in unstable patients. Only with such monitoring can a rational approach to the use of inotropes, vasopressors, vasodilators and fluid therapy be achieved (Barnard & Linter, 1993). Hypotension may require the administration of fluid and/or inotropic agents. Hypertension may be related to inadequate sedation, analgesia or hypercapnoea.

Prevention of raised intracranial pressure by positioning, avoidance of hypotension or hypertension and correction of hypercapnoea are essential. Routine intracranial pressure monitoring is not indicated. Fitting (seizure) leads to hypoxaemia, increases intracranial pressure and cerebral oxygen demand and can result in hyperthermia. Fits should be controlled with diazepam, phenytoin or barbiturates, recognizing the potential for depression of respiration by these drugs. Patients requiring neuromuscular blockade to permit ventilation will need continuous EEG monitoring.

In the immediate postresuscitation phase, high circulating catecholamine and corticosteroid levels lead to hyperglycaemia (Steen et al., 1992). This may aggravate cerebral damage and reperfusion injury by increasing the degree of lactic acidosis (Longstreth & Inin, 1984; Lundy et al., 1987). In contrast, hypoglycaemia will cause neuroglycopenia and also adversely affect cerebral function. Therefore plasma glucose levels should be closely monitored and kept within the normal range. The view that the brain cannot withstand more than 4–5 min of complete normothermic ischaemia and anoxia has been challenged, and there is some evidence that recovery may occur up to 20 min after complete circulatory standstill. This may be related to the degree of cerebral blood flow and perfusion produced during CPR. Normothermic patients with cardiac arrest who have survived following up to 2 h of CPR have been reported (Mackay et al., 1987). It is possible that total ischaemia may actually be less injurious than inadequate blood flows in which reperfusion injury may occur. During the reperfusion phase, complex neuronal interactions develop including calcium ion shifts, free radical generation and raised levels of excitatory amino acids (Siesjo, 1988, 1992). The normal intracellular/extracellular calcium gradient is disturbed during ischaemia and reperfusion. Intracellular calcium ion levels rise due to influx into the ischaemic cell. This leads to a cascade of adverse intracellular events affecting intracellular proteins, phospholipids and cell membrane stability. Anaerobic metabolism also leads to the production of lactic acid and excitatory amino acid (EAA) neurotransmitters such as glutamic, gamma-aminobutyric and aspartic acids. EAAs bind to receptors in areas of the brain particularly susceptible to ischaemia (Gustafson et al., 1992). These receptors are located on the neuronal cell surface and when activated can lead to structural damage. The NMDA (N-methyl-D-aspartate) receptor is closely involved in calcium ion influx into the ischaemic cell. Release of free fatty acids also follows cell membrane dysfunction. When metabolized, these free fatty acids lead to the generation of superoxide radicals which may cause further injury by producing vasoconstriction and platelet aggregation (McCord, 1985).

Many agents affecting various components of these complex interrelated mechanisms have been used to prevent or ameliorate ischaemic/anoxic cerebral injury. These include corticosteroids, barbiturates, aminosteroids, haemoperfusion, EAA receptor blockers and calcium channel blockers. Some agents have shown promise in a variety of animal models, but none has convincingly been shown to be of any benefit in man (Aitkenhead, 1991a, b; Steen et al., 1992). At present it seems overly simplistic to expect a single agent which may block one or more of these pathways to prevent the complex interactions involved in ischaemic brain damage.

THE CARDIAC ARREST TEAM

The major difference between in-hospital and accident and emergency (A&E) resuscitation attempts is the paucity of knowledge of the previous history and preceding events for patients brought to the A&E. Therefore, it is important to commence resuscitation while these details are being obtained from members of the ambulance crew, relatives or friends.

The key individual in the management of a cardiac arrest is the team leader. In most A&E departments this is the senior A&E doctor. This individual must have sufficient seniority, knowledge and experience to direct the arrest procedure in a controlled and competent fashion. The optimal size of the team involved in the resuscitation is the team leader, three members of the medical staff and two members of the nursing staff (see Fig. 6). All the team members should have a full understanding of their role during the resuscitation. The team leader's role is to coordinate the activity of all the members of the team and not to become physically involved with practical procedures unless difficulties occur. This enables the team leader to objectively assess the priorities and requirements while controlling the activities of the team and receiving appropriate input and feedback from the team members.

The management of the resuscitation attempt is conducted following the guidelines above. The introduction of nationally recognized and accredited Advanced Life Support Courses by the Resuscitation Council (UK) is a major step in the education and training of all staff who will be involved in CPR.

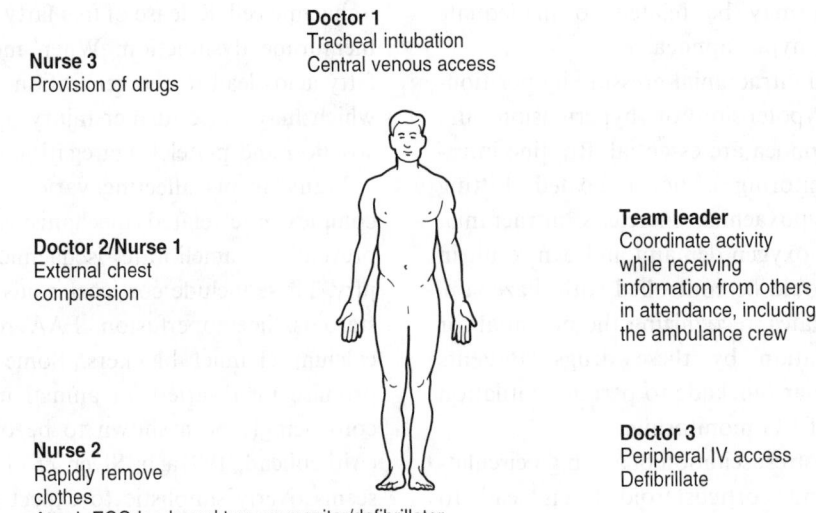

Doctor 1
Tracheal intubation
Central venous access

Nurse 3
Provision of drugs

Doctor 2/Nurse 1
External chest
compression

Team leader
Coordinate activity
while receiving
information from others
in attendance, including
the ambulance crew

Nurse 2
Rapidly remove
clothes
Attach ECG leads and turn on monitor/defibrillator

Doctor 3
Peripheral IV access
Defibrillate

Fig. 6. Suggested roles of team leader and team members at cardiac resuscitation. (Adapted, by permission of Oxford University Press, from Skinner & Vincent, 1993.)

With a team of five individuals under the direction of an experienced team leader, simultaneous performance of tasks should be performed such that within 30 sec of the patient's arrival in the resuscitation room, BLS will be continued, the patient's upper clothing cut off or removed, ECG monitoring instituted and, if indicated, the first defibrillating shock applied. After 60 sec, if not already performed, advanced airway management and venous access will be secured. The standard algorithms are followed under the team leader's direction.

In the excitement of a resuscitation attempt, there can be a tendency for basic safety procedures to be forgotten. It is the responsibility of the team leader to ensure that all members of his team act in an appropriate and safe manner, particularly in relation to aspects of defibrillation and protective precautions for sharps disposal and blood and other body fluid contamination.

Where the patient responds to resuscitation with restoration of spontaneous output, the team leader then liaises with the in-hospital specialist teams regarding the admission of the patient and postresuscitation care. Where unsuccessful, a brief review of the event by the members of the team should be performed under the direction of the team leader. At this time, positive aspects of the attempts should be highlighted and appropriate praise given. Deficiencies or mistakes can be discussed in a non-judgemental manner and education and strategems highlighted to prevent repetition. In those situations where the patient dies, the team leader, together with a senior nurse, should be the individuals involved in speaking directly to the relatives and arranging appropriate liaison with general practitioners, officers of the law, etc. These tasks should not be delegated to junior medical or nursing staff members.

OUTCOME PREDICTION

The accurate prediction of outcome following the successful immediate management of cardiac arrest is fraught with difficulty, and no single factor can reliably lead to an accurate prognosis in the early stages of patient management (Marwick et al., 1991; Martens et al., 1992). Two separate clinical situations can be considered: the prediction of those patients in relation to restoration of a spontaneous cardiac output, and prediction for these individuals as to full recovery. The single most important determinant of success in restoration of spontaneous circulation is the primary rhythm. Up to 40–50% of patients with VF will have restoration of spontaneous circulation with hospital discharge rates of up to 30%. Delay, particularly in delivery of the first defibrillating shock, is associated with marked reduction in the chance of successful outcome. In contrast, while up to 10–15% of patients with EMD or asystole may have a rhythm and output restored, less than 5% will survive to hospital discharge (Cobbe et al., 1991; Tunstall-Pedoe et al., 1992).

The primary cause of death amongst the initial survivors of cardiac arrest is related to recurrent arrhythmias and cardiogenic shock, followed by cerebral injury. Age alone is a relatively poor prognostic indicator, although the presence of underlying cardiac or other serious prearrest pathologies are. Attempts at determining outcome have used the Glasgow Coma Score or the Glasgow Pittsburgh Coma Score (Mullie *et al.*, 1988; Niskanen *et al.*, 1991). These should be performed and recorded twice daily, taking into account the effects of drug therapy. After 48 h these tools are strongly predictive of the chances of successful outcome. Nuclear magnetic resonance imaging and CSF enzyme analysis and evoked potentials are promising new techniques in the attempt to provide earlier accurate prediction (Steen *et al.*, 1992; Madl *et al.*, 1993).

Bibliography

AITKENHEAD, A.R. (1991b). Cerebral protection after cardiac arrest. *Resuscitation*, **22**, 197–202.

AITKENHEAD, A.R. (1991a). Drug administration during CPR: what route? *Resuscitation*, **22**, 191–5.

ALS WORKING PARTY OF THE ERC (1992). Guidelines for advanced life support. *Resuscitation*, **24**, 111–22.

AYLWARD, P.E., KIESO, R., HITE, P. *et al.* (1985). Defibrillator electrode–chest wall coupling agents: influence on transthoracic impedance and shock success. *J. Am. Coll. Cardiol.*, **6**, 682–6.

BARNARD, M.J. & LINTER, S.P.K. (1993). Acute circulatory support. *Br. Med. J.*, **307**, 35–41.

BARNETT, W.M., ALIFINOFF, J.K., PARIS, P.M. *et al.* (1986). Comparison of open chest cardiac massage techniques in dogs. *Ann. Emerg. Med.*, **15**, 408–11.

BAYES DE LUNA, A., GUINDO, J. & RIVER, I. (1989). Ambulatory sudden death in patients wearing Holter devices. *J. Ambul. Monit.*, **2**, 3–14.

BERENYI, K.J., WOLK, M. & KILLIP, T. (1975). Cerebrospinal fluid acidosis complicating therapy of experimental cardiopulmonary arrest. *Circulation*, **52**, 319–24.

BJORK, R.J., CAMPION, B.C., SNYDER, B.D. *et al.* (1980). Medical complications of cardiopulmonary arrest. *Circulation*, **62** (Suppl. 3), 338.

BLS WORKING PARTY OF THE EUROPEAN RESUSCITATION COUNCIL (1992). Guidelines for basic life support. *Resuscitation*, **24**, 103–10.

BOSSAERT, L. & KOSTER, R. (1992). Defibrillation: methods and strategies. *Resuscitation*, **24**, 211–25.

BRIGGS, B.D., SHELDON, D.G. & BEECLES, H.K. (1956). Cardiac arrest. *JAMA*, **160**, 1439–44.

BROWN, C.G. & WERMAN, H.A. (1990). Adrenergic agonists during cardiopulmonary resuscitation. *Resuscitation*, **19**, 1–16.

BROWN, C.G., MARTIN, D.R., PEPE, P.E. *et al.* (1992). A comparison of standard dose and high-dose epinephrine in cardiac arrest outside the hospital. *N. Engl. J. Med.*, **327**, 1051–55.

CALDWELL, G., MILLER, G., QUINN, E. *et al.* (1985). Simple mechanical methods for cardioversion: defence of the precordial thump and cough version. *Br. Med. J.*, **291**, 627–30.

CALLAHAN, M., MADSEN, C.D., BARTON, C.W. *et al.* (1992). A randomized clinical trial of high dose epinephrine and norepizephrine vs standard dose epinephrine in prehospital cardiac arrest. *JAMA*, **268**, 2667–72.

CAMPBELL, R.W.F. (1993). Ventricular ectopic beats and non-sustained ventricular tachycardia. *Lancet*, **341**, 1454–8.

CARDIAC ARRHYTHMIA SUPPRESSION TRIAL II (1992). Effect of the antiarrhythmic agent moticizine on survival after myocardial infarction. *N. Eng. J. Med.*, **327**, 227–33.

CARLI, P., HAPNES, S.A. & PASQUALUCCI, V. (1992). Airway management and ventilation. *Resuscitation*, **24**, 205–10.

CHAMBERLAIN, D.A. (1991). Lignocaine and bretylium as adjuncts to electrical defibrillation. *Resuscitation*, **22**, 153–7.

CIPOLOTTI, G., PACCAGNELLA, A. & SIMINI, G. (1991). Successful CPR using high doses of epinephrine. *Int. J. Cardiol.*, **33**, 430–1.

CLARK, D.T. (1962). Complications following closed chest cardiac massage. *JAMA*, **181**, 127.

CLAYTON, R.H., MURRAY, A., HIGHAM, P.D. *et al.* (1993). Self-terminating ventricular tachyarrhythmias – a diagnostic dilemma. *Lancet*, **341**, 93–5.

COBBE, S., REDMOND, M., WATSON, J. *et al.* (1991). 'Heartstart Scotland' – initial experience of a national scheme for out of hospital defibrillation. *Br. Med. J.*, **302**, 1517–20.

COHEN, T.J., TUCKER, K.J., LURIE, K.G. *et al.* (1992a). Active compression decompression: a new method of cardiopulmonary resuscitation. *JAMA*, **267**, 1916–23.

COHEN, T.J., TUCKER, K.J., REDBERG, R.F. *et al.* (1992b). Active compression–decompression resuscitation: a novel method of cardiopulmonary resuscitation. *Am. Heart J.*, **124**, 1145–50.

CRILE, G. & DOLLEY, D.H. (1906). Experimental research into resuscitation of dogs killed by anaesthetics and asphyxia. *J. Exp. Med.*, **8**, 713–20.

CRILEY, J.M., BLAUFUSS, A.H. & KISSEL, G.L. (1976). Cough induced cardiac compression self administered form of CPR. *JAMA*, **2336**, 1246–50.

DALZELL, G.W. & ADGEY, A.A.J. (1991). Determinants of successful transthoracic defibrillation and outcome in ventricular fibrillation. *Br. Heart J.*, **61**, 311–6.

DAVIES, M.J. & THOMAS, A. (1984). Thrombosis and acute coronary artery lesions in sudden cardiac ischaemic death. *N. Engl. J. Med.*, **310**, 1137–40.

DEBEHNKE, D.J., ANGELOS, M.G. & LEASURE, J.E. (1991). Comparison of standard external CPR, open-chest CPR and cardiopulmonary bypass in a canine myocardial infarct model. *Ann. Emerg. Med.*, **20**, 754–60.

DEL GUERCIO, L.M.R., COOMARASWANY, R. & STATE, D. (1963). Cardiac output and other haemodynamic variables during external massage in man. *N. Engl. J. Med.*, **269**, 1398–401.

DEMBO, D.H. (1981). Calcium in advanced life support. *Crit. Care Med.*, **9**, 358–9.

DEWOOD, M.A., SPORES, J., NOTSTE, R. *et al.* (1980). Prevalence of total coronary occlusion during the early hours of transmural myocardial infarction. *N. Engl. J. Med.*, **303**, 897–902.

DICKEY, W., DALZELL, G.W.N., ANDERSON, J.McC.C. *et al.* (1992). The accuracy of decision making of a semiautomatic defibrillator during cardiac arrest. *Eur. Heart J.*, **13**, 608–15.

DITCHLEY, R.V., WINKLER, J. & RHODES, C.A. (1982). Relative lack of coronary blood flow during closed chest resuscitation in dogs. *Circulation*, **66**, 297–303.

DORIAN, P., FAIN, E.S., DAVEY, J.M. *et al.* (1986). Lidocaine causes a reversible, concentration-dependent increase in defibrillation energy requirements. *J. Am. Coll. Cardiol.*, **8**, 327–32.

ECHT, D.S., LIEBSON, P.R., MITCHELL, B. *et al.* (1991). Mortality and morbidity in patients receiving encainide, flecainide or placebo. *N. Engl. J. Med.*, **324**, 781–5.

FISHER, J., VAGHAIWALLA, F., TSITLIK, J. *et al.* (1982). Determinants and clinical significance of jugular venous competence. *Circulation*, **65**, 188–96.

FORNEY, J. & ORNATO, J.P. (1980). Blood flow with ventilation alone in a child with cardiac arrest. *Ann. Emerg. Med.*, **9**, 624–6.

GARNETT, A.R., ORNATO, J.P., GONZALEZ, E.R. *et al.* (1987). End-tidal carbon dioxide monitoring during CPR. *JAMA*, **257**, 512–5.

GEEHR, E.C. & AUERBACK, P.S. (1985). Open chest cardiac massage for victims of medical cardiac arrest. *Ann. Emerg. Med.*, **14**, 499.

GULY, U.M., PELL, A.C.H. & ROBERTSON, C.E. (1993). Blood flow mechanisms during cardiopulmonary resuscitation. In *1993 Yearbook of Intensive Care and Emergency Medicine*, ed. J.-L. Vincent, pp. 444–51. Berlin: Springer-Verlag.

GUSTAFSON, I., EDGREN, E. & HULTINH, J. (1992). Brain-orientated intensive care after resuscitation from cardiac arrest. *Resuscitation*, **24**, 245–61.

HALPERIN, H.R., GUERCI, A.D., CHANDRA, N. *et al.* (1986). Vest inflation without simultaneous ventilation during cardiac arrest in dogs. *Circulation*, **74**, 1407–15.

HAPNES, S.A. & ROBERTSON, C.E. (1992). CPR – drug delivery routes and systems. *Resuscitation*, **24**, 137–42.

HEDGES, J.R., BARSON, W.B., DOAN, L.A. *et al.* (1982). Central vs peripheral intravenous routes in CPR. *Am. J. Emerg. Med.*, **2**, 383–90.

HESS, D. & BARAN, C. (1985). Ventilatory volumes using mouth-to-mouth, mouth-to-mask and bag–valve–mask techniques. *Am. J. Emerg. Med.*, **3**, 292–6.

HIGANO, S.T., OH, J.K., EIVY, G.A. *et al.* (1990). The mechanism of blood flow during closed chest cardiac massage in humans: transoesophageal echocardiographic observations. *Mayo Clin. Proc.*, **65**, 1432–40.

JESUDIAN, M.C., HARRISON, R.R., KEENAN, R.L. *et al.* (1985). Bag–valve–mask ventilation: two rescuers are better than one. *Crit. Care Med.*, **13**, 122–3.

JOHANNIGMAN, J.A., BRANSON, R.D., DAVIS, K. *et al.* (1991). Techniques of emergency ventilation. *J. Trauma*, **31**, 93–8.

KAGSTROM, E., SMITH, M.-L. & SIESJO, B.K. (1983). Cerebral circulatory responses to hypercapnia and hypoxia in the recovery period following complete and incomplete ischaemia in the rat. *Acta Physiol. Scand.*, **118**, 281–91.

KERBER, R.E., GRAYZEL, J., HOYT, R. *et al.* (1981). Transthoracic resistance in human defibrillation: influence of body weight, chest size, serial shocks, paddle size and contact pressure. *Circulation*, **63**, 676–82.

KOSCOVE, E.M. & PARADIS, N.A. (1988). Successful resuscitation from cardiac arrest using high dose epinephrine therapy. *JAMA*, **259**, 3031–4.

KOSTER, R. & CARLI, P. (1992). Acid–base management. *Resuscitation*, **24**, 143–6.

KOUWENHOVEN, W.B., JUDE, J.R. & KNICKERBOCKER, G.G. (1960). Closed chest cardiac massage. *JAMA*, **173**, 1064–7.

KRIJNE, R. (1984). Rate acceleration of ventricular tachycardia after a precordial chest thump. *Am. J. Cardiol.*, **53**, 964–5.

KUHN, G.J., WHITE, B.C., STRETNAN, R.E. *et al.* (1981). Peripheral vs central circulation times during CPR. *Ann. Emerg. Med.*, **10**, 417–9.

LEACH, A., ALEXANDER, C.A. & STONE, B. (1993). The laryngeal mask in CPR in a district general hospital: a preliminary communication. *Resuscitation*, **25**, 245–8.

LERMAN, B.B. & DEALE, O.C. (1990). Relation between transcardiac and transthoracic current during defibrillation in humans. *Circ. Res.*, **67**, 1420–6.

LIE, K.I., WELLENS, J.H.H., VAN CAPELLE, F.J. *et al.* (1974). Lidocaine in the prevention of primary ventricular fibrillation. *N. Engl. J. Med.*, **291**, 1324–6.

LINDNER, K.H. & KOSTER, R. (1992). Vasopressor drugs during cardiopulmonary resuscitation. *Resuscitation*, **24**, 147–54.

LINDNER, K.H., AHREFELD, F.W. & BOWDLER, I.M. (1991). Comparison of different doses of epinephrine on myocardial perfusion and resuscitation during CPR in a pig model. *Am. J. Emerg. Med.*, **9**, 27–31.

LITTLE, R.A., FRAYN, K.N., RANDALL, P.E. *et al.* (1985). Plasma catecholamines in patients with acute myocardial infarction and cardiac arrest. *Q. J. Med.*, **214**, 133–40.

LONGSTRETH, W. & ININ, T.S. (1984). High blood glucose level on hospital admission and poor hemological recovery after cardiac arrest. *Ann. Neurol.*, **15**, 59–63.

LONGSTRETH, W., DIEHR, P. & ININ, T.S. (1983). Prediction of awakening after out of hospital cardiac arrest. *N. Engl. J. Med.*, **308**, 1378–82.

LUCE, J.M., ROSS, B.K., O'QUINN, R.J. *et al.* (1983). Regional blood flow during CPR in dogs using simultaneous and non-simultaneous compression and ventilation. *Circulation*, **67**, 258.

LUNDY, E.F., KUHN, J.E., KWON, J.M. *et al.* (1987). Infusion of 5% dextrose increases mortality and morbidity following 6 minutes of cardiac arrest in resuscitated dogs. *J. Crit. Care*, **2**, 4–14.

MACKAY, J., McAREAVEY, D. & ROBERTSON, C.E. (1987). Prolonged mechanical CPR. *Br. J. Accid. Emerg. Med.*, **2**, 15.

MADL, C., GRIMM, G., KRAMER, L. *et al.* (1993). Early prediction of individual outcome after CPR. *Lancet*, **341**, 855–8.

MARTENS, P.R., MULLIE, A., BUYLAERT, W. *et al.* (1992). Early prediction of non-survival for patients suffering cardiac arrest – a word of caution. *Intens. Care Med.*, **18**, 11–14.

MARWICK, T.H., CASE, C.C., SISKIND, V. *et al.* (1991). Prediction of survival from resuscitation: a prognostic index derived from multivariate logistic model analysis. *Resuscitation*, **22**, 129–38.

McCORD, J.M. (1985). Oxygen-derived free oxygen radicals in post-ischaemic tissue injury. *N. Engl. J. Med.*, **312**, 159–63.

MICHAEL, J.R., GUERCI, A.D., KOEHLER, R.C. *et al.* (1984). Mechanisms by which epinephrine augments cerebral and myocardial perfusion during CPR in dogs. *Circulation*, **69**, 822–35.

MULLIE, A., BUYLAERT, W., MICHEM, N. *et al.* (1988). Predictive value of GCS for awakening after out of hospital cardiac arrest. *Lancet*, **i**, 137–40.

NAGEL, E.L., FINE, E.G., KRISCHNER, J.P. *et al.* (1981). Complications of CPR. *Crit. Care Med.*, **9**, 424.

NEMOTO, E.M. (1978). Pathogenesis of cerebral ischaemia-anoxia. *Crit. Care Med.*, **6**, 203–14.

NIEMANN, J.T. (1989). Alternatives to standard CPR in cardiopulmonary resuscitation. In *Cardiopulmonary Resuscitation*, ed. W. Kaye & N.G. Bircher, pp. 103–16. Edinburgh: Churchill Livingstone.

NIEMANN, J.T., CRILEY, J.M., ROSBOROUGH, J.P. *et al.* (1985). Predictive indices of successful cardiac resuscitation after prolonged cardiac and experimental CPR. *Ann. Emerg. Med.*, **14**, 521–8.

NISKANEN, M., KARI, A., NIKKI, P. *et al.* (1991). APACHE II and GCS as predictors of outcome from intensive care after cardiac arrest. *Crit. Care. Med.*, **19**, 1465–73.

PARADIS, N.A. & KOSCOVE, E.M. (1990). Epineph-rine in cardiac arrest: a critical review. *Ann. Emerg. Med.*, **19**, 1288–301.

PARADIS, N.S., MARTIN, G.B., GOETTING, M.G. *et al.* (1981). Simultaneous aortic, jugular bulb and tight atrial pressures during CPR in humans: insights into mechanisms. *Circulation*, **80**, 361–8.

PARADIS, N.A., MARTIN, G.B., GOETTING, M.G. *et al.* (1992). Aortic pressure during human cardiac arrest. *Chest*, **101**, 123–8.

PARASKOS, J.A. (1992). Biblical accounts of resuscitation. *J. Hist. Med. Allied Sci.*, **47**, 310–21.

PEDERSEN, A., JESPERSEN, H. & TORP-PEDER-SEN, C. (1991). The place of intracardiac injections in the treatment of cardiac arrest. *Drugs*, **42**, 915–8.

PENNINGTON, J.E., TAYLOR, J.& LOWN, B. (1970). Chest thump for reverting ventricular tachycardia. *N. Engl. J. Med.*, **22**, 1192–5.

PETERS, J. & IHLE, P. (1990). Mechanics of the circulation during CPR (parts I and II). *Intens. Care Med.*, **16**, 11–27.

POWER, D.J., HOLCOMB, P.A. & MELLO, L.A. (1984). Cardiopulmonary resuscitation related injuries. *Crit. Care Med.*, **12**, 54.

QUINTON, D.N., O'BYRNE, G. & AITKENHEAD, A.R. (1987). Comparison of endotracheal and peripheral intravenous adrenaline in cardiac arrest. *Lancet*, **i**, 828–9.

ROBERTSON, C. (1992). The precordial thump and cough techniques in advanced life support. *Resuscitation*, **24**, 133–6.

ROBERTSON, C.E. & HOLMBERG, S. (1992). Compression techniques and blood flow during cardiopulmonary resuscitation. *Resuscitation*, **24**, 123–32.

ROSSEN, R., CABAT, H. & ANDERSON, J.P. (1943). Acute arrest of the cerebral circulation in man. *Arch. Neurol.*, **30**, 510–28.

RUBEN, H., KNUDSEN, E.J. & CARUGATI, G. (1961). Gastric inflation in relation to airway pressure. *Acta Anaesthesiol. Scand.*, **5**, 107–14.

SABIN, H.I., COGHILL, S.B., KHUNTI, K. *et al.* (1983). Accuracy of intracardiac injection determined by a post mortem study. *Lancet*, **ii**, 1054–5.

SAFAR, P. (1989). History of cardiopulmonary–cerebral resuscitation. In *Cardiopulmonary Resuscitation*, ed. W. Kaye & N.G. Bircher, pp. 1–53. Edinburgh: Churchill Livingstone.

SAFRANEK, D.J., EISENBERG, M.S. & LARSEN, M.P. (1992). The epidemiology of cardiac arrest in young adults. *Ann. Emerg. Med.*, **21**, 1102–6.

SANDERS, A.B., EWY, G.A., BRAGG, S. *et al.* (1985). Expired pCO_2 as a prognostic indicator of successful resuscitation from cardiac arrest. *Ann. Emerg Med.*, **14**, 948–52.

SCHOTT, E. (1920). Uber Ventrikelstillstand (Adams-Stokes'sche Anfalle) nebst Bemerlemgen uber andersantige arhthmien Passagerer. *Dtsch. Arch. Klin. Med.*, **131**, 211–29.

SIESJO, B.K. (1988). Mechanisms of ischaemic brain damage. *Crit. Care Med.*, **16**, 954–63.

SIESJO, B.K. (1992). Pathophysiology and treatment of focal cerebral ischaemia. *J. Neurosurg.*, **77**, 169–84.

SIRNA, S.J., FERGUSON, D.W., CHARBONNIER, F. *et al.* (1988). Factors affecting transthoracic impedance during electrical cardioversion. *Am. J. Cardiol.*, **62**, 1048–52.

SKINNER, D.V. & VINCENT, R. (1993). *Cardiopulmonary Resuscitation* (Oxford Handbooks in Emergency Medicine). Oxford: Oxford University Press.

STEEDMAN, D.J. & ROBERTSON, C.E. (1990). Measurement of end-tidal carbon dioxide concentration during cardiopulmonary resuscitation. *Arch. Emerg. Med.*, **7**, 129–34.

STEEDMAN, D.J. & ROBERTSON, C.E. (1992). Acid–base changes in arterial and central venous blood during cardiopulmonary resuscitation. *Arch. Emerg. Med.*, **9**, 169–76.

STEEN, P.A., EDGREN, E., GUSTAFSON, I. *et al.* (1992). Cerebral protection and post-resuscitation care. *Resuscitation*, **24**, 233–7.

STEUVEN, H.A., THOMSON, B.M., APRAHAM-IAN, C. *et al.* (1984). Calcium chloride: reassessment of use in asystole. *Ann. Emerg. Med.*, **13**, 820–2.

STEVENSON, H.E., REID, L.C. & HINTON, J.W. (1953). Some common denominators in 1200 cases of cardiac arrest. *Ann. Surg.*, **137**, 731–44.

STIELL, I.G. *et al.* (1992). High dose epinephrine in adult cardiac arrest. *N. Engl. J. Med.*, **327**, 1045–9.

TENAGLIA, A.N., CALIFF, R.M., CANDELA, R.J. *et al.* (1991). Thrombolytic therapy in patients requiring CPR. *Am. J. Cardiol.*, **68**, 1015–9.

THOMASSEN, A. & WERNBERG, M. (1979). Prevalence and prognostic significance of coma after cardiac arrest outside intensive care and coronary units. *Acta Anaesth. Scand.*, **23**, 143–8.

TUNSTALL-PEDOE, H., BAILEY, L., CHAMBER-LAIN, D.A. *et al.* (1992). Survey of 3765 cardiopulmonary resuscitations in British hospitals (The Bresus Study). *Br. Med. J.*, **304**, 1347–51.

TZIVONI, D., KEREN, A. & STERN, S. (1983). Torsade de pointes vs polymorphic ventricular tachycardia. *Am. J. Cardiol.*, **52**, 639–40.

URBAN, P., SCHIEDEGGER, D., BUCHMANN, B. *et al.* (1988). Cardiac arrest and blood ionized calcium levels. *Ann. Intern. Med.*, **109**, 110–13.

VINCENT, J.-L., THYS, L., WEIL, M.H. *et al.* (1981). Clinical and experimental studies on electromechanical dissociation. *Circulation*, **64**, 18–27.

VISKIN, S., BELHASSEN, B., ROTH, A. *et al.* (1993). Aminophylline for bradyasystolic cardiac arrest refractory to atropine and epinephrine. *Ann. Intern. Med.*, **118**, 279–81.

VON PLANTA, M. & CHAMBERLAIN, D.A. (1992). Drug treatment of arrhythmias during cardiopulmonary resuscitation. *Resuscitation*, **24**, 227–32.

VON PLANTA, M., WEIL, M.H., GASMUN, R.J. *et al.* (1989). Myocardial acidosis associated with CO_2 production during cardiac arrest and circulation. *Circulation*, **80**, 684–92.

WALLER, D.G. (1991). Treatment and prevention of ventricular fibrillation: are there better agents? *Resuscitation*, **22**, 159–66.

WALLER, D.G. & ROBERTSON, C.E. (1991). Role of sympathomimetic amines during CPR. *Resuscitation*, **22**, 181–90.

WEIL, M.H. & NOC, M. (1992). Cardiopulmonary resuscitation: state of the art. *J. Cardiothor. Vasc. Anaesth.*, **6**, 499–503.

WEISER, F.M., ADLER, A.N. & KUHN, L.A. (1962). Haemodynamic effects of closed and open chest cardiac resuscitation in normal dogs and those with acute myocardial infarction. *Am. J. Cardiol.*, **10**, 55.

WOODHOUSE, S.P., CASE, C., COX, S. *et al.* (1993). Trial of large dose adrenaline vs placebo in cardiac arrest. *Resuscitation*, **25**, 89 (Abstract).

WRENN, K. (1990). The hazards of defibrillation through nitroglycerin patches. *Ann. Emerg. Med.*, **19**, 1327–8.

YIN, F.C.P., COHEN, J.M., TSITLIK, J. *et al.* (1982). Role of carotid artery resistance to collapse during high intrathoracic pressure CPR. *Am. J. Physiol.*, **243**, H259.

4 Cardiopulmonary resuscitation in children

Department of Anaesthesia, Great Ormond Street Hospital for Children, London, UK

Chapter plan

Aetiology
Basic life support
Advanced life support
Resuscitation at birth

AETIOLOGY

In adults, cardiac arrest is commonly a result of primary cardiac disease, usually ventricular fibrillation (VF) resulting from ischaemic heart disease. The heart stops suddenly and unexpectedly. Because the circulation has been previously normal, there is little arterial hypoxaemia or acidosis. It is difficult to anticipate this type of cardiac arrest and treatment can only be started after the event.

The exact causes of cardiac arrest in children vary from study to study depending on whether the arrest occurred in hospital (Lewis *et al.*, 1983; Gillis *et al.*, 1986; Innes *et al.*, 1993) or outside (Eisenberg *et al.*, 1983; O'Rourke, 1986). The commonest causes result in respiratory or circulatory insufficiency, leading to cardiorespiratory

---

Causes of cardiac arrest in children

- Sudden infant death syndrome (<1 year old)
- Trauma (particularly head injury)
- Upper airway obstruction
- Respiratory infections
- Hypovolaemia
- Congenital cardiac disease
- Sedative drug overdose

---

failure. The heart stops as a result of myocardial hypoxia/ischaemia, and usually slows progressively prior to arrest in asystole. VF is uncommon in paediatric cardiac arrest (Eisenberg *et al.*, 1983; Innes *et al.*, 1993; Stopfkuchen *et al.*, 1989). At the time of the arrest there is generally profound arterial hypoxaemia and acidosis. Hypoxic tissue damage is likely and outcome after asystolic arrest is consequently poor, particularly for out-of-hospital arrests (O'Rourke, 1986) or resuscitation attempts lasting over 30 min (Innes *et al.*, 1993). In contrast, the outcome from respiratory arrest, if it is detected before the heart has stopped, is good (Lewis *et al.*, 1983; Innes *et al.*, 1993).

There are several implications for the practice of paediatric resuscitation resulting from these differences in aetiology.

- Cardiac arrest in children is not sudden and unexpected. It should be possible to identify children at risk at an early enough stage to institute treatment aimed at preventing its occurrence.
- There is no 'period of grace' before the onset of neurological damage and therefore no time for prior evaluation; basic life support (BLS) must be instituted immediately.
- The underlying hypoxaemia must be treated before the heart can be restarted. Indeed, clearing the airway and instituting effective pulmonary ventilation is often all that is required.
- There is likely to be a profound metabolic acidosis which may have a number of adverse effects, including a reduction in the effectiveness of exogenously administered adrenaline.
- A precordial thump is unlikely to be of any benefit unless the child is known to be in VF.

The BLS sequence for infants and children is consequently different from that for adults in that assessment

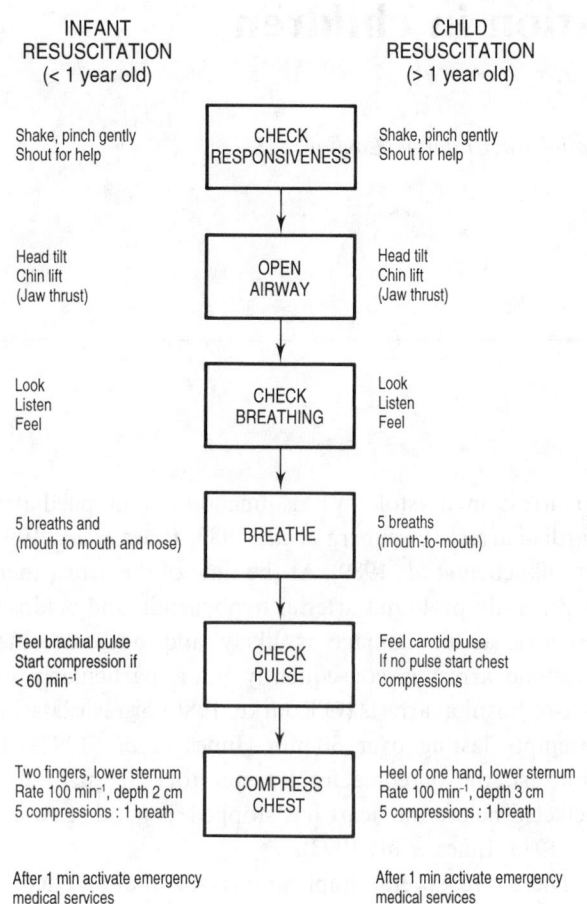

INFANT
RESUSCITATION
(< 1 year old)

CHILD
RESUSCITATION
(> 1 year old)

| | CHECK RESPONSIVENESS | |
Shake, pinch gently
Shout for help

Shake, pinch gently
Shout for help

| | OPEN AIRWAY | |
Head tilt
Chin lift
(Jaw thrust)

Head tilt
Chin lift
(Jaw thrust)

| | CHECK BREATHING | |
Look
Listen
Feel

Look
Listen
Feel

| | BREATHE | |
5 breaths and
(mouth to mouth and nose)

5 breaths
(mouth-to-mouth)

| | CHECK PULSE | |
Feel brachial pulse
Start compression if
< 60 min⁻¹

Feel carotid pulse
If no pulse start chest
compressions

| | COMPRESS CHEST | |
Two fingers, lower sternum
Rate 100 min⁻¹, depth 2 cm
5 compressions : 1 breath

Heel of one hand, lower sternum
Rate 100 min⁻¹, depth 3 cm
5 compressions : 1 breath

After 1 min activate emergency
medical services

After 1 min activate emergency
medical services

Fig. 1. Algorithm for basic life support in infants and children. (European Resuscitation Council.)

and treatment are performed concurrently in order to avoid any delay.

BASIC LIFE SUPPORT

The BLS algorithms are shown in Fig. 1.

Points

Airway

The head tilt chin lift manoeuvre is usually effective in clearing airway obstruction due to the tongue. In small children the protuberant occiput causes flexion of the cervical spine and moderate extension of the head at the atlanto-occipital joint results in the optimum 'sniffing' position. Overextension of the head should be avoided (Fig. 2). It is essential to lift the chin with the fingers on the bony mandible only, in order to avoid compressing the soft tissues under the jaw as this pushes the tongue

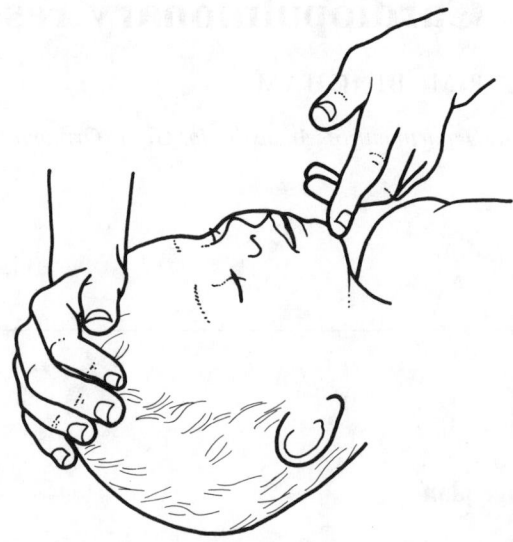

Fig. 2. Simple airway manoeuvre in a child. Note the position of the finger on the tip of the mandible, avoiding compression of the soft tissues under the jaw.

backwards into the pharynx and increases obstruction. The jaw thrust manoeuvre is useful if the head tilt is not effective, or there is a suspected cervical spine injury. If a correctly applied jaw thrust manoeuvre fails to clear the airway, it is unlikely that the obstruction is due to the tongue alone, and another cause should be considered.

Look, listen, feel

If there are chest excursions and air movement can be heard and felt, the child should be placed in the recovery position, the pulse should be checked and, if possible, oxygen should be administered. Chest excursions without air movement suggest airway obstruction and further measures should be applied to clear the airway (see later). If there is no chest movement, positive pressure ventilation is required.

Expired air respiration (EAR)

In small infants both the mouth and nose should be covered by the rescuer's lips. In older children, when this is physically difficult it is also unnecessary. Five initial breaths should be given before checking the pulse as these may provide sufficient oxygenation to prevent an imminent cardiac arrest, or even to restart an hypoxic heart. The volume should be sufficient to make the child appear to take a big breath. It should be given reasonably slowly (over 1–1.5 sec) in order to avoid gastric distension. If there is a pulse present but there is no respiratory effort, EAR should continue at a rate of about 20 min^{-1} (i.e. 1 breath every 3 sec).

Check pulse

The carotid pulse is the easiest to feel in older children and adults, but the short infant neck makes it difficult in this age group and the brachial pulse (on the inner aspect of the upper arm) or the femoral pulse should be sought. Palpate for about 5 sec to ensure that a faint or very slow pulse will be detected. If the pulse is less than 60 min^{-1} in infants or absent in older children, external chest compressions (ECC) will be necessary.

External chest compressions (ECC)

In infants the compression should be at a point one finger's breadth below an imaginary line joining the nipples (Orlowski, 1984; Phillips & Zideman, 1986). It is best applied using the index and middle fingers of one hand but rescuers with large hands may be able to encircle the infant's chest with both their hands and perform the compressions with both thumbs. If the latter method is used particular care should be taken to ensure that the chest is allowed to completely re-expand. The depth of compressions should be 2 cm, at a rate of 100 min^{-1}. There should be 1 breath to every 5 compressions. Simultaneous ventilation/compression cardiopulmonary resuscitation is not advocated in children because of concern over increased risks of barotrauma, and lack of evidence of its efficacy. In older children the heel of one hand should be used at a point two fingers' breadth above the xiphisternum. The depth of compression is approximately 3 cm but the same rate and ratio to ventilation should be used. It is useful to check for a pulse during ECC. If a pulse is present it does not necessarily imply an adequate cardiac output but an absent pulse should prompt a search for causes such as incorrect technique or hypovolaemia.

Upper airway obstruction

If there is chest and/or abdominal movement and no expired air can be heard or felt, then upper airway obstruction is present and further manoeuvres to clear the airway are urgently required. If the obstruction is due to the tongue alone (by far the commonest cause) it can almost always be cleared by using either the chin lift or

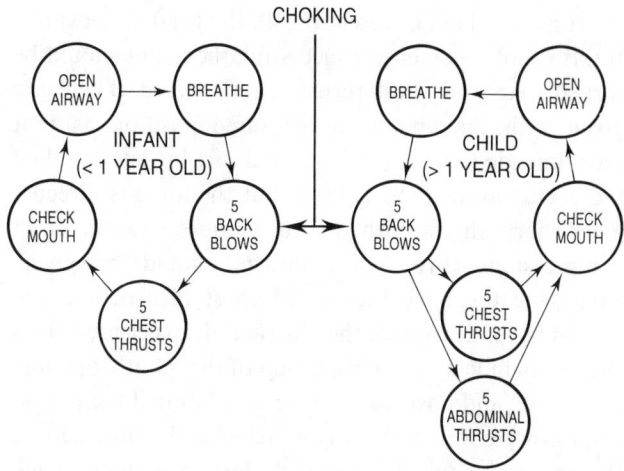

Fig. 3. Algorithm for dealing with choking in infants and children. (European Resuscitation Council.)

jaw thrust. If obstruction persists after using these techniques correctly another cause should be sought. The most likely is foreign body obstruction or inflammation due to upper airway infection.

Foreign body obstruction (Fig. 3)

This should be suspected in the circumstances described above, or if there is a history of sudden onset of airway obstruction, particularly if accompanied by paroxysmal coughing. If the victim is making efforts to clear the obstruction, these should be encouraged.

There should be no intervention unless complete obstruction is imminent, spontaneous efforts are clearly ineffective or consciousness is lost.

The infant larynx is cone-shaped, with the narrowest part at the level of the cricoid cartilage. Foreign bodies above the glottis are therefore liable to be impacted in the cricoid region if blind finger sweeps are employed in an effort to remove them. Blind finger sweeps should not therefore be used. Fortunately, because of the conical shape it is possible to expel an impacted foreign body by producing an abrupt increase in the pressure in the thorax by means of back blows or chest thrusts.

Back blows and chest thrusts

Five firm blows should be delivered with the heel of a hand to a point between the infant's shoulder blades. This should be performed with the infant face down on the rescuer's thigh or forearm with the head downwards. If this is not immediately successful, the infant should be turned over and chest thrusts administered. These are given with the fingers in the same position as that recommended for ECC (if the hands are big enough then the encircling method is best), but the force is directed as a sharp thrust rather than a squeeze as in chest compressions. Five chest thrusts should be given. Following the back blows and chest thrusts, a check should be made to see if the obstruction has cleared. This should include a visual inspection of the mouth, opening the airway and positive pressure ventilation if there is no respiratory effort. If there is no relief of the obstruction, the process should be repeated starting with the back blows. In older children (>1 year) abdominal thrusts can be used instead of chest thrusts after the second round of back blows. These can take the form of a Heimlich manoeuvre if the child is conscious. If unconscious, the child should be laid supine on a hard surface and the heel of one hand should be placed in the middle of the upper abdomen and five thrusts directed upwards towards the diaphragm. Abdominal thrusts are not used in infants because of the danger of hepatic or splenic damage. The above sequences are repeated, with inspection and intermittent attempts at positive pressure ventilation, as the foreign body may be dislodged sufficiently to allow air to be forced past.

Obstruction due to upper airway infections

This should be suspected in any case of upper airway obstruction accompanied by fever or a preceding upper respiratory tract infection. The history is usually that of steadily increasing obstruction (over hours or minutes) rather than sudden unheralded obstruction as with a foreign body.

If this diagnosis is suspected it is vital not to intervene in any way unless complete obstruction occurs.

Calm but urgent preparation should be made to get the child into a location where tracheal intubation can be safely performed if necessary. Should complete obstruction occur, positive pressure ventilation (EAR or bag–valve–mask) may be effective and should be the first intervention.

ADVANCED LIFE SUPPORT

Advanced life support (ALS) encompasses the use of drugs and equipment to continue the resuscitation process. It does not replace BLS and effective BLS is an essential prerequisite to the following techniques.

Oxygen administration

Children, particularly infants, are predisposed to hypoxaemia for the following reasons:

- Terminal airway closure is likely during tidal respiration. There is mismatching of pulmonary ventilation and perfusion, allowing desaturated pulmonary arterial blood to be shunted past unventilated alveoli. Infants consequently have a lower resting arterial oxygen tension than young adults.
- The lung volume at the end of expiration (i.e. the functional residual capacity) is relatively low. There is consequently a low reserve of oxygen within the lungs.
- Oxygen consumption is approximately twice that of an adult.

The onset of hypoxaemia in infants with pulmonary disease or airway obstruction is thus extremely rapid and this underlines the importance of early oxygen administration.

There are no contraindications to the use of high concentrations of oxygen in the resuscitation of acutely ill infants and children.

There are a number of ways in which oxygen can be administered to children: head box, oxygen tent, masks, nasal cannulae, 'anaesthetic circuits', or just blown over the child's face. The most appropriate method is that which the child tolerates best, as an anxious and struggling child may consume more additional oxygen than is being delivered.

Monitoring

Monitoring is vital in order to anticipate and therefore treat any deterioration in the child's condition and therefore prevent cardiac or respiratory arrest.

Clinical observation

Level of consciousness and demeanour is an extremely valuable and simple observation. Unless there is specific central nervous system (CNS) disease (e.g. meningitis, head injury) or drug administration, depression of consciousness or confusion and disorientation in a child imply that there is failure of delivery of sufficient substrate (e.g. oxygen, glucose) to the CNS to maintain its function. In either event it is a sign of profound physiological disturbance and should not be ignored. Children are naturally curious and interested in their environment; absence of curiosity, apathy and particularly lack of response to parental presence or absence are non-specific indicators of serious illness.

Simple charting of respiratory rate and pulse rate can yield valuable information. Both tend to rise with deteriorating respiratory and cardiovascular function until, as a preterminal event, they fall acutely. Other valuable respiratory observations include assessment of respiratory work such as intercostal recession and the use of accessory muscles of respiration. Early signs of cardiovascular deterioration include tachycardia and peripheral vasoconstriction. The latter can be assessed by examining capillary refill, peripheral pulses and peripheral temperature.

Blood pressure measurement

This is simple to perform but there may be problems with its interpretation in children.

- An inaccurate measurement may result from using a cuff of the wrong size. The correct cuff width should be two-thirds of the length of the upper arm.
- Normal blood pressure varies with age. The lower limits of normal can be estimated from Table 1.
- Homeostatic mechanisms in children are capable of maintaining a normal blood pressure in the face of considerable physiological disturbance. In haemorrhagic shock, for example, blood pressure may remain relatively unchanged until up to half the circulating volume is lost. Consequently, a normal blood pressure should not be taken to mean that all is well. Conversely, hypotension is a late and extremely worrying sign.

Table 1. *Lower limits of normal for systolic blood pressure in children*

Newborn	60 mmHg
Infant	70 mmHg
Older children	$70 + 2 \times$ age mmHg

Pulse oximetry

Any area which is likely to have to deal with sick children should have access to pulse oximetry. The measurement of peripheral oxygen saturation has considerably simplified the continuous monitoring of children with respiratory compromise, although it must be remembered that it only provides information about oxygenation and not carbon dioxide elimination. In addition to facilitating the early detection of falls in oxygenation, pulse oximetry allows oxygen therapy to be given in a controlled manner and may also provide useful information about peripheral perfusion, although its accuracy is questionable if this is poor.

ECG monitoring

Although children are far less likely to have arrhythmias than adults, electrocardiographic (ECG) monitoring is still useful, if only to provide a continuous monitor of heart rate. Should cardiac arrest occur, an ECG is mandatory since further treatment will depend on the rhythm found.

Advanced airway management

This involves the use of airway adjuncts. Since these are also described in Chapter 2, only the differences between adults and children are highlighted here.

Oropharyngeal airways

These are available in a number of sizes (000–4). The most suitable size is best gauged by holding the airway against the child's face. With the flange at the lips, the end of the airway should be level with the angle of the jaw. Although oropharyngeal airways are useful in unconscious children, they may provoke vomiting or laryngospasm in the semiconscious and should be removed if they are rejected during insertion. They are inserted in the same way as in adults, initially upside down and then rotated through 180° whilst being advanced into their final position.

Nasopharyngeal airways

Nasopharyngeal airways are better tolerated in semiconscious children. The correct size airway will have the same internal diameter as the appropriately sized endotracheal tube (Table 2), and the length should be

Table 2. *Paediatric tracheal tube sizes*

Age	Tube size (ID)
Newborn	3.0 mm
6 months	3.5 mm
1 year	4.0 mm
>1 year	Age/4 + 4 mm

estimated from the distance between the external nares and the angle of the jaw. Because nasopharyngeal airways are prone to cause bleeding during insertion, they are best avoided during acute resuscitation. Their use is contraindicated if a basal skull fracture is suspected.

Endotracheal intubation

Endotracheal intubation is the 'gold standard' of airway management. It provides a clear airway, affords protection against the aspiration of gastric contents and allows positive pressure ventilation to be performed without gastric distension, even in the presence of low pulmonary compliance. Unfortunately, it is a technique associated with many complications, both during the insertion of the tube and once it is in place.

Because the narrowest section of a child's larynx is the cricoid ring, which is circular in cross-section, a plain uncuffed tracheal tube of the correct size will form a seal which will allow positive pressure ventilation and protect the lungs from the aspiration of gastric contents. Not only is a cuff unnecessary on a paediatric tracheal tube but it may cause mucosal damage, resulting in swelling and narrowing of the already small trachea following extubation.

Since the resistance to gas flow through a tube is inversely proportional to the fourth power of its radius (Poiseuille's Law), even a small amount of mucosal oedema will result in a large increase in resistance to flow and thus work of breathing. Selecting the correct size of tube is therefore vital: too small and effective ventilation may not be possible, too large and the mucosa may be damaged. Table 2 gives guidelines for tube sizes. Once the tube is in place the size should be confirmed by listening for a small leak around it during a positive pressure inflation of between 20 and 30 cmH$_2$O. The correct length of the tube should also be confirmed at this time by carefully auscultating both lung fields. The trachea of a newborn baby is approximately 4–5 cm long,

so between 2 and 3 cm of tube should be passed through the vocal cords to place the tip of the tube in midtrachea.

The technique of tracheal intubation in children is described below. It is important to remember that intubation is only a means to an end and that the ultimate goal is oxygenation. Intubation attempts should always be preceded by preoxygenation with the highest possible inspired oxygen concentration and prolonged attempts should not be made without frequent interruptions for further oxygen. In most circumstances, oral intubation is the easiest method and should be the first choice for resuscitation. If nasal intubation is required for further management, the tubes can be exchanged electively after the initial stabilization of the child.

Because of the small sizes of paediatric tracheal tubes, they are prone to blocking, kinking or misplacement. An acute deterioration in an intubated child should prompt a careful examination of the tracheal tube.

If the child continues to deteriorate and there is any doubt about the tube, it should be removed and the child oxygenated with a bag–valve–mask system.

TECHNIQUE

Tracheal intubation with straight blade laryngoscope

Indications
- To bypass upper airway obstruction.
- To facilitate positive pressure ventilation.
- To protect against the aspiration of gastric contents.

Contraindications
There are no absolute contraindications to tracheal intubation, but particular care must be taken in patients with suspected cervical spine injury.

Anatomy
The infant airway differs from that of the adult and older child in the following ways:

- The tongue is relatively large.
- The larynx is higher in the neck and more anterior.
- The glottic opening is angled posteriorly.
- The epiglottis is relatively long, U-shaped and floppy.

These anatomical differences make intubation with a conventional curved blade laryngoscope relatively difficult (but not impossible) and most operators feel that a straight bladed laryngoscope facilitates intubation in the first year or two of life.

Equipment
- Bag–valve–mask system with oxygen supply.

- Suction equipment with Yankauer end and selection of suction catheters.
- Laryngoscope (a spare should also be available).
- Selection of appropriately sized tracheal tubes with connectors (see Table 2).
- Stylets.
- Adhesive tape for fixation.
- Stethoscope.

There are a number of different patterns of straight blade available. There are two main types: those with relatively flat blades (Seward, Robertshaw) and those which are C-shaped in cross-section (Magill–Anderson, Miller). The latter are more efficient at keeping the lips apart, which helps to provide a better view, but the former leave more space in the mouth for manipulation of the tube. This is particularly useful when changing from an oral to a nasal tube.

Procedure
- Ensure the infant is adequately oxygenated before starting.
- The head is positioned in a neutral position. Overextension of the neck should be avoided. Pillows or neck rolls are usually unnecessary.
- The jaws are parted with the fingers of the right hand, the laryngoscope advanced into the right-hand side of the mouth taking care to sweep the entire tongue to the left. The blade is advanced, keeping the tip in contact with the tongue, until the epiglottis is seen. Until this point the technique is the same as that for tracheal intubation using a curved blade.
- The tip of the blade is placed underneath the laryngeal surface of the epiglottis and the larynx exposed by lifting the laryngoscope upwards along the axis of its handle (not levering on the upper jaw). An alternative is to deliberately pass the laryngoscope into the oesophagus and then withdraw it slowly, keeping the tip elevated, until the larynx drops into view.
- The vocal cords should now be visible and the tube can be passed under direct vision. Visualisation of the larynx can be facilitated by gentle pressure on the cricoid cartilage. The use of a tracheal tube introducer to produce a curve in the tip of the tracheal tube may also be helpful, but care must be taken to prevent it protruding beyond the end of the tube and damaging the tracheal mucosa. In infants, 2-3 cm of the tube should be passed through the cords.
- The position should be confirmed by careful auscultation of both lung fields. The child's condition should improve. Any deterioration following intubation should be presumed to be a misplaced tube unless proven otherwise.
- The tube should be carefully secured (usually with adhesive tape) and a further check made to confirm correct positioning.

Artificial airways

Even in the best of circumstances, tracheostomy in children is a difficult procedure with many potential complications (Myers & Stool, 1985). Performed outside the operating theatre by inexperienced personnel in an emergency, it is nearly impossible. The preferred method of securing an emergency artificial airway is to perform a needle cricothyroidotomy. It is important to appreciate that it is not possible to achieve satisfactory ventilation by this method and that it should only be used as a last resort when other methods of maintaining the airway have either failed or are clearly not possible.

TECHNIQUE
Needle cricothyroidotomy

Indications
- To bypass upper airway obstruction which cannot be relieved by any other means (e.g. in facial trauma or massive upper airway oedema). Conventional airway management techniques should be tried first.

Contraindications
This is a technique of last resort. It should only be used if other methods of securing an airway have either failed or are clearly impossible.
  Caution should be exercised if cervical spine injury is suspected. In particular, neck extension should be avoided.

Anatomy
The cricothyroid membrane lies between the cricoid and thyroid cartilages. In older children it is as easy to feel as in adults. In infants, however, the laryngeal anatomy is poorly defined and it may be difficult to locate. In this case the highest palpable tracheal ring may be used as an alternative site. Palpation can be facilitated by extension of the head and neck over a bag of fluid or sand bag (not in suspected neck injury).

Equipment
- Intravenous cannula (largest possible, e.g. 12 or 14 SWG, depending on size of child).
- 5 ml syringe.
- 3.5 mm (Portex) or 3.0 mm (other manufacturers) tracheal tube connector.
- Bag–valve–mask system with oxygen supply and reservoir.

Procedure
- The space is located and the skin prepared with a suitable antiseptic solution.
- The larynx is immobilized by placing the finger and thumb of one hand on either side.
- The intravenous cannula with syringe attached is

advanced toward the trachea with the other hand at right-angles to all planes.

- A loss of resistance should be felt when the needle enters the trachea.
- Gentle suction on the syringe should be applied to confirm that air can be freely aspirated.
- When satisfied that the lumen of the trachea has been entered, the needle is withdrawn slightly and the cannula is advanced off the needle, as in venous cannulation, in a caudal direction.
- Another aspiration test is performed with a syringe attached directly to the cannula to confirm that it is still in the lumen of the trachea.
- Once in place the cannula is attached to a 3.5 mm (Portex) or 3.0 mm (other manufacturers) tracheal tube connector which can be connected to a self-inflating bag delivering 100% oxygen.

Ventilation in this manner is extremely inefficient, and high inspiratory pressures are necessary. Any pressure-limiting devices must be overridden. Expiration is passive and usually occurs via the upper airway which is not normally completely obstructed. If there is total upper airway obstruction, great care must be taken to avoid overdistension of the lungs.

An alternative ventilation system requires the connection of the cannula to an oxygen flowmeter via a three-way tap or Y-connector with one of the three limbs left open to the atmosphere. The flowmeter is set at an initial flow of 1 litre min^{-1} for each year of age, and inflation is accomplished by intermittent occlusion of the open end. This system allows more effective ventilation but is more likely to result in barotrauma or, should the cannula be misplaced, surgical emphysema.

The preferred site for this technique in adults is the cricothyroid membrane as it is relatively avascular and easily identified. In infants and small children, however, the cricoid and thyroid cartilages are not clearly demarcated and it may be difficult to locate (Rood, 1985) (Fig. 4). In addition, the cricothyroid membrane is above the narrowest portion of the airway (the cricoid ring). Therefore, although it should be the preferred site of puncture in older children, it may be necessary to use a prominent upper tracheal ring in infants and in some types of upper airway obstruction such as impacted foreign body or subglottic stenosis. When the cannula has been introduced it may be connected to a bag and valve device by means of a 3.0 or 3.5 mm (depending on the make of tube) tracheal tube connector. Even with the pressure relief valve occluded, ventilation by this means will be inadequate for carbon dioxide elimination, but if the largest possible cannula and high concentrations of oxygen are used (preferably 100%) it should be possible

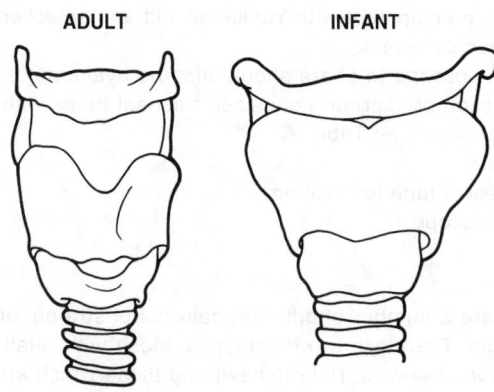

Fig. 4. Comparison of laryngeal morphology between infants and adults.

to provide sufficient oxygenation to allow time for more definitive airway management (Cote *et al.*, 1988). Although inspiration will be under positive pressure, expiration is passive and care must be taken to avoid overdistension of the lungs. This is particularly likely if there is complete obstruction of the upper airway. If available, the recently introduced paediatric sizes of the Seldinger technique cricothyroidotomy sets claim to offer advantages.

Other airway adjuncts

The oesophageal obturator airway should not be used in children. The laryngeal mask airway is useful in paediatric anaesthesia but the child needs to be deeply unconscious to tolerate its presence. This will limit its use in paediatric resuscitation and there are insufficient data to recommend it for this purpose at present.

Positive pressure ventilation

If there is apnoea or the respiratory rate or depth is inadequate, positive pressure ventilation is necessary. The presence of a tracheal tube will facilitate this, but is not essential, as bag and mask ventilation is effective. There are a number of different types of mask available for paediatric use. The main consideration is that the mask fits the child's face well, forming an airtight seal. Without this, positive pressure ventilation is impossible. The semitransparent, floppy-rimmed masks are the most efficient in this respect.

There are two main types of bag systems for positive pressure ventilation in children. The T-piece (or anaesthetic) circuit and the self-inflating bag. The former is useful in experienced hands but requires an oxygen supply and considerable practice if it is to be effective. It is also possible for the transmission of extremely high pressures directly to the lungs to occur with this type of system.

Self inflating bags are much easier to use and can be used without an additional oxygen supply. They are available in different sizes, usually 300, 500 and 1500 ml. The two smaller bags are designed for use in infants but the 300 ml bag is probably too small to allow the effective delivery of a sustained breath (Milner *et al.*, 1984). A pop-off valve, which vents the bag if high pressures (>30–$40\,cmH_2O$) are generated, is often incorporated into the small bags. This should have an override facility since higher inflation pressures may be needed if ventilating with a mask or if the lungs are very stiff. It is possible to use the largest bag on the smallest baby provided it is used with care and the chest excursions are carefully observed.

Self-inflating bags deliver room air, and added oxygen should always be used if available. The simple attachment of an oxygen flow into the port provided can increase the inspired oxygen to about 40%. To achieve higher levels it is necessary to add a reservoir bag to the air inlet of the bag. This will allow the delivery of almost 100% oxygen.

When performing positive pressure ventilation on a child who is making some spontaneous respiratory effort, the positive pressure breaths should be synchronized with the child's own inspiratory efforts. If the child is apnoeic, the respiratory rate should be approximately 20 breaths min^{-1} in children, although it can be faster in small infants. The chest excursions should be carefully monitored, both to ensure that ventilation is effective and to avoid overdistension of the lungs. The child should appear to take a deep breath with each inflation. If the minute ventilation needs to be increased it is best to increase the respiratory rate rather than the tidal volume.

Vascular access

Circulatory access is essential for the effective delivery of resuscitation drugs and fluids. Although adrenaline, atropine and lignocaine can all be given by the tracheal route, this is an inferior method of delivery and should only be used if vascular access is delayed.

A clear order of priorities should be formed when approaching vascular access in a child undergoing acute resuscitation. This should be as follows.

- If there is a functioning peripheral or central venous line *in situ*, initial drug administration should be by this route.
- If there is no intravenous access, brief attempts should be made at peripheral venous cannulation. If no suitable superficial hand or foot veins can be seen, the long saphenous, femoral or external jugular veins are often available. These attempts should be limited to three in number or approximately 90 sec in time.
- If there is no access after this time an intraosseous cannula should be inserted (Fiser, 1990) (see p. 1209). All resuscitation drugs and fluids may be given by this route.
- The endotracheal route should not be used unless there is a delay in achieving circulatory access. If it is used, the appropriate intravenous dose of the drug should be given in addition once venous access is available.

There is no absolute consensus on the appropriate drug dosage for the tracheal route. The recommended dose of endotracheal adrenaline is $0.1\,mg\,kg^{-1}$ ($10\times$ the intravenous dose) because there is evidence that the blood levels of adrenaline delivered tracheally are only 10% of those found after intravenous administration (Quinton *et al.*, 1987). It has been shown that a satisfactory response can be obtained to a tracheal dose of atropine of double the intravenous dose (Howard & Bingham, 1990). This can be repeated as necessary. Lignocaine toxicity is a potential problem when delivering large doses endotracheally and since this drug is now only given late in the VF algorithm, it should probably be kept in reserve until circulatory access is available.

Any endotracheal drug administration should deliver the drug as deep into the bronchial tree as possible in 2–3 ml of 0.9% saline. This can be facilitated by administering the drug via a long catheter. Dispersion is aided by giving several large positive pressure breaths.

Drugs given into peripheral or intraosseous cannulae should always be followed with 5–10 ml of 0.9% saline both to facilitate their delivery into the central circulation and to avoid physical drug interactions.

The central venous route of administration is the most effective, but insertion of an internal jugular or subclavian catheter during acute resuscitation carries an unacceptably high complication rate and is best avoided until the phase of postresuscitation stabilization. A femoral cannula can easily be exchanged for a long catheter using a Seldinger wire if one is available.

PAEDIATRIC ADVANCED LIFE SUPPORT

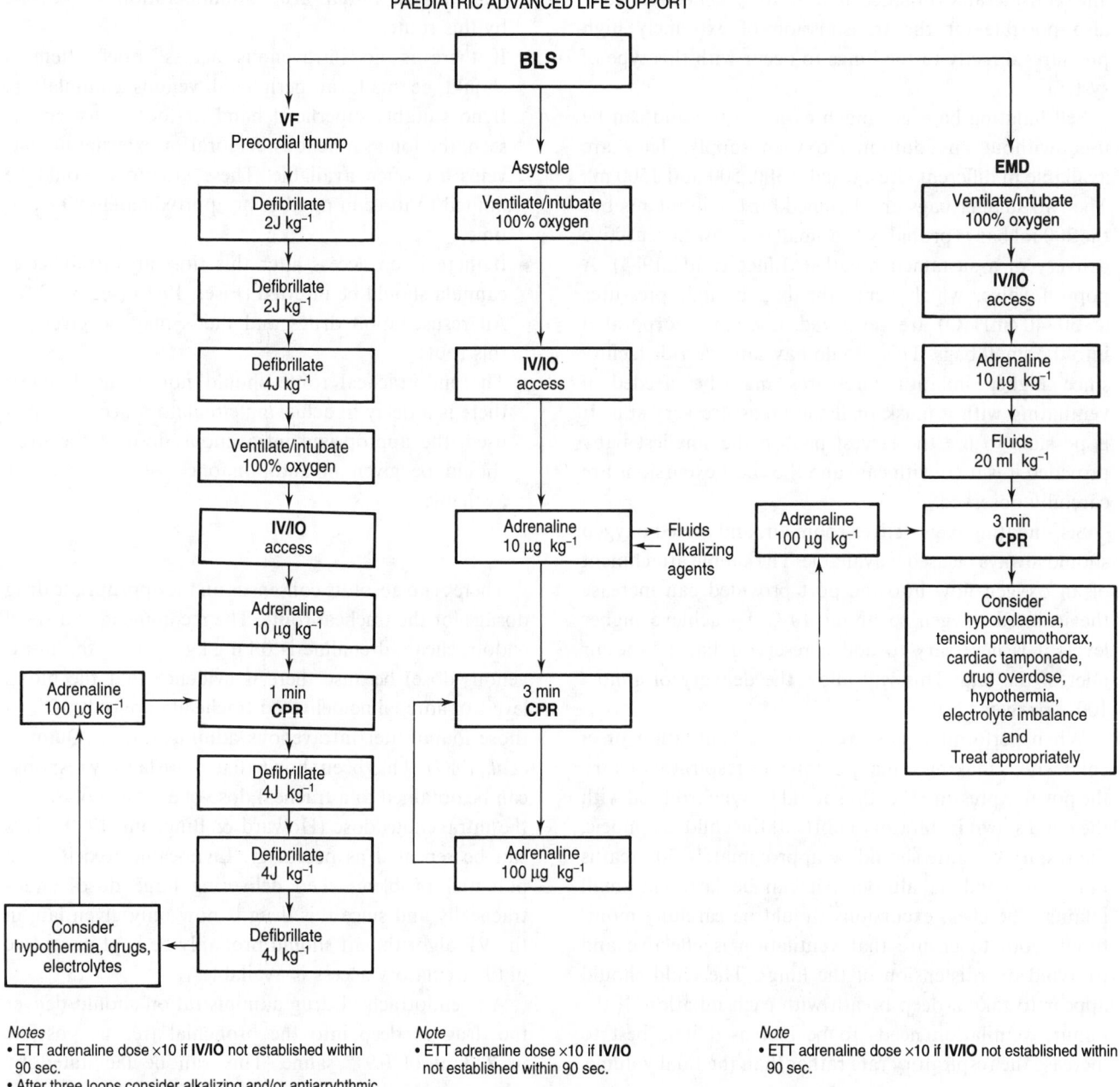

Fig. 5. Paediatric advanced life support algorithm. For abbreviations, see text. (European Resuscitation Council.)

Treatment of cardiac arrest

The initial management of cardiac arrest in children is effective BLS, irrespective of the cause. Further specific management will depend on the underlying rhythm (Fig. 5). As in adults, there are three possibilities: asystole, ventricular fibrillation (VF) and electromechanical dissociation (EMD).

Asystole

This is the commonest arrhythmia seen in children suffering cardiac arrest and is usually the final result of a progressive bradycardia secondary to hypoxaemia. The priority is thus oxygenation. This is initially achieved by effective BLS with as high an inspired oxygen concentration as possible. If there is no response to oxygenation, adrenaline $(0.01 \, \text{mg kg}^{-1})$ is the drug of first choice. If this is ineffective, a further dose of adrenaline at $10\times$ the initial dose should be given. The administration of sodium bicarbonate $(1 \, \text{mmol kg}^{-1})$, and a fluid bolus $(20 \, \text{ml isotonic fluid kg}^{-1})$ should also be considered at this point, depending on the suspected aetiology. Although CPR and adrenaline administration should be continued until treatable precipitating causes can be excluded, the absence of a response to the second round of drugs in asystolic cardiac arrest signals a very poor outcome (Barzilay et al., 1988; Zimmermann & Schmalz, 1990).

Ventricular fibrillation

VF is an uncommon arrhythmia in children and there is often a precipitating cause such as an electrolyte disturbance (particularly hypokalaemia), drug toxicity, or hypothermia. Irrespective of the cause, the treatment of VF is defibrillation, although a precordial thump is worth trying in witnessed (monitored) VF if a defibrillator is not immediately available. The energy level for defibrillation should be $2 \, \text{J kg}^{-1}$ for the initial two shocks and $4 \, \text{J kg}^{-1}$ for subsequent shocks (Gutgesell et al., 1976). The first three shocks should be delivered in quick succession. The appropriate paddle size is that which fully contacts the chest wall, and is usually 4.5 cm in small infants and 8 cm in older children. If small paddles are not available, front-to-back defibrillation can be performed using standard paddles. It is essential to ensure that there is no possibility of arcing of current between the electrodes. For this reason care must be taken to prevent the spreading of electrode jelly on the chest wall. If there is no response to the initial succession of three shocks, adrenaline $(0.01 \, \text{mg kg}^{-1})$ should be given, with BLS to allow the drug to circulate before a further three defibrillation attempts (at $4 \, \text{J kg}^{-1}$). If there is still no response, any precipitating cause should be identified and, if possible, treated. A further dose of adrenaline $10\times$ greater than the first should also be given at this point. Other measures which may be considered are the administration of lignocaine or other antiarrhythmic drugs such as bretylium. Because VF results in a primary cardiac arrest, the outcome may be better than that for secondary cardiac arrest as in asystole and every effort should be may to restore sinus rhythm. Adrenaline should be continued at regular intervals in order to maintain cerebral perfusion.

Electromechanical dissociation or pulseless electrical activity

In children, this is often the result of a physical cause such as hypovolaemia, tension pneumothorax or cardiac tamponade, and these should be considered and treated as appropriate. General treatment involves BLS, adrenaline $(0.01 \, \text{mg kg}^{-1})$ and fluid administration $(10-20 \, \text{ml kg}^{-1})$ because these are useful irrespective of the cause. Further, larger doses of adrenaline $(0.1 \, \text{mg kg}^{-1})$ should be given if there is no response to the initial dose. If hypovolaemia is considered likely repeat fluid boluses should be given depending on the response.

Other arrhythmias

Although primary arrhythmias are uncommon in children, severe tachycardia or bradycardia may result in a low cardiac output and require emergency treatment. Bradycardias in children are usually secondary to arterial hypoxaemia and thus the most important aspect of treatment is oxygenation. Some bradycardias, particularly those associated with vagal stimulation, respond to atropine administration $(0.02 \, \text{mg kg}^{-1})$. Adrenaline $(0.01 \, \text{mg kg}^{-1})$ should be the first line drug in bradycardia associated with shock.

There can be some confusion in differentiating between a supraventricular tachycardia resulting in poor peripheral perfusion and a sinus tachycardia secondary to hypovolaemia, pyrexia or pain. The two can usually be distinguished by means of history, examination, ECG and chest X-ray (Table 3). The treatment of sinus tachycardia is directed at the underlying condition (usually hypovolaemia). The treatment of supraventricular tachycardia depends on its severity. In a stable, conscious child with reasonable peripheral perfusion, time is available to perform further investigations and obtain a specialist opinion. In an unconscious child with profound circulatory disturbance the treatment of choice is synchronized DC cardioversion (initially $0.5-1 \, \text{J kg}^{-1}$). In children with circulatory impairment but who are still conscious, general anaesthesia and DC cardioversion may be avoided by chemical cardioversion with adenosine $(0.05-0.25 \, \text{mg kg}^{-1}, \text{rapid IV bolus})$ (Till et al., 1989). Other agents used for the treatment of supraventricular tachycardia in adults are associated with a high incidence of adverse effects in children and should be avoided (Epstein et al., 1985).

Table 3. *Characteristics of supraventricular and sinus tachycardia*

	SVT	Sinus tachycardia
History	Sudden onset, breathlessness	Preceding illness, progressive deterioration
Examination	Pulmonary congestion, large liver, raised JVP	Clear lung fields, low JVP, small liver
ECG	Rate >220 beats min^{-1}	Rate <220 beats min^{-1}
Chest X-ray	Large heart, pulmonary plethora	Small heart, pulmonary oligaemia

JVP, jugular venous pressure; SVT, supraventricular tachycardia.

Drug points (Zaritsky, 1993)

Adenosine

Dose 0.05--0.1 kg^{-1}. Adenosine produces a transient atrioventricular nodal block which interrupts the re-entry circuits involved in the majority of paediatric tachy-arrhythmias. It has an extremely short duration of action (about 10 sec) as it is metabolized by erythrocyte adenosine deaminase. Because of this it must be given by rapid bolus injection and larger doses (up to 0.25 mg kg^{-1}) may be required if it is administered by a peripheral rather than central venous route because of the increased transit time.

Adrenaline

Initial dose: 0.01 mg kg^{-1}. The first-line drug in paedi-atric resuscitation is adrenaline. As in adults, the rationale for its use is primarily to increase aortic diastolic pressure and therefore promote coronary and carotid perfusion and thus myocardial and cerebral oxygen delivery. Since a common denominator of all the pulseless rhythms is poor myocardial oxygenation, adrenaline is appropriate in all cardiac arrests.

There is some evidence that the chances of restoring spontaneous cardiac output are improved by the use of very large doses of adrenaline (0.1 mg kg^{-1}), and this may possibly be translated into an improved neurological outcome (Goetting & Paradis, 1991). It is therefore recommended that following cardiac arrest the second and subsequent doses of adrenaline should be 10 times the initial dose.

Atropine

Dose: 0.02 mg kg^{-1}. A minimum dose of 0.1 mg should be used as central effects of very small doses may result in a paradoxical bradycardia (Koltmeier & Gravenstein,

1968). The universal response of the young heart to hypoxaemia is bradycardia. This can often be partially ameliorated by the administration of atropine but this should not allow attention to be diverted from the correction of the underlying cause. Atropine is particu-larly useful to prevent or treat bradycardias associated with high vagal tone such as occur with intubation and tracheal suction. There is no evidence that atropine is effective in the management of asystole but it is unlikely to be harmful.

Bretylium

Dose: 5 mg kg^{-1}. There are only isolated anecdotal reports on the use of bretylium in childhood (Mong-kolsmai *et al.*, 1984), but in the context of VF refractory to treatment with adrenaline and lignocaine it should be considered.

Sodium bicarbonate

Dose: 1 mmol kg^{-1} or according to blood gas analysis. Since tissue hypoxia commonly precedes cardiac arrest in children, a profound acidosis is common. Sodium bicarbonate may therefore have a greater place in paediatric than in adult resuscitation, particularly if a profound acidosis is felt to be inhibiting the action of adrenaline. As in adults, it should only be administered after the ventilation has been controlled and circulation established so that the evolved carbon dioxide can be eliminated. If possible the correct dose should be established following blood gas analysis. There may be a place for a dose of sodium bicarbonate prior to the second dose of adrenaline in the management of asystole This is because lack of response to adrenaline at this stage is associated with a particularly poor outcome. The injection port should always be flushed with saline following sodium bicarbonate administration.

Calcium chloride

Dose: 0.2 ml of 10% calcium chloride kg^{-1}. Calcium may be useful in the treatment of cardiac arrest in children associated with hyperkalaemia, calcium channel blocker overdose or hypocalcaemia. Since hypocalcaemia is common in critically ill children, calcium administration should be considered in refractory EMD.

Glucose

Dose: 0.5 g kg^{-1}. Both lowered and raised blood glucose levels are capable of adversely prejudicing the neurological outcome after resuscitation, and a bedside reagent strip test should be performed at the first possible opportunity. Resuscitation fluids should not contain glucose and glucose should only be administered if hypoglycaemia has been demonstrated or is strongly suspected. If glucose administration is necessary, an infusion of 25% dextrose (2 ml kg^{-1}) is preferable to bolus administration.

Lignocaine

Dose: 1 mg kg^{-1}. Lignocaine is used in the treatment of ventricular arrhythmias. Because it stabilizes the existing rhythm, it is most useful in the treatment of ventricular extrasystoles that are considered likely to progress to a more serious arrhythmia, or of VF which is easily defibrillated but quickly reverts. There is an increasing body of evidence in the adult literature that the cardiovascular depressant effects of lignocaine outweigh its advantages in the initial treatment of VF (p. 70). It is therefore no longer recommended as a first-line drug in this rhythm and, as in adults, it should be reserved for consideration with other antiarrhythmic drugs in the management of intractable VF.

Fluids

Dose: 10 ml kg^{-1}, repeated depending on the response. Hypovolaemia is a common precipitant of, or accompaniment to, cardiorespiratory failure in children and volume expansion is commonly required. Although there is much debate on the merits or otherwise of crystalloid versus colloid solutions the most important features of initial resuscitation fluids in children are that they should be isotonic and not contain glucose; 0.9% saline, Hartmann's solution, and 4.5% or 5% albumin are all acceptable. There are few data on the safety of artificial colloids, but they are widely used in older children (Huskisson, 1992).

Dosages

Irrespective of the type of drug administered, it is vital that the correct dose is chosen, and calculations based on mental arithmetic without reference to charts are likely to be inaccurate. It is vital that standard paediatric emergency drug dosage charts are easily available in all areas in which acutely ill children may be encountered (Oakley, 1988).

RESUSCITATION AT BIRTH

This section is directed at the resuscitation of a newborn baby outside the delivery suite (e.g. in an A&E department). Although the fundamental principles do not vary significantly with location, there are some differences in approach which are due to the lack of specialist equipment and staff.

Neonatal physiology

The transition from fetus to newborn involves profound physiological changes. Those that are most relevant to the resuscitation of the newborn are discussed below.

Respiratory system

In utero the lungs are collapsed and fluid-filled. Most of the fluid is expelled during birth or absorbed shortly afterwards. The expansion and aeration of the lungs require a very large transpulmonary pressure gradient during the first few breaths. This is usually generated by the gasping respirations which occur when the baby is subjected to the sudden increase in stimuli which accompanies birth. If the lungs are not expanded when resuscitation is attempted sustained positive pressure inflation at higher than usual pressures may be initially necessary, and intubation may be required to achieve this effectively. This is particularly likely in preterm infants (<32 weeks) in whom surfactant deficiency may exacerbate the problem.

Cardiovascular system

In utero, oxygenation is provided by the placenta. Blood bypasses the lungs via the foramen ovale and ductus arteriosus. These fetal channels normally close at birth but may be capable of reopening, allowing desaturated systemic venous blood to enter the aorta. This is particularly likely in the presence of arterial hypoxaemia, hypercapnoea and acidosis. Particular care must be taken in the postresuscitation phase to avoid these precipitating factors.

Central nervous system

The brain of a newborn baby, particularly a premature one, has a delicate system of blood vessels in the region of the cerebral ventricles (germinal matrix). These vessels are particularly prone to bleeding if exposed to sudden swings in serum osmolarity or blood pressure (Finberg, 1977; Hambleton & Wigglesworth, 1976).

Temperature control

Newborn infants are particularly susceptible to hypothermia because of their high surface area and thin dermis. In addition there is a large heat loss from the evaporation of liquor amnii from the baby's skin. Hypothermia exacerbates both hypoxaemia and acidosis and inhibits the production of surfactant (Roberton, 1986). The newborn baby should therefore be dried and wrapped in warm covering as soon as possible. Since it may be necessary to expose the baby for the purpose of resuscitation, the room should be warmed in advance (to approximately 25°C) and an overhead radiant heater should be available for use (Scopes & Ahmed, 1966).

Preparation

It is usually possible to predict the delivery of a baby, if only by a few minutes. During this time it should be possible to warm the room and prepare the necessary equipment and drugs in advance (see Table 4).

If there is time to elicit a history from the mother it should be possible to predict babies at high risk for requiring resuscitation (Table 5).

Assessment

The assessment score devised by Virginia Apgar (Apgar, 1953) is widely used for the evaluation of the newborn infant. Whilst this is an extremely valuable tool, especially for audit purposes, time should not be wasted in its computation, particularly by those unfamiliar in its use. It is far easier to quickly evaluate respiratory activity, heart rate, colour and tone superficially than to

Table 4. *Equipment for resuscitation at birth*

Overhead heater
Clock
Stethoscope
Umbilical vein catheter set
Bag–valve system
Oropharyngeal airways (00 and 0)
Oxygen supply
Suction apparatus
Suction catheters (6, 8 and 10 FG)
Face masks
Laryngoscope and blade (×2)
Tracheal tubes (2, 2.5, 3.0 and 3.5 mm ID)

Drugs
Adrenaline (1:10 000), naloxone (0.2 mg ml^{-1}), sodium bicarbonate (8.4% or 4.2%), glucose (10% and 20%), access to plasma expanders (see text)

Table 5. *High-risk deliveries*

Maternal factors
Heavy sedation
Drug addiction
Severe hypertension
Diabetes mellitus
Chronic illness

Fetal factors
Multiple
Preterm (< 34 weeks)
Small for dates
Rhesus incompatibility
Abnormal baby

Others
Meconium-stained liquor, abnormal presentation, antepartum haemorrhage

go through the full score. Heart rate can be assessed by either listening to the apex beat or palpating the brachial or femoral pulse. Using this method it is usually possible to categorize the baby into one of three groups within the initial 30 sec.

- Fit and healthy, crying lustily with a heart rate above 100 min^{-1}. (By far the majority.)
- In need of help, some respiratory effort present but inadequate. Usually cyanosed with reduced tone. Heart rate above 80 min^{-1}.

- Flat baby, pale with little if any tone, no respiratory effort and heart rate less than 60 min^{-1}. (Less than 0.5% of all deliveries).

Management

First group

For the first group, little or no intervention is required. The baby should be quickly wrapped in a warm dry cover and given directly to the mother (remember to check that the umbilical cord is securely clamped).

Second group

The second group do require some attention. The initial steps involve positioning, suction, tactile stimulation and the administration of oxygen.

Positioning

The baby should be initially placed on its side in a slightly head down position if possible. The airway should, if necessary, be maintained as in infant and child resuscitation by extending the head slightly and supporting the tip of the jaw. Oxygen should be blown over the baby's face.

Suction

A variety of suction devices are available, both hand-operated and mechanical. The maximum negative pressure should be limited to 100 mmHg. Most babies need little if any suction at birth. If suction is required it should be confined to clearing obvious secretions from the front of the mouth and, since newborns are obligatory nose-breathers, the external nares. Deep nasal or pharyngeal suction should be avoided as it may cause vagal stimulation with bradycardia and laryngospasm (but see meconium aspiration).

Stimulation

The onset of respiration is partially mediated by the sudden increase in stimulation accompanying birth. This can be augmented by gentle tactile stimulation. In most cases drying the baby is sufficient but the infant's feet can be slapped or tickled or its back can be rubbed in addition. If these methods fail to establish the onset of respiration within the first minute, or the

heart rate starts to fall below 80 min^{-1}, they should be abandoned in favour of full basic, and if necessary, advanced life support.

Third group

The third group of babies will need full resuscitation immediately.

Resuscitation

Airway

For resuscitation the infant will need to be supine. Because of the large infant occiput it is sometimes helpful to place a small roll underneath the shoulders in order to prevent overflexion of the neck. In most cases the newborn airway will be maintained by simple manoeuvres described above. Occasionally an oropharyngeal airway is necessary, particularly if there is nasal airway obstruction (e.g. choanal atresia) or micrognathia (e.g. Pierre Robin syndrome).

Breathing

There are several variations on the circuits used for ventilation during newborn resuscitation. Outside the delivery suite it is best to use a 500 ml self-inflating bag with a pop-off valve, as the other systems such as the anaesthetic T-piece circuit require continual practice for effective use. Smaller self-inflating bags are available but with these it is difficult to maintain the sustained inflation pressure which is occasionally required to produce the initial expansion of the lungs (Milner et al., 1984). Since higher than normal inflation pressures are sometimes helpful, it may also be necessary to override the pop-off valve on the bag. This should only be done with caution and careful monitoring of the chest expansion. If, despite this, the baby is not improving and the chest does not seem to be expanding adequately, proceed immediately to tracheal intubation. This is more likely in babies who have never taken a breath or cried and in those of less than 32 weeks' gestation. If the chest is moving well it is best to maintain high respiratory rates (up to 60 min^{-1}) in order to minimize inflation pressures. If the baby is making respiratory effort, try to synchronise inflation with spontaneous inspiration.

Intubation

Intubation allows much more efficient expansion of the lungs at the expense of an increased risk of pulmonary barotrauma. The technique for intubating newborns is the same as that for infants. Although many units use standard plain tracheal tubes, some use Cole pattern tubes. The latter are slightly easier to pass and they have a shoulder which is supposed to prevent them from entering a bronchus. This should not be relied upon, and a careful check on the air entry to both lungs should always be made after intubation. Most newborn babies take a 3.0 mm ID tube but a size 2.5 and a size 3.5 mm should also be available.

Circulation

Should the heart rate drop below 60 min^{-1} ECC should be performed. The technique is the same as that described previously for infants. An alternative involves encircling the baby's chest with the hands and compressing the lower third of the sternum with the thumbs (Todres & Rogers, 1975; David, 1988). The rate should be slightly faster than for older infants (120 min^{-1}) and the ratio of compression/ventilation ratio should be 3:1. An intermittent pulse check should be made and ECC should be continued until the pulse rate is above 80 min^{-1}.

Vascular access

If the baby does not respond immediately to the above measures, vascular access will be needed. If peripheral veins are present, they may be cannulated, but prolonged searches should not be made because the umbilical vein is easily available.

TECHNIQUE

Umbilical vein cannulation

Indications
- Vascular access in the newly born (usually <1 week of age).

Contraindications
- Local infection of umbilical stump.

Anatomy
When the cut end of the umbilicus is inspected there are usually two arteries which have thick walls and a relatively small lumen, and one vein which has a large irregular lumen. Occasionally there is a small amount of clot in the end of the vein which should be removed before catheterization.

Equipment
- Skin preparation.
- 5FG PVC catheter preflushed with heparinized saline.
- Two pairs of fine forceps.
- Ligatures.
- Tape for fixation.

Procedure
- Under full sterile conditions, place a loose ligature around the base of the umbilical cord.
- Transect the end of the stump at least 1 cm from the abdominal wall and identify the vein.
- The stump should be held either with a gloved hand or a pair of forceps and the preflushed catheter advanced gently into the vein with a second set of forceps until it is judged to be just below the abdominal wall level. There should be free return of blood on aspiration.
- There is usually very little resistance to insertion. If this is encountered, the catheter should be withdrawn slightly and the cord angled caudally and put under gentle traction before gently advancing the catheter again.
- Once inserted the catheter should be carefully secured.

Complications
The complications of the technique include infection, portal vein thrombosis, pulmonary embolus and air embolus. Thrombosis is more likely if hypertonic solutions are infused into the vein without careful flushing afterwards.

Drugs

As in infants and children, adrenaline (0.01 mg kg^{-1}) is the first-line drug; it is required if the heart rate does not rise above 80 min^{-1} despite adequate BLS. It may be given intravenously or, if this route is not available, endotracheally. There is concern that hypertension may cause periventricular haemorrhage in newborns so the tracheal dose should be the same as the intravenous dose, although it may be repeated if there is no response. For similar reasons, high-dose intravenous adrenaline is not recommended in newborns. If there is no response to the initial adrenaline, 1–2 mmol sodium bicarbonate kg^{-1} (as 2–4 ml of 4.2% solution kg^{-1}) or an equivalent dose of another base may be given prior to a second dose of adrenaline. Hypoglycaemia is common because of low hepatic glycogen stores and glucose adminstration should be considered, preferably after performing a bedside reagent strip test. It is particularly likely in infants of diabetic mothers.

The rapid administration of hyperosmolar solutions such as 50% glucose or 8.4% sodium bicarbonate may be detrimental, particularly in the preterm infant. Such solutions should be diluted with an equal volume of water and administered slowly.

Meconium-stained liquor

This is an indicator of fetal distress and, in addition, the aspiration of meconium may cause mechanical obstruction of the bronchi and a serious chemical pneumonitis. The best form of defence is prevention and the presence of all but the most trivial of meconium staining should prompt full nasopharyngeal and oropharyngeal suction. This should take place before the baby has taken a breath if possible (i.e. immediately the head is delivered). If there is any doubt that all the meconium has been removed, suction under direct vision with a laryngoscope should be performed. If there is meconium below the vocal cords it should be removed by intubation followed by the application of suction directly to the tracheal tube since meconium is too sticky to be effectively aspirated up a fine-bore suction catheter.

Problems with resuscitation

If there is a poor response to resuscitation, the most likely causes are those associated with the tracheal tube and equipment. These should be checked carefully. In particular, oesophageal and bronchial intubation or an obstructed tube should be excluded. If there is doubt it is better to remove the tube and perform bag–mask ventilation for a few breaths before replacing it. Pneumothorax is a common problem. There is not usually sufficient time to confirm the diagnosis with a chest X-ray but transillumination of the chest with a cold light source may be helpful if one is immediately available. Treatment should not be delayed, however, and if a pneumothorax is suspected a needle should be passed into the suspect side in the 2nd intercostal space in the midclavicular line. The sound of escaping air or clinical improvement confirms the diagnosis and a formal chest drain should then be sited.

Other causes of difficulty with resuscitation are those related to conditions affecting the baby:

- Babies who quickly become pink and well perfused with a reasonable heart rate following ventilation but do not start spontaneous breathing may be under the influence of narcotic analgesics administered to the mother. If this is suspected, naloxone ($0.1 \, \text{mg} \, \text{kg}^{-1}$) should be administered. Since the duration of action of intravenous naloxone may be less than that of the narcotic, the infant should be closely observed and the dose may need to be repeated. In babies of narcotic-dependent mothers, naloxone may precipitate an acute withdrawal and should be avoided.

- Hypovolaemia should be suspected in infants with a history suggestive of blood or fluid loss, or who are particularly pale or poorly perfused despite an adequate heart rate. In this case 10 ml of a suitable volume expander kg^{-1} (e.g. 5% human albumin solution) should be given. This may be repeated, depending on the response. If a transfusion of greater than $20 \, \text{ml} \, \text{kg}^{-1}$ is necessary, or anaemia is suspected, consideration should be given to blood transfusion. Group O negative blood cross-matched against maternal serum should be used.

- Persistent central cyanosis has several causes. The mnemonic COPS is useful in separating them.

C	Congenital cardiac disease (including transitional circulation)
O	Obstruction of the airway (e.g. choanal atresia)
P	Pulmonary parenchymal disease (e.g. hyaline membrane disease)
S	Space occupying lesions (e.g. pneumothorax, diaphragmatic hernia).

Prematurity

Although the treatment of preterm babies is substantially the same as for others, there is a very high incidence of surfactant deficiency in babies of less than 30 weeks. Consequently it may be difficult to expand the lungs adequately. Tracheal intubation should be performed early if there is difficulty ventilating with a bag–mask system. Special care should be taken to maintain body temperature as these babies are particularly liable to hypothermia. Because of the greater likelihood of periventricular haemorrhage, care should be taken with the administration of hyperosmolar solutions and rapid changes in arterial pressure should be avoided if possible.

Although one of the causes of retinopathy of prematurity is raised arterial oxygen tensions, high inspired oxygen concentrations can be safely used in the short term for resuscitation, even in the most premature.

When to stop

The decision to stop resuscitating is one of the most difficult to make. Good neurological recovery is likely in pulseless and apnoeic newborns who respond to resuscitative measures within the first 5–10 min (Scott, 1976) but if there is no spontaneous cardiac activity by 15 mins despite maximum treatment the outcome is likely to be very poor indeed. Babies who have spontaneous cardiac activity but no respiratory movement need further investigation before firm prognostic conclusions can be drawn.

There is increasing evidence that extremely small or premature (<28 weeks) babies who do not respond rapidly to simple measures such as intubation, ventilation with oxygen and ECC are very likely to have a poor neurological outcome (Sims *et al.*, 1994).

Bibliography

APGAR, V. (1953). Proposal for a new method of evaluation of newborn infants. *Anaesth. Analg.*, **32**, 260–7.

BARZILAY, Z., SOMEKH, E., SAGY, M. *et al.* (1988). Paediatric cardiopulmonary resuscitation outcome. *J. Med.*, **19**, 229–41.

COTE, C.J., EAVEY, R.D., TODRES, D. *et al.* (1988). Cricothyroid membrane puncture: oxygenation and ventilation in a dog model using an intravenous catheter. *Crit. Care Med.*, **16**, 615–19.

DAVID, R. (1988). Closed chest cardiac massage in the newborn infant. *Pediatrics*, **81**, 552–4.

EISENBERG, M., BERGNER, L. & HULLSTROM, A. (1983). Epidemiology of cardiac arrest and resuscitation in children. *Ann. Emerg. Med.*, **12**, 672–4.

EPSTEIN, M., KIEL, E. & VICTORIA, B. (1985). Cardiac decompensation following verapamil in infants with supraventricular tachycardia. *Pediatrics*, **75**, 737–40.

FINBERG, L. (1977). The relationship of intravenous infusions and intracranial hemorrhage: a commentary. *J. Pediatr.*, **91**, 777–8.

FISER, D.H. (1990). Intraosseous infusion. *N. Engl. J. Med.*, **322**, 1579–81.

GILLIS, J., DICKSON, D., RIEDER, M. *et al.* (1986). Results of inpatient paediatric resuscitation. *Crit. Care Med.*, **14**, 469–71.

GOETTING, M.G. & PARADIS, N.A. (1991). High dose epinephrine improves outcome from pediatric cardiac arrest. *Ann. Emerg. Med.*, **20**, 22–6.

GUTGESELL, H.P., TACKER, H.A., GEDDES, L.A. *et al.* (1976). Energy dose for ventricular defibrillation of children. *Pediatrics*, **58**, 898–901.

HAMBLETON, G. & WIGGLESWORTH, J.S. (1976). Origin of intraventricular haemorrhage in the preterm infant. *Arch. Dis. Child.*, **51**, 651–9.

HOWARD, R. & BINGHAM, R.M. (1990). Endotracheal vs intravenous administration of atropine. *Arch. Dis. Child.*, **65**, 449–50.

HUSKISSON, L. (1992). Intravenous volume replacement. Which fluids and why? *Arch. Dis. Child.*, **67**, 649–53.

INNES, P.A., SUMMERS, C.A., BOYD, I.M. *et al.*

(1993). Audit of paediatric cardiopulmonary resuscitation. *Arch. Dis. Child.*, **68**, 487–91.

KOLTMEIER, C. & GRAVENSTEIN, J. (1968). The parasympathomimetic activity of atropine and atropine methylbromide. *Anesthesiology*, **29**, 1125–33.

LEWIS, J.K., MINTER, M.G., ESHELMAN, S.J. *et al.* (1983). Outcome of paediatric resuscitation. *Ann. Emerg. Med.*, **12**, 297–9.

MILNER, A.D., VYAS, H. & HOPKIN, I.E. (1984). Efficacy of facemask resuscitation at birth. *Br. Med. J.*, **289**, 1563–5.

MONGKOLSMAI, C., DOVE, J. & KYROUAC, J. (1984). Bretylium tosylate for ventricular fibrillation in a child. *Clin. Pediatr.*, **23**, 696–8.

MYERS, E.N. & STOOL, S.E. (1985). Complications of tracheotomy. In *Tracheostomy*, ed. E.N. Myers, S.E. Stool & J.T. Johnson. New York: Churchill Livingstone.

OAKLEY, P.A. (1988). Inaccuracy and delay in decision making in paediatric resuscitation and a proposed reference chart to reduce errors. *Br. Med. J.*, **290**, 817–19.

ORLOWSKI, J.P. (1984). Optimal position for external cardiac massage in infants and children. *Crit. Care Med.*, **12**, 224.

O'ROURKE, P.P. (1986). Outcome of children who are apnoeic and pulseless in the emergency room. *Crit. Care Med.*, **14**, 466–8.

PHILLIPS, G.W. & ZIDEMAN, D.A. (1986). Relation of infant heart to the sternum: its significance in cardiopulmonary resuscitation. *Lancet*, **i**, 1024–5.

QUINTON, D.N., O'BYRNE, G. & AITKENHEAD, A.R. (1987). Comparison of endotracheal and peripheral venous intravenous adrenaline in cardiac arrest: is the endotracheal route reliable? *Lancet*, **i**, 828–9.

ROOD, S.R. (1985). Anatomy for tracheotomy. In *Tracheotomy*, ed. E.N. Myers, S.E. Stool & J.T. Johnson. New York: Churchill Livingstone.

ROBERTON, N.R.C. (1986). Temperature control. In: *A Manual of Neonatal Intensive Care*, ed. N.R.C. Roberton. London: Edward Arnold.

SCOPES, J.W. & AHMED, I. (1966). Range of critical temperatures in sick and premature newborn babies. *Arch. Dis. Child.*, **41**, 417–9.

SCOTT, H.M. (1976). Outcome of very severe birth asphyxia. *Arch. Dis. Child.*, **50**, 712–16.

SIMS, D.G., HEAL, C.A. & BARTLE, S.M. (1994). Use of adrenaline and atropine in neonatal resuscitation. *Arch. Dis. Child.*, **70**, F3–F10.

STOPFKUCHEN, H., STEIN, G., QUEISSER-LUFT, A. *et al.* (1989). Results of cardiopulmonary resuscitation in children. *Klin. Pediatr.*, **201**, 373–6.

TILL, J., SHINEBOURNE, E.A., RIGBY, M.L. *et al.* (1989). Efficacy and safety of adenosine in the treatment of supraventricular tachycardia in infants and children. *Br. Heart J.*, **62**, 204–11.

TODRES, I.D. & ROGERS, M.C. (1975). Methods of external cardiac massage in the newborn infant. *J. Pediatr.*, **86**, 781–2.

ZARITSKY, A. (1993). Pediatric resuscitation pharmacology. *Ann. Emerg. Med.*, **22**, 445–55.

ZIMMERMANN, R. & SCHMALZ, A.A. (1990). Cardiopulmonary resuscitation of children and adolescents in the prehospital stage. *Monatsschr. Kinderheilkd.*, **138**, 326–30.

Further reading

EMERGENCY CARDIAC CARE COMMITTEE AND SUBCOMMITTEES, AMERICAN HEART ASSOCIATION (1992). Guidelines for cardiopulmonary resuscitation. Part V. Pediatric basic life support. *JAMA*, **268**, 2251–61.

EMERGENCY CARDIAC CARE COMMITTEE AND SUBCOMMITTEES, AMERICAN HEART ASSOCIATION (1992). Guidlines for cardiopulmonary resuscitation. Part VI. Pediatric advanced life support. *JAMA*, **268**, 2262–75.

EMERGENCY CARDIAC CARE COMMITTEE AND SUBCOMMITTEES, AMERICAN HEART ASSOCIATION (1992). Guidelines for cardiopulmonary resuscitation. Part VII. Neonatal resuscitation. *JAMA*, **268**, 2276–81.

PAEDIATRIC LIFE SUPPORT WORKING PARTY OF THE EUROPEAN RESUSCITATION COUNCIL (1994). Guidelines for paediatric life support. *Resuscitation*, **27**, 91–105.

SEIDEL, J. (1993). Pediatric cardiopulmonary resuscitation: an update based on the new American Heart Association guidelines. *Pediatr. Emerg. Care*, **9**, 98–103.

5 Early management of the multiply injured patient

K.I. MAULL

Department of Surgery, Stritch School of Medicine, Loyola University, Maywood, Illinois, USA

Chapter plan

Introduction
Preparation
Assessment
Resuscitation
Stabilization
Documentation

INTRODUCTION

The first rule of trauma care is 'Do no harm'.

This is not a principle to be taken lightly. Everything done to and for an injured patient has potential risks and potential benefits. In caring for the injured, aggressive action is sometimes needed when the diagnosis is not totally clear. However, the risks are real, to patient and physician alike. In the multisystem trauma patient, the physician, often hampered by an incomplete database, must deal rapidly with a life-threatening situation. While there is no substitute for experience in such difficult circumstances, it is helpful to have an organized approach to the injured patient that seeks first to identify and treat life-threatening problems quickly yet detect other significant injuries before they cause additional morbidity. In this chapter, an approach to the early management of the injured patient will be described which adheres to the first rule of trauma care by emphasizing assessment, resuscitation and safe application of life-saving interventions. The goal is to improve outcome. The separation into assessment, resuscitation and stabilization is both arbitrary and somewhat contrived. In fact, in some instances, the physician will have to resuscitate before the assessment is completed and intervene before the patient can be stabilized. As the reader proceeds, maintaining an organized approach to the trauma patient will prove to have merit.

PREPARATION

Management of the multiply injured patient is facilitated by having qualified personnel and the necessary equipment in a state of readiness. Each individual involved in the trauma resuscitation should have a defined role. Except for learners, individuals not involved in the management of the patient should be restricted from the immediate area. In the typical trauma centre, participants in the early management of the multiply injured patient are members of a *trauma team*, a cohesive group which works together using an organized approach (Fig. 1). In real life, most injured patients are initially evaluated at the closest hospital. Therefore, it is important for *any* hospital with an emergency unit to be prepared to provide immediate assessment and resuscitation of injured patients. While it may not be possible to gather all the resources available at a level 1 trauma centre, most general hospitals can function cost-effectively as a level 3 trauma centre, which is, by definition, a hospital committed to providing assessment, resuscitation and stabilization of the injured patient on a priority basis.

Protective equipment for all rescuers is essential. Greater awareness of the risks of diseases transmitted through body fluids has led to the concept of total body fluid isolation, previously characterized as universal precautions. As a minimum, individuals having direct contact with the injured patient should wear gloves, impermeable gowns and protective eyewear. Because certain subgroups of injured patients constitute a high-risk group for hepatitis and AIDS (acquired immunodeficiency syndrome), additional measures may sometimes be indicated.

In addition to the necessary personnel and protective equipment, specific equipment is required to aid in early

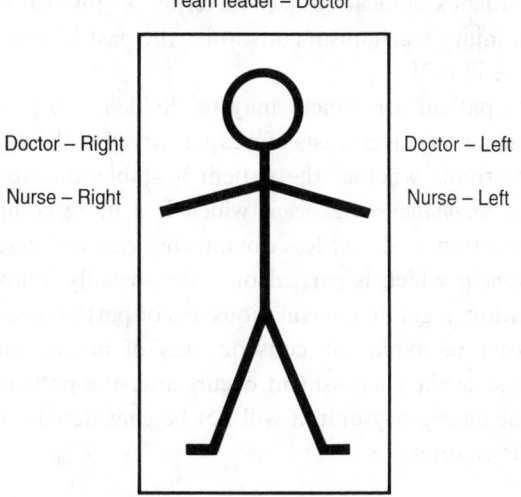

Fig. 1. Diagram of typical trauma resuscitation, including essential medical personnel and their roles.

- *Team leader – doctor*
  - Receives historical information from the prehospital providers.
  - Directs the management of the patient and actions of team members.
  - Decides the treatment and diagnostic priorities.
  - Supervises the interventions.
  - Discusses treatment plan with consultants and family.
  - Maintains close communication with the primary nurse.

- *Doctor on right*
  - Achieves venous access on right side.
  - Obtains central venous access unless contraindicated.
  - Performs emergency procedures needed on right side.
  - Draws arterial blood gases.
  - Maintains arm traction for cervical spine films.
  - Inserts urinary and gastric tubes.
  - Assists with diagnostic peritoneal lavage.
  - Acts on the instructions of the team leader.

- *Doctor on left*
  - Achieves venous access on left side.
  - Performs emergency procedures needed on left side.
  - Cultures open fracture sites and applies dressings.
  - Closes lacerations.
  - Records history and physical examination.
  - Acts on the instructions of the team leader.

- *Nurse on left (primary nurse)*
  - Coordinates nursing care and assessment.
  - Assists team leader with airway management.
  - Monitors vital signs and fluid infusions.
  - Gives nursing report to appropriate units.
  - Administers medications.
  - Acts on the instructions of the team leader.

- *Nurse on right*
  - Verifies cervical spine immobilization.
  - Draws routine trauma blood work.

  - Assists physicians with interventions.
  - Prepares peritoneal lavage tray.
  - Sends urine for analysis.
  - Prevents hypothermia by covering patient.
  - Assists primary nurse.

- *Other personnel*
  - Recorder.
  - Laboratory and X-ray technicians.
  - Respiratory therapist.
  - Unit secretary.
  - Chaplain.

Table 1. *Recommended resuscitation equipment for emergency unit*[a]

- Airway control and ventilation equipment including laryngoscopes and tracheal tubes of all sizes, bag–mask resuscitator, pocket masks, and mechanical ventilator
- Suction devices
- Cardiac monitor/defibrillator
- Central venous manometer
- Standard intravenous fluids, administration sets and catheters
- Sterile surgical trays for commonly performed invasive procedures
- Gastric lavage equipment
- Specific drugs and supplies appropriate for emergency care
- X-ray capability immediately available
- Two-way radio linkage with prehospital emergency vehicles
- Skeletal traction device for cervical injuries
- Swan–Ganz catheters
- Arterial catheters
- Thermal control equipment for administered blood and fluids and for the patient

[a] Recommended by Committee on Trauma, American College of Surgeons.

patient management (Table 1). Of critical importance are laryngoscopes with selected blades (adult and paediatric), suction with rigid suction tip, an orderly arranged array of variously sized tracheal tubes, warm infusion fluids and prepacked sterile surgical trays suitable for placement of cricothyroidostomy, tube thoracostomy and other emergency procedures. Not only must the equipment be available but personnel must know where the equipment is and must ensure that it is operational and replenished following each use. In practice, resuscitation equipment is best placed on open labelled shelves where it can be immediately reached.

Preparation is also enhanced by knowing what is coming and when. This implies reliable radio communication with emergency vehicles. A 'trauma alert' allows time to gather the resuscitation team, double-check the availability of appropriate equipment and alert support services. There is no substitute for good communication between field personnel and the hospital. Unfortunately, not only does this communication occasionally fail but not all injured patients arrive by ambulance! Therefore, an immediate response capability is essential.

ASSESSMENT

The assessment of the patient provides the basis for all subsequent management, whether the patient is observed, subjected to extensive diagnostic studies or rushed to theatre for direct operative intervention. Just as the detective seeks to solve a crime by searching for clues, so the physician searches for signs and symptoms of serious injury. These clinical tips become more apparent if the physician knows what to look for and where. In the uninjured emergency patient, the history constitutes the primary basis for diagnosis. Physical examination serves a somewhat lesser role – to confirm the clinical impression arrived at through a careful chronological review of the patient's complaints. Certain characteristics of the trauma patient render such an approach unworkable, perhaps even dangerous. For example, trauma is a time-sensitive disease. On many occasions the physician must treat before firmly establishing the diagnosis. Often a history is unobtainable, at least from the patient, and family or friends may not be forthcoming with information that might compromise the patient socially or legally. The physician must listen, but also recognize that it is the nature of trauma patients to volunteer information of questionable reliability. Substantiation of historical data should be sought for it may significantly affect subsequent management.

Impaired ventilation, severe haemorrhage and head injury, alone or in combination, account for the vast majority of deaths at the scene of road crashes. The patient who sustains these injuries and survives to reach hospital requires immediate assessment and interventions. The treating physician has a major ally in the prehospital provider. It is the ambulance personnel who assess the incident scene, establish baseline parameters and perhaps speak to the only witnesses. It is the ambulance personnel who are experienced in defining mechanism of injury, the principal historical finding. By knowing the likely mechanism of injury, the physician can fine-tune the assessment, determine the value of certain diagnostic tests and selectively monitor trends in the patient's clinical course. In terms of physical diagnosis, injury mechanism constitutes the past history and present illness!

The patient assessment may be divided into *primary assessment* which consists of a rapid survey of the patient to determine whether the patient is stable, unstable or dying; *secondary assessment* which is a more complete examination to detect less obvious injuries; and *tertiary assessment* which is carried out later, usually following operation, regaining of consciousness or partial recovery, in order to avoid the consequences of missed injury. Because tertiary assessment occurs after the patient has left the emergency unit, it will not be considered further in this chapter.

Primary assessment

The primary assessment is done quickly to prevent an immediate death in a dying patient, to determine the urgency of resuscitative measures in an unstable patient and to begin an organized approach to the stable patient so that injuries can be discovered, prioritized and treated. It is done according to the alphabetical mnemonic: ABC. The Airway is assessed first. If the airway is unobstructed, the patient should be assessed for adequacy of Breathing. Although discussed separately below, the airway and breathing should be considered as a unit during assessment and if interventions are needed. Circulation is judged by the presence of palpable peripheral pulses. If the patient has an open airway, is breathing spontaneously and has a palpable pulse, immediate death is not likely. However, the patient may indeed be unstable. Stability implies a steady-state over time. Injured patients may exist in a fragile equilibrium, appear less ill than they really are, and become moribund in minutes if not closely managed. This is a pitfall for the inexperienced. Unlike the British and American judicial systems where one is innocent until proven guilty, the injured patient must always be considered guilty until proven innocent – i.e. must be presumed to have a serious injury until excluded by clearly defined diagnostic protocols. Deviation from defined protocols is a recognized cause for missed injury.

The alphabetical mnemonic can be continued with D and E. Disability is a convenient term to emphasize the early determination of responsiveness or level of consciousness. It is essential to Expose the patient for further evaluation. This is true for all trauma patients but especially for the unresponsive who cannot direct the physician to sites of injury. Once examined, the patient should be covered to prevent loss of body heat.

Mnemonic for primary assessment
A Airway
B Breathing
C Circulation
D Disability
E Expose

Airway

All multiply injured patients are at risk of cervical spine injury. During airway manoeuvres, proper alignment of the neck must be maintained.

Obstruction of the airway is a common cause of early death in injured patients. Because a compromised airway kills quickly, the physician's first priority is to determine if an obstruction is present and, if it is, to clear the obstruction. In the injured patient, the causes of airway obstruction are finite:

- Facial fractures.
- Mechanical obstruction by dentures, loose teeth or foreign body.
- Mechanical obstruction by tongue.
- Aspiration of blood or vomitus.
- Injuries to the larynx or trachea.

Bleeding into the airway may follow injuries to the face, ncluding facial lacerations, lacerations to the tongue, oral and nasal cavities, disruption of the sinuses and fractures of the facial bones. Bleeding may be profuse and uncontrollable, especially from branches of the external carotid artery. Bleeding into the airway may also follow direct trauma to the upper (supraglottic) or lower (subglottic) airway with or without loss of airway integrity. When the patient cannot clear their own airway and bleeding into the airway is the principal cause of obstruction, high-flow oxygen should be provided and the posterior oropharynx suctioned. Suction should be vigorous but intermittent with the goal of maintaining a patent airway and allowing oxygen-enriched air to reach the alveoli. Be mindful that this setting predisposes rescue personnel to contamination from airborne blood as the patient attempts to clear the airway by coughing. In this circumstance there is no substitute for properly worn protective eyewear. Foreign bodies may also obstruct the airway. Loose teeth, denture fragments and food are most commonly seen. Suction may help but manual removal is usually required. This can be accomplished by sweeping the posterior oropharynx with the gloved finger or using a Magill forceps or other similar instrument to extract the obstructing substance. Unless the patient is flaccid or intentionally paralysed, a bite block should be carefully inserted to maintain an open mouth prior to inserting one's finger. If the patient is conscious, tell the patient what you are doing and why and solicit their cooperation. While most conscious patients should be able to clear their own airway, the patient with a high spinal injury may asphyxiate from an easily remediable problem while fully awake. Patients with altered levels of consciousness are also at risk.

Vomiting is an ever-present danger to the injured patient. One deep inhalation with the posterior pharynx awash in vomit may be fatal to a patient already suffering from multiple trauma. Anticipation is essential. Manoeuvres used to open the airway, such as removal of blood or other secretions and foreign bodies, may stimulate the gag reflex, resulting in the sudden appearance of large amounts of vomitus in the mouth. Vomiting also occurs spontaneously and during placement of endotracheal and nasoenteric tubes. Depending on when and what the patient last ate, vomitus may not be retrievable via suction. Particulate matter may obstruct (and reobstruct) the suction tube as the patient struggles to get air. This is a particularly difficult and not uncommon situation in the multiply injured patient. Because aspiration of vomitus can rapidly lead to hypoxaemia, chemical pneumonitis and death, immediate measures to protect the airway must be instituted. The patient should be tipped head down or turned as a unit to the exaggerated lateral or semiprone position to allow the vomit to drain out of and away from the airway. This is facilitated by proper backboard immobilization. If the patient is properly immobilized, the backboard can be lifted and rotated, thereby protecting the spine from undue motion. If the patient is not confined to a backboard, assistance should be sought to safely turn and maintain the patient in a position with spinal alignment. The upper airway should be suctioned and further vomiting anticipated. While in a protected position, a nasogastric tube should be passed and the stomach emptied. If the vomitus is thick and particulate, passage of a nasogastric tube at this point is superfluous and only likely to stimulate further vomiting. If aspiration is suspected, immediate tracheal intubation is indicated to aid retrieval of the offending fluid.

The airway may also be directly injured by either blunt or penetrating forces. If the patient survives to reach the hospital but is in respiratory distress, high-flow oxygen should be provided through a non-rebreather mask and preparation made to gently place an endotracheal tube under direct vision. Means for placement of a surgical

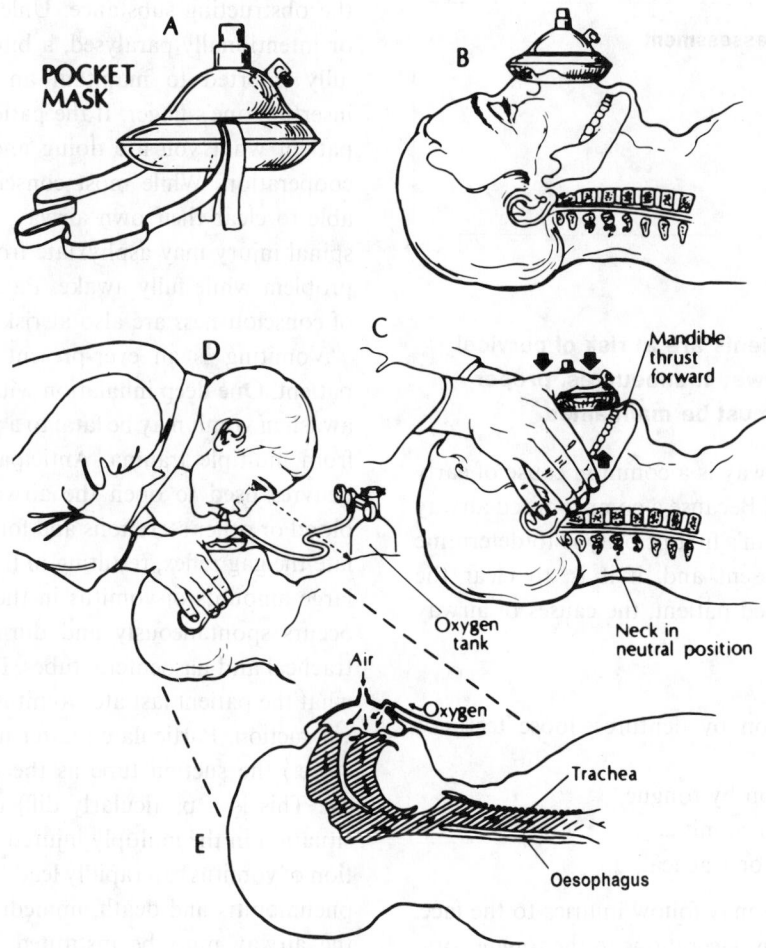

Fig. 2. Diagram demonstrating the combination of the jaw thrust manoeuvre and mouth-to-mask breathing – an excellent technique to open the airway, maintain cervical spine immobilization and provide adequate volumes of oxygen-enriched ventilation.

airway should be at hand. Ideally, patients with suspected airway injury should be managed in the operating room where definitive repair of the injury may be necessary and life-saving.

All of the potential threats to the airway cited thus far can occur regardless of the level of responsiveness of the patient. However, in the unresponsive patient, the airway is most commonly obstructed by the tongue dropping posteriorly and occluding the posterior oropharynx. This may lead to complete or partial obstruction to the flow of air into the trachea. In either situation, the patient is in jeopardy and the problem can be readily corrected by bringing the mandible forward. In the injured patient the safest technique is to use the jaw thrust manoeuvre while maintaining cervical alignment (Fig. 2). If this relieves the obstruction as measured by the return of adequate ventilatory effort, a patent upper airway may be sustained by use of an oropharyngeal or nasopharyngeal tube. Both tubes are effective but must be placed properly.

The oropharyngeal tube is especially hazardous if inserted incorrectly. Lacerations to the palate and posterior impaction of the tongue can occur. Both of these complications may be avoided by placing the oropharyngeal tube under direct vision with the tongue brought forward and depressed. If breathing is still difficult, the device should be immediately removed. In order to further protect the airway from induced vomiting, oropharyngeal tubes should not be placed in patients with an intact gag reflex. The nasopharyngeal tube is less hazardous but must be well lubricated and passed gently along the floor of the nasopharynx. Passage is not possible in some patients with nasal septal deviation.

In some trauma patients, these basic airway measures supplemented by high-flow (15 litres min^{-1}) oxygen via a reservoir mask will be sufficient to ensure an airway and adequate oxygenation. In others, placement of a definitive airway will be required. A *definitive airway* is defined as an inflated cuffed tube in the trachea.

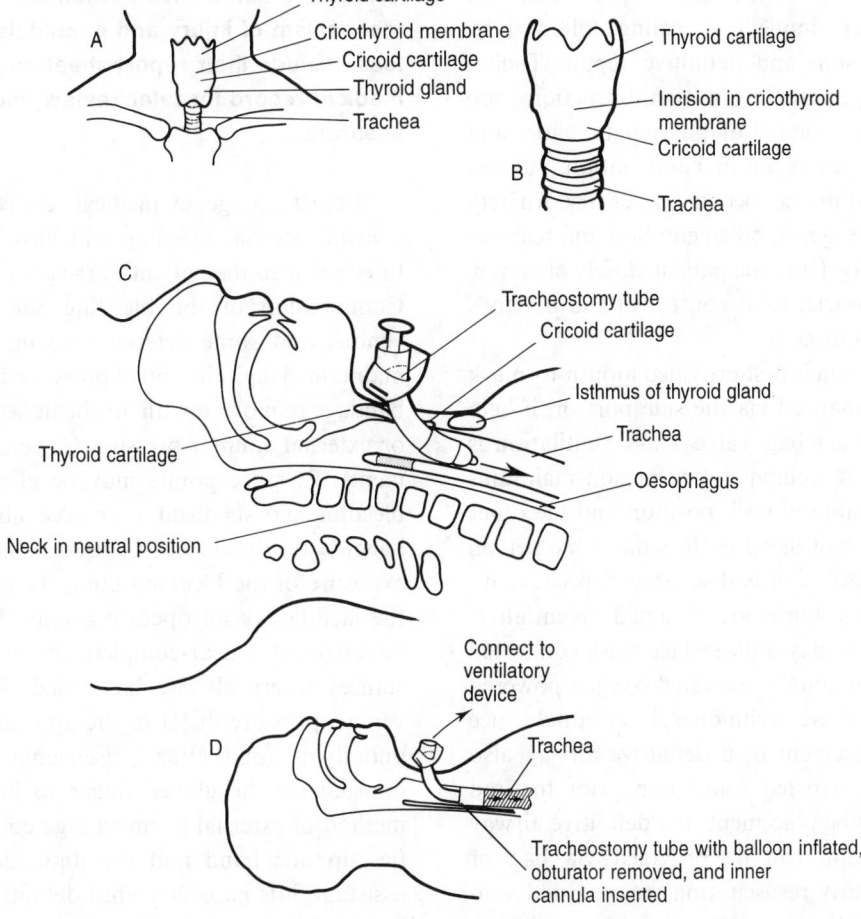

Fig. 3. Diagram showing sequential steps in performing surgical cricothyroidostomy.

Definitive airways may be placed orally, nasally or surgically through the cricothyroid membrane or trachea. The selection of the oral or nasal route depends first and foremost on the skill and confidence of the physician. In general, nasotracheal intubation is restricted to breathing patients and is contraindicated in patients with significant facial injury. It is especially useful in a patient with known unstable cervical spine fracture because passage of the tube is facilitated by maintaining a neutral position of the neck. Nasotracheal intubation may be readily accomplished in an awake patient without the need for muscle relaxants. The same is not always true for the oral route, especially if the patient is uncooperative. The oral route is safe provided in-line immobilization of the cervical spine is preserved by an assistant. Following the placement of either an oral or nasal tube, the tube must be properly positioned and secured in place. Breath sounds should be audible in both hemithoraces and absent over the epigastrium. Tube placement should be confirmed by chest radiography.

Occasionally the physician will need to secure a surgical airway. Cricothyroidotomy is the preferred emergency surgical airway. Provided that the external landmarks are properly identified, the technique is quick and safe (Fig. 3). Need for a definitive airway and inability to place one via the oral or nasal route constitute the sole indication for emergency cricothyroidotomy.

Breathing

Ensuring oxygenation of the patient is a two-step process. Opening the airway of an apnoeic patient does little unless ventilation is provided!

The most urgent determination made in the primary survey is whether or not the patient is breathing. If the answer to this question is affirmative, adequacy of ventilation must be immediately assessed. The chest is observed for the characteristic rise and fall, and the rate and labour of breathing are identified. Open wounds of the chest wall require immediate sealing, followed by early lung re-expansion and definitive repair. Tachypnoea, asymmetry, paradoxical motion, retractions, use of accessory muscles, isolated diaphragmatic effort and peripheral cyanosis, alone or in combination, suggest that assisted ventilation may become necessary. Anxiety is often profound. Oxygen supplementation and reassurance should be provided and the patient closely observed. If the patient is apnoeic, total control of the patient's ventilation is mandatory.

Immediate ventilation is best provided mouth-to-mask with oxygen flow enhanced via the side port or, if help is available, two-rescuer bag–valve–mask ventilation is recommended. In this technique, one person maintains mask seal and neutrality of neck position and the other person squeezes the bag using both hands. One-person bag–valve–mask ventilation is discouraged because insufficient ventilatory volumes are obtained. As an alternative, a single rescuer may utilize a face mask connected to a flow-restricted manually operated oxygen-powered device. Mastery of these techniques is essential since patients needing placement of a definitive airway also need either total or assisted ventilation prior to (and sometimes during) tube placement. If a definitive airway is in place, ventilation can be provided via bag or ventilator. During early resuscitation, bag-assisted ventilation is favoured because the physician can more readily detect changes in airway resistance.

Circulation

Shock is a state of impaired perfusion. In the injured patient, the physician's concern relates to the loss of integrity of the vascular system. Although there are several types of shock and all can be seen in the multiply injured patient at one time or another, control of bleeding and volume replenishment are paired very much as airway and breathing are. Just as a clear airway is a precondition to providing effective ventilation, similarly one must stop the bleeding if volume replenishment is to succeed. Bleeding can be arbitrarily divided into *external bleeding* and *internal bleeding*. It is easy to underestimate external blood loss in a hypotensive patient arriving in the emergency unit with major lacerations. Bleeding is often minimal and evidence of active haemorrhage remains at the scene. While it is sometimes difficult to accurately determine the amount of blood lost at an incident, field providers can estimate severity of haemorrhage in general terms.

Talk to the ambulance personnel to define mechanism of injury and quantitate external blood loss. Include their report sheet as part of the medical record for later review and quality assurance.

In most emergency medical service systems, efforts to control external bleeding will have already been instituted prior to the patient's arrival in the emergency unit. Compression of the bleeding site will control most venous and some arterial bleeding. Pressure may be maintained digitally with a pressure dressing (plain gauze bandage reinforced with an elastic wrap), with air splints or external counter-pressure (pneumatic antishock garment). Pressure points may be effective when arterial bleeding persists distal to an accessible pulse. Clamps or haemostats should not be used without careful surgical exposure of the bleeding point. Generally, this requires the facilities of an operating suite. Tourniquets should be restricted to near-complete amputations or to circumstances where all else has failed. Tourniquets elevate venous pressure distal to the application site and crush underlying (and already ischaemic) tissues. It is not unusual for the gloved finger to be the only effective method of external haemorrhage control. Although this ties up one hand and the undivided attention of an assistant, it is necessary until definitive control of bleeding can be rendered.

External and internal bleeding may coexist. There are two pitfalls in this circumstance. The physician may underestimate the severity of bleeding and/or attribute the patient's blood loss strictly to external sources, thereby delaying diagnosis and management of internal injury. The converse is also true. The physician may overestimate the magnitude of internal bleeding by failing to appreciate the actual volume of external blood loss, leading to overaggressive management of the internal bleeding. With the exception of pelvic fracture haemorrhage, which may require external fixation or angiographic embolization, most internal bleeding requires operative management. Therefore, it is not only important to be able to estimate accurately the amount of blood lost but it is also helpful to distinguish the likely sites of bleeding. However, a definitive diagnosis is not established during the primary assessment. Instead, the physician seeks the early signs of shock to guide resuscitation. The rate and quality of the pulse, the temperature, colour and condition of the skin and the patient's responsiveness provide initial signals. Tachycardia and a weak thready pulse are reliable compensatory signs. Pallor and cool moist skin confirm impaired perfusion. While most injured patients are distressed, the anxiety of the patient in shock cannot be easily relieved.

Shock in the injured patient is not always due to blood loss. While hypovolaemia is common enough to be regarded as a 'working diagnosis' in the hypotensive patient, shock from other sources kills just as quickly. The status of the neck veins is a clinical sign which can assist in distinguishing between the potential aetiologies of shock and should be looked for early. The cervical immobilization collar is removed to allow visualization of the anterior surface of the neck. If awake, the patient is instructed to remain still during the inspection. In the combative patient, an assistant manually immobilizes the neck during this part of the examination. Neck vein distension reflects increased venous pressure and, when present in a hypotensive patient, is strongly suggestive of a cause other than hypovolaemia. Tension pneumothorax elevates venous pressure by increasing intrathoracic pressure and displacing the mediastinum to the side opposite the pneumothorax, creating torsion of the major veins in the superior mediastinum. In pericardial tamponade and blunt cardiac injury, venous return is impeded by compression of the cardiac chambers and by loss of myocardial contractility, respectively. Tension pneumothorax and pericardial tamponade require immediate decompression.

If shock is confirmed, suspected or anticipated, intravascular volume is restored promptly and the patient's response to therapy is monitored. Baseline vital signs are recorded before, during and after intravenous fluids are administered. Vascular access is gained via forearm veins unless ipsilateral axillary or supraclavicular injury exists. Alternative sites include the opposite upper extremity and/or external jugular vein, lower extremity (saphenous) veins by direct catheterization or cut-down, or proximal femoral, subclavian or internal jugular approaches by Seldinger or other practised technique. In general, peripheral venous access sites are favoured because they are safer and readily available. In children peripheral sites should be sought first and accessed by cut-down if necessary. Intraosseous cannulation is an alternative technique in the infant and young child. Large-bore catheters (14 gauge) should be used in the adult; the selection of catheters in children should be age-specific.

Central venous cannulation may be used as a primary route for volume resuscitation. Experience with the technique is the principle determinant of both successful placement and incidence of complications. While many physicians favour centrally placed high-flow (8Fr) catheters because they can serve as both resuscitation and monitoring lines, it is recommended that all lines placed in an emergency setting be changed within 24 h to avoid intravenous line sepsis. High-flow lines can also be placed through a peripheral vein. The incidence of pneumothorax is reduced if the central line is placed after intravascular volume is restored.

At the time of vascular access, blood is drawn for blood bank use and baseline laboratory studies. Infusion rates, types of fluid and the need for blood and/or blood products depend on the patient's clinical status, especially the estimated blood loss. In turn, this calculation is based on the physician's initial clinical impression, the vital signs and the mechanism of injury, if known. Because significant blood loss can occur before there is a reduction in blood pressure, it is important to recognize the early signs of shock and to institute treatment accordingly. This is particularly true in the pregnant patient where the mother's condition may appear stable while placental flow is curtailed through compensatory mechanisms. Tachycardia, peripheral vasoconstriction and narrowed pulse pressure are early manifestations of hypovolaemia. In the adult, a rapid initial 2 litre fluid bolus is provided (20 ml kg^{-1} in the child). Further therapy is guided by clinical response.

Determination of level of responsiveness

This assessment is performed early and forms part of the physician's initial impression. The talking patient declares a clear airway, adequate ventilation and intact cerebral perfusion. While nothing is implied about stability by having the patient talk, other priorities can be assessed. The patient who is not talking at the time of arrival in the emergency unit must be evaluated for level of responsiveness. The most critical determination is whether the patient is able to follow commands. This confirms that high cerebral integrative function is intact. The mnemonic AVPU is a useful matrix to translate level of responsiveness. If the patient is Alert the patient is talking and following commands. The patient who is not spontaneously responsive but reacts to the spoken voice is defined as responsive to Vocal stimulus. If the patient does not react to the spoken voice, reaction to a Painful stimulus is determined and described. The description should include what painful stimulus is being applied and where. In the motionless patient, the painful stimulus should be applied above and below the clavicles. Failure to react to a painful stimulus confirms that the patient is Unresponsive.

Mnemonic for level of responsiveness

A	Alert
V	Vocal stimulus
P	Painful stimulus
U	Unresponsive

Determination of level of responsiveness is done early in the initial assessment and repeated during the subsequent course of management. If responsiveness is impaired at any level, it must be accounted for. Close monitoring is essential to follow trends and determine effectiveness of resuscitation.

Evaluation

At this point, the physician has formed an initial impression and taken steps to address life-threatening problems detected during the initial assessment. The patient is undressed completely to expose additional injuries. Leads are attached to the patient and connected to an appropriate cardiac monitor. A pulse oximeter is attached to a convenient site. Provided suitable precautions are taken, this is often a convenient time to place the nasogastric tube and urinary catheter. Radiographs of the cervical spine, chest and pelvis are obtained for later review. Thus far, much of what has been done to and for the patient was based on physical assessment and mechanism of injury. Additional historical information may be pertinent to the interpretation of physical findings and guide further therapy.

The history may be obtained from the patient, family, friends or bystanders. If the patient is unresponsive or under the influence of alcohol or other drugs, it may not be possible to elicit an accurate history from the patient. Anyone who accompanied the patient to the hospital should be requested to remain until they can be debriefed. When there are no witnesses and the patient cannot communicate, efforts should be made to contact family members for both notification and information. Injuries occur in a multiplicity of settings, both lawful and unlawful. Circumstances of the trauma incident must be taken into account in determining the reliability of the history, regardless of the source. The history follows the mnemonic AMPLE. Because medications may need to be administered early in the management of the patient, it is important to know whether the patient has any Allergies or is taking any Medications.

The Past history, both medical and surgical, should be described in detail. The time of the Last meal should be noted. Circumstances surrounding the Event – the trauma incident – should also be described in detail, including the condition of the patient immediately before and after the trauma incident, injuries or deaths of others, and information that clarifies the mechanism of injury.

Mnemonic for history taking

A	Allergies
M	Medications
P	Past history
L	Last meal
E	Event – circumstances surrounding the trauma incident

Secondary assessment

The secondary assessment is an organized approach to the injured patient that provides a rapid and reproducible physical examination to detect and follow injuries to all body systems. It is easy for the clinician to get distracted by spectacular injuries yet it is often the subtle findings that have the more important implications for the well-being of the patient. If one deviates from a standardized method of assessment, omissions may occur and lead to missed diagnoses. Radiological studies supplement the clinical assessment and are specific to the patient's symptoms and physical signs elicited by the examining physician. While films of the cervical spine, chest and pelvis are recommended in all multiply injured patients, the 'shotgun' approach to X-ray studies is neither useful nor cost-effective. During the secondary assessment, careful reassessment of the airway, adequacy of ventilation and response to volume loading should be performed in all unstable patients.

Each body system is considered to be injured until injury is excluded by appropriate examination.

The secondary assessment utilizes the skills of inspection, palpation and auscultation. Inspection requires total exposure of the patient, good lighting and access to the back of the patient as well as the front. Injuries have been missed simply by failing to look at the patient's posterior surface. It is also easy to misinterpret minor external wounds which may belie deeper more serious injury. Palpation should be done gently and is used to detect tenderness in the responsive patient, responsiveness in the unconscious patient and instability of the body part. Careful palpation can define the nature and extent of the injury and direct further analysis. Auscultation is used for determining blood pressure and examining the lungs and vascular system.

Secondary assessment begins at the top of the patient and proceeds inferiorly. Although the patient's condition dictates the rapidity of the secondary assessment, in general the secondary assessment is time well spent.

Head

The head is inspected for external signs of injury. Contusions over the skull indicate direct trauma and increase the likelihood of underlying brain injury. Contusion over the mastoid (Battle's sign) indicates basilar skull fracture. A tender swelling in the scalp most commonly represents a subgaleal haematoma with or without an underlying skull fracture. Scalp lacerations bleed profusely and quickly saturate the hair. Copious amounts of blood may emanate from a relatively small laceration and obscure the bleeding site. This is particularly problematic in long-haired individuals. Nonetheless, the laceration should be identified and palpated carefully with the gloved finger to detect interruption in the continuity of underlying bone. If bleeding is incompletely controlled by a compression dressing applied tightly to the skull, clips may be applied to the edges of the laceration to control persistent haemorrhage. The potential blood loss from an uncontrolled major scalp laceration is great. A few moments spent to stop scalp bleeding will pay dividends later. The ears are checked closely for signs of injury. Bleeding from the external auditory meatus with or without Battle's sign suggests a fracture through the base of the skull. Unilateral deafness of acute onset is also suggestive. Otoscopic examination may differentiate internal disruption from laceration of the external canal but is often inconclusive. Leakage of cerebrospinal fluid (CSF) should be suspected in all patients with bloody otorrhoea. If CSF is present, a drop of discharge placed on filter paper will demonstrate a central dense red area surrounded by a lighter zone (ring sign). Pinnal lacerations may result in significant morbidity if they become infected. A sterile dressing should be applied and early definitive repair is indicated.

Face

The function of the face is to appear normal. Injuries to the face range from the subtle, obvious only to the patient, to the dramatic with life-threatening consequences. The face is inspected for symmetry and external signs of injury. Contusions may indicate underlying fracture. Periorbital ecchymosis commonly accompanies orbital or other facial fracture, or basilar skull fracture. If injury has occurred about the eyes, vision is checked individually by having the patient read anything with large print while covering one eye and then the other. The eyes are inspected for pupillary size and symmetry and any abnormality is noted. Direct and consensual reactivity to light is recorded. If abnormality is present, a fundoscopic examination is indicated to seek evidence of direct ocular injury or papilloedema. At times, periorbital swelling may close the eye and make examination difficult. Nonetheless, it is essential to determine vision status, which may require an assistant to gently separate the eyelids. Unilateral drooping of the eyelid may indicate Horner's syndrome and point toward blunt neck injury. The nose is inspected and palpated for swelling and deformity. Haemorrhage from the nares has the same significance as otorrhoea and may reflect dural tear with CSF leakage (CSF rhinorrhoea). However, nasal bleeding is commonly from other sources. The oropharynx is inspected and palpated with the proviso that the awake patient is cooperative. The patient is requested to put the teeth together and asked whether occlusion is normal. The patient will readily determine any difference from their preinjury state. Mucosal disruptions usually indicate underlying bony injury and bleeding is often brisk. The patient is asked to extrude the tongue to detect injury or deviation. Tongue lacerations do not have the same significance as mucosal defects but also bleed actively. Be mindful that oropharyngeal and nasopharyngeal bleeding put staff at risk from blood spraying from the patient. Lacerations of the face also tend to bleed actively and may require direct pressure for control. If branches of the facial nerve are at risk, the patient should be asked to raise the brow, squint, smile and contract the platysma by example to document possible nerve injury.

The face should be palpated carefully, moving from orbit to zygoma to maxilla to mandible, palpating both sides simultaneously to detect palpable differences in the bony landmarks. Tenderness, irregularity, crepitus and motion imply underlying fracture. Although facial injuries cause anxiety in the patient, definitive management can usually be safely delayed until other priorities have been addressed.

Neck

The neck occupies a small area in size but contains structures of vital importance to the patient's survival. The neck is also a tightly contained space with limited potential to accommodate added volume or pressure. The neck is assessed by inspection, palpation and auscultation. The first impediment to neck assessment is the cervical immobilization collar. This must be removed to perform an adequate neck examination. Measures to sustain cervical spine immobilization during the neck examination include patient cooperation or manual stabilization by an assistant. The neck is visualized to detect swelling, asymmetry and other external signs of trauma. Neck vein fullness indirectly reflects response to volume replacement or may be a more ominous telltale sign. Neck swelling of even modest extent should be regarded as potentially life-threatening and airway compromise anticipated. The neck is palpated, beginning at the posterior midline superiorly and moving inferiorly. Each vertebral level is gently felt to determine the existence of tenderness or irregularity. If present, a cervical spine fracture is presumed. The lateral and anterior neck are palpated in sequence, and the position of the trachea is determined. The stethoscope is placed directly over each carotid artery to determine the presence or absence of bruits. An audible bruit detected after a deceleration crash may be the only early sign of a carotid artery injury. At the completion of the examination, the cervical immobilization collar is replaced.

Radiographs of the lateral cervical spine provide valuable initial screening information but do not constitute a complete examination. If pain, tenderness and neurological signs are lacking, the likelihood of a significant cervical spine injury is remote. In the unresponsive patient and the patient with multiple other painful injuries, completion of the cervical spine series (anteroposterior and odontoid views) is recommended. Presence of a cervical spine fracture increases the likelihood of other spinal injury and complete spinal radiographic studies are indicated.

Chest

The chest is reassessed for adequacy of ventilation, symmetry, paradoxical motion and external signs of trauma. Determine whether there has been any progression of earlier findings and re-check the cardiac monitor. Paradoxical chest wall motion indicates underlying flail chest. The larger the unstable segment, the more severe the injury it represents. Although a chest radiograph may show multiple fractures, this diagnosis is based strictly on clinical findings. These patients almost always worsen as they tire. Anticipate the possible need for tracheal intubation and positive pressure ventilation. Also anticipate the presence of associated pulmonary contusion. Volume replacement must be carefully adjusted in patients with pulmonary contusion to address actual needs from volume loss. Overzealous fluid administration during resuscitation may lead to significant and potentially fatal consequences later.

Look for the deepened hue over the upper chest, neck and face from traumatic asphyxia. Facial petechiae and proptosis offer a frightening presentation and represent consequences of sudden thoracic compression with a closed glottis. Other intrathoracic injuries may coexist. The chest wall should be gently palpated for tenderness and/or crepitus and, if present, rib fracture suspected. Placement of the palms of both hands over the chest wall is useful to determine equality of chest wall expansion and tactile signs of retained secretions. Breath sounds should be compared side-to-side for uniformity. The presence of adventitious sounds signifies difficulty in handling secretions, lower airway obstruction or direct injury to the lung or bronchi. If breath sounds are absent or significantly diminished on one side, pneumothorax and/or haemothorax may be present. Percussion of the chest wall may help distinguish between pneumothorax (hyper-resonant percussion note) and haemothorax (dull percussion note). Unless tension pneumothorax is suspected or the patient's clinical condition warrants, treatment follows radiographic confirmation.

Tension pneumothorax is treated by needle decompression and tube thoracostomy based strictly on clinical suspicion. The patient with increasing respiratory distress, absent breath sounds, distended neck veins, displaced or absent point of maximum cardiac intensity and shock warrants immediate decompression. All of these signs need not be present to institute treatment. Because collapse of the lung and bleeding into the pleural space often coexist, lateral chest tube placement is the approach of choice in the injured patient (Fig. 4). A large-bore tube (32Fr or larger in the adult) is selected and placed at the nipple level between the anterior and midaxillary lines. If the tube is placed too far posteriorly, it may kink or become dislodged and the patient experiences added discomfort. This is already a painful procedure and well remembered by patients after the event. Consistent with the patient's condition, take time to administer sufficient local anaesthesia and reassure the patient prior to tube insertion.

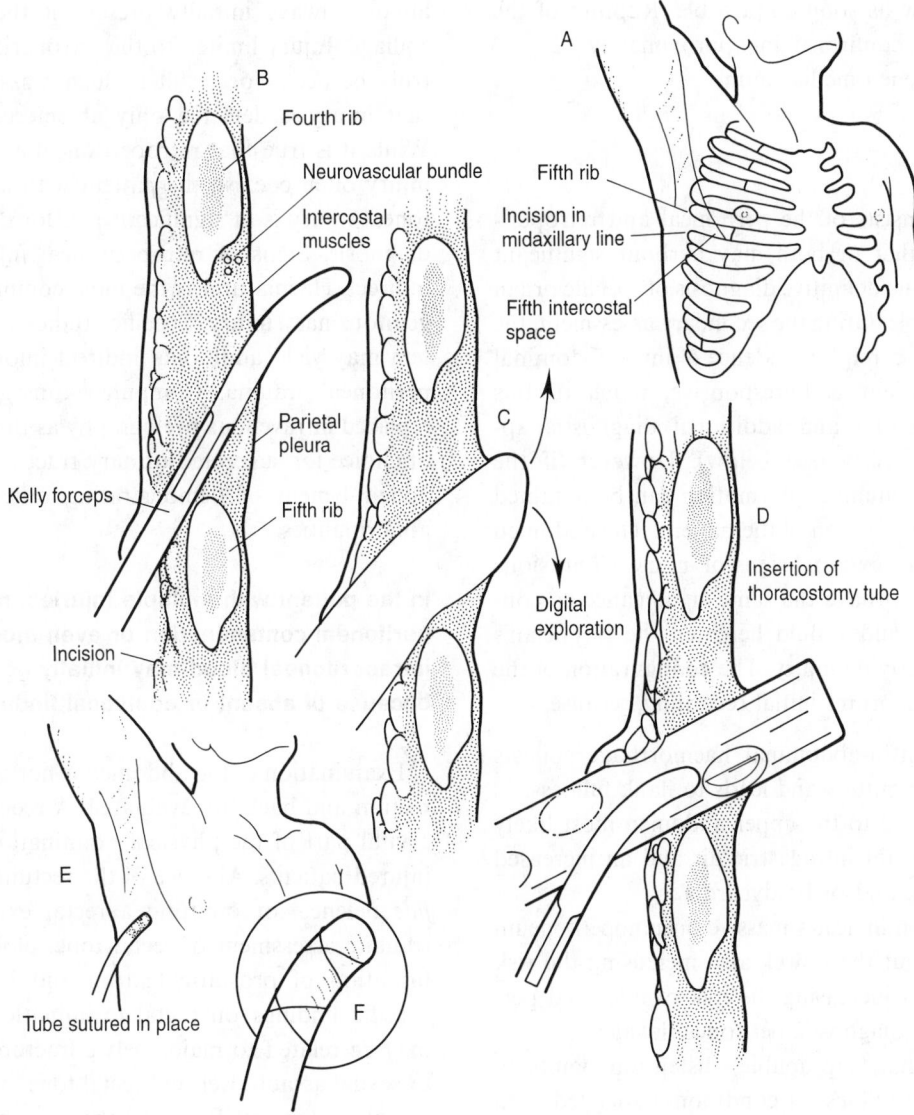

Fig. 4. Diagram showing preferred technique for performing tube thoracostomy.

If the chest tube is placed for haemothorax, the rate of egress of blood and the initial and ongoing loss determine the need for definitive operative management. Blood in the pleural space is analogous to external haemorrhage and is lost to the vascular compartment. Volume replacement must be just as vigorous for haemothorax as for bleeding elsewhere. Although most patients with haemothorax do not require further invasive management beyond evacuation of pleural blood and pulmonary re-expansion, intrapleural blood signifies injury within the thorax and an explanation should be sought. Rib fracture(s) with laceration of intercostal vessels account for the majority of significant haemothoraces. Bleeding from the pulmonary parenchyma usually ceases spontaneously because pulmonary vascular pressure is comparatively low. However, more serious trauma may be present. The initial supine chest film, while far from definitive, serves as an early guide. The mediastinum warrants careful inspection in all trauma patients. Suspicion of a widened mediastinum on a supine film should first be confirmed on an upright film if the patient's condition allows. Rupture of the thoracic aorta occurs most commonly following deceleration. Therefore, patients injured in high-speed automobile crashes are at risk for this injury and, if they reach the hospital alive, are at grave risk of sudden death. Although transoesophageal echography has advocates, most physicians believe prompt aortography is necessary to diagnose the injury. Operation should follow as soon as possible. Rupture of the thoracic aorta is confirmed in approximately 15% of patients with widened mediastinum.

Abdomen

The abdomen consists of the peritoneal and retroperitoneal spaces. Either or both may harbour significant haemorrhage. While definitive diagnosis of specific organ injury is not possible during the secondary assessment, the physician should search for evidence of intra-abdominal injury. If the patient is unresponsive, much of this evidence is inferential and additional diagnostic approaches are necessary (see below). However, if the patient is awake, valuable information can be obtained from a careful examination of the patient. The abdomen is first inspected for external signs of injury. Contusions across the abdomen have the same significance as contusions elsewhere and should heighten the physician's awareness of underlying injury. The configuration of the abdomen is an important initial recording because:

- Uncontrolled intra-abdominal haemorrhage collects in the paracolic gutters and leads to flank fullness.
- Distension limited to the upper abdomen most likely indicates significant intragastric air and an increased risk of vomiting and/or bradycardia.
- Global distension indicates massive pneumoperitoneum or air throughout the bowel, also increasing the risk of vomiting and increasing the risk of intestinal perforation during diagnostic peritoneal lavage.
- Lower abdominal (suprapubic) distension points to urinary bladder fullness, a condition associated with spinal injury or disruption at the bladder neck or urethra.

Scars confirm previous wounds and/or operations and may limit or alter the diagnostic approach.

Intra-abdominal air or gas can be readily distinguished from fluid by percussion. The latter yields a dull percussion note while air or gas is tympanitic. Percussion is also useful for the detection of intra-abdominal tenderness. Percussion tenderness, whether diffuse or limited to a specific area or quadrant, indicates underlying peritoneal irritation and has the same significance as rebound tenderness. The abdomen is palpated to determine the presence of direct tenderness. Blood is an irritant to the peritoneum but it may not be manifest immediately, especially if the patient has multiple other painful injuries. By contrast, disruption of a hollow viscus leads to immediate peritoneal inflammation and tenderness is almost always initially present if there is significant spillage. Injury limited to the retroperitoneal space may truly be occult or result in such massive haemorrhage that injury is detected only at emergency coeliotomy. While it is true that retroperitoneal and intraperitoneal injury often coexist, the patient with isolated retroperitoneal injury is at significant risk for delayed or missed diagnosis. Signs of retroperitoneal injury are, at best, indirect. Haematuria is the most common and indicates genitourinary injury. Specific studies of the urinary system may yield additional indirect information of retroperitoneal trauma. Computed tomography (CT) has replaced intravenous pyelography as the diagnostic study of choice for suspected urinary tract injury and has the added benefit of demonstrating other retroperitoneal abnormalities.

In the patient with multiple injuries, minimal peritoneal contamination or even moderate intraperitoneal blood may initially go undetected because of absent or equivocal findings.

Examination of the abdomen is not complete until the rectum and back are evaluated. A rectal examination is a vital part of the physical examination of all multiply injured patients. Absence of the rectum is the only *bona fide* defence for omitting a rectal examination. Local trauma, assessment of rectal tone, blood, and the confirmation of prostatic texture and location comprise specific findings on rectal examination. Local trauma may be related to major pelvic fracture, straddle injury or sexual assault. Relaxed rectal tone may signify serious spinal cord injury. Blood on the examining gloved finger is a significant finding. It should alert the physician to the possibility of injury to the rectum or more proximal bowel. This is not an uncommon finding in patients with penetrating trauma or pelvic fractures. Regardless of the aetiology, the finding of rectal blood calls for further study to elucidate the site and cause. Anoscopy and proctosigmoidoscopy may disclose the nature of the problem. A rectal examination should be performed prior to insertion of the urinary catheter and, if urethral injury is suspected, a gentle retrograde urethrogram should guide the method of establishing urinary drainage. In women, a pelvic examination is also essential. Bleeding from the vagina should not be dismissed as menses until direct injury to the vagina has been excluded by an adequate speculum examination.

The posterior surface of the patient can hide significant physical findings. While this is especially true in patients

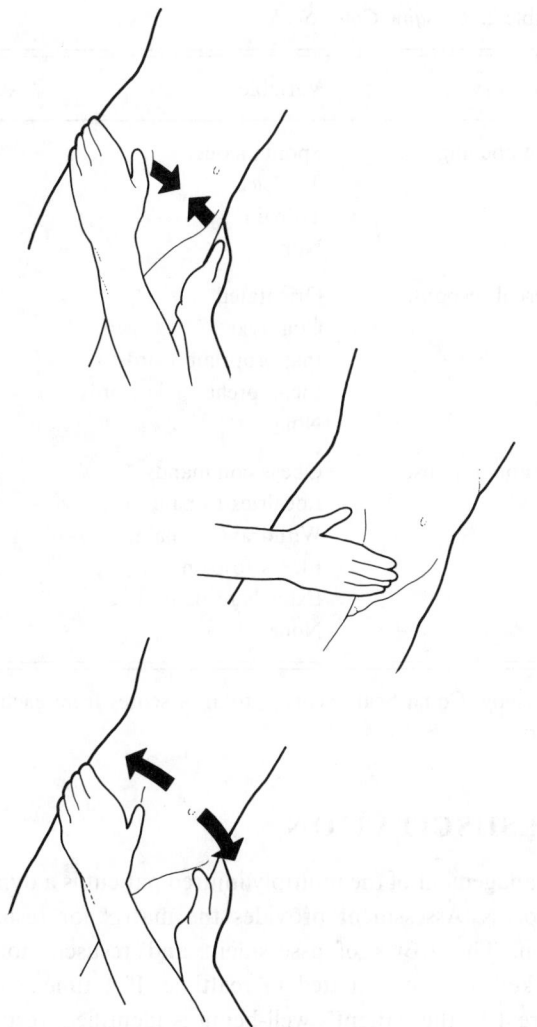

Fig. 5. Examination for pelvic stability. This method includes gentle manual compression and distraction of the iliac wings and ballottement of the pubis.

with penetrating injuries (e.g. entrance or exit wounds), it is also true for other injured patients as well. The patient should be carefully rolled as a unit, first to one side, then to the opposite side. The back should be inspected and palpated for indications of injury. If an unstable spinal injury is identified, this part of the examination may be limited to careful palpation in the supine position until stabilization of the spinal injury is accomplished.

Injuries to the pelvis are seen following motor vehicle/pedestrian impacts, motorcycle and motor vehicle crashes, falls and crush injuries. These injuries may be severe and associated with massive bleeding. The patient will complain of pain in the region of the pelvis and tenderness will be elicited by the compression–distraction manoeuvre (Fig. 5). This must be done gently and, once confirmed,

the unstable pelvis should be protected from further motion. All unstable pelvic fractures are accompanied by venous bleeding and some by bleeding from both venous and arterial sources. Undue motion aggravates bleeding regardless of origin. Laceration of the perineum indicates an open pelvic fracture until proven otherwise. Such patients are at added risk of blood loss and later complications.

Because of the limitations of the physical examination of the injured patient, additional diagnostic techniques have emerged to provide confirmation if injury is suspected. These diagnostic techniques include diagnostic peritoneal lavage, abdominal ultrasonography, CT, angiography and, most recently, diagnostic laparoscopy. In turn, each have their own limitations and/or complications.

Extremities

Musculoskeletal injuries account for over 50% of injuries following blunt trauma. Although less likely than torso injuries to pose an immediate threat to life, extremity injuries cause considerable morbidity, especially if missed or managed improperly. As with trauma to other systems, the unresponsive patient is at particular risk for missed musculoskeletal injuries. In order to maximize the opportunity for diagnosis, each extremity should be closely inspected and palpated for abnormality and compared level-by-level with the opposite extremity. Tenderness, swelling, deformity, contusion, laceration, abnormal or absent sensation, pain with motion and abnormal positioning all signify the possibility of injury. Pulses should be assessed both proximally and distally and reassessed if realignment of a deformed extremity is performed. Obvious fractures should be immobilized, protected from further injury and stabilized early by the appropriate method. Compartment syndrome should be suspected if significant crush, comminution or compression occurred. Intact distal pulses do not exclude progressive muscle ischaemia.

Following clinical assessment of the injured part, radiographic evaluation is almost always indicated. While there is often debate about when in the scheme of things it is best to X-ray the extremities, there is no argument that taking appropriate and adequate films the first time can save valuable time. It is essential to survey the extremity from the proximal joint through the joint distal to the injury and to take views best suited to the type of injury. Occasionally, the standard radiographic approach to an injury will be insufficient to guide treatment and special views or additional diagnostic adjuncts may be necessary. Knowing the mechanism of injury can assist in identifying associated musculoskeletal injuries:

- Joints above and below a long bone fracture.
- Fall on outstretched hand – fractures from wrist to shoulder.
- Fall from height – calcaneal fracture and lumbar spine compression fracture.
- Femoral shaft fracture and pelvic fracture.

Although there is a tendency to dismiss or delay both the assessment and the definitive management of extremity injuries until internal injuries have been excluded, early involvement of the orthopaedic team is important in order to prioritize treatment of musculoskeletal trauma, reduce pain and prevent morbidity.

Neurological

Brain and spinal cord injuries are common, frequently life-threatening and, if survived, may lead to serious and life-long impairments. Therefore, not only is early diagnosis important, but prevention of secondary neurological injury assumes increasing relevance. Since hypotension and hypoxia are the greatest enemies of the neurologically impaired trauma patient, careful monitoring of the patient's blood pressure and level of oxygenation is essential.

Central nervous system or peripheral nerve injuries may be suspected at various points during the performance of the secondary assessment but it is necessary to complete a focused neurological examination and document the findings. The neurological assessment of the injured patient begins with determination of responsiveness by the AVPU method (see above). Nowhere in the assessment of the patient is the concept of *reassessment* more important than in the determination of neurological impairment. Progressive impairment, whether in level of consciousness, level of paralysis, or other parameter, increases the priority for definitive neurological intervention. Therefore, defining objective neurological change and correcting its causation is a critical feature of trauma management. The focused neurological assessment of the injured patient consists of quantifying the level of responsiveness, pupillary examination and determining motor function in each extremity. In the unresponsive patient, the patient should be inspected for posturing. These observations, when considered together and weighted, constitute the Glasgow Coma Scale and have prognostic significance (Table 2).

Table 2. *Glasgow Coma Scale*

Category	Variable	Score
Eye opening	Spontaneous	4
	To voice	3
	To pain	2
	None	1
Verbal response	Orientated	5
	Confused	4
	Inappropriate words	3
	Incomprehensible words	2
	None	1
Motor response	Obeys commands	6
	Localizes to pain	5
	Withdraws to pain	4
	Flexes to pain	3
	Extends to pain	2
	None	1

Glasgow Coma Scale Score = total of scores from each category.

RESUSCITATION

Management of the multiply injured patient is a dynamic process. Assessment provides the matrix for resuscitation. The ABCs of assessment and resuscitation are linked and coordinated in realtime. If a time-sensitive threat to the patient's well-being is identified, resuscitative measures are begun immediately to address the threat. If the patient is not in immediate danger, the primary assessment is completed and resuscitation begun as the secondary assessment proceeds. Reassessment, monitoring and meticulous attention to the patient's therapeutic response guide modifications to the various resuscitative initiatives. It is the patient's clinical response that provides the key to whether resuscitative measures are right or wrong, adequate or inadequate, and whether the physician has time to complete the diagnostic work-up or must institute prompt definitive trauma care. It is useful to develop a mental checklist in order to stay organized and prevent omissions. At the completion of resuscitation, all patients should have specific minimal interventions in place (Table 3). Additional interventions may be indicated depending on the injuries. Confirming the effectiveness of these specific interventions is an important element of resuscitation. The clinician's checklist should include specific questions:

Table 3. *Basic interventions for resuscitation*

Open airway
Positioning
Airway adjuncts
Suction
Definitive airway

Ventilate
High-flow oxygen
Mouth-to-mask
Bag–valve–mask (two people)
Bag-to-tube (two hands)
Ventilator

Stop external bleeding
Compression
Pressure points
(Tourniquet)

Restore intravascular volume
Two 14 gauge IV catheters
High-flow (8Fr) lines
Cut-downs
Warmed crystalloids and blood

Prevent complications
Maintain immobilization
Insert nasogastric or orogastric tube
Insert urinary catheter
Maintain core temperature

Monitor
Vital signs
Urine output
Responsiveness
Central venous and/or pulmonary wedge pressure

IV, intravenous.

- Is the airway secure?
- Is the patient receiving adequate volumes of oxygen-enriched air?
- Are both lungs being ventilated?
- Is the effectiveness of the airway and ventilation reflected in the patient's overall condition and confirmed by arterial blood gas determinations and pulse oximetry?
- Is all external haemorrhage controlled?
- Is volume replenishment complete or is further fluid therapy needed to achieve the desired result?
- Are all tubes (urinary, nasogastric, etc.) in place and functional?

- Have baseline radiographs been completed, reviewed, and follow-up studies ordered?
- Most importantly, is the patient adequately monitored and improving?

While confirmation of airway and ventilatory manoeuvres is objectively assessed by laboratory parameters and oximetry, determining the response to volume replacement may not be quite as easy. The normalization of vital signs provides some reassurance but it is often useful to estimate blood loss by recognizing the signs of shock and classifying the hypovolaemic state according to the potential volume loss they represent. This serves as an important reminder that a drop in systolic blood pressure is actually a late sign of shock. For example, the previously normotensive anxious patient with a normal blood pressure but a narrowed pulse pressure and a heart rate of 110 min^{-1} may not alarm the casual observer. However, it is quite possible that the patient is 1.5 litres deficient and 4.5 litres is needed to reach baseline. Continuing blood loss increases the fluid needs. Replacement using the 'three-for-one' rule is based on the empirical observation that approximately 300 ml of crystalloid is needed for every 100 ml of blood loss. Clearly, the patient who responds to an initial fluid bolus only to have hypotension return is most likely to be bleeding and in need of definitive care.

Under most circumstances, definitive trauma care means operative care, in an operating room that is fully staffed and equipped to handle any and all unanticipated emergencies. Failure to respond to resuscitative measures dictates the need for early operation just as clearly as identifying an anatomical injury requiring surgical correction. At times, it is entirely appropriate for assessment and resuscitation to take place in the operating room.

There are pitfalls for the unwary. Whenever a resuscitative measure is followed by an unexpected or opposite response, the physician should suspect missed or mistaken diagnosis. For example, a patient intubated for airway obstruction who fails to improve and then regresses following the application of positive pressure ventilation may have an undetected tension pneumothorax worsened by assisted ventilations. The hypotensive patient who deteriorates while receiving vigorous volume replenishment for suspected exsanguination may have progressive pericardial tamponade unintentionally aggravated by fluid therapy. The physician must be equally dynamic in adjusting their thinking whenever the clinical reality does not fit with the working diagnosis. Another pitfall in resuscitation relates to the technical complications that may follow certain interventions. It is wise to remember that the physician who fails to admit to one mistake will be condemned to making many. What is important is to recognize that complications do occur, to learn from them and seek means to avoid them in the future. Steps taken to save time often cost time (and more!) if associated with increased patient risk. Pneumothorax following central line insertion is a case in point. This is a common emergency intervention. It is well established that the complication rate for central line insertion falls with experience. Since placement of the central catheter is easier if the veins are full, placement of central venous catheters should be limited to volume-resuscitated patients whenever possible. Since this is not always possible, added precautions should be taken to avoid pleural laceration in emergency situations. Because the physician is guided by the principle to do no further harm to the patient, the safe way is preferred.

Resuscitation merges imperceptibly with definitive care and, in many patients, continues throughout the specific interventions needed to stop haemorrhage, decompress expanding lesions, control contamination and the like.

STABILIZATION

The initial goal of assessment and resuscitation is to reach a steady-state in which the patient is no longer in immediate danger. This state is called stabilization and presents an opportunity to reassess the patient's post-injury course and response to treatment and begin to make decisions critical to subsequent trauma management. Careful monitoring is essential during stabilization to recognize injuries that may not have been apparent during the resuscitative phase. It is during the stabilization phase that treatment priorities are defined, consultation is sought for injuries in specific specialty areas, and decisions are made regarding the possible need for transfer. The decision to transfer a patient to another facility is based on the condition and specific needs of the patient, the hospital's capability and the availability of its staff. This is not always an easy question and the answer is not consistently obvious. The physician must make a judgement regarding the patient's ultimate outcome, do so often without definitive information and incur the added risk of transporting the injured patient long distances for specialized care. Therefore, the physician must decide whether specialty care and the unavoidable delay in providing such care defines prognosis or if immediate surgical care is of greater consequence. This decision varies from patient to patient but the

decision matrix is the same for all patients. It is important that the physician understand the capabilities of their own hospital and know the capabilities of the receiving facility as well.

In some trauma patients, stabilization without operation is unattainable. The decision in such patients is dictated by the urgency of the situation and the nature of the injuries. As a rule, unstable patients should not be transferred until measures have been taken to control whatever difficulty is causing the instability. In the small rural hospital this presents a dilemma, especially if the surgical capability is limited by lack of blood and other support services. Surgical input in these situations is mandatory.

A stable postoperative trauma patient is safer to transfer than an unstable patient in need of an operation.

Occasionally, a stable patient becomes unstable en route to a receiving facility. Although this circumstance cannot be predicted with certainty, it is often possible to anticipate the potential for in-transit problems and send a prepared crew.

DOCUMENTATION

The importance of timely and accurate record-keeping cannot be overstated. Although the circumstances of a trauma resuscitation tend to be rushed and involve numerous individuals performing many and varied activities to and for the patient, preplanning can overcome most of these problems. First, obtain as much information as possible before the patient arrives. Establish radio contact with ambulance personnel and obtain pertinent information. Appoint one person to serve as recorder during the resuscitation. Develop a form or flowsheet separate from the emergency unit record that follows the resuscitation protocols. This 'trauma resuscitation' form must have space for times (including prehospital times), mechanism of injury, nursing assessment, scoring, primary assessment parameters (multiple entries), intake and output, medications, laboratory data (requested and results), consultations (when called, when arrived) and disposition of the patient. Data and times entered on the trauma resuscitation form become part of the permanent medical record and, when completed appropriately, provide an accurate account of what happened, when and in which order.

It may also be useful to develop an in-patient form,

the 'trauma admission record'. This form may be completed in lieu of a handwritten or dictated history and physical examination. The trauma admission record follows the primary assessment/secondary assessment format and is completed by the physician. By preprinting each body region and potential abnormality on the record, the physician is reminded of what needs to be evaluated, checks off those that are normal and describes in detail specific injuries. When followed conscientiously, this approach significantly reduces incomplete medical records, provides more accurate data, and facilitates trauma registry data entry and quality assurance.

Bibliography

APRAHAMIAN, C. & MATEER, J.R. (1989). Prehospital trauma care. In *Advances in Trauma*, Vol. 4, ed. K. Maull, H. Cleveland, G. Strauch *et al.*, pp. 1–18. Chicago: Mosby Year Book.

BOYD, C.R. & MERRIMAN, S.J. (1990). Airway management in trauma. In *Advances in Trauma and Critical Care*, ed. K. Maull, H. Cleveland, D. Feliciano *et al.*, pp. 49–72. Chicago: Mosby Year Book.

COMMITTEE ON TRAUMA (1993). *Advanced Trauma Life Support Program for Physicians*, 5th edn. Chicago: American College of Surgeons.

COMMITTEE ON TRAUMA (1994). *Resources for Optimal Care of the Injured Patient*. Chicago: American College of Surgeons.

DUTKY, P.A., STEVENS, S.L. & MAULL, K.I. (1989). Factors affecting rapid fluid resuscitation with large-bore introducer catheters. *J. Trauma*, **29**, 856–60.

ENDERSON, B.L. & MAULL, K.I. (1991). Missed injuries: the trauma surgeon's nemesis. *Surg. Clin. North Am.*, **71**, 399–418.

ENDERSON, B.L., REATH, D.B., MEADORS, J. *et al.* (1990). The tertiary trauma survey: a prospective study of missed injury. *J. Trauma*, **30**, 666–70.

GENTILELLO, L.M. (1994). Practical approaches to hypothermia. In *Advances in Trauma and Critical Care*, ed. K. Maull, H. Cleveland, D. Feliciano *et al.*, pp. 39–79. Chicago: Mosby Year Book.

KIRBY, J. (1992). Kinematics. In *Trauma Update for the EMT*, ed. K. Maull, J. Kirby & D. Rowe, pp. 1–16. Englewood Cliffs: Prentice Hall.

MARTIN, R.W. & RHODES, R.S. (1994). Protective surgical wear. In *Advances in Trauma and Critical Care*, ed. K. Maull, H. Cleveland, D. Feliciano *et al.*, pp. 81–8. Chicago: Mosby Year Book.

MAULL, K.I., ENDERSON, B.L. & FRAME, S.B. (1993). Comprehensive management of the trauma patient. In *Current Practice of Surgery*, Vol. IV, ed. B. Levine, E. Copeland, R. Howard *et al.*, pp. 1–18. New York: Churchill Livingstone.

RHODES, M. & BRADER, A.H. (1989). Organization of a trauma resuscitation system. In *Advances in Trauma*, Vol. 4, ed. K. Maull, H. Cleveland, G. Strauch *et al.*, pp. 19–42. Chicago: Mosby Year Book.

TRUNKEY, D.D. (1991). Initial treatment of patients with extensive trauma. *N. Engl. J. Med.*, **324**, 1259–63.

6 Shock

I.McA. LEDINGHAM

Department of Emergency and Critical Care Medicine, Faculty of Medicine and Health Sciences, United Arab Emirates University, Al-Ain, U.A.E.

Chapter plan

Definition
Classification
General clinical aspects
Pathophysiology
Assessment, monitoring and investigations
Hypovolaemic shock
Septic shock

DEFINITION

Shock may be defined as an acute pathophysiological disturbance of oxygen transport which, in the absence of appropriate treatment, will culminate in tissue hypoperfusion and cellular destruction. The condition remains common and the resulting mortality considerable. Awareness of the circumstances leading to shock, detection of its early clinical features and prompt, adequate remedial action are mandatory if morbidity and mortality are to be reduced. Development of expertise in the management of the shocked patient is important in the training of all clinicians and a *sine qua non* for those working in the acute care environment.

In this chapter the reader will find a commonly used classification of the shock syndrome and an outline of the general clinical aspects and systemic manifestations of the subgroups. This is followed by a summary of the current views of the pathophysiology of shock including mediators, neurohumoral responses and effects upon specific organs. A description of assessment, monitoring and investigations deals principally with those relevant to the prehospital and emergency (A&E) department situations. Finally, more specific detail will be provided concerning hypovolaemic and septic shock.

CLASSIFICATION

It is convenient to consider shock under four primary aetiological headings (Table 1), always accepting that overlap between the different catergories is common in clinical practice and factors such as age, pre-existing disease, duration of the acute illness and previous treatment will modify the clinical presentation.

Table 1. *Classification of shock*

Hypovolaemic shock
- Haemorrhage, oedema
- Burns
- Salt and water deficits
    e.g. Addison's disease
         Gastrointestinal losses
         Diabetes insipidus

Cardiogenic shock
- Primary myocardial failure
    e.g. Ischaemia
         Arrhythmias
         Valvular damage
         Cardiomyopathy
- Secondary myocardial failure
    e.g. Drugs
         Hypoxia
         Acute rise in afterload

Obstructive shock
- Pulmonary embolism
- Tamponade
- Aortic dissection

Distributive shock
- Sepsis
- Anaphylaxis
- Late stages of hypovolaemic shock

GENERAL CLINICAL ASPECTS

The syndrome of cold, pale (and occasionally cyanotic) skin, sweating, tachycardia, hypotension, hyperventilation, clouding of consciousness and oliguria is characteristic of most forms of shock (volume-repleted septic shock is exceptional in this respect, the details of which will be presented later). The full-blown clinical presentation is almost always preceded by more subtle physiological and metabolic disturbances which are not so easily detected but which are of major significance from the point of view of effective treatment. While changes in arterial blood pressure, heart and respiratory rate, for example, are readily recognized and routinely recorded, earlier alterations are likely to have occurred in blood volume, blood flow and oxygen delivery and consumption, correction of which may lead to rapid restoration of normal cardiovascular and respiratory status. In the absence of appropriate early treatment, shock leads to a progressively widening gulf between oxygen supply and demand, the ultimate effect of which is irreversible injury to cellular function. Death may result acutely from cardiovascular collapse or later from multiple organ failure.

As the classification of shock described above testifies, almost any insult to the body can lead to shock and when the syndrome is fully developed few physiological processes remain unaffected. For these reasons any *general* description of the syndrome inevitably tends to emphasize the final common pathway of tissue hypoxia rather than the earlier, more readily reversible, stages. The duration of onset of the shock state is variable, and its initial pattern and character are influenced not only by the primary aetiology but also by the age and pre-existing condition of the patient and by the nature of coincidental treatment. Interpretation of these various factors is not always easy in the individual patient. Futhermore, uncertainty about the precise sequence of pathophysiological events in shock in general has been the source of academic debate for many years. Within the past decade or so, a combination of unparalleled technological advance, burgeoning scientific knowledge, intensive study of relevant experimental models and, lastly, increasingly high-quality clinical investigations has resulted in vastly improved understanding of the shock state. Thus far, however, these gratifying developments have yet to be translated into uniformly impressive reductions in morbidity and mortality in clinical practice.

Hypovolaemic shock follows acute loss of whole blood, plasma or interstitial fluid. Clinical examples include haemorrhage due to medical or surgical causes, extensive burns and severe gastrointestinal fluid losses. Fluid replacement is the backbone of treatment but controversy exists as to how this is best achieved. Prevention of further fluid loss is clearly mandatory.

In non-survivors, death usually occurs within the first 24–48 h and is attributable to the severity and nature of the primary insult; the few late deaths are predominantly from sepsis.

Cardiogenic shock results from pump failure due to a variety of causes. *Primary myocardial dysfunction* is usually attributable to coronary artery disease and shock follows acute myocardial ischaemia. The condition complicates the clinical course of between 5% and 10% of patients admitted with acute myocardial infarction (Forrester *et al.*, 1976 a,b). Predominantly left ventricular mechanical dysfunction occurs in myocardial infarction (usually involving more than 40% of the ventricle); rupture of a papillary muscle or a ventricular septal defect further interferes with the normal forward flow of blood. Less commonly, depressed right ventricular contractility from right ventricular infarction leads to underfilling of the left ventricle and reduced left ventricular compliance.

The clinical picture is similar to hypovolaemia with clouding of consciousness, tachypnoea and orthopnoea, hypotension, tachycardia, poor peripheral perfusion, an elevated jugular venous pressure and oliguria.

Pulmonary oedema may cause hypoxia, coronary perfusion pressure and time are reduced, and coronary vessel lesions decrease myocardial oxygen supply further. Tachycardia and peripheral vasoconstriction increase myocardial oxygen demand and the worsening myocardial oxygen supply/demand ratio may lead to further deterioration of myocardial function and increase the size of myocardial infarction, resulting in a downward spiral of clinical deterioration.

Hypoperfusion results in cellular dysfunction and the effects are liable to be worsened by critical stenotic lesions in major vessels (e.g. the carotid and renal arteries), such that ischaemia occurs at a higher mean pressure than would otherwise be the case. As major organ dysfunction supervenes, the metabolic derangement and hypoxia worsens, endotoxaemia may occur from gut hypoperfusion, and secondary myocardial depression exacerbates the physiological derangement.

Aggressive treatment by medical means including thrombolytic agents, selective fluid administration and pharmacological support of the myocardium has not altered the very high mortality associated with this condition (more than 80%; Forrester *et al.*, 1976 a,b). As in hypovolaemic shock, most deaths occur early and are related to the extent of myocardial infarction.

Secondary myocardial dysfunction is seen in severe hypoxia, metabolic derangement (especially acidosis) and following negatively inotropic drugs; sepsis also leads to this condition.

Obstructive shock occurs in the presence of an obstruction affecting the cardiovascular system, such as a large pulmonary embolism, tension pneumothorax, pericardial tamponade, aortic dissection or vena caval compression in pregnancy.

Treatment in this heterogeneous group of conditions varies markedly and outcome is clearly influenced by the availability and institution of prompt and appropriate intervention.

Distributive shock is a condition in which cardiac output may exceed normal. Despite this, alterations in microvascular blood flow may cause cellular hypoperfusion. The prime example is septic shock in which a patient with infection displays hypotension, vasodilatation and unexplained metabolic acidosis. Gram-negative bacteraemia is the commonest cause and shock develops in approximately 40% of instances. Mortality has remained between 30% and 60% during the past two decades in spite of the regular introduction of new and powerful antibiotics, more sophisticated monitoring and steadily improving critical care techniques.

The clinical picture in volume-repleted septic shock is one of variable confusion, tachypnoea associated with a characteristic 'white-out' pattern on the chest radiograph consistent with pulmonary oedema, warm, dilated extremities with tachycardia and bounding pulse, hypotension and oliguria.

Treatment consists of general resuscitative measures combined with elimination of sepsis. The initial response to prompt resuscitation is such that early mortality is low. Often, cardiovascular stability can be restored and outcome is determined by the effectiveness of procedures to eradicate sepsis and by avoidance of multiple organ failure. Recurring cycles of recovery and relapse may occur; later mortality is related to the number of organs or systems that become involved and death may be delayed for days or weeks.

Anaphylactic shock – a subset of distributive shock – is the extreme manifestation of an allergic reaction when a previously sensitized individual is exposed to a specific antigen; bronchospasm, angioedema and pulmonary oedema are common coincidental features. Arteriolar and capillary dilatation is the main early pathological change followed by increased capillary permeability characteristic of histamine release.

Early treatment with adrenaline and intravenous fluids is mandatory in this situation. The route and dose of adrenaline are dependent on the severity of the condition; colloid rather than crystalloid solutions appear to be preferred for volume loading (Fisher, 1992). The role of H_2 receptor blocking agents in the presence of hypotension remains to be determined. The small number of deaths occur early and are usually attributable to individual sensitivity and delayed treatment.

PATHOPHYSIOLOGY

An outline of the often overlapping inter-relationship between the four previously described categories of shock and the final common pathway of microcirculatory disturbances and cellular dysfunction leading to cell death is represented in Fig. 1. Unless the primary insult promptly resolves or responds to treatment, it is common clinical experience that patients suffering from hypovolaemic, obstructive or cardiogenic shock sooner or later fall victim to the sequence of pathophysiological changes normally associated with septic shock. The speed of these events is very variable but is probably more rapid than was previously recognized. In the subset of hypovolaemic shock attributable to trauma, this phenomenon may be almost coincident with the primary insult. It is known, for example, that the incidence of early bacteraemia and endotoxaemia increases with the severity and duration of the shock in traumatized patients. Whether this is caused by contamination at the time of injury, during resuscitation or by secondary gut mucosal injury is uncertain. Whatever the mechanism, multiple organ failure and late deaths from sepsis in these circumstances can, in many instances, be traced back to the initial period of shock, irrespective of its cause (Fig. 2).

In the case of shock associated with infection, there is almost invariably an important component of hypovolaemia. Only when this has been corrected can the causal relationship between the septic process and the haemodynamic disturbances be ascertained. In a recent publication seeking to settle the perennial terminological disputes relating to shock, septic shock is defined as sepsis-induced hypotension, persisting despite adequate fluid resuscitation, along with the presence of hypoperfusion abnormalities or organ dysfunction (Bone *et al.*, 1992). This clarification may help to disentangle some

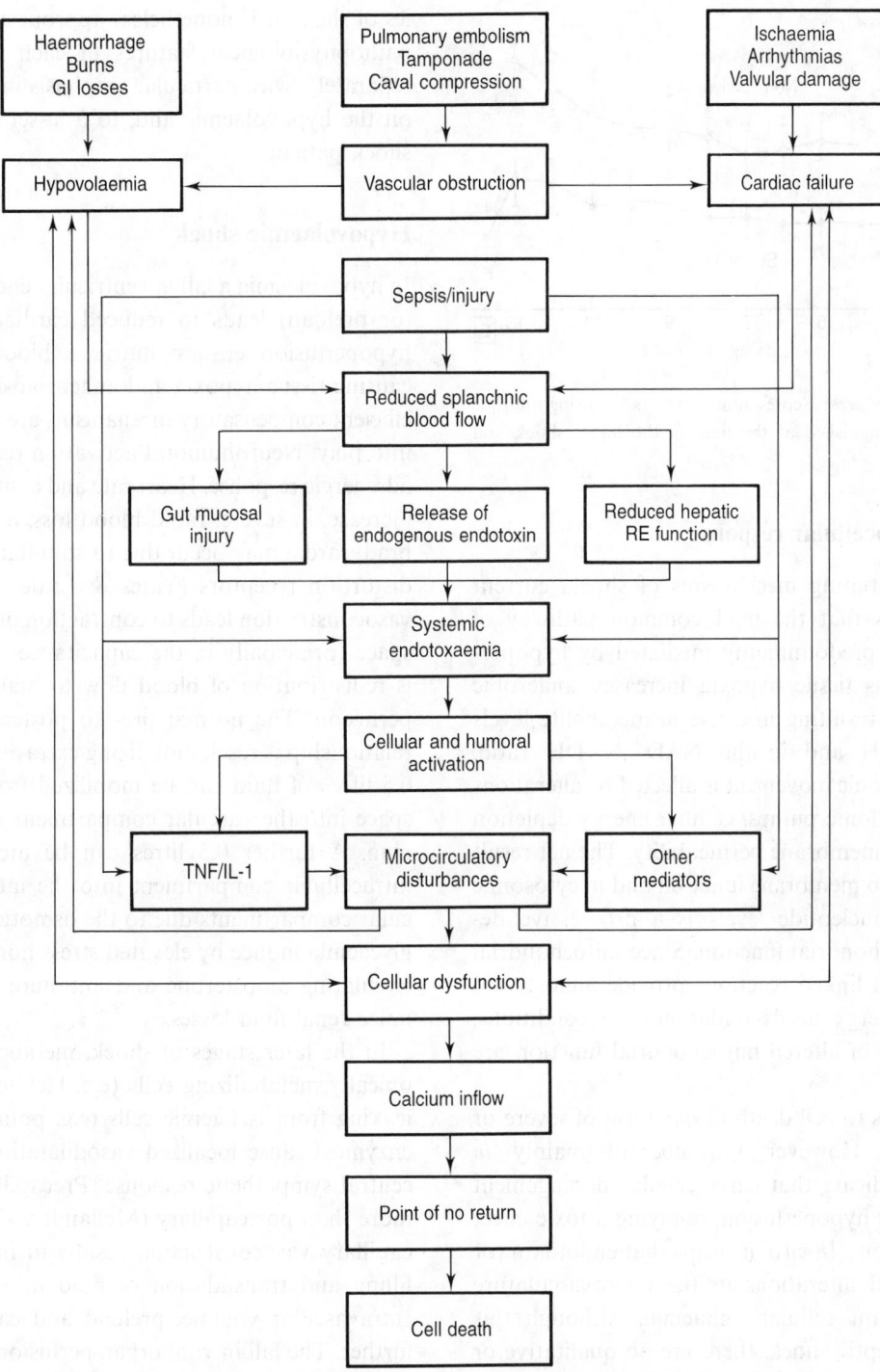

Fig. 1. A schematic representation of the pathogenesis of shock, demonstrating the interrelationship between the four commonly described categories. RE, reticuloendothelial; TNF, tumour necrosis factor; IL-1, interleukin-1; GI, gastrointestinal.

of the confusion that bedevils interpretation of the effects of new therapeutic agents in the treatment of the shocked patient.

In a small proportion of patients with cardiogenic shock, stroke volume may be reduced because of reduced preload or because of primary right wall infarction. This important clinical entity can be easily recognized by the absence of signs and symptoms of pulmonary congestion and may be successfully treated with volume loading and inotropic agents.

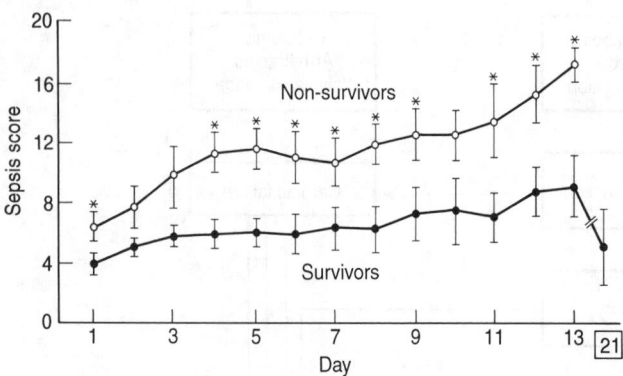

Fig. 2. On the basis of sepsis scores, non-survivors following multiple trauma may be distinguished at the time of the initial shock and certainly by day 4.

Cellular and subcellular response

Whatever the initiating mechanisms of shock, current evidence suggests that the final common pathway of cellular injury is predominantly mediated by hypoperfusion. Initially as tissue hypoxia increases, anaerobic glycolysis occurs resulting in a rise in metabolite levels and a fall in pH and in the NAD^+:NADH ratio. Transmembrane ionic movement is affected by alterations in the activity of ionic pumps, cellular energy depletion or an increase in membrane permeability. The net result of these changes to membrane function and in cytosomic electrolyte and nucleotide levels is a progressive depression of mitochondrial function. Since mitochondrial electron transport linked reactions provide almost 95% of the body's energy needs under normal conditions, the consequences of altered mitochondrial function are obvious.

Ischaemia leads to cell death in *any* form of severe or prolonged shock. However, a number of (mainly '*in vitro*') studies indicate that early cellular derangement in sepsis precedes hypoperfusion, implying a toxic effect of endotoxin action. '*In vivo*' it seems that endotoxin (or mediator)-induced alterations in the microvasculature result in significant cellular ischaemia. Although this occurs early in septic shock, there are no qualitative or quantitative differences in the dysfunction, whatever the aetiology of shock. Haljamäe (1987) has reviewed this topic and stresses the role of alterations in nutritive blood flow (due to microvascular failure) in the aetiology of cellular damage. He concludes that 'there are no data indicating that the sepsis-induced impairment (of cellular ion regulation) is different from that induced by any other form of shock.'

Accepting that overlap occurs in the clinical categor-ies of shock it is nonetheless appropriate to describe the pathophysiological features of each of the categories separately, with particular emphasis in this presentation on the hypovolaemic and, to a lesser extent, the septic shock patient.

Hypovolaemic shock

In hypovolaemia a fall in ventricular end-diastolic volume (or preload) leads to reduced cardiac output. Global hypoperfusion ensues; nutritive blood flow decreases causing tissue hypoxia and anaerobiosis. In early shock, efficient compensatory mechanisms are normally brought into play. Neurohumoral activation results in a massive adrenergic response. Heart rate and contractility normally increase; in severe, rapid blood loss, a vagally mediated bradycardia may occur due to stimulation of ventricular distortion receptors (Yates & Little, 1985). Peripheral vasoconstriction leads to contraction of the intravascular space (principally in the capacitance system) and there is redistribution of blood flow to maintain vital organ perfusion. The normal pre- to postcapillary resistance relationship is reset, mobilizing extravascular fluid; up to 0.5 litres of fluid can be mobilized from the interstitial space into the vascular compartment in an adult 70 kg man. A further 0.5 litres can be mobilized from the intracellular compartment into the interstitial and vascular compartments due to the osmotic action of hyperglycaemia induce by elevated stress hormones. Increased circulating aldosterone and antidiuretic hormone minimize renal fluid losses.

In the later stages of shock, metabolites from anaerobically metabolizing cells (e.g. lactate) and substances leaking from ischaemic cells (e.g. potassium, lysosomal enzymes) cause localized vasodilatation, overriding the central sympathetic response. Precapillary vessels dilate more than postcapillary (Mellander, 1978). Loss of precapillary vasoconstriction results in increased capillary filling and transudation of fluid into the interstitium. Intravascular volume, preload and cardiac output fall further. The fall in vital organ perfusion thus engendered will be exacerbated by the release of myocardial depressant substances (including, for example, angiotensin II, myocardial depressant factor and endothelium-derived nitric oxide), increased capillary permeability and the initiation of cellular and humoral enzyme cascades. In the absence of appropriate treatment the scene is set for adhesion of activated polymorphonuclear leucocytes to the vascular endothelium which, together with endothelial cell swelling, results in progressive deterioration in microvascular flow. In addition, the white cell–endothelial interaction promotes the release of vasoactive mediators and toxic oxygen species leading to further redistribution of tissue perfusion, macromolecular capillary leakage into the interstitial space and further obstruction to nutritive flow (Messmer, 1990). Patients with hypovolaemic shock who survive the primary insult may later develop systemic sepsis and the multiple organ dysfunction syndrome (Bone et al, 1992).

In addition to the derangements caused by the initial disease process, resuscitation from shock may itself have deleterious effects. The importance of injury during reperfusion is now well recognized. The effects of reperfusion and reoxygenation have been separated and it is apparent that restoration of oxygen to the tissues is the trigger for further cellular damage. In experimental studies, allopurinol, a xanthine oxidase inhibitor, (McCord, 1985), and free-radical scavengers have been shown to exert a protective effect, although they have no proven clinical role.

Septic shock

In septic shock the primary insult appears to be a disturbance in peripheral vascular reactivity. This is reflected in the fall in systemic vascular resistance commonly observed in septic shock patients undergoing resuscitation (Parker et al., 1984a). The anatomical site of this vasodilation is unknown but is probably caused by the accumulation of products of anaerobic metabolism and locally released vasoactive mediators in the microcirculation. Initially, cardiac output is maintained or increased by cardiac dilation and tachycardia, although there is evidence of coincidental intrinsic myocardial depression (Parker et al., 1984b; Parillo et al., 1985). The reasons for the myocardial depression remain obscure but alterations in both diastolic and systolic function have been demonstrated. Possible causes include myocardial oedema, segmental coronary hypoperfusion, right ventricular dilation, circulating myocardial depressant factors and altered myocardial metabolism. However, in the majority of non-surviving septic patients cardiac output is maintained until death occurs (Parker et al, 1984a). In the later stages of septic shock, reduced 'capillarity' is demonstrable in a number of organs; 'capillarity' is defined as the amount of capillary system in the tissues available for oxygen delivery. In skeletal muscle this takes the form of an increase in both spatial heterogeneity of capillary blood flow and the number of stop-flow capillaries (Morisaki & Sibbald, 1993).

Septic shock occurs commonly in the presence of Gram-negative bacteraemia, but it is now generally accepted that an identical pattern of physiological and biochemical disturbances may also occur in association with other groups of organisms or even in the absence of organisms. The latter finding may be explained in some instances by the technique of bacteriological sampling or by the presence of antibiotics, but in others no such explanation is appropriate and the concept of 'abacterial sepsis' has gained increasing popularity. Current attempts to link these disparate observations are at best tentative and likely to require modification as new information comes to hand. Endotoxin may play an important but not necessarily exclusive role in this process and three possible sequences are envisaged.

First, endotoxin may be released in small quantities from Gram-negative bacteria derived from foci of infection, frequently intra-abdominal or genitourinary in origin. Systemic endotoxaemia ensues, its effects mediated by, for example, Kupffer cell activation in the liver or local release of mediators in other areas such as the lung.

Second, endotoxin may be derived from the reservoir of Gram-negative organisms within the gut. The barrier function of the gut is disrupted in a wide spectrum of disorders, resulting in systemic endotoxaemia (Cahill, 1983). Splanchnic blood flow falls markedly during hypovolaemia and cardiogenic shock and, although hepatic blood flow rises in early sepsis (Fish et al, 1986), hepatic oxygen supply (assessed by tissue electrodes) is markedly reduced. Thus, in shock of whatever aetiology, gut permeability is increased whilst hepatic clearance is reduced and systemic endotoxaemia may occur.

Third, two recently isolated proinflammatory cytokines, tumor necrosis factor (TNF) and interleukin-1 (IL-1), have been shown to play a central role in the modulation and amplification (Fig. 3) of immune responses to infection (Shapiro & Gelfand, 1993). These two cytokines synergistically orchestrate all of the haemodynamic and metabolic effects of septic shock. At end-organ level, specific final common mediators, adhesion molecules and activated polymorphonuclear leucocytes combine to contribute to tissue damage. A pivotal role for TNF and/or IL-1 is supported by the protection afforded by pre-treatment with specific antibodies in various experimental animal models. However, TNF and/or IL-1 may be stimulated by factors other than endotoxin, including antigen–antibody complexes, complement activation products and necrotic tissues (Fig. 3), thus explaining the presence of the 'sepsis syndrome' in the absence of any obvious infecting organism.

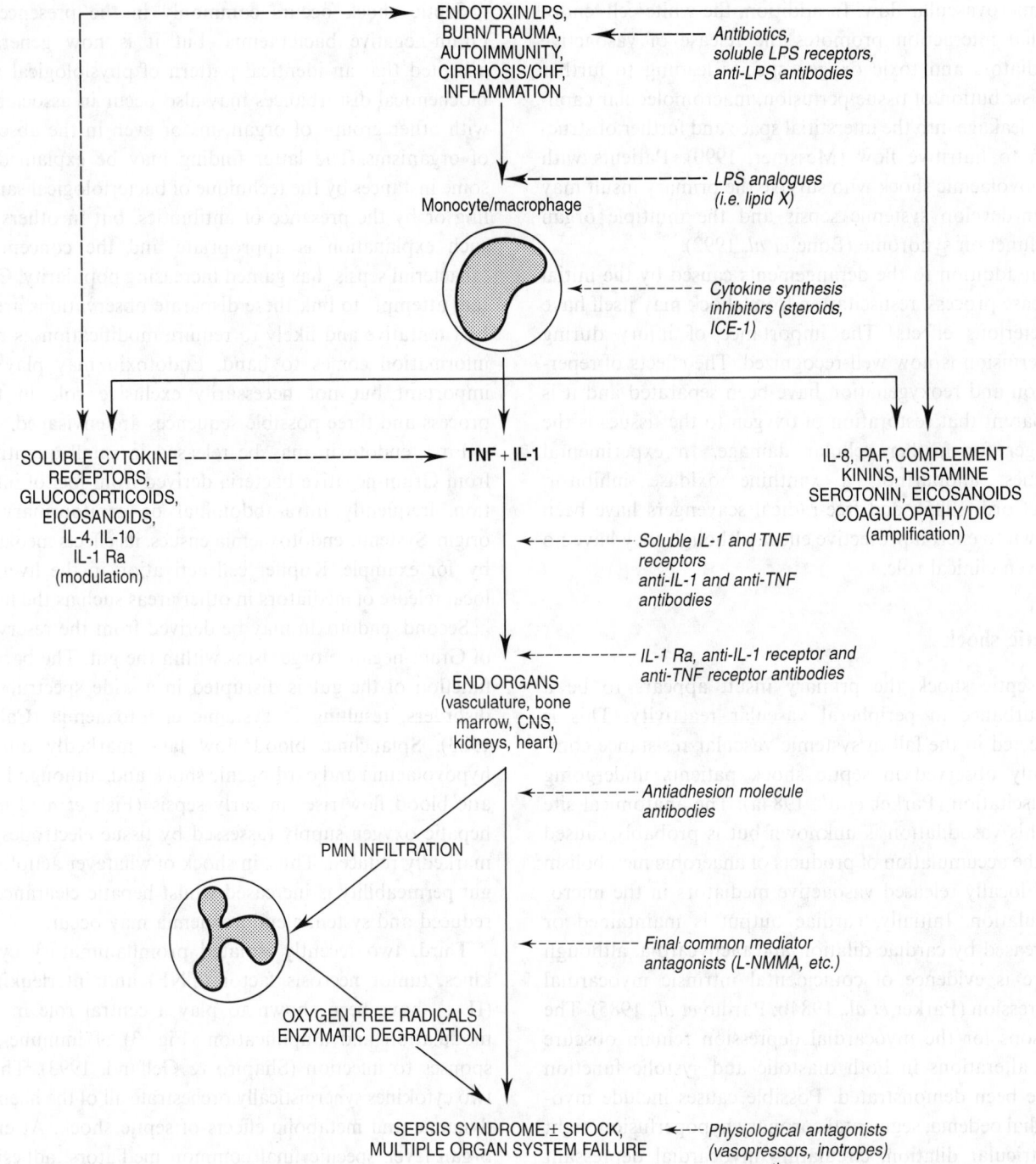

Fig. 3. Multiple initiating factors interacting with mononuclear leucocytes and stimulating secretion of proinflammatory cytokines. The response of end-organs and interaction with polymorphonuclear leucocytes may lead to multiple organ system failure. Possible targets for intervention are shown.

Conditions associated with shock

Supply-dependent oxygen consumption

All the above processes may affect the delivery of oxygen to the tissues. Recently, much interest has emerged in the

relationship between oxygen delivery (DO_2) and tissue oxygen consumption (VO_2); DO_2 is the product of arterial oxygen content (CaO_2) and the volume of blood perfusing a tissue, organ or the whole body (Q) (i.e. $DO_2 = CaO_2 \times Q$ ml min^{-1}), while VO_2 is expressed as

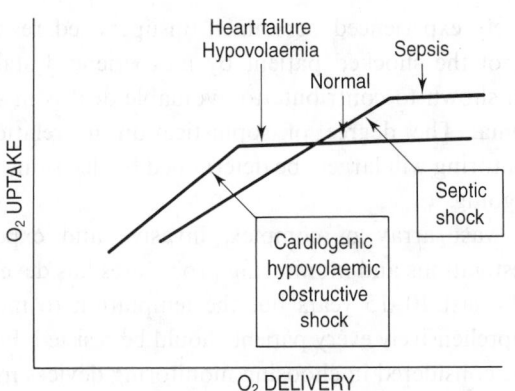

Fig. 4. Oxygen delivery/consumption relationships in normal patients and in those with shock.

$(CaO_2 - CvO_2)Q$, where CvO_2 is mixed venous oxygen content. In a healthy person, as DO_2 falls, VO_2 remains constant due to capillary recruitment, which lessens the mean diffusion distance between the capillaries and the cells, thus increasing the oxygen extraction ratio, $(CaO_2 - CvO_2)/CaO_2$. A critical point is reached when no further capillary recruitment can occur, and VO_2 then becomes supply-dependent (Fig. 4). In numerous conditions, such as adult respiratory distress syndrome (ARDS), liver failure and septic shock, VO_2 appears to be supply-dependent over a much greater range. In addition, the oxygen extraction is typically not constant, and maximum VO_2 is often greatly increased. On the basis of recent experimental evidence, the most likely explanation for the foregoing observations is reduced capillary reserve rather than direct depression of cellular metabolism.

Refractory shock and multiple organ dysfunction syndrome

Whatever the cause of cellular injury, prompt resuscitation may abort the decline in cellular function. If rapid and appropriate treatment is applied, it is rare to succumb to shock *per se* in its early stages. However, prolonged shock leads to organ dysfunction and certain organs are particularly susceptible. The vulnerability of the lung to shock is due not only to perfusion related factors but also to others, notably oxygen toxicity and abnormal fluid distribution. ARDS is dealt with elsewhere (see Chapter 44).

Even those organs whose perfusion is preserved are not immune to ischaemia. The ascending limb of the loop of Henle in the kidney, for example, normally functions in a borderline hypoxic state due to a countercurrent

exchange of oxygen, and it is easy to imagine the effect of reduced oxygen transport in these cells. Subendocardial perfusion may also be compromised during hypotension and prolonged diminished coronary perfusion pressure may ultimately affect cardiac performance. In sepsis, the microvascular changes outlined above affect all organs. Although initial resuscitation may mitigate the haemodynamic deterioration, MODS (multiple organ dysfunction syndrome), may occur. Prognosis is related to the number of organs involved and death usually occurs in association with endogenously acquired infection (Marshall, 1992).

ASSESSMENT, MONITORING AND INVESTIGATIONS

Appropriate assessment and monitoring of the shocked patient need to be instituted as rapidly as possible after the primary insult. In the first instance, investigations should be limited to those critical to the success of resuscitation. Elsewhere in this volume prehospital management will be dealt with in detail, particularly in relation to trauma and cardiac arrest (Chapter 14). For the purposes of this presentation only brief mention will be made of this phase in the continuum of patient care although its importance in relation to outcome cannot be exaggerated. Those responsible are usually members of the professional rescue services but occasionally medical or nursing staff may be involved. Admission to hospital permits more sophisticated monitoring and laboratory investigations.

Prehospital phase

An adequate history must always be part of the initial assessment, but clearly the degree of detail and accuracy will vary with the circumstances; some or all of the information may have to be obtained from eye witnesses or relatives. Interruption or delay may be necessary in the interests of prompt resuscitation. Physical examination of the patient should be as complete as possible.

The level of monitoring will depend on local policy and the skill and experience of the attendants. As a minimum, observations would include conscious state, respiratory effort, capillary refill, eye opening, verbal response and motor response. Information should be recorded on the use of any therapeutic manoeuvres, such as oropharyngeal airway, artificial ventilation, oxygen administration and cardiac massage. Increasingly sophisticated monitoring includes electrocardiography (ECG), body temperature measurement and pulse oximetry (see below). The administration of intravenous fluids and drugs is part of the professional paramedic's therapeutic armamentarium and complementary monitoring is appropriate. In this context, it should be appreciated that non-invasive arterial blood pressure measurement in transit is notoriously difficult and inaccurate.

Technological advances are such that the full range of routine monitoring procedures conventionally used in the intensive care setting may be deployed in the field or in transit but are only relevant in special circumstances – most notably secondary transport (Runcie *et al*, 1992) (by which time shock should not be a problem although its prevention is obviously essential). Nonetheless, it is important to appreciate that there are practically no technical limitations to the use of these procedures outside hospital. The real question relates to their indications and cost-effectiveness in a wide range of different circumstances.

Hospital reception

A more detailed history and assessment of the shocked patient is usually possible in the emergency room setting. Physical examination is best done in a logical sequence (e.g. in systems or anatomical regions) in order to avoid serious oversights. A checklist or prepared form is of great value for inexperienced or experienced clinicians alike, and reduces time spent on clerking. The aims of the initial examination are to identify the likely cause of shock and to determine which systems in particular need to be monitored during resuscitation. In the case of trauma, arrangement of the injuries in order of priority in management permits monitoring and resuscitation to proceed methodically and efficiently. Physical examination should be regularly repeated. This has the dual function of stimulating a fresh assessment of each system, allowing early identification of new problems or review of the existing complaint. It also ensures that the patient is treated as a whole.

Delays in resuscitation may be prevented by the use of a management protocol or algorithm; reduction in mortality and morbidity may result. It is an important matter of overall hospital policy (as well as individual patient care) to determine the extent to which resuscitation should be conducted in the emergency room and at what stage other sites would be more appropriate (e.g. the intensive care unit or operating theatre). An equally, if not more important, issue is the deployment of appropriately experienced personnel; unsupervised resuscitation of the shocked patient by inexperienced staff has been shown to contribute to avoidable deaths in severe trauma. The degree of sophistication in relation to monitoring will largely be determined by decisions in the foregoing.

A vast array of complex, invasive and expensive investigations and monitoring procedures has developed in the last 10–15 years but the temptation to monitor comprehensively every patient should be resisted. Factors to be considered in choosing monitoring devices include accuracy, reliability, safety, ease of operation, convenience, cost of purchase, cost and ease of maintenance, patient comfort, invasiveness and the skill of the operator (Phillips *et al.*, 1989). It should be remembered that, in the case of invasive monitoring, there is a risk/benefit ratio for every procedure. Monitoring of shock may include invasive and non-invasive monitoring of haemodynamic parameters, and monitoring of the biochemical consequences of hypoperfusion.

In practice, monitoring of the shocked patient should be simple and adequate. In the majority of instances, and in all seriously shocked patients, a series of procedures are recommended as a basis for initial management.

Procedure for initial management of shocked patients

- Large-bore intravenous cannulae
- Central venous catheter ⎰ for pressure monitoring
- Arterial catheter   ⎱ and blood sampling
- Pulse oximetry (for oxygen saturation)
- ECG monitoring
- Core/peripheral thermometry
- Bladder catheter (in absence of urethral injury)

Cardiovascular parameters may be displayed conveniently and continuously using simple monitoring apparatus. The ECG is useful for detecting arrhythmias and myocardial ischaemia but it is not a reliable indicator of myocardial function. Non-invasive arterial blood pressure measurement in the shocked patient may involve errors up to 30%. Automated devices are not more accurate than the standard clinical auscultatory method; their advantage is that they leave the attendant's hands free for other tasks. Intravascular measurement of arterial and central venous pressure (CVP) has greatly facilitated management; the catheter systems are easy to set up, reliable and accurate. The incidence of complications is low in centres where the techniques are in regular use. The radial artery is the preferred site for cannulation and has the lowest complication rate. Monitoring of CVP provides a rough index of venous return (right ventricular preload) and is thus helpful in determining the appropriate volume of fluid required for restoration of haemodynamic stability. The catheter should be inserted through a peripheral vein unless the attending physician is experienced, in which case the subclavian or internal jugular route is preferable (Trunkey *et al.*, 1988). It should be remembered that in certain conditions CVP measurement gives no guidance as to left ventricular filling pressures (e.g. myocardial infarction, hypoxia, sepsis, or pulmonary embolism). In these circumstances left heart pressure may have to be measured directly using a pulmonary artery flotation catheter (see below). Absolute values of either right- or left-sided filling pressures should be regarded with caution. Trends in response to a fluid challenge are more useful in resuscitation. An index of preload is plotted against an index of ventricular function to construct a ventricular function curve. A bolus of 50–200 ml of colloid is infused rapidly (say over 10 min), and may be repeated until a further rise in preload is not matched by a rise in output. At this point, further fluid challenge should be delayed.

When the manoeuvres described above are completed, a series of measurements may be obtained which include:

- Conscious level.
- Heart rate and rhythm, arterial and central venous blood pressure.
- Respiratory rate and rhythm, arterial blood gas analysis, oxygen saturation.
- Core/peripheral temperature difference.
- Urine output.
- Haemoglobin/haematocrit.
- Electrolytes/acid–base balance.
- Chest radiograph.

Arterial blood gas analysis may signal the early development of respiratory complications, particularly when used in conjunction with the inspired oxygen concentration from which an estimation may be made of the alveolar/arterial oxygen tension gradient. Oxygen saturation may be determined by pulse oximetry from the absorption of light in a finger tip or ear lobe, intermittent (i.e. arterial) absorption being electronically distinguished from constant (i.e. capillary and venous) absorption. It can reflect accurately the arterial oxygen tension, but errors occur in low-flow states, in anaemic (<5 g%) and hypothermic patients, in strong sunlight and bumpy movement (e.g. in ambulances), and in the presence of methaemoglobin and carboxyhaemoglobin (Hutton & Clutton-Brook, 1993). Skin pigmentation and jaundice

do not appear to be sources of error. A serious pitfall of pulse oximetry is failure to detect hypoventilation in patients receiving supplementary oxygen (Davidson & Hosie, 1993). It is important to appreciate that, because of the alinearity of the oxygen dissociation curve above approximately 90% saturation, small changes in saturation reflect large changes in oxygen tension. Its main use is probably to identify acute hypoxic episodes associated with physiotherapy, suctioning and similar patient care manoeuvres (Taylor & Whitwam, 1988). More sophisticated respiratory gas monitoring techniques include those to determine transcutaneous oxygen and carbon dioxide tension, and end-tidal carbon dioxide. While the first two are unlikely to play a major role in emergency medicine, end-tidal carbon dioxide measurement is useful in the shocked patient (see below) and gives immediate warning of misplacement of an endotracheal tube.

The core/peripheral (or peripheral/environmental) temperature gradient is a useful non-invasive indicator of the adequacy of peripheral perfusion and, in certain circumstances, closely reflects changes in cardiac output. However, the previously claimed close relationship between these two variables has been challenged (Woods *et al.*, 1987). Urine output is a simple and sensitive indicator of total renal blood flow and its distribution. An output of 50 ml h^{-1} should be achieved in an adult patient. The information obtained from all those measurements may be a reasonable guide during the early phase of resuscitation but it is vital to remember that normal initial measurements (e.g. of CVP or chest radiography) may be misleading and that their real value lies in simultaneous and constant re-evaluation.

In a small number of instances, hardly ever in emergency medicine, catheterization of the pulmonary artery is indicated. In patients with protracted hypovolaemic shock, or with suspected cardiac or pulmonary disease, or in whom management includes the use of mechanical ventilation, the use of a pulmonary artery flotation catheter (PAFC) is of value. Once in position, the catheter can be used to measure pulmonary artery pressures, pulmonary capillary wedge pressure, cardiac output by thermodilution and mixed venous oxygen saturation. The composite information may be used to construct a physiological profile consisting of pulmonary and systemic vascular resistances, right and left ventricular stroke work, and DO_2 and VO_2. In the complex haemodynamic circumstances of protracted shock the PAFC may aid:

- Fluid management.
- Evaluation of both right and left ventricular function.
- Vasoactive drug administration.
- Management of acute interstitial pulmonary oedema.
- Diagnosis of pulmonary embolism.

Thus the PAFC provides a wealth of data, but its use is by no means always selective and its ability to aid in clinical decision-making has been challenged (Ontario Intensive Care Study Group, 1992).

Complications associated with the use of the pulmonary artery flotation catheter

- Complicated venous insertion (bleeding, haemo-pneumothorax, nerve injury)
- Arrhythmias (ventricular tachycardia or fibrillation, atrioventricular block, etc.)
- Catheter knotting
- Pulmonary thrombosis or infarction
- Endothelial/endocardial damage
- Catheter-related infection
- Pulmonary artery rupture

Laboratory investigations

The function of the cardiovascular system is to provide sufficient perfusion such that the cells are provided adequately with oxygen and substrates and metabolic products are removed. Haemodynamic monitoring provides diagnostic information but does not usually reflect tissue perfusion directly. This function is performed better using biochemical monitoring which measures substrate supplied to and metabolites derived from the respiring tissues.

Blood gas analysis is the most common form of biochemical monitoring. The arterial oxygen tension may fall as a result of cardiovascular failure (e.g. due to pulmonary oedema) or may reveal the cause of secondary myocardial depression. Acid–base analysis (from pH, standard bicarbonate and base deficit values given by most blood gas machines) may likewise show an acidosis as a result of poor tissue perfusion leading to anaerobic metabolism. The hormonal and substrate changes in shock have been characterized but unfortunately are of limited clinical value. For example, serial measurement of serum lactate, a product of anaerobic metabolism, has shown good correlation with outcome in shock (Cowan et al., 1984; Bakker et al., 1991). Similarly, a number of experimental and clinical studies have shown that the VO_2/DO_2 dependency phenomenon is associated with

elevated blood lactate levels (Bakker & Vincent, 1991). However, the interpretation of blood lactate levels can be complicated by the fact that they are not synonymous with lactic acidosis (Pinsky, 1993) and also reflect both production and elimination of lactate. The latter can be protracted, especially in patients with liver dysfunction. Attempts to construct more complex biochemical profiles have proved to be of value as a research tool but so far are not used routinely in clinical practice.

Determination of gastric intramucosal pH (pHi) can be useful to assess the degree of gut hypoxia (Gutierrez et al., 1992). pHi measurements have been shown to be of prognostic value in critically ill patients (Gutierrez et al., 1992). Moreover, the combination of blood lactate levels and pHi may be useful in monitoring tissue hypoxia (Friedman & Vincent, 1993). However, the two parameters are not entirely independent.

In the assessment of the patient with hypovolaemic shock, initial haemoglobin and haematocrit values do not help to quantify the magnitude of acute blood loss. These values, however, provide important baseline information and should be obtained on admission. Subsequent measurements will help to indicate the need for whole blood or red cell transfusion. Serum electrolyte concentrations are often measured but interpretation of the results can be difficult. For example, hyponatraemia is only seen if sodium losses are severe and hypernatraemia is seldom observed other than as a sequel to iatrogenic misadventure (e.g. overindulgence in hypertonic saline administration during resuscitation). Hyperkalaemia is a feature of prolonged severe ischaemia, and hypokalaemia may follow profuse vomiting, diuretic therapy and, again, primary resuscitation with hypertonic solutions. In recent years, the simultaneous measurement of serum and urine electrolytes and osmolality has helped interpretation of data and rationalization of treatment. Reduced total protein content and colloid oncotic pressure reflect massive protein loss (e.g. following burn injury or during septic shock).

Knaus et al. (1985) derived a scoring system (APACHE II), recently updated to APACHE III (Wagner et al., 1989), which ascribes a weighed value to derangements of haemodynamic and metabolic parameters from normal. When measured as a single value on admission to the intensive therapy unit, a close correlation with outcome has been demonstrated. The difficulty is that overlap between different score bands makes it impossible to apply to the individual patient although it is valuable as a research and audit tool. In addition, although the general relationship that increasing APACHE

Table 2. *Classification of hypovolaemic shock according to blood loss (after Baskett, 1990)*

	Class I	Class II	Class III	Class IV
Blood loss				
Percentage	<15	15–30	30–40	>40
Volume (ml)	750	800–1500	1500–2000	>2000
Blood pressure				
Systolic	Unchanged	Normal	Reduced	Very low
Diastolic	Unchanged	Raised	Reduced	Very low or unrecordable
Pulse (beats min^{-1})	Slight tachycardia	100–120	120 (thready)	>120 (very thready)
Capillary refill	Normal	Slow (>2 sec)	Slow (>2 sec)	Undetectable
Respiratory rate	Normal	Normal	Tachypnoea (>20 min^{-1})	Tachypnoea (>20 min^{-1})
Urinary flow rate (ml h^{-1})	>30	20–30	10–20	0–10
Extremities	Colour normal	Pale	Pale	Pale and cold
Complexion	Normal	Pale	Pale	Ashen
Mental state	Alert	Anxious or aggressive	Anxious, aggressive, or drowsy	Drowsy, confused, or unconscious

II score is associated with increasing mortality is true, the precise correlation varies with different categories of disease.

HYPOVOLAEMIC SHOCK

The following text will deal with the subdivisions of hypovolaemic shock as listed in Table 1, but it must be appreciated that most patients demonstrating the classical features of shock, whatever its cause, will respond favourably to intravenous fluid administration. Thus, selected patients suffering from shock attributable to sepsis, drug overdose and even myocardial infarction manifest increased cardiac output and improved tissue perfusion in response to fluids. Hypovolaemia, either relative or absolute, is therefore a universal accompaniment of all forms of shock and its identification and elimination is fundamental to the success of treatment.

The effects of *haemorrhage* vary with the nature, duration and severity of blood loss, the patient's age and general health, and with the speed, adequacy and nature of resuscitation. In previously healthy young adults, the acute loss of 10% of total blood volume has been shown to reduce arterial pressure by 7% and cardiac output by 21%; the loss of 20% of the blood volume reduced arterial pressure by 15% and cardiac output by 41% (Hinshaw *et al.*, 1961). Thus in most cases the signs and symptoms

can be related to the amount of blood loss which can be classified in four broad groups (Table 2). However, individual response is remarkably variable and reduction in plasma volume of as much as 25% may occur without arterial hypotension (Hardaway, 1979). The presence of cardiovascular disease or anaemia can be expected to alter this pattern of response, increasing the risk of a critical reduction in tissue oxygen availability and subsequent complications. In patients with acute upper gastrointestinal haemorrhage, for example, the presence of hypovolaemic shock, age over 60 years, and haemoglobin concentration at admission to hospital of less than 10 g dl^{-1} were associated with increased mortality (Macleod & Mills, 1982). Not surprisingly, the additional insult of trauma augments the endocrine and metabolic effects of hypovolaemia.

The reduction in blood volume following *thermal injury* results from loss of plasma at the site of burn, and the rate and volume of plasma deficit are roughly proportional to the extent of the area burned (Goodwin, 1984). The increase in capillary permeability and subsequent sequestration of intravascular fluid in the extravascular space lead to the formation of tissue oedema and an increase in haematocrit, packed cell volume often reaching 70–80% in the absence of rapid, adequate fluid replacement. The composition of the oedema fluid closely resembles that of plasma with respect to sodium and potassium concentrations.

Hypovolaemia may be a consequence of *dehydration* from either a primary deficit of water or a primary deficit of salt. A primary deficit of water generally results from reduced intake rather than from increased loss. The commonest cause in clinical practice is inability of the patient to acquire an adequate volume of fluid either because of exhaustion or disturbance of consciousness (as in the case of intrinsic brain pathology or the effects of drugs – e.g. sedatives) or because drinking is forbidden (as in the case of upper gastrointestinal operations). Causes of increased loss include pituitary and nephrogenic diabetes insipidus. A primary deficit of salt arises not from reduced intake but from increased loss. The deficiency may be of salt alone if the patient loses both salt and water and replaces the water by drinking, as may happen in diarrhoea, copious sweating or Addison's disease. A deficiency of both salt and water occurs most commonly when fluid is lost from the gastrointestinal tract, for instance in intestinal obstruction, severe diarrhoea and biliary and pancreatic fistula. Sodium loss in excess of water also arises in a proportion of patients with chronic renal failure and in uncontrolled diabetes mellitus.

A primary deficit of water leads to cellular dehydration as a result of the increase in tonicity of the extracellular fluid and the metabolic response to stress. By contrast, a primary deficit of salt leads to a reduction in the volume of extracellular fluid (including a reduction in blood volume) but not to cellular dehydration. As blood volume contracts there is increasing difficulty in maintaining an adequate circulation.

Assessment and measurement of fluid loss

Detection of the presence of hypovolaemia would seem a relatively simple task and, in many instances, the combination of overt fluid loss with inadequate replacement makes for an easy diagnosis. In a proportion of patients, however, the clinical presentation may be less clear-cut. Even when the existence of hypovolaemia is not in doubt, accurate quantification of volume deficit is often difficult. Subjective visual estimation of fluid loss is fraught with problems and may be grossly inaccurate. Blood loss may be assessed on the basis that a hand represents 500 ml, but the method takes no account of loss from major vessels. In thermal injury, the figure of 4 ml of plasma loss per kg body weight for each per cent of body surface burned is widely accepted but in some cases it may be a significant underestimate (Goodwin *et al.*, 1983). Clinical features of dehydration are important

for diagnostic purposes but cannot be used to quantify extracellular losses. Thirst is an insensitive measure of water deprivation and becomes obvious only after a deficit of 1.5 litres has occurred. Moderate to severe water deprivation is associated with deficits of 4–10 litres. Slight to moderate salt depletion, associated with lassitude and orthostatic fainting, implies a deficit of up to 4 litres of isotonic saline. Moderate to severe salt depletion is associated with deficits of 6–10 litres.

Although a number of methods are available for measuring blood volume, they have not become widely popular or practised outside a few committed centres.

Treatment

The principal objectives of treatment are to prevent further fluid losses, restore oxygen delivery to meet the metabolic requirements of the tissues and minimize reperfusion injury.

The importance of prompt and adequate resuscitation in the early stages of hypovolaemia is clear, often before the diagnosis can be confirmed. In practice, acute resuscitation of a patient suffering from *any* form of shock is influenced more by the nature of the associated physiological disturbances than by specific aetiological factors. Success of subsequent treatment, on the other hand, is largely dependent on detection and elimination of the underlying cause. In many patients, considerable overlap will exist between the two processes.

Initial resuscitation

The immediate aims are to augment intravascular volume, optimize cardiac output and its distribution, and ensure adequate pulmonary gas exchange. These aims are achieved by:

- Minimizing further fluid loss and replacing estimated loss with colloid solutions, crystalloid solutions and transfusion with concentrated red cells to a haematocrit of 30–35%.
- The judicious use of pharmacological agents.
- The administration of oxygen together with mechanical ventilation when indicated.

Whether in the prehospital phase or in the emergency room, reducing the risk of further fluid loss in the hypovolaemic patient is imperative. The avoidance of unnecessary movement, immobilization of broken limbs, gentle handling of damaged tissues and maintenance of pressure dressings are as important in the A&E depart-

Table 3. *Intravenous fluid replacement in haemorrhagic shock* (after Baskett, 1990)

Class I (haemorrhage 750 ml, 15%)	2.5 litres Ringer-lactate solution or 1.0 litre polygelatin
Class II (haemorrhage 800–1500 ml, 15–30%)	1.0 litre polygelatin plus 1.5 litres Ringer-lactate solution
Class III (haemorrhage 1500–2000 ml, 30–40%)	1.0 litre Ringer-lactate solution plus 0.5 litre polygelatin plus 1.0–1.5 litres equal volumes of concentrated red cells and polygelatin
Class IV (haemorrhage >2000 ml, >40%)	1.0 litre Ringer-lactate solution plus 1.0 litre polygelatin plus 2.0 litres whole blood or 2.0 litres equal volumes concentrated red cells and polygelatin or hetastarch

ment, operating theatre and intensive therapy unit as during prehospital transport. The role of the pneumatic antishock garment is uncertain. This three-compartment inflatable suit applies compression to the lower abdomen, pelvis and lower limbs. Used at low pressure, the device may be a useful splint and reduce venous pooling; at higher pressure, compression of the inferior vena cava and increase in afterload may result, together with respiratory embarrassment. At best, it may serve as a temporary expedient in the field (Holcroft, 1982) or in gaining time in selected patients with severe abdominal or pelvic haemorrhage. A recent randomized trial of this modality in the prehospital management of penetrating abdominal injuries in an urban setting showed no benefit as regards admission trauma scores or ultimate survival (Bickell et al, 1987). Whatever its role, there is no doubt that sudden deflation of this support (>5 mmHg min^{-1}) before adequate fluid replacement can lead to dangerous hypotension. The practice of tilting the hypovolaemic patient headdown in an attempt to augment venous return is less frequently utilized than formerly. There is certainly no evidence that this manoeuvre achieves any consistent haemodynamic improvement (Sibbald et al, 1979) and adverse pulmonary and cerebral effects have been reported. Raising the legs is an adequate and safe first aid procedure.

Optimizing oxygen delivery

The initial aim of this aspect of treatment is normally achieved using a combination of intravenous fluids and increased inspired oxygen concentration. Further sophistication of this process involves improving microvascular flow, pulmonary ventilation/perfusion ratios and individual organ perfusion. Finally, judicious control of factors leading to increased oxygen consumption (e.g. pain and fever) is important.

The standard approach

Cardiac output is increased in the first instance by adjusting intravascular volume such that end-diastolic volume (i.e preload) is optimal. The use of inotropic and/or vasodilator drugs may be indicated in the event of a poor response to the use of fluids alone.

Successful resuscitation is dependent more on the rapidity and adequacy of fluid repletion than on the composition of the regimen. The principal dispute as to the selection of fluids for resuscitation (the colloid versus crystalloid controversy) centres mainly on issues relating to the perceived nature of the underlying physiological disturbance, side-effects and economics (Ledingham & Ramsay, 1986; Ledingham & Wright, 1988). Important as these issues are, it is clear that a variety of colloid and crystalloid solutions (or combinations of solutions) will provide successful resuscitation in the majority of patients. An example of a typical intravenous fluid replacement regimen is illustrated in Table 3. A judicious mixture of colloids to augment intravascular volume and crystalloids to replace interstitial fluid losses seems to produce optimum results as judged by tissue oxygen consumption data, and it is commonly used in clinical practice. Although it is logical to proceed with volume replacement as rapidly as possible, a recent study (Kaweski et al, 1990) examining the effect of the administration of fluids in the prehospital phase in a large series of trauma patients revealed no benefit by comparison with a group not receiving fluids. Early mortality rate appeared to be related to the severity of the underlying injuries rather than to fluid administration in these patients. The mean prehospital time in this series was short (36 min) and crystalloid solutions were used. Whether alternative fluid regimens (Mattox et al, 1991) or longer transport times would reveal convincing benefit remains to be demonstrated. Whichever regimen is chosen, the importance of rigorous, frequent and comprehensive monitoring cannot be overstated. At all times, careful judgement is required in striking the optimal balance between the volume of fluid per unit time needed for adequate tissue perfusion and that which will induce overload. The value of the 'fluid challenge' technique to detect exhaustion of preload reserve has been emphasized (Wood & Hall, 1985).

The optimum haemocrit in shock resuscitation has not until recently been a source of much controversy, the prevailing wisdom being that a value of between 30% and 35% (corresponding to a haemoglobin range of $10-11.5 \text{ g dl}^{-1}$) is an appropriate therapeutic target. Recently, however, Dietrich et al. (1990) found that raising the haemoglobin value from 8.3 g dl^{-1} to 10.5 g dl^{-1} did not improve the shock state in a group of volume-resuscitated, critically ill, non-surgical patients. The authors concluded that, after appropriate volume replacement and the use of inotropic agents, red cell transfusion did not further improve tissue oxygen metabolism. Since other studies have shown a similar lack of appreciable improvement in circulatory parameters, including cardiac output and (inferentially) splanchnic perfusion, following blood transfusion in low-flow states (Morisaki & Sibbald, 1993), the previously held views on optimum haemocrit will have to be revised, at least to some extent. Possible explanations for these observations might include an increase in the blood viscosity at the microcirculatory level (large vessel haemocrit does not closely reflect microvascular haemocrit) and the relatively low oxygen-carrying capacity of transfused bank blood which is not corrected for many hours.

Many shocked patients manifest hypoxaemia of varying degree and multifactorial aetiology. Rapid correction of disturbed pulmonary gas exchange is an important component of primary care and in the first instance arterial oxygen content may be increased by augmenting the inspired oxygen fraction (FiO_2). Early mechanical ventilation is often used with the aim of averting subsequent pulmonary complications, although the evidence for this remains subjective. Unequivocal indications for ventilatory assistance include failure of adequate oxygenation – PaO_2 less than 8.7 kPa (65 mmHg) – when breathing oxygen spontaneously (15 litres min^{-1} through a high-flow mask), excessive respiratory work or ventilatory inadequacy with hypercapnia. Techniques which increase mean intrathoracic pressure, such as positive end-expiratory pressure (PEEP) and constant positive airway pressure should be used with caution in hypovolaemic patients and the optimum increased pressure should be selected to provide maximum oxygen delivery. Continuous measurement of mixed venous oxygen saturation during the application of PEEP will indicate changes in arterial (although not necessarily tissue) oxygen delivery. PEEP improves gas exchange in patients with pulmonary oedema, not by reducing lung water content but by increasing alveolar volume. Adverse effects of PEEP include hepato-renal dysfunction and pulmonary barotrauma (Sha et al, 1987).

If restoration of blood volume and correction of pulmonary gas exchange disturbance fail to restore cardiovascular stability, early consideration should be given to pharmacological assistance. The drugs most commonly used in these circumstances are the inotropic agents (to increase myocardial contractility), with or without the use of vasodilators (to decrease afterload). Dopamine has proved attractive for its effects on both cardiac output and renal function. If administered by intravenous infusion at a rate ($2-20 \text{ } \mu\text{g/kg}^{-1}/\text{min}^{-1}$) such that systolic arterial pressure does not increase above 80–100 mmHg, dopamine will normally induce a gratifying diuresis. If the rate is increased, the alpha-adrenergic agonist action of the drug emerges and arrhythmias occur. The risk of intrapulmonary shunting should also be noted. Toxic side-effects increase with the passage of time although withdrawal of this agent has been successfully achieved after many days of administration. Dobutamine, acting directly on beta$_1$-adrenergic receptors, may have a more pronounced inotropic action on the heart than dopamine, with less marked effects on heart rate and excitability. A beneficial effect of dobutamine on oxygen consumption has been reported in a mixed population of shocked patients (Shoemaker et al, 1986), suggesting improved peripheral perfusion consequent on vasodilation. A manoeuvre which is gaining popularity is to use dopamine by low-dose infusion during the early stages of resuscitation to maintain renal perfusion and, if cardiac output requires to be augmented, either to increase the dose of dopamine or to add dobutamine (with the aim of achieving the best combination of pharmacological actions).

Commonly used vasodilators are chlorpromazine, nitroprusside and nitroglycerin. Selection should be based on the predominant cardiovascular disturbance (Ledingham & Wright, 1988). In all cases caution should be exercised since the risk of reduction in cardiac filling pressures and/or systemic hypotension is always present. The number of vasoactive drugs increases steadily and both new adrenergic (e.g. dopexamine) and noradrenergic (e.g. amrinone) agents have appeared. All are undergoing evaluation in various forms of shock.

Acid–base imbalance rarely requires pharmacological

correction. Non-respiratory acidosis associated with perfusion failure is rapidly self-correcting once cardiac output is improved and its disappearance may be used as a marker of the adequacy of resuscitation. Furthermore, recent studies have suggested that sodium bicarbonate may exert detrimental metabolic and circulatory effects in patients with hypoxaemia and an unstable circulation (Mizock & Falk, 1992).Occasionally, however, bicarbonate may be required when pre-existing hyperkalaemia is exacerbated by a decreasing extracellular pH as a result of non-respiratory acidosis. Respiratory acidosis demands correction of ventilation. Electrolyte balance is calculated from knowledge of input, serial serum estimations and analysis of 24-h urinary output and other measurable external losses. Diuretics may be required in the later stages of resuscitation, usually to minimize the risk of pulmonary overload; in this context both frusemide and dopamine may be administered by intravenous infusion.

New approaches

The inconsistent response to standard resuscitation as outlined above has encouraged continuing exploration of novel approaches to treatment, including the concept of achieving 'supranormal' levels of cardiorespiratory function, manipulation of the microcirculation and control of individual organ blood flow.

In spite of its logicality, treatment aimed at restoration of normal haemodynamic and respiratory values does not consistently lead to recovery (Shoemaker et al, 1973). In a group of critically ill, postoperative patients, improved survival was noted to be associated with a hyperdynamic circulatory and metabolic response to resuscitation (Shoemaker et al, 1983), an observation in keeping with the 'delivery-dependent oxygen consumption' phenomenon described earlier. This has led over the past decade to the view that the conventional ABC (airway, breathing, circulation) principles of resuscitation should be extended to include D (increased oxygen delivery) and E (normalization of oxygen extraction) (Fiddian-Green et al, 1993). The pathophysiological justification for this approach is seen to be three-fold:

1. Tissue oxygen debt consequent on hypoperfusion needs to be repaid.
2. Increased metabolic activity associated with recovery from low-flow states demands increased DO_2.
3. Disturbed microcirculatory flow necessitates a 'supranormal' cardiac index to provide adequate tissue oxygenation, even if some regions are overperfused.

The protagonists of this approach point to the evidence that prospective clinical trials in surgical and septic shock patients confirm the association between improved survival and the achievement of the revised targets for DO_2. (The use of the term 'supranormal' has been challenged on the grounds that the chosen minimum target value for DO_2 of 600 ml/min^{-1} per m^2 is, in fact, normal for a resting, unstressed individual; (Edwards, 1993a). A measure of satisfactory normalization of tissue oxygen extraction is stated to be a pHi value exceeding 7.35 (Gutierrez et al, 1992).

Support for this therapeutic philosophy is slow in developing, partly because of conflicting evidence and the possible risks of the regimen and partly because its accomplishment requires the use of extensive invasive monitoring and the deployment of highly skilled and experienced personnel.

Few studies are available to demonstrate the effect of treatment on nutritive flow in the microcirculation, but the observations of Velasco et al. (1980) and De Felippo et al. (1980) and their colleagues suggest that altering the osmolar and oncotic properties of the fluid regimen used in resuscitation may be rewarding. These authors demonstrated that the short-term infusion of hypertonic saline solution (2400 mOsm^{-1}/l) can restore cardiovascular function within minutes when given in volumes of 4 ml^{-1}/ kg^{-1}. Similar effects have been described using dextran solution (Kreimeier & Messmer, 1987) and prompt restoration of nutritive blood flow was demonstrated even after prolonged hypotension. The additional possible effect of reducing reperfusion injury has also been highlighted. The potential advantages of combined hyperosmolar/hyperoncotic fluid regimens as an integral part of primary resuscitation are becoming recognized. The possible adverse side-effect of such solutions are likely to be minimal since only small volumes are used over limited periods. A recent clinical study in prehospital management of trauma patients confirms the essential safety of the technique while leaving its efficacy to be further evaluated (Mattox et al., 1991).

The concept of manipulating the microcirculation by pharmacological means has attracted considerable recent interest. Of the available agents, prostacyclin has been examined in greatest detail. Unlike conventional vasodilators such as nitroprusside, prostacyclin appears to restore the normal pattern of microcirculatory flow following shock and may have a selective effect in reducing postcapillary resistance. This may be of relevance in the later stages of shock and help to attenuate the associated 'capillary leak' effect. Like dopamine, prostacyclin substantially increases splanchnic blood flow, thus reducing the potential for ischaemic damage to the gut mucosa and the attendant risk of endotoxin absorption. In addition to its vascular effects, prostacyclin inhibits white cell and platelet activation – actions whose importance in clinical shock remain to be evaluated. In a recent study of critically ill, predominantly septic patients, Bihari et al (1987) used an infusion of prostacyclin as a test of the adequacy of oxygen delivery – the 'oxygen flux test'. Whereas survivors increased their oxygen consumption by only 5%, the equivalent figure in the non-survivors was 19%. Non-survivors therefore had a discrepancy between their actual and potential oxygen consumption, implying that a proportion of their cells were functioning anaerobically. Studies of the effects of long-term infusion of prostacyclin on mortality are awaited.

One of the weaknesses of existing strategy in the treatment of shock is that it is based on the assumption that the observed microcirculatory disturbances are uniform throughout the body. Clearly, this is unlikely to be true. Organs vary in their susceptibility to shock and interpatient variation is also significant, depending on such factors as age and pre-existing disease. For these reasons, methods are being developed in an attempt to direct oxygen transport to where it is most required in individual patients. Hepatic hypoperfusion secondary to sepsis, general anaesthesia and the use of PEEP may be ameliorated by the administration of low-dose dopamine (Maestracci et al, 1981) and hepatocyte oxygenation may be improved by infusion of prostacyclin. Similar benefits may accrue from the use of these two agents in the case of renal hypoperfusion, where the cells of the ascending limb of the loop of Henle in the renal medulla are the most susceptible to hypoxic injury. The subsequent risk of acute tubular necrosis may be further reduced using mannitol, which promotes an osmotic diuresis and may limit reperfusion injury, and frusemide, which increases renal prostaglandin production and renal blood flow. Recent work suggests that the latter agents should be reserved until urine flow has been restored, in which case they may decrease the period of oliguria and render dialysis less necessary (Parsons, 1988). In the case of the lung, both prostacyclin and prostaglandin E_1 have been administered to improve regional parenchymal blood flow but neither is of proven efficacy.

Control of oxygen consumption

While the first priority in the treatment of shock is augmentation of oxygen delivery, interventions that decrease oxygen demand are occasionally appropriate. Analgesic and sedative drugs are not only for the relief of pain and distress but may well beneficially reduce total body oxygen consumption (Wallace et al, 1988; Van der Linden & Vincent, 1993). Mechanical ventilation is used to improve pulmonary gas exchange, but additional benefit may accrue from reducing the oxygen demands of the increased work of breathing commonly associated with shock. Finally, while decreased body temperature is associated with a lowered metabolic rate (if shivering is prevented), induced hypothermia has not been shown to be of value in the clinical setting. Nevertheless, avoidance of sustained extreme elevations of core temperature ($>40°C$) is rational.

SEPTIC SHOCK

Septic shock is a convenient term used to describe a condition in which severe haemodynamic instability is attributable principally or wholly to infection. Although bacteria are clearly involved in this process, interpretation of their role has changed in recent years, and it is now generally accepted that host defence and environmental factors also exert a major influence on the development of this syndrome.

Two major types of infection lead to this condition – pre-existing and acquired. In a number of critically ill patients, the existence of severe infection is the primary reason for hospital admission. The principal sites of this type of infection are shown in Table 4. On the other hand, most patients suffering from septic shock who are admitted to the intensive care unit develop infection following admission to hospital, typically as a consequence of severe trauma, burns and major abdominal or pelvic surgery. The causative organisms reflect the different sources of infection although it is now accepted that the type of organism is not a major determinant of the pathophysiological disturbances of septic shock. Humoral and cellular mediators of the inflammatory response are the primary determinants and these may be triggered by any organisms or indeed by a variety of non-septic insults.

In the A&E department, septic shock patients may present a diagnostic dilemma, especially if admission has been delayed and hypovolaemia has become a significant problem. Rapid and adequate fluid repletion generally unmasks the underlying problem and the bacteriological diagnosis may then be ascertained. In this situation, the characteristic hyperdynamic cardiovascular features are

Table 4. *Principal sites of infection*

Site	Nature of infection	Comment
Head/neck	Meningitis Encephalitis Brain abscess Epiglottitis	Commonly children
Thorax	Pneumonia	Community Ward } acquired (often HDM)
	Empyema Mediastinitis	Prolonged pulmonary sepsis Oesophageal surgery/injury
Abdomen/pelvis	Peritonitis	Perforated viscus
	Abscess (single/multiple)	{ Prolonged intra-abdominal sepsis Pelvic inflammatory disease Pancreatitis
Genitourinary system	Pyelonephritis Abscess	} Prolonged sepsis
	Toxic shock syndrome Septic abortion	Commonly associated vaginal tampon
Soft tissues	Necrotizing fasciitis	Commonly abdomino/pelvic
	Tetanus Fulminating cellulitis Gas gangrene	} Usually post-traumatic
	Miscellaneous wound	Post-traumatic
Bone	Osteomyelitis Septic arthritis	Children Prolonged joint disease
Blood	Septicaemia	Varied primary source
Miscellaneous	Burns	Associated { Smoke inhalation Carbon monoxide poisoning
	AIDS	Drug abuse

AIDS, acquired immunodeficiency syndrome; HDM, host defence mechanisms.

obvious and appropriate treatment may be instituted. It must be appreciated that the evolution of some forms of 'primary' septic shock in newly admitted patients may be very rapid and delay can be fatal. Infections such as pneumococcal pneumonia, toxic shock syndrome, necrotizing fasciitis, clostridial myositis and meningococcal and streptococcal bacteraemias can be lethal within hours unless aggressive resuscitation and appropriate definitive treatment is promptly instituted. Antibiotics are usually administered on a 'best guess' basis in the first instance until a definitive bacteriological diagnosis has been made. Fortunately, the clinical history is normally helpful in this regard.

Resuscitation

It is pertinent to ask whether the resuscitation of a patient suffering from septic shock should differ from that of hypovolaemic shock. The short answer is that in the acute phase, the crystalloid versus colloid controversy is just as relevant or irrelevant in both forms of shock. The important points are that a surprisingly large volume of fluid may be required to restore adequate circulatory performance in septic shock and that three to four times the volume of crystalloids will have to be administered to achieve the same end results as with colloids. The longstanding concern that vascular permeability in septic shock is an important factor determining the choice of resuscitation fluid has recently resurfaced (Morisaki & Sibbald, 1993). The relevant studies have suggested that, notwithstanding the lack of superiority of either solution in acute resuscitation, there may be a long-term (>48 h) beneficial effect of colloid solutions. This took the form of a greater capillary luminal area and less endothelial swelling and parenchymal injury. These observations could be attributed to the hyperoncotic action of the colloid solution and a possible oxygen scavenging effect.

The previously mentioned investigations of optimum haematocrit in shock resuscitation are also relevant in major sepsis. In brief, red blood cell transfusion is frequently advocated in increasing DO_2 to levels associated with raised tissue VO_2 as part of the supply dependency phenomenon. There is no doubt that in some cases DO_2 is raised, but this is not a consistent finding and the effect cannot be predicted on the basis of individual haemodynamic or metabolic variables. Furthermore, there is increasing evidence that microcirculatory oxygen availability may be adversely affected, particularly if the transfused blood is not fresh.

Pharmacological manipulation

In septic shock, dopamine is probably the most widely used agent and has similar haemodynamic effects to those previously described in protracted hypovolaemic shock – i.e. improvement in cardiac output and stroke volume, and a variable increase in arterial blood pressure. Even at low dosage, however, vasoconstriction may occur and result in reduced microcirculatory oxygen availability. Dobutamine does not demonstrate a vasoconstrictive effect and also has the ability to reduce pulmonary capillary wedge pressure, thereby allowing increased fluid volume infusion. For these reasons dobutamine, either alone or in conjunction with noradrenaline to counteract hypotension, is becoming increasingly popular (Edwards, 1993b). To be of value, the dose of catecholamine(s) should be adjusted to meet the needs of the individual patient, and therefore management of the septic shock patient, other than in the earliest phase, demands that the patient be transferred to the intensive care unit and extensively monitored, often with a PAFC (pulmonary artery flotation catheter). Vasodilators may be indicated when cardiac failure is present, but low mean arterial blood pressure limits their use in septic shock. Treatment directed at attaining high levels of oxygen delivery and oxygen consumption is under investigation but the value of high dose inotropic support in septic shock remains uncertain (Hinds et al, 1993).

One further drug is worthy of mention, if only for historic reasons. Until recently, high-dose corticosteroids were recommended in the early management of shock, particularly of septic origin. Their use was advocated to preserve endothelial integrity, interfere with leucocyte degranulation, inhibit prostaglandin synthesis, exert an anticoagulant effect, inhibit the release of adrenocorticotrophic hormone and endorphins from the pituitary gland, increase cellular oxygen uptake and inhibit the febrile response (Hartvig-Jensen & Andersen, 1988). Additional advantages of this group included their positive inotropic and vasodilatory actions, the latter particularly affecting the pulmonary circulation. In spite of these apparently beneficial effects, two recent controlled clinical trials (Bone et al, 1987; The Veterans Administration System Cooperative Study Group, 1987) have shown disappointing results, with no improvement in mortality and an increase in infection attributable to the corticosteroids. The present understanding is that the case for steroids in septic shock has passed from the category of 'not proven' to that of 'not indicated'. It is worth commenting that such clinical trials do have their limitations and corticosteroids may well re-emerge in the future as one of a cocktail of agents with complementary actions. Since high circulating levels of cortisol are normally a feature of the stress response, few shocked patients require steroids in physiological dosage.

Adjunctive treatment

A number of therapeutic modalities are under review.

A series of clinical trials involving the administration of antilipopolysaccharide antibodies have been concluded but the results have not been consistently encouraging and at present these agents have been withdrawn in some countries pending the acquisition of additional experimental data. Alternative immunomodulation therapy is being investigated and some beneficial effects have been reported. For instance, antibodies directed at TNF appear to improve myocardial contractility in experimental studies (Heard et al, 1992) and in early clinical experiences (Vincent et al, 1992). The IL-1 receptor antagonist also seems to improve cardiac function during septic shock in primates (Fischer et al, 1992). Antagonists to platelet activating factor may also improve cardiac function (Anderson et al, 1991). Nitric oxide, which is released in greater amounts in severe sepsis, may contribute to the myocardial depression as well (Brady et al, 1992).

Other forms of pharmacological treatment are directed towards the underlying metabolic and host defence disturbances: cryoprecipitate to correct opsonic deficiency (as measured by plasma fibronectin), a mixture of agents to restore protease/antiprotease balance, and heparin and supplementary coagulation factors to ameliorate severe disseminated intravascular coagulation.

A largely unavoidable risk of prompt, aggressive resuscitation, particularly in septic or cardiogenic shock, is a variable degree of pulmonary and systemic oedema – generally considered to be one of the factors presaging infection. If the underlying cause of shock has been eliminated, this problem will resolve spontaneously, but in some instances additional measures may be required. Mechanical ventilation will combat the worst effects of pulmonary oedema but systemic interstitial fluid may have to be removed by dialysis and ultrafiltration, or by the newer, simpler and safer technique of haemofiltration. Continuous arteriovenous haemofiltration (with or without pump assistance) is particularly suitable for the patient with a labile blood pressure since it causes minimal haemodynamic disturbance and can be readily adapted to individual patient requirement without the constant presence of specially trained staff. An additional, recently discovered advantage is that circulating middle molecular weight substances, (e.g. myocardial depressant factor) may also be removed (Coraim et al, 1986).

Bibliography

ANDERSON, B.O., BENSARD, D.D. & HARKEN, A.H. (1991). The role of platelet activating factor and its antagonists in shock, sepsis and multiple organ failure. *Surg. Gynecol. Obstet.*, **172**, 415–24.

BAKKER, J. & VINCENT, J.L. (1991). The oxygen supply dependency phenomenon is associated with increased blood lactate levels. *J. Crit. Care*, **6**, 152–9.

BAKKER, J., COFFERNILS, M., LEON, M. et al. (1991). Blood lactate levels are superior to oxygen derived variables in predicting outcome in human septic shock. *Chest*, **99**, 956–62.

BASKETT, P.F.J. (1990). Management of hypovolaemic shock. *Br. Med.. J.*, **300**, 1453.

BICKELL, W. H., PEPE, P.E., BAILEY, M.L. et al. (1987). Randomized trial of pneumatic antishock garments in the prehospital management of penetrating abdominal injuries. *Ann. Emerg. Med.*, **16**, 653–8.

BIHARI, D., SMITHIES, M., GRIMSON, A. et al. (1987). The effects of vasodilation with prostacyclin on oxygen delivery and uptake in critically ill patients. *N. Engl. J. Med.*, **317**, 397–403.

BONE, R.C., FISHER, C.J., CLEMMER, T.P. et al. (1987). A controlled clinical trial of high-dose methylprednisolone in the treatment of severe sepsis and septic shock. *N. Engl. J. Med.*, **317**, 653–8.

BONE, R.C., BALK, R.A., CERRA, F.B. et al. (1992). Definitions for sepsis and organ failure and guidelines for the use of innovative therapies in sepsis. *Chest*, **101**, 1644–55.

BRADY, A.J., POOLE-WILSON, P.A., HARDING, S.Z. et al. (1992). Nitric oxide production within cardiac myocytes reduces their contractility in endotoxaemia. *Am. J. Physiol.*, **32**, H1963–6.

CAHILL, C.J. (1983). Prevention of postoperative renal failure in patients with obstructive jaundice – the role of bile salts. *Br. J. Surg.*, **70**, 590–5.

CORAIM, F.J., CORAIM, H.P., EBERMANN, R. et al. (1986). Acute respiratory failure after cardiac surgery: clinical experience of continuous arteriovenous hemofiltration. *Crit. Care Med.*, **14**, 714–18.

COWAN, B.N., BURNS, H.J.G., BOYLE, P. et al. (1984). The relative prognostic value of lactate and haemodynamic measurements in early shock. *Anaesthesia*, **39**, 750–5.

DAVIDSON, J.A.H. & HOSIE, H.E. (1993). Limitations of pulse oximetry: respiratory insufficiency – a failure of detection. *Br. Med. J.*, **307**, 372–3.

DE FELIPPO, JR., J., TIMONER, J., VELASCO, I.T. et al. (1980). Treatment of refractory hypovolaemic shock by 7.4% sodium chloride injections. *Lancet*, **ii**, 1002–4.

DIETRICH, K.A., CONRAD, S.A., HERBERT, C.A. et al. (1990). Cardiovascular and metabolic response to red blood cell transfusion in critically ill volume-resuscitated nonsurgical patients. *Crit. Care Med.*, **18**, 940–4.

EDWARDS, J.D. (1993a). Clinical controversies concerning oxygen transport principles: more apparent than real? In *Yearbook of Intensive Care and Emergency Medicine*, ed. J.L. Vincent, pp. 385–405. Berlin: Springer-Verlag.

EDWARDS, J.D. (1993b). Management of septic shock. *Br. Med. J.*, **306**, 1661–4.

FIDDIAN-GREEN, R.G., HAGLUND, U., GUTIERREZ, G. et al. (1993). Goals for the resuscitation of shock. *Crit. Care Med.*, **21**, S25–S31.

FISCHER, E., MARANO, M.A., VAN ZEE, K.J. et al. (1992). Interleukin-1 receptor blockage improves survival and hemodynamic performance in *Escherichia coli* septic shock, but fails to alter host responses to sublethal endotoxemia. *J. Clin Invest.*, **89**, 1551–7.

FISH, R.E., LANG, C.H. & SPITZER, J.A. (1986). Regional blood flow during continuous low-dose endotoxin infusion. *Circ. Shock*, **18**, 267–75.

FISHER, M. (1992). Treating anaphylaxis with sympathomimetic drugs. *Br. Med. J.*, **305**, 1107–8.

FORRESTER, J.S., DIAMOND, G., CHATTERJEE, K. et al. (1976a). Medical therapy of acute myocardial infarction by application of hemodynamic subsets (Part 1). *N. Engl. J. Med.*, **295**, 1356–62.

FORRESTER, J.S., DIAMOND, G., CHATTERJEE, K. *et al.* (1976b). Medical therapy of acute myocardial infarction by application of hemodynamic subsets (Part 2). *N. Engl. J. Med.*, **295**, 1404–13.

FRIEDMAN, P.J. & VINCENT, J.L. (1993). Comparison of blood lactate levels and pHi in septic patients. *Am. Rev. Respir. Dis.*, **147**, A623.

GOODWIN, C.W. (1984). Burn shock. In *Clinical Surgery International*, Vol. 9, *Shock and Related Problems*, ed. G.T. Shires, p. 71. London: Churchill Livingstone.

GOODWIN, C.W., DORETHY, J., LAM, V. *et al.* (1983). Randomized trial of efficacy of crystalloid and colloid resuscitation on hemodynamic response and lung water following thermal injury. *Ann. Surg.*, **197**, 520.

GUTIERREZ, G., PALIZAS, F., DOGLIO, G. *et al.* (1992). Gastric intramucosal pH as a therapeutic index of tissue oxygenation in critically ill patients. *Lancet*, **339**, 195–9.

HALJAMÄE, H. (1987). Cellular function. In *Update in Intensive Care and Emergency Medicine*, Vol. 4, *Septic Shock*, ed. J.L. Vincent & L.G. Thijs, pp. 13–25. Berlin: Springer-Verlag.

HARDAWAY, R.M. (1979). Monitoring of the patient in a state of shock. *Surg. Gynecol. Obstet.*, **148**, 339.

HARTVIG-JENSEN, T. & ANDERSEN, L.W. (1988). Are steroids useful in septic shock? *Intensive Care World*, **5**, 23–4.

HEARD, S.O., PERKINS, M.W. & FINK, M.P. (1992). Tumor necrosis factor-alpha causes myocardial depression in guinea pigs. *Crit. Care Med.*, **20**, 523–7.

HINDS, C.J., WATSON, J.D., HAYES, M. *et al.* (1993). High dose inotropic support in septic shock (Letters). *Br. Med. J.*, **307**, 446.

HINSHAW, L.B., PETERSON, M., HUSE, W.M. *et al.* (1961). Regional blood flow in hemorrhagic shock. *Am. J. Surg.*, **102**, 224.

HOLCROFT, J.W. (1982). Impairment of venous return in hemorrhagic shock. *Surg. Clin. North Am.*, **62**, 17.

HUTTON, P. & CLUTTON-BROOK, T. (1993). The benefits and pitfalls of pulse oximetry. *Br. Med. J.*, **307**, 457–8.

KAWESKI, S.M., SISE, M.J. & VIRGILIO, R.W. (1990). The effect of prehospital fluids on survival in trauma patients. *J. Trauma*, **30**, 1215–18.

KNAUS, W.A., DRAPER, E.A., WAGNER, D.P. *et al.* (1985). APACHE II: a severity of disease classification system. *Crit. Care Med.*, **13**, 818–29.

KREIMEIER, U. & MESSMER, K. (1987). New perspectives in resuscitation and prevention of multiple organ system failure. In *Surgical Research: Recent Concepts and Results*, ed. A. Baethmann & K. Messmer, pp. 39–50. Berlin: Springer-Verlag.

LEDINGHAM, I.McA. & RAMSAY, G. (1986). Hypovolaemic shock. *Br. J. Anaesth.*, **58**, 169–89.

LEDINGHAM, I.McA. & WRIGHT, I. (1988). Treatment of cardiovascular failure in the intensive therapy unit. In *General Anaesthesia*, 5th edn., ed. J.F. Nunn, J.E. Utting & B.R. Brown, pp. 1256–71. London: Butterworth.

McCORD, J.M. (1985). Oxygen-derived free radicals in post-ischaemic tissue injury. *N. Engl. J. Med.*, **312**, 159–63.

MACLEOD, I.A. & MILLS, P.R. (1982). Factors identifying the probability of further haemorrhage after acute upper gastrointestinal haemorrhage. *Br. J. Surg.*, **69**, 256.

MAESTRACCI, P., GRIMAUD, D., LIVRELLI, N. *et al.* (1981). Increase in hepatic blood flow and cardiac output during dopamine infusion in man. *Crit. Care Med.*, **9**, 14–16.

MARSHALL, J.C. (1992). Multiple organ failure and infection: cause, consequence or coincidence. In *Yearbook of Intensive Care and Emergency Medicine*, ed. J.L. Vincent, pp. 3–13. Berlin: Springer-Verlag.

MATTOX, K.L., MANINGAS, P.A., MOORE, E.E. *et al.* (1991). Prehospital hypertonic saline/dextran infusion for post-traumatic hypotension. *Ann. Surg.*, **213**, 482–91.

MELLANDER, S. (1978). On the control of capillary fluid transfer by precapillary and postcapillary vascular adjustments. A brief review with special emphasis on myogenic mechanisms. *Microvasc. Res.*, **15**, 319–30.

MESSMER, K.F.W. (1990). Mechanisms of traumatic shock and their consequences. In *Blunt Multiple Trauma – Comprehensive Pathophysiology and Care*, ed. J.R. Border, M. Allgower, S.T. Hansen & T.P. Ruedi, pp. 39–49. New York: Marcel Dekker.

MIZOCK, B.A. & FALK, J.L. (1992). Lactic acidosis in critical illness. *Crit. Care Med.*, **20**, 80–93.

MORISAKI, H. & SIBBALD, W.J. (1993). Issues in colloid and transfusion therapy of sepsis. In *Yearbook of Intensive Care and Emergency Medicine*, ed. J.L. Vincent, pp. 357–72. Berlin: Springer-Verlag.

ONTARIO INTENSIVE CARE STUDY GROUP (1992). Evaluation of right heart catheterisation in critically ill patients. *Crit. Care Med.*, **20**, 928–33.

PARKER, M.M., SHELHAMER, J.H., NATANSON, C. *et al.* (1984a). Serial hemodynamic patterns in survivors and non-survivors of septic shock in humans. *Crit. Care Med.*, **12**, 311.

PARKER, M.M., SHELHAMER, J.H., BACHARACH, S.L. *et al.* (1984b). Profound but reversible myocardial depression in patients with septic shock. *Ann. Intern. Med.*, **100**, 483–90.

PARRILLO, J.E., BURCH, C., SHELHAMER, J.H. *et al.* (1985). A circulating myocardial depressant substance in humans with septic shock. *J. Clin. Invest.*, **76**, 1539–43.

PARSONS, V. (1988). Recent advances in management of acute renal failure. In *Recent Advances in Critical Care Medicine*, No. 3, ed. I.McA. Ledingham, pp. 195–209. Edinburgh: Churchill Livingstone.

PHILLIPS, G.D., RUNCIMAN, W.B. & ILSLEY, A.H. (1989). Monitoring in emergency medicine. *Resuscitation*, **18**, S21–S35.

PINSKY, M.R. (1993). Oxygen delivery and uptake in septic patients. In *Yearbook of Intensive Care and Emergency Medicine*, ed. J.L. Vincent, pp. 373–84. Berlin: Springer-Verlag.

RUNCIE, C.J., REEVE, W.R. & WALLACE, P.G.M. (1992). Preparation of the critically ill for interhospital transfer. *Anaesthesia*, **47**, 377–81.

SHA, M., SAITO, Y., YOKOYAMA, K. *et al.* (1987). Effects of continuous positive pressure ventilation on hepatic blood flow and intra-hepatic oxygen delivery in dogs. *Crit. Care Med.*, **15**, 1040–3.

SHAPIRO, L. & GELFAND, J.A. (1993). Cytokines and sepsis: pathophysiology and therapy. New horizons. *Sci. Pract. Acute Med.*, **1**, 13–22.

SHOEMAKER, W.C., MONTGOMERY, E.S., KAPLAN, E. *et al.* (1973). Physiologic patterns in surviving and non-surviving shock patients. *Arch. Surg.*, **106**, 630–6.

SHOEMAKER, W.C., APPEL, P. & BLAND, R. (1983). Use of physiologic monitoring to predict outcome and to assist in clinical decisions in critically ill postoperative patients. *Am. J. Surg.*, **146**, 43–50.

SHOEMAKER, W.C., APPEL, P. & KRAM, H.B. (1986). Hemodynamic and oxygen transport effects of dobutamine in critically ill general surgical patients. *Crit. Care Med.*, **14**, 1032–7.

SIBBALD, W.J., PATERSON, N.A.M., HOLLIDAY, R.L. *et al.* (1979). The Trendelenburg position: haemodynamic effects in hypotensive and normotensive patients. *Crit. Care Med.*, **7**, 218–24.

TAYLOR, M.B. & WHITWAM, J.G. (1988). The accuracy of pulse oximeters. *Anaesthesia*, **43**, 229–32.

THE VETERANS ADMINISTRATION SYSTEM COOPERATIVE STUDY GROUP (1987). Effect of high-dose glucocorticoid therapy on mortality in patients with clinical signs of systemic sepsis. *N. Engl. J. Med.*, **317**, 659–65.

TRUNKEY, D.D., CATALANO, R. & CARMONA, R.H. (1988). Hypovolemic and traumatic shock. In *Shock: The Reversible Stage of Dying*, ed. R.M. Hardaway, pp. 158–72. Littleton, MA: PSG Publishing.

VAN DER LINDEN, P. & VINCENT, J.L. (1993). The effects of sedative drugs. In *Oxygen Transport. Principles and Practice*, ed. J.D. Edwards, W.C. Shoemaker & J.L. Vincent, pp. 209–25. London: W.B. Saunders.

VELASCO, I.T., PONTIERI, V., ROCHA E SILVA, JR., M. *et al.* (1980). Hyperosmotic NaCl and severe hemorrhagic shock. *Am. J. Physiol.*, **239**, 664–73.

VINCENT, J.L., GRIS, P., COFFERNILS, M. *et al.* (1992). Myocardial depression and decreased vascular tone characterize fatal course from septic shock. *Surgery*, **111**, 660–7.

WAGNER, D., DRAPER, E. & KNAUS, W. (1989). Development of APACHE III. *Crit. Care Med.*, **17**, S199–S203.

WALLACE, P.G.M., BION, J.F. & LEDINGHAM, I.McA. (1988). The changing face of sedative practice. In *Recent Advances in Critical Care Medicine*, No. 3, ed. I.McA. Ledingham, pp. 69–94. Edinburgh: Churchill Livingstone.

WOOD, L.D.H. & HALL, J.B. (1985). Hemodynamic measurements and interpretations in critical illness. In *Proceedings of the 4th World Congress on Intensive and Critical Care Medicine*, p. 125. London: King & Wirth.

WOODS, I., WILKINS, R.G., EDWARDS, J.D. *et al.* (1987). The danger of using peripheral/core temperature gradient as a guide to therapy in shock. *Crit. Care Med.*, **15**, 850–2.

YATES, D. & LITTLE, R.A. (1985). Hypovolaemic shock. *Surgery*, **98**, 608–12.

7 Fluid, electrolyte and acid–base balance

J. HARRIS, S. HARROD and D. WATSON

Department of Anaesthesia and Intensive Care Medicine, St Bartholomew's Hospital, London, UK

Chapter plan
H^+ homeostasis
Water and electrolyte homeostasis

H^+ HOMEOSTASIS

Introduction

This section will outline the physiological principles and homeostatic mechanisms which dictate the volume and composition of body fluids and form the basis for diagnosis and rational treatment of fluid and electrolyte imbalance.

Basic physiology

An acid is a substance that tends to donate a hydrogen ion (H^+, proton). A base is a substance that tends to accept an H^+. The stronger the tendency to lose an H^+ (dissociate) the stronger the acid, and vice versa.

By definition, acids and bases exist in a state of equilibrium:

$$Acid \rightleftharpoons base^- + H^+$$

$$H_2SO_4 \rightleftharpoons HSO_4^- + H^+$$

$$H_2CO_3 \rightleftharpoons HCO_3^- + H^+$$

A substance may behave as an acid or as a base depending on the circumstances. Thus, bicarbonate is the conjugate base of carbonic acid but the conjugate acid of carbonate ions.

$$HCO_3^- \rightleftharpoons H^+ + CO_3^{2-}$$

The conventional measure of acid-base is $[H^+]$ (hydrogen ion concentration), which has now superseded pH.

$$pH = -\log_{10}[H^+]$$

$$Normal\ [H^+] = 40 \times 10^{-9}\ mol\ l^{-1}$$

$$= 40\ nmol\ l^{-1}$$

This corresponds to a pH value of 7.40 (Fig. 1).

Note that with the logarithmic notation, small changes in pH represent large changes in $[H^+]$ (Table 1).

By convention, a patient is:

ACIDOTIC if pH < 7.35, $[H^+]$ > 45 nmol l^{-1}
ALKALOTIC if pH > 7.45, $[H^+]$ < 35 nmol l^{-1}

Life is an acidogenic process. During normal (aerobic) metabolism, there is a net production of greater than 1000 mmol H^+ per day, largely from the oxidation of sulphur-containing amino acids plus approximately 15 000 mmol of carbon dioxide from the oxidation of carbon during tissue respiration. There is also an internal

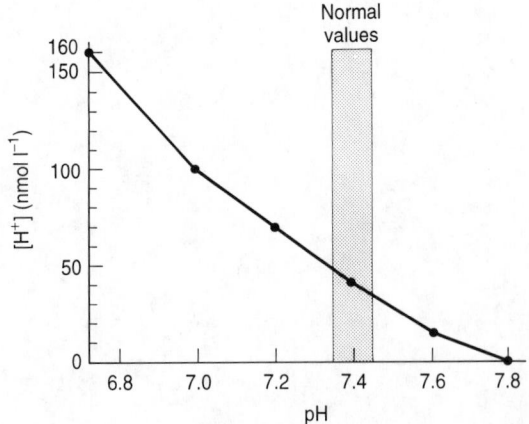

Fig. 1. The relationship between hydrogen ion concentration and pH.

Table 1. *pH and [H$^+$]*

pH (units)	[H$^+$] (nmol l^{-1})	
3	10^6	
6	10^3	
7	100	
7.1	80	
7.35	45	⎫
7.4	40	⎬ Normal range
7.45	35	⎭
7.7	20	
8	10	
9	1	

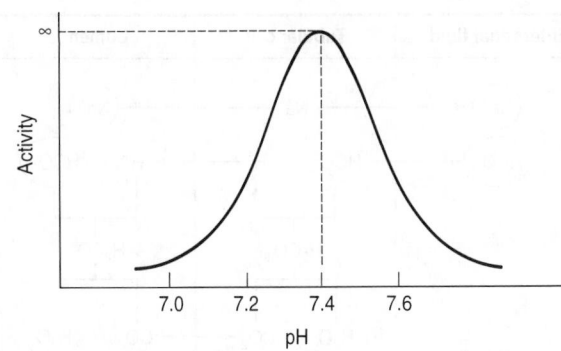

Fig. 2. Enzyme activity curve and acid–base balance.

transfer of organic acids such as lactic, hydroxybutyric and acetoacetic acids (from intermediate metabolism of fats, carbohydrates and amino acids) which are metabolized by the liver.

Carbon dioxide (CO_2) is not an acid *per se*, but in the presence of carbonic anhydrase it can combine with water to form carbonic acid:

$$CO_2 + H_2O \rightleftharpoons H_2CO_3 \rightleftharpoons H^+ + HCO_3^-$$

Assuming adequate pulmonary ventilation, carbon dioxide is eliminated in expired air. H$^+$ can only be eliminated by the kidney.

Table 2 indicates the amount of H$^+$ that is produced daily. Not surprisingly, the body has intrinsic mechanisms which maintain an integral 'status quo' without which life would not be possible. More than 100 years ago, Claude Bernard recognized the need for electrolyte homeostasis and H$^+$ is no exception to the rule.

The homeostatic mechanisms for H$^+$ are efficient and, in health, balance the rates of production and excretion. Any imbalance is offset by buffering, which keeps [H$^+$] within narrow limits so as to provide a suitable environment for enzyme reactions without which the metabolic machinery would grind to a halt. Enzymes are complex proteins whose catalytic activity is both dependent on and exquisitely sensitive to [H$^+$]. They have an optimal [H$^+$] range and are readily denatured by excessively acidic or basic conditions (Fig. 2). Furthermore, acidosis diminishes myocardial performance, reduces vascular reactivity to catecholamines and ultimately produces depression of the central nervous system. Although a modest degree of acidosis is an integral part of the physiological response to stress/trauma, extreme values are associated with profound metabolic derangement and are the precursor to cell death. Acidosis occurs when excess quantities of H$^+$ are generated and/or renal function and the buffer systems are suboptimal.

Alkalosis results from an excessive intake of bases (e.g. bicarbonate) or a loss of acid (e.g. prolonged vomiting or selective renal excretion of H$^+$ in the face of hypokalaemia). It is associated with a shift of the oxyhaemoglobin dissociation curve to the left and impaired oxygen delivery to the tissues. These changes are compensated for by parallel and sequential changes in circulating buffer systems (almost instantaneous), pulmonary ventilation (rapid) and renal exchanges (slow, i.e. up to 72 h) (Fig. 3). Buffers represent the first line of defence against an H$^+$ insult and play a crucial role in the homeostatic process.

Table 2. *H$^+$ flux*

Source	Daily output (mol)	Nature	Elimination
Aerobic respiration	15.0	Carbon dioxide	Lungs
Liver/muscle/brain	1.5	Organic acids, e.g. lactate	Liver
Diet	0.1	Inorganic acids, e.g. sulphuric acid	Kidney

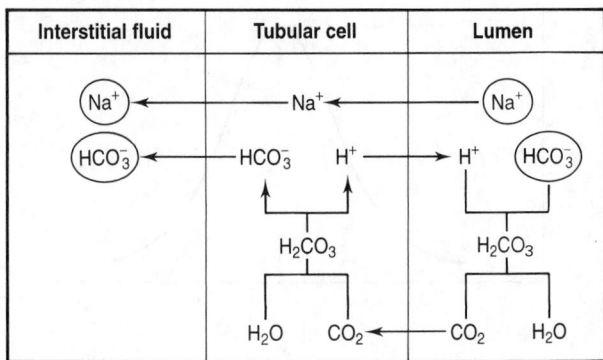

Interstitial fluid	Tubular cell	Lumen

Fig. 3. Renal reabsorption of HCO_3^-.

Buffers

A buffer, in this context, is defined as a compound which opposes change in $[H^+]$. Physiological buffers consist of a weak acid in equilibrium with its conjugate base:

$$Acid \rightleftharpoons conjugate\ base^- + H^+$$

$$K_a = ([H^+] \times [conjugate\ base^-])/[acid]$$

where K_a is the dissociation constant. H^+ added to this system will combine with the conjugate base to form the undissociated acid (lowering the $[H^+]$). If $[H^+]$ falls, the acid will dissociate to generate more H^+.

The body's main buffer systems are:

- Intracellular:
  - Protein.
  - Phosphate.
  - Haemoglobin.
- Extracellular:
  - Bicarbonate.

The efficiency of a buffer is represented by its concentration and its equilibrium position. It is most efficient at a $[H^+]$ that results in equal concentrations of acid and conjugate base (i.e. when $[H^+] = K_a$). Thus the most efficient buffers are those whose K_a approximates to the $[H^+]$ of its environment; for example:

$$K_a\ (protein) = 100, corresponding\ to\ an\ intracellular$$
$$[H^+]\ of\ 100\ nmol\ l^{-1}$$

$$K_a\ (haemoglobin) = 40, corresponding\ to\ an\ intravascular$$
$$[H^+] of\ 40\ nmol\ l^{-1}$$

Paradoxically, the principal extracellular buffer is bicarbonate whose K_a ($\approx 1000\ nmol\ l^{-1}$) should make it relatively inefficient. However, its strength lies in the large quantities available plus the fact that its component

HCO_3^- and carbonic acid (dissolved carbon dioxide) are easily manipulated by the kidneys and lungs respectively, assuming adequate haemodynamic renal and pulmonary function.

The bicarbonate system

Consider the dissolution of carbon dioxide in blood:

$$CO_2 + H_2O \rightleftharpoons H^+ + HCO_3^-$$

The dissociation of carbonic acid is described by the constant K_a (law of mass action):

$$K_a = ([H^+] \times [HCO_3^-])/H_2CO_3]$$

The pH of this solution is given by the Henderson–Hasselbach equation:

$$pH = (pK_a + log_{10}[HCO_3^-])/(0.03 \times Pa_{CO_2})$$

where $[H_2CO_3]$ has been replaced by $Pa_{CO_2} \times$ constant (Henry's law).

Under normal circumstances, the ratio of $[HCO_3^-]$ to Pa_{CO_2} is 20:1. Irrespective of the individual values, if the ratio remains the same the pH (or $[H^+]$) will not change.

In general, H^+ released into the circulation will combine with HCO_3^- to form carbonic acid which will then dissociate into carbon dioxide and water. Carbon dioxide is then delivered to the lungs and eliminated in the expired air. A prerequisite for this is therefore:

- Adequate cardiopulmonary circulation.
- Adequate pulmonary ventilation.

Carbon dioxide removal requires:

- Cardiopulmonary circulation ☑
- Pulmonary ventilation ☑

Acid–base disturbance: clinical considerations

Arterial blood gas sampling

When taking an arterial blood gas sample, the following points should be considered:

- Date and time of sample.
- Current therapy.
  - Oxygen.
  - Bicarbonate.

- Ventilatory status.
- Heparin: $Paco_2$ and $[HCO_3^-]$ show an inverse relationship to the volume of heparin used, especially if the volume is greater than 10% of the sample volume. Heparin $5000\,IU\,ml^{-1}$ is acidic and may influence $[H^+]$ reading.
- Air bubbles: greater than 0.5–1% of sample volume will introduce error.
- Machine calibration must be carried out at least once a day against standardized solutions.
- Remember to record patient temperature (e.g. cardiopulmonary bypass).
- Indices will deteriorate with time ($Paco_2$ and $[H^+]$ will rise). Any sample that cannot be measured in less than 10 min must be sealed, packed in ice and measured within 2 h.

Arterial blood gas indices

NB: $mmHg = kPa \times 7.5$.

Measured (electrode) indices

Hydrogen ion concentration ($[H^+]$)
Normal value: 34–$45\,nmol\,l^{-1}$.
pH < 7.35 ($[H^+] > 45\,nmol\,l^{-1}$) is defined as acidotic.
pH > 7.45 ($[H^+] < 35\,nmol\,l^{-1}$) is defined as alkalotic.

Abnormalities of the $[H^+]$ are described as respiratory, metabolic or mixed in origin.

Partial pressure of oxygen, arterial Pao_2
Normal value: 9.3–$13.1\,kPa$.

The Pao_2 represents the partial pressure of oxygen in an arterial sample; it gives no indication of the oxygen content of the blood or delivery to cells.

The Fio_2 (fraction of oxygen in inspired air) must be recorded for valid interpretation. A normal Pao_2 in the face of an Fio_2 of 0.8 indicates advanced lung pathology.

Partial pressure of carbon dioxide, arterial $Paco_2$
Normal value: 4.5–$6.0\,kPa$.

The $Paco_2$ indicates the adequacy of alveolar ventilation. A raised $Paco_2$ ($>6.0\,kPa$) is defined as respiratory acidosis, irrespective of $[H^+]$. A low $Paco_2$ ($< 4.5\,kPa$) is defined as respiratory alkalosis, irrespective of $[H^+]$.

Derived indices (microprocessor)

Actual bicarbonate ($[HCO_3^-]$)
Normal value: 23–$28\,mmol\,l^{-1}$.

This can be calculated from the Henderson–Hasselbach equation provided $[H^+]$ and $Paco_2$ are known:

$$[HCO_3^-] = (24 \times Paco_2)/[H^+]$$

Although primarily influenced by metabolic derangements, $[HCO_3^-]$ is also changed by respiratory disorders (e.g. $[HCO_3^-]$ will fall with respiratory alkalosis).

Standard bicarbonate ($[HCO_3^-]$)
Normal value: 23–$28\,mmol\,ml^{-1}$.

This is the bicarbonate concentration of plasma that has been fully equilibrated with a normal $Paco_2$ at standard temperature and pressure and thus reflects only non-respiratory (i.e. metabolic) effects.

Base excess
Normally $0.0 \pm 2.0\,mmol\,l^{-1}$.

Base excess is defined as the titratable base to a $[H^+]$ of $40\,nmol\,ml^{-1}$ and a $Paco_2$ of $5.3\,kPa$ at $37°C$. It represents the deviation from normal of the buffering capacity of the body and is calculated from a nomogram (Sigaard Anderson). A deficiency of buffer base or negative base excess (synonymous with base deficiency) implies a non-respiratory (metabolic) acidosis; a positive base excess implies metabolic alkalosis.

Note: Standard bicarbonate and base excess, being *in vitro* calculations, are inherently flawed as they take no account of *in vivo* interstitial and intracellular buffering.

Finally, it must be remembered that, as with all measured variables, it is the trend which may be as important as an individual result.

Acid–base disturbances

Recognizing the central role of bicarbonate in H^+ regulation, we can use a graphical representation of the Henderson–Hasselbach equation to depict the serial events in the four main acid–base perturbations. Fig. 4 shows a series of $[H^+]$ isopleths (lines of constant $[H^+]$) plotted against $Paco_2$ and $[HCO_3^-]$. Any deviation from the $[H^+] = 40\,nmol\,l^{-1}$ (pH 7.40) line represents a change in the $[HCO_3^-]/Paco_2$ ratio and a movement to another $[H^+]$ isopleth. Any compensation will tend to return the $[H^+]$ towards normal but at a different point on the line bearing in mind the simple rule:

COMPENSATION IS NEVER COMPLETE

An acidosis remains an acidosis
An alkalosis remains an alkalosis

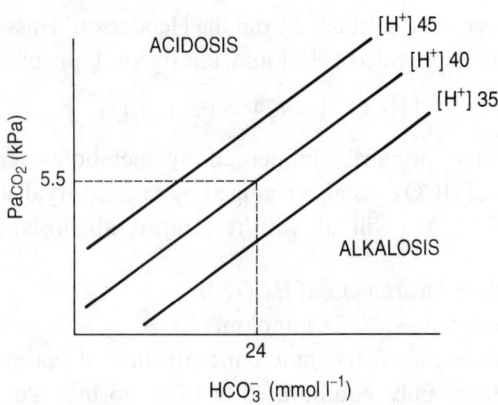

Fig. 4. Graphical representation of the Henderson–Hasselbach equation.

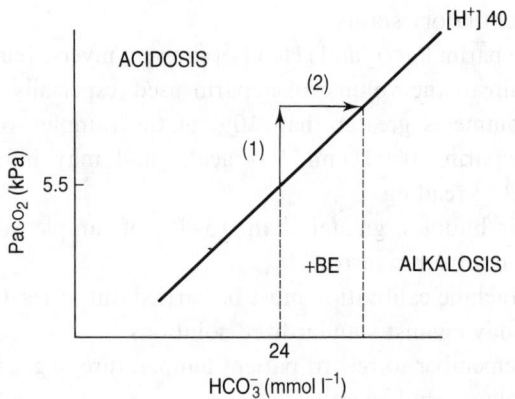

Fig. 5. Schematic depicting the development of a primary respiratory acidosis (1) and a secondary compensatory metabolic alkalosis (2).

Respiratory acidosis

Definition

- $Paco_2 > 6.0\,kPa$.

Pathology

- See Fig. 5.

Aetiology: causes of respiratory acidosis

Carbon dioxide production normal, reduced alveolar ventilation

- Depression of respiratory centre:
  - Anaesthetics.
  - Sedatives, including opioids.
  - Muscle relaxants.
  - Trauma.
  - Space-occupying lesions:
     Tumour.
     Blood.
     Pus.
     Fluid.
- Airway obstruction:
  - Chronic airflow limitation.
  - Bronchospasm.
  - Laryngospasm.
  - Foreign body.
  - Epiglottitis.
- Pulmonary disease:
  - Fibrosis.
  - Pneumonia.
  - Adult respiratory distress syndrome (ARDS).
- Extrapulmonary disease:
  - Kyphoscoliosis.
  - Flail chest.
  - Pneumothorax.

- Neuromuscular disease:
  - Polio.
  - Motor neurone disease.
  - Guillain–Barré syndrome.
  - Tetanus.
  - Botulism.

Carbon dioxide production increased, normal alveolar ventilation

- Malignant hyperpyrexia.
- Catabolism.

Increased $Fico_2$

- Closed-circuit anaesthesia.

Features of respiratory acidosis

- Central nervous system effects:
  - Increased intracranial pressure secondary to cerebral vasodilation.
  - Tachypnoea.
  - Headache.
  - Impaired cerebration.
  - Loss of consciousness.
  - Apnoea.
  - Convulsions.
- Cardiovascular effects:
  - Catecholamine release.
  - Increased heart rate ⎫ Warm dry skin, bounding
  - Increased pulse pressure ⎬ pulse, increased surgical
  - Peripheral vasodilation. ⎭ bleeding
  - Increased blood pressure.
  - Arrhythmias.
  - Conduction defects.

- General effects:
  - Increased serum potassium.
  - Displacement of the oxyhaemoglobin dissociation curve to the right.

Treatment

This should be directed at the primary cause and aim to decrease $Paco_2$ by increasing alveolar ventilation. If a high $Paco_2$ persists, then a compensatory metabolic alkalosis develops through increased renal elimination of H^+ and reabsorption of HCO_3^-. This can take days to develop. Mechanical ventilation may be necessary in severe cases.

Respiratory alkalosis

Definition

- $Paco_2 < 4.5\,kPa$.

Pathology

- See Fig. 6.

Aetiology: causes of respiratory alkalosis

- Hypoxia:
  - Altitude.
  - Anaemia.
  - Pulmonary disease:
    Embolus.
    Fibrosis.
    Oedema.
    Pneumonia.

- Increased respiratory drive:
  - Respiratory stimulants:
    Salicylates.
    Doxapram.
    Trauma.
    Infection.
  - Cerebral pathology:
  - Hepatic failure.
  - Septicaemia.
- Mechanical hyperventilation.
- Physiological:
  - Pain.
  - Anxiety.
  - Pregnancy.

Features of respiratory alkalosis

- Specific effects:
  - Euphoria/confusion (secondary to cerebral vaso-constriction).
  - Increased neuromuscular excitability ⎫ Secondary to
  - Carpopedal spasm. ⎬ decreased
  - Circumoral tingling. ⎭ Ca^{2+}
- General effects:
  - Shift of oxyhaemoglobin curve to the left.
  - Hypokalaemia.

Therapy

This should be directed towards the primary cause for hyperventilation. Respiratory alkalosis is not unusual in the anaesthetized and (hyper)ventilated patient. This is no threat to the young and fit but significant hypocarbia ($Paco_2 < 3.8\,kPa$) may compromise cerebral circulation in the elderly. Compensation occurs slowly and is characterized by renal excretion of bicarbonate and the development of a metabolic acidosis.

Metabolic acidosis

Definition

- $[H^+] > 45\,nmol\,l^{-1}$ and decrease in $[HCO_3^-]$ in the presence of a normal $Paco_2$.

Pathology

- See Fig. 7.

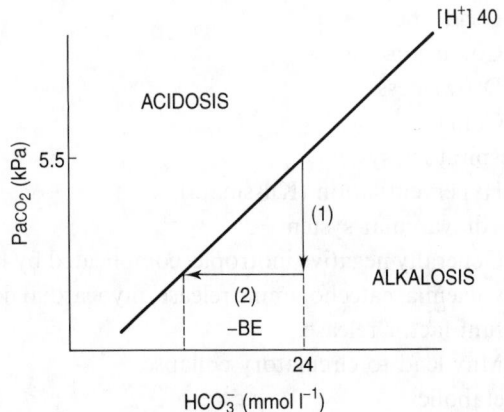

Fig. 6. Schematic depicting the development of a primary respiratory alkalosis (1) and a secondary compensatory metabolic acidosis (2).

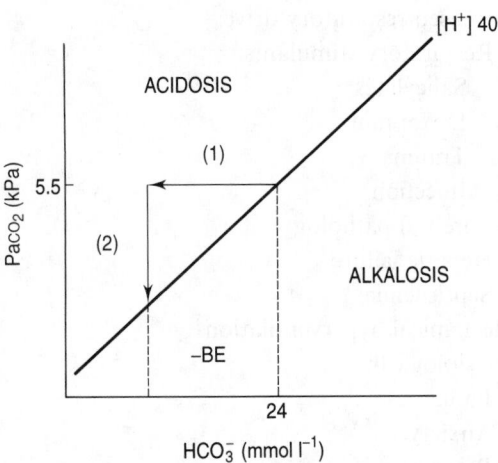

Fig. 7. Schematic depicting the development of a primary metabolic acidosis (1) and a secondary compensatory respiratory alkalosis (2).

Aetiology

Metabolic acidosis involves acid accumulation with a corresponding fall in serum bicarbonate, the anionic moiety being retained to maintain neutrality. Diagnosis can be difficult but may be classified by consideration of the anion gap.

Anion gap

In order to maintain electrical neutrality the sum of the plasma cations (Na^+ and K^+) must equal the sum of the anions (Cl^- and HCO_3^-). Normally the former outweigh the latter by approximately $10–15$ mmol l^{-1}. This is the anion gap and represents (unmeasured) proteins, phosphate, sulphate or exogenous anions. An elevated anion gap is usually synonymous with a metabolic acidosis provided antibiotic treatment (sodium load) and dehydration are excluded (Table 3).

Metabolic acidosis can also occur with a normal anion gap. This may follow loss of bicarbonate from the kidney or gut, the loss being compensated by retention of chloride.

Causes of metabolic acidosis with a normal anion gap:

- Gastrointestinal bicarbonate loss:
  - Pancreatic fistulae.
  - Diarrhoea.
  - Ureteric diversion.
- Hyperalimentation.
- Drugs:
  - Carbonic anhydrase inhibitors.
  - Ammonium chloride.
  - Hydrochloric acid.

Table 3. *Causes of metabolic acidosis with an increased anion gap*

Abnormality	Unmeasured anions
Lactic acidosis	Lactate
Ketoacidosis	Acetoacetate
Uraemia	–
Drugs	–
– Salicylates	
– Methanol	
– Paraldehyde	
– Ethylene glycol	

Lactic acidosis

Definition: $[H^+] > 45$ nmol l^{-1}, serum lactate > 5 mmol l^{-1}.

This remains an important cause of metabolic acidosis and, in the absence of serum lactate measurements, should be considered in any patient with a large anion gap or acidosis in the absence of uraemia or ketoacidosis.

Causes of lactic acidosis:

- Inadequate tissue perfusion:
  - Shock.
- Drugs:
  - Ethanol, methanol.
  - Biguanides.
  - Fructose, sorbitol.
- Congenital:
  - Glucose-6-phosphate dehydrogenase deficiency.
- Inadequate hepatic perfusion:
  - Hepatic failure.
  - Reye's syndrome.

Features of metabolic acidosis

- Central nervous system:
  - Headache.
  - Confusion.
  - Drowsiness.
  - Coma.
- Respiratory system:
  - Hyperventilation (Kussmaul).
- Cardiovascular system:
  - Generally negative inotropic, complicated by hypervolaemia, catecholamine release, myocardial depressant factor release.
  - May lead to circulatory collapse.
- Metabolic:
  - Decreased gluconeogenesis.
  - Decreased hepatic uptake of lactate.

- Decreased glycolysis.
- Increased urinary ammonium.
- Decreased urea synthesis.
- General:
  - Hyperkalaemia.
  - Shift of oxyhaemoglobin dissociation curve to the right.

Therapy

This should be directed at the primary cause but should generally be supportive to cardiorespiratory performance:

- Maintain Pao_2.
- Treat hypovolaemia.
- Support the cardiovascular system to maintain cardiac output and tissue perfusion (i.e. renal and hepatic), if necessary by pharmacological/mechanical means.
- Treat hyperkalaemia.
- Treat hyperglycaemia.
- If $[H^+]$ is less than 20 nmol l^{-1} with adequate cardiac index, then consider:
  - Sodium bicarbonate (NB: the use of bicarbonate is controversial unless the primary pathology is one of bicarbonate loss; see cardiopulmonary resuscitation below).
  - Dialysis.

Metabolic alkalosis

Definition

- Increase in plasma $[HCO_3^-]$ in the presence of normal $Paco_2$.

Pathology

- See Fig. 8.

Aetiology: causes of metabolic alkalosis

- Gastrointestinal:
  - High-volume gastric aspirates or vomiting.
  - Pyloric stenosis.
- Renal:
  - Mineralocorticoid excess:
    Cushing's syndrome.
    Conn's syndrome.
- Alkali treatment:
  - Chronic ingestion.
  - Overtreatment of acidosis.

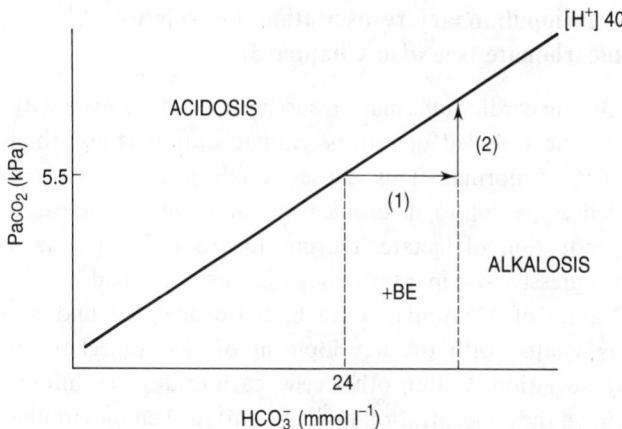

Fig. 8. Schematic depicting the development of a primary metabolic alkalosis (1) and a secondary compensatory respiratory acidosis (2).

Features of metabolic alkalosis

- Volume depletion, which can be severe.
- Hypokalaemia:
  - Muscle weakness.
  - Lethargy.
  - Arrhythmias.

Therapy

Requires correction of the primary defect. The amount of hydrochloric acid lost in vomitus can be considerable (e.g. pyloric stenosis). Treatment includes normal saline with potassium supplementation. The compensation is the development of a respiratory acidosis. In the intensive therapy unit, a common cause of metabolic alkalosis is hypokalaemia. Efflux of K^+ from the cells to correct the extracellular fluid deficit causes an influx of H^+, thereby generating the metabolic alkalosis. The resulting hypoventilation may complicate weaning from mechanical ventilation.

Table 4. *Summary of the primary acid-disturbances* (1) *and their secondary compensatory adjustments* (2) *(see Figs 5–8)*

	Respiratory acidosis	Respiratory alkalosis	Metabolic acidosis	Metabolic alkalosis
$[H^+]$	↑	↓	↑	↓
$Paco_2$	↑ (1)	↓ (1)	↓ (2)	↑ (2)
HCO_3^-	↑ (2)	↓ (2)	↓ (1)	↑ (1)
Base excess (BE)	Positive	Negative	Negative	Positive

Cardiopulmonary resuscitation: the role of bicarbonate (see also Chapter 3)

During cardiopulmonary resuscitation (CPR), even with the most skilled operators, cardiac output is less than 30% of normal. This causes a fall in tissue oxygen delivery, a shift to anaerobic metabolism and an increased production of lactate. During anaerobiosis there is a progressive rise in intramyocardial carbon dioxide levels. Values of 475 mmHg have been documented and are associated with the development of electromechanical dissociation. Within other cells, carbon dioxide diffuses down the concentration gradient into the venous circulation such that during CPR mixed venous blood samples may be profoundly acidotic (pH 7.15) and hypercarbic ($Pv_{CO_2} > 74$ mmHg). Blood passing through the heart into the arterial circulation is easily 'purged' of carbon dioxide. The net result is arterial blood with a pH that may be normal or even alkalotic in the face of venous blood that remains acidotic. This scenario is termed the 'venous paradox' and raises important questions about:

1. The validity of arterial blood gas measurements during CPR.
2. The routine use of bicarbonate therapy during CPR.

Pharmacological buffers

Sodium bicarbonate (NaHCO₃)

Traditionally 8.4% sodium bicarbonate (1 ml = 1 mmol) has been recommended as an intervention to buffer the increased amount of H^+ during CPR and maintain the arterial pH greater than 7.25. However, sodium bicarbonate solutions contains a large amount of dissolved carbon dioxide ($P_{CO_2} = 260–280$ mmHg) which has been shown to penetrate cells more quickly than the bicarbonate ion (HCO_3^-). Paradoxically, this produces a rise in intracellular P_{CO_2} and $[H^+]$. These effects have been demonstrated in the central nervous system where cerebrospinal fluid acidosis may explain the impaired cerebration following cardiac resuscitation. In experimental animals, an elevated intramyocardial P_{CO_2} is associated with decreased myocardial contractility.

Sodium bicarbonate may cause other problems, including:

- Hyperosmolality (circulation overload).
- Alkalosis.
- Hypernatraemia.
- Venous hypercarbia.
- Intracellular acidosis.
- Tissue hypoxia.

To date, its use has not been shown to improve survival. Current protocols do not recommend its routine use in the management of cardiac arrest until other interventions have been employed; i.e.:

- Effective external chest compression.
- Effective intermittent positive pressure ventilation.
- Defibrillation.
- Pharmacological support.

Bicarbonate therapy may nevertheless be indicated in some situations:

- Pre-existing metabolic acidosis.
- Hypercalcaemia.
- Prolonged CPR.

If sodium bicarbonate is used, an initial dose of 1 mmol kg^{-1} is recommended, with no more than half the original dose subsequently. Repeat doses must be guided by arterial blood gas measurements, recognizing that this is a poor index of cellular acidosis.

Calculations may be based on the base excess (BE), assuming that extracellular fluid is 30% of body mass. Therefore the dose required (mmol) is 0.3 × body weight (kg) × BE.

Alternative agents

Other agents are currently being assessed, some of which appear promising by not exacerbating intracellular acidosis. None, however, have been shown to improve survival:

- Tromethamine (THAM) – a potent amine which binds H^+ intracellularly.
- Dichloroacetate (DCA) – reduces serum lactate by stimulation of pyruvate dehydrogenase.
- CARBICARB (sodium carbonate and bicarbonate) – a carbon dioxide consuming agent.

Conclusion

Intracellular acidosis is a significant factor affecting survival from shocked states or cardiac arrest. To date, the only proven corrective intervention is adequate restoration of circulating volume and effective CPR. Pharmacological buffers have not been shown to increase survival. The unacceptable risk/benefit ratio of bicarbonate only supports its use in selected circumstances and not for routine management of profound metabolic acidosis. Alternative agents have potential but cannot be recommended to date. Greater understanding may lead to earlier ventilatory support to maintain or augment respiratory compensation.

WATER AND ELECTROLYTE HOMEOSTASIS

Body fluids

In health, water accounts for two-thirds of body mass, varying with sex, age and build, and is greater in males and infants. A 75 kg adult contains approximately 45 litres of water, distributed as follows:

- Intracellular fluid (ICF): approx. 30 litres.
- Extracellular fluid (ECF): approx. 15 litres, comprising:
  – Vascular compartment: approx. 5 litres.
  – Interstitial compartment: approx. 10 litres.

Distribution of water

Water is not actively transported but moves between the ICF and ECF in response to two influences:

- Osmotic pressure.
- Oncotic pressure.

Osmotic pressure

The osmolality of a solution is dependent on the total number of dissolved particles within it. In the human body the major determinants of osmolality are:

- In the ECF: Na^+, Cl^-, HCO_3^-, glucose, urea.
- In the ICF: K^+.

The two compartments exist in a state of equilibrium such that a change in solute concentration in one will elicit a movement of water to restore equal osmolality (isotonicity).

Oncotic pressure

Water distribution between the vascular and interstitial spaces is further influenced by the oncotic pressure of non-diffusible plasma proteins (albumin). Transcapillary movement of water is governed by the balance of hydrostatic and oncotic forces identified by Starling in 1896:

$$Q = K_F[(HP_{cap} - HP_{int}) - \sigma(\pi_p - \pi_{int})]$$

where Q is fluid flux, K_F is the filtration coefficient, HP is hydrostatic pressure, σ is the reflection coefficient, π is oncotic pressure; cap, int and p indicate capillary, interstitial fluid and plasma, respectively.

Electromechanical neutrality

In a system where an electrolyte solution is separated by a semipermeable membrane, the product of diffusible cations and anions on one side of the membrane must equal the sum of the same ions on the other side (Gibbs–Donnan law). In view of the higher plasma protein (anionic) content, the concentration of plasma cations is higher and the concentration of inorganic anions is lower than in the ICF.

Table 5 illustrates the predominance of Na^+ and Cl^- in the ECF and K^+ in the ICF. This distribution results from the action of ion pumps in the cell wall which actively remove Na^+ from inside the cell, and has implications for fluid distribution and circulating blood volume.

ECF osmolality – the role of water

In health, the volume of the ECF is kept remarkably constant. Regulation operates primarily through control of ECF osmolality and, as sodium is the major influence of ECF tonicity, it is this, with its accompanying water, that determines compartmental volume.

Plasma osmolality is calculated from the formula: $2 \times ([Na^+] + [urea] + [glucose])$. The normal value is 280–295 mOsmol kg^{-1}. As water is conserved, plasma osmolality returns to normal. A contraction in the circulating volume of 10% is a potent stimulus for antidiuretic hormone (ADH) release via:

- Volume receptors in the great veins.
- The renin–angiotensin axis.

Table 5. *Electrolyte and protein content of intracellular fluid, extracellular fluid and interstitial fluid*

	Intracellular fluid	Extracellular fluid (plasma)	Interstitial fluid
Na^+	10	142	144
K^+	160	4	4
Cl^-	2	102	114
HCO_3^-	8	26	30
Mg^{2+}	13	1.0	0.5
Ca^{2+}	1.5	2.5	1.25
SO_4^{2-}	10	0.5	0.5
PO_4^{3-}	57	1.0	1.0
Protein	55	60	0

Conversely, a fall in ECF osmolality inhibits ADH release and causes dilute urine production, permitting water loss and a return of osmolality to normal.

ECF volume – the role of sodium

ECF volume is directly related to its Na^+ content, control of which is mediated by at least two renal mechanisms:

- *Aldosterone.* Elimination of sodium in the urine is a trade-off between glomerular filtration and tubular reabsorption in the kidney. Normally, 75% of filtered sodium is reabsorbed. Expansions of the ECF causes an increase in the glomerular filtration rate, stimulation of receptors in the afferent arterioles of the glomerulus, activation of the renin–angiotensin system and release of aldosterone. This results in increased sodium reabsorption and an expansion (ultimately) of the vascular compartment.
- *Atrial natriuretic peptide (ANP).* Volume receptors in the atrial walls control the release of ANP in response to an increase in ECF volume. ANP increases sodium excretion by inhibiting reabsorption in the distal nephron.

Recognizing the importance of ECF osmolality, it follows that expansion of the vascular compartment is more easily achieved by an isosmolar saline solution (e.g. 0.9% $NaCl = 300$ mOsmol kg^{-1}) than by the hypotonic 0.18% saline. (The more dilute solution will distribute between the ECF and ICF to maintain osmotic equilibrium). Conversely, loss of an isotonic solution from the ECF will have more impact on the plasma volume.

Table 6. *Twenty-four-hour water balance*

Loss	ml	Gain	ml
Skin	500	Diet minimum	1100
Renal	500	Metabolism	400
Gastrointestinal	100		
Pulmonary	400		
Total	1500	Total	1500

In the clinical context, a primary disturbance of sodium or water flux occurs less commonly than a disturbance where both are implicated. Both, however, have distinct features and will be considered separately.

Water balance

Water is gained from food, fluid and basal metabolism. In health, intake is balanced by losses from the gut, kidneys, skin and lungs (Table 6). The minimum dietary input to achieve a balance is 1100 ml per 24 h. Assessment of water balance in the clinical setting requires meticulous fluid charting and serial clinical examination, including measurements of body weight (1 litre of water weighs 1 kg).

Water excess

Causes of water excess:

- Increased intake:
  - Polydipsia.

– Iatrogenic:
Parenteral fluid
Bladder irrigation (TURP).
● Decreased excretion:
– Syndrome of inappropriate ADH secretion.
– Renal failure.
– Cortisol deficiency.
– Drugs, e.g. chlorpropamide (potentiates ADH).

Water intoxication is usually related to diminished water excretion. The additional water distributes across the ECF/ICF with only a modest expansion of the vascular space. Water intoxication is usually asymptomatic unless $[Na^+]$ is less than 120 mmol l^{-1}. However, hyponatraemia accounts for the clinical features which relate to cerebral oedema:

● Early:
– Nausea/vomiting.
– Headache.
– Confusion.
● Late:
– Drowsiness.
– Convulsions.
– Coma.
– Death.

Management should be directed at the primary cause, but definitive treatment will involve water restriction. In time, obligatory water losses will allow the osmolality of the body compartments to normalize. In more severe cases, twice normal saline can be administered.

Water depletion

Water depletion in isolation is uncommon but will occur when intake is inadequate and/or losses are excessive. Causes include:

● Increased excretion:
– Skin: sweating.
– Renal: diuretics, diabetes insipidus.
– Gastrointestinal: fistulae, diarrhoea.
– Pulmonary: mechanical ventilation.
● Decreased intake:
– Impaired conscious level.
– Age:
Very young.
Elderly.
– Perioperative starvation.
– Dysphagia.

Loss of water from the ECF causes a rise in serum osmolality and stimulation of ADH release and thirst. Features of a reduced plasma volume are absent except 'in extremis' as the water loss is 'buffered' by redistribution from within the cells. An inexorable increase in oncotic pressure will aid fluid retention in the vascular compartment and make circulatory failure a late feature. Diabetes insipidus should be managed by replacement therapy with the vasopressin analogue desmopressin (e.g. DDAVP 0.5–1 µg by subcutaneous injection, repeated as necessary).

The features of water depletion are:

● Early:
– Thirst.
– Oliguria.
– Dry mucous membranes.
– Poor skin turgor.
● Late:
– Weakness.
– Confusion.
– Drowiness.
– Collapse.

Management should be directed at the primary defect and its replacement. Water should be replaced enterally if possible or intravenously if necessary, using 5% dextrose or hypotonic saline. In cases of severe dehydration (e.g. plasma $[Na^+]$ greater than 160 mmol l^{-1}), judicious rehydration over 24–48 h is indicated to avoid rapid changes in plasma $[Na^+]$.

Sodium balance

A 75 kg adult contains approximately 4000 mmol of sodium distributed as 2100 mmol Na^+ in the ECF and 400 mmol Na^+ in the ICF. A further 1500 mmol Na^+ are found in bone.

As cell membranes are permeable to sodium, Na^+ is actively transported across the cell wall in order to maintain the transcellular gradient.

A typical Western diet contains approximately 150 mmol Na^+, representing ten times the daily losses from gut, skin and kidneys. Dietary sodium is small compared to the substantial production by the gut. Normally the kidneys retain more than 95% of filtered sodium and play a pivotal role in homeostasis.

Sodium excess

The causes of primary sodium excess are:

- Increased intake:
  - Iatrogenic, e.g. total parenteral nutrition, sodium bicarbonate therapy.
- Decreased excretion:
  - Renal failure:
    - Acute.
    - Chronic.
  - Cushing's syndrome.
  - Conn's syndrome.
  - Congestive cardiac failure.
  - Nephrotic syndrome.
  - Cirrhosis.

Hypernatraemia occurs most commonly in situations of predominant water depletion. It may also occur in association with impaired renal excretion when it is invariably associated with retention of chloride and water. Symptoms are then a result of an expansion of plasma and interstitial volumes producing oedema, and include:

- Peripheral oedema.
- Weight gain.
- Dyspnoea.
- Hypertension.
- Pulmonary oedema.
- Effusions.

Management should be directed at the primary cause. Loop diuretics may be used to expedite sodium excretion. Dialysis may be necessary to support compromised renal function and/or in the event of volume overload. Otherwise treatment is with hypotonic intravenous fluids.

Sodium depletion

Causes of primary sodium depletion:

- Decreased intake:
  - Rare.
- Increased excretion:
  - Skin: sweating, burns, cystic fibrosis.
  - Renal diuresis:
    - Drugs
    - Acute tubular necrosis.
  - Gastrointestinal: diarrhoea, ileus, fistulae.

Sodium depletion is associated with loss of both water and chloride. Symptoms result from a contraction in the vascular space, including:

- Weakness.
- Dizziness.
- Syncope.
- Tachycardia. ⎫
- Hypotension. ⎭ Impending circulatory failure.

Thirst is not a feature of sodium depletion. Compensation involves renal sodium conservation via aldosterone and urinary concentration through ADH release. Cardiovascular decompensation occurs earlier than in primary water depletion as fluid loss from the ECF is not 'buffered' by the ICF.

Management should be directed at the primary cause. Severe plasma volume deficits warrant prompt intravenous replacement with isotonic fluids, colloid or plasma to restore cardiovascular stability.

Assessment of sodium/water status

Serum $[Na^+]$ is not indicative of ECF sodium content, only the relative amounts of sodium and water. It can thus be normal, raised or lowered in states of both sodium excess and depletion.

Accurate assessment requires:

- *History:* to identify relevant features of gastrointestinal disturbance.
- *Examination:* noting hydration, circulatory status and presence of oedema. Serial fluid charts, including body weight, are invaluable for the in-patient.
- *Investigations:*
  - Haemoglobin, urea and serum proteins.
  - Serum and urine chemistry: measurements of urine volume, electrolyte content and osmolality provide essential information when related to clinical status and the biochemical profile of the serum.

Hyponatraemia

This is common, particularly in hospital in-patients.

Aetiology

- Sodium depletion.
- Water excess.
- Combination of sodium depletion and water excess.
- 'Sick cell' syndrome.

- Syndrome of inappropriate ADH secretion.
- Pseudohyponatraemia (secondary to hyperlipidaemia).

Features

- These depend on the predominant pathology.

Management

This is aimed at the primary defect. Asymptomatic patients may not need treatment. Aggressive correction of salt and water imbalance is rarely justified and may be hazardous. Judicious correction over 24–48 h is appropriate.

Hypernatraemia

This occurs less commonly.

Aetiology

- Pure water depletion.
- Water depletion greater than sodium depletion: usual.
- Sodium excess: rare.

Features

Depend on overriding pathology, usually water depletion.

Management

This must address the primary cause. Hypotonic fluids should be given slowly. A sudden fall in serum [Na$^+$] may precipitate cerebral oedema.

Potassium balance

Body potassium is distributed predominantly (98%) as an intracellular cation, with only 2% present in the ECF. In view of the volume of plasma (5 litres) compared to interstitial fluid (10 litres), only one-third of the ECF potassium is in the plasma. Clearly, therefore, serum [K$^+$] is a poor index of total body potassium content.

Homeostasis

The normal serum [K$^+$] of 3.5–5.0 mmol l^{-1} contrasts with the ICF [K$^+$] of approximately 160 mmol l^{-1}. This concentration gradient is responsible for the resting membrane potential necessary for the function of excitable cells (nerve, muscle, myocardium).

A typical diet contains 150 mmol K$^+$, which easily exceeds the obligatory daily losses from the kidneys (10–20 mmol) and gut (10–20 mmol). Nevertheless, gastro-intestinal secretions are rich in potassium, and substantial losses (through diarrhoea and vomiting) can compromise extracellular potassium balance. In the kidneys, most filtered K$^+$ is passively reabsorbed. In the distal nephron, K$^+$ and Na$^+$ are actively exchanged under the influence of aldosterone.

Serum [K$^+$] is dependent upon its distribution across the ICF/ECF, which in turn is predominantly a result of the Na$^+$/K$^+$ pump. Further influences include insulin, which augments cellular uptake, and acid–base balance. A reciprocal relation exists between H$^+$ and K$^+$. In situations where the Na$^+$/K$^+$ pump is deranged (sick cell syndrome), there will follow progressive hyponatraemia and hyperkalaemia.

Hypokalaemia

This results from inadequate intake, increased excretion or redistribution:

- Decreased intake:
  - Oral.
  - Parenteral.
- Increased excretion:
  - Diuresis.
  - Conn's syndrome.
  - Cushing's syndrome.
  - Diarrhoea.
  - Vomiting.
  - Laxative abuse.
  - (Rectal) villous adenoma.
- Redistribution:
  - Insulin.
  - Alkalosis.

Features

Hypokalaemia may be asymptomatic. Symptoms relate to excitable cell dysfunction:

- Weakness.
- Areflexia.
- Ileus (pseudo-obstruction).
- ST/T wave depression.
- U wave.
- Metabolic alkalosis.
- Polyuria.

Table 7. *Treatment for hypokaelaemia*

$[K^+] = 2.5–3.5$ mmol l^{-1}	$[K^+] \leqslant 2.5$ mmol l^{-1}
Conservative: supplementation oral potassium	Intravenous potassium Monitor ECG
Measure serum $[K^+]$ daily	Measure serum $[K^+]$ hourly

Management (see Table 7)

This should be directed at the primary cause (e.g. withdrawal of diuretics and increasing oral potassium supplementation). In severe cases (e.g. serum $[K^+] <$ 2.5 mmol l^{-1}) or in the presence of arrhythmias, intravenous therapy may be needed. As the vascular compartment is small and easily overloaded, intravenous replacement must be carried out with extreme caution after noting renal function.

As a guide, potassium should only be given in diluted form, limited to 40 mmol h^{-1}. Continuous ECG monitoring and hourly serum $[K^+]$ measurements are mandatory to avoid complications.

Hyperkalaemia

Definition: $[K^+] > 7.0$ mmol l^{-1}.

This is less common, but is more serious in view of the potential for dangerous arrhythmias. Causes include decreased potassium excretion, excessive intake or intracellular displacement:

- Increased intake:
  - Oral.
  - Parenteral:
    Total parenteral nutrition.
    Blood transfusion.
- Decreased excretion:
  - Renal failure.
    Acute.
    Chronic.
  - Drugs, potassium-sparing diuretics.
  - Mineralocorticoid deficiency.
  - Addison's disease.
- Redistribution:
  - Acidosis.
  - Tissue damage, crush injury.
  - Catabolism.
- Others:
  - Haemolysed blood sample.

Features

Hyperkalaemia may be asymptomatic, but cardiac arrest can occur without warning. Ominous ECG changes include peaked T waves, broad QRS complex and prolonged P-R interval.

Management

Hyperkalaemia is an emergency. Treatment must be immediate.

Options:

1. Calcium gluconate: 10 ml of a 10% solution intravenously over 5 min.
   - May stabilize the myocardium if ECG changes are present.
   - Has no influence on plasma $[K^+]$.
2. Glucose: 50 ml of a 50% solution intravenously over 5 min with 20 units of soluble insulin.
3. Sodium bicarbonate: 100 ml of an 8.4% solution intravenously over 5 min.
   - Useful if acidosis is present.

The above are temporary measures which merely displace K^+ into the cells. Additional measures may be necessary to expedite potassium elimination or prevent further K^+ release, including:

- Ion-exchange resins (oral, rectal). ⎫
- Dialysis (peritoneal, haemodialysis). ⎬ Renal failure
- Salbutamol infusion.
- Surgical debridement of devitalized tissue (e.g. following crush injury).

Calcium

The body contains approximately 25 000 mmol of calcium, 99% of which is complexed within bone. Only a small fraction (<25 mmol) is confined to the ECF. A typical diet contains approximately 25 mmol of calcium, two-thirds of which is eliminated in the faeces, and one-third in the urine. It is essential to maintain serum calcium between the limits 2.25–2.6 mmol l^{-1} in view of its central role in:

- Neuromuscular function.
- Coagulation.
- Intracellular messengers.

Serum calcium exists in three forms:

1. Ionized (active): 50%.
2. Protein-bound (albumin): 45%
3. Complexed (citrate/phosphate): 5%.

The ionized fraction is influenced by $[H^+]$ which determines the equilibrium of the reaction between ionized and unionized calcium. Total serum calcium is also affected by plasma protein (albumin) concentration. Corrective formulae are used routinely.

Control of ECF calcium (Ca^{2+}) and phosphate (PO_4^{2-}) depends on a complex interplay between two hormones:

1. Parathyroid hormone (PTH).
2. Calcitriol (1,25-dihydroxycholecalciferol).

These hormones exert their effect through gut absorption, bone reabsorption and renal elimination. The role of a third hormone, calcitonin, is uncertain.

Hypercalcaemia

Aetiology: causes of calcium excess

- Malignant disease $\pm$ metastasis.
- Primary hyperparathyroidism.
- Tuberculosis.
- Sarcoidosis.
- Vitamin D excess.
- Thyrotoxicosis.
- Milk alkali syndrome ⎫
- Immobilization   ⎬ Rare
- Lithium treatment   ⎭

Features

Clinical features of calcium excess:

- Weakness.
- Lethargy.
- Nausea.
- Vomiting.
- Constipation/abdominal pain.
- Polyuria.
- Mental disturbance.
- Arrhythmias (QT interval varies inversely with $[Ca^{2+}]$).

Management

This should be directed at the primary cause. Malignancy should be excluded as this is a likely precipitant. Treatment options include:

- Rehydration with intravenous crystalloid.
- Diuretics to promote calcium elimination.
- Drug treatment:
  - Corticosteroids.
  - Calcitonin.
  - Biphosphonates.
  - Mithramycin.
- Dialysis.
- Surgery (e.g. parathyroidectomy).

Hypocalcaemia

Aetiology

- Vitamin D deficiency, diet, malabsorption, inadequate UV light exposure.
- Renal failure.
- Hypoparathyroidism.
- Surgery of the parathyroid, thyroid glands.
- Pancreatitis.
- Alkalosis.

Features of calcium deficiency

- Confusion.
- Numbness, paraesthesia.
- Laryngeal spasm.
- Tetany:
  - Trousseau + ve (peripheral nerves).
  - Chvostek + ve (facial nerve).
- Convulsions.
- Arrhythmias (prolonged QT).

Management

This is directed at the primary cause. If symptomatic, it may be treated with intravenous calcium gluconate (10 ml of 10% solution, slowly). Oral supplements may be required long term.

Magnesium

Total body magnesium constitutes approx. 1000 mmol distributed between muscle and bone. Magnesium is predominantly an intracellular ion, only a small fraction being confined to the ECF. The normal serum range of $0.8–1.2 \, \text{mmol} \, l^{-1}$ is controlled through renal mechanisms. Mg^{2+} plays a role in:

- Muscle contraction.
- Protein synthesis (enzyme cofactor).

A primary disturbance is uncommon and usually develops in parallel with other electrolyte abnormalities.

Hypermagnesaemia

This is uncommon but may be seen in renal failure exacerbated by magnesium-containing antacids/enemas.

Features

- Central nervous system depression.
- Arrhythmias (similar to hyperkalaemia).

Treatment

The acute effects of magnesium can be temporarily antagonized by intravenous calcium. Dialysis may be necessary.

Hypomagnesaemia

This is more common and results from increased gut or urinary loss or impaired intake. Hypocalcaemia is an important consequence of hypomagnesaemia since PTH secretion is Mg^{2+}-dependent.

Definition: $[Mg^{2+}] < 0.7 \, \text{mmol} \, l^{-1}$.

Aetiology

Causes of magnesium deficiency:

- Decreased intake:
  - Starvation.
  - Malabsorption.
  - Total parenteral nutrition.
- Increased excretion:
  - Renal tubular acidosis.
  - Diuretic treatment.
  - Diarrhoea.
  - Vomiting/nasogastric loss.
  - Fistulae.
- Other:
  - Acute pancreatitis.
  - Cardiopulmonary bypass.

Features

Clinical features of magnesium deficiency:

- Confusion.
- Agitation.
- Ataxia.
- Tremor.
- Tetany.
- Convulsions.
- Arrhythmias (increased QT interval).

Management

This should be directed at the primary cause. Mild deficiency may be treated with oral supplements. In severe cases, magnesium may be given by slow intravenous infusion.

Fluid requirements

Maintenance

In order to achieve homeostasis in the face of obligatory losses, the average adult requires approximately 2.5 litres of water plus approximately $2 \, \text{mmol} \, \text{kg}^{-1} \, Na^+$ and approximately $1 \, \text{mmol} \, \text{kg}^{-1} \, K^+$ on a daily basis. For adults, and children heavier than 10 kg, this volume can be estimated by application of the '4, 2, 1 rule'.

'4, 2, 1 rule' for estimating adult fluid requirements

For body weight = 75 kg:

Maintenance fluid volume = $4 \, \text{ml} \, \text{kg}^{-1} \, \text{h}^{-1}$
            for the first 10 kg
    + $2 \, \text{ml} \, \text{kg}^{-1} \, \text{h}^{-1}$
            for the second 10 kg
    + $1 \, \text{ml} \, \text{kg}^{1} \, \text{h}^{-1}$
            for the remainder

    = 4×10
    + 2×10
    + 1×55

    = $115 \, \text{ml} \, \text{h}^{-1}$

For children weighing less than 10 kg (especially premature infants), requirements may be higher (e.g. 4–6 $\text{ml} \, \text{kg}^{-1} \, \text{h}^{-1}$).

Replacement

Rational fluid therapy requires consideration of three factors:

1. Maintenance fluid.
2. Pre-existing deficit (e.g. preoperative fluid deprivation).
3. Current losses (e.g. haemorrhage, burn transudate, intestinal fistulae).

If losses are excessive (e.g. fistulae) it is advisable to measure their electrolyte content as well as volume to allow accurate replacement calculations.

Hypovolaemia: choice of fluid

It is recognized that volume requirements in hypovolaemia exceed measured losses. Endothelial permeability increases in hypovolaemic shock causing reduced oncotic pressure and cellular/interstitial oedema. Furthermore, a 'third compartment' to indicate sequestration of fluid within damaged tissue following surgery or trauma has been described. Volume replacement is not just concerned with the vascular compartment but must also address the intracellular and interstitial compartments whose deficits cannot be measured. The aim of fluid therapy is to replenish but not overload these compartments and much of the current controversy relates to these issues. The choice of fluid will be dictated by the type of loss that has occurred (e.g. haemorrhage, burns, etc.). In the treatment of hypovolaemia, rapid volume expansion takes precedence over consideration of the type of fluid being used in the restoration of tissue perfusion. Oxygen delivery can be improved by dilution of the remaining red blood cells and a reduction in viscosity. Below a haematocrit of 0.25, diminishing red cell availability becomes a limiting factor mandating immediate blood transfusion.

The choice between crystalloid and non-blood colloid continues to generate controversy. Crystalloids are attractive transfusion agents which rapidly distribute between the ICF/ECF. They do not possess the oncotic effect of colloids with the attendant problems of tissue fluid overload, and in particular pulmonary oedema.

Table 8 shows some of the currently available intravenous electrolyte solutions. Physiological saline (0.9%) continues to be popular for both maintenance and initial management of hypovolaemia.

Colloids have the advantage of volume expansion by affecting the intrinsic oncotic pressure. However, sequestration of high molecular weight complexes in the pulmonary interstitium may produce ventilatory impairment. The use of high-quality colloid (e.g. albumin) is expensive and should be restricted to specific indications. Although the choice of resuscitation fluids continues to be debated, the American College of Surgeons currently supports the use of balanced electrolyte solutions (with blood) in the management of hypovolaemia. Despite this, an emerging consensus is that resuscitation fluid requirements (greater than 3–4 litres in an adult) should feature both crystalloid and colloid, with emphasis on the latter as resuscitation volume increases. Oxygen transport can be achieved by maintaining a haematocrit greater than 0.25 by appropriate use of blood products.

Limitations of conventional therapy have generated renewed interest in hypertonic saline and formulations combining hypertonic saline with hypertonic colloid (Table 9). The rationale includes improved haemodynamics with a small volume challenge and reduced interstitial oedema. Whether this translates to improved survival has yet to be shown. Such therapy may have a role in the management of combined haemorrhagic shock and neurological injury.

Table 8. *Intravenous electrolyte solutions (mmol l^{-1})*

	Na$^+$	K$^+$	HCO$_3^-$	Cl$^-$	Ca^{2+}	Dextrose (mg ml^{-1})
Normal saline	150			150		
Dextrose saline (0.18% saline + 4% dextrose)	30			30		40
5% dextrose						50
Sodium lactate (Hartmann's)	131	5	29	111	2	
Ringer's solution	147	4		156	2.2	

Table 9. *Osmolarity and oncotic pressure of intravenous fluids*

	Osmolarity (mOsm l^{-1})	Oncotic pressure (mmHg)
Isotonic crystalloid Physiological saline (0.9%)	308	0
Hypertonic crystalloid Sodium chloride (7.5%)	2400	0
Isotonic colloid 6% HES (hydroxyethyl starch, hetastarch)	310	31
Hyperoncotic colloid 20% HES	312	>100
Combination solutions 7.5% sodium chloride/20% HES	2400	25

Recognizing the importance of oxygen transport, the hazards of blood transfusion and the limitation of administering blood stored for more than 2 weeks, the search for an alternative resuscitation fluid continues. Modified haemoglobin solutions, perfluorochemicals and encapsulated haemoglobin are currently being investigated. It is possible that a substitute may be available within the decade.

Further reading

HINDS, C. J. and WATSON, D. (1996). *Concise Textbook of Intensive Care*. W. B. Saunders, London.

8 Anaphylaxis

A.G. BIRD

Department of Immunology, Oxford Radcliffe Hospital NHS Trust, Oxford, UK

Chapter plan

Introduction
Epidemiology
Pathogenesis
Clinical features
Differential diagnosis
Acute management
Hereditary angioedema
Management on discharge and later assessment
Causes of anaphylaxis
Prognosis

INTRODUCTION

Anaphylaxis (literally 'reverse protection') is a clinical diagnosis characterized by a constellation of manifestations.

Principal manifestations of anaphylaxis

- Acute onset of urticaria
- Cutaneous or mucosal angioedema
- Bronchospasm
- Nausea
- Vomiting
- Cramping abdominal pain and watery diarrhoea
- Hypotension
- Collapse

Classical clinical descriptions of anaphylaxis preceded the understanding of the pathophysiology of the condition by many decades. Anaphylaxis is now known to be the result of the rapid systemic release of large quantities of pharmacologically active mediators from mast cells and basophils and represents the most severe and potentially fatal form of immediate hypersensitivity. Most early descriptions of the condition were associated with the administration of foreign proteins (particularly horse serum for passive protection). It was apparent that previous exposure was required and that subsequent re-exposure weeks or months later caused the risk of anaphylaxis. Subsequent scientific developments allowed the nature of these reactions to be ascribed to the production of antigen-specific IgE (immunoglobulin E) against the protein or drug involved. However, other clinical reactions did not apparently involve prior sensitization and yet showed a similar or identical clinical course in situations where there was no evidence of IgE involvement.

More recent descriptions of anaphylaxis have restricted the use of the term to true allergic reactions known to be triggered by allergen binding to specific IgE on mast cells. The term 'anaphylactoid' has been applied to clinical reactions that are indistinguishable from anaphylaxis but which result from the non-specific degranulation of mast cells and release of mediators by drugs, chemicals or other triggers which do not involve IgE-based sensitivity.

In the acute clinical situation, attempts at such discrimination are meaningless and potentially counterproductive. The term 'anaphylaxis' is probably best used to describe all relevant clinical events, and to direct appropriate and effective acute therapy, which is *identical* for all forms. Differentiation of reactions into IgE-based allergic reactions and non-allergic reactions can only be made later following full clinical and laboratory assessment when anaphylaxis can be described as IgE-mediated, non-IgE-mediated or truly idiopathic (Table 1). Such later assessment is essential so that possible provoking agents can be identified and avoided and therapeutic advice can be given to control unexpected re-exposure.

Table 1. *Classification of immediate generalized reactions*

IgE-mediated

Chemicals and drugs
Penicillins
Cephalosporins
Tetracyclines
Sulphonamides
Macrolides
Quinolones
Streptokinase
Thiopentone and propofol
Suxamethonium and other depolarizing muscle relaxants
Ethylene oxide
Dextran

Foreign proteins
Heterologous serum: horse, mouse, etc.
IgA in IgA-deficient subjects (blood, blood products)
Insulin
Insect venoms
Protamine sulphate
Latex
Desensitizing allergen extracts

Foods
Fish and shellfish
Nuts, especially peanuts
Milk
Eggs
Fruits
Meats
Seeds and spices

Director/mediator release (non-IgE-mediated)
Opiates
Radiocontrast media
Pentamidine

Unknown (anaphylactoid)
Radiocontrast media
Aspirin and other non-steroidal analgesics
ACE inhibitors

Idiopathic

ACE, angiotensin-converting enzyme.

EPIDEMIOLOGY

The apparent incidence of anaphylaxis has varied widely in this century as a result of different approaches to medical therapy and other factors. In the early part of the century, anaphylaxis resulting from the parenteral use of animal sera was the predominant cause of severe reactions. This cause was virtually eliminated with the introduction of antibiotic therapy, but it was replaced by penicillin which was associated with a number of fatal reactions in the early years of its use. Even today, penicillin is associated with fatal reactions at a frequency of between 1 and 7.5 per million treatments and remains the major cause of in-patient anaphylaxis which occurs in about 1 in 3000 hospitalized patients. Amongst in-patients, severe reactions to intravenous anaesthetic agents are the second major cause of anaphylaxis, occurring in between 1 in 5000 and 1 in 25000 anaesthetic inductions (Fisher & Moore, 1981). Intravenous contrast media are also a prominent cause of severe reactions, occurring in 1 in 1000 procedures.

Good data about the frequency of severe or fatal reactions to foods are not available and further epidemiological studies are required. Nevertheless, food-induced anaphylaxis is a significant cause of morbidity and mortality and probably exceeds insect venom anaphylaxis as a cause of death in the UK. In the USA, insect venom sensitivity sufficient to pose a risk of anaphylaxis is present in 0.4% of the population (Settipane & Boyd, 1970).

No surveys have suggested that age, sex or race are factors, and the incidence of anaesthetic, drug and insect venom anaphylaxis is not increased in atopic individuals, although there is evidence that some of the more severe complications (e.g. bronchospasm) are more common in such patients.

PATHOGENESIS

Tissue mast cells and blood basophils contain a number of preformed mediators and upon stimulation are capable of *de novo* synthesis of an even broader range. A full list of the relevant mediators and their biological activities is given in Table 2. The classical activation of the mast cell results from the cross-linking of adjacent specific IgE molecules passively bound to membrane receptors specific for the invariant region of IgE. In a sensitized person, the drug, protein or food will be responsible for the cross-linking of specific IgE molecules on the mast cell membrane. Why only certain exposed individuals form IgE antibodies is not understood and sensitization is *not* restricted to atopic individuals who have a known predisposition to form IgE to environmental allergens. In addition to the classical IgE trigger for mast cell degranulation, a number of other stimuli, including complement-derived split products C3a and C5a (anaphylatoxins), heat and cold, pressure and exercise, can

Table 2. *Mast cell and basophil mediators involved in anaphylaxis*

Preformed mediators: immediate release
Histamine
Heparin
Chondroitin sulphate
Tryptase
Chymase

Secondary, newly synthesized, mediators: delayed reactions
Prostaglandin D$_2$
Leukotrienes, especially C4
Platelet-activating factor
Cytokines

induce mediator release directly by a variety of different mechanisms resulting in similar clinical presentations in some exposed individuals. Finally, certain drugs and chemicals, including aspirin and tartrazine and hyperosmolar solutions (particularly radiocontrast dyes), can induce mast cell degranulation in a small proportion of the population by unknown mechanisms which do not involve IgE.

Hypotensive reactions seen during anaphylaxis are directly related to the release of mast cell mediators, including histamine and tryptase, into the systemic circulation. These mediators act directly on vessel endothelium to induce vasodilation and increase capillary permeability. Recent studies in induced bee-sting anaphylaxis also suggest that activation of plasminogen can be a feature and may result in the further cleavage of biologically active peptides, including C3a and C2 peptide, which may contribute to the pathogenesis of the vascular events of anaphylactic shock (Van der Linden *et al.*, 1993).

CLINICAL FEATURES

Individual patients present with a range of features of varying severity resulting from individual organ sensitivity to the systemic mediator release that characterizes anaphylaxis. The route of exposure, quantity of antigen and rate of administration, as well as coexistent features such as exercise or alcohol (in the case of food sensitivity), can all be important in determining the pattern of an individual attack. However, if an individual suffers repeated attacks, each attack tends to display a similar constellation of features although the overall severity of each attack may vary.

Symptoms in the vast majority commence within minutes of exposure to an identified trigger factor, but occasionally occur with a delay of hours. If a food is responsible, then local oral or oesophageal dysaesthesia, swelling or discomfort may precede the onset of the systemic reaction. However, once the first features of the latter appear, the attack usually evolves with explosive tempo.

First features of a systemic reaction may comprise generalized pruritus, skin flushing, tingling, altered hearing, blurred vision or a feeling of detachment. Such non-specific features rapidly evolve into generalized urticaria and/or angioedema, feelings of foreboding, bronchospasm and stridor resulting from laryngeal oedema. Loss of consciousness can result from hypotension and shock or from direct cardiac effects. Abdominal colic, nausea and diarrhoea are prominent in some individuals and females may experience pelvic pain from uterine contraction.

Fatalities are usually associated either with hypoxia resulting from acute bronchospasm, acute laryngeal obstruction secondary to angioedema or from cardiac collapse or arrhythmias. These cardiac effects may be the direct consequence of anaphylaxis in a minority of individuals (Wasserman, 1986).

In patients undergoing anaesthesia who experience anaphylactic reactions to parenterally administered drugs, some or most of the features of anaphylaxis may be masked or overlooked. Such reactions may present merely as apparently unexplained hypotension or bronchospasm, unless other more subtle features are identified. However, in such clinical situations confirmation of a reaction is of critical importance and its significance appreciated so that full assessment and investigation of the reaction may be undertaken later. Only in this way can a plan of management for future anaesthesia be organized which will avoid the use of agents to which the individual is sensitized.

Following appropriate management of an acute episode, a small proportion of subjects will experience a late second-phase reaction 8–10 h after the initial remission of symptoms. Such late-phase reactions are reminiscent of the second phase of bronchoconstriction that may follow inhalent allergen provocation in an IgE allergic subject. The mechanism of such reactions is probably similar and reflects the release of newly synthesized mediators from mast cells. Experience derived from bronchial challenge suggests that such late-phase reactions can be blocked by corticosteroid administration. This knowledge strengthens the rationale for the routine use of corticosteroids in acute anaphylaxis even though such agents have little immediate benefit in the acute emergency situation.

DIFFERENTIAL DIAGNOSIS

A number of the clinical features of anaphylaxis are similar or identical to manifestations of other local or systemic diseases. Accurate clinical assessment is essential since the management of some of these other conditions may differ significantly from that of acute anaphylaxis.

Other causes of acute loss of consciousness, including vasovagal syncope, arrhythmias and acute myocardial infarction, can mimic features of anaphylaxis, including some of the prodromal sensations that can precede the latter condition. Acute severe asthma, acute bacterial epiglottitis and acute foreign-body upper airways obstruction can cause confusion with acute anaphylaxis since they present with upper or lower respiratory tract obstruction. Some systemic disorders characterized by mediator release, including systemic mastocytosis or the carcinoid syndrome, can reproduce the urticaria or flushing which is a feature of many anaphylactic attacks.

Finally, hereditary angioedema, a non-irritant inflammatory condition resulting from the dominantly inherited condition of C1 esterase inhibitor deficiency, produces recurrent attacks of subcutaneous and submucosal oedema. These episodes are not accompanied by urticaria and are associated with progressive evolving swelling which may involve the upper airway due to tracheal obstruction. Asthma and urticaria are *never* a feature of C1 esterase inhibitor deficiency. Acute attacks require a completely different approach to management and are refractory to all acute therapy used for anaphylaxis. Acute abdominal pain is a further feature that can be shared between anaphylaxis and hereditary angioedema. However, in the latter condition it would be unusual for abdominal symptoms, which are the result of bowel mucosal oedema, to be accompanied by skin or mucosal swelling as part of a single acute attack.

The potential difficulty of correct diagnosis of an acute attack, combined with the need to assess accurately and exclude provoking factors for future anaphylaxis, highlights the importance of full assessment and design of future management strategies for all patients who have undergone previous severe allergic or anaphylactic events. Failure to undertake such assessments and implement management strategies have been a recurring theme in the audit of subsequent deaths from anaphylaxis.

ACUTE MANAGEMENT

Anaphylaxis is an acute medical emergency which, in the absence of appropriate acute medical management, carries a significant mortality. Rapid and appropriate treatment can minimize morbidity and even eliminate mortality. Recent mortality surveys of anaphylaxis series in the USA have highlighted the importance of parenteral adrenaline therapy in acute management. In two recent surveys, mortality was principally seen in adults and children who had not received adrenaline in the course of an acute attack (Yunginger et al., 1988; Sampson et al., 1991). Although anaphylactic attacks are uncommon, their serious and preventable nature means that every A&E doctor, physician, surgeon and anaesthetist should be fully confident of the treatment required. A recent report by the Association of Anaesthetists (1990) has highlighted the need for members to be aware of the procedures for managing an acute attack and to practise them at regular intervals.

Effective management of a severe reaction requires the administration of drugs and intravenous fluids and a sequence of action events.

Immediate action

Faced with an evolving acute anaphylactic reaction, the administration of oxygen and adrenaline are the most critical interventions (Table 3). The adult patient should first be placed flat and 0.3–0.5 ml of 1/1000 adrenaline solution should be given subcutaneously or intramuscularly if the patient is hypotensive but has a systolic blood pressure greater than 80 mmHg. This drug should always be given to a recumbent patient to minimize the risk of hypotensive collapse following administration. This dose may be repeated at 10–20 min intervals if required. In cases of reactions to intravenous anaesthetic agents or with severe hypotension (systolic blood pressure less than 80 mmHg) or, of course, cardiac arrest (Handley & Swain, 1994), 1 mg adrenaline should be given intravenously. Immediate attention to the airway may also be required and, in the case of oral mucosal angioedema, may require immediate tracheal intubation, cricothyroid puncture or tracheostomy to overcome acute upper respiratory tract obstruction. Following establishment of the airway, 100% oxygen should be given with ventilation if necessary.

Establishment of venous access is the next major priority and, in cases of hypotension, saline or colloid fluid replacement should be initiated at a dosage of 10 ml kg^{-1}; dopamine, antiarrhythmic drugs and other

Table 3. *Summary of management principles in an acute attack*

Immediate action

Attention to airway

Adrenaline	0.3–0.5 ml 1/1000 solution subcutaneously in mild anaphylaxis; IM if patient hypotensive but systolic BP >80 mmHg; 1 mg IV if patient hypotensive with systolic BP <80 mmHg, or in cardiac arrest. Repeat at 10–20 min intervals if no response
Oxygen	100%

Venous access

Fluid replacement	Saline or colloid 10 ml kg^{-1}
Bronchodilators	Salbutamol 250 µg IV stat., followed by 5–20 µg min^{-1}
Steroids	Hydrocortisone 500 mg IV or methylprednisolone 2 g IV
Antihistamines	Chlorpheniramine 20 mg IV stat.

Secondary management

- Identification of causative agents if possible and exacerbation factor, e.g. asthma
- Avoidance of exposure, dietary or occupational advice if necessary
- Provision of self-injectable adrenaline and instructions for use
- Optimal management of asthma and cardiac disease and review of current drug therapy, especially ACE inhibitors, beta-blockers, NSAIDs, aspirin
- Consider desensitization if insect venom sensitivity
- Medic-Alert bracelet with appropriate documentation

IM, intramuscular; IV, intravenous; ACE, angiotensin-converting enzyme; NSAIDs, non-steroidal anti-inflammatory drugs.

management of acute hypotension may be required in severe cases (Table 3).

Secondary management

Bronchospasm is a frequent accompaniment of anaphylaxis, particularly in patients with pre-existing asthma or hyper-responsive airways. Its appearance is a frequent source of mortality, particularly in food-allergic subjects and in patients undergoing allergic reactions to intravenous anaesthetic reagents. Parenteral adrenaline, nebulized β-adrenergic agonists and parenteral aminophylline may all be required to overcome acute bronchospasm. Salbutamol 250 µg IV as a loading dose, followed by 5–20 µg min^{-1} as intravenous maintenance or aminophylline 6 µg kg^{-1} IV should be given over a 20-min period. Acute therapy should be supplemented with intravenous hydrocortisone 500 mg IV or methylprednisolone 2 g IV to prevent the development of late-phase reactions in such patients. Urticaria may benefit from antihistamine (H1) blockers symptomatically (chlorpheniramine 20 mg IV diluted and given slowly), but these agents have little or no effect on the other life-threatening features of an acute anaphylactic episode and play little role in its acute management. They are no substitute for adrenaline in the management of anaphylaxis.

Patients with a major anaphylactic episode involving respiratory obstruction or breathing difficulty should not be discharged home immediately after recovery but must be observed for a minimum of 16 h to ensure that there is no late-phase reappearance of symptoms requiring further management. Mortality has been described as a result of such delayed reactions (Yunginger *et al.*, 1988).

HEREDITARY ANGIOEDEMA

As already indicated, features of this genetic deficiency can mimic acute anaphylaxis but differentiation from the latter condition is important since all the drugs conventionally used to manage anaphylaxis (adrenaline, steroids and H1 blockers) are ineffective in terminating an acute attack. The infusion of purified C1 inhibitor concentrate (if available) or fresh frozen plasma can be life-saving in acute attacks and is rapidly effective. However, intubation, cricothyrotomy or tracheostomy may still be required if patients present late in an attack with acute upper respiratory tract obstruction.

The key to management of this condition is its accurate diagnosis and the subsequent long-term administration of prophylactic therapy with anabolic steroids or protease inhibitors. These will largely prevent sporadic attacks or their more predictable appearance following trauma or dental extraction in affected patients (Sheffer *et al.*, 1987).

MANAGEMENT ON DISCHARGE AND LATER ASSESSMENT

All subjects who have experienced anaphylaxis from whatever apparent cause should be referred to an allergist or clinical immunologist with experience in the assessment and management of this condition. However, pending future assessment, all cases except those in which the provocation is obvious and re-exposure totally avoidable (e.g. antibiotic or anaesthetic drugs) should be immediately equipped with self-injectable adrenaline and full instructions about its use (Wynn *et al.*, 1993).

The aim of later assessment is to determine the aetiology of the anaphylaxis where possible and to educate the patient (parents if relevant) and general practitioner regarding future avoidance of a specific trigger and appropriate management of any future reactions.

Assessment of IgE-based triggers is reliant on an accurate allergy history, use of skin-prick tests and/or specific IgE estimations in an attempt to confirm specific sensitivities and consideration for specific desensitization in the case of insect venom anaphylaxis. Interpretation of skin-prick test and specific IgE estimations requires experience since both false negative and false positive results can be seen. In suspected allergy to venoms, antibiotics or anaesthetic reagents, intradermal skin challenge techniques are preferable to prick tests because of their greater sensitivity and quantitated challenge dose. However, such re-exposure carries a significant risk of further anaphylaxis which can be fatal (Lockey *et al.*, 1987).

Anaphylactoid reactions to drugs such as aspirin or radiocontrast media do not involve specific IgE-based mechanisms and cannot be assessed by skin testing or specific antibody measurement.

CAUSES OF ANAPHYLAXIS

Food-induced anaphylaxis

Foods are widely recognized as a definite cause of anaphylaxis. However, there has been little attempt to collect data systematically on the incidence or prevalence of fatal or non-fatal food-induced episodes. Interpretation is confused because of the increasing attribution of distant and probably unrelated symptoms such as epilepsy, headaches or behavioural disorders, particularly in children, to food sensitivity or intolerance. Most examples of the latter are not confirmed on double-blind food challenge but have served to draw attention away from the genuine, important and potentially life-threatening examples of food-induced sensitivity or anaphylaxis.

Most cases of food-induced anaphylaxis are associated with a clear history of immediate urticaria and mucosal angioedema followed by severe bronchospasm or collapse, usually occurring within minutes of ingestion of the relevant food. Confirmation of a direct association is strengthened if the association between a specific food and local or generalized reaction has been documented on more than one occasion.

Assessment is primarily dependent on the history but confirmatory data can be obtained by skin or specific IgE (RAST, radioallergosorbent test) tests to individual foods. Food withdrawal or challenge may be required to give definitive confirmation of the food responsible. Food challenge carries the risk of reinduction of anaphylaxis and should only be conducted with full resuscitation facilities available and by investigators confident of the management of acute attacks.

In children, anaphylactic reactions resulting from milk or egg sensitivity are often transient below the age of 5 years but nut and shellfish sensitivity is usually persistent and may cause serious or life-threatening reactions in both adults and children.

Latex sensitivity and anaphylaxis

IgE-based sensitivity to latex is being increasingly described in the medical literature. A problem particularly for the healthcare professions, the rise in prevalence appears to parallel the increasing routine use of gloves as part of the regimen for universal precautions against bloodborne infections. Recent studies suggest that the prevalence of latex allergy may be as high as 10% amongst healthcare workers who routinely use latex gloves (Hunt, 1993). Atopic subjects appear to be particularly prone to sensitization, perhaps because of the increased opportunity for sensitization via eczematous skin. Children or young adults with spinal abnormalities also appear to be at high risk of sensitization because of frequent latex re-exposure during urinary catheterization.

Once sensitized, an individual can produce local or systemic reactions to minute re-exposures with latex, including during radiographic procedures (Sussman *et al.*, 1992) or surgery (Leynadier *et al.*, 1988) when cases of anaphylaxis have been well described. Confirmed reactions have also been reported to cause confusion during the assessment of suspected anaphylactic reactions to intravenous anaesthetic agents.

Latex allergy should be considered in individuals, particularly healthcare workers, who experience episodes of unexplained anaphylaxis or localized angioedema. Many patients will report a history of local mucosal reactions after latex contact when blowing up balloons or during use of condoms. Some individuals report coexisting allergies to fruits, especially banana or avocado pear.

No standardized skin test preparations for latex are available in the UK. Specific IgE (RAST) detection can help confirm a clinical diagnosis, although false negative results have been reported (Turjanmaa *et al.*, 1988). Elimination of latex exposure can prove more difficult in healthcare workers. Advice to healthcare attendants for subsequent surgical or dental care of sensitized individuals requires considerable thought and care.

Anaphylaxis to anaesthetic agents and other drugs

Anaphylaxis to agents used during intravenous anaesthesia is being increasingly reported and is replacing penicillin as the major cause of drug-induced anaphylaxis. True prevalence of severe reactions is unknown but current estimates range from 1 in 5000 to 1 in 15 000 operations (Moscicki *et al.*, 1990). Prevalence is probably largely determined by agents in current use and opportunities for previous sensitization amongst the population undergoing anaesthesia. Severe reactions are reported more frequently in females but the role of atopy is uncertain as conflicting evidence has been reported. Muscle relaxants and barbiturates, particularly thiopentone, are most frequently incriminated although severe or fatal reactions to a range of other agents have been reported (Fisher & Moore, 1981).

Allergic reactions to intravenously administered drugs during anaesthesia can induce a wide variety of forms of anaphylaxis ranging from generalized urticaria to acute bronchospasm and profound hypotension and cardiac arrhythmias.

Accurate diagnosis of the reaction at the time, followed by careful appraisal at follow-up to identify the drug(s) responsible, is the key to prevention of recurrence. Skin testing has proved valuable in later assessment. Care in its interpretation is required, however, since some agents, including opiates and some muscle relaxants, have direct histamine-releasing properties and can produce false positive results at high concentrations.

Elimination of incriminated drugs has been found to be successful and in one recently published study no patients developed anaphylaxis again after agents producing positive skin tests had been eliminated from a subsequent anaesthetic regimen (Moscicki *et al.*, 1990).

Other causes

Despite rigorous investigation, some anaphylactic reactions remain genuinely idiopathic or are induced by physical factors, including exercise. If recurrent, such idiopathic reactions require prompt therapy and, in some, long-term prophylaxis with oral corticosteroid therapy may be partially effective (Patterson *et al.*, 1993) and be required to control episodes. Beta-adrenergic blockers exacerbate anaphylaxis (Jacobs *et al.*, 1981) and should be avoided in patients with a history of repeated attacks. Angiotensin-converting enzyme inhibitors and non-steroidal analgesics can exacerbate angioedema or anaphylactoid reactions and should be discontinued (Orfan *et al.*, 1990; Slater *et al.*, 1988).

The mainstay of future management of allergic patients with a previous history of anaphylaxis is avoidance of re-exposure to foods, insect stings or drugs. However, even highly motivated individuals are subject to accidental re-exposure. Unknowing exposure to nuts in foods eaten away from home are a recurring feature of reports of fatal or near-fatal anaphylaxis (Yunginger *et al.*, 1988; Sampson *et al.*, 1991).

This experience means that it is essential that such subjects continue to carry self-injectable adrenaline and know how to use it. Such preloaded syringes are distributed by International Medical Systems (Daventry, Northamptonshire, UK). Such patients should also carry a Medic-Alert tag or pendant indicating the nature of their sensitivity, the fact that they carry adrenaline and simple instructions about its use. These identifiers are obtainable in the UK from the Medic-Alert Foundation (12 Bridge Wharf, 156 Caledonian Road, London, N1 9UU; tel. 0171-833 3034; 2323 Colorado Avenue, Turlock, CA 95382-2018, USA). Patients with concomitant asthma should have this well controlled since a superimposed anaphylactic reaction is more likely to prove fatal in the presence of increased bronchial reactivity (Yunginger *et al.*, 1988). In situations of drug sensitivity in which there is a significant risk of anaphylaxis upon re-exposure and yet use of that agent is deemed clinically essential, protocols exist for short-term desensitization to minimize the risk of systemic reactions following administration (Weiss and Adkinson, 1988).

Patients should be instructed that any reaction severe enough to necessitate the use of adrenaline should be followed by immediate transfer to an A&E department.

There, steroids can be given and observations made so that late-phase reactions can be managed appropriately or avoided.

PROGNOSIS

The natural history and prognosis of anaphylaxis is variable. Many cases are not solitary and recurrence is common and should be anticipated, re-emphasizing the need for accurate assessment and follow-up. In children, many will grow out of early food-induced adverse reactions, particularly to milk, but peanut sensitivity is usually life-long and may be associated with fatal reactions later in life (Bock and Atkins, 1989).

Insect venom stings rarely cause anaphylactic fatality in children but are a significant cause of mortality in adults, in whom desensitization should be seriously considered in individuals with a history of severe reactions.

Idiopathic anaphylaxis, like idiopathic angioedema, may enter a period of spontaneous remission following repeated exacerbations which may last from months to years. However, in some cases of whatever cause, anaphylaxis can result in severe or even fatal reactions, even after many years of remission. The condition, therefore, remains a source of potential fatality which indicates the need for persistent vigilance for those patients at risk.

Bibliography

ASSOCIATION OF ANAESTHETISTS (1990). *Report: Anaphylactic Reactions Associated with Anaesthesia.* Association of Anaesthetists.

BOCK, S.A. & ATKINS, F.M. (1989). The natural history of peanut allergy. *J. Allergy Clin. Immunol.*, **83**, 900–4.

FISHER, M.M. & MOORE, D.E. (1981). The epidemiology and clinical features of anaphylactic reactions in anaesthesia. *Anaesth. Intensive Care*, **9**, 226–34.

HANDLEY, A.J., SWAIN, A.H. *et al.* (1994). Resuscitation in special circumstances. In *Advanced Life Support Manual.* Resuscitation Council, UK.

HUNT, L.W. (1993). The epidemiology of latex allergy in health care workers (Editorial). *Arch. Pathol. Lab. Med.*, **117**, 874–5.

JACOBS, R.L., RAKE, G.W., FOURNIER, D.C. *et al.* (1981). Potentiated anaphylaxis in patients with drug-induced beta adrenergic blockade. *J. Allergy Clin. Immunol.*, **68**, 125–7.

LEYNADIER, F., PECQUET, C. & DRY, J. (1988). Anaphylaxis to latex during surgery. *Anaesthesia*, **44**, 547–50.

LOCKEY, R.F., BENEDICT, L.M., TURKELTAUB, P.C. *et al.* (1987). Fatalities from immunotherapy (IT) and skin testing (ST). *J. Allergy Clin. Immunol.*, **79**, 660–77.

MOSCICKI, R.A., SOCKIN, S.A., CORSELLO, B.F. *et al.* (1990). Anaphylaxis during induction of general anaesthesia: subsequent evaluation and management. *J. Allergy Clin. Immunol.*, **86**, 325–32.

ORFAN, N., PATTERSON, R. & DYKEWICZ, M.S. (1990). Severe angioedema related to ACE inhibitors in patients with a history of idiopathic angioedema. *JAMA*, **264**, 1287–9.

PATTERSON, R., STOLOFF, R.S., GREENBERGER, P.A. *et al.* (1993). Algorithms for the diagnosis and management of idiopathic anaphylaxis. *Ann. Allergy*, **71**, 40–4.

SAMPSON, H.A., MENDELSON, L. & ROSEN, M.D. (1991). Fatal and near-fatal food anaphylaxis reactions in children. *J. Allergy Clin. Immunol.*, **87**, 176.

SETTIPANE, G.A. & BOYD, O.K. (1970). Prevalence of bee sting allergies in 4992 boy scouts. *Acta Allergol.*, **25**, 286–91.

SHEFFER, A.L., FEARON, D.T. & AUSTEN, K.F. (1987). Hereditary angioedema: a decade of management with stanozolol. *J. Allergy Clin. Immunol.*, **80**, 855–60.

SLATER, E.E., MERRILL, D.D., GUESS, H.A. *et al.* (1988). Clinical profile of angioedema associated with angiotensin converting-enzyme inhibition. *JAMA*, **260**, 967–70.

SUSSMAN, G.L., TARLO, S. & DOLOVICH, J. (1992). The spectrum of IgE-mediated responses to latex. *JAMA*, **265**, 2844–7.

TURJANMAA, K., RUELANA, T. & RASANEN, L. (1988). Comparison of diagnostic methods in latex surgical glove contact urticaria. *Contact Dermatitis*, **19**, 241–7.

VAN DER LINDEN, D.-W.G., HACK, C.E., STRUYVENBERG, A. *et al.* (1993). Controlled insect-sting challenge in 55 patients: correlation between activation of plasminogen and the development of anaphylactic shock. *Blood*, **82**, 1740–8.

WASSERMAN, S.I. (1986). The heart in anaphylaxis (Editorial). *J. Allergy Clin. Immunol.*, **77**, 663–5.

WEISS, M.E. & ADKINSON, N.F. (1988). Immediate hypersensitivity reactions to penicillin and related antibodies. *Clin. Allergy*, **18**, 515–40.

WYNN, S.R., FRAZIER, C.A., MUNOZ-FURLONG, A. *et al.* (1993). Anaphylaxis at school: etiologic factors, prevalence and treatment. *Pediatrics*, **91**, 516.

YUNGINGER, J.W., SWEENEY, K.G., STURNER, W.Q. *et al.* (1988). Fatal food-induced anaphylaxis. *JAMA*, **260**, 1450–2.

9 Coma: initial assessment and management

C. GRANGE and D. WATSON

Department of Anaesthesia and Intensive Care Medicine, St Bartholomew's Hospital, London, UK

Chapter plan

Definition
Causes and pathophysiology
Prehospital treatment
Initial accident and emergency management
Assessment
Early management
Conclusion

DEFINITION

The term 'coma', derived from the Greek meaning 'deep sleep', has traditionally been used rather loosely to describe a wide spectrum of neurological conditions in which the main feature is depression of conscious level. However, it should be more correctly defined as a state of total absence of awareness of both self and the external environment (i.e. total unresponsiveness to all internal and external stimuli) with only residual reflex activity remaining. It is the final stage of brain failure in the continuum of conciousness from alert to drowsy to unconscious. Unrousable unresponsiveness is equivalent to coma. Patients who do not open their eyes to pain, do not obey commands and do not utter recognizable words are by definition in coma.

CAUSES AND PATHOPHYSIOLOGY

Coma is a failure of arousal and lack of awareness of one's surroundings. Arousal is mediated by the reticular activating system (RAS) and can be expressed as eye opening. Awareness consists of complex memory, analytical, emotional and language functions which depend on the integrity of the cerebral cortex and can be tested by verbal and motor responses to command or stimulation (Miller, 1987).

The RAS is a diffuse brainstem structure extending from the caudal medulla to rostral midbrain, with projections to the diencephalon and cerebral cortex. It has a vast sensory input mainly from the spinoreticular and spinothalamic pathways, cerebellum, basal ganglia, hypothalamus and cerebral cortex (Guyton, 1991). In order to be in the state of arousal or responsiveness the cerebral cortex requires constant input from the RAS necessary for its integrating function. Therefore any interruption of this stimulation is likely to result in coma (Moruzzi, 1949).

Coma occurs when both cerebral hemispheres and/or the brainstem RAS are grossly impaired. An important exception is the temporary coma that can occur with acute extensive damage to the dominant hemisphere (Albert *et al.*, 1976). Lesions causing coma can be classified as follows:

Classification of lesions causing coma

- Diffuse metabolic abnormalities that impair the function of both cerebral hemispheres and/or the brainstem.
- Supratentorial lesions that either compress or destroy the RAS.
- Subtentorial lesions that either compress or destroy the RAS.

Table 1 lists the disorders causing coma on the basis of this classification. The metabolic encephalopathies make up the largest category of illnesses causing coma. In adults, coma is caused by diffuse metabolic encephalopathies in approximately 66% of cases and by structural lesions in the remaining 33% (20% supratentorial, 13% subtentorial) (Plum & Posner, 1980). However, in children, diffuse metabolic causes account for 95% of the cases and the residual 5% are caused by structural lesions (Advanced Paediatric Life Support, 1993).

Table 1. *Disorders causing coma*

Diffuse (metabolic) abnormalities	Supratentorial (cerebral) lesions	Subtentorial (brainstem and cerebral) lesions

1. *Substrate lack*
  Hypoxia
  Ischaemia (decreased cardiac output, cardiac arrest, occlusion
  Hypoglycaemia
  Vitamin deficiency (thiamine – Wernicke's encephalopathy)
	1. *Haemorrhage*
	  Extradural
	  Subdural
	  Subarachnoid
	  Intracerebral
		1. *Haemorrhage*
		  Pontine
		  Cerebellar
		  Posterior fossa extradural and subdural (rare)

2. *Drugs*
  Sedatives (hypnotic, anaesthetics, alcohol, anticholinergics)
  Analgesics (opioids, salicylates)
  Poisons (paraldehyde, methyl alcohol)
	2. *Tumours*	2. *Tumours*

3. *Infective*
  Encephalitis
  Meningitis
  Sepsis
	3. *Infective*
	  Abscess
		3. *Infective*
		  Abscess

4. *Electrolyte disturbances*
  Na^+, Ca^{2+}, Mg^{2+}
  Acidosis
  Hyper/hypo osmolar state
	4. *Infarction*	4. *Infarction*
		  Basilar artery occlusion
		  Cerebellar

5. *Fits/postictal*	5. *Trauma* Contusion	5. *Trauma*

6. *Organ failure*
  Respiratory (carbon dioxide narcosis)
  Kidney (uraemic coma)
  Liver (hepatic coma)
  Endocrine (thyroid, parathyroid, pancreas, pituitary, adrenals)		

7. *Physical injury*
  Hypo/hyperpyrexia
  Diffuse axonal injury		

8. *Hydrocephalus*		
9. *Hypertensive encephalopathy*		

It is important to remember that single focal lesions in the cerebral cortex do not produce coma unless the lesion compresses the brainstem RAS. Also, unlike small supratentorial lesions, small lesions in the brainstem can cause coma because of the discrete location of the RAS. It is worth reiterating the fact that the cause of coma may be multifactorial; for example, an alcoholic patient may be intoxicated, hypoglycaemic or have incurred an intracranial bleed from a fall.

With the exception of hypothermia and drug neuro-depression, all causes of coma are produced by one or more of the following mechanisms:

- Trauma causing shearing forces and neuronal disruption either as a diffuse axonal injury of the cerebral hemispheres or a focal lesion affecting the RAS. The shearing forces can also affect the vasculature, producing tears with resultant intracranial haematoma.

- Mass lesions causing increases in intracranial contents in a fixed volume container (the skull) resulting in intracranial pressure increases causing brain tissue shifts and compression of crucial brain areas.
- Lack of subtrates, either globally or focally, leading to energy failure. Neurones have high energy requirements for synaptic transmission and functioning of Na^+/K^+ ion pumps at the cell membranes (Astrup, 1982; Siesjo, 1984). As a result, if energy production is disrupted, neuronal dysfunction and death will occur rapidly. This produces a potassium (K^+) shift extracellularly and a sodium (Na^+), chloride (Cl^-) and calcium (Ca^{2+}) shift intracellularly. The net result is the activation of metabolic cascades, phospholipid degeneration and proteolysis (Seisjo & Wieloch, 1985).

Each of these mechanisms can lead to cerebral oedema, which may be localized or generalized depending on the nature, dose, duration and site of action of the causative agent. Cerebral oedema can be caused by two mechanisms (Klatzo, 1967): vasogenic due to the breakdown of the blood/brain barrier resulting in increased extracellular water, or cytotoxic due to neuronal death resulting in increased intracellular water.

The disastrous effects of an increase in intracranial pressure (ICP) are due to reductions in cerebral perfusion pressure (CPP) and the effects of herniation/compression of brain tissue. Following brain injury as autoregulation is usually disrupted, the CPP becomes the major determinant of cerebral blood flow:

$$mCPP = mAP - (mICP + mCVP)$$

where m denotes mean, AP is systemic arterial pressure and CVP is central venous pressure.

A reduction in mAP or an increase in either mICP or mCVP will produce a reduction in mCPP with the potential for secondary ischaemic brain damage.

The intracranial contents include 80–85% brain tissue, the remainder being cerebrospinal fluid (CSF), blood and interstitial fluid. Initially, the patient is able to compensate for increases in ICP by driving CSF out of the intracranial compartment and also by reducing blood volume in the cerebral capacitance vessels. The infant has a further compensatory mechanism if the fontanelles are still open. However, after a critical volume is reached, no further compensation can occur and any further increases in ICP will produce a reduction in CPP (and ischaemia) and also cause brain shifts. The brain tissue will tend to decompress through the tentorial aperture or foramen magnum. Successive regions are therefore compressed against more rigid intracranial structures, injured and reactively swollen. Two clinical syndromes are described: the uncal syndrome and the central syndrome. Both result in acute compression of the brainstem and require immediate action before irreversible brainstem dysfunction and cardiac arrest occur.

Uncal syndrome

This syndrome can occur if there is a lateral supratentorial mass lesion (i.e. in the temporal or parietal lobes). The uncus, part of the hippocampal gyrus, is forced through the tentorial aperture and compresses against the fixed edge of the tentorium. The herniating temporal lobe directly compresses the third cranial nerve producing ipsilateral pupillary dilation and paralysis of medial extraocular movements. Further herniation can cause hemiparesis/hemiplegia on both or either side of the body.

If the supratentorial mass is medial (i.e. frontal, occipital or at the vertex), it exerts a more central pressure downwards so that the diencephalon is forced through the tentorium and oculomotor signs are not seen.

Central syndrome

This is caused by the compression of the medulla by the cerebral tonsils as the whole brain is pressed down towards the foramen magnum.

PREHOSPITAL TREATMENT

A comatosed patient is unable to perceive or respond adequately to a changing environment (i.e. is unable to demonstrate protective responses). Therefore the patient must be protected from airway obstruction, hypoxia, hypoventilation, aspiration of stomach contents and hypothermia. As the primary insult to the brain has already occurred, the main aim of prehospital treatment is to recognize and correct factors producing secondary brain damage (Fig. 1). This will provide the best conditions for recovery of the dysfunctional or damaged brain tissue (Miller, 1990). The secondary insults of most concern are hypoxaemia (Gordon, 1986; Miller, 1982), hypercapnia, arterial hypotension and brain compression from haematoma or increased ICP (Miller & Becker, 1982).

The aims of prehospital care are:

1. Rapid initial assessment and simultaneous management of life-threatening conditions enabling stabilization for transportation.

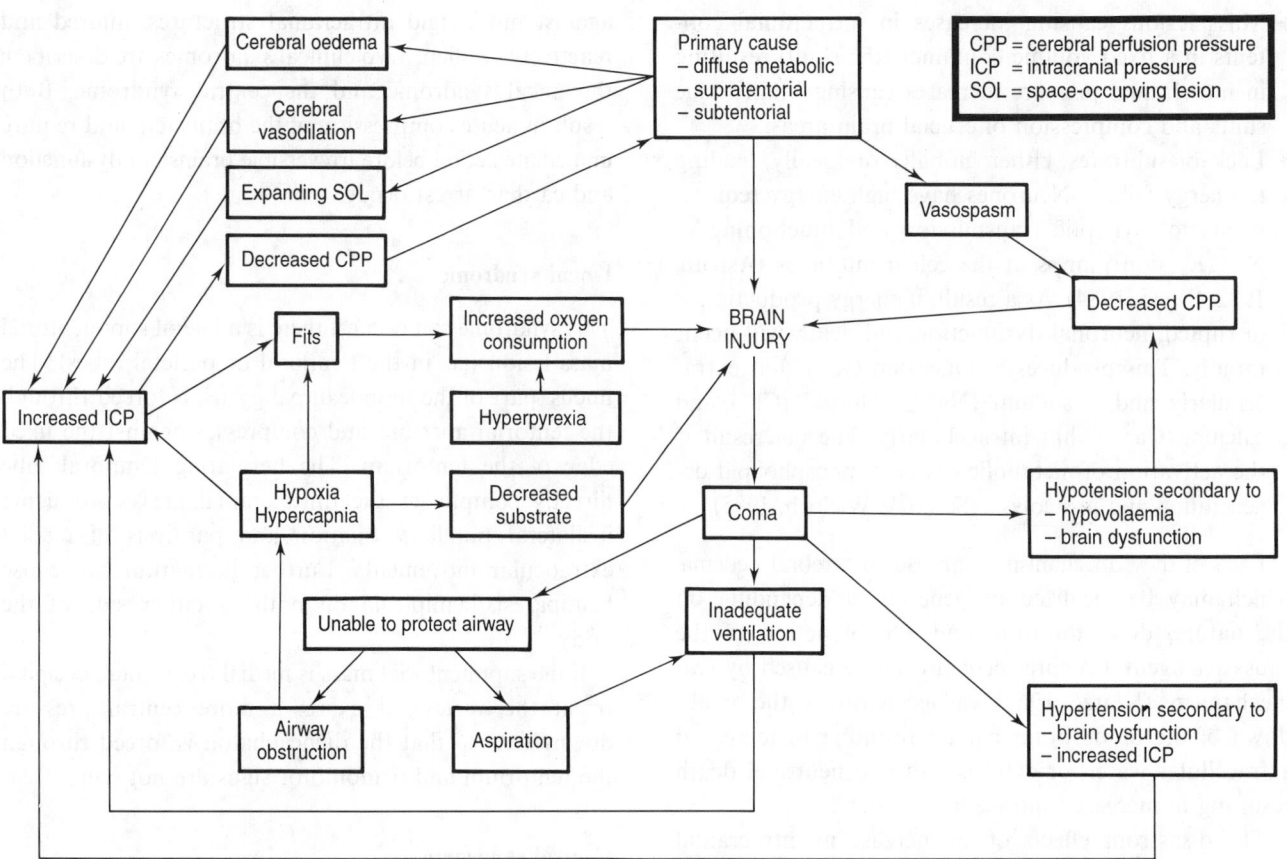

Fig. 1. Primary and secondary causes of coma.

2. Prevention or reversal of factors producing secondary brain damage.
3. Adequate monitoring, reassessment and further management as necessary during transportation.

It is vital that the airway, breathing and circulation have been secured as quickly as possible with the most simple and effective method.

Prior to transportation it is important to confirm that the airway is clear and secured, the cervical spine is immobilized, breathing is not compromised, intravenous access has been obtained, monitoring is adequate and that drugs and equipment are readily available (Fig. 2). In order to minimize the risk of aspiration in a spontaneously breathing patient, suction and a Trendelenberg tilt on the stretcher should be available. During transportation, airways and intravenous lines may become disconnected or removed so anticipation of the worst scenario is essential. Unnecessary movement of the head should be minimized (Wilson & Driscoll, 1991).

INITIAL ACCIDENT AND EMERGENCY MANAGEMENT

Initial management in the accident and emergency department (A&E) is similar to prehospital care, albeit with more highly qualified medical staff and investigative equipment.

The initial aims of A&E management are prevention of secondary brain injury by maintaining cerebral fuels – oxygen and glucose (Fig. 3) – and early diagnosis of remediable medical and surgical conditions such as hypoglycaemia or opioid overdose. Patient management must consist of rapid primary evaluation, resuscitation of vital functions, a more detailed secondary assessment and finally the initiation of definitive care. As ever, the initial steps are control of the airway and cervical spine, breathing and circulation (Fig. 2). High-concentration oxygen should be given to all coma patients. Intubation, if necessary (Table 2), should be undertaken by experienced staff. Adequate sedation and muscle relaxation should be provided to prevent adverse rises in ICP during intubation and a rapid neurological assessment should be made before these drugs are given. Prior to intubation,

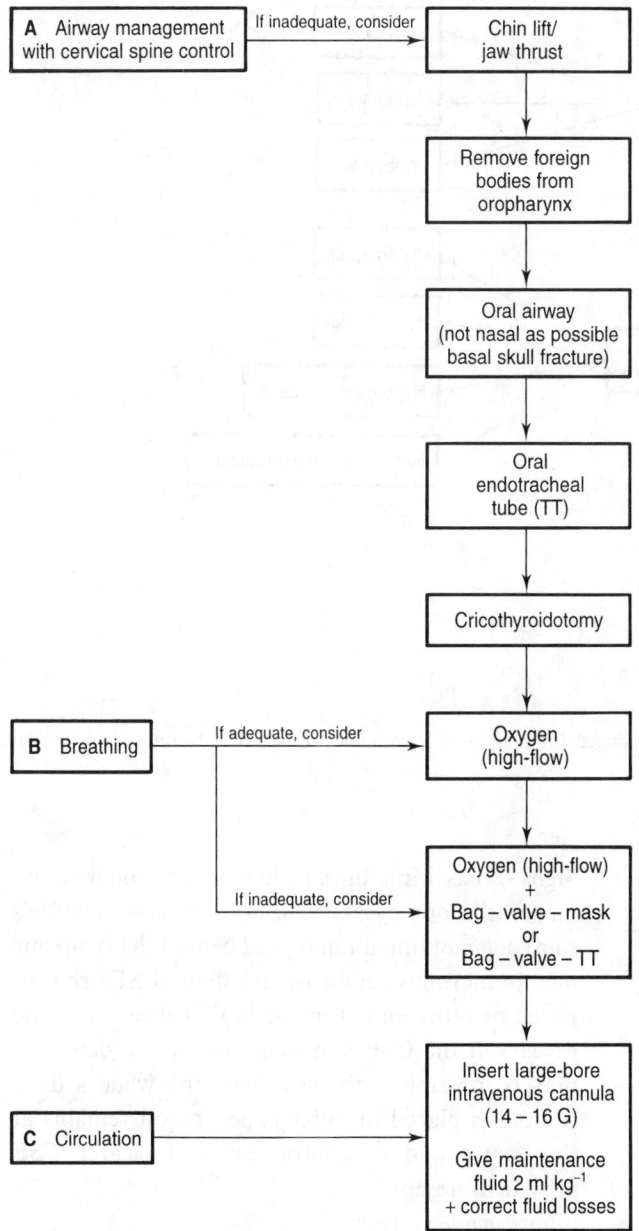

Fig. 2. Initial management.

Table 2. *Indications for tracheal intubation*

Maintenance of airway
– Upper airway obstruction
– Absence of protective laryngeal reflexes (cough/gag) precipitating danger of lower airway soiling
– Impending or potential compromise of airway, e.g. status epilepticus

Need for ventilation

• Respiratory
  – Apnoea
  – Excessive respiratory work (e.g. respiratory rate > 40 min^{-1})
  – Ventilatory insufficiency (PaCO$_2$ > 6 kPa)
  – Failure of adequate oxygenation (PaO$_2$ < 9 kPa) on 60% oxygen

• Neurological
  – Uncontrolled fits
  – Evidence of raised ICP/deterioration of neurological signs

• Others
  – To facilitate adequate analgesia or control of fits without producing respiratory compromise
  – To allow safe transport (Gentleman, 1993)

the patient should be preoxygenated, the cervical spine immobilized, and cricoid pressure applied to prevent aspiration of gastric contents. Orotracheal tubes are preferred because of the potential risk of misplacing nasal tubes into the brain substance should basal skull fractures be present.

Hypovolaemia should be aggressively treated with intravenous fluids until losses have been replaced, followed thereafter by judicious fluid replacement (e.g. 1 ml/kg^{-1} h^{-1}) to prevent overhydration and increases in ICP. It should be remembered that isolated head injuries rarely cause shock and therefore other causes for hypotension should be found.

Although mean systemic blood pressure should normally be maintained between 60 and 110 mmHg (i.e. the limits of cerebral autoregulation), hypertension may occasionally be the result of increased ICP. In this situation, the hypertension is protective (maintaining CPP) and treatment should be aimed at ICP control and not lowering the blood pressure. Hypoglycaemia, thiamine deficiency, hypo/hyperthermia should be excluded or corrected. Prolonged or repetitive fits must be controlled (Bean, 1986) because of the risk of secondary brain damage. The paralysed patient may show no external signs of fitting but brain injury can occur if the fits are not terminated. Once life-threatening conditions are stable, a thorough investigation can be undertaken to find the cause of the coma. Consideration should be given to specific antidotes (e.g. naloxone, flumazenil) and screening blood tests obtained. If the patient remains unstable or deteriorates, further primary assessment and management should be instigated.

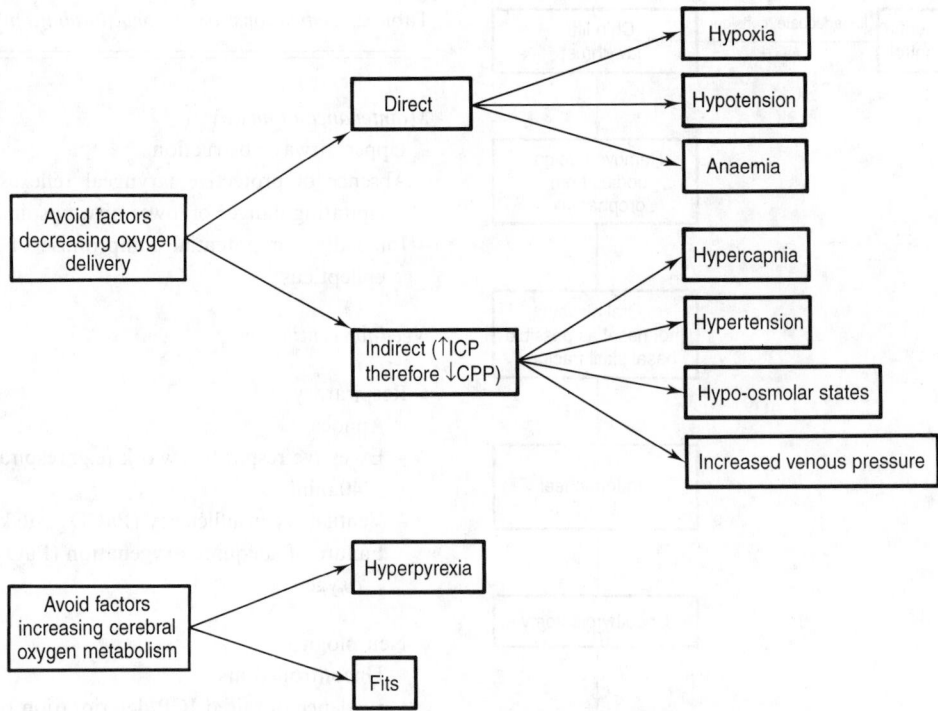

Fig. 3. Preventing secondary injury to brain from hypoxia. Note that damaged brain is more susceptible to lack of substrates than normal brain, therefore deprivation causes worse damage than in uninjured brain.

ASSESSMENT

History

As usual the diagnosis depends on a good history and examination, backed up with sensible investigations. The history, although unobtainable from the patient, can be obtained from relatives, friends, witnesses, police and ambulance crews. Information concerning previous illnesses, medication and hospital admissions can be sought from the general practitioner or old hospital notes. Any drugs, prescriptions, syringes or medical alert bracelets on the patient should be noted. The most immediately relevant questions are recent symptoms, recent trauma, speed of onset of coma, previous episodes of coma, medication available to the patient, and predisposing conditions (Table 3).

General examination

A detailed general and neurological examination should be performed when vital functions (ABCs) are secured. Specific attention should be directed toward the following:

- *Signs of head trauma*:
  - Cuts/abrasions/swelling.
  - Depressed skull fractures on palpation.

- Signs of basal fractures, including periorbital ecchymoses (raccoon eyes), mastoid ecchymoses (Battle's sign), haemotympanum (blood behind the tympanic membrane) and cerebrospinal fluid (CSF) rhinorrhoea or otorrhoea (leakage of CSF from the nose or ear). If the CSF is mixed with blood, detection may be possible with the 'ring sign': when a drop of fluid is placed on filter paper, blood remains at the centre and concentric rings of clearer CSF appear if present.
- *Cardiovascular system*:
  - Bradycardia (seen with raised ICP), hypoxia (late sign), drug effects (e.g. beta-blockers), arrhythmias (e.g. complete heart block).
  - Tachycardia, seen with hypoxia, shock, anticholinergic poisoning, fast atrial fibrillation (possible embolic ischaemic events).
  - Hypertension, may be:
    - Longstanding hypertension predisposing to intracranial haemorrhage.
    - The rare condition of hypertensive encephalopathy.
    - The protective response of the brain to coma-causing process (e.g. intracranial , subarachnoid haemorrhage or rarely brainstem stroke).

Table 3. *Specific points in the patient's history and their possible implications*

History	Implications	History	Implications
Recent symptoms	Headache/focal symptoms – mass lesions/ raised ICP TIA's, vertigo Chest pain, arrhythmias – brain ischaemia. Fever – infective causes, pontine lesion	Predisposing factors (general) medical disorders) (*contd.*)	Pulmonary disease – hypoxia Metabolic disease – diabetes – renal failure – Addison's disease – hypercalcaemia (secondary to metabolic carcinoma) Epilepsy – fit – postictal Clotting disorder – intracranial haematoma Psychiatric – depression/suicide Immunocompromised – sepsis Foreign travel – cerebral malaria Location found – carbon monoxide poisoning
Recent head trauma	Immediate – concussion/contusion Hours – raised ICP/intracranial haematoma Days to weeks – chronic subdural		

Speed of onset of coma	Sudden – head injury
	   – fit/postictal
	   – vascular
	     – subarachnoid haemorrhage
	     – brainstem infarction
	     – cardiac arrest/arrhythmia
	Slow (hours to days)
	– infective
	– metabolic
	   – hyper/hypoglycaemia
	   – acidosis
	   – hypoxia
	   – drug overdose
	– mass lesion
	   – tumour
	   – haematoma (subdural)		

		Recurrent coma episodes	Endocrine Epilepsy Inborn errors of metabolism (children)
Predisposing factors (general medical disorders)	Cardiovascular disease – cerebrovascular – arrhythmias – hypotension/myocardial infarction – hypertension	Drugs (known medication or drug access)	Overdose Toxic effect Anticoagulation – intracranial haematoma

ICP, intracranial pressure;
TIA's, transient ischaemic attacks.

- Hypotension, seen with shock or drug-depressant effects.
- Carotid bruits, indicating arterial stenosis/thrombosis.
- *Respiratory system*:
  - Hyperventilation
    - Metabolic acidosis (diabetic ketoacidosis, sepsis).
    - Salicylates.
    - Aspiration of foreign body or gastric contents.
    - Pneumonia.
    - Coincidental chest problems in a multiple injured patient.
    - Neurogenic pulmonary oedema (rare, in severe brain injury).
  - Pontine lesion.
  - Hypoventilation
    - Drugs.
    - Severe head injury.
    - Brainstem dysfunction.

Varying ventilatory patterns are seen in brain lesions as well as metabolic disturbances and are therefore unhelpful for anatomical localization of disorders producing coma.

- *Abdomen*:
  - Hepatosplenomegaly – liver failure.
  - Peritonitis – sepsis/shock.

- *Breath*:
  - Characteristic breath odours of alcohol, diabetic ketoacidosis, hepatic failure, kidney failure and ingested organophosphates.
- *Evidence of recent fit*:
  - bitten tongue/mouth or incontinence during fit produced by epilepsy, hypoglycaemia, hypocalcaemia or hypokalaemia.
- *Neck stiffness*:
  - Meningitis, subarachnoid haemorrhage.

  Neck stiffness is lost in deep coma. Obviously the neck should not be moved unless a cervical spine lesion has been excluded. Other signs of meningeal irritation include Brudzinski's sign (flexion at the knee and hip in response to forward flexion at the neck) and Kernig's sign (inability to completely extend the legs).
- *Skin*:
  - Pallor – shock/hypothyroidism (dry, rough skin).
  - Central cyanosis – hypoxia.
  - Peripheral cyanosis – hypoxia or hypoperfusion.
  - Warm/flushed skin – sepsis/hypercarbia.
  - Spider naevi/jaundice – liver failure.
  - purpura – clotting disorder/excessive anticoagulation or meningococcal septic rash.
  - Non-specific erythema/urticaria on pressure points.
  - Injection scars – drug abusers, diabetic patients.
  - Hypopituitarism – loss of hair, pallor, skin depigmentation.
  - Addison's disease – hyperpigmentation of hand creases and buccal mucosa.
  - Carbon monoxide poisoning – classical cherry red skin (pallor also seen).
- *Temperature*:
  Coma present if:
  - < 26°C (Greenberg, 1993).
  - > 43°C (increased metabolic demand).
- *Sweating*:
  - Fever.
  - Hypoglycaemia.
  - Drug withdrawal

Neurological examination

The goals of the neurological examination are to assess the degree of coma, to detect focal neurological deficit and brainstem function, and to recognize any remediable cause of the coma. The initial neurological examination provides a baseline with which to compare subsequent examinations and determine whether the patient is deteriorating or improving. All previous efforts will be pointless

if signs of neurological deterioration are not appreciated. Due to lack of volition, the neurological examination is limited to:

- Assessing depth of coma (Glasgow Coma Scale).
- Assessing brainstem function:
  - Pupillary light reflex.
  - Spontaneous eye movements.
  - Oculocephalic/oculovestibular reflexes.
  - Gag/cough reflex.
- Fundi (for signs of increased ICP).
- Motor responses and lateralizing signs.

Assessing depth of coma–the Glasgow Coma Scale

The Glasgow Coma Scale (GCS) is an internationally accepted, quantitative measure of depth of coma (Table 4). The scale numerically scores three different areas of assessment: a 4-point best eye opening response, a 5-point best verbal response and a 6-point best motor response. The summed score ranges between 3 and 15.

Although originally developed for the neurological assessment of head-injured patients (Teasdale & Jennett, 1974), it has also proved useful in assessing patients with other causes of coma (Bates *et al*, 1977). The uses of the GCS are as follows:

- A quantitative measure of coma depth.
- Monitoring trends in deterioration/improvement in clinical conditions.
- Categorizing patients for auditing in and between centres.
- Predicting outcome. The motor response score accounts for almost all the predictive power of the GCS (Jagger *et al*, 1983). The prognostic value of the GCS is greatest in the immediate postinjury phase (Lyle *et al*, 1986). The predictive ability can be improved by combining the GCS with a score for brainstem reflexes (Born, 1987).
- Triage by creating arbitrary thresholds for management decisions. Thus, severe head injury (GCS ≤ 8) has a mortality of 40%, moderate head injury (GCS 9–12) has a mortality of 4% and minor head injury (GCS 13–15) has a mortality of 0.4%.

However, there are problems with the GCS, and patient deafness or inability to speak the native language means assessment can be deficient. Responses in all three areas may be impossible if the patient has been sedated and paralysed for ventilation (residual paralysis can be confirmed with a nerve stimulator). Sedation and paralysis will also interfere with the ability to measure

Table 4. *Glasgow Coma Score* (Teasdale & Jennett, 1974)

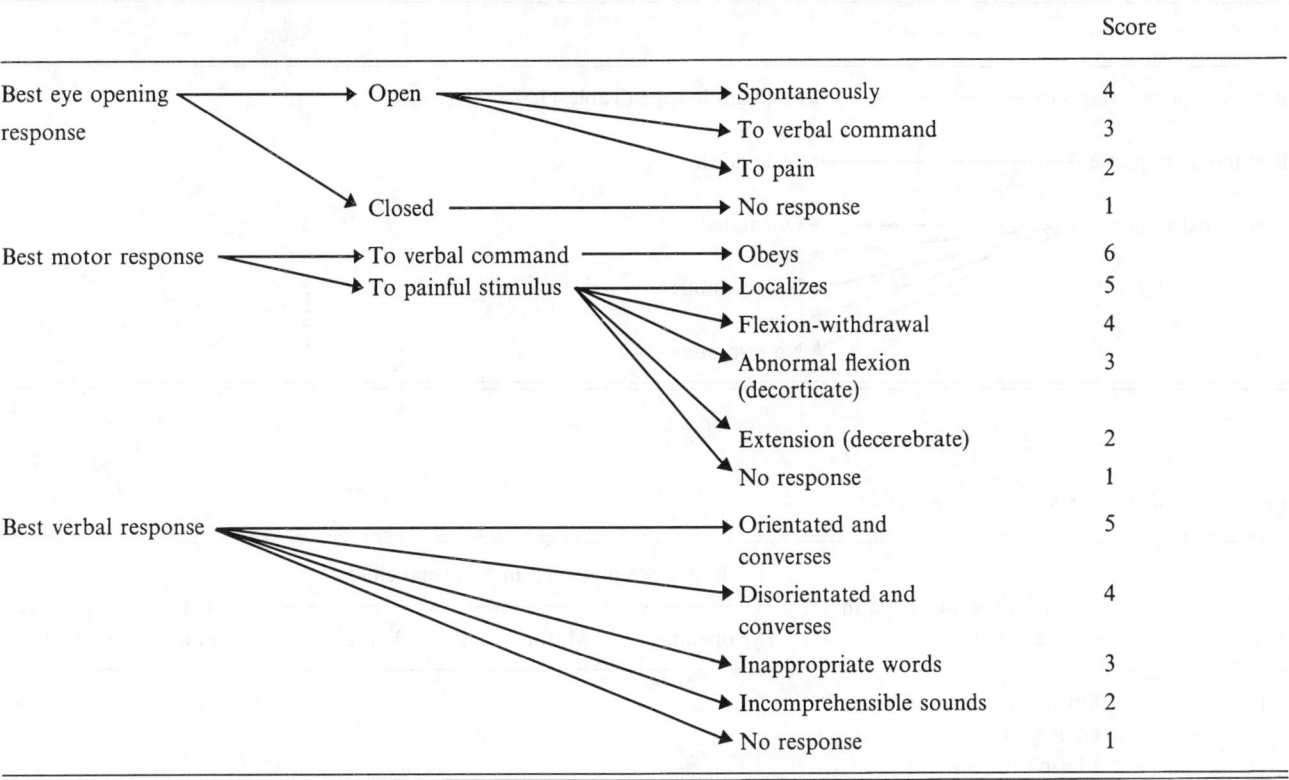

			Score
Best eye opening response	Open	Spontaneously	4
		To verbal command	3
		To pain	2
	Closed	No response	1
Best motor response	To verbal command	Obeys	6
	To painful stimulus	Localizes	5
		Flexion-withdrawal	4
		Abnormal flexion (decorticate)	3
		Extension (decerebrate)	2
		No response	1
Best verbal response		Orientated and converses	5
		Disorientated and converses	4
		Inappropriate words	3
		Incomprehensible sounds	2
		No response	1

- Localizing means localizing to painful stimuli and is best tested by a painful stimulus on the supraorbital ridge producing flexion/abduction of upper limbs.
- Abnormal flexion means flexion at elbow and wrist, pronation of forearm and adduction of thumb into palm of hand.
- Extension means extension at elbow, pronation of forearm and flexion of wrist. Occasionally supination of the forearm is present.

changes in level of coma over a time period. The eye opening response may not be possible with gross periorbital oedema, as with the verbal response if the patient has a tracheal tube or tracheostomy. Assessment of the motor response may not be possible if the limbs are immobilized for fracture reduction. Spinal cord lesions from trauma or anoxia/ischaemia may result in motor/sensory disturbances and therefore it is important to apply painful stimuli above the neck (e.g. the supraorbital ridge). When one area of assessment cannot be evaluated the total score becomes misleading. Another criticism of the GCS is that it lacks sensitivity as the same score can be achieved by different combinations.

Children present a further problem as a classical GCS assessment is not possible. A 6-month-old infant will not be able to obey commands or verbalize in order to be assessed as 'orientated'. Therefore, a paediatric variant of the GCS (Table 5) takes into account that verbal and motor responses are scored lower in the scale

in normal children than corresponding normal adults (Reilly *et al.*, 1988).

The paediatric scale correlates reasonably well with standard development screening tests (Table 6), but the predicted normal responses have been placed slightly low to take into account the effect of a frightened child's sudden admission to hospital.

Assessing brainstem function

Pupillary light reflex (Table 7)

The pupillary light reflex is assessed by flashing a bright light into the eye. The normal response is for the pupil on the stimulated side, as well as that on the opposite side, to constrict (direct and consensual light reflexes, respectively). If the pupil is very small, magnification may be necessary to see any reaction. As well as reactivity

Table 5. *Paediatric Glasgow Coma Scale* (Simpson & Reilly, 1982)

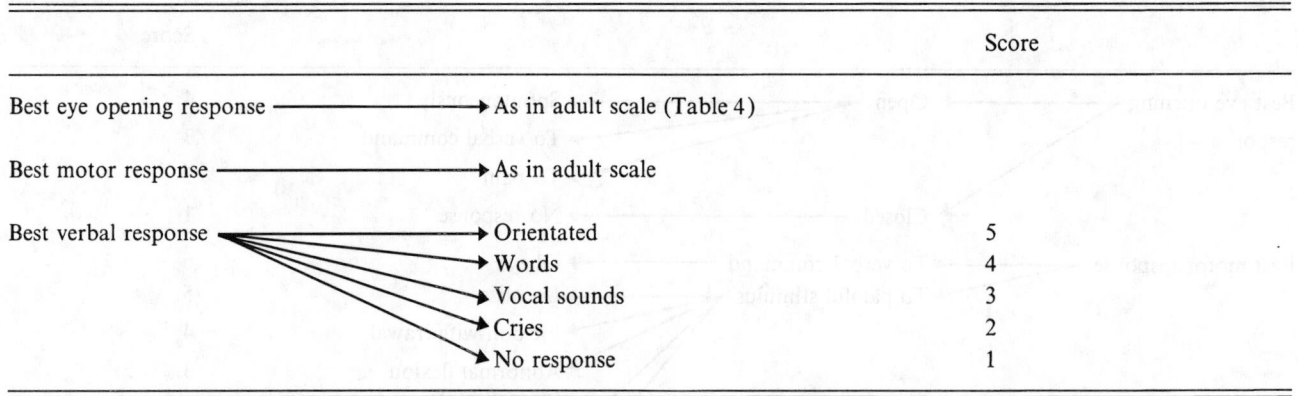

		Score
Best eye opening response ⟶	As in adult scale (Table 4)	
Best motor response ⟶	As in adult scale	
Best verbal response ⟶	Orientated	5
	Words	4
	Vocal sounds	3
	Cries	2
	No response	1

Table 6. *Paediatric GCS in the normal child*

Age	Best response predicted in normal child	Best score predicted in a normal child			Total aggregate score in a normal child
		Eye opening	Motor	Verbal	
< 6 months	Opens eyes spontaneously Cries/grunts Flexion to pain	4	4	2	10
6–12 months	Opens eyes spontaneously Babbles/vocal sounds Localizes to pain	4	5	3	12
1–2 years	Opens eyes spontaneously Recognizable words Localizes to pain	4	5	4	13
2–5 years	Opens eyes spontaneously Recognizable words Obeys commands	4	6	4	14
> 5 years	Opens eyes spontaneously Orientated and converses Obeys commands	4	6	5	15

to light, the size and equality of pupils must be noted. Pupillary size is dependent on a balance between parasympathetic (constrictor) tone and sympathetic (dilator) tone. The light reflex is mediated solely through the parasympathetic system via the optic nerve, optic tract, lateral geniculate nuclei, the Edinger–Westphal nucleus (cranial nerve III) and the ciliary ganglion (i.e. the cortex is not involved). Spurious changes in size/reaction to light may be seen in iris disease, with mydriatic or cycloplegic agents or pre-existing disorders (e.g. Holmes–Adie syndrome).

Spontaneous eye movements

Conjugate lateral gaze is controlled by cerebral (frontal and occipital) and pontine gaze centres. Unless there is a structural injury, the eyes of a comatose patient are directed straight ahead or are slightly divergent. Full horizontal roving eye movements exclude brainstem lesions as the cause of coma and further testing of oculocephalic or oculovestibular reflexes are unnecessary (Sigsbee & Plum, 1979). A lesion in the frontal cerebrum will result in conjugate lateral deviation of the eyes to

Table 7. *Summary of pupillary response*

Pupil size and reactivity to light	Cause
Pinpoint, fixed (1–2 mm)	Miotic drugs
	Injection of organophosphates
Pinpoint, reactive (1–2 mm)	Opioids
	Pontine lesion
	Anticholinesterase (e.g. neostigmine)
Small, reactive (2–3 mm)	Metabolic disorders
	Medullary lesion
Mid-size, fixed (5 mm)	Midbrain lesion
Dilated, fixed (> 7 mm)	Severe hypoxia/ischaemia
	Hypothermia
	Barbiturates (late sign)
	Anticholinergics (atropine)
	Sympathomimetics
	Hypoglycaemia
	Fit/postictal
	Brainstem lesion
Unilateral dilated, fixed	Uncal herniation
	Cranial nerve III lesion (fixed to direct/consensual)
	Cranial nerve II (fixed to direct, not to consensual)
	Fit
Unilateral constricted, fixed	Horner's syndrome (a Horner's syndrome of recent onset may indicate central transtentorial herniation)

- In metabolic coma the pupillary light reflex is usually preserved except with severe hypoxia/ischaemia or barbiturate and anticholinergic overdoses. In contrast, the reflex is lost early in transtentorial herniation.
- Muscle relaxants have no effect on pupillary light reflex.
- 20% of the normal population has asymmetric pupils (1 mm difference in size).

the affected side, whereas a lesion in the pons will direct eyes away from the affected side. It is important to note there will be no eye movements if the patient has been given a muscle relaxant. Ocular bobbing (eyes intermittently jerk down and then slowly return to midposition) is pathognomonic of an extensive lesion of the pons (Critchley, 1988).

Oculocephalic and oculovestibular reflexes

These reflexes detect the integrity of cranial nerves VIII (afferent), III, IV and VI (efferent) and the median longitudinal fasciculus. Although more time-consuming, the end-point of the oculovestibular reflex is easier to observe. It should be performed instead of the oculocephalic reflex if spinal cord trauma is suspected. Both reflexes can be lost with bilateral middle ear disease and drugs such as muscle relaxants, barbiturates, phenytoin and tricyclic antidepressants.

The *oculocephalic reflex* is elicited by holding open the patient's eyes and turning the head from side to side in the horizontal plane. The reflex is present if, as the patient's head is turned, there is conjugate movement of the eyes to the opposite side; i.e. it appears as if the patient is maintaining a fixed gaze ahead. The absence of the reflex occurs in a conscious patient or a comatose patient with a damaged brainstem. Although metabolic causes can be responsible for the absence of the reflex, it will then tend to be symmetrical (unlike that due to a focal brainstem lesion). Presence of the reflex indicates an intact brainstem.

The *oculovestibular reflex* is elicited by squirting 50 ml of ice-cold water into the auditory canal over 30 sec. The canal should be free of wax and the ear drum intact. Raising the patient's head 30° above the horizontal maximizes the reflex. Cold caloric stimulation of the left ear is equivalent to turning the head to the right in oculocephalic testing. Conjugate deviation of the eyes toward the irrigated ear (opposite if warm water is used) indicates intact brainstem pathways. No response from one ear only indicates an ipsilateral lesion (either vestibular or brainstem) and similarly no response from either ear indicates a bilateral lesion (Bleck & Klawans, 1986).

Gag/cough reflexes

The gag and cough reflexes test the integrity of cranial nerves IX and X. Their absence or depression increase the likelihood of aspiration, necessitating intubation to protect the airway.

Fundi

Papilloedema is the most important finding in fundal examination. Although it is the hallmark of raised ICP, it takes time to develop (> 6 h) and in some individuals never occurs. Therefore lack of papilloedema does not exclude raised ICP.

Motor response

Information from the GCS can be compounded with an assessment of lateralizing/asymmetric differences in muscle power and tone. Flaccidity with no response to pain may be caused by a pontine/medullary lesion, but should be differentiated from peripheral nerve paralysis or 'spinal shock'. Asymmetry of motor function is invariably caused by a structural lesion in the contralateral cerebral hemisphere or contra/ipsilateral brainstem (beware hypoglycaemia) (Cartlidge, 1984).

Proprioceptive (deep tendon) reflexes are not particularly useful in coma assessment as they are only tests of peripheral nerve, root, and spinal cord function and not of cerebral/brainstem function. However, plantar reflexes retain their localizing value (Samuels, 1992).

Investigations

The order of investigations depends on the clinical situation. Uses include initial diagnosis, exclusion of diagnosis and baseline result.

Blood

- Complete blood cell count
  - baseline reading.
  - excludes anaemia (which reduces oxygen-carrying capacity of blood).
  - leucocytosis in sepsis.
- Urea and electrolytes
  - excludes abnormalities of Na^+, K^+, Ca^{2+}, Mg^{2+}.
  - indication of renal function.
- Osmolality – excludes hypo/hyperosmolar states.
- Glucose – excludes hypo/hyperglycaemia.
- Liver function tests (LFTs) and ammonia
  - in hepatic failure LFTs can be normal but ammonia is usually raised.
- Thyroid function tests – if appropriate.
- Blood culture – if appropriate.
- Arterial blood gases
  - need to be corrected for temperature.
  - identifies need for oxygen therapy and/or ventilation.
- Clotting screen – baseline.

Toxicology screen

- Blood/urine/gastric contents
  - if other investigations do not produce a diagnosis for the cause of coma, consider urgent toxicology screening (Helliwell *et al*, 1979).

Urine

- Glucose/ketones – exclude diabetic ketoacidosis.

X-rays

The patient should be accompanied by suitably experienced medical staff and be adequately monitored (Association of Anaesthetists, 1988).

- Chest X-ray – aspiration.
- Skull X-ray – consider in head trauma if it will alter management (e.g. to transfer patient or do CT scan; head injury plus skull fracture increases risk of intracranial haematoma).
- Cervical spine series.
- CT scan (head)
  - to diagnose cerebral oedema, midline shift, hydrocephalus, intracranial haematoma, infarction, intracranial mass, tumour and abscess. It should be noted that a unilateral supratentorial lesion which does not cause midline shift is unlikely to be a cause of coma.
  - Indications for CT scan include:
    - Uncertain cause of coma.
    - Raised ICP.
    - Focal signs.
    - Deterioration in depth of coma.
    - Status epilepticus.
    - Severe head injury (GCS < 8 gives 40% risk of intracranial haematoma; Miller, 1990).

Miscellaneous investigations

- Lumbar puncture – to diagnose meningitis and identify the organism and sensitivity.
Contraindications:
- Evidence of raised ICP.
- Focal signs.
- Coagulation disorder.
- Local infection at lumbar puncture site.
- ECG – to diagnose arrhythmias and myocardial infarction which may have caused the initial hypoxic/ischaemic episode responsible for coma.

EARLY MANAGEMENT

After resuscitation and full investigation of the cause of coma, further management must continue to support vital functions, maintain homeostasis (Table 8) and

Table 8. *Aims of patient homeostasis*

Mean BP	$>60 < 110$ mm Hg
CPP	>60 mm Hg
Temperature	$<38°C$
Pao_2	>10 kPa
$Paco_2$	<4.5 kPa
$Paco_2$	3.3–4 kPa if hyperventilating for increased ICP
Hb	>10 g dl^{-1}
Osmolality	$>290 < 310$ mosm kg^{-1}
Na$^+$	$>130 < 150$ mmol l^{-1}
Glucose	$>5 < 15$ mmol l^{-1}

Table 9. *Causes of raised intracranial pressure*

Structural
- Intracranial mass/haematoma
- Hydrocephalus

Physiological
- Cerebral oedema
- Increased intracranial blood volume
  - Hypercarbia
  - Hypoxia
  - Hyperpyrexia
  - Systemic hypertension when autoregulation lost
  - Fits
  - Poor venous drainage
    - Raised intrathoracic pressure
    - Venous obstruction below head
    - Trendelenberg (head down)

Table 10. *Signs of raised intracranial pressure*

- Brainstem compression
  - Abnormal brainstem reflexes
  - Decorticate/decerebrate posturing
  - Abnormal pupillary signs
- Fundi
  - Papilloedema
  - Absence of venous pulsation in retinal vessels
- Bulging fontanelle (infants)
- Non-cardiogenic pulmonary oedema (rare)
- Systemic hypertension
- Reflex bradycardia ⎬ Cushing's Triad
- Abnormal breathing patterns ⎭ (late sign)

Table 11. *Medical treatment of raised intracranial pressure*

Reduction in cerebral blood volume
- Hyperventilation (to reduce $Paco_2$)
- Avoid hypoxia/hyperpyrexia
- Maintain mean systemic blood pressure within limits of autoregulation
- Control fits
- Improve venous drainage
  - Reverse Trendelenberg (head up 30°)
  - Avoid extremes of flexion/extension of neck
- Avoid increased intrathoracic pressure i.e. avoid
  - Coughing/straining
  - PEEP (positive end-expiratory pressure)

Prevent/reduce cerebral oedema
- Diuretics
- Fluid restriction
- Steroids only for vasogenic oedema (see text)

prevent secondary brain insults from increases in ICP (Tables 9 and 10). Structural causes of raised ICP mandate surgical intervention, but physiological causes require medical treatment. Medical treatment may also be useful for 'buying time' until operative procedures or neurological improvement takes place. Treatment focuses on reducing cerebral blood flow or cerebral oedema (Table 11).

Methods of reducing cerebral blood flow

The principal method of acutely reducing cerebral blood flow is by hyperventilation, causing a reduction in $Paco_2$, cerebral blood volume, and ICP. Optimal cerebral vasoconstriction probably occurs at $Paco_2$ 3.3–4.0 kPa. Further hyperventilation may lead to detrimental effects by reducing cerebral blood flow to such an extent that ischaemia occurs, or by shifting the oxygen dissociation curve so that less oxygen is released to the brain tissue. Optimal hyperventilation is probably the best emergency treatment for raised ICP, as a significant fall in ICP occurs within 10–15 sec of acutely reducing $Paco_2$ (Gordon, 1986).

As long as systemic arterial blood pressure remains within the limits of cerebral autoregulation (i.e. mean arterial pressure 60–110 mmHg), cerebral blood flow/

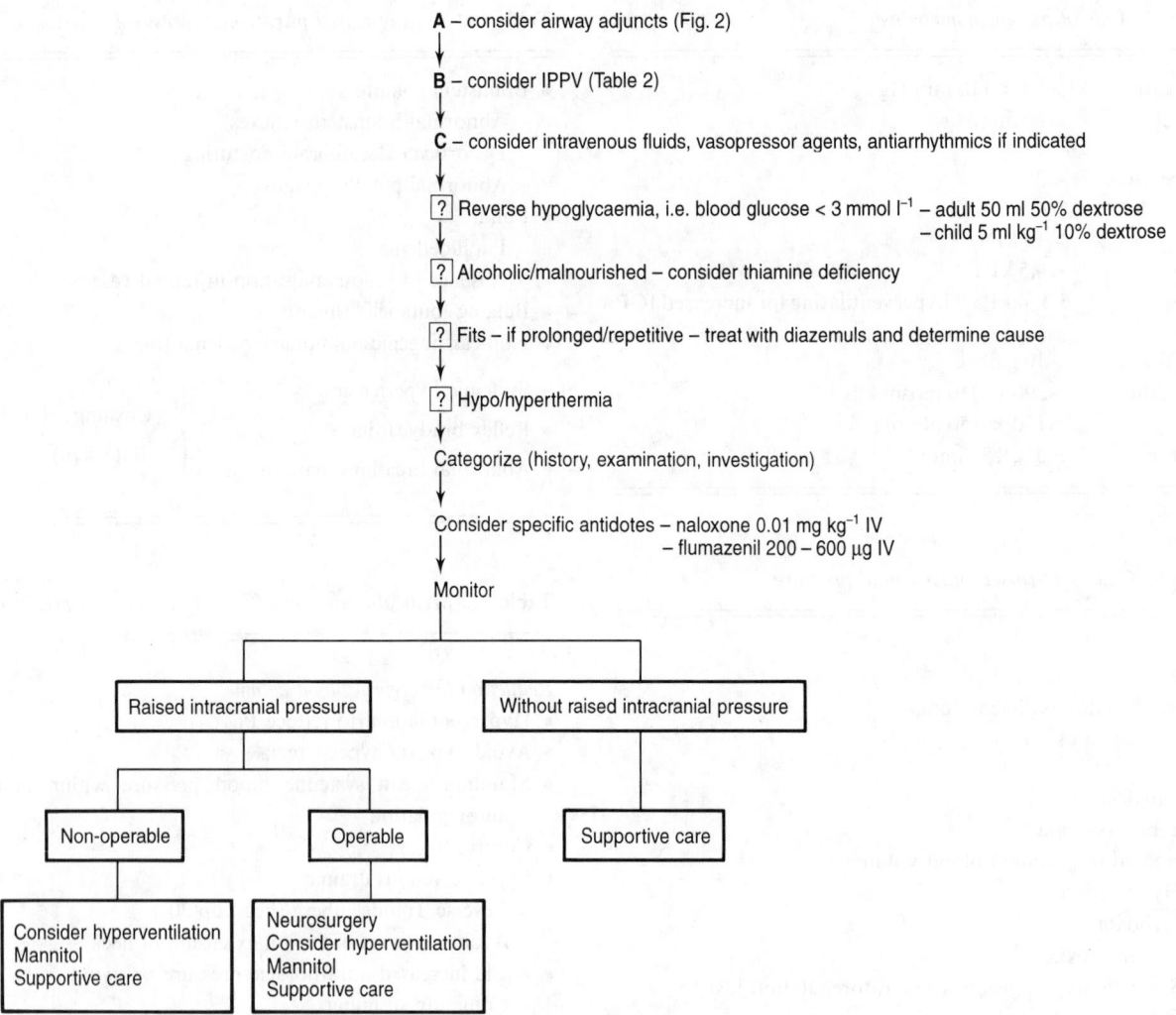

A – consider airway adjuncts (Fig. 2)

B – consider IPPV (Table 2)

C – consider intravenous fluids, vasopressor agents, antiarrhythmics if indicated

[?] Reverse hypoglycaemia, i.e. blood glucose < 3 mmol l⁻¹ – adult 50 ml 50% dextrose
– child 5 ml kg⁻¹ 10% dextrose

[?] Alcoholic/malnourished – consider thiamine deficiency

[?] Fits – if prolonged/repetitive – treat with diazemuls and determine cause

[?] Hypo/hyperthermia

Categorize (history, examination, investigation)

Consider specific antidotes – naloxone 0.01 mg kg⁻¹ IV
– flumazenil 200 – 600 µg IV

Monitor

Raised intracranial pressure | Without raised intracranial pressure

Non-operable | Operable | Supportive care

Consider hyperventilation
Mannitol
Supportive care

Neurosurgery
Consider hyperventilation
Mannitol
Supportive care

Fig. 4. Initial management of coma.

volume can be kept constant. However, above the limits of autoregulation, cerebral blood flow becomes pressure-dependent and ICP can increase. Therefore by reducing the systemic pressure to within this range, ICP can be reduced. Beta-blockers are the logical choice as they do not induce vasodilation which would cause the cerebral blood volume to increase.

Methods of reducing cerebral oedema

Cerebral oedema is chiefly treated with diuretics, both osmotic (mannitol) and loop types (frusemide).

Mannitol acts intravascularly and removes fluid from the brain tissue across the blood/ brain barrier. Its peak action occurs within 2 h and lasts 4–6 h (Sigsbee & Plum, 1979).

Mannitol is contraindicated in renal failure and congestive cardiac failure because it increases intravascular volume. Some authors believe mannitol is no longer effective after 48 h as it eventually crosses the blood/brain barrier and pulls fluid into brain tissue causing an increase in ICP ('rebound phenomenon').

The dual action of *frusemide* acutely reduces ICP firstly by initiating a diuresis and secondly by a direct effect in reducing CSF production. Frusemide is the agent of choice in congestive cardiac failure and it has a synergistic action with both mannitol and steroids.

Steroids have been shown to reduce vasogenic oedema associated with primary and metastatic brain tumours and abscesses. However, no improvement is produced in oedema associated with head injuries (Cooper et al, 1979), anoxia, stroke and metabolic encephalopathies (Shapiro, 1975).

CONCLUSION

The aim of this chapter is to emphasize the importance of the initial assessment and early management of the comatose patient (Fig. 4) so as to provide the best conditions for optimal recovery. Outcome after coma ranges from death, persistent vegetative state (awake but not cognitive), severe disability (conscious but dependent), moderate disability (independent but disabled) and good recovery (no disabling sequelae). Although some patients continue to improve after 6 months, most reach their ultimate outcome within 3 months. Post-traumatic coma patients have a better prognosis, in relation to their neurological abnormality, than patients in non-traumatic coma. Jennett et al. (1979) found the outcome of traumatic coma patients at 6 months to be 49% dead, 2% persistent vegetative state, 10% severely disabled, 17% moderately disabled, 22% good recovery. In contrast, the outcome of non-traumatic coma patients at 1 year was 60% dead, 12% persistent vegetative state, 11% severely disabled, 16% moderately disabled/good recovery (Levy et al, 1981). The most important predictors of neurological outcome, particularly in head injured patients, are duration of coma, age and Glasgow Coma Scale (Macpherson et al., 1992; Bullock & Teasdale, 1991). Although treatment enables many patients who would have previously died to make a good recovery, the converse is that some patients will survive with severe brain damage or die after lengthy hospitalization. Treatment is therefore only justifable if there is reasonable probability of 'a decent life in which a patient can reasonably be thought to have a continued interest' (BMA Medical Ethics Committee, 1992; Jennett, 1992).

Bibliography

ADVANCED PAEDIATRIC LIFE SUPPORT (1993). London: BMJ Publishing.

ALBERT, R.D., SILVERBERG, R., RECHES, A. et al. (1976). Cerebral dominance for consciousness. Arch. Neurol., 33, 453–54.

ASSOCIATION OF ANAESTHETISTS OF GREAT BRITAIN AND IRELAND (1988). Recommendations for Standards of Monitoring during Anaesthesia and Recovery.

ASTRUP, J. (1982). Energy requiring cell functions in ischaemic brain. J. Neurosurg., 56, 482–97.

BATES, D., CARONNA, J.J., CARTLIDGE, E.F. et al. (1977). A prospective study of non-traumatic coma, methods and results in 310 patients. Ann. Neurol., 2, 211–20.

BEAN, S.C. (1986). Emergency medicine for the primary care physician—Convulsions. Primary Care, 13, 77–82.

BLECK, T.P. & KLAWANS, H.L. (1986). Neurological emergencies. Med. Clin. North Am., 70, 1167.

BMA MEDICAL ETHICS COMMITTE (1992). Discussion Paper on Treatment of Patients in Persistent Vegetative State. London: British Medical Association.

BORN, J.D. (1987). Assessment of impaired consciousness. Acta Anaesthesiol. Belg., 38, 381–86.

BULLOCK, R. & TEASDALE, G. (1991). Head injuries. In ABC of Major Trauma, ed. D. Skinner, P. Driscoll, R. Earlam, pp. 25–32. London: BMJ Publishing.

CARTLIDGE, N.E.F. (1984). Coma and disorders of consciousness after trauma. In Trauma and the Anaesthetist, ed. J.C. Stoddart, pp. 130–49. Baillière Tindall, Oxford.

COOPER, P.R. et al., (1979). Dexamethasone and severe head injury, a prospective double blind study. J. Neurosurg., 51, 307–16.

CRITCHLEY, E.M.R. (1988). Coma. In Neurological Emergencies, pp. 21–95. London: W.B. Saunders.

GENTLEMAN, D., DEARDEN, M., MIDGLEY, S. et al. (1993). Guidelines for resuscitation and transfer of patients with serious head injuries. Bri. Med. J., 307, 547–52.

GORDON, E. (1986). Care at the accident site and during transport. Acta Neurochir. Suppl., 36, 56–7.

GREENBERG, D., AMINOFF, M. & SIMON, R. (1993). Clinical Neurology, pp. 281–98, Appleton and Lange.

GUYTON, A.C. (1991). The nervous system. Motor and integrative neurophysiology. In Textbook of Medical Physiology, 8th edn, pp. 589–685. Philaedelphia: W.B. Saunders.

HELLIWELL, M., HAMPEL, G., SINCLAIR, E. et al. (1979). Value of emergency toxicological investigations in differential diagnosis of coma. Bri. Med. J., 2, 819–21.

JAGGER, J., JANE, J. & RIMEL, R. (1983). The Glasgow Coma Scale: to sum or not to sum? Lancet, ii (8341), 97.

JENNETT, B., TEASDALE, G., BRAAKMAN, R. et al. (1979). Prognosis of patients with severe head injury. Neurosurgery, 4, 283–9.

JENNETT, B. (1992). Letting vegetative patients die. Bri. Med. J., 305, 1305–6.

KLATZO, I. (1967). Neuropathological aspects of brain oedema. J. Neuropathol. Exp. Neurol., 26, 1–14.

LEVY, D., BATES, E., CARONNA, J.J. et al., (1981). Prognosis in non traumatic coma. Ann. Intern. Med., 94, 293–301.

LYLE, D.M., PIERCE, J.P., FREEMAN, E.A. et al., (1986). Clinical course and outcome of severe head injury in Australia. J. Neurosurg., 65, 15–18.

MACPHERSON, V., SULLIVAN, S.J. & LAMBERT J. (1992). Prediction of motor status 3 and 6 months post severe traumatic brain injury: a preliminary study. Brain Injury, 6, 489–98.

MILLER, J.D. & BECKER, D.P. (1982). Secondary insults to the injured brain. J. R. Coll. Surg. Edinb., 27, 292–8.

MILLER, J.D. (1987). Neurological evaluation of the unconscious patient. *Prog. Neurol. Surg.* **12**, 1–14.

MILLER, J.D. (1990). Assessing patients with head injury. *Br. J. Surg.* **77**, 241–2.

MORUZZI, G.M. (1949). Brain stem reticular formation and activation of the EEG. *Electroencephalog. Clin. Neurophysiol.*, **1**, 455.

PLUM, F. & POSNER, J.B. (1980). In *Stupor and Coma*. Philadelphia: F.A. Davis.

REILLY, P.L., SIMPSON, D.A., SPROD, R. *et al* (1988). Assessing the conscious level in infants and young children; a paediatric version of the Glascow Coma Scale. *Childs Nerv. Syst.*, **4**, 30–3.

SAMUELS, M. (1992). A practical approach to coma diagnosis in the unresponsive patient. *Cleve. Clin. J. Med.*, **59**, 257–61.

SHAPIRO, H.M. (1975). Intracranial hypertension, therapeutic and anaesthetic considerations. *Anaesthesiology*, **43**, 445–71.

SIESJO, B.K. (1984). Cerebral circulation and metabolism. *J. Neurosurg.*, **60**, 883–908.

SIESJO, B.K. & WIELOCH, T. (1985). Cerebral metabolism in ischaemia: neurochemical basis for therapy. *Br. J. Anaesth.*, **57**, 47–62.

SIGSBEE, B. & PLUM, F. (1979). The unresponsible patient, diagnosis and early management. *Med. Clin. North Am.*, **63**, 813–34.

SIMPSON, D. & REILLY, P. (1982). Pediatric coma scale (letter). *Lancet*, **ii** (8295), 450.

TEASDALE, G. & JENNET, B. (1974). Assessment of coma and impaired conciousness, a practical scale. *Lancet*, **ii**, 81–3.

WILSON, A. & DRISCOLL, P. (1991). Transport of injured patients. In *ABC of Major Trauma*, ed. D. Skinner, P. Driscoll, R. Earlam, pp. 91–5. London: BMJ Publishing.

10 Analgesia and anaesthesia

J.P. NOLAN[a] and P.J.F. BASKETT[b]

[a]Department of Anaesthesia, Royal United Hospital, Bath, UK
[b]Department of Anaesthesia, Frenchay Hospital, Bristol, UK

Chapter plan

Introduction
What is pain?
Analgesics
Routes of analgesic administration
Local anaesthesia
General anaesthesia in the A&E department
Relationship between anaesthetic and A&E departments

INTRODUCTION

In the UK and continental Europe, the anaesthetist has a recognized important role in the accident and emergency (A&E) department (Association of Anaesthetists of Great Britain and Ireland, 1991). Along with colleagues in accident and emergency medicine, surgery and cardiology, the anaesthetist is an integrated member of the team involved in the resuscitation of seriously ill or injured patients. Furthermore, the anaesthetist has particular skills in the provision of pain relief and anaesthesia, both of vital importance in the A&E department.

Analgesia should be regarded as part of the resuscitation process for it brings with it not only compassionate relief but also cardiovascular stability and restoration of organ and tissue perfusion (Rady *et al.*, 1991). Effective relief of severe pain in the compromised patient requires not only knowledge and experience of the wide variety of analgesic agents but also the skill to support the vital functions involved in respiration and the circulation which may be depressed by effective analgesic doses. Therefore, sophisticated airway and ventilation control and support of arterial pressure in the patient whose catecholamine response has been modified are essential skills needed to provide reliable and effective analgesia. Indeed, it is becoming recognized practice to fully anaes-thetize patients with major trauma soon after admission to the A&E department (Stene, 1992) to ensure a secure airway and adequate ventilation (hyperventilation is often required to correct the patient's lactic acidosis). It is generally easier to obtain X-rays and to stabilize spinal, pelvic or limb fractures with patients anaesthetized, particularly if they are drunk or otherwise uncooperative. Thus, haemorrhage and other complications are reduced, and an adequate circulation and oxygen delivery will be restored more rapidly.

This chapter will cover control of mild to severe pain together with anaesthetic techniques ranging from those for simple procedures in the A&E department to those required as part of the resuscitation process.

WHAT IS PAIN?

Pain has been defined by the International Association for the Study of Pain as 'an unpleasant sensory and emotional experience associated with actual or potential tissue damage, or described in terms of such damage'. Most pain originates when specific nerve endings (nociceptors) are stimulated, producing nerve impulses which are transmitted to the brain. There are two types of nociceptor:

1. Mechanoceptors, which are present mainly in the skin and respond rapidly to pinprick or heat via $A\delta$, myelinated, afferent neurones.
2. Polymodal nociceptors are the nerve endings of unmyelinated C type afferent neurones and are widely distributed throughout most tissues; they respond to tissue damage caused by mechanical, thermal, or chemical insults and are responsible for the slow in onset, prolonged, poorly localized, aching pain following an injury.

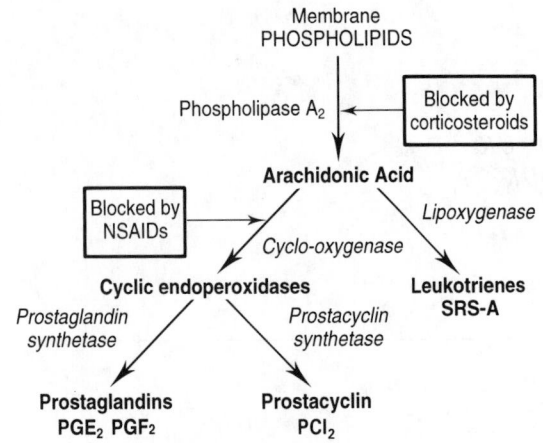

Fig. 1. Cyclo-oxygenase is inhibited by non-steroidal anti-inflammatory agents (SRS-A).

Both $A\delta$ and C fibres enter the spinal cord through the dorsal root and terminate in the grey matter of the dorsal horn. Here a number of chemicals are involved in the transmission of pain to the ascending pathways in the spinothalamic tract. The principal neurotransmitter is thought to be the peptide, substance P, but many others have been identified. Pain transmission can be inhibited at the spinal cord level by inhibitory inter-neurones or from descending inhibitory fibres. Opioid receptors are present in the dorsal horn and it is thought that enkephalins (endogenous opioid peptides) are neuro-transmitters in the inhibitory interneurones.

Phospholipids released from damaged cell membranes trigger a cascade of reactions culminating in the produc-tion of prostaglandins which sensitize nociceptors to other inflammatory mediators such as histamine, sero-tonin and bradykinin (Fig. 1). Cyclo-oxygenase acts on arachidonic acid, producing reactive superoxide inter-mediates in the generation of endoperoxides. Prosta-glandins and prostacyclin are in turn generated from the endoperoxides. Non-steroidal anti-inflammatory drugs (NSAIDs) inhibit cyclo-oxygenase, prevent prostaglan-din synthesis and superoxide generation, and therefore prevent sensitization of the peripheral nociceptors.

ANALGESICS

Pain-killing drugs (analgesics) may be directed at the peripheral nociceptor, at conduction in peripheral or central neural afferent pathways, at areas of pain modu-lation in the central nervous system (CNS), or at efferent pathways. In the periphery, blockade of formation of the relevant chemical mediators by NSAIDs will prevent

activation of the nociceptors. Nerve conduction can be blocked by local anaesthetics and CNS processing can be modulated by opioids. A classification of analgesics is given in Table 1.

ROUTES OF ANALGESIC ADMINISTRATION

Effective analgesia can be provided by a variety of routes. The route chosen will depend on a number of factors, which include:

- Patient cooperation and preference.
- The nature and intensity of the pain.
- The potential side-effects of the analgesic and the ability to overcome and counteract them.
- The patient's vital signs.
- The patient's prior medical status including history of allergy and sensitivity.
- The uptake and distribution from the site of adminis-tration of the analgesic.

The following routes for analgesic administration will be discussed:

- Oral.
- Sublingual.
- Rectal.
- Topical.
- Inhalational.
- Intramuscular.
- Intravenous.

Oral analgesia

The oral route is the most commonly used method for administering analgesic drugs and is generally appro-priate for mild to moderate pain, though more severe chronic pain can be treated effectively with oral opioids. Headache, toothache and pain from inflamed soft tissues are examples of pain that may be treated adequately with oral analgesia. Patients with major fractures will require opioids given parenterally.

The efficacy of analgesic drugs given orally depends on gastric emptying and absorption from the small intestine. Acute, severe pain will reduce gastric emptying and render oral analgesics ineffective. Nausea and vomit-ing also will contraindicate the oral route, as will of course the unconscious or uncooperative patient.

Analgesics given orally will inevitably be slow in onset. For example, after taking aspirin by mouth, plasma

Table 1. *Classification of analgesics with available routes for administration*

Non-opioids
Simple analgesics
Paracetamol (PO, PR)

Non-steroidal anti-inflammatory drugs (NSAIDs)
Salicylates
Aspirin (PO, PR)

Propionic acid derivatives
Ibuprofen (PO)
Ketoprofen (PO, PR, IM)
Fenoprofen (PO)
Flurbiprofen (PO, PR)
Naproxen (PO, PR)
Fenbufen (PO)

Indene derivatives
Indomethacin (PO, PR)
Sulindac (PO)
Tolmetin (PO)

Fenamates
Mefenamic acid (PO)

Oxicams
Piroxicam (PO, PR, IM)
Tenoxicam (PO)

Acetic acid derivatives
Diclofenac (PO, PR, IM)
Ketorolac (PO, IM, IV)

Opioids
Codeine phosphate (PO, IM)
Dihydrocodeine tartrate (PO, IM)
Pethidine (PO, IM, IV)
Papavaretum (IM, IV)
Morphine (PO, SC, IM, IV, PR)
Diamorphine (PO, SC, IM, IV)
Buprenorphine (SL, IM, IV)
Meptazinol (PO, IM, IV)
Nalbuphine (IM, IV)
Fentanyl (IV)
Alfentanil (IV)
Methadone (PO, SC, IM)

Combinations
Paracetamol 500 mg + codeine 8 mg (Co-codamol)
Paracetamol 500 mg + dihydrocodeine 10 mg (Co-dydramol)
Paracetamol + dextropropoxyphene (Co-proxamol)
Paracetamol + aspirin (Benorylate)
Aspirin + papavaretum (Aspav)

Inhalational analgesia
Nitrous oxide/oxygen mixture

PO, per os; PR, per rectum; IM, intramuscular; IV, intravenous; SC, subcutaneous; SL, sublingual.

Table 2. *Adult doses of paracetamol and commonly used oral non-steroidal anti-inflammatory drugs*

Drug	Usual daily dose (mg)	Usual single dose (mg)	Usual dose interval (h)	Time to peak effect (h)
Paracetamol	2000–4000	500–1000	4	1
Aspirin	1800–3600	300–600	4	0.5–1
Ibuprofen	1200–2400	300–600	6–8	0.5–1.5
Fenoprofen	1800–2400	600	6–8	1–2
Ketoprofen	100–200	25–50	6–8	0.5–2
Naproxen	500–750	250	12	1–2
Indomethacin	75–150	25–50	6–12	1–2
Diclofenac	75–150	50–75	8	1–3
Piroxicam	20–30	10–20	12–24	2

concentrations reach effective levels from about 30 min, and a peak value at approximately 2 h.

There are vast numbers of oral analgesics available and the most sensible approach is to become familiar with just a few, preferably one or two from each group. The five properties that might be used to influence the choice of an oral analgesic are: efficacy, safety, tolerance, convenience, cost. Generally, analgesics with anti-inflammatory properties are particularly good for mild to moderate musculoskeletal pain while opioids are appropriate for severe visceral pain. The NSAIDs are valuable because they do not cause respiratory or cardiovascular depression. Doses of commonly used oral NSAIDs are given in Table 2.

Paracetamol is an inexpensive, simple analgesic of similar efficacy to aspirin but without the gastrointestinal side-effects. It has replaced aspirin as the analgesic and antipyretic agent of choice in children. Although paracetamol exerts no peripheral anti-inflammatory activity, it is thought to act by the inhibition of prostaglandin synthesis in the CNS; this is also likely to be the mechanism for its antipyretic activity. Paracetamol is ideal for mild pain without an inflammatory component (e.g. headache). An oral suspension or solution is available for children and may be given as 10 mg kg^{-1} 4 hourly as required. Paracetamol is absorbed rapidly from the small intestine and peak plasma concentrations are reached in 30–60 min. Side-effects from paracetamol taken within the recommended dose range are rare. However, in overdose paracetamol may cause serious liver damage.

Aspirin is the most commonly used NSAID; is the least expensive, and is an appropriate drug for headache, dysmenorrhoea and mild musculoskeletal pain. The most common complication of aspirin is gastrointestinal irritation and a history of gastric ulceration contraindicates its use. A variety of formulations, such as effervescent or timed-release tablets, have been introduced in an attempt to reduce the gastrointestinal side-effects. Aspirin is contraindicated in children under 12 years of age because of its links with Reye's syndrome. Like other NSAIDs, it may provoke bronchospasm in asthmatic patients. Other side-effects associated with the NSAIDs include sodium and water retention, impaired renal function, reduced platelet aggregation, and idiosyncratic reactions such as rashes and photosensitivity.

Ibuprofen is the most widely used propionic acid derivative. It has only weak anti-inflammatory activity but is said to be associated with fewer side-effects than many of the other NSAIDs and is ideal for mild musculoskeletal pain. Ibuprofen can be bought across the counter without prescription. Other propionic acid derivatives include fenoprofen, ketoprofen and naproxen.

Indomethacin is the most well known of the indene derivatives and has potent anti-inflammatory properties. However, its use is associated with a high incidence of adverse effects, in particular gastric irritation.

Diclofenac, an acetic acid derivative, is available in rectal and parenteral formulations as well as oral. The rectal preparation is particularly useful for postoperative pain relief (see below), but the oral form would seem to have little advantage over ibuprofen.

Piroxicam has a prolonged duration of action which may be an advantage in patients with poor compliance. However, once again, it is associated with a higher incidence of side-effects in comparison to ibuprofen.

Patients with moderate to severe acute pain are likely to require more potent analgesics in the form of opioids. There are oral formulations for many of the opioids but in the A&E department a parenteral preparation is likely to be more appropriate. There are a few 'weak' opioids which may be useful in oral form for moderate pain, particularly where NSAIDs are contraindicated.

Codeine occurs naturally in opium and is closely related structurally to opium. Unlike morphine, codeine does not undergo extensive first-pass metabolism by the liver so its oral bioavailability is 50% compared with only 20% for morphine. Given as a single parenteral dose, codeine is less than one-twelfth as potent as morphine but between one-third and one-fourth as potent by mouth. About 10–20% of a dose of codeine is converted to morphine and its analgesic effect probably results entirely from this metabolite. The usual oral dose of codeine is 30–60 mg; it has a plasma half-life of 2.5–3 h and the useful duration of effect is 4–6 h. In equianalgesic doses codeine is a more potent cough suppressant than morphine. Codeine shares the adverse effects (e.g. respiratory depression) of the other opioids, but, in standard dose constipation is a particular problem. Dihydrocodeine is about one-third more potent than codeine but is identical in other respects.

Dextropropoxyphene is less potent than codeine and the combination of dextropropoxyphene with paracetamol (co-proxamol), though very popular, provides little more analgesia than paracetamol alone. Furthermore, if co-proxamol is taken in overdosage the patient will be exposed to the side-effects of dextropropoxyphene (respiratory depression and acute heart failure) as well as those of paracetamol (hepatic failure).

Pethidine can reasonably be given orally since it will still have 50% bioavailability by this route. Many paediatricians prescribe oral pethidine to provide potent analgesia in children with severe pain.

Sublingual analgesia

Buprenorphine is a potent semisynthetic analgesic with both opioid agonist and antagonist properties. Its main advantage over the other opioids is that it can be given by the sublingual route. Administration by this route avoids first-pass metabolism of the drug, avoids the need for injections, and its efficacy is unaffected by impaired gastric emptying, gastrointestinal immotility or vomiting. The patient must be cooperative enough not to chew or swallow the tablet and it may be slow to dissolve if there is reduced saliva production.

Buprenorphine produces analgesia and other CNS effects that are qualitatively similar to those of morphine. A sublingual dose of 0.4 mg is equianalgesic with morphine 10 mg given intramuscularly. Peak plasma levels are reached at 2 h and the duration of analgesia is 6–8 h. The respiratory depression produced by buprenorphine may only be partially reversed by naloxone.

Rectal analgesia

Like the sublingual route, rectal administration reduces the rate of first-pass metabolism and is independent of gastric emptying and nausea and vomiting. However, absorption, and therefore onset, is slow and, in contrast to the French, this route has still to gain widespread acceptance amongst British patients. A number of analgesic preparations can be given rectally, in particular paracetamol, a number of NSAIDs, and morphine. There is said to be less risk of gastrointestinal side-effects when NSAIDs are administered rectally. The rectal route is particularly useful for the maintenance of analgesia, and diclofenac 100 mg administered rectally every 18 h is very effective for postoperative pain.

Topical analgesia

EMLA cream

Intact skin is a major barrier to the diffusion of local anaesthetics. A topically applied local anaesthetic will be effective only if there is a high concentration of the uncharged base form of the local anaesthetic, and a high water content to enhance penetration. Since the base form of a local anaesthetic dissolves poorly in water, the only way to combine the active base with water is to make an 'oil-in-water' emulsion. However, under normal conditions the maximum concentration of local anaesthetic which can be obtained in a droplet of the emulsion is only 20%, too low for effective penetration of intact skin.

Lignocaine and prilocaine bases each have melting points well above room temperature, but when crystals of these bases are mixed in equal amounts their melting point is lowered to 18°C and at room temperature they form an oil. This is a eutectic mixture (hence eutectic mixture of local anaesthetic, EMLA), comparable to the production of water after salt is added to ice. If the lignocaine/prilocaine oil is used to form an emulsion, the concentration of local anaesthetic in each droplet is 80%, even though the total concentration of local anaesthetic is only 5%. If a thick layer of EMLA cream is applied to the skin and covered with an occlusive dressing, effective anaesthesia of the underlying skin will be produced in about 1 h. This will allow painless needle penetration.

The most obvious indication for EMLA cream is to ensure painless venepuncture in children for obtaining blood samples or cannulation. The very slow onset of effective anaesthesia precludes its use if venepuncture is required urgently. EMLA cream has been used also to provide anaesthesia during harvesting of small skin grafts and during excision of small skin lesions. It should not be applied to wounds, mucous membranes or eczematous skin.

Local anaesthetic gels

Local anaesthetics are effectively absorbed from mucous membranes and a number of topical preparations, in particular lignocaine, are available. 2% lignocaine gel is used for anaesthetizing the male urethra before catheterization. The maximum dose is calculated using the same criteria as described below; thus, for a 70 kg man, 10 ml of 2% lignocaine gel is the maximum dose. Lignocaine gel is an ideal lubricant for nasal airways and should always be used if inserting a nasal airway in a conscious patient.

Topical NSAIDs

Topical NSAIDs have been developed in an attempt to reduce the risks of systemic treatment, while preserving the analgesic and anti-inflammatory properties. Whether they achieve this goal is controversial. The majority of those drugs that are able to penetrate the skin are taken up rapidly into the systemic circulation which prevents them from accumulating locally. However, topically applied salicylates and some NSAIDs can achieve high local tissue concentrations relative to plasma levels and this has prompted a number of manufacturers to produce NSAID gels or creams for the treatment of localized soft tissue trauma and inflammatory musculoskeletal conditions. Examples currently available include ibuprofen 5% gel or cream, piroxicam 0.5% gel, felbinac 3% gel, and diclofenac 1% gel. These preparations can be applied to the affected area three to four times daily and result in plasma levels about 5% of those that follow a standard oral dose. Unfortunately, despite the low plasma levels of drug, topical application does not eliminate the risk of NSAID side-effects. The Committee on the Safety of Medicines has received reports of asthma and dyspepsia in association with topical NSAIDs. The evidence that any of the topical NSAIDs give useful benefit is tenuous and the conclusions drawn by reviews in the *Drug and Therapeutics Bulletin* were that their use was hard to justify (Consumers' Association, 1990, 1991).

Inhalational analgesia

The inhalational route has formed the basis for general anaesthesia since its inception almost 150 years ago. It was first introduced for analgesia in the 1930s in obstetric patients when Minnit used a mixture of nitrous oxide and air (Minnit, 1934). Later apparatus was designed to deliver trichloroethylene and methoxyflurane in air. The hypoxic nitrous oxide and air mixtures were replaced with 50% nitrous oxide and oxygen with the introduction of Entonox which contains both gases premixed in a single cylinder. The inhalational route was extended to include analgesia for dental procedures and the general relief of pain associated with trauma, myocardial ischaemia and other conditions (Baskett & Bennett, 1971; Baskett, 1972).

With the demise of trichloroethylene and methoxyflurane, nitrous oxide and oxygen is the prevalent inhalational analgesic in current use. Nitrous oxide is a potent analgesic and sedative which, in a 50% mixture with oxygen, equates to 10 mg morphine in an average adult ($0.16 \, mg \, kg^{-1}$). It has a low blood and fat solubility which ensures a rapid onset and a speedy recovery once inhalation stops. In the UK and certain other countries, it is available in a single cylinder of premixed gases and in the USA as a two-cylinder apparatus delivering a fixed concentration of the gases in equal proportions (Nitronox). Both systems use a preferential inhalational demand arrangement for self-administration although in certain circumstances this can be overridden to produce a continuous flow of gas.

In the UK and Australia the use of Entonox has gained widespread acceptance for the relief of pain in trauma and medical and surgical emergencies, in the prehospital phase and in the A&E department.

Advantages of nitrous oxide/oxygen analgesia using a self-administration demand inhalational system

These include:

- *Effective analgesia in the majority of patients.* Studies show that some 66% of patients achieve good pain relief, 30% fair pain relief and only 4–5% have minimal pain relief (Baskett & Bennett, 1971; Thal *et al.*, 1979; Stewart *et al.*, 1983).
- *Inherent safety.* The self-administration demand flow system requires the patient to generate a negative pressure at the inspiratory port. In essence, this requires an airtight fit between the mask or mouth piece and the face or lips. As the patient holds the mask himself, should he become drowsy his grip will relax, the airtight seal will be lost and the gas flow will stop.
- *Freedom from side-effects.* In over 25 years of clinical practice in the A&E field, Entonox has not been associated with reports of significant depression of protective reflexes, ventilation or cardiovascular function. Myocardial depression has not been recorded in

patients in pain in the prehospital or A&E department setting. The relatively short period of use (up to 2 h) is not associated with bone marrow depression. Nausea and vomiting are rare and drowsiness, while not unwanted, is controlled by the self-administration system. Carbon dioxide retention and narcosis in patients with chronic obstructive pulmonary disease is prevented also by the self-administration demand system.

- *Adequate oxygen therapy.* The demand system ensures that the patient receives a guaranteed fractional inspired oxygen concentration (FiO_2) of 0.5 which is similar to the FiO_2 delivered by continuous flow apparatus available in the majority of ambulances.
- *Ease of use.* The apparatus is simple to use and 'fails safe'. In the event of cylinder exhaustion the patient breathes atmospheric air. There is no possibility of hypoxic gas mixtures being inhaled. The Nitronox apparatus is designed with an immediate nitrous oxide cut-off should the oxygen supply run out. The self-administration system can be supervised by an ambulance technician or nurse, bringing the availability of powerful analgesia to prehospital care and hospital departments without physician intervention.

Real and potential disadvantages of nitrous oxide analgesia

These include:

- *Barotrauma.* Nitrous oxide can diffuse into gas filled spaces 25 times as fast as nitrogen can diffuse out. Thus, it will increase the volume of a pneumothorax, a pneumopericardium, or a pneumoencephalus and will tend to cause gastric and intestinal distension. Pressure in the ears and sinuses may be increased as will the volume of any gas emboli (in divers with the bends, for example). Such conditions represent absolute contraindications to the use of nitrous oxide/oxygen mixtures.

  With prolonged use, nitrous oxide will gradually diffuse into the cuff of a tracheal tube causing expansion and subsequent excessive compression of the tracheal mucous membrane.

- *Extremes of temperature.* Premixed nitrous oxide and oxygen in 50% proportions (Entonox) remains stable as a single-phase gas when compressed to almost $140 \, kg \, cm^{-2}$ at temperatures above $-6°C$. Below this temperature the gas mixture separates and the nitrous oxide falls to the bottom of the cylinder. If the cylinder is then used, oxygen in high concentration is delivered at first, but as the cylinder empties increasing proportions of nitrous oxide are delivered. The stable mixture can be reconstituted after warming to above 0°C and inverting the cylinder several times. Thus, cylinders of Entonox should be stored and used only in environments above −6°C. This limitation does not apply to the Nitronox apparatus. Entonox, while not inflammable or explosive, will support combustion vigorously and should therefore be used with caution, in the same way as oxygen, when there is a possibility of ignition with cutting apparatus, etc.

- *Patient cooperation.* The use of the self-administration demand system requires a certain amount of patient involvement and cooperation. this may be lacking in the very old, the very young, and the confused and bewildered. In such patients the apparatus may be converted to a continuous flow mode provided the attendant is fully conversant with the potential sequelae of loss of consciousness and protective reflexes which may occur when the safeguards of the demand system are lost.

- *Pollution.* Some concern has been expressed as to the possibility of pollution by nitrous oxide in confined spaces such as the inside of ambulances. In practice this has not proved to have been a problem; the recorded levels have been very low because ambulances tend to be well ventilated. If concern is still present, a scavenging system can simply be incorporated into the apparatus.

- *Abuse.* There is a theoretical danger of abuse and addiction occurring in attendants, nurses and, indeed, physicians. Although isolated anecdotal incidents have occurred, this has not been a significant problem in extensive practice over 25 years. Nevertheless, all personnel involved should be warned of the hazards of abuse.

Parenteral analgesia

Patients requiring parenteral (intramuscular (IM) or intravenous (IV)) analgesia include those with acute moderate or severe pain or those who are unable or unwilling to take oral analgesics. The majority of analgesics given parenterally are opioids but an increasing number of NSAIDs are becoming available in parenteral form. In addition, ketamine, a phencyclidine derivative, is a valuable parenteral analgesic.

Advantages of the intramuscular route are that the drug can be given by a nurse and, in comparison with the intravenous route, the duration of action is longer. However, the rate of absorption of an analgesic from an intramuscular site will depend on the vascular perfusion and blood flow to muscle, resulting in a variable onset and quality of analgesia. In comparison with the intravenous route, the analgesia provided by intramuscular opioids is delayed. In patients with a low cardiac output, as a result of hypovolaemia or myocardial dysfunction for example, onset of analgesia after intramuscular injection will be extremely slow. Furthermore, if the lack of effect results in a second intramuscular dose being given, effective resuscitation of the patient may then be followed by respiratory depression as muscle blood flow is restored. This complication was noted in battle casualties during the Falklands campaign (Jowitt, 1993). In the patient with multiple injuries do not give analgesics by the intramuscular route; instead, give analgesics by careful intravenous titration (see below).

The intravenous route is the most precise, rapid and effective method of relieving severe pain. The drug reaches the appropriate receptors directly without being dependent on uptake into the blood stream from muscle, mucous membrane, or alveolus. Analgesia, and of course, depressant side-effects, occur rapidly.

In any individual patient the response to a parenteral opioid will vary widely according to age, prior medical status and medication, current cardiovascular and respiratory status and the performance of degradation and excretory systems; there may be a ten-fold difference in the dose per kg required between a 20-year-old man and a 90-year-old lady. Thus, the inexperienced doctor may find it difficult to estimate the appropriate dose of opioid. The intramuscular route makes it very difficult to titrate the dose of drug to produce the required analgesia. Additional disadvantages of the intramuscular route include the pain caused by the injection and the risk of serious bruising in patients with bleeding disorders. The sciatic nerve is at risk from injections placed too medially in the buttocks.

Intravenous analgesia may be given in small divided bolus doses titrated to effect or by continuous infusion, or a combination of both. Continuous infusions of opioid, given by programmed infusion pumps, are more likely to be used in other areas of the hospital. In the A&E department, the bolus doses would usually be given by an attendant, but in other areas of the hospital patient-controlled analgesia (PCA) systems allow the patient to administer their own analgesia.

The PCA system offers considerable safeguards, being a fail-safe system in that patient drowsiness ensures a cut-off. In the routine postoperative field the PCA system works well when the patient has been coached in the use of the system beforehand. In the majority of cases the patient is satisfied with the pain relief provided by the PCA system and tends to require less analgesic in comparison with the intramuscular route. However, some patients, such as those who are confused or agitated or unable to comprehend simple instructions, are unsuitable for PCA. Such conditions prevail in many trauma patients in the early stages after injury. Thus, the best plan for pain relief in the trauma patient is to give small divided doses intravenously, titrated until the desired effect is achieved. At a later stage on the ward, conscious patients may receive a low-dose continuous infusion supplemented by patient-controlled boluses. On the intensive care unit, unconscious, ventilated patients requiring analgesia may receive a low-dose continuous infusion supplemented by bolus doses given by attendants as required.

Opioid analgesics

Terminology and classification

The term 'narcotic', derived from the Greek 'narco-' meaning to deaden, is now outdated although it is still found in legal terminology. The constituents of opium (from the Greek 'opion', meaning poppy juice) were known as opiates and this term was applied also to synthetic analogues of morphine. More recently it has been recognized that a wide variety of synthetic chemical structures may cause morphine-like effects and this led to the adoption of 'opioids' as a term applying to all naturally occurring and synthetic drugs producing morphine-like effects. Thus opioids may be classified according to their origin:

- Naturally occurring opium derivatives, e.g. morphine, codeine.
- Semisynthetic derivatives of morphine, e.g. diamorphine, papavaretum.
- Synthetic opioids, e.g. pethidine, fentanyl, alfentanil, sufentanil, buprenorphine, nalbuphine.

All opioids act through specific receptors located in the brain and spinal cord. A variety of receptors have been discovered and each is associated with a specific action. The action of a particular drug depends on its affinity for a given receptor and whether it exerts an agonist or antagonist action.

The current list of receptors include mu, delta, kappa, sigma, and epsilon. They are responsible for a variety of effects such as: analgesia, euphoria, respiratory depression (mu); cough suppression, sedation (kappa); dysphoria, hallucinations (sigma); nausea and vomiting, pruritus (delta).

Side-effects

All potent opioid analgesics carry the potential to depress levels of consciousness, protective reflexes and vital functions and it is mandatory that these are closely monitored during and after administration. Specifically, side-effects of opioid drugs include:

- *Respiratory depression*. Minute ventilation and respiratory rate are reduced, although tidal volume is increased.
- *Nausea and vomiting*. Caused by direct stimulation of the chemoreceptor trigger zone for emesis in the area postrema of the medulla. There is also a vestibular component; nausea and vomiting are relatively uncommon in recumbent patients given therapeutic doses of morphine, but nausea will occur in approximately 40% and vomiting in 15% if the patients are ambulatory.
- *Hypotension*. Many opioids, particularly pethidine and morphine, provoke the release of histamine and this may cause hypotension.
- *Constipation*.
- *Spasm of the sphincter of Oddi*. The pressure in the common bile duct may rise more than ten-fold in 15 min, lasting up to 2 h. Therefore, patients with biliary colic may experience exacerbation rather than relief of pain when given opioids. All of the opioids can produce this effect but it is said to be less common with pethidine.
- *Miosis*. Opioids cause constriction of the pupil due to an excitatory action on the autonomic segment of the nucleus of the oculomotor nerve.

Prescribing opioids in the A&E department

Opioids prescribed commonly by parenteral routes in the A&E department include pethidine, morphine, diamorphine, papavaretum, codeine, and nalbuphine. Unfortunately, a popular approach is to select a dose of one of these drugs (e.g. pethidine 75 mg IM) and give that same dose to all adult patients, regardless of age or medical condition. This practice is to be deplored. Intramuscular opioids should be on the basis of weight, taking

Table 3. *Doses and dose intervals for commonly used intramuscular opioids*

Drug	Intravenous dose[a]	Intramuscular dose ($mg\,kg^{-1}$)	Dosing interval (h)	Equianalgesic dose (mg)[b]
Pethidine	10–25 mg	0.5–2	2–3	100
Morphine	2–5 mg	0.1–0.2	3–4	10
Diamorphine	1–2.5 mg	0.05–0.15	3–4	5
Papavaretum	2–5 mg	0.15–0.3	3–4	20
Codeine	N/A	0.5–1	4	120
Nalbuphine	2–5 mg	0.1–0.3	3–4	10–15
Buprenorphine	N/A	0.003–0.006	6–8	0.4
Fentanyl	0.5 µg	N/A	Duration of effect 0.75	0.075

[a] Suggested intravenous bolus doses for an adult, given every 5–10 min until desired effect is achieved.
[b] Equivalent to morphine 10 mg.

into account also the patient's age and physical condition. Approximate doses and dose intervals for intramuscular opioids, are given in Table 3. Intravenous opioids should be titrated in small doses (Table 3) given at 5–10 min intervals until appropriate analgesia is achieved.

Morphine

Morphine represents the analgesic yardstick by which others are judged. Arguably it remains the most effective analgesic for the management of severe acute pain. It stimulates the mu-receptors producing profound analgesia, euphoria and respiratory depression. It also produces nausea and vomiting by virtue of binding with the delta-receptors. All actions are dose related commensurate with the patient's previous health and current vital signs. Thus, cardiovascular and respiratory depression occur with even small doses in the hypovolaemic patient with obtunded reflexes. Onset of action is 5 min after an intravenous dose and 15–20 min after an intramuscular dose, and its duration of action is 3 h.

Diamorphine

This drug is produced when two hydroxyl groups on the morphine molecule are replaced by acetyl groups. These increase the lipid solubility of diamorphine, giving it a slightly shorter time for onset of action (5–10 min after intramuscular injection, 2–5 min after intravenous injection). Diamorphine is metabolized to morphine, thus the duration of action is similar. Diamorphine is said to

produce less nausea and vomiting and more euphoria than morphine, but whether these represent clinically significant advantages over morphine is controversial. It produces the same degree of respiratory depression as morphine. Diamorphine is not available for therapeutic use in the USA. In the UK, many consider diamorphine the analgesic of choice for cardiac pain for which it is generally administered in 2.5 mg aliquots until the desired effect is achieved.

Pethidine

Pethidine was developed from a phenylpiperidine molecule in Germany between the 1st and 2nd World Wars, as the first truly synthetic opioid. In equianalgesic doses it produces as much sedation, respiratory depression and euphoria as does morphine. Unlike morphine, pethidine has atropine-like effects at cholinergic nerve endings and does not cause bradycardia. Relative to its analgesic actions, pethidine causes less smooth muscle constriction than morphine and thus less rise in common bile duct pressure. CNS excitation and hypertension or hypotension may occur if pethidine is given to patients taking monoamine oxidase inhibitors. Pethidine may be given in 25 mg IV increments, at 5–10-min intervals, until the desired effect is achieved. Onset of analgesia by the intramuscular route is within 15 min, reaching a peak at 1 h. The duration of action of pethidine is 2–3 h. This is significantly shorter than morphine. For some reason pethidine is a popular choice of opioid analgesic for children. This may be because the appropriate dose ($1–2\,mg\,kg^{-1}$) is easy to remember!

Papavaretum

This has been a commonly prescribed drug for post-operative pain and for premedication. Papavaretum is a mixture of alkaloids of opium comprising anhydrous morphine 47.5–52.5%, anhydrous codeine 2.5–5%, noscapine 16–22%, and papavarine 2.5–7%. Thus, 20 mg of papavaretum is equivalent to 12.5 mg of morphine sulphate and its onset time and duration are the same as morphine. Like morphine, papavaretum can be given intravenously in 2–5 mg increments. Not surprisingly, it has very similar effects to morphine and is associated with pronounced euphoria. The use of papavaretum declined suddenly in 1991 following a report that noscapine can induce polyploidy in mammalian cell lines maintained *in vitro*. Consequently, the Committee on Safety of Medicines (CSM) recommended that all products containing papavaretum should be contraindicated in woman of child-bearing potential. Recently, Roche have reformulated their brand of papavaretum (Omnopon) to exclude noscapine.

Codeine

Given orally this drug provides useful analgesia for mild to moderate pain. However, it is a very weak opioid and there is little point in selecting it for parenteral use. Although still licensed for intravenous use, codeine by this route is never clinically indicated, and bolus injection may be associated with a significant risk of severe hypotension (Parke *et al.*, 1992). Codeine 120 mg IM is said to be equivalent to morphine 10 mg. Historically, codeine is the analgesic selected for patients with head injuries, ranging from a minor bump to those who are semiconscious. In head-injured patients, intramuscular codeine has no advantages over most other opioids. In equianalgesic doses it is a more potent histamine releaser than morphine and has the same other side-effects as morphine, including the ability to induce respiratory depression and miosis. This is hardly surprising since its effects are brought about by the 10–20% that is metabolized to morphine. The percentage converted to morphine varies considerably due to the genetic polymorphism that governs the enzymatic process. On occasions we have seen codeine 30–60 mg IM given as the sole analgesic to patients with multiple injuries, simply because there was a vague history of head injury. Under these circumstances, this dose of codeine will do nothing to relieve pain. The correct approach is to titrate slowly a suitable opioid by the intravenous route. Later, if intramuscular analgesia is required, it is better to use a small dose of morphine with relatively predictable effects than the more unreliable codeine.

Buprenorphine

The chief advantage of this drug over the other opioids is that it can be given by the sublingual route (see above). In comparison with morphine, buprenorphine is associated with a high incidence of nausea, vomiting and dysphoria, but a lower incidence of respiratory depression. Although an intramuscular preparation of buprenorphine is available, it offers little advantage over morphine.

Nalbuphine

This is a synthetic *N*-allyl derivative of oxymorphone. Like buprenorphine it is a partial agonist and therefore is associated with a ceiling to its depressant effect on respiration and antagonism of the analgesic actions of pure agonist opioids (e.g. morphine). Nalbuphine 10 mg is said to be equianalgesic with morphine 10 mg and its onset time and duration of action are similar also. It can be titrated intravenously in 5 mg increments, up to 20 mg. It causes relatively little myocardial depression and has even been suggested to improve cardiovascular haemodynamics after myocardial infarction. It has less emetic and dysphoric effects than buprenorphine and because it is not subject to such legal controls as the morphine and pethidine groups it is currently recommended for use by paramedics in the prehospital phase.

Fentanyl, alfentanil, sufentanil

Like pethidine, these three agents are phenylpiperidine derivatives. All are very potent analgesics associated with pronounced respiratory depression and are generally used by anaesthetists only. They are given intravenously only and have a very rapid onset of action and provide analgesia for a relatively short duration. They do not cause histamine release and are less likely to cause hypotension than morphine. Alfentanil is too short-acting (10 min) to be useful in the A&E department and sufentanil is not available in the UK. After an intravenous bolus of fentanyl 1 μg kg^{-1}, onset of analgesia is within 2 min and lasts approximately 30–45 min. These characteristics make the accurate titration of fentanyl relatively easy and safe, and in the hands of a clinician experienced in its use it is an excellent analgesic for use during the resuscitation of the multiply injured patient. Of course, its duration of action is short and doses need to be repeated; this, however, allows continuous reassessment of the patient. Later, when the patient is more stable, a longer acting opioid (e.g. morphine) can be substituted. In the trauma patient who has been intubated and ventilated mechanically, fentanyl is the analgesic of choice.

Phencyclidine derivatives

The principal phencyclidine derivative used as an analgesic is ketamine. Ketamine was originally developed as an anaesthetic but in smaller doses ($0.25-0.5$ mg kg^{-1}) is a most effective analgesic and sedative. At this dose level the unwanted side-effects of dysphoria and hallucinations associated with sigma-receptor activity are almost absent. Respiratory and cardiovascular depression are minimal except in profoundly hypovolaemic patients. However, its use in head-injured patients is controversial because of the potential risk of increasing intracranial pressure. Ketamine can be given intravenously or intramuscularly. In adults, intravenous doses should be given in 20 mg aliquots until the desired effect is achieved.

Parenteral non-steroidal anti-inflammatory drugs

Parenteral NSAIDs may provide useful analgesia in situations where there is a significant inflammatory component, but where the patient is unable to take an oral preparation. They are particularly useful for renal colic. The NSAIDs may usefully be combined with opioids since they provide analgesia by completely different mechanisms and the addition of an NSAID will reduce the dose of opioid required for effective analgesia (an opioid-sparing effect).

Diclofenac

This has been available as an intramuscular preparation (75 mg in 3 ml) for number of years. By this route peak plasma concentrations are achieved within 30 min, compared to 1 h after a suppository. The recommended dosage is 75 mg by deep intramuscular injection once or twice a day. Intramuscular diclofenac is associated with the same adverse effects as oral NSAIDs but, in addition, there are complications related to the injection *per se*: first, the 3 ml volume can be very painful and, second,

the solvent (propylene glycol, benzyl alcohol and mannitol) can cause muscle damage resulting in a marked rise in plasma creatine phosphokinase and occasional sterile abscess formation.

Ketorolac

Ketorolac is structurally and pharmacologically related to indomethacin (Kenny, 1990). It is available as 10 mg tablets and in ampoules of 10 mg for intramuscular and intravenous use. It is relatively more effecttive as an analgesic than as an anti-inflammatory agent. The time to onset of analgesic effect following both intramuscular and intravenous administration is 30 min, with maximum analgesia occurring within $1-2$ h. The duration of analgesia is $4-6$ h. Ketorolac 30 mg provides similar analgesia to morphine 10 mg (Power *et al.*, 1990). Following a number of reports of adverse reactions (gastrointestinal haemorrhage, postoperative bleeding, anaphylaxis, and renal failure), the dosing recommendations for ketorolac have been recently revised. The starting intravenous/intramuscular dose has been reduced to 10 mg, with subsequent $10-30$ mg doses $4-6$ h as required. The maximum daily dosage has been reduced to 60 mg for the elderly and 90 mg in non-elderly patients. The principal advantages that ketorolac has over diclofenac are: the solvent is not associated with local muscle damage, the 1 ml volume is not particularly painful after intramuscular injection, and it is now licensed for intravenous use.

LOCAL ANAESTHESIA

Local anaesthesia is a cheap, simple, relatively safe and highly effective method of removing the discomfort from many procedures that are performed in the A&E department. The techniques described in this section can be performed well by properly trained A&E doctors, though for reasons of safety intravenous regional anaesthesia is ideally performed by a trained anaesthetist. Although the use of local anaesthesia is simple, certain precautions must be taken to prevent rare, though potentially fatal, complications. These are likely to result from overdose or faulty technique, such as intravenous injection. Anyone giving a local anaesthetic should be adequately trained in basic resuscitation and should have immediate access to oxygen and a means of ventilating the patient's lungs and securing venous access.

Pharmacology of local anaesthetic drugs

A local anaesthetic is a drug which temporarily blocks the transmission of peripheral nerve impulses by blocking membrane depolarization. The drug is injected into tissue in the ionized form (usually as acid solutions of the hydrochloride salt), but a percentage will dissociate to become free base. This lipid-soluble free base form of the drug penetrates the nerve membrane to reach the interior of the axon where a portion of the drug will reionize and block the sodium ion channels. Inactivation of the sodium channels prevents transmission of nerve impulses. Nerve function recovers once the drug has diffused back out into the tissues.

All local anaesthetics have a three-part structure, with either an ester or amide bond at the centre. The ester drugs (e.g. cocaine, procaine, amethocaine) tend to have shorter half-lives and are more likely to produce allergic reactions than the amide drugs (e.g. lignocaine, prilocaine, bupivacaine). The more lipid-soluble drugs will tend to be more potent, while the degree of protein binding will determine duration of action. The pK_a determines the portion of a drug dissociating to the free base, and is therefore responsible for the speed of onset.

Lignocaine is a more potent vasodilator than either prilocaine or bupivacaine, and its duration of action and maximum safe dose can be extended significantly by the addition of adrenaline $1:200\,000$ (e.g. adrenaline 0.1 mg in 20 ml solution). Adrenaline will also extend the duration of action of prilocaine but has little effect on bupivacaine (Table 4). A vasoconstrictor should never be used near end arteries (e.g. fingers, toes, penis, nose).

Local anaesthetic toxicity

The effects of local anaesthetics are not unique to peripheral nerves; they will have a similar effect on the cells of the CNS and the heart if significant systemic drug levels are attained. Severe toxicity may result from accidental intravascular injection or overdose. The maximum safe doses for lignocaine, prilocaine and bupivacaine are given in Table 4, along with their duration of action. Lignocaine is a vasodilator; consequently, the addition of adrenaline reduces significantly the vascular uptake of the drug and increases the maximum safe dose. This does not apply to bupivacaine or prilocaine which are very weak vasodilators only.

The CNS is most sensitive to local anaesthetics, but the rich blood supply to the tongue may mean that circumoral numbness slightly precedes light-headedness as the initial symptom of systemic toxicity. The progression of symptoms and signs of local anaesthetic toxicity with increasing plasma levels of lignocaine is depicted in Table 5. If a large dose of local anaesthetic has been injected intravenously, the patient is likely to lose consciousness and convulse immediately. The respiratory depression and hypoxia resulting from convulsions and coma will impair myocardial performance and this is a greater problem than the direct depressant effect of local anaesthetic on the heart. Amide local anaesthetics, such as lignocaine or bupivacaine, are group 1b anti-arrhythmic agents (Vaughn-Williams classification) and as such will reduce the rate of depolarization, the duration of the action potential, and the effective refractory period.

Table 4. *Maximum doses and duration of action of lignocaine, prilocaine and bupivacaine, with plain solutions and with adrenaline*

| | Infiltration | | | | Minor nerve block | |
| | Plain solution | | Adrenaline | | Plain solution | Adrenaline |
	Dose (mg kg^{-1})	Duration (min)	Dose (mg kg^{-1})	Duration (min)	Duration (min)	Duration (min)
Lignocaine	3	30–60	7	120–360	60–120	120–180
Prilocaine	7	30–90	8	120–360	60–120	120–180
Bupivacaine	2	120–240	2	180–420	180–360	240–480

Note: a 1% solution contains 10 mg of drug ml^{-1}.

Table 5. *Signs and symptoms of systemic local anaesthetic toxicity*

	Plasma lignocaine (μg ml^{-1})
Circumoral numbness	3
Light-headedness	4
Tinnitus	5
Visual disturbance	6
Slurred speech	7
Muscular twitching (especially facial)	8
Irrational conversation	9
Unconsciousness	10
Grand mal convulsions	12
Coma	15
Apnoea	20
Severe direct cardiovascular depression	25

Table 6. *Differential diagnosis of local anaesthetic reactions*

Aetiology	Clinical features
Local anaesthetic toxicity	
Intravascular injection	Immediate convulsion
Relative overdose	Onset of irritability in 5–15 min, progressing to convulsions
Reaction to vasoconstrictor	Tachycardia, hypertension, headache, apprehension
Vasovagal	Rapid onset of bradycardia, hypotension, pallor and faintness
Allergy	
Immediate	Anaphylaxis with hypotension, bronchospasm and oedema
Delayed	Urticaria

Local anaesthetic toxicity must be differentiated from other reactions to local anaesthetic, such as reaction to a vasoconstrictor, a vasovagal reaction, or true allergy (see Table 6).

The goal in the treatment of severe local anaesthetic toxicity is to reverse the hypoxia and acidosis which tends to keep the local anaesthetic ionized, thus preventing it leaving the CNS and myocardium. Clear the patient's airway and give high-concentration oxygen by face mask or by bag–valve–mask device if the patient requires assisted ventilation. Obtain intravenous access and if the patient is convulsing give Diazemuls 0.15 mg

kg^{-1} IV. If the convulsions continue, thiopentone 1–4 mg kg^{-1} IV can be given, though this is done ideally by an anaesthetist. The anaesthetist may also elect to paralyse (suxamethonium 1.5 mg kg^{-1} IV) and intubate the patient to guarantee an airway and ease of ventilation. If the patient is hypotensive, elevate the legs and infuse rapidly 500 ml of gelatin solution. After this, if the systolic blood pressure is less than 90 mmHg give ephedrine 5 mg IV. In the event of severe cardiovascular collapse use instead 1 ml IV increments of adrenaline 1:10 000.

Local anaesthetic techniques

TECHNIQUES

Local infiltration of the skin

This is the simplest of local anaesthetic techniques and the one most commonly used in the A&E department.

Indications
- Suturing lacerations.
- Minor surgical procedures (e.g. excision of sebaceous cyst).
- Debriding wounds.
- Supplementing a peripheral nerve block.

Contraindications
- A large wound or laceration requiring more than the maximum permitted dose.

Technique
Use 0.5% or 1% lignocaine, up to 3 mg kg^{-1}, to provide a rapid onset. The addition of 1:200 000 adrenaline will increase the duration of action, increase the maximum permitted dose to 7 mg kg^{-1}, and reduce bleeding, but should not be used if near an end artery. Onset time will be approximately 2 min. For maximal patient comfort use the smallest needle possible, usually a 25G or 23G. Inject the local anaesthetic subcutaneously around the required area. If the needle is kept moving there is no need for repeated aspiration since small amounts only of dilute local anaesthetic will be entering veins. If more than one entry into the skin is required, always reintroduce the needle through skin that has already been anaesthetized.

Digital nerve block

Each digit is supplied by four nerve branches (two dorsal and two palmar) which accompany the digital vessels. Fingers and toes are easily and effectively anaesthetized by blocking these nerves.

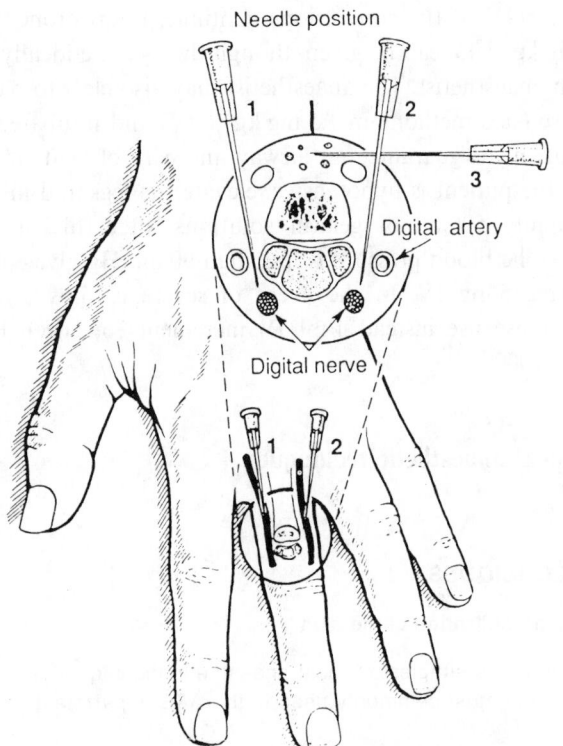

Fig. 2. Digital nerve block. (Reproduced, with permission, from Illingworth, K.A. (1989). Anaesthesia and pain control. In *Accident and Emergency Medicine*, ed. W.H. Rutherford, R.N. Illingworth, A.K. Marsden, P.G. Nelson, A.D. Redmond and D.H. Wilson. Edinburgh: Churchill Livingstone.)

Indications

- Suturing lacerations or debriding wounds on fingers and toes.
- Simple operations on fingers and toes (e.g. removal of toe nail).

Technique

Use 2–5 ml of 2% lignocaine or 0.5% bupivacaine. Bupivacaine will provide effective analgesia for a few hours. Do not use adrenaline-containing solutions for digital nerve blocks. Using a 23G needle, approach the nerves from dorsal aspect at each side of the base of the digit (Fig. 2). Inject 1.5 ml of local anaesthetic around each palmar digital nerve. The dorsal branches can be blocked by injecting another 1.5 ml across the dorsum of the base of the digit.

Potential complications

Unnecessarily high volumes of local anaesthetic (e.g. above 5 ml in an adult) will create very high pressures at the base of the digit and may impair the local circulation. It will be also very uncomfortable for the patient.

Peripheral nerve blocks

The cutaneous distribution of peripheral nerves to the hand is shown in Fig. 3. Suitable local anaesthetics for peripheral nerve blocks include bupivacaine 0.5%, lignocaine 1%, lignocaine 1% with adrenaline.

Median nerve block

The median nerve can be blocked at either the elbow or the wrist, but the latter is the more usual and will be described here. At the wrist the median nerve lies quite superficially, just under and on the radial side of palmaris longus tendon.

Indications

- Minor surgery to those areas of the hand innervated by the median nerve.

Contraindications

- A history of carpal tunnel syndrome.
- Neuritis.

Technique

Use 5 ml of 0.5% bupivacaine or 1% lignocaine and a 25G needle. Make the tendons of palmaris longus and flexor carpi radialis become more prominent by getting the patient to flex the wrist against resistance. Insert the needle at right-angles to the skin at the proximal skin crease of the wrist between the tendons of palmaris longus and flexor carpi radialis (Fig. 4). The nerve is about 1 cm deep at this point and paraesthesia may be obtained by moving the needle fanwise in an ulnar direction. Once paraesthesia is elicited, withdraw the needle slightly and inject the local anaesthetic. Allow 15 min for onset of anaesthesia.

Ulnar nerve block

The ulnar nerve can be blocked at either the wrist or the elbow. The approach at the wrist involves two needle insertions and is more difficult to perform. At the elbow the ulnar nerve lies tightly bound in fibrous tissue in a groove behind the medial epicondyle. In the distal forearm the ulnar nerve is medial to the ulnar artery. About 5 cm proximal to the wrist the ulnar nerve divides into a sensory dorsal branch and a mixed palmar branch.

Indications

- Minor procedures on the little finger and ulnar aspect of the hand.

Contraindications

Ulnar nerve neuritis.

Technique (at elbow)

With the patient supine, flex the elbow 90°. Palpate the ulnar nerve 2–3 cm proximal to the medial epicondyle

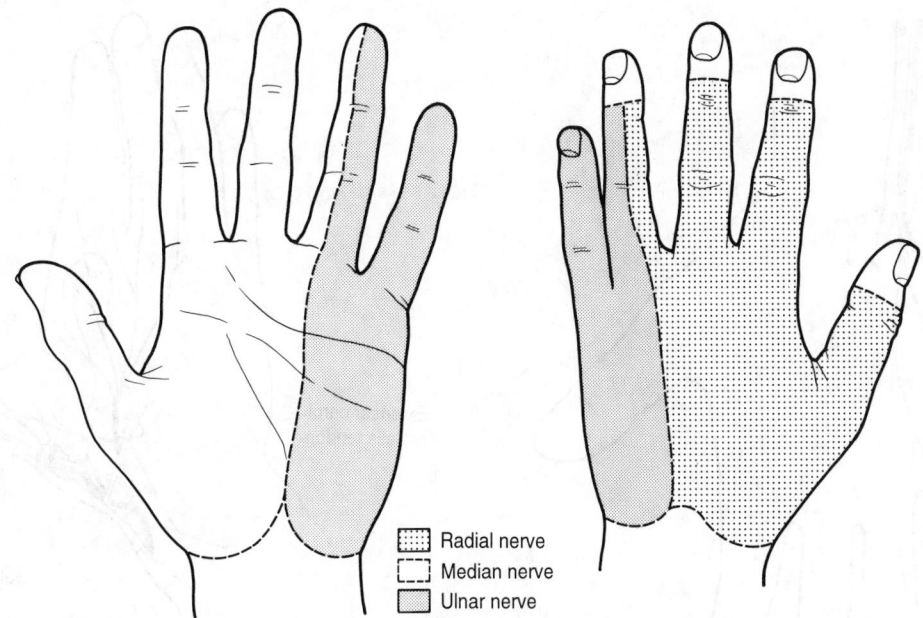

Fig. 3. Cutaneous distribution of peripheral nerves to the hand.

Radial nerve
Median nerve
Ulnar nerve

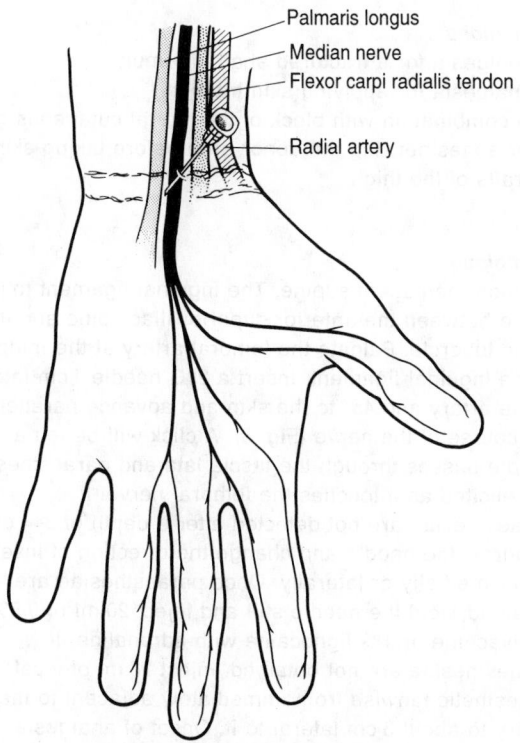

Palmaris longus
Median nerve
Flexor carpi radialis tendon
Radial artery

Fig. 4. Median nerve block.

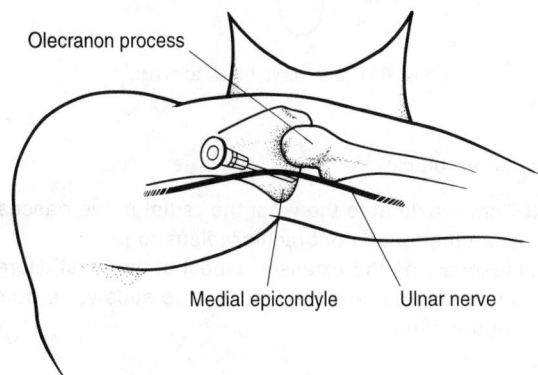

Olecranon process
Medial epicondyle   Ulnar nerve

Fig. 5. Ulnar nerve block at elbow.

(Fig. 5). Using a 23G needle inject 5 ml of 0.5% bupivacaine alongside the nerve. There is a risk of neuritis if paraesthesiae are sought with this approach. A successful block of the ulnar nerve at the elbow may provide anaesthesia for many hours.

Technique (at wrist)
Flex the wrist against a resistance to help identify flexor carpi ulnaris. The palmar branch of the ulnar nerve is blocked at the level of the ulnar styloid process by inserting a 25G needle at right-angles to the skin between the tendon of flexor carpi ulnaris and the ulnar artery (Fig. 6). If paraesthesia is obtained, inject 5 ml of 0.5% bupivacaine at that point. If bone is encountered instead, inject 10 ml of 0.5% bupivacaine while the needle is withdrawn into the subcutaneous tissue. The dorsal branch of the ulnar nerve is blocked by subcutaneous infiltration of 5 ml of 0.5% bupivacaine along the ulnar border of the wrist from flexor carpi ulnaris to the styloid process of the ulna. Anaesthesia of the palmar branch is likely to last twice as long as that of the dorsal branch.

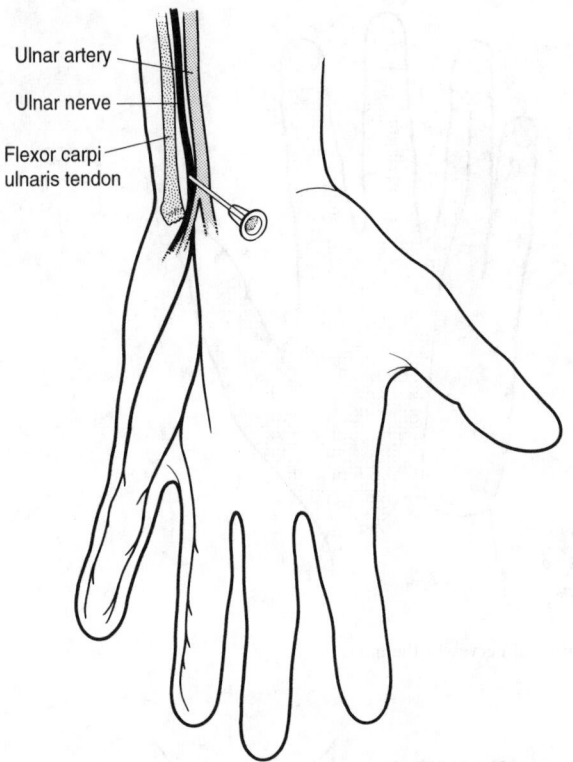

Fig. 6. Ulnar nerve block at wrist.

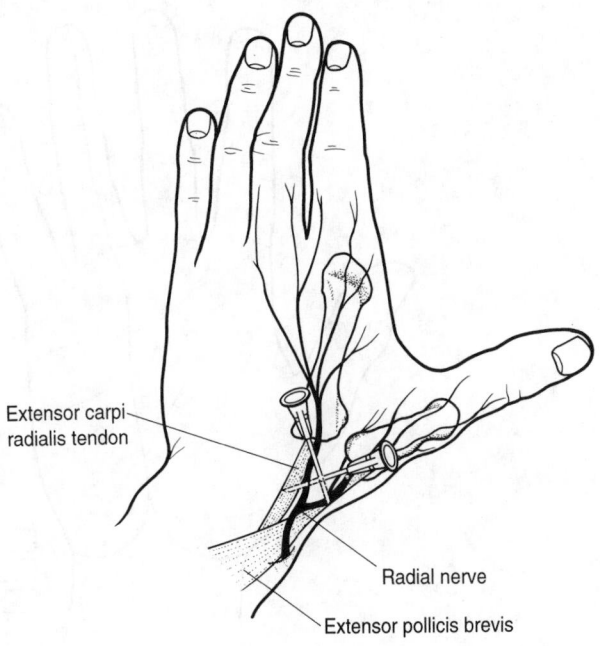

Fig. 7. Radial nerve block.

Radial nerve block

About 7 cm proximal to the wrist the radial nerve passes underneath the tendon of brachioradialis to lie subcutaneously on the extensor aspect of the wrist. Here it divides into several terminal branches to supply the dorsal aspect of the hand.

Indications

● Minor surgery to areas of the hand innervated by the radial nerve.

Technique

Starting at the 'anatomical snuffbox', infiltrate subcutaneously 5–10 ml of 1% lignocaine with adrenaline around the radial border of the wrist from the skin overlying the tendon of extensor carpi radialis to the skin overlying the radial pulse (Fig. 7). This block should last about 1 h.

Femoral nerve block

Femoral nerve block can provide excellent, safe analgesia for patients with fractures of the upper or midfemoral shaft. The femoral nerve lies lateral to the femoral vessels as they pass under the inguinal ligament to enter the thigh. The nerve is outside the fascial sheath which invests the femoral artery and vein.

Indications

● Analgesia for a fractured shaft of femur.
● Analgesia for applying skin traction.
● In combination with block of the lateral cutaneous nerve, for anaesthetizing the donor area before taking skin grafts of the thigh.

Technique

Position the patient supine. The inguinal ligament follows a line between the anterior superior iliac spine and the pubic tubercle. Palpate the femoral artery at the midpoint of the inguinal ligament. Insert a 21G needle 1 cm lateral to the artery and 45° to the skin and advance parallel with the course of the nerve (Fig. 8). A click will be felt as the needle passes through the fascia lata and paraesthesiae are elicited as it touches the femoral nerve. If paraesthesiae are not detected after a depth of 3–4 cm, withdraw the needle and change the direction of insertion either medially or laterally. Once paraesthesiae are obtained, hold the needle still and inject 20 ml of 0.5% bupivacaine or 1% lignocaine with adrenaline. If paraesthesiae are not obtained, inject 20 ml of local anaesthetic fanwise from immediately adjacent to the artery to about 3 cm lateral to it. Onset of analgesia should be within 10 min and will last up to 4 h, depending on the accuracy of the injection and the local anaesthetic used.

Complications

The commonest complication of femoral nerve block is puncture of the femoral artery. If this occurs apply direct pressure for 5 min before reattempting the block.

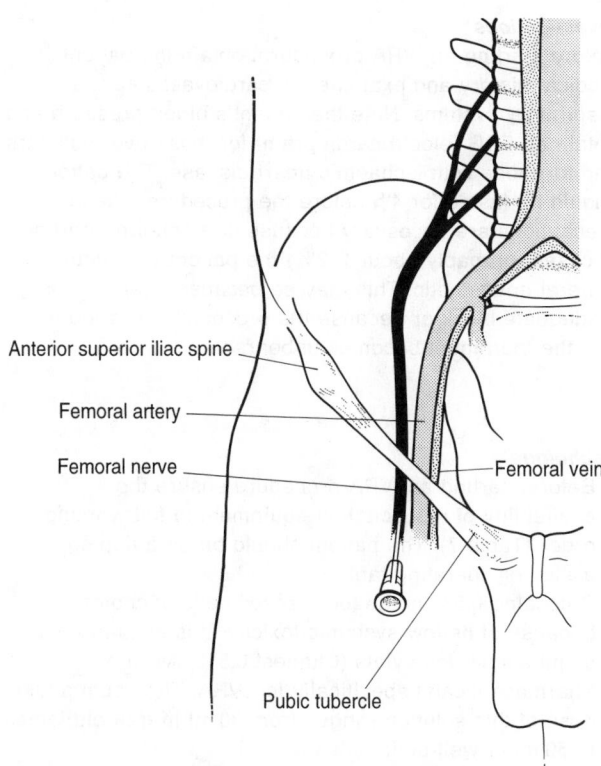

Fig. 8. Femoral nerve block.

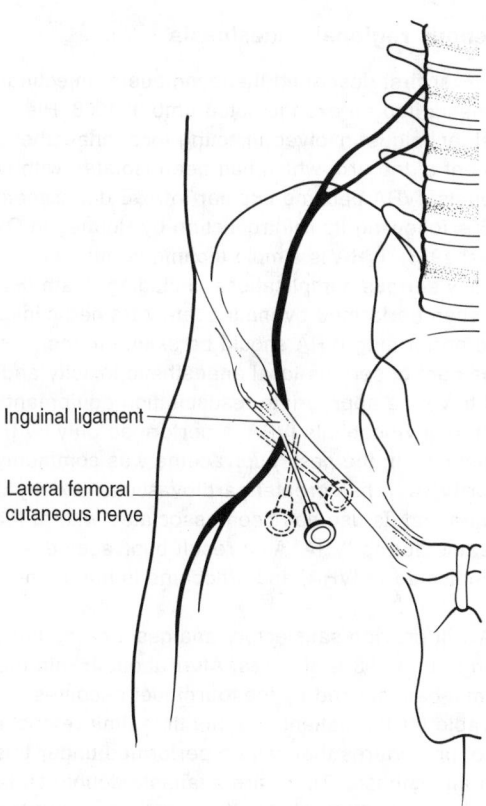

Fig. 9. Lateral cutaneous nerve of thigh block.

Lateral cutaneous nerve of thigh

The lateral cutaneous nerve of the thigh passes behind the inguinal ligament and enters the thigh 1–2 cm medial to the anterior superior iliac spine (Fig. 9). It supplies the skin of the lateral aspect of the thigh.

Indications

• In combination with femoral nerve block for anaesthetizing the donor area before taking skin grafts of the thigh.

Technique

With the patient in the supine position, insert a 23G needle perpendicularly through the skin 1 cm medial and 2 cm below the superior iliac spine. A slight click is felt as the needle pierces the fascia lata, deep to the subcutaneous tissue. Inject 2 ml of 1% lignocaine with adrenaline. Repeat this manoeuvre, slightly laterally and then medially to this point, injecting 2 ml of local anaesthetic on each occasion.

Haematoma block

Although some clinicians favour the use of haematoma blocks as a means of providing analgesia for fracture manipulation, it is not a technique that we can recommend. It is used generally for anaesthetizing Colles' fractures in those accident departments that have difficulty in obtaining anaesthetists to perform intravenous regional anaesthesia (IVRA) (see below). The advantages of haematoma blocks are simplicity and convenience.

The nerves supplying the soft tissue, periosteum and bone around the fracture site are blocked by infiltration of local anaesthetic.

Indications

• Reduction of wrist fractures where IVRA or general anaesthesia is not possible or advisable.

Technique

Use 15–20 ml 1% prilocaine and a 23G needle. Prepare the skin with antiseptic, drape the area and, under aseptic conditions, insert the needle into the fracture haematoma. Confirm the correct position by aspiration of blood and inject the local anaesthetic slowly. Onset of analgesia occurs within 5 min and lasts up to 1 h.

Complications

• This technique converts a closed fracture into one which is technically open. Thus, sepsis is a theoretical risk.
• The analgesia provided by this method is often inadequate and is likely to be completely ineffective in fractures more than 24 h old (the organized haematoma prevents spread of the local anaesthetic).
• Rapid absorption of local anaesthetic from the fracture haematoma or from accidental intravenous injection may cause toxicity.

Intravenous regional anaesthesia

August Bier first described the technique of injecting local anaesthesia into an exanguinated limb in 1908. His original technique involved injecting local anaesthetic into a segment of the arm which had been isolated with two tourniquets. IVRA became popular in A&E departments in the 1960s following its reintroduction by Holmes in Oxford (Holmes, 1963). IVRA is simple technique but has potentially serious complications, including death (Heath, 1982), when performed by inadequately trained clinicians. Anyone performing IVRA should be skilled in the management of serious local anaesthetic toxicity and should have the appropriate resuscitation equipment at hand. In many hospitals IVRA is performed only by trained anaesthetists. In the past, bupivacaine was commonly used for IVRA. It has greater cardiovascular toxicity than prilocaine and its use has been associated with at least four deaths during IVRA. As a result bupivacaine is contraindicated in IVRA, and prilocaine is the agent of choice.

IVRA will provide satisfactory analgesia of the hand and forearm in up to 98% of cases. After about 45 min the ischaemic pain caused by the tourniquet becomes unbearable for the patient and this time limit restricts the range of procedures that can be performed under this form of anaesthesia. There are available double cuffs which are designed to enable the duration of the block to be extended comfortably. The upper cuff is inflated first and the anaesthetic injected. The arm just below this cuff should be anaesthetized, allowing the lower cuff to be inflated about 20 min later without causing discomfort to the patient. The upper cuff is then deflated. Unfortunately, this system does not always reduce the ischaemic pain and there is a risk of accidental release of the wrong cuff with ensuing local anaesthetic toxicity. Therefore, we recommend the simplicity of the single cuff tourniquet.

The mode of action of IVRA is controversial. It is likely that the local anaesthetic acts on the nerve trunks at the elbow where the median, ulnar and radial nerves are close to large veins.

Although IVRA can be used on the arm or the leg, the latter site requires very large volumes of local anaesthetic and is less frequently used.

Indications
- Reduction of fractures below the elbow, in particular Colles' fractures.
- Operations on the hand or forearm.

Contraindications
- Inadequate resuscitation equipment.
- Known hypersensitivity to amide local anaesthetics.
- Procedures expected to exceed 45 min.
- Uncooperative patient.
- Children under age 8 years (will depend on the individual child).
- Sickle cell disease or trait.

Investigations
Before starting an IVRA procedure, obtain the patient's medical history and examine the cardiovascular and respiratory systems. Note the patient's blood pressure and obtain an ECG (electrocardiogram) for those over 60 years and for those with ischaemic heart disease. The patient should be fasted for 4 h before the procedure. These precautions are necessary because in a small proportion of cases (probably about 1–2%) the patient will require a general anaesthetic. This may be because of an inadequate block or because the procedure lasts too long and the tourniquet becomes unbearable.

Technique
- Before starting an IVRA procedure ensure the availability of resuscitation equipment in full working order (Table 7). The patient should be on a tipping trolley or operating table.
- Prilocaine 0.5% is the local anaesthetic of choice because of its low systemic toxicity. It is available in 50-ml single dose vials (Citanest 0.5%; Astra Pharmaceuticals) specifically for IVRA. The usual adult dose of this solution ranges from 30 ml in frail old ladies to 50 ml in well-built males.
- Explain the procedure to the patient.
- Place a small cannula (e.g. 20G) in the hand on the opposite side to the arm to be operated on; this will be used to inject drugs if required during the procedure. Do not use 'butterfly cannulae' – these have a tendency to cut-out the vein.
- Place a similar 20G cannula in the hand of the affected arm.
- Elevate the affected arm for 3 min to assist venous drainage. Exsanguination is enhanced by simultaneously occluding the brachial artery at the elbow. Alternatively, in the absence of a fracture, an Esmarch bandage or Rhys Davies exsanguinator can be used. While elevating the limb an assistant can wrap some wool and the tourniquet around the upper arm.
- Inflate the tourniquet to a pressure 50 mmHg above systolic and note the time.

Table 7. *Resuscitation equipment to be available during procedures performed under sedation or intravenous regional anaesthesia*

- Oxygen
- Bag–valve–mask device
- Defibrillator
- Full range of resuscitation drugs, in particular adrenaline
- Intravenous fluids
- Diazemuls, thiopentone, suxamethonium
- Laryngoscope, tracheal tubes, laryngeal mask

- Lower the arm and inject slowly the appropriate volume of 0.5% prilocaine. Adequate analgesia should be established within 5 min. If not, a further 5–10 ml may be injected.
- Remove the cannula on the affected side before starting the procedure.
- The tourniquet must remain inflated for at least 15 min. After this time, release of the tourniquet will result in less than half of the original dose of local anaesthetic being released into the circulation.
- Immediate reinflation of the tourniquet (within 30 sec) for a further 2 min may reduce the size of the local anaesthetic bolus entering the circulation.
- If adverse reactions are going to occur they are most likely to happen during the first few minutes after tourniquet release. Monitor the patient particularly carefully during this time. The patient should be observed for at least 30 min before being discharged from the hospital.

Modification of the IVRA technique for the foot

The same principles, as described above, apply for IVRA for the foot. The tourniquet should be applied well below the knee to avoid compressing the peroneal nerve on the neck of the fibula.

Complications

Cuff failure accompanied by CNS and cardiovascular toxicity, and rarely death.
- Methaemoglobinaemia, associated with prilocaine in doses of greater than 600 mg.
- Peripheral nerve damage from the tourniquet is very rare, provided that inflation pressures are not excessive, since during IVRA it is rarely inflated for longer than 60 min.

GENERAL ANAESTHESIA IN THE A&E DEPARTMENT

The Association of anaesthetists of Great Britain and Ireland have published a monograph on appropriate standards of anaesthetic care and safety in the A&E department (Association of Anaesthetists of Great Britain and Ireland, 1991).

Indications for general anaesthesia in the A&E department

- General anaesthesia may be induced during the resuscitation of a patient with major injuries.

Under these circumstances, induction of anaesthesia should be undertaken by an experienced anaesthetist. Inappropriate doses of

any of the intravenous anaesthetic agents can cause severe hypotension in hypovolaemic patients.

In combination with intubation and positive pressure ventilation, the airway will be secured and oxygenation and carbon dioxide elimination will be optimized. General anaesthesia provides 'definitive' analgesia.
- Minor, semiurgent procedures may be performed in the A&E department under general anaesthesia. These include reduction of dislocated shoulder, manipulation of minor fractures (e.g. Colles' fracture), incision and drainage of small abscesses (e.g. axillary abscess), exploration for and removal of foreign bodies (e.g. needle in foot), suturing of lacerations.
- Minor but very urgent procedures, such as: reduction of ankle dislocation or reduction of traumatic hip dislocation.

Contraindications to anaesthesia in the A&E department

- Inexperienced anaesthetist.
- Inadequate anaesthetic and resuscitation equipment.
- Inadequate monitoring facilities.
- Inadequate space.
- No suitable anaesthetic assistant (operating department technician or trained anaesthetic nurse).
- Lack of a suitably equipped and staffed area for recovery.
- The patient cannot be supervised at home (assuming he is to be discharged from the department on the same day).
- Patients in poor health (American Society of Anesthesiologists (ASA) categories III, IV, or V; see Table 8), except of course those requiring general anaesthesia as part of resuscitation. For urgent, short procedures, it may be reasonable to anaesthetize an ASA III or IV patient in the A&E department.

Facilities required for general anaesthesia

With the exception of dire emergencies, no anaesthetist should undertake general anaesthesia without adequate assistance from a trained anaesthetic nurse or operating department technician. If suitable assistance is not available in the A&E department, the procedure must be performed in the operating suite.

A 'quick whiff of gas' was a term bandied about in the past; it should now be recognized that patients are

Table 8. *American Society of Anesthesiologists (ASA) classification*

Class[a]	Physical status
I	Normal, healthy
II	Mild systemic disease
III	Severe systemic diseases that limits activity but is not incapacitating
IV	Incapacitating systemic disease that is a constant threat to life
V	Moribund; not expected to survive 24 h with or without an operation

[a] In the event of an emergency operation, precede the class number with an E.

exposed to virtually the same risks whether the anaesthetic is short or whether it is long. Minimum standards of monitoring during general anaesthesia have been published by the Association of Anaesthetists of Great Britain and Ireland (1988). Essential monitoring can be divided into that for the anaesthetic machine and that for the patient. The oxygen supply to the anaesthetic machine should contain a low-pressure warning device and the system should include an oxygen concentration analyser. If mechanical ventilation is to be used, airway pressure and end-tidal carbon dioxide should be monitored. In any case, in our opinion, an end-tidal carbon dioxide monitor should be present in the A&E department for use during resuscitation following cardiac arrest or after major trauma. The patient is monitored, to a large extent, by the clinical observations of the anaesthetist (patient's colour, movements of the reservoir bag, pulse, etc.), but these should be supplemented by continuous ECG and pulse oximetry, and intermittent measurements of arterial pressure. Monitoring should be continued throughout induction, anaesthesia and recovery.

Patient preparation

With the exception of extreme emergencies, a complete patient medical history and appropriate examination should be performed before general anaesthesia, by the A&E doctor. The anaesthetist also should perform a full preoperative assessment. The patient history should include:

- *Past surgical and anaesthetic history* – previous operations, anaesthetic problems.

- *Past medical history* – particularly myocardial infarction, angina, hypertension, stroke, asthma, chronic pulmonary disease, diabetes, epilepsy, family history of anaesthetic problems.
- *Present illness.*
- *General* – exercise tolerance, teeth.
- *Allergies.*
- *Systems review* – detailed cardiovascular and respiratory review, heartburn (risk of regurgitation), allergies.
- *Drugs.*
- *Social history* – following day case general anaesthesia the patient must be supervised at home by a responsible person.

The examination should include:

- *Airway* – restricted mouth opening or neck movement, awkward teeth.
- *Cardiovascular system* – pulse rate, rhythm, blood pressure.
- *Respiratory system.*

Some investigations may be indicated:

- *Haemoglobin estimation* – some anaesthetists will request this on every patient due to undergo general anaesthesia. However, it is probably unnecessary in healthy male patients.
- *Serum electrolytes and urea* – required in patients taking diuretics, antihypertensives, or digoxin, and patients with metabolic disease.
- *Chest X-ray* – this should not be required before general anaesthesia in the A&E department. Preoperative chest X-rays are obtained to assess the chest before major abdominal surgery or in patients with severe cardiovascular or respiratory disease (contraindications to general anaesthesia in the A&E department).
- *ECG* – indicated in all patients over 60 years and in any patient with cardiovascular and/or respiratory disease.

With the exception of emergencies, patients should not have eaten for at least 6 h, or drunk water for 2 h before induction of general anaesthesia. Patients at particular risk of delayed stomach emptying include those injured soon after eating, those who have consumed alcohol, those who are in pain, or those who are frightened (particularly children). The anaesthetist will need to take precautions to prevent pulmonary aspiration of gastric contents for up to 24 h after injury.

In general, anaesthetists prefer not to premedicate patients undergoing day case general anaesthesia.

A suitably equipped area for recovery, staffed by designated, appropriately trained staff, is required. the recovery staff should give any postoperative analgesic prescribed. Before being discharged, the patient or relative should be given written instructions for postoperative care including a telephone contact number at the hospital. The patient should be advised not to drive, operate machines, or consume alcohol for 24 h.

Drugs used during general anaesthesia

The anaesthetist will induce general anaesthesia in a patient with either an intravenous injection (e.g. thiopentone, propofol, etomidate) or, less frequently, by inhalation of a volatile anaesthetic agent (e.g. halothane, enflurane or isoflurane). Inhalational inductions are more frequently used for children or for patients with potentially very difficult airways (e.g. airway burns). Induction of anaesthesia may be supplemented by small doses of intravenous opioids (e.g. fentanyl or alfentanil). General anaesthesia is maintained usually by a combination of a volatile agent carried in a mixture of nitrous oxide and oxygen.

Patients at risk of regurgitation will need their airways secured by tracheal intubation. This is performed usually after the patient has been paralysed by a neuromuscular blocking drug. Under these circumstances, the most commonly used agent is suxamethonium, a drug which produces a depolarizing block within 1 min and wears off in most patients in less than 5 min. Rocuronium, a non-depolarizing neuromuscular blocking drug, is almost as fast in onset but has a duration of approximately 30 min. If the anaesthetist wishes to keep the patient paralysed for more than 5 min (e.g. a head-injured patient en route to the CT (computed tomography) scanner), he has the choice of a number of non-depolarizing neuromuscular blockers which have durations of action of 30–45 min (e.g. vecuronium, rocuronium, atracurium, alcuronium).

Sedation

Indications for sedating a patient in the A&E department may include the manipulation of fractures, reduction of a dislocated shoulder, anxiolysis during other minor surgical procedures such as suturing a laceration. Sedation should be used only by those with suitable training and experience. Remember, there is a fine line between sedation and general anaesthesia and this can easily be crossed accidentally, particularly in elderly patients. Sedated patients with full stomachs are at significant risk of regurgitation and pulmonary aspiration. Ideally, the patient should be starved (2 h for clear fluids and 6 h for solids) before being sedated; if not, ensure minimal sedation only. Full resuscitation equipment must be immediately available (Table 7). Sedated patients can become hypoxic easily and the use of supplementary oxygen and pulse oximetry is strongly recommended (Association of Anaesthetists of Great Britain and Ireland, 1991).

Benzodiazepines are the most commonly use drugs for sedation, although some anaesthetists will use propofol. The latter is a very short-acting, general anaesthetic agent and under no circumstances should this be used by the non-anaesthetist. Benzodiazepines act by stimulating the activity of the inhibitory transmitter gamma-aminobutyric acid (GABA), causing presynaptic inhibition in various areas of the CNS, particularly in the midbrain reticular formation. In addition to sedation, other effects of benzodiazepines on the CNS are anterograde amnesia, anxiolysis and anticonvulsant properties. Large doses of benzodiazepines will obtund laryngeal reflexes and depress respiration. In the elderly this effect is exaggerated and a number of deaths have occurred in this age group from oversedation during endoscopic procedures. As a rough guide the appropriate dose of a benzodiazepine reduces by 10% for each decade of life after 20–30 years old. Benzodiazepines decrease cardiac output and systemic arterial pressure, particularly in the elderly and in hypovolaemic patients. The cardiorespiratory effects of benzodiazepines are exaggerated by the addition of opioids and this combination must be used with great care.

The most commonly used benzodiazepines for intravenous sedation are diazepam and midazolam; recommended sedation doses are given in Table 9. Diazepam is available as an emulsion of 10 mg in 2 ml lipid

Table 9. *Pharmacological data for diazepam and midazolam*

	Dose (mg kg^{-1})	Onset^a (min)	Half-life (h)	Concentration (mg ml^{-1})
Diazepam	0.15–0.2	1–2	36	5
Midazolam	0.03–0.1	<1	2	2 or 5

^{a} After intravenous bolus.

(Diazemuls); this preparation is ideal for intravenous sedation and has an onset time of 1–2 min after intravenous bolus. Midazolam has a faster onset time and much shorter elimination half-life than diazepam though the latter makes minimal difference to the recovery time after a single dose. Midazolam is approximately twice as potent as diazepam and is relatively even more potent in the elderly. Unfortunately, midazolam is available in the same concentration as Diazemuls (10 mg in 2 ml) and this tends to lead to relative overdosage by the inexperienced. Although midazolam is available also as 10 mg in 5 ml, we recommend routinely diluting midazolam with saline to $1\,mg\,ml^{-1}$, thus making accurate titration easier. When using benzodiazepines for intravenous sedation, always titrate slowly, carefully watching the effect on the patient. In the elderly, for example, it is appropriate to give midazolam in 1 mg increments waiting 3–4 min after each.

Flumazenil is a specific benzodiazepine antagonist with a half-life of 45 min. An accidental overdose of benzodiazepine during attempted sedation can be reversed immediately by giving up to 0.5 mg (given in up to three increments: 0.1 mg, 0.2 mg, 0.2 mg). The duration of action of flumazenil may be significantly less than that of the benzodiazepine, resulting in resedation. For this reason, we do not recommend using flumazenil routinely to expedite a patient's discharge from the A&E department after intravenous sedation.

RELATIONSHIP BETWEEN ANAESTHETIC AND A&E DEPARTMENTS

In any hospital there should be, and generally are, strong cooperative links between the anaesthetic and A&E departments. Although this is true for the UK, in the USA emergency physicians rarely call for assistance from anaesthetists except for very complex airway problems. In the operating theatres, anaesthetists manage airways, ventilation, and venous and arterial access many times each day, so it would seem sensible to make use of these skills in the A&E department. Anaesthetists and A&E physicians share many similarities (Oakley, 1993). Both deal with a wide spectrum of critically ill patients, use invasive techniques, and tend to deal with patients in the short term only, leaving long-term follow-up to other physicians.

In each hospital one consultant anaesthetist should be responsible for coordinating anaesthetic services in the A&E department (Association of Anaesthetists of Great Britain and Ireland, 1991). This person's role is to:

- Liaise with the A&E consultant and other staff.
- Liaise with other members of the department of anaesthesia to ensure that equipment is compatible with those areas such as the intensive therapy unit, high-dependency units and operating theatres.
- Direct anaesthetic services both inside and outside the hospital.
- Be involved with major accident plans and responses.
- Organize training for trainee anaesthetic and other medical staff, nurses, paramedics and others in the A&E department.

Thus, anaesthetists play an important role in the training of A&E medical and nursing staff and provide patient resuscitation and pain relief in conjunction with their A&E colleagues, in addition to giving a regional local and general anaesthesia service. They may also become involved in integrated research studies and audit programmes.

Bibliography

ASSOCIATION OF ANAESTHETISTS OF GREAT BRITAIN AND IRELAND (1988). *Recommendations for Standards of Monitoring During Anaesthesia and Recovery.* London: Association of Anaesthetists of Great Britain and Ireland.

ASSOCIATION OF ANAESTHETISTS OF GREAT BRITAIN AND IRELAND (1991). *The Role of the Anaesthetist in the Emergency Service.* London: Association of Anaesthetists of Great Britain and Ireland.

BASKETT, P.J.F. (1972). Use of Entonox in the ambulance service. *Proc. R. Soc. Med.,* **65**, 7–8.

BASKETT, P.J.F. & BENNETT, J.A. (1971). Pain relief in hospital: the more widespread use of nitrous oxide. *Br. Med. J.,* **2**, 509–11.

CONSUMERS' ASSOCIATION (1990). More topical NSAIDs: worth the rub? *Drug Ther. Bull.,* **28**, 27–8.

CONSUMERS' ASSOCIATION (1991). Diclofenac gel – topical NSAIDs and science. *Drug Ther. Bull.,* **29**, 95–6.

HEATH, M. (1982). Deaths after intravenous regional anaesthesia. *Br. Med. J.,* **288**, 913–14.

HOLMES, C.M. (1963). Intravenous regional analgesia. *Lancet,* **i**, 245–6.

JOWITT, M.D. (1993). Falkland campaign. In *Textbook of Trauma Anesthesia and Critical Care,* ed. C.M. Grande, pp. 1310–18. St Louis: Mosby-Year Book.

KENNY, G.N.C. (1990). Ketorolac trometamol: a new non-opioid analgesic (Editorial). *Br. J. Anaesth.,* **65**, 445–7.

MINNIT, R.J. (1934). Self-administered anaesthesia in childbirth. *Br. Med. J.,* **1**, 501.

OAKLEY, P.A. (1993). Interface of anesthesiology and emergency medicine in trauma management. In *Textbook of Trauma Anesthesia and Critical Care*, ed. C.M. Grande, pp. 106–19. St Louis: Mosby-Year Book.

PARKE, T.J., NANDI, P.R., BIRD, K.J. et al. (1992). Profound hypotension following IV codeine phosphate. *Anaesthesia*, **47**, 852–4.

POWER, I., NOBLE, D.W., DOUGLAS, E. et al. (1990). Comparison of IM ketorolac trometamol and morphine sulphate for pain relief after cholecystectomy. *Br. J. Anaesth.*, **65**, 448–55.

RADY, M.Y., LITTLE, R.A., EDWARDS, J.D. et al. (1991). The effect of nociceptive stimulation on the changes in haemodynamic and oxygen transport induced by haemorrhage in anesthetized pigs. *J. Trauma*, **31**, 617–21.

STENE, J.K. (1992). Analgesics in emergency medicine. In *Emergency Medicine and the Anaesthetist*, ed. H.H. Delooz, pp. 107–17. London: Baillière Tindall.

STEWART, R.D., PARIS, P.M., STOY, W.A. et al. (1983). Patient-controlled inhalational analgesia in prehospital care: a study of side-effects and feasibility. *Crit. Care Med.*, **11**, 851–5.

THAL, E.R., MONTGOMERY, S.J., ATKINS, J.M. et al. (1979). Self-administered analgesia with nitrous oxide. Adjunctive aid for emergency medical care systems. *JAMA*, **242**, 2418–19.

Further reading

PARK, G. & FULTON, B. (1991). *The Management of Acute Pain*. Oxford: Oxford University Press.

11 Poisoning

J.A. HENRY

Medical Toxicology Unit, Guy's Hospital, London, UK

Chapter plan

Introduction
Aetiology of poisoning
Diagnosis and assessment
Pathophysiology and mechanisms of poisoning
Management principles
Antidotes
Agents responsible for poisoning
Cardiopulmonary resuscitation in poisoning
Contacting and using poisons centres
Appendix: National Poisons Information Service – UK

INTRODUCTION

Acute poisoning is common and accounts for approximately 3% of accident and emergency (A & E) attendances and up to 10% of acute medical admissions. The most important thing to remember is that the great majority of poisoned patients will make a full recovery provided they receive adequate supportive care. Only a small proportion will require specialized investigations and treatments. Commonsense application of the basic principles of care is thus of great importance, but it is also essential to be aware of poisons and circumstances which require particular knowledge in diagnosis and management. This chapter highlights the general principles of management and covers the main causes and types of poisoning. The psychiatric aspects of deliberate self-harm are dealt with in Chapter 55. Further information on toxicity and management may be obtained from poisons centres, which may also be able to provide analytical support or supply specialized antidotes.

AETIOLOGY OF POISONING

There are many different causes of poisoning (Table 1) and the risks and management may each vary according to the aetiology.

Before birth

Many drugs, including alcohol, are teratogenic but this does not result in acute medical presentation. There is little evidence that drug overdose during pregnancy causes damage to the fetus, and the management is no

Table 1. *Common causes of poisoning at different ages*

Before birth
- Teratogenic drugs, smoking and alcohol
- Drug overdose during pregnancy

Neonatal period
- Iatrogenic overdose

Infants
- Accidental
- Non-accidental

Children
- Volatile substance abuse
- Alcohol
- Drug overdose

Adults
- Deliberate self-harm
- Accidental
- Effects of illicit drug use
- Iatrogenic (prescribed and alternative medication)
- Homicidal

different from that of overdose in non-pregnant women. The use of antidotes such as acetylcysteine (Riggs *et al.*, 1989) or desferrioxamine (McElhatton *et al.*, 1991) should not be withheld because the patient is pregnant.

Neonates

During the neonatal period, particularly in premature infants, there is a risk of iatrogenic overdose because of the poor metabolic and excretory capacity relative to body weight. However, the commonest cause of serious toxicity is dosage error (most often ten times the dose). Particular care should be taken with drugs such as theophylline, digoxin, chloramphenicol and morphine.

Infants

The commonest cause of poisoning between the ages of 1 and 4 years is accidental poisoning, associated with the natural exploratory activities of children at this stage of life. Each year this results in 20 000 admissions to hospitals in Britain, but only about ten fatalities. The commonest agents involved are paracetamol and oral contraceptives, but most fatalities occur from tricyclic antidepressants, salicylates, iron, opioids and quinine.

Another cause of poisoning in this age group is non-accidental injury, which is usually inflicted by a carer such as the mother. The child may present with repeated episodes of floppiness and collapse depending on the substance, which is most commonly a drug prescribed for the mother.

Childhood

During childhood, volatile substance abuse ('glue sniffing') can cause serious problems. There are about 150 deaths each year in Britain from this cause (Anderson, 1990). Acute and chronic alcohol toxicity are often underestimated in this age group. Intentional drug overdose is common but suicide is rare.

Adult life

In early adult life, particularly in females, drug overdose in the form of parasuicidal gestures is common. Fatalities are uncommon. In later adult life, suicidal intent is commoner and parasuicidal gestures are less frequent. The commonest causes of suicidal poisoning in England are carbon monoxide, analgesic drugs and tricyclic antidepressants. Male suicides outnumber female suicides by

about 3:1. Drug abuse is an increasing cause of medical complications in young adults. Accidental poisoning in adults is usually domestic, where the commonest agent is carbon monoxide, or industrial, where a wide range of chemicals may be involved. Homicidal poisoning, though rare, may go undetected if it is not suspected; the emergency team should take close note of suspicious inconsistencies.

DIAGNOSIS AND ASSESSMENT

Most poisoned patients are awake, cooperative, and able to provide a reasonable history. Some publications indicate that the history is highly unreliable, but this is not generally true. Only rarely does the poisoned patient consciously provide a misleading history. If the patient is unconscious or unable to give the history and poisoning is a possibility, a rapid working diagnosis must be made and treatment urgently provided (Figure 1). Resuscitation will be required for a cardiorespiratory arrest or severe shock and medical assistance should be called if necessary. An intravenous line must be established and endotracheal intubation may be needed. Witnesses, family members, friends and ambulance personnel should be detained and questioned concerning the time and details of exposure, the probable agents involved and the progression of symptoms. The first priorities in examination are to make a rapid cardiovascular, respiratory and neurological assessment (Olson *et al.*, 1987).

Respiratory assessment

A patent airway is the first priority. The next consideration is whether the patient requires mechanical ventilation. The patient's colour, depth of coma and the pattern and depth of respiration should be carefully noted. If there is any doubt, the minute volume should be measured, and if it is less than 4 litres min^{-1} in an adult, intubation and ventilation are likely to be required. Arterial blood gases should also be measured in the very ill patient; a $PaCO_2$ of over 6.5 kPa usually means that mechanical ventilation will be needed; an anaesthetist should be consulted without delay. Auscultation of the lungs may reveal localized crackles following aspiration of vomit or signs of pulmonary oedema or bronchospasm.

Cardiovascular assessment

The patient's cardiovascular status should be assessed. Pulse rate and blood pressure should be noted and the

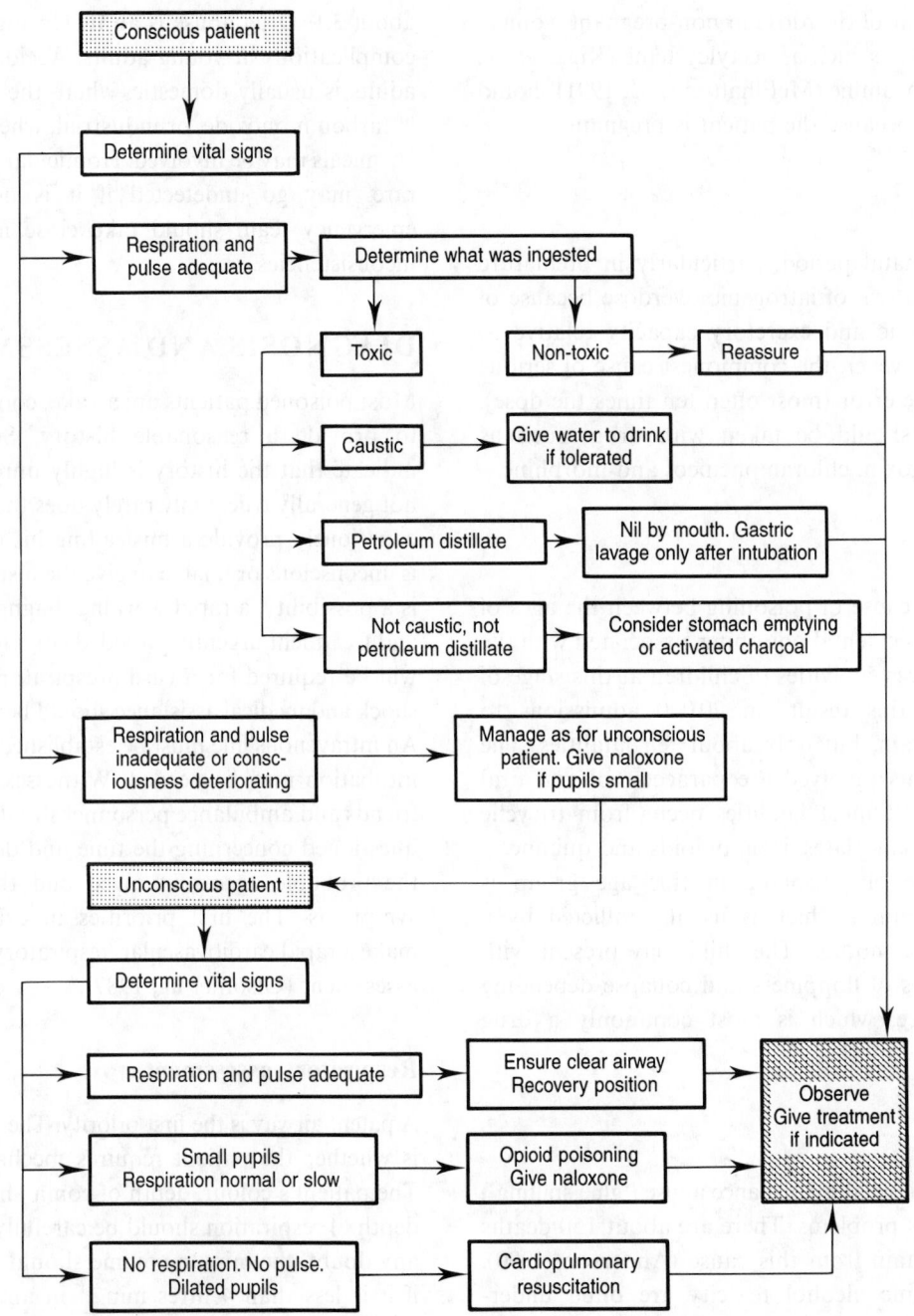

Fig. 1. Immediate management.

central venous pressure should be measured if the patient is hypotensive.

Neurological assessment

Neurological complications of poisoning include hallucinations, depressed conscious level, seizures, cerebral oedema and peripheral nerve injuries resulting from prolonged pressure in the comatose patient. The conscious level should be observed and recorded using a coma grading such as the Glasgow Scale. The size and the reaction of the pupils should be noted. Causes of changes in pupil size are given in Table 2. Convulsions are most commonly due to hypoxia but may also be due to the effect of the poison on the central nervous system (CNS).

Table 2. *Clinical signs in the poisoned patient*

System	Symptom	Possible cause
Gastrointestinal	VOMITING	Many causes
	HAEMATEMESIS	Corrosives Iron Salicylate Theophylline
	DIARRHOEA	*Amanita phalloides* Carbamates Food poisoning Opioid withdrawal Organophosphates
	SALIVATION, DYSPHAGIA, ABDOMINAL PAIN	Caustics Corrosives
Cardiovascular	TACHYCARDIA	Amphetamines Anticholinergic agents Cocaine Sympathomimetics Theophylline Tricyclic antidepressants
	BRADYCARDIA	Beta-blocking drugs Calcium channel blockers Carbamates Digoxin Organophosphates
	HYPOTENSION	Antihypertensive drugs All drugs under coma (see below)
Neurological	COMA	Alcohols Anticonvulsants Antidepressants Sedative and hypnotic drugs Opioids Solvent abuse Tricyclic antidepressants
	CONVULSIONS	Antihistamines Carbamazepine Carbon monoxide Cyanide Hypoglycaemic agents Isoniazid Lead Lithium Mefenamic acid Phenothiazines Theophylline Tricyclic antidepressants

Table 2. *Continued*

System	Symptom	Possible cause
	DYSTONIC SPASMS	Metoclopramide
		Phenothiazines
	HALLUCINATIONS, AGITATION	Amphetamines
		Antidepressants
		Antihistamines
		Atropine
		Drug withdrawal
		LSD
		Phenothiazines
		Psilocybe mushrooms (magic mushrooms)
	AGITATION, HYPER-REFLEXIA	Amphetamines (inc. MDMA)
	PYREXIA	Anticholinergic agents
		Amphetamines (inc. MDMA)
		Cocaine
		Monoamine oxidase inhibitors
		Phencyclidine
		Tricyclic antidepressants
	PUPILS: DILATED	Amphetamines
		Antihistamines
		Atropine
		Botulism
		Cocaine
		Glutethimide
		Hypothermia
		Hypoxia
		Hypoglycaemia
		LSD
		Psilocybe mushrooms (magic mushrooms)
		Sympathomimetics
		Tricyclic antidepressants
	PUPILS: CONSTRICTED	Carbamates
		Opioids (including Lomotil)
		Organophosphates
	BLINDNESS	Methanol
		Quinine
Metabolic	METABOLIC ACIDOSIS	Ethanol
		Ethylene glycol
		Iron
		Isoniazid
		Methanol
		Salicylates
		Tricyclic antidepressants

(*continued*)

Table 2. *Continued*

System	Symptom	Possible cause
	HYPOGLYCAEMIA	Ethanol
		Insulin
		Oral hypoglycaemic agents
		Paracetamol
		Salicylates
	RENAL FAILURE	Essential oils
		Ethylene glycol
		Inorganic mercurials
		Paracetamol
		Paraquat
		Phenols
		Salicylates (children)
	HEPATIC FAILURE	*Amanita phalloides*
		Chlorinated hydrocarbons
		Paracetamol

History

A detailed history should be taken from the patient or if necessary from others who may be able to provide bottles, tablets, syringes, plant material, suicide note or other evidence. In childhood poisoning it is often difficult to know whether the patient has ingested the suspected substance or not.

Major points for history-taking in poisoning

- Poison(s) involved or suspected
- Time of exposure and duration of exposure
- Mode of exposure: oral, intravenous, inhaled
- Has there been any contact with skin or eyes?
- Has the patient vomited or had any other symptoms?
- Has the patient taken alcohol?
- Past medical history and current drug treatment

Further examination

A full physical examination should be completed. The body temperature should be measured accurately. In all unconcious patients, the rectal temperature should be taken with a low-reading thermometer. The mouth and skin should be inspected for corrosive burns or coloured stains in the mouth, blisters, injection marks, or other evidence of poisoning or drug abuse. The smell of the breath may be characteristic for solvents, ketones, and other substances. A smell of alcohol gives no guidance to the concentration in the blood. Any vomit produced should be inspected for tablet residues or other evidence of ingestion. A chest X-ray and an electrocardiogram (ECG) should be obtained in severely poisoned patients.

Laboratory analyses

Blood should be taken for haematological examination, measurement of urea, electrolytes and glucose, and also for toxicological analyses. In unconscious patients, plasma paracetamol and salicylate should be measured in case of ingestion. Further toxicological analyses may be necessary. Some of these may be obtained from the local pathology laboratory while others may have to be obtained through a specialized poisons laboratory. It is customary to save 10 ml of heparinized blood, 20 ml of vomit or gastric aspirate, and 20 ml of the first sample of urine passed so that they are available later if required for diagnostic, scientific or medicolegal purposes. Whole blood should be taken into an EDTA (ethylenediaminetetraacetic acid) tube for carboxyhaemoglobin (carbon monoxide), methaemoglobin, and metals such as lead and mercury. A fluoride tube should be used for glucose, alcohol, formate and cocaine.

Diagnosis

The history, examination and laboratory investigations as above should enable an accurate diagnosis as to the substance and severity. However, the diagnosis is not always apparent because the patient's state could be due to another illness, or because the poison is unusual or the features are atypical. There are several syndromes which are typical of poisoning. Certain biochemical changes such as a metabolic acidosis are characteristically caused by poisons; these are reviewed in Chapter 7. Major disasters may be complicated by release of a toxin; see Chapter 13. When there is difficulty in making a diagnosis, a poisons centre should be consulted (see Appendix).

PATHOLOGY AND MECHANISMS OF POISONING

Most acute poisonings which require immediate attention involve disruption of the oxygen pathway from the inspired air to cellular respiration. A reduction in the oxygen content of the inspired air may cause acute hypoxia producing collapse and coma. Interference with the mechanics of respiration by poisons may result in hypoxia and hypercapnia. Disturbance of oxygen transfer may produce hypoxaemia. Even if the oxygen content of the air is not diminished and respiration is functioning adequately, disturbances to other processes may prevent oxygen reaching its intracellular site of action. The oxygen-carrying capacity of the blood may be reduced by the presence of carboxyhaemoglobin or methaemoglobin, or more rarely by acute haemolysis. Cardiac output may be reduced by a number of poisons which cause cardiac arrhythmias, depress the contractility of the heart or cause extreme vasodilation. The final step where poisons may interfere with the oxygen pathway is blockage of the cytochrome enzyme chain by toxins such as cyanide and hydrogen sulphide. These effects and the main poisons involved are outlined in Fig. 2. Understanding of this pathway is essential for the intelligent resuscitation of the acutely poisoned patient and is useful for teaching trainees at all levels.

Many types of poisoning involve a highly specific interaction between a toxin and a particular receptor or tissue. Examples include paracetamol, cholinesterase inhibitors and cardiac glycosides. In other instances, the type of toxicity may be less clearly definable. The acute effects of ethanol are due to a central nervous depressant effect. The tricyclic antidepressants, many volatile sub-stances, some beta-adrenergic blocking drugs and dextro-propoxyphene can produce cardiotoxicity due to a quinidine-like effect; the precise mechanism may be an effect on sodium channels. This produces cardiac depression and cardiac arrhythmias (Figure 3).

MANAGEMENT PRINCIPLES

The most important aspect of management is to provide adequate supportive care, in order to prevent complications. Resuscitation should be prompt and effective, as described at the end of this chapter and in Chapter 3. The comatose patient should be managed as in Chapter 9; specific causes of coma are dealt with later in this chapter.

Preventing intestinal absorption

All of the methods used in preventing absorption of ingested poisons have limited effectiveness, and the topic is controversial (Wheeler-Usher et al., 1986). Five methods of gastrointestinal decontamination can be considered

- Emesis.
- Gastric aspiration and lavage.
- Administration of activated charcoal.
- Catharsis.
- Whole bowel irrigation.

Emesis

Only two methods of inducing emesis deserve consideration. All other methods, including saline emesis, are now considered outdated, useless and possibly harmful. Stimulation of the pharynx can be used out of hospital but is not very effective in inducing vomiting. Syrup of ipecacuanha is an emetic which acts locally by irritation of the gastric mucosa and centrally by stimulation of the chemoreceptor trigger zone. It has long been used almost routinely in the management of ingested poisons but is now viewed much more critically. Although it is undoubtedly effective in inducing emesis within 30 min in over 90% of cases, there is little evidence that it effectively empties the stomach of its contents or reduces the severity of poisoning (Saetta & Quinton, 1991). Its use is therefore no longer recommended apart from special circumstances such as a recent potentially severe ingestion of a sustained release preparation or of plant material. There is no place for its 'routine' use in adults or children. The doses and contraindications are given in

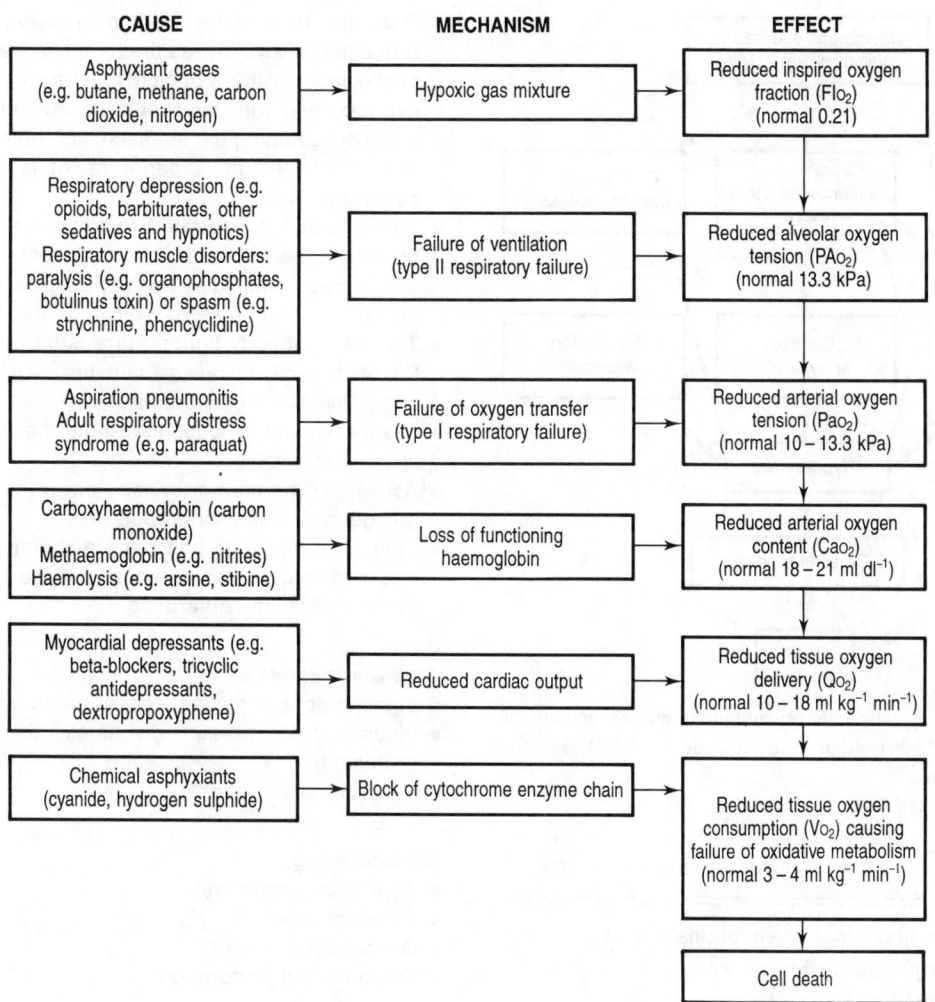

CAUSE	MECHANISM	EFFECT
Asphyxiant gases (e.g. butane, methane, carbon dioxide, nitrogen)	Hypoxic gas mixture	Reduced inspired oxygen fraction (FIo$_2$) (normal 0.21)
Respiratory depression (e.g. opioids, barbiturates, other sedatives and hypnotics) Respiratory muscle disorders: paralysis (e.g. organophosphates, botulinus toxin) or spasm (e.g. strychnine, phencyclidine)	Failure of ventilation (type II respiratory failure)	Reduced alveolar oxygen tension (PAo$_2$) (normal 13.3 kPa)
Aspiration pneumonitis Adult respiratory distress syndrome (e.g. paraquat)	Failure of oxygen transfer (type I respiratory failure)	Reduced arterial oxygen tension (Pao$_2$) (normal 10 – 13.3 kPa)
Carboxyhaemoglobin (carbon monoxide) Methaemoglobin (e.g. nitrites) Haemolysis (e.g. arsine, stibine)	Loss of functioning haemoglobin	Reduced arterial oxygen content (Cao$_2$) (normal 18 – 21 ml dl^{-1})
Myocardial depressants (e.g. beta-blockers, tricyclic antidepressants, dextropropoxyphene)	Reduced cardiac output	Reduced tissue oxygen delivery (Qo$_2$) (normal 10 – 18 ml kg^{-1} min^{-1})
Chemical asphyxiants (cyanide, hydrogen sulphide)	Block of cytochrome enzyme chain	Reduced tissue oxygen consumption (Vo$_2$) causing failure of oxidative metabolism (normal 3 – 4 ml kg^{-1} min^{-1})
		Cell death

Fig. 2. Scheme showing some major causes of blockade of the oxygen pathway due to poisoning, with mechanisms and typical values.

Table 3. The delay in production of emesis (usually 20–30 mins) is a major disadvantage. It is contraindicated if deterioration of consciousness is anticipated; other contraindication are given in Table 3.

Gastric aspiration and lavage

If there is evidence that the patient has ingested a potentially toxic amount of a drug or poison, there is a body of opinion that it is useful to empty the stomach by gastric lavage. Gastric aspiration and lavage should only be used when there is a clearly thought-out rationale in each case. It should never be performed on a routine basis or for 'medicolegal' reasons or as a deterrent. It may be of benefit in adults presenting within 2 h of ingestion or 12 h in the case of salicylates, carbamazepine or tricyclic antidepressants, or at any time in the unconscious patient. If the patient is comatose, has swallowed petroleum distillate or the gag reflex is absent, gastric lavage can only be carried out after endotracheal intubation. Consent can be assumed in the unconscious patient.

TECHNIQUE

Method of gastric aspiration and lavage

Procedure
- The procedure should be explained carefully to the patient and consent obtained. Consent should be assumed in the unconscious patient.
- A large-diameter stomach tube should be chosen ensuring that the hole size is adequate for insoluble or sustained-release preparations or for large recent ingestions of tablets or capsules. The end of the tube may be lubricated with water-soluble jelly.

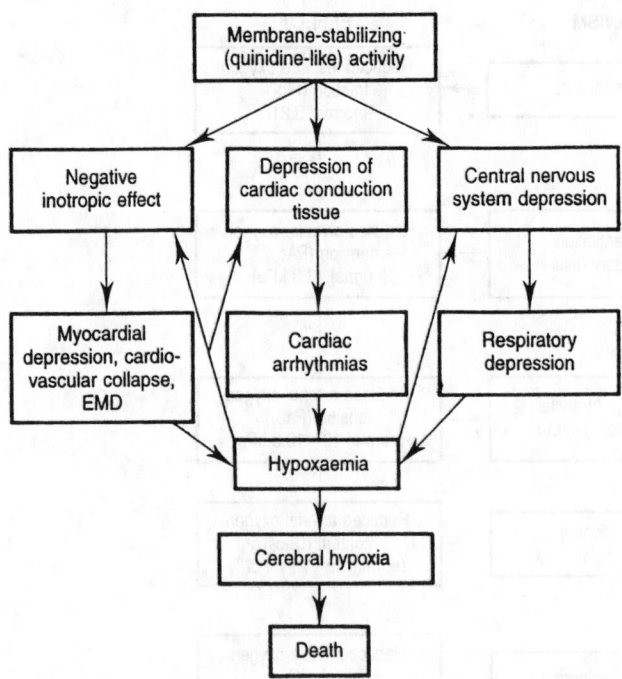

Fig. 3. Mechanisms by which the membrane-stabilizing activity of antidepressants and other drugs can cause death. EMD, electro-mechanical dissociation.

Table 3. *Guidelines for syrup of ipecacuanha administration*

- Ipecacuanha should never be given routinely; it is only rarely required in clearly defined circumstances
- Contraindications
  - Age under six months
  - Late pregnancy
  - Severe cardiac or respiratory disease
  - Cardiac dysrhythmias
  - Shock
  - Corrosive ingestions
  - Petroleum distillate ingestions
  - Depressed level of consciousness
- Dosage regime
  - Children 6–8 months: 10 ml
  - Children over 18 months: 15 ml
  - Adults: 30 ml
  - Given with water or fruit juice
  - Repeat the dose once if no result within 30 min

- If the patient has an impaired gag reflex or is unconscious, the airway should be protected by passing a cuffed endotracheal tube.
- The patient should be lying on the left side, tilted so that the head is higher than the body. The orogastric route is preferable.

- Once the tube is inserted the patient (if conscious) is requested to swallow as the tube is advanced. Placement of the tube in the stomach must be confirmed. A 50 ml syringe filled with air should be emptied down the tube while auscultating the stomach; aspiration of the fluid and testing it with litmus paper (acid) is a further way of confirming this.
- The stomach is aspirated to remove any contents. Part of this is saved in a universal container for possible toxicological analysis. The aspirate should be inspected for tablets, plant material, etc.
- Tap water at body temperature is introduced: 50 ml kg^{-1} for each cycle of lavage can be used for children and about 200–400 ml for adults.
- Lavage should be continued until the fluid returns clear for several cycles.
- Activated charcoal may be left in the stomach after lavage has been carried out.
- Epigastric massage has been recommended to enhance return of particulate poisons, but there is no evidence that it makes any difference.

Contraindications
- Ingestion of corrosives (concentrated acid or alkalis).
- Ingestion of petroleum distillates (unless the airway is protected).
- Uncooperative patient.

Complications
- Aspiration pneumonitis.
- Laryngospasm.
- Oesophageal spasm.
- Oesophageal perforation.

Major problems with gastric lavage include incomplete removal of toxins (Saetta & Quinton, 1991) and the possibility of washing ingested poisons further down the gut (Saetta *et al.*, 1991). Complications include laryngospasm, cyanosis and arrhythmias during intubation and lavage, aspiration pneumonia, intestinal perforation and water intoxication.

Uses of laxatives and cathartics

Laxatives and cathartics reduce the intestinal transit time. Substances used include lactulose, mannitol, sorbitol, magnesium sulphate and magnesium hydroxide. There is no evidence that they reduce toxicity following ingestion of overdoses of slowly absorbed drugs or sustained release formulations. They are therefore not recommended for use alone but may have a place in conjunction with repeated doses of activated charcoal. Their use must be set against the risk of excessive diarrhoea leading to volume depletion, hypotension and electrolyte disturbances. The main contraindications are extremes of age, caustic ingestions and disorders of bowel motility (Shannon et al., 1986).

Whole bowel irrigation

Whole bowel irrigation is induced following ingestion of potentially toxic substances which are not adsorbed by activated charcoal (iron, lithium salts, packets of illicit drugs, large doses of sustained-release preparations and possibly after some heavy metal ingestions) (Tenenbein, 1988). Because it is isosmotic, the solution is safely used for drug and other ingestions which have passed through the pylorus. The technique is incompatible with the use of multiple dose activated charcoal and it should not be used after syrup of ipecacuanha has been given. The fluid is usually administered through a nasogastric tube at the rate of 2 litres h^{-1} in adults (25 ml kg^{-1} h^{-1} in children). The end-point is the passage of clear rectal effluent (usually 4–6 h) or when tablets or packages cease to be passed. In the case of iron tablet ingestion, clearance can be checked by X-ray.

Activated charcoal

Activated charcoal is fine, granular, heat-treated charcoal with a very large surface area for non-specific adsorption of drugs and chemicals. It is the most effective and least traumatic method of managing ingested poisons (Kulig et al., 1985). The accepted charcoal/poison weight ratio of 10:1 is a useful guide to the dose required. Its main use in A&E medicine is as a single dose given as soon as possible after potentially toxic ingestion. Effectiveness is greatest up to 1 h and may be less after this as absorption of the poison occurs. Activated charcoal can be given after gastric lavage or after emesis. Substances not effectively adsorbed by activated charcoal include acids, alkalis, cyanide, iron, ethanol, methanol, ethylene glycol and lithium salts.

Repeated doses of activated charcoal are sometimes used to create a concentration gradient across the gut. Absorbed drugs may then diffuse back into the gut to be adsorbed by the charcoal. This process may be effective in drugs that have small volumes of distribution such as salicylates, barbiturates and theophylline. Repeated doses of charcoal may also be indicated for sustained-release or enteric coated preparations.

Complications of this technique include vomiting and constipation. Ileus, intestinal obstruction and pulmonary aspiration have been reported rarely. Activated charcoal turns the stools black so the patient or parents should be warned that this may occur. The main contraindications to activated charcoal are emetics (such as ipecacuanha) or oral antidotes (such as methionine) which may be adsorbed and rendered ineffective.

Because it has been demonstrated as effective and very safe, activated charcoal is gaining increasing acceptance as a first line treatment for the management of ingested poisons (Palatnick & Tenenbein, 1992; Vale & Proudfoot, 1993).

Skin and eye decontamination

The skin or the eyes may be the major area exposed, or part of more general contamination. These problems are dealt with in detail in Chapter 21.

Promoting excretion

There are few indications now for increasing the excretion of poisons. The most important is salicylate poisoning where urine alkalinization is used in mild to moderate poisoning and haemodialysis is indicated in severe poisoning. Acidification of the urine is recommended for enhancing excretion of phenoxyacetates (Flanagan et al., 1990) in cases of severe poisoning. Charcoal haemoperfusion is rarely required but may be indicated in severe calcium antagonist or theophylline poisoning. The methods and indications for promoting elimination of poisons are summarized in Table 4.

ANTIDOTES

Only a relatively small number of antidotes can be considered of immediate use in A&E departments. These are listed in Table 5.

AGENTS RESPONSIBLE FOR POISONING

Gaseous agents

The history may indicate that the victim has been exposed to toxic gases, fumes, smoke or vapour. When this is suspected, 100% oxygen should be administered while blood is assayed for carbon monoxide and other possible agents, as well as arterial gases, haematology and blood chemistry. It is important to establish the

Table 4. *Enhancing elimination*

Urinary alkalinization	Salicylate
Urinary acidification	Amphetamines Phencyclidine Phenoxyacetates
Haemodialysis (peritoneal dialysis is two to three times less efficient)	Barbiturates Ethylene glycol Lithium Methanol Salicylates
Charcoal haemoperfusion	Theophylline
Repeat dose activated charcoal	Barbiturates Carbamazepine Quinine Salicylates Sustained-release preparations Theophylline
Whole bowel irrigation	Drug packets Iron Lithium Sustained-release preparations

causative agent as soon as possible, as treatments differ. Poisoning by carbon monoxide and cyanide should be treated as described below.

Carbon monoxide

Carbon monoxide exposure produces cerebral hypoxia secondary to its reversible combination with haemoglobin to form carboxyhaemoglobin and with cytochrome enzymes in cell walls. Symptoms are poorly related to the blood carboxyhaemoglobin concentration and depend also on the duration of exposure, time since exposure and the treatment given. Lethargy, throbbing headache, vomiting without diarrhoea, mental slowness and hyperventilation are typical in the early stages and these may progress to convulsions, coma, hypoventilation, bradycardia and cardiovascular collapse. Where there is a history of exposure the diagnosis presents little difficulty, but in many cases the diagnosis may not be apparent and the possibility of carbon monoxide poisoning should be borne in mind, especially when several people are affected with headache, vomiting and collapse. Symptoms are

often minimal or mild even after severe exposure; the patient may speak slowly with a monotonous voice and have impaired cerebellar signs but no other evidence of neurological damage. In the elderly, carbon monoxide toxicity may present as a cerebrovascular accident or as myocardial infarction. The source of exposure is usually inhalation of products of combustion. In domestic incidents there may be a faulty appliance or a blocked flue (Crawford *et al.*, 1990). Motor exhaust gas inhalation is the cause of many suicidal deaths. The prognosis is grave in severe poisoning. Because of the high affinity of carbon monoxide for haemoglobin, a few breaths at high concentrations can be fatal; 1% carbon monoxide in air can kill within minutes. This cause of suicidal poisoning is decreasing with the compulsory use of catalytic converters.

Treatment consists of removal from the source of exposure and administration of 100% oxygen immediately, after taking an anticoagulated whole blood sample for carboxyhaemoglobin estimation. The pregnant patient or any patient who has had symptoms suggestive of severe poisoning should be treated with hyperbaric oxygen if available (Weiss & Van Meier, 1992). In addition to shortening the half-life of carboxyhaemoglobin, hyperbaric oxygen may prevent late neurological sequelae (Mathieu *et al.*, 1985; Norkool & Kirkpatrick, 1985). Poisons centres can provide details of establishments currently providing this service.

Cyanide

Cyanide can be rapidly fatal. It may be inhaled as hydrogen cyanide gas (from an industrial accident or as a product of combustion), ingested as cyanide salts or as cyanogenic glycosides (for example, following massive ingestion of stone fruit kernels or apple pips) which release cyanide following intestinal hydrolysis. Cyanide salts are also absorbed through the skin.

Cyanide acts as a chemical asphyxiant, rapidly blocking cellular oxygen utilization so that cerebral function and circulation are rapidly impaired with the development of a metabolic acidosis. Early signs include hyperventilation and tachycardia, but coma, cyanosis and convulsions soon supervene. The prospects for success with cardiopulmonary resuscitation are high. Mouth-to-mouth resuscitation may be given for hydrogen cyanide inhalation, but care should be taken with this procedure if cyanide salts have been ingested: the lethal dose may be as low as 100 mg and the victim's vomitus could thus be hazardous. A high concentration of inspired oxygen is an effective treatment (Bismuth *et al.*, 1984).

Table 5. *Commonly used antidotes in poisoning.* Adult doses are given unless indicated

Poison	Antidote	Mechanism of action	Dosage regime
Anticholinergic agents	PHYSOSTIGMINE	Cholinesterase inhibitor	2 mg IV over 5 min; continue with an infusion of 4–6 mg hourly
Anticoagulants (warfarin type)	VITAMIN K (phytomenadione)	Competitive antagonist at site of prothrombin manufacture in liver	2–5 mg IV adult, 0.4 mg kg^{-1} child
Benzodiazepines	FLUMAZENIL	Competitive antagonist at benzodiazepine receptors	Initially 0.2 mg IV over 30 sec; further doses of 0.5 mg can be given over 30 sec at 60-sec intervals to a total dose of 3 mg
Beta-blockers	GLUCAGON	Stimulates myocardial adenyl cyclase	5 mg IV over 1 min followed by an infusion of 1–10 mg hr^{-1}
	ISOPRENALINE	Competitive antagonist at beta-receptors	10–50 mg min^{-1} IV
Carbon monoxide	OXYGEN (normobaric or hyperbaric)	Competitive displacement of carbon monoxide from haemoglobin and cytochrome molecules	Administer as high an inspired oxygen as possible until carboxyhaemoglobin concentration falls below 5%; consider hyperbaric oxygen in severe cases
Cyanide	DICOBALT EDETATE	Chelates cyanide ions	300 mg IV over 3 min
	SODIUM NITRITE	Forms methaemoglobin which combines with cyanide	10 ml of 30% solution IV
	SODIUM THIOSULPHATE	Substrate for enzymatic detoxification of cyanide	50 ml of 25% solution IV
	HYDROXOCOBALAMIN	Combines with cyanide to form cyanocobalamin	May be up to 4 g IV
	OXYGEN	Competitive substrate binding	Administer a high inspired oxygen until clinical recovery occurs
Digoxin and digitoxin	Fab ANTIBODY FRAGMENTS	Antidote forms an inert complex with poison	Dose should match the estimated dose of ingested digoxin
Ethylene glycol	ETHANOL	Competitive substrate for alcohol dehydrogenase, slows toxic metabolite production	Dose given should be sufficient to maintain plasma ethanol level at 1–2 g l^{-1}
Heavy metals (lead, mercury, arsenic) NB: the latter three chelating agents are now seldom used, in favour of DMSA and DMPS	DMSA (2, 3–dimercaptosuccinic acid)	Chelating agent	30 mg kg^{-1} 8-hourly for 5 days, then 20 mg kg^{-1} 12-hourly for 14 days

(*continued*)

Table 5. *Continued*

Poison	Antidote	Mechanism of action	Dosage regime
Heavy metals (*contd*)	DMPS (2,3-dimercaptopropane sulphonic acid)	Chelating agent	Acute: 250 mg every 4 h for 24 h then 250 mg every 6 h for the next 24 h Chronic: 100 mg three times a day
	SODIUM CALCIUM EDETATE	Chelating agent	Up to 40 mg kg^{-1} twice daily by IV infusion, repeated every 48 h until lead level falls below toxic range
	DIMERCAPROL	Chelating agent	Mercury: 2.5–3 mg kg^{-1} deep IM injection 4 hourly for 2 days; 2–4 times on third day; 1–2 times for up to 10 days
	PENICILLAMINE	Chelating agent	Lead: 0.5–1.5 g per day orally for 1–2 months or until lead level falls below toxic range
Hydrofluoric acid	CALCIUM GLUCONATE	Forms an inert complex (calcium fluoride)	For burns: calcium gluconate (10%) 0.25–0.5 mmol kg^{-1}, up to 25 mmol kg^{-1}
Iron salts	DESFERRIOXAMINE	Chelating agent	In severe iron poisoning (>90 mmol l^{-1}) up to 15 mg kg^{-1} h^{-1} reduced to keep the total IV dose under 80 mg kg^{-1} in each 24 h
Methanol	ETHANOL	Competitive substrate for alcohol dehydrogenase, slows toxic metabolite production	As for ethylene glycol
Methaemoglobin	METHYLENE BLUE	Cofactor for reduction of methaemoglobin by NADPH	0.2 ml kg^{-1} 1% solution (i.e. 2 mg kg^{-1}) slowly IV over 5 min, repeated as necessary, to a maximum of 6 mg kg^{-1}
	ASCORBIC ACID	Reducing agent	1 g per 24 h IV or orally
Opioids	NALOXONE	Competitive antagonist at opioid receptors	0.8–1.2 mg IV (children 0.2 mg); repeat if respiratory depression is not reversed within 1–2 min; continue with half the amount required to produce a response as an infusion over 30 min
Organophosphates	ATROPINE	Competitive antagonist at acetylcholine receptors	2 mg IV (IM or SC in less severely poisoned patients) followed by further 2 mg doses at 5–10 min intervals until clinical features of full atropinization become apparent (dry mouth is the most reliable sign)

(continued)

Table 5. *Continued*

Poison	Antidote	Mechanism of action	Dosage regime
Organophosphates (*contd*)	PRALIDOXIME	Cholinesterase reactivator	1 g IV (in 100 ml saline over 30 min) repeated every 4 h for 24 h in severe cases
Paracetamol	ACETYLCYSTEINE	Replenishes hepatic glutathione stores	150 mg kg^{-1} over 15 min, then 50 mg kg^{-1} over 4 h, then 100 mg kg^{-1} over 16 h
	METHIONINE	Replenishes hepatic glutathione stores	2.5 g orally every 4 h for 12 h (total 10 g)
Thallium	BERLIN BLUE	Chelating agent	250 mg kg^{-1} per day in divided doses; ideally given until thallium level is <10 mg l^{-1} in blood and urine

Symptoms of anxiety and panic may mimic those of early cyanide toxicity. When the diagnosis is certain, and the patient has symptoms of toxicity, dicobalt edetate 300 mg in 20 ml is an effective antidote and should be given intravenously over 3 min, repeated as necessary. Although relatively non-toxic when administered to the cyanide poisoned patient, dicobalt edetate can produce severe anaphylactoid reactions with laryngeal oedema and convulsions if given to a non-poisoned patient. The safest course of action is to give the antidote only if the patient's level of consciousness is deteriorating. Another group of antidotes (amyl nitrite and sodium nitrite) act by producing methaemoglobin which binds cyanide ions. Sodium thiosulphate acts by providing a substrate for the enzyme rhodanese to produce sodium thiocyanate. Although slower acting, sodium thiosulphate is non-toxic and should be given whenever there is a suspicion of cyanide poisoning (see Table 5). It is important to have a good understanding of the mechanism of cyanide toxicity and modes of action of antidotes (Marrs, 1988).

Subacute cyanide toxicity can also occur during prolonged nitroprusside therapy. The main clinical feature is a metabolic acidosis; if none is present then cyanide toxicity can be ruled out. Cyanide measurement is not usually necessary; a rapid improvement should occur after administration of sodium thiosulphate intravenously. Other cyanide antidotes are not indicated.

Gas and smoke inhalation

Exposure to asphyxiant gases demands full resuscitation and measures to prevent the sequelae of hypoxia. Simple asphyxiants act by reducing the proportion of oxygen in the inspired air. Many gases may be responsible such as hydrogen, helium, methane, petroleum vapour, carbon dioxide and nitrogen. The duration and severity of hypoxia plays a critical part in determining the symptoms and outcome. An atmosphere of less than 6–8% oxygen will rapidly produce coma and cardiorespiratory collapse due to cerebral hypoxia. With gases heavier than air there may be several victims, as each tries to rescue the others without using breathing apparatus.

Fire victims may have cutaneous burns, but attention should also be paid to the possibility of sytemic poisoning by products of combustion and to the possibility of burns in the upper respiratory tract. Patients may be suffering from the effects of hypoxia or of carbon monoxide or cyanide toxicity. Carboxyhaemoglobin levels and a careful clinical assessment are important in deciding the severity of smoke exposure. Cyanide toxicity may occur in fire victims; an elevated plasma lactate concentration may indicate cyanide toxicity in patients without severe burns (Baud *et al.*, 1991). Water-insoluble gases such as acrolein or phosgene tend to reach the lungs and may cause bronchoconstriction and pulmonary oedema, often after a latent interval, so that the patient should be observed for 24 h. Pateints with circumferential neck burns, dysphonia, soot in the oropharynx or a blood carboxyhaemoglobin of over 12% are at risk of delayed pulmonary damage. They should have a baseline chest X-ray and their respiratory function should be monitored; if necessary, they should be transferred to a centre with facilities for ventilation. Use of an algorithm can facilitate management decisions following smoke inhalation (Langford & Armstrong, 1989).

Exposure to other gases should be treated on their merits. Inhalation of water-soluble irritant gases (such as CS or CN gas or ammonia) produces severe lacrimation and upper respiratory tract irritation and coughing, but resuscitation is not usually needed and symptomatic measures are sufficient. Gases such as arsine and stibine can cause minimal symptoms on inhalation but may produce severe haemolysis and haemoglobinuria, sometimes presenting as renal failure 24 h after exposure. Accidental or intentional inhalation of volatile substances may result in deep coma, hyporeflexia and cardiac arrhythmias which may progress to ventricular fibrillation. Treatment is symptomatic; a beta-blocking drug such as esmolol may help to control arrhythmias.

Liquid agents

Corrosive ingestion

Strong acids and alkalis are corrosive. The main symptom following ingestion is pain, but shock and coma can develop rapidly. If the patient is able to swallow, three or four cups of water or milk (adult) should be given immediately by mouth and the face and hands if contaminated should be washed with copious amounts of water. If the patient is unable to swallow and saliva accumulates in the mouth, there are usually pharyngeal burns. Acids or alkalis should not be neutralized since the reaction is exothermic. Acids tend mainly to damage the oesophagus and alkalis the stomach.

Stomach emptying is contraindicated as it may produce further upper gastrointestinal damage. Opioid analgesics should be given as required for pain, and plasma and saline should be given for shock. Where there is an experienced endoscopist, endoscopy should be performed early to assess the extent of damage (Ali Zagar et al., 1991). If perforation has occurred, urgent surgical intervention is essential. Time should not be wasted attempting to improve the metabolic or cardiovascular state.

Hydrocarbons, petroleum distillates and essential oils

These are found in the home as white spirit, petroleum jelly, polishes, waxes, window cleaners, turpentine substitute, paraffin, petrol, and solvents for garden pesticides. Ingestion of petroleum distillates and hydrocarbon oils and waxes causes two main problems:

1. If aspirated during ingestion or subsequent vomiting, they can cause chemical pneumonitis.
2. If absorbed via the lungs or the gut they can cause CNS system depression.

It should be remembered that many pesticides contain hydrocarbons which may contribute to toxicity.

Clinical features

Hydrocarbon ingestion can cause irritation of mucous membranes, producing nausea, vomiting and diarrhoea. The hydrocarbons destroy pulmonary surfactant properties so that aspiration of even small amounts of paraffin or petrol can cause an acute pneumonitis developing 12–24 h after exposure. Mineral oils and waxes cause low-grade chronic inflammation. Clinical signs include cough, a rapid respiratory rate, cyanosis and crackles. Radiological signs consist of dense patchy shadowing, usually in the lower lobes. Many cases (especially in children) may be asymptomatic. If sufficient is absorbed, CNS involvement can lead to restlessness, drowsiness, confusion and coma. Essential oils such as oil of turpentine (not turpentine substitute), camphorated oil and oil of eucalyptus are highly toxic and can also cause convulsions and renal failure.

Treatment

The patient should be admitted for at least 24 h after ingestion. A chest X-ray should be performed on admission and at 12–24 h after exposure. Emesis is contraindicated because of the risk of aspiration. If a large amount (over 10 ml kg^{-1}) has been ingested (within the last 2 h) or if the patient is losing consciousness, the patient should be intubated in order to prevent aspiration of gastric contents, and gastric lavage should be performed. In the case of essential oils, gastric lavage is indicated if over 10 ml have been swallowed by a child or 25 ml by an adult. Activated charcoal should be given. Oxygen and bronchodilators should be used as required if aspiration is suspected or if lung damage has occurred. Recovery should take place within 1–2 weeks but may take longer with waxes and polishes. There is no specific treatment and no evidence that high-dose steroids will help to prevent damage or hasten recovery. If other organs are involved, management is symptomatic and supportive.

Chlorinated hydrocarbons and dry-cleaning agents

Dry-cleaning agents are usually chlorinated hydrocarbons such as trichloroethylene or trichloroethane. Poisoning can occur from accidental inhalation, from inhalation by abuse and from ingestion. Carbon tetrachloride is no longer used as a dry-cleaning agent. Chlorinated solvents are in general highly toxic causing marked gastrointestinal irritation, central nervous depression, and potentially serious hepatic damage.

Management

Chlorinated hydrocarbons are radio-opaque (Dally *et al.*, 1987) and significant amounts recently ingested should appear on an abdominal X-ray. This type of solvent is not an aspiration risk so the stomach may be emptied after first ascertaining the ingredients since some formulations also contain petroleum distillates. Acetylcysteine should be given as in paracetamol poisoning as the mechanism of hepatic toxicity appears to be similar.

Methanol (methyl alcohol) and ethylene glycol

Methanol and ethylene glycol are constituents of some antifreezes. Ethylene glycol tastes sweet and red antifreezes may be mistaken for alcoholic or soft drinks. Model aircraft fuel contains methanol as does screen-wash fluid and some varnishes and thinners. Ten millilitres of pure methanol can be fatal in a child and 50 ml in an adult, causing profound metabolic acidosis, coma, convulsions and blindness. Ethylene glycol tends initially to cause signs similar to mild alcohol intoxication, followed later by convulsions, tachycardia, pulmonary oedema and acure renal failure. There is no smell of alcohol on the breath.

Both of these substances have relatively low toxicity but are metabolized via alcohol dehydrogenase to toxic metabolites (Fig. 4) which are responsible for the major clinical features of poisoning. The main principles of treatment are to correct acidosis, delay the metabolism of methanol or ethylene glycol to toxic metabolites by administering ethyl alcohol (ethanol) orally or intravenously as appropriate, and to hasten elimination by increasing the fluid output by the kidneys or by using haemodialysis in severe cases to remove the substance from the blood stream (Jacobsen & McMartin, 1986).

Gastric aspiration and lavage should be used to empty the stomach up to 1 h after ingestion. The dyes in antifreezes help to confirm ingestion but their colour is changed by gastric acid (blue dyes become green/yellow, red dyes become orange/yellow).

Arterial blood gases, plasma electrolytes, urea and osmolality should be measured. Acidosis should be corrected immediately with intravenous sodium bicarbonate. If plasma omolality is normal, treatment will not be required. It may be necessary to consult a poisons centre for measurement of levels and for the regime of ethyl alcohol administration. The aim is to keep the blood ethanol level in the range $1-2$ g l^{-1}. Haemodialysis is indicated if plasma methanol is over 500 mg l^{-1}.

Occupational hazards

Chronic occupational exposure is monitored by authorities in each country, to prevent toxicity in employees. A wide range of substances may be involved in occupational poisoning: these may include corrosive chemicals, adhesives, volatile substances, metal salts, pesticides, phenols and hydrofluoric acid (Proctor *et al.*, 1988). Many of these are dealt with in Chapter 35.

Accidental ingestion of plants, mushrooms and berries

Young children often ingest plants and berries, but this seldom gives rise to serious problems. Generally a mild gastrointestinal disturbance is the most that will occur and symptomatic and supportive treatment is all that is required. It is important to identify the plant in case it is capable of causing significant or serious toxicity. Although emesis with syrup of ipecacuanha is of little use in managing most types of poisoning, it may have a place for recent (less than 1 h) plant ingestions, both to remove and to enable identification of ingested plant material. Table 6 lists the more commonly found toxic plants in the British Isles together with indications for emesis; the toxic amounts are much larger. After emesis, treatment is supportive. Further information may be obtained from the reference texts (Lang, 1987; Cooper & Johnson, 1984).

The management of suicidal or accidental ingestion by an adult depends on the case and amount taken. Large accidental ingestions of toxic plants in mistake for edible species, unusual suicide attempts and also homicidal

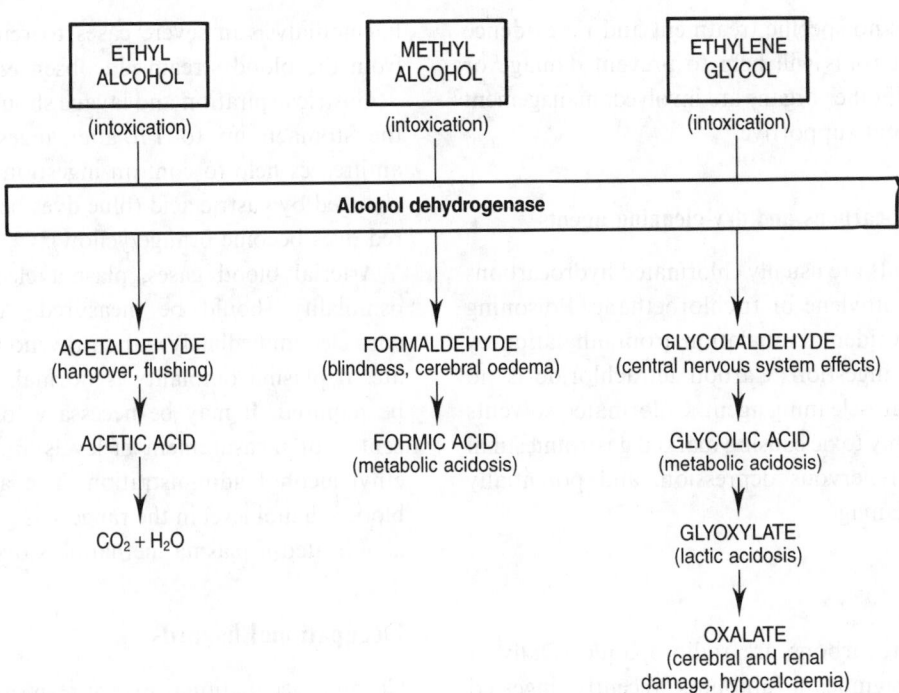

Fig. 4. Metabolic pathways for ethyl alcohol, methyl alcohol and ethylene glycol. Since ethyl alcohol has a higher affinity for alcohol dehydrogenase than methyl alcohol, it can delay their metabolism, thus reducing their toxicity.

poisoning due to plant ingestion occur occasionally. Symptoms may be severe. Poisons centres will be able to advise on the appropriate management.

Envenomation (See Chapter 43)

Bee and wasp stings may cause local swelling and pain, and rarely anaphylaxis, which should be dealt with as described in Chapter 8. Snake envenomation is unusual in Europe, the only toxic species being the adder (Vipera berus). Other toxic snakes, scorpions, fish and spiders are outside the scope of this chapter; a poisons centre should be consulted. (See Chapter 43.)

Ethanol (ethyl alcohol)

Ethanol is possibly the best known of all toxins. It is taken in about 50% of cases of self-poisoning with other substances. There are over 150 deaths each year in England and Wales from acute alcohol toxicity but the numbers of deaths from other causes including chronic hepatic damage and accidents on the road and in the workplace is considerably greater than this, with the total toll being over 25 000 deaths each year in Britain.

Acute effects of alcohol

Severe alcohol intoxication can occur in infants from accidental ingestion of alcoholic beverages, mouthwashes or perfumes and aftershave lotions, or in young people from drinking large amounts of spirits, sometimes as deliberate self-harm. Dilute ethanol enhances gastric emptying but high concentration (of the strength found in spirits) may cause gastric irritation and can delay stomach emptying; it may be worth aspirating the stomach contents through a narrow tube to shorten the duration of intoxication (Pollack et al., 1992).

Intellectual performance, judgement and coordination are progressively impaired at increasing blood concentrations. The legal limit in the UK for being in charge of a motor vehicle is 80 mg dl^{-1}. At 150 mg dl^{-1} most people have cerebellar ataxia with marked impairment of coordination and are obviously drunk. However, tolerant individuals may have a blood alcohol concentration as high as 500 mg dl^{-1} (5.0 g l^{-1}) without apparent intoxication (Urso et al., 1981). By contrast, death from acute alcohol toxicity may occur in non-tolerant individuals with blood ethanol levels in the range 200–400 mg dl^{-1} (2–4 g l^{-1}), from cardiac or respiratory depression or asphyxiation.

Table 6. *Plant ingestion*:

Amounts for which emesis or activated charcoal administration is indicated (this is not an exhaustive list but includes the more common British poisonous plants and mushrooms).

Plant	Amount ingested
Deadly nightshade: all parts	Any amount
Other species containing atropine-like compounds, e.g. *Datura stramonium* (thorn-apple)	Any amount
Woody nightshade: all parts	Any amount of unripe berries; over 5 ripe berries (child)
Christmas/Jerusalem cherry: leaves or unripe berries	5 unripe berries
Yew: leaves and seeds (the red fleshy part is not toxic)	Any amount
Snowberry	More than 3 berries
Holly berries	More than 10 berries
Foxglove: all parts	Any amount
Privet: leaves and berries	More than 1 berry
Bryony	Any amount
Daffodil bulbs	Any amount
Amanita phalloides	Any amount
Gyromitra esculenta (poisonous if eaten raw)	Any amount
Laburnum: all parts	Any amount
Cuckoo pint or lords and ladies (*Arum maculatum*)	More than 10 berries
Cherry laurel	Any amount
Daphne (*laureola* and *mezereum*): all parts	Any amount
Mistletoe	More than 10 berries

Clinical pitfalls

Deep coma may occur in a patient who has taken subtoxic amounts of alcohol plus a sedative or hypnotic drug or an opioid. Alcohol intoxication may mask the presence of a head injury or another agent which has been ingested, particularly salicylate or paracetamol which tend to cause few symptoms in early stages. In children, convulsions and hypoglycaemia may follow acute intoxication. Alcohol potentiates rebound hypoglycaemia. At all ages severe depression of consciousness may lead to loss of protective reflex, aspiration of vomit, accumulation of secretions, or blockage of the airway by the tongue. Although there is sometimes a small rise in serum enzyme levels, there is no evidence that a single acute massive ingestion of alcohol causes long-term hepatic damage.

Management of acute toxicity

Management is supportive, aiming at maintaining respiration and circulation. Although death can occur with a blood alcohol level of over 2.0 g l^{-1}, severe intoxication with levels of 5 or 10 g l^{-1} may be managed conservatively. Measurement of alcohol levels is helpful but not essential; the clinical state is more important. Haemodialysis may rarely be required for the management of profound hypotension or respiratory depression.

Late and chronic effects of alcohol

Alcohol ketoacidosis may follow bouts of heavy drinking. Heavy beer drinkers may suffer from alcohol potomania, with mental disturbance and hyponatraemia. Very heavy ingestion of alcohol may lead to the clinical picture of alcohol hepatitis, with fever, leucocytosis and hepatomegaly. Chronic ingestion can lead to a type IV hyperlipidaemia with raised serum triglyceride levels, and hyperuricaemia with gout is common in chronic heavy alcohol drinkers. A pseudo-Cushing's syndrome occurs in alcoholics and may be accompanied by a myopathy. The commonest sequal of long-term alcohol abuse is cirrhosis, which is accompanied by typical physical signs and the biochemical changes of hepatic impairment. Acute bleeding may occur from ruptured oesophageal varices.

When chronic abuse is diagnosed for the first time in the A&E department, the opportunity should be taken to help the patient. Questionnaires (e.g. CAGE) are available for establishing the diagnosis. Apart from an exceptional binge the night before, the presence of alcohol in a morning blood or urine sample is diagnostic of alcoholism. The other important tests for chronic abuse are a raised gamma-glutamyltranspeptidase and a raised mean corpuscular volume.

The alcohol-dependent patient who discontinues drinking following an accident or hospital admission may develop an alcohol withdrawal syndrome in which there is a risk of convulsions and death. Initial agitation may develop into frank hallucinations, and sedation with diazepam or infusion of a sedative drug such as chlormethiazole may be needed. Tremor may respond to a beta-blocking drug such as atenolol. The patient should never be discharged with chlormethiazole tablets.

Drugs

Salicylates

Salicylates can cause severe poisoning with relatively few symptoms and every case of ingestion should therefore be taken seriously. The fatal adult dose is 500 mg kg^{-1}. They are more toxic in infants and small children than in adults, and salicylate-containing preparations should never be given to children under 12 months. They are also contraindicated in children under 12 years because of the risk of precipitating Reye's syndrome. Salicylates are found in aspirin (acetylsalicylic acid), benorylate, oil of wintergreen, liniments, and some teething preparations, although the latter rarely cause poisoning as the amount of salicylate is small.

Clinical features

Salicylates cause irritability, tinnitus, deafness, nausea, vomiting and hyperventilation. Uncoupling of oxidative phosphorylation leads to mitochondrial heat production. In adults this leads to sweating, with the body temperature usually remaining normal, while in children pyrexia may occur. The combination of vomiting, hyperventilation and sweating may lead to severe volume depletion and electrolyte disturbances. The mechanism of toxicity of salicylates has been reviewed by Krause et al., (1992).

Respiratory alkalosis, metabolic acidosis, ketosis, hypoglycaemia and hyperglycaemia may all occur. The patient usually presents with a combined respiratory alkalosis and metabolic acidosis, with a blood pH in the range 7.40–7.46. Later, as metabolic compensation fails, the arterial pH may fall below 7.40. The most important clinical signs of serious toxicity are a falling plasma pH, hypoxaemia, or the development of pulmonary oedema. Confusion and depressed consciousness are serious signs.

Management

Every patient suspected of salicylate toxicity should be detained until the severity has been assessed biochemically. The plasma salicylate level should be measured on presentation and repeated after 3 h in case it is rising. At the same time, arterial blood gases and plasma biochemistry should be checked. Gastric decontamination should be performed with repeat dose activated charcoal because salicylate may be retained in the stomach for many hours after ingestion. Central venous pressure should be measured early and the patient should be rehydrated with intravenous fluids and metabolic acidosis or hypoglycaemia corrected.

If there are severe metabolic changes, or the salicylate level is over 800 mg l^{-1} (5.76 mmol l^{-1}), haemodialysis is indicated and the patient should be referred urgently for treatment. If the level is over 600 mg l^{-1} (4.32 mmol l^{-1}) urinary alkalinization (intravenous sodium bicarbonate 8.4%) should be commenced. The aim is to produce a urinary pH of over 7.5 as this enhances renal salicylate elimination. In infants, salicylate levels of over 300 mg l^{-1} should be regarded as potentially toxic and a poisons centre should be consulted. The management of salicylate poisoning has been reviewed by Notarianni (1992).

Paracetamol (acetaminophen)

Paracetamol (acetaminophen) overdose is common (up to 40% of A&E attendances for poisoning). Serious toxicity is rare in children because they do not usually ingest large amounts and possibly also because they are more resistant to the effects of the drug.

Mechanisms

Although paracetamol is a very safe analgesic when taken in the recommended dose, it is potentially very toxic in overdose. This is because a small proportion (approximately 4%) is metabolised by cytochrome P450 to produce a highly reactive chemical, N-acetyl-p-benzoquinoneimine (NABQI). This reactive metabolite can be metabolized by conjugation to form non-toxic mercapturic acid conjugates, provided glutathione is present in the liver cell. An overdose of paracetamol may exhaust glutathione stores. In this case NABQI covalently binds to sulphhydryl groups in hepatocytes forming an irreversible complex which can produce acute centrilobular necrosis. Paracetamol is also metabolized in the cells of the renal tubule where a similar process can occur leading to acute tubular necrosis.

An increase in oxidative metabolism of paracetamol resulting from enzyme induction by alcohol in chronic alcoholics or by phenobarbitone or phenytoin in epileptics can generate large amounts of NABQI. Glutathione reserves are then rapidly depleted so that hepatoxicity may occur following a relatively small overdose of paracetamol. Severe toxicity is also more likely in people whose intracellular stores of glutathione are depleted by a starvation diet or protein malnutrition. Chronic alcoholics have been shown to have low hepatic glutathione

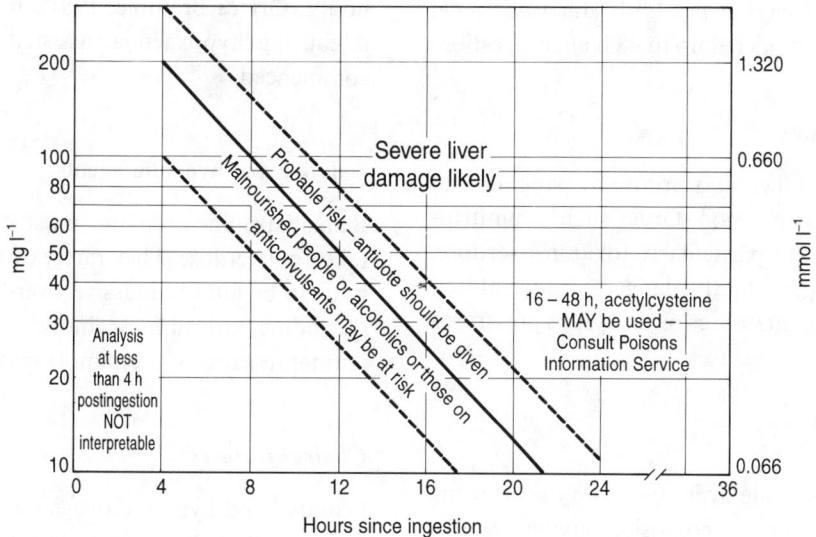

Fig. 5. Recommendations for treatment of paracetamol poisoning.

reserves. Thus, in these at-risk groups, the widely accepted nomogram of paracetamol concentration at a given time after an overdose (Fig. 5) may be unreliable and it is prudent to lower the line to one which starts at 100 mg l^{-1} at 4 h after ingestion.

Clinical features

The symptoms of paracetamol poisoning usually follow a well-defined time course (Table 7). In the first 24 h after ingestion, the patient is most commonly symptomless, but may have nausea, vomiting, dizziness, or sweating. In the late stages there may be hepatic tenderness, and jaundice may become apparent. Prolongation of the prothrombin time by 15–18 h is an early sign of hepatic damage; the prognosis is poor if it is over 20 sec at 24 h or 44 sec at 48 h or rising after 48 h. Serum transaminases start to rise by 18–24 h and peak about 3 or 4 days after ingestion, returning to normal within 7–10 days in those who recover. Levels which may be very high (several thousand units) are not a good guide to prognosis. Liver histology returns to normal by 3 months even after serious poisoning. The patient should be monitored for hypoglycaemia, coagulation disturbances and renal impairment. Renal tubular necrosis can occur, sometimes with minimal evidence of liver damage.

Management

Blood should be taken not less than 4 h after ingestion for plasma paracetamol measurement and treatment

Table 7. *Symptoms and biochemical changes following paracetamol overdose*

Day 1	May be anorexia, nausea, vomiting
Day 2	Abdominal pain Prolonged prothrombin time Plasma enzyme levels rising
Day 3	Hypoglycaemia Jaundice
Day 4	Deteriorating renal function Hepatic encephalopathy
Day 5–7	Hepatic coma progressing to death or beginning to recover

should be guided by reference to a treatment nomogram. The stomach should be emptied if the patient presents within 2 h. If a large overdose is suspected and the patient presents within 12 h, treatment should be commenced with antidotes at once without waiting for blood paracetamol results. Treatment is much less likely to be effective after 12 h. Oral methionine may be given if the patient presents within 8–10 h and is able to swallow. Intravenous acetylcysteine should be given if the patient is comatose or vomiting, or presents more than 8–10 h after ingestion. The blood paracetamol level will indicate whether treatment needs to be continued or not. Acetylcysteine may be of benefit in late presenting patients with evidence of toxicity (Keays et al., 1991; Harrison et al., 1990) and should be considered up to 48 h after ingestion.

Tricyclic antidepressants

These are likely to be taken in overdose by patients who are being treated for depression. Drugs such as amitriptyline and dothiepin are particularly toxic in overdose. Tricyclic drugs are particularly dangerous in children who may take their parents' drugs or the syrups prescribed for enuresis.

Clinical features

The patient may deteriorate over several hours following ingestion, with agitation or confusion giving way to deepening coma. Convulsions are common and muscle tone is often increased with brisk tendon reflexes and extensor plantar reflexes. Dilated pupils and tachycardia are caused by the anticholinergic effects of the drug. The most dangerous problem is cardiac toxicity which may be associated with widened QRS complexes (Boehnert & Lovejoy, 1985), ventricular arrhythmias, severe hypotension, metabolic acidosis, heart block and asystole. Respiratory depression is also common in severe cases. Death occurs mainly from hypotension and cardiac arrhythmias (Pentel & Benowitz, 1986).

Management

Oral activated charcoal for a conscious child, and gastric lavage followed by active charcoal for an adult or an unconscious child, should be preformed up to 12 h after ingestion. Plasma electrolytes and arterial blood gases should be measured and the ECG monitored. Sodium bicarbonate should be given intravenously to correct any metabolic acidosis and to raise the arterial pH to 7.5 in severe cases irrespective of whether the patient is acidotic or not (Molloy et al., 1984). This often produces a marked improvement. Hypokalaemia should be corrected. Intravenous esmolol or atenolol should be given for arrhythmias and repeated as necessary. Lignocaine is contraindicated. Phenytoin can also be used (18 mg kg^{-1} intravenously over 20 min). Intravenous diazepam can be given for convulsions. Inotropic agents usually have little effect on tricyclic-induced hypotension, but glucagon may be effective. If there is severe unresponsive hypotension or if a cardic arrest occurs, the circulation should be supported by external cardiac massage for as long as necessary as recovery can occur after long periods, even

hours (Orr & Bramble. 1981). If respiratory depression is causing hypoxaemia, assisted ventilation should be commenced.

Sedative and hypnotic agents

Benzodiazepines are the most common sedative drug taken in overdose. They rarely cause severe complications but can be fatal in massive overdose. Many other drugs (including barbiturates, chloral hydrate, opioids, tricyclic antidepressants and ethanol) may produce deep coma.

Clinical features

Sedative and hypnotic drugs may cause excitability and occasionally hallucinations but drowsiness usually supervenes and larger doses cause flaccid coma. Aspiration of vomit and respiratory depression are the most important complications. Hypothermia may occur.

Management

Drowsy or comatose patients should be placed in the recovery position to protect the airway. Blood gas tensions should be measured and ventilation assisted if respiratory depression is suspected or present. If the patient is comatose and has no gag reflex, gastric lavage should be performed after first passing an endotracheal tube. Activated charcoal should be left in the stomach. It is customary to measure plasma paracetamol and salicylate in case these have also been ingested.

Use of flumazenil in benzodiazepine poisoning

Flumazenil is a competitive benzodiazepine antagonist licensed for reversal of benzodiazepine sedation but not overdose (Votey et al., 1991). Owing to the low toxicity of benzodiazepines and the high cost of flumazenil, its role for the routine reversal of benzodiazepine overdose is limited. It is contraindicated in benzodiazepine-dependent patients (especially epileptics) and those who have also taken tricyclic antidepressants because of the risk of convulsions. However, it may have diagnostic or therapeutic value in some cases (Lheureux & Askenasi, 1988). The typical dosage is 0.2 mg IV over 15 sec. If there is a minimal or absent response within 60 sec, a further 0.3 mg can be administered over 30 sec. After 60 sec, further doses of 0.5 mg can be given over 30 sec at 60 sec intervals to a total dose of 3 mg. Its elimination half-life is 52 min so repeated doses or an infusion may be needed ($0.1–0.5$ mg h^{-1} according to response).

Drugs and substances of abuse

Many drugs and chemicals are widely abused and some cause serious medical complications. There are approximately 200 deaths from opioid abuse and 150 deaths from volatile substance abuse each year in Britain. Although other abused substances cause fewer deaths, they remain an important cause of morbidity. Apart from opioid toxicity, management is mainly symptomatic. Confirmation of exposure is often necessary for diagnostic or medicolegal reasons. Detection in plasma is often difficult. Urine tests remain positive for most drugs of abuse for 36 h or more after exposure.

Amphetamines

The amphetamines are frequently abused for their stimulant effects. Amphetamine sulphate may be injected, inhaled or taken orally. Methylamphetamine ('ice') comes in the form of crystals which are smoked and is about twenty times more potent as amphetamine sulphate but has similar effects. The main complications of amphetamine toxicity include agitation, convulsions, hyperthermia and myoglobinuric renal failure which can be aggravated by volume depletion. Cerebral haemorrhage may occur. There is no specific pharmacological antidote and management is generally supportive. Sedation and anticonvulsants will be needed for the patient who is agitated or convulsing. Ensuring an acid urine markedly increases the excretion of amphetamine and shortens its elimination half-life. However, if there is a suspicion of rhabdomyolysis, for example following repeated seizures, or if the plasma creatine kinase activity is raised or myoglobinuria is present, then alkalinization of the urine is recommended in order to prevent myoglobinuric renal failure. Management has been reviewed by Linden et al., (1985).

MDMA (3, 4-methylenedioxymethamphetamine) MDMA (3, 4-methylenedioxymethamphetamine), also known as 'ecstasy' or 'E', is an amphetamine derivative with different properties from amphetamine. In the usual doses (tablets or capsules contain 50–200 mg and most users take 1–5 orally during the course of an evening), it has few adverse effects in the majority of people. The commonest are trismus, tachycardia, sweating and agitation. A small proportion develop muscle pain and stiffness which may persist for a week. When the drug is used as a 'dance drug', continuous exertion with inadequate fluid replacement may lead to collapse, convulsions and acute hyperthermia, rapidly followed by disseminated intravascular coagulation and rhabdomyolysis. Deaths have occurred after a single dose (Henry et al., 1992). Overdose or ingestion without hyperactivity tends to produce a more amphetamine-like symptom pattern. Management initially should be directed to restoring fluid volume and reducing body temperature. Intravenous dantrolene may help to limit damage in severe hyperthermia ($>41°C$).

Opioids

As well as heroin, morphine and pethidine, the narcotic analgesics dihydrocodeine, diamorphine pentazocine, dextromoramide and dextropropoxyphene are potentially fatal in overdose. Proprietary cough mixtures and pain relievers contain amounts of opioids which are potentially toxic in children and the antidiarrhoea preparation Lomotil (diphenoxylate combined with atropine) can cause respiratory depression.

Heroin (diamorphine) abuse is common in the UK, causing 200 deaths per year. Many of these are due to respiratory failure after the first use of the drug, but experienced users may die from acute respiratory depression or aspiration of vomit following a change in supplier (in Britain the purity of street heroin may vary between 10% and 80%) or loss of tolerance after a period of abstinence. The dose requirement may fall by 10- to 50-fold over a period of 2–3 weeks of abstinence, so that the dose which previously produced euphoria may prove fatal. The signs of opioid toxicity consist of depressed consciousness, which may amount to profound coma, small or 'pinpoint' pupils and respiratory depression. Hypotension, convulsions, vomiting and pulmonary oedema may also occur. The pupils may not constrict with pethidine, and may dilate due to cerebral hypoxia or hypothermia or other drugs taken. The pattern of opioid-induced respiratory depression is characteristic and consists of a slowing of respiration, whereas other respiratory depressants tend to decrease depth of respiration with little effect on rate.

Management Acute ingestion of opioids requires gastric emptying and activated charcoal. If the patient is cyanosed or convulsing, or if naloxone is not available, assisted ventilation should be started immediately. Naxolone is the antidote of choice and should be given intravenously

in doses of 0.8–2.0 mg as required. A response should occur within 30–60 sec, with reversal of signs of toxicity. A partial or short-lived response may be explained by the size of the overdose, the type of opioid or the presence of another sedative or hypnotic agent, and further doses of naloxone should be given. Since the duration of response may be less than 10 min, the patient should be detained and observed closely for signs of deterioration. However, in mild poisoning, permanent recovery may follow a single dose of naloxone.

Once the diagnosis of opioid toxicity has been confirmed by the response to naloxone, the choice can be made between continuing reversal with an infusion of naloxone sufficient to maintain adequate spontaneous respiration (this can be started at half the dose sufficient to produce initial reversal over each 30 min), or ventilating the patient until the drug is metabolized. Diamorphine has a short elimination half-life of 2–4 h but other opioid drugs such as buprenorphine, methadone and dextropropoxyphene have considerably longer elimination half-lives and a longer period of recovery should be anticipated.

Complications of heroin overdose include a chemical pneumonitis following aspiration of vomit, non-cardiogenic pulmonary oedema and non-traumatic rhabdomyolysis. The question of provoking heroin withdrawal symptoms in an addict by administration of naloxone is often raised; this should not prevent the use of naloxone since withdrawal is a non-fatal condition which is short-lived because of the duration of a single dose of naloxone (10–30 min). In any case, withdrawal symptoms can be treated by sedation.

LSD (lysergic acid diethylamide)

LSD is a synthetic hallucinogen, which may be associated with behavioural disturbances, accidents or suicide attempts. Effects often last 8–12 h. There is no specific antidote. If the patient is hallucinating or violent, diazepam or haloperidol are the most suitable drugs to use.

Cocaine

Cocaine abuse produces marked mental and cardiovascular effects. Patients may present with confusion, agitation, aggression, convulsions, myocardial infarction, acute heart failure or cerebral haemorrhage. 'Crack' smokers may get acute lung damage (most commonly a short-lived pneumonitis) from direct inhalation of smoke from flamed crystals of free-base cocaine, especially if their supply is contaminated. There is no specific antidote

but control of blood pressure with agents such as intravenous nitrates is essential. Other management is supportive. Cocaine 'body-packers' may be managed by whole gut lavage which should rapidly speed the packets through the gut. If it can be set up quickly this is preferable to activated charcoal.

Cardioactive drugs

Cardiac glycosides

Acute poisoning with cardiac glycosides such as digoxin, digitoxin or plants such as foxglove, *Thevetia spp.* or oleander can produce cardiac arrhythmias and hyperkalaemia, both of which can be fatal. If the patient presents within 4 h of ingestion, gastric lavage should be performed and activated charcoal left in the stomach. Clinical features of toxicity include cardiac arrhythmias, heart block or a high or rising plasma potassium. The important investigations are ECG, digoxin assay and plasma potassium; a potassium concentration of over 5 mmol l^{-1} is a strong indicator of potential toxicity. Plasma digoxin levels can only be interpreted 6 h after ingestion. In plant poisonings, a measured digoxin concentration by immunoassay, although of no help in quantifying the toxin, may be used to confirm ingestion. Where necessary, arrangements should be made to obtain digoxin-specific Fab antibodies urgently in case life-threatening toxicity should develop. These Fab fragments of sheep antidigoxin immunoglobulin molecules bind with high affinity to digoxin and other cardiac glycosides, removing the poison from tissue sites.

Beta-adrenoceptor antagonists, lignocaine, amiodarone or phenytoin may be useful in treating cardiac arrhythmias, and insulin with glucose can be used as a short-term measure for hyperkalaemia. A pacing wire should be inserted if second or third degree heart block develops. Direct current countershock should be used for ventricular fibrillation. If these measures fail to restore an adequate cardiac output, the circulation can be supported with external chest compression pending the arrival of Fab antibodies, which should reverse the clinical features of cardiac glycoside poisoning within 20–30 min (Zucker *et al.*, 1982; Smith *et al.*, 1982). The dose (in mg) of antibody can be calculated from the amount of digoxin ingested (dose in mg × 60) or the plasma digoxin concentration (concentration in $\mu g \, l^{-1}$ or ng ml^{-1} × 0.34 × weight of patient in kg). If the dose required cannot be calculated and treatment is indicated, a speculative dose of 200 mg (5 ampoules) can be given, and further doses of 200 mg added depending on the response. Overdosage with the antibody is at worst likely to cause hypokalaemia if treatment for hyperkalaemia has already been given or may precipitate fast atrial fibrillation or cardiac failure if the patient was taking digoxin for control of these disorders. Allergic reactions do not appear to be a problem. Once Fab antibodies have been given, plasma digoxin assay results are likely to be unreliable (Gibb *et al.*, 1983).

Beta-blocking drugs

In overdose, beta-adrenergic antagonists can cause hypotension, bradycardia, cyanosis, coma and convulsions (Weinstein, 1984). Deaths can occur with propranolol, oxprenolol, sotalol and acebutolol, but are extremely rare with other beta-adrenergic blocking drugs. In severe cases hypotension may be marked and electromechanical dissociation may occur. Electrical conduction disturbances (first degree atrioventricular block and widened QRS complexes) are common. Sotalol is atypical and can also cause ventricular arrhythmias, which respond to infusion of isoprenaline.

After correction of hypovolaemia, the most appropriate treatment is to give either an intravenous bolus of glucagon 10 mg, followed by an infusion of $1-5$ mg h^{-1}, or an intravenous infusion of isoprenaline $10-100$ µg min^{-1}. The response should be assessed by the improvement in blood pressure, rather than by change in the pulse rate and the isoprenaline infusion rate should be increased until the blood pressure responds. High doses may be needed (Critchley & Ungar, 1989). Where asystole occurs, external chest compressions should be used to maintain the circulation. Once the patient comes under medical care full recovery should be the rule, provided hypoxic cerebral damage has not occurred.

Anticonvulsants

Anticonvulsant overdose is most commonly encountered in epileptics. In this case, serial measurements of plasma concentrations of the drug should be made, so that therapy can be restarted when the plasma concentrations of the drug have fallen into the therapeutic range, in order to prevent seizures.

Phenytoin

This drug has dose-dependent elimination kinetics, and phenytoin toxicity can occur after regular therapy on inappropriately high doses, or from acute overdose. Clinical features are prolonged and include cerebellar ataxia, confusion and vomiting. Deep coma and respiratory depression are rare. Excessively rapid intravenous administration of phenytoin can cause cardiac arrest due to the propylene glycol vehicle. Gastric lavage, repeated doses of activated charcoal (Mauro *et al.*, 1987) and supportive care are the best means of treatment. Forced diuresis, haemodialysis and haemoperfusion are not necessary.

Phenobarbitone

Phenobarbitone overdose causes prolonged deep coma and its elimination half-life in overdose may be from 50 to over 100 h. Pupil size fluctuates. There may be respiratory depression, vasodilatation and hypotension. Cardiac output is proportional to the depth of coma. Ileus ('intestinal narcosis') may cause further absorption of drug and deepening of coma as signs of recovery become apparent. Treatment with repeated doses of activated charcoal may shorten the elimination half-life of phenobarbitone. Alkaline diuresis with dopamine has been used, but, in severe poisoning, haemodialysis or haemoperfusion is the most effective way of removing the drug and shortening toxicity.

Sodium valproate

Overdose of this drug causes gastrointestinal symptoms, ataxia, irritability, drowsiness and coma. Pupils are constricted. If over 25 g has been taken (adult), or plasma concentrations exceed 1000 mg l^{-1}, there is a possibility of convulsions and cerebral oedema. Management is supportive (Dupuis *et al.*, 1990).

Iron

Iron is a common cause of childhood poisoning. It is not difficult for a child to ingest a toxic amount, except in the case of multivitamins with iron which contain only a small amount of iron. Deaths have occurred from iron poisoning, and all overdoses should be regarded as potentially serious. Treatment is required for >20 mg elemental iron kg^{-1} body weight (Proudfoot *et al.*, 1986; Schauber *et al.*, 1990). The fatal dose of ferrous sulphate is 0.9 g kg^{-1}.

Clinical features

Vomiting is an early symptom. Haematemesis and severe, possibly bloody, diarrhoea may occur. Shock may develop within 6 h of ingestion. There may be an apparent recovery between 12 and 24 h, but hepatic and renal failure are late sequelae appearing 24–48 h after ingestion and accompanied by metabolic acidosis, hypoglycaemia and hypotension. Perforation of the bowel is a possibility, and intestinal stricture may occur after 2–6 weeks.

Management

All symptomatic patients should be admitted and resuscitated if shocked. Iron is radio-opaque. An early abdominal X-ray may confirm ingestion and show the position of iron tablets in the gut. Absence of opaque material does not exclude iron ingestion. Whole gut lavage should be considered following a potentially serious ingestion. Gastric lavage with 5% sodium bicarbonate should be performed if the patient is shocked or comatose. Oral administration of desferrioxamine is not recommended. Serum iron levels and iron-binding capacity should be measured if possible 4–6 h postingestion. A serum iron above $55 \, \mu mol \, l^{-1}$ is usually toxic and a serum iron considerably greater than serum iron-binding capacity indicates serious toxicity. If there are only minimal symptoms by 6 h after ingestion, the patient can be sent home and late sequelae should not be anticipated.

If the plasma iron is in the toxic range or the patient is symptomatic, 1 g of desferrioxamine in 5 ml of water should be injected intramuscularly and desferrioxamine $15 \, mg \, kg^{-1} \, h^{-1}$ is given by infusion. Adequate urine flow should be ensured, otherwise the ferrioxamine chelate is not excreted and may cause toxicity. Haemodialysis or peritoneal dialysis are therefore required if the patient is developing renal failure. Ferrioxamine chelate gives the urine a red or *vin rosé* colour so a test dose may be used to confirm the presence of toxic amounts of drug and the need for continued treatment. The management of iron poisoning has been well reviewed.

Theophylline

Most formulations are sustained-release. The patient may be asymptomatic or mildly symptomatic on presentation, but treatment is urgent, because deterioration is common (Goldberg *et al.*, 1986).

Clinical features

Symptoms may develop over several hours and include vomiting, abdominal pain, haematemesis, irritability, hyperventilation, convulsions, hypokalaemia and hyperglycaemia. Cardiovascular signs include sinus tachycardia, hypotension and cardiac arrhythmias (most commonly supraventricular tachycardia).

Management

If vomiting has not occurred, activated charcoal (10 g for a child and 50 g for an adult) should be given and repeated after 4 h; severe vomiting should be suppressed by metoclopramide 10–40 mg IV or ondansetron. In an adult, a dose of over 5 g should be considered life-threatening and may well exceed the adsorbent capacity of activated charcoal. Haemodialysis or haemoperfusion should be considered.

A plasma theophylline level should be obtained where possible. Over $40 \, mg \, l^{-1}$ is a potentially severely toxic plasma level after acute overdose. Plasma potassium and blood glucose should also be measured. Hypokalaemia should be treated with a potassium chloride infusion in asthmatic patients, but propranolol can reverse both the haemodynamic and metabolic changes in non-asthmatic patients. An infusion of 5–10 mg can be given intravenously over 1 h, and may be repeated if necessary. The patient must be monitored. Esmolol, a short-acting beta-blocker, may be indicated to control intractable arrhythmias even in asthmatic patients.

Convulsions should be treated with intravenous diazepam. If there are serious symptoms (such as convulsions or cardiac arrhythmias), charcoal haemoperfusion or haemodialysis should be considered to remove theophylline from the bloodstream.

Chloroquine

This antimalarial and antirheumatic drug can cause serious toxicity in overdose (Jaeger *et al.*, 1987), with cardiovascular collapse, hypoxic convulsions and hypokalaemia. Serious and possibly fatal toxicity may occur following a dose of over 5 g (adult) or a blood chloroquine concentration over $25 \, mol \, l^{-1}$ producing a systolic blood pressure less than 85 mmHg, QRS complex duration over 0.12 sec.

The patient should be resuscitated and given external chest compression for cardiac support if necessary. A regimen of adrenaline and diazepam has been effective in resuscitating potentially fatal cases (Riou *et al.*, 1988).

CARDIOPULMONARY RESUSCITATION IN POISONING

In the patient who is apnoeic or pulseless, the most urgent measure is to re-establish ventilation and circulation by cardiopulmonary resuscitation (CPR). Once this is done effectively, the opportunity may be taken to treat the cause of the problem. In some cases certain antidotes can be given which will reverse the effects of the poisoning during the course of CPR. Examples include naloxone, atropine, cyanide antidotes or digoxin-specific Fab antibodies (Table 5). Other poisons are capable of producing cardiac arrest, intractable arrhythmias or electromechanical dissociation which cannot be reversed by the usual resuscitative measures. In these cases it may be worth persisting with resuscitation if necessary for several hours until spontaneous cardiac output returns as the drug or poison is metabolized by the body. There have been several case reports of the successful use of prolonged external chest compression in tricyclic antidepressant poisoning, where the patient had severe hypotension or asystole (Orr & Bramble. 1981). Prolonged CPR has also been used successfully in poisoning by beta-blockers, quinine, chloroquine and digoxin, local anaesthetics and also in hypothermia, which may complicate poisoning. The hypothermic poisoned patient can usually be re-warmed relatively quickly (see Chapter 38). Prolonged resuscitative efforts are therefore indicated in many types of poisoning which are refractory to other treatments.

If the patient is profoundly hypotensive, the response to a fluid challenge (500 ml of saline given rapidly intravenously) may indicate that hypovolaemia is the major problem and further volume replacement should be given as required. In other cases the problem may be a negative inotropic effect depressing the heart, and inotropic agents will be indicated (dopamine, dobutamine and glucagon). If the blood pressure is very low or unrecordable, it may be necessary to support cardiac output with external chest compressions until the cardiac output can be restored by other means. Respiratory depression due to sedative and hypnotic agents produces shallow respiration; that from opioids produces slow or irregular respiration. Intravenous naloxone can be used to reverse opioid poisoning but, in other cases, assisted ventilation may be required urgently to prevent hypoxic cerebral damage.

CONTACTING AND USING POISONS CENTRES

In Britain and many other countries there is a network of poisons centres which provide information and advice on the toxicity, symptoms and management of poisoning. Several centres in the UK provide a 24-h service. Enquiries may be answered in the first instance by trained information staff with physicians available when a medical opinion is needed. Some centres also provide a laboratory analytical service, while others stock specialized antidotes.

Telephone calls to a poisons centre

The caller should be ready to give the name of the suspected agent(s) involved as accurately as possible. Since the manufacturer's name or other details may also be needed, container(s) should if possible be at hand. In addition, the following information is usually required:

- The patient's name, age and weight (in kg).
- Time of exposure.
- Any apparent signs or symptoms.
- Treatment already given.

In Britain, the emergency information service answers inquiries only from hospitals, general practitioners, and other emergency services. The caller may subsequently receive a follow-up questionnaire requesting information regarding the outcome of the poisoning. This should be filled in and returned to the information service as it is essential for improving our knowledge and understanding of acute poisoning in man, especially where new or uncommon compounds are involved.

APPENDIX: National Poisons Information Service–UK

Poisons Information Centre
Royal Group of Hospitals
Grosvenor Road
BELFAST BT12 6BA

Tel. 01232 240503
Fax. 01232 249261

National Poisons Information Service (London)
Medical Toxicology Unit
Avonley Road
LONDON SE14 5ER
Tel. 0171 635 9191
Fax. 0171 635 1056

West Midlands Poisons Unit
City Hospital NHS Trust
Dudley Road
BIRMINGHAM
B18 7QH

Tel. 0121 554 3801
Fax. 0121 523 652

Leeds Poisons Information Service
Pharmacy Department
The General Infirmary
Great George St
LEEDS
LS1 3EX

Tel. 0113 243 0715
Fax. 0113 244 5849

Welsh National Poisons Unit
Ward West 5
Llandough Hospital
PENARTH
S GLAMORGAN
CF6 1XX

Tel. 01222 709901
Fax. 01222 704357

Scottish Poisons Information Bureau
The Royal Infirmary
Lauriston Place
EDINBURGH
EH3 9YW

Tel. 0131 229 2477
Fax. 0131 228 3332

Northern Regional Drug and Therapeutics Centre
Wolfson Unit
Claremont Place
NEWCASTLE-UPON-TYNE
NE1 4LP

Tel. 0191 232 5131
Fax. 0191 232 3613

Bibliography

ALI ZAGAR, S., KOCHLAR, R., MEHTA, S. *et al.* (1991). The role of fibreoptic endoscopy in the management of corrosive ingestion and modified endoscopic classification of burns. *Gastrointest. Endosc.,* **37**, 165–9.

ANDERSON, H.R. (1990). Increase in deaths from deliberate inhalation of fuel gases and pressurised aerosols (Letter). *Br. Med. J.,* **301**, 6742.

BAUD, F.J., BARRIOT, P., TOFFIS, V. *et al.* (1991). Elevated blood cyanide concentrations in victims of smoke inhalation. *N. Engl. J. Med.,* **325**, 1761–66.

BISMUTH, C., CANTINEAU, J.P., PONTAL, P. *et al.* (1984). Cyanide poisoning. Priority to symptomatic treatment. 25 cases. *Presse Med.,* **13**, 2493–7. (in French).

BOEHNERT, M.T., & LOVEJOY, F.N. (1985). Value of the QRS duration versus the serum drug level predicting seizures and ventricular arrhythmias after an acute overdose of tricyclic antidepressants. *N. Engl. J. Med.,* **313**, 474–9.

BROWN, T.C., BARKER, G.A. & DUNLOP, M.G. (1973). The use of sodium bicarbonate in the treatment of tricyclic antidepressant-induced arrhythmias. *Anaesth. Intensive Care,* **1**, 203–10.

COOPER, M.R. & JOHNSON, A.W. (1984). *Poisonous plants in Britain and their effects on animals and man.* (MAFF Reference Book 161.) London: HMSO.

CRAWFORD, R., CAMPBELL, D.G.D. & ROSS, J. (1990). Carbon monoxide poisoning in the home: recognition and treatment. *Br. Med. J.,* **301**, 977–9.

CRITCHLEY, J.A. & UNGAR, A. (1989). The management of acute poisoning due to beta-adrenergic antagonists. *Med. Toxicol.* **4**, 32–45.

CROUZETTE, J., VICAUT, E., PALOMBO, S. *et al.* (1983). Experimental assessment of the protective activity of diazepam on the acute toxicity of chloroquine. *J. Clin. Toxicol.* **20**, 271–9.

DALLY, S., GARNIER, R. & BISMUTH, C. (1987). Diagnosis of chlorinated hydrocarbon poisoning by X-ray examination. *B. J. Indust. Medi.,* **44**, 424–5.

DUPUIS, R.E., LICHTMAN, S.N. & POLLACK, G.M. (1990). Acute valproic acid overdose–clinical course and pharmacokinetic disposition of valproic acid and metabolites. *Drug Safety,* **5**, 65–71.

FLANAGAN, R.J., MEREDITH, T.J., RUPRAH, M. *et al.* (1990). Alkaline diuresis for acute poisoning with chlorophenoxy herbicides and ioxynil. *Lancet,* **335**, 454–60.

GIBB, I., ADAMS, P.C., PARNHAM, A. J. *et al.* (1983). Plasma digoxin: assay anomalies in Fab-treated patients. *B. J. Clin. Pharmacol.* **16**, 445–7.

GOLDBERG, M.J., PARK, G.D. & BERLINGER, W. G. (1986). Treatment of theophylline overdose. *J. Allergy Clin. Immunol.,* **78**, 811–17.

HALL, A.H., KULIG, K.W. & RUMACK, B.W. (1986). Drug and chemical induced methaemoglobinaemia. Clinical features and management. *Med. Toxicol.,* **1**, 253–60.

HARRISON, P.M., KEAYS, R., BRAY, G.P. *et al.* (1990). Improved outcome of paracetamol-induced fulminant hepatic failure by late administration of acetylcysteine. *Lancet,* **335**, 1572–3.

HENRY, J.A., JEFFREYS, K.J. & DAWLING, S. (1992). Toxicity and deaths from 3,4-methylenedioxymeth-amphetamine ('ecstasy'). *Lancet*, **ii**, 384–7.

JACOBSEN, D. & McMARTIN, K.E. (1986). Methanol and ethylene glycol poisonings. Mechanism of toxicity, clinical course, diagnosis and treatment. *Med. Toxicol.*, **1**, 309–34.

JAEGER, A., SAUDIER, P., KOPFERSCHMITT, J. *et al.* (1987). Clinical features and management of poisoning due to antimalarial drugs. *Med. Toxicol.*, **2**, 242–73.

KEAYS, R., HARRISON, P.M., WENDON, J.A. *et al.* (1991). Intravenous acetylcysteine in paracetamol induced fulminant hepatic failure: a prospective study. *Br. Med. J.*, **303**, 1026–9.

KRAUSE, D.S., WOLF, B.A. & SHAW, L.M. (1992). Acute aspirin overdose: mechanisms of toxicity. *Ther. Drug. Monit.*, **14**, 441–51.

KULIG, K., BAR-OR, D., CANTRILL, S.V. *et al.* (1985). Management of acutely poisoned patients without gastric emptying. *Ann. Emerg. Med.*, **14**, 562–7.

LANG, D.C. (1987). *The Complete Book of British Berries*. London: Threshold Books.

LANGFORD, R.M. & ARMSTRONG, R.F. (1989). Algorithm for managing injury from smoke inhalation. *Br. Med. J.*, **299**, 902–5.

LHEUREUX, P. & ASKENASI, R. (1988). Specific treatment of benzodiazepine overdose. *Hum. Toxicol.*, **7**, 165–70.

LINDEN, C.H., KULIG, K.W. & RUMACK, B.H. (1985). Amphetamines. *Trends Emerg. Med.*, **7**, 18–32.

MARRS, T.C. (1988). Antidotal treatment of acute cyanide poisoning. *Adverse Drug React. Acute Poisoning Rev.*, **4**, 179–206.

MATHIEU, D., NOLF, M., DUROCHER, A. *et al.* (1985). Acute carbon monoxide poisoning. Risk of late sequelae and treatment by hyperbaric oxygen. *Clin. Toxicol.*, **23**, 315–24.

MAURO, L.S., MAURO, V.F., BROWN, D.L. *et al.* (1987). Enhancement of phenytoin elimination by multiple-dose activated charcoal. *Ann. Emerg. Med.*, **16**, 1132–5.

MCELHATTON, P.R., ROBERTS, J.C. & SULLIVAN, F.M.(1991). The consequences of iron overdose and its treatment with desferrioxamine in pregnancy. *Hum. Exp. Toxicol.*, **10**, 251–9.

MOLLOY, D.W., PENNER, S.B., RABSON, J. *et al.* (1984). Use of bicarbonate to treat tricyclic antidepressant-induced arrhythmias in a patient with alkalosis. *Can. Med. Assoc. J.*, **130**, 1457–9.

NORKOOL, D.M. & KIRKPATRICK, J.N. (1985). Treatment of acute carbon monoxide poisoning with hyperbaric oxygen: a review of 115 cases. *Ann. Emerg. Med.*, **14**, 1168–71.

NOTARIANNI, L. (1992). A reassessment of the treatment of salicylate poisoning. *Drug Safety*, **7**, 292–303.

OLSON, K.R., PENTEL, P.R. & KELLEY, M.T. (1987). Physical assessment and differential diagnosis of the poisoned patient. *Med. Toxicol.*, **2**, 52–81.

ORR, D.A. & BRAMBLE, M.G. (1981). Tricyclic antidepressant poisoning and prolonged external massage during asystole. *Br. Med. J.*, **283**, 1107–8.

PALATNICK, W. & TENENBEIN, M. (1992). Activated charcoal in the treatment of drug overdose. An update. *Drug Safety*, **7**, 3–7.

PENTEL, P.R. & BENOWITZ, N.L. (1986). Tricyclic antidepressant poisoning: management of arrhythmias. *Med. Toxicol.*, **1**, 101–21.

POLLACK, C.V., JORDEN, R.C., CARLTON, F.B. *et al.* (1992). Gastric emptying in the acutely inebriated patient. *J. Emerg. Med.*, **10**, 1–5.

PROCTOR, N.H., HUGHES, J.P. & FISCHMAN, M.L. (1988). *Chemical Hazards of the Workplace*, 2nd edn. Philadelphia: J.B. Lippincott.

PROUDFOOT, A.T., SIMPSON, D. & DYSON, E.H. (1986). Management of acute iron poisoning. *Med. Toxicol.*, **1**, 83–100.

RIGGS, B.S., BRONSTEIN, A.C., KULIG, K. *et al.* (1989). Acute acetaminophen overdose during pregnancy. *Obstet. Gynecol.*, **74**, 247–53.

RIOU, B., BARRIOT, P., RIMAILHO, A. *et al.* (1988). Treatment of severe chloroquine poisoning. *N. Engl. J. Med.*, **318**, 1–6.

SAETTA, J.P. & QUINTON, D.N. (1991). Residual gastric content after gastric lavage and ipecacuanha-induced emesis in self-poisoned patients: an endoscopic study. *J. R. Soc. Med.*, **84**, 35–8.

SAETTA, J.P., MARSH, S., GAUNT, M.E. *et al.* (1991). Gastric emptying procedures in the self-poisoned patients: are we forcing gastric contents beyond the pylorus? *J. R. Soc. Med.*, **84**, 274–6.

SCHAUBEN, J.L., AUGENSTEIN, L., COX, J. *et al.* (1990). Iron poisoning: report of three cases and a review of therapeutic intervention. *J. Emerg. Med.*, **8**, 309–19.

SHANNON, M., FISH, S.S. & LOVEJOY, F.H. (1986). Cathartics and laxatives. Do they still have a place in the management of the poisoned patient? *Med. Toxicol.*, **1**, 247–52.

SMITH, T.W., BUTLER, V.P. JR., HABER, *et al.* (1982). Treatment of life-threatening digitalis intoxication with digoxin-specific Fab antibody fragments. Experience in 26 cases. *N. Engl. J. Med.*, **307**, 1357–62.

SWARTZ, C.M. & SHERMAN, A. (1984). The treatment of tricyclic antidepressant overdose with repeated charcoal. *J. Clin. Psychopharmacol.*, **4**, 336–40.

TENENBEIN, M. (1988). Whole bowel irrigation as a gastrointestinal decontamination procedure after acute poisoning. *Med. Toxicol.*, **3**, 77–84.

URSO, T., GAVALER, J.S. & VAN-THIEL, D.H. (1981). Blood ethanol levels in sober alcohol users seen in an emergency room. *Life Sci.*, **28**, 1053–6.

VALE, J.A. & PROUDFOOT, A.T. (1993). How useful is activated charcoal? *Br. Med. J.*, **306**, 78–9.

VOTEY, S.R., BOSSE, G.M., BAYER, M.J. *et al.* (1991). Flumazenil – a new benzodiazepine antagonist. *Ann. Emerg. Med.*, **20**, 181–8.

WEINSTEIN, R.S. (1984). Recognition and management of poisoning with beta adrenergic blocking agents. *Ann. Emerg. Med.*, **13**, 1123–31.

WEISS, L.D. & VAN METER, K.W. (1992). The applications of hyperbaric oxygen therapy in emergency medicine. *Am. J. Emerg. Med.*, **10**, 558–68.

WHEELER-USHER, D.H., WANKE, L.A. & BAYER, M.J. (1986). Gastric emptying. Risk versus benefit in the treatment of acute poisoning. *Med. Toxicol.*, **1**, 142–53.

ZUCKER, A.R., LACINA, S.J., DAS-GUPTA, D.S. *et al.* (1982). Fab fragments of digoxin-specific antibodies used to reverse ventricular fibrillation induced by digoxin ingestion in a child. *Pediatrics*, **70**, 468–71.

12 Wound care

J. HEYWORTH

Accident and Emergency Department, Southampton General Hospital, Southampton, UK

Chapter plan

Introduction
History
Examination
Wound healing
Wound management
Cross-infection of healthcare workers
Special wounds

INTRODUCTION

Wound care should prevent infection and achieve rapid healing with minimal scarring allowing early return to normal function. This chapter will discuss the early management of wounds commonly seen in emergency medicine.

Approximately 3 million patients with wounds are seen annually in UK accident and emergency (A&E) departments and 10 million patients in US emergency departments. Wound infection occurs in less than 10% but has a detrimental effect on healing, tissue strength and cosmesis (Lammers *et al.*, 1992). A standardized approach to wound care has yet to be established, in part because of the lack of statistically powerful clinical studies. Many practitioners rely on personal experience and preference using a variety of practices contrary to current literature and recommendations. These include using 10% povidone-iodine or hydrogen peroxide to cleanse wounds, irrigating wounds under the 5–8 p.s.i. necessary for adequate tissue cleansing, infrequent use of delayed primary closure, inappropriate antibiotic usage, and a variety of dressings (Berk *et al.*, 1992; Howell & Chisholm, 1992).

HISTORY

When did the wound occur?

Bacteria proliferate during the first 6 h, but the time from injury should never be the sole determinant of management. A facial laceration from a knife wound may be safely closed 36 h after injury but a blunt injury to the foot of an elderly diabetic may be unsafe to suture even 1 h after injury.

The question of whether a simple wound presenting for care later than 12–24 h after injury can be closed safely is unresolved. Orthodox teaching suggests a period ranging from 6 to 24 h, during which primary closure may be accomplished with a high degree of success, after which should follow serial dressing changes and antibiotics.

A 19-h golden period has been suggested for repair of simple wounds involving body areas other than the head, after which sutured wounds are significantly less likely to heal. Clean simple wounds involving the head are unaffected by the interval between injury and repair (Berk *et al.*, 1988).

All wounds should be evaluated individually with treatment based on the mechanism and circumstances of injury, degree of contamination and the clinician's evaluation of the wound. (Batchelor, 1988; Edlich *et al.*, 1988).

What was the mechanism of injury?

This indicates risk factors for damage to underlying structures, infection or retained foreign body. Saliva, faeces and organic soils deliver concentrated bacterial inocula. Clay-containing soils impair host defence mechanisms but sandy soils present low risk.

Age of the patient

Children heal rapidly although the appearance of the final scar is critical, particularly with facial wounds. In elderly patients looser skin allows wound apposition for closure but infection is more common.

General health

Patients with pretibial lacerations who have malnutrition, lower limb oedema, diabetes, etc., heal slowly with increased risk of infection.

Current medication

Steroids disrupt macrophage function, collagen synthesis and cause immune suppression. Immunosuppressive therapy prolongs healing time and increases susceptibility to infection.

EXAMINATION

Nature of the wound

Wounds are tidy or untidy depending on the degree of contamination. Wounds colonized by fewer than 10^5 organisms g^{-1} wound tissue have a favourable prognosis while those above this are at high risk of infection.

A method for rapidly identifying wounds contaminated by greater than 10^5 bacteria g^{-1} has been described, using microscopic examination of a slide specimen of wound biopsy sample (Robson & Heggers, 1969). Wounds contaminated with pus, faeces, saliva and vaginal secretions invariably become infected. Silk sutures dramatically reduce the number of bacteria necessary to produce infection.

Wound Classification

- *Laceration*
  - Incised lacerations – heal well with low risk of infection, but damage to vessels, tendons or nerves may occur.
  - Flap laceration, e.g. pretibial wounds.
- *Contused Wound.* Wounds with crushed and devitalized tissue have an increased susceptibility to infection. Blunt injuries result in microvascular disruption, oedema and devitalization of tissue (Rutherford & Spence, 1980). Lower bacterial loads ($<10^4$ organisms g^{-1} tissue) may cause infection. Devitalized tissue must be excised and ragged skin edges trimmed. Stellate

---

Nature of wounds.

Tidy Wound
- Clean incision
- Uncontaminated
- Less than 6 h old
- Low-energy trauma

Note: May be deep

Untidy Wound
- Ragged edge
- Contaminated
- More than 12 h old
- High-energy trauma
- Crushed tissue
- Burns

Note: High risk of infection if treatment inadequate

---

lacerations with abrasions of the skin adjacent to the wound are prone to infection, especially those greater than 5 cm in length.
- *Puncture Wound.*
- *Bites*–animal or human.
- *Degloving wounds*, e.g. ring finger injuries.
- *Abrasions.* Embedded dirt will cause tattooing unless removed.

Site of the wound

The infection rate is least in head and neck wounds, worst in the legs and feet and intermediate in the arms and hands (Cruse, 1973).

Wounds of the face heal well but optimal cosmetic outcome must be ensured in all age groups. Wounds over extensor surfaces of joints (e.g. the elbow and knee) will dehisce if the sutures are removed before healing has occurred and the joint is allowed to return to a full range of movement. Longitudinal wounds over the flexor aspects of joints, in particular the fingers, may develop contracture as the scar matures, requiring surgery to release the contracture and restore movement and function.

Scalp

The scalp is extremely vascular and haemostasis difficult. Elevate the head of the bed, apply pressure and infiltrate with lignocaine and adrenaline. Clips may be required or closure with interrupted 3/0 or 4/0 synthetic monofilament non-absorbable sutures.

Face

Minimize scarring by avoiding uneven wound edges and using layered closures. Failure to approximate the vermilion curve of the lip leaving a step of even 2 mm gives a poor cosmetic result. Repair should only be undertaken by experienced staff in optimal conditions; refer if necessary.

Mouth

Only gaping or actively haemorrhaging mucosal or tongue lacerations need be closed.

Damage to underlying structures

The key to assessment is the mechanism of injury. A laceration to the palm on broken glass, for example, poses a risk of damage to tendons, nerves and vessels. Function in all nerves and tendons which could conceivably have been involved must be tested and documented for future reference.

Function in a partially divided tendon may be present on initial examination but when the tendon is stressed later, division is completed and function lost. Division of a digital nerve is not always followed by immediate loss of sensation, although altered sensation occurs within a few hours. For these patients consider exploration of the wound in theatre by senior staff to ensure that significant injury is not missed and that the potential for further harm is avoided.

Penetrating wounds may involve underlying joints (e.g. the knee or human closed-fist bite injuries involving metacarpophalangeal joints). Examination may give little indication of the extent of the injury. Diagnosis depends on the mechanism of injury and its precise location, and it may be confirmed by intracapsular air on X-ray. These wounds should be referred to orthopaedic surgeons for exploration and irrigation to prevent infection and septic arthritis.

WOUND HEALING

There are three types of wound healing.

In *first intention* or *primary healing* wound edges are reapproximated immediately. The gap across the wound is small so little granulation tissue forms and a thin scar results with minimal deformity (Dimick, 1988). This is ideal wound healing. The fibrin network initially bonds the wound and is invaded by fibroblasts on about the fifth day after injury. Epidermal continuity is restored after 48–72 h. Platelets produce growth factors which summon fibroblasts and smooth muscle cells to wounded tissue, stimulate fibroblasts and facilitate both epithelialization and the formation of new blood vessels. Macrophages, lymphocytes, fibroblasts, smooth muscle cells and endothelial cells produce small peptide growth factors. Fibroblast growth factor combined with a collagen carrier has been used topically to stimulate wound repair. Healing times of skin graft sites treated with epidermal growth factor were significantly shorter (Howell, 1992).

In *second intention healing* the wound is left open because of gross contamination or a soft tissue defect which precludes closure. The wound fills with granulation tissue – capillary vessels, fibroblasts and collagen. Contraction of the edges of the wound by myofibroblasts and migration of the epithelium from the wound margin occur by up to 80% over 2 weeks in an attempt to cover the granulation tissue bed. A lag phase of 2–3 days is followed by a period of rapid contraction which is almost complete by 14 days. The combination of contraction and epithelialization ultimately results in closure of the wound. The resulting scar is larger than in primary healing and the deformity is greater. Once the wound is healthy skin grafts can be used to cover the residual defect. (Hunt, 1988; Rigby, 1992).

Third intention healing or *delayed primary closure* occurs when the wound is left open for 4–5 days. When oedema has subsided, no infection is present and all debris and exudates have been removed, the wound can be closed primarily as in first intention healing leaving minimal tissue defect. The final scars are identical to those following primary closure.

Factors to be considered in the decision to close primarily or delay repair

Host factors
- Age
- General health/nutritional state
- Presence of immunocompromising conditions
- Medication

Likelihood of significant bacterial contamination
- Degree of contamination by soil or other organic debris
- Time since injury
- Mechanism of injury
- Site of wound

Abnormal healing

Keloid is a large, thick scar exceeding the size of the original wound. Keloids are more frequent in adolescents, pregnant women and patients with deeply pigmented skin. Collagen formation exceeds collagen breakdown, possibly because of melanocyte stimulating hormones.

Hypertrophic scars are abnormally thick but do not extend beyond the limits of the original injury and tend to occur over joints (e.g. knees and shoulders) or in wounds overlying the sternum (as do keloids). Hypertrophic scars involute with time.

WOUND MANAGEMENT

Local anaesthesia

Most wounds in the A & E department can be managed with local anaesthesia although for some procedures this is impractical or impossible (e.g. cleansing and debridement of extensive or complicated lacerations and abrasions) (Norris, 1992).

Local anaesthetics

Lignocaine

Lignocaine is the most widely used local anaesthetic. It acts more rapidly and is more stable than other local anaesthetics.

The addition of a vasoconstrictor such as adrenaline diminishes local blood flow, slows the rate of absorption of the local anaesthetic, and prolongs the local effect (Todd *et al.*, 1992). However, adrenaline has undesirable potential effects; for example, the infection rate in contaminated wounds is increased, presumably due to vasospasm-induced local ischaemia (Table 1).

Subcutaneous injection of lignocaine is amongst the safest procedures in emergency medicine. The maximum dose of $5–7$ mg kg^{-1} appears virtually completely safe with no reported dose-dependent fatalities (see Table 2). Trauma-induced vasoconstriction decreases lignocaine absorption.

Toxicity is manifested first by the central nervous system (CNS) with light-headedness, dizziness, nystagmus, sensory disturbance, slurred speech and seizures. At higher blood levels, cardiovascular changes occur, with hypotension, bradycardia, prolonged ECG (electrocardiographic) intervals and cardiac arrest. The most common complication is hypotension and bradycardia – a vasovagal reaction. Lignocaine should always be

Table 1. *Complications of adrenaline*

Increases
– infiltration pain
– wound inflammation
– wound infection   DO NOT USE IN
                      CONTAMINATED WOUNDS

Tissue ischaemia
  digits
  tip of nose
  pinna   } NEVER USE HERE
  penis

Palpitations, tremor, syncope

CAUTION
  Elderly
  Coronary artery disease
  Hypertension
  Hyperthyroidism
  Phaeochromocytoma
  Beta-blockers

Table 2. *Maximum dose mg kg^{-1} (and maximum adult dose, mg) of local anaesthetics*

	Lignocaine	Bupivacaine
Plain	4 (300)	2 (175)
With adrenaline	7 (500)	3 (250)
Duration (mins)	90–200	180–600

administered when the patient is supine. If there is a true history of allergy, subcutaneous infiltration of injectable diphenhydramine $0.5–1\%$ solution provides brief adequate analgesia for some procedures.

Lignocaine depresses the cellular synthesis of mucopolysaccharides and collagen. Fibroblast growth and motility are inhibited by lignocaine and bupivacaine (Sturrock & Nunn, 1979). Lignocaine in a concentration of 0.5% does not impair wound healing to any greater extent than water (Morris & Tracey, 1977).

Bupivacaine

The duration of local anaesthesia induced by bupivacaine is nearly four times longer than for lignocaine (Table 2) but it takes 30 min for full effect (Reichl & Quinton, 1987; Spivey et al, 1987). Bupivacaine is useful for facial wounds where duration of anaesthetic is diminished compared to other sites.

Techniques of local anaesthesia

Infiltration anaesthesia

Infiltration anaesthesia is the simplest and most practical technique. Pain is minimized by applying pressure to the site undergoing injection, injecting slowly, anaesthetizing as much tissue as possible through a single site and, on extremities, starting proximally and moving distally. Injecting from within the wound is less painful than injection of subcutaneous tissue through intact skin, but the latter is preferable when the wound is untidy. Rapid injection (less than 2 sec) into the dermal or subdermal tissue causes significantly more pain than when the same volume of anaesthetic is instilled slowly over 10 sec. The flow rate can be limited by using large-bore syringes (over 10 ml) and the smallest internal diameter needles (25 gauge or smaller). Long needles decrease the number of times tissues must be punctured.

Buffering the lignocaine with sodium bicarbonate (1 ml to 10 ml of 1% lignocaine) further enhances pain reduction (McGlone & Bodenham, 1990). Local anaesthetics are manufactured with an acidic pH to enhance shelf-life. Buffered lignocaine remains effective for at least 1 week, maintaining a pH of 7.38–7.41 when stored at room temperature. Buffering does not affect the degree or duration of anaesthesia (Bartfield et al., 1990, 1993).

Reduce pain of injection

- Apply local pressure
- Inject slowly within wound
- Small-gauge long needles
- Buffer lignocaine
- Avoid adrenaline

Topical anaesthesia

Topical anaesthesia is an attractive alternative, particularly in the management of children with simple wounds of 5 cm or less on the face or scalp (Grant & Hoffman, 1992). The effects are less in trunk or extremity wounds and in adults. A solution containing 0.5% tetracaine, 1:2000 adrenaline and 11.8% cocaine (TAC) is used in the U.S.A. Compared with lignocaine infiltration it provides equivalent anaesthesia, reduction in time required for repair of paediatric wounds, enhanced patient acceptance and less tissue distortion allowing accurate repair (Anderson et al., 1990; Hegenbarth et al., 1990). Discomfort associated with injection and the need for sedation in children are avoided. The solution (maximum 5 ml in adults) is applied for 15–20 min or until visible blanching occurs – indicating adequate anaesthesia. On extremities, TAC may be used as an adjunct to lignocaine (Bonadio & Wagner, 1992).

The inclusion of vasoconstricting adrenaline and cocaine is a contraindication to the use of TAC in contaminated wounds because of the risk of infection (Martin et al., 1990). Cocaine overdose may occur secondary to mucosal absorption causing CNS toxicity or death (Fitzmaurice et al., 1990). Therefore TAC should not be used on mucosal surfaces, denuded or burned skin, or in areas that can be reached by children's mouths. Eye contact can produce corneal damage. TAC is contraindicated in regions of end artery flow (i.e. digits, nose, pinna and penis) because of the intense vasoconstriction. The solution is not approved by the US Food and Drug Administration (FDA).

Anaesthesia for burns and abrasions can be achieved using 2% lignocaine gel. Care must be taken to avoid toxicity from absorption.

Nerve blocks

Regional, digital or field blocks avoid wound distortion and facilitate approximation of wound edges.

Techniques for anaesthesia of fingers include:

- Transthecal digital nerve block by palmar percutaneous injection of local anaesthetic into the flexor tendon sheath resulting in rapid total anaesthesia of the digit (Morrison, 1993).
- Digital and metacarpal blocks – each are equally painful although digital nerve block is more efficacious and requires significantly less time to anaesthesia.
- Transcutaneous electrical nerve stimulation significantly reduced the pain of lancet-induced trauma to the fingertip by stimulation of the digital nerve (Webster, et al., 1992).

Sedation

Anxiety occurs in all age groups, especially in young children, from needle phobia, fear of pain, separation from parents or physical restraint to prevent sudden movement. Lacerations requiring sutures account for one-third of all childhood injuries presenting to A&E

departments (Proudfoot *et al.*, 1993; Berman & Graber, 1992).

Local anaesthesia and a calm, reassuring manner in a quiet, dedicated treatment area often attenuate fears. The ideal drug should provide ease of administration, rapid onset, effective analgesia and sedation, minimal cardiac and respiratory effects, stable airway maintenance and a broad margin of safety with rapid, smooth recovery. Parenteral administration should be intravenous, not intramuscular – which is painful with variable onset of clinical effect.

Sedatives commonly used for children in the UK include oral promethazine 15–25 mg or trimeprazine up to 2 mg kg^{-1}. Adequate sedation to allow optimal wound repair, especially of complex facial lacerations or large wounds, is difficult and general anaesthesia in theatre is recommended.

Benzodiazepines provide excellent sedation, hypnosis, amnesia and muscle relaxation. In the past diazepam (administered intravenously or rectally) has been the most widely used benzodiazepine but midazolam causes less pain on injection, a significantly greater degree of early sedation and more rapid return to baseline function (Wright *et al.*, 1993). Midazolam is a safe and effective anxiolytic agent. The intravenous dose is 0.07 mg kg^{-1}, although under 2 mg may provide adequate sedation in adults. Sedation occurs within 3–5 min and lasts 20–30 min (Taiwo *et al.*, 1992).

Although available only for intravenous or intramuscular use in the UK, studies from the USA report safe and effective oral, rectal and intranasal administration of midazolam (Hennes *et al.*, 1990; Yealy *et al.*, 1992). Respiratory depression can occur, leading rapidly to hypoxaemia in young children because of their small functional residual capacity and high oxygen consumption. Pulse oximetry and heart rate should be monitored continuously. The benzodiazepine reversal agent flumazenil must be available.

Oral midazolam 0.6 mg kg^{-1} (in 20–30 mls of clear juice to mask the bitter taste) provides sedation in 10–15 min and lasting 60 min.

Hypnosis, nitrous oxide and intramuscular meperidine with promethazine and chlorpromazine (MPC) have proved unreliable. Nitrous oxide is a safe sedative and analgesic which may reduce pain during laceration repair only in children more than 8 years old. Analgesia begins 20 seconds after the onset of inhalation.

Fentanyl is an opioid of rapid onset (within 90 sec) and short duration of action (30–60 min) when given intravenously in children (1–3 µg kg^{-1}) and in adults (100–250 µg kg^{-1}). Adverse effects include bradycardia and respiratory depression, which can be reversed by naloxone (Lind *et al.*, 1991).

Intranasal administration is safe and non-invasive; 95% of children had significant sedation (mean duration 62 min) and analgesia (Essells & Jones, 1993). Intranasal sufentanil and midazolam were as effective as MPC for sedation with more rapid recovery (Bates *et al.*, 1993).

Ketamine has been reported as a safe and effective analgesic and sedative agent for paediatric sedation whilst maintaining airway reflexes. Potential side effects, however, include respiratory arrest, laryngospasm, muscular hypertonicity and emergence reactions (Smith & Santer, 1993). These frightening hallucinations are more common with rapid intravenous use in patients over 10 years of age but they can be averted with benzodiazepines. The common dose used for paediatric sedation, 1–2 mg kg^{-1} I/V, provides sedation in 30 sec, lasting for 5–10 min. Ketamine may be useful for children with wounds of the tongue, lip or ear, dirty abrasions, burns or foreign bodies (Green *et al.*, 1990).

Music played through headphones during laceration repair in adults provides a safe, inexpensive and effective adjunct to lower pain by distracting from the pain stimulus, but does not affect anxiety (Menegazzi *et al.*, 1991). The possibility of inserting a subliminal message (e.g. 'I feel no pain') may be beneficial.

TECHNIQUE

SEDATION IN CHILDREN

1. Calm the child
   - parents present
   - quiet pleasant room
   - minimise pain of local anaesthetic infiltration
   - gentle but firm restraint
2. Consider general anaesthesia – large or complex wounds/facial lacerations.
3. Sedation
   - ORAL: Promethazine.
            Trimeprazine.
   - INTRAVENOUS: Midazolam – ensure monitoring and resuscitation facilities are available.

Prevent contamination

Hair is a source of contamination and should be removed. This also facilitates wound repair by preventing hair from becoming entangled in the suture and wound during closure. Razor preparation increases wound infection in surgical wounds, presumably due to transection of the infundibula of the hair follicles providing access for bacteria. Shaving has not been shown to increase infection in wounds treated in the A&E department. Surgical clippers are recommended for hair removal. Eyebrows must not be shaved as regrowth may be slow and irregular, and landmarks for repair are lost.

Cleansing

Of minor wounds sutured in A&E departments, 10% become infected. Effective antiseptic prophylaxis is required. Historically, cleansing agents have included cobwebs and faeces, milk and honey, urine, resins and Lister's carbolic acid.

All wounds should undergo some form of cleansing to decrease the bacterial inoculum to levels that can be managed by host defences. Successful management of the contaminated wound must remove contaminants while inflicting minimal injury to the tissue (Chisholm, 1992).

Preparation of skin surrounding simple wounds with antiseptic (e.g. povidone-iodine or chlorhexidine) prior to suture closure is a generally accepted practice. The wound should be protected from the inadvertent entry of detergents which are toxic to fibroblasts.

The application of antiseptics within the wound is debated because of the potential of some agents to damage tissue (Gruber et al., 1975). Hypochlorite and 5% povidone-iodine stop blood flow in the capillary circulation of granulation tissue and repair is delayed (Brennan & Leaper, 1985). Saline and 1% povidone-iodine solution are innocuous.

Hydrogen peroxide has no role as a wound irrigant. It impairs wound healing and has poor bactericidal activity. Chlorinated solutions (e.g. Eusol and Chlorasol) also delay healing due to fibroblast toxicity, delay epithelialization and are irritant (Moore, 1992). The antiseptic effect is lost in the presence of blood, pus and slough.

Irrigation

Irrigation lowers the infection rate in contaminated wounds. Probably the most commonly used wound irrigant is 0.9% saline solution – a safe, inexpensive, non-irritant solution which has no adverse effects on the wound healing. It has no antiseptic qualities, but is an efficient cleaning agent and decreases bacterial loads for all types of wounds. It is ineffective against infection except to dilute the concentration of bacteria (Platt & Bucknall, 1984)

Irrigation fluid is delivered through a 19 gauge needle from a 35 ml syringe to produce 8 p.s.i., which successfully cleanses wounds of small particulate matter, bacteria and soil fractions. Lower pressures will remove larger particulate matter only. High pressures damage tissue defences making the wound more susceptible to infection, and are reserved for heavily contaminated wounds. Lacerations should be irrigated with 250 ml of saline for each 5 cm of laceration, increasing the amount as host or wound risk factors increase. Splatter must be minimized.

Iodine compounds

Iodine compounds have a wide range of bactericidal activity and act rapidly (Gravett et al., 1987). The antibacterial effect is reduced by contact with blood, pus and exudate (Oberg, 1987).

Povidone-iodine 5% solutions are toxic for phagocytic cells and suppress lymphocyte response. However, 1% povidone-iodine irrigation prior to suturing demonstrated no difference in tensile strength or wound histology compared with controls (Mulliken et al., 1980). Povidone-iodine diluted to 1% appears to be effective and safe with no effect on wound healing, microcirculation or fibroblast activity. This should be used in situations of high host or wound risk (Howell et al., 1992).

Povidone-iodine dry powder spray as prophylaxis against wound infection in minor wounds of the forearm and hand showed a statistically significant reduction in infection rate (Bickerstaff & Regnard, 1984; Morgan, 1979).

Initial irrigation with saline, then instillation of 1% povidone-iodine into the wound and gentle cleansing with a sterile gauze swab reduces infection in contaminated wounds significantly. In busy departments this should be done as soon as possible by the triage nurse.

Chlorhexidine

Chlorhexidine is a safe and highly effective agent for wound treatment; 0.5% chlorhexidine has a rapid and wide range of antibacterial activity for Gram-positive and Gram-negative bacteria. It is relatively free from toxicity, has no inhibitory effect on healing of experimental wounds and has a low potential for skin irritation. It maintains the antiseptic effect in the presence of blood and pus.

Antibiotics

Antibiotics may be used topically or to irrigate contaminated wounds, especially if povidone-iodine is contra-indicated (Lindsey, *et al.*, 1982). Penicillin irrigation is superior to saline in lowering the incidence of infection in wounds flooded with 10 ml of 5% solution of sodium benzylpenicillin.

Debridement

Debridement is the most important single factor in the management of the contaminated wound (Haury *et al.*, 1978). Debridement removes tissue heavily contaminated by dirt and bacteria. Macroscopic debris is removed with forceps. Mechanical scrubbing increases wound inflammation and should be avoided unless there is an overwhelming amount of foreign debris. Devitalized tissue is removed by careful excision. When the wound contains specialized tissues (e.g. nerves or tendons), complete excision of the wound may not be feasible. In such cases high-pressure irrigation followed by excision of all fragments of tissue which are not clearly viable is indicated. Devitalized tissue acts as a culture medium promoting bacterial growth and inhibits leucocyte phago-cytosis. Identification of the exact limit of devitalized tissue in a wound may be difficult, especially in muscle. Contractility, the ability of the muscle to bleed, and the colour and consistency of muscle are commonly used. Extensive wound debridement should be performed in an operating theatre.

Closure

Immediate primary closure with complete haemostasis and precise restoration of anatomy should be the aim. Haematoma or the inclusion of dead material in a wound will lead to inflammation, painful slow healing and poor anatomical restoration with an increased volume of scar tissue. The blood supply to the wound tissue is the key to success and repair must not jeopardize blood supply to the wound edges.

Layered closure and elimination of dead space have been advocated to reduce infection. The incidence of infected wounds is, however, consistently proportional to the number of sutured layers, and leaving dead space results in lower rates of infection. Subcutaneous fat stitches also fail to reduce infection rates and placement of subcutaneous sutures result in higher rates of wound infection (De Holl *et al.*, 1974). Deep absorbable sutures

---

Factors which increase scarring

- Healing by secondary intention
- Wound direction perpendicular to lines of static and dynamic skin tension, crease lines or Langer's lines
- Infection
- Wound tension
- Suture marks
- Uneven wound edges
- Inversion of wound edges
- Tattooing secondary to retained dirt
- Tissue necrosis
- Haematoma formation
- Hyperpigmentation of scar or abraded skin
- Failure to align landmark, eg vermilion border.

---

may be placed to repair periosteum, muscle or fascia, and to minimize tension on skin wounds. For cosmesis in deep facial wounds, the wound should be closed in layers.

In most wounds, however, leaving potential dead space appears preferable to attempting to obliterate it. For function, as in hand and foot lacerations, the wound should be closed with a minimal number of sutures in a single layer left in place for up to two weeks.

Sutures

The use of thread for wound closure was described in 1500 BC.

Non-absorbable sutures

Non-absorbable sutures are made from natural braided fibres (e.g. silk), or synthetic monofilaments such as nylon (Ethilon, Dermalon), polypropylene (Prolene) and polybutester (Novafil) (Markovchick, 1992). Silk is easy to tie, has excellent knot security and good initial tensile strength, but it allows the passage of bacteria into the wound by capillary action and excites a local in-flammatory response resulting in red wounds and visible stitch marks. Silk should be avoided in wounds with known bacterial contamination. It has been replaced, except for the closure of oral mucosal lacerations.

Synthetic monofilaments have low infection potential, are relatively non-reactive with excellent tensile strength, and pass easily through tissue. However, knot tying is difficult, particularly under tension. A synthetic mono-filament should be used routinely for skin suturing.

Polybutester has superior handling qualities, greater knot security, easy removal and it produces a cosmetically better scar. It stretches with increasing wound oedema and resumes the original shape once oedema subsides, being particularly useful for lacerations secondary to blunt trauma (Bang & Mustafa, 1989).

Absorbable sutures

Absorbable sutures are natural products (e.g. catgut) or synthetic, such as polyglycolic acid (Dexon), polyglactin (Vicryl) and polydioxanone (PDS), which are made from collagen or synthetic polymers. Collagen sutures are derived from the submucosa of sheep or bovine small intestine, or from tendon collagen of beef.

Chromic gut is treated in chromium trioxide to increase resistance to absorption (Start et al., 1989). Catgut has poor tensile strength, rapid and variable absorption, it excites brisk inflammation and increases infection potential. Only tradition and handling commend it.

Synthetic absorbable sutures are less reactive with greater tensile strength and excellent knot security. They gradually lose strength retaining 70% of their breaking strength for 28 days.

Suture techniques

All sutures reduce local tissue defences against infection. Tight sutures impair blood supply causing tissue necrosis. Sutures penetrating intact skin provide an avenue for wound contamination through the perisutural cuff. The presence of the suture material itself increases the susceptibility to infection.

Sutures are used to appose wound edges only until this is achieved by the increasing strength of the repaired tissue. A suture should only be tight enough to bring the wound edges into contact and allowance must be made for later swelling. Sutures which are tied too tightly cause necrosis and result in untidy scars. Skin tension can be reduced by undermining the wound edges, but this may damage the skin blood supply.

There are many suturing techniques. Simple interrupted stitches are the most versatile and appropriate for use in A&E departments. Care is necessary to avoid inversion of a skin edge leading to a step in the healed wound. Mattress sutures eliminate this problem but double the number of skin punctures and may result in excess tension in the stitches. Subcuticular closure eliminates stitch marks but requires practice before accurate and even skin apposition can be achieved.

In general 3/0 sutures are appropriate for skin on the trunk and lower limb, 4/0 for the hand and arm and 5/0

Table 3. *Sutures used for wound closure in A&E departments*

Wound site	Suture size	Suture removal (days)
Face	6/0	4–5
Arms Legs Feet Trunk	3/0, 4/0	10 (up to 14 over joints and sole)
Hands	4/0	Dorsum 8–10 Palm 10–14
Scalp	3/0	7
(blue sutures are easier to find in hair)		

or 6/0 for the thinner skin of the face (Table 3). The fine atraumatic cutting needles accompanying these sutures cause minimal skin damage.

The timing of suture removal ranges from 48 h for eyelids up to 3 weeks in palmar or plantar skin and will vary according to stresses on the wound. Skin sutures which remain in place for more than 5–7 days leave scars. This is necessary in some wounds but should be avoided wherever possible.

Sutures should be removed early enough to prevent suture marks but avoid wound dehiscence. For facial wounds and in children, wounds heal faster and suture marks form earlier. Following early suture removal, protect the wound with skin tape.

Absorbable sutures for children's scalp wounds avoid the trauma of suture removal. Sutures fall out at 2–4 weeks. Hair tying for suitable scalp wounds is cheap, effective, less painful and less distressing than suturing for children under 8 years old. The twists of hair are tied in a surgical knot and sprayed with Nobecutane or touched with tissue glue (Davies, 1988).

The patient should be advised to use sun block with a protection factor of 15 whenever the wound is exposed to sunlight over the following 6 months to prevent hyperpigmentation.

Skin staples

Skin stapling is up to six times faster than suturing and it evokes less tissue reaction. (McGregor et al., 1989). Staples project above the skin so surface cross-hatching associated with sutures is avoided and cosmetic results are improved. Staples are more expensive than sutures but less painful, simpler to use and safer, with no risk of needlestick injury (Ritchie & Rocke, 1989).

Infection rates are lower than with sutures. Injuries most amenable to closure with staples are linear lacerations of the scalp, trunk and extremities (George & Simpson, 1985).

Glue

This is absorbable monomeric *n*-butyl-2-cyanoacrylate. Suitable wounds are clean, superficial lacerations less than 6 cm long. The wound is cleaned and swabbed dry. The skin edges must be carefully apposed as poor alignment cannot be corrected. Wounds longer than 3 cm and those under tension should be supported with stitches or staples. Application takes between 5 and 30 sec with an overall treatment time averaging 2–5 min (Morton *et al.*, 1988). A light dressing is optional but the patient should avoid washing the wound for 5 days. The glue absorbs and gently rubs off. A mild burning sensation associated with evaporation is minimized by applying the adhesive thinly and intermittently (spotting). Advantages include speed, ease of application and avoidance of the pain associated with suture placement and removal.

A potential problem is glue trickling into the eye with risk of corneal injury. If adhesive does enter the eye no attempt should be made to force the lids apart because if the cornea becomes stuck to the palpebral conjunctiva major corneal damage may result. Patients should be referred to an ophthalmologist (McCabe *et al.*, 1989).

For paediatric facial lacerations tissue adhesive is a faster and less painful method of repair than sutures and produces similar cosmetic results. However, glue may be less beneficial for lacerations subject to movement with changes in facial expression (Quinn *et al.*, 1992; Watson, 1989). Adhesives do not perform well in wounds under significant static or dynamic tension.

Glue may be used with hair ties for simple scalp lacerations. A few strands from each side of the wound carried across the wound and glued together provide sufficient tension to appose skin edges (Gordon, 1989).

In rats, sutures and tissue glue showed similar wound strength, stretch and histology. Time to closure was significantly less using glue. No physiological differences were seen regarding cellularity, collagen fibres, proteoglycans or epithelial response. Glued wounds were cosmetically superior.

Adhesive tape

Tape can be used alone or with staples or sutures. Its application is easy and atraumatic, achieving good cosmetic results, reduced potential for infection and optimal tensile strength. Indications include the primary closure of incisions, finger tip injuries and pretibial flap lacerations in the elderly. Tapes are useful to stabilize wounds closed with absorbable subcuticular sutures, or after suture removal.

There is no discomfort, suture removal, or suture marks. However, wound edges may invert. Tapes are easy to apply on the lax skin of the face and abdomen and in the obese patient. Skin of the extremities subject to frequent movement requires sutures. The moist environment of the axillae, palms and soles impairs tape adherence. Total haemostasis is required. Compound benzoin tincture is a good adhesive adjunct.

Dressings

In primarily closed wounds the dressing acts as a barrier to exogenous bacteria during the first 3 days. The dressing may be removed at 48 hours to allow inspection for signs of infection and wound cleansing to minimize coagulant separating the wound edges. Wounds heal best in a moist environment conducive to epithelial migration from the wound edges across the surface of the wound. When epidermis is lost, water evaporates and the exudate on the surface dries. Progressive drying of the dermis and scab formation causes resistance to the migration of epidermal cells which are restricted to deeper layers of the dermis where there is enough moisture to maintain cellular viability. The wound should therefore be covered by a dressing that prevents or delays evaporation of water from the surface. Permeable dressings, however, may allow the moist exudate to become a suitable culture medium for microorganisms.

Semipermeable film dressings (e.g. Op-site, Tegaderm) allow water vapour permeability and provide a moist wound healing environment. The wound is protected from outside contamination allowing the patient to bathe. The dressings are useful for the management of lacerations, abrasions and minor burns where wound exudate is absent or very limited. The transparent nature allows observation of the wound site and flexibility allows freedom of movement.

Hydrocolloid dressings are water-resistant and used for the management of moderately exuding wounds including abrasions and burn injuries.

Calcium alginate dressings are derived from seaweed and used for wounds that produce copious exudate including partial-thickness burns.

Dressings should be non-adherent as dressing changes are painful and injure viable tissue, retarding epithelial resurfacing by stripping off delicate newly formed epithelial cells (Malone, 1987). A non-adherent layer should be applied first (e.g. paraffin gauze). A film of silver sulphadiazine can prevent drying out and adherence.

Occlusive dressings are not adherent, they speed healing and improve the cosmetic appearance. Gauze and other non-occlusive dressings are adherent, inhibit epithelial cell metabolism and are not a barrier to bacteria.

Dressings exert pressure on underlying tissue to minimize the accumulation of intercellular fluid and limit the dead space. These dressings also immobilize the site of injury, improving resistance to bacterial growth. The wound should be elevated to limit oedema and allow rehabilitation.

Topical application of antibiotics (e.g. neomycin) to the suture line after wound closure to prevent exogenous bacterial contamination is useful if a dressing cannot be applied (e.g. face or scalp wounds) in providing protection until epithelialization is complete in approximately 2 days (Dire *et al.*, 1991). Topical antimicrobials are ineffective if administered more than 3 h after injury due to protective wound coagulant. Topical proteolytic enzymes may extend this period.

Elemental zinc is important in wound healing (Maitra & Dorani, 1992). Zinc is involved in protein synthesis and cellular metabolism. Epithelialization may be delayed by zinc deficiency. This is reversed by zinc-based adhesive dressings which have been used for treating pre-tibial flap lacerations, finger tip injuries and burns (Hughes & McLean, 1988). Zinc oxide tape is easy to apply, cheap and readily accepted.

Finger tip injuries often appear minor but cause difficulties in convalescence and absence from work.

Discharge instructions to wound patients

- Elevate for 48 h
- Immobilize extremity wounds
- Review after 48 h
  - infection-prone wounds
  - borderline perfusion, e.g. flap lacerations
  - ? missed nerve/tendon injury
- Sunscreen to avoid differential pigmentation for 6 months

Table 4. *Summary of dressings used in A & E departments*

Type of wound	Dressing
Sutured	Non-adhesive gauze/film
Lips, eyelids, face, scalp	Antibiotic ointment
Clean open, e.g. delayed suture	Paraffin gauze
Abrasions	Film dressings
Necrotic/infected/sloughy	Hydrocolloid
Finger tip injury ⎫ Burns ⎭	Silver sulphadiazine/ paraffin gauze

Silver sulphadiazine applied to the finger tip, which is then placed in a non-sterile surgical glove, results in marked reduction of infection and rapid epithelialisation with early return of active and passive movements (Arbel *et al.*, 1989).

Table 4 summarizes the dressings used in A&E departments.

Antibiotics

Wound infection bacteria

- *Staphylococcus aureus*
- *Streptococcus* spp.
- Clostridia
- Enterobacteria

- Faeces/manure
  - gram-negative coliforms
  - obligate anaerobes
- Fresh water
  - *Aeromonas hydrophilia*
- Animal bites
  - *Pasteurella multocida*

The therapeutic value of antibiotics in preventing wound infection is controversial. Indiscriminate use of prophylactic antibiotics continues, but does not replace correct wound care (Rodgers, 1992).

The interval between the time of wounding and the delivery of antibiotics is critical. There is an initial period of 3 h during which developing infections may be suppressed by antibiotics. These should be present in the wound tissue fluid in an effective concentration at the time of wound closure and should therefore be administered intravenously (Edlich *et al.*, 1986). Studies of simple wounds of all body areas, including the hand, indicate that oral antibiotic administration has no benefit (Worlock *et al.*, 1980).

Antibiotic treatment of uninfected wounds may paradoxically increase infection as the more virulent bacteria survive, a rebound increase of the bacterial population may occur and antibodies impair host defences.

Factors which influence infection include:

- Anatomical site.
- Wound appearance.
- Time since injury.
- Subcutaneous closure.
- Wound contamination.
- Host immune status.
- Local tissue milieu.

Impaired host defences:
- Compromised immune system.
- Diabetes mellitus.
- Chronic malnutrition – vitamins A and C, iron, zinc deficiency.
- Alcoholism.
- Hepatic/renal insufficiency.
- Asplenism.
- Malignancies.
- Obesity.
- Extremes of age.
- Medication – steroids, chemotherapy, radiotherapy.

Antibiotic prophylaxis is recommended for:

- Wounds at high risk of infection, for example:
  - foot lacerations,
  - dirty or contaminated wounds
  - delay to wound cleansing and repair longer than 6 h
  - contamination with pus, saliva, faeces, or vaginal secretions.
- Minor soft tissue lacerations in patients with orthopaedic prostheses or with valvular heart disease at risk of endocarditis.
- Immunocompromised patients.
- Fresh water lacerations at risk of infection with *Aeromonas hydrophilia* – a problem with water-based leisure activities (Grant & Hoddinott, 1993).
- Extensive intraoral lacerations.

Use:

1. Flucloxacillin 250 mg q.d.s. for 5 days (erythromycin if allergic to penicillin). To be effective, give intravenously within 3 h of injury.
   or
2. Co-amoxiclav 250 mg t.d.s. for 5 days.

CROSS-INFECTION OF HEALTHCARE WORKERS

Viruses transmitted by blood

Hepatitis B, C and D
HIV I, II
Cytomegalovirus
Epstein–Barr
HTLV (human T-cell lymphotropic virus) I, II

Human immunodeficiency virus and hepatitis B virus

Healthcare workers have a low but measurable risk of transmission of HIV and hepatitis B virus (HBV) (Dwyer *et al.*, 1991). Occupational HIV infection has been recorded in 32 healthcare workers worldwide, of which 63% were nurses, 14% doctors and 11% laboratory staff. Of these infections, 28 followed needlestick injuries and four followed mucocutaneous exposure. Transmission of HIV and HBV can occur with less than 2 ml of blood.

There are an estimated 20 000 HIV-positive patients in the UK. In the USA, the HIV antibody seroprevalence rate is up to 19% amongst A&E department patients, although it varies (Sturm, 1991; Baraff *et al.*, 1991) with rates of 2.6% for HBV and 3.4% for HIV in injured patients in California (Rhee *et al.*, 1992). Ease of travel demands increased awareness that seropositive patients may present in any A&E department and staff must use precautions for all patients.

The prevalence of HBV and HIV-positive patients varies (Zalut *et al.*, 1990), but if risk factors are adequately elicited (intravenous drug use, homosexuality, known positive HIV and blood transfusion prior to 1985) the risk of encountering an unknown positive patient is lowered. The majority of individuals infected with HBV and HIV are asymptomatic and unaware. Serological testing of random or selected groups remains controversial (Doyle & Taylor, 1992).

For emergency physicians in high prevalence areas not using universal precautions, assuming HIV seroprevalence increases to a steady state, the median estimate of cumulative risk of HIV infection over a 30-year career is 1.4%. For low-prevalence A&E departments, the median is 0.1% (Wears *et al.*, 1991).

Hepatitis B immunization is essential for all staff. Increasing awareness and safety of the vaccine have raised uptake of immunization programmes in the UK (Heyworth, 1988). In the USA, 30–60% of health care workers are not immunized.

The risks of HIV and HBV transmission by inoculation with a contaminated needle are less than 0.5% and 3–16%, respectively. Resheathing of needles must be avoided (Schneider *et al.*, 1993). The needle may, for example, be embedded into the rubber syringe plunger through the nozzle (Prior, 1993).

Blood splashes and needlestick injuries occur during wound management. In wound irrigation, local anaesthesia and suturing there is contact between the patient's blood and the doctor's hands, face, body and feet (Marcus *et al.*, 1990). The American College of Emergency Physicians recommends that all patients treated in the A&E department should be considered potentially infected and precautions be universally applied, including gloves, mask, protective eyewear or complete face shield, gown, boots and apron.

Universal precautions are often ignored by A&E department personnel; gloves are worn most frequently (74%) followed by goggles, gowns and masks (1%). Reasons for non-compliance include time, dexterity and appearance (Henry *et al.*, 1992; Go *et al.*, 1991).

Precautions are often only taken for patients with large blood spillage and not for minor injuries (Todd & Berk, 1992). Breaches in glove integrity, not visible on inspection occur during common procedures subjecting doctors to the risk of exposure. The leakage incidence for suturing is 9.5% (Hansen *et al.*, 1992).

Prevention

- All at-risk staff must be immunized against hepatitis B.
- Assume *all* patients carry bloodborne infection. Wear protective clothing (gloves at least) with *any* exposure to blood.
- Cover abrasions/cuts.
- Wash off any body fluid on skin immediately.
- Have protocols for care of the bleeding patient and phlebotomy.
- Use safe blood collection systems.
- Do not resheath needles.
- *Concentrate* at the time of potential exposure.

Post exposure

- Immediate consultation.
- Source and donor status.
- Hepatitis B immunization status – ?accelerated vaccination/immunoglobulin.
- Take baseline bloods.

- ? Zidovudine (AZT) prophylaxis – commence within 2 h; efficacy not yet proven.
- Follow-up.

SPECIAL WOUNDS

Foreign bodies

Foreign bodies increase the infectivity of bacterial inoculants. If foreign bodies are irritant or near vital structures, morbidity may include delayed wound healing, infection, functional impairment and destruction of adjacent soft tissues. Complications of retained foreign bodies include:

- Chronic sinus.
- Sterile abscess.
- Granuloma.
- Cyst.
- Monoarticular septic arthritis.
- Periosteal reactions.
- Osteomyelitis.
- Pseudotumours of bone.
- Delayed nerve/tendon injury.

Chronic, delayed or recurrent infections resistant to antibiotics are associated with unsuspected foreign bodies.

Not all foreign bodies, however, need to be removed. Those that are inert or inaccessible and causing no damage to underlying structures may be left in place. Glass and metal are relatively inert and removal is not urgent. Toxic substances (e.g. plant and animal spines) require early removal.

Methods of detection

Demonstration by plain radiography depends on the density, configuration, size and orientation of the foreign body. X-rays will identify all retained glass and most metallic fragments. The assumption that only some glass is radio-opaque is mistaken (DeLacey *et al.*, 1985). All glass commonly found on motor vehicles and in the house will be radio-opaque. Radio-opacity does not depend on lead content but on the relative density. Many highly reactive organic fibres, including wood splinters, thorns, cactus spines and vegetable matter, are not seen. Aluminium, some plastics and fish bones are not visible.

Radio-opaque foreign bodies include:

- Metal.
- Bone, teeth.
- Pencil graphite.
- Glass.

- Gravel.
- Some plastics.
  (Non radio-opaque foreign bodies may show a radio-lucent filling defect.)

The wounds most likely to have retained glass are puncture wounds and head or foot wounds. Wounds caused by stepping on glass or by motor vehicle accidents and patients who have the perception of glass retention are likely to harbour foreign bodies. (Montano *et al.*, 1992).

Plain radiography is the diagnostic tool of choice for confirming the presence of a glass foreign body. False negative reports occur especially when the foreign body is adjacent to bone or deep within soft tissues. Only 8% of X-rays taken to detect the presence of a glass foreign body are positive (Courter, 1990).

The size of the glass foreign body, not the type of glass, is usually the limiting factor. Overlying bone may completely obscure fragments as large as 2 mm. Thin slivers of glass may be difficult to detect but should be visualized with good radiographic technique (e.g. oblique views and careful scrutiny). Underpenetrated soft tissue techniques will reveal fragments less than 0.5 mm in diameter (Lammers & Magill, 1992).

Retained wood and plastic are often detectable only by computed tomography, xerography or wound exploration.

Xerographs may show thorns and spines, wood, plastic, rubber and graphite better than X-rays. The radiation dose is 20 times that of plain X-rays.

Computed tomography (CT) has been used for wood splinters and thorns but, because of cost and higher radiation dose, it has limited use.

Magnetic resonance imaging (MRI) is superior to CT for the detection of plastics. MRI cannot be used for metallic foreign bodies, gravel or other ferromagnetic substances.

Ultrasound is being used increasingly for non-radio-opaque material, 1×2 mm or larger, with a sensitivity of 95% and specificity of 89%. A percutaneous ultrasound-guided extraction technique allows minimal dissection. Potential problems arise with scarring from previous procedures or large incisions with artifacts due to blood or air. Ultrasound allows accurate compartment localization (Humphrey *et al.*, 1993; Bradley *et al.*, 1992).

Other authors have used a metal detector to aid removal of metallic foreign bodies (West & Glucksman, 1987) or a hand held image intensifier, the Lixiscope

---

> **Foreign body–diagnosis**
>
> - Radiography – detects 80–90%
>   - Deep glass wound
>   - Patient believes foreign body present
>   - Infection
>   - Swelling
>   - Delayed healing
>   - Unexplained pain
>   - Neurological deficit
> - Ultrasound or CT
>   - Radiolucent foreign body
>   - Equivocal X-rays

(Daniels & Mason, 1985), but practical problems arose with peri-operative localization because of the laterally reversed image and difficulty in screen visualization in bright light.

Embedded blackthorn or acacia thorn may cause bone lesions resembling osteomyelitis. The foreign bodies are not visible on X-ray. Given a history of thorn injury, treatment must be surgical with a wide exposure if necessary to ensure removal of a migrated thorn. The thorn with surrounding inflamed tissue should be excised. If no thorn can be found, the wound is left open to granulate and the limb is splinted (Vaishya, 1990).

Removal

Foreign bodies in feet are usually symptomatic and require removal. In hands and elsewhere, small inert asymptomatic foreign bodies may be left in place. Foreign bodies deep in hands and feet should be referred to appropriate specialists.

The attempted removal of small, deep foreign bodies may cause more damage than leaving the object in place. Accurate localization is essential, using ultrasound, fluoroscopy, paper clips on the skin or inserting 2–3 needles at 90° to each other. Having identified the needle closest to the foreign body, the others are removed and the tissue is dissected along the path of the closest needle.

Adequate anaesthesia, good lighting and haemostasis are essential. A time limit should be set. After removal of the foreign body the wound should be irrigated and debrided, and delayed closure used if the wound is heavily contaminated.

Bites

Animal bites

Dog and cat bites comprise 1% of A&E department visits. More than 80% in most series are dog bites.

Most dog and cat bite injuries are minor wounds that require only local care and a check for tetanus and rabies immunoprophylaxis. For larger wounds, primary or delayed primary closure can be performed safely. When antibiotics are necessary inexpensive penicillins or cephalosporins are adequate for initial therapy (Dire, 1992).

Dog bites

In adults most bites are to the extremities, but in children 80% are to the face and scalp following face-to-face proximity. Most (except puncture, crushed or old wounds) can be safely sutured, do not need prophylactic antibiotics or initial wound cultures and have an infection rate of 5–10%. Hand wounds are more likely to become infected, face and scalp wounds are low risk. Suturing wounds does not increase infection except on the hand. Sutured dog bites of the head and neck without antibiotics have an infection rate of only 1.4%. Additional complications include cosmetic disfigurement with scars or keloid, development of epidermal inclusion cysts, functional impairment and psychological trauma (Table 5). Two per cent of patients require admission with massive lacerations. Deeper injury may occur including arterial injuries, particularly in the upper limbs, diagnosed by angiography (Snyder & Pentecost, 1990). Ten to 20 dog bite related fatalities occur each year in the USA, 42% from pit bull terriers.

Treatment should include wound exploration, toilet, debridement, trimming devitalized skin edges, irrigation and closure (Maimaris & Quinton, 1988). Debridement reduces the infection rate 30-fold. If there is any suspicion that the presentation of the wound has been delayed, then delayed primary closure should be considered. Exceptions to this general advice include facial/scalp wounds. Puncture wounds may be extensive and have twice the infection rate as thorough irrigation is difficult and may cause bacterial infiltration.

More than 64 species of bacteria are part of the normal flora of a dog's mouth and up to 36% of dog bite wounds culture more than one species. No single organism accounts for more than 15% of infections.

Culture of infected dog bites frequently isolates *Staphylococcus aureus, Pasteurella, Streptococcus* spp. and enterobacteria. Culture of non-infected wounds is of no benefit in predicting the source of later infection. Wounds due to *Pasteurella multocida* develop an intense inflammatory reaction within a few hours. Infection developing after 24 h is more likely to be caused by staphylococcus or streptococcus (Callaham, 1988).

Initial antibiotic therapy must cover the broad range of potential pathogens, which includes both aerobic and anaerobic bacteria; for example, amoxycillin/clavulanic acid, or penicillin with flucloxacillin (erythromycin if penicillin-allergic). In wounds presenting 9–24 h after injury the infection rate is reduced significantly with amoxycillin/clavulanic acid but not in wounds less than 9 h old (Brakenbury & Muwanga, 1989). Prophylactic penicillin decreases the incidence of infection in high-risk wounds only. Prophylactic antibiotics are therefore recommended for puncture wounds and bites to the hand. There is no benefit for wounds of the face or scalp.

Cat bites

Pasteurella multocida is found in 80% of infections. Tetracycline is effective against pasteurella but should only be used for proven pasteurella infection resistant to initial treatment.

Septic arthritis may follow (Table 5). Cat bites can also transmit cat scratch fever, tularaemia, rat bite fever, rabies, toxoplasmosis, or Q fever.

Human bites

Human bites of the hand (closed-fist injuries) have a poor prognosis because of their location and initial neglect by the patient. Human bites elsewhere have no higher risk of infection than animal bites, and on the face, lips and ears this is under 3%. At least 42 species of bacteria have been reported in human saliva. In the hand, streptococci are found in 15%, *Staphylococcus aureus* in 38% and *Eikenella corrodens* in 29% of infected human bite wounds. Anaerobes are also present.

Any penetrating injury in the vicinity of the metacarpophalangeal joint should be considered a human bite until proven otherwise. X-rays should be obtained to look for foreign bodies, bone fragments and air in joints as up to 70% of patients may have positive findings. Subtle radiological findings include soft tissue swelling, and small defects in the subchondral bone plate of the metacarpal head. In late presentations there may be soft tissue swelling, periarticular osteoporosis, narrowing of the joint space, bony erosions and periostitis.

Treatment must be aggressive with thorough irrigation using 1% povidone-iodine solution and the wound left open, dressed and elevated. Prophylactic antibiotics (penicillin) are recommended. Patients presenting with any degree of infection beyond very limited and superficial cellulitis should be admitted for intravenous

Table 5. *Complications of bites*

- Sepsis
- Septic arthritis
- Tenosynovitis
- Fractures
- Osteomyelitis
- Peritonitis
- Endophthalmitis
- Meningitis
- Disfiguring wounds
- Damage to deep structures
- Psychological trauma

antibiotic treatment. Penetration of the joint or tendon sheath, presence of a foreign body or bone involvement warrant admission whether there is infection or not. In patients presenting late with infection, the average duration of morbidity is 87 days.

There is no indication for prophylactic antibiotics in human bites other than in the hand. Microbiology of human hand bite wounds must always include anaerobic cultures. Transmission of actinomycosis, syphilis, tuberculosis and hepatitis B have been documented. Human bites are not considered by the American Centre for Disease Control to carry a risk of transmission of HIV (human immunodeficiency virus). However, bites from infected or high risk persons should receive thorough wound irrigation and consider obtaining a baseline HIV blood test for medicolegal purposes and reassurance.

TECHNIQUE

Wound care–bites

- Exclude injury to deep structures.
- X-ray – if swollen/tender or suspected bony involvement/foreign body.
- Wound toilet – debridement/irrigation with saline and 1% povidone-iodine.
- Primary closure, e.g. face.

NOT – puncture wounds
 – extensive crush injury
 – hand bites ⎱ Use delayed primary closure
 – immunosuppressed patients
 – delay to treatment

- Ensure tetanus immunization.
- Assess rabies risk.
- Prophylactic antibiotics: 5 days

Indications for prophylactic antibiotics

- Hand or lower extremity bites.
- Wounds requiring surgical debridement.

– Wounds involving joints, tendons, ligaments or fractures.
– Full thickness puncture wounds *especially* cats.
– High risk hosts.

 – Dog ⎱ Flucloxacillin (250 mg q.d.s.) + Penicillin V (250 mg q.d.s.) ⎰ *or* Co-amoxiclav (250 mg t.d.s.)
 – Cat ⎰

 – Human: Flucloxacillin (250 mg q.d.s.) and penicillin V (250 mg q.d.s.) (erythromycin 250 mg q.d.s. if allergic to penicillin).
 or Co-amoxiclav 250 mg t.d.s.

- Infection within 24 h (*P. multocida*)
 – Penicillin V 500 mg q.d.s. ⎱ 7 days
 Amoxycillin 500 mg t.d.s. ⎰
 (if high-risk host, intitial dose intravenously)
 – Tetracycline if allergic to penicillin (over 8 years old)
- Infection after 24 h (*staphylococcus/streptococcus*)
 – Co-amoxiclav 250–500 mg t.d.s: 7 days
- Admit for intravenous antibiotics If lymphangitis, lymphadenitis, tenosynovitis, septic arthritis or fever.

Puncture wounds

Puncture wounds of the foot comprise 0.1% of all conditions presenting to UK A & E departments, and, in the USA, 7.4% of lower extremity diagnoses (Schwab & Powers, 1993). There is high potential for infection from the introduction of pathogens and debris into the deep tissue (e.g. fragments of epidermis or clothing). Cellulitis develops in up to 8% of patients within 4 days, and osteomyelitis, septic arthritis or deep tissue abscesses may follow. The organisms are usually streptococcus, staphylococcus, or pseudomonas. *Pseudomonas aeruginosa* infection of bone or cartilage is the most serious complication of plantar puncture wounds caused by a nail penetrating a shoe (Reichl, 1989).

Complications can be prevented by careful attention to the wound. Any foreign body must be removed. Superficial wounds are cleaned with iodine, but deep wounds should ideally be surgically debrided. Irrigation of the deep part of the wound is otherwise impossible. Tetanus prophylaxis must be ensured. Antibiotics are recommended for deep wounds, especially those involving bone or joints, and older infected wounds (Chudnofsky & Sebastian, 1992).

Treatment of puncture wounds of foot

- If contaminated excise rim.
- Irrigate with saline.
- Apply povidone-iodine.
- Antibiotics for deep wounds.

- Elevate.
- Review if any signs of infection.

Pretibial lacerations

Lacerations over the shin are common and may take many weeks to heal, especially in older patients, those with circulatory problems or those on steroid treatment. Three-quarters of patients are women over the age of 50 years (Jones & Sanders, 1983).

Frequently, a flap of skin and subcutaneous tissue is raised and this may be attached proximally or distally. The vascular supply of the pretibial skin is by vessels which perforate the deep fascia and branch into a small area of skin. When a flap is raised these vessels are torn and the skin becomes ischaemic. Suture of such a wound will fail. The tissues are always bruised and soon become oedematous resulting in increased tension. If this is compounded by suturing there will be necrosis, infection, enlargement of the defect and greatly delayed healing (Sutton & Pritty, 1985).

Treatment should avoid if possible hospital admission, general anaesthesia and immobilization. Debridement and anchorage of the flap with adhesive strips produces a mean healing time of 39 days. Glue is an alternative to strips for the fixation of pretibial flap lacerations (Burchett, 1989). Immediate debridement and skin grafting under general anaesthesia has a mean healing time of 27 days but the length of time in hospital is considerable (Haiart et al., 1990). This may be shortened if early mobilization is encouraged. Debridement and delayed skin grafting under regional anaesthesia or immediate meshed skin grafting under local anaesthesia as an out-patient produces good results (Shankar & Koo, 1987).

The skin flap may be used as a full-thickness fenestrated skin graft. The healing time is shorter than with conservative methods and similar to that of meshed split-skin grafting but without the disadvantage of a donor site (Foroughi & Nouri, 1990).

Rabies

Rabies is a fatal viral acute encephalomyelitis. Once clinical signs develop there is no known cure and death is almost certain. Rabies has been recorded in most species of warm-blooded animals. Suspicious characteristics in animals include aggression, indifference, ataxia, unresponsiveness or even an overfriendly demeanour. In Europe it is mostly the red fox and in domestic animals, the dog and cat that carry rabies. There have been no cases of rabies in animals outside quarantine in the UK since 1970. In the USA, rabies is mostly found amongst raccoons, skunks, bats and foxes, with 0–5 human cases each year (Harrigan et al, 1993).

Transmission is by the introduction of infectious saliva through animal bites and scratches. However, any break in the skin or intact mucous membrane exposed to infectious saliva can lead to viral inoculation. The virus travels along peripheral nerves to the CNS. The incubation period varies with the age of the patient, size of inoculant and location of the bite. Young patients generally have shorter incubation times and a direct relationship exists between the distance of the bite from the CNS and the length of incubation.

There is a prodromal phase with pain, paraesthesia or pruritus radiating proximally from the site of viral entry, with non-specific accompanying symptoms including fever, malaise, fatigue, myalgia. This may last from 24 h to 10 days following which the illness may progress to classic rabies (80%) or paralytic rabies (20%).

Classic rabies features the pathognomonic finding of hydrophobia with vigorous irregular contractions of the diaphragm and accessory muscles of respiration, terror, anxiety, agitation and facial grimacing. Later autonomic hyperactivity emerges with arrhythmias and seizures. The differential diagnosis includes tetanus, delirium tremens, hysteria and other viral encephalitides.

Preventive treatment of rabies includes meticulous cleansing of the wound with soap solution, which is a potent viricidal agent. The wound should not be sutured.

Rabies prophylaxis is by human diploid cell rabies vaccine 1 ml injected into the deltoid muscle on days 0, 3, 7, 14, 30 and 90. The antibody response develops in 7–10 days and persists for over 2 years. For post exposure treatment a course of injections should be started immediately whenever a patient has been attacked by an animal in a country where rabies is endemic, even if there is no direct evidence of rabies in the attacking animal. The biting animal should be confined and observed for 10 days. If the animal becomes ill it is sacrificed and the brain examined for negri bodies.

Human rabies immunoglobulin (dose 20 international units kg^{-1}) provides immediate antibodies until the vaccine can promote an adequate host antibody response. Up to 50% is infiltrated around the wound and the remainder of the dose is given intramuscularly in the gluteal region.

Table 6. *Immunization against tetanus*

	Clean wound	Tetanus-Prone Wound
Course or reinforcing dose within last 10 years	Nil	Nil (unless especially high-risk)
More than 10 years	Dose of adsorbed vaccine	Dose of adsorbed vaccine
Non-immune or immunization status not known	Three-dose course of adsorbed vaccine	Three-dose course of adsorbed vaccine plus immunoglobulin (different site)

Tetanus

The bacterium *Clostridium tetani* is an obligatory anaerobe which thrives in the bowel of herbivorous mammals and is profuse on manured ground and farmland. Spores are resistant to dehydration and are found in dust or dirt. There are 20–60 cases of tetanus annually in the UK. The disease is rare but the organism is widespread (British Association for Accident and Emergency Medicine, 1992).

The overall level of immunity against tetanus in the UK is probably higher than assumed, regardless of age group or immunization history. In one study, no patient fell below the accepted protective level of 0.01 units of antitoxin ml^{-1} and this includes patients whose last booster was over 10 years previously (Chikhani & Kumar, 1988).

The elderly are more vulnerable; 45% of elderly patients lack a protective level of antitoxin and after immunization 44% fail to seroconvert within 14 days (Gareau *et al.*, 1990).

Infection is only acquired via wounds. The key in the prevention of tetanus is meticulous surgical cleansing of the wound. If the wound is fresh (less than 6 h old), clean, superficial and cleanly incised or abraded, this is a low-risk wound.

The wound is tetanus-prone if it is any of the following:

- Not fresh.
- Deep and penetrating.
- Contaminated.
- Involves crushing or bruising of tissue.
- Infected.
- Associated with farming, gardening, field sports or unclean water.

Active immunization is performed by injection of adsorbed tetanus vaccine 0.5 ml (tetanus toxoid). A primary course consists of three doses at 1-month intervals. The first dose has no protective effect. The course leaves the patient protected for at least 10 full years.

Reinforcing boosters on wounding are necessary if the primary course was greater than 10 years previously.

Passive immunization is achieved using human anti-tetanus immunoglobulin 250 international units IM.

Wound management–Summary

History
- Patient
  - Age
  - Medical history
  - Medication
- Injury
  - Mechanism
  - Time
  - Potential for contamination, retained foreign body

Examination
- Site
- Wound–contamination, crushed or devitalized tissue
- Injury to underlying nerves, tendons, vessels, joints

CONSIDER REFERRAL IF EXPERIENCE OR CONDITIONS INADEQUATE

Treatment
- ? Local anaesthetic/sedate/general anaesthetic
- Cleanse
  - Surrounding skin
  - Wound – irrigation
- Debridement
- Close
  - Sutures
  - Staples
  - Paper strips
  - Glue
- If contaminated – delayed primary suture
- ? Prophylactic antibiotics
- ? Tetanus/rabies prophylaxis
- Dress
- Elevate/immobilize
- Discharge instructions

PROTECT ALL STAFF FROM HBV/HIV TRANSMISSION

Absolute indications are a patient with a wound which is tetanus-prone who has never been actively immunized, or a patient who is immunocompromised.

The strategy for immunization against tetanus is summarized in Table 6.

Tetanus vaccine quite often causes painful local reactions which are not dangerous and need symptomatic treatment only. All immunization procedures occasionally cause serious generalized anaphylactic reactions and treatment for anaphylaxis must be available.

Bibliography

ANDERSON, A., COLECCHI, C., BARONSKI, R. *et al.* (1990). Local anaesthesia in paediatric patients: topical TAC v lidocaine. *Ann. Emerg. Med.*, **19**, 519–22.

ARBEL, R., GOODWIN, D. & OTREMSKI, I. (1989). Treatment of finger tip injuries with silver sulphadiazine occlusion dressing. *Injury*, **20**, 161–3.

BANG, R. & MUSTAFA, M. (1989). Comparative study of skin wound closure with polybutester and polypropylene. *J. R. Coll. Surg. Edin.* **34**, 205–7.

BARAFF, F. L., TALAN, D. & TORRES, M. (1991). Prevalence of HIV antibody in a non-inner city university hospital emergency department. *Ann. Emerg. Med.*, **20**, 782–6.

BARTFIELD, J., GENNIS, P., BARBERA, J. *et al.* (1990). Buffered versus plain lidocaine as a local anaesthetic for simple laceration repair. *Ann. Emerg. Med.*, **19**, 1387–9.

BARTFIELD, J., FORD, D. & HOMER, P. (1993). Buffered versus plain lidocaine for digital nerve block. *Ann. Emerg. Med.*, **22**, 216–19.

BATCHELOR, A. (1988). Wound management. *Surgery*, **54**, 1281–5.

BATES, B., SHUTZMAN, S. & FLEISHER, G. (1993). Comparison of intranasal sufentanil and midazolam, to meperidine, promethazine and chlorpromazine for sedation during laceration repair in children. *Ann. Emerg. Med.*, **22**, 899.

BERK, W., OSBOURNE, D. & TAYLOR, D. (1988). Evaluation of the golden period for wound repair: 204 cases from a Third World emergency department. *Ann. Emerg. Med.*, **17**, 496–500.

BERK, W., WELCH, R. & ROCK, B. (1992). Controversial issues in clinical management of the simple wound. *Ann. Emerg. Med.*, **21**, 72–80.

BERMAN, D. & GRABER, D. (1992). Sedation and analgesia. *Emerg. Med. Clin. North Am.*, **10**, 691–705.

BICKERSTAFF, K. & REGNARD, C. (1984). Prophylactic povidone iodine spray in accidental wounds. *J. R. Coll. Surg. Edin.*, **29**, 234–6.

BONADIO, W. & WAGNER, V. (1992). Adrenaline–cocaine gel topical anaesthetic for dermal laceration repair in children. *Ann. Emerg. Med.*, **21**, 1325–38.

BRADLEY, M., KADSZOMBE, E., SIMMS, P. *et al.* (1992). Percutaneous ultrasound guided extraction of non-palpable soft tissue foreign bodies. *Arch. Emerg. Med.*, **9**, 181–4.

BRAKENBURY, P. & MUWANGA, C. (1989). A comparative double blind study of amoxycllin/clavulanate vs placebo in the prevention of infection after animal bites. *Arch. Emerg. Med.*, **6**, 251–6.

BRENNAN, S. & LEAPER, D. (1985). The effect of antiseptics on the healing wound: a study using the rabbit ear chamber. *Br. J. Surg.*, **72**, 780–2.

BRITISH ASSOCIATION FOR ACCIDENT AND EMERGENCY MEDICINE (1992). *Guidelines for the Prevention of Tetanus.* London.

BURCHETT, N. (1989). Cyanocrylate tissue adhesive. *Arch. Emerg. Med.*, **6**, 155–6.

CALLAHAM, M. (1988). Controversies in antibiotic choices for bite wounds. *Ann. Emerg. Med.*, **17**, 1321–30.

CHIKHANI, C. & KUMAR, K. (1988). Tetanus booster every 5 years: an unnecessary routine? *Arch. Emerg. Med.*, **5**, 4–11.

CHISHOLM, C. (1992). Wound evaluation and cleansing. *Emerg. Med. Clin. North Am.*, **10**, 665–71.

CHUDNOFSKY, C. & SEBASTIAN, S. (1992). Special wounds: nail bed, plantar puncture and cartilage. *Emerg. Med. Clin. North Am.*, **10**, 801–22.

COURTER, B. (1990). Radiographic screening for glass foreign bodies – what does a negative foreign body series really mean? *Ann. Emerg. Med.*, **19**, 997–1000.

CRUSE, P. (1973). A five-year prospective study of 23,649 surgical wounds. *Arch. Surg.*, **107**, 206–10.

DANIELS, R. & MASON, A.M. (1985). The lixiscope portable imaging device: an assessment of its use in the accident and emergency department. *Arch. Emerg. Med.*, **2**, 100–3.

DAVIES, N. (1988). Scalp wounds. An alternative to suture. *Injury*, **19**, 375–6.

DE HOLL, D., RODEHEAVER, G., EDGERTON, N. *et al.* (1974). Potentiation of infection by suture closure of dead space. *Am. J. Surg.*, **127**, 716–20.

DELACEY, G., EVANS, R. & SANDIN, B. (1985). Penetrating injuries: how easy is it to see glass and plastics on radiographs? *Br. J. Radiol.*, **58**, 27–30.

DIMICK, A. (1988). Delayed wound closure: indications and techniques. *Ann. Emerg. Med.*, **17**, 1303–4.

DIRE, D. (1992). Emergency management of dog and cat bite wounds. *Emerg. Med. Clin. North Am.*, **10**, 719–36.

DIRE, D., COPPOLA, N., DWYER, D. *et al.* (1991). A prospective evaluation of topical antibiotics for uncomplicated soft tissue lacerations. *Ann. Emerg. Med.*, **20**, 451.

DOYLE, M. & TAYLOR, R. (1992). Prevalence of human immunodeficiency virus risk factors in patients attending an Accident & Emergency department. *Arch. Emerg. Med.*, **9**, 196–202.

DWYER, B., WEINSTEIN, L. & HOWARD, W. (1991). HIV in the second decade: new trends in epidemiology, updated pathogenesis, occupational exposure risks and prevention. *Emerg. Med. Rep.*, **12**, 161–70.

EDLICH, R., KENNEY, J., MORGAN, R. *et al.* (1986). Antimicrobial treatment of minor soft tissue lacerations: a critical review. *Emerg. Med. Clin. North Am.*, **4**, 561–80.

EDLICH, R., RODEHEAVER, G., MORGAN, R. *et al.* (1988). Principles of emergency wound management. *Ann. Emerg. Med.*, **17**, 1284–302.

ESSELLS, S. & JONES, J. (1993). Intranasal sufentanil for sedation and analgesia in paediatric patients. *Ann. Emerg. Med.*, **22**, 899.

FITZMAURICE, L., WASSERMAN, G., KNAPP, J. *et al.* (1990). TAC use and absorption of cocaine in a paediatric emergency department. *Ann. Emerg. Med.*, **19**, 515–18.

FOROUGHI, D. & NOURI, D. (1990). Grafting without a donor site: an easy approach to pretibial lacerations. *J. R. Coll. Surg. Edinb.*, **35**, 235–47.

GAREAU, A., EBY, R., McCLELLAN, B. *et al.* (1990). Tetanus immunisation status and immunologic response to a booster in an emergency department's geriatric population. *Ann. Emerg. Med.*, **19**, 1377–81.

GEORGE, T. & SIMPSON, D. (1985). Skin wound closure with staples in the Accident and Emergency department. *J. R. Coll. Surg. Edin.*, **30**, 54–6.

GO, G., BARAFF, L. & SCHRIGER, D. (1991). Management guidelines for health care workers exposed to blood and bodily fluids. *Ann. Emerg. Med.*, **20**, 1341–50.

GORDON, G. (1989). The use of histoacryl tissue adhesive for the primary closure of scalp wounds. *Arch. Emerg. Med.*, **6**, 160.

GRANT, A. & HODDINOTT, C. (1993). Aeromonas hydrophilia infection of a scalp laceration (with synergistic gas gangrene). *Arch. Emerg. Med.*, **10**, 232–4.

GRANT, S. & HOFFMAN, R. (1992). Use of tetracaine, epinephrine and cocaine as a topical anaesthetic in the emergency department. *Ann. Emerg. Med.*, **21**, 987–95.

GRAVETT, A., STERNER, S., CLINTON, J. *et al.* (1987). A trial of povidone iodine in the prevention of infection in sutured lacerations. *Ann. Emerg. Med.*, **16**, 167–71.

GREEN, S., NAKAMURA, R. & JOHNSON, E. (1990). Ketamine sedation for paediatric procedures. *Ann. Emerg. Med.*, **19**, 1024–32.

GRUBER, R., VISTNES, L. & PARDOE, R. (1975). The effect of commonly used antiseptics on wound healing. *Plast. Reconstr. Surg.*, **55**, 472–6.

HAIART, D., PAUL, A., CHALMERS, R. *et al.* (1990). Pretibial lacerations: a comparison of primary excision and grafting with defatting of the flap. *Br. J. Plast. Surg.*, **43**, 312–14.

HANSEN, K., KORNIEWCZ, E., LARSON, E. *et al.* (1992). Loss of glove integrity during common ED procedures. *Ann. Emerg. Med.*, **21**, 599.

HARRIGAN, R., KAUFFMAN, F., BINDER, L. *et al.* (1993). Current issues in rabies: epidemiology, clinical management and post-exposure prophylaxis. *Emerg. Med. Rep.*, **14**, 37–44.

HAURY, B., RODEHEAVER, G., VENSKO, J. *et al.* (1978). Debridement: an essential component of traumatic wound care. *Am. J. Surg.*, **135**, 238–42.

HEGENBARTH, N., ALTIERI, N., HAWK, W. *et al.* (1990). Comparisons of topical tetracaine, adrenaline and cocaine anaesthesia with lidocaine infiltration for repair of lacerations in children. *Ann. Emerg. Med.*, **19**, 63–7.

HENNES, H., WAGNER, V., BONADIO, W. *et al.* (1990). The effect of oral midazolam on anxiety of pre-school children during laceration repair. *Ann. Emerg. Med.*, **19**, 1006–9.

HENRY, K., CAMPBELL, S. & MAKI, M. (1992). A comparison of observed and self reported compliance with universal precautions among emergency department presonnel at a Minnesota public teaching hospital: implications for assessing infection control programmes. *Ann. Emerg. Med.*, **21**, 940–6.

HEYWORTH, J. (1988). Hepatitis B vaccination in United Kingdom Accident & Emergency departments. *Arch. Emerg. Med.*, **5**, 59–68.

HOWELL, J. (1992). Current and future trends in wound healing. *Emerg. Med. Clin. North Am.*, **10**, 655–63.

HOWELL, J. & CHISHOLM, C. (1992). Outpatient wound preparation and care: a national survey. *Ann. Emerg. Med.*, **21**, 976–81.

HOWELL, J., STAIR, T., HOWELL, A. *et al.* (1992). Cefazolin and povidone iodine as irrigants of contaminated wounds. *Ann. Emerg. Med.*, **21**, 603.

HUGHES, G. & McLEAN, N. (1988). Zinc oxide tape: a useful dressing for the recalcitrant finger tip and soft tissue injury. *Arch. Emerg. Med.*, **5**, 223–7.

HUMPHREY, G., SUPER, P., DALTON, M. *et al.* (1993). Retained glass foreign bodies: configuration and localisation by computerised tomography and ultrasonography. *Injury*, **24**, 493–4.

HUNT, T. (1988). The physiology of wound healing. *Ann. Emerg. Med.*, **17**, 1265–73.

JONES, B. & SANDERS, R. (1983). Pre-tibial injuries: a common pitfall. *Br. Med. J.*, **286**, 502.

LAMMERS, R. & MAGILL, T. (1992). Detection and management of foreign bodies in soft tissue. *Emerg. Med. Clin. North Am.*, **10**, 767–81.

LAMMERS, R., HUDSON, D. & SEAMAN, M. (1992). Predictors of infection in uncomplicated, traumatic wounds. *Ann. Emerg. Med.*, **21**, 604.

LIND, G., MARCUS, M., MEARS, S. *et al.* (1991). Oral transmucosal fentanyl citrate for analgesia and sedation in the emergency department. *Ann. Emerg. Med.*, **20**, 1117.

LINDSEY, D., NAVA, C. & MART, M. (1982). Effectiveness of penicillin irrigation in control of infection in sutured lacerations. *J. Trauma*, **22**, 186–9.

MAIMARIS, C. & QUINTON, D. (1988). Dog bite lacerations: a controlled trial of primary wound closure. *Arch. Emerg. Med.*, **5**, 156–61.

MAITRA, A. & DORANI, B. (1992). Role of zinc in post-injury wound healing. *Arch. Emerg. Med.*, **9**, 122–4.

MALONE, W. (1987). Wound dressing adherence: a clinical comparative study. *Arch. Emerg. Med.*, **4**, 101–5.

MARCUS, R., BELL, D. & CULVER, D. (1990). Frequency of emergency care providers contact with blood of patients infected with human immunodeficiency virus. *Ann. Emerg. Med.*, **19**, 454.

MARKOVCHICK, V. (1992). Suture material and mechanical after care. *Emerg. Med. Clin. North Am.*, **10**, 673–89.

MARTIN, J., DOEZEMA, D., TANDBERG, D. *et al.* (1990). The effect of local anaesthetics on bacterial proliferation: TAC versus lidocaine. *Ann. Emerg. Med.*, **19**, 987–90.

McCABE, M., NASH, P. & BHIDE, A. (1989). The use of histoacryl tissue adhesive for the primary closure of scalp wounds. *Arch. Emerg. Med.*, **6**, 159.

McGLONE, R. & BODENHAM, A. (1990). Reducing the pain of intradermal lignocaine injection by pH buffering. *Arch. Emerg. Med.*, **7**, 65–8.

McGREGOR, F., McCOMBE, A., KIND, P. *et al.* (1989). Skin stapling of wounds in the accident department. *Injury*, **20**, 347–8.

MENEGAZZI, J., PARIS, P., KERSTEEN, C. *et al.* (1991). A randomised controlled trial of the use of music during laceration repair. *Ann. Emerg. Med.*, **20**, 348–50.

MONTANO, J., STEELE, M. & WATSON, W. (1992). Foreign body retention in glass caused wounds. *Ann. Emerg. Med.*, **21**, 1360–3.

MOORE, D. (1992). Hypochlorites: a review of the evidence. *J. Wound Care*, **1**, 44–53.

MORGAN, W. (1979). The effect of povidone iodine aerosol spray on superficial wounds. *Br. J. Clin. Practic.*, **33**, 109–10.

MORRIS, T. & TRACEY, J. (1977). Lignocaine: its effects on wound healing *Br. J. Surg.*, **64**, 902–3.

MORRISON, W., (1993). Transthecal digital block. *Arch. Emerg. Med.*, **10**, 35–8.

MORTON, R., GIBSON, M. & SLOAN, J. (1988). The use of histoacryl tissue adhesive for the primary closure of scalp wounds. *Arch. Emerg. Med.*, **5**, 110–12.

MULLIKEN, J., HEALEY, N. & GLOWACKI, J. (1980). Povidone iodine and tensile strength of wounds in rats. *J. Trauma*, **20**, 323.

NORRIS, R. (1992). Local anaesthetics. *Emerg. Med. Clin. North Am.*, **10**, 707–17.

OBERG, N. (1987). Povidone iodine solutions in traumatic wound preparation. *Am. J. Emerg. Med.*, **5**, 553–5.

PLATT, J. & BUCKNALL, R. (1984). An experimental evaluation of antiseptic wound irrigation. *J. Hosp. Infect.*, **5**, 181–8.

PRIOR, A. (1993). Minimising needlestick injury after venesection. *Hosp. Update*, **12**, 653–4.

PROUDFOOT, J., ROBERTS, N. & MELLICK, L. (1993). Providing safe and effective sedation and analgesia for paediatric patients. *Emerg. Med. Rep.*, **14**, 207–17.

QUINN, J., DRZEWIECKI, A. & LI, M. (1992). A clinical trial comparing *N*-2-butyl-cyanoacrylate with suturing facial lacerations in children. *Ann. Emerg. Med.*, **21**, 591.

REICHL, M. (1989). Septic arthritis following puncture wound of the foot. *Arch. Emerg. Med.*, **6**, 277–9.

REICHL, M. & QUINTON, D. (1987). Comparison of 1% lignocaine with 0.5% bupivacaine in digital ring blocks. *J. Hand Surg.*, **12-B**, 375–6.

RHEE, K., ALBERTSON, T., KIZER, K. *et al.* (1992). A comparison of HIV-1, HBV, and HTLV-1/2, sero prevalence rates of injured patients admitted through California emergency departments. *Ann. Emerg. Med.*, **21**, 397–400.

RIGBY, H. (1992). Tissue healing. *Surgery*, **10**, 261–4.

RITCHIE, A. & ROCKE, L. (1989). Staples versus sutures in the closure of scalp wounds: a prospective, double blind, randomised trial. *Injury*, **20**, 217–18.

ROBSON, M. & HEGGERS, J. (1969). Bacterial quantification of open wounds. *Milit. Med.*, **134**, 19–24.

RODGERS, K. (1992). The rational use of anti-microbial agents in simple wounds. *Emerg. Med. Clin. North Am.*, **10**, 753–65.

RUTHERFORD, W. & SPENCE, R. (1980). Infection of wounds sutured in the Accident and Emergency department. *Ann. Emerg. Med.*, **9**, 350–2.

SCHNEIDER, S., TALAN, D. & PANACEK, E. (1993). Emergency department management of needlestick injuries. *Emerg. Med. Rep.*, **14**, 200–6.

SCHWAB, R. & POWERS, R. (1993). Conservative therapy of plantar puncture wounds. *Ann. Emerg. Med.*, **22**, 941.

SHANKAR, S. & KHOO, C. (1987). Lower limb skin loss: simple outpatient management with meshed skin graft with immediate mobilisation. *Arch. Emerg. Med.*, **4**, 187–92.

SMITH, J. & SANTER, L. (1993). Respiratory arrest following intramuscular ketamine injection in a 4-year-old child. *Ann. Emerg. Med.*, **22**, 613–15.

SNYDER, K. & PENTECOST, M. (1990). Clinical and angiographic findings in extremity arterial injuries secondary to dog bites. *Ann. Emerg. Med.*, **19**, 983–6.

SPIVEY, W., McNAMARA, R., MacKENZIE, R. *et al.* (1987). A clinical comparison of lidocaine and bupivacaine. *Ann. Emerg. Med.*, **16**, 752–7.

START, N., ARMSTRONG, A. & ROBSON, W.J. (1989). The use of chromic catgut in the primary closure of scalp wounds in children. *Arch. Emerg. Med.*, **6**, 216–19.

STURM, J. (1991). HIV prevalence in a mid-western emergency department. *Ann. Emerg. Med.*, **20**, 276–8.

STURROCK, J. & NUNN, J. (1979). Cytotoxic effects of procaine, lignocaine and bupivacaine. *Br. J. Anaesth.*, **51**, 273.

SUTTON, R. & PRITTY, P. (1985). Use of sutures or adhesive tapes for primary closure of pre-tibial lacerations. *Br. Med. J.*, **290**, 1627.

TAIWO, B., FLOWERS, M. & ZOLTIE, N. (1992). Reducing children's fear when undergoing painful procedures. *Arch. Emerg. Med.*, **9**, 306–9.

TODD, K. & BERK, W. (1992). Infection control for health care workers caring for critically injured patients: a national survey. *Ann. Emerg. Med.*, **21**, 589.

TODD, K., BERK, W. & HUANG, R. (1992). Effect of body locale and addition of epinephrine on the duration of action of a local anaesthetic agent. *Ann. Emerg. Med.*, **21**, 723–6.

VAISHYA, R. (1990). A thorny problem: the diagnosis and treatment of acacia thorn injuries. *Injury*, **21**, 97–100.

WATSON, D. (1989). Use of cyanoacrylate tissue adhesive for closing facial lacerations in children. *Br. Med. J.*, **299**, 1014.

WEARS, R., VUKICH, D., WINTON, C. *et al.* (1991). An analysis of emergency physicians cumulative career risk of HIV infection. *Ann. Emerg. Med.*, **20**, 749–53.

WEBSTER, D., PELLEGRINI, L. & DUFFY, K. (1992). Use of transcutaneous electrical nerve stimulation for finger tip analgesia: a pilot study. *Ann. Emerg. Med.*, **21**, 1472–5.

WEST, A. & GLUCKSMAN, E. (1987). The use of a metal locator in an accident and emergency department. *Arch. Emerg. Med.*, **4**, 57–61.

WORLOCK, P., BOLAND, P., DARRELL, J. *et al.* (1980). The role of prophylactic antibiotics following hand injuries. *Br. J. Clin. Pract.*, **39**, 290–2.

WRIGHT, S.W., CHUDNOFSKY, C., DRONEN, S. *et al.* (1993). Comparison of midazolam and diazepam for conscious sedation in the emergency department. *Ann. Emerg. Med.*, **22**, 201–5.

YEALY, D., ELLIS, J., HOBBS, G. *et al.* (1992). Intranasal midazolam as a sedative for children during laceration repair. *Ann. Emerg. Med.*, **21**, 619.

ZALUT, T., COOPER, M., WAINSTEIN, J. *et al.* (1990). Prevalence of HIV positive patients in multiple emergency department settings. *Ann. Emerg. Med.*, **19**, 611.

13 Hospital response to disasters in the UK

M.C. GAVALAS[a] and S.A.D. MILES[b]

[a]Accident and Emergency Department, University College Hospital, London, UK
[b]Accident and Emergency Department, Royal Hospitals' NHS Trust, London, UK

Chapter plan

Introduction
Types and causes of major disasters
Hospital major incident plan

INTRODUCTION

Major disasters, with the potential to overwhelm emergency services and hospitals, occur infrequently and for this reason concern about the chaos they may produce may with time be replaced by complacency amongst those whose responsibilities it will be to care for the victims. Postdisaster assessment of recent tragedies has naturally included a great deal of praise for personnel working under great strain and in adverse conditions (Rowlands, 1990); the feeling is generated that those involved have undoubtedly 'done their best'.

More realistic examination of the conduct of such incidents has frequently shown major deficiencies (New, 1992). Poor training of personnel, lack of communication between emergency services and hospitals, poor communication technology and inadequacies of equipment have all been identified. Such deficiencies may only be remedied by detailed planning and investment in training and equipment.

The UK is fortunate not to be plagued by natural catastrophes such as the earthquakes which devastated Armenia and Mexico City, but the activities of man produce a steady stream of disasters. These are characterized by their great variability, rendering the preparation of a universal plan for responding to these incidents virtually impossible (Sharpe et al., 1985).

Although individual hospitals will rarely experience such disasters it is essential that all hospitals dealing with major trauma have a general multidisciplinary response plan which can be tailored to local circumstances and occurrences.

Preparation of a well-researched and frequently revised Hospital Major Incident Plan (HMIP) incorporates:	
PLANNING	Taking into account local resources
PREDICTION	Special risk factors, e.g. Nuclear/Chemical/Airports
PREVIOUS INCIDENTS	Studied and lessons learnt, e.g. Communications
PRACTICE	Table-top and full-scale exercises
POTENTIAL FOR IMPROVEMENT	Implementation of changes
PARTICIPANTS	Training of staff and familiarization with HMIP
PRESS AND PUBLIC	Control/Assistance/Security

It should be recognized by hospital authorities that the detailed planning and training required for major incident capability are time-consuming and may be expensive, particularly if realistic exercises are conducted (Rutherford, 1990). They may need to be reminded of the provisions contained in the guidance issued by the Department of Health (HC(90)25) which makes regional health authorities responsible for ensuring that all districts have comprehensive plans for disasters. Such plans must pay attention to the possibility that the disaster may involve the hospital itself.

TYPES AND CAUSES OF MAJOR DISASTERS

Natural disasters

Destructive climatic incidents occur infrequently (Table 1) and when they do occur they rarely reach disaster proportions; however, the potential for injuring humans in large numbers can never be ignored.

Table 1. *Natural disasters in the UK*

East coast floods	February 1953	Widespread destruction and 280 deaths
Aberfan	October 1966	Coaltip loosened by rain. Landslip covered junior school and many houses, killing 116 children and 28 adults
South-East Britain	October 1987	Hurricane havoc and devastation

Man-made disasters

Man-made calamities in peacetime caused by travel, terrorism, fire and industrial accidents are sudden events causing a variable number of deaths but a predictable pattern of survivors.

```
Types of man-made major incidents

FIRES

TRANSPORT
- Air
- Rail     (a) Underground   (b) Overground
- Road
- Water    (a) River   (b) Sea

EXPLOSIONS
- Chemical, Gas, Mines,
- Munitions, Terrorism, Nuclear

CROWD
- Civil riots
- Sports events

BUILDING COLLAPSE

SHOOTING INCIDENTS

FOOD AND WATER CONTAMINATION

EPIDEMICS

WAR
```

However, the Gulf conflict, due to the large number of British troops involved (30 000) and the need to plan for what was anticipated to be a long conflict, proved to be a milestone in understanding major incident planning and the problems inherent in the multi-disciplinary response required to treat seriously injured patients (Yates, 1991). The mass casualties anticipated never materialized, but the lessons learnt in the UK proved an invaluable experience for peacetime.

Transport disasters

Road traffic accidents

The ever-increasing use of our roads, particularly motor-ways, inevitably leads to major accidents and multiple casualties (Fig. 1).

Irrespective of numbers, if the severity of injuries requires extraordinary measures to be taken for their reception and management, this constitutes a major incident; e.g. M4 multiple vehicle accident March 1991, 45 vehicles involved, 10 dead, 25 injured.

The initiative of the Department of Health, 'The Health of the Nation', with its emphasis on prevention, must be taken seriously by the specialty of accident and emergency (A&E) medicine, which must exert pressure for the introduction (and legislation) of accident prevention measures.

Airport/aircraft accidents

These attract wide media interest and coverage in spite of the superior safety record of air travel. Excluding acts of terrorism (e.g. Lockerbie; Fig. 2), the majority of such accidents are caused by human error; only rarely are mechanical faults to blame (Table 2).

Table 2. *Air travel incidents*

Cardiff	March 1950	80 dead	Human error
Manchester Ringway	August 1985	54 dead	Design fault
Kegworth – M1 (Fig. 3)	January 1989	38 dead	Mechanical fault/ Pilot error

The chances of survival in accidents occurring at an airport outweigh those occurring during flights which are generally non-survivable. If there are survivors on board they usually outnumber the dead (e.g. Kegworth; Fig. 3) (Fahey, 1988).

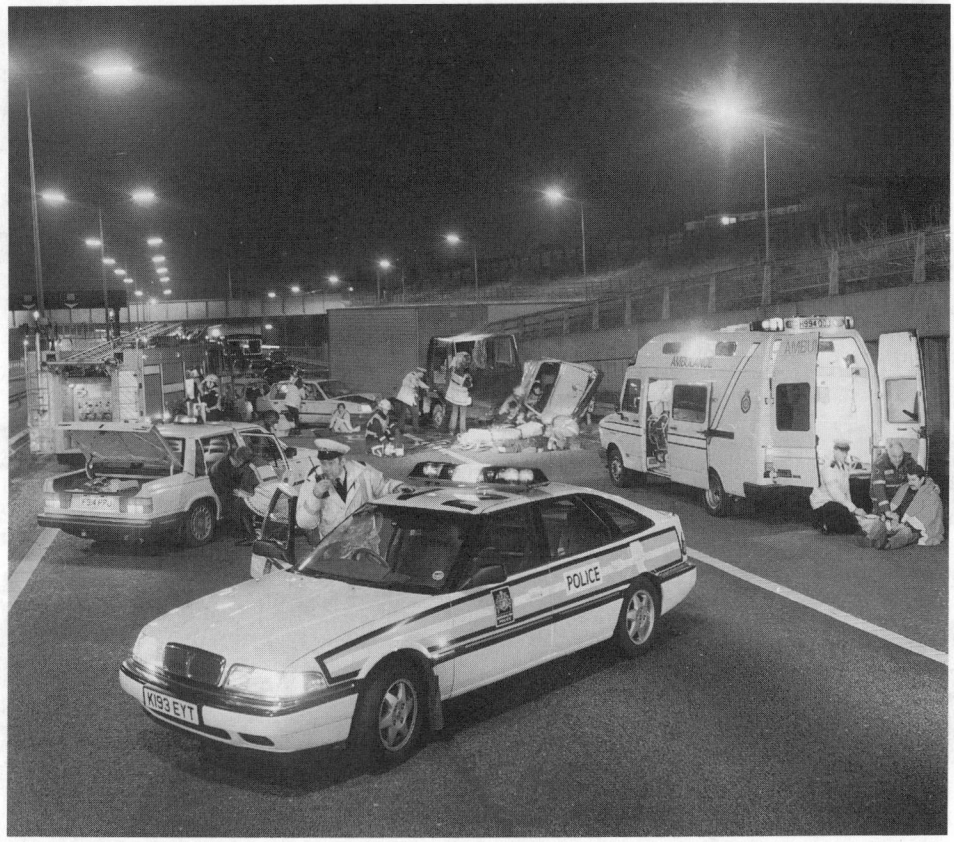

Fig. 1. Training exercise of a multiple vehicle crash. (Courtesy of the Metropolitan Police New Scotland Yard.)

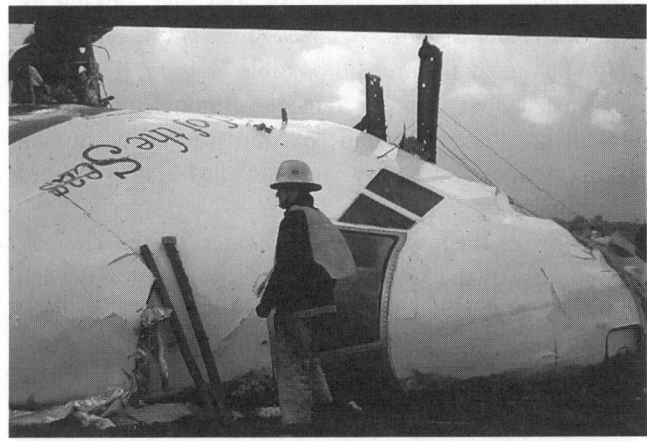

Fig. 2. The Lockerbie disaster. (Courtesy of Dr Brian Roberts, BASICS.)

In planning for aircraft accidents, the possibility of ground casualties must be borne in mind and the proximity of high-rise residential or office blocks to airports be taken into account.

Spectators at airshows are also at risk; e.g, Farnborough disaster September 1952 – 26 dead, 65 injured, and Ramstein August 1988 – 33 dead, hundreds injured.

Helicopter crashes are also responsible for a number of major incidents which may paralyse an unprepared local hospital and emergency services; e.g. Scilly Isles July 1983 – 20 dead, and Shetland Islands November 1986 – 45 dead.

Rail and tunnel accidents

Derailments, often caused by vandalism or failure of railway equipment or structure, and crashes caused by signalling faults, or other direct impact collisions, will regrettably continue to occur (Table 3 and Fig. 4).

The disaster at Moorgate (Fig. 5) was unique in its morphology (Winch et al., 1976) but the difficulties of tunnel rescue (entrapment, poor access and environmental factors) will always exist. In the future, the Channel Tunnel could become the site for such an incident.

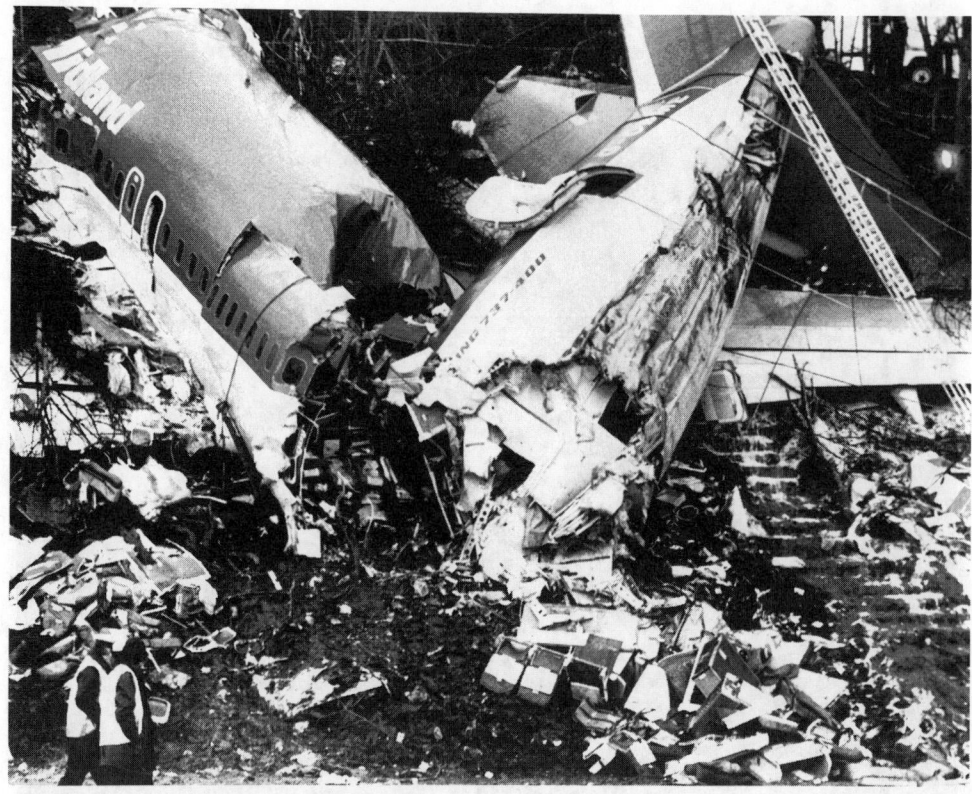

Fig. 3. The crash at Kegworth. (Courtesy of the Guardian.)

Table 3. *Recent UK rail accidents*

Underground and tunnel accidents		
Moorgate crash	February 1975	43 dead, 74 injured
Cannon Street crash[a]	January 1991	2 dead, 277 injured
Overground		
Nuneaton derailment	June 1975	6 dead, 30 injured
Falkirk crash	July 1984	13 dead, 33 injured
Clapham Junction crash	December 1988	35 Dead, hundreds injured
Purley rail crash	March 1989	5 Dead, 87 injured

[a] Although a British Rail station, Cannon Street is actually situated underground (Fig. 4).

The inaccessibility of the scene of many rail accidents (well illustrated by the Clapham Junction disaster; Fig. 6) and the risk to rescuers from electricity are problems peculiar to rail crashes (Stevens & Partridge, 1990).

River/sea travel

Disasters on rivers or at sea are not uncommon and can cause major loss of life. The capsizing of the *Estonia* and the *Herald of Free Enterprise* and the sinking of the *Marchioness* in the Thames (Fig. 7) are reminders that such incidents are still possible.

Capsizing or sinking due to criminal negligence, unseaworthiness and from collisions caused by human error or poor visibility are not just Third World phenomena.

Following the loss of the *Marchioness* on the Thames, the enquiry by the Marine Accident Investigation Branch resulted in strict regulations controlling all aspects of river traffic. The possibility of a collision on the rivers and in the ports remains, in spite of these safety measures.

Fires

Fire disaster medicine is very complex due to the unique association of fires with explosions, road and rail accidents, terrorism and airline incidents. Apart from burns, patients often sustain other serious injuries including fractures and pulmonary inhalation (Griffiths, 1985).

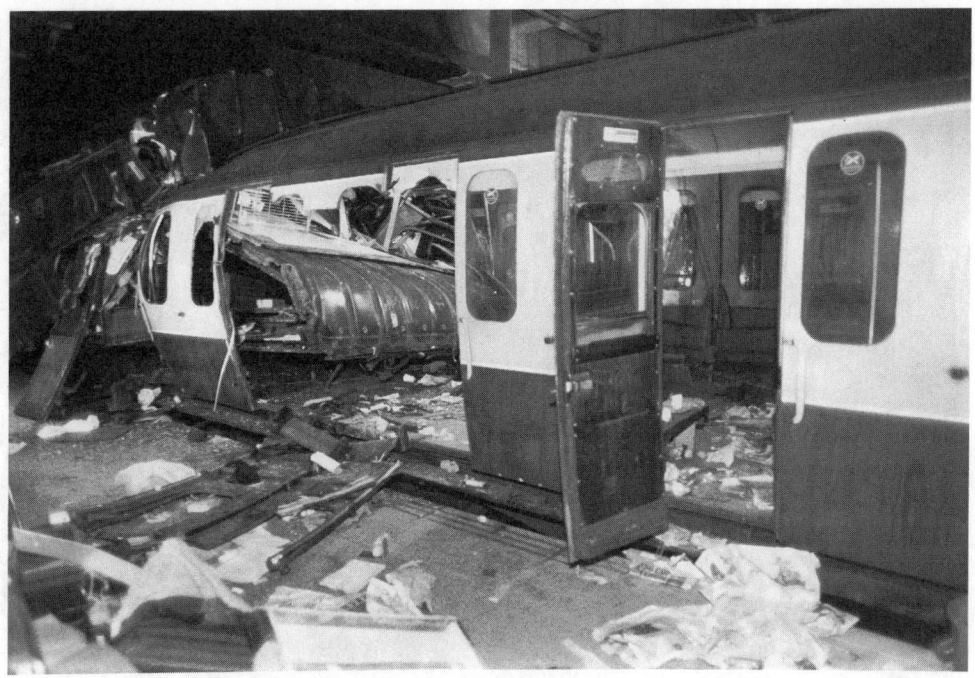

Fig. 4. Crash at Cannon Street. (Courtesy of the Guardian.)

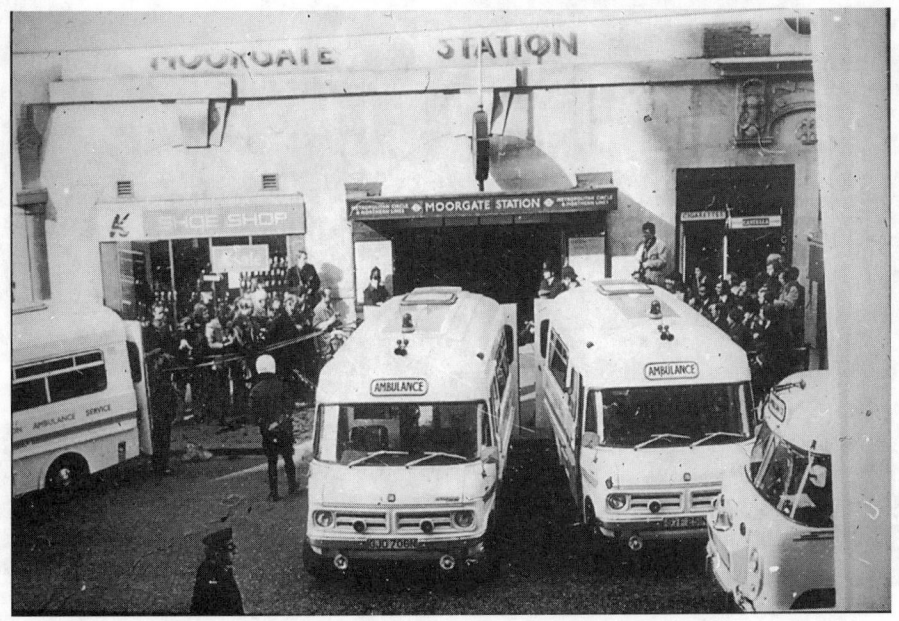

Fig. 5. Crash at Moorgate. (Courtesy of Dr Ken Hines, BASICS.)

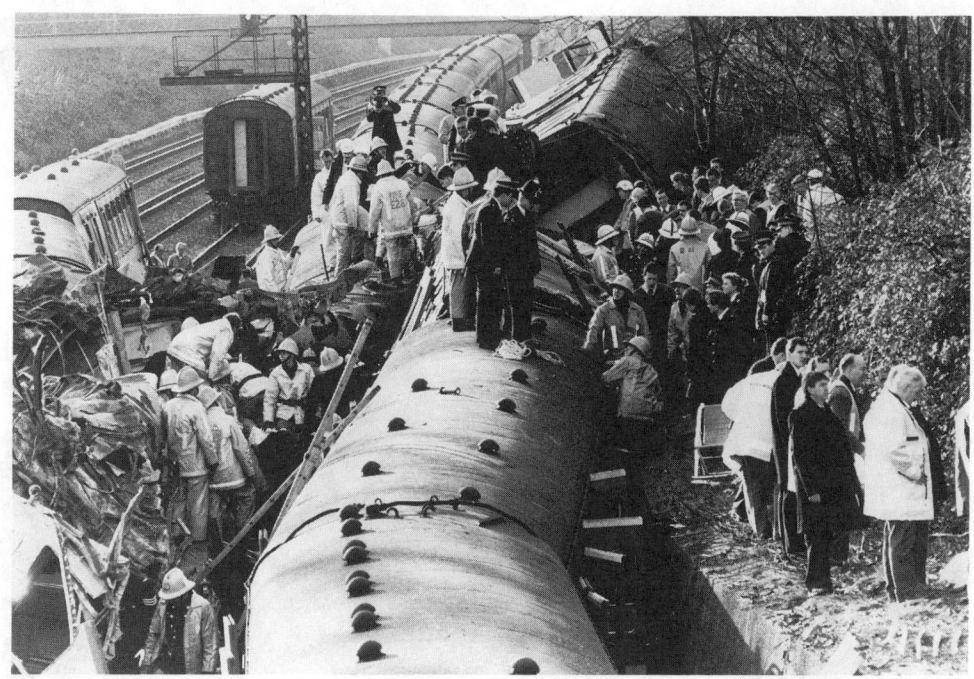

Fig. 6. The Clapham Junction disaster. (Courtesy of the Guardian.)

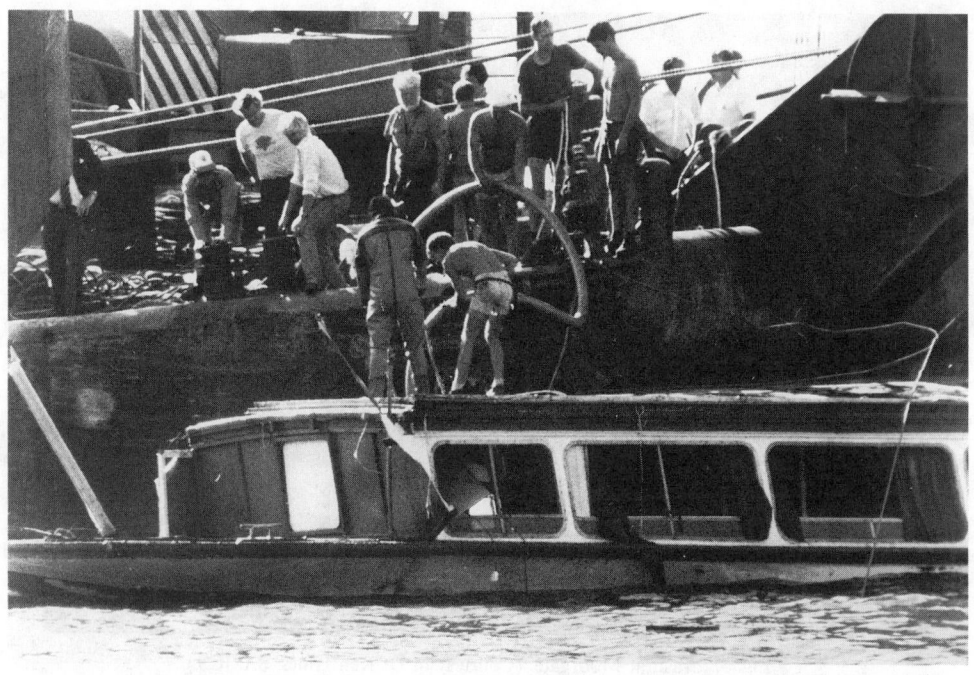

Fig. 7. The *Marchioness* disaster. (Courtesy of the Guardian.)

Table 4. *Recent fire disasters in the UK*

London	August 1980	37 dead, 62 injured
		– Inadequate fire escapes
Stardust Club, Dublin	February 1981	49 dead, 130 injured
	(St Valentine's Day disaster)	– Emergency exits blocked
Bradford football ground	May 1985	56 dead, 55 burnt, hundreds injured
		– Turnstile exit doors locked
Manchester Ringway Airport	August 1985	54 dead, 40 injured
		– Fatalities due to toxic fumes
King's Cross underground	November 1987	32 dead, 37 injured
		– Emergency equipment and plans non-existent
Piper Alpha oil rig	July 1988	167 Dead

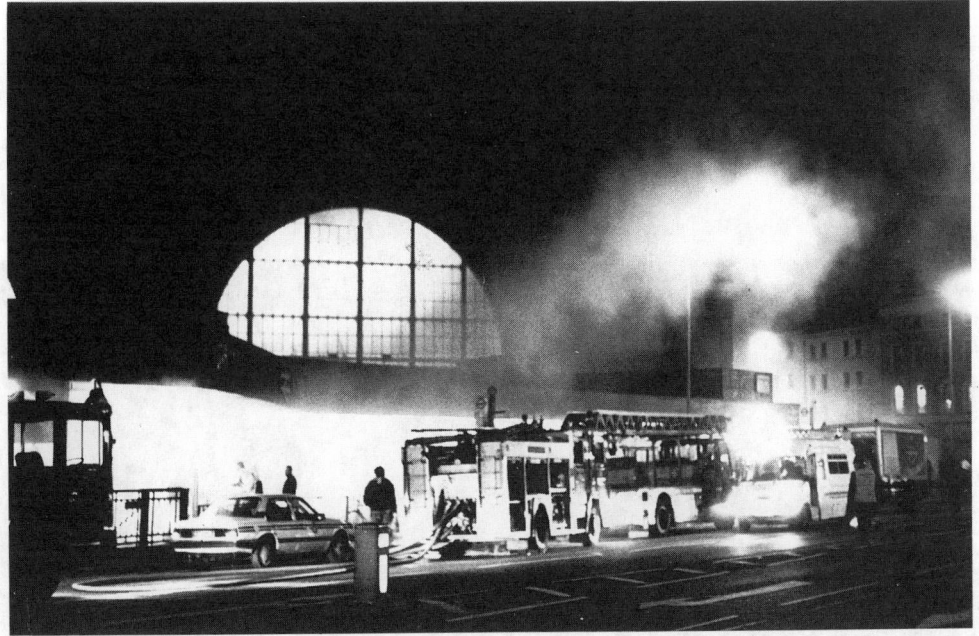

Fig. 8. The fire at King's Cross Station. (Courtesy of the Guardian.)

These disasters generally occur in confined and enclosed areas and it is easily understood how large numbers of people die trapped, unable to escape an inferno, e.g. King's Cross fire (Fig. 8). However, fire disasters may occur in open air stadia, killing spectators who may be trapped behind obstructions such as fences or gates (Sharpe *et al.*, 1985) (Table 4).

With the exception of deaths caused by critical burns and multiple injuries seen following desperate jumps from burning buildings, many fatalities associated with fire disasters are preventable (Fig. 9).

Carbon monoxide poisoning, toxic fume and smoke inhalation, and direct thermal pulmonary injury (leading later to sepsis or adult respiratory distress syndrome) need early intensive care management. This may, unfortunately, be the limiting factor as the number of intensive care beds is restricted.

The wooden stands in less glamorous football clubs and the breaches of legislation regarding locking of exits and access to the pitch are a potential recipe for disaster. A repetition of the stadium fire at Bradford (Fig. 10) is a remote but frightening possibility.

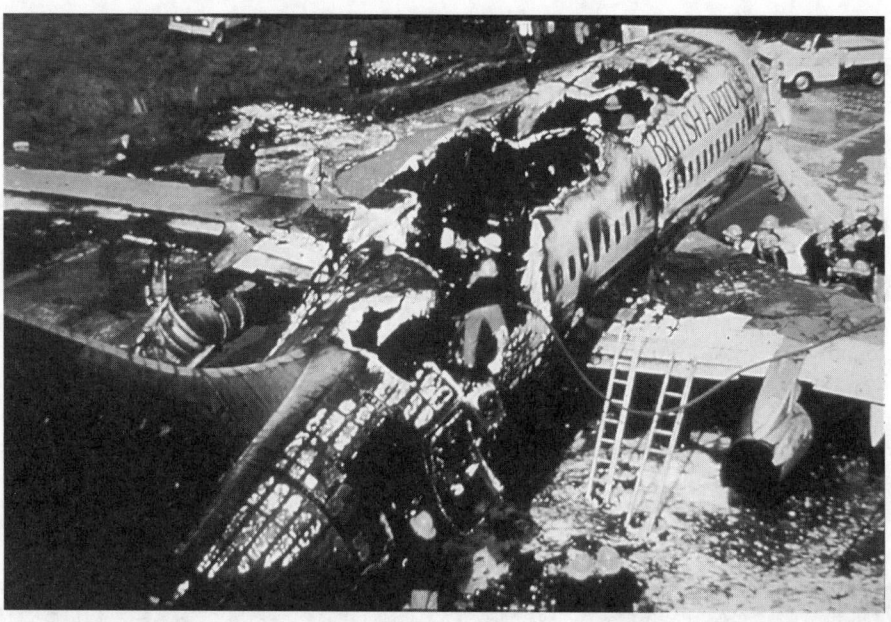

Fig. 9. The Manchester Airport disaster. (Courtesy of Dr Brian Roberts, BASICS.)

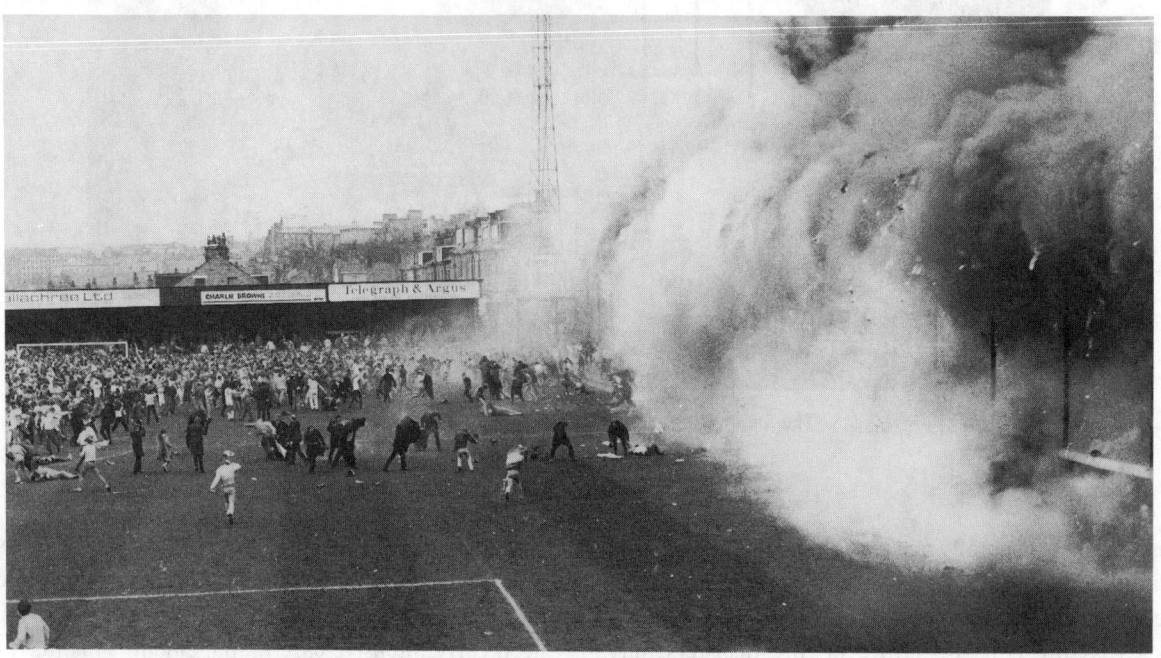

Fig. 10. The Bradford diaster. (Courtesy of Express Newspapers.)

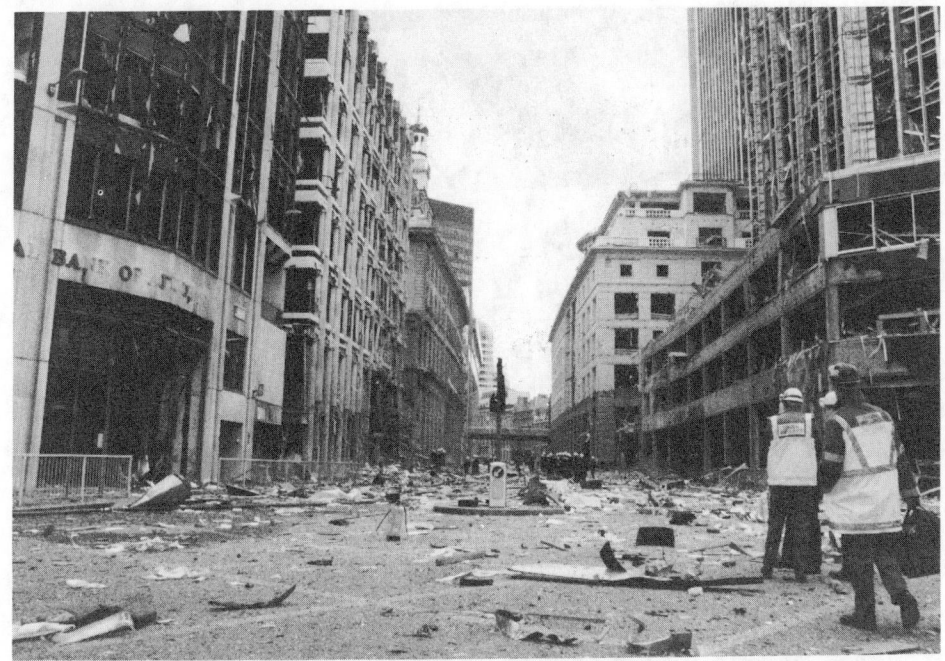

Fig. 11. Bomb explosion in the City of London. (Courtesy of the London Ambulance Service.)

Table 5. *UK bomb incidents*

Birmingham	November 1974	17 dead
		120 injured
Chelsea Barracks	October 1981	2 dead
		72 injured
Regent's Park	July 1982	6 dead
		30 injured
Harrods	December 1983	5 dead
		90 injured
Brighton, Conservative Convention	October 1984	15 dead
		30 injured
Lockerbie, Scotland	December 1988 (foreign terrorists)	270 dead (inc. 11 on ground)
Deal Barracks	September 1989	11 dead
		30 injured
St Mary Axe, London, Baltic Exchange	April 1992	3 dead
		93 injured
Bishopsgate (City of London)	April 1993	1 dead
		31 injured
Belfast, Shankhill Road	October 1993	9 dead
		55 injured

It is ironic that television programmes expose continental hotels for their lack of fire precautions whereas in the UK there are guest houses which lack basic fire and safety measures.

Terrorism

Terrorism is defined as peacetime acts of intimidatory violence against civilians or military personnel.

London (Fig. 11) and other big cities have been targeted for financial reasons and to embarrass the authorities (Brighton bomb attack; Fig. 12).

Doctors, nurses and members of the emergency services have an ethical and moral obligation to care for all patients without bias. Casualties may include members of terrorist groups involved in the incident who will have to be treated despite the feelings of staff.

Bombs have been responsible for the great majority of casualties associated with terrorism in this country and they are generally used in densely populated areas with the intention of maximizing destruction (Table 5). Rescue operations are hampered by the possibility of further explosives left on the scene by the terrorists (Haywood, 1988).

Rupture of the tympanic membrane due to the blast effect may produce walking but disorientated casualties who add further to the problem.

The psychological consequences affecting all those involved in the incident, including the rescue teams, is a crucial element of major incident planning that needs to be taken into account.

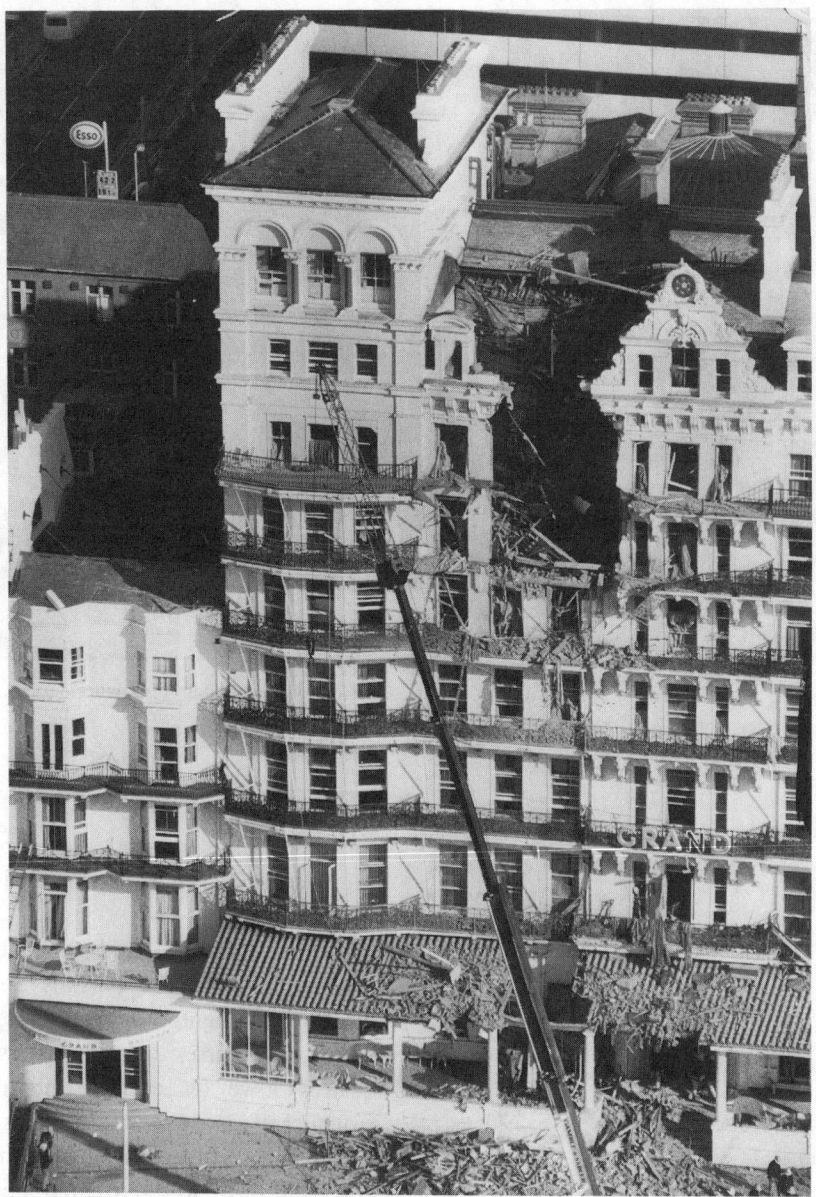

Fig. 12. The Brighton bomb explosion. (Courtesy of Express Newspapers.)

Chemical incidents

Chemicals are hazardous materials and can easily cause vapour or flammable gas explosion, fires, and release of toxins. Disasters involving chemicals are uncommon occurrences in the UK in spite of the enormous size of the industry (80 million tonnes of chemicals are distributed annually by river, sea, road, rail and pipeline).

Stringent efforts in the UK to control and regulate the production, storage, transport and use of these dangerous materials are encapsulated in legislation, 'Control of

Industry Major Accident Hazard Regulations, 1984' (CIMAH), which requires planning to be undertaken for on-site and off-site incidents and has resulted in co-operation between the emergency services and the medical profession in planning for chemical incidents (Fig. 13).

Although disasters of the catastrophic dimensions of Bhopal and Mexico City are never expected to be seen in this country, there are serious doubts regarding the health service's readiness to deal with major chemical incidents (Baxter 1991), expressed at a symposium at the

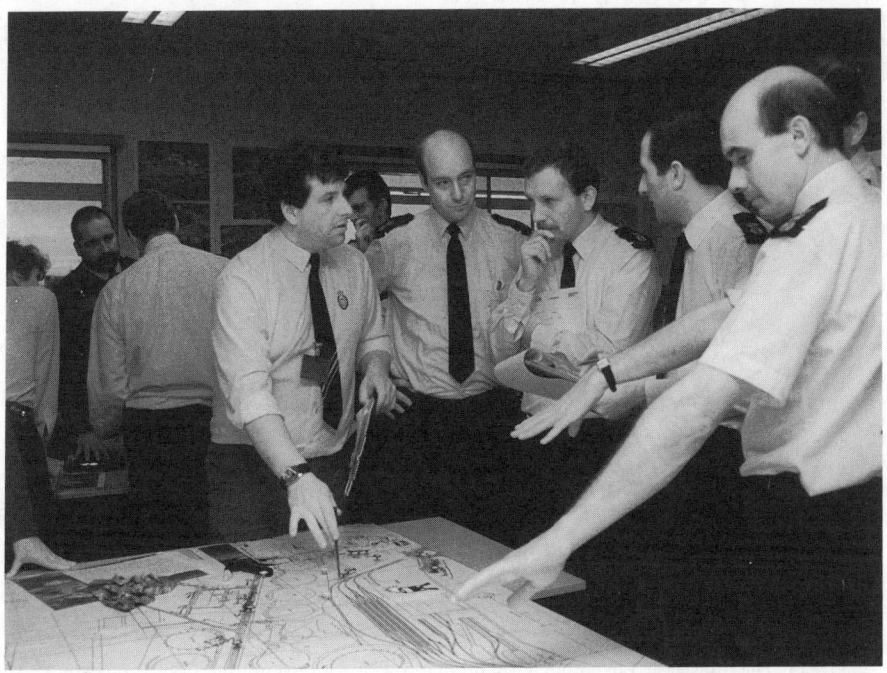

Fig. 13. CIMAH exercise at Beckton gas works, London. (Courtesy of the Emergency Planning Department, LFCDA.)

Royal Society of Medicine in London 1990. Serious chemical incidents have occurred and will continue to do so, constantly putting the emergency services' readiness and organization to the test.

The disaster at Flixborough (Humberside) in 1974, in which an industrial explosion wrecked 100 stone-built houses (29 dead, hundreds injured), was the worst incident of this sort that has occurred in the UK (Fig. 14). The incidents on the A4 in North London in 1990 (which injured 12 following a leak of ethyl dichlorosilane) (Thanabalasmgham et al., 1991) and at the Bank underground station in 1992 (which injured 24, two of whom were critical) were potentially very serious accidents.

The accident at Castleford (Wakefield) in 1992 (which killed two and injured 15) was a critical incident which highlighted the real risk of contamination of hospital staff.

Planning must always take into consideration that the majority of chemical plants and other hazardous industrial complexes have until recently been built in densely populated areas, and are a constant threat to life (Cassidy, 1990).

The 'chain of rescue' for a major chemical incident consists of five links with communication between them and a source of toxicological expertise being of vital importance (Fig. 15).

The emergency services have standard procedures for dealing with chemical incidents and through training have acquired proficiency in dealing with them (Fig. 13).

Like any chain, this one is only as strong as its weakest link; A&E departments and staff are experienced in dealing with trauma but regrettably generally lack protocols for managing multiple casualties exposed to chemicals (Baxter, 1991). A&E departments may lack protective clothing, facilities for decontamination and access to antidotes. Most staff are not trained for this type of disaster medicine.

Lack of local toxicological and epidemiological expertise contributes to the complexity of problems associated with major chemical incidents. Patients may be suffering concurrently from trauma caused by blast, road traffic accidents and burns.

Gas explosions/building collapses

Most of the casualties have crush injuries caused by collapse of buildings or asphyxiation associated with entrapment (Table 6). Victims buried in rubble may only have had access to small pockets of air for lengthy periods of time.

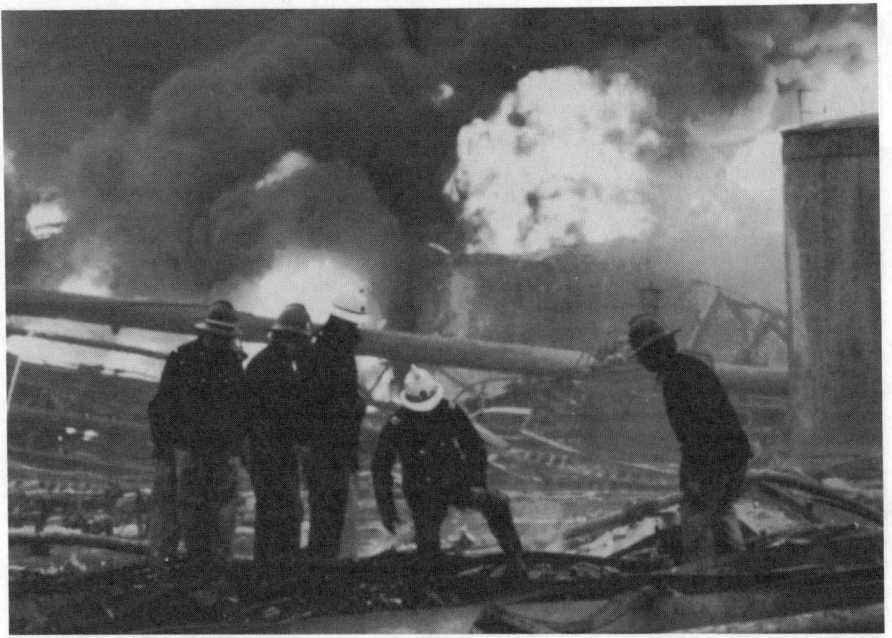

Fig. 14. The disaster at Flixborough. (Reproduced with permission from Civil Protection.)

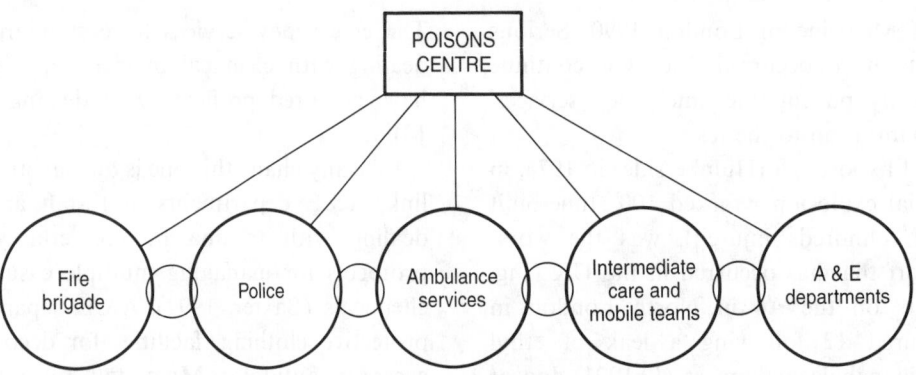

Fig. 15. 'Chain of rescue' for a major chemical incident.

Table 6. *Incidents of gas explosion in the UK*

Ronan Point, Newham, London	May 1968	3 dead 32 injured	Tower block collapse after gas explosion
Clarkston, Scotland	October 1971	20 dead 110 injured	Leak of household gas
Abbeystead, Lancashire	May 1984	13 Dead 60 injured	Underground gas explosion
Putney, London[a]	January 1985	8 dead 17 injured	Gas explosion

[a] Fig. 16.

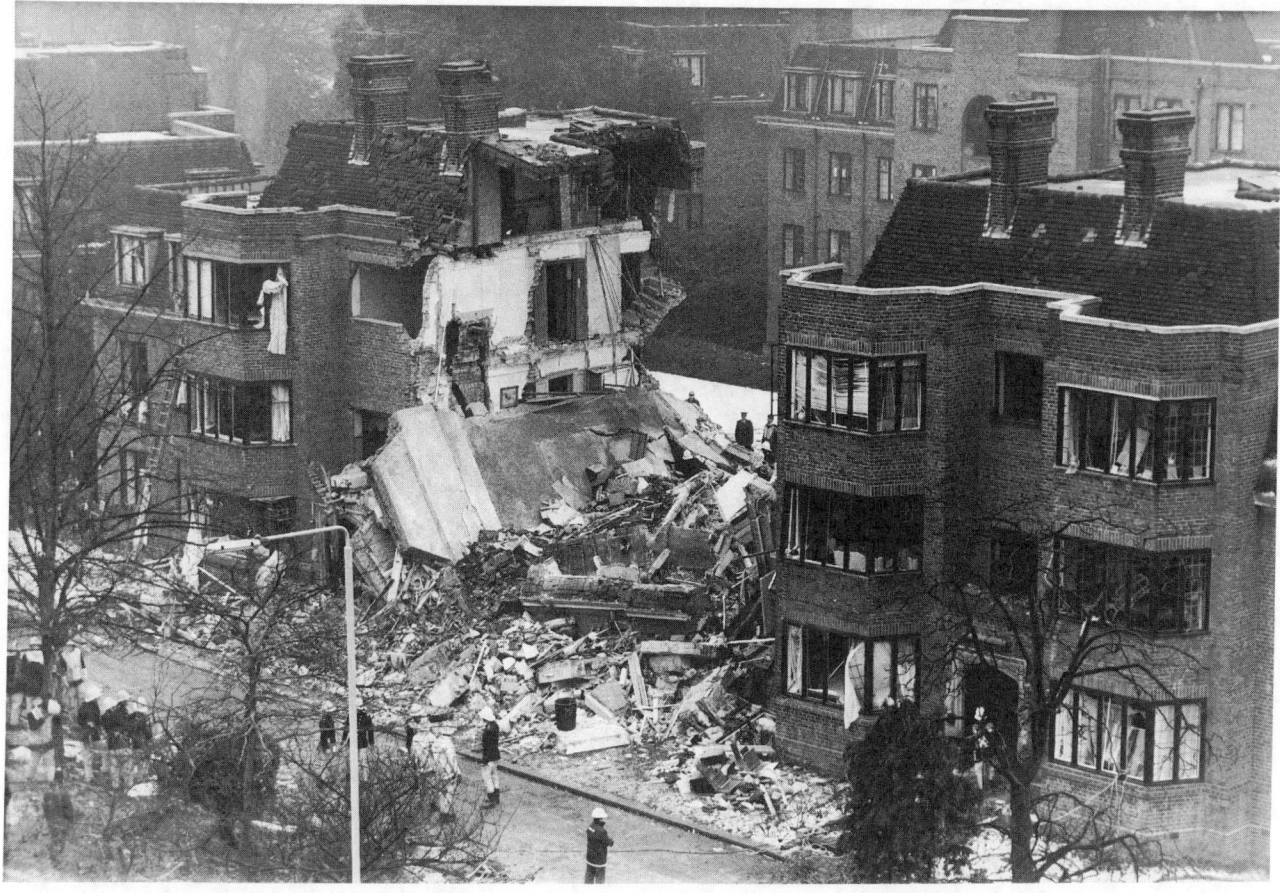

Fig. 16. The Putney explosion. (Courtesy of the Evening Standard.)

Thermal imaging devices (Fig. 17) can now pin-point buried victims, and this factor must influence the cessation of the hospitals' major incident response.

It is rare for buildings to collapse spontaneously or from overcrowding in this country. The Ronan Point Disaster (caused by an engineering fault) was an exception; although tower blocks remain socially and aesthetically disliked, they offer safe dwellings to thousands of people.

Many of the major and minor injuries that occur when buildings collapse are caused by flying glass fragments; therefore the use of structural glass should be controlled (Fig. 18).

Mine explosions and collapses

With the decline in the coal industry, there has been a parallel decline in accidents and, although isolated incidents which claim lives still occur (e.g. Derbyshire 1950 – 80 dead), they rarely reach the proportion of a disaster.

Shooting incidents

There are three types of shooting incidents:

1. Criminal: armed robbery, often drug related.
2. Terrorism.
3. Psychopathic violence.

In spite of strict legislation forbidding the carrying or selling of firearms, with the increase in drugs-related crimes there has been an explosion of shooting incidents involving firearms. Contract killings and the creation of 'no go areas' and ghettos in our inner cities are regrettably increasingly common.

The availability of sophisticated firearms has increased the potential for gang warfare between drug 'barons' as well as the shooting of individuals. This is a challenge to A&E departments near high-risk sites such as Moss Side in Manchester.

Unpremeditated massacres occur, involving deranged

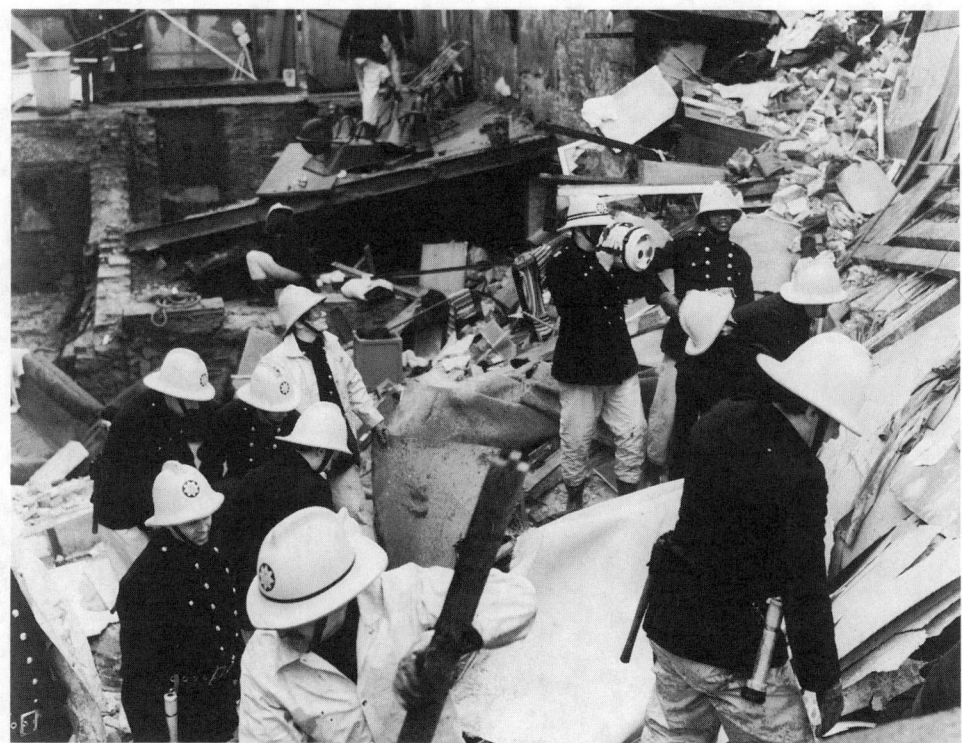

Fig. 17. Thermal imaging device in use. (Courtesy of the London Fire Brigade.)

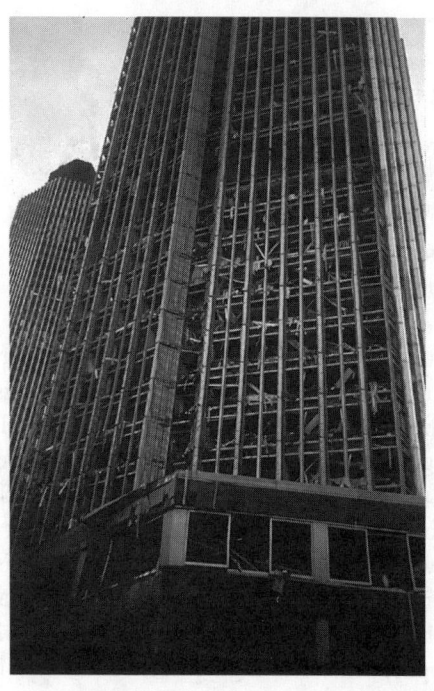

Fig. 18. Extensive damage in a glass tower (Bishopsgate) following a terrorist attack. (Courtesy of Dr Ken Hines, BASICS.)

individuals, often licensed to keep guns and rifles. A repeat of the 'Hungerford' and 'Dunblane' incidents could occur unless more stringent legislation is able to control the use of firearms.

Sports and other public venues

It is easy to understand how a disaster can occur when a panic-stricken crowd rushes through a bottleneck to a perceived area of safety, especially when the exits leading to safety are blocked, obstructed or locked with steel gates. This was exemplified by the tragedy in Bethnal Green in March 1943 when, during a false air raid alarm, a total of 178 people died and ironically not a single bomb fell.

The Hillsborough (Fig 19) and Ibrox disasters (Table 7) were caused by a catalogue of errors, misjudgement and poor terrace design.

Such inadequacies at stadia and other sporting venues may be aggravated by deficiencies in the personnel and equipment necessary for the provision of advanced life support. Even small-scale emergencies such as cardiac arrests are often poorly dealt with (Wardrope et al., 1991).

Twenty years after Ibrox, and following the report of the public inquiry into the Hillsborogh disaster (Taylor,

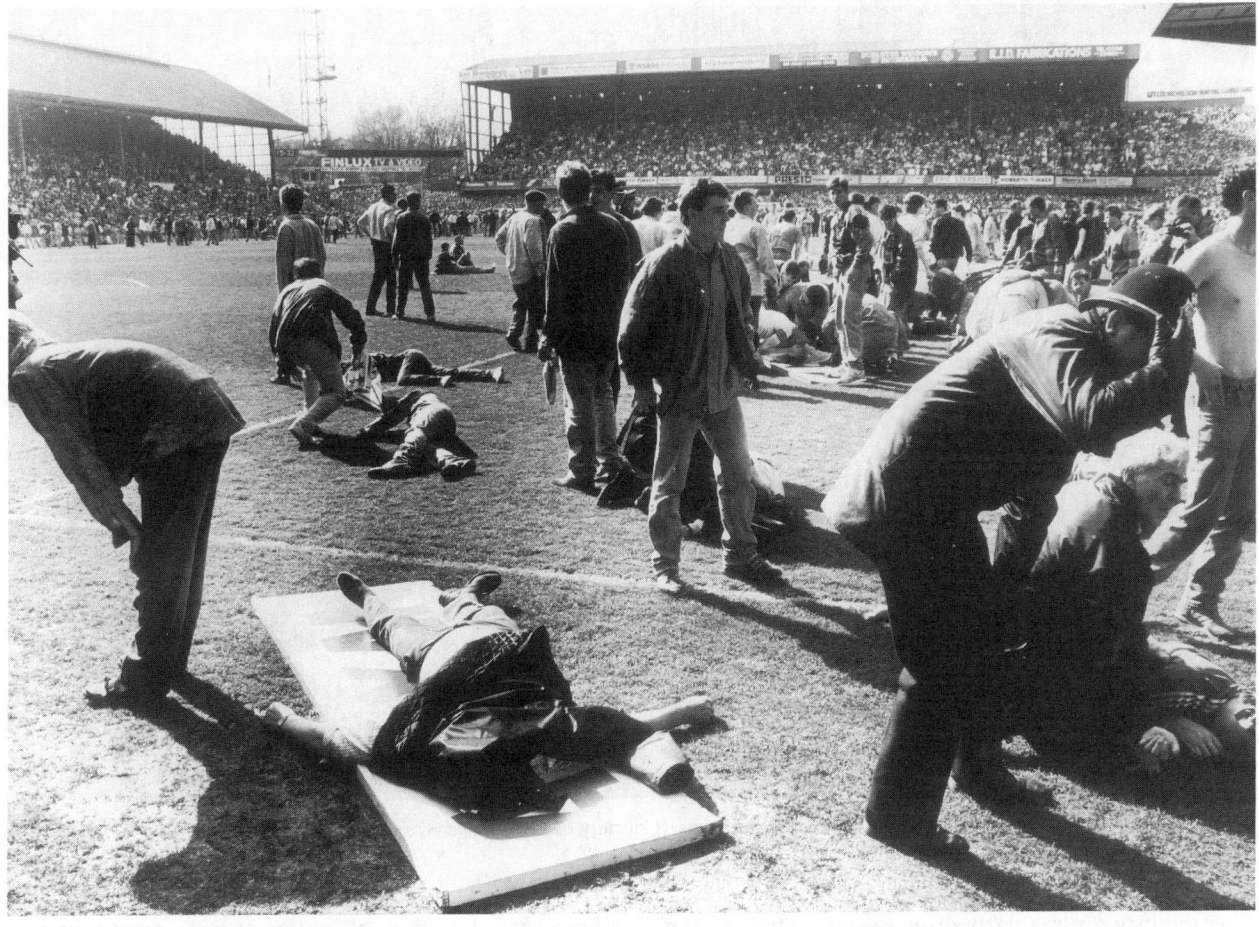

Fig. 19. Chaos and tragedy of Hillsborough. (Courtesy of the Sun.)

Table 7. *Incidents at sports venues in the UK*

Ibrox, Glasgow	January 1971	66 dead
		100 injured
Hillsborough, Sheffield	April 1989	95 dead
		200 injured

1989), the likelihood of an incident of similar dimensions should now be remote. Important lessons were also learnt which have implications for disaster planning (e.g. communications and dealing with the media and distressed relatives) (Wardrope *et al.*, 1990).

Civil disturbances

Socioeconomic discontent, homelessness, unemployment and racial conflict have all been blamed for a series of riots and civil unrest that shook the UK in the 1980s. Brixton (April 1981) (Fig. 20), Liverpool and Birmingham (July 1981), the miners' dispute (1984–1985), the Tottenham riots (October 1985) and the Trafalgar Square Riot (March 1990) are examples.

When civil unrest is close to a designated hospital, rescue arrangements can be hampered and it may be necessary for victims to be treated in other hospitals (Haywood, 1988), with segregation of the 'warring factions' and police casualties (antiracism protests, East London 1993).

Nuclear accidents, epidemics and public health incidents

Nuclear accidents

There is always potential for accidents at nuclear installations, which is enhanced by the increasing age of many of these. Incidents may also occur during the transport of nuclear fuel.

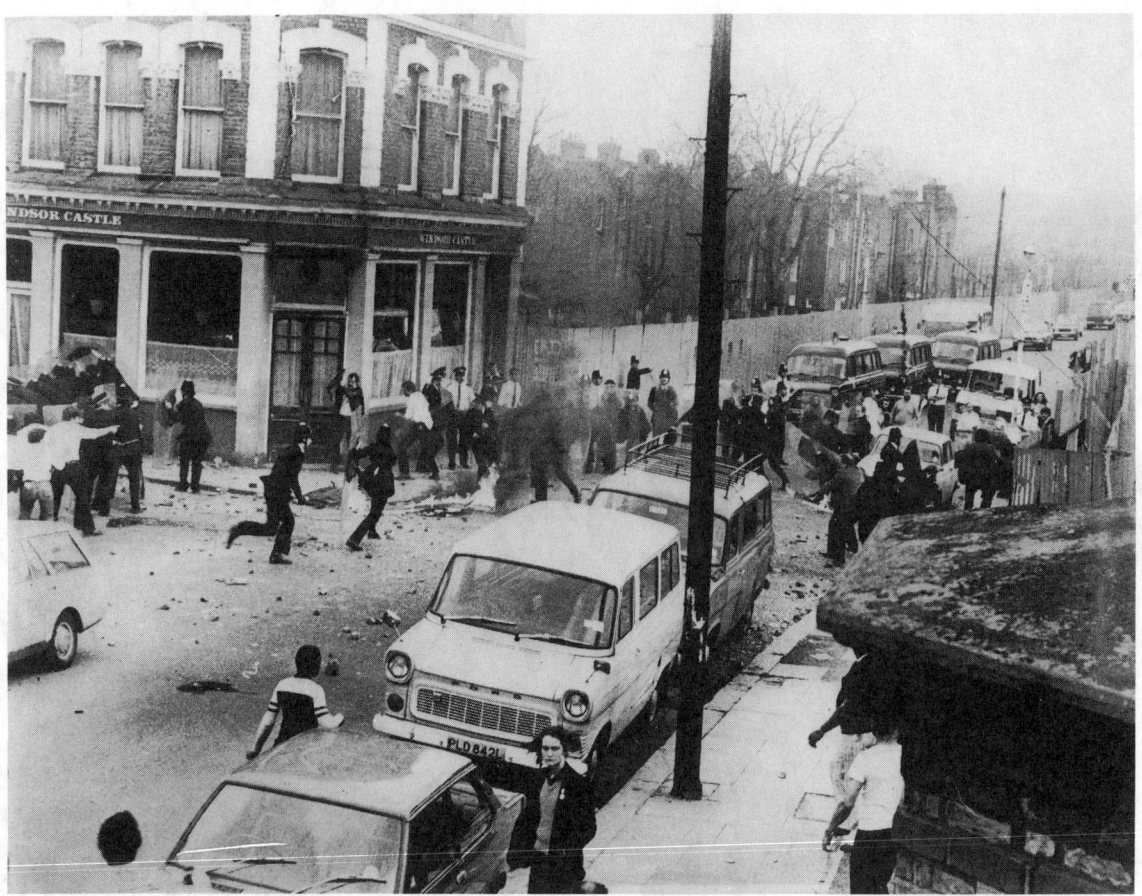

Fig. 20. The Brixton riots. (Courtesy of Express Newspapers.)

The military are regularly drilled in decontamination procedures, but staff in A & E departments may lack basic training in the medical management of nuclear incidents.

Stringent contingency plans cover the risks of transporting nuclear fuel. This is not the case with a convoy of nuclear weapons or incidents at power stations in which contamination of a wide area and long-term morbidity and mortality may well occur (Weller, 1988).

Public health incidents

Outbreaks of food poisoning may result from a breakdown in food handling or storage or an overall lack of hygiene in institutions catering for large numbers of people.

These outbreaks may have catastrophic effects on the young, weak or infirm (Wakefield August 1984, *Salmonella* outbreak – 26 dead, 16 seriously ill; London September 1985, *Escherichia coli* outbreak – 15 dead, 69 seriously ill).

Epidemics rarely reach major incident proportions;

however, the flow of patients may create immense problems for ill-prepared staff, especially when the infectivity is unknown (e.g. Legionnaire's disease outbreak, Staffordshire May 1985 – 31 dead).

The Lowermoor incident (July 1988) in which 20 tonnes of concentrated aluminium sulphate was accidentally discharged into the water treatment works near Camelford had fortunately no long-term effects; it illustrated that such contamination incidents differ from other chemical accidents and need specific planning (Volans, 1990).

HOSPITAL MAJOR INCIDENT PLAN

The key to successful management of a major incident is the operation (both on site and in hospital) of an integrated command and control structure involving the emergency services and listed hospitals. The Hospital Major Incident Plan (HMIP) must always be fully integrated with those of the emergency services (Miller, 1980), be well tested and have an effective communications plan (Yates, 1991). The provision of a medical incident officer (MIO) is essential but who should take on this role is a contentious issue. Taking resources into consideration, this plan should provide for:

- Storage of predetermined equipment and supplies.
- On-site emergency care through mobile medical teams
- Facilities for the reception, treatment and disposal of a specific number of casualties that the hospital is able to deal with.
- Transfer of casualties to other hospitals (Allen *et al.*, 1989).

Provision for the care of in-patients unrelated to the incident should be included in the HMIP, as should an effective system for notification of personnel. Clearly defined areas for the treatment of patients should include decontamination sites (a vital component of planning for chemical/nuclear incidents).

Security procedures for the safety and privacy of patients, staff, relatives and their property should be specified. The comfort and care of distressed relatives and friends and cooperation with the press are vital.

'Action cards' summarizing the roles of personnel involved in dealing with the incident should be provided (Miller, 1980; Miles, 1991) but are no substitute for familiarity with the HMIP. Action cards should be updated regularly and be accessible.

The Department of Health's guidelines for major incidents are regularly revised and should be incorporated into all HMIPs.

Planning should anticipate civilian incidents with mass burn casualties and make provisions for the sharply differing needs of these patients who may be suffering from major injuries (Sharpe *et al.*, 1985).

Putting the HMIP into action

Initiation of major incident procedure

Notification of a major incident is essentially undertaken by the Ambulance Services (Wardrope *et al.*, 1991) via a direct communication link (which should be foolproof and frequently tested) with the A&E departments of receiving and supporting hospitals. Ideally, messages should be taken by the senior doctor or nurse on duty in the A&E department and conveyed to the hospital switchboard where the operator should activate the major incident call-out procedure. Alternatively, the hospital switchboard may be notified directly, in which case their first action should be to notify A&E.

The alerting message should be one of two standard phrases:

1. 'Major incident standby'
2. 'Major incident declared – activate plan'

'*Major incident standby*' warns the hospital that a serious incident may have occurred, or that there is a chance that it will do so.

On receiving this message duty medical, nursing and administrative personnel are alerted to form a coordination team; they establish the control centre and initiate 'warming-up' procedures.

Designated hospitals near major airports which are frequently on standby come under the umbrella of a well-rehearsed AIRPORT MAJOR DISASTER PLAN and should therefore be proficient in initiating specific major incident standby procedures (Malone, 1990). Similar principles apply to hospitals with chemical/ nuclear installations in their catchment areas, and of necessity to hospitals in London and other city centres where false bomb alerts are a frequent phenomenon.

Other hospitals should not limit the extent of their standby procedure but take forward the plan and mobilize their in-hospital response to high levels of operational activity, especially if they receive major incident alerts infrequently. This offers the distinct advantage that, if the incident turns out to be a false alarm, invaluable experience has been gained; if patients start pouring in unexpectedly, the hospital is at maximum readiness to receive them.

If after accepting the major incident standby it is found not to be required, it should be rescinded using the message 'MAJOR INCIDENT CANCELLED'

'*Major incident declared – activate plan*' indicates clearly that a major incident has occurred.

Information on the timing, site and type of incident plus an approximate number of casualties should be clearly supplied and it is essential to know whether the hospital is the first receiving hospital.

Call-out procedure

The HMIP should clearly state how this complex operation is undertaken both in and out of office hours. If names and telephone numbers of key contacts are included in 'action cards' this may inadvertently and inappropriately delegate the responsibility of a so-called cascade call-out system to clinical personnel (Wardrope et al., 1991). Experience from Hillsborough shows that this task should be assigned to administrative personnel and the hospital switchboard.

The HMIP must provide a comprehensive call-out list compiled in order of priority, and should identify two groups. The first group is contacted in standby alerts, and the call-out is extended to the second group if a major incident is declared. The system requires an internal bleep system for resident staff and sophisticated long-range message pagers or home telephone numbers for non-resident staff. Conversation between the contacting and the contacted should be brief and to the point.

Establishment of the control centre

This is essentially a command control with medical leadership provided by the medical incident coordinator. During a major incident all clinical staff will come under his or her authority. This is vital and should be reinforced well in advance to all staff. The medical coordinator liaises with the nursing and administrative coordinators, who in turn supervise the staff under their control.

The control centre should be strategically positioned in close relationship to the A&E department. It should be equipped with special stationery, and patient control boards, signs for hospital use, major incident role tabards and communications equipment.

Medical incident officer

There is no disagreement on what the role of the MIO should be. Their duties are largely concerned with the deployment of medical and nursing personnel at the scene and communication with the receiving hospitals. These are administrative duties and there is no clinical responsibility to care for individual casualties (Miller,

1980). It is mandatory that the MIO is experienced with the emergency services' command structure and communications system and knows in some detail the facilities of the receiving hospitals.

The MIO needs access to a good communication system to liaise with the emergency services and receiving hospitals (New, 1992). The MIO assesses the scene (type of incident, number of casualties, severity of injuries) and the need for medical teams. Other responsibilities include establishing a casualty clearing station, ensuring efficient triage at the scene, transport of patients to appropriate hospitals, and supplies. The MIO should be aware of the physical and psychological state of all medical and nursing staff on the scene and replace them if necessary. The MIO conveys to the ambulance incident officer (AIO) in the ambulance control point (ACP) up-to-date information about the capacity of receiving hospitals to accept more patients.

The HMIP should always designate a MIO and ensure that only trained and experienced clinicians undertake this role. When summoned, the MIO should collect a special uniform from the major incident store room (in A&E) and report to the control centre to be dispatched in an emergency ambulance with police escort to the site of the incident. On arrival the MIO should report to the ACP which is the 'nerve centre' of all activities at the scene (Fig. 21).

Some complex incidents (e.g. underground accidents) may require the support of more than one MIO – one remaining at the ACP and another working closer to the medical teams under his/her supervision. It should be stressed, however, that there should only be one senior MIO in overall charge.

Whatever scheme is employed, all MIOs require instruction in their role. Some groups, such as the British Association for Immediate Care (BASICS), are practised and interested in providing support at the scene of major

---

Once the control centre has been established top priorities are:

Major incident standby
- Summon the medical incident officer (MIO) and medical team
- Start preparations in A&E for the reception of casualties
- Warn ITU*/theatres/clinics about possible disruption of activities
- Commence call-out procedure

Major incident declared
- Dispatch the appropriately uniformed and equipped MIO and mobile teams to the scene (if needed)
- Clear A&E of existing patients, establish triage point, and designate the role of triage officer to a senior surgeon

* Intensive therapy unit.

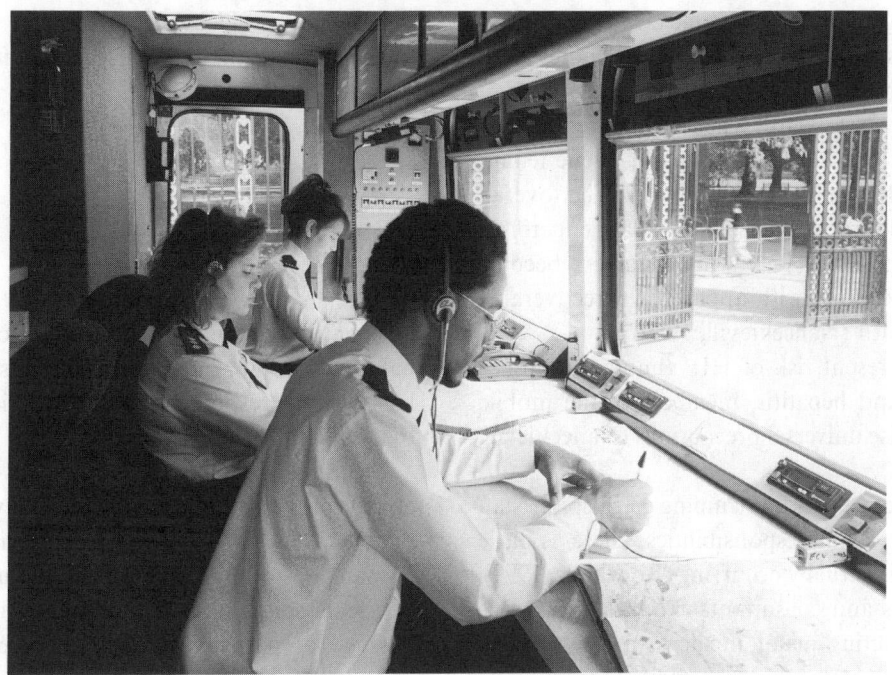

Fig. 21. The ambulance control point (emergency control vehicle). (Courtesy of the London Ambulance Service.)

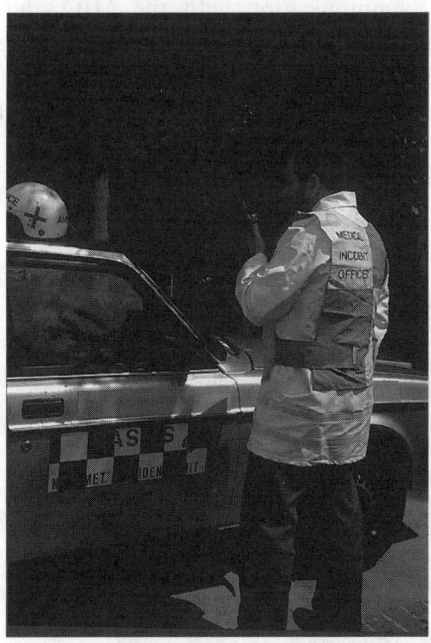

Fig. 22. A BASICS doctor acting as MIO. (Courtesy of Dr Ken Hines, BASICS.

incidents (Fig. 22). It may be appropriate (with the agreement of the appropriate authorities) for hospitals with small numbers of resident staff to write members of such groups into the HMIP as the hospital's designated MIO. Groups of interested A&E consultants may act in a similar way.

Mobile medical team

Like the MIO, team members should wear appropriate protective uniforms (which are now standardized and colour-coded) and carry tabards displaying 'DOCTOR', 'NURSE', etc. They should also wear helmets with headlamps, and robust footwear.

This team (usually made up of one to two doctors and two to four nurses) should be dispatched only on request and it is crucial that provision of this team should not deplete the receiving hospital. Their equipment should be checked regularly and items replaced as necessary. Collaboration with the ambulance services ensures compatibility of equipment and avoids unnecessary duplication.

It is vital that the packing and equipment is user-friendly, sturdy and truly portable (Miller, 1980) and that the staff are familiar with it (usually in **A**irway – **B**reathing – **C**irculation order).

Although mobile teams vary in their constitution, their function is always the same: to report to the MIO at the ACP and follow instructions concerning resuscitation, triaging and removal of casualties by the ambulance services. Speedy medical confirmation of fatalities is crucial to ensure that rescue workers can concentrate efforts on survivors (Edwards, 1989). The dead and the mortally wounded should be photographed to help identification (some HMIPs now include a medical photographer for this gruesome duty) (Wardrope, 1991), but there is no need to remove the bodies until major incident personnel have been stood down.

Medical teams go forward when there are trapped casualties to assist and advise the fire and rescue teams, and offer medical care to these victims. The overall aim is to provide rapid life-saving treatment to as many victims as possible; only when numbers become manageable should those with apparently irrecoverable injuries be dealt with (Nancekievill, 1989).

With the ever-present risk of HIV (human immuno-deficiency virus) and hepatitis, members of the mobile team should practise universal precautions (Nancekievill, 1992).

In spite of guidelines on the training of hospital staff to assume mobile team responsibilities, there is little evidence that this is actually occurring (Rowlands, 1990). Hospital managers and consultants should address this or consider contracting major incident on-site services to specially trained groups (Cooke, 1992). These may be regional teams with previous experience (Redmond, 1989) or teams based on 'Trauma Centres' (Nancekievill, 1992). An alternative is the development of a system similar to that in France (Service d'aide Médicale Urgente – SAMU) whose success depends of the participation of a specialized physician in the mobile medical team.

The role of helicopter services (Fig. 23), if available, should be included in the HMIP.

Personal accident insurance for the members of the medical teams is essential but often ignored in the HMIP.

Hospital coordination team

Medical incident coordinator

As mentioned, the medical incident coordinator (MIC) liaises with senior nursing and administrative officers and has overall responsibility for the implementation of the HMIP.

The duties of the MIC should be well defined and are chiefly organizational, with no involvement in treating patients. The MIC ensures that triaged patients are despatched to appropriate and adequately staffed areas of the hospital in an organized fashion and that the passage of patients through the A&E department is expedited.

The MIC summons extra medical help if necessary and organizes shifts if the incident is prolonged, keeps in constant communication with the MIO and decides when the hospital can accept no more casualties. Other responsibilites are coordination with the hospital ambulance liaison officer, casualty bureau, police, and hospital management to maximize the use of resources and assist with the issuing of press statements.

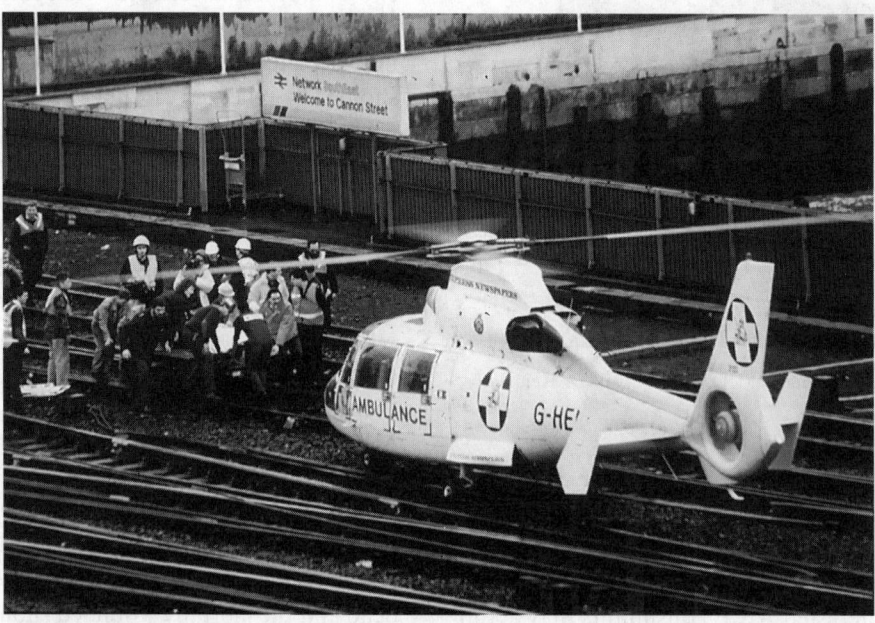

Fig. 23. The helicopter emergency medical services in action. (Courtesy of Dr Gareth Davies.)

Nursing incident coordinator

Like the MIC, the nursing incident coordinator's role is the management of personnel and resources. This includes the organization of beds (not just for the incoming casualties but also for those who have had to be moved to make way for the victims of the incident) and making available appropriate theatre and intensive care facilities (Walsh, 1989).

Administrative coordinator

This role is taken by the most senior manager available whose main responsibility is to mobilize resources. Readiness is achieved through planning and training (Miles, 1991). It is a complex job which demands skills in interpersonal communications, motivating staff, and improvisation.

Through delegation, the administrative coordinator is responsible for the setting up of a hospital information centre, dealing with the press and the police, and ensuring that non-clinical hospital and voluntary personnel are available. Overall responsibilities include organization of medical equipment, duty officers, porters, clerical staff, security, telephonists and catering.

The administrative coordinator liaises with other key personnel (pharmacy, blood transfusion and central sterile supply department), maintaining the momentum of the hospital response.

Communications

To date, effective communications (which include initiation of the major incident response and call-out procedures) have been singled out in every postdisaster assessment to be the *major weakness* in major incident management (Malone, 1990). Being an integral part of operational activities (Fig. 24), a communications system that fails to deliver is a recipe for chaos both at the site of the incident and at the receiving hospitals (Sharpe *et al.*, 1985).

Communications between the disaster site and the receiving hospital should only be made via the ACP and the MIO (New, 1992). The ACP must be the only vehicle with flashing lights (Malone, 1990), and it should have direct radio links with the hospital. It is essential that the MIO and AIO do not give conflicting information or repeat messages which could result in confusion and duplication of items requested.

It is crucial that the MIO has constant communication with incident officers in the other emergency services and relays accurate information to the hospital, (e.g. on chemical incidents and the identification of toxic substances).

The MIO and support hospitals should be in direct communication using cellular telephones (Allen *et al.*, 1989) or radio, with interhospital communications and links clearly identified in the HMIP (of value in 'cross-boundary incidents') (Malone, 1990).

Links between the MIO and the mobile medical team on site must be established using hand-held radios (Nancekievill, 1992). These will generally be issued by the ambulance service at the ACP.

Hospital switchboards are often the weakest link of the communications chain. They may be jammed by worried relatives and friends and representatives of the press, or even staff (Wardrope *et al.*, 1990). This problem may be ameliorated in several ways:

- Directly or indirectly alerted staff should not phone the hospital seeking information and out-going calls should be restricted to an absolute minimum.
- There is no need to contact the site for regular updates.
- Use of direct lines and public phones in the hospital will limit traffic through the switchboard.
- Communication within the hospital between key personnel should ideally be established with hand-held two-way radios which put no extra pressure on an already overstretched telephone system.

Irrespective of the equipment used (telephones, cellular phones, radiopagers and fax machines) it is vital to ensure that channels of communication are available for the free flow of information, taking into consideration that unless a special facility is established, the cellular network may become saturated by the members of the public and the press.

The HMIP should set out (depending on availability) the precise location of all communications equipment and arrangements for its regular servicing. This includes rooms and telephones designated for use by the police, media and relatives.

Good communications are essential to the management of any disaster.

Triage

Efficient triage procedures are fundamental in managing mass casualties (Edwards, 1989). They should be

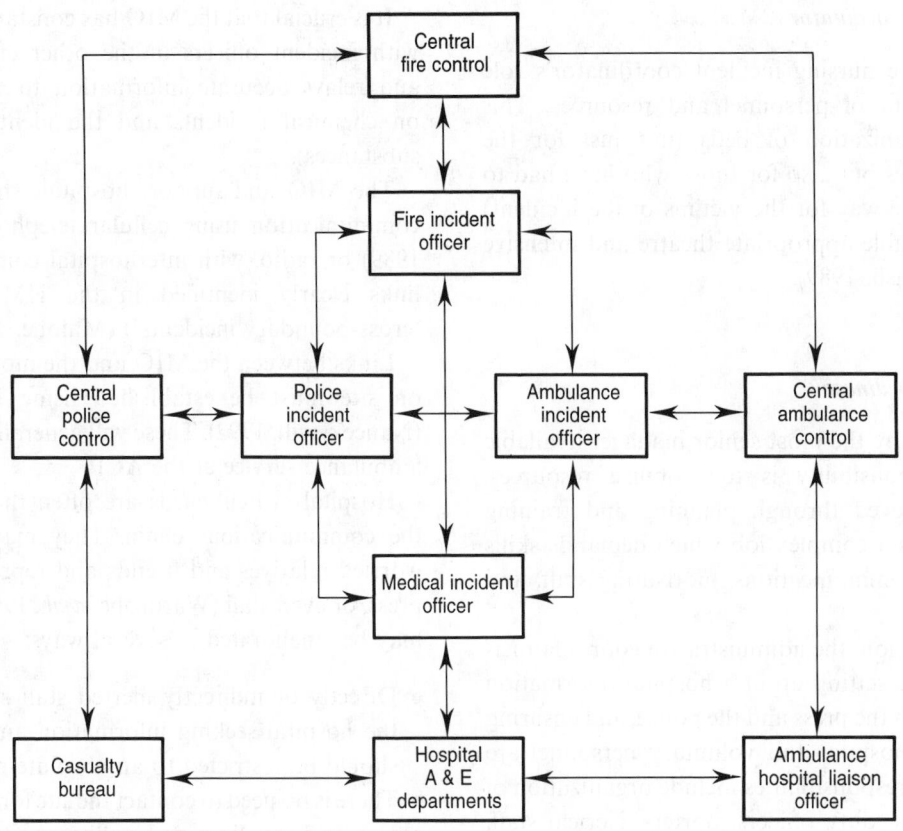

Fig. 24. Interservice communication at a major incident. (Courtesy of Dr Ken Hines, BASICS.)

undertaken by trained and experienced staff (Yates, 1979; Dilliner, 1992) and be employed for as long as an imbalance exists between demand and resources.

Triage at the scene is essential to ensure that the most seriously injured and treatable victims are transported to hospital first. A single nationally agreed system of labelling patients according to triage category has been developed.

Triage should be dynamic: priorities are constantly changing and a low-priority case may suddenly become critical. Reassessment of these priorities may well dictate a different order of transport and treatment from that originally envisaged.

The same system of triage should continue in the receiving hospital where a single triage officer in conjunction with the MIC should ensure that there is only one entrance to the A&E department, and that all patients are triaged at that point (Yates, 1979).

The ambulance entrance to A&E is usually the triage point where the patients are given treatment priorities and then rapidly despatched to the appropriate areas.

Treatment priorities allocated at triage		
IMMEDIATE – FIRST PRIORITY		
	– resuscitation bays	(Red)*
URGENT – SECOND PRIORITY		
	– Trolley cubicles	(Yellow)
DELAYED – THIRD PRIORITY		
	– Minor injuries area	(Green)
DEAD – Mortuary		(White)
* Colour of priority label.		

Those who have clearly suffered mortal injuries from which they will not recover should be treated in a cubicle designated for this purpose and made as comfortable as possible.

Early clinical decisions will determine who is in need of immediate surgery, who needs surgery within hours, and those for whom it may be safely postponed. Local resources will determine if casualties in need of less urgent surgery are transferred elsewhere or whether outside staff are drafted in.

Fire incidents

For fire incidents the HMIP should make special provision. A plastic surgeon (if available) should adopt the role of triage officer (Sharpe *et al.*, 1985; Griffiths, 1985). Burn casualties may be sorted into four categories.

1. *Non-salvageable*: sometimes a decision that only an expert can make, by identifying certain patterns of burns which make survival impossible. This group needs admission but no special treatment facilities.
2. *Life-threatening*: often first or second priority who need airway management and resuscitation prior to transfer to specialized areas with a high ratio of staff to patients.
3. *Disabling but <20% burns*: often third priority (but occasionally second) who need hospital admission and specialized treatment (e.g. hand and perineum injuries).
4. *Small burns*: third priority casualties who are treated and reassured prior to discharge and out-patient follow-up.

Provision of medical care

Primary treatment areas

Care in A&E should be delivered by teams of staff who should wear identification tabards indicating specialty, grade or role in the major incident. These groups of doctors and nurses from A&E and other specialties must team up at short notice. This task can be made easier if A&E staff who are familiar with the department and the environment are easily identified (Stevens & Partridge, 1990) and take the lead.

The HMIP should define the use of universal precautions and make them compulsory for all teams working in resuscitation and high-dependency bays, and where spillage of blood and body fluids has occurred.

There is great benefit in resuscitating the critically injured in resuscitation rooms and high-dependency areas within the A&E department, as in normal A&E work. These areas are fully operational at all times. During a major incident they must be under the supervision of a designated intensivist or a senior A&E doctor.

As the number of casualties with minor injuries always exceeds the seriously injured group, the 'walking wounded' should be directed to larger areas identified in the HMIP. It should be borne in mind that their comparatively 'trivial' injuries may be complicated by considerable psychological and emotional trauma, and the HMIP should specify provisions for counselling and follow-up where these problems may be calmly and sympathetically dealt with.

As the disaster develops, it may be necessary to expand the primary treatment areas to prevent overcrowding and this should be addressed in the HMIP. As time goes by, more and more staff may arrive to assist with the incident and the MIC must take measures to prevent too many staff becoming involved.

A senior A&E doctor must lead a team of juniors in the minor treatment area. His role is to ensure that the triage category of patients has not changed. Patients with apparently minor injuries may deteriorate in X-ray departments or whilst awaiting treatment for their minor wounds.

Soft tissue injuries and fractures must be treated rapidly but be fully documented. The fact that there are gravely injured patients in close proximity must not be allowed to impact on the quality of care delivered to the walking wounded. It should be remembered that some of these patients will have relatives and loved ones injured or missing.

The role of the nurse in charge in A&E is crucial and this person is often the first to take charge of the incident, make decisions and take on responsibilities that can influence the outcome considerably.

Junior doctors and nurses need guidance, support, supervision and encouragement to ensure that time is deployed appropriately, efficiency is maximized and that they are coping physically and psychologically.

Secondary treatment areas

A difficult scenario in a disaster is the need to ventilate large numbers of casualties simultaneously (Edward, 1989). ICU (intensive care unit) beds are limited and are occupied by critically ill patients unrelated to the incident. The HMIP should identify how the available equipment and ICU resources should be used. In particular, coronary care patients may be transferred to designated general beds to release ICU beds for major incident victims who require ventilation.

As in the ICU, theatres treat the most seriously injured. The HMIP allocates the responsibility of managing theatre space to the theatre manager and a senior surgeon who must constantly ensure that all aspects of surgical care are efficiently delivered (Bliss, 1984) without undue staff fatigue or psychological stress.

Preoperative and recovery bays are usually in close proximity to the ICU so that they can easily become

'ICU areas' looked after by teams of ICU/general nursing staff and junior anaesthetists.

A key element of any HMIP is the creation of a casualty reception ward (CRW) which accommodates all patients who require admission regardless of age, sex, or type of injury. It has the advantage of allowing resources to be concentrated in one area.

The CRW is created by the vacation of an entire ward (Walsh, 1989). This often has adverse effects elsewhere which should be dealt with by the nursing coordinator.

Immediate discharges from other wards need to be made to make room for the admitted patients. An in-patient holding area should be designated in the HMIP to facilitate this discharge programme.

As the creation of a CRW can only begin when other wards have cleared their beds, it is important that contingency plans for this exist. The CRW should be optimally situated for security purposes. It should be fully equipped and adequately sized, allowing partitioning for nursing different groups of patients. The patients should be able to communicate with each other easily to share their experiences (Walsh, 1989).

Hospital information centre

This is set up by the administrative coordinator and should remain open for at least 24 h following the incident. The major incident information officer receives information about incident victims, checks its accuracy, then categorizes and disseminates information to interested parties.

The administrative coordinator is responsible for ensuring that medical records staff register all casualties, and should provide translators when casualties are foreign nationals or speak very little English.

The maintenance of up-to-date information and its supply on request to the press officer, major incident coordinator, police and relatives reception officer is vital and often an indicator of how well the HMIP is being implemented.

The HMIP must include facilities for a police documentation team to relay crucial information to the police casualty bureau concerning identity of victims.

Major incident documentation should be standardized, and provision of a *unique* 'major incident number' to all casualties is a fundamental prerequisite (Malone, 1990). This number should be adhered to on all documentation including labelling of specimens. Ideally the major incident number and police number should be the same for each patient.

Other information on the major incident document should be charted by ticking boxes (Allen, 1989). These data will be used in postdisaster audit assessment which is an essential educational and research exercise.

Patient discharge area

This area allows staff to ensure that investigations, treatment and documentation are completed prior to discharge. In this area, casualties are reunited with their relatives or friends, assisted with transportation home and offered social and psychiatric support.

The relatives' waiting area – relatives' reception officer

The relatives' reception officer (RRO) is designated by the administrative coordinator, and supervises the care given to friends and relatives who are under considerable stress. In a designated room away from A&E and the press, counselling and comfort are provided by staff and volunteers. Through the information officer, the RRO obtains answers to enquiries regarding casualties and, in conjunction with the police, distressing news is conveyed to relatives, and escorts to various destinations are arranged.

Volunteers

The role that volunteers play in major disasters is invaluable. Under the control of a designated member of staff they are registered, issued with identity documentation and given duties to assist with the comforting of relatives and friends, and numerous other errands.

Patient affairs officer

This person collects property and property record forms and liaises with the RRO to inform relatives about property held. Relatives are assisted with formalities regarding deceased victims and deaths are registered with the police and Her Majesty's Coroner.

Supporting departments

A senior radiologist is included in the HMIP to manage all radiological investigations and interventions, ensuring the appropriate utilization of resources (Yates, 1979; Allen, 1989). Results of investigations should be reported immediately by a team of radiologists and made available to the clinical areas.

The Blood Transfusion Service is assisted by carefully screening requests for cross-matching of blood and ensuring that adequate details are included on request forms, so that issuing of blood is not delayed. Numbered patient identification tags are very helpful.

The central sterile supply department (CSSD) and pharmacy managers are in constant touch with the control centre ensuring that extra supplies are available.

The assistance offered by the social work department to discharged patients and their relatives is invaluable and should be defined in the HMIP. Similarly, offering religious and psychiatric support should always be part of the care given to casualties and their relatives in a major disaster and every attempt should be made to accommodate all religions.

The catering manager is responsible for calling in additional staff and maintaining food and beverage services for the wards, staff restaurant and A&E. Additional services should be provided for the relatives' waiting area, discharged patients' area and press room.

Media

A press room with direct telephone lines should be made available away from patients and relatives but near enough for designated staff to give short statements to the media without disrupting their work.

If disruption of hospital routines by action-seeking press and TV and radio crews is to be avoided, arrangements must be made for information to be given effectively.

The press officer should be a senior hospital manager who can ensure that press releases are made at appropriate times for stations and newspapers.

TV interviews on the medical condition of patients are best left for the MIC, thus diverting undesirable press attention away from individual members of the staff or patients.

Casualties and fatalities should be named in conjunction with the police press liaison officer and only when the next of kin have been informed.

Police

The police documentation centre conveys information from the hospital to the police casualty bureau, and also assists in communications between the site and supporting hospitals. The police casualty bureau's numbers are released very early by the media and callers to the hospital should be referred to these numbers.

Collection of forensic evidence is becoming increasingly important (Haywood, 1988), therefore the HMIP must identify an area where police forensic staff can operate.

Nursing staff should be made aware that patients' property does not necessarily need to be listed and that items can be released directly to the police.

Planning should include arrangements at local level to guarantee staff access to the hospital, as roadblocks, check-points and diversions are established by the police trying to seal off areas for security and safety reasons.

Police and security officers must be located at vital points and should request evidence of identity if it is required.

This right to challenge individuals should be practised courteously so that authorized personnel and others take no offence. The police also make provision for additional temporary mortuaries and ensure these are protected from unauthorized personnel.

Ambulance liaison officer

The ALO deployed to the hospital must report to the MIC and should stay in constant communication with the ACP, keeping the AIO informed of the hospital's status.

The ALO is responsible for maximizing the efficiency of ambulance transport to the hospital and for arranging secondary interhospital transport. In chemical incidents, potentially contaminated vehicles must not be used again until decontaminated.

Visits by distinguished persons

Following any major incident, it is likely that senior health officials, ministers of State and even royalty may wish to visit victims. The HMIP should designate an officer responsible for these arrangements so that these visits do not disrupt the hospital's activities but raise the morale of patients and staff (Stevens & Partridge, 1990).

Incident stand-down

When all casualties have been removed from the scene or have been accounted for, the AIO and MIO in conjunction with their colleagues from the police and fire services issue the message 'MAJOR INCIDENT STAND-DOWN' together with the time of the declaration.

The hospital stand-down may occur when the message is received but if large numbers of casualties are still being cared for in the A&E department, it may be wise to maintain major incident status until the backlog has been cleared.

Debriefing and psychological aftermath of major incidents

If lessons are to be learnt, deficiencies must be pin-pointed objectively in postdisaster assessments. The HMIP should be regularly scrutinized and recommendations for changes drawn up and implemented in a revised plan.

The necessity of providing psychological counselling to victims and relatives of the disaster has long been identified and should be an essential component of all HMIPs; but the emotional and psychological trauma inflicted on rescue workers and hospital staff may be underestimated, because stress is often suppressed in an attempt to 'cope' with the situation.

This makes rescue workers vulnerable to a wide variety of symptoms of both acute and insidious onset (disaster syndrome) which can range from mild sleeping disturbances, fatigue, decreased efficiency, irritability, depression, psychoses and even suicidal tendencies.

To minimize these deleterious effects, mental health services need to tackle spiritual and emotional problems in a short-term and long-term support programme. Information about services, counselling, crisis-intervention, psychological debriefing and post-traumatic therapy must be provided for victims and staff (Dyregrov, 1989).

In the UK, this is achieved by enthusiastic groups from A&E, psychiatry, social services and the clergy, but the creation of a national centre for crisis psychology (like Norway, where teams of experts are available to assist those involved) is long overdue. If performed by expert personnel, psychological debriefing has been shown to prevent much of the psychological morbidity experienced by rescuers.

Training

Although this is known to be essential, most hospital staff simply do not receive training to prepare them for major incidents and the health service response to disasters remains confused (Dilliner, 1992). Specialized courses have been organized (London and Manchester), but only a relatively small number of enthusiasts can be trained on these.

Individual hospitals should arrange for senior and permanent members of staff, (e.g. A&E consultants) to be sent on such courses, following which they will be in a position to direct training efforts in the hospital.

Bibliography

ALLEN, M.J. (1989). Coping with the early stages of the M1 disaster: at the scene and on arrival at hospital. *Br. Med. J.*, **298**, 651–4.

BAXTER, R.J. (1991). Major chemical disasters: Britain's health services are poorly prepared. *Br. Med. J.*, **302**, 61.

BLISS, A.R. (1984). Major disaster planning. *Br. Med. J.*, **288**, 1433–4.

CASSIDY, K. (1990). National and international legislation on major chemical hazards. In *Major Chemical Disasters – Medical Aspects of Management*, ed. V. Murray. London: Royal Society of Medicine Services.

COOKE, M.W. (1992). Arrangements for on-scene medical care at major incidents. *Br. Med. J.*, **305**, 478

DEPARTMENT OF HEALTH (1990). *Emergency Planning in the NHS*. HC (90) 25 NHS Management Executive. London: HMSO.

DILLINER, L. (1992). Health service response to disasters is confused. *Br. Med. J.*, **305**, 1384.

DYREGROV, A. (1989). Caring for helpers in disaster situations: psychological debriefing. *Disaster Manage.*, **2** (1), 25–30.

EDWARDS, J.D. (1989). Mass casualties. *Br. J. Hosp. Med.*, **42**, 99.

FAHEY, M. (1988). Airport and aircraft accidents. In *Medicine for Disasters*, ed. P. Basket & R. Weller. London: Butterworth.

GRIFFITHS, R.W. (1985). Management of multiple casualities with burns. *Br. Med. J.*, **291**, 917–18.

HAYWOOD, I. (1988). Terrorism management and forensic aspects. In *Medicine for Disasters*, ed. P. Basket & R. Weller. London: Butterworth & Co.

MALONE, W.D. (1990). Lessons to be learnt from the major disaster following the civil airliner crast at Kegworth in January 1989. *Injury*, **21**, 49–52.

MILES, S.A.D. (1991). Major accidents. In *ABC of Major Trauma*, ed. D. Skinner, P. Driscoll & R. Earlam. London: BMJ Publications.

MILLER, P.J. (1980). The Nuneaton derailment. *Injury*, **12**, 130–8.

NANCEKIEVILL, D.G. (1989). Disaster management; practice makes perfect. *Br. Med. J.*, **298**, 477.

NANCEKIEVILL, D.G. (1992). On-site medical services at major incidents. *Br. Med. J.*, **305**, 726–7.

NEW, B. (1992). 'Too many cooks'. The response of health-related services to major incidents in London. *Kings Fund Institute Research Report* No. 15.

REDMOND, A.D. (1989). Disaster management. *Br. Med. J.*, **298**, 962.

ROWLANDS, B.J. (1990). Are we ready for the next disaster? *Injury*, **21**, 61–2.

RUTHERFORD, W.H. (1990). Place of exercises in disaster management. *Injury*, **21**, 58–60.

SHARPE, D.T., ROBERTS, A.H.N., BARCLAY, T.L. *et al.* (1985). Treatment of burns casualties after fire at Bradford City football ground. *Br. Med. J.*, **291**, 945–8.

STEVENS, K.L.H. & PARTRIDGE, R. (1990). The Clapham rail disaster. *Injury*, **21**, 37–40

TAYLOR, P. (1989). *The Hillsborough Stadium Disaster*. London: HMSO.

THANABALASMGHAM, T., BECKETT, M.W. & MURRAY, V. (1991). Hospital response to a chemical incident. *Br. Med. J.*, **302**, 101.

VOLANS, G.N. (1990). Medical management of chemical disasters involving food or water. In *Major Chemical Disasters – Medical Aspects of Management*, ed. V. Murray. London: Royal Society of Medicine Service.

WALSH, M. (1989). Coping with catastrophe. *Nursing Times*, **85**, 19, 27–31

WARDROPE, J., HOCKEY, M.S., CROSBY, A.C. *et al.* (1990). The hospital response to the Hillsborough tragedy. *Injury*, **21**, 53–4.

WARDROPE, J., RYAN, F., CLARK, G. *et al.* (1991). The Hillsborough tragedy. *Br. Med. J.*, **303**, 1381–4.

WELLER, R. (1988). Nuclear accidents. In *Medicine for Disasters*, In ed. P. Basket–R. Weller. London: Butterworth & Co.

WINCH, R.D., HINES, K.C., BOOKER, H.T. *et al.* (1976). The Moorgate train crash. *Injury*, **7**, 288–91.

YATES, D.W. (1979). Major disaster surgical triage. *Br. J. Hosp. Med.*, 323–6.

YATES, D.W. (1991). The NHS prepares for war. *Br. Med. J.*, **302**, 130.

14 Prehospital care

M. WARD and M. WILLIS (A: Prehospital care and the ambulance service)

M. EISENBERG (B(i): Prehospital cardiac care I: An overview)

R.O. CUMMINS and J.R. GRAVES (B(ii): Prehospital cardiac care II: European and American perspectives)

P.L. LANE (C(i): Prehospital care of the trauma patient)

P.L. LANE (C(ii): Interhospital transport of the trauma patient)

Chapter plan

A: Prehospital care and the ambulance service

B(i): Prehospital cardiac care I: An overview

Sudden cardiac death in the community

Factors associated with successful resuscitation

Prehospital cardiac care

Recommended guidelines for uniform reporting of data from out-of-hospital cardiac arrest. The Utstein style

Improving survival from sudden cardiac death

B(ii): Prehospital cardiac care II: European and American perspectives

The importance of prehospital cardiac care

Perspective of this chapter

Organization and description of EMS systems

Description of selected EMS systems surveyed in Europe and the USA

Conclusions and recommendations

Appendix: The Utstein Consensus Conferences

C(i): Prehospital care of the trauma patient

Introduction

System features

Field assessment of the trauma patient

Field treatment of the trauma patient

Quality management and research

C(ii): Interhospital transport of the trauma patient

Introduction

Why transport trauma patients?

Who to transport?

When to refer and transport?

How to transport?

Quality management and research

A: Prehospital care and the ambulance service

M. WARD[a] and M. WILLIS[b]

[a]Nuffield Department of Anaesthetics, John Radcliffe Hospital, Oxford, UK

[b]Norfolk Ambulance NHS Trust, Norwich, UK

The days of the modern ambulance service in the UK began with the introduction of the 1946 National Health Act, which was implemented in 1947. This required local authorities to ensure that free ambulance transport was available to take patients to and from the various treatment centres. At that time, the ambulance service in England and Wales was provided by 59 county council services and 85 county borough services. Authorities had an option to employ their own staff or to use one of the recognized voluntary agencies such as St John or St Andrews Ambulance, or the British Red Cross. By the early 1960s all authorities had decided to employ their own staff, phasing out the volunteers who had supported the service during holiday times, weekends, and at night. During the late 1960s ambulance training was still primarily based on the voluntary societies' handbooks, and ambulance staff were trained only in the most basic life-support skills. Public expectation was for a service of a significantly higher standard than that which was being provided.

In 1966 a Government Working Party, chaired by Mr E. L. M. Miller, produced a report which set out the desired standard of training and equipment for the modern ambulance service. The backbone of this report was the establishment of a number of national training centres together with a nationwide training programme.

It was not until April 1974 that the next significant change in the ambulance service took place when, with the reorganization of the National Health Service (NHS) as a whole, responsibility for the ambulance services moved from local authorities to health authorities, either at the area level (equivalent to county in the USA) or regional level (equivalent to a North American state). This direct association between ambulance service and health authority brought about the integration of the ambulance service with the health organization for which it provided. The advantage was a much closer link with healthcare professions, and for the first time the users of the service were directly responsible for the standards and the demands placed upon it.

The equipment carried on ambulances during the early years of the modern ambulance service varied considerably from service to service, ranging from blankets and dressings only, the inclusion of (ineffective) splints, oxygen and Entonox (premixed oxygen and nitrous oxide). Standardization began during the late 1960s and early 1970s but progress varied from service to service.

Ambulance provision in Europe and America is more difficult to summarize as it differs from country to country and within each country, particularly in the USA.

In mainland Europe, no country has introduced ambulance paramedics as understood by the UK or American concept. The most significant emergency ambulance service in Europe is the French SAMU (Service d'Aide Médicale Urgente) system, for which a control room is located in each of the 101 'départements' (counties). Not only are the ambulances staffed by doctors and nurses but so are the control centres, a situation not found in the UK, with the possible exception of a single medical controller in the HQ control of London. Within this sophisticated system, the ambulance men or women make up the third member of the crew. The nurse/doctor system is the predominant one in other European countries such as Germany and Belgium. In many cases the local service is supported by mobile intensive care units and a comprehensive helicopter network, not necessarily to move the patient but to provide clinical expertise rapidly at the scene. However, whilst the SAMU and associated systems provide a high standard of care, much of the local emergency provision is of a basic standard with minimally trained crews and no purpose-built vehicles.

The USA, regarded by many as the birth place of ambulance paramedics, does not have a common national standard and services vary from state to state. Paramedic and ambulance care is provided by diverse agencies ranging from the police and fire departments to numerous private emergency medical service (EMS) companies. Even in states where care is provided to a high standard, the cover may be patchy with rural communities being served by volunteers.

One of the significant differences between the American and UK system is the USA's rigorous adherence to protocols and external clinical control. This control, often administered via a communications network, has drawbacks including a lack of flexibility for paramedics. The failure or reluctance of the paramedic to establish the communication link may delay clinical discussion until after the event. The UK approach to paramedic training has consciously avoided this approach, as its everyday use is flawed and leads to frustration on all sides. Therefore, whilst the advent of paramedic training is attributed to the USA, the initial concept is practised in the British Isles.

The development of the ambulance vehicle has also been one of evolution. At present the Technical Committee of the European Standards Commission is preparing a draft European standard for ambulances, stretchers and equipment. This will bring with it the advantage of additional equipment but the disadvantage of what may be a less flexible vehicle for use in the UK.

At the beginning of the 1990s the ambulance service of the UK reached a pinnacle. At this time the British government decided to take a positive view of care provided by the ambulance service and entered into an undertaking to ensure that all front-line (emergency) vehicles would carry at least an advisory defibrillator and that by the year 1994 that there would be one paramedic on every front-line ambulance. Great improvements are taking place and the spreading of 'prehospital trauma life support' ideals and their introduction into the UK has led to a better understanding of the importance of more aggressive prehospital treatment.

Paramedic training largely started as a result of the influx to North America of the returning battle paramedics from Vietnam. These individuals found themselves without a role to play in civilian life and were successful in persuading some of the American fire services to employ them to provide similar medical field management at the scene of 'battles' in their high streets. The good results of work performed by such personnel in Orange County (California) and elsewhere gradually spread across the USA. Once the concept had become accepted, the North American fear of the threat of litigation became an imperative for medical directors and ensured the spread of paramedic training.

In the UK, observers of the American experience could see the value of improving prehospital care from the simple first-aid applied by the old-style ambulance attendant. Dr Peter Baskett in Avon and Dr Douglas Chamberlain in Brighton adopted different lines of approach. The Brighton scheme was set up to provide cardiac prehospital care very similar to that which was started in Belfast but based on paramedics as opposed to medical attendants. The Avon scheme has always concentrated on a more aggressive approach to the management of trauma. Oxford, at the end of the 1970s, chose to take elements of these schemes to develop an integrated programme that could introduce a comprehensive prehospital care scheme based upon a relatively short training period. At this time, however, the spread of extended training was officially regarded very differently from the way it was perceived in North America, with concern from the British government about the ability of non-physicians to manage acute medical and surgical emergencies. The alternative to such paramedic interventions in the UK was the development of the British Association of Immediate Care Scheme (BASICS) based upon general practitioners who would respond at the request of ambulance services. In the rural areas this was a great success but, with one or two exceptions, urban parts of the country were poorly served.

Ambulance personnel campaigned to provide extended care, and eventually this was accepted after prehospital care was given to Government ministers, including the Prime Minister Margaret Thatcher, as a result of the bombing of the Grand Hotel in Brighton during the Conservative Party Conference in October 1984. This event brought the ambulance service and paramedic training into the public eye. Also at this time there were a number of major incidents and the part played by the prehospital attendants, other than medical personnel, became increasingly relevant to planners of major incident procedures. In 1984 a letter advised services that, following a report by York University, the standing Medical Advisory Committee was supporting the development of paramedic training schemes but the decision to proceed or not would be left to each local authority. It was not until 1987 with the introduction of the first paramedic training syllabus by the NHS Training Directorate (NHSTD) that paramedic training achieved a national perspective.

Following a dispute in the late 1980s, a new pay structure was introduced which recognized extended training. In 1990 the Government demanded that training should be properly controlled and statutory bodies were set up for the approval of training schemes. This became the responsibility of the NHS Training Executive, later to become the Training Directorate (NHSTD). The Royal College of Anaesthetists took up the role of promoting training for the trainers. All ambulance training schools in the UK are now visited at least every 3 years by representatives of the NHSTD's Approvals Executive, and their training schemes must conform to the minimum standard set by the Approvals Executive body. The Joint Colleges Ambulance Liaison Committee was set up in 1989, with representation from all the medical colleges and ambulance senior personnel, to discuss innovations and standard setting. This is now seen as a major forum for discussion of new developments in prehospital care in the UK. The present training scheme for ambulance paramedics has been so effective because those responsible for the training standards are those who receive the patients treated by ambulance staff. A totally revised manual was issued in 1991 and included a new section on the management of obstetric emergencies as a result of the decision of the Royal College of Obstetrics and Gynaecology to accept the provision of 'obstetric flying squad' services by paramedics alone.

It is at the door of the accident and emergency (A&E) department that the two services meet. It is therefore essential that there is respect and understanding by all involved. Whilst this is the case in the majority of areas, there are still pockets of resistance to progressive changes in prehospital care. This, by its very nature, is often a barrier to effective communication and inevitably affects patient care. In most authorities, the clinical and nursing staff are involved in the training of ambulance paramedics. A number of clinicians are involved in preclinical paramedic training and also in the hospital departments where the theoretical and practical skills acquired in the training school are put into practice. It is the relationships that are established during this important period that normally provide the basis for effective understanding between the paramedic, clinician and nursing staff. It is often during this time that there is an appreciation of each other's needs and the problems both groups face. In a number of services the reciprocal provision of experience for clinicians and nurses in the prehospital environment has promoted mutual appreciation. It is now recognized that those responsible for providing tuition must be exposed to the environment in which the paramedic and general practitioner apply their skills. It is only on the basis of such experience that practical skills can be adapted from the hospital environment.

The position of the medical profession in prehospital care is still unsatisfactory. BASICS trained doctors continue to provide an excellent standard, particularly in those rural areas where ambulances may be delayed. Also in these areas their contribution to medical incident management is largely unrecognized. The Royal College of Surgeons of Edinburgh has established a Diploma of Immediate Care, for medical practitioners. In Germany, Denmark and France the medical contribution to the first-line response is so great as to make the need for paramedic training almost non-existent. Why is there this enormous difference in attitude? It is tempting to blame it all upon the availability of medical staff. Philosophies in both France and Germany with respect to the number of medical graduates have been different. To provide a doctor on every front-line ambulance in the UK would be impossible logistically and prohibitive financially. These restrictions do not apply in either Germany or France. Whilst European standards are being set for medical equipment in ambulances, it is increasingly difficult to cater for vehicles which carry medical staff as well as vehicles that carry only paramedical staff.

What then of patient transport? Ambulance vehicles have developed significantly over the last few years. Cost is no longer the only determinant. The changing role of the crew has necessitated the creation of an environment where skills can be applied to best effect and the patient can be conveyed in a safe and comfortable manner. Many services have moved away from the true multipurpose vehicle and there is now a clear distinction between vehicles used for the conveyance of out-patients and those used for prehospital emergency care. In recent years, air-conditioning and floating stretchers (which isolate the patient from vehicle movement) have become a more common feature of the modern ambulance. Whilst these items are not yet basic equipment on all ambulances, the fact that some services now provide such facilities is a sign of progress. These aspects become even more important as the journey to hospital is extended, either by a move towards regional trauma centres or because of a reduction in local treatment centres.

The future of trauma centres is yet to be determined. Ambulance staff, however, still face the dilemma of whether or not to bypass a local unit and proceed directly to a major treatment unit. Clearly the number of patients who require transfer from a major unit to a trauma centre are minimal. One problem facing ambulance crews is that, whilst they may feel they wish to go directly to the trauma centre, the presence of a general practitioner at the scene may influence the decision to use a closer A&E department. It would be difficult for the crew to disregard such a request, for, if the patient deteriorates in transit, the crew and the service would be open to criticism, and litigation may arise. Use of agreed transport protocols may guide their decision and offer staff some legal protection.

Triage at the scene of an accident is paramount and, with the increasing number of major and multiple casualty situations, the triage process takes on greater importance. Whilst the arrival of an ambulance activates a paramedical cascade arrangement, the stabilization and transfer of casualties to an appropriate centre must be coordinated and planned. It is at this scenario that the interface between paramedic, general practitioner and immediate care physician may have the greatest influence.

The patient's transfer from the scene can be by land or air ambulance. The latter, however, are still subject to trial in the UK, with their effectiveness yet to be fully evaluated. Factors influencing the decisions to use helicopter transport are availability, i.e. night flights, bad weather, inappropriate landing areas at scene, combined with the lack of appropriate landing facilities at the receiving hospital. All of these significantly reduce the effectiveness of air transport. At present no rotary or fixed wing aircraft, other than in Scotland and London, are funded by the state. The majority are funded by public subscription, the most notable of which is the Cornwall helicopter. Another initiative is a combined project which is coordinated with the police, and as such the paramedic may also be trained as a police observer.

The most controversial helicopter service at the time of writing is London-based and operates out of the Royal London Hospital. The HEMS (helicopter emergency medical system) aircraft has been funded partly by the Express Newspaper Group, and more latterly supported by the NHS in order to complete the agreed trial period. This trial may well form the basis of further decisions on air transport as an integral part of an emergency service. However, this service and many others involve medical personnel both in planning and in manning. The Royal London Hospital's helicopter carries both a doctor and a paramedic. It is still too early to say what the correct level of manning should be.

In all cases, the provision of or access to communication is essential. The recent report on A&E departments by the Royal College of Surgeons of England emphasized the need for effective communication between the scene and the receiving unit. Whilst this exists in many services, maximum advantage is not always made of the facility, and, if it is, it is not always the most appropriate individual in the A&E unit who receives the message. The target of ensuring that all staff transmit the trauma score to the hospital in advance of the patient arriving will enhance the patient's reception. Telemetry is not used at present in the UK due to the level of interference. A review of the present radio specification and the use of improved technology could facilitate the introduction of this system, not to take the decision away from those at the scene but to provide important information for those at the receiving unit. Communication difficulties between land ambulances and air transport have still not been fully resolved but it is essential that this is rectified.

The introduction into the UK of 'criteria based dispatching' may further improve the provision of the thinly spread, high-quality service. Modification of the USA protocols and adaptation to British needs was completed at the end of 1994. Trial areas have been identified and will report the efficiency of this system. Whether it becomes apparent that the absence of medical presence in the control rooms (unlike USA and European practice) is important, may be a useful finding from this experiment.

What more could be achieved by prehospital paramedical care? In essence, it is important that the simple ABCs are properly managed and restored. Recognition of the need for airway care, ventilation and support of the circulation are the major thrusts of prehospital care. Maintenance of the patient's life during the early part of the 'golden hour' must be the aim. Recent developments to this end have been the introduction, even in the UK, of needle thoracotomy and cricothyroid puncture. The introduction of new skills is monitored at a local level by the medical advisory panel and, at a national level, by the Joint Colleges Ambulance Liaison Committee. The spread of 'prehospital trauma life support' courses in the UK – imported like advanced trauma life support (ATLS) from America – should further cement the principles of correct care in the field. Furthermore, this course emphasizes the importance of deciding when to abandon support in-the-field in favour of rapid evacuation to hospital. This time the decisions will be based on experience and a good understanding of physiology.

B(i): Prehospital cardiac care I: An overview

M. EISENBERG

Emergency Medicine Service, University of Washington Medical Center, Seattle, Washington, USA

SUDDEN CARDIAC DEATH IN THE COMMUNITY

Prehospital cardiac care was established by Pantridge and Geddes in Belfast, Northern Ireland in 1966 (Pantridge & Geddes, 1967). Since then, hundreds of prehospital programmes have been established throughout Europe and the USA for the management of cardiac and other emergencies (Eisenberg *et al.*, 1990). Since sudden cardiac death is the leading cause of death in industrialized nations, this critical emergency is the major condition which requires prehospital emergency care (Kuller, 1980; Kuller *et al.*, 1975). If sudden death victims can be reached in time with the proper level of care, there is a reasonable chance of survival (Eisenberg *et al.*, 1984).

The types of prehospital emergency care and reported survival rates from various communities differ widely throughout the world (Eisenberg *et al.*, 1990). The purpose of this chapter is to discuss the reasons for these differences, and to describe actions which can be taken to improve survival from cardiac arrest. Emergency physicians working in communities should ask themselves the following questions: 'What kind of prehospital emergency system exists in my community?' 'What is the likelihood of successful resuscitation from cardiac arrest in my community?' 'How can this likelihood increase?' 'What can I do to bring about improved emergency services for sudden cardiac death?'

Aetiology

The causes of sudden cardiac death are many. The most common cause, accounting for up to 90% of all sudden cardiac deaths, is coronary artery disease. Other aetiologies include valvular heart disease, myocarditis, coronary artery spasm, cardiomyopathy, and prolonged QT syndrome. Most patients with sudden death have underlying coronary artery disease, usually involving major pathological changes in two or more arteries (Reichenbach *et al.*, 1977). Since the major aetiology for sudden death is coronary artery disease, the risk factors

Table 1. *Syndromes of sudden cardiac death* (Eisenberg, 1978)

	Infarction	Ischaemia	Electrical
Pathophysiology	Infarcted area causes pump failure or may lead to rhythm disturbance	Ischaemic area may trigger rhythm disturbance	Rhythm disturbance triggered by poorly understood mechanisms
SCD percentage	20–30%	Unknown	Unknown
Autopsy	Coronary artery occlusion with resultant myocardial infarction	Evidence of ischaemia	'Normal' heart – usually evidence of underlying coronary artery disease
Most common rhythm	Ventricular fibrillation and other rhythms	Ventricular fibrillation	Ventricular fibrillation
Warning prior to collapse	Minutes to hours	Minutes	None or seconds
Mortality within 1 year after discharge	5%	Unknown	30%

SCD, sudden cardiac death.

for coronary artery disease are the same risk factors as those for sudden cardiac death (Weaver *et al.*, 1976). These include male gender, cigarette smoking, high cholesterol, high blood pressure, and diabetes. In addition, high-grade ventricular ectopy and underlying congestive heart failure are additive risk factors (Ruberman *et al.*, 1981). While these risk factors point to individuals at higher risk of experiencing sudden cardiac death, they do not define when the event is likely to occur. There is no simple, non-invasive way to identify a subset of patients at imminent danger of experiencing sudden death. Thus, interventions must focus on programmes and services to deal with the problem in the community since the event is likely to happen in any place at any time (Cobb & Werner 1982).

Clearly, prevention is the only means to definitively solve the problem of sudden cardiac death. Regrettably, at this time, prevention is not a realistic possibility. Although it is possible to reduce risk factors, and thus the incidence of sudden death, such an approach will only lead to a gradual decline in the incidence of sudden cardiac death and will not eliminate the problem.

Syndromes of sudden cardiac death

There is no single trigger for sudden death. Possible triggers which have been studied include ischaemia, electrolyte imbalances, stress, neurochemical transmitters, and clotting abnormalities. While there is no single

aetiology, it is possible to describe several syndromes of sudden cardiac death. These syndromes are based on prodrome, pathological findings, prognosis, and likely trigger events. Table 1 describes the syndromes of sudden cardiac death

FACTORS ASSOCIATED WITH SUCCESSFUL RESUSCITATION

The outcome following sudden cardiac death in the community is determined by factors and circumstances associated with that particular event. Some of these factors relate to the patient, and some relate to the system responding to the emergency. It is convenient to group these factors into fate and system factors. Fate factors refer to characteristics unique to the patient, or chance events. These include, for example, the prior medical condition of the patient, the cardiac rhythm associated with the collapse, and whether the collapse was witnessed or unwitnessed. System factors, on the other hand, describe characteristics of the emergency medical services (EMS) system. System factors include the type of system, whether a bystander initiated cardiopulmonary resuscitation (CPR), and the various time intervals from collapse to CPR and defibrillation (Eisenberg *et al.*, 1984).

Gender is not related to outcome following cardiac arrest, and age is only weakly associated with outcome. For patients discharged alive after out-of-hospital arrest, the average age is 61 years compared to an age of

Table 2. *Cardiac rhythm and outcome for paramedic-treated cases of sudden cardiac death*

Rhythm (upon arrival)	Number	%	Discharged	%
Ventricular fibrillation	1238	58	385	31
Ventricular tachycardia	50	2	23	46
Asystole	576	27	11	2
Idioventricular	162	8	5	3
Other or unknown	125	6	19	15
Total	2151	101[a]	443	97

Source: Center for Evaluation of Emergency Medical Services, Division of Emergency Medical Services, King County Health Department, Seattle, Washington.
[a]Does not equal 100% due to rounding out of figures.

66 years for non-survivors. Patients with a prior history of congestive heart failure have a lower likelihood of survival compared to patients without congestive heart failure. The strongest fate factors predictive of successful resuscitation are the rhythm associated with the collapse and whether the collapse was witnessed. Patients with ventricular fibrillation (VF) or ventricular tachycardia have the highest likelihood of admission and discharge. Patients with other rhythms, such as asystole or pulseless electrical activity, have a much poorer likelihood of survival. Survival rates associated with various rhythms noted at the time of cardiac arrest are shown in Table 2. Patients with a witnessed collapse have a much higher likelihood of survival compared to patients with unwitnessed cardiac arrest. Survival following unwitnessed cardiac arrest is close to zero. This is not surprising given the unknown period of time the patient had to wait before being discovered.

System factors

The system factors most predictive of outcome are the time from collapse to CPR, and the time from collapse to defibrillation and definitive care. Early CPR can most easily be accomplished through initiation of this procedure by bystanders at the scene. Cummins has demonstrated that bystander CPR has a dramatic effect on the likelihood of successful resuscitation (see Chapter 14B(ii)). Table 3 shows the results of 17 controlled studies comparing patients with early bystander CPR versus those with later CPR. In all of the studies except one, the odds ratio for the probability of survival following out-of-hospital cardiac arrest was

significantly greater than 1. The one location which did not demonstrate a beneficial effect of bystander CPR probably had a very fast aid unit response time. Since the average response time was 2.1 min, there was little difference in time between bystander CPR and aid unit CPR (Cummins & Eisenberg, 1985; Cummins et al., 1985; Cummins & Graves, 1989; Thompson et al., 1985; Stueven et al., 1986).

The other important critical time factor, namely time from collapse to definitive care, is intimately related to time from collapse to CPR. Studies of cardiac arrest suggest that CPR prolongs the duration of VF and, therefore, prevents the deterioration from coarse VF to fine VF, and ultimately asystole. Thus, rapid-onset CPR increases the likelihood that VF will last longer and that the response to defibrillation will be positive. The relationship from time to collapse to CPR and time from collapse to definitive care is shown in Fig. 1.

Definitive care encompasses all interventions of advanced life support, including defibrillation, medications, and endotracheal intubation. While the independent benefit of defibrillation is clear, there have been no studies which have quantified the individual benefit of medications or intubation. Such studies would be impossible to perform since the combination of all these treatments defines the standard of care for cardiac arrest.

The outcome following cardiac arrest is determined by the combination of fate and system factors. For example, if the cardiac arrest is unwitnessed and the rhythm is asystole, it makes little difference how rapidly CPR or defibrillation is provided. On the other hand, if the collapse is witnessed and the rhythm is VF, then every minute of delay to CPR and to defibrillation will lower the likelihood of survival.

PREHOSPITAL CARDIAC CARE

The first programme designed to deliver prehospital cardiac care was the mobile coronary care unit (MCCU) established by Pantridge and Geddes in Belfast, Northern Ireland, in 1966. Their unit was staffed by a physician and nurse, and provided early treatment, primarily antiarrhythmic drugs, for suspected acute myocardial infarction. They were also able to defibrillate patients who went into cardiac arrest after arrival of the unit. The first MCCUs in the USA were based on the Belfast model and were started in the late 1960s by Grace in New York City, Crampton in Charlottesville, Virginia, and Warren in Columbus, Ohio. In the early 1970s a model of prehospital care substituting paramedics for physicians

Table 3. *Controlled studies of survival (discharged alive) from out-of-hospital cardiac arrest: bystander cardiopulmonary resuscitation compared with late cardiopulmonary resuscitation* (Cummins & Chamberlain, 1991)

Location/system	Witnessed arrest	Rhythm	Number of patients	Discharged alive (n)	Odds ratio[a]
Oslo, Norway EMTs only	Not reported	Not reported	Bys CPR = 75 Late CPR = 556	36% (27) 8% (43)	6.7
Birmingham Paramedics only	Implied yes	VF or VT	Bys CPR = 7 Late CPR = 12	86% (6) 50% (6)	6.0
Seattle EMTs and paramedics	76% overall witnessed	VF only	Bys CPR = 109 Late CPR = 207	43% (47) 21% (43)	2.9
Winnipeg EMTs only	Not reported	VF or VT	Bys CPR = 65 Late CPR = 161	25% (16)	6.2
Iceland EMTs only	Not reported	All rhythms	Bys CPR = 38 Late CPR = 84	42% (16) 2% (2)	11.5
Vancouver EMTs and paramedics	77% overall witnessed	All rhythms	Bys CPR = 43 Late CPR = 272	21% (9)	4.0
Los Angeles Paramedics	41% overall witnessed	All rhythms	Bys CPR = 93 Late CPR = 150	22% (20) 5% (7)	5.6
		VF only	Bys CPR = 45 Late CPR = 70	27% (12) 6% (4)	6.0
King County EMTs and paramedics	Not reported	All rhythms	Bys CPR = 108 Late CPR = 379	23% (25) 2% (45)	2.2
Pittsburgh Paramedics	Not reported	VF/VT only	Bys CPR = 25 Late CPR = 59	24% (6) 7% (4)	4.3
Milwaukee EMTs and paramedics	Witnessed only	All rhythms	Bys CPR = 1248 Late CPR = 252	15% (182) 15% (38)	1.0
		Coarse VF	Bys CPR = 628 Late CPR = 151	24% (148) 23% (35)	1.0
Michigan/Ohio communities EMTs and paramedics	Not reported	All rhythms	Bys CPR = 472 Late CPR = 1367	13% (56) 5% (64)	2.7
King County EMT-Ds and paramedics	Both	All rhythms	Bys CPR = 726 Late CPR = 1317	27% (196) 13% (177)	2.4
	Witnessed only	All rhythms	Bys CPR = 579 Late CPR = 718	32% (186) 22% (158)	1.7
York/Adams EMTs and paramedics	Witnessed only	VF only	Bys CPR = 157 Late CPR = 225	22% (34) 6% (13)	4.5
Tucson EMTs and paramedics	Witnessed only	All rhythms	Bys CPR = 65 Late CPR = 130	20% (13) 9% (12)	2.5
West Yorkshire Ambulance personnel	Not reported	All rhythms	Bys CPR = 47 Late CPR = 50	15% (7) 8% (4)	2.0
Belgium Ambulance Personnel	Not reported	All rhythms	Bys CPR = 985 Late CPR = 2036	10% (98) 5% (109)	1.9
Houston EMTs and medics	Both	Unmonitored VF/VT	Bys CPR = 53 Late CPR = 133	30% (16) 14% (9)	2.1

EMT, emergency medical technican; EMT-D, emergency medical technician trained to defibrillate; VF, ventricular fibrillation; VT, ventricular tachycardia; Bys, bystander; CPR, cardiopulmonary resuscitation.

[a]Odds ratio is not a simple ratio of survival rates. It is calculated as the odds of surviving with bystander CPR (number discharged alive divided by number who die) divided by the odds of discharge alive for people who received late CPR (number discharged alive divided by number who die).

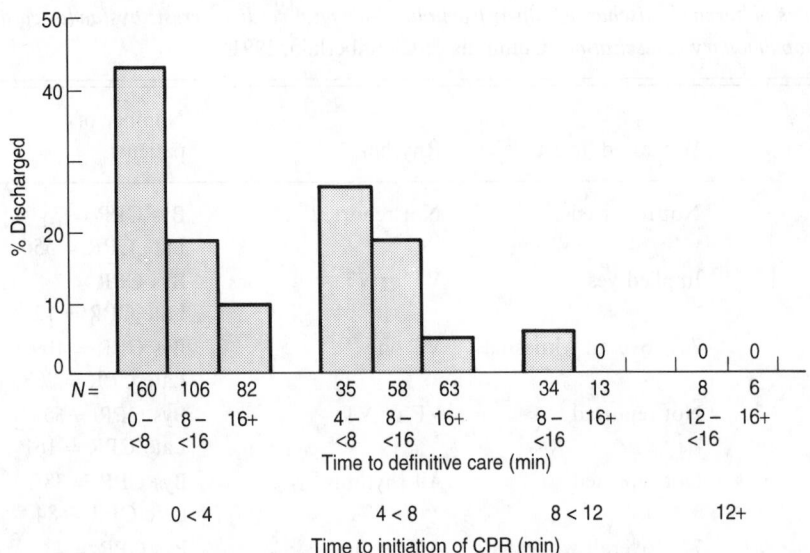

Fig. 1. Relationship of discharge following out-of-hospital cardiac arrest to time to definitive care and time to initiation of cardiopulmonary resuscitation (CPR). (Reproduced, with permission, from Eisenberg, M.S., Bergner, L. & Hallstrom, A. (1979). Cardiac resuscitation in the community: the importance of rapid delivery of care and implication for program planning. *JAMA*, **241**, 1905. Copyright 1979, American Medical Association.)

was begun by Nagel in Miami, Cobb in Seattle, and Criley in Los Angeles. Although established initially to provide emergency coronary care, these programmes soon began to encompass all types of prehospital emergencies (Cobb *et al.*, 1980; Cobb & Hallstrom, 1982).

Five types of systems

Virtually all prehospital EMS systems in the USA can be characterized as one of five types. Systems using physicians in prehospital units are not found in the USA, although this is a popular model in Europe and Israel. The following are definitions of the five systems. Table 4 provides details.

1. *Basic EMT* (emergency medical technician): ambulance or aid response unit staffed with personnel trained in basic cardiac life support.
2. *EMT-D*: basic EMTs also trained in the use of defibrillators.
3. *Paramedic*: personnel trained in advanced cardiac life support capable of providing defibrillation, medication, and endotracheal intubation.
4. *Basic EMT/paramedic*: a double response system with the first responding unit staffed with basic EMTs, and the second responding units staffed with paramedics.
5. *EMT-D/paramedic*: a double response system with the first responding unit staffed with EMT-D personnel, and the second response unit staffed with paramedics.

The survival experience from these five types of prehospital systems have been described in 29 communities (Eisenberg *et al.*, 1990). The range of discharge rates for all rhythms and VF is shown in Fig. 2. The EMT-D/paramedic system had the highest survival rate with 29% for VF. The lowest survival rate was found in the basic EMT system – 12% from VF.

Model to predict outcomes from the five types of systems

It is clear that the more sophisticated the system the higher the survival. The main reason some systems have higher survivals than others is their ability to deliver CPR, defibrillation, and definitive care rapidly. From the moment of collapse, the probability of survival decreases with every minute of delay to initiation of these interventions. Prehospital interventions generally occur in a sequence with CPR being the first (started by bystanders or ambulance personnel), followed by defibrillatory shocks administered by EMT-Ds or by paramedics, followed by advanced care given by paramedics or at the hospital in situations without paramedics. The average time to performance of each of these critical interventions determines the survival rate following cardiac arrest in a community. A graphical model demonstrating these relationships is shown in Fig. 3. Based upon a study of 1667 witnessed cardiac arrest patients with VF in King County, Washington, a linear regression model, taking

Table 4. *Types of emergency medical systems*

The times shown are average; actual times may vary from location to location. The average time from collapse to CPR will be shorter if bystanders initiate CPR at the scene prior to emergency agency arrival.

Type of system	Number of vehicles responding	Training of emergency personnel	Skills	Survival rate following VF[a]	Time to CPR[b]	Time of defibrillation	Time of advanced life support[c]
Emergency medical technician	1	EMT 110 h	CPR	12%	4 min	20 min (at hospital)	20 min (at hospital)
Emergency medical technician-defibrillation (EMT-D)	1	EMT 120 h (110 h + 10 h in defibrillation skills)	CPR Defibrillation	15%	4 min	6 min	20 min (at hospital)
Paramedic	1	Paramedic 400–1500 h	CPR Defibrillation Medication Airway intubation	17%	8 min	10 min	10 min
EMT plus paramedic	2	EMT 110 h Paramedic 400–1500 h	As above	25%	4 min	10 min	10 min
EMT-D plus paramedic	2	EMT-D 120 h Paramedic 400–1500 h	As above but earlier defibrillation by EMT-D	29%	4 min	6 min	10 min

[a]Reported hospital discharge rate following sudden cardiac death associated with ventricular fibrillation (VF).
[b]Measured from patient collapse to start of CPR.
[c]Includes emergency drugs and advanced airway control.

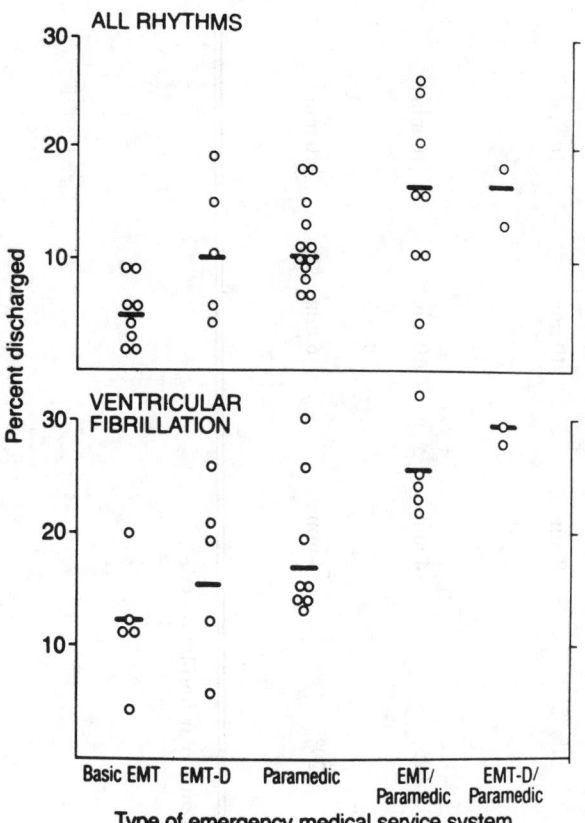

Fig. 2. Percentage discharged from out-of-hospital cardiac arrest in all rhythms (top panel) and in ventricular fibrillation (bottom panel) from five emergency medical service (EMS) systems. The circles represent the percentage discharged from individual communities; the horizontal bars represent the weighted mean discharge rate. (Reproduced, with permission, from Eisenberg, M.S., Horwood, B. T., Cummins, R. O. *et al.* (1990). Cardiac arrest and resuscitation: a tale of 29 cities. *Ann. Emerg. Med.*, **19**, 179–86.

into account time to CPR, time to defibrillation, and time to definitive care, was developed. The model predicted that approximately 70% survival would be likely if all three interventions were to occur immediately upon collapse. The decline in survival without treatment is 5.5% per min. For every minute of delay in time to CPR, approximately a 2.5% fall in survival occurs, 1.1% per min of delay to defibrillation, and 2.1% per min of delay to definitive care. Graphically, the interventions of CPR, defibrillation and advanced care can be considered to alter the survival curve after cardiac arrest. Since the survival curve for cardiac arrest is defined in minutes, an intervention, if given in a timely enough fashion, can alter the slope of the survival curve. Once definitive care can be provided, the survival curve is stabilized and reaches a plateau. Admittedly this is a model, but it does graphically present the effect of each intervention and the relationship

between time delay and ultimate survival (Larson *et al.*, 1993).

Chain of survival

A metaphor used to describe the sequence of events from calling for help to delivery of definitive care is defined in the 'chain of survival'. There are four links in the chain of survival: 'early access', 'early CPR', 'early defibrillation', and 'early advanced care' (see Chapter 14B(ii)). A community with integrated links along this chain will have a high survival from cardiac arrest, and communities with weak links, or even missing links, will have very poor outcomes (Cummins *et al.*, 1991b).

Options to improve early access

Communities with universal access numbers such as 911 or 119 are able to shorten dispatch time because of community awareness of the proper phone number. Other factors which are related to early access involve specific protocols for the identification of cardiac arrest, and immediate dispatching of units before full information is obtained. Once the unit is en route, it is possible to provide more information as it is obtained.

Improving the link of early CPR

Programmes to achieve widespread training of CPR by the general population have been successful in achieving early CPR. Citizen CPR programmes were first initiated by Cobb and his colleagues in 1971 and have become an important part of many EMS systems over the last two decades. Training, which can be as brief as 3 h, is usually provided by public agencies or local fire departments, free or for a small fee. The American Red Cross and American Heart Association have been actively involved in training of citizens in CPR (Cobb & Hallstrom, 1982).

The mass media may play a useful role in public education in CPR. Whether shown on television or displayed in widely used items such as phone books, efforts to demonstrate the techniques of CPR are likely to have a beneficial affect. A programme in King County has mailed free video tapes to households with individuals over the age of 50 years in an effort to allow them to watch a 10-min video on how to do CPR.

Yet another approach is for the emergency dispatcher to provide telephone instruction in CPR to the person calling the cardiac emergency. Such a programme has been in place in King County, Washington, since 1981.

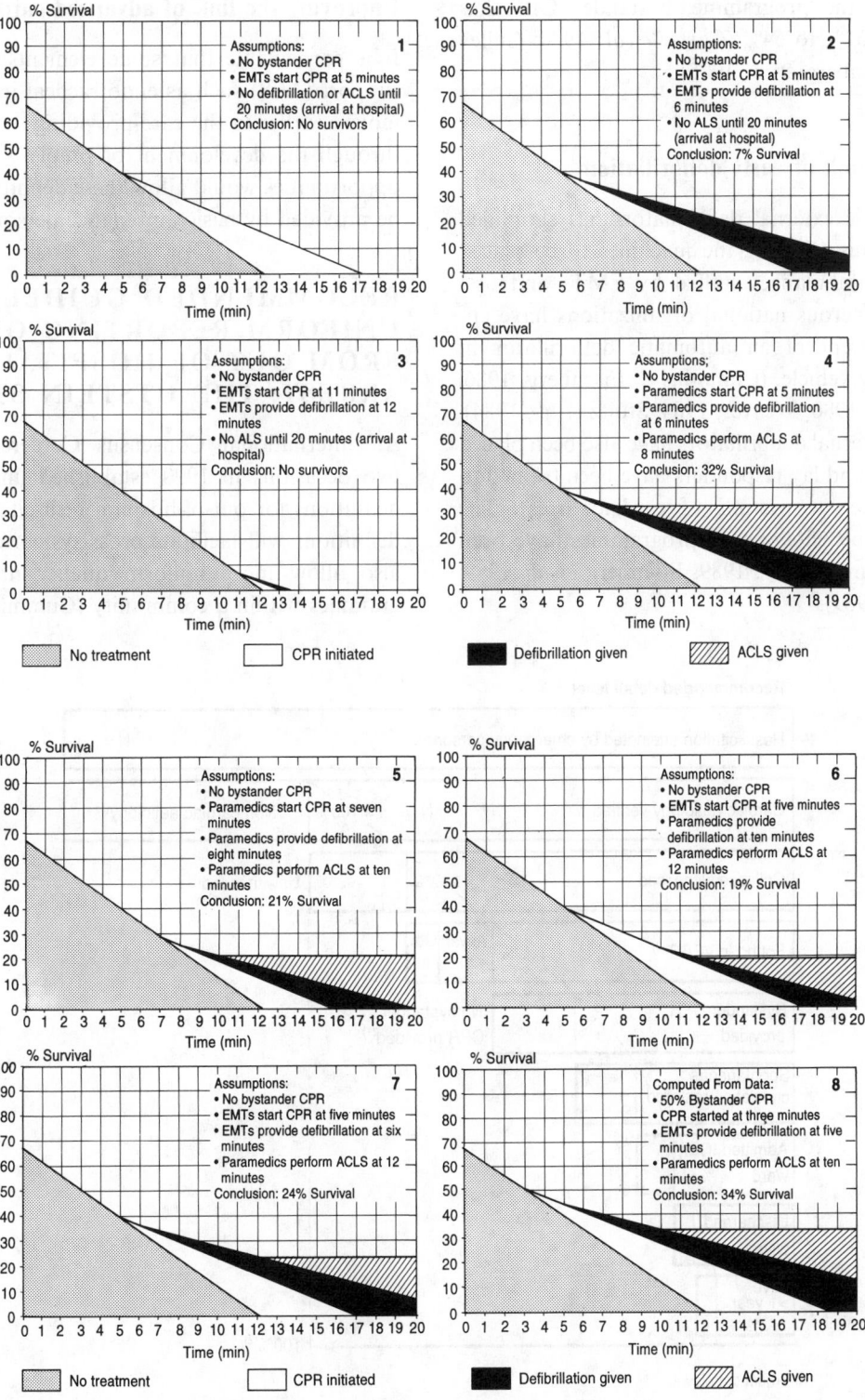

Fig. 3. Survival from cardiac arrest for different types of prehospital emergency medical services (EMS) systems. (1) EMT system with response time of 4 min. (2) EMT-D system with a response time of 4 min. (3) EMT-D system with a response time of 10 min. (4) Paramedic system with a response time of 4 min. (5) Paramedic system with a response time of 6 min. (6) EMT/paramedic system with response times of 4 and 9 min respectively. (7) EMT-D/paramedic system with response times of 4 and 9 min respectively. (8) King County with an EMT-D/paramedic system with response times of 4 and 9 min respectively and 50% bystander CPR. (Reproduced, with permission, from Larson, M. P., Eisenberg, M. S., Cummins, R. O. *et al.*, (1993). Predicting survival from out-of-hospital cardiac arrest. *Ann. Emerg. Med.*, **22**, 1652–8.)

As a result of the programme, bystander CPR has increased from 32% to 54% (Carter *et al.*, 1984; Culley *et al.*, 1991; Eisenberg *et al.*, 1985).

Improving the link of early defibrillation

Use of automatic external defibrillators has simplified defibrillation, thus allowing the machines to be placed in more basic ambulances staffed by EMTs and first responders. Numerous national organizations have endorsed the concept of an automatic defibrillator in every emergency vehicle, (Cummins & Eisenberg, 1986; Eisenberg *et al.*, 1980; Weaver, 1984; Stultz *et al.*, 1984).

Automatic external defibrillators have also been placed in public places and lay responders have been trained to attach the device to victims of cardiac arrest. The limitations and benefits of such programmes have been described (Cummins *et al.*, 1989; Eisenberg *et al.*, 1989; Weaver *et al.*, 1989).

Improving the link of advanced cardiac life support

It is conceivable that some elements of advanced life support (ALS) such as endotracheal intubation may be moved earlier in the care-providing sequence – perhaps through the development of simple, safe devices. Such opportunities would allow these definitive procedures to be provided by basic ambulance personnel.

RECOMMENDED GUIDELINES FOR UNIFORM REPORTING OF DATA FROM OUT-OF-HOSPITAL CARDIAC ARREST: THE UTSTEIN STYLE

An international Consensus Conference meeting on two occasions in 1990 established uniform terms and definitions for out-of-hospital resuscitation. Using such definitions will facilitate cross-system comparisons and also allow more uniform quality improvement programmes within a community (Cummins *et al.*, 1991a).

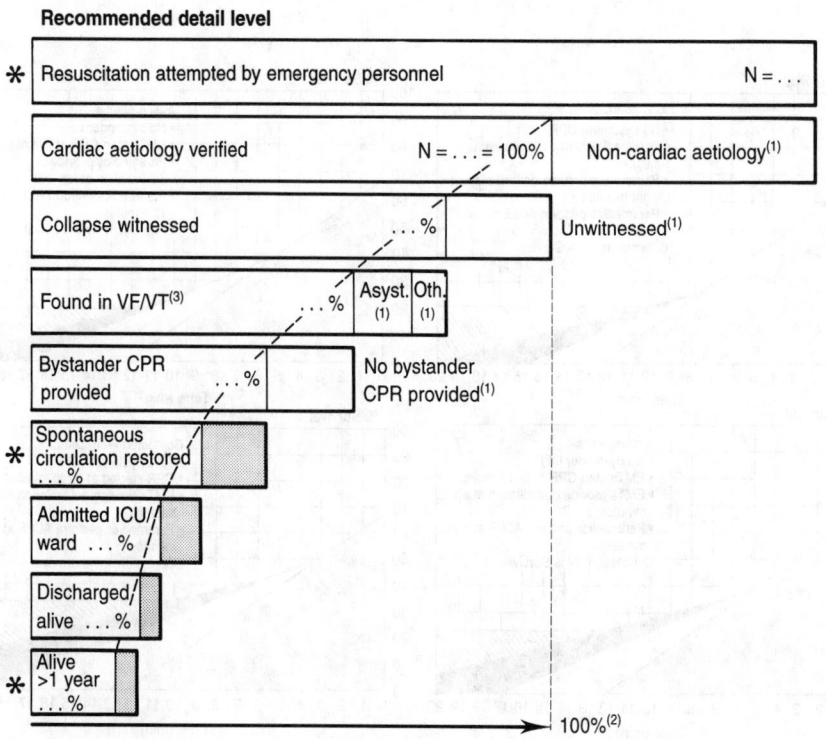

* Minimum data level

(1) Subgroups with an additional survival potential which may be analyzed using an identical pattern, i.e. broken into the lower steps in the template

(2) For purposes of uniform reporting the recommended '100%', or denominator group, is resuscitations attempted on cardiac arrests of cardiac aetiology

(3) VT should be reported as a separate group

Fig. 4. Utstein II recommendations on data to be reported on cardiac arrest resuscitation. (Reproduced with permission. © Recommended guidelines for uniform reporting of data from out-of-hospital cardiac arrest: the Utstein Style. *Circulation*, **84**, August 1991. Copyright American Heart Association.)

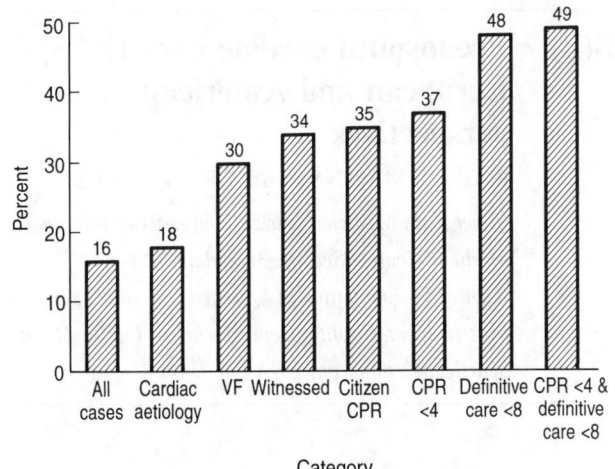

Fig. 5. Percentage discharged from out-of-hospital cardiac arrest in King County, Washington, for different subgroups of all cardiac arrests. (Reproduced, with permission, from Eisenberg, M. S., Cummins, R. O. & Larsen, M. P. (1991). Numerators, denominators, and survival rates: reporting survival from out-of-hospital cardiac arrest. *Am. J. Emerg. Med.*, 9, 544–6.)

The Consensus Conference recommended that a template approach be used for reporting data from pre-hospital resuscitations. Fig. 4 provides a graphic representation of the information that should be collected in various communities. The actual Utstein Style Template for the recommended full data collection on cardiac arrest is shown in Chapter 14B(ii). The template calls for numbers to be inserted at each level. Each level serves two functions: the numerator for the level above, and the denominator for the level below. The importance of defining numerators and denominators is shown in Fig. 5 with data from King County, Washington. Changing the definition of cases in the denominator dramatically changes resulting survival rates (Eisenberg *et al.*, 1991).

IMPROVING SURVIVAL FROM SUDDEN CARDIAC DEATH

Emergency physicians are pivotal in improving a community's survival rate from sudden cardiac death. They frequently supervise the prehospital EMS system and they have a unique clinical perspective. Emergency physicians should be able to define survival as well as key factors and time intervals in their community. This information can then be used to improve the system and allow more people to survive cardiac arrest.

Bibliography

CARTER, W.B. *et al.* (1984). Development and implementation of emergency CPR instruction by telephone. *Ann. Emerg. Med.*, **13**, 695.

COBB, L.A. & HALLSTROM, A.P. (1982). Community-based cardiopulmonary resuscitation: what have we learned? *N.Y. Acad. Sc*, **382**, 330–42.

COBB, L.A. & WERNER, J.A. (1982). Predictors and prevention of sudden cardiac death. In *The Heart*, 5th edn ed. J. W. Hurst. New York: McGraw-Hill.

COBB, L.A., WERNER, J. & TROBOUGH, G. (1980). Sudden cardiac death: 1. A decade's experience with out-of-hospital resuscitation. *Mod. Concepts Cardiovasc. Dis.*, **49**, 31.

CULLEY, L., CLARK, J., EISENBERG, M.S. *et al.* (1991). Dispatcher assisted telephone CPR: standards and time requirements. *Ann. Emerg. Med.*, **20**, 362–6.

CUMMINS, R.O. & EISENBERG, M.S. (1985). Prehospital cardiopulmonary resuscitation: is it effective? *JAMA*, **253**, 2408.

CUMMINS, R.O. & EISENBERG, M.S. (1986). Automatic external defibrillators: clinical issues for cardiology. *Circulation*, **73**, 381.

CUMMINS, R.O. & CHAMBERLAIN, D.A. (1991). Recommended guidelines for uniform reporting of data from out-of-hospital cardiac arrest: The Utstein Style. *Circulation*, **84**, 960–75.

CUMMINS, R.O. & GRAVES, J. (1989). Clinical results of standard CPR: prehospital and in hospital. In *Cardiopulmonary Resuscitation*, ed. W. Kaye & N. G. Bircher. New York: Churchill Livingstone.

CUMMINS, R.O., EISENBERG, M.S., HALLSTROM, A.P. *et al.* (1985). Survival of out-of-hospital cardiac arrest with early initiation of cardiopulmonary resuscitation. *Am. J. Emerg. Med.*, **3**, 114–18.

CUMMINS, R.O., EISENBERG, M.S., LITWIN, P.E. *et al.* (1987). Automatic external defibrillators use by emergency medical technicians: a controlled clinical trial. *JAMA*, **257**, 1605.

CUMMINS, R.O., SCHUBACH, J.A., LITWIN, P.E. *et al.* (1989). Training lay persons to use automatic external defibrillators: success of initial training and one year retention of skills. *Am. J. Emerg. Med.*, **7**, 143.

CUMMINS, R.O., ORNATO, J.P., THIES, W. *et al.* (1991). Improving survival from cardiac arrest: the chain of survival concept. *Circulation*, **83**, 1832–47.

EISENBERG, M.S. (1978). Sudden cardiac death and resuscitation: the results. In *Critical Care: State of the Art*, Vol. 8, ed. F. B. Cerra. Fullerton, CA: Society of Critical Care Medicine.

EISENBERG, M.S., COPASS, M. & HALLSTROM, A. (1980). Treatment of out-of-hospital cardiac arrest with rapid defibrillation by emergency medical technicians. *N. Engl. J. Med.*, **302**, 1379.

EISENBERG, M.S., BERGNER, L. & HALLSTROM, A. (1984). *Sudden Cardiac Death in the Community.* p. 34. New York: Praeger.

EISENBERG, M.S., HALLSTROM, A. & CARTER, W. (1985). Emergency CPR instruction via telephone. *Am. J. Public Health*, **75**, 47.

EISENBERG, M.S., MOORE, J. & CUMMINS, R.O. (1989). Use of the automatic external defibrillators in homes of survivors of out-of-hospital ventricular fibrillation. *Am. J. Cardiol*, **63**, 443.

EISENBERG, M.S., HORWOOD, B.T., CUMMINS, R.O. *et al.* (1990). Cardiac arrest and resuscitation: a tale of 29 cities. *Ann. Emerg. Med.*, **19**, 179–86.

KULLER, L.H. (1980). Sudden death: definition and epidemiologic considerations progress. *Prog. Cardiovasc. Dis.*, **23**, 1.

KULLER, L.H., PERPER, J. & COOPER, M. (1975). Demographic characteristics and trends in arteriosclerotic heart disease mortality: sudden death and myocardial infarction. *Circulation*, **52**, (Suppl. III), 1–11.

LARSON, M.P., EISENBERG, M.S., CUMMINS, R.O. *et al.* (1993). Predicting survival from out-of-hospital cardiac arrest. *Ann. Emerg. Med.*, **22**, 1652–8.

PANTRIDGE, J.F. & GEDDES, J.S. (1967). A mobile intensive care unit in the management of myocardial infarction. *Lancet*, **ii**, 271.

REICHENBACH, D.D., MOSS, N.S. & MEYER, E. (1977). Pathology of the heart in sudden cardiac dealth. *Am. J. Cardiol.*, **39**, 865.

RUBERMAN, W., WEINBLATT, E., GOLDBERG, J.D. *et al.* (1981). Ventricular premature beats and mortality after myocardial infarction. *Circulation*, **64**, 297–305.

STUEVEN, H. TROIANO, P., THOMPSON, B. *et al.* (1986). Bystander first responder CPR: ten years experience in a paramedic system. *Ann. Emerg. Med.*, **15**, 707–10.

STULTS, K.R., BROWN, D.D., SCHUG, V.L. *et al.* (1984). Prehospital defibrillation performed by emergency medical technicians in rural communities. *N. Engl. J. Med.*, **310**, 219.

THOMPSON, B. M., STUEVEN, H.A., MATEER, J.R. *et al.* (1985). Comparison of clinical CPR studies in Milwaukee and elsewhere in the United States. *Ann. Emerg. Med.*, **14**, 750–4.

WEAVER, W.D. (1984). Improved neurologic recovery and survival after early defibrillation. *Circulation*, **69**, 943–8.

WEAVER, W.D., LORCH, G.S., ALVAREZ, H.A. *et al.* (1976). Angiographic findings and prognostic indicators for patients resuscitated from sudden cardiac death. *Circulation*, **54**, 895.

WEAVER, W.D., SUTHERLAND, K., WIRKUS, M. *et al.* (1989). Emergency medical care requirements for large public assemblies and a new strategy for managing cardiac arrest in this setting. *Ann. Emerg. Med.*, **18**, 155–60.

B(ii): Prehospital cardiac care II: European and American perspectives

R.O. CUMMINS[a] and J.R. GRAVES[b]

[a]*Emergency Medicine Service, University of Washington Medical Center, Seattle, Washington, USA*
[b]*Center for Evaluation of Emergency Medical Services, Seattle-King County Department of Public Health, Seattle, Washington, USA*

THE IMPORTANCE OF PREHOSPITAL CARDIAC CARE

Sudden cardiac arrest remains the most dramatic and demanding problem in emergency medicine (American Heart Association, 1993). The magnitude of sudden cardiac death assumes the proportions of an epidemic in all major developed nations. In the USA an estimated 1 600 000 people each year have heart attacks because of coronary artery disease; 600 000 of them die, 450 000 die outside the hospital. This incidence rate is 1.8 out-of-hospital deaths per year for every 1000 adults in a community. *No other medical problem approaches this magnitude.* And yet many communities have failed to organize their emergency medical system in a manner that effectively reduces this huge toll on life and productivity.

The problem of sudden cardiac arrest has exerted a profound influence on all aspects of the organization of emergency care. 'Resuscitation', primarily from sudden cardiac death, is an important multidisciplinary branch of emergency medicine, calling for a spectrum of skills and attracting a plethora of specialties and organizations. Efforts to improve the management of sudden cardiac arrest in the community have driven much of the development of prehospital emergency care. Pantridge's and Adgey's mobile coronary care units in Ulster stimulated the creation of paramedics in the USA and doctor-manned ambulances in Europe (Pantridge &

Disclaimer: This chapter presents analyses of information gathered from 13 different EMS systems. These interpretations, analyses and commentaries are solely those of the authors of this chapter and do not reflect necessarily the viewpoints of the EMS systems surveyed, nor the opinions of the task force members and organizations that participated in the development of the Utstein Guidelines.

Geddes, 1966). Although the duties and roles of these personnel now encompass more than just the treatment of cardiac arrest, much of emergency care originated to treat sudden cardiac death. The successes observed led to improvements in all aspects of emergency care including, in the USA, emergency medical technicians, first responders and early defibrillation programmes and, in Europe, doctor-manned ambulances and emergency medical technicians.

Increased understanding of the mechanism and therapy of sudden death helped everyone realize that a rapid response with personnel capable of a narrow range of specific skills could save lives. Getting these skilled personnel to a patient in sudden cardiac arrest as fast as possible has become a driving force in the organization of emergency care throughout the world. This principle has led to the development of dispatch systems, public awareness schemes, community cardiopulmonary resuscitation (CPR) training programmes, the entire early defibrillation movement with the development of automated external defibrillators, and the development of paramedic- and doctor-manned ambulances schemes.

PERSPECTIVE OF THIS CHAPTER

This chapter provides an overview of how a number of systems in Europe and the USA are organized to provide effective emergency care. This description will help emergency physicians understand better the range of activities now occurring in Europe and the USA, and will help provide new ideas on how every system can solve problems and improve emergency cardiac care.

In addition, the Appendix to this chapter reviews in detail the recommendations of the Utstein Consensus Conference on uniform reporting of data from out-of-hospital cardiac arrest. This conference, and the subsequent publication of its recommendations in several journals, is a landmark event in emergency medicine for it reflects one of emergency medicine's first international consensus conferences. The general thrust of the recommendations should be understood by everyone involved in emergency medicine, particularly people interested in resuscitation and prehospital emergency care.

ORGANIZATION AND DESCRIPTION OF EMS SYSTEMS

The organization of a community's emergency medical services (EMS) systems has a major effect on cardiac arrest outcomes (Cobb & Hallstrom, 1982; Cobb et al.,

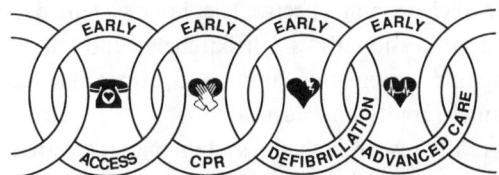

CHAIN of SURVIVAL

Fig. 1. The chain of survival. (Reproduced with permission. Cummins, R.O., Ornato, J.P., Thies, W. et al. (1991). Improving survival from cardiac arrest: the 'Chain of Survival' concept. *Circulation*, **83**, 1832–47. Copyright 1991 American Heart Association.)

1980, 1990; Cummins et al., 1991a). An EMS system's organization for cardiopulmonary emergencies can be described using two overlapping concepts. The first is the 'chain of survival' metaphor which states that the divisions of an EMS system can be likened to the links in a chain (Fig. 1) (Cummins et al., 1991a). Each division requires separate attention, even separate programmes; weaknesses in any one link will condemn an entire system to poor survival rates.

The other conceptual approach is to consider an EMS systems' 'tiers' or layers of responders to a prehospital emergency. Using the 'tiers' concept one can describe an EMS system in terms of the therapeutic skill levels of the responders in each tier, and evaluate the system in terms of the speed with which personnel deliver these interventions.

There is considerable overlap among the features of the 'chain of survival' concept and the 'tiered response' concept. Both concepts can be used together to evaluate, describe and compare EMS systems. The 'chain of survival' concept is valuable for it adds elements that EMS organizers and directors frequently neglect; for example, the role that lay rescuers play by recognizing an emergency, calling the emergency number, and then initiating CPR. The most sophisticated dispatch centre in the world, teamed with the most advanced ambulance personnel, will achieve little if it is not combined with an alert, well-trained and involved citizenry.

The 'chain of survival' concept and the 'tiered response' concept

The 'early access' link: recognition, alerting and dispatch

'Early access' starts the chain of survival and gets trained help to the patient as quickly as possible. The goal of early access is to have people recognize an emergency quickly, know how to get help, and then be able to rapidly and effectively communicate that emergency to the EMS system. Early access requires the combination of trained citizens, an effective telephone system, personnel trained professionally as dispatchers, and an efficient dispatching system that alerts and dispatches response personnel rapidly and accurately.

Currently researchers and system managers are paying much closer attention to this 'forgotten link' in the chain of survival. Emergency medical dispatchers in some systems are required to have special skills such as previous emergency medical technician (EMT) or paramedic experience and training. Other systems require that only nurses perform the dispatch role, or that 24-h physician consultation be available. In many systems no professional criteria must be met other than several months of on-the-job training and supervision. Some dispatch systems are dedicated to EMS only, whereas in others the dispatch system must also cover fire and police. A variety of communication numbers and systems are used, such as a three-digit number, enhanced three-digit number systems with caller location, seven-digit numbers, or computer-aided dispatch.

Some systems may employ formal protocols for dispatching while others, mainly those employing experienced paramedics and EMTs, depend on the 'background knowledge and experience' of the dispatchers to know what to do. The most advanced and successful systems provide 'prearrival' instructions to the callers. The dispatcher keeps the caller on the telephone, calming the caller down, soliciting additional information, and often advising specific actions to take, such as control of bleeding, relief of obstructed airways, and mouth-to-mouth ventilation and chest compressions. Dispatcher-assisted CPR instruction offered to callers has been adopted by many systems and several studies have confirmed its effectiveness in increasing the number of arrests with bystander-CPR and in improving survival (Eisenberg et al., 1985, 1986a; Carter et al., 1984; Kellerman et al., 1989).

Several other features of the dispatching system can affect the success of prehospital treatment of sudden cardiac arrest. Does the system use *simultaneous dispatching* for cardiac arrest patients? This important approach helps assure better cardiac arrest survival. Once the dispatcher gathers enough information to recognize a potential cardiac arrest, they use simultaneous dispatching to send not only the first responding tier but also the more advanced second and third tiers. These latter tiers can involve paramedics, nurses and even doctor-manned ambulances. When witnesses call to

report a sudden cardiac arrest they will not often state the problem as 'sudden cardiac arrest' but rather will use terms such as 'collapsed', 'not breathing', 'turning blue', 'unconscious' or 'not responsive'. Advanced EMS systems employ protocols by which the dispatchers activate the first response vehicle during the interrogation, based simply on the initial complaint.

EMS systems must never require the first responding units to confirm a suspicious collapse as a sudden cardiac death before dispatching the advanced tier. This will produce unacceptable delays before arrival of the secondary and more advanced personnel. The EMS systems with the best survival rates use the first-addressed operator to activate the EMS system – usually on the basis of just a few words of complaint – and will not require the call to be routed to other operators. For example, a dispatcher, upon hearing a crying, distressed caller state 'my husband just collapsed and is turning blue' should be able to immediately activate the EMS response of not only the first responding tier, but also the more advanced paramedic- or doctor-manned vehicles.

The operation and success of the EMS dispatching system depends heavily upon the witnesses to a cardiac emergency. Strength can be gained in the early access link by education of the public, specifically those individuals most likely to witness a cardiac arrest. Persons uninformed about chest pain and respiratory distress may fail to comprehend the signs of an impending cardiac arrest. When a person collapses, such witnesses may take an excessively long time to call the emergency dispatch centre. Witnesses may call neighbours, relatives or even their local doctors before calling the emergency dispatch number. Educational and public service programmes, such as those developed by the American Heart Association, the British Heart Foundation, the Red Cross, and the European Resuscitation Council attempt to inform the public of what to do in the event of a cardiac arrest. In CPR classes and in school and worksite training, people learn to recognize the warning signs of a heart attack and the signs of a person who collapses.

The early CPR link: citizens versus the first tier

The goal of the early CPR link is to have someone start basic CPR as soon as possible after a cardiac arrest (less than 1 min). This almost always means lay witnesses to the collapse must start CPR. This action should occur as soon as the witnesses recognize a cardiac arrest, and simultaneously with efforts to contact and activate the EMS system. The best statistic to evaluate whether this goal is achieved is simple: in what percentage of witnessed arrests in a community have one of the witnesses started CPR? Many programmes have been distracted by less important data such as the number of people trained in CPR in a community, or the percentage of a population trained. The important question is the direct one: if a sudden cardiac arrest is witnessed, does someone start CPR?

In the past, many EMS systems depended upon the 'first tier' in the system to initiate CPR. Leonard Cobb, in Seattle, Washington, quickly demonstrated that this 'first tier' really must be the lay witnesses to the event and not the late-responding emergency personnel (Cobb & Hallstrom, 1982; Cobb et al., 1980). Other EMS systems, especially in Europe, were quick to adopt Cobb's ideas, but encountered numerous barriers to implementation. Many EMS systems continue to operate from the narrow perspective of depending on the first tier of emergency responders to start CPR, rather than the lay witnesses.

Many reports provide data that compare the survival rates of cardiac arrest victims who receive 'early' CPR (defined as CPR initiated by citizens or bystanders) with the survival rates of those who received 'late' CPR (i.e. CPR initiated by emergency responders). 'Early' CPR usually differed from 'late' CPR by about 4 min. In all but one system, comparisons between early and late CPR reveal a significant positive benefit from early CPR. The magnitude of this contribution may be considerable. Odds ratios for improved survival with early CPR can range as high as 11.5 (a person is 11.5 times more likely to survive with early CPR than with late CPR) (Cummins & Eisenberg, 1985; Cummins et al., 1985, 1991a). Two methods for achieving early CPR performed by lay bystanders include wide spread community-based CPR programmes and 'targeted' CPR programmes. In 'targeted CPR', instructors identify and teach basic CPR to middle-aged people, residents and staff of senior centres, and the family members of survivors of a myocardial infarction, or to other patients identified as having cardiac arrest risk factors.

A final method to achieve early CPR is 'dispatcher-assisted' CPR instruction. This refers to programmes in which emergency telephone dispatchers offer CPR instructions to people at the time they call to report a cardiac arrest. Dispatchers can focus panicked bystanders and encourage and instruct them to perform CPR when

they 'draw a blank' at the sudden sight of a cyanotic and breathless loved one.

One of the key points in evaluating EMS systems is to consider whether the system managers think the major responsibility of the first tier is to perform CPR. The predominant viewpoint now endorsed by the American Heart Association and the European Resuscitation Council is that the lay witnesses should be the major providers of early CPR (not the EMS system) and that the first responding EMS personnel should concentrate on being the major providers of early defibrillation as well as taking on responsibility for continued CPR.

The early defibrillation link: the key purpose of the first tier of professional EMS responders

Much research in prehospital care of sudden cardiac arrest now focuses on early defibrillation (Bocka, 1989; Bossaert & Koster, 1992; Calle et al., 1992; Cobbe et al., 1991; Colquhoun, 1988, 1993; Cummins, 1989; Cummins et al., 1987; Fonsmark et al., 1989, 1993; Gallehr & Vukov, 1993; Hargarten et al., 1990; Offstad et al., 1992; Richless et al., 1993; Scott & Fitzgerald, 1993; Sedgwick et al., 1992; Silfvast, 1990). A reductionist viewpoint is widespread because of two understandings supported by extensive research. First, almost all people who have the potential to survive sudden unexpected death are in ventricular fibrillation (VF). Second, the only effective therapy for VF is early defibrillation – not endotracheal intubation, not intravenous medications – just defibrillation. The key operative word here is 'early'. Multiple studies demonstrate that a person in VF must be defibrillated within 10 min of their collapse or their probability of survival approaches zero (Cobb & Hallstrom, 1982; Cobb et al., 1990; Eisenberg et al., 1990a). The decline in the probability of survival, however, is continuous, declining with each minute that passes. Some studies estimate that the probability of being successfully defibrillated from VF to a rhythm that produces effective contractions drops 7% with each minute (Eisenberg et al., 1990a,b). Since the best possible survival from VF is 70% if the shock is delivered in less than a minute, a 7% decline per minute leaves a victim with a 0% survival chance at the end of 10 min. Bystander CPR will help slow this rate of decline significantly, but will not prevent the decline. The advanced tier in only a few systems can achieve a median 10-min interval between the patient's collapse and personnel arrival at the patient's side.

Two events, however, have combined to brighten this bleak outlook for treating sudden cardiac death. First, research projects confirmed that defibrillation was a skill that should not be reserved only for use by paramedics and physicians on ambulances. Defibrillation can be performed with equal effectiveness by any first tier responder including ambulance drivers and EMTs. Second, modern engineering gave us the new technology of automated external defibrillators (AEDs) in the 1980s and greatly simplified training, continuing education, supervision, and the success of defibrillation by first responding personnel.

There is now widespread endorsement of the concept that early defibrillation can best be achieved by allowing personnel in the first tier emergency response to use and operate AEDs. Some countries have displayed a reluctance to have ambulance staff with basic training operate AEDs. This reluctance, however, cannot be based on an argument that the personnel cannot be trained or that the technology does not work. Numerous publications confirm that first tier ambulance staff can be trained successfully to operate AEDs and to save lives. Entire countries (such as Scotland) have embraced the principle of early defibrillation by equipping every ambulance with an AED and training all personnel to use the devices. The great success of this approach is well documented. Even greater successes are expected when Scotland's objective of a paramedic on every ambulance is achieved.

While many EMS systems have adopted early defibrillation programmes in which the first responding EMS personnel are allowed to defibrillate, some communities have not observed an improvement in cardiac arrest survival rates. While we lack a full explanation for their lack of success, most of these systems have two shortcomings: first, few victims have received early CPR prior to defibrillation; second, the defibrillation delivered is not truly 'early', often falling outside the critical 10-min limit. Consequently, the Utstein Guidelines recommend recording the median (not mean) call response interval for the various tiers of the response system. Those systems not achieving more than 50% of their first tier calls with less than 10-min response intervals have little expectation of achieving anything more than occasional successful resuscitations.

The early advanced cardiac life support link: intubation, medications, diagnosis and stabilization

Advanced cardiac life support (ACLS) has traditionally been defined as the provision of three interventions: defibrillation, endotracheal intubation and intravenous medications. A major conceptual change has occurred, however, in that defibrillation should now be delegated to the first responding personnel. In many locations this delegation of defibrillation to non-ACLS personnel poses a major policy problem, usually because defibrillation was formerly considered a 'restricted medical act' that could only be performed by physicians. Numerous research projects have confirmed that this restriction of defibrillation to only medical personnel is harmful. Defibrillation must be performed by the first arriving emergency personnel – not delayed until more highly trained personnel arrive. Policies that restrain early defibrillation programmes must be changed because we now possess incontrovertible evidence that early defibrillation is the major way to significantly improve survival rates.

Thus the advanced life support tier is defined as the personnel who perform endotracheal intubation and who are authorized to gain access to the vascular system to administer intravenous medications. They are, of course, not prohibited from cardiac monitoring and defibrillation. In most locations in the USA paramedics comprise the second tier of emergency personnel to arrive, and no third tier exists. In Europe there is often a second or third tier that consists of emergency physicians who respond outside the hospital. These variations are discussed below.

The idea of doctor-staffed ambulances has stimulated considerable discussion. Doctor-staffed ambulances have never been adopted in the USA, and yet in many European countries such ambulances have become the model for the highest quality advanced emergency care. The most obvious explanation lies with the more limited physician resources in the USA. The physician/population ratio is much higher in Europe than in the USA, and consequently more European physicians have been available to provide physician care in the prehospital setting. In the USA emergency medical care outside the hospital has long been a prized and sought-after professional role for non-physicians. This trend was facilitated by the practice, starting in the 1970s, of transferring more and more skills to non-physicians in the prehospital setting. While Europe has possessed a long tradition of sophisticated ambulance services staffed by non-physicians, many European ambulance services restrict defibrillation, drug administration and intubation to physicians in the ambulances.

Another explanation for why the USA lacks physician-staffed ambulances lies with the rapid growth of emergency medicine as a recognized specialty in the USA starting in the late 1970s. Active emergency physicians have created a high level of quality care in US emergency departments. The expectation for prehospital care was to provide immediate stabilization and rapid transport to the emergency department for more definitive care. Not all hospitals in mainland Europe have placed a strong emphasis on the care delivered in their emergency departments. The trend to take physician-based emergency care out to the patients was a natural effort to supplement less than optimal hospital emergency departments, as well as an effort to render physician-provided advanced care as quickly as possible. The differences are simply the setting for providing the physician-based emergency care – at the patient's side in the community or at the patient's side in the emergency department. Examples of these trends are provided in the discussion below.

DESCRIPTION OF SELECTED EMS SYSTEMS SURVEYED IN EUROPE AND THE USA

The following section and Table 1 describe 12 leading EMS systems in Europe and one from the USA. The description uses the headings of the links in the chain of survival (Cummins *et al.*, 1991a), and presents descriptive elements recommended in the Utstein Guidelines (Chamberlain *et al.*, 1991, 1992; Cummins *et al.*, 1991b). Individuals associated with each of these systems graciously responded to a survey questionnaire based on the Utstein Guidelines, as well as numerous conversations and several visits. This discussion provides an overview of the many innovative ways that EMS systems approach the problem of out-of-hospital cardiac arrest, and where these systems have identified opportunities for improvement.

Comments and observations that emerge from this overview

Response intervals

Most EMS systems in this survey use a two-tiered response to cardiac emergencies. Personnel in the first tiers are more numerous, more highly concentrated, with smaller geographic areas to which they must respond. The first tier brings basic CPR, positive pressure ventilation using a pocket face mask or bag–valve mask or an automatic positive pressure ventilator and, in many systems, AEDs. The first tier personnel respond faster

with median call-to-arrival-at-scene-of-the-emergency intervals that are remarkably similar, with a narrow, 4-min range from the most rapid to the slowest:

- 4–5 min (Copenhagen, King County, Paris, Göteborg).
- 5–6 min (Mainz).
- 6–7 min (Antwerp, Brussels, Helsinki, Stavanger).
- 7–8 min (Northumbria, Scotland, Tromsø).

Second tier personnel are more skilled, but less plentiful and therefore fewer in number and location. The second tier personnel by definition and organization of system are going to have longer response times. This leads to the tiered system paradox: systems are organized to give the longest response intervals for the level of care that should by definition have the shortest response intervals. All EMS systems attempt to reduce this problem by the technique of *simultaneous dispatching*, which means both personnel tiers are dispatched at the moment dispatchers suspect the problem of sudden cardiac arrest. In practice, however, while the first tier personnel are dispatched during the call, second tier dispatching may be delayed until further questioning.

The median call-to-arrival-at-scene-of-the-emergency intervals for the second tier are considerably longer than for the first tier:

- <10 min (Scottish Ambulance, Stavanger, Göteborg, Paris SAMU).
- 10–11 min (King County).
- 11–12 min (Antwerp, Brussels, Helsinki, Mainz).
- 12–13 min (Paris Fire Brigade).

Early access: dispatching

All survey EMS systems are aware that delays can occur at all steps in the early access/dispatching tier: from the moment of the collapse to the initial call, and from the initial call to the ambulance moving towards the victim. Each survey system has taken one or more steps to provide remedies.

One concern is caller knowledge of the proper emergency number. In Paris and in Mainz, callers have to know a different number each for medical, police and fire emergencies. Despite the recommendations of the European Resuscitation Council to have a single European medical emergency number there remain a variety of numbers used in Europe, though most numbers were the same throughout a single country as noted in Table 2.

Table 1. *The chain of survival in 13 EMS systems: activities in each link*

Country/city/system	Early access	Early CPR	Early defibrillation	Early ACLS
1. Belgium: Antwerp Uses three tier system: • 1st tier = EMT & EMT-D • 2nd tier = nurse/MD • Special 2nd tier = MUG (medical urgency group in auto) • Mixed EMS fire service	• Number used: 100 • 21 medical emergency calls per 1000 pop'n • Physician role in dispatch process is experimental • No special training or requirements • Enhanced = partly; addresses retrievable	• Dispatcher-CPR = NO • Percent of witnessed arrests with bys-CPR = 33% of witnessed arrests in one study • National CPR training effort	• Early defibrillation = about half of 1st tier defibrillates • 1st tier = 100 h training • Response interval = 7 min urban, 12 min rural	• Simultaneous dispatching • No paramedics • Doctor-staffed vehicles with nurse/doctor/driver • Sometimes uses MUG- (1 nurse/1 doctor/1 driver in automobiles) • Thrombolytics in field
2. Belgium: Brussels Uses two tier system: • 1st tier = EMT • 2nd tier = nurse + MD • Pop'n = 1.1 million • Mixed EMS/fire service	• Number used: 100 • Dispatchers = 5–10 years in ambulance service; 2–3 months training • Enhanced = NO	• Dispatcher-CPR = NO • Percent of witnessed arrests with bys-CPR = unknown • 'Friends of SAMU' programme teaches CPR for high schools and families of high-risk patients	• Early defibrillation = some AED use; no manual • Response interval = 6–7 min • First tier gets 100 h of training	• No paramedics • Doctor-staffed vehicles (called 'MICU') = 1 MD, 1 nurse, 2 EMTs • MDs at night respond from ICUs causing delays • Thrombolytics in field • Response interval = 11:22
3. Denmark: Copenhagen • Pop'n = 1.5 million Uses two tier system • 1st tier = EMT • 2nd tier = EMTs + MD Mixed fire service/EMS	• Number used: 000 • Dispatchers must be EMTs with 6 months training • Enhanced = NO	• Percent of witnessed arrests with bys-CPR = unknown • Dispatcher CPR = YES	• Early defibrillation = NO, but pilot projects some areas • 300 EMTs per 460 000 pop'n (1 EMT per 1500 pop'n) • 3.5 months training • 12 vehicles in service by day and 8 by night • Response interval = 78% of calls < 4 min	• No paramedics • Doctor-staffed vehicles often not available • Usually anaesthesiologists + driver only • 4500 responses; 16 MDs per 460 000 pop'n (1 MD per 29 000 pop'n)
4. England: Northumbria • Pop'n = 1.4 million • EMS-only system • Uses one tier system • 1st tier = EMT-D	• Number used: 999 • 142 000 calls per year • Call receipt to vehicle mobile <3 min 98% of time • Enhanced = NO	• Percent of witnessed arrests with bys-CPR = unknown • Dispatcher CPR = NO • Median response interval = 8 min	• Early defibrillation = YES (AED and manual) • 272 technicians (1 EMT per 5100 pop'n)	• Paramedics (1 per ambulance by 1993–1994) • 44 vehicles 7 a.m.–7 p.m., 28 vehicles 7 p.m.–7 a.m. • 160 paramedics (1 paramedic per 8750 pop'n)

5. Finland: Helsinki
Uses variable three tier system
- 1st tier = EMT
- 2nd tier = EMT-paramedics
- 3rd tier = full-time emergency physician always available

- Number used: 000 (this number often not first one called)
- Little EMD training

- Percent of witnessed arrests with bys-CPR = unknown
- Dispatcher-CPR = SOME
- Requires all CPR trainers to be registered nurses

- Early defibrillation = YES (AED used in all units)
- Median response interval = $6\frac{1}{2}$–7 min
- About 7 ambulances make 29 000 responses per year

- One doctor-staffed vehicle 24 h per day as first ACLS response
- Median response interval = 11–12 min
- Paramedics respond when MDs busy. Happens 1–2 times per day
- Paramedics can give drugs and ETT if no MD

6. France: Paris (Brigade de Sapeurs Pompiers de Paris)
- Pop'n = 6 million
Uses two tier system
- 1st tier = firemen
- 2nd tier = ambulance MDs (some are SAMU physicians)

- Dispatch system has MD present 24 h per day; 150 000 calls
- 1 year training
- Simultaneous dispatching = YES
- Enhanced = NO

- Dispatcher-CPR = YES
- Percent of witnessed arrests with bys-CPR = unknown (rare)
- <5% of pop'n trained in CPR

- Early defibrillation = NO
- 4100 technicians with 160 h training (1 technician per 1500 pop'n)
- 3–5 team members
- 243 vehicles in service; 150 000 calls
- Median response interval = 4–5 min

- Doctor-staffed vehicles with nurse + driver
- Median response interval = 13 min
- Physicians = full-time with fire service
- 250 personnel; 7 vehicles with 9 belonging to SAMU
- 11 000 responses per year

7. France: Paris (SAMU; Service d'Aide Médicale Urgente)
- SAMU provides anaesthesiologists in a doctor-manned ambulance system

- Number used: 15 (medical emergency); 17 (police); 18 (fire)
- 1st dispatcher determines nature of call and priority
- 2nd dispatcher = MD gives precise analysis of call.
- Simultaneous dispatching = YES

- Dispatcher CPR = YES
- Percent of witnessed arrests with bys-CPR = unknown (rare)
- <5% of pop'n CPR-trained
- Unique MD dispatcher system gives more options; e.g. phone advice; home GP visit; simple transport to hospital by regular ambulance; critical cases get SAMU

Early defibrillation = NO
- For ACLS: has 2 year programme for anaesthesiologists or EM MDs to become fully trained as SAMU physicians

- Doctor-staffed vehicles with nurse and 2 personnel; MICU (mobile intensive care unit) for all life-threatening emergencies
- Median response interval = 8 min
- 7 full-time anaesthetists
- 15 part-time MDs
- 10 vehicles per day per 3 000 000 pop'n

(continued)

Table 1—(continued). The chain of survival in 13 EMS systems: activities in each link

Country/city/system	Early access	Early CPR	Early defibrillation	Early ACLS
8. Germany: Mainz Uses variable three tier approach • 1st tier = EMTs • 2nd tier = MD + 2 paramedics ambulance • 3rd tier = 'rendezvous' auto with MD and paramedic	• Number used: 19222 (medical emergency); 110 (police); 112 (fire) • median collapse to call receipt = 4 min • Ambulance dispatch can take 2–3 min especially if wrong number called first	• Dispatcher CPR = YES • Percent of witnessed arrests with bys-CPR = 26% • Rare citizen CPR • Trying to get CPR required before driver's licence • Median collapse to EMS CPR = 7 min	• Early defib programme exists but as pilot study projects in 15–20 cities • 1 EMT per 8000 people • 20000 responses: 22 vehicles • Median response interval = 5 min • Median collapse to defibrillation = 8.9 min	• 2 ACLS approaches: 1 MICU = stationary ALS units based at hospitals with MD and 2 paramedics 2 A 'rendezvous' system with fast car + MD + paramedic to meet MICU at the scene • Median response interval = 9 min • Median collapse to ACLS = 11.3 min
9. USA: King County. WA Uses a two tier approach • 1st tier = EMT-D • 2nd tier = paramedics	• Number used: 911 • Prearrival = YES • Enhanced = YES • Simultaneous = YES • EMD training	• Dispatcher CPR = YES • Percent of witnessed arrests with bystander CPR = 50–60% • CPR offered and taught in most public schools twice in 12 years	• Early defib = YES • Median response interval = 4–6 min	• 9–11 min responses • Paramedics follow strict protocols after extensive (>2000 h) training
10. Norway: Stavanger Uses a variable three tier approach • 1st tier = EMT-D • 2nd tier = paramedics only or with MDs • 3rd tier = doctor-manned ambulance or helicopter • EMS-only system	• Number used: 003 • Prearrival = YES • Enhanced = YES • Simultaneous = YES • EMD training • Nurses are used to provide instructions • MDs on duty for consultation	• Dispatcher-CPR = YES • 5–10% of country's pop'n trained in CPR • CPR training mandated in schools and military service	• Early defib = YES (AED only) • 100 EMTs in 15 vehicles make 13000–14000 responses for 240000 (1 EMT per 2400 pop'n) • Median response time = 5–7 min urban, 7–10 min rural • Of all VF patients more than 95% shocked by 1st tier	• 8 MDs (anaesthesiologists) and 4 paramedics (1 MD per 30000 pop'n) • 2 MD cars, 1 helicopter and 1 ambulance; 1100 responses per year • Response interval < 10 min for 6/9 areas. Rendezvous system used in some areas (car or helicopter + ambulance); 80% of patients reached in 16 min flying

11. Norway: Tromsø

Uses a variable three tier approach

- 1st tier = EMT-D (some locations)
- 2nd tier = paramedics only or with MDs (some locations)
- 3rd tier = doctor-manned ambulance or doctor-manned helicopter

- Number used: 003
- Working on direct access telephone systems linked with radio transmission to ambulances and MD on call in each district (Emergency Medical Communication Centres)

- Dispatcher CPR = YES
- CPR training in schools, and military service
- New communication system will combine with public CPR education
- Targeted CPR training with fishermen and their families in Nordland, Troms, Finnmark, and with district doctors

- Early defib = growing use of AEDs with ambulances
- All PHC (public health care) doctors are equipped with defibrillators
- Ambulance system not fully organized with no widespread standards

- 90% of pop'n served with 1st responder-technicians + ambulance drivers
- No paramedic system in many areas
- No permanent doctor-manned ambulances system yet but hospital-based doctor may staff ambulances in some locations

12. Scotland: Scottish Ambulance Service

Uses single-tiered system

- 1st tier = EMT-D (will add paramedic to every ambulance)

- Number used: 999
- Enhanced and computer-aided under development
- Mean dispatching interval = 1.4min

- Dispatcher CPR = YES
- Citizen CPR = 50% of witnessed arrest (20–30% survival if CPR for witnessed arrest)
- National newspaper and, telephone directory campaigns

- Early defib = YES
- 1347 ambulance technicians serve 5 102 000 pop'n (1 EMT per 3800 pop'n)
- Median response interval = 8 min

- Rare responses with paramedics or doctors
- Recent plans to add paramedic to every ambulance
- Phases = 1 per station; 1 per shift; 1 per ambulance

13. Sweden: Göteborg

Uses two-tiered system

- 1st tier = EMT-D
- 2nd tier = nurses + ambulance personnel

- Number used: 90000
- 10–12 weeks training; 6 months on-job training
- Dispatcher CPR = YES
- 2–3 min call-processing

- Extensive public CPR training and campaigns throughout the country, especially in the Göteborg area
- Unique system where citizen CPR providers mail in card whenever they do CPR. Many successes

- Early defib = YES
- 450 EMTs ('ambulance personnel') in 10 vehicles, make 15 526 responses to 500 000 pop'n (1 EMT per 1200 pop'n).
- Median response interval = 4–5 min

- 2 vehicles with 4 people per shift make 3800 responses to 500 000 pop'n
- Nurses staff ambulance plus 2 ambulance men
- 8–9 min response time

Table 2. *EMS systems survey: early access and dispatching*

Survey EMS system	Number to call for medical emergency	'Enhanced dispatching'	Dispatcher-assisted CPR instructions
Antwerp	100	No	No
Brussels	100	No	No
Copenhagen	000	No	Yes
Helsinki	112	Yes	Some
Göteborg	90 000	No	Yes
Paris	15	No	Yes
Mainz	19 222	No	Yes
King County	911	Yes	Yes
Stavanger	003	Yes	Yes
Tromsø	003	Yes	Yes
Scotland	999	In development	Yes
Northumbria	999	No	No

- Four systems (Helsinki, King County, Stavanger, Tromsø) had what is referred to as 'enhanced emergency telephone 911 systems' (even though the number 911 is only used in the USA). These are sophisticated computer-based systems linked to the telephone system. 'Enhanced dispatching' provides immediate display of the name and address of the owner of the telephone. Most other systems are planning to instal enhanced dispatching. Computerized enhancement of dispatching does, however, have the potential to cause problems.

- All systems acknowledge some failure of dispatchers to identify every cardiac arrest and thus simultaneously dispatch the appropriate second tier. For example, a percentage of all cardiac arrests (5–10% depending on the system) are not identified until *after* the first tier personnel arrives. This represents poorly articulated complaints from often panicked callers, as well as deficiencies in the interrogation skills and protocols followed by the dispatchers. Callers may misidentify a cardiac arrest as a 'collapse', a 'faint', a 'seizure', or use a variety of misleading terms like 'spells', 'unconscious episodes' or 'acting funny'. In addition, agonal respirations in a cardiac arrest victim can confuse both witnesses and dispatchers and lead to failure to recognize that severe cardiac compromise exists (Clark *et al.*, 1992). King County has reported that up to 30% of the calls reporting cardiac arrest also report agonal respirations (Clark *et al.*, 1992), and the Belgium resuscitation database has observed that 17% of all arrest victims had agonal respirations ('were gasping') at the time of arrival of EMS personnel.

These problems with identification of an arrest could be presenting an unidentified problem in many other systems as well.

- Often patients or witnesses call other numbers first. In Mainz, Germany, an analysis of the calling done to report cardiac arrests revealed that calling and dispatching was plagued with inaccurate reporting. The EMS number (19222) was called first only 27% of the time; family medical doctors were called first in 17% of the arrests; police were called 36% of the time; the fire department was called 20% of the time. Sometimes the family physician is at the scene first and calls the emergency system.

- Specific curriculum-based emergency medical dispatch training does not exist other than in Norway (which is the most advanced), England and Scotland (which are just getting started), and King County, Washington. Most survey systems depended largely upon on-the-job training. The background training required to become an emergency dispatcher varied greatly. In King County no specific experience is required. In Paris, the chief dispatchers are required to be physicians, and a doctor must be available immediately to provide telephone consultations 24 h a day. The Paris system is elaborate, with the dispatch physicians frequently providing detailed medical advice, dispatching other levels or ambulances, and even ordering home visits by general physicians. Other locations use registered nurses (Tromsø, Stavanger), or EMTs or ambulancemen (Brussels, Copenhagen, Northumbria)

- All the survey EMS systems are giving serious consideration to installation of dispatcher-assisted emergency prearrival instructions. The systems that are currently providing prearrival instructions are Stavanger, Tromsø, King Country, Scottish Ambulance Service, and Northumbria. Helsinki is beginning to develop prearrival instructions.

Early CPR

EMS systems should examine two variables related to early CPR. The first is to determine whether people with witnessed cardiac arrest who receive bystander CPR have a better outcome than the people who do not receive bystander CPR. Following the recommendations of the Utstein Style the systems in this survey are gathering appropriate data. At least seven Belgian centres and King County, Stavanger, Scottish Ambulance Service and Göteborg have already published related results.

The second variable, and the more telling information, is to determine how often witnesses to a sudden cardiac collapse start basic CPR. This, in essence, should be the most legitimate outcome of citizen-based CPR training. A programme that trains people to know when and how to perform CPR should result in more people actually taking that action when the indications are present. So many other factors, it can be argued, affect ultimate survival that it is probably unfair to ask whether citizen CPR produced more survivors (it does, however, according to most studies). In King County, Washington, the combination of widespread community CPR training plus dispatcher-assisted CPR instructions has produced an annual percentage of 60–70% of bystander-witnessed sudden deaths receiving basic CPR. In Belgium, 13% of the adult population have at some point had CPR training. About half of all cardiac arrests are witnessed; of these, bystanders performed CPR in 33%.

Few of the EMS systems in this survey, other than King County, Scotland, and Mainz, could identify the percentage of witnessed arrests with bystander CPR. None of the systems could identify the percentage of the population trained in CPR, though this figure will always be confused by people 'ever' trained compared to people 'currently' trained and people 'retrained'. Part of the problem is that EMS systems and managers often ignore activities that may increase citizen CPR. The EMS systems in Europe displayed little activity in CPR training with the notable exceptions of Belgium, Norway and Sweden, whose efforts in community CPR training are well known (Bossaert *et al.*, 1989a, b; Holmberg &

Wennerblom, 1984). The reasons most often cited for why the people in various EMS systems seldom attended CPR training or initiated CPR during witnessed arrests include:

- Fear of contracting a disease.
- Fear of malpractice accusations.
- Societal prohibitions against touching a stranger or getting involved.
- A sense that it is really the government's or the emergency system's responsibility.

EMS systems in Europe did, however, display considerable interest in *mandating* a CPR programme in some required manner rather than depending on volunteerism. For example, several European countries have initiated a number of plans where CPR training is required before getting a driver's licence, before high school graduation, or prior to completion of military service. Several of the more intriguing CPR schemes reported are:

- Innovative public education campaigns in Sweden and Belgium involving advertisements on all forms of public transportation, public telephone books, grocery store bags, and bill boards.
- Requirement, in Finland, that only registered nurses can serve as CPR instructors. This is described as a successful quality-control technique.
- A 'CPR by VCR' programme in King County that distributes a videotape of a brief training lesson in basic CPR skills. New, simplified training mannikins are also distributed with the videotape to provide immediate hands-on practice.
- The growing trend, stimulated by new simplified CPR mannikins, towards CPR training with higher instructor/student ratios and longer hands-on mannikin practice time.
- A targeted CPR training programme for fishermen and their families in remote areas of northern Norway.
- School site CPR training classes in Rogaland County, Norway, in which the instructors arrive via air ambulance helicopters near the school yard.
- National newspaper and telephone directory education campaigns conducted by the Scottish Ambulance Service.
- Swedish programme to give everyone who completes CPR training a preaddressed card to mail in if they ever perform CPR. This allows identification and follow-up of people who experienced a cardiopulmonary emergency and then performed lay CPR.

Table 3. *EMS systems survey: first tier defibrillation programmes*

Survey EMS system	First tier defibrillation programme in place
Antwerp	Some pilot projects
Brussels	Some pilot projects
Copenhagen	Some pilot projects
Helsinki	Yes
Göteborg	Yes
Paris	No
Mainz	Some pilot projects
King County	Yes
Stavanger	Yes
Tromsø	In planning
Scotland	Yes
Northumbria	Yes

Early defibrillation

Both the American Heart Association and the European Resuscitation Council have now published guidelines for emergency cardiac care which clearly endorse the principle of early defibrillation. This principle states that the first responding EMS unit should be able to defibrillate. In Scotland this principle first was achieved by mandating, as a national policy, that there should be an AED on every ambulance, and personnel trained to defibrillate (Cobbe *et al.*, 1991). England and Wales are also working actively to implement the same policy.

Elsewhere in Europe innovative leaders in other systems like Stavanger, Helsinki and Göteborg have long ago instituted early defibrillation programmes without controversy and with documented success. Pilot programmes are now underway, thanks to effective leadership in parts of Belgium, Germany and Denmark. In other systems surveyed, such as Paris, considerable interest has not yet been followed with practical implementation. Table 3 displays the current status of first tier defibrillation programmes in the surveyed EMS systems.

Early ACLS

The ACLS link can be provided by the first, second or third tier, depending on the system. Three levels of personnel provide the advanced care – physicians, paramedics, and registered nurses; but many types of vehicles provide transportation – mixed EMT/physician-manned ambulances, paramedic-only ambulances and special doctor-staffed cars and ambulances, as well as helicopters and even motor cycles. King County, for example, always uses specially trained paramedics transported in a special

paramedic-only, second-responding vehicle. In England and Scotland, paramedic-level ambulance staff are placed in each first-responding ambulance. In France, Belgium, Germany and Finland, doctor-staffed ambulances are used as well as specially equipped 'doctor-cars' that follow a rendezvous system. In Sweden, ACLS is provided by specially trained intensive care nurses rather than physicians. The pattern of staffing may change within the same system depending on the time of day and day of week, with less frequent use of doctor-staffed ambulances at night and on weekends.

In fact, staffing patterns are an important question in regard to the ACLS tier. The Utstein Guidelines recommend identification of staff/population ratios. This would be valuable information to use to compare different EMS staffing approaches; for example, physician-staffed ambulances compared to staffing with nurses or paramedics. Even the most superficial review of data supplied by the surveyed EMS systems demonstrates immense variation in the ratio of advanced personnel such as emergency physicians, emergency nurses or paramedics to population. In this survey it became impossible to determine basic service/population ratios for the various tiers of care.

Most EMS systems simply lack these data. For example, what is the optimal vehicle/population ratio? How many ambulances are required to provide proper service to a defined population (e.g. 100 000 people)? What is the population of an urban area where hundreds of thousands of people migrate in and out during a typical working day? Should the determining factor be response intervals rather than service/population ratios? If response intervals were the major way to determine staffing then rural areas would require a much greater personnel/population ratio because of the larger distances to cover. In urban areas greater concentrations of people in a limited geographic area mean response distances are relatively short. Problems of actually locating and getting to patients in urban areas, however, can be considerable. Busy EMS units will often find themselves engaged in the care of one patient when yet another emergency occurs.

Another feature that makes accurate staffing patterns difficult to determine is that almost all surveyed systems vary their staffing patterns according to the hour of the day and the day of the week. For example, in many surveyed systems the hours 7 a.m. to 6 p.m. on weekdays will find physician-manned ambulances available. On weekends and nights, however, there is much more frequent use of paramedics and EMTs who have received additional training. The demanding solution in King

County of two-paramedic-staffed ambulances 24 h a day, 7 days a week is just not practical in many European systems (and even in many US systems). Physicians may be located specifically in emergency departments during the weekdays in some locations, but at night the ambulance physicians may have to respond from hospital intensive care units, and even from operating rooms. A few of the surveyed systems revealed that despite a goal of always providing a physician-staffed ACLS response there were times during the night and on weekends when physicians just were not available on the ambulances. How frequently this problem occurs is unknown; the situation does not apply to all systems included in this survey.

Some additional observations about the ACLS response in this survey:

- Almost all non-physician-staffed systems use standing-order protocols for the first stages in resuscitation. No system required radio contact permission to initiate therapy for cardiac arrest patients, though they did need to make contact to continue or discontinue further efforts.
- Historically, physician-manned ambulances were advocated to fulfil the mandate that 'the doctor has to come to the wounded, not the wounded to the doctor'. Though this reflected a worthy goal, there was little objective evidence provided to support physician-staffed ambulances over paramedic-staffed ambulances with rapid transport to well-equipped and well-staffed emergency departments.
- One value of physician-manned units is the elimination of the need to transport every patient with ongoing CPR. Ambulance doctors could cease resuscitation efforts in the field and eliminate the need to conduct futile transportation with continuing CPR. In most systems, for example Scotland and Northumbria, the absence of physicians in the prehospital setting necessitated transport of all cardiac arrest patients to hospital, a well-documented futile and expensive approach.
- All the systems that use ambulances manned by physicians, especially anaesthesiologists and emergency physicians, point out the value of general anaesthesia administered in the field. Anaesthesiologists and emergency physicians working in field ambulances can often identify those patients with severe trauma who will need exploratory surgery for definitive diagnosis and treatment. These physicians can initiate intubation and even administer general anaesthesia; they can obtain appropriate central vein access, and can diminish markedly the time from original injury to operating room treatment.

- An additional argument put forward for doctor-staffed ambulances is the superior diagnostic and decision-making skills of the physicians, compared to the superb technical skills, but often limited diagnostic skills, of EMTs and paramedics.
- A major consideration with regard to ambulance staffing became apparent during this survey: the quality of the receiving hospitals and emergency departments. It can be argued that doctor-manned ambulances are a comment on the quality of care provided in A&E departments. In many locations in Europe the quality of staffing and care in local hospitals and emergency departments has been highly suspect, sometimes non-existent. Emergency medicine, as a specialty, is not yet widespread in Europe, and emergency-trained physicians, other than in the UK, are rare. Since emergency patients are not being met by specially trained physicians in many emergency departments, why not solve the problem by sending emergency physicians out in the ambulance? This rationale was directly responsible for the development of the SAMU system in France, and it applies to many other European areas as well. In contrast, emergency medicine, as a specialty, has been a strong force in the USA, such that the receiving hospitals for prehospital emergencies are staffed 24 h a day with well-trained emergency specialists. These physicians are so readily available at the receiving hospitals that they see no advantages (and many disadvantages!) to leaving the hospitals and delivering care in prehospital settings. This situation is rapidly changing in Europe with much growth in the number of physicians trained in emergency medicine as well as increases in the number of emergency physicians trained in other specialties (surgery, anaesthesiology, internal medicine).
- Doctor-manned ambulances can perform hyperventilation for head-injured patients, start antibiotics for patients with meningococcal sepsis (Norway), and administer a variety of other medications and procedures not available in paramedic-based systems.
- Several locations use a 'rendezvous' system in which a specially equipped automobile takes physicians to the scene to meet with the ambulance team. (In Norway, the rendezvous vehicle may actually be a helicopter.) This brings a high skill level of ACLS to the scene, but their arrival can be delayed if the physician has to be picked up at a hospital where the physician may normally be working in the emergency department or critical care unit.
- The air ambulance system in Norway (Stavanger and

Tromsø) represents a unique approach to a challenging geography in which land travel to many areas is indirect and difficult or even impossible. This also demonstrates a powerful sense of responsibility where cost concerns take second place to an attitude that all citizens deserve the best level of emergency care. The interval from scramble to lift-off is 3–5 min in the bases where helicopter and crew are located together.

- A number of locations still use general practitioners (Kupio region in Finland, Grampian region in Scotland) to answer emergency calls. This is understandable from the standpoint that patients are used to calling their general practitioner for their problems. This practice, however, affects treatment times, and is not the best approach for cardiopulmonary emergencies unless the general practitioners, equipped with defibrillators, can consistently arrive before the ambulances (Colquhoun, 1988).

CONCLUSIONS AND RECOMMENDATIONS

Our survey of representative EMS systems in Europe and the USA reveals the rich variety of approaches used to address the modern epidemic of sudden cardiac death. There is no such thing as 'the best' EMS organization. Local practices, conditions, resources and even traditions have combined in every location to shape a system's organization. Nevertheless, there are always opportunities for improvement. Every system regularly must ask the question, how can we improve? How can we provide better care for the people we serve? The critical acts are to ask these questions and to be interested in improvement. The Utstein Guidelines and this survey of EMS systems provide several observations that can help in these quality improvement examinations.

1. The Utstein Uniform Guidelines on reporting of data from out-of-hospital cardiac arrest will help many EMS systems to develop and improve their programmes. A new community-wide CPR programme or a new early defibrillation programme must be carefully inserted as one of the links in the EMS continuum. Some systems, however, find it difficult to plan for reorganization or the addition of new components because they lack information on the incremental value of these additional programmes. Communities that hope to develop a reasonably effective approach will be able to review the published materials on system organization with confidence. EMS systems can avoid duplication of unnecessary activities and repetition of avoidable errors.

They can learn quickly, given their local resources, which of several EMS approaches will be most effective. The Utstein Guidelines should support the performance of intra- and intersystem evaluations: *intrasystem* evaluations would support local quality improvement programmes; *intersystem* comparisons would help identify the relative benefits of different system approaches.

2. The generally accepted and widely endorsed 'chain of survival' concept has expanded the complexity of our thinking about the organization of EMS systems (Eisenberg *et al.*, 1990b). This concept has led people to alter traditional views about the management of pre-hospital cardiac arrest in the following ways:

- Witnesses to the cardiac emergency initiate the entire EMS system response. No level of training, equipment or staffing will succeed if lay people fail to recognize the signs and symptoms of a cardiac emergency, fail to decide to take action, or fail to take the right action.
- Witnesses to the cardiac emergency learn to recognize the emergencies and to take appropriate action primarily from citizen CPR training. EMS systems must, therefore, place much greater emphasis on citizen CPR training, not just to increase the chances that someone will perform CPR, but also to increase the chances that the emergency will be recognized and the system will be activated in a timely fashion. These goals will require, in most locations, a change in the way CPR is taught. There should be less emphasis on the theory of the technique, more hands-on practice time, and more emphasis on the proper overall response. Both the American Heart Association and the European Resuscitation Council are moving in these directions.
- Dispatching – part of the early access link – merits much closer attention in almost every EMS system. This includes the performance of the telephone system, the training of the dispatchers, the protocols they follow, the ability to perform simultaneous dispatching, the implementation of enhanced communication and the provision of dispatcher-assisted CPR. Complicated call-routing, prolonged caller interrogation, or failure to permit decision-making by the initial dispatcher are problems that consume long periods of time. Inefficiencies in the dispatching/access link can destroy the benefit of citizen CPR training, early defibrillation programmes and expensive paramedic/physician training.
- The quality of citizen CPR training should be evaluated by asking how often do witnesses of a cardiac arrest start CPR. Has a community supported enough citizen CPR training to ensure that most witnessed cardiac

arrests will be seen by someone who has learned how to do CPR? Was the nature of that training such that the witness will start CPR attempts and feel capable of making a difference?

- Early defibrillation—with the emphasis on early—must be recognized as the most important intervention in resuscitation. Certainly intubation and intravenous medications contribute to some resuscitations, and undoubtedly some people who are not in VF are resuscitated successfully. But the majority of successful resuscitations, more than 80% in most EMS systems, are people in VF who were defibrillated early. *This is the single most important step for EMS systems to take to improve survival.* The first responding EMS personnel in every EMS system must be allowed to defibrillate. Success in these programmes depends on effective training and continuing professional education. Remaining legislative or regulatory barriers to the use of defibrillators by non-physicians must be removed. Scarce resources should be allocated to purchase defibrillators above other equipment. Systems with paramedic-staffed or physician-staffed ambulances must abandon any opposition they have towards AEDs used by first tier personnel. Several studies have documented the superiority of AEDs to conventional defibrillators when used by non-physicians and non-paramedics. Preferences for conventional defibrillators over automated defibrillators represent matters of personal taste rather than technical superiority.
- ACLS, in relation to sudden cardiac death, comprises endotracheal intubation and intravenous medications. Who delivers these interventions, like who delivers defibrillation, is less important than performing these interventions early. The advantages (and disadvantages) of doctor-staffed ambulances and paramedic-staffed ambulances can be debated endlessly. The debate, however, must never lose sight of the principle of *early* defibrillation, *early* intubation and *early* medication. How a system is organized in terms of personnel is less important than how it is organized to assure that these interventions occur early.

APPENDIX: The Utstein Consensus Conferences

In two meetings, June and December 1990, representatives from the American Heart Association, the European Resuscitation Council, the Heart and Stroke Foundation of Canada, and the Australian Resuscitation Council met to establish uniform terms and definitions for out-of-

hospital resuscitation. Members of all these organizations attended an International Resuscitation Meeting at the historic Utstein Abbey, on a small island off Stavanger, Norway (Cummins & Chamberlain, 1991). Participants discussed the widespread nomenclature problem and the lack of standardized language in reports. The recommendations of the Utstein Conference have been widely disseminated in Europe (Chamberlain *et al.*, 1991a–d, 1992a, b) and in the USA (Cummins *et al.*, 1991b, c). A number of articles have appeared commenting on the Utstein style, endorsing it, or making recommendations for revisions (Gallehr & Vukov, 1993; Allen, 1991; Jastremski, 1993; Valenzuela *et al.*, 1992, 1993; Swanson, 1991; Cummins, 1993a, b).

The Utstein Conference presented:

1. A glossary of terms.
2. A reporting template for resuscitation studies that will ensure comparability.
3. Definitions for time points and time intervals related to cardiac resuscitation.
4. A listing and definitions of individual clinical items and outcomes that systems should gather.
5. Recommendations for the description of emergency medical resuscitation systems.

The Ulstein glossary of terms

Cardiac arrest Cardiac arrest is the cessation of cardiac mechanical activity, confirmed by the absence of a detectable pulse, by unresponsiveness, and by apnoea (or agonal, gasping respirations) (Cobb *et al.*, 1980; Greene *et al.*, 1989; Goldstein, 1982; Greene, 1990). For the purposes of the Utstein style no comment on time or 'suddenness' is recommended (Greene *et al.*, 1989; Greene, 1990). Previous definitions of 'suddenness' have ranged from death within less than a minute of symptoms to death within 24 h of symptoms.

Bystander CPR, Lay responder CPR, Citizen CPR These are synonymous terms; the Consensus Conference prefers 'bystander CPR'. Bystander CPR is any attempt to perform basic CPR by someone who is NOT part of an organized response system. In general this will be the person who witnessed the arrest. In certain situations, therefore, physicians, nurses and paramedics may perform 'bystander', or, more properly, 'professional first responders', CPR.

Emergency personnel Emergency personnel are individuals who respond to a medical emergency in an official capacity as part of an organized response team. By this definition, physicians, nurses or paramedics who witness a cardiac arrest in a public setting and initiate CPR, but who have *not* responded to the event as part of an organized team, are *not* 'emergency personnel'.

Cardiopulmonary resuscitation ('CPR') Cardiopulmonary resuscitation ('CPR') is a broad term meaning the *act of attempting* to achieve restoration of spontaneous circulation. CPR is an action; it can be either successful, or unsuccessful, *basic* or *advanced* (see below).

Basic CPR Basic CPR is the act of attempting to restore an effective circulation using *external* compressions of the chest wall, plus *expired* air inflation of the lungs. Rescuers can provide the ventilation through airway adjuncts and barrier devices (face shields, etc.) appropriate for use by the lay public. This definition excludes the bag–valve–mask, invasive techniques of airway maintenance such as intubation of the airway, and any airway devices that pass the pharynx.

Basic cardiac life support This term, especially in the USA, has an expanded meaning beyond the term 'basic CPR'. It includes an entire educational programme that provides information about access to the EMS system and recognition of a cardiac arrest, as well as basic CPR (Cummins & Eisenberg, 1985).

Advanced CPR, also known as advanced cardiac life support or ACLS (Bocka, 1989; Bossaert *et al.*, 1992). These terms refer to the act of attempting to restore spontaneous circulation by using basic CPR *plus* advanced airway management and ventilation techniques, defibrillation, and intravenous or endotracheal medications. There are several possible intermediate levels of care defined by the number and types of interventions provided. The Consensus Conference participants saw little value in providing specific titles for this entire list of possibilities. Instead they recommend specific descriptions of the interventions that are permitted.

Cardiac aetiology (presumed) It is impractical for researchers to determine accurately the specific cause of cardiac arrest for all attempted resuscitations. The biological model of sudden cardiac death, which is receiving growing acceptance, places little value in attempts to discriminate between thrombotic and electrophysiological cardiac arrest (Myerburg, 1986; Myerburg *et al.*, 1989). In this model, multiple functional factors may interact with a host of underlying structural abnormalities to initiate lethal arrhythmias. For the purposes of the Utstein Reporting Template, observers should classify cardiac arrests as presumed cardiac aetiology if this is likely on the basis of all available information. In the best of circumstances, this can include autopsy data

and hospital records. Frequently, however, this becomes a diagnosis of exclusion. Consequently, included in this category are the patients who do not fit in the more readily defined category of *cardiac arrest of non-cardiac aetiology*.

Non-cardiac aetiology While this is a disparate collection of causes, they are often obvious and easy to determine. Specific subcategories include sudden infant death syndrome, drug overdose, suicide, drowning, hypoxia, exsanguination, cerebrovascular accident, subarachnoid haemorrhage, and trauma. When necessary for specific purposes (for example, a study of drowning) separate categories can be identified.

Call–response interval This term should replace 'response time', one of the most frequently, and yet inconsistently, used terms in resuscitation. Call–response interval is the period from receipt of call by the emergency response dispatchers to the moment when the emergency response vehicle stops moving (see Figs A2 and A3). Note that this interval does *not* begin when the emergency response vehicle begins to move. Call–response interval should include the time required for processing the call, dispatching the emergency personnel, personnel movement from quarters to emergency vehicle, getting the vehicle in motion, and the interval required for travel to the scene. Note that this interval does not extend to arrival at the patient's side nor to the time of defibrillation. Recent data demonstrate that the additional intervals from when the vehicle stops to arrival at the patient's side and to delivery of first defibrillatory shock may be excessively long, and may play a major role in determining survival (Becker *et al.*, 1991; Campbell *et al.*, 1992).

Automated external defibrillators (AEDs) Automated external defibrillator is a generic term that refers to defibrillators that perform some degree of rhythm analysis of the patient's surface electrocardiogram (ECG). This rhythm analysis is dichotomous – either ventricular fibrillation/ventricular tachycardia or non-ventricular fibrillation. AEDs provide information to the operator whenever the device detects VF or ventricular tachycardia. This information provided to the operator is usually dichotomous as well – either 'shock' or 'no shock indicated'.

Times versus intervals Imprecision and inconsistency in the use of *times* and *intervals* has produced much confusion and misunderstanding in publications about cardiac arrest. A precise distinction between 'time' and 'interval' has been one of the major contributions of the Utstein Style. The word 'interval', not 'time', refers to the period between two events. The definition of the interval should be clear from the expression used, and not be dependent on EMS jargon. The format for expression of intervals should be *event-(to)-event interval*, with an explicit statement of the two anchor events. For example, authors of various publications have used *downtime* to refer to either the *collapse-to-start of CPR* interval, the *collapse-to-first defibrillatory shock* interval, or the *collapse-to-return of spontaneous circulation* interval. As another example, numerous authors have used *time-to-definitive care* to establish the importance of short intervals between collapse and interventions. In practice, however, this term has meant only the arrival at the scene of advanced life support personnel with the capability to deliver *definitive care*. The true times of delivery (and the related intervals) for the specific elements of definitive care (defibrillatory shocks, intubation, vasoactive medications) remain unknown in most published studies.

The Utstein Template for reporting cardiac arrest data

The template approach

The Utstein style recommends a template approach to reporting data, especially outcome data, relating to cardiac arrest. Fig. A1 presents the Utstein Style Template for data collection on cardiac arrest. The template requires that a specific number be inserted for each level. These numbers permit calculation of multiple rates, because the number at each level serves two functions: the denominator for the levels above, and the numerator for all levels below.

The template begins with the population served by the EMS system and displays how various exit points occur before arrival at the *cardiac aetiology* patients. Use of this scheme by an EMS system will permit immediate comparisons with all other systems that have used the template and have published or distributed their results.

The shaded exit points to the left have no further divisions displayed below them. Nevertheless, all downstream subsets remain possible. The template does not display all outcomes that are possible even though collection of the recommended individual clinical data would permit detailed analyses and presentations.

The issue of outcomes

Evaluators can calculate a large variety of outcomes from the reporting template because multiple combinations of denominators and numerators are possible. Reports should present outcomes as rates or percentages. An example would be the rate of successful admissions per total resuscitations attempted. The *best* outcome to report may be different for different systems and locations. Most authors recommend reporting number discharged alive divided by number of people with witnessed cardiac arrest, in VF, of cardiac aetiology (Eisenberg *et al.*, 1990a, b; Cummins *et al.*, 1991b; Cummins, 1993a, b; Becker & Pepe, 1993; Becker *et al.*, 1993). This single rate would be most practical for intersystem comparisons, and was recommended for use by the Utstein Task Force. This rate, while a *core* piece of information, reports only a small proportion of the total activities of a system, and thus fails to capture the full complexity of EMS resuscitation activities.

Utstein Template Sections

1. *Population served.* The starting point in the template is the population served. This permits calculation of population-based incidence, as well as population-based survival rates. The total population of a community is a useful figure *only* when the entire population resides within the specific service area of the EMS system. Daily movement of large numbers of people between residential areas and commercial areas present severe complexities to an accurate estimation of the 'population served' especially in urban/suburban areas. The methodology section of any manuscript or report on cardiac arrest outcomes should include some description of the community served. The core data recommended for out-of-hospital cardiac arrests are: total population served by the EMS system, geographic area served (in square kilometres), and the percentage of the population over age 65 years. The supplementary data should include special problems or unique circumstances within a community. For example, authors should describe the presence of many high-rise residential buildings, multiple languages, unusual geography or climate, narrow roads, and unique traffic regulations or other conditions (Becker *et al.*, 1991).

2. *Confirmed cardiac arrests considered for resuscitation.* These include *all* unresponsive, breathless and pulseless patients for whom the emergency personnel are called. The emergency personnel must confirm the cardiac arrests. Notation should also be made of the number of patients in whom resuscitation was attempted by lay rescuers (either ventilation attempts,

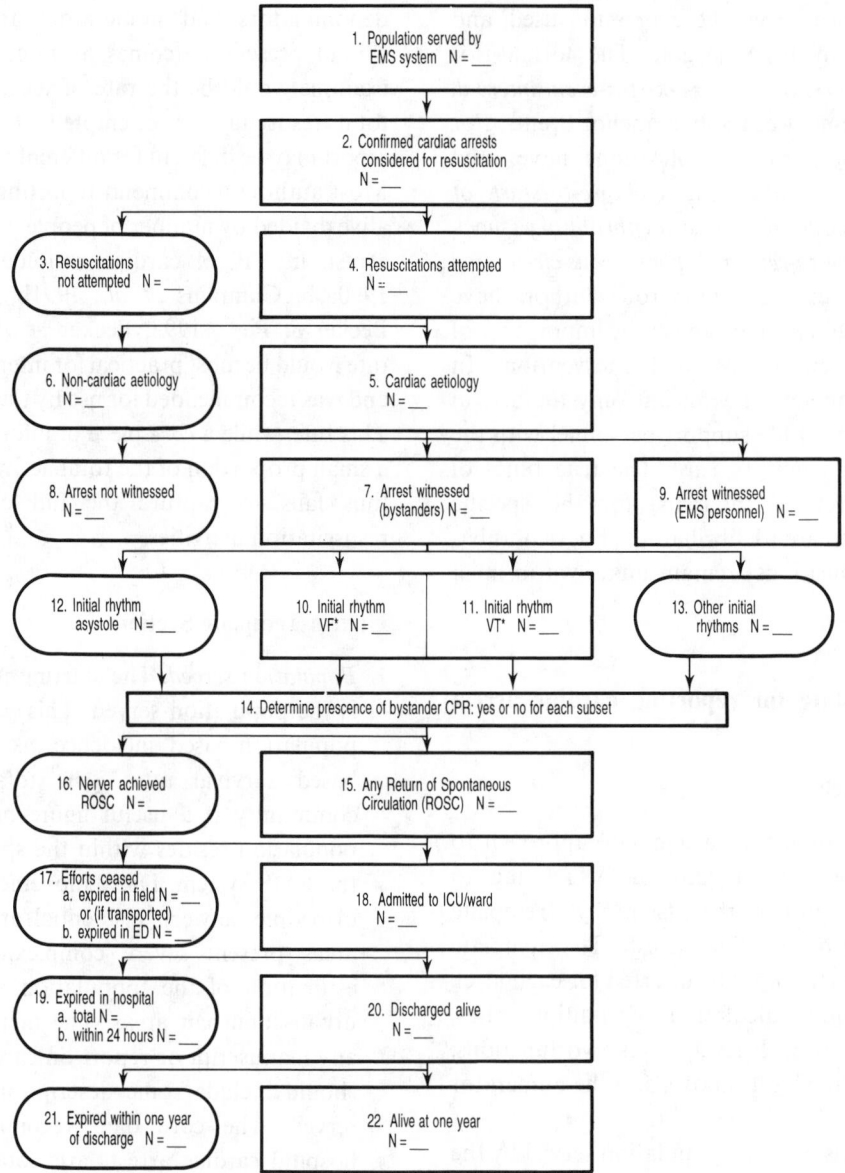

* VF and VT should be reported separately through template

Fig. A1. Recommended Utstein Style Template for reporting data on cardiac arrest. (Reproduced with permission. Cummins, R., Chamberlain, D., Abramson, N. *et al.* (1991). Recommended guidelines for uniform reporting of data from out-of-hospital cardiac arrest: the Utstein Style. *Circulation*, **84**, 960–75. Copyright 1991 American Heart Association.)

chest compressions or both) but whom the emergency personnel observe to have a pulse upon arrival. This additional subgroup permits an assessment of possible lay person 'saves', but may include 'false positive cardiac arrests' and 'respiratory arrests'. Reports should tabulate this group separately, and not in the total of confirmed cardiac arrests considered for resuscitation.

3. *Resuscitations not attempted.* Resuscitation attempts for some patients in cardiac arrest are inappropriate

and should not be initiated. Reports should state the local criteria for such patients. In most locations these individuals have obvious evidence of irreversible death such as decapitation, incineration, decomposition, rigor mortis, or dependent livido. This group also includes people with 'do not resuscitate orders' (DNR), or living wills, provided that no resuscitation efforts were made.

4. *Resuscitations attempted by emergency personnel.* This group includes all people for whom any emergency

system personnel made attempts at resuscitation (other than basic assessment). A resuscitation attempt means at least some effort at basic CPR. This definition mandates that this section of the template will contain people who have DNR status or living wills, or for whom more senior attendants halt resuscitation efforts upon their arrival. With its goal of precision and standardization, the Utstein Style recognizes that overall success rates will be lowered slightly by having the denominator include people who have no possibility of success.

5. *Cardiac aetiology* (see Glossary). Emergency personnel should determine the presence and duration of antecedent signs and symptoms of ischaemia. This would permit some discussion of the 'suddenness' of the cardiac arrest and some consideration of mechanisms of arrest such as primary electrical events in contrast to ischaemic or thrombotic events. The boundaries between these groups, however, are often blurred both clinically and physiologically, and are not *required* for reported cardiac arrest data.

6. *Non-cardiac aetiology* (see Glossary). The template shows 'non-cardiac aetiology' as an exit event. The Consensus Conference strongly recommended, however, that additional detailed data be acquired about this group. This would permit recording and reporting all features of the template listed below *cardiac aetiology* (e.d., witnessed, rhythms, outcomes).

7. *Witnessed* and 8. *Unwitnessed arrests.* The recommended focus of the Utstein Template is arrests that are witnessed. These are arrests in which a bystander or emergency personnel or both saw or heard the patient collapse. The Utstein Template displays unwitnessed arrests, as well as arrests of non-cardiac aetiology, as 'exit' categories. Supplementary recording and reporting, however, includes rhythm identification, presence of bystander CPR, and clinical outcomes for the unwitnessed arrests.

9. *Arrests after arrival of emergency personnel.* Most reports of cardiac arrest observe that approximately 10% of out-of-hospital cardiac arrests occur after the arrival of emergency personnel (Becker *et al.*, 1991; Iseri *et al.*, 1977; Eisenberg *et al.*, 1986b; Roth *et al.*, 1984). The Utstein Style recommends that these arrests after arrival patients be separated from the unwitnessed arrests, and from the bystander witnessed arrests (see Fig. A1). There are two reasons for this separation. First, the presence or absence of bystander CPR and the length of the call–response intervals do not apply to these patients. To include these patients would distort tabulation of the percentage of patients who receive bystander CPR and measurement of the call–response interval. Second, the arrests after arrival subgroup contains important information that should be analysed and reported separately. For example, some researchers have suggested that survival rates for this subgroup are the best current outcome measures to judge the performances of ACLS personnel (Becker *et al.*, 1991; Eisenberg *et al.*, 1986b). This is because time delays are not a factor in their resuscitation effort. Others suggest that the underlying pathophysiology of this group is different from those persons with sudden unexpected collapse (Eisenberg *et al.*, 1986b). Arrests after arrival patients have developed pain and symptoms that led them to call for emergency help, thus suggesting a thrombotic event. The patient with sudden collapse, in contrast, may have experienced an electrical dysrhythmic arrest. The biological model of sudden cardiac death, however, would suggest that both mechanisms are operative (Myerburg *et al.*, 1989). Additional description of the arrest after arrival group should include rhythm identification, the time intervals indicated in Fig. A3, and the clinical outcomes indicated in the lower portions of the Utstein Template.

10. *Ventricular fibrillation* (VF) and 12. *Asystole.* Subdivisions of VF, such as fine, moderate or coarse are of limited clinical usefulness (Hargarten *et al.*, 1990; Weaver *et al.*, 1985). A specific distinction, however, between fine VF and asystole, while clinically and physiologically indeterminate, should be made for the purposes of uniform reporting (Weaver *et al.*, 1985; Cummins *et al.*, 1988). The Utstein Style recommends a specific discrimination point between asystole and fine VF: a deflection on the surface electrocardiogram of less than 1 mm amplitude (calibrated at $10 \, \text{mm} \, \text{mV}^{-1}$) is asystole; 1 mm or greater is VF (Cummins *et al.*, 1991). Automated external defibrillators already use this criterion (Cummins, 1989).

11. *Ventricular tachycardia* (VT). Because it has a different outcome spectrum, the Utstein Style recommends that pulseless VT not be grouped with VF but should have a separate template pathway. These patients are, however, such a small proportion of the out-of-hospital cardiac arrests that they are often combined with the much larger number of VF patients.

13. *Other rhythms.* This category includes the rhythms

in which some electrical activity is observed in a patient in cardiac arrest. The activity usually appears as ventricular escape complexes that probably represent the last electrical activity of a dying heart. For people in confirmed cardiac arrest, there is little to be gained by detailed refinement of this category. 'Electromechanical dissociation', a poorly defined term that is undergoing redefinition (Bocka, 1989; Berryman, 1986), should, at this time, be grouped with 'other rhythms'. The American Heart Association now uses the term 'pulseless electrical activity' to encompass idioventricular rhythms, bradyasystolic rhythms, pseudoelectromechanical dissociation, as well as electromechanical dissociation (Emergency Cardiac Care Committee, 1992b).

14. *Determine presence of bystander CPR.* This allows calculation of the percentage of cardiac arrests in which bystanders have initiated CPR. A high percentage of early bystander-initiated CPR effort is associated with improved survival from cardiac arrest (Cobb & Hallstrom, 1982; Cobb et al., 1980, 1990; Cummins & Eisenberg, 1985; Cummins et al., 1985; 1991a). These data also assess other aspects of an EMS system's 'chain of survival' and are important information to gather for programme evaluation (Cummins et al., 1991a). Note that the way the template is arranged allows multiple analyses to occur. For example, researchers can determine the survival outcomes for those people in witnessed VF who received early bystander CPR compared to those who received only late CPR from the emergency personnel.

15. *Return of spontaneous circulation (ROSC).* The Utstein Template accepts return of any spontaneous palpable pulse. The template requires no specific 'duration' of a pulse; for example, 'more than 5 min'. A 'palpable pulse' would be one detectable by manual palpation of a major artery, usually the carotid. This pulse implies a systolic blood pressure of approximately 60 mmHg. ROSC is clearly an intermediate outcome which may be evanescent. While ROSC is of less clinical importance than hospital admission or eventual discharge, it may prove useful in clinical trials and other intervention studies. Reports should note the number of patients who 16. *never achieve ROSC.*

17. *Efforts ceased:* a. *died in the field, or* (*if transported*) b. *died in the ED* (emergency department). Multiple studies have confirmed the futility of transporting cardiac arrest patients who have never achieved ROSC

to emergency departments (Bonnin & Swor, 1989; Bonnin et al., 1993; Kellermann, 1993; Kellermann et al., 1988, 1993). Successful outcomes for these patients are rare. Nevertheless, a number of systems, especially in the USA, require emergency personnel to transport victims with unsuccessful field resuscitations to the emergency department. The reporting template allows these patients to be recorded, and will permit assessment of their outcomes. The template also allows notation of the patients for whom emergency personnel terminate resuscitation efforts in the field without hospital transport. This practice is slowly spreading throughout the USA and is endorsed in the Guidelines of the American Heart Association (American College of Emergency Physicians, 1988; Aprahamian et al., 1986; Emergency Cardiac Care Committee, 1992a).

18. *Admit to intensive care unit or other hospital unit.* This level of the template refers to patients who had ROSC sustained long enough to merit admission to the intensive care unit or another hospital unit. For the purposes of standardization, the Utstein Style defines a successful hospital admission as a patient who is admitted to the hospital with spontaneous circulation, and a measurable blood pressure, with or without vasopressors. Patients may or may not be breathing spontaneously, and they may or may not be intubated. The need for continuing CPR or mechanical CPR devices implies the absence of spontaneous circulation and such patients should be excluded. Artificial circulatory assists, such as emergency cardiopulmonary bypass and intra-aortic balloon pumps, imply spontaneous circulation is present, and such patients should be included. The recommendations place no duration requirement on 'successful admission'.

19. a. *Died in hospital,* b. *died in first 24 hours.* Researchers should tabulate the number of people who die in the hospital. Special notation should be made of those patients who die within the first 24 h of admission. Patients who experience additional cardiac arrests *during the index hospitalization* are counted as a single person in the data analysis, whether or not they are successfully resuscitated.

20. *Discharged alive.* Reports should note the number of patients discharged from the hospital alive, and the discharge destination: home, prearrest residence, rehabilitation facility, extended care facility (nursing home) or other duration of hospitalization should be recorded. If possible and practical, researchers

should record the 'best-ever achieved' cerebral performance category (CPC) and overall performance category (OPC). If 'best-ever achieved' presents collection difficulties, researchers should note the OPC and CPC at the time of discharge.

21. *Death within 1 year after discharge.* As core data, record the date and cause if death occurs in the first year after discharge. This allows calculation of length of survival. Record the OPC and CPC near the time of death. As supplementary data, record the best OPC and CPC *ever achieved* between discharge and death, though as noted above this may be difficult to determine.

22. *Alive at 1 year.* For those patients who survive for more than 1 year, note the OPC and CPC near the 1-year mark. As supplementary data, optimally, record the best OPC and CPC ever achieved in that year. The recommendation for people who experience additional *out-of-hospital* cardiac arrests during their first year of survival is to treat each cardiac arrest and resuscitation attempt as separate events (Eisenberg *et al.*, 1982). Thus a second cardiac arrest in the year after the index cardiac arrest marks the end of survival for the index event, and counts as a 'death' regardless of whether the person survived or not. If emergency personnel attempted to resuscitate this person in the later events, the template would count that person as an additional 'resuscitation attempted'. If they lived to hospital discharge again, they would continue to be counted as a completely separate person.

Utstein time points and time intervals

Treatment delays are one of the most critical issues in prehospital emergency care. This is particularly true in cardiopulmonary emergencies because only a few minutes can make the difference between a good neurological outcome and severe deficits and even death. Delay until treatment determines the immediate, intermediate and overall outcomes in cardiac arrest (Cummins *et al.*, 1991a). The most powerful determinants of restoration of a beating heart are time intervals; specifically, the time interval from collapse to initiation of resuscitative efforts. Concomitantly, this interval is the major determinant of ultimate survival (Mullie *et al.*, 1989; Delooz & Lewi, 1989; Cerebral Resuscitation Group, 1989). Research about cardiac arrest and all evaluations of system performance depend on accurate

determination of when specific events occurred and the time intervals between these events.

Systematic recording of event times should be an integral part of cardiac arrest management, delegated to a recognized member of the team. As such it should figure prominently in training and testing of personnel. Citizens in CPR classes should be encouraged to memorize when witnessed arrests occurred and when they started basic CPR. Researchers should aspire to as much precision as possible in recording time events, and should explore new technologies and methods that will increase accuracy (Bradley, 1993; Bock, 1993; Ornato, 1993a) Improved data collection, however, must not interfere with care or impose non-clinical activities on field personnel (Spaite *et al.*, 1990).

Fig. A2 displays the complexity associated with recording time intervals of cardiac arrest. Instead of one, there are four different clocks running once a cardiac arrest occurs and the EMS response begins. First, there is the *patient clock*, which begins with the collapse and runs until effective circulation and respirations are restored. Second, there is the *clock of the dispatch centre*. This clock begins with the receipt of the emergency call that reports the collapse, and ends after prearrival instructions, especially telephone-assisted CPR instructions, are delivered to the caller. Third, is the *clock of the ambulance* and the emergency response personnel. This clock begins to run when the response vehicle starts to move, and ends when the patient arrives at the hospital. Fourth, is the *hospital clock*, which begins with patient's arrival at the emergency department and ends when the patient is discharged from the hospital, or dies during hospitalization.

Fig. A3 depicts the major events associated with resuscitation attempts after cardiac arrest. These are the recommended time events that an emergency system should record. Each of these events occurs at a single moment. The period between two time events is the 'event-to-event' interval. Researchers should always use the term 'interval' and not 'time' to refer to the time that passes between any two events (see Glossary). The label for the interval should state the two anchor events. Reports should avoid neologisms, jargon and non-specific terms that mistakenly use 'time' instead of 'interval'. Examples of these include 'downtime' or 'response time' or 'time to definitive care'. A 'stacked index card' design in Fig. A3 conveys that these events can be shuffled about, with events occurring in different sequences with different patients. In addition, there can

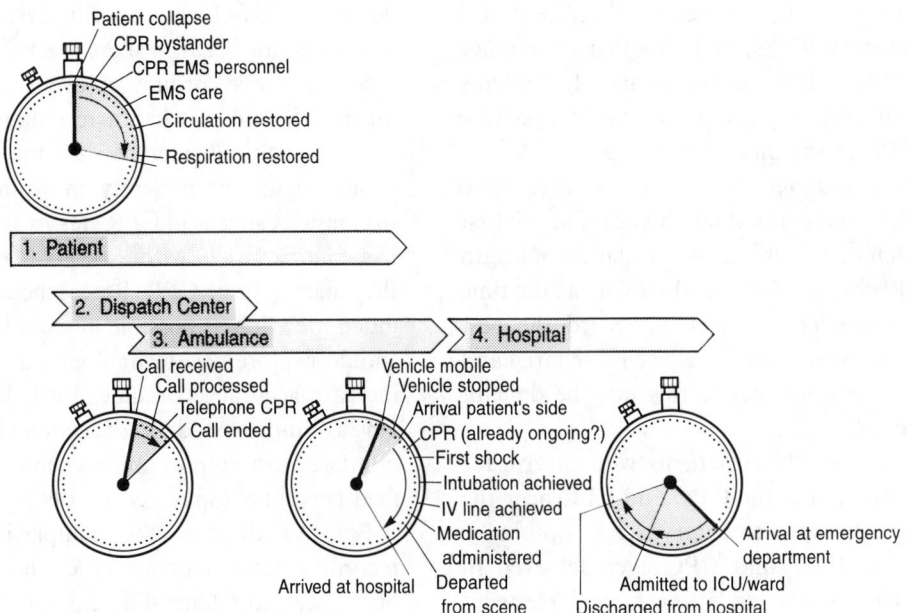

Fig. A2. The four clocks of sudden cardiac arrest. (Reproduced with permission. Cummins, R., Chamberlain, D., Abramson, N. *et al.*, (1991). Recommended guidelines for uniform reporting of data from out-of-hospital cardiac arrest: the Utstein Style. *Circulation*, **84**, 960–75. Copyright 1991 American Heart Association.)

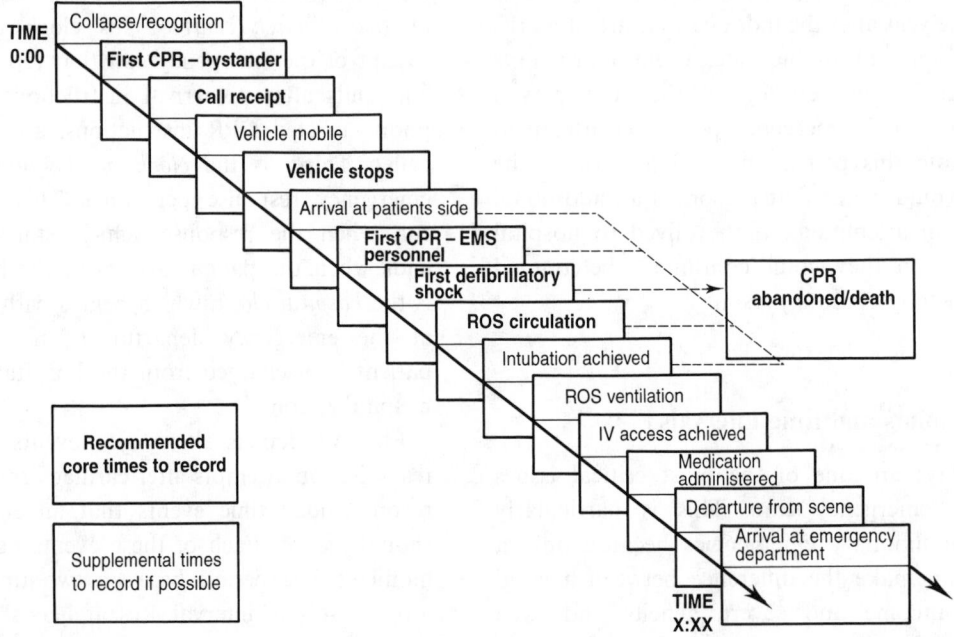

Fig. A3. Events associated with out-of-hospital cardiac arrest resuscitation attempts. (Reproduced with permission. Cummins, R., Chamberlain, D., Abramson, N. *et al.* (1991). Recommended guidelines for uniform reporting of data from out-of-hospital cardiac arrest: the Utstein Style. *Circulation*, **84**, 960–75. Copyright 1991 American Heart Association.)

be variable space (intervals) between the cards for different patients.

Recording the time events depicted in Fig. A3 permits a large variety of intervals to be tabulated. Many of these, such as 'call receipt' to 'arrival at patient's side' interval, are essential to quality assurance plans and system evaluation. The two most important intervals, however, from the perspective of patient survival, are the 'collapse' to 'first CPR attempt' interval and 'collapse' to 'first defibrillatory shocks' interval (Cummins *et al.*, 1991a; Chamberlain *et al.*, 1992a).

Many EMS systems may not participate in multicentre

research projects and shared data registries. Thus they will not need the complete supplementary detail recommended in Fig. A3. These systems and responsible physicians, however, will want to know the core data they should collect to obtain an assessment of how well they perform when compared to similar communities. Fig. A3 indicates the core times to record: first CPR by bystanders, receipt of dispatch call, vehicle stops, first CPR by EMS personnel, first defibrillatory shock, return of spontaneous circulation, CPR abandoned/death.

Utstein recommendations related to event timing in cardiac arrest

- Time of collapse/time of recognition. The time of collapse is recommended as core datum, but the time of this event is inherently imprecise. The emergency personnel must ask additional questions of the bystanders to identify this time. This information is key, however, to understanding the ischaemic interval (Safar *et al.*, 1988). Note that time of collapse can ONLY be obtained for witnessed cardiac arrests. The recommendations define a *witnessed arrest* as one in which the collapse or signs of distress are seen (or heard) by an identifiable witness. Time of recognition is the time at which an unwitnessed arrest is discovered.
- Time of call receipt (core). Modern emergency dispatching records this event automatically. If multiple routings of the message occur, passing the call from dispatcher to dispatcher, use the first operator contacted as the 'time of call receipt'.
- Time first emergency response vehicle is mobile. For precise data collection this is defined as the moment when the emergency response vehicle begins to move. Prolonged intervals between time of call receipt and time vehicle mobile begins to move may be due to long 'call-processing intervals' or to slowness of personnel.
- Time vehicle stops (core). This is the time when the emergency response vehicle stops moving, at a location as close as it can come to the patient. This replaces the commonly used term 'time of scene arrival', an imprecise term with meaning that has ranged from 'destination visually spotted' to 'personnel at patient's side'.
- Time of arrival at patient's side. If at all possible, systems should record the moment of arrival at the patient's side. It is difficult, however, to determine the time interval from leaving the emergency response vehicle to beginning the resuscitation attempt, though new defibrillator features now make this possible.

- Time of first CPR attempts (core). The Glossary defines 'CPR'. The time of first CPR attempts should be recorded both for CPR initiated by bystanders and for CPR initiated by emergency personnel. Note that personnel should also record the time when further CPR is considered futile, and they cease performing chest compressions and ventilations. While in general this would be the time of death, some systems require that a physician officially pronounce death.
- Time of first defibrillatory shock (core). Early defibrillation is the foundation for success in resuscitation of patients in VF. Systems should focus attention towards recording the moment when personnel deliver the first defibrillatory shock. The time interval from collapse to the first defibrillatory shock serves as a key evaluative measure for many other components of an emergency system. It is reduced by the competence of bystanders who can recognize a cardiac arrest and respond with a rapid telephone call, the efficiency of the dispatch system that can process calls quickly and activate the appropriate responding unit, and the skills of early defibrillation teams that can gain access to the patient and perform their defibrillation protocols rapidly. The best method to obtain this information is through automated external defibrillators or through conventional defibrillators with automated event documentation. These devices provide precise details on initial rhythm, times, and responses of heart rhythm to therapy. The value of such technology is obvious. There should be more widespread use of devices with these capabilities.
- Time of return of spontaneous circulation (core). (See Template Section, No. 15.)
- Time intubation achieved. As with defibrillation, airway management is a critical intervention for CPR. Emergency personnel should record the time of intubation if they can do so accurately and without interfering with patient care. Return of spontaneous ventilation occurs when voluntary respiratory efforts, including agonal-like gasping, begin. This may be extremely difficult for field emergency personnel to record accurately, often because agonal-like gasping may not have ceased before intubation.
- Time intravenous access achieved and time medications administered. Research has not yet established the true incremental value of the intravenous or endobronchial medications used in cardiac resuscitation (Brown *et al.*, 1992; Callaham *et al.*, 1992; Hoekstra *et al.*, 1993; Ornato, 1993b; Paradis & Koscove, 1990). Nevertheless, the effectiveness that does exist for these

agents is certainly time-dependent. Recent evidence suggests that assignment of defibrillation tasks to the first responding EMTs not only shortens the interval from collapse to defibrillation for those patients in VF, but also reduces significantly the intervals to intubation and medication administration (Hoekstra *et al.*, 1993).

- Time CPR abandoned/death (core). Emergency personnel should record the time at which they terminate resuscitation efforts outside the hospital, specifically the chest compressions and ventilation efforts of CPR.

- Departure from scene and arrival at the emergency department. Emergency personnel can record these times easily and accurately. Various related intervals are key components for an effective quality assurance and general management programme. These include 'vehicle stops' to 'departure from scene' interval, 'departure from scene' to 'arrival at hospital' interval, and 'vehicle rolling' to 'departure from hospital' interval (so-called 'personnel out-of-service interval' – meaning they are not available for other care activities).

Utstein Recommendations: individual clinical data

Recommended clinical data

The Utstein Task Force recommended that responsible personnel should attempt to record the clinical data listed below for each attempted resuscitation.

- *Location of person's arrest* (core). Home, street, public place, workplace, mass gatherings, in the ambulance, nursing home or other long-term care facility.

- *Prearrest clinical status* (supplementary). Overall performance category (OPC) and the cerebral performance category (CPC).

- *Witnessed arrest prior to arrival of emergency personnel* (core): yes or no.

- *Precipitating insult* (supplementary) (as determined as best as possible at the scene). Acute cardiac event, trauma, exsanguination, hypoxia, intracranial event, intoxication (drug ingestion), metabolic, drowning, sepsis, sudden infant death syndrome. As core data, an attempt should be made to classify the arrest as 'cardiac', or 'non-cardiac'.

- *Clinical status of patient when ambulance arrives* (core). Breathing (yes/no), palpable pulse (yes/no), bystander CPR (yes/no).

- *Arrest after arrival of emergency personnel* (core). yes or no.

- *Initial recorded rhythm* (core). Ventricular fibrillation (VF), ventricular tachycardia (VT), asystole, and other.

- *Treatment* (core). The specific protocols used by a system should be listed when the emergency medical system is described. For individual patients, however, personnel should record the specific interventions they used. As core information, the personnel should record: the type of respiratory support provided (mouth-to-mouth or mask breathing, endotracheal intubation, other type of airway management), whether the intubation was successful, the number of defibrillatory shocks given, and the medications administered. The strong association between unsuccessful resuscitation attempts and numerous interventions is obvious – the more difficult a resuscitation the more interventions that are used. Consequently, an account of interventions in unsuccessful attempts provides little information of value. Researchers must emphasize, therefore, all the interventions used for people who regained a spontaneous circulation.

- *Final patient status at the scene* (core). This refers to the condition of the patient when either transport commences or efforts terminate. The recommended categories are ROSC, continuing CPR, or death (CPR efforts stopped; record specific time).

- *Status on arrival at emergency department* (supplementary). This information would reflect a change in status during transport. The possibilities here are continuing CPR, pronounced dead on arrival (record specific time), or the presence of spontaneous circulation (ROSC). If the ROSC lasts longer than 5 min, personnel should record the blood pressure, respiratory rate, and the Glasgow Coma Score (GCS). In addition, the personnel should record the patient's temperature, especially in arrests associated with hypothermia.

- *Status after treatment in the emergency department* (core). The possibilities are admission to the hospital intensive care unit or alternative location, or pronounced dead with termination of efforts (record specific time).

- *Status on admission to hospital unit* (supplementary). Personnel should record the GCS, the blood pressure, the rate of spontaneous respirations, if any, and basic brainstem reflexes.

- *Discharged alive* (core). If the patient died in the hospital, personnel should record the time and date of death and the length of survival after ROSC. They should note those patients who die within 24 h, including exact time. Also record the OPC and CPC at time of discharge (supplementary). If the person dies before surviving 1 year then record the best score achieved in the week prior to death. The supplementary data to record would include the 'best-ever' outcome achieved during hospitalization and in the year following the arrest, though these data may be difficult to gather in a practical manner.

- *Discharge destination* (supplementary). If the patient is discharged, researchers should record the discharge destination: home (or prearrest residence), rehabilitation facility, extended care facility (nursing home) or other.
- *Alive at 1 year* (*yes or no*) (core). If yes, then record the OPC and CPC score at 1 year. Personnel can often obtain these scores via telephone interviews with family members. If the person dies in the first year, then record the date of death and the length of survival.

ACKNOWLEDGEMENTS

The material presented in the Appendix to this chapter was adapted from 'Recommended guidelines for uniform reporting of data from out-of-hospital cardiac arrest: the Utstein Style' which was prepared by a Task Force of the American Heart Association, the European Resuscitation Council, the Heart and Stroke Foundation of Canada, and the Australian Resuscitation Council. Figures are reproduced with the permission of the American Heart Association.

The Utstein report was published in the August 1991 issue of *Circulation*, the August 1991 issue of *Resuscitation*, and in translation in the German journals *Notfallmedizin* and *Intensivmedizin und Notfallmedizin*, and the French journal *JEUR*. Members of the Utstein Task Force included: Douglas A. Chamberlain and Richard O. Cummins (Co-chairmen), and Norman S. Abramson, Mervyn Allen, Peter Baskett, Lance Becker, Leo Bossaert, Herman Delooz, Wolfgang Dick, Mickey Eisenberg, Thomas Evans, Stig Holmberg, Richard Kerber, Arsene Mullie, Joseph P. Ornato, Eric Sandoe, Andreas Skulberg, Hugh Tunstall-Pedoe, Richard Swanson, William H. Thies.

In addition, this chapter contains special information on the Utstein description of EMS systems from 13 different locations. The Laerdal Foundation for Acute Medicine helped support the collection of information from these 13 EMS systems. The following individuals cooperated with the Utstein survey of their EMS systems and graciously supplied information: Judy Reid Graves (King County, Washington); Leo Bossaert (Antwerp, Belgium); Pierre Mols (Brussels, Belgium); Lise Fonsmark and Eric Sandoe (Copenhagen, Denmark); Laurie M. Caple and Thomas Evans (Northumbria); M. C. Julien (Paris, France); Pierre Carli (Paris, France); Svein Arne Hapnes and Kristian Lexow (Stravanger, Norway); Ragnar Hotvedt and Mads Gilbert (Tromsø, Norway); Johan Herlitz, Stig Holmberg and Marianne Blom (Göteborg, Sweden); Wolfgang Dick and Dietmar Mauer (Mainz, Germany); David J. Carrington and Stuart Cobbe (Scottish Ambulance Service).

Bibliography

ALLEN, M. (1991). Review of the Utstein Style. *J. Aust. Med. Assoc.*, **27**, 281–3.

AMERICAN COLLEGE OF EMERGENCY PHYSICIANS (1988). Guidelines for 'do not resuscitate' orders in the prehospital setting. *Ann. Emerg. Med.*, **17**, 1106–8.

AMERICAN HEART ASSOCIATION (1993). *1992 Heart and Stroke Facts Statistics*. p. 44. Dallas: American Heart Association.

APRAHAMIAN, C., THOMPSON, B. & GRUCHOW, H. (1986). Decision making in prehospital sudden cardiac arrest. *Ann. Emerg. Med.*, **15**, 445–9.

BECKER, L. & PEPE, P. (1993). Ensuring the effectiveness of community-wide emergency cardiac care. *Ann. Emerg. Med.*, **22**, 354–65.

BECKER, L.B., OSTRANDER, M. P., BARRETT, J. et al. (1991). Survival from cardiopulmonary resuscitation in a large metropolitan area: where are the survivors? *Ann. Emerg. Med.*, **20**, 355–61.

BECKER, L., SMITH, D. & RHODES, K. (1993). Incidence of cardiac arrest: a neglected factor in evaluating survival rates. *Ann. Emerg. Med.*, **22**, 86–91.

BERRYMAN, C.R. (1986). Electromechanical dissociation with a directly measurable arterial blood pressure. *Ann. Emerg. Med.*, **15**, 625–6.

BOCK, H. (1993). Field verification methodology using bar coding to record data. *Ann. Emerg. Med.*, **22**, 75–9.

BOCKA, J. (1989). Automatic external defibrillators. *Ann. Emerg. Med.*, **18**, 1264–8.

BONNIN, M. & SWOR, R. (1989). Outcomes in unsuccessful field resuscitation attempts. *Ann. Emerg. Med.*, **18**, 507–12.

BONNIN, M., PEPE, P., KIMBALL, K. et al. (1993). Distinct criteria for termination of resuscitation in the out-of-hospital setting. *JAMA*, **270**, 1457–62.

BOSSAERT, L. & KOSTER, R. (1992). Defibrillation: methods and strategies. A statement for the Advanced Life Support Working Party of the European Resuscitation council. *Resuscitation*, **24**, 211–25.

BOSSAERT, L., VANHOEYWEGHEN, R. et al. (1989a). Bystanders cardiopulmonary resuscitation (CPR) in out-of-hospital cardiac arrest. *Resuscitation*, **17** (Suppl.), S55–S69.

BOSSAERT, L., VANHOEYWEGHEN, R. et al. (1989b). Evaluation of cardiopulmonary resuscitation techniques. *Resuscitation*, **17**, S99–S109.

BRADLEY, K. (1993). Use of a cassette recorder for data collection in prehospital cardiac arrest research. *Ann. Emerg. Med.*, **22**, 80–4.

BROWN, C., MARTIN, D., PEPE, P. et al. (1992). A comparison of standard-dose and high-dose epinephrine in cardiac arrest outside the hospital. *N. Engl. J. Med.*, **327**, 151–5.

CALLAHAM, M., MADSEN, C., BARTON, C. et al. (1992). A randomized clinical trial of high-dose epinephrine and norepinephrine versus standard-dose epinephrine in prehospital cardiac arrest. *JAMA*, **268**, 2776–72.

CALLE, P., VANACKER, P., BUYLAERT, W. et al. (1992). Should semi-automatic defibrillators be used by emergency medical technicans in Belgium? The Belgian Cerebral Resuscitation Study Group. *Acta Clin. Belg.*, **47**, 6–14.

CAMPBELL, J., GRATTON, M., SALOMONE, III, J. et al. (1992). Time-to-patient interval: the hidden component of response time. *Ann. Emerg. Med.*, **21**, (Abstract).

CARTER, W.B., EISENBERG, M.S., HALLSTROM, A. P. et al. (1984). Development and implementation of emergency CPR instructions via telephone. *Ann. Emerg. Med.*, **13**, 695–700.

CEREBRAL RESUSCITATION STUDY GROUP (1989). The Belgian Cardiopulmonary Cerebral Resuscitation Registry. Form Protocol. *Resuscitation*, **17** (Suppl.), S5–S10.

CHAMBERLAIN, D., CUMMINS, R., EISENBERG, M. et al. (1991a). Recommended guidelines for uniform reporting of data from out-of hospital cardiac arrest: the Utstein Style. *Resuscitation*, **22**, 1–26.

CHAMBERLAIN, D., CUMMINS, R., EISENBERG, M. et al. (1991b). Empfehlungen zur einheitlichen Daten-erfassung bei Herzstillstand – Teil I. Der 'Utstein-Style' (translated by A. Schmidt & W. Dick.) *Notfallmedizin*, **17**, 510–18.

CHAMBERLAIN, D., CUMMINS, R., EISENBERG, M. et al. (1991c). 'Recommandation pour une description uniforme des donnees concernant l'arret cardiaque extra-hospitalier: le style d'Utstein (Translated by P. Carli, B. Riou, P. Barriot & Y. Lambert). *JEUR (Eur. J. Emerg.)*, **4**, 402–23.

CHAMBERLAIN, D., CUMMINS, R., EISENBERG, M. et al. (1991d). Recommended guidelines for uniform reporting of data on out-of-hospital cardiac arrest: the Utstein Style. *Intensivmed. Notfallmed.*, **12**, 20–8.

CHAMBERLAIN, D., CUMMINS, R., EISENBERG, M. et al. (1992a). Recommended guidelines for uniform reporting of data from out-of-hospital cardiac arrest (new abridged version): the 'Utstein style'. *Br. Heart J.*, **67**, 325–33.

CHAMBERLAIN, D., CUMMINS, R., ABRAMSON, N. et al. (1992b). Recommended guidelines for uniform reporting of data from out-of-hospital cardiac arrest (new abridged version): the 'Utstein Style'. *Eur. J. Anaesthesiol.* (Special Supplement.)

CLARK, J.J., LARSEN, M.P., CULLEY, L.L. et al. (1992). Incidence of agonal respirations in sudden cardiac arrest. *Ann. Emerg. Med.*, **21**, 1464–7.

COBB, L.A. & HALLSTROM, A.P. (1982). Community-based cardiopulmonary resuscitation: what have we learned? *Ann. N.Y. Acad. Sci.*, **382**, 330–42.

COBB, L.A., WERNER, J.A. & TROBAUGH, G.B. (1980). Sudden cardiac death: I. A decade's experience with out-of-hospital resuscitation. *Mod. Concepts Cardiovasc. Dis.*, **49**, 31–6.

COBB, L.A., WEAVER, W.D., HALLSTROM, A.P. et al. (1990). Cardiac resuscitation in the community. The Seattle experience. *Cardiologia.* (Supplement II). 42–7.

COBBE, S., REDMOND, M., SATSON, J. et al. (1991). 'Heartstart Scotland' – initial experience of a national scheme for out of hospital defibrillation. *Br. Med. J.*, **302**, 1517–20.

COLQUHOUN, M. (1988). Use of defibrillators by general practiconers. *Br. Med. J.*, **297**, 336–7.

COLQUHOUN, M. (1993). Automated external defibrillation. *Br. J. Gen. Pract.*, **43**, 95–6.

CUMMINS, R. (1989). From concept to standard-of-care? Review of the clinical experience with automated external defibrillators. *Ann. Emerg. Med.*, **18**, 1269–75.

CUMMINS, R. (1993a). Moving towards uniform reporting and terminology. *Ann. Emerg. Med.*, **22**, 33–6.

CUMMINS, R. (1993b). The Utstein Style for uniform reporting of data from out-of-hospital cardiac arrest. *Ann. Emerg. Med.*, **22**, 37–40.

CUMMINS, R. & CHAMBERLAIN, D. (1991). The Utstein Abbey and survival from cardiac arrest: what is the connection? *Ann. Emerg. Med.*, **20**, 918–19.

CUMMINS, R.O. & EISENBERG, M.S. Prehospital cardiopulmonary resuscitation: is it effective? *JAMA*, **253**, 2408–12.

CUMMINS, R.O., EISENBERG, M.S., HALLSTROM, A. P. et al. (1985). Survival of out-of-hospital cardiac arrest with early initiation of cardiopulmonary resuscitaiton. *Am. J. Emerg. Med.*, **3**, 114–18.

CUMMINS, R.O., EISENBERG, M.S., LITWIN, P. E. et al. (1987). Automatic external defibrillators used by emergency medical technicians. A controlled clinical trial. *JAMA* **257**, 1605–10.

CUMMINS, R.O., STULTS, K.R., HAGGER, B. et al. (1988). A new rhythm library for testing automatic external defibrillators: performance of three devices. *J. Am. Coll. Cardiol.*, **11**, 597–602.

CUMMINS, R.O., ORNATOR, J.P., THIES, W. et al. (1991a). Improving survival from cardiac arrest: the 'Chain of Survival' concept. *Circulation*, **83**, 1832–47.

CUMMINS, R., CHAMBERLAIN, D., ABRAMSON, N.

et al. (1991b). Recommended guidelines for uniform reporting of data from out-of-hospital cardiac arrest: the Utstein Style. *Circulation*, **84**, 960–75.

CUMMINS, R., CHAMBERLAIN, D., EISENBERG, M. *et al.* (1991c). Recommended guidelines for uniform reporting of data from out-of-hospital cardiac arrest: the Utstein Style. *Ann. Emerg. Med.*, **20**, 861–74.

DELOOZ, H., LEWI, P.J. & CEREBRAL RESUSCITATION STUDY GROUP (1989). Early prognostic indices after cardiopulmonary resuscitation (CPR). *Resuscitation*, **17** (Supp.), S149–S155.

EISENBERG, M., HALLSTROM, A. & BERGNER, L. (1982). Long term survival after out-of-hospital cardiac arrest. *N. Engl. J. Med.*, **306**, 1340–3.

EISENBERG, M.S., HALLSTROM, A.P., CARTER, W.B. *et al.* (1985). Emergency CPR via telephone. *Am. J. Public Health*, **75**, 47–50.

EISENBERG, M.S., CARTER, W., HALLSTROM, A. *et al.* (1986a). Identification of cardiac arrest by emergency dispatchers. *Am. J. Emerg. Med.*, **4**, 299–301.

EISENBERG, M.S., CUMMINS, R.O., LITWIN, P.E. *et al.* (1986b). Out-of-hospital cardiac arrest: significance of symptoms in patients collapsing before and after arrival of paramedics. *Am. J. Emerg. Med.*, **4**, 116–20.

EISENBERG, M., HORWOOD, B., CUMMINS, R. *et al.* (1990a). Cardiac arrest and resuscitation: a tale of 29 cities. *Ann. Emerg. Med.*, **19**, 238–43.

EISENBERG, M.S., CUMMINS, R.O., DAMON, S. *et al.* (1990b). Survival rates from out-of-hospital cardiac arrest: recommendations for uniform definitions and data to report. *Ann. Emerg. Med.*, **19**, 1249–59.

EMERGENCY CARDIAC CARE COMMITTEE AND SUBCOMMITTEES, AMERICAN HEART ASSOCIATION (1992a). Guidelines for cardiopulmonary resuscitation and emergency cardiac care. *JAMA*, **268**, 2171–95.

EMERGENCY CARDIAC CARE COMMITTEE AND SUBCOMMITTEES, AMERICAN HEART ASSOCIATION (1992b). Guidelines for cardiopulmonary resuscitation and emergency cardiac care, Part III: Adult Advanced Cardiac Life Support. *JAMA*, **268**, 2199–241.

FONSMARK, L., SANDOE, E., KASTRUP, J. *et al.* (1989). Treatment of cardiac arrest outside hospital with a semiautomatic defibrillator, Heartstart 2000. *Ugeskr. Laeger*, **151**, 1048–51.

FONSMARK, L., LEIKERSFELDT, G., MOLLER, J. *et al.* (1993). Influence of various therapeutic models on survival after prehospital cardiac arrest. *Ugeskr. Laeger*, **155**, 1953–8.

GALLEHR, J.E. & VUKOV, L.F. (1993). Defining the benefits of rural emergency medical technician – defibrillation. *Ann. Emerg. Med.*, **22**, 108–12.

GOLDSTEIN, S. (1982). The necessity of a uniform definition of sudden coronary death: witnessed death within 1 hour of the onset of acute symptoms. *Am. Heart J.*, **103**, 156–9.

GREENE, H.L. (1990). Sudden arrhythmic cardiac death – mechanisms, resuscitation and classification. *Am. J. Cardiol.*, **65**, 4B–12B.

GREENE, H.L. *et al.* (1989). The Cardiac Arrhythmia Suppression Trial. Classification death after MI as arrhythmic or nonarrhythmic. *Am. J. Cardiol.*, **63**, 1–6.

HARGARTEN, J., STUEVEN, H., WAITE, E. *et al.* (1990). Prehospital experience with defibrillation of coarse ventricular fibrillation: a ten-year review. *Ann. Emerg. Med.*, **19**, 157–62.

HOEKSTRA, J., BANKS, J., MARTIN, D. *et al.* Effect of first-responder automated defibrillation on time to therapeutic interventions during out-of-hospital cardiac arrest. *Ann. Emerg. Med.*, **22**, 1247–53.

HOLMBERG, S. & WENNERBLOM, B. (1984). Out-of-hospital cardiac arrest. *Am. J. Emerg. Med.*, **2**, 222–4.

ISERI, L., SINER, E., HUMPHREY, S. *et al.* (1977). Prehospital cardiac arrest after arrival of the paramedic unit. *J. Am. Coll. Emerg. Physicians*, **6**, 530–5.

JASTREMSKI, M. (1993). In-hospital cardiac arrest. *Ann. Emerg. Med.*, **22**, 113–17.

KELLERMANN, A.L. (1993). Criteria for dead-on-arrivals, prehospital termination of CPR, and do-not-resuscitate orders. *Ann. Emerg. Med.*, **22**, 47–51.

KELLERMANN, A., STAVES, D. & HACKMAN, B. (1988). In-hospital resuscitation following unsuccessful prehospital advanced cardiac life support: 'heroic efforts' of an exercise in futility? *Ann. Emerg. Med.*, **17**, 589–94.

KELLERMAN, A.L., HACKMAN, B.B. & SOMES, G. (1989). Dispatcher-assisted cardiopulmonary resuscitation: validation of efficacy. *Circulation*, **80**, 1231–9.

KELLERMANN, A., HACKMAN, B. & SOMES, G. (1993). Predicting the outcome of unsuccessful prehospital advanced cardiac life support. *JAMA*, **270**, 1433–6.

MULLIE, A., VANHOEYWEGHEN, R. & QUETS, A. (1989). Influence of time intervals on outcome of CPR. *Resuscitation* **17** (Suppl.), S23–S33.

MYERBURG, R. (1986). Sudden cardiac death: epidemiology, causes, and mechanisms. *Cardiology* **74** (Suppl. II), 2–9.

MYERBURG, R., KESSLER, K., BASSETT, A. *et al.* (1989). A biological approach to sudden cardiac death: structure, function and cause. *Am. J. Cardiol.*, **63**, 1512–16.

OFFSTAD, J., HELDAL, D., AKSNES, E. *et al.* (1992). The Nord Gudrandsdal Project – results of treatment of circulatory collapse in sparsely populated regions. *Tidsskr. Nor. Laegeforen.*, **112**, 2874–8.

ORNATO, J. (1993a). Methodology in cardiac arrest research: newer concepts for data collection. *Ann. Emerg. Med.*, **22**, 62–3.

ORNATO, J. (1993b). Use of adrenergic agonists during CPR in adults. *Ann. Emerg. Med.*, **22**, 411–16.

PANTRIDGE, J. & GEDDES, J. (1966). Cardiac arrest after myocardial infarction. *Lancet*, **i**, 807–8.

PARADIS, N.A. & KOSCOVE, E.M. (1990). Epinephrine

in cardiac arrest: a critical review. *Ann. Emerg. Med.*, **19**, 1288–301.

RICHLESS, L.K., SCHRADING, W.A., POLANA, J. *et al.* (1993). Early defibrillation program: problems encountered in a rural/suburban EMS system. *J. Emerg. Med.*, **11**, 127–34.

ROTH, R., STEWART, R.D., ROGERS, K. *et al.* (1984). Out-of-hospital cardiac arrest: factors associated with survival. *Ann. Emerg. Med.*, **13**, 237–43.

SAFAR, P., KHACHATURIAN, Z., KLAIN, M. *et al.* (1988). Recommendations for future research on the reversibility of clinical death. *Crit. Care Med.*, **16**, 1077–84.

SCOTT, I.A. & FITZGERALD, G.J. (1993). Early defibrillation in out-of-hospital sudden cardiac death: an Australian experience. *Arch. Emerg. Med.*, **10**, 1–7.

SEDGWICK, M., WATSON, J., DALZIEL, K. *et al.* (1992). Efficacy of out of hospital defibrillation by ambulance technicians using automated external defibrillators. The Heartstart Scotland Project. *Resuscitation*, **24**, 73–87.

SILFVAST, T. (1990). Prehospital resuscitation in Helsinki, Finland. *Am. J. Emerg. Med.*, **8**, 359–64.

SPAITE, D.W., HANLON, T., CRISS, E.A. *et al.* (1990). Prehospital data entry compliance by paramedics after institution of a comprehensive EMS data collection tool. *Ann. Emerg. Med.*, **19**, 1270–3.

SWANSON, R. (1991). Recommended guidelines for uniform reporting of data on out-of-hospital cardiac arrests: the Utstein style (Editorial). *Can. Med. Assoc. J.*, **145**, 407–10.

VALENZUELA, T. & WEAVER, W. (1993). Cardiac arrest research methods. Prehospital Disaster *Med.*, **8** (Suppl. 1), S41–S44.

VALENZUELA, T., SPAITE, D., MEISLIN, H. *et al.* (1992). Case and survival definitions in out-of-hospital cardiac arrest: effect on survival rate caculation. *JAMA*, **267**, 272–4.

WEAVER, W., COBB, L., DENNIS, D. *et al.* (1985). Amplitude of ventricular waveform and outcome after cardiac arrest. *Ann. Intern. Med.*, **102**, 53–5.

C(i):   Prehospital care of the trauma patient

P. L. LANE

Trauma Services, Victoria Hospital, London, Ontario, Canada

INTRODUCTION

The assessment and management of the injured patient provide prehospital personnel with perhaps the most challenging and rewarding aspects of their practice. Challenges abound as the environment is almost always dangerous and hostile, diagnoses are rarely apparent, clinical conditions change rapidly, and the decisions made can and do have a profound influence on outcome. Yet for precisely these same reasons, care of injured patients in the field can be extremely rewarding – lives can be saved, and outcomes improved substantially.

This chapter will essentially complement the preceding comments regarding trauma care generally, and those regarding prehospital care. System design features specific to the trauma population will be discussed, particularly from the point of view of medical directors of prehospital care systems. The essential components of the field assessment and management of the injured patients will be outlined. A final section will then present a system of quality management for prehospital trauma care, and discuss opportunities for research in the area.

SYSTEM FEATURES

Much of the very rich history of prehospital care stems from systems designed to care for injured soldiers during armed conflict. Napoleon's medical corps utilized the first air ambulance in the form of a hot air balloon. The introduction of femoral traction splints on the field of battle dramatically improved the outcome of injured soldiers during the First World War. Dr. Norman Bethune used blood transfusions in the field during the Spanish Civil War. Field medics and surgical units at the front during the Korean and Vietnam conflicts further improved results and many of the medics trained during these wars returned to become the paramedics of today.

The orientation of civilian prehospital care systems changed during the 1960s with the advent of cardiopulmonary resuscitation (CPR) and protocols for advanced cardiac life support (ACLS). The goals became the provision of CPR within the crucial 4–6-min interval following cardiac arrest, and ACLS within 10–12 min. The training of prehospital workers was enhanced to provide ACLS to the cardiac arrest patient and the emphasis was on stabilization at the scene before transport. Systems designed to those specifications have shown significant gains for cardiac patients.

The work of trauma 'pioneers' such as West, Trunkey and Cowley in the 1970s began to suggest that severely injured patients did better if cared for in hospitals specially equipped and staffed for this purpose. Cales furthered this and showed that outcomes improved and no preventable deaths occurred if severely injured patients were taken directly to trauma hospitals, by-passing local facilities. Further work in the 1980s by Mattox, Jacobs and others debated the trade-off between stabilizing trauma patients at the scene, as had proven beneficial in the cardiac population, and a 'load and go' or 'scoop and run' approach, emphasizing rapid transport to the trauma centre with minimal or no advanced procedures being performed in the prehospital setting. Some systems, particularly in Europe, suggest potential benefits from the involvement of physicians in the provision of care to severely injured patients in the field.

Although much work remains to be done, and improvements will continue to be made, some conclusions regarding the design of prehospital care systems for trauma are possible. Prehospital procedures and protocols must take into account the environment and transport times, the type of trauma occurring in the region, the prehospital resources available, and the location and capabilities of medical facilities. If trauma centres exist, then assessment protocols should include triage criteria by which the prehospital worker can identify severely injured patients in order to transport them directly to the trauma centre. Treatment protocols should take into account the training and capabilities of the personnel involved, with an emphasis on essential interventions that require a minimum of time to perform, yet will have a positive impact on outcome. Medical control efforts and quality management activities should similarly focus on minimal time delays and improved outcomes.

Environment and transport times

From the perspective of trauma, prehospital care systems strive to assess and transport the severely injured patient to a trauma facility within 1 h of injury. Services responsible for regions with a largely rural population face substantially different considerations from those in inner city urban areas. This has a particular bearing on the location of ambulance stations, whether or not inactive crews are best situated in a station or mobile, whether or not a helicopter ambulance is the best option for more remote locations, and whether or not it is practical to use hospital-based crews of physicians, nurses and/or ambulance attendants. Some rural services strive to minimize on-scene time and to provide airway stabilization and shock management interventions en route. Urban services with short transport times tend to place more emphasis on rapid assessment and transport, with no advanced interventions until the patient arrives at hospital.

Types of injuries

A knowledge of the types and frequencies of injuries occurring within the region also influences system design. Areas with a higher incidence of violent crime require mandatory police accompaniment on all such calls. Services with a higher incidence of motor vehicle crash calls requiring extrication have the fire or rescue service attend all calls. The prehospital care system in the former West German Republic has achieved particular success with the response of a physician via helicopter to motor vehicle crash victims. Higher frequencies of farming, boating and industrial injuries all bear implications for response patterns and equipment needs.

Prehospital resources available

A particular challenge in system design is to match resources to needs. Dispatch has an important role, in that decisions about the deployment of resources must often be made on the basis of minimal information. In services with only one response option – a basic life support (BLS) or emergency medical technician (EMT) ambulance – the dispatcher must make an estimate based on available information of the number of patients requiring transport from the scene of an incident and dispatch an appropriate number of vehicles. Increasingly, however, services provide a spectrum of response capabilities such as BLS vehicle, paramedics, helicopter, physician-staffed vehicles, etc. These options must be matched with the dispatcher's best estimation of needs at the scene. Protocols and algorithms have been developed in many systems to assist the dispatcher in these almost instantaneous decisions. An example of a

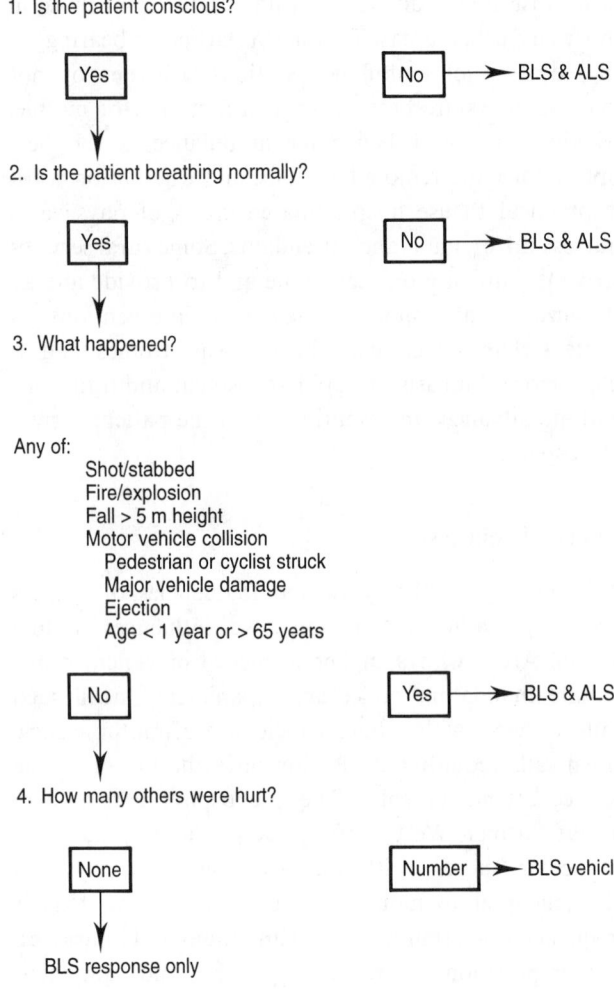

1. Is the patient conscious?

Yes →

No → BLS & ALS

2. Is the patient breathing normally?

Yes →

No → BLS & ALS

3. What happened?

Any of:
    Shot/stabbed
    Fire/explosion
    Fall > 5 m height
    Motor vehicle collision
        Pedestrian or cyclist struck
        Major vehicle damage
        Ejection
        Age < 1 year or > 65 years

No →

Yes → BLS & ALS

4. How many others were hurt?

None →

Number → BLS vehicles

BLS response only

Fig. 1. Dispatch algorithm.

dispatch algorithm is provided in Fig. 1. Such protocols should consider not only the number of potential patients and the nature of their injuries, but also the quality of the information, (i.e. from a bystander, police officer, or ambulance crew). Often, the response options will be modified based on more reliable information subsequently provided by professionals on the scene.

Triage criteria

Numerous studies have now shown the benefits of transporting severely injured patients to the nearest *appropriate* hospital. In his seminal article (Trunkey, 1983), Trunkey noted that, while more than 50% of fatalities occur in the first few minutes after the injury, the bulk of the preventable 'early' deaths do not occur until 2–6 h postinjury. This provides a very narrow 'window of

opportunity' for the trauma care system. The important time interval is that between injury and definitive surgical care. This 1–2 h period should provide enough time to get severely injured patients to trauma hospitals directly from the scene, particularly within urban settings.

Efforts over the past two decades have centred on defining field criteria for the identification of those most likely to benefit from care at hospitals specializing in the treatment of severely injured patients. Criteria have been based on anatomical and physiological parameters, and on the circumstances surrounding the injury including its mechanism. Anatomical scales are of limited use because of the impracticality of making an anatomically precise diagnosis in the field. Physiological scores, depending upon deteriorations in respiratory, circulatory and neurological function, can be misleading because of the rapid changes in these parameters in the first few minutes postinjury. Some examples of physiological scores proposed or in use include the Trauma Score, the Revised Trauma Score, the Pre-hospital Index, the CRAMS Scale, the Paediatric Trauma Score, and the Trauma Triage Rule. To date, criteria based on the mechanism of injury have not been precise enough. A list of some of the more commonly cited incident characteristics and mechanisms associated with more severe injury are included in the triage algorithm example shown in Fig. 2. The challenge in developing any triage system is to minimize both overtriage – transporting too many patients with minor injuries to trauma hospitals – and undertriage – inadvertently transporting severely injured patients to hospitals not equipped to care for them. Recent work by Champion *et al.* suggests that involving a physician in these decisions, either via radio or at the local emergency department, may significantly improve both sensitivity and specificity. A more comprehensive discussion of the advantages and disadvantages of various scales and criteria can be found in the references provided.

FIELD ASSESSMENT OF THE TRAUMA PATIENT

Injury is a time-dependent disease, and this principle underlies all aspects of the systems designed to care for trauma patients. Prehospital personnel have a number of crucial tasks to perform in a very short time span in their assessment of the trauma patient. Their relevance varies somewhat depending on the circumstances.

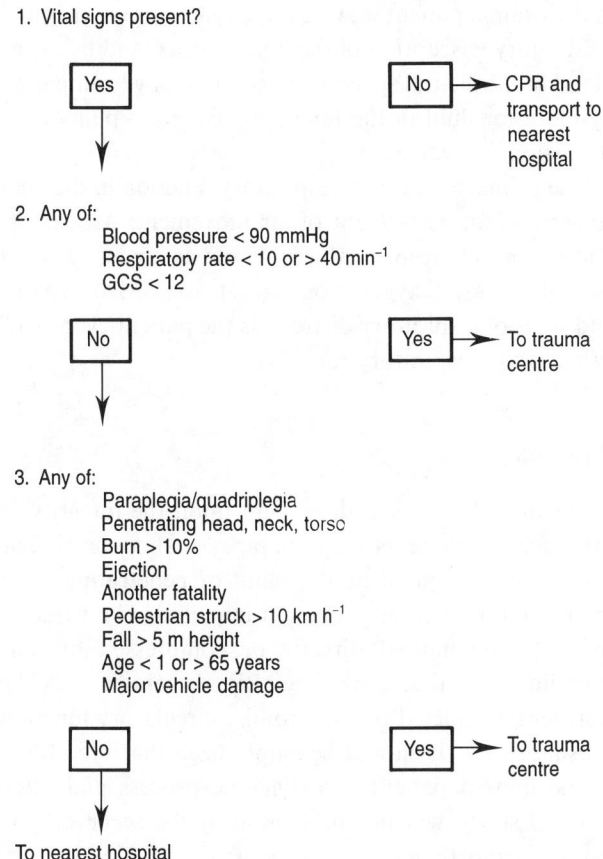

1. Vital signs present?

Yes   No → CPR and transport to nearest hospital

2. Any of:
    Blood pressure < 90 mmHg
    Respiratory rate < 10 or > 40 min^{-1}
    GCS < 12

No   Yes → To trauma centre

3. Any of:
    Paraplegia/quadriplegia
    Penetrating head, neck, torso
    Burn > 10%
    Ejection
    Another fatality
    Pedestrian struck > 10 km h^{-1}
    Fall > 5 m height
    Age < 1 or > 65 years
    Major vehicle damage

No   Yes → To trauma centre

To nearest hospital

Fig. 2. Prehospital triage algorithm. CPR, cardiopulmonary resuscitation; GCS, Glasgow Coma Score.

Crucial tasks in assessing the trauma patient

- Secure the scene
- Assess the ABCs – Airway, Breathing, Circulation, Consciousness
- Assess the mechanism of injury
- Reach a triage decision
- Secondary survey

Each task will be discussed sequentially, but in reality they are performed simultaneously, along with treatment and extrication. Because of the time factor and the realities of the field, the attendant makes decisions critical to the outcome of the patient based on the minimal data that are immediately available.

Secure the scene

The attendant will be of no assistance to the patient if he/she undertakes an unacceptable risk and becomes another victim. Securing the scene therefore requires an immediate assessment of that risk upon arrival and will depend upon prearrival information received by radio, a quick 360° visual inspection, and reports from bystanders or other emergency response personnel already on the scene. If possible, the role of scene commander should be assumed by another emergency responder – police or firefighter – in order to allow ambulance personnel to assess and care for the patient. If not possible, ambulance personnel must assume this role and summon other resources. Similarly, the visual scan and on-scene reports allow a rapid assessment of the ambulance resources necessary. Further crews and vehicles are summoned at this point, before the ambulance attendants become directly involved with the patients.

The wide variety of scenarios encountered is almost limitless and each brings special needs and requirements in terms of securing the scene. A few of the more frequent scenarios, however, are worthy of discussion. Motor vehicle crash scenes are by definition high-risk situations. The scene commander must never assume that the flashing lights of the rescue vehicle are enough to warn oncoming traffic. The ambulance as well as the crash scene are tremendous distractions to the curious driver. The scene commander should ensure that appropriate warning triangles or flares are placed well in advance of the crash scene. Traffic should be safely diverted around the crashed vehicles and the ambulance.

Situations involving interpersonal violence are particularly dangerous. Ambulance attendants should not attempt to access such a patient until a police commander has declared it safe. At a fire scene, fighting the fire and rescuing victims is the job of the firefighters, and ambulance attendants and their equipment should remain well clear. The responsibility for rescue from remote or difficult locations varies among different jurisdictions and ambulance personnel must be familiar with their own service's protocols and responsibilities.

Assess the ABCs – Airway, Breathing, Circulation, Consciousness

Once the scene is secure, the attendant's first priority becomes Airway, Breathing, Circulation and Consciousness. Time is crucial and a quick primary survey is conducted at this point to identify any immediately life-threatening conditions. While it is discussed separately below, initial treatment priorities follow the same rubric and are conducted simultaneously; for example, when an airway obstruction is identified, it is cleared before breathing is assessed. Details of the prehospital primary survey are well covered in other sources, such as the Basic Trauma Life Support (BTLS), so only the essential principles will be outlined here.

Airway – with cervical spine control

Ensuring an adequate airway while maintaining control of the cervical spine is paramount in the field assessment of the trauma patient. The two questions that the field worker must answer are: Is the airway patent? and Can the patient control it? If the answer to either question is 'no' or 'maybe', then invasive manoeuvres must be taken to secure the airway.

The commonest cause of airway obstruction in the injured patient is the tongue, as it falls posteriorly as a result of loss of tone or integrity in the musculature and bony structure of the floor of the mouth. Blood, foreign bodies, stomach contents, soft tissue swelling and direct laryngeal injury are all potential causes of airway obstruction that must be considered. If adequate air movement cannot be ensured, then the airway must be secured.

The ability to cough is essential to airway control – the patient who cannot cough cannot clear secretions and/or foreign material. Hence, any patient who does not cough in response to foreign material in the airway such as blood, secretions, or deep suctioning cannot control the airway.

Cervical spine injuries, while relatively uncommon, can have disastrous long-term consequences if not adequately managed. The ancient medical admonition 'above all else, do no further harm' is particularly relevant here. The neck can be injured in motor vehicle crashes, falls, assaults, industrial and sporting injuries, and even penetrating trauma, and the signs and symptoms are not apparent in the field. An injury must be assumed to be present until proven otherwise in the hospital. Cervical spine control is therefore maintained throughout the prehospital assessment and management of the trauma patient.

Breathing

Respiratory function depends on the two components of air movement and gas exchange – ventilation and oxygenation. Air movement depends on the integrity of neuromuscular factors, of the bony thorax, and the thoracic cavity itself. Gas exchange depends on the integrity of the capillary/alveolar membrane. Ventilation in the trauma patient may be impaired by brain or spinal cord injury, disruption of the bony thorax, and by air or blood in the pleural space. Oxygenation may be impaired by blood or fluid in the lung parenchyma – pulmonary contusion or oedema.

The primary survey of respiratory function in the field consists of an assessment of air movement: Are respirations normal, deep, or shallow? and Is air entry equal on both sides? Oxygenation is best assessed by colour and signs of respiratory distress: Is the patient cyanosed? What is the respiratory rate?

Circulation

Circulatory function is dependent upon the integrity of the three components – pump, pipes, and contents. The heart may be injured in any blunt or penetrating chest injury and its pumping function impaired. The vascular tree may be injured directly or compressed by surrounding soft tissue swelling. Blood volume may be sufficiently depleted to compromise circulatory function causing shock. It should be emphasized that blood loss in the injured patient is a dynamic process and often signs of shock will not be present at the scene despite major haemorrhage.

Circulatory function in the field consists of a quick visual haemorrhage check – Is there major external bleeding? – and an assessment of output – What is the pulse rate and blood pressure?

Often, the presence of clothing or injuries will preclude the normal assessment of a blood pressure at the brachial artery. Blood pressure can be roughly approximated in the adult by palpating the best available pulse (Table 1).

Consciousness

Brain function depends on the delivery of adequate oxygen and nutrients to intact neural tissue. Therefore, airway, breathing and circulatory compromise can all

Table 1. *Blood pressure estimation*

Best pulse	Systolic blood pressure (mm Hg)
Carotid	60
Femoral	70
Brachial	80

impair consciousness. Focal or diffuse brain injury can also occur and is very common among blunt multisystem trauma patients.

Brain function is best assessed by the level of consciousness. The Glasgow Coma Scale (GCS) developed by Teasdale & Jennett (1974), is the most practical and reliable means with which to assess level of consciousness. Indeed, a comparison of the GCS on arrival at hospital with that noted in the field is very valuable to the neurosurgeon or trauma team leader caring for the patient. The ambulance attendant should also assess pupillary size and reactivity. The field assessment then consists of: What is the Glasgow Coma Score? and What is the size and reactivity of the pupils?

Assess the mechanism of injury

An understanding of the basic mechanisms of injury can assist at all levels of trauma care. Time is of the essence and knowing how the patient was injured can guide the

assessment and provision of care in both the prehospital and in-hospital phases. The physician's best information source as to the direction and magnitude of the forces involved is the report of the ambulance attendant from the scene. Standardized report forms aid greatly in the retrieval and reporting of such information. The nature of the injuries sustained is related to the type of energy transferred. In the case of kinetic energy, injuries can be anticipated with a knowledge of the direction and magnitude of the energy involved. In practical terms in the field, this means a report that includes both direction and velocity.

An understanding of the mechanism of injury can also aid in triage decisions because of the association with severity of injury (see below). The velocity of the vehicles involved, whether or not the patient was ejected, the degree of deformation of the vehicle, the type of weapon used, whether or not the explosion was within an enclosed space, are all important details, only available to prehospital workers (see Fig. 3).

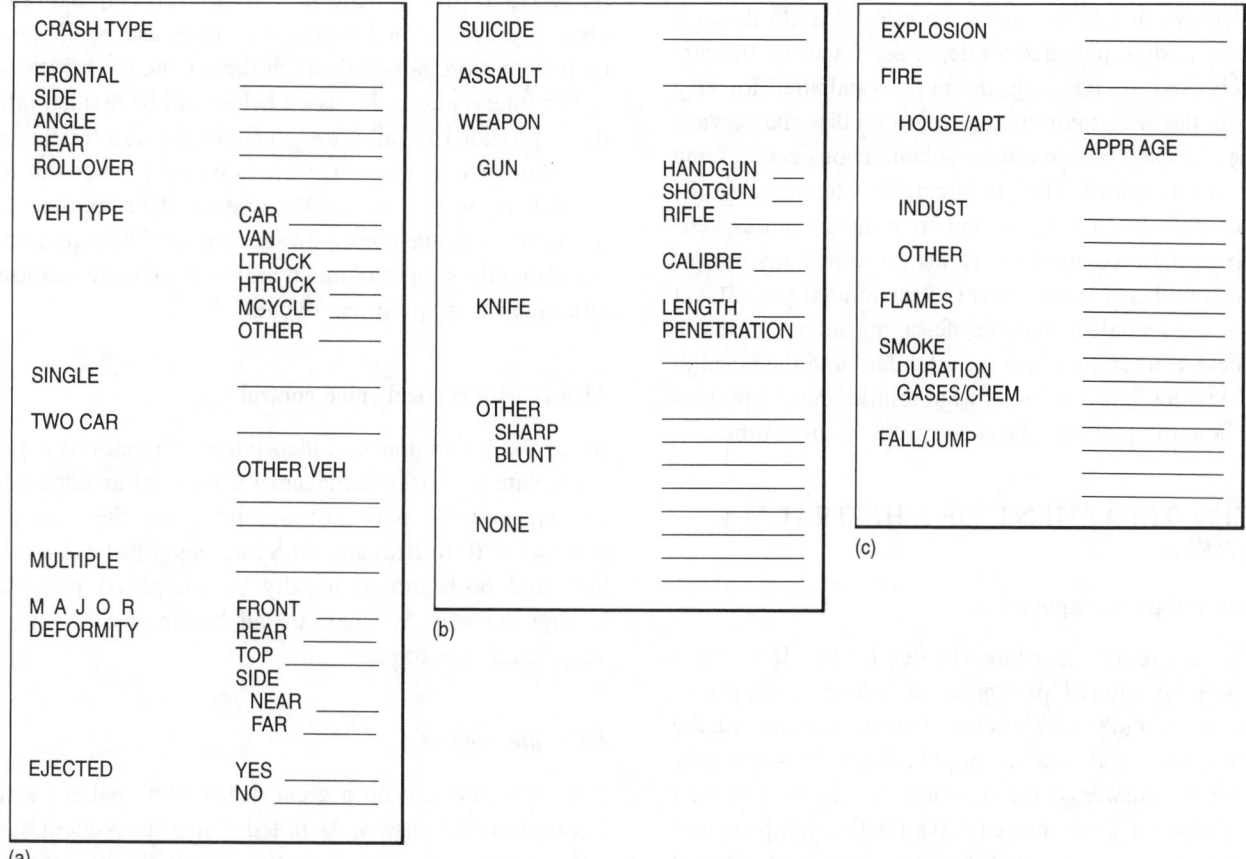

Fig. 3. Examples of standardized reporting forms in cases of (a) motor vehicle crash, (b) assault/suicide, (c) fire/explosion. for completion by prehospital personnel.

Reach a triage decision

In systems where trauma centres and triage criteria exist, the next task in the prehospital phase is to reach a decision regarding the transport destination (i.e. to the nearest hospital or to the trauma centre). This decision will depend on the criteria defined by the local medical control authority. Most protocols call for diversion to the nearest hospital if the patient develops a cardiac arrest or an obstructed airway. Otherwise, severely injured patients are transported to the trauma facility. The criteria take into account the type and location of injuries, physiological parameters (such as level of consciousness, heart rate, respiratory rate and blood pressure), and incident characteristics including mechanism of injury. An example of a triage algorithm is provided in Fig. 2.

Secondary survey

The secondary survey is completed en route if the patient requires transport to a trauma facility and at the scene if they are not severely injured. The secondary survey is a head-to-toe system-by-system assessment of the patient to identify non-life-threatening injuries. It is at this stage that the scalp is palpated for depressed fractures, the ears are checked for bleeding, the neck is palpated for step deformities whilst continuing to immobilize the cervical spine, the chest is assessed for subcutaneous emphysema and rib fractures, the abdomen for tenderness, the extremities for fractures and peripheral pulses, etc. Each of these components forms an important part of the comprehensive assessment of the injured patient, yet none is essential in making life-saving interventions in the field. Rather, they give the attendant and the hospital staff a better appreciation of what injuries may be present and how the patient's status may change over time.

FIELD TREATMENT OF THE TRAUMA PATIENT

Treat versus transport

Debate continues regarding whether it is best to stabilize the severely injured patient at the scene or simply to transport rapidly to a trauma facility. Because of the heterogeneity of the trauma population, there is probably no correct answer to the question. It may well be best to stabilize the brain injured patient with a compromised airway when transport times are long and trained personnel are available. It may well be appropriate to rapidly transport the patient with penetrating chest trauma from an inner city. However, the vast majority of trauma patients and circumstances fall between these two extremes, and clear guidance from the literature is elusive. Smith *et al.* (1985) noted that ALS interventions in the field delayed care significantly whereas Jacobs *et al.* (1984) concluded that well-trained paramedics working under protocols could perform a variety of interventions resulting in more favourable outcomes. Local protocols and procedures must be based on capabilities, patterns and locations of injuries, transport times, effective medical control, and active quality management/improvement programmes.

Treatment protocols and options

Prehospital treatment protocols follow the same sequence as the clinical assessment protocols outlined above – the ABCs. Indeed, life-saving interventions are performed simultaneously with the assessment phase. After the ABCs of assessment and treatment are completed or at least commenced, the patient must be extricated and prepared for transport by immobilizing the spine and extremities. If the patient is not severely injured and appears stable, some interventions may also be dictated by information gained through the secondary survey.

The interventions discussed below will be divided into those provided by all crews, including BLS attendants, and those ALS procedures provided by paramedics or physicians on the scene. Because of their more controversial and time-consuming nature, ALS interventions have been the subject of much more extensive evaluation, although many questions remain.

Airway with cervical spine control

By far the most important life-saving interventions in the field relate to airway management. Without an adequate airway, patients may not survive even the shortest transports. Both BLS and ALS interventions have a role here and both should usually be completed prior to leaving the scene as they are all but impossible in an ambulance or aircraft.

Basic life support

The BLS crew can do a great deal for the patient with a compromised airway. As noted above, assessment and interventions are always undertaken with the cervical spine controlled. The issue of positioning is somewhat controversial. The 'recovery' position, with the patient on the side and slightly head down, is no doubt best to prevent aspiration but adequate cervical spine control is impossible. As a result, it should only be utilized in the awake, sober patient with no neck pain and no other significant injuries. Such situations are so exceedingly rare among trauma patients with airway problems that they will not be discussed further.

The challenge for the BLS crew is to maintain an adequate airway in the supine position, with the neck immobilized. In the assessment section, we identified two issues with respect to the airway – patency and control. In the unconscious patient, the tongue falling back onto the posterior pharyngeal wall is usually the major problem in terms of patency. Because of the possibility of neck injury, the BCLS manoeuvre of extending the head and neck is contraindicated in the trauma patient. Furthermore, the manual techniques of chin lift and jaw thrust are both difficult with a collar in place and impractical to maintain for any length of time. An oropharyngeal or nasopharyngeal airway can assist in displacing the tongue anteriorly but in the semiconscious patient this may stimulate a gag reflex and subsequent vomiting. Most patients who tolerate a pharyngeal airway cannot by definition control their own airway. Foreign bodies and aspirated material may also compromise patency but standard BLS procedures of 'finger sweep' and suctioning should be sufficient. The more complex problems of oedema, soft tissue swelling with airway occlusion, and loss of airway integrity due to direct trauma are beyond the scope of BLS procedures but they are thankfully exceedingly rare in the first hour.

Airway control is a significant problem in many severely injured patients, whether due to unconsciousness or to significant bleeding into the area. Constant vigilance by the attendant to suction blood and secretions is necessary. This is particularly true during transport when the motion of the vehicle may precipitate vomiting. Suction equipment should be portable and attendants must be familiar with it. The suction source should be sufficiently powerful to remove very thick vomitus and the reservoir should be sufficiently large to accommodate large quantities of blood. Spare reservoirs should be available in the vehicle, particularly for longer transfers. Both pharyngeal and deep suction catheters must be available. The rigid pharygeal or 'tonsil tip' suction device is needed for oropharyngeal suctioning and the apertures should be sufficiently large to accept particulate matter. Suction catheters of various sizes will be needed for deep pharyngeal suctioning, especially via the nasopharyngeal airway. Pressure on the cricoid cartilage should be discouraged as it may be transmitted to the carotid sinuses causing a vagotonic response. It could also displace an extremely unstable neck injury or cause oesophageal rupture from increased pressure during retching.

Advanced life support

Advanced airway control procedures are arguably the first and most important skills that should be acquired by prehospital personnel caring for a significant volume of seriously injured patients. The skills of oral and nasal endotracheal intubation can be successfully taught to prehospital non-medical personnel. An appropriately trained paramedic should be able to intubate a trauma patient within the first minute, without significantly delaying care and transport. The adverse effects of transporting a severely injured patient with a compromised airway far outweigh the possible complications of intubation in the field.

To control the airway, a wide variety of techniques and devices have been described and utilized. Some of these, such as the oesophageal obturator airway, seem to have developed because of the initial reluctance of the medical community to train and delegate tracheal intubation to non-physicians. Some devices have largely been abandoned as historical relics. Others such as the oesophageal gastric tube airway, the pharyngotracheal airway and the lighted airway stylet have been described but have found little acceptance. Techniques such as digital intubation have been described. However, without doubt the gold standard against which all airway management techniques must be measured are oro- and nasotracheal intubation. Both can and have been successfully taught to and used by prehospital personnel. Both techniques are essentially the same as those employed by emergency physicians in hospitals.

In the rare circumstance when definitive control of the airway in the field is essential and intubation is impossible, the physician or paramedic may consider a surgical airway. This can be accomplished via the cricothyroid membrane which is preferred as it is relatively avascular, is sufficiently superior to avoid the isthmus of the thyroid gland, and is usually readily palpable. Airway access for the insufflation of oxygen may be achieved by the percutaneous insertion of a large-bore plastic cannula through the membrane until air is aspirated. A 3 mm paediatric endotracheal tube adapter may then be attached to the cannula and oxygen insufflated from, a 50 litre min^{-1} flow source. Because of the high resistance to flow, no air will be exhaled through the cannula, so for each second of insufflation 3 sec is allowed for passive exhalation through the upper airway. This technique does not provide definitive airway control but allows a temporary route for the insufflation of oxygen until a more permanent airway can be established.

Breathing

A significant proportion of preventable trauma deaths occur as a result of inadequate ventilation and/or oxygenation. As noted in the assessment section, there are a variety of injuries and clinical problems that may compromise breathing but the actual diagnosis is rarely relevant in the prehospital setting.

Basic life support

Oxygen is probably the most useful and the least toxic drug in our armamentarium, yet there is still a reluctance to use it at times. Every severely injured patient should have oxygen and the more the better. The concern regarding carbon dioxide narcosis is not relevant in the back of an ambulance. Transport times are relatively short and these patients are under constant surveillance. If they hypoventilate because of rising Po_2, then the attendant can either remove the oxygen temporarily or bag the patient until arrival at hospital. Oxygen is life-saving to patients with pulmonary injuries and consequent ventilation/perfusion mismatch. Hypotensive patients experience peripheral vasoconstriction and reduced perfusion of skin and many other tissues – oxygen helps to preserve aerobic metabolism in minimally perfused tissue. Patients who have bled significantly have reduced oxygen carrying capacity and hence need an increased Po_2 to satisfy cellular requirements. Patients with reduced cerebral blood flow due to increased intracranial pressure similarly need an increased Po_2 to satisfy cellular requirements in the central nervous system. There is no clinical circumstance in the severely injured patient in which oxygen is contraindicated, provided the patient is under constant observation.

Assisted ventilation with a bag–valve–mask system is an important skill that should be within the capability of BLS attendants. Patients who hypoventilate because of a spinal cord or brain injury and those in respiratory distress because of thoracic injuries will benefit from assisted ventilation. This skill involves achieving an effective seal with an appropriately sized mask, providing well-timed positive pressure 100% oxygen as the patient breathes in, and being sensitive to the 'feel' of airway resistance. Only the bag system should be used, never the oxygen-powered breathing device, as this may inflate the stomach or worsen an existing pneumothorax. Care must be taken even with the bag to avoid inflating the stomach. Significant resistance sensed when the bag is squeezed means that there is obstruction of some sort either because the timing is wrong and the patient is exhaling, or that the airway is obstructed or a pneumo/haemothorax exists. Attempting to squeeze firmly against resistance may well inflate the stomach and lead to aspiration. The skill is often not well taught in prehospital care training programmes and is best demonstrated and practised in the clinical setting. Yet it can greatly assist the severely injured patient in the prehospital setting.

The management of an open pneumothorax is another area in which the BLS crew can play an important role. An open chest wound, often termed a sucking chest wound, renders ventilation inefficient. With each inspiration, the negative intrathoracic pressure generated draws air into the pleural space, compressing the lung. The simple application of an occlusive dressing, taped on three sides, creates a one-way valve preventing worsening of the pneumothorax. The occlusive dressing can be of vaseline-impregnated gauze or something as simple as a plastic bag or latex glove.

Attempts to stabilize flail segments of the chest wall in the field are not appropriate. First aid courses and prehospital care training manuals are replete with descriptions of various techniques designed to prevent the segment from flailing. However, if recognized in the field a flail chest should alert the BLS attendant to the fact that a life-threatening injury exists; the patient should be provided with oxygen and transported to a trauma facility as soon as possible. Sandbags, positioning, or 'compression strapping' are time-consuming and may well further reduce ventilation in an already compromised patient. The patient in severe respiratory distress due to a flail segment can be best aided by gentle assisted respiration with the bag–valve–mask. This will serve to provide positive intrathoracic pressure with inspiration, and thus negate the deleterious mechanical effects of the flail. It also will help to alleviate pain. The principal cause of respiratory distress in this situation is usually the underlying pulmonary contusion, and ventilation with 100% oxygen is an effective treatment.

Advanced life support

Physicians or paramedics at the scene should be skilled at the interventions listed above which are likely to be sufficient in the vast majority of injured patients at the scene. In particular, assisted ventilation via bag or endotracheal tube is an important and potentially life-saving skill. The decision to ventilate must be based on the degree of respiratory distress, its probable cause and the transport time. Ventilation with positive pressure in the setting of rib fractures deserves a note of caution as this may precipitate or aggravate a pneumothorax. Similarly, if significant airway resistance is encountered while ventilating via an endotracheal tube, the possibility of a pneumo- or haemothorax must be urgently considered and treated.

Subtle or small pneumothoraces need not be treated in the field. However, the patient in severe respiratory distress with asymmetrical air entry poses a true emergency. Such a patient will usually have already been intubated and the tube should be checked to ensure that it has not been advanced down the right mainstem bronchus. If this is not the case, then the possibility of a large pneumothorax or haemothorax should be considered. Chest percussion is of little value in the field setting to distinguish the two and in fact there is no need to make an accurate diagnosis. The hemithorax should be decompressed if it is judged that the patient cannot survive the journey without it. The benefits of decompression must be weighed against the delays involved in performing the procedure. It it always preferable and safer to insert a chest tube in hospital but, in rare circumstances, field decompression may be life-saving.

Needle thoracostomy involves the insertion of a large bore (12–14 gauge) catheter-over-needle into the pleural space. The needle is advanced just above the lower rib, to avoid damage to the neurovascular structures. Once air or blood is aspirated freely in the syringe, the catheter is passed, the needle is removed, and a one-way valve is attached to the hub. The finger cot of a latex glove, a punctured latex condom, or even the three-sided occlusive dressing described above will all suffice. A chest tube will need to be inserted immediately upon arrival at hospital and the emergency department should be alerted to this effect. Physicians or paramedics with appropriate training may prefer to insert a chest tube in the field. This can be very difficult and time-consuming and should only be used if transport times are prolonged and the patient is in severe distress.

Circulation

Of those preventable trauma deaths occurring in the first few hours after injury, many are due to inadequately treated hypovolaemic shock. It should be noted at the outset that the definitive treatment for hypovolaemic shock is almost always surgical. In this sense, the most effective and life-saving treatment available to prehospital personnel is rapid safe transport to an appropriate facility. Excessive on-scene times can be deadly. Prehospital care systems must continually monitor scene and transport times and interventions to ensure that patient outcomes are improving.

Basic life support

The BLS crew has an important role to play in reducing blood loss by doing a rapid external haemorrhage check and applying pressure dressings. Any site of continuing and significant bleeding should have a pressure dressing applied at the scene or in transit. The pressure need only be sufficient to overcome the intravascular pressure. Usually this is venous so a firmly taped gauze dressing is satisfactory. In the case of bright red pulsatile bleeding, arterial pressure must be overcome. Again, however, a tight dressing or a firm hand can usually exert 100–150 mmHg pressure with no difficulty. There is no role for tourniquets or clamps which will cause vascular damage and tissue ischaemia. Inflatable air splits and 'antishock' garments have not been shown to be effective in controlled trials and should be avoided.

Advanced life support

The ALS interventions to treat shock are responsible for much of the controversy regarding prehospital trauma care. The debates centre around at least three issues:

1. Do the time delays involved in starting one or more intravenous lines outweigh the benefits?
2. What is the most appropriate resuscitation fluid?
3. Does restoring blood pressure in fact increase blood loss?

Complicating the assessment of these issues are the great differences between penetrating and blunt trauma and the important influence of transport times. If the administration of intravenous fluids in the field is to benefit a severely injured patient, the time taken to start the intravenous line must not result in an unacceptable degree of further blood loss. Lewis (1986), using a computer model, suggested that fluids would be of benefit if prehospital times were greater than 30 min, bleeding rates between 25 and 100 ml min^{-1}, and the infusion rate was at least equal to the bleeding rate. Presumably, less severely injured patients would show no benefit at all and more severely injured patients require immediate surgical intervention. Kaweski *et al.* (1990) conducted an extensive retrospective review of 6855 trauma patients transported in San Diego County. Using a variety of analyses, and stratifying by injury severity and by probability of survival, they could demonstrate no benefit from prehospital intravenous fluid administration in terms of mortality rates. The mean prehospital time in those receiving fluids and those given no fluids was 36 min.

Early in the debate on these issues, concern was expressed that on-scene intravenous therapy delays care. Smith *et al.* (1985) reviewed 52 cases of hypovolaemic shock in trauma victims and found that on-scene intravenous start times (11.3 min) exceeded transport times (10.7 min) and concluded that this was unacceptable. Subsequently, Pons *et al.* (1988), in the Denver system, showed that intravenous start times averaged only 90 sec, whereas Slovis *et al.* (1990) found a 95% success rate among intravenous starts in hypotensive trauma patients in a moving ambulance.

The selection of the most beneficial intravenous fluid for use in the prehospital setting is no easier than in hospital. The debate regarding the use of crystalloid versus colloidal solutions is beyond the scope of this chapter. Because of the practical considerations of dealing with bulky and heavy volumes of fluid in an inhospitable environment, interest has been expressed in the use of smaller volumes of hypertonic solutions. Animal model work suggested the possibility of benefit in trauma, and a preliminary study from Houston (Maningas *et al.*, 1989) evaluated the prehospital use of 7.5% saline in 6% dextran 70 (HSD). In 1991, Mattox *et al.* reported the results of a three-centre trial using the same protocol of HSD versus normal saline. This trial showed no overall effect on mortality, but in the group requiring surgical intervention HSD patients did somewhat better in terms of improved survival and fewer complications. The study demonstrated the safety of HSD in the prehospital setting.

Neurological disability

The assessment of the patient's level of consciousness in the field and the changes that occur over time are an extremely important tool in subsequent clinical decisions about the management of the patient in hospital. There is little, however, that either the BLS or the ALS prehospital crew can do in the field directly to control or reverse conditions leading to impaired consciousness. Managing the ABCs by maximizing oxygenation and perfusion, and undertaking prompt transport to an appropriate facility, are of paramount importance.

Other basic skills

A number of other basic skills of prehospital care are essential in the management of the injured patient in the field – bandaging, splinting, spinal immobilization, extrication – and these are described elsewhere. Training and quality improvement efforts should emphasize that, while important, none of these techniques and efforts should significantly delay treatment and transport. Indeed, many of the more complex bandaging procedures can be accomplished in transit.

Spinal immobilization should be routine for all seriously injured patients. The only patients who do not require complete spinal immobilization are those who are fully awake, not intoxicated, have no neck or back pain or tenderness, and no other significant injuries which might distract their appreciation of pain from a spinal injury. Since this essentially eliminates the vast majority of injured patients, the safest policy is to undertake spinal precautions in all. Spinal precautions include the use of a semirigid collar, sand bags or rolls beside the head, and securing the head and torso with tape and belts to a full-length spinal board.

QUALITY MANAGEMENT AND RESEARCH

Quality improvement is exceedingly important in prehospital trauma care and it can and does have significant measurable effects on outcome. Quality management projects in the area are often reported to advance knowledge in the field and to contribute to research.

One approach to quality management is outlined below. An essential component of whichever model is followed is to involve the staff at all stages of project planning, implementation, evaluation and reporting. Quality management must be seen as a corporate responsibility that will contribute to better outcomes for patients, rather than as a punitive 'witch hunt' to identify and discipline poor performers.

Identify the patient population

The first task of the quality management team is to identify the patient population to be studied. Projects are best limited to well-defined groups of patients rather than the entire population served. This allows a more accurate description of the pathways of care and changes in quality indicators will be more readily apparent.

Define the pathway of care

The pathway of care describes all of the components of prehospital care for the defined population, in the order in which they occur. It is worthwhile attempting to identify all internal and external factors that may influence the pathway so that the causes of changes in the quality indicator(s) can be determined. For some projects, it is useful to identify components and steps in the pathway as being 'pre-event', 'event', and 'postevent'. Pre-event components include factors relating to the availability of appropriate equipment and trained personnel, as well as factors leading to the injury producing the event itself. Event steps in the pathway begin with the incident and access to emergency services, and continue until the patient is transferred to the care of hospital personnel, and records are completed. Postevent components include factors influencing subsequent phases of hospital care, as well as the record review, quality management, and continuing education activities of the ambulance service.

Select a quality indicator

A quality indicator is a measure of the process or outcome of care provided to the patient population as a result of the defined pathway of care. The indicator should fairly reflect the results of the care provided and should be readily available and quantifiable. As far as possible, indicators are selected that are wholly or largely dependent on the pathway of care. Mortality rates, while available and quantifiable, are usually dependent on too many variables to be useful. On the other hand, time measures such as time-at-scene or response times are clear reflections of prehospital care. Successful procedural rates such as intubations or intravenous start times are useful, as are cost analyses. Indicators should have both intuitive and scientific validity; they should be acceptable to those involved to represent a fair and reasonable measure of the care provided, and ideally should be selected from indicators or measures already validated in the literature.

Evaluate baseline

With the indicator selected, a baseline evaluation is conducted. The results for the defined patient population within a representative time frame are analysed and reported.

Select component and implement change

With the baseline results available, the team then selects a component or step in the pathway for change. If the project is also to be utilized for research purposes, a research hypothesis can be established at this stage. The hypothesis postulates that the change(s) in the component selected will result in a measurable improvement in the indicator selected; i.e. that a new laryngoscope will result in more successful intubations, or that a new dispatch algorithm will improve response times. The proposed change is then implemented.

Evaluate results

The indicator is monitored on a prospective basis, to identify changes. Usually, results should not be reported to personnel until the study period is completed as this may introduce bias and confounding variables.

Report

Once the study and analysis are completed, the results should be widely shared so that the personnel involved can see the positive results of the changes that they have made. If possible and appropriate, the report should be published. This not only helps to recognize quality improvements but also contributes to knowledge and may help other services to improve the quality of care they are providing.

Bibliography

BAKER, S.P., O'NEILL, B., HADDON, W. et al. (1974). The injury severity score: a method for describing patients with multiple injuries and evaluating emergency care. J. Trauma, 14, 187.

BAXT, W.G., BERRY, C.C., EPPERSON, M.D. et al. (1989). The failure of prehospital trauma prediction rules to classify trauma patients accurately. Ann. Emerg. Med., 18, 1–8.

BAXT, W.G., JONES, G. & FORTLAGE, D. (1990). The trauma triage rule: a new resource based approach to the prehospital identification of major trauma victims. Ann. Emerg. Med., 19, 1401–6.

BORDER, J.R., LEWIS, F.R., APRAHAMIAN, C. et al. (1983). Panel: prehospital trauma care – stabilize or scoop and run. J. Trauma, 23, 708–11.

BOYD, C.R., TOLSON, M.A. & COPES, W.S. (1987). Evaluating trauma care: the TRISS method. J. Trauma, 27, 370–8.

CALES, R.H. (1984). Trauma mortality in Orange County: the effect of implementation of a regional trauma system. Ann. Emerg. Med., 13, 1–10.

CALES, R.H. (1985). Trauma scoring and prehospital triage (Editorial). Ann. Emerg. Med., 14, 1005.

CALES, R.H. (1986). Injury severity determination: requirements, approaches, and applications. Ann. Emerg. Med., 15, 1427.

CALES, R.H., ANDERSON, P.T. & HEILIG, R.W. (1985). Utilization of medical care in Orange County: the effect of implementation of a regional trauma system. Ann. Emerg. Med., 14, 853–8.

CAMPBELL, J.E. (1988a). BTLS: Basic Prehospital Trauma Care. Englewood Cliffs, NJ: Prentice-Hall.

CAMPBELL, J.E. (1988b). Basic Trauma Life Support: Advanced Prehospital Care. Englewood Cliffs, NJ: Prentice-Hall.

CAYTEN, G., LONGMORE, W., KUEHL, A. et al. (1985). Prolongation of scene time by advanced life support (ALS) in an urban setting. J. Trauma, 25, 679.

CHAMPION, H.R. (1982). Field triage of trauma victims. Ann. Emerg. Med., 11, 160.

CHAMPION, H.R., SACCO, W.J., HANNAN, D.S. et al. (1980a). Assessment of injury severity: the triage index. Crit. Care Med., 8, 201.

CHAMPION, H.R., SACCO, W.J., LEPPER, R.L. et al. (1980b). An anatomic index of injury severity. J. Trauma, 20, 188.

CHAMPION, H.R., SACCO, W.J., CARNAZZO, A.J. et al. (1981). Trauma score. Crit. Care Med., 9, 672–6.

CHAMPION, H.R., SACCO, W.J., GAINER, P.S. et al. (1988). The effect of medical direction on trauma triage. J. Trauma, 28, 235–9.

CHAMPION, H.R., SACCO, W.J., COPES, W.S. et al. (1989). A revision of the trauma score. J. Trauma, 20, 188.

COWLEY, R.A., HUDSON, F., SCALAN, E. et al. (1973). An economical and proved helicopter program for transporting the emergency critically ill and injured patient in Maryland. J. Trauma, 13, 1029–38.

CWINN, A.A., PONS, P.T., MOORE, E.E. et al. (1987). Prehospital advanced trauma life support for critical blunt trauma victims. Ann. Emerg. Med., 16, 399–403.

EICHELBERGER, M.R., GOTSCHALL, C.S., SACCO, W.J. et al. (1989). A comparison of the Trauma Score, the Revised Trauma Score and the Paediatric Trauma Score. Ann. Emerg. Med., 18, 1053–8.

EMERMAN, C.L., SHADE, B., KUBINCANEK, J. (1991). A comparison of EMT judgement and prehospital trauma triage instruments. J. Trauma, 31, 1369–75.

GORMICAN, S.P. (1982). CRAMS scale: field triage of trauma victims. Ann. Emerg. Med., 11, 132.

GUSS, D.A., MEYER, F.T., NEUMAN, T.S. et al. (1989). The impact of regionalized trauma system on trauma care in San Diego County. Ann. Emerg. Med., 18, 1141.

HEDGES, J.R., SACCO, W.J. & CHAMPION, H.R. (1982). An analysis of prehospital care of blunt trauma. J. Trauma, 22, 989–93.

HEDGES, J.R., FERRO, S., MOORE, B. et al. (1988). Factors contributing to paramedic on scene time during evaluation and management of blunt trauma. Am. J. Emerg. Med., 6, 443–8.

JACOBS, L.M., SINCLAIR, A., BEISER, A. et al. (1984). Prehospital advanced life support: benefits in trauma. J. Trauma, 24, 8–13.

KAWESKI, S.M., SISE, M.J. & VIRGILIO, R.W. (1990). The assessment of prehospital fluids on surgical in trauma patients. J. Trauma, 30, 1215–19.

KILBERG, L., CLEMMER, T.P., CLAWSON, J. et al. (1988). Effectiveness of implementing a trauma triage system on outcome: a prospective evaluation. J. Trauma, 28, 1493.

KNOPP, R., YANAGI, A., KALISEN, G. et al. (1988). Mechanisms of injury and anatomic injury as criteria for prehospital trauma triage. Ann. Emerg. Med., 17, 895.

KOEHLER, J.J., BAER, L.J., MALAFA, S.A. et al. (1986). Prehospital Index: a scoring system for field triage of trauma victims. Ann. Emerg. Med., 15, 178–82.

KOEHLER, J.J., MALAFA, S.A., HILLESLAND, J. et al. (1987). A multi-centre validation of the prehospital index. Ann. Emerg. Med., 16, 380.

LEWIS, F.R. (1986). Prehospital intravenous fluid therapy: physiological computer modelling. J. Trauma, 26, 804–11.

MACKENZIE, E.J. (1984). Injury severity scales: overview and directions for future research. Am. J. Emerg. Med., 2, 527.

MACKENZIE, E.J., SHAPIRO, S. & EASTHAN, J.

(1985). Rating AIS severity using emergency department sheets vs. in-patient charts. *J. Trauma*, **25**, 984.

MANINGAS, P.A. & BELLAMY, R.F. (1986). Hypertonic sodium chloride solutions for the prehospital management of traumatic hemorrhagic shock: a possible improvement in the standard of care? *Ann. Emerg. Med.*, **15**, 1411.

MANINGAS, P.A., MATTOX, K.L., PEPE, P.E. *et al.* (1989). Hypertonic saline–dextran solutions for the prehospital management of traumatic hypotension. *Am. J. Surg.*, **157**, 528–34.

MASLANKA, A.M. (1993). Scoring systems and triage from the field. *Emerg. Med. Clin. North Am.*, **11**, 15–27.

MATTOX, K.L., BICKELL, W.H., PEPE, P.E. *et al.* (1986). Prospective randomized evaluation of anti-shock MAST in post traumatic hypotension. *J. Trauma*, **26**, 779–86.

MATTOX, K.L., BICKELL, W.H., PEPE, P.E. (1989). Prospective MAST study in 911 patients. *J. Trauma*, **29**, 1104–12.

MATTOX, K.L., MANINGAS, P.A., MOORE, E.E. *et al.* (1991). Prehospital hypertonic saline–dextran infusion for post traumatic hypotension: The USA Multi-Centre Trial. *Ann. Surg.*, **213**, 482.

MOREAU, M., GAINER, P.S., CHAMPION, H. *et al.* (1985). Application of the trauma score in the prehospital setting. *Ann. Emerg. Med.*, **14**, 1049–54.

MORRIS, J.A., AUERBACH, P.S., MARSHALL, G.A. *et al.* (1986). The trauma score as a triage tool in a prehospital setting. *JAMA*, **256**, 1319–25.

O'GORMAN, M., TRABULSY, P., PILCHER, D.B. (1989). Zero-time prehospital. IV. *J. Trauma*, **29**, 84.

ORNATO, J., MLINEK, Jr., E.A. & CRAREN, E.J. (1985). Ineffectiveness of the trauma score and the CRAMS scale for accurately triaging patients to trauma centres. *Ann. Emerg. Med.*, **14**, 1061.

POLLACK, C.V. (1993). Prehospital fluid resuscitation of the trauma patient: an update on the controversies. *Emerg. Med. Clin. North Am.*, **11**, 61–70.

PONS, P.T., MOORE, E.E., CUSICK, J.M. *et al.* (1988). Prehospital venous access in an urgan paramedic system – a prospective on scene analysis. *J. Trauma*, **28**, 1460–3.

POTTER, D., GOLDSTEIN, G., FUNG, S.C. *et al.* (1988). A controlled trial of prehospital advanced life support in trauma. *Ann. Emerg. Med.*, **17**, 588.

SACCO, W.J., CHAMPION, H.R., GAINER, P.S. *et al.* (1984). The Trauma Score as applied to penetrating trauma. *Ann. Emerg. Med.*, **13**, 415.

SCHWAB, C.W., CIVIL, I. & SHAYNE, J.P. (1986a). Saline-expanded group O uncrossmatched packed red blood cells as an initial resuscitation fluid in severe shock. *Ann. Emerg. Med.*, **15**, 1282.

SCHWAB, C.W., SHAYNE, J.P. & TURNER, J. (1986b). Immediate trauma resuscitation with type O uncrossmatched blood: a 2-year prospective experience. *J. Trauma*, **26**, 897.

SHACKFORD, S.R., MACKERSIE, R.C., HOYT, D.B. *et al.* (1987). Impact of a trauma system on outcome of severely injured patients. *Arch. Surg.*, **122**, 523–7.

SHATNEY, C.H., DEEPIKA, K., MILLIPELLO, P.R. *et al.* (1983). Efficacy of hetastarch in the resuscitation of patients with multi-system trauma and shock. *Arch. Surg.*, **118**, 804.

SLOVIS, C.M., HERR, E.W., LONDORF, D. *et al.* (1990). Success rates for initiation of intravenous therapy en route by prehospital care providers. *Am. J. Emerg. Med.*, **8**, 305–7.

SMITH, P., BODAI, B., HILL, A. *et al.* (1985). Prehospital stabilization of critically injury patients: a failed concept. *J. Trauma*, **25**, 65–70.

SPAITE, D.W. & JOSEPH, M. (1990). Prehospital cricothyrotomy: an investigation of indications, technique, complications, and patient outcome. *Ann. Emerg. Med.*, **19**, 279–85.

SPAITE, D.W., TFE, D.J., VALENZUELA, T.D. *et al.* (1991). The impact of injury severity and prehospital procedures on scene time in victims of major trauma. *Ann. Emerg. Med.*, **20**, 1299–305.

TEASDALE, G. & JENNET, B. (1974). Assessment of coma and impaired consciousness: a practical scale. *Lancet*, **ii**:81.

TRUNKEY, D. (1983). Trauma. *Sci. Am.*, **249**, 28.

TRUNKEY, D. (1984). Is ALS necessary for prehospital trauma care? *J. Trauma*, **24**, 86–7.

WALSH, J.C., ZHUANG, J. & SHACKFORD, S.R. (1991). A comparison of hypertonic to isotonic fluid in the resuscitation of brain injury and hemorrhage shock. *J. Surg. Res.*, **50**, 284.

WEST, J.G., TRUNKEY, D.D. & LIM, R.C. (1979). Systems of trauma care: a study of two counties. *Arch. Surg.*, **114**, 455.

WEST, J.G., CALES, R.H. & GAZZANIGA, A.G. (1983). Impact of regionalization: the Orange County experience. *Arch. Surg.*, **118**, 740.

C(ii): Interhospital transport of the trauma patient

P.L. LANE

Trauma Services, Victoria Hospital, London, Ontario, Canada

INTRODUCTION

The definitive care of severely injured patients requires specialized expertise and equipment beyond the capabilities of most facilities. Concerns for both the quality of care and for cost-efficiency have led to the rationalization of trauma care to specialized facilities such as the Baltimore Shock Trauma Unit, and the Sunnybrook Regional Trauma Unit. One of the consequences of this trend to regionalized care has been an increasing need to transport acutely injured patients from community hospitals where they are resuscitated to the regional facility. With the trend to regionalization has come the understanding that trauma care is a continuum with several components. Regional centres play a lead role in coordinating and improving all components along the continuum, including the interhospital transport of critically injured patients. Fig. 1 provides an overview of the 'journey of the trauma patient', identifying many of these components.

The interhospital transport of trauma patients places different demands on the system than the transport of other categories of critically ill patients. Systems developed primarily to serve the needs of perinatal patients or patients with overwhelming sepsis and multiple organ system failure must be adapted to meet the requirements of the acutely injured. Patients with complex medical illnesses typically require highly specialized care in transit and extensive intervention by the escort team prior to transportation. Critically injured patients, on the other hand, require rapid and effective stabilization of the 'ABCs' – Airway, Breathing and Circulation – with a minimal degree of intervention and rapid transport.

Delays can significantly compromise the outcome, and the goal must be to get the patient to definitive care at the trauma centre within the first few hours after injury in order to take advantage of the 'window of opportunity'. The commonest causes of delays are:

- Overzealous resuscitation in the referring hospital – performing too many X-rays, investigations or procedures.
- Prolonged response times to mobilize transport teams and equipment.

Regional trauma centres play an essential leadership role in ensuring that the critical care transport system meets the special needs of trauma patients in their region.

WHY TRANSPORT TRAUMA PATIENTS?

Simply stated, a trauma patient should be transported when the anticipated patient care requirements exceed the capacity of the hospital.

These requirements can be assessed in terms of space, equipment, personnel, and expertise.

Space is becoming an increasingly precious commodity in cost-constrained health delivery systems. Both community hospitals and tertiary care centres face the issue on a regular basis. In terms of trauma patients, transport may be necessary because of the lack of availability of beds in the intensive care unit, the surgical ward, or lack of operating room availability. Trauma systems need to ensure that medical information systems are in place to allow the resuscitating physician in the emergency department to know, on a minute-to-minute basis, the current resource status of the hospital. Similarly, physicians charged with the responsibility of receiving referrals from community hospitals need to know the current resource status of their institution so that immediate decisions can be made when the referring phone call or radio transmission is received, avoiding the necessity of 'calling back'.

Equipment needs may be a determining factor. Many injured patients require specialized imaging such as computed tomography (CT), magnetic resonance imaging (MRI), angiography, or other facilities not available in the community hospital. Specialized therapeutic equipment such as membrane oxygenators, jet ventilators, intracranial pressure monitors and orthopaedic fixation devices may not be available either.

Personnel shortages, such as the lack of critical care nurses, may be a factor. This is increasingly a problem with cost-containment efforts of hospitals. Also, the hospital may be overwhelmed by work, resulting in staff shortages. Again, this information must be available in the emergency department so that appropriate referral decisions can be made without delay.

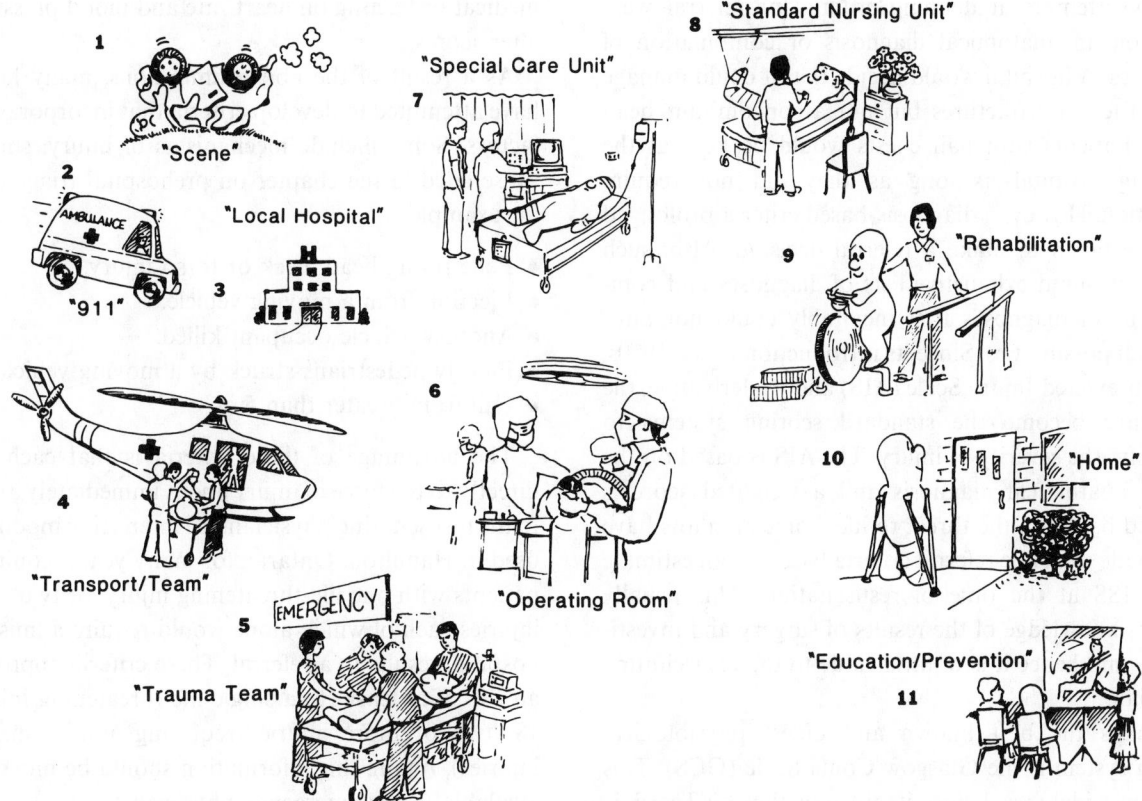

Fig. 1. Journey of the trauma patient. (Reproduced by permission of Director of Corporate Communications, Victoria Hospital.)

The *expertise* required to care for the severely injured patient is the commonest reason for referral. Community hospitals will not normally have the necessary medical, surgical, nursing and allied health expertise to manage the complex acute and subsequent needs of the severely injured patient. With system rationalization, many tertiary care centres will have recruited staff and developed expertise in other areas – transplantation, oncology, geriatrics, cardiac surgery – and will not be staffed to meet the needs of trauma patients.

WHO TO TRANSPORT?

The decision of a hospital to define the care of severely injured patients as a primary mission implies a significant commitment. By the same token, the decision of an institution not to care for the trauma population requires a commitment to define which patients will be cared for and which will be referred. The medical staff of the hospital, in conjunction with the regional referral centre, should define criteria by which referral decisions can be made. The emergency physician in the midst of a complex and stressful resuscitation should not have to 'guess'

whether or not the hospital can care for the patient. Trauma referral criteria should be developed so that the information required to make the decision is available within the first few minutes of the resuscitation; i.e. the decision should not be dependent upon the results of complex and time-consuming investigations such as a CT scan, or the results of surgical exploration. Criteria should be sufficiently sensitive to identify all severely injured patients in need of trauma centre care. This will result in an expected false positive referral rate, i.e. patients referred who ultimately are determined not to have suffered severe injury. Some systems define severe injury in terms of the Injury Severity Score (ISS), with an ISS greater than 15 being considered severe injury needing referral. If at least 10–15% of referrals do not have an ISS less than 15, the criteria used are not sensitive enough and severely injured patients are probably being missed.

Several different criteria have been proposed and are in use. They may be based on anatomical criteria, physiological scoring methods, or a combination of both. The accuracy of these criteria should be monitored and improved continuously.

Early attempts at defining criteria for referral were based on an anatomical diagnosis or combination of diagnoses. A hospital would decide that it could manage isolated femoral fractures but not a concomitant head injury. Patients with flail chests would be kept at the receiving hospital as long as they did not require intubation. However, diagnosis-based criteria prolonged the time taken to make a referral decision. Also, such criteria required exhaustive lists of diagnoses and combinations of diagnoses that inevitably could not anticipate all possibilities. Since its introduction in the 1970s, the Abbreviated Injury Scale (AIS) and its derivative, the ISS, have become the standard scoring systems to 'quantify' the severity of injury. The AIS is based on the precise anatomical diagnosis and a weighted score is assigned based on the threat to life. Some attempts have been made to define referral criteria based on an estimate of the ISS at the time of resuscitation. This usually requires knowledge of the results of surgery and investigations and hence it is of little value to the resuscitating physician.

Perhaps the best known and oldest physiological scoring system is the Glasgow Coma Scale (GCS). This has been widely used since its introduction by Teasdale & Jennett in 1974 as a measure of the level of consciousness. Some hospitals have incorporated this into referral criteria in the sense that patients with a GCS of less than a predefined cut-off point, usually 10 or 12, should be referred to a trauma centre for possible neurosurgical intervention. A number of other physiological scoring systems have been proposed and tested, notably the Trauma Score (TS), the Revised Trauma Score (RTS), the Paediatric Trauma Score (PTS), and the CRAMS scale (Circulation, Respiration, Abdomen, Motor, and Speech). Each of these systems has its advocates and more or less measures the same thing. Any significant compromise of respiratory, circulatory and/or neurological function results in a score that is correlated with severe injury and mandates referral to a trauma centre. Unfortunately, all of the systems noted produce relatively high rates of false positive and false negative decisions. Physiological parameters depend on a variety of factors other than the severity of injury. Assessments performed too early may not identify patients with significant hypovolaemia while they may overestimate the severity of brain injury. These parameters are clearly affected by the treatment provided; paradoxically, effective treatment may result in an underestimation of the severity of injury. Comorbid factors such as the presence of intoxicants, heart and lung disease, or medications acting on heart rate and blood pressure can alter scores.

As a result of the above limitations, many hospitals have attempted to develop criteria that incorporate other factors. Some include mechanisms of injury, similar to those cited in the chapter on prehospital triage criteria; for example:

- Penetrating head, neck or torso injury.
- Ejection from a moving vehicle.
- Another vehicle occupant killed.
- Elderly pedestrians struck by a moving vehicle.
- Fall from greater than 5 m.

The advantage of these criteria is that each relates directly to the force of injury and is immediately available to the resuscitating physician. An interesting modification used in Hamilton, Ontario, for many years requires that patients with one life-threatening injury, or two or more injuries each of which alone would require admission to hospital, results in a referral. These criteria approximate an ISS of at least 16 (a single life-threatening injury) or 18 (two or more injuries requiring admission, AIS 3 injuries). Again, this information should be immediately available to the emergency physician.

Ultimately, each hospital and its medical staff must consult with their regional trauma hospital and develop criteria. These should be monitored and modified continuously to best serve the needs of their trauma patients.

WHEN TO REFER AND TRANSPORT?

The call to the trauma centre is ideally made as soon as the decision to refer is taken. Often, the information necessary to make the decision is available within a few minutes of the patient's arrival and this is when the call should be made. Unlike other categories of patients referred, it is not necessary to make a precise diagnosis and to fully complete the assessment and stabilization before contacting the referral centre. The early call to the trauma centre allows several things to occur. The receiving physician, surgeon, or trauma team leader may be able to provide advice regarding resuscitation and can begin to mobilize trauma centre staff and resources to prepare for the arrival of the patient. It may be necessary to mobilize transport vehicles and escort staff and this can be done while the resuscitation continues.

While the initial attempt to contact may be made by clerical or nursing personnel, referrals are always made physician-to-physician. It is inappropriate and potentially detrimental to delegate this to other staff. Trauma centre staff should be immediately available to take a phone call from a referring physician at all times and the physician taking the call should have the authority to make the decision to accept immediately, without checking hospital status or consulting a more senior physician. The referral call or transmission should include a brief report of the mechanism of injury, the patient's clinical status, injuries identified, and interventions performed. The receiving physician may make some suggestions about further investigations or interventions in preparation for transport but these should be limited to only those tests and interventions needed to ensure safe rapid transport. The two physicians should then discuss and agree upon the mode of transport, escorts required, medical responsibility in transport, and the estimated time of arrival at the trauma centre.

When to transport might seem to be a relatively simple matter – the patient should be transported as soon as possible once the airway is secured, respiratory and circulatory states are stable, lines and tubes are inserted and secured, and the vehicle and escorts are available. Unfortunately, it is rarely that simple. Severely injured patients are rarely, by definition, 'stable'. Hence, considerable judgement is required on the part of the referring physician regarding the safest moment to leave. This judgement will be based on weighing the risks of delay and further intervention against the risks of deterioration of the patient prior to arrival at the trauma centre. It should be possible to secure an airway and adequate respiratory function in any emergency department with the insertion of endotracheal and chest drainage tubes if indicated. However, haemodynamic and neurological instability pose much more difficult problems. As a rule, patients in persistent shock should not be tranported. However, if the sending institution lacks the surgical capability to operate to identify the cause and repair the problem, then occasionally it may be necessary to leave with a patient in shock while fluid and blood infusions continue. Similarly, patients with deteriorating neurological status, particularly if accompanied by lateralizing signs, may require surgical intervention before transport. Such decisions should be made in conjunction with the surgical consultants at the trauma centre.

HOW TO TRANSPORT?

The question of how to transport the severely injured patient can be best understood by addressing the components involved: vehicles, equipment, personnel,

and protocols. In addition, the special considerations and restrictions imposed by the form of transportation will be discussed.

Vehicles

The choice of vehicle depends largely on availability, response time, and travel time. The goal of interhospital transport must be to minimize the time between hospitals, and to avoid complications in transit, i.e. safe rapid transport. It follows then that the preferable vehicle is a fixed wing aircraft for longer journeys (more than 500 km), a rotary wing aircraft for intermediate journeys (100–500 km), and a land vehicle for short transfers. Each of the three can be configured to safely transport the patient and escorts. However, aircraft are an expensive resource and are not usually based in rural or small urban communities. Consequently, their response times become crucial – how long it takes to fly to the smaller community to pick up the patient. In North America, helicopters tend to be based in the larger urban areas where the trauma centre is located. As a rule, therefore, it usually takes approximately the same length of time to mobilize and fly to the referring hospital as it would to travel the distance by land in a regular ambulance. The advantage of the helicopter then is to minimize interhospital time, allowing more time at the referring institution to stabilize the patient. This reinforces the benefits of making the call to the trauma centre as early as possible to allow the vehicle to be mobilized and arrangements to be made while the resuscitation continues. With fixed wing aircraft, this is less of a consideration because travel time for jet or turboprop aircraft is faster and the distances are sufficiently long to make land travel not a viable option. An important consideration in the overall time equation with fixed wing aircraft is the land travel time between the airports and the hospitals at both ends of the trip.

Equipment

The ambulance environment poses special considerations with respect to the trauma patient. Basic ambulance equipment is of course necessary, including:

- Suction with sufficient capacity to last the duration of the journey.

Table 1. *Trauma transport jump kit*

Airway
- Endotracheal tubes – paediatric and adult
- Scalpel, haemostats, and tracheostomy tube

Breathing
- Chest drainage tubes
- Plastic underwater drainage reservoir
- Transport ventilator
- Oxygen saturation monitor

Circulation
- Intravenous fluids – saline and Ringer's lactate
- Intravenous tubing sets
- Intravenous catheters
- Pressure infusion cuffs/devices
- automatic BP cuff monitor
- Multichannel ECG and VS monitor
- Defibrillator

Drugs
- Lignocaine
- Adrenaline
- Atropine
- Fentanyl
- Vecuronium
- Diazepam
- 20% mannitol
- Naloxone
- Diphenhydramine
- Lignocaine spray
- Lignocaine 1% local anaesthetic
- 50% dextrose

BP. blood pressure; ECG, electrocardiogram; VS, vital signs.

- An adequate supply of high-flow oxygen for the entire trip.
- Bag–valve–mask ventilation equipment.
- Spinal splints including semirigid collars and spinal boards.
- Extremity splints.
- Bandages.
- Gloves.
- Urine containers.

In addition, it is essential that the patient, the stretcher, and all attendants and escorts are appropriately restrained at all times. Unfortunately, crashes involving land and air ambulances are not rare.

Advanced life support (ALS) is also necessary. Dedicated air ambulances should normally be stocked with the appropriate equipment and drugs. However, when basic life support (BLS) land vehicles or non-dedicated aircraft are used, the equipment and drugs will need to be obtained from the hospital. It is recommended that community hospitals have a prestocked 'jump kit' (Table 1) for such transfers. Before departure, any special needs should be considered and the kit augmented accordingly. As a general rule, anticipate disaster and be equipped to deal with it when it occurs. A frequent example is the need for extra intravenous fluids and uncross-matched blood if there is any potential for the patient to become hypotensive in transit.

Personnel/escorts

Who to send as an escort depends on the patient's needs and the personnel available. At the outset it should be stated that patients who have been so severely injured that they require transport to a trauma centre need more than a BLS ambulance attendant as an escort. By definition, these patients have sustained severe if not life-threatening injuries and accompanying personnel need to be prepared to intervene in transit. The referring physician is in the best postion to determine what clinical complications or deteriorations may arise en route and which type of escort would be most appropriate based on the 'worst case scenario'.

Given what has happened to this patient and the injuries that they may have suffered, what is the worst thing that could happen in transit?

With that in mind, personnel with sufficient skills and judgement to intervene must be sent. Patients with isolated extremity fractures who are and have been stable can be accompanied by a nurse alone. However, patients with head and neck, chest, abdominal, or back injuries or who have been unstable in any way should be accompanied by escorts who can recognize deterioration and intervene – intubate, give drugs, start another intravenous infusion, administer blood, etc. This requires either a physician or an appropriately trained ALS provider (e.g. paramedic or transport nurse with extended training).

BLS ambulance attendant

The basic ambulance attendant does not have the skills, judgement, or the authority to care for the severely injured patient in transit between hospitals. To resuscitate patients in a hospital, define that they are severely injured and require trauma centre care, and then send them in an ambulance with a basic crew is a significant step down in care. It would have been wiser to transport directly to the trauma centre in the first place because the crew cannot intervene if the patient deteriorates en route. However, as BLS attendants are more familiar with the vehicle, its equipment, and its limitations, their role in support of ALS escorts is important.

Nurse

The accompanying nurse, if alone, assumes considerable responsibility. She/he should ensure that all the necessary equipment for patient monitoring and care is available. The referring physician should formally transfer care to the nurse, discuss problems which may occur in transit, give 'prn' orders to intervene if problems arise, and be available throughout to give advice or further orders by radio or phone. If possible, contingency plans should be made to divert to a closer hospital if significant deterioration occurs. The nurse should be prepared to give a formal report to the waiting team on arrival at the trauma centre.

ALS provider

Each jurisdiction has its own regulations and requirements regarding training, certification, procedural skills and medical responsibility for ALS providers. The designations used vary greatly as well – paramedics, EMT-P (emergency medical technician), critical care transport technician, extended role nurse, to name only a few. Usually, ALS providers will have begun their training and career in another role before their advanced training – nurse, ambulance attendant, respiratory therapist, etc. To be useful in the setting of the interhospital transport of trauma patients, these ALS personnel must have, as a minimum, advanced assessment and procedural skills including endotracheal intubation, ventilation, intravenous infusion and maintenance, blood administration, intravenous drug therapy including all ACLS (advanced cardiac life support) drugs plus the use of paralytic agents and mannitol, and gastric tube and Foley catheter insertion. In many jurisdictions, this skill set will need to be expanded in the light of the transport times involved, the types of vehicles used, the degree of stabilization usually required in the referring hospitals prior to departure, the equipment and drugs

available, and whether or not paediatric and neonatal patients are transported. With appropriate training, protocols, and medical control, ALS personnel are usually the most appropriate personnel to send with trauma patients as they have all the skills necessary to intervene and are familiar with the transit environment. In many ways, they are more appropriate and better suited to care for the trauma patient in transit than many physicians.

Physician

For most physicians, the transfer of a trauma patient is one of the most difficult and stressful roles that they may undertake in their careers. The patients are unstable, their clinical course in transit is unpredictable, and the environment imposes severe restrictions on the physician's ability to monitor and intervene. Accompanying physicians should be sufficiently senior and skilled to make decisions in the vehicle without having to radio to a senior for advice. Most physicians find it helpful to also be accompanied by a nurse or ALS provider, preferably one familiar with the vehicle and the transport environment. The physician should, before leaving, familiarize him/herself with the equipment and drugs available and fully understand the patient's condition, clinical course and injuries. Again, before leaving, the physician should anticipate disaster and be prepared for it.

Pretransport checklist

- Check position and secure all tubes
- Ensure at least two intravenous lines
- Tape all lines securely
- Ensure chest X-ray to rule out pneumothorax
- Ensure gastric tube and Foley catheter and secure
- Use full spinal precautions, secure firmly to the board
- Secure all dressings
- Get a full report and any orders
- Get all records, X-rays and lab results
- Check transport equipment, drugs and intravenous fluids

Protocols for transport

Physician-to-physician

The referral of a severely injured patient is made from the physician in the community hospital to the physician in the trauma centre. Before any transport can take place, there should be direct communication between the two. The severely injured patient should *not* be loaded into the ambulance before the call is made. It is the responsibility of the trauma centre to have a senior or consultant-level physician, capable and authorized to make the decision to accept and to give advice about resuscitation. Staff in the referring hospital are busy resuscitating the patient and cannot afford to spend time making several calls. The receiving physician or surgeon on call should not be unavailable in the operating room or clinic. The referring physician and staff in the community hospital should be familiar with how to access the appropriate physician in the regional trauma centre so that frustrating delays are avoided.

Medical responsibility for care in transit

In most cases, the medical responsibility for care in transit lies with the referring physician until the patient arrives at the trauma centre. As such, the referring physician needs to think through the care that may be needed and give appropriate orders to escorting personnel. The physician should be available for radio or telephone consultation in the event that the patient's clinical status changes and the escorts need advice or new orders. If ALS providers are to accompany the patient then medical responsibility for care in transit reverts to the ALS control authority, or base hospital once the patient leaves. Of course, a physician accompanying the patient in transit bears medical responsibility.

Communications in transit

Efforts should be made to ensure a communications link is maintained throughout the transfer. This is particularly important if the escorts are non-physicians as a secure link with the responsible physician is essential. As a minimum, it is important to inform the trauma centre either directly or through a link with the radio dispatch centre of the time of departure and, a few minutes later, to give an accurate estimate of the time of arrival. The second call should also inform the trauma centre staff of the patient's clinical condition and of any immediate needs upon arrival.

When disaster strikes

Despite the best preparation and care, disaster will strike eventually. Trauma patients are severely injured and often unstable and their clinical course cannot always be predicted. Vehicles travelling rapidly, usually at night and often in poor weather, do break down and occasionally crash. Communications systems seem particularly prone to failure just when they are needed most. Protocols should be in place for the different types of disaster that can and will occur. The worst is a cardiac arrest. If this occurs, there is very little that can be done for the trauma patient in a land ambulance or an aircraft. Protocols should be established whereby, if the patient does arrest, the ambulance diverts to the nearest hospital. If anything is to be done for the patient, it will usually require immediate surgical intervention so diversion should occur to the nearest hospital with that capability. A sudden deterioration in the patient's condition may also necessitate such a diversion. In this instance, the responsible physician should be contacted for orders. If communications fail, the escort personnel must then determine whether to continue or to divert. Usually, as long as the patient is stable, it is safe to continue. Communication systems failures are often temporary. However, if the escorts determine the urgent need for medical contact and intervention because of a change in the patient's status, then diversion will be necessary. In the case of air transports, protocols should be in place to guide the crew if the aircraft goes down. At least one crew member should be trained in survival techniques in hostile environments. Survival equipment should be routinely carried aboard aircraft used for such transfers. Escort personnel should bear responsibility not only for the patient but for any other injured crew as well.

Special considerations of the transport environment

Ambulances, particularly land vehicles, are almost the worst environment in which to care for a critically injured patient. Space limitations, movement, noise, power sources, lighting and, if flying, atmospheric pressure all impose restrictions.

Space limitations, particularly in land and rotary wing vehicles, mean that access to the patient is severely restricted. Escorts must position themselves so that they can ensure access to the head and upper torso of the patient. Most patient transport compartments have a very low roof as well so that pressure infusion devices will be necessary to ensure the flow of intravenous fluids and blood.

Vehicle movement makes the performance of even the most routine medical procedures challenging. If the patient requires in intravenous line or the insertion of an endotracheal tube, it is usually safest to stop the vehicle. This, of course, is not an option with air transport. Movement can induce motion sickness in staff as well as patients. The patient, secured in the supine position to a board with only the ceiling to look at, will in all likelihood become nauseated so a gastric tube is mandatory. Staff should be prepared for motion sickness; some are more affected than others. Vehicle movement also renders much hospital-based monitoring equipment useless. Movement artefact can make an ECG monitor or arterial pressure monitor unreadable. Fortunately, some manufacturers are now producing very good electronic equipment for use in transit.

The noise level in most vehicles makes the use of a stethoscope almost impossible. Some other technique for measuring blood pressure is needed. Even the palpation of a normal pulse can be very difficult. Chest auscultation is not possible unless the vehicle has stopped or some sort of electronically augmented stethoscope is used.

Vehicles depend upon battery sources for electric power. As a result, hospital-based equipment which requires alternating current (AC) cannot be used without either its own battery or a DC/AC converter. The lighting in vehicles can often be frustrating and an alternative light source is useful – even the simple flashlight.

The changes in atmospheric pressure which result from flying at altitude can have significant effects on patient, equipment and staff. Fortunately helicopters can fly at low altitude if necessary and many fixed wing air transport vehicles have pressurized cabins. Several other sources describe the effects of atmospheric pressure changes more comprehensively than required here but a special note should be made regarding trapped gases. As atmospheric pressure falls with ascent, the volume occupied by a gas increases. Clinically, this means that any trapped gases will expand. This is of particular relevance in the trauma patient. If the patient has a small or moderate pneumothorax at ground level, this will expand upon ascent and further compromise breathing. Similarly, air trapped in the gut will expand. This underscores the need for a chest X-ray prior to transfer, and a chest drainage tube if there is any question of a pneumothorax. It also justifies a gastric tube for all trauma patients.

QUALITY MANAGEMENT AND RESEARCH

Interhospital transfer is an extremely important step in the 'journey of the trauma patient'. It must be accomplished both safely and rapidly. Care given at this stage has a profound effect on the outcome of the patient. Improvements made in the interhospital phase are important and have measurable consequences. The quality management methodology outlined in the previous part of this chapter facilitates this. Research continues to further knowledge in this area. Some examples are cited in the references listed.

Bibliography

ASSOCIATION FOR THE ADVANCEMENT OF AUTOMOTIVE MEDICINE (1990). *Abbreviated Injury Scale (AIS) – 1990 Revision*. Des Plaines, IL: Association for the Advancement of Automotive Medicine.

BAXT, W.G. & MOODY, P. (1983). The impact of a rotorcraft aeromedical emergency care service on trauma mortality. *JAMA*, **249**, 3047–51.

BAXT, W.G. & MOODY, P. (1987a). The impact of advanced prehospital emergency care on the mortality of severely brain-injured patients. *J. Trauma*, **27**, 365–9.

BAXT, W.G. & MOODY P. (1987b). The impact of a physician as part of the aeromedical prehospital team in patients with blunt trauma. *JAMA*, **257**, 3246–50.

BAXT, W.G., MOODY, P., CLEVELAND, H.C. et al. (1985). Hospital based rotorcraft aeromedical emergency care services and trauma mortality: a multi-centre study. *Ann. Emerg. Med.*, **14**, 859–64, 1985.

BAXT, W.G., BERRY, C.C., EPPERSON, M.D. et al. (1989). The failure of prehospital trauma prediction rules to classify trauma patients accurately. *Ann. Emerg. Med.*, **18**, 1–8.

BURNEY, R.E. & FISCHER, R.P. (1986). Ground vs. air transport of trauma victims: medical and logistical considerations. *Ann. Emerg. Med.*, **15**, 1491–5.

CAMPBELL, J.E. (1988a). *BTLS: Basic Prehospital Trauma Care*. Englewood Cliffs, NJ: Prentice-Hall.

CAMPBELL, J.E. (1988b). *Basic Trauma Life Support: Advanced Prehospital Care*. Englewood Cliffs, NJ: Prentice-Hall.

CLEVELAND, H.C., BIGELOW, D.B. et al. (1976). A civilian air emergency service: A report of its development, technical aspects, and experience. *J. Trauma*, **16**, 452–63.

EHRENWERTH, J., SORBO, S. & HACKEL, A. (1983). Transport of critically ill adults. *Crit. Care Med.*, **14**, 543–7.

EICHELBERGER, M.R., GOTSCHALL, C.S., SACCO, W.J. et al. (1989). A comparison of the Trauma Score, the Revised Trauma Score, and the Paediatric Trauma Score. *Ann. Emerg. Med.*, **18**, 1053–8.

FARNELL, M.B. & SACHS, J.L. (1989). Mayo clinic's hospital based emergency air medical transport service. *Mayo Clin. Proc.*, **64**, 1213–25.

GIROTTI, M.J. & PAGLIARELLO, G. (1988). Transport of critically ill adult patients. *Am. J. Surg.*, **31**, 319–22.

KANTER, R.K. & TOMPKINS, J.M. (1989). Adverse events during interhospital transport: physiological deterioration associated with pretransport severity of illness. *Pediatrics*, **84**, 43–8.

LEICHT, M.J., DULA, D.J., BROTMAN, F. *et al.* (1986). Rural interhospital helicopter transport of motor vehicle trauma victims: causes for delays and recommendations. *Ann. Emerg. Med.*, **15**, 450–3.

MacNAB, A.J. (1991). Optimal escort for interhospital transport of pediatric emergencies. *J. Trauma*, **31**, 205–9.

MASLANKA, A.M. (1993). Scoring systems and triage from the field. *Emerg. Med. Clin. North Am.*, **11**, 15–27.

McMURTRY, R.Y. & McLELLAN, B.A. (1990). *Management of Blunt Trauma*. Baltimore, MD: Williams & Wilkins.

McMURTRY, R.Y., NELSON, W.R. & DeLaROCHE, M.R.P. (1989). Current concepts in trauma: 1. Principles and directions for development. *Can. Med. Assoc. J.*, **141**, 529–33.

SCHILLER, W.R., KNOX, R. *et al.* (1988). Effective helicopter transport of trauma victims on survival in an urban trauma centre. *J. Trauma*, **28**, 1127–34.

SCHMIDT, U., FRAME, F.B., NERLICH, M.L. *et al.* (1992). En scene helicopter transport of patients with multiple injuries – comparison of a German and an American system. *J. Trauma*, **33**, 548–55.

SCHWARTZ, R.J., JACOBS, L.M. & YAEZEL, D. (1989). Impact of pretrauma centre care on length of stay and hospital charges. *J. Trauma*, **29**, 1611–15.

SHACKFORD, S.R., MACKERSIE, R.C., HOYT, D.B. *et al.* (1987). Impact of a trauma system on outcome of severely injured patients. *Arch. Surg.*, **122**, 523–7.

15 Radiology – emergency imaging

J.G. MURRAY, J.J. CURTIN and G.J. de LACEY

Radiology Department, Northwick Park Hospital, Harrow, UK

Chapter plan

Introduction
Terminology of bone injuries
Paediatric fractures
Head injury radiology
Cervical spine trauma
Chest
Upper limb
Lower limb
The acute abdomen
Abdominal trauma
Pelvis
The testis
Foreign bodies

INTRODUCTION

Diagnostic and interventional radiology have changed markedly during the past two decades primarily as a result of the rapid development of new imaging modalities. These include ultrasound, computed tomography (CT), digital subtraction angiography and magnetic resonance imaging (MRI). These new techniques have had an effect on the investigation of patients attending the accident and emergency (A&E) department. For this reason it is important that those working in A&E are not only familiar with routine plain radiographs, but are also aware of the potential role and usefulness of the other imaging modalities.

This chapter describes the place of imaging in diagnosis and management in some areas where confusion may arise. The description is not comprehensive because many conditions are extensively covered in other chapters. Guidelines are suggested to assist clinicians make the best use of the modalities currently available.

Errors in interpretation

Recent surveys have found that over one-third of clinically significant injuries shown on plain radiographs are misinterpreted by junior doctors in A&E departments (Swain, 1986; Vincent *et al.*, 1988). The most commonly missed abnormalities are those involving the skull, spine, ankle, hand and foot. Equally disturbing was the finding that there was no improvement in performance during the junior doctors' 6-month rotation in A&E. Based on these results Vincent *et al.* (1988) and Guly (1992) believe that it is unrealistic to expect junior doctors in A&E to acquire interpretative skills simply through experience, and that more formal training and guidance is necessary. In the meantime, how might errors in interpretation be kept to a minimum? When all A&E radiographs are assessed by a radiologist the error rate is significantly reduced (Guly, 1992), yet this simple safeguard is not always put in place. In a recent review of 360 cases of radiological litigation, 278 related to trauma (Craig, 1989). In 32% of these there was no radiological report, and the films were interpreted only by junior doctors in A&E.

Unnecessary radiography

Diagnostic radiology provides 90% of the total man-made radiation exposure to the population (RCR Working Party, 1993). Doctors have thus a greater scope than any other group in reducing unnecessary radiation exposure. It has been estimated that some 20% of radiographic examinations carried out in the UK have no clinical justification (RCR Working Party, 1993). Between 30% and 70% of new patients attending an A&E department are referred for radiography (de Lacey, 1979). This wide variation in referral rates may well be due to different local approaches to investigation, occasionally compounded by confusing medicolegal perceptions, rather than being solely due to differences in case mix. In order to rationalize the use of radiological tests, the Royal College of Radiologists has published a booklet: 'Making the Best Use of a Department of Clinical Radiology: Guidelines for Doctors' (RCR Working Party, 1993). The booklet emphasizes that diagnostic radiology should only be used as an adjunct to clinical examination. The medical defence societies repeatedly stress that the best defence against litigation is proper clinical assessment, adequate clinical notes and good communication with patients. Pilling (1976), a coroner, made the role of imaging absolutely clear when stating that the law is on the side of those who, after a careful clinical examination, reasonably decide that radiographs are not necessary, even if later this is proved by events to have been wrong.

Selecting the appropriate imaging modality

Plain radiographs remain the mainstay of radiological investigation. They are readily available, and in most cases provide the clinical information required by the A&E clinician. Plain radiographs are of little value in the assessment of soft tissue injuries. Ultrasound is much more sensitive in the investigation of abdominal, pelvic and soft tissue trauma; furthermore, it is ideally suited to A&E because it is portable, and an adequate examination can rapidly be performed even on a restless patient. Recent developments including colour duplex and high resolution scanning have expanded its role to include the diagnosis of deep venous thrombosis, tendon injuries and non-opaque foreign bodies. Nuclear medicine has a limited role in the A&E department as these examinations are generally performed in a non-emergency setting. Emergency angiography is particularly useful in the assessment of the thoracic aorta, and vascular injuries associated with fractures. CT offers the most comprehensive evaluation of severe trauma to the head, thorax, abdomen and pelvis. MRI has not yet developed an established role in the assessment of acute trauma with the exception of spinal cord injury. However, the multiplanar imaging capability of MR, coupled with superb soft tissue contrast and recent reductions in scan time, will almost certainly soon result in its increased use in A&E departments. Interventional radiological procedures, including arterial embolization and percutaneous abscess drainage, have expanded in parallel with the newer imaging modalities and now commonly offer an alternative to surgery.

TERMINOLOGY OF BONE INJURIES

It is important to be familiar with the terminology used to describe bony injuries. The features of a fracture or dislocation that need to be recorded are outlined below.

Site

Record the bone or joint involved, and the location of the fracture within the bone (proximal, mid or distal third).

Alignment

It is conventional to describe malalignment of the axial skeleton by relating the upper vertebral body at the site of injury to the one below. In the peripheral skeleton it is standard practice to describe the alignment of the distal portion of the fracture (normal, medial/varus, lateral/valgus, anterior or posterior) with respect to the proximal portion (Fig. 1). Bony displacement, rotation and overlap should also be noted (Fig. 2).

Type

Open, comminuted and pathological fractures should be specified. A distracted fracture is an unstable injury in which the fracture margins are separated either as a result of soft tissue interposition or muscle contraction (Fig. 3). This contrasts with an impacted fracture which is a stable injury because of compression (Fig. 1).

Articular involvement

The presence of a lipohaemarthrosis is a useful indicator of an intra-articular fracture (Fig. 4). A step in the articular margin, a loose intra-articular body or joint subluxation/dislocation should all be reported (Figs 2 and 5).

Degenerative change

Pre-existing degenerative bony changes seen at the time of injury should be recorded. This is important medicolegally to ensure that on subsequent radiographs

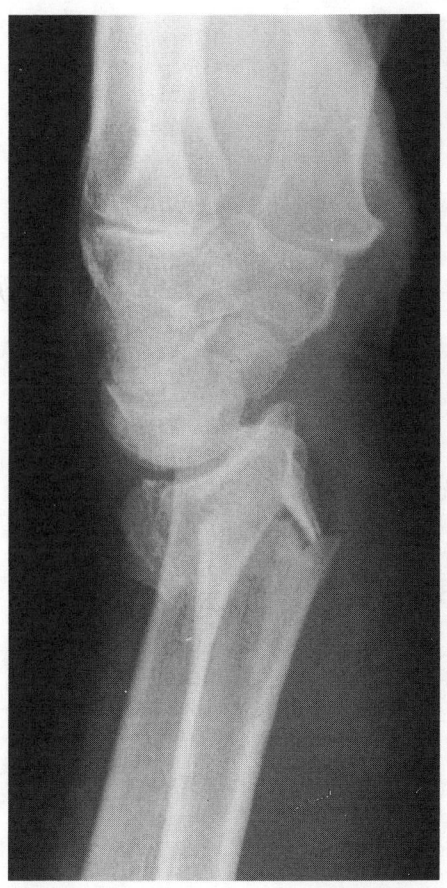

(a)

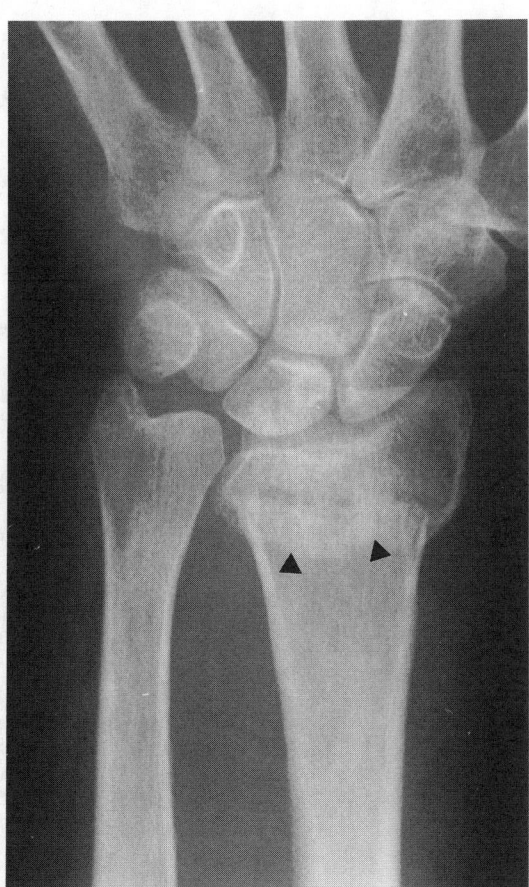

(b)

Fig. 1. Colles' fracture. Posterior angulation and impaction are seen on the lateral view (a). Impaction is identified on the frontal radiograph (b) by the sclerotic line (arrowheads) resulting from bony overlap.

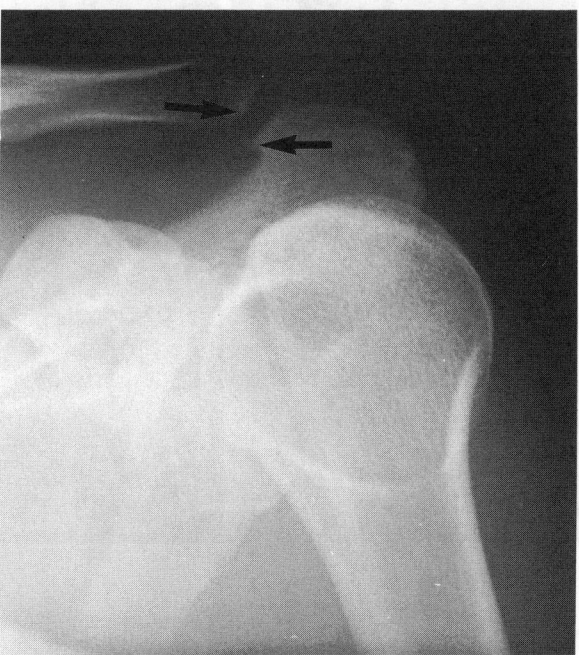

Fig. 2. Acromioclavicular subluxation indicated by malalignment along the inferior margins of the clavicle and acromion (arrows).

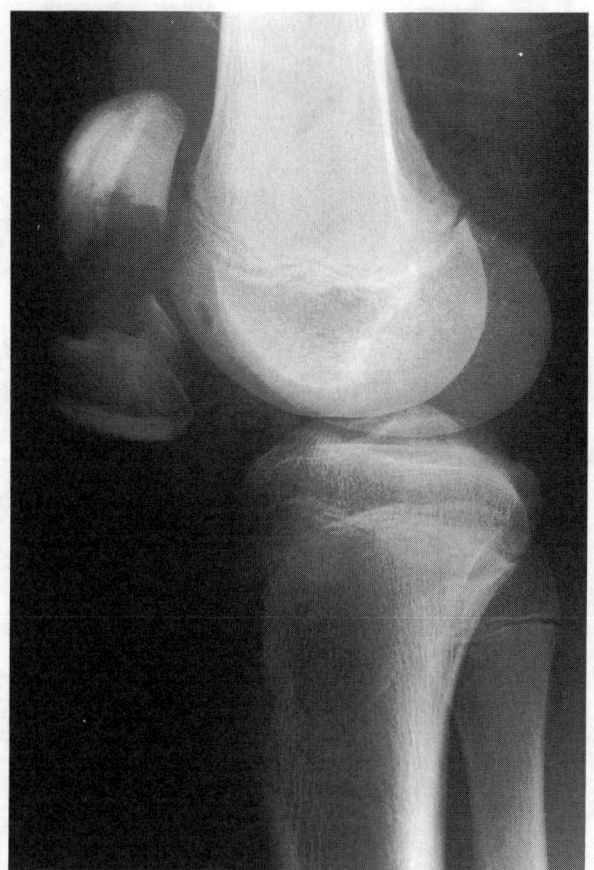

Fig. 3. Comminuted transverse fracture of the patella with wide distraction of fragments due to contraction of the quadriceps muscle.

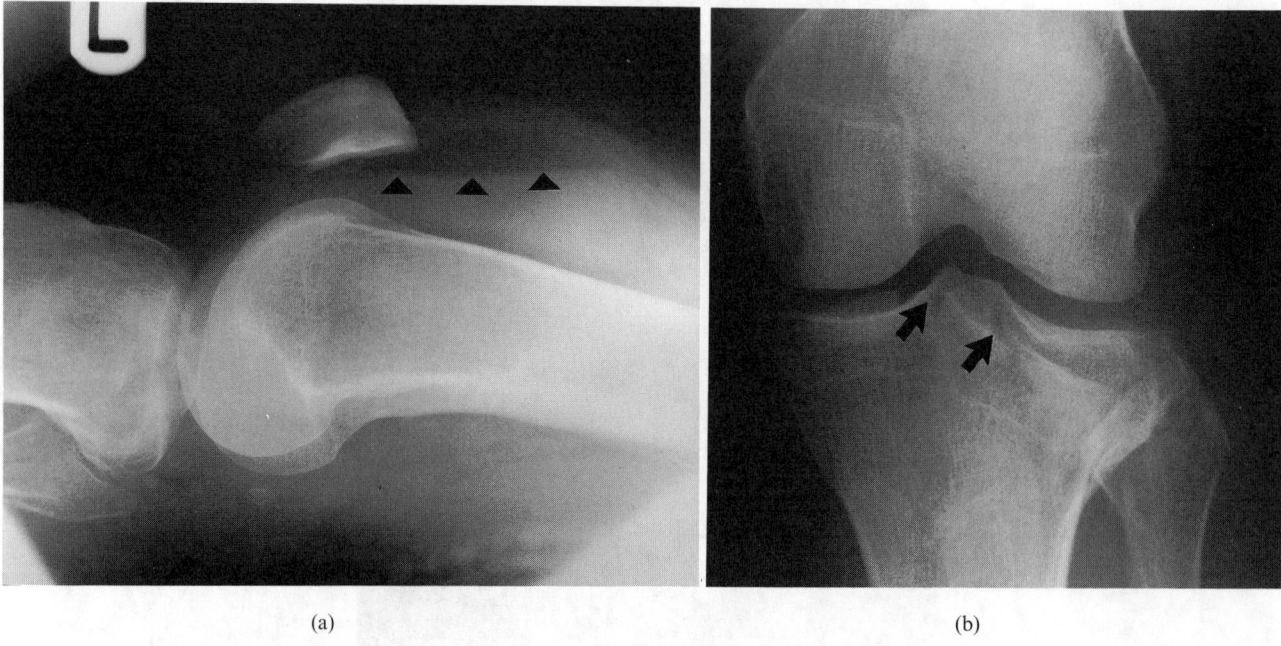

(a)   (b)

Fig. 4. (a) The horizontal beam lateral radiograph shows a fat/fluid level (arrowheads). Marrow fat within the joint indicates an intra-capsular fracture. (b) The anteroposterior radiograph reveals a fracture of the lateral tibial plateau. The fracture involves the articular surface (arrows).

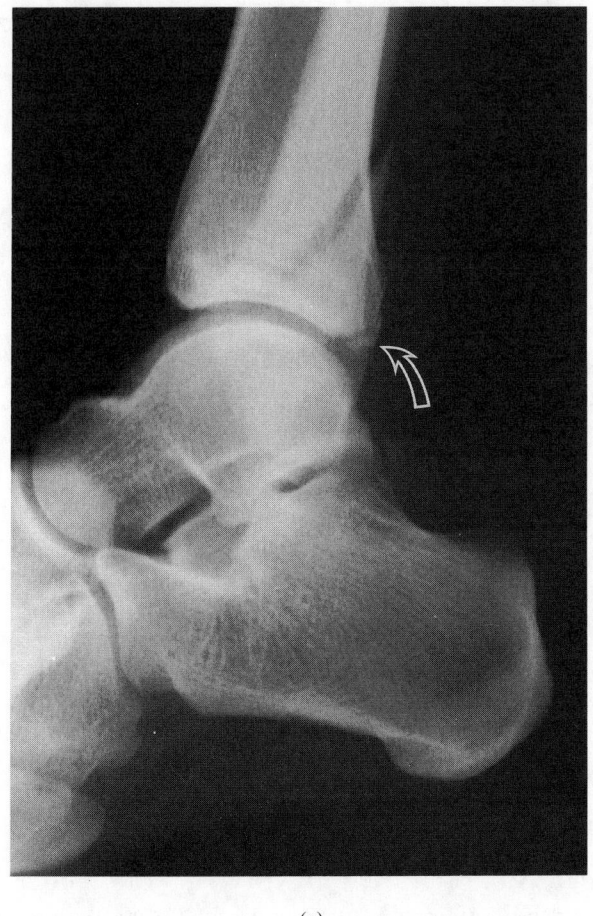

(a)

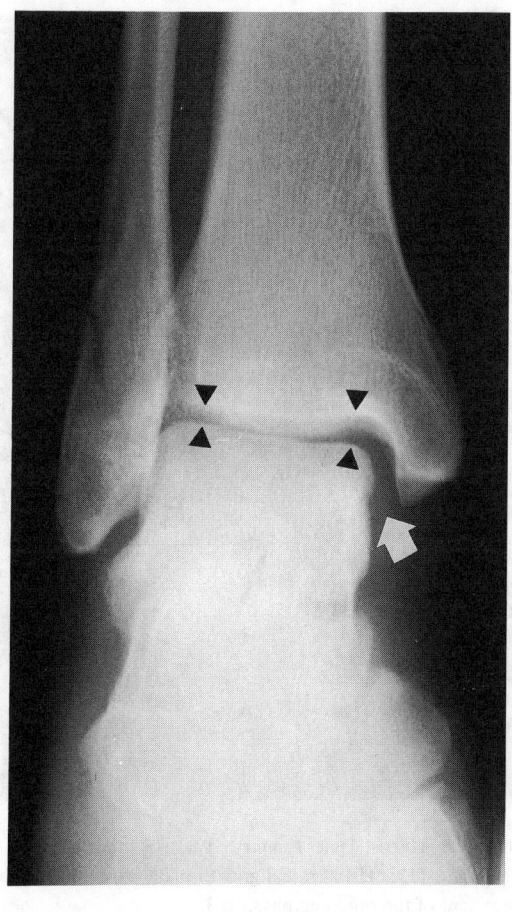

(b)

Fig. 5. Lateral (a) and anteroposterior (b) views of the ankle. The lateral view shows an oblique fracture of the distal fibula, with an additional fracture through the posterior aspect of the tibia (arrow). On the anteroposterior view there is widening of the space between the talus and the medial malleolus (white arrow). There is also asymmetry of the superior aspect of the ankle joint (arrowheads). These appearances are caused by a tear of the medial collateral ligament permitting lateral subluxation of the talus. This is an unstable injury.

these degenerative changes are not mistakenly attributed to the injury.

PAEDIATRIC FRACTURES

Classification

Fractures of the paediatric skeleton (epiphyses open) can be divided for descriptive purposes into those involving the growth plate (physis), and those of the bony shaft.

Growth plate injuries

These fractures are most commonly classified using the system first described by Salter & Harris (1963). This system divides fractures into five types depending on the pattern of involvement of the growth plate and adjacent epiphysis and metaphysis.

- *Type I* (6%) injury represents a fracture of the growth plate without involvement of the adjacent bone, and most commonly occurs in children under 5 years of age. It is difficult to diagnose unless there is epiphyseal displacement (Fig. 6).
- *Type II* injury (75%) represents a fracture through most of the growth plate which also extends through the adjacent metaphysis. The size of the metaphyseal fragment, and degree of displacement are variable (Fig. 7).
- *Type III* injury (8%) represents a fracture through a variable portion of the growth plate that extends through the epiphysis to involve the articular margin (Fig. 8).
- *Type IV* injury (10%) represents a vertical fracture through the metaphysis, growth plate and epiphysis (Fig. 9).

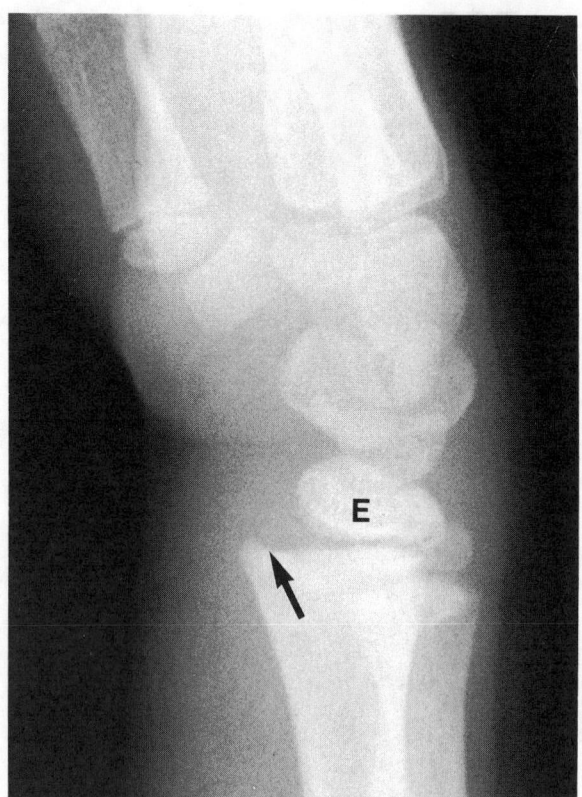

Fig. 6. Salter–Harris Type I injury. There is malalignment at the palmar aspect of the distal radial growth plate (arrow), with posterior displacement of the radial epiphysis (E).

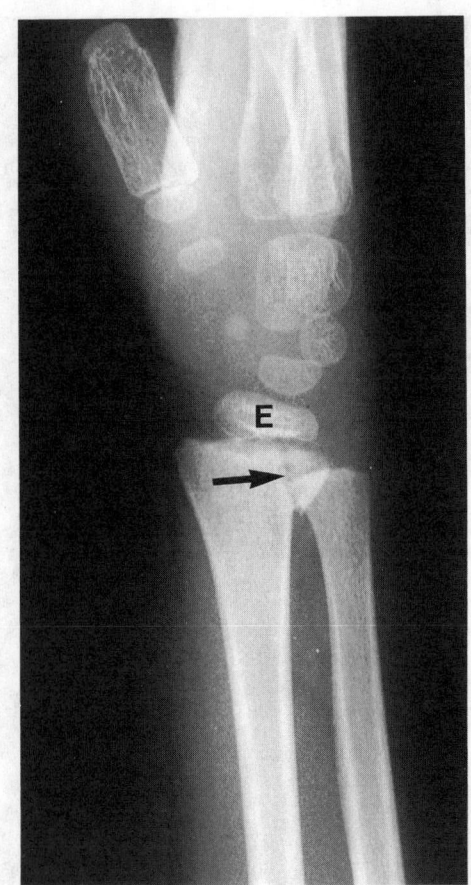

Fig. 7. Salter–Harris Type II injury. Fracture of the dorsal aspect of the distal radial metaphysis (arrow), with posterior displacement of the epiphysis.

- *Type V* injury (1%) represents a crush injury of the growth plate. This is very difficult to diagnose radiographically as there is no bony displacement or fracture line visible. Prognosis is poor because it is likely to lead to developmental growth disturbance.

Shaft Fractures

Because of the elasticity of the paediatric skeleton, fractures of the shafts of long bones often do not traverse the entire bony diameter. Three fracture patterns are well recognized.

- A torus fracture appears as a buckling of the cortex on the side of the compressive force (Fig. 10).
- A greenstick fracture is seen as a disruption of the bony cortex on the side of the bone undergoing tensile force, while the opposite cortex (undergoing compression) remains intact (Fig. 11).
- A plastic bowing injury appears when the cortex is intact, but microscopic fractures lead to a bowed or bent appearance (Fig. 12).

Paediatric elbow fractures

Supracondylar fractures

Supracondylar fractures account for up to 60% of all paediatric elbow fractures, and generally result from a fall on an outstretched hand. The majority of cases result in posterior displacement of the distal humeral fragment. In approximately 25% of cases a fracture line is not seen. The diagnosis is then inferred by the presence of a joint effusion and an abnormal anterior humeral line (Pitt & Speer, 1990). This line is drawn along the anterior cortex of the humerus, and generally intersects the capitellum in its middle third (Fig. 13). When a supracondylar fracture is present this line will either not pass through the capitellum or will project through its anterior aspect (Pitt & Speer, 1990; Karasick *et al.*, 1991) (Fig. 14).

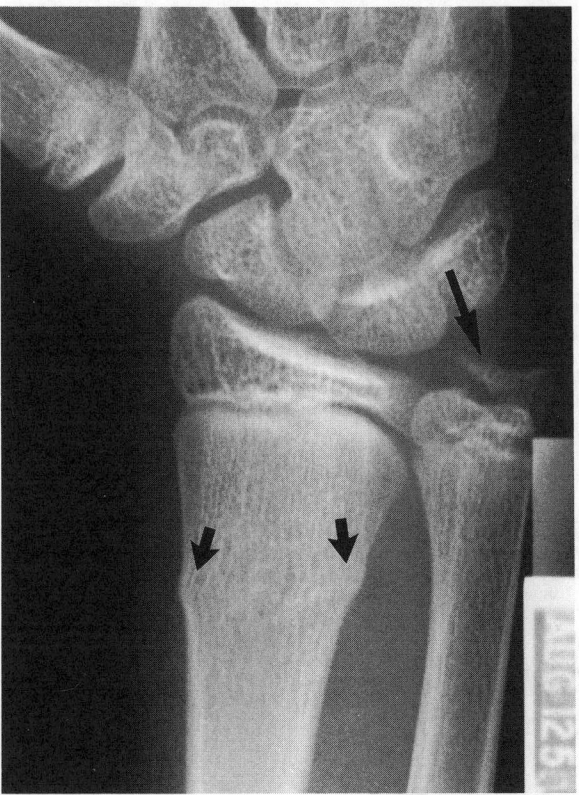

Fig. 8. Salter–Harris Type III injury. Widening of the growth plate with fragmentation of the ulnar epiphysis (long arrow). [Note also the torus fracture of the distal radius (short arrows).]

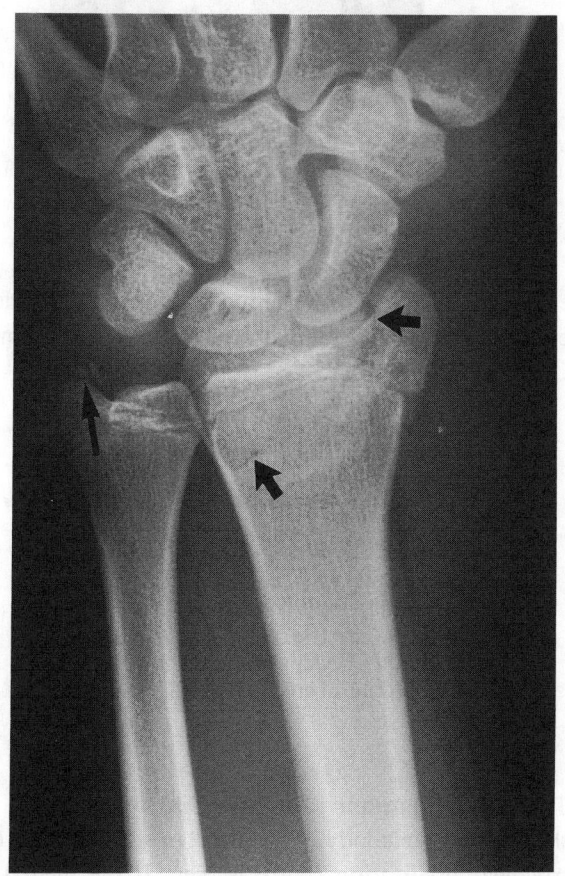

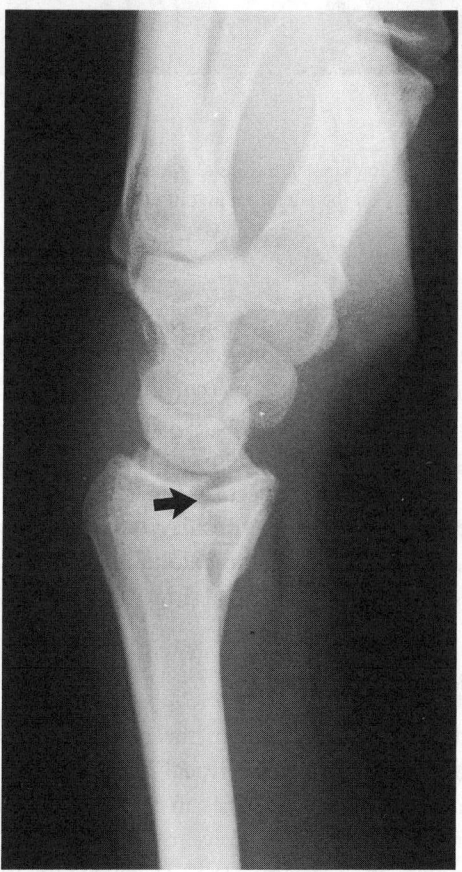

(a)   (b)

Fig. 9. (a, b) Salter–Harris Type IV injury. Fracture extending through the radial metaphysis and epiphysis (short arrows). [Note also the fracture of the tip of the ulnar styloid (long arrow).]

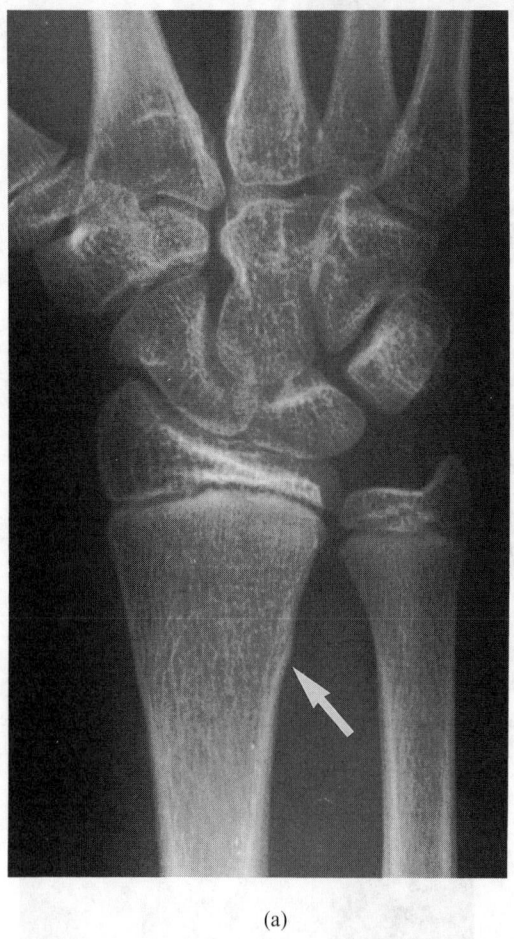

(a)

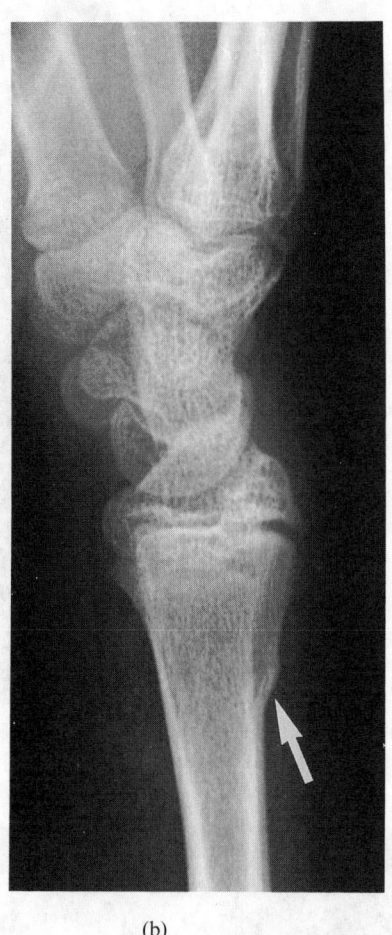

(b)

Fig. 10. Torus fracture of the distal radius. This is easily overlooked on the frontal radiograph (a), but is clearly visible as a buckling of the bony cortex on the lateral radiograph (b).

Radial head dislocation

Radial head dislocations can be differentiated from supracondylar fractures of the humerus using another line: the radiocapitellar line. This line extends through the central long axis of the proximal radial head and neck and it should intersect the middle third of the capitellum on all views (Resnik, 1989; Karasick et al., 1991). The normal radiocapitellar alignment is preserved with supracondylar fractures (Fig. 15).

Ossification centres

The maturation sequence of the ossification centres of the paediatric elbow is of critical importance in trauma. The Capitellar centre ossifies in the first year, followed by the Radial head (3–6 years), the Internal/medial epicondyle (4–7 years), the Trochlea (9–10 years), the Olecranon (6–10 years) and the External/lateral

epicondyle (11 years) (Rogers, 1982). The usual order of ossification can be remembered using the mnemonic CRITOE.

Mnemonic for order of ossification in paediatric elbow		
C	Capitellar centre	1 year
R	Radial head	3–6 years
I	Internal/medial epicondyle	4–7 years
T	Trochlea	9–10 years
O	Olecranon	6–10 years
E	External/lateral epicondyle	11 years

The most important relationship to remember is that the medial epicondyle should be seen whenever a trochlear ossification centre is seen. If the medial epicondyle ossification centre is not seen on a radiograph

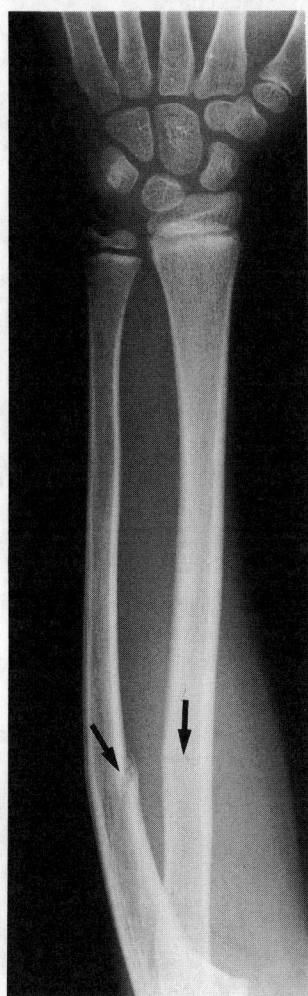

Fig. 11. Greenstick fracture of the ulna. Transverse fracture of the radius.

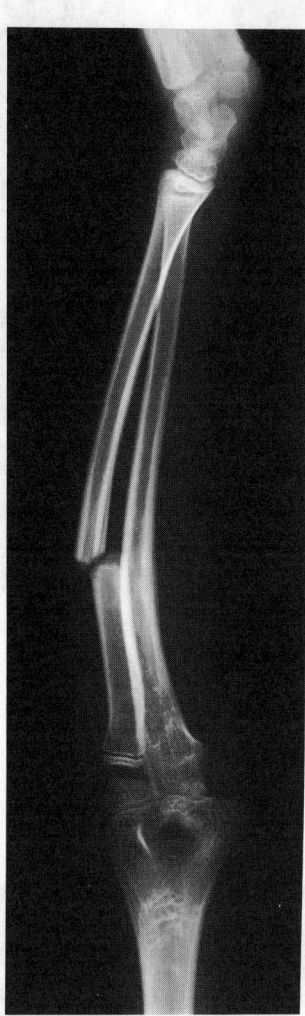

Fig. 12. Transverse fracture of the radius. The ulna is bent; this is a plastic bowing fracture.

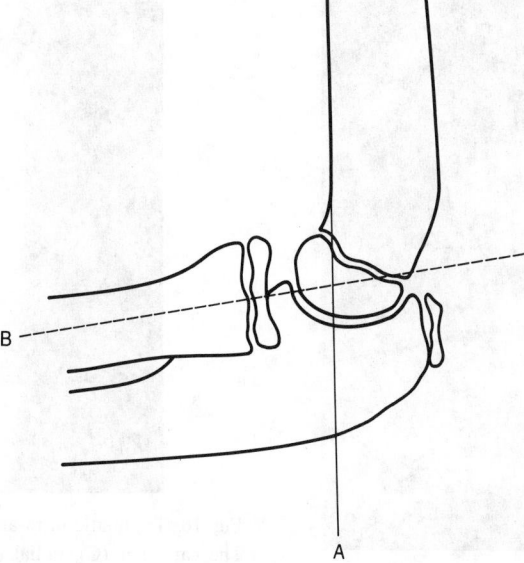

Fig. 13. The anterior humeral line (solid line A) and the radiocapitellar line (broken line B). Both lines normally intersect the capitellum in its middle third.

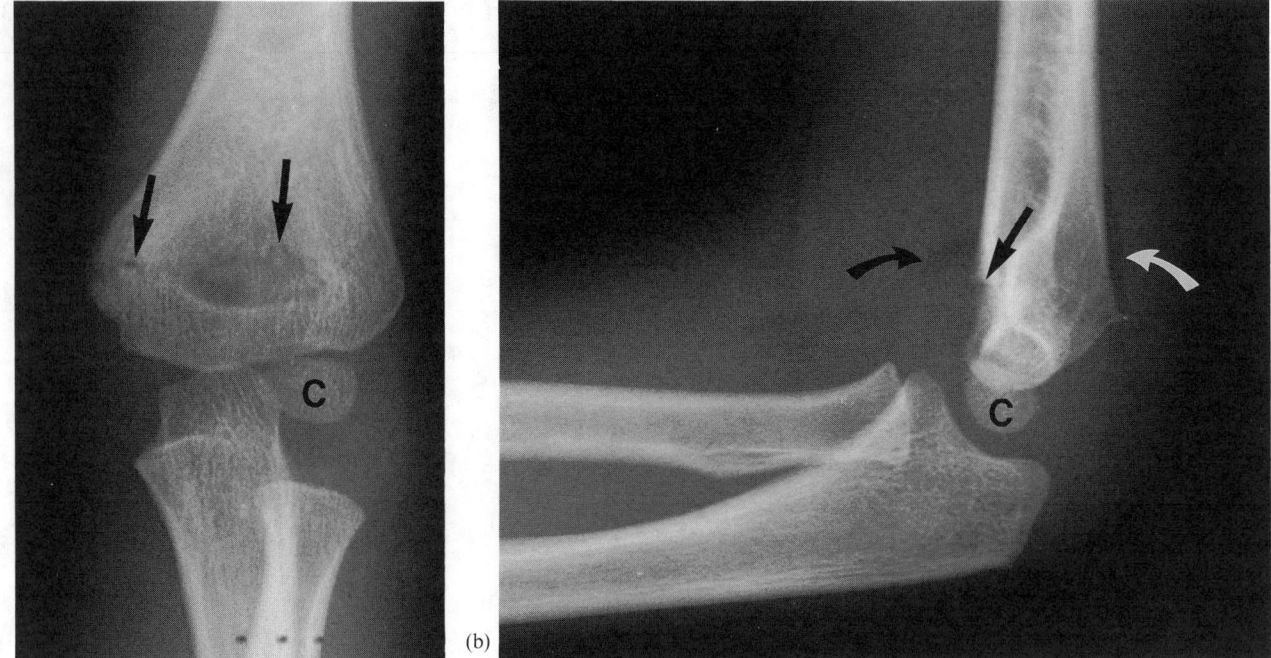

(a)

(b)

Fig. 14. anteroposterior (a) and lateral (b) radiographs of the elbow in a child. The anterior humeral line fails to intersect the capitellum (C) on the lateral view. This raises the possibility of a supracondylar fracture. The supracondylar fracture is visible (straight arrows). The posterior fat pad is visible (radiolucent stripe, curved white arrow), and the anterior fat pad is bowed anteriorly (radiolucent stripe, curved black arrow). These fat pad appearances indicate a joint effusion

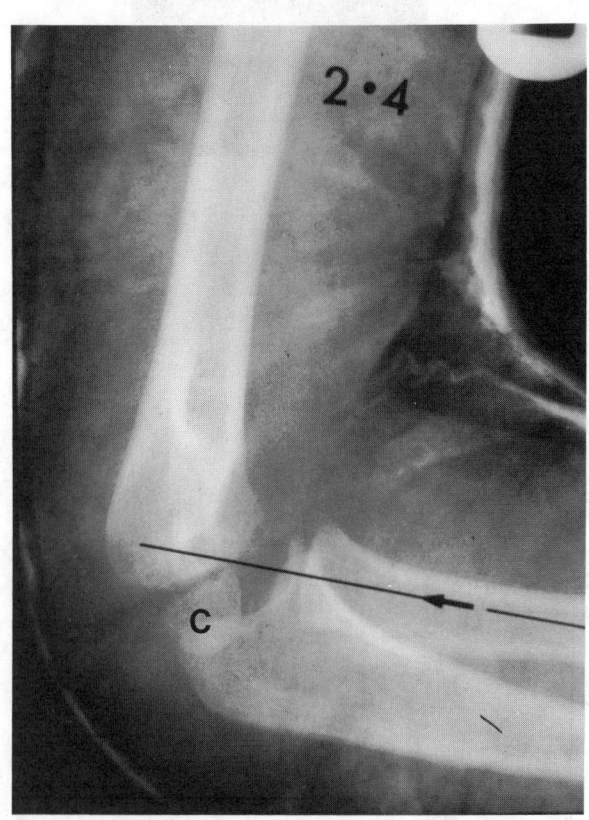

Fig. 15. Lateral radiograph of the elbow in plaster demonstrating a radial head dislocation. The radiocapitellar line fails to intersect the capitellum (C).

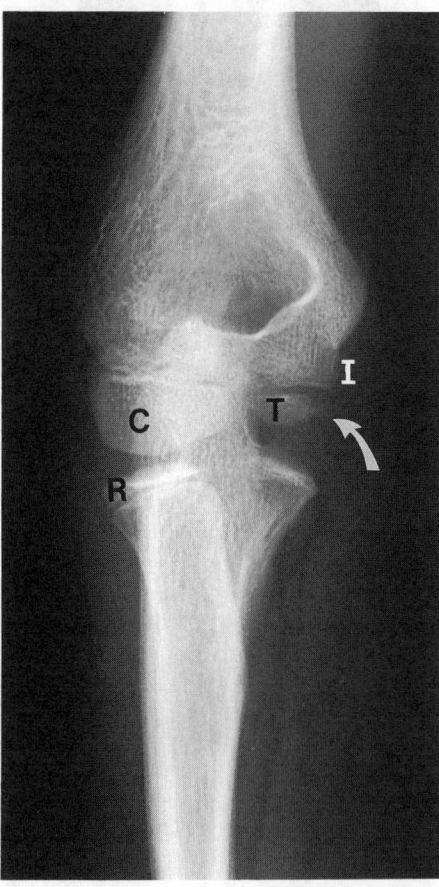

Fig. 16. Traumatic intra-articular avulsion of the medial epicondyle. The capitellar (C), radial (R) and trochlear (T) ossification centres are visible. The ossification centre for the internal epicondyle should be present at this stage, but is not seen at its normal site (I). This centre is seen inferiorly (arrow) adjacent to the trochlea.

in which the trochlea is visible, then an avulsion injury with intra-articular entrapment of the medial epicondyle should be suspected (Fig. 16). This is a serious injury often requiring operative reduction. Irregular or fragmented ossification centres are normal variants. These may even be unilateral (Resnik, 1989).

HEAD INJURY RADIOLOGY

Head injuries are extremely common. Much has been written on the optimum protocol for investigation. The indications for skull radiography continue to be debated (Brocklehurst et al., 1987; Masters et al., 1987; Lancet Editorial, 1990). The Harrogate Seminar on the Management of Acute Head Injury (Harrogate Seminar Report, 1983) made recommendations which provide a starting point for a balanced approach to the use of the skull X-ray. As a result of this symposium and taking into account the recommendations of the Royal College of Radiology Working Party (1983) de Lacey et al. (1990) proposed a system which links a policy for obtaining skull radiography with admission policy (Fig. 17). This eliminates the need for skull films in many patients who are admitted for observation.

A simple skull fracture is only important as a marker for more serious intracranial pathology (Figs 18–20). However, intracranial haematoma is often present without a concomitant fracture, particularly in children (Teasdale et al., 1990). Patients with a depressed level of consciousness, focal neurological signs, or who have had a penetrating injury require a CT scan, regardless of the skull radiography findings, and in these cases the skull X-ray series can usually be omitted. The CT provides accurate information on cerebral contusion, cerebral haemorrhage and intracranial haematoma (Figs 21–23) which is essential for management but which is, at best, only crudely inferred from the plain film findings.

CERVICAL SPINE TRAUMA

Guidelines as to when to request cervical spine radiography are summarized in Fig. 24 and some important facts regarding radiographic interpretation are presented in Fig. 25. Note that any patient with severe multisystem trauma must be assumed to have a cervical injury until proved otherwise (American College of Surgeons Committee on Trauma, 1993). A cross-table lateral cervical spine view is obtained in these patients in the first instance while immobilization is maintained, supple-

mented by other views as necessary. Note that films obtained in this way are often suboptimal and the clinical evaluation takes priority over the radiographic findings as the films may be falsely negative.

A technically adequate set of films is essential. Injuries occurring at the cervicothoracic junction and atlantoaxial level pose particular difficulty – usually because inadequate views have been obtained (Fig. 26). The C7/T1 junction must be visible on the lateral view on order to assess the alignment between these two vertebrae. In some patients additional views will be required to demonstrate this region and the 'swimmer's' view is commonly performed. This does, however, require adjustment in patient position. Recent reports suggest that if an unstable injury is suspected the 'trauma oblique' view may be a satisfactory alternative to the swimmer's view (Murphey et al., 1989).

Alignment is assessed on the lateral view by means of lines which provide important clues to ligamentous and bone injury (Fig. 27). On the frontal view the spinous processes and lateral vertebral borders should be in a straight line or curve gently. If facet dislocation or subluxation is suggested on the anteroposterior or lateral views then oblique views should be obtained (Fig. 28). The open mouth view shows the lateral masses of C1 lying on the superior articular facets of C2 (Fig. 29).

Sometimes delayed views are indicated. Patients with minor degrees of antero- or retrolisthesis, or marked straightening of the cervical lordosis, may have an unstable injury which is initially masked by muscle spasm (Fig. 30). These patients, if considered fit for discharge, should be booked for flexion and extension views when the spasm has settled down. The patient should be alert and cooperative and flex and extend the spine himself under close supervision.

Careful plain film imaging provides sufficient information in most patients (Figs 31 and 32) but further investigation is occasionally required. Conventional tomography images axially orientated fractures (e.g. the dens) (Fig. 33). Computed tomography can clearly demonstrate the extent of bone injury (Fig. 34), the location of fracture fragments, and spinal canal morphology. However, the axial imaging plane can make detection of some abnormalities, such as axially orientated fractures and facet subluxation or dislocation, difficult.

MRI is especially helpful when the plain films are either normal or only mildly abnormal in the presence of signs of cord injury. It is excellent for imaging spinal cord

1 Head Injury
Policy in A & E

Skull films if depressed* fracture *likely,*
or a large haematoma

If not, do you still intend to admit?
(See Card A)

YES — NO

Immediate SXR **not** necessary

Is SXR indicated on clinical grounds?
(Card B)

NO

HOME

(*ACTA CHIR SCAND 1973, 139:605...Risk of infection)

2 Head Injury
Policy if admitted for observation

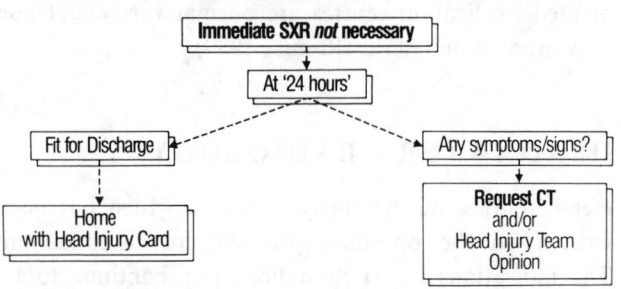

Immediate SXR *not* necessary

At '24 hours'

Fit for Discharge

Home
with Head Injury Card

Any symptoms/signs?

Request CT
and/or
Head Injury Team
Opinion

Head Injury
A Clinical Criteria for admission*

1. Confusion or depression of level of consciousness *at time of examination*
2. Focal Neurological Signs
3. Signs of raised Intracranial Pressure
4. Difficult to assess (e.g. Alcohol, Epilepsy)
5. CSF from Nose or CSF/Blood from Ear
6. Other important medical conditions
7. Poor social conditions or lack of responsible adult

NOTE: Amnesia for *the event* or transient loss of consciousness is not an indication for admission

(*HARROGATE CRITERIA. **rph** MODIFICATION)

Head Injury
B Clinical criteria for SXR*

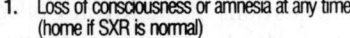

1. Loss of consciousness or amnesia at any time (home if SXR is normal)
2. Suspected penetrating injury
3. Difficult to assess (e.g. Alcohol, Epilepsy)... **Unless you intend to admit**

NOTE:
(A) Simple scalp laceration is **not** a criterion for skull X-ray
(B) Cervical spine X-rays should **not** be routine in mild head injury

Do not X-ray patients who are to be admitted

(*HARROGATE CRITERIA. **rph** MODIFICATION)

Fig. 17. Guidelines on head injury policy will vary between centres. These guidelines link skull radiography to the local admission policy. SXR, skull radiography; CT, computed tomography; CSF, cerebrospinal fluid. (Courtesy of Kodak UK.)

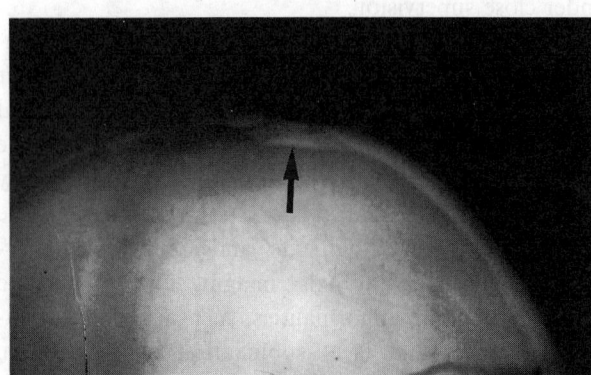

Fig. 18. Depressed skull fracture. The depressed fragment is clearly seen on this tangential view.

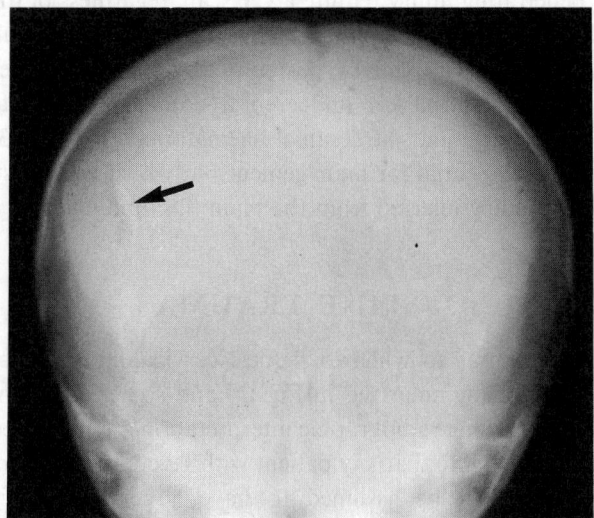

Fig. 19. A depressed fracture is seen as a focal area of increased density.

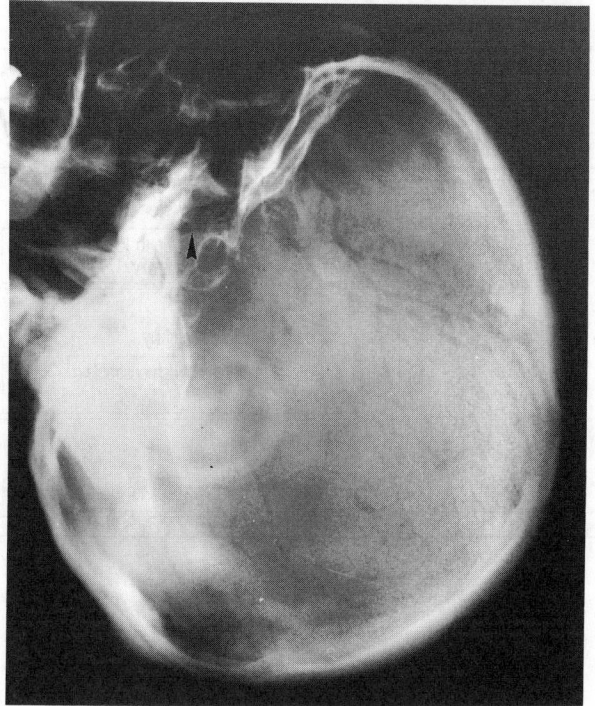

Fig. 20. Horizontal beam lateral skull radiograph. There is an air/fluid level in the sphenoid sinus (arrowhead). This indicates that a basal skull fracture is present.

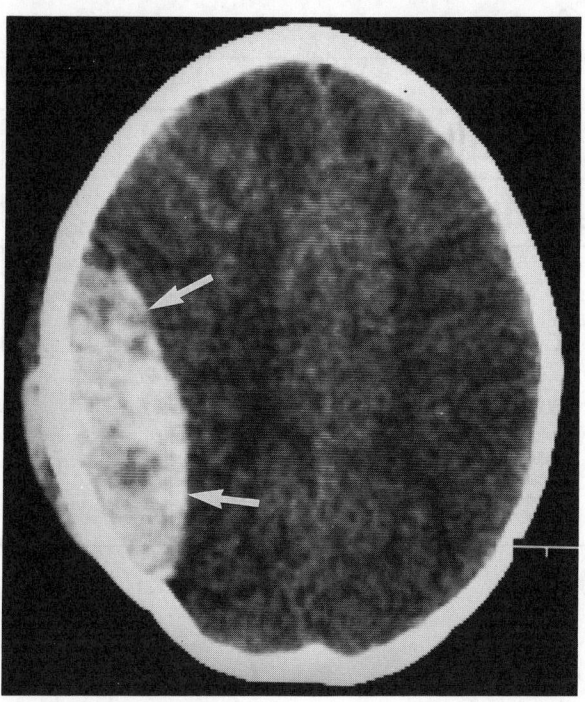

Fig. 22. CT section demonstrating a large extradural haematoma (arrows).

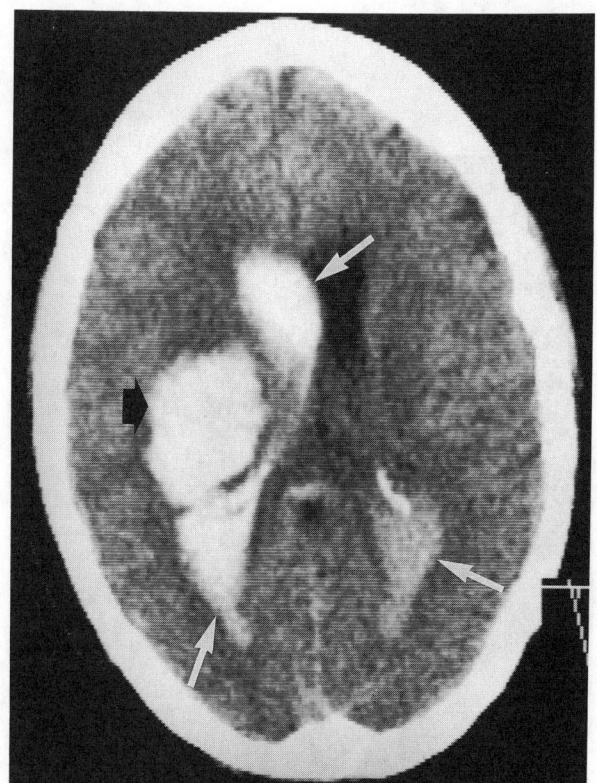

Fig. 21. CT section demonstrating intracerebral haemorrhage. A large haematoma (black arrow) is seen in the area of the right internal capsule. There is an associated intraventricular haemorrhage (white arrows).

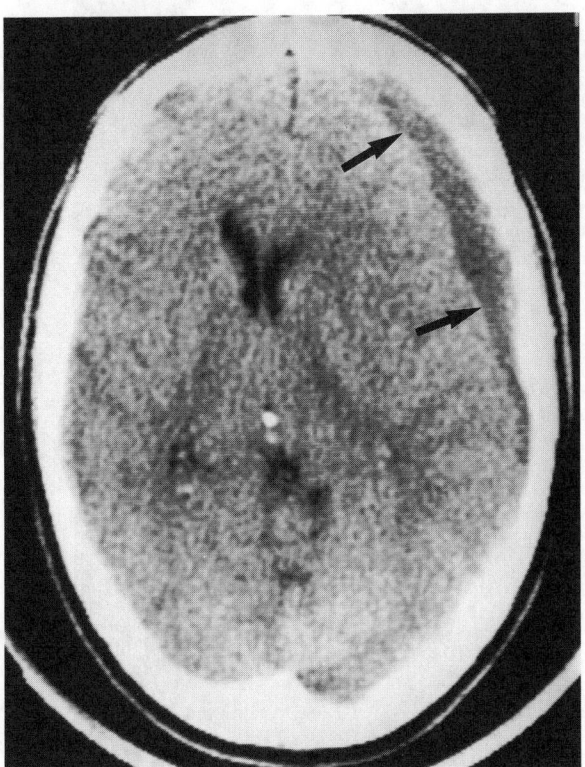

Fig. 23. CT section in a patient presenting with confusion and a deteriorating level of consciousness. Crescentic low density area on the left (arrows) indicates a chronic subdural haematoma. There is associated midline shift.

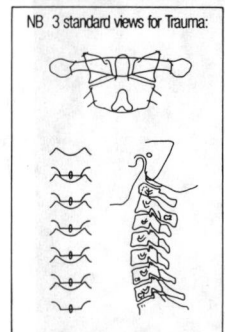

Adult Cervical Spine
Trauma...When to X-ray

1. Neck injury *with pain*
2. Severe head injury
3. Patient unconscious

SOME *'NORMAL'* PATIENTS NEED FURTHER X-RAYS :

Initial X-rays 'normal' but severe spasm or pain then
request flexion and extension views (carefully supervised)
because of possible hidden/delayed instability.

(N.B. If not possible because of spasm, then put in a collar and book
for X-rays in 3/7).

Fig. 24. (Courtesy of Kodak UK.)

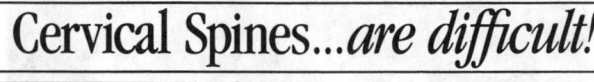

Cervical Spines...*are difficult!*

NB 3 standard views for Trauma:

1 Scrutinise the
LATERAL VIEW

2 Are you sure you have
seen C7/T1?

up to ⅓ of fractures
involve C7/T1*

3 Examine the AP VIEWS carefully

up to 20% of fractures not demonstrable on
lateral view*

Any queries pass the X-ray buck to your *Radiologist!*

(* BRIT. J. RAD. 1987, 60: 1059)

Fig. 25. (Courtesy of Kodak UK.)

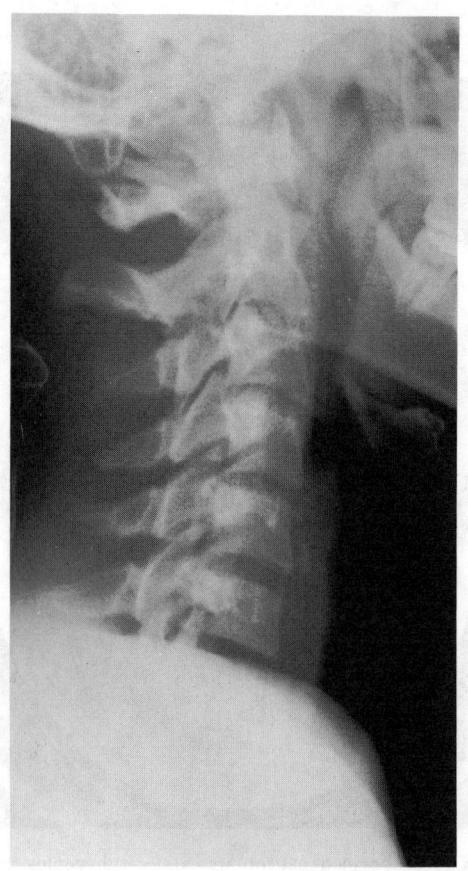

(a)

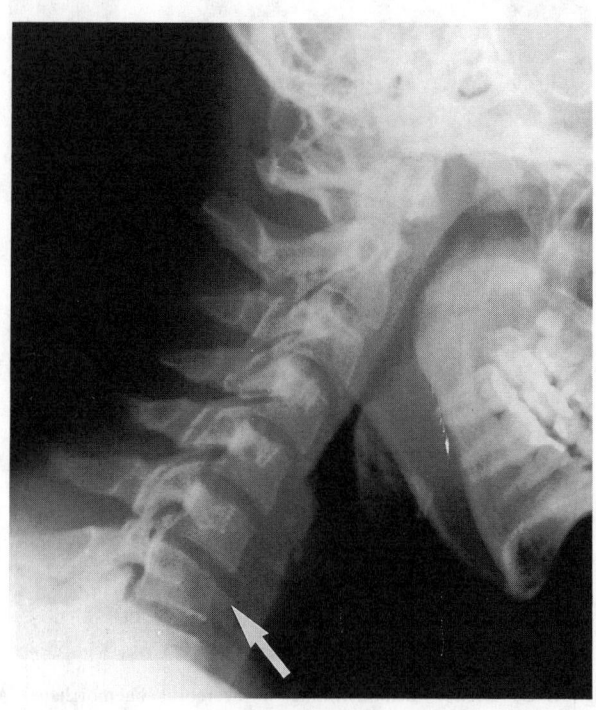

(b)

Fig. 26. It is important to visualize all the cervical vertebrae on the lateral view. The initial film (a) does not include the C7–T1 disc
space. A repeat radiograph (b) reveals a fracture of the anterior aspect of C7 (arrow).

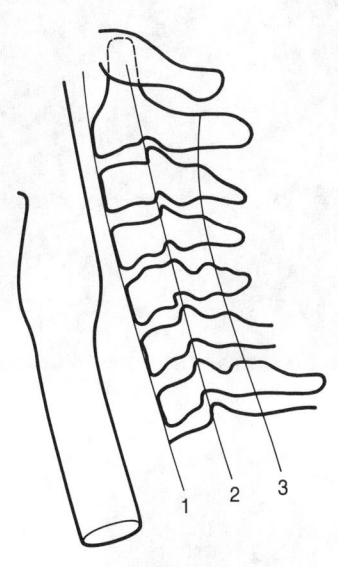

(a)

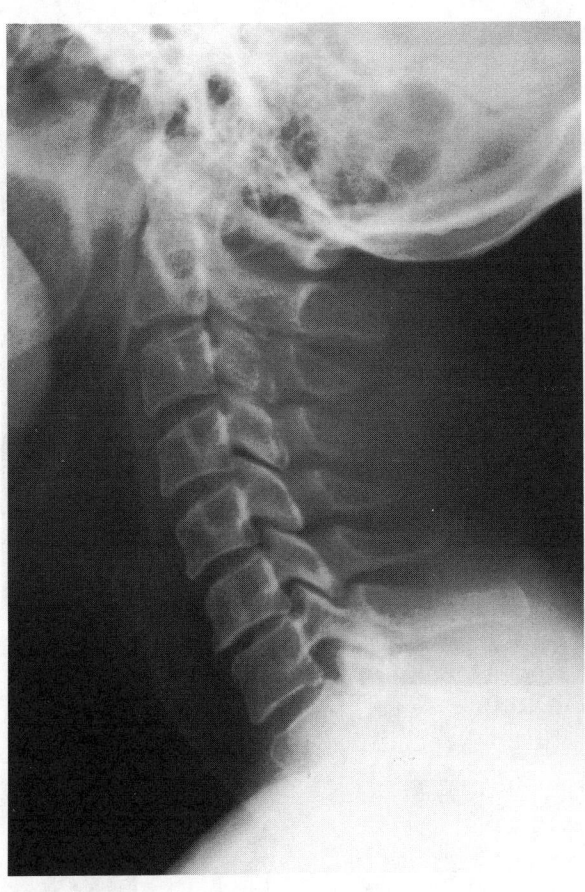

(b)

Fig. 27. (a) Diagram illustrating the three important lines in assessing vertebral alignment on the lateral view: 1, the anterior vertebral line; 2, the posterior vertebral line; 3, the spinolaminar line. These lines should form smooth curved arcs. Some variation is, however, acceptable; the spinolaminar junction of C2 may lie up to 2 mm posterior to the line derived from the spinolaminar junctions of the other cervical vertebrae. In children it can be normal for there to be slight anterior subluxation of C2 on C3, but in these cases the spinolaminar line will be normal. (b) Lateral cervical spine view showing normal alignment.

damage, ligamentous injury, acute intervertebral disc disease, epidural and soft tissue haematomata, and it will often identify fractures.

CHEST

Trauma

There is often poor correlation between the presence or absence of external signs of chest wall injury and the seriousness of the intrathoracic injury. In addition, the chest radiograph will often underestimate the severity of the intrathoracic injury (Fig. 35) (Stark, 1993; Greene 1992).

When the patient's condition permits, an erect chest X-ray should be obtained as it has several advantages over a supine radiograph. Pleural air and fluid collections are easier to detect and to quantify, and difficulties in interpretation resulting from mediastinal magnification are fewer. The supine film may cause apparent mediastinal widening because of geometric factors and this can lead to unnecessary investigation in an ill patient.

Bones

Rib fractures may be difficult to demonstrate, particularly when they overlie the axillary region or the soft tissues of the abdomen. A fracture of the 1st or 2nd rib usually results from violent trauma, and this finding increases the likelihood of a fatal outcome from injuries to the head, neck, aorta, or tracheobronchial tree (Richardson et al., 1975). Fractures of the lower ribs should lead to consideration of a possible liver, spleen or renal laceration (Fig. 36).

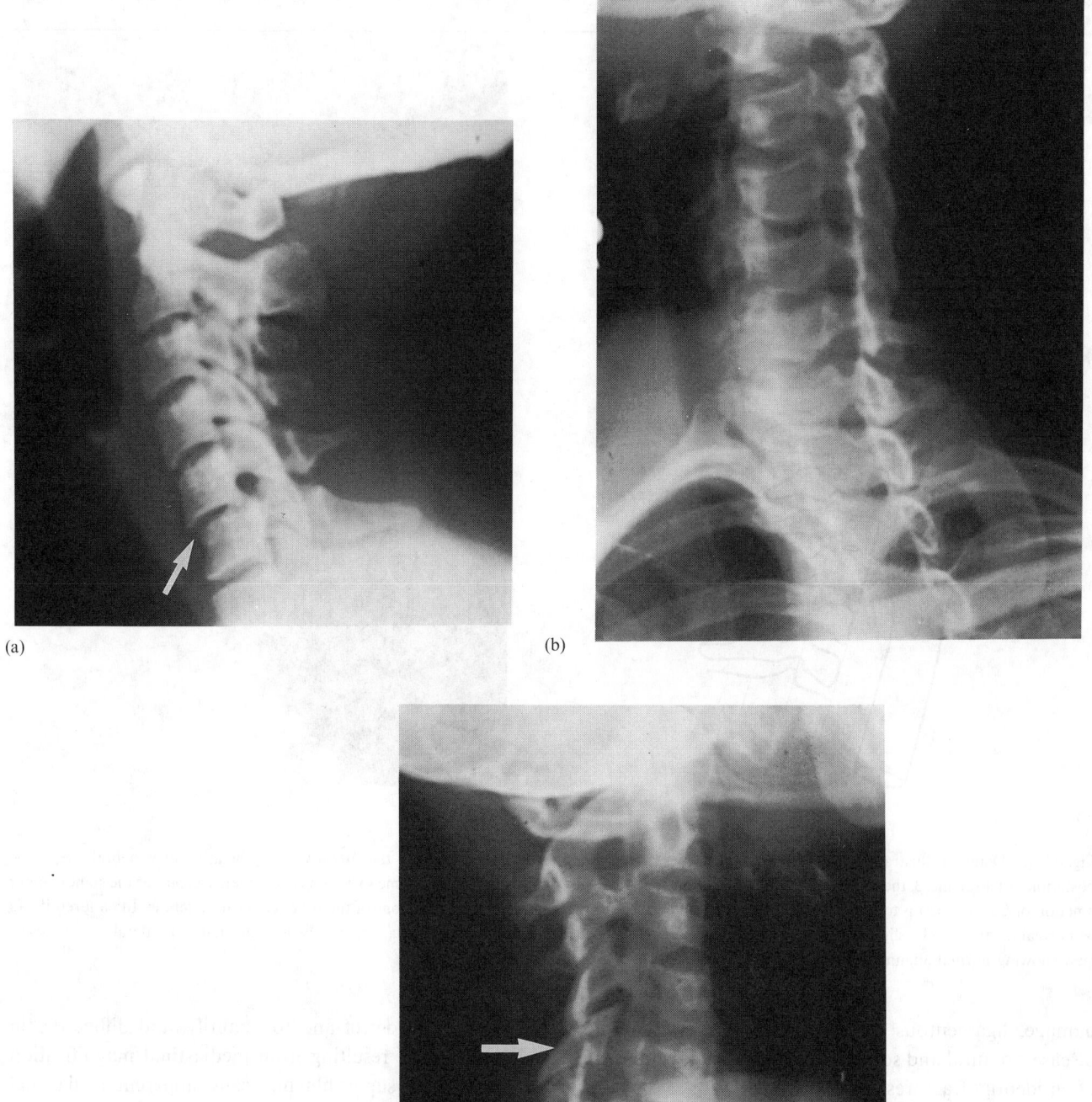

Fig. 28. Unilateral facet joint dislocation. (a) Lateral view shows forward slip of C5 on C6. (b) Right posterior oblique view. This demonstrates the left intervertebral canals. These are normal. (c) Left posterior oblique view. This demonstrates the right intervertebral canals. There is an abnormality at C5 due to anterior dislocation of the C5 facet (arrow). Compare this appearance with (b).

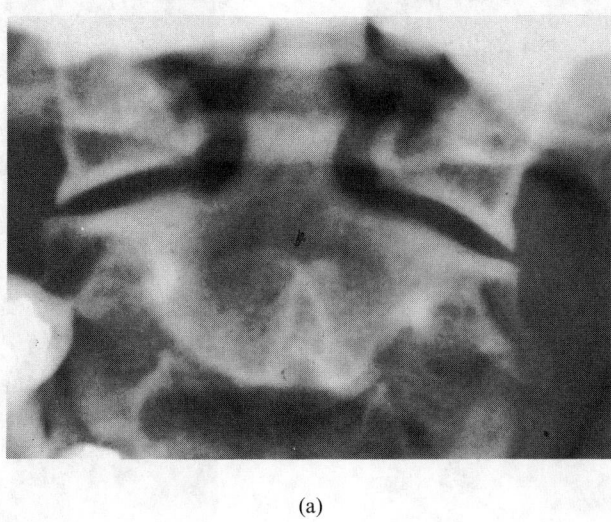

(a)

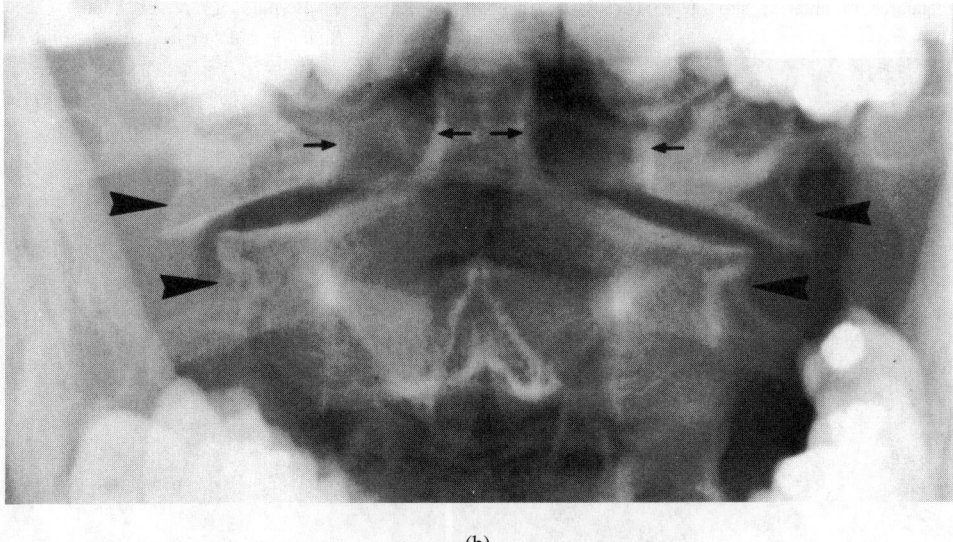

(b)

Fig. 29. (a)Normal 'open mouth' odontoid peg view. Note that the lateral margins of the C1 lateral masses are aligned with the C2 lateral masses. Overhang of the C1 lateral masses relative to C2, if it occurs, is less than 2 mm in the normal adult patient. The lateral masses of C1 ossify more rapidly than C2, so that in children this rule cannot be strictly applied. In general the distance between the dens and the medial aspects of the C1 lateral masses should be equidistant, as in this case, but slight inequalities are usually due to rotation rather than pathology. (b) Jefferson fracture. This occurs when the ipsilateral anterior and posterior arches of C1 are fractured. It can be bilateral, as in this case. Note: (1) the lateral masses of C1 have moved laterally relative to those of those of C2; (2) the dens to lateral mass distances are abnormally increased bilaterally. (Courtesy of Raby, N., Berman, L. & de Lacey, G. (1994). *Accident and Emergency Radiology: A Survival Guide*. London: W.B. Saunders.)

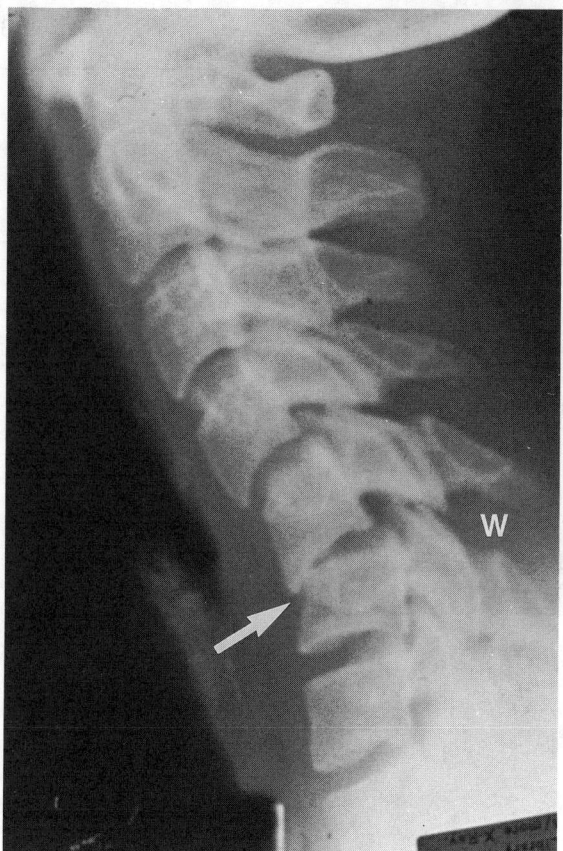

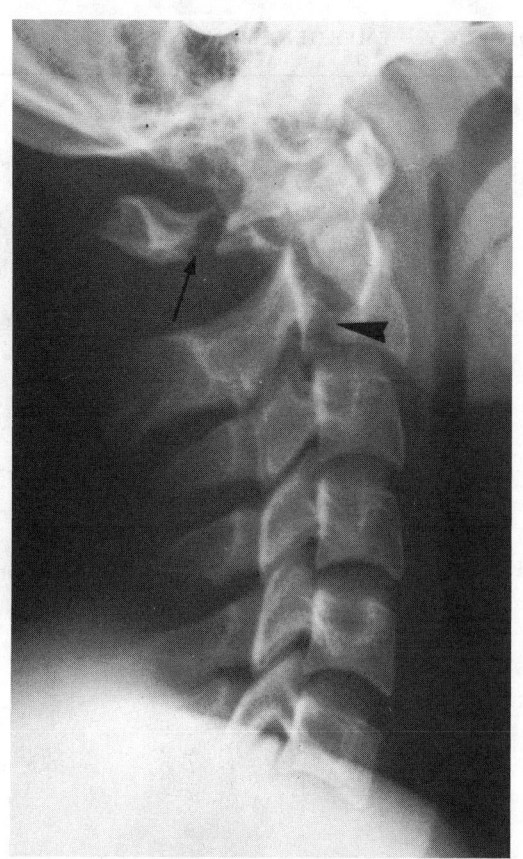

Fig. 30. Hyperflexion sprain. Disruption of the posterior ligaments leads to an abnormally wide interspinous space (W) and forward slip of C5 on C6 (arrow). This is clearly an unstable injury. Note: although the C5 facets have slipped forward on those of C6, this does not represent bilateral facet dislocation. With the latter there would be a greater degree of anterior slip of C5 (>50% of the vertebral body width).

Fig. 31. Hangman's fracture of C2 (arrowhead). This occurs when there is separation of the body of C2 from its pedicles (arrowhead). Note: the body of C2 has slipped forward on C3 and there has been posterior movement of the posterior vertebral elements. A fracture through the posterior arch of C1 is also present (arrow). (Courtesy of Raby, N., Berman, L. & de Lacey, G. (1994). *Accident and Emergency Radiology: A Survival Guide*. London: W.B. Saunders.)

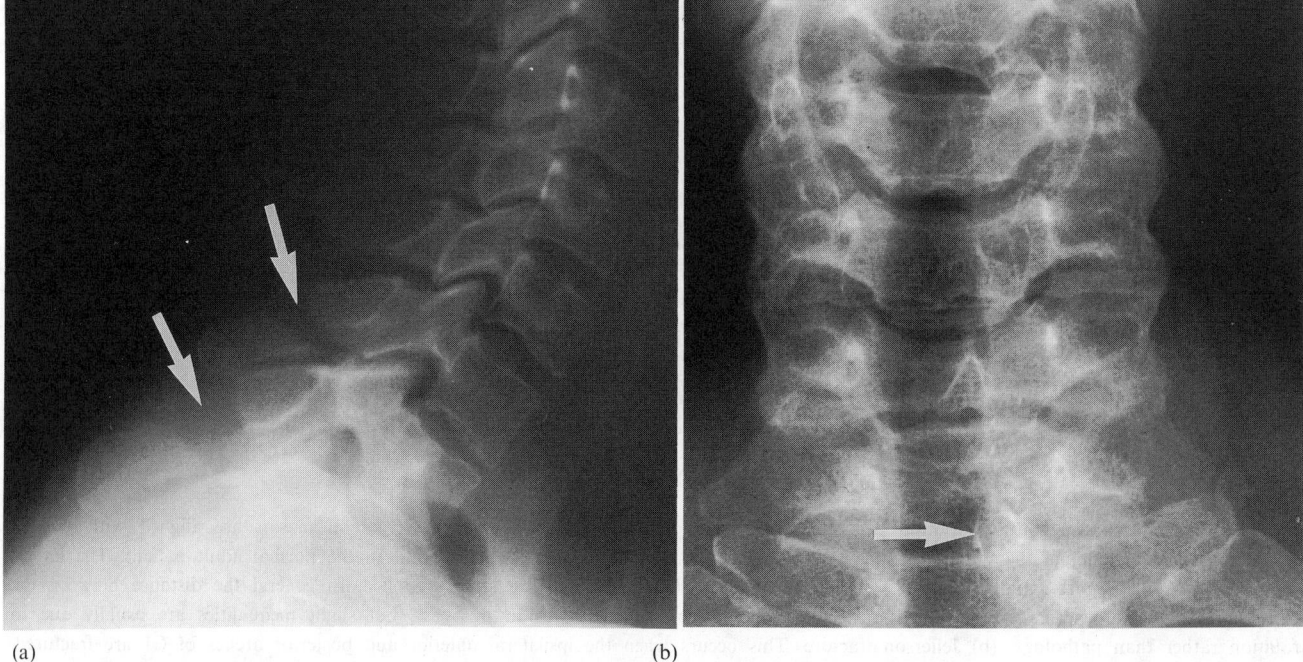

(a)

(b)

Fig. 32. 'Clay shoveller's' fractures of the spinous processes of both C7 and T1 (a). This occurs when a sudden load is applied to the flexed spine. It is a stable injury. Note on the anteroposterior film (b) that the spinous process of C7 has moved to the left out of alignment relative to the other cervical spinous processes.

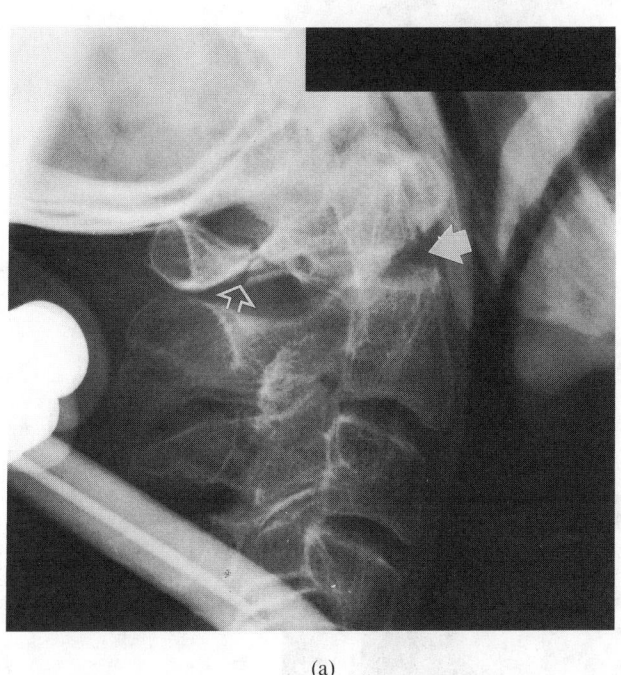
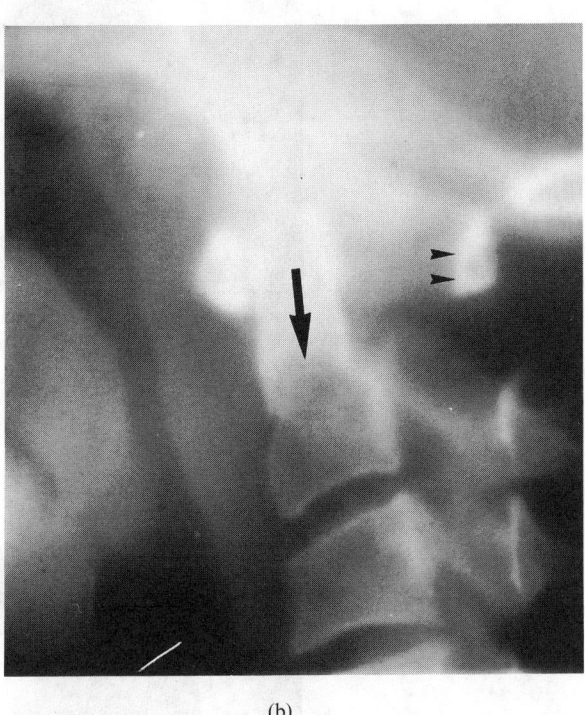

(a) (b)

Fig. 33. (a) Fracture through the dens (closed arrow) and the posterior arch of the C1 (open arrow). (b) Different patient. Lateral tomogram through the dens which is fractured (arrow). Note the forward displacement of C1 on C2 as demonstrated by the abnormal step of the spinolaminar line at this level (arrowheads).

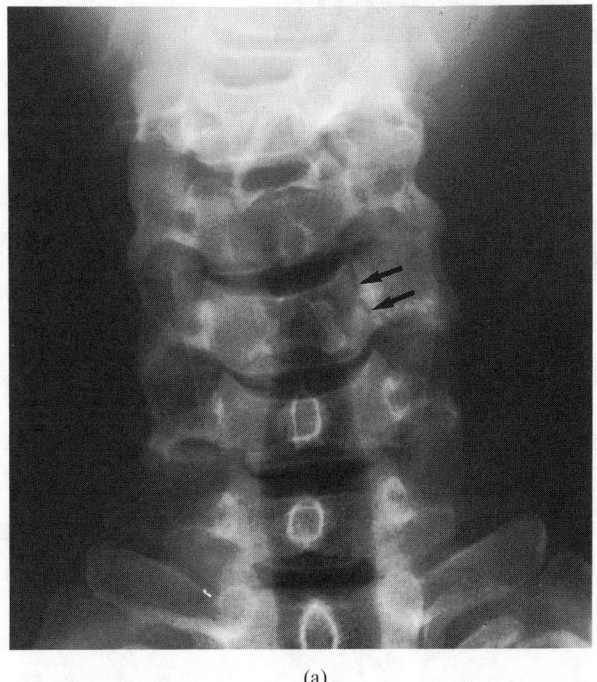
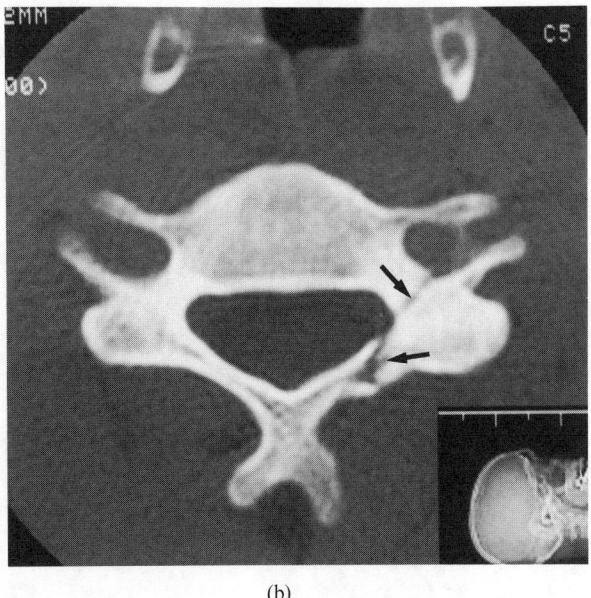

(a) (b)

Fig. 34. (a) Pillar fracture through the left side of C5 (arrows). This was not visible on the lateral view. (b) CT section defines the injury more clearly (arrows). This is a stable fracture; it may sometimes cause radicular pain.

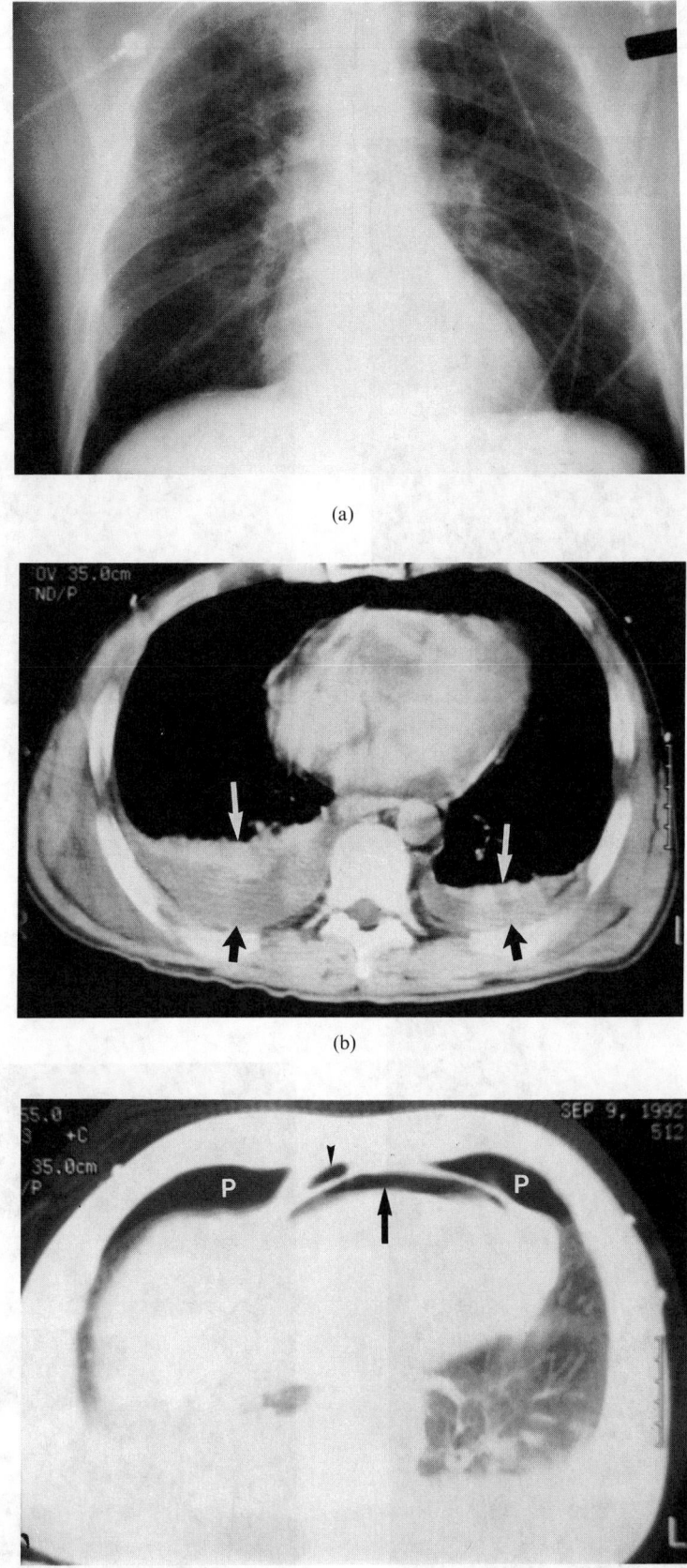

(a)

(b)

(c)

Fig. 35. (a) Supine chest X-ray in a patient who had been involved in a collision with a train. The appearances are unremarkable. (b, c) CT sections obtained within 30 min of the chest X-ray. There are bilateral pleural effusions (black arrows) and consolidation (white arrows). In addition there are bilateral pneumothoraces (P), a pneumomediastinum (arrowhead), and a pneumopericardium (arrow).

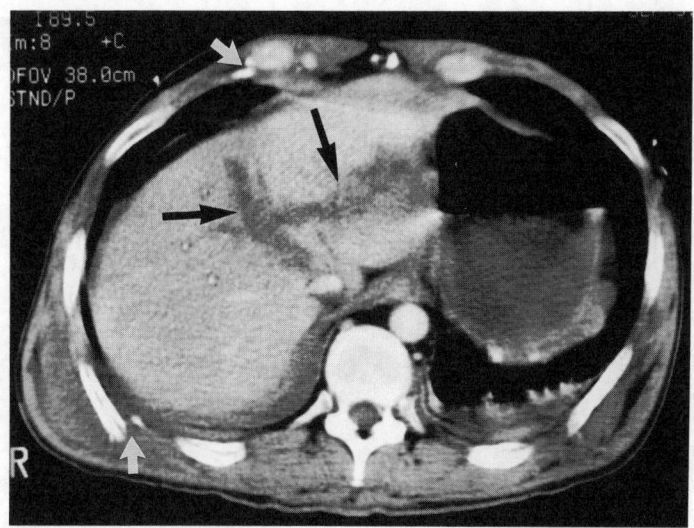

Fig. 36. Contrast-enhanced CT section through the upper abdomen in a patient who had been involved in a road traffic accident. There is a laceration of the liver (black arrows) and fractures through the lower ribs (white arrows).

Diaphragm

Diaphragmatic rupture results from blunt trauma to the abdomen or pelvis, or to direct penetrating injury. It is much more common on the left (Fig. 37). There is often a significant delay between the time of injury and the passage of abdominal contents through the defect, with the result that the injury is not detected at initial presentation in up to 50% of patients. If there is gross herniation of gas-filled bowel loops into the chest this may occasionally lead to confusion with pneumothorax and inappropriate tube thoracostomy (Brown & Richardson, 1985).

Aorta

Mediastinal widening on the chest X-ray can be caused by mediastinal haemorrhage, fat, vascular ectasia, adjacent pleural or pulmonary disease, and spurious widening on the supine film (thus the need to obtain an erect chest film if at all possible). Mediastinal widening is associated with aortic rupture in 25% of cases and necessitates an urgent aortogram to establish or exclude this important diagnosis (Fig. 38). In clinically stable patients there may be a place for rapid screening by high-quality CT to determine which patients really do have mediastinal haemorrhage and thereby reduce the number of unnecessary angiograms by 30–60% (Morgan *et al.*, 1992).

Medical

Acute dyspnoea and/or chest pain are the common presentations. History, clinical examination and simple tests such as electrocardiography (ECG), peak flow rate, and arterial blood gases will lead to a confident and correct diagnosis in the majority of patients. The chest X-ray is usually of secondary importance, and most useful in confirming the suspected clinical diagnoses of pulmonary oedema (Fig. 39), pneumothorax (Fig. 40), pleural effusion, or pneumonia.

Aortic dissection

Aortic dissection is not excluded by a normal chest X-ray (Slater and DeSanctis, 1976). When clinically suspected, a further test is required to establish the diagnosis, to classify the dissection, and to assist in management. Aortography is now being replaced by less invasive imaging. Echocardiography, particularly by the trans-oesophageal route, can establish the diagnosis in a large proportion of patients and may be especially useful in those who are extremely ill (Nienaber *et al.*, 1993). An alternative is contrast-enhanced CT which is an excellent confirmatory test (Fig. 41). MRI is also very accurate for the diagnosis of dissection but may be unsuitable for patients who require close monitoring and life-support equipment (Nienaber *et al.*, 1993).

Pulmonary embolism

Although a commonly encountered condition, there continue to be difficulties confirming or excluding the diagnosis of pulmonary embolism. The chest X-ray is

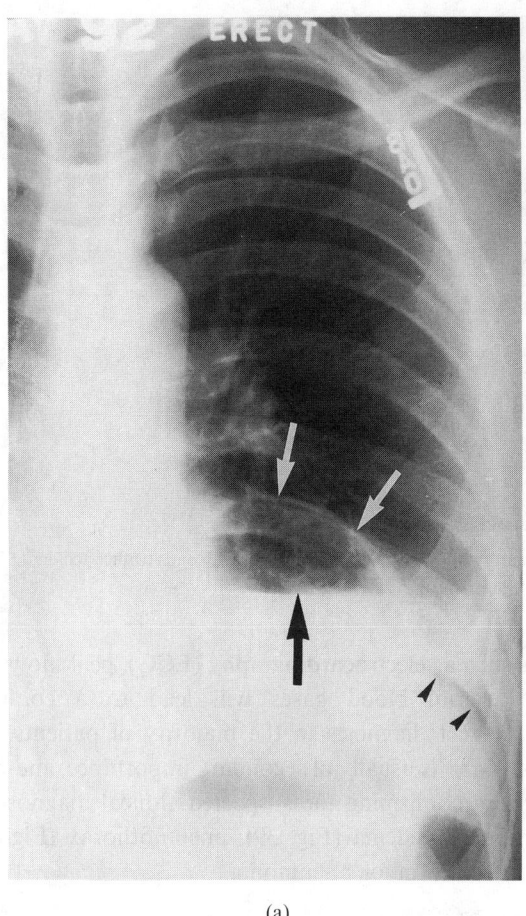
(a)

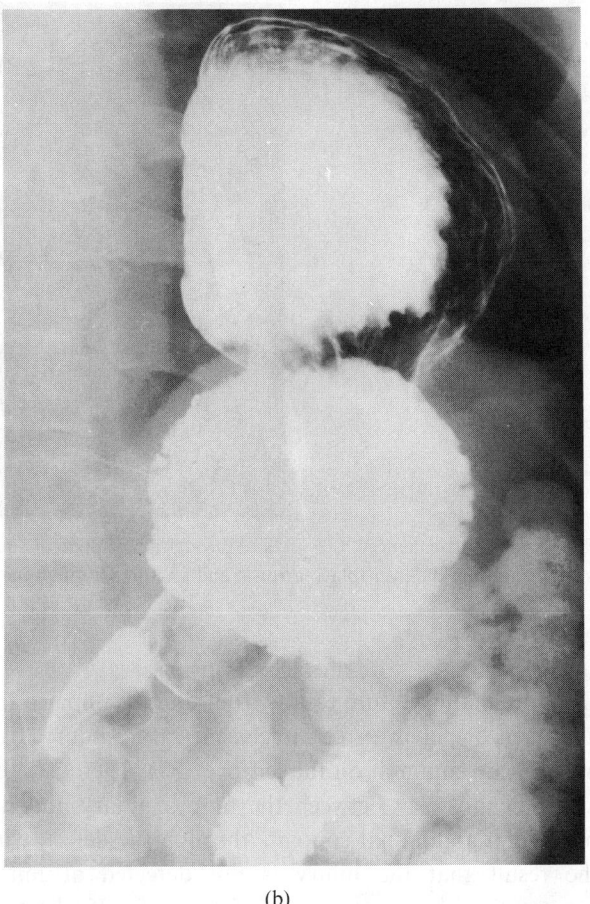
(b)

Fig. 37. Diaphragmatic rupture. (a) Thin-walled structure (white arrows) containing an air/fluid level (black arrow) at the left base in a patient who had suffered blunt abdominal trauma. (b) Barium examination demonstrates that the structure is in fact the stomach which has herniated into the thorax through a tear in the left hemidiaphragm. Note: free intraperitoneal air is visible under the diaphragm on film (a) (arrowheads), and water-soluble contrast rather than barium should have been used in view of the risk of causing barium peritonitis.

often normal or shows a non-specific abnormality. Sometimes an enlarged hilar artery, focal oligaemia, a wedge-shaped pleural based consolidation (Hampton's hump), or a pleural effusion may be present and lend support to the diagnosis. These findings, however, have a low sensitivity and specificity.

The clinical suspicion based on the history, examination, ECG and arterial blood gases, combined with the results of ventilation/perfusion isotope studies and, if necessary, imaging of the lower limb veins (venography, duplex doppler ultrasound or impedance plethysmography) (Fig. 42), will elucidate the diagnosis in most patients, without the need for pulmonary angiography (Stein *et al.*, 1993). Spiral CT angiography may prove to be a useful non-invasive tool for the detection of pulmonary emboli in the future (Remy-Jardin *et al.*, 1992) (Fig. 43).

UPPER LIMB

Shoulder dislocations

The shoulder joint is the most mobile and least stable joint in the body. Anterior dislocations account for the majority of shoulder dislocations. Posterior dislocations represent approximately 3% (Neustadter and Weiss, 1991).

An anterior dislocation occurs when the arm is forcibly externally rotated and abducted. Radiographically the diagnosis is obvious on an anteroposterior film, as the humeral head lies inferomedial to the glenoid (Fig. 44). During dislocation a compression fracture of the postero-superior aspect of the humeral head (Hill Sachs deformity) may occur as a result of impaction against the antero-inferior rim of the glenoid fossa (Fig. 44). A fracture of the anteroinferior glenoid labrum (Bankhart injury) may

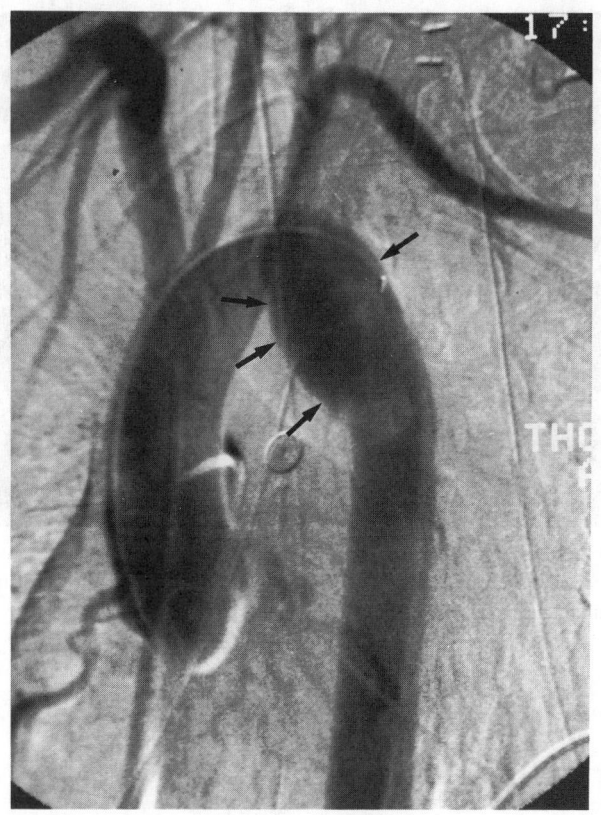

Fig. 38. Aortogram (digital subtraction image) of the driver of a vehicle which had been involved in a high speed accident. Typical appearance and site of a traumatic aortic rupture (arrows).

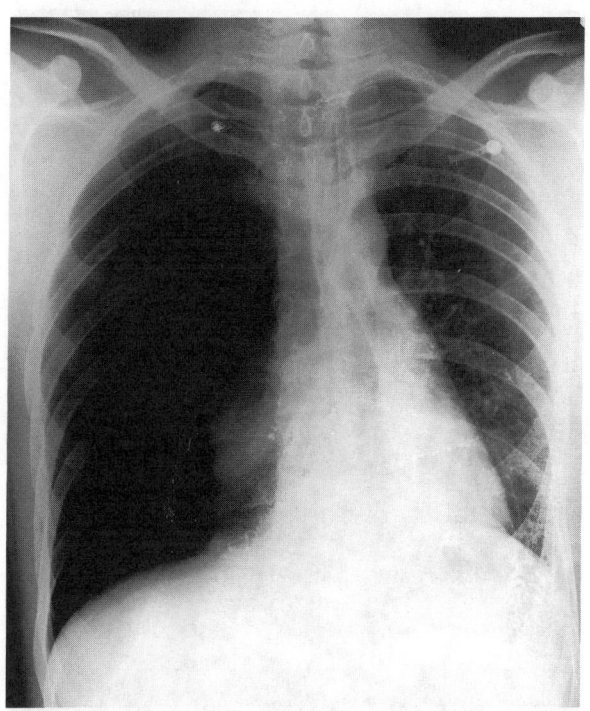

Fig. 40. Right tension pneumothorax causing depression of the right hemidiaphragm and mediastinal shift to the left.

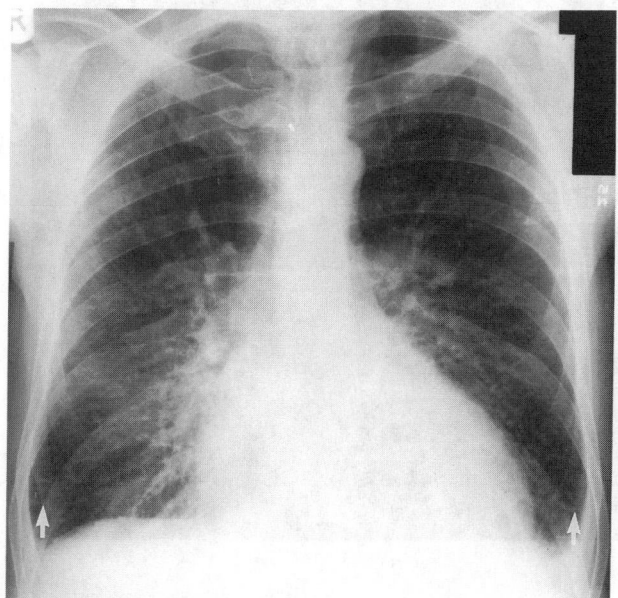

Fig. 39. Acute dyspnoea. There is cardiomegaly, increased density in the perihilar areas, septal lines (arrows), and small bilateral effusions. Left ventricular failure with pulmonary oedema.

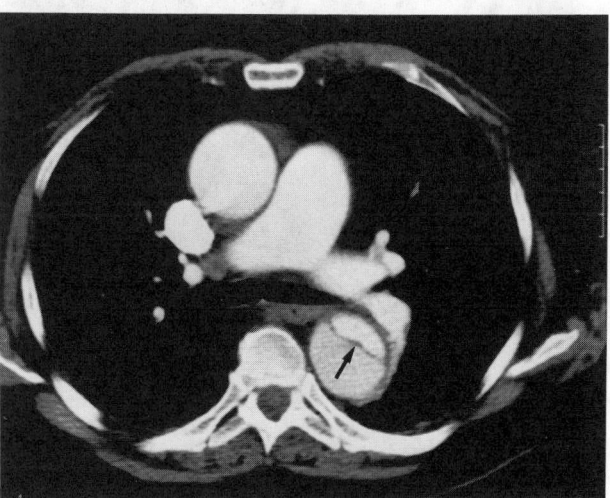

Fig. 41. Contrast-enhanced CT clearly demonstrating an intimal flap (arrow) in the descending aorta. Aortic dissection.

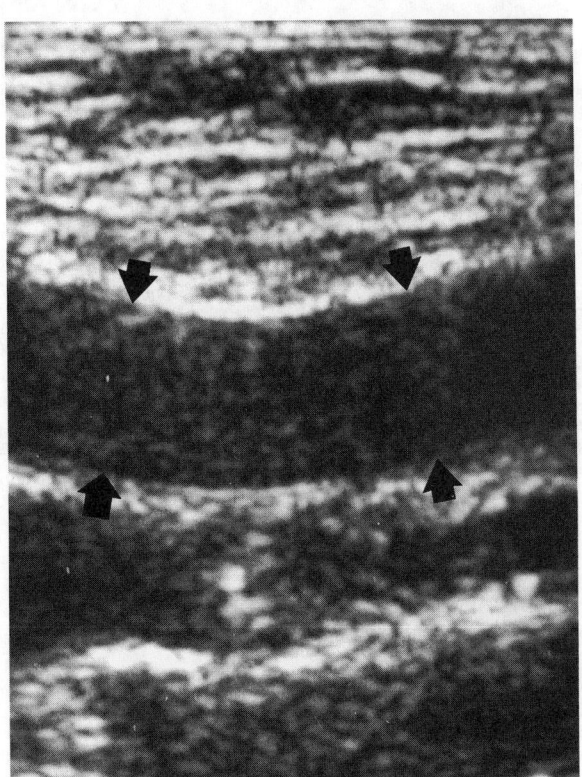

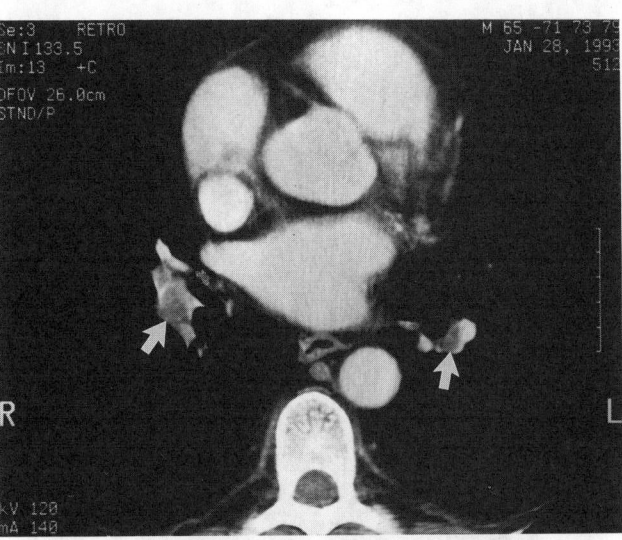

Fig. 43. Contrast-enhanced spiral CT section in a patient with suspected pulmonary embolism. Extensive thrombus is seen as low-density filling defects in the pulmonary arteries (arrows).

Fig. 42. Ultrasound of the left superficial femoral vein with compression. The vein (arrows) is full of weakly echogenic thrombus and cannot therefore be made to collapse by compression.

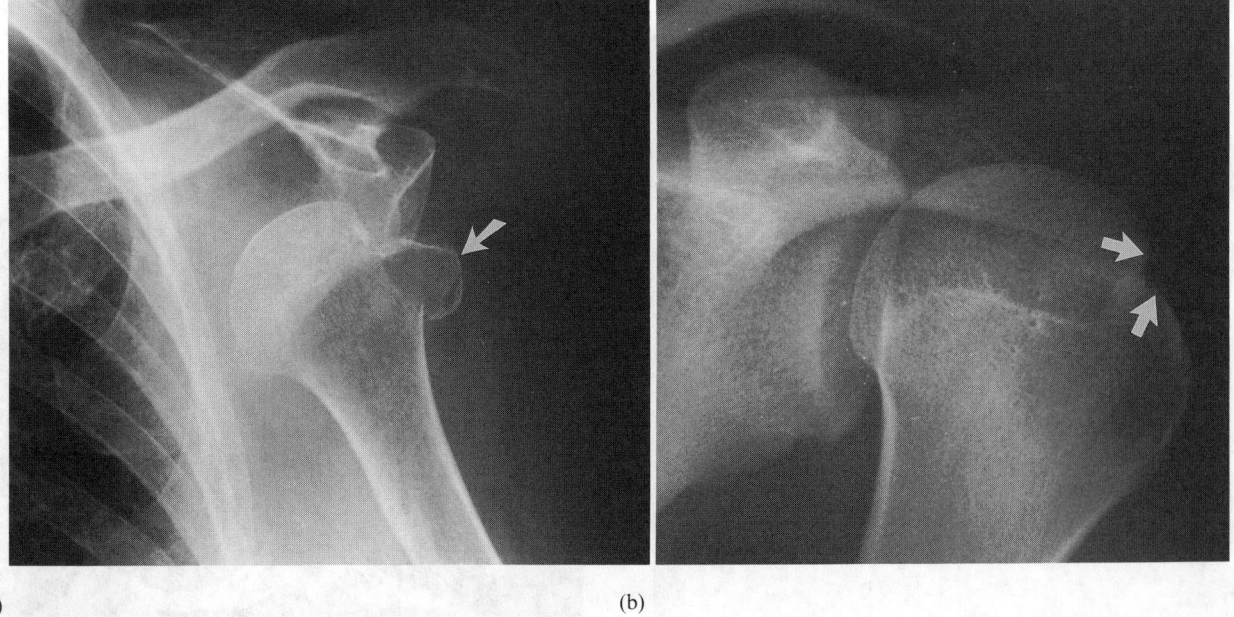

(a)   (b)

Fig. 44. Anteroposterior radiograph of the shoulder (a) demonstrating an anteroinferior dislocation, with an associated avulsion fracture of the posterosuperior aspect of the humeral head (arrow). Anterior dislocations may also result in compression of the posterosuperior aspect of the humeral head; known as a Hill Sachs (Hatchet) deformity (b, arrows).

also result but is less common. Bankhart injuries are generally cartilaginous, are associated with recurrent dislocations, and are best seen on CT arthrography.

Posterior dislocation is caused by forcible internal rotation of the humerus. Appearances are subtle on anteroposterior radiographs and approximately 50% are initially overlooked on this view. The best way to diagnose a posterior dislocation is to obtain an axial or trans-scapular radiograph. Axial views require the patient to move the arm and shoulder which can be extremely painful, and we therefore recommend the trans-scapular or Y view (Fig. 45).

Elbow

One of the most helpful indicators of significant trauma to the elbow is the presence of a joint effusion (Helms, 1989) (Fig. 14). This is seen on a lateral radiograph as elevation of the anterior and posterior fat pads. The posterior fat pad is not normally visible since it lies deep within the olecranon fossa. The anterior fat pad is seen in many normal patients as a vertically oriented radiolucent stripe close to the distal humeral diaphysis. In the presence of an effusion the posterior fat pad will become visible; the anterior fat pad will become elevated and bowed anteriorly resembling a spinnaker sail (sail sign). In the setting of trauma a visible posterior fat pad indicates an intracapsular fracture even if the fracture itself is not seen. In adults the fracture site is almost always through the radial head, while in children it usually indicates a supracondylar fracture (Helms, 1989; Resnik, 1989; Karasick *et al.*, 1991).

Forearm

When only one of the forearm bones is fractured, the wrist and elbow joints should be examined for the presence of an associated dislocation. Two types of fracture dislocation occur. The most common is the Monteggia fracture in which there is a fracture of the ulna and dislocation of the radial head (Reckling, 1982) (Fig. 46). The dislocated radial head is easy to overlook clinically, and misdiagnosis may lead to aseptic necrosis with subsequent elbow dysfunction. The Galeazzi fracture involves a fracture of the radius with dislocation of the distal radioulnar joint (Fig. 47). The deformity of the wrist joint is usually obvious clinically.

Wrist

Fractures of the carpal bones are less common than those of the distal radius. They are particularly rare in children.

Scaphoid

Scaphoid fractures account for approximately 80% of carpal fractures and generally occur between the ages of 15 and 40 years; 70% involve the waist, 20% the proximal pole and 10% the distal pole (Meyer, 1991). Most scaphoid fractures are undisplaced and many are difficult to detect radiographically at time of injury. Specific scaphoid views should be requested, and if the radiographs are normal then the wrist should be immobilized and repeat films obtained after 10–14 days. A fracture line is then usually seen due to adjacent bony resorption resulting from disuse and hyperaemia (Meyer, 1991) (Fig. 48). Radioisotope bone scanning is an alternative means of investigation. This technique is highly sensitive and can be used to exclude a fracture as early as 24–48 h after injury (Meyer, 1991).

Lunate / perilunate

Lunate and perilunate dislocations are serious injuries. These dislocations can be suspected on an anteroposterior view of the wrist by noting a triangular or pie-shaped lunate. In practice, they are much easier to diagnose by assessing the lateral view. With a perilunate dislocation the lunate maintains its alignment with the radius, whilst the capitate and remainder of the carpal bones are displaced dorsally. With a lunate dislocation the lunate is dislocated anteriorly but the capitate and carpal bones maintain a normal alignment with the radius (Fig. 49). Associated injuries are common, and include fractures of the scaphoid, radial styloid, capitate and triquetrum (Helms, 1989).

Triquetrum

Bony chips seen posteriorly on lateral wrist radiographs are virtually pathognomonic of triquetral avulsion fractures (Fig. 50).

LOWER LIMB

Hip and proximal femur

Fractures and dislocations

Femoral head dislocations (anterior, posterior and central) are classified according to their relationship to the

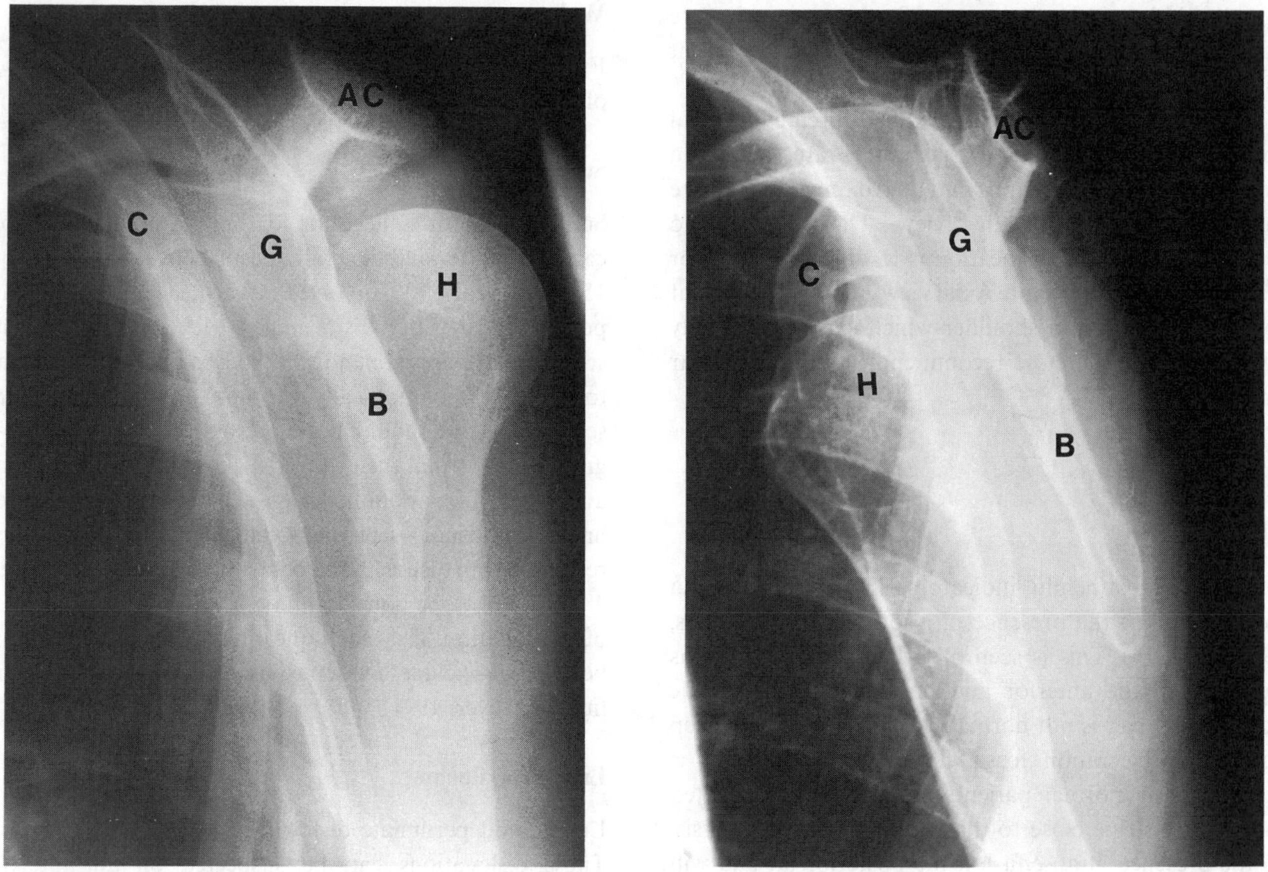

Fig. 45. (a, b) Anterior and posterior dislocations. Trans-scapular views of shoulder. On the normal trans-scapular view the acromion (AC), coracoid (C) and blade of the scapula (B) should all form a Y with the glenoid (G) at its axis. The coracoid lies anteriorly, whereas the acromion is seen posteriorly. The humeral head (H) normally overlies the glenoid. Posterior dislocation (a) is diagnosed when the humeral head is displaced from the glenoid in the direction of the acromion. Anterior dislocation (b) is seen as displacement of the humeral head in the direction of the coracoid.

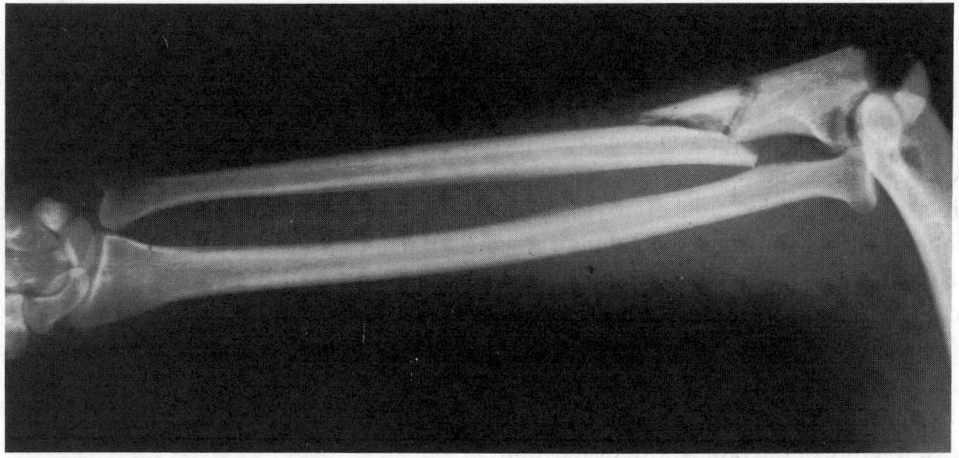

Fig. 46. Lateral view of the forearm demonstrating a comminuted fracture of the proximal ulna with dislocation of the radial head (Monteggia fracture). (There is also a vertical fracture through the olecranon.)

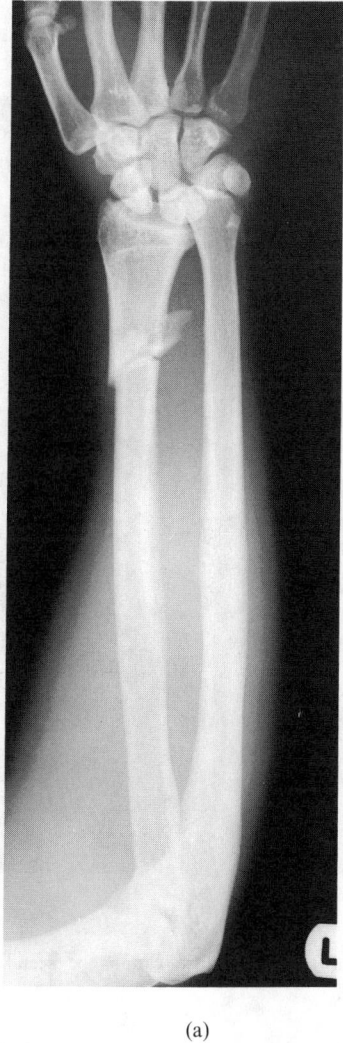

(a)

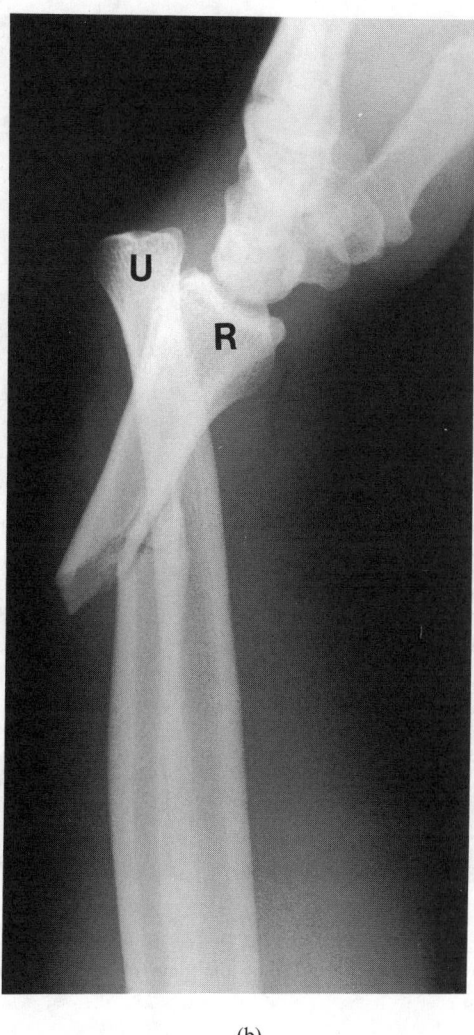

(b)

Fig. 47. Galeazzi fracture. Anteroposterior (a) and lateral (b) views of the forearm showing a comminuted fracture of the shaft of the radius (R) with posterior dislocation of the ulna (U).

acetabulum. Posterior dislocations are the commonest type (80%), and are associated with fractures of the posterior acetabular rim, femoral shaft, patella and knee (Fig. 51). If there is persistent joint widening following reduction, this raises the possibility of bony or cartilaginous fragments within the joint. CT can precisely define the extent of the bony fracture, and is useful in identifying intra-articular bony fragments (Fig. 51).

Fractures of the proximal femoral neck are classified by the position of the fracture: capsular (subcapital and transcervical), and extracapsular (basicervical and trochanteric) (Fig. 52). Intracapsular fractures are the most common (63%), and are associated with delayed/non-union, or avascular necrosis in up to 25% of cases. This is due to disruption of the blood supply to the femoral head (Resnick *et al.*, 1988). Anteroposterior and

lateral radiographs are sufficent to identify the majority of injuries. In some cases there is difficulty in diagnosis and then either linear tomography or radionuclide bone scanning can be helpful. The latter should be delayed until at least 24 h postinjury, as sensitivity increases from 80% at 24 h, to almost 100% at 72 h (Matin, 1983).

Children

Hip pain with restricted movement and a limp is a frequent clinical presentation in childhood. All patients should be referred to either a specialist orthopaedic or paediatric team. Possible diagnoses include slipped epiphysis, Perthes' disease, irritable hip (transient synovitis) and septic arthritis (Fig. 53). The only way to exclude septic arthritis is to obtain synovial fluid for

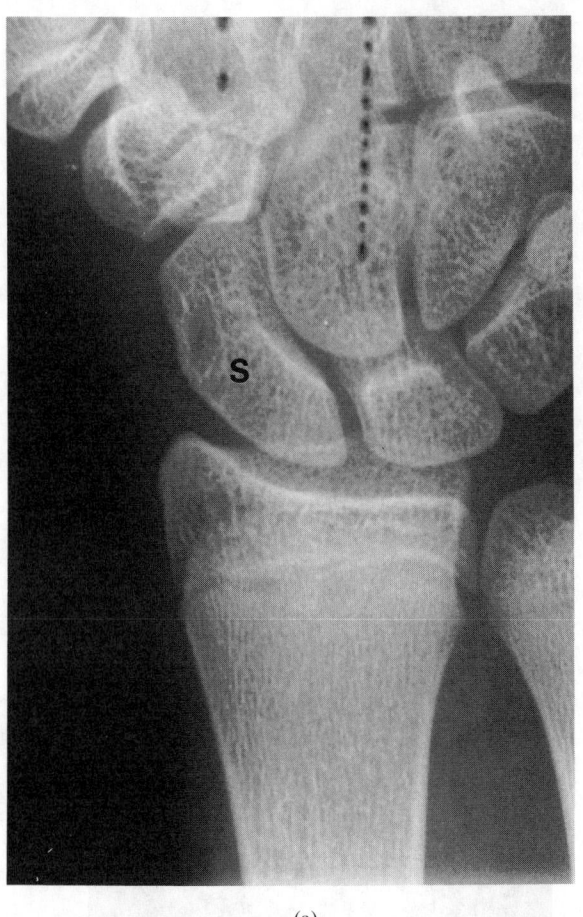

(a)

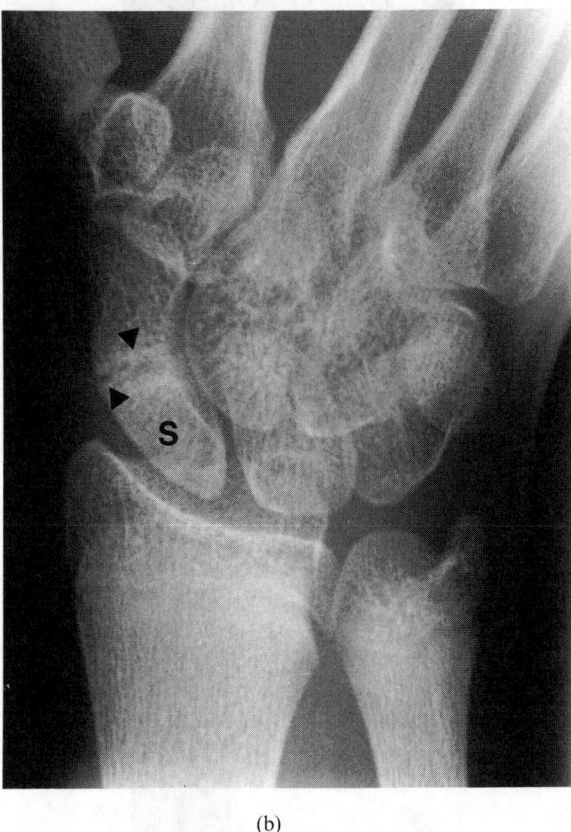

(b)

Fig. 48. The scaphoid bone (S) at the time of initial trauma (a) and 10 days later (b). The fracture cannot be seen on the initial radiograph.

Gram stain and culture as clinical history, physical examination and haematological tests are often inconclusive. The following is a protocol that can be followed in all cases (Fink *et al.*, 1993; Raby *et al.*, 1994).

TECHNIQUE

Investigation of hip pain in a child

- When the child presents to the A&E department local anaesthetic cream is applied to the hip skin crease and a plain radiograph is obtained.
- If the plain radiograph reveals obvious Perthes' disease or a slipped capital femoral epiphysis no further investigations are required.
- When the radiograph is normal then the child is referred for an immediate hip ultrasound.
- If a joint effusion is found it is aspirated and a sample sent for immediate Gram stain and culture.
- Therapy is commenced if the gram stain is positive, but if negative, then the child can be safely

discharged home while cultures are awaited provided the family can be easily contacted by telephone.
- All children are reviewed 1 week later at the orthopaedic or paediatric clinic, and if pain persists an isotope bone scan is ordered to exclude early Perthes' disease.

Hind/Midfoot

Fractures of the mid and hindfoot are commonly misinterpreted on plain radiographs.

The calcaneus is the most frequently injured tarsal bone. In 75% of cases the fracture is compressive and extends to involve the subtalar joints (Mitchell *et al.*, 1989); 10% are bilateral 10% also and involve the thoracolumbar spine. Calcaneal fractures can be difficult to diagnose on lateral views, and Böhlers angle is a useful measure to aid diagnosis (Fig. 54). If this angle measures less than 20° a compressive calcaneal fracture can be diagnosed (Fig 55).

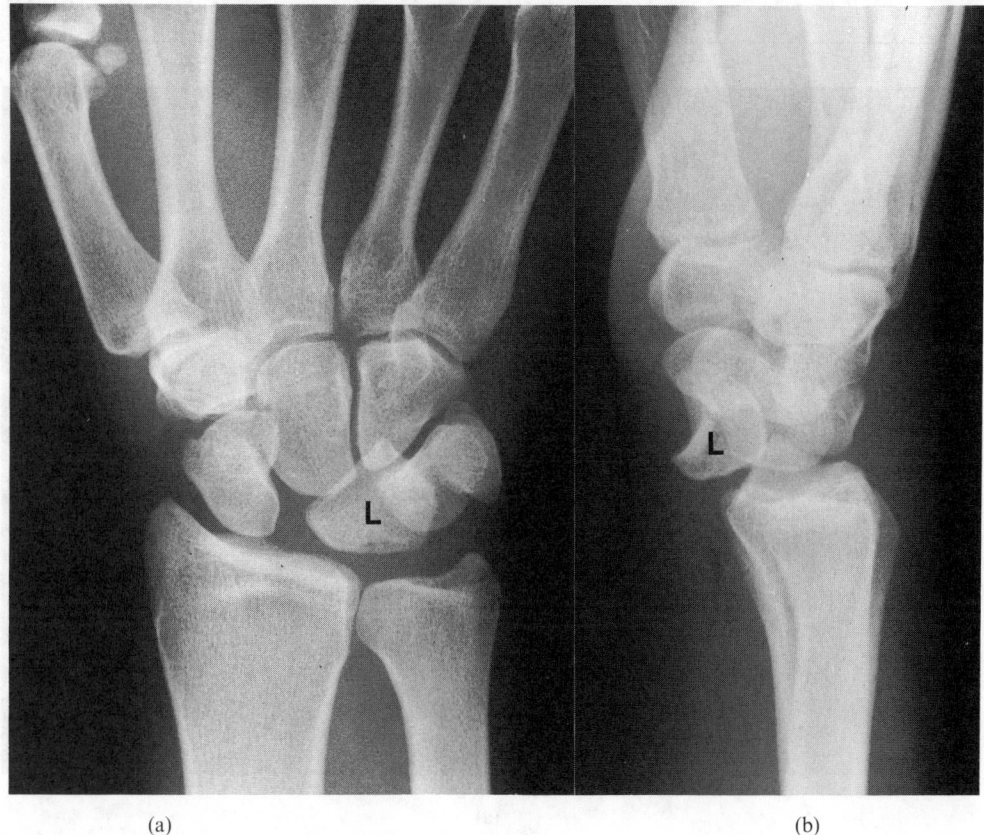

(a)   (b)

Fig. 49. Anteroposterior (a) and lateral (b) radiographs of the wrist demonstrating a lunate dislocation. On the anteroposterior view the lunate (L) appears 'piece of pie' shaped and there is widening of the scapholunate articulation (Terry Thomas sign) due to ligamentous rupture. On the lateral view the lunate has tipped anteriorly but the capitate and radius maintain their normal alignment. (Courtesy of Raby, N., Berman, L. & de Lacey, G. (1994). *Accident and Emergency Radiology: A Survival Guide.* London. W.B. Saunders.)

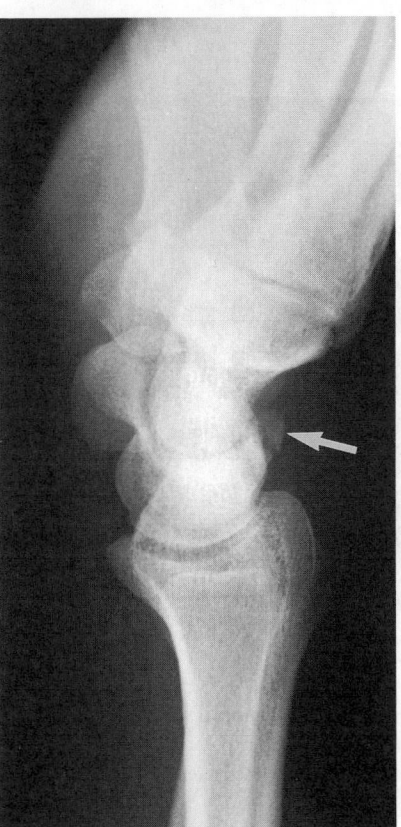

Fig. 50. Lateral view of the wrist in which an avulsed bony fragment is seen posteriorly (arrow). This appearance on the lateral view is virtually pathognomonic of a triquetral fracture.

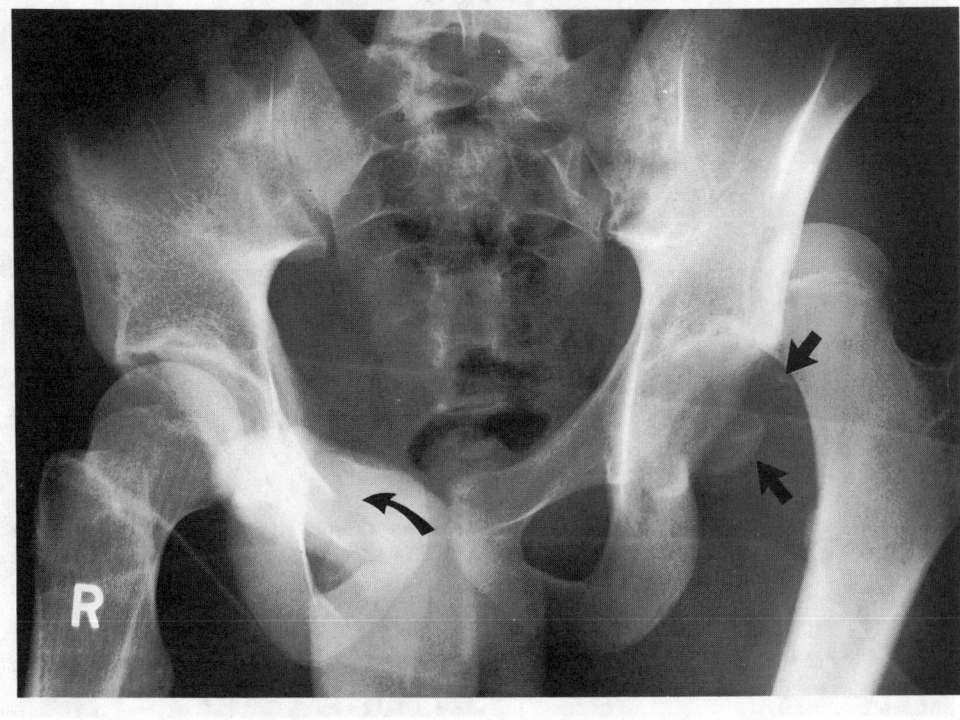

(a)

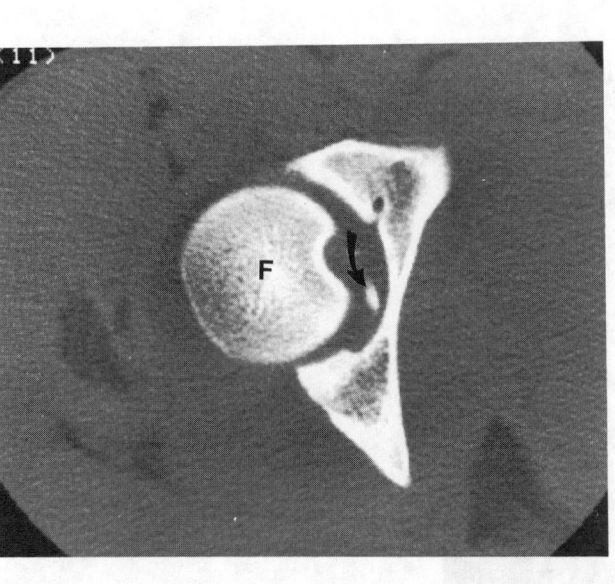

(b)

Fig. 51. (a) Plain radiograph demonstrating a posterior dislocation of the left hip with two fragments (solid straight arrows) detached from the posterior acetabular margin. There is also a comminuted fracture of the right superior pubic ramus (curved arrow). (b) CT scan in a different patient after reduction of a hip dislocation. This shows a small bony fragment (curved arrow) lying in the joint space medial to the femoral head (F).

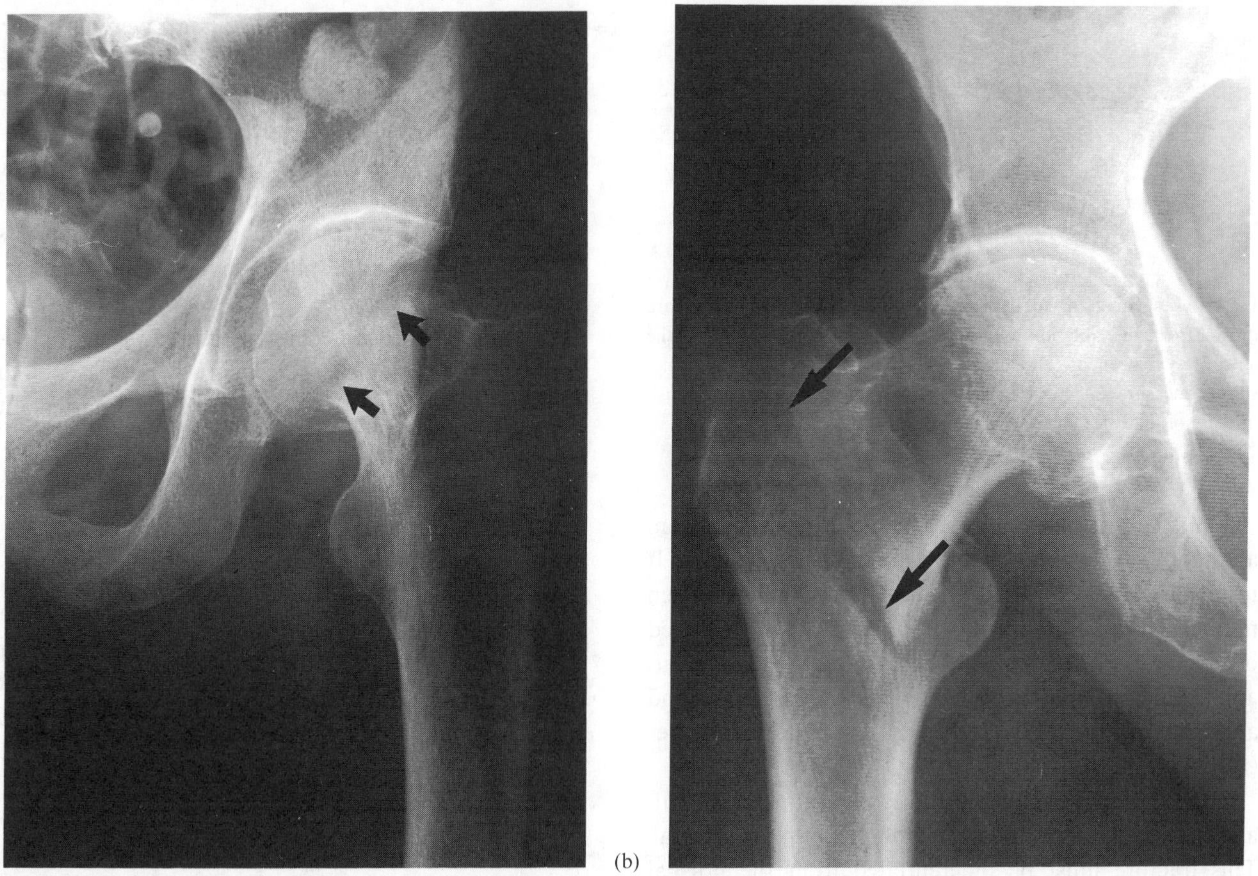

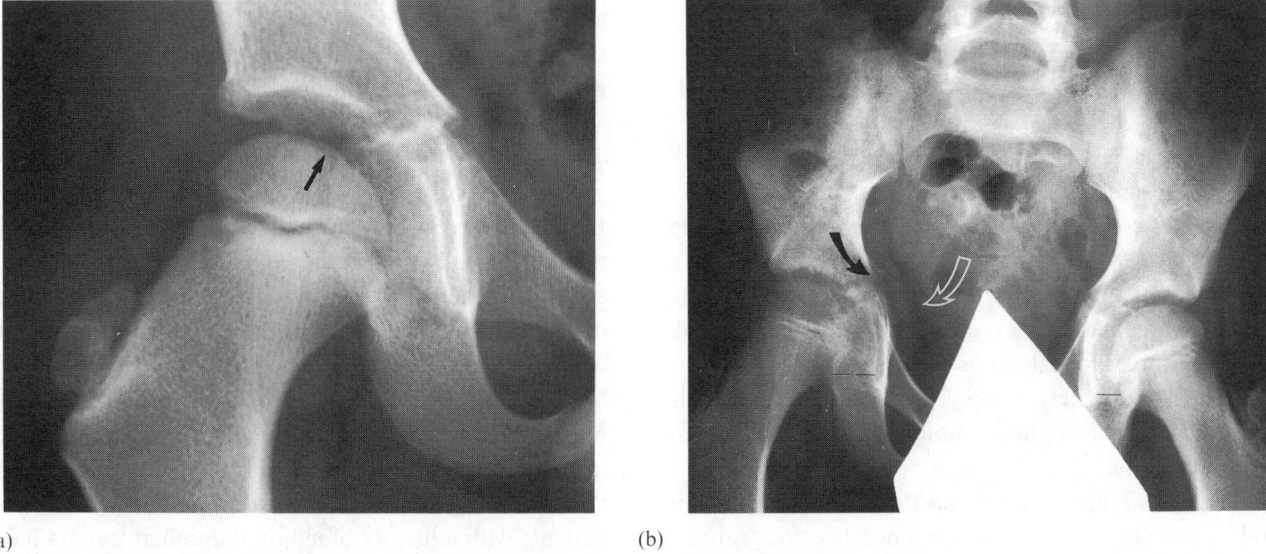

Fig. 52. (a) Anteroposterior radiograph of an impacted subcapital fracture (arrows) of the left femoral neck. (b) Anteroposterior radiograph of a basicervical fracture (arrows) of the right femoral neck.

Fig. 53. (a) Subtle crescent shaped lucency in the capital femoral epiphysis (arrow). This is diagnostic of an early Perthes disease. (b) Eight-year-old boy with a history of a sore right hip for 6 weeks. There is extensive disuse osteopenia of the right hemipelvis, with a soft tissue mass (open arrow) and some bony destruction (solid arrow). The presence of an effusion can be inferred from the increased distance between the medial margin of the femur and the adjacent acetabulum (compare with the normal left side). The effusion was confirmed at ultrasound and 10 ml of pus were aspirated. Tuberculosis was diagnosed.

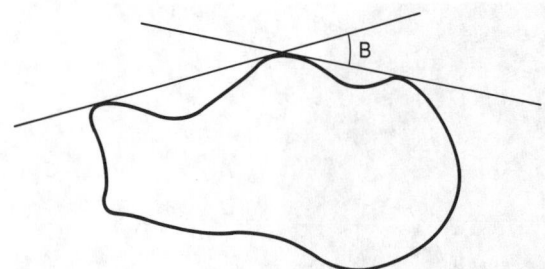

Fig. 54. Line diagram to demonstrate Böhler's angle B. Lines are drawn from the anterior and posterior calcaneal processes to the apex of the calcaneus. The angle between these lines (Böhler's angle) should measure 20–40°; when it is less than 20° degrees a crush fracture of the calcaneus can be diagnosed.

The Lisfranc fracture is a serious injury resulting from a fracture dislocation at the tarsometatarsal joints. It results from severe forefoot abduction. There is often minimal dislocation and the injury is easily overlooked on plain radiographs. The key to diagnosis is malalignment of the medial borders of the bases of the second and third metatarsals with the adjacent cuneiform bones (Fig. 56).

Inversion injuries of the ankle are associated with avulsion fractures of the base of the fifth metatarsal. This fracture must be differentiated from the normal apophyses that occur at this site. Fractures are typically transversely orientated with an irregular margin, whereas the apophysis is longitudinally orientated with a smooth well-corticated margin (Fig. 57).

THE ACUTE ABDOMEN

Plain radiographs have a well-defined role in a number of acute abdominal conditions, but in others they usually provide no useful information (Mirvis *et al.*, 1986; de Lacey *et al.*, 1980; Alford and McIlhenny, 1992) (Fig. 58). Bowel obstruction (Fig. 59), toxic megacolon (Fig. 60), caecal volvulus and sigmoid volvulus are well demonstrated.

Free intraperitoneal air is best imaged by a well-penetrated erect chest X-ray (Fig. 61). If the patient is unable to stand or sit a left decubitus view of the abdomen is also accurate.

Field *et al.* (1985) recommend that only a supine film and erect chest X-ray be obtained as the routine abdominal series. They suggest that an erect abdominal film is only necessary when an intra-abdominal abscess is suspected (Fig. 62). Although it is contentious, we would recommend that in suspected intestinal obstruction an erect film also be obtained.

In suspected acute renal colic an intravenous urogram is the preferred investigation (Fig. 63). The high false negative rate of ultrasound in this condition makes it an unsuitable option in most patients.

Acute cholecystitis is often a difficult clinical diagnosis and here ultrasound can be very helpful (Fig. 64). If the ultrasound is negative and the clinical suspicion is still high then cholescintigraphy is indicated (Shuman *et al.*, 1982) (Fig. 64).

Abdominal aortic aneurysm rupture is usually obvious clinically. Radiological investigation in these circumstances may simply delay the urgently required intervention. If there is genuine uncertainty about the diagnosis then ultrasound, if necessary followed by CT, will establish or exclude the diagnosis.

ABDOMINAL TRAUMA

Radiological investigation of abdominal trauma is primarily determined by the patient's haemodynamic status. If clinical examination indicates that emergency surgery is essential then imaging is unnecessary, and it may delay treatment with fatal consequences. In the overall setting of major trauma, a lateral radiograph of the cervical spine, and supine chest and pelvic radiographs are first performed in accordance with the ATLS guidelines (American College of Surgeons Committee on Trauma, 1993). Further investigations are determined by the patient's clinical status, the severity of the trauma, and the modalities available. It is beyond the scope of this discussion to cover all the eventualities. Instead, some general principles are outlined.

Ultrasound versus CT scanning

Ultrasound is widely available and portable and is therefore ideally suited to the initial imaging of acute abdominal trauma. Ultrasound is, however, highly operator-dependent and less likely to be definitive in obese patients, or in those with abdominal lacerations or lower rib fractures. If the operator feels that the examination has been inadequate then referral for CT scanning is advised.

CT is undoubtedly the imaging modality of choice in the assessment of severe abdominal trauma; 25–50% of patients with a history of major abdominal trauma have associated injuries to the thorax, pelvis, spine or head. Imaging is these patients is best achieved by a single CT examination, and other modalities such as abdominal ultrasound can be bypassed. In experienced hands, CT has a similar sensitivity to diagnostic peritoneal lavage,

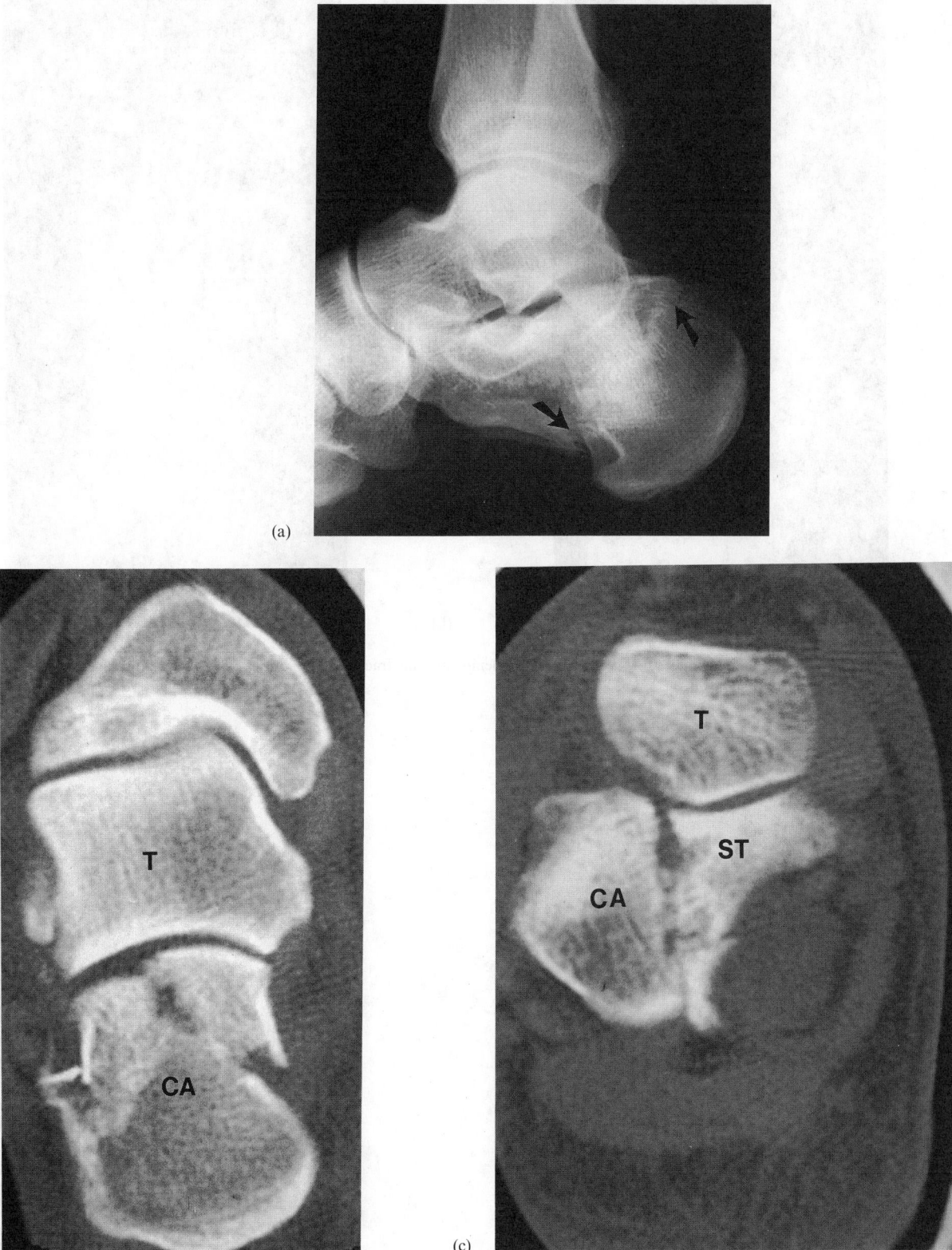

Fig. 55. (a) Lateral radiograph of the calcaneus in which Böhler's angle is almost zero. This indicates a crush fracture. Note that the fracture line is seen posteriorly (arrows). (b, c) CT scans define the extent of the fracture. There is a comminuted fracture of the calcaneus (CA) which extends to the articular margin with the talus (T). At a more anterior level (c) the fracture line is seen to extend through the base of the sustentaculum tali (ST).

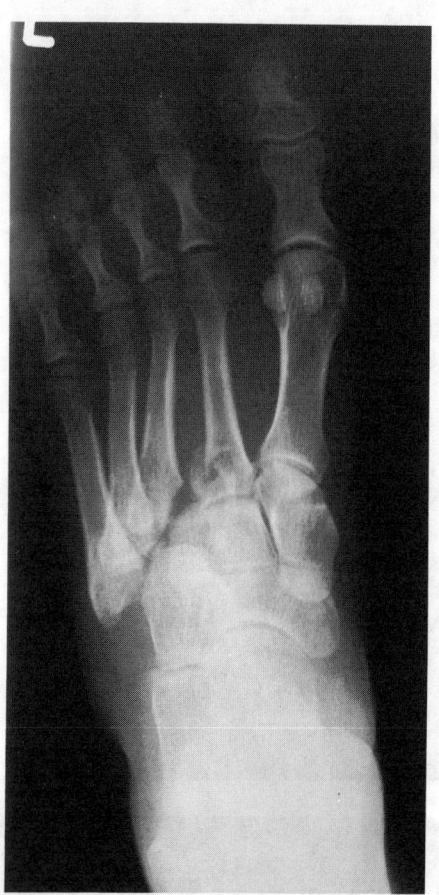

(a)

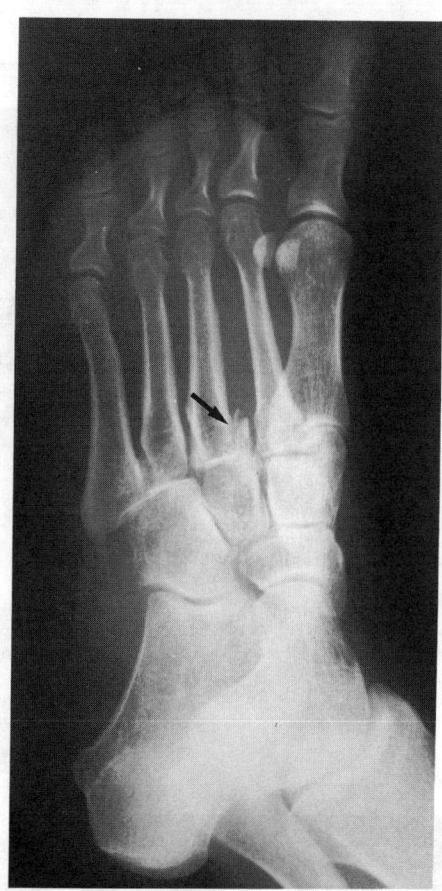

(b)

Fig. 56. Anteroposterior (a) and oblique (b) views of the foot demonstrating fracture dislocations with lateral displacement at the bases of the second, third and fourth metatarsals.

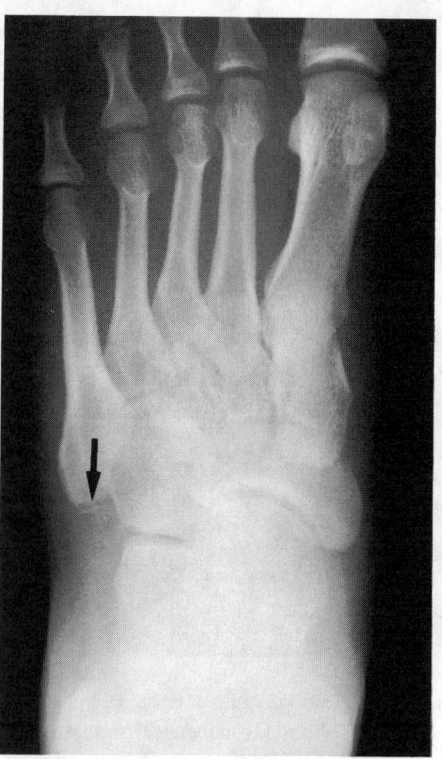

(a)

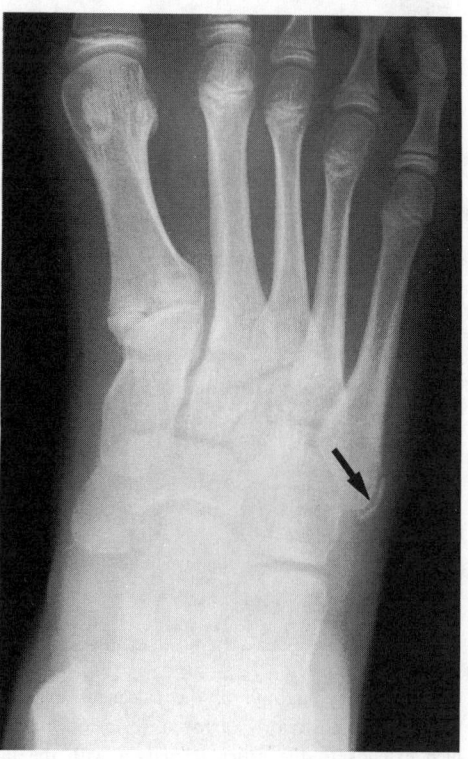

(b)

Fig. 57. (a) Normal linear apophysis at the base of the fifth metatarsal (arrow). (b) Transverse avulsion fracture.

1 Abdominal pain
'When NOT to X-ray'

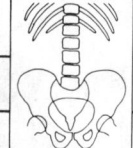

'Non-specific' abdominal pain
Constipation
Haematemesis/melaena
Urinary retention
Acute urinary tract infection
Acute peptic ulceration
Biliary disease … *request ultrasound*
Acute appendicitis
Pancreatitis

rarely helpful!

2 Acute Abdominal pain
When to X-ray

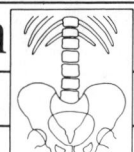

	Supine	Erect	CXR
Obstruction	YES	YES	YES
Perforation	YES	**NO**	YES
Renal colic	YES	**NO**	**NO**

But *only* as part of a 2 film IVU

Fig. 58. IVU, intravenous urography. (Courtesy of Kodak UK.)

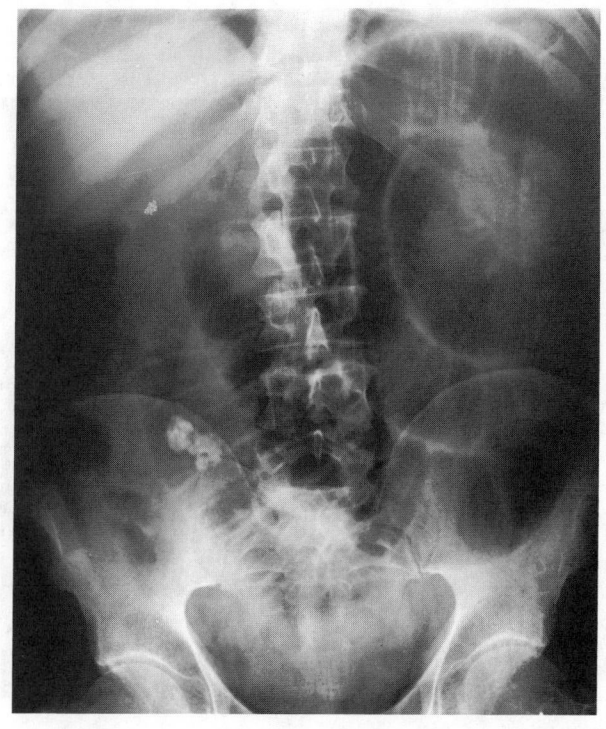

(a)

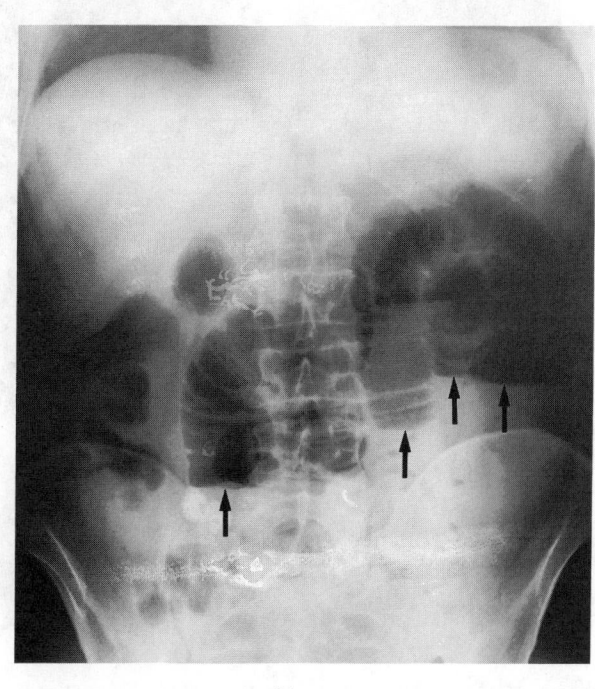

(b)

Fig. 59. Small bowel obstruction. (a) Supine film: multiple dilated small bowel loops. (b) Erect film: multiple air/fluid levels in the small bowel (arrows).

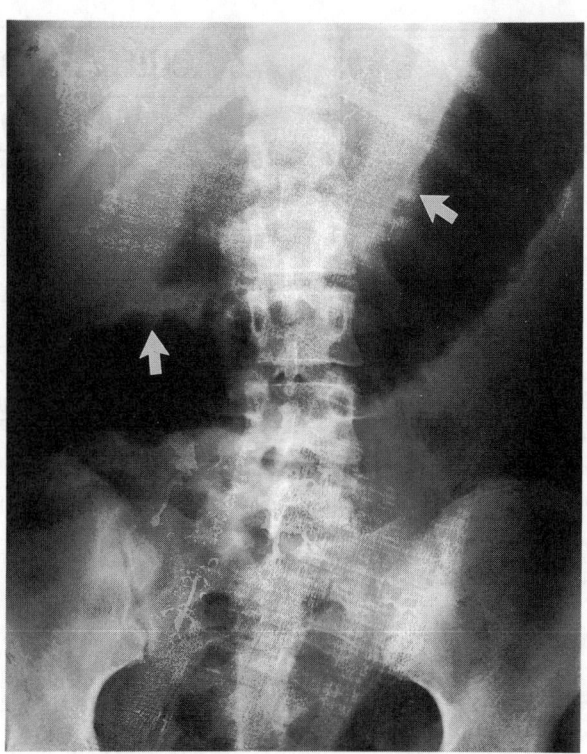

Fig. 60. Toxic megacolon in a patient with Crohn's disease. Islands of mucosal oedema (arrows) are seen in the dilated transverse colon, giving rise to the appearance of 'thumbprinting'.

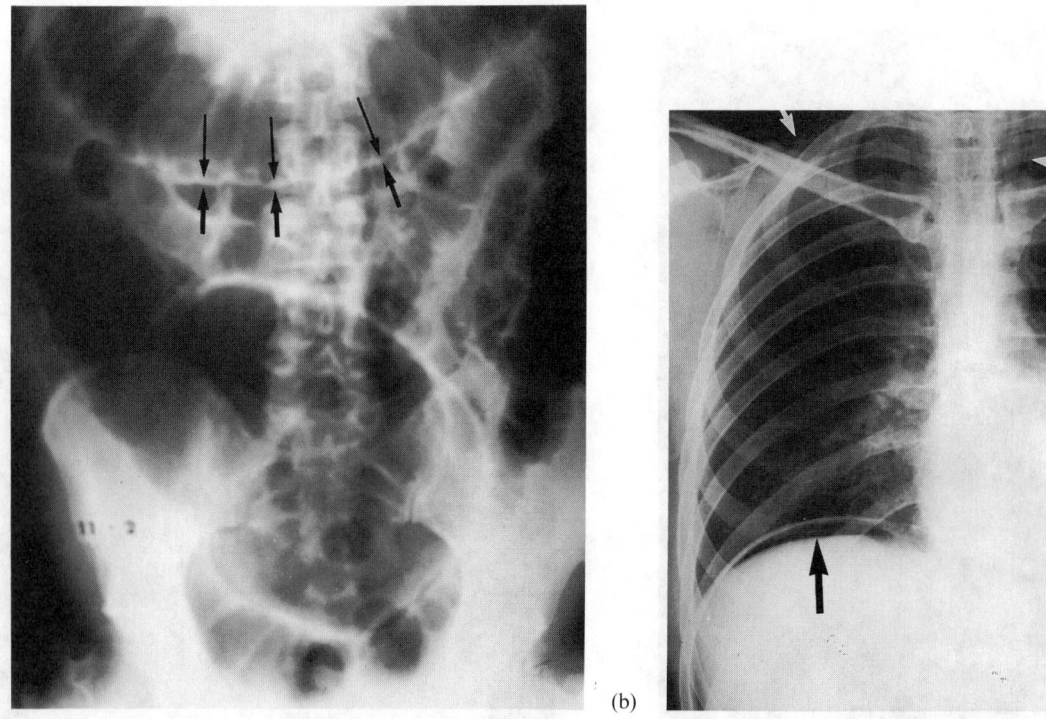

(a)   (b)

Fig. 61. Free intraperitoneal air. (a) Patient A: supine film. Both walls of the colon are clearly visible (arrows) due to the presence of air within the lumen and in the peritoneal space. (b) Patient B: erect chest X-ray demonstrating free intraperitoneal air beneath both hemidiaphragms (black arrows). Note that in this patient air has tracked into the mediastinum and subcutaneous tissues of the neck (white arrows).

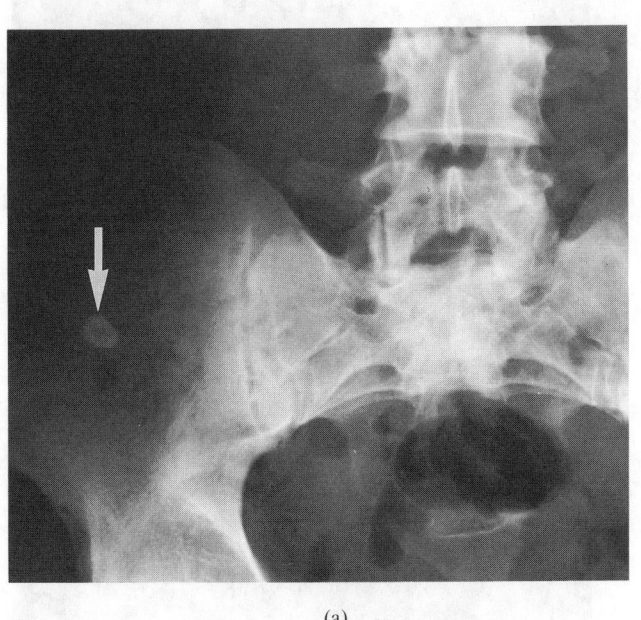

(a)

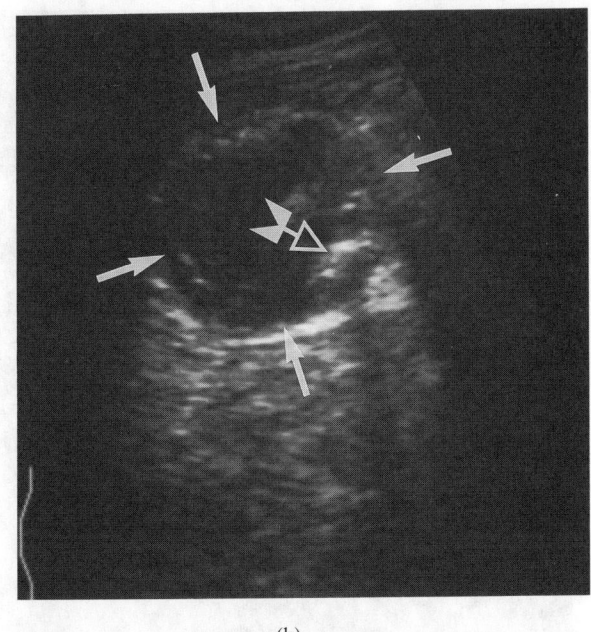

(b)

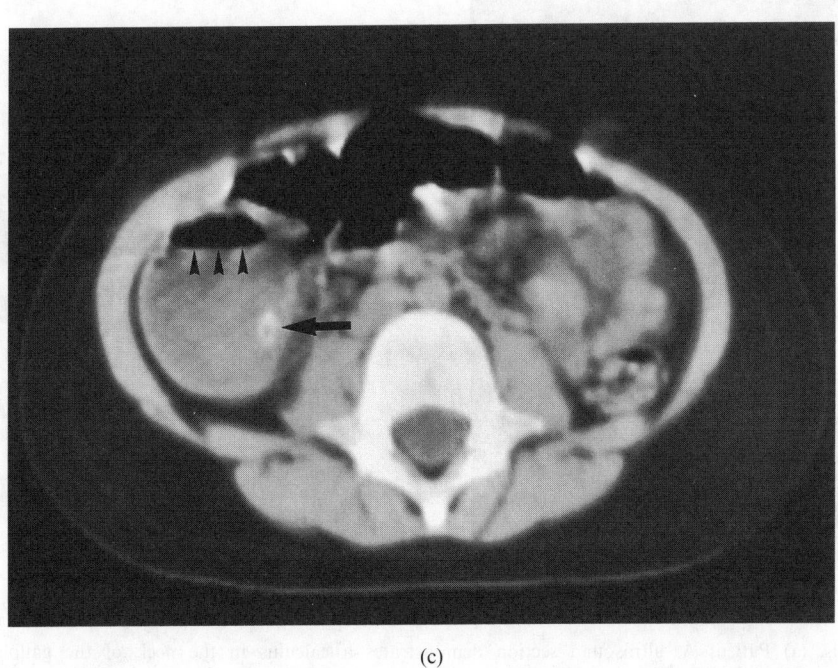

(c)

Fig. 62. Appendicolith and appendix abscess. (a) Plain film demonstrating an appendicolith in the right iliac fossa. (b) Ultrasound section showing a well circumscribed abscess (closed arrows) and the appendicolith (open arrow). (c) CT section shows the abscess and appendicolith (arrow). Gas is present within the abscess (arrowheads).

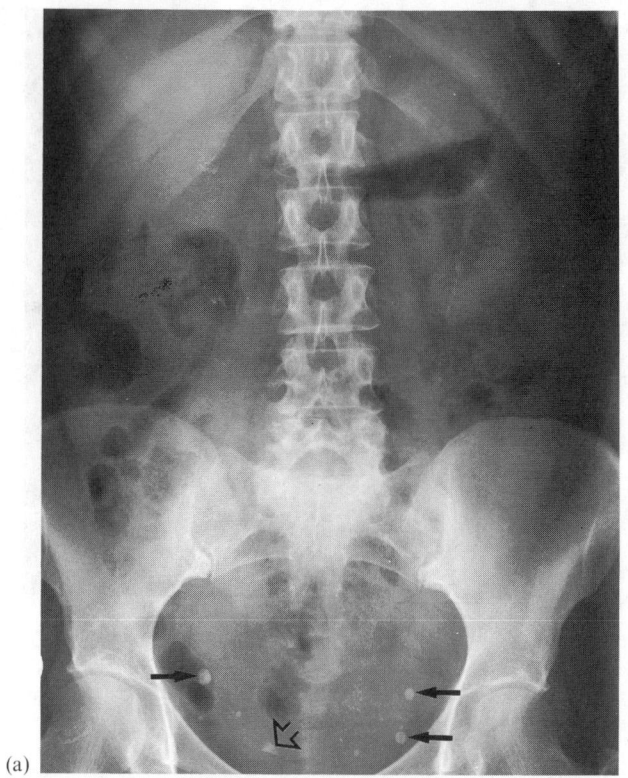 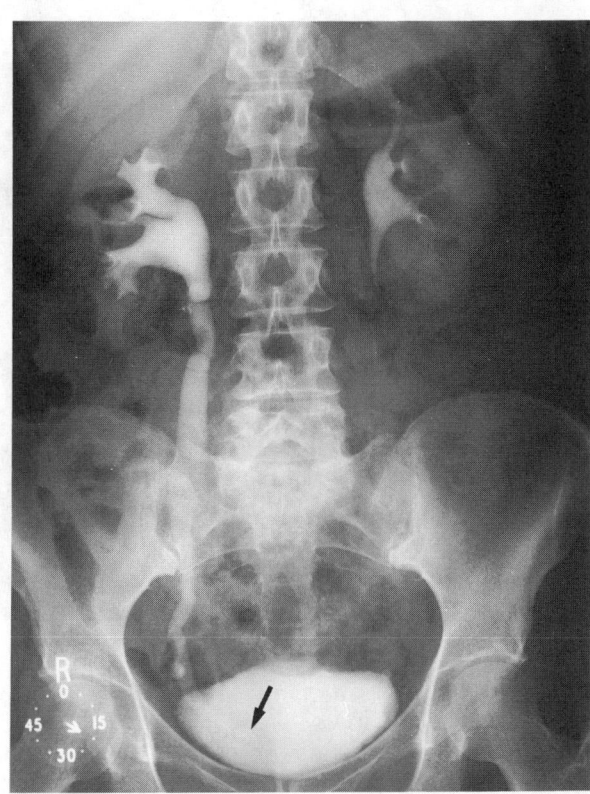

(a)   (b)

Fig. 63. Right renal colic. (a) Multiple phleboliths are seen within the pelvis on the plain film. These are rounded and have lucent centres (closed arrows). An additional triangular opacity is present on the right (open arrow). (b) 20 min after injection of contrast medium. Right hydronephrosis and hydroureter to the level of the triangular calculus at the vesicoureteric junction (arrow).

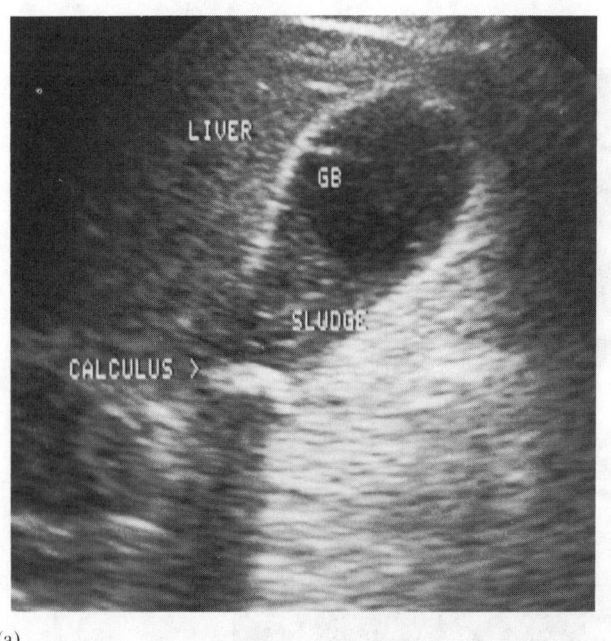 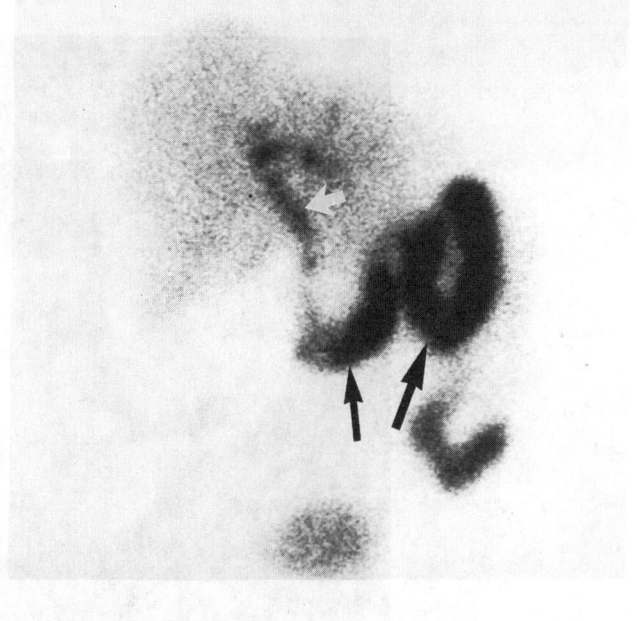

(a)   (b)

Fig. 64. Acute cholecystitis. (a) Patient A: ultrasound section demonstrates a calculus in the neck of the gallbladder with sludge lying superior to it. The patient was exquisitely sensitive to pressure applied by the ultrasound probe over the fundus i.e. an ultrasound positive Murphy's sign. (b) Patient B: right upper quadrant pain. HIDA (hepatic iminodiacetic acid) scan showing radiopharmaceutical in the common bile duct (white arrow) and in small bowel loops (black arrows). There is no gallbladder filling. This confirms the clinical diagnosis of acute cholecystitis.

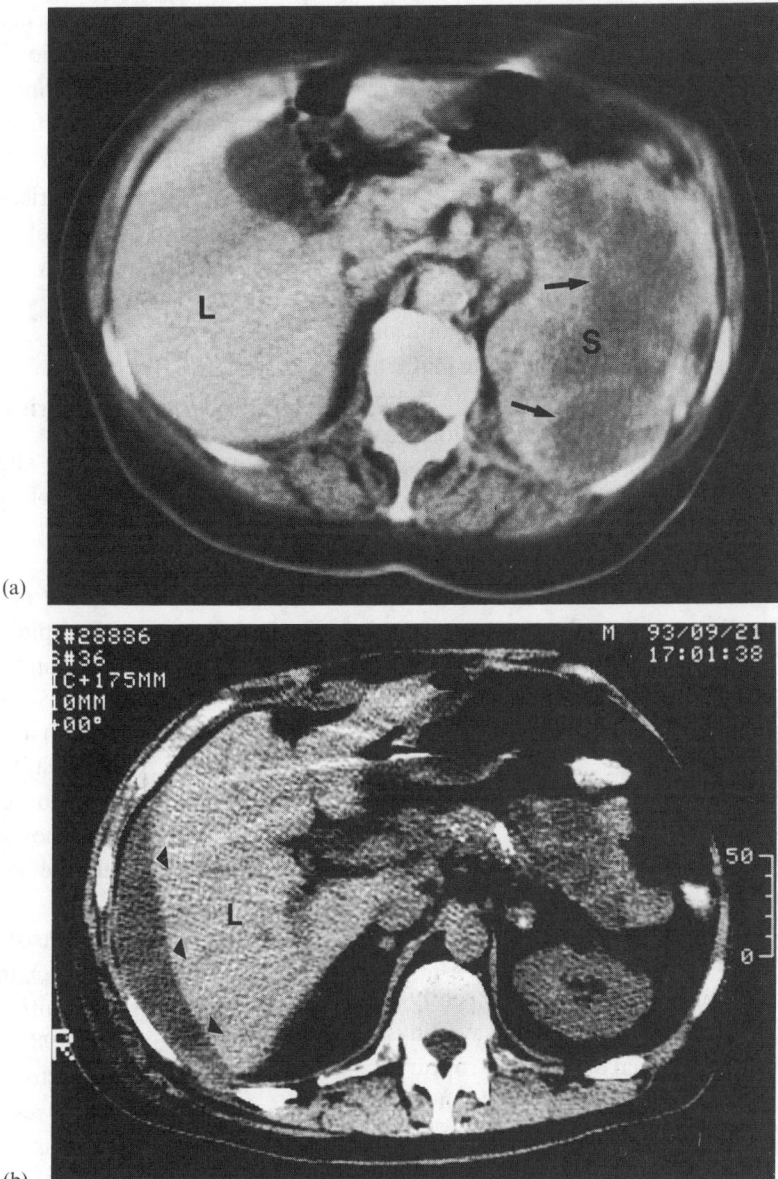

Fig. 65. (a, b) CT scans of the upper abdomen following blunt abdominal trauma. In (a) the spleen (S) contains multiple confluent areas of haemorrhagic contusion (arrows). In (b) there is a large subcapsular haematoma of the liver (L) (arrowheads).

but it is more specific in defining the site and extent of injury (Gay & Sistrom, 1992). Using CT it is possible to diagnose retroperitoneal, and subcapsular injuries that may be missed by diagnostic peritoneal lavage (Figs 36 and 65). In addition, it is possible to monitor injuries which are treated conservatively.

Visceral trauma

In splenic injury, overlying rib fractures are present in less than 50% of cases, and are an insensitive sign of serious splenic injury. The liver and spleen are most comprehensively imaged using CT which has an accuracy of almost 100% (Fig. 65). The diagnosis of pancreatic injury is particularly difficult even with CT, and is generally self-limiting. Pancreatic laceration with ductal disruption is, however, an indication for immediate laparotomy. Bowel and mesenteric injuries also occur in approximately 5% of blunt abdominal injuries. Early recognition is essential as delay increases mortality from 5% to 65%. The diagnosis of intraperitoneal bowel rupture can be made if free gas is seen below the diaphragm on an erect chest radiograph.

Retroperitoneal bowel (duodenum and colon) rupture is difficult to diagnose on plain radiographs, but can be diagnosed on CT as extravasated oral contrast or free gas in adjacent soft tissues. Most patients with injuries to the abdominal aorta and inferior vena cava are haemodynamically unstable and require operative intervention rather than radiological investigation.

The radiology of renal trauma deserves special mention. Although microscopic haematuria is commonly present after minor trauma, it is only associated with significant renal injury in 0.1% of cases (Mirvis and Shanmuganathan, 1992). These patients do not routinely warrant radiological investigation. A protocol for the radiological management of patients with renal trauma is outlined in Fig 66.

PELVIS

Fractures

Plain radiographs remain the mainstay in the radiological
evaluation of acute pelvic trauma. Over 90% of pelvic
fractures can be diagnosed from an anteroposterior radiograph. A systematic approach to interpretation of this view has been outlined by Driscoll *et al.* (1993). If a fracture or diastasis is found it is important to check for a second break as the bony pelvic ring is frequently disrupted at more than one site. If the pubic symphysis is wider than 2.5 cm there is partial or complete rupture of the sacroiliac ligaments. Assess for abnormal soft tissue opacities, which may indicate haematoma or soft tissue oedema. CT superbly demonstrates pelvic anatomy, and is useful to plan definitive therapy, but should be reserved for complex injuries once haemodynamic stability has been achieved.

Pelvic haemorrhage

The acute treatment of pelvic ring disruptions is designed to control pelvic vascular haemorrhage. The mortality and incidence of vascular laceration and retroperitoneal haematoma is highest with posterior pelvic injuries. Blood loss from fractured cancellous bone and venous plexuses is best treated by surgical immobilization of the pelvis (Heare *et al.*, 1989). Arterial injury is a common but potentially treatable cause of lethal haemorrhage. There are two main indications for arteriography:

- Patients with persisting haemodynamic instability despite external fixation.
- Patients in whom complex fractures (e.g. disrupted iliac wing) make external fixation impossible.

Most arterial bleeding arises from branches of the internal iliac artery on the side of pelvic disruption, and this can be successfully treated by embolization (Heare *et al.*, 1989: Pitt *et al.*, 1992).

Urethral/bladder injuries

Urethral injuries occur almost exclusively in men, and complicate some 14% of pelvic fractures. Clinical signs include:

- Blood at the urethral meatus.
- Inability to void despite a full bladder
- Elevation of the prostate on rectal examination.

Bladder catheterization in these circumstances is contraindicated. After consultation with the urologists, the patient can be referred for retrograde urethrography (Fig. 67). If urethrography shows the urethra to be intact, then the bladder should be catheterized and cystography performed.

Bladder injuries consist of contusion (36%), extraperitoneal rupture (26%), intraperitoneal rupture (15%), and a combination of intra- and extraperitoneal rupture (21%) (Heare *et al.*, 1989). Contusion generally causes no abnormality on cystography. Extraperitoneal injury is caused by a fracture resulting in a bladder laceration and is seen as extravasated contrast in the perineum and along the anterior abdominal wall. Intraperitoneal rupture occurs as a result of a direct blow to a distended urinary bladder which generally ruptures at its dome. It is diagnosed at cystography when free intraperitoneal contrast is seen surrounding bowel loops and extending to the paracolic gutters (Fig. 68). Immediate surgical repair is advised due to the risk of peritonitis, hyperkalaemia and uraemia.

THE TESTIS

The role of imaging in the evaluation of acute scrotal pain is to differentiate those conditions that represent acute surgical emergencies (testicular rupture and torsion), from those conditions that are best managed conservatively (testicular contusion and epididymo-orchitis).

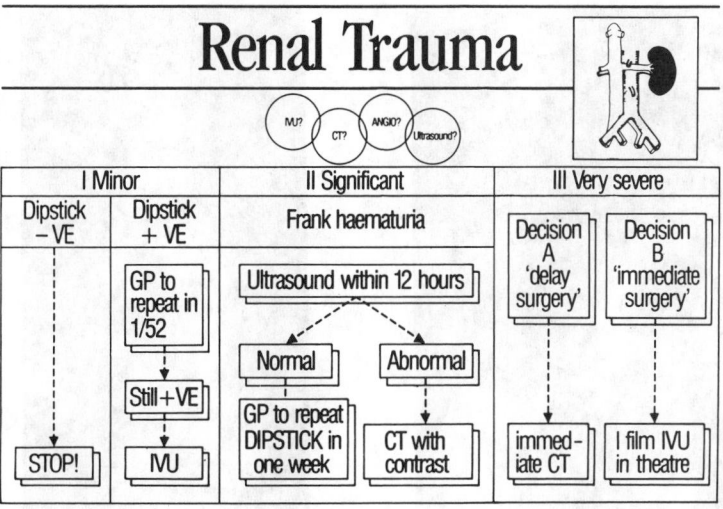

Fig. 66. (Courtesy of Kodak U.K.)

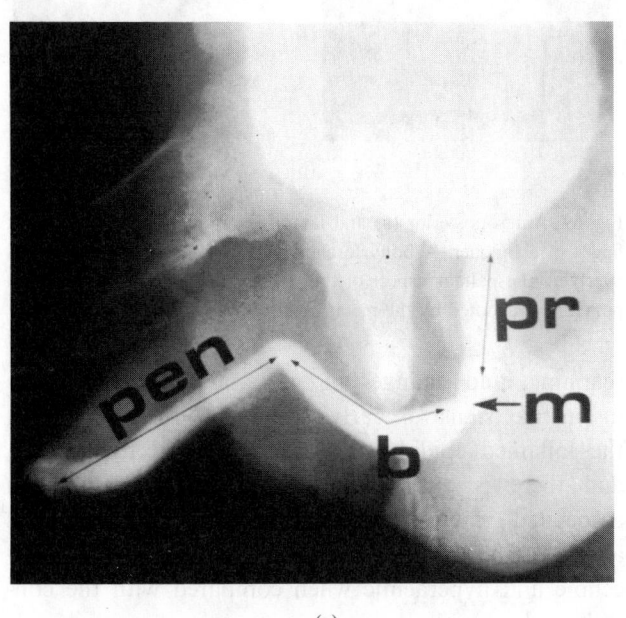

(a)

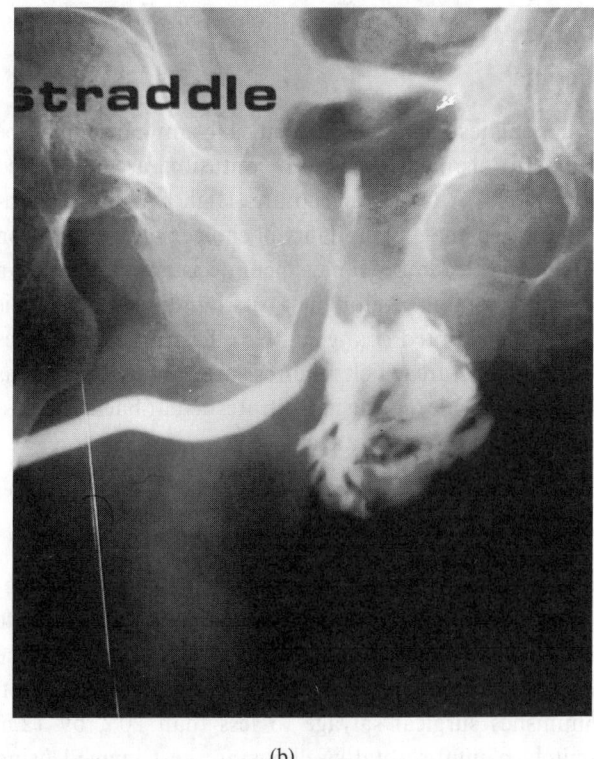

(b)

Fig. 67. (a) Normal retrograde urethrogram demonstrating the four anatomical divisions of the male urethra. The penile (pen) and bulbous (b) urethra form the anterior urethra, whilst the membranous (m) and prostatic (pr) urethra form the posterior urethra. (b) Straddle injury: retrograde urethrogram demonstrating a rupture of the urethra with contrast seen entering the perineal soft tissues and scrotum. (Courtesy of deLacey, G.J., Wilkins, R.A., Small, M.D., *et al.* (1973). *Am. J. Roentgenol.*, **199**, 822–31.)

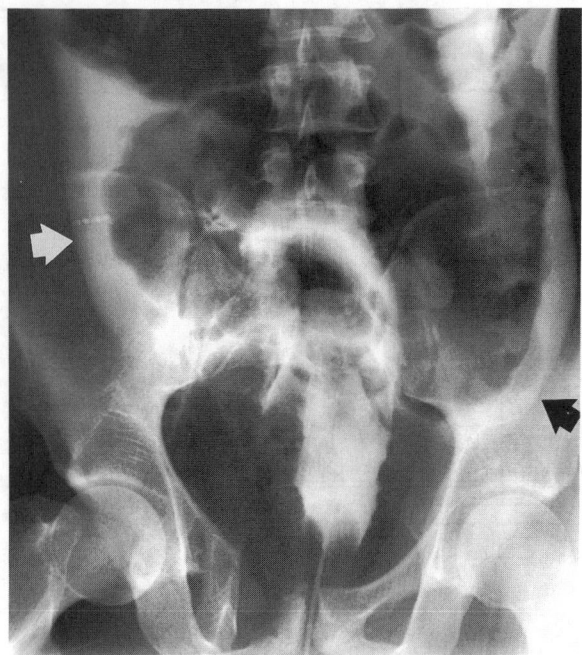

Fig. 68. Cystogram demonstrating intraperitoneal bladder rupture. There is free intraperitoneal contrast in the paracolic gutters (arrows). A foley catheter can be seen in the bladder which is displaced to the left of the midline by a pelvic haematoma resulting from the fracture of the right superior pubic ramus.

Trauma

Following testicular trauma clinical examination may be unable to distinguish between contusion, a complicated hydrocoele, or testicular rupture. High-resolution ultrasound is the imaging modality of choice in the evaluation of testicular trauma. Management decisions are based on whether the tunica albuginea surrounding the testis is intact or disrupted (Langer, 1993). Disruption indicates testicular fracture which requires surgical repair, whereas an intact capsule (contusion, intratesticular haematomas) can be treated conservatively.

Torsion/epididymo-orchitis

In the absence of trauma, testicular torsion and epididymo-orchitis are the major differential diagnoses for acute painful scrotal swellings. It is critical to make the diagnosis of torsion within 4–6 h of onset as infarction diminishes surgical salvage to less than 20% by 12 h. Acutely painful scrotal swellings are best imaged using colour doppler ultrasound (Langer, 1993). The most common finding in torsion is complete absence of detectable blood flow in the symptomatic testicle. The testis may, however, appear normal on grey scale

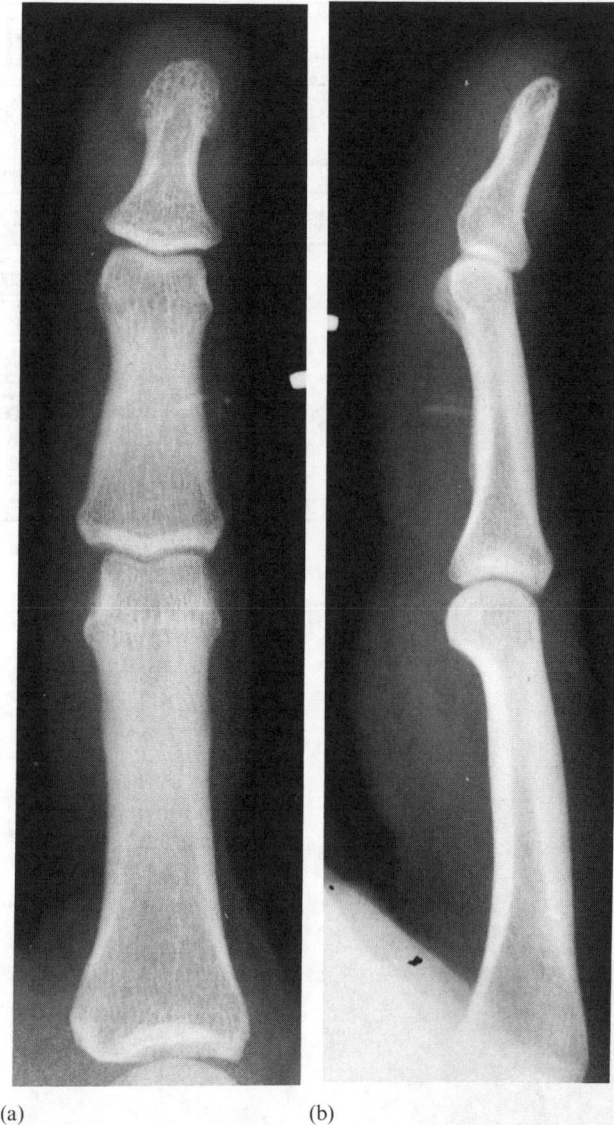

(a)   (b)

Fig. 69. Anteroposterior (a) and lateral (b) radiographs of the index finger of a butcher. A bony foreign body is seen in the soft tissues overlying the palmar aspect of the middle phalanx. The site of skin puncture is denoted by the metal pointer.

scanning, and changes in size and echogenicity are insensitive signs of early ischaemia. In epididymitis the inflamed epididymis is enlarged and hypoechoic, and there is often scrotal wall thickening and an associated reactive hydrocoele. When the testicle is affected (epididymo-orchitis) it appears enlarged, hypoechoic and hyperaemic when compared with the contralateral normal testis.

Scrotal scintigraphy is an alternative accurate means of differentiating testicular torsion and epididymo-orchitis if colour doppler ultrasound is not readily available (Kim *et al.*, 1993).

FOREIGN BODIES

Foreign bodies (FBs) are a common clinical problem, and a regular cause of medicolegal malpractice suits. The role of radiology is to confirm or exclude a suspected FB, and to provide accurate localization if removal is indicated.

Soft tissues

Detection

The commonest sites for soft tissue FBs are the extremities, particularly the fingers of the dominant hand (Fig. 69). Two-thirds of cases are in men, and 80% present within 24 h. The most frequent FBs are wood, glass and metallic splinters. The appropriate imaging modality is determined by the composition of the FB. Glass is always radio-opaque (Remedios *et al.*, 1993). Clinical examination including wound exploration is inadequate to exclude a glass FB, and as a result plain radiographs are indicated in all suspected cases. Metallic FBs are adequately assessed on plain radiographs. Almost all wood is radiolucent, and wooden FBs are best detected using high-resolution ultrasound (Fig. 70) (Remedios *et al.*, 1993).

Localization

Geometric localization of most superficial radio-opaque FBs can be adequately achieved by two radiographs taken at right-angles to each other (Fig. 69), supplemented if necessary by tangential views. However, since most radio-opaque FBs lie within 2 cm of the skin, high-resolution ultrasound is the most useful imaging technique (Fig. 70), with reported sensitivity and specificity of 95% and 89%, respectively.

Gastrointestinal foreign bodies

Ingested FBs occur most frequently in children, with most occurring in the first decade.

Coins

Coins may impact in the oesophagus (Fig. 71), a few of these will be asymptomatic, and occasionally impaction will be prolonged with necrosis of the adjacent mucosa. It is recommended that radiographic evaluation in these children should be limited to a well-penetrated frontal radiograph of the the chest and neck (RCR Working Party, 1993). Abdominal films are rarely necessary as coins passing beyond the cardia tend to pass without incident, and the practice of obtaining routine abdominal radiographs represents unjustified radiation exposure of the gonads.

Fish/chicken bones

Bony spicules from fish or fowl are among the commonest ingested FBs in adults (Fig. 72). Diagnostic difficulty may arise in distinguishing these FBs from normal irregular calcification in the laryngeal, cricoid, arytenoid and hyoid cartilages. It is useful to remember that bony FBs generally have an orderly structure with a visible cortex, and usually lodge just below the level of the cricoid cartilage. If perforation or abscess formation have ocurred, a soft tissue swelling, sometimes containing gas, may be seen. In cases in which the diagnosis remains in doubt, direct laryngoscopy is indicated. If oesophageal rupture is suspected then an oesophagogram using non-ionic, low osmolar contrast agent should be requested as barium is contraindicated.

Other objects

Suspected ingestion of a sharp or pointed object (e.g. a razor blade, a nail or glass) is an indication for abdominal radiography. If this film is normal then frontal and lateral chest radiographs (to include the neck) are indicated. Swallowed button (e.g. watch) batteries are also an indication for abdominal radiographs (Fig. 73), as their contents (mercury and potassium hydroxide) may leak. Signs of battery disintegration or delayed bowel transit beyond 48 h are indications for endoscopic or surgical removal (Remedios *et al.*, 1993).

Airway foreign bodies

Inhalation of FBs occurs most often in children and anaesthetized patients, with 77% of patients being less than 3 years old. Small FBs usually migrate to the lower lobe bronchi, particularly on the right. Peanuts and other foods are the most frequent causes. Peanuts are radiolucent: they may, however, produce secondary pulmonary changes (distal atelectasis or obstructive emphysema) which are evident on the plain chest X-ray or at fluoroscopy. Chest radiographs have a sensitivity of only 68% in the detection of inhaled FBs, and therefore

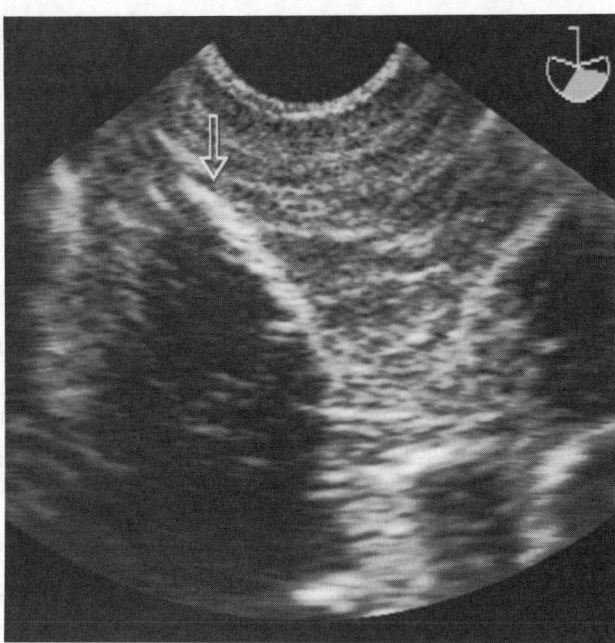

Fig. 70. Ultrasound demonstrates a wooden splinter (arrow). This would not be visible on a plain radiograph.

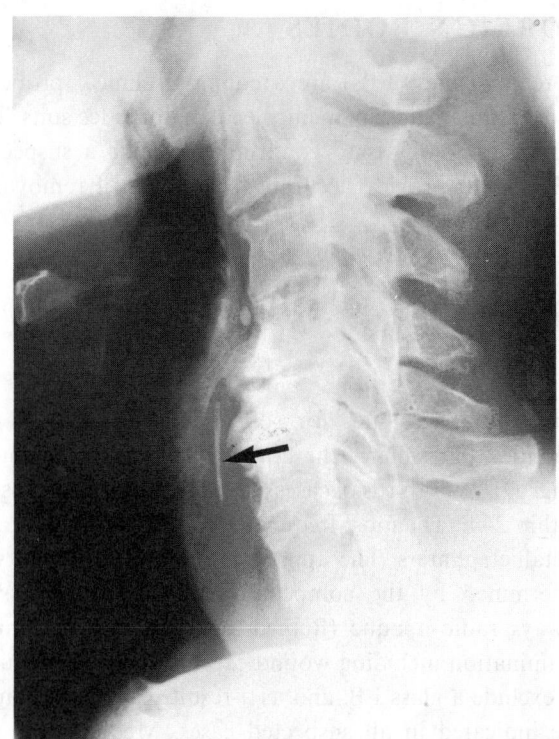

Fig. 72. Lateral radiograph of the neck demonstrating a fish bone in the soft tissues of the upper oesophagus (arrow).

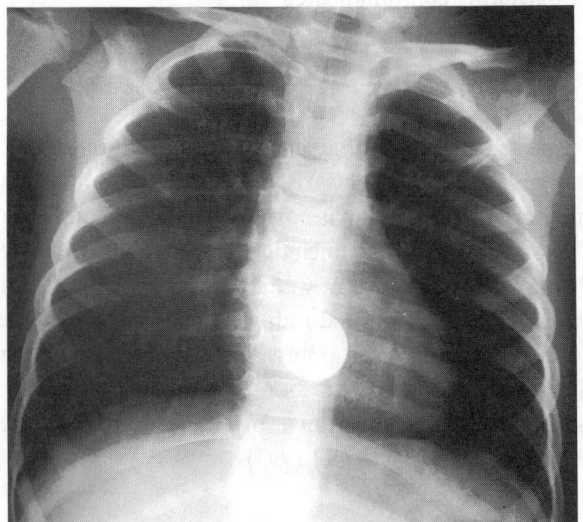

Fig. 71. Plain radiograph of the chest demonstrating an impacted coin in the lower oesophagus in an asymptomic patient.

it is important that management decisions are based on clinical suspicion not normal radiographs. Early bronchoscopy is indicated in all suspicious cases.

Orbital foreign bodies

Plain radiographs should always be taken if there is a history suggesting the possibility of a penetrating radio-

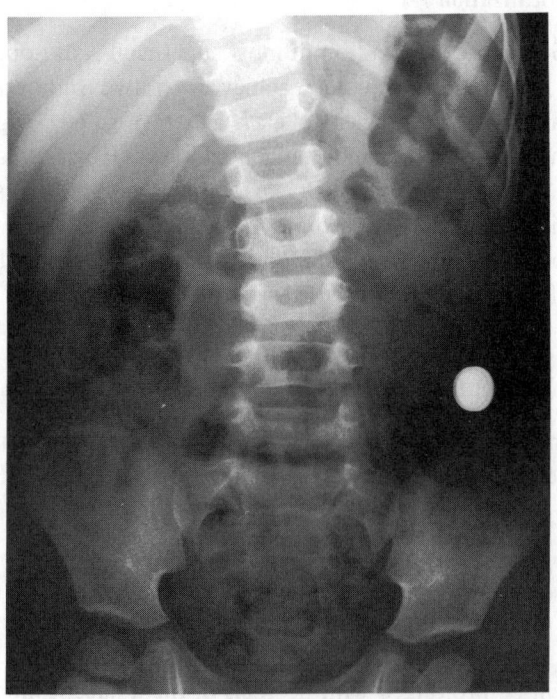

Fig. 73. Plain radiograph of the abdomen demonstrating a button (disc) battery in the descending colon.

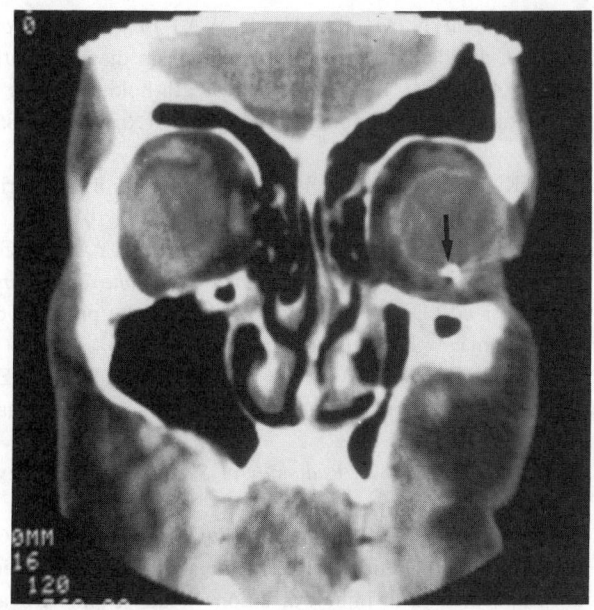

Fig. 74. CT scan of a patient with a metallic foreign body (arrow) in the orbit. The relationship of the foreign body to the orbital globe and inferior rectus muscle is well shown.

opaque FB. Standard views include a frontal projection (with upward and downward gaze) and a lateral projection. From these radiographs it is generally possible to determine whether an orbital FB lies within the globe (altered position with eye movement), or outside (generally posterior and unaffected by eye movement). High-frequency ultrasound is particularly sensitive in diagnosing FBs within the globe, and can detect associated complications such as vitreous haemorrhage or retinal tears. Although CT delivers a high radiation dose to the lens, it is the most definitive imaging modality to assess orbital FBs, and demonstrates the retrobulbar space better than ultrasound (Fig. 74).

Bibliography

ALFORD, B.A. & McILHENNY (1992). The child with acute abdominal pain and vomiting. *Radiol. Clin. North Am.*, **30**, 441–53.

AMERICAN COLLEGE OF SURGEONS COMMITTEE ON TRAUMA (1993). *Advanced Trauma Life Support Course.* American College of Surgeons, Chicago.

BROCKLEHURST, G., GOODING, M. & JAMES, G (1987). Comprehensive care of patients with head injury. *Br. Med. J.*, **294**, 345–7.

BROWN, G.L. & RICHARDSON, J.D. (1985). Traumatic diaphragmatic hernia: a continuing challenge. *Ann. Thorac. Surg.*, **39**, 170–3.

CRAIG, J.O.M.C. (1989). Radiology and the law. *Clin. Radiol.*, **40**, 343–6.

DE LACEY, G. (1979). Number of casualty attenders referred for X-ray examination. *Br. J. Radiol.*, **52**, 332–3.

DE LACEY, G., WIGNALL, B.K., BRADBROOKE, S. *et al.* (1980). Rationalising abdominal radiography in the accident and emergency department. *Clin. Radiol.*, **31**, 453–5.

DE LACEY, G., Mc CABE, M., CONSTANT, O. *et al.* (1990). Testing a policy for skull radiography (and admission) following mild head injury. *Br. J. Radiol.*, **63**, 14–18.

DRISCOLL, P.A., ROSS, R.A. & NICHOLSON, D.A. (1993). ABC of emergency radiology: the pelvis. *Br. Med. J.*, **307**, 927–31.

FIELD, S., GUY, P.J., UPSDELL, S.M. *et al.* (1985). The erect abdominal radiograph in the acute abdomen: should its use be abandoned? *Br. Med. J.*, **290**, 1934–6.

FINK, M., BERMAN, L., EDWARDS, D. *et al.* (1993). Irritable hips – is there need for hospital admission. *Br. J. Radiol.*, **66**, 787.

GAY, S.B. & SISTROM, C.L. (1992). Computed tomographic evaluation of blunt abdominal trauma. *Radiol. Clin. North Am.*, **30**(2), 367–88.

GREENE, R. (1992). Blunt thoracic trauma. In *Syllabus: A Categorical Course in Diagnostic Radiology: Chest Radiology.* pp. 297–309. RSNA Publications, Oak Brook, IL, USA.

GULY, H.R. (1992). *Diagnostic Errors in Trauma Care.* Bristol: Clinical Press.

HARROGATE SEMINAR REPORT, No. 8 (1983). *The Management of Acute Head Injury.* London: Department of Health and Social Security.

HEARE, M.M., HEARE, T.C., GILLESPY, III, T. (1989). Diagnostic imaging of pelvic and chest wall trauma. *Radiol. Clin. North Am.*, **27**(5), 873–89.

HELMS, C.A. (1989). Trauma. In *Fundamentals of Skeletal Radiology*, ed. C.A. Helms. pp. 91–125. Philadelphia: W.B. Saunders.

KARASICK, D., LAWRENCE, Jr., B. & GROSS, G.W. (1991). Trauma to the elbow and forearm. *Semin. Roentgenol.*, **26**, 318–30.

KIM, C.H., ZUCKIER, L.S. & ALAVI, A. (1993). The role of nuclear medicine in the evaluation of the male genital tract. *Semin. Roentgenol.*, **28**, 31–42.

LANCET EDITORIAL (1990). Head to head over Harrogate. *Lancet*, **335**, 695–6.

LANGER, J.E. (1993). Ultrasound of the scrotum. *Semin. Roentgenol.*, **28**, 5–18.

MASTERS, S.J., McCLEAN, P.M., ARCARESE, J.S. *et al.* (1987). Skull x-ray examinations after head trauma; recommendations by a multidisciplinary panel and validation study. *N. Engl. J. Med.*, **316**, 84–91.

MATIN, P. (1983). Bone scintigraphy in the diagnosis and management of traumatic injury. *Semin. Nucl. Med.*, **13**, 104–22.

MEYER, S. (1991). Radiographic evaluation of wrist trauma. *Semin. Roentgenol.*, **26**, 300–17.

MIRVIS, S.E. & SHANMUGANATHAN, K. (1992). Abdominal computed tomography in blunt trauma. *Semin. Roentgenol.*, **27**, 150–83.

MIRVIS, S.E., YOUNG, J.W., KERAMATI, B. *et al.* (1986). Plain film evaluation of patients with abdominal pain: are three radiographs necessary? *Am. J. Radiol.*, **147**, 501–3.

MITCHELL, M.J., HO, C., RESNICK, D. *et al.* (1989). Diagnostic imaging of lower extremity trauma. *Radiol. Clin. North Am.*, **27**(5), 909–28.

MORGAN, P.W., GOODMAN, L.R., ABRAHAMIAN, C. *et al.* (1992). Evaluation of traumatic aortic injury: does dynamic contrast-enhanced CT play a role? *Radiology*, **182**, 661–6.

MURPHEY, M.D., BATNITZKY, S. & BRAMBLE, J.M. (1989). Diagnostic imaging of spinal trauma. *Radiol. Clin. North Am.*, **27**, 855–72.

NEUSTADTER, L.M. & WEISS, M.J. (1991). Trauma to the shoulder girdle. *Semin. Roentgenol.*, **26**, 331–43.

NIENABER, C.A., VON KODOLITSCH, Y., NICOLAS, V. *et al.* (1993). The diagnosis of thoracic aortic dissection by non-invasive imaging procedures. *N. Engl. J. Med.*, **328**, 1–9.

PILLING, H.H. (1976). A coroner's view of routine radiography. *Proc. R. Soc. Lond. Ser. B*, **69**, 760–2.

PITT, M.J. & SPEER, D.P. (1990). Imaging of the elbow with an emphasis on trauma. *Radiol. Clin. North Am.*, **28**, 293–305.

PITT, M.J., RUTH, J.T. & BENJAMIN, J.B. (1992). Trauma to the pelvic ring and acetabulum. *Semin. Roentgenol.*, **27**, 299–318.

RABY, N., BERMAN, L. & DE LACEY, G.J. (1994). *Accident and Emergency Radiology: A Survival Guide*. London: W.B. Saunders.

RCR WORKING PARTY (1993). *Making the Best Use of a Department of Clinical Radiology: Guidelines for Doctors*. London: Royal College of Radiologists.

RECKLING, F.W. (1982). Unstable fracture dislocations of the forearm. (Monteggia and Galeazzi lesions). *J. Bone Surg.*, **64A**, 857–63.

REMEDIOS, D., CHARLESWORTH, C. & DE LACEY, G. (1993). Imaging of foreign bodies. *Imaging*, **3/4**, 171–9.

REMY-JARDIN, M., REMY, J., WATTINNE, L. *et al.* (1992). Central pulmonary thromboembolism: diagnosis with spiral volumetric CT with the single breath-hold technique – comparison with pulmonary angiography. *Radiology*, **185**, 381–7.

RESNIK, C.S. (1989). Diagnostic imaging of pediatric skeletal trauma. *Radiol. Clin. North Am.*, **27**(5), 1013–22.

RESNICK, D., GOERGEN, T.G. & NIWAYAMA, G. (1988). Physical injury. In *Diagnosis of Bone and Joint Disorders*, ed. D. Resnick & G. Niwayama, pp. 27–56. Philadelphia: W.B. Saunders.

RICHARDSON, J.D., McELVEIN, R.B. & TRINKLE, J.K. (1975). First rib fracture: a hallmark of severe trauma. *Ann. Surg.*, **181**, 251–4.

ROGERS, L.F. (1982). *Radiology of Skeletal Trauma*. New York: Churchill Livingstone.

ROYAL COLLEGE OF RADIOLOGISTS WORKING PARTY (1983). Patient selection for skull radiography in uncomplicated head injury: a national study by the Royal College of Radiologists. *Lancet*, **i**, 115–18.

SALTER, R.B. & HARRIS, W.R. (1963). Injuries involving the epiphyseal plate. *J. Bone Joint Surg.*, **45A**, 587.

SHUMAN, W.P., MACK, L.A., RUDD, T.G. *et al.* (1982). Evaluation of acute right upper quadrant pain: sonography and 99mTc-PIPIDA cholescintigraphy. *Am. J. Radiol.*, **139**, 61-4.

SLATER, E.E. & DeSANCTIS, R.W. (1976). The clinical recognition of dissecting aortic aneurysm. *Am. J. Med.*, **60**, 625.

STARK, P. (1993). *Radiology of Thoracic Trauma*. Oxford: Butterworth-Heinemann.

STEIN, P.D., HULL, R.D., SALTZMAN, H.A. *et al.* (1993). Strategy for diagnosis of patients with suspected acute pulmonary embolism. *Chest*, **103**, 1553–9.

SWAIN, A.H. (1986). Radiological audit – change in casualty officer performance during tenure of post. *Br. J. Accid. Emerg. Med.*, June, 5–9.

TEASDALE, G.M., MURRAY, G., ANDERSON, E. *et al.* (1990). Risks of acute traumatic intracranial haematoma in children and adults: implications for managing head injuries. *Br. Med. J.*, **300**, 363–7.

VINCENT, C.A., DRISCOLL, P., AUDLET, R.J. *et al.* (1988). Accuracy of detection of radiographic abnormalities by junior doctors. *Arch. Emerg. Med.*, **5**, 101–9.

16 Deaths

C. McLAUCHLAN

Accident and Emergency Department, Royal Devon and Exeter Hospital, Exeter, UK

Chapter plan

Introduction
Management of the deceased patient
Management of the relatives
Staff support
Multiple deaths
Organ donation

"Men fear death as children fear to go in the dark; and as that natural fear in children is increased with tales, so is the other." (Francis Bacon, *Essays,* 1625).

INTRODUCTION

Death in the accident and emergency (A&E) department is usually sudden and unexpected. Relatives and staff alike are unprepared, there is no time to get to know the patient or the relatives, and staff, including doctors, are often poorly trained in dealing with bereavement. A department seeing 40 000 new patients a year can expect over 40 deaths a year (with a similar number being dead on arrival).

The commonest single cause of death is a cardiac event, usually secondary to ischaemic heart disease; approximately two-thirds of all patients have a medical condition, less than one-third trauma and a minority a surgical condition. Medical causes will usually be greater in an urban setting. In one urban study, 6% of deaths in A&E were due to carcinomatosis which is sad and inappropriate (Shalley & Cross, 1984). Training in bereavement care and follow up can reap rewards for relatives and health professionals alike.

MANAGEMENT OF THE DECEASED PATIENT

Brought in dead/dead on arrival

The ambulance service will bring in bodies from public places or private houses if death has not been confirmed at the scene by a doctor. The A&E doctor is required to confirm death, usually in the back of the ambulance before the body is taken to the mortuary. The doctor should first obtain any history from the emergency crew and then make an examination to confirm that vital functions have ceased (Table 1). Fixed, dilated pupils are not a reliable sign of death on their own. Broken columns of blood in the retinal vessels (cattle trucking), seen with an ophthalmoscope, are difficult to detect and not essential.

The deceased's details, history and examination should be recorded in the medical notes and clearly signed, timed and dated. The Coroner's Officer (or Procurator Fiscal in Scotland) should be routinely notified. If there are any suspicious circumstances the police must be informed immediately.

Table 1. *Confirmation of death*

- Circumstances of death
- General appearance and colour
- Absent major pulse
  Absent heart sounds
  Absent respiratory efforts — For at least 0.5–1 min in warm patient
  Absent breath sounds over trachea
- Eye signs
- Consider heart monitoring

If there is any doubt about death the patient must be assumed to be alive and taken into the department for further assessment. Patients suffering from hypothermia or severe poisoning may cause particular difficulty. The back of an ambulance is not an easy or appropriate place for junior doctors to decide if resuscitation should be continued. Indeed, it has been recommended that all patients who are thought to be dead on arrival should be taken into the department for further examination (e.g. to exclude foul play) and confirmatory heart monitoring (Christian *et al.*, 1980). Unfortunately this practice is still not widespread and the facilities rarely exist. Rigor mortis is apparent after about 6 h and up to 48 h.

Died in the A & E department

Once the most senior doctor present has decided to stop resuscitation, death needs to be confirmed as described, but with the assistance of monitoring equipment. The Coroner's Officer must always be notified.

Legal procedure and notifying Coroner

The legal procedure following a death may be summarized as follows:

1. The cause of death must be known and certified by death certificate or determined by investigation by the Coroner, including postmortem examination.
2. The details will be recorded by the Registrar of Births and Deaths.
3. The body must be disposed of by any lawful means such as burial or cremation.

The object of a death certificate is to prevent concealment of crime and to obtain statistical information. A doctor may only issue a death certificate if he or she knows the cause of death *and* attended the deceased during the last illness (within 14 days of death in England or 28 days in Northern Ireland and Eire). The Coroner may find that the general practitioner or hospital doctor (but rarely the A & E doctor) is able to issue a certificate. Under these circumstances the completed death certificate is taken by the informant, usually a relative, to the Registrar who will then issue a certificate for disposal by burial or cremation as shown in the sequence in Fig. 1.

Strangely, it is not a legal responsibility of the doctor to notify the Coroner's Officer of unexpected deaths, but it is usual practice and indeed highly desirable usually by telephone or sometimes by facsimile. Outside office hours the police are notified by telephone. There is no proscribed list, but generally the types of deaths which must be reported to the Coroner are:

1. Deaths in any way related to violence, accident or industrial disease.
2. A death which is unexplained or uncertain.
3. Death within 24 h of hospital admission, or related to an anaesthetic or operation.

If there is any doubt it is always best to discuss the case with the Coroner's Officer and thereby avoid further distress to the relatives from unexpected investigations or autopsy. In the case of violent deaths, particularly if homicide is suspected, then the Coroner's Officer and the police must be notified urgently. Once the Coroner is notified the procedures outlined in Fig. 1 are followed. This applies to England and Wales, with minor variations in Northern Ireland and Eire.

In Scotland, the Procurator Fiscal replaces the Coroner and the same types of death should be referred to him as are to the Coroner in England (generally all deaths in the A & E department). Unlike England, the death certificate can be issued by any doctor who knows the cause of death, even if not in attendance during the last illness.

Forensic evidence

If death involves suspicious circumstances or a known assault (Gee & Watson, 1989), the police and Coroner's Officer will need to be notified immediately. Staff should be aware of the evidential needs to ensure that their actions do not obstruct any criminal investigation. When victims die, their clothes and all evidence becomes the property of the Coroner. Forensic investigation is based on the concept that every contact leaves a trace (Locard's Principle). Trace material such as fibres, hairs or body fluids may be anywhere on the victim or clothing and should be sampled as soon as possible. In suspicious cases the body and property should therefore be handled as little as possible before the police, police surgeon or forensic pathologist attend.

In forensic cases staff should avoid unnecessary handling of body and property.

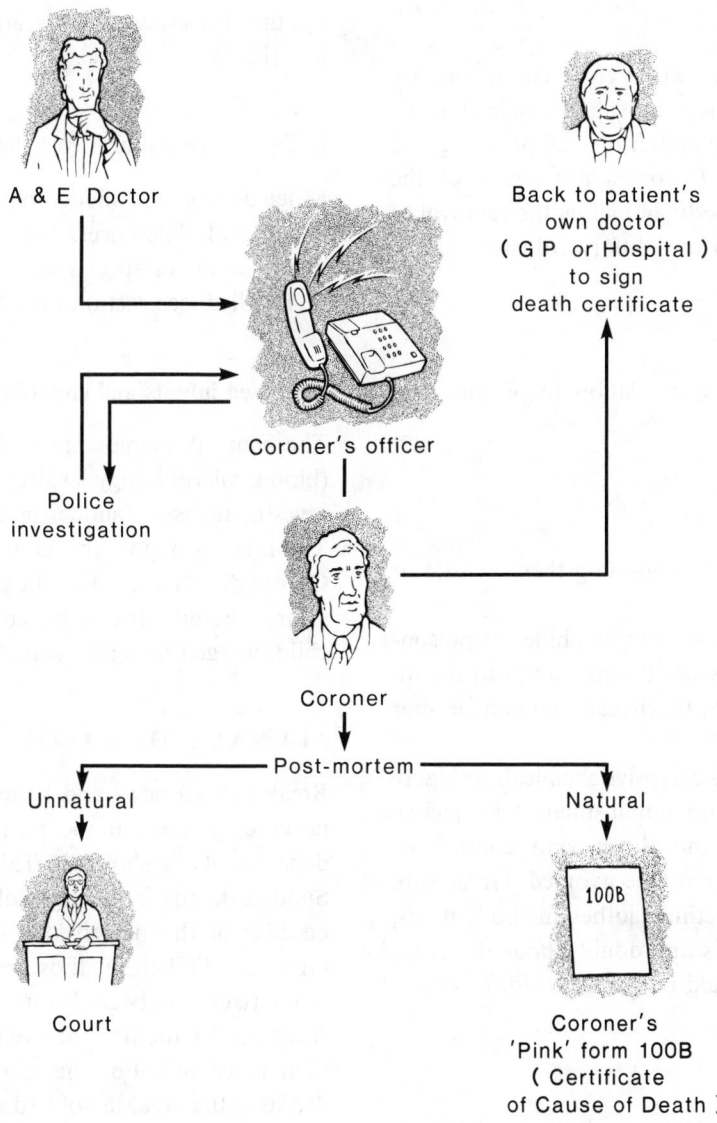

Fig. 1. Death certification – the Coroner's procedure following deaths in A&E.

Forensic considerations in major assaults or suspicious cases

- Save all material, including the paper trolley liner, and throw nothing away.
- Avoid stab and bullet holes when cutting clothes off during resuscitation.
- Items of clothing removed before death should be kept in separate bags. If damp use paper bags to avoid decomposition.
- If blood is being taken keep a further sample for forensic analysis.
- Clearly document who packed and labelled the property.

- Wounds and injuries need to be clearly documented (e.g. on a diagram) and differentiated from medical interventions such as chest drain or peritoneal lavage wounds.

It is inappropriate to treat every sudden death as a potential murder, but quiet suspicion is needed to avoid missing the unsuspected stab wound in the back. It cannot be predicted which items may become important evidence; for example, after a road traffic accident, forensic examination of the patient's shoes may be able to tell if they were pressing on the brake or the accelerator at the time of the 'accident'.

Handling the deceased

First consider if there are any forensic considerations. In unsuspicious deaths the removal of tracheal tubes and other invasive lines is a matter of local policy agreed with the Coroner. Most Coroners are aware of the relatives' need to see the body and allow the removal of resuscitation equipment in straightforward cases.

Risks to the staff

Rarely, there may be risks in relation to poisons and infection.

Poison

In most cases of death from poisoning there is little or no risk to the staff.

Hydrogen cyanide and hydrogen sulphide gas poisoning could be a risk to a rescuer during mouth-to-mouth ventilation, but there would be virtually no danger after death.

When poisoning involves corrosive chemicals or highly toxic substances (such as organophosphates), protective clothing must be worn and direct skin contact or inhalation of toxic fumes must be avoided. Great care should be taken with the victim's clothes and body fluids, especially vomit. If there is any doubt about the risks, the local poisons unit should be contacted for advice.

Infection

Simple measures (gloves, gowns and thorough hand-washing) will prevent transmission of infection. Great care should be taken with sharps, particularly in the debris left by resuscitation attempts. Advice from pathologists or infection control specialists may be sought concerning notifiable diseases and other circumstances.

Hepatitis B virus and human immunodeficiency virus (HIV) given rise to concern, although the risk of transmission of infection is very small, especially for HIV. All patients should be assumed to be potential carriers. Blood is the single most important source of these viruses. Staff should always cover any wounds or abrasions and be particularly careful to avoid direct contact with any bloodstained body fluids. In high-risk cases it would be reasonable to wear two pairs of gloves and eye protection in addition to the routine measures listed above. Other body fluids which may carry the virus are semen, vaginal secretions, and pleural, peritoneal and pericardial fluids.

Sputum, faeces, sweat, urine and vomit carry an extremely low risk.

Religious and cultural considerations

Much distress and offence may be caused by an ignorance of cultural differences. Staff should therefore enquire about rituals or special ways in which the body should be handled (see section on ethnic minority groups).

Deceased infants and children

The same principles apply. Samples may be required (blood, microbiology swabs, and cerebrospinal fluid) to investigate cases of sudden infant death syndrome (SIDS). The infant's nappy and clothes should be kept for the Coroner's Officer. The possibility of non-accidental injury should always be considered, especially when children aged under 5 years die from trauma.

MANAGEMENT OF THE RELATIVES

Breaking bad news and handling distressed relatives is never easy and can be particularly difficult in A&E departments as shown in Table 2 (McLauchlan, 1992). Sudden deaths involving violence, fire and the young, because of the perceived suffering of the victims, are especially difficult for those left (Parkes, 1975). The care of relatives may begin before they arrive at hospital and carry on for months, or even years, after the death of their loved one. For the relative or close friend of the deceased the breaking of bad news may be the beginning of the worst time in their lives. Appropriate and skilled handling of the bereaved in A&E helps to prevent long-term problems and will ease their journey through the bereavement process.

Table 2. *Problems associated with breaking bad news in A&E*

- Death is often sudden and unexpected
- Victim may be young
- Severe trauma or disfigurement may be involved
- Relatives may already have been notified in an unskilled manner
- The patient may have recently been discharged from hospital
- The victim may have committed suicide
- There may have been multiple trauma or deaths from the same accident
- Staff are often very busy

Dealing with death and talking to distressed relatives is one of the main causes of emotional distress in junior house officers (Firth-Cozens, 1987), yet death remains a neglected topic. In spite of its import, medical students and junior doctors do not usually receive adequate training in care of the bereaved. Despite inclusion in the curriculum, a study of preregistration house officers in the UK showed that 75% felt that they had never received adequate guidance or support on breaking bad news, either at medical school or during their preregistration training (Field, 1984; Dent *et al.*, 1990). Most newly qualified doctors know about rare syndromes which they will probably never see, yet few know about handling death which they will meet frequently. Senior nursing staff in A&E have often led the way in the care of distressed relatives, but there is a wide variation in training (Field & Kitson, 1986). Hopefully the publication of a report on bereavement care in A&E departments will help to improve services and facilities nationally. Useful guidelines and recommendations are provided in the report (Working Group of BAEM/RCN on behalf of the Department of Health, 1995).

Notification and initial contact of relatives

The initial contact with the next of kin should not be left to chance. Resuscitation takes priority, but once the victim is identified the closest relative or friends should be notified.

Initial contact with relatives

- Telephone information should be given by experienced staff
- Full details are usually best explained at hospital
- Relatives should not drive to hospital
- The police may be able to help

Communication with the emergency services will provide information about the incident and probably any relatives so that their arrival at hospital may be anticipated. It may be preferable for a sympathetic police officer to make initial contact with the nearest relative. Many police forces now provide appropriate training and may be able to help with transport.

If the telephone has to be used to break bad news this should be done by an experienced doctor or nurse. The lone relative should be advised against driving to hospital alone and should be encouraged to obtain local support.

It may be helpful to telephone someone for them. The information given on the telephone will depend on the circumstances and whether resuscitation attempts are being made. Rather than saying that victims are dead or dying it may be better to say that they are in a 'critical' condition. The word unconscious may emphasize the seriousness of the situation and suggest that the patient is not suffering. Details can then be explained at the hospital. Giving the relatives some warning in this way will give them time to prepare. Some situations, such as overseas or long-distance separation, call for more detailed information, including news of the death given over the telephone. Local support is then especially important and a senior nurse or doctor should ring back later to answer questions, provide further information and a contact point. The doctor or nurse may have to make quick decisions and this is why it should not be left to the inexperienced. By not saying that the victim is dead the relative may feel guilt for not arriving at hospital in time. It is important to dispel any self-recrimination by providing full information and the time of death when the relatives arrive.

Arrival at hospital

The arrival of relatives should be expected and co-ordinated by the nurse in charge. They should be greeted by a named link nurse who will look after them and provide information. The relatives should not be kept waiting in busy areas or quiet corridors, and they should not be made to feel in the way. In some cases it may be a friend of either sex who is closest to the victim and they should be handled in the same way. For this section, 'relatives' includes close friends, regardless of their official relationship.

The A&E department should have a private room or office where relatives can wait and be seen. Privacy is important and ideally this room should be solely for relatives and furnished comfortably (Table 3). Facilities such as a telephone and drinks should be readily available to allow some autonomy. The relatives' room should be near to the resuscitation room; if it is away from the emergency area the relatives will feel distanced from their loved one (although it may suit the staff!). Lack of windows can increase the feeling of isolation and fear. Privacy and accessibility are both valued (Wright, 1991). It is a myth that distressed relatives should be 'protected' from events; exposure to resuscitation will be discussed later.

Table 3. *Important features of a relatives' room*

- PRIVACY
- Telephone with outside line
- Appropriate decor and furniture
- Hand basin and mirror
- Tea set
- Tissues
- Easy access to toilets
- Window with outside view and optional view to corridor

The vigil

The time relatives spend waiting will seem like an eternity. The named link staff member is usually a nurse, but some hospitals successfully use a chaplain or a social worker, although they will have less access to the emergency room and its procedures. Compassion is unrelated to seniority and certain lay or junior staff may have the skills to sit with relatives in an emergency.

If the relative was not involved in the emergency, the victim will need to be identified and this will remove the lingering uncertainty. This early identification of the dead or dying patient helps the relative to accept reality and reduce the denial reaction, 'It can't be him, can it?...', which can also be difficult for the carer to handle.

The link nurse or other carer has a clear duty to provide clear and honest information and some warning of the severity of the situation. Regular updates are important and help the bereaved to prepare themselves for the eventual outcome. The nurse may be able to use a senior member of the resuscitation team to help with progress reports.

This is also an opportunity to obtain information about the patient (medical history, medication and quality of life) for the resuscitation team and make the relative feel involved.

Breaking the news

There are no hard rules as to whether a doctor, nurse or other carer breaks the news; it may depend on the situation and staff available. Ideally this should be done by a senior member of staff with authority, communication skills, warmth and time. In reality it is often left to a junior doctor. Relatives, however, expect and need a doctor to provide medical details and answer questions at an early stage. There is great advantage in the doctor and nurse working as a team to help the relative and support each other.

Practical points

The following principles apply when breaking bad news, although the details have to be tailored to the situation.

- The accuracy of the news should be confirmed before going to the relatives. Devastating mistakes and misinterpretation have occurred.
- Physical and mental preparation. Take a few moments while washing and removing bloodstains to compose yourself and think of what you will say. Take the link nurse so that she is able to continue where you leave off. Ask the link nurse to check your appearance while she briefs you on the relatives.
- In the relatives' room confirm again who's who, their relationship with the patient and what is known already. Much upset and embarrassment can be avoided.
- Enter the room and sit down at eye level with the person who is emotionally closest to the victim. Eye contact is important, as is acknowledgement of other friends and family in the room. This especially applies to children and adolescents who may feel left out and unsure how to react. This should be addressed later.
- Give the impression that you have plenty of TIME.
- Give direct honest information and get to the point quickly. If death has occurred then you must say so, using the word 'dead' or 'death'; euphemisms such as 'She has gone to a better place' or 'We have lost her' are open to misinterpretation by the distraught relative. If death seems likely you must say so. If the severity of the situation is not appreciated it should be re-emphasized and relatives should be taken to see the patient or body as soon as possible.
- Beware of false optimism; it is easy for the relative to seize on an investigation or procedure as a sign of hope.
- Allow silence. After breaking the news, it is important to allow the relatives time to assimilate the devastating information and to react in their own way. You can show more feeling with silence than by any number of supposedly well-chosen expressions.
- Be prepared for any reaction. Common reactions (Table 4) can be expressed in a wide variety of ways, dependent on factors such as personality and culture. By your words and actions allow people to cry, scream or roll on the floor kicking. If allowed the bereaved will do whatever they feel is appropriate, which is usually easier to handle than the relative who shows denial, guilt or the 'business as usual' approach.
- Touching or holding the bereaved person is a natural comfort and can say more than any words. Social and

Table 4. *Common initial grief reactions*

- Numbness – apparent understanding but no feeling
- Denial
- Acute distress
- Anger – including blame against themselves, the staff or even the deceased
- Guilt
- Relief (less common)
- Acceptance – although this may never be total

cultural factors will influence this, but generally if it feels right then it probably is right.

- Avoid platitudes. In moments of natural silence it is all too easy for the stressed staff to chip in with unhelpful expressions such as 'You still have your other sons' or 'He has had a good innings'. It is the dead person they want back and nothing else will do.
- Wherever possible give a clear explanation of the cause of death. The timing depends on the situation, but complicated explanations should not be given initially.
- The question of suffering during the terminal stages commonly arises and should be dealt with routinely. It is nearly always possible to give strong reassurance on this point, but if there was apparent suffering then this should be talked through.
- Staff should not completely conceal their own feelings. The quiver in your voice or the tear in your eye shows that you are human and that death is not a routine event. (The bereaved often misconceive it is a commonplace activity for staff.) Conversely, distressed staff should not dominate the proceedings!

The above practical points are not exhaustive, but they indicate problem areas; it is often the simple and practical skills which are not done well.

When breaking bad news:	
DO	DO NOT
– give time	– rush
– give direct, honest information	– use euphemisms
	– use platitudes
– allow any reaction or silence	– completely conceal your feelings
– allow questions	

Further care

Tea shared with the bereaved gives an opportunity for questions from which a measure of understanding can be gauged. Questions vary and some may be unanswerable or philosophical. If they are answered at all these questions are best reflected back as in 'Why, indeed ... it seems very unfair'. Do not allow false sympathy to slip out as in 'I know what it's like', you probably do not! Categorizing responses can lead to problems as reactions are not always what is expected. The nature of the relationship is usually unknown and death may even be a great relief! It is much safer to reflect back the emotions and empathize, as in 'It must be an awful shock ...'.

Complicated blame and guilt reactions are more difficult to deal with. Do not get involved in taking sides; simply listen and reassure if you can. There may be blame against a doctor; for example if the deceased had just seen the general practitioner. Difficult problems with blame arise if death is due to assault or carelessness – as with a drunk driver, or suicide. Sometimes a minor squabble with the deceased may take on major proportions and complicate feelings with self-recrimination and even anger against the dead person.

The 'If only ...' rumination is a common feeling which should be listened to, but actively discouraged with medical explanation of the inevitability of events. First aid attempts may need talking through with assurance, when appropriate, that 'Everything was done'.

The bereaved may suffer from a loss of autonomy which is regretted later. It is easy for them to be 'taken over' by the hospital system or their own dominant, but well-meaning, relatives. Older relatives may inappropriately advise against seeing the body as in '... remember him how he was'. With the use of open questions the situation must be tactfully manipulated so that the bereaved can remain autonomous.

Children should not be excluded from the proceedings in the mistaken belief that they need protection. Their fears and fantasies need more attention rather than less. If left out of the grieving process they may feel that they were somehow to blame. To involve them they could, for example, be asked if they want to bring back a small token or drawing to put with the body. Older children may feel the need to be alone or express themselves differently to adults. This is normal and parents may need reassurance or help with this later.

The relative should be allowed, and even encouraged,

to see the patient who is still alive, albeit briefly, and especially before a long procedure or investigation. It may be the last time they will. Reality is usually preferable to cruel fantasy. Relatives are less concerned about equipment and tubes than the staff believe and are sometimes reassured. Early contact helps to make the relative feel more involved.

It is common for parents to remain present when their child is being resuscitated and paediatricians have become accustomed to this. The same opportunity should be considered for relatives of adult patients. A study in the USA (Doyle et al., 1987) concluded that relatives felt more involved, which helped them. It does depend on a member of staff being available to support them and explain procedures. This is not yet common practice but may become so. Staff may have negative feelings and without their agreement this arrangement could adversely affect their performance in the resuscitation room.

Prepared relatives may like to be with the patient as they die after stopping resuscitation. Equipment should be removed, including the cardiac monitor which can cause distress as the complexes fade away. Warning should be given concerning agonal gasps.

Seeing the deceased person

The bereaved should always be offered the chance to see the body as soon as possible. It is a natural thing for them to want to see their loved one and say 'goodbye'. If there is any doubt then they should be actively encouraged, although the final decision and timing must be theirs. Many people have regretted not seeing the body; painful reality is preferable to unreality. The relative will often want to see the body at the place of death but in a busy A & E department it may be necessary to use a separate cubicle or special room. Nursing staff usually prepare the body but some relatives like to help, particularly parents and certain religions. The relatives should be warned of any discoloration, disfigurement or remaining tubes. Even in the presence of trauma to the face or neck they are usually better off seeing the body as their own fantasies may be far worse than reality. Bad injuries can be covered and the patient positioned to expose the good side. Relatives should be allowed to touch, hold and say goodbye. Babies and children may be picked up and given to the parents to hold and cuddle. Often one hand is left exposed, but touching and holding should not be confined to this. The bereaved should always be offered the chance to be left alone; this will

give them the opportunity to speak to the deceased and even apologize for not being present at their death. Unfortunately facilities for this are inadequate in many hospitals.

Formal identification for official purposes should be regarded separately from this valuable time and should never delay or replace it. The Coroner's Officer may witness this subtly or simply accept the staff as witnesses.

Rarely forensic matters, under the direction of the police or Coroner's Officer, influence time spent with the body. In law, once referred, a body belongs to the Coroner although emotionally it is still part of the family.

The hospital should provide a 24-h system to allow the bereaved repeated visits to the deceased person, and delayed visits from family or friends further afield. It is unacceptable for the bereaved to wait over the weekend because there is no one to clean the body or prepare the viewing area. In practice it is often the A & E nurses who arrange this, in spite of deficient facilities.

Other actions

The small touches

"Death can make triviality momentous" (Edward le Comte).

It is a myth that the relatives are too stunned to remember details and it is often the small touches of care that they will appreciate and remember. The offer of a mounted lock of hair from the dead person, in adults as well as in children, always seems to be appreciated. Other apparently small gestures such as providing toys and drinks for children are valued.

Providing more support

Ask if there is anyone else whom the relatives would like contacted. This may be a close friend or a minister. Hospital chaplains, sometimes used routinely, or other religious ministers from an on-call list can be a source of great support to both the relatives and staff, as well as a link with the community. The family do not have to be strictly religious to benefit. Other counselling services should be contacted at an early stage (e.g. the paediatric service concerning 'cot deaths').

Legal and practical matters

Relatives also need information on practical matters such as the role of the Coroner's Officer, death registration, arranging the funeral and collecting property. There is a

NOTIFY		
* Coroner's Officer Fax ☐ Phone ☐		
* GP		
FOR RELATIVES		
* Information leaflet, with staff names		
* Arrangements to see body		
* Further support/follow-up		
* Appointment with consultant		
* Property/valuables		
* Other, e.g. lock of hair/photograph		
INFANTS/CHILDREN		
* Local paediatric follow-up system		
* Notify health visitor		
* Ensure removal from local authority immunization reminder list		

Fig. 2. A & E deaths: example of a checklist.

lot to absorb, and information is best given in the form of a department booklet which warns them of possible reactions and emotions, and can also list support organizations such as CRUSE. A Department of Health leaflet, 'What to Do After Death' (leaflet D49) can also be slipped into the relative's pocket for later perusal as it explains official procedures and how to obtain financial assistance.

Organ donation should be considered and discussed when appropriate. It may comfort the relatives if handled sensitively (see below).

Sedation for a distressed relative may be requested, often by a third party, and generally should be gently refused. They may need a clear head and grief cannot be escaped so easily; the delay may make it worse.

Notifying the general practitioner is important and the bereaved should be told that this is happening, to facilitate contact and prevent later embarrassment. It is useful to have a department checklist as in Fig. 2.

Deaths in infants and children

Deaths in the young are even more difficult to deal with in A&E; the main causes are trauma and the SIDS.

The same general principles apply, with some specific points. A crib or bedding arrangement and suitable clean baby clothes will be needed. The parents should be offered

the chance to bring in the infant's own clothes and a favourite toy. A photograph may be very important to the family and is best taken professionally, perhaps later with the parents. An alternative is a polaroid picture but this cannot mask the baby's discoloration and tends to fade. The parents may have difficulty 'letting go' and so may need time in the department and at return visits to see and hold their child.

In SIDS a parent puts to bed a healthy baby and when next seen it is dead. Relatives often blame themselves and others such as the health visitor, doctor or babysitter. Careful explanation is needed that the death was not predictable and that a cause is rarely found. Further information about unsuspected disease may be available later. Parents should be reassured that any vomit was not the main cause of death. The role of the Coroner's Officer must be explained at this sensitive time (see Chapter 60).

Ethnic minority groups

A&E staff need to have some awareness of cultural and religious beliefs as much distress and offence can be caused by ignorance (Black, 1987). The patient or the relatives should always be asked if there are any religious considerations. This applies to all religions, but most difficulties and misunderstandings occur with Asian patients whose culture and beliefs differ widely from Western religions (Table 5). Problems are compounded by linguistic difficulties. Staff cannot be expected to know all religious practices, but the important point is to be aware and to ask.

Table 5. *Practical points for staff when handling Asian cultures*

- Grief often uninhibited – need privacy
- Avoid/remove inappropriate religious symbols in viewing chapel and on shrouds (use plain sheets with no hospital stamp for all deaths)
- Only essential handling and wear gloves. Hindus and Muslims (but not Sikhs) believe that only members of their faith should touch the body
- Do not remove jewellery or possible religious insignia from body; ask relatives first
- Allow family the chance to wash and lay out body
- Variation in beliefs on organ donation, postmortems and funeral arrangements

Awareness of possible ethnic differences can avoid much distress.

With ethnic minorities, seek help from a religious representative and/or an interpreter. Hospital lists of these should be available. Young children of the family are inappropriate to act as interpreters in serious situations.

Leaving the hospital, concluding process

Leaving the hospital, possibly with a plastic bag of possessions, can take on great significance for the bereaved and is a difficult time for staff. The way this is done may be perceived as a reflection of the overall care. They are handing back their baby or spouse to the hospital and understandably find it difficult. They should be allowed to take home items of special significance such as a wedding ring. This needs sensitivity as the bereaved may feel a dustbin bag of property is all that is left after 50 years of marriage. This emotion can be acknowledged, as in 'It must hard to go home without him'. Stained and cut clothing may not be wanted but should always be offered to the relatives. Staff can express their own sorrow at this time. The bereaved must know the next step and that they have some written information, including the names of staff for later contact. A follow-up appointment with the A&E consultant or other senior doctor in 2–3 weeks should be offered when details of the postmortem will be available; alternatively this can be arranged with their general practitioner. It is useful to document something of the encounter, and plans. It would more truly reflect the department's workload if the bereaved were booked in with their own A&E card.

Relatives must have transport and someone to accompany them home.

Follow-up and aftercare

Arrangements for early follow-up may be needed. Except after paediatric deaths and some major incidents, a glaring gap exists in the aftercare of the suddenly bereaved. Paediatric aftercare systems provide a model that should ideally be applied to all bereavements. Although most A&E departments in the UK provide good immediate care, subsequent management is almost invariably inadequate (Cooke *et al.*, 1992). It is therefore especially important that there is liaison with the general practitioner and community services. A few departments have liaison or follow-up arrangements, via a special

social worker, bereavement officer or chaplain. Details should be in the department's bereavement booklet.

Many A&E nurses make themselves available to the bereaved on an informal basis and partially fill the gap in care.

The bereaved in the first weeks may have feelings of isolation exacerbated by the unhelpful reactions of neighbours and associates who avoid them and the difficult subject of death. This may need explanation, as well as reassurance of their sanity when they imagine that they see or hear the deceased in familiar settings. The amount of support needed varies greatly, depending on personality, availability of family and friends and the need to talk. They must be encouraged to express their feelings with the avoidance of cliches. Information on the post-traumatic stress disorder (PTSD) may need to be given with an explanation of the symptoms which include anxiety, depression, intrusive flashbacks and nightmares. If the death was due to a road traffic accident – particularly when avoidable, as in victims of drunk or dangerous driving – the relatives usually find the word 'accident' particularly inappropriate. A word such as 'collision' is better. In any road 'incident' the relatives may appreciate information on contacting the traffic police. Some relatives, if not progressing, may need referral to specialized counselling services or a psychiatrist. It may take some months to recognize abnormal grief, but early referral is beneficial before the pathology is well established. A good start to the bereavement process with early support will help to reduce many of the long-term problems.

Good early management of the bereaved will improve their long-term prognosis.

STAFF SUPPORT

Every department should ensure a mechanism exists for the support of ALL staff.

The carers should not be forgotten as they may have given much of themselves, physically and emotionally (including ambulance personnel, bystanders and lay staff). There are well-described difficulties for staff in breaking bad news (Buckman, 1984). These include the fear of:

- Being blamed.
- The unknown and untaught.
- Unleashing a reaction.

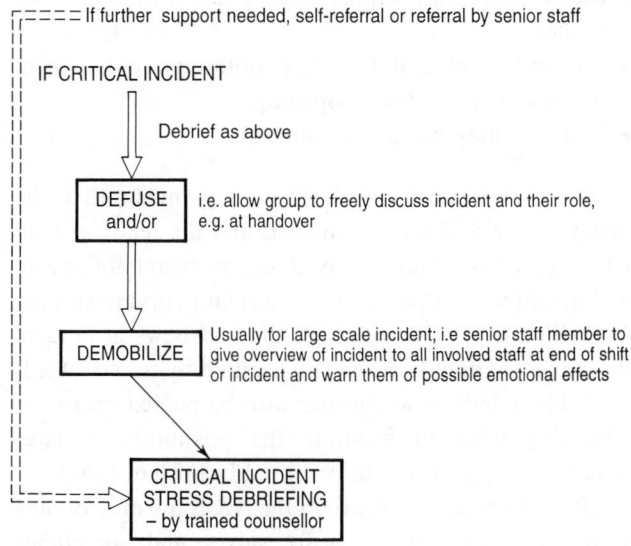

All stages must be completely confidential

AFTER EVERY DEATH

DEBRIEF — Senior staff should create mechanism to debrief all staff
– informally, e.g. in coffee room or while clearing up
or
– Formally, e.g. at handover/report or with senior colleague
as soon as possible. (ancillary staff should not be forgotten)

If further support needed, self-referral or referral by senior staff

IF CRITICAL INCIDENT

Debrief as above

DEFUSE
and/or — i.e. allow group to freely discuss incident and their role,
e.g. at handover

DEMOBILIZE — Usually for large scale incident; i.e senior staff member to
give overview of incident to all involved staff at end of shift
or incident and warn them of possible emotional effects

CRITICAL INCIDENT
STRESS DEBRIEFING
– by trained counsellor

Fig. 3. Suggested structured approach to staff support in A&E.

- Expressing an emotion.
- Not knowing the answers.
- Personal illness or death.

Staff may also suffer from the fear of having personally failed the patient or his family with feelings of inadequacy. Awareness of these fears may help understanding and lead to improved training.

A&E staff may identify with particular cases or they may have suffered their own recent bereavement. Repeated stress, overinvolvement with bereavement and isolation can lead to loss of efficiency and 'burnout', when the carer becomes physically tired, anxious, depressed and emotionally labile. Staff in emergency specialties may find it particularly difficult to discuss their feelings and emotions as they fear it may be perceived as a sign of weakness.

Mechanisms for staff support

Every A&E department should have a policy for staff support. The National Association for Staff Support Charter (1992) provides a useful framework. A suggested structure for staff support in the A&E department is shown in Fig. 3.

Debriefing

Soon after every death, or indeed any stressful incident, all staff involved should be encouraged by senior staff to talk about it and express their feelings as in 'that was awful, wasn't it?...'. This may be informal to formal and must be confidential, individually or to the group. Staff may also need reassurance as to their own performance. If senior staff hide their feelings in excessive 'professionalism' their juniors may follow their bad example. Pressure is often applied to the junior doctor to continue seeing patients. It is particularly important that the doctor takes at least 10 min to unwind (this also benefits the next patient!). Ancillary staff and ambulance crews involved in resuscitation should be included in debriefing. Humour can help, if it comes naturally, but care must be taken as the relatives would not appreciate black jokes!

"Life does not cease to be funny when people die, any more than it ceases to be serious when people laugh". (George Bernard Shaw, *The Doctor's Dilemma*, 1913)

Postmortem results and other feedback should be given to staff later and can be reassuring. Care should be taken when reviewing audit videos of resuscitations to avoid overt individual criticism.

Critical Incidents

A critical incident is any incident causing an unusually strong emotional reaction (see also section on multiple deaths, below). This may be anything from a single event to a major incident. Along with early debriefing there should be a chance for groups to 'defuse' and 'demobilize', particularly after larger incidents. These mechanisms all encourage the expression and sharing of emotions (see Figure 3). Staff are warned of possible distress but reassured that it is a normal reaction to an abnormal event. Later trained help from outside the department may be required and referral systems should be in place.

Training

Most doctors have had inadequate training in breaking bad news and handling distressed relatives. Training reduces the level of stress, the staff feel more competent and the load can be shared. There is much to teach junior doctors in A&E but they should have at least one tutorial in their induction programme to cover basic, practical aspects and local policy, including staff

support. Senior nurses can help greatly with this and
follow-up training. Outside agencies can also help with
staff training and this can be a useful way of establishing
contact for referring relatives or staff in the future. A
permanent member of staff should have responsibility for
training and coordination of the bereavement service.

MULTIPLE DEATHS

Fortunately multiple deaths are uncommon in any one
A & E department, but regularly occur nationally (i.e.
following multiple road traffic accidents or house fires
when whole families can be killed or seriously injured).
Multiple deaths may also occur as a result of a major
incident when a special response is required.

The relatives

Such events are usually sudden and involve trauma and
destruction which makes it especially difficult for the
relatives. They may not be able to cope initially and will
have exaggerated grief responses, particularly denial. The
denial response is a self-protection device and should be
handled gently during the first few hours. Free access to
return to the department for more information and to
see the bodies is important in the first few days. The
relatives may have witnessed, or been involved in the
incident and may develop long-term problems with their
grief. They must be encouraged to express their feelings
and share them with others from the same incident. PTSD
is becoming increasingly recognized and may need
specialist intervention via a local referral mechanism.

The staff

It is important to check carefully the identity of the
deceased and the relatives to prevent unnecessary distress
from misinformation. The facilities for relatives may
become overwhelmed and help should be sought from
outside the department. The staff involved should be
thanked for their work in difficult conditions and they
will benefit from debriefing exercises as for a 'critical
incident' (see section on staff support and Fig. 3). Staff
involved in major incidents may also be prone to PTSD,
particularly those involved at the scene of a disaster.
Counselling may be required later from an outside agency
and is usually available after major incidents (Mitchell,
1983).

ORGAN DONATION

There is a national shortage of organs and if any good
can come out of a sudden tragedy it may be by organ
donation. Although major organ donation is uncommon
in A & E, the possibility of donation may arise in a number
of ways:

- the relatives may express the patient's, or their own
  wishes.
- the finding of a donor card (although not a legal
  document) provides an opening.
- The staff may broach the subject.

If donation is not considered it may mean that the
deceased's wishes are not fulfilled and the relatives may
later regret this. Many bereaved parents regret not having
had the chance to donate their dead child's organs (Finlay
& Dallimore, 1991). Although the bad news is sudden,
the subject of donation can still be aired by trained A & E
staff. The relative's wishes can also be passed on to the
admitting team to facilitate the possibility of later
donation in patients with potential brainstem death.

After a hypotensive death in the A & E the only organs
viable are the corneas, heart valves and sometimes
kidneys. For details of retrieval see Table 6 (King, 1991).
Ten millilitres of blood are required from all potential
donors for screening purposes. In cases of potential
brainstem death, organs such as the heart, lungs, liver
and pancreas can be considered for transplant if the
relatives are agreeable and life-support facilities are
available. A & E departments should maintain close links
with their local transplant centre and ophthalmologists.
In addition, A & E departments should keep consent
forms and written information on support groups for
donor families (e.g. BODY, British Organ Donor
Society).

The Coroner's or Procurator Fiscal's permission
should be sought via his officer for all cases where the
death would be notified to them (all A & E deaths). After
a hospital death the person in lawful possession of the
body is the Health Authority or Trust until such time as
it is claimed by the person with the right of possession,
usually the Coroner, Procurator Fiscal or next-of-kin.
Rarely it may be appropriate to initiate organ donation
in A & E without the relative's permission, but this would
only be in exceptional circumstances to fulfil a patient's
clearly stated wish when the next-of-kin is not contactable
(Working Party on behalf of the Health Departments of
Great Britain and Northern Ireland, 1983). To consider
organ donation in A & E is not easy, but if dealt with

Table 6. *Retrieval of corneas, heart valves and kidneys*

	Corneas	Heart valves	Kidneys
Notes	Provides two corneas Race, blood group and tissue type irrelevant	Aortic and pulmonary valves Descending aorta Accidental death preferred	Depends on cardiac massage continuing after unsuccessful arrest until preserving fluid infused via catheter
Age limits	Nil, but adults preferred	3 months to 60 years	1–70 years
Main contraindications	Obvious scarring, infection of eye, invasive eye tumours	Sepsis, HIV, hepatitis B, Marfan's syndrome	Major sepsis, HIV, hepatitis B, malignancy
Death to retrieval time	Keep to minimum. Up to 12 h if moist	Keep to minimum. Up to 48 h if refrigerated	To retrieve in theatre within 4 h of renal perfusion with preserving fluid
Approximate preservation time	1-month	Long-term storage	Keep to minimum – but 12–24 hours at 4°C

sensitively there can be benefit for both relatives and recipients.

Conclusion

Although improving, death is still a neglected ethic. In A&E the sudden, unexpected and often violent nature of the death makes the situation more difficult for relatives and staff. The principles of management are:

- Give the relatives, or close friend, direct and honest information and avoid 'protecting' them from the truth.
- Help the relatives to accept the painful reality, e.g. encourage them to see the patient or body.
- Support the relatives and arrange follow-up and further help as needed and so share the load.
- Remember staff training; support and encourage them to encounter their feelings later; consider formal debriefing.

Bibliography

BLACK, J. (1987). Broaden your mind about death and bereavement in certain ethnic groups in Britain. How to do it. *Br. Med. J.*, **2**, 29–38.

BUCKMAN, R. (1984). Breaking bad news: why is it still so difficult? *Br. Med. J.*, **288**, 1597–9.

CHRISTIAN, M.S., GOSNOLD, J.K. & KERSLEY, P.N. (1980). Confirmation of death. *Br. Med. J.*, **281**, 717–19.

COOKE, M.W., COOKE, H.M. & GLUCKSMAN, E.E. (1992). Management of sudden bereavement in the A&E Department. *Br. Med. J.*, **304**, 1207–9.

DENT, T.H.S., GILLARD, J.H., AARONS, A.J. *et al.* (1990). Pre-registration house officers in the four Thames regions: survey of education and workload. *Br. Med. J.*, **300**, 713–16.

DOYLE, C.J., POST, H., BURNEY, R.E. *et al.* (1987). Family participation during resuscitation: an option. *Ann. Emerg. Med.*, **16**, 6.

FIELD, D. (1984). Formal instruction in the United Kingdom medical schools about death and dying. *Med. Educ. J.*, **18**, 429–34.

FIELD, D. & KITSON, C. (1986). Coping with death: the practical reality. *Nursing Times*, 19 March, 33–4.

FINLAY, I. & DALLIMORE, D. (1991). Your child is dead. *Br. Med. J.*, **302**, 1524–5.

FIRTH-COZENS, J. (1987). Emotional distress in junior house officers. *Br. Med. J.*, **295**, 533–5.

GEE, D.J. & WATSON, A.A. (1989). *Lecture Notes of Forensic Medicine*, 5th edn. Oxford: Blackwell Scientific.

KING, C. (1991). *The Future of Life After Death.* Information leaflet on organ transplantation in A&E. A&E Department, Leicester Royal Infirmary.

McLAUCHLAN, C.A.J. (1992). ABC of major trauma – Handling distressed relatives and breaking bad news. *Br. Med. J.*, **301**, 1145–9.

MITCHELL, J.T. (1983). When disaster strikes – the critical incident stress debriefing process. *J. Emerg. Serv.*, January.

PARKES, C.M. (1975). *Bereavement: Studies of Grief in Adult Life*, 2nd edn. Harmondsworth: Penguin.

SHALLEY, M.J. & CROSS, A.B. (1984). Which patients are likely to die in an Accident and Emergency Department? *Br. Med. J.*, **289**, 419–21.

WORKING GROUP OF THE BAEM/RCN FOR
THE DEPARTMENT OF HEALTH (1995). Bereavement care in A&E departments.

WORKING PARTY ON BEHALF OF THE HEALTH
DEPARTMENTS OF GREAT BRITAIN AND
NORTHERN IRELAND. CADAVERIC ORGANS
FOR TRANSPLANTATION (1983). A code of practice,
including the diagnosis of brain death.

WRIGHT, B. (1991). *Sudden Death, Intervention Skills.*
Edinburgh: Churchill Livingstone.

BROADSHEET (1987). Guidelines for the Management
of Assault Victims. Joint paper from Casualty Surgeons'
Association (now BAEM), Association of Police Surgeons
of Great Britain, and Royal College of Nursing A&E
Forum.

PART II TRAUMA

17 Concepts of trauma management – epidemiology, mechanisms and prevention

P.E. COLLICOTT

Department of Surgery, University of Nebraska Medical Center, Lincoln, Nebraska, USA

Chapter plan

Introduction
Kinematics and patterns of injury
Prevention
Summary
Appendix

INTRODUCTION

Trauma has been defined by Presswalla (1978) as a wound or injury characterized by a structural alteration or physiological imbalance that results when energy is imparted during interaction with physical or chemical agents. This rather inclusive definition encompasses a vast array of injuries, of which some may require urgent diagnosis and treatment.

In Chapter 5, a detailed description and analysis has been presented outlining the proper initial approach to the multiply injured patient. This chapter will present an overview of the general management of the trauma patient from an analysis of the problems facing the medical profession and the public to some proposed solutions to these problems.

Since the beginning of time, man's encounters with environmental energy resulting in injury have been dutifully recorded. Unfortunately, the ubiquitous presence of injuries has diluted their importance and fostered an acceptance of their occurrence. In other words, apathy. That attitude began to change with the report to the United States Congress by the National Academy of Sciences (1985) entitled 'Injury in America'. This report cited the dearth of data exposing the inadequacies in dealing with this epidemic disease, trauma. The Royal College of Surgeons of England (1988) in its report, 'The Management of Patients with Major Injuries', extensively reviewed this public health issue in the UK.

Trauma data today are being compiled by the World Health Organization, based upon the International Classification of Disease (ICD) and E-Codes. Accidental death rates vary widely from a low of 14.3/100 000 population in Hong Kong to 84.5/100 000 in Hungary (Table 1). Aetiological factors regarding these ICD codes are further categorized by the use of E-Codes (Appendix).

Accidents are the leading cause of death among all persons aged 1–37 years. Among persons of all ages, accidents are the fourth leading cause of death. In the 15–24 age group, injuries claim almost three times more lives than the next leading cause of death. More than three out of four victims in this age group are males.

Accidents in the USA alone resulted in costs of over $177 billion in 1991 due to lost wages ($48.5 billion), insurance administration ($35.4 billion), uninsured work loss ($29.7 billion), medical expenses ($29.6 billion), motor vehicle damage (29 billion) and fire loss ($7.7 billion). The Medical Commission on Accident Prevention estimated that the total cost of road accidents to the British economy in 1985 was £2.8 billion. The World Health Organization considers that in economic terms the cost of all accidents is approximately 1% of the Gross National Product of a country. Injuries are not only initially costly but the total cost is beyond comprehension in regard to future earning power, production capacity, scientific and industrial advances. Motor vehicle injuries in the USA alone accounted for 1.3 million years of productive life lost per year, more than three times that for either malignant neoplasms or disease of the heart (Table 2).

Table 1. *Accidental deaths and death rates by nation*

Nation	Year	Deaths	Rate[a]
Hong Kong	1989	825	14.3
Singapore	1989	392	14.6
Egypt	1987	8 919	18.2
Chile	1987	3 038	24.2
Netherlands	1990	3 629	24.3
United Kingdom	1990	14 008	24.4
Japan	1990	32 122	26.2
Israel	1989	1 345	29.8
Ireland	1989	1 108	31.5
West Germany	1990	20 653	32.3
Australia	1988	5 751	34.8
Sweden	1989	2 975	35.0
Canada	1989	9 436	36.0
Spain	1987	13 921	36.0
United States of America	1989	95 028	38.3
Italy	1988	22 638	39.4
New Zealand	1988	1 351	40.6
Bulgaria	1990	3 881	43.2
East Germany	1989	7 289	43.8
Greece	1989	4 448	44.3
Denmark	1990	2 301	44.8
Portugal	1990	4 560	46.2
Austria	1990	3 584	46.4
Norway	1989	2 053	48.6
Switzerland	1990	3 505	52.2
Mexico	1986	43 448	53.5
Finland	1990	2 815	56.5
Poland	1990	21 857	57.3
Czechoslovakia	1990	9 280	59.3
France	1990	33 933	59.8
Cuba	1988	8 278	81.5
Hungary	1990	8 760	84.5

Source: World Health Organization.
Note: Differences in reporting among nations affect comparison.
[a] Per 100 000 population.

Road accident statistics

The world's first motor vehicle death probably occurred in London, England, on 17 August 1896. The first motor vehicle death in the USA reportedly occurred in New York City on 13 September 1899. Trinca *et al.* (1988) estimate that approximately 500 000 people die and 15 000 000 people are injured annually from road traffic accidents worldwide. It is estimated by the World Health Organization that this figure may be doubled by the end of this century. In the UK, France, Switzerland and

Table 2. *Years of potential life lost (YPLL) before age 65 by major cause of death, 1988*

Cause of death	Persons dying before age 65	YPLL	Average YPLL per death
Malignant neoplasms	160 842	1 628 184	10.1
Motor vehicle traffic crashes	41 006	1 345 274	32.8
Diseases of the heart	137 547	1 310 037	9.5

Based on data provided by the National Center for Health Statistics.

Germany, road traffic increases 2–3% per year and by 2–5% per year in the USA. It is difficult to compare motor vehicle traffic deaths amongst different nations due to differences in population densities, volume and kinds of traffic, vehicle miles travelled and other factors (Table 3).

One of the most detailed data collection systems available to individuals and institutions regarding motor vehicle mortality data is the Fatal Accident Reporting System (FARS). The National Highway Traffic Administration of the US Department of Transportation operates FARS. Some interesting data and trends of interest from FARS relating to 1990 US fatal crashes are:

- Average years of potential life lost per fatal accident = 32.8.
- Fatal crashes on the interstate system accounted for 10.6% of fatal crashes and 22.3% of all vehicle miles travelled (VMT) with a rate of 0.9 fatal crashes per 100 million VMT, the lowest rate of all classes of roads.
- Arterial highways accounted for almost one-half of all fatal crashes with a rate of 2 per 100 million VMT.
- 67% of fatal crashes occurred on undivided highways with 88% of these on two-lane undivided roadways.
- Weather was not a factor in 86.7% of the fatal crashes; but, of those that occurred in adverse weather conditions, rain was the predominant factor 75% of the time.
- The number of fatalities per 100 million VMT was 2.1, the lowest in the history of FARS.
- Four out of five persons dying from motor vehicle accidents were occupants. Fatally injured passenger car occupants were almost twice as likely to be unrestrained. Uninjured occupants involved in fatal crashes were three times more likely to be restrained.

Table 3. *Motor vehicle deaths and death rates by nation*

Nation	Year	Number	Rate[a]
Syrian Arab Republic	1985	176	1.7
Hong Kong	1989	309	5.4
Egypt	1987	3 248	6.6
Singapore	1989	226	8.4
Netherlands	1990	1 290	8.6
Israel	1989	439	9.7
United Kingdom	1990	5 628	9.8
Sweden	1989	857	10.1
East Germany	1989	1 909	11.5
West Germany	1990	7 435	11.6
Japan	1990	14 398	11.7
Denmark	1990	617	12.0
Finland	1990	628	12.6
Ireland	1989	456	13.0
Czechoslovakia	1990	2 127	13.6
Switzerland	1990	930	13.9
Mexico	1986	12 288	15.1
Italy	1988	8 885 (1)[b]	15.5
Canada	1989	4 210 (2)	16.1
Spain	1987	6 681 (3)	17.3
France	1990	10 006 (4)	17.6
Austria	1990	1 408	18.2
Australia	1988	3 078	18.6
United States	1989	46 586 (1)	18.8
Greece	1989	2 066	20.6
Belgium	1986	2 057 (2)	20.9
New Zealand	1988	725	21.8
USSR	1990	66 092	22.9
Hungary	1990	2 609	25.2
Portugal	1990	2 784	28.2

Source: World Health Organization.

[a]Deaths per 100 000 population.

[b]Death definition: In general, deaths are included if they occur within 30 days after the accident, but other time periods are as follows: (1) 1 year; (2) at accident scene only; (3) 24 h; (4) 3 days.

- Pedestrians accounted for 86.8% of non-motorist fatalities with 43% being killed between 18:00 and 23:59 hours.
- Most pedestrians are killed on the roadway with those aged over 70 years having twice the mortality of those aged under 70 years.
- Mean age of pedal cyclists fatally injured was 28. One-third of the deaths occurred between ages 5 and 15 with a male/female ratio of 6:1.
- 49.5% of fatal crashes were alcohol-related (12.9% decrease since 1982).

- Average elapsed time between arrival of prehospital unit at the scene and its arrival at the hospital nationwide for fatal crashes occurring in urban areas was 24.34 min and in rural areas 34.66 min.
- Highest number of fatal crashes occurred in July and August, on the weekends, and between 14:00 and 02:00 hours.

The National Safety Council (1992) reports that accidental deaths in the USA in 1991 were the lowest since 1924. The death total was 88 000, a decrease of 5% from the total deaths of 93 000 recorded in 1990. Motor vehicle deaths in 1991 were at their lowest since 1962. The population death rate in 1991 for all accidents was also at its lowest, 34.9/100 000, down 6% from 1990s rate of 37.3/100 000. These figures are truly encouraging and speak well for the continued efforts to develop nationwide trauma systems in the USA. Unfortunately a true 'network' of trauma systems has not yet developed and, in those areas without trauma systems, evidence still exists that there is a 20–25% preventable trauma mortality directly related to this deficit.

Accidental deaths from causes other than motor vehicles in 1990 have remained fairly static in the USA except for those due to firearms in which there has been a 25% increase since 1989 with a death rate of 0.2/100 000 population. While these deaths receive a great deal of publicity because of their concentration in the large metropolitan areas, the rate per 100 000 population from drownings (1.2) and falls (1.9) is much higher. While these latter problems do not get the publicity, they are in fact the leading cause of death at the extreme ends of the age spectrum.

Knowledge regarding the magnitude of the trauma problem and facts regarding its epidemiology will provide the medical profession and the public with the knowledge that is required to defeat this worldwide epidemic.

KINEMATICS AND PATTERNS OF INJURY

Introduction

In order to become a complete professional in the management of a multiply injured patient, one must know the type of physical force, environment, position of the patient at the time of injury and the wounding agent involved in the incident.

The major patterns of injury are brought about by either blunt or penetrating mechanisms. Occasionally thermal injuries coexist as well as manmade (e.g. nuclear) or natural (e.g. venomous) threats to life. Wound ballistics, thermal factors and other aetiological agents are discussed in detail in other chapters.

Penetrating trauma, although more common in the USA than in Europe, accounts for only approximately 15% of trauma incidents from which patients present themselves to accident and emergency (A&E) departments. The majority of these injuries are caused either by intentional assaults (knives, handguns, rifles, and shotguns) or are 'accidental'. By and large, penetrating injuries caused by gunshots are surgical emergencies with the extent of the injuries being related to the calibre of the weapon, the distance at which the victim was shot, and the number of missiles which penetrated the various body regions. Stab wounds, on the other hand, may be treated expectantly dependent upon the attending surgeon's philosophy, the length of the blade and the bodily habitus of the patient.

Blunt trauma, however, is by far the most frequent (up to 90% in some series) and often most challenging injury seen by A&E personnel. The majority of these patients have been involved in motor vehicle or car/pedestrian crashes. Frequently they will have been motorcyclists, pedal cyclists, or have fallen. It is of the utmost importance to interview prehospital personnel for details of the incident.

Important details of traffic incident that should be elicited from prehospital personnel

- The type of vehicle involved
- The patient's position at the scene – e.g. ejected, lying face down, entrapped, etc.
- Unrestrained versus restrained
- Position of the patient in the vehicle – front seat versus back seat, passenger versus driver
- Site of impact on the vehicle or person – head-on, side, rear-end
- Conscious versus unconscious
- Speed of vehicle(s) involved
- Condition of the environment – temperature, noxious fumes, fire, etc.

Comorbid factors such as concomitant disease and the age of the patient are also very important.

The significance of this interview in the further assessment of the patient will become evident once the reader understands the kinematics of the incident and the expected pattern of injuries.

Road trauma

In global terms, pedestrians represent the largest group of fatalities on the road. In the USA only 1.6% of traffic fatalities are in this group while in the UK they represent 36% of the total (Table 4). The vast majority of pedestrians are struck by cars (75%), especially the front of the car. Initially the victim is struck on one or both legs depending on whether he is facing the vehicle or is turning to avoid the impact. Adults tend to turn away while children tend to 'freeze' and take the impact frontally. Additionally, if the vehicle is braking, the point of impact with the bumper will be lower on the leg than if the vehicle had not attempted to brake at all. The impact with the bumper then is the first collision. As the force of impact continues forward, the pedestrian may then strike the leading edge of the bonnet depending on the victim's height. The second collision occurs as the pedestrian is angled and thrown onto the bonnet, windscreen and frame of the vehicle, striking his shoulder, chest, abdomen and, occasionally, head. As the vehicle continues to move forward, he then slides off the vehicle onto the road striking his head and face or other body parts, depending on the speed of the vehicle, until all energy from the impact has dissipated. Therefore, these trauma patients are most likely to present with lower extremity fractures, blunt torso trauma and craniofacial injuries. If a patient is found to have two such injuries, the third must be ruled out by appropriate evaluation. Mackay (1992) has shown that the severity of injury from the first collision is directly proportional to the speed of the vehicle but that the contact with the ground is not. Additionally, there is an overall relationship between the exterior design of the vehicle and the severity of injury. For example, a rigid bonnet ornament as opposed to a flexible or indeed absent ornament has impaled more than one pedestrian. The shape of the bonnet such as that of the Volkswagen 'Beetle' versus the large Cadillac

Table 4. *Categories of fatalities*

Class	Fatalities range (%)
Car and light truck occupants	38–66
Pedestrians	16–36
Motorcyclists	10–20
Pedal cyclists	2–5
Large truck and bus occupants	2–4

Source: MacKay (1992).

Table 5. *Fatal crashes by speed limit, crash type and manner of collision*

Posted speed limit (m.p.h)	Non-motorist	Single vehicle	Multiple vehicle				Total
			Rear-end	Head-on	Angle	Other	
None	23	74	2	5	4	3	111
5–15	28	40	0	4	5	0	77
20–25	741	821	28	90	324	30	2 034
30–35	2 557	2 673	198	611	1 499	177	7 715
40–45	1 440	2 366	307	997	1 734	219	7 063
50	336	741	117	335	462	52	2 043
55	1 842	8 063	846	3 227	2 921	621	17 520
60	1	12	1	2	0	2	18
65	248	1 239	253	204	108	125	2 177
Unknown	275	465	27	82	148	24	1 021
Total	7 491	16 494	1 779	5 557	7 205	1 253	39 779

bonnet and grille has accounted for 30% less severe injuries according to Mackay (1992). However, victims vary in height. The present bumper standard for vehicles in the USA has diminished physical damage to the vehicle but increased the number of severe knee injuries. In order to achieve the strength requirements for a 5 m.p.h. impact, a rigid beam has been placed across the front of the vehicle at a standard 50 cm above the ground, corresponding to the height of the average knee joint!

Mackay (1992) defines five types of vehicle impact:

1. Frontal.
2. Side.
3. Sideswipe.
4. Rear.
5. Rollover.

Each is unique in the kinematics of the impact and the subsequent associated injury patterns.

The position of the victim within the vehicle, and whether restraints were applied also are important to the health professional assessing the patterns of injury in the casualty patient. Most collisions involve frontal impact in which airbags and seat belts are most effective. Viano (1992) states that a driver airbag provides an 18% reduction in fatality and a three-point restraint 42%. According to FARS 1990, fatalities are equal if not higher in the angled collisions which tend to occur in the younger age group who drive more aggressively and tend to lose control of the vehicle (Table 5). In these crashes, the crash worthiness of the vehicle may be just as important as the use of restraints. The pattern of injury is not the same for the driver, front seat occupant or rear seat occupant (Nygen, 1984). Each occupant has a different risk of striking the steering column, dashboard, 'A' pillar (between windscreen and side window), 'B' pillar (between front and rear door), rearview mirror, back of front seat, or other passengers within the vehicle during a 'second collision'.

If not ejected, the unrestrained driver in a frontal impact has sequential loads applied to his feet from the forward bulkhead, to his knees from the instrument panel, to his chest from the steering wheel and column, and to his head from the windshield or 'A' frame. If the driver survives to reach hospital, the following injury patterns may be found (Daffner et al., 1988):

- Fracture of the femur (56%), about the knee (19%), tibia/fibula (32%), ankle (39%), foot (32%) – floorboard and dashboard.
- Fracture of the pelvis (46%), hip (10%), posterior hip dislocation (7%) – instrument panel.
- Fracture of ribs and/or sternum, pulmonary contusion, laceration or rupture, cardiac contusion or rupture (steering wheel or column), transection of aorta distal to left subclavian artery (46%) – deceleration.
- Maxillofacial injuries (37%) – windscreen or steering wheel. Fractures of cervical spine (10%) – windscreen.
- Fracture of the radius/ulna (46%), wrist (23%), humerus (15%) – windscreen or steering wheel.
- Cranial injuries (16%) – windscreen or rearview mirror.
- Laceration of spleen or liver or rupture of small bowel (5%) – deceleration.

The unrestrained front seat occupant presents with an injury pattern somewhat different from the driver. Forces are first applied to the feet and knees as with the driver but then the head strikes the windscreen or the 'A' pillar since no steering wheel is present. This lack of contact between the chest and the steering wheel diverts a greater load to the head and neck producing more serious injuries, In Daffner's studies (Daffner *et al.*, 1988), the major difference in injury patterns observed in the unrestrained front seat passenger as opposed to the unrestrained driver were as follows:

- More cranial injuries (24% vs 16%) and more facial fractures (41% vs 37%).
- Fewer thoracic or rib injuries (33% vs 46%).
- More abdominal visceral injuries (13% vs 5%).
- Fewer fractures of femurs (41% vs 65%), about the knee (7% vs 19%), in the tibia/fibula (23% vs 32%) and in the ankle or foot (0% vs 39% or 32%).
- More fractures of the clavicle (16% vs 0.4%) and humerus (30% vs 15%).

The unrestrained rear seat occupant presents an additional hazard to the front seat occupants during the 'second collision'. Nygen (1984) states that 'the risk of injury to a front seat occupant is doubled in a frontal impact if an unrestrained rear seat occupant is in the vehicle'. The pattern of injuries, however, differs little from that of the unrestrained front seat passenger.

The restrained driver or occupant in a frontal collision will still have knee contact with the forward super-structure. If no airbag is in the vehicle then the head and face may make contact with the steering wheel. Viano (1992) states that the head flexes forward until the chin touches the sternum (about 46–72 cm in a 30 m.p.h. collision). The steering wheel in most cars is placed about 40 cm from the chest for driving convenience, thus head contact is inevitable. Further-more, improperly worn seat belts can cause injuries. Abdominal injuries can occur if the lap portion of the three-point restraint system is positioned above the iliac spines of the pelvis. If the shoulder strap is too tight, rib and sternal fractures with their associated vascular injuries may occur. Use of the 'automatic seat belt' without the lap component will lead to 'submarining' or 'up and over' action of the body leading to a higher incidence of femoral shaft, pelvis and craniofacial injuries. Underarm placement of the shoulder belt component results in more significant cardiopulmonary and upper abdominal injuries.

In a sideswipe or angled collision, the occupant tends to move toward the position from which the principle force is applied. For example, as a lateral component begins to exert its influence in a frontal collision the occupant's trajectory changes. A crash at the 10 or 11 o'clock position results in the front seat occupant's path angling across the interior so that the head of the occupant sitting on the left would strike the 'A' pillar and the head of the occupant on the right would strike the rearview mirror. Three-point restraints are very effective in angled collisions.

Lateral collisions account for approximately one-quarter of all fatalities and serious injuries. The pattern of injuries present will depend upon the occupant's position in the vehicle and from which side of the vehicle the impact occurred. For the occupant on the side of impact, restraints have little benefit but will protect the adjacent passenger – an important mechanism of injury in severe lateral collisions.

The occupant in a rear collision is initially propelled back against the seat as the vehicle is accelerated forward. The head lags behind the thorax causing extension over the top of the seat followed by flexion as the occupant springs forward. This rapid extension of the neck followed by flexion brings about the condition of 'whiplash' or cervical sprain. A properly adjusted head restraint (occipital level), if strong enough, will prevent the initial extension but will not protect against sub-sequent flexion. Restrained occupants may have more flexion of the neck than unrestrained occupants but the latter will impact on the forward compartment. With this type of crash, the physician must carefully examine the cervical spine.

Crash studies have shown that, if the occupant of a rollover crash is not ejected or if the vehicle does not strike any rigid objects, injuries sustained are not as serious as described in other types of crashes. The kinetic energy of the crash is absorbed more by the vehicle than the occupant. The advantages of being restrained compared with unrestrained are obvious but not proven scientifically because of the random motion and contacts of the occupant that occur. If the occupant is ejected, the incidence of serious injuries is high.

Finally, the patterns of injuries observed in cycle and motorcycle crashes are somewhat random but closely resemble the injury patterns seen with pedestrian/vehicle collisions. Two classes of collision occur. First, the single vehicle crash where the rider loses control and impacts against the road surface sustaining damage from angular forces. Second, the vehicle/cyclist injury pattern where the rider strikes either his own or the other vehicle or both. Injury patterns observed are influenced by the exterior design of the other vehicle and the presence or absence of a helmet. In comparison to other vehicle types, motorcycles are substantially more likely to be involved in a fatal fixed-object crash. Most pedal cyclist deaths occur on the road away from junctions.

Falls

Falls are second only to vehicle collisions as a major cause of traumatic deaths and injuries. Most injuries are focal since falls usually involve short distances or occur from a standing position. A free fall is defined by Buckman & Buckman (1991) as a 'fall from a known point to a known impact point'. The patterns of injury depend upon the impact velocity, the material struck, body orientation, age and environment. The orientation of the body is extremely important – affecting the probability of survival Whereas 50% of adults succumb to falls of 15 m, children have a 50% mortality with falls of 22 m despite a higher frequency of head-first landings. In those patients who reach hospital alive following an urban free fall, head injuries are present approximately 20% of the time. Thoracic and abdominal injuries are not uncommon. Whilst thoracic aortic disruption is common in autopsy series, the majority of patients who reach hospital alive have pulmonary contusion, bronchial disruption and rib fractures. Abdominal injuries usually involve a hollow viscus with shearing of the bowel at the junction between its fixed and mobile portions. Fractures of the spine, pelvis and lower extremities are common. Three types of vascular injury may be encountered: aortic disruption is rarely seen in hospital, but peripheral vascular injuries associated with fractures of the lower extremities and the compartment syndromes are; a third type of vascular injury is the rupture of lumbar, superior gluteal, and internal pudendal arteries from spine and pelvic fractures.

Summary

The astute clinican will be able to avoid missing an occult injury in the multiply injured patient if he is familiar with the different patterns of injury. Knowledge of the kinematics of vehicle collisions, ballistics and environmental conditions in which the traumatic incident occurred will prove invaluable in the initial evaluation and management of these difficult patients.

PREVENTION

McLoughlin & McGuire (1991) in their review established three categories of trauma prevention:

1. Primary – before the injury occurs.
2. Secondary – minimizing the damage when an injury occurs.
3. Tertiary – minimizing the long-term damage caused by an injury.

Primary measures to reduce the incidence of injury must include modifications of the environment, products or the behaviour of people at risk. In order to assess these problems we must have an adequate knowledge base for these modifications. This must include the use of E-Codes and the development of trauma registries. Injury epidemiology is the foundation of good injury prevention, and the medical profession is responsible for collecting and documenting detailed information.

Epidemiological data on injuries that need to be documented by the medical profession

- Nature, type and brand names of products causing injury
- The involvement of alcohol and other drugs contributing to the injury
- Motor vehicle collision incidents – location, presence or absence of restraints, position of injured occupant in the vehicle, type of crash, etc.
- Sharing of registry data

National medical organizations must recognize that this aspect of trauma care is much more cost-effective than the treatment which is rendered after the injury. The hospitals and organizations then can become lead advocacy groups in legislative and press forums. Only if public opinion is changed can the devastating effects of this epidemic begin to be addressed.

Secondary injury prevention is designed to minimize the damage to the person once the injury has occurred. This is the area on which most medical personnel have traditionally focused their efforts. Examples include:

- The training of prehospital personnel and development of treatment protocols for them.
- The establishment of an effective communication system.
- The development of regionalized trauma systems.

- Training of personnel in trauma care by the use of standardized educational programmes – e.g. Advanced Trauma Life Support, Advanced Cardiac Life Support, Advanced Burn Life Support, Advanced Trauma Nursing Course.
- Biomedical research on physiological responses to injury and the biomechanics of injury.
- Trauma fellowships.
- Appropriate funding to achieve these goals.

Tertiary prevention is synonymous with rehabilitation. Greater emphasis must be placed upon the earlier involvement of rehabilitation specialists during the acute phase of injury management. Early involvement ensures that the patient, family and clinical staff can effectively work together to achieve optimal results, thus returning the patient to society as an active and productive participant. Development of regional rehabilitation centres for the complete care of the injured patient is needed.

Advances in injury prevention have been made over the past few decades. Motor vehicles are now design more for their 'crash worthiness' than economy. The installation of seat belts, airbags, antilock brakes, headrests, collapsible steering columns, padded dashboards, reinforced side panels, elimination of rigid bonnet ornaments and side mirrors and recessed door handles are just a few of the improvements in vehicle design. Better roads with reflective divider markers, collapsible utility poles, grooved roadways and lower speed limits have also reduced the number of crashes. Legislative mandates regarding helmet and seatbelt use, restriction of firearms sales, stricter drink/driving laws and, in some states in the USA, mandated trauma centre designations have diminished the death toll. The establishment of standards in trauma education and facility resourcing by the American Association for the Surgery of Trauma and the American College of Surgeons Committee on Trauma have been very effective.

There is no expeditious solution to control this epidemic disease called trauma. The most effective preventative strategies will require decades of social change, public policy development and political will.

SUMMARY

Management of the trauma patient must begin before the injury occurs and continue until the patient re-enters society. Trauma is an international disease. Its implications and costs to society are enormous. Much has been accomplished but a great deal more needs to be done. The preventable mortality from this epidemic remains unacceptably high. A better understanding of the disease and effective mechanisms for its treatment are needed.

Medical personnel must understand the epidemiology of trauma, the patterns of injury observed, effective means of prevention, and its impact. Numerous chapters in this book address specific areas of concern and management of the trauma patient but one must not just focus on initial or subsequent patient care.

APPENDIX

International Classification of Diseases, environmental events, circumstances, and conditions as the cause of injury, poisoning, and other adverse effects

E800–807 Railway Accidents
E810–819 Motor Vehicle Traffic Accidents
E820–825 Motor Vehicle Nontraffic Accidents
E826–829 Other Road Vehicle Accidents
E830–838 Water Transport Accidents
E840–845 Air & Space Transport Accidents
E846–848 Vehicle Accidents Not Elsewhere Classifiable, e.g. Cable Cars Not On Rails
E849   Place of Occurrence
    849.0 Home
    849.1 Farm
    849.2 Mine & Quarry
    849.3 Industrial Place & Premise
    849.4 Place for Recreation or Sport
    849.5 Street or Highway
    849.6 Public Building
    849.7 Residential Institution
    849.8 Other (Forest, Beach, Parking Lot, etc.)
E850–858 Accidental Poisonings by Drug, Medicinal Substances, and Biologicals
E860–869 Accidental Poisonings by Other Solid and Liquid Substances, Bases, and Vapors
E870–879 Surgical and Medical Procedures as the Cause of Abnormal Reaction of Patients or Later Complications Without Mention of Misadventure at the Time of Procedure
E880–888 Accidental Falls
E890–899 Accidents Caused by Fire and Flames
E900–909 Accidents Due to Natural & Environmental Factors
E910–915 Accidents Caused by Submersion, Suffocation, & Foreign Bodies
E916–928 Other Accidents
E929   Late Effects of Accidental Injury

E930–949 Drugs, Medicinal & Biological Substances Causing Adverse Effects in Therapeutic Use

E950–959 Suicide & Self-Inflicted Injury

E960–969 Homicide, and Injury Purposely Inflicted by Other Persons

E970–978 Legal Intervention

E980–989 Injury Undetermined Whether Accidentally or Purposely Inflicted

E990–999 Injury Resulting from Operations of War

Bibliography

BUCKMAN, Jr., R.F. & BUCKMAN, P.D. (1991). Vertical deceleration trauma. *Surg. Clin. North Am.*, **71**, 331–44.

CAMPBELL, B.J. (1992). Reducing traffic injury: size of the problem and lack of research resources. *World J. Surg.*, **16**, 410–19.

COMMISSION ON THE PROVISION OF SURGICAL SERVICES (1988). *Report of the Working Party on the Management of Patients with Major Injuries.* London: Royal College of Surgeons of England.

COMMITTEE ON TRAUMA RESEARCH, NATIONAL RESEARCH COUNCIL AND THE INSTITUTE OF MEDICINE (1985). *Injury in America,* Washington, DC: National Academy Press.

DAFFNER, R.H., DIEB, Z.L., LUPETIN, A.R. *et al.* (1988). Patterns of high-speed impact injuries in motor vehicle occupants. *J. Trauma,* **28**, 498–504.

FELICIANO, D.V. & WALL, Jr., M.J. (1991). Patterns of injury. In *Trauma,* ed. E. Moore, K. Mattox & D. Feliciano. pp. 81–96. Norwalk: Appleton & Lange.

MACKAY, M. (1992). Mechanisms of injury and biomechanics: vehicle design and crash performance. *World J. Surg.*, **16**, 420–7.

McLOUGHLIN, E. & McGUIRE, A. (1991). Injury prevention. In *Current Therapy of Trauma,* ed. D. Trunkey & F. Lewis, Jr. pp. 4–8. Philadelphia: Decker.

NATIONAL HIGHWAY TRAFFIC SAFETY ADMINISTRATION (1991). *Fatal Accident Reporting System 1990.* Washington, DC: US Department of Transportation.

NATIONAL SAFETY COUNCIL (1992). *Accident Facts 1992.* Itasca, IL: National Safety Council.

NYGEN, A. (1984). Injuries to car occupants – some aspects of the interior safety of cars. *Acta Otoloaryngol. Scand.*, **395** (Suppl.), 1–8.

PRESSWALLA, F.B. (1978). The pathophysics and pathomechanics of trauma. *Med. Sci. Law,* **18**, 239–45.

RICE, D.P. & MacKENZIE, E.J. (1989). *Cost of Injury in the United States: A Report to Congress.* Institute for Health & Aging, University of California, San Francisco, and Injury Prevention Center, The Johns Hopkins University.

RYAN, G.A. (1992). Improving head protection for cyclists, motorcyclists, and car occupants. *World J. Surg.*, **16**, 398–402.

TRINCA, G.W., JOHNSTON, I.R., CAMPBELL, J.R. *et al.* (1988). *Reducing Traffic Injury – A Global Challenge.* Melbourne: Royal Australasian College of Surgeons, A. H. Massina & Co.

VIANO, D.C. (1992). Causes and control of spinal cord injury in automobile crashes. *World J. Surg.*, **16**, 410–9.

18 Head injuries

D. GENTLEMAN[a], R. BRADFORD[b] and G. DUNWOODY[b]

[a] *Department of Neurosurgery, Dundee Royal Infirmary, Dundee, UK*
[b] *Department of Neurosurgery, Royal Free Hospital, London, UK*

Chapter plan

Introduction
The pathophysiology of traumatic brain injury
The assessment of head-injured patients in the resuscitation room
Investigating a head-injured patient
Deciding on a plan of management
Emergency management before transport
Safe transfer to the neurosurgical unit
Management at the neurosurgical unit
Conclusion

INTRODUCTION

Head injury is a major public health problem in the UK as in other countries. One million people with head injury are seen each year in accident and emergency (A&E) departments, 100 000 are admitted to hospital, and 10 000 are transferred to neurosurgical units. At one end of the spectrum of severity 5000 patients die after a head injury and many more are permanently disabled. The lives of survivors and their families can be ruined by the effects of brain damage, and the economic cost is reflected in the scale of the personal injury settlements which many survivors receive (Krause, 1987; Goldstein, 1990).

After a serious head injury the chain of early management runs from the scene of injury to the A&E department, referral and transfer to a specialist facility, and definitive treatment of the head injury there. Accurate assessment, thorough resuscitation, timely referral of selected cases, and safe transfer to the neurosurgical unit are all vital to minimize mortality and morbidity, and there is plenty of evidence of the dire consequences when these are not done well. Jennett's group in Glasgow showed in the 1970s that the commonest preventable cause of death was delay in identifying and treating raised intracranial pressure (ICP) from an expanding haematoma or brain swelling (Reilly *et al.*, 1975; Rose *et al.*, 1977; Jennett & Carlin, 1978). In the 1980s they showed that inadequate attention to resuscitation and safe transfer was translated into poorer outcome after serious head injury (Gentleman & Jennett, 1990; Gentleman, 1992). Actions and omissions before head-injured patients ever reach the neurosurgical unit can cast a long shadow over their future.

THE PATHOPHYSIOLOGY OF TRAUMATIC BRAIN INJURY

Most serious head injuries are caused by road accidents, falls and assaults. Injury to the brain is classified as immediate (primary) or delayed (secondary), a distinction which is clinically important. Little can be done to modify the course of primary brain damage once an injury has occurred, but secondary brain damage is at least potentially preventable, and the degree of success with which this is done influences outcome profoundly.

Primary brain injury

The mechanical forces applied to the brain at the moment of injury transfer energy to it. Neurones (and especially their axons) throughout the brain are damaged, but some areas are particularly susceptible, causing a pattern of damage often termed 'diffuse axonal injury'. Glial cells are more robust but are also affected, as is the cerebral microvasculature. The clinical hallmark of primary brain injury is an immediate change in conscious level, the depth and duration of which reflect the magnitude of the neuronal damage.

So much brain tissue may be destroyed that death is instantaneous. At the other end of the spectrum of severity is the clinical syndrome of concussion: a brief loss of consciousness, followed by a period of discontinuous memory (post-traumatic amnesia) before an apparently full recovery. In cases of intermediate severity some neurones die at the moment of injury but others, though damaged and functionally silent for a time, can recover if conditions are favourable.

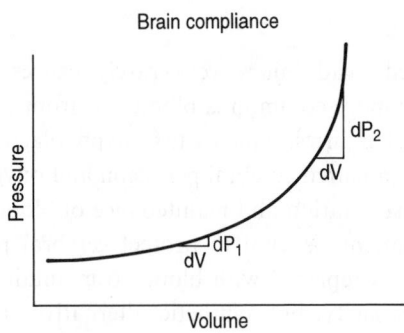

Fig. 1. Pressure–volume relationship.

Secondary brain injury

Primary injury to the brain can be followed by events which add further insult to the already injured brain and cause clinical deterioration. Minimizing secondary brain damage can avert a poor outcome, and is the key to the optimal management of head-injured patients (Miller & Becker, 1982; Gentleman, 1990).

Table 1 lists the causes of secondary brain damage. Their common denominator is a failure of adequate oxygen supply at neuronal level. Mechanically injured neurones are exquisitely sensitive to the effects of cerebral ischaemia or hypoxaemia, which can damage them beyond hope of recovery (Jenkins et al., 1989). The aim of treatment is to restore their oxygen supply by controlling intracranial pressure (ICP), maintaining cerebral blood flow (CBF) and cerebral oxygen delivery, and minimizing the increased metabolic requirements for oxygen seen in the injured brain.

Normal ICP is 5–10 mmHg and mean arterial blood pressure (MAP) is 80–90 mmHg; the difference between

these is the cerebral perfusion pressure (CPP). In health the brain maintains a constant CBF by reducing arteriolar tone when CPP falls, but this 'autoregulation' is impaired after head injury. CBF and hence cerebral oxygen delivery then become critically dependent on CPP, and are vulnerable to any rise in ICP or fall in MAP, both of which tend to lower CPP.

Rising pressure inside the rigid box of bone which is the skull damages injured and normal brain tissue alike. An increase in the volume of the intracranial contents (e.g. by an expanding haematoma or hypoxic brain swelling) causes little rise in pressure until the critical point when no more CSF (cerebrospinal fluid) or venous blood can be squeezed out of the cranial cavity. Beyond this point ICP rises steeply as the volume continues to rise (Fig. 1). The result is a fall in CPP, CBF and cerebral oxygen delivery, with progressive secondary brain damage.

Table 1. *Causes of secondary brain damage after head injury*

- Extracranial
  —Systemic hypoxaemia
  —Hypercarbia
  —Shock
  —Posthaemorrhagic anaemia
- Intracranial
  —Haematoma or contusion
  —Diffuse brain swelling (intra/extracellular)
  —Seizures
  —Intracranial infection
  —Neurochemical damage

Hypoxia and hypercarbia

Systemic hypoxaemia is the commonest correctable cause of secondary brain damage, and can occur at any stage after injury. Preventing and treating it is of fundamental importance in early head injury management. Airway obstruction and inadequate pulmonary gas exchange lower PaO_2, and also raise $PaCO_2$. This leads to inadequate cerebral oxygen delivery not only directly but also indirectly, because ICP is raised by hypoxic cell swelling and carbon dioxide induced cerebral vascular engorgement. Preventing and correcting hypoxaemia and hypercarbia depend on a clear airway, adequate pulmonary ventilation, and giving high-flow supplemental oxygen from the earliest possible moment.

Shock

An isolated head injury very rarely causes systemic shock. Far more common is blood loss from associated extracranial injuries, which cause hypovolaemic shock and hence impaired cerebral perfusion and oxygenation. Prompt resuscitation and maintenance of blood volume in these patients is vital to protect cerebral perfusion. Blood loss is replaced with blood to maintain oxygen-carrying capacity, but synthetic alternatives are being sought.

Intracranial haematoma and contusion

Most intracranial haematomas are supratentorial and unilateral. As a haematoma expands it increases the ICP and also compresses and distorts the brain within the skull, causing characteristic clinical features which are discussed later. If a large haematoma is not evacuated promptly the rise in ICP lowers CPP, CBF and cerebral oxygen delivery below critical levels, causing progressive secondary brain damage. A small haematoma may not do this at first but only later, as it enlarges or as other factors like brain swelling add to its effects.

Brain swelling

The brain can swell focally or generally because of mechanical or hypoxic damage to the blood/brain barrier and to cell membranes. Water then accumulates in the cerebral interstitial space and enters cells down ionic gradients, and the ICP rises. This complication of head injury is refractory to treatment, and is much better prevented or limited by prompt correction of hypoxia and hypercarbia and by surgically removing areas of badly contused brain.

Infection

A breach of the skull and meninges allows pathogenic bacteria to enter the brain and cause meningitis or an abscess, days or weeks after the injury. These complications increase morbidity and mortality, and are a particular risk with skull base fractures, compound depressed fractures of the skull vault with dural tears, and other penetrating wounds of the brain. Intracranial infection after trauma is eminently preventable by antibiotic prophylaxis and by applying sound surgical principles to wound treatment.

Epilepsy

All seizures reflect disordered electrical activity in the cerebral cortex. Most of those which follow head injury involve generalized tonic–clonic muscle contractions. In the acute phase they increase the cerebral metabolic requirement for oxygen ($CMRO_2$), further threatening injured neurones. In the presence of an already swollen brain whose CBF and oxygen delivery are at critical levels, seizures can be devastating. Prolonged or repeated fits also threaten the airway, causing hypoxaemia and hypercarbia. Anticonvulsant drugs may be needed to abolish or prevent fits.

Neurochemical damage

It has been increasingly recognized in the last 10 years that much of the continuing damage to neurones after head injury is the result of chemicals which accumulate around them after injury and swamp the mechanisms which inactivate them in health. For example, 'excito-toxic' neurotransmitters derived from damaged neurones cause inappropriate depolarization and so raise $CMRO_2$ (Faden *et al.*, 1989), while free oxygen radicals damage cell membranes by lipid peroxidation and disrupt membrane transport and ionic gradients (Chan *et al.*, 1982). Much interest is being shown in the possibility of developing 'neuroprotective' drugs to protect the injured brain from such toxic chemicals (Fadden & Salzmann, 1992; Scatton *et al.*, 1991).

THE ASSESSMENT OF HEAD-INJURED PATIENTS IN THE RESUSCITATION ROOM

The history

Most patients seen at hospital after a head injury are conscious and can give a history. Others have more serious head injuries and are unable to do so, and it then becomes particularly important to question witnesses and ambulance crew about the details of what happened, the time of injury and the patient's condition since then. Vital information can be obtained in this way. For example, being told that a crash victim was ejected from the vehicle should increase the index of suspicion for serious extracranial injury. Knowing that a patient who is unconscious on arrival at hospital was able to talk at the scene of the accident indicates that primary brain injury was not severe, and demands urgent action to identify and correct the cause of the secondary deterioration. Information about past medical history often emerges only when relatives appear at hospital, and can take days to piece together.

Initial priorities: the ATLS system

When a patient is known or suspected to have serious injuries the standard ATLS sequence of priorities is followed in the resuscitation room (American College of

---

Order of priorities for the resuscitation of a seriously injured patient—the ATLS system

A Airway (with cervical spine control)
B Breathing
C Circulation (with haemorrhage control)
D Disability (neurological assessment)
E Exposure of the whole body and environmental considerations

---

Surgeons Committee on Trauma, 1993). An initial assessment (primary survey) is done at the same time as the patient is resuscitated from life-threatening injuries and complications. This is followed by a detailed head-to-toe assessment of injuries (secondary survey). The patient is transferred to the CT (computed tomography) scan suite or the neurosurgical unit only when stable; surgery may be needed to control exsanguinating trunk or extremity haemorrhage.

The primary survey and resuscitation

The purpose of this is to identify and correct life-threatening injuries and complications at the earliest possible moment.

Airway

The first priority in a seriously head-injured patient is always to clear and maintain the airway, while protecting the cervical spine. Simple manoeuvres are tried first: suction of the mouth and pharynx, chin lift or jaw thrust, insertion of an oral airway. Every patient receives high-flow oxygen via a reservoir bag.

Early endotracheal intubation may be needed (Table 2), and should not be delayed simply to allow a more detailed neurological examination later; good cerebral oxygenation is the higher priority. The decision to

Table 2. *Indications for establishing a definitive airway in a seriously head-injured patient*

- Coma (not obeying, not speaking, not eye opening), i.e. GCS 8 or less
- Loss of the protective laryngeal reflexes
- Ventilatory insufficiency (as judged by blood gases)
    Hypoxaemia ($Pao_2 < 9$ kPa on air or < 13 kPa on oxygen)
    Hypercarbia ($Paco_2 > 6$ kPa)
- Spontaneous hyperventilation causing $Paco_2 < 3.5$ kPa
- Respiratory arrhythmia
- The aim is to achieve:
    $Pao_2 > 15$ kPa (on 100% oxygen)
    $Paco_2$ 4.0–4.5 kPa

---

intubate a head-injured patient is also a decision to ventilate, in order to control ICP, and this is likely to need short-acting sedative and muscle relaxant drugs.

The cervical spine is injured in 5% of severely head-injured patients. It should be regarded as unstable until proven otherwise, and immobilized—especially during manoeuvres to protect the airway such as intubation.

Breathing

When serious head and chest injuries occur together this traditionally carries a poor prognosis, underlining how important it is to identify and stabilize life-threatening chest injuries before sending the patient for definitive neurosurgical care. For example, an untreated pneumothorax causes blood gas disturbances and shock and threatens cerebral oxygen delivery.

Circulation

Venous access is established with at least two wide-bore cannulae, of such a calibre that blood can be infused rapidly through them. Samples are sent for emergency cross-match of type-specific blood and baseline measurement of haematology and biochemistry indices. There should be no hesitation in infusing a fluid bolus of 2 litres to replace blood loss and maintain the circulating volume; concern that the brain will be waterlogged by overenthusiastic fluid infusion is overstated. The far greater hazard is that the brain will be underperfused because hypovolaemic shock has not been corrected. Initially the state of the circulation is monitored by clinical assessment (pulse rate and volume, peripheral colour and temperature, blood pressure), pulse oximetry and urine volumes. Invasive monitoring of blood pressure and central venous pressure can be useful at a later stage.

External haemorrhage is controlled by pressure and a search is made for sources of internal haemorrhage. Patients with severe head injuries often have occult injuries which can lose much blood—ruptured spleen or liver, haemothorax, pelvic fracture—and particular care is needed to identify these. As well as clinical assessment, three films are taken during the primary survey to look for extracranial injuries: anteroposterior films of the chest and pelvis, and a lateral film of the cervical spine showing the C7/T1 junction.

Disability (neurological assessment)

The most important part of the neurological examination is the measurement of conscious level, as this is the most sensitive guide to intracranial conditions. A rapid assessment is made during the primary survey, using the

---

AVPU system of neurological assessment

A Alert
V responding to Voice
P responding to Pain
U Unresponsive

AVPU system, and the pupils are checked for size, equality and reaction to light. A more detailed neurological assessment is deferred until the secondary survey.

Exposure

The patient is fully undressed to allow a complete examination during the secondary survey. Clothes are cut off to avoid injudicious movement of body parts. An Identiband label becomes crucial in a naked unconscious patient.

Secondary survey: the neurological assessment

A thorough but concise neurological assessment is made after the primary survey and resuscitation: conscious level, the pupils, and the limb responses.

Conscious level

This is recorded using the Glasgow Coma Scale (GCS) (Teasdale & Jennett, 1974). Table 3 shows how the

Table 3. *The Glasgow Coma Scale and score in adults*

Eye opening response	
Spontaneous	4
To speech	3
To pain	2
None	1
Best motor response in (upper limbs)	
Obeys commands	6
Localizes to painful stimuli	5
Withdraws to painful stimuli	4
Abnormally flexes to painful stimuli	3
Extends to painful stimuli	2
None	1
Best verbal response	
Orientated	5
Confused	4
Inappropriate words	3
Incomprehensible sounds	2
None	1

The normal score in an adult is 15

---

scale describes conscious level in terms of three variables: the eye opening response, best motor response in the upper limbs, and best verbal response. Each feature is graded from best to worst, and each grade is given either a short carefully defined descriptive term or a number. The numbers can be added to give a GCS score from 3 to 15, but the descriptive words are more useful when managing an individual patient. The GCS was devised for use by doctors, nurses and paramedics of all levels of experience, and as it is simple yet reliable it has become the universal means of communication worldwide for describing conscious level—not only after head injury. Measurements are repeated at frequent intervals and recorded on a chart, so that trends—especially deterioration—can be identified as early as possible.

A patient who does not open the eyes to any stimulus, does not obey commands, and does not speak is by definition in coma (GCS 8 or less out of 15). A head-injured patient who remains in coma for at least 6 h can be defined as having had a severe head injury. This term is now also used to describe patients who undergo surgical intervention for acute intracranial haematomas or injuries which penetrate the brain, whatever their conscious level.

The best motor response is assessed in the upper limbs. A flexor response to stimulation in the lower limbs can result from a spinal reflex arc, even after brain death. First, the patient is asked to obey simple commands: 'squeeze my hand', 'lift up your arm', 'stick out your tongue'. If the patient cannot do this, a painful stimulus is applied with the thumb over a branch of the trigeminal nerve in the supraorbital notch, to see if he can 'localize' to the stimulus by bringing up one or both upper limbs above the level of the clavicle. If not, pressure on a fingernail bed may produce a motor response at the elbow: withdrawal or 'normal' flexion, abnormal or 'spastic' flexion, or extension. Flexion at the elbow can have both normal and spastic elements, which can be difficult for non-specialists to distinguish, so that observation charts in many hospitals do not distinguish between these.

The verbal response is assessed by asking the patient questions to test orientation. 'Do you know where you are?' 'What day is it?' 'What happened to you?' An alert and apparently well patient who is talking in sentences may prove to be confused rather than orientated when tested in this way—a key distinction when deciding on a plan of management (see below). The patient may speak but only inappropriately, using disjointed phrases or single words (often Anglo-Saxon monosyllables!), or may utter no recognizable words but only incomprehensible sounds (groaning, crying, or muttering). Special problems are presented by young children, those who do not speak English, and the very deaf.

Focal neurological signs: the pupils and limbs

After a head injury the symmetry of the pupils and their response to a light stimulus are repeatedly assessed and recorded. A dilating pupil which reacts more and more sluggishly to light can indicate an intracranial mass lesion on the same side. The symmetry of the limb responses to standard stimuli is also repeatedly assessed and recorded. Unilateral limb weakness (hemiparesis) can reflect intracranial damage on the opposite side, or spinal cord injury.

These focal neurological deficits are relatively late signs of rising ICP. Changes in conscious level occur first, and must be acted upon early.

INVESTIGATING A HEAD-INJURED PATIENT

Since the early 1980s it has been well understood that early identification and surgical treatment is the key to improving haematoma management (Teasdale *et al.*,

1982), and that skull fracture and abnormal conscious level are powerful predictors of intracranial haematoma (Mendelow *et al.*, 1983). Guidelines for skull radiology, admission to hospital, and referral to a neurosurgeon after head injury in adults were published in 1984 (Briggs *et al.*, 1984) and rationalized UK practice. They were later refined and extended to children (Teasdale *et al.*, 1990). These guidelines may now need revision, for two reasons. First, CT scanning facilities are no longer exclusive to neurosurgical centres, and in many general hospitals the decisions to scan and to refer are not now identical. What matters is not whether a scan precedes or follows referral, but to agree on which patients need neurosurgical help. Second, significant intracranial damage can often be seen on scans in patients with little or no neurological impairment (Servadei *et al.*, 1989; Miller *et al.*, 1990). In countries more generously endowed than the UK with scanners (and malpractice lawyers) this has already lowered the threshold for scanning (Stein & Ross, 1992; Servadei *et al.*, 1993), and this will come to affect UK practice too.

Magnetic resonance imaging (MRI) shows greater detail of structural change than CT (Jenkins *et al.*, 1986), but practical considerations (availability, cost, patient support during image acquisition) limit its usefulness in acute assessment after head injury.

It must be emphasized again that action to clarify the intracranial diagnosis begins only after the primary survey and all life-saving interventions.

External signs of head injury

The extent of scalp injury can reflect the extent of intracranial damage. Lacerations can involve the galea as well as the skin, and can be extensive. Its rich blood supply often makes scalp blood loss profuse, but a pressure dressing will control this and also keep the wound clean.

Definitive scalp repair should be delayed until more pressing matters are resolved, and may need the help of a plastic surgeon if there is loss of tissue.

Skull fractures and their significance

Skull fractures are important markers of possible intracranial damage. A linear fracture greatly increases the risk that a clinically important haematoma is already present or will develop. A depressed or basal fracture carries a risk of delayed intracranial infection. No patient with a skull fracture should ever be sent home from the A&E department, however well he is neurologically.

Despite the significance of finding a fracture, skull films are redundant when on clinical grounds a head injury is judged serious enough to warrant a CT scan. They will remain useful as a screen for less seriously injured patients until CT scanning guidelines relax. Clinical judgement is necessary, but the following criteria for X-rays are helpful:

- History of high-velocity injury (road accident, fall from a height).
- History of assault with a weapon.
- Unconsciousness at any time since injury.
- Any alteration of consciousness at hospital.
- Difficulty in assessment, e.g. intoxication, epilepsy.
- Focal neurological signs.
- Skull penetration (CSF leak, obvious skull depression, stab/shot).
- Marked bruising or laceration of the scalp.

Three views are taken: anteroposterior, lateral, and a Towne's view (to show the occipital bones). Films of poor diagnostic quality should never reassure, and are reasons to err on the side of caution: repeat the films, arrange a CT scan, or admit the patient to hospital.

Fractures of the skull vault are either linear or depressed, and are either closed or open (compound). Most are linear and closed, and appear on skull films as roughly straight sharp lines crossing normal anatomical features like sutures and vascular markings (Fig. 2). Any linear fracture carries an increased risk of intracranial damage, but some have particular notoriety. A temporal fracture can tear the middle meningeal artery and cause an extradural haematoma, and an occipital fracture (seen best on the Towne's view) from falling on to the back of the head can be associated with 'contracoup' contusions of the frontal lobe and delayed neurological deterioration.

A depressed fracture is a fragment of skull vault displaced inwards by a blow to the head, commonly from a blunt weapon. Most are compound, and the main risk is that bacteria can penetrate the brain unless the wound is surgically debrided and closed. The fracture is best seen in a radiographic projection tangential to the fracture site (Fig. 3), and it causes a 'double density' on a plain film when the bone fragment is projected through overlying bone.

A fracture of the skull base is likely to tear adjacent mucous membranes (e.g. in the paranasal air sinuses), and is therefore always regarded as compound. The fracture may be visible on plain films but usually is not, as the anatomy of this area is complex. However, films may show free intracranial gas or an air–fluid level in the sphenoid sinus. A basal fracture can usually be diagnosed clinically:

- CSF leak from nose or ear; often bloodstained in the initial stages, the leak may not appear until soft tissue swelling subsides.

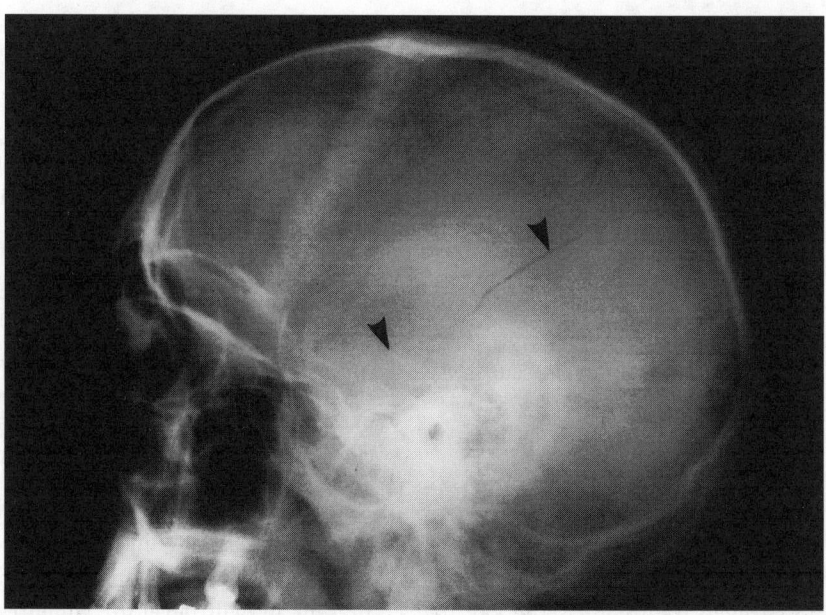

Fig. 2. Linear fracture of the skull vault.

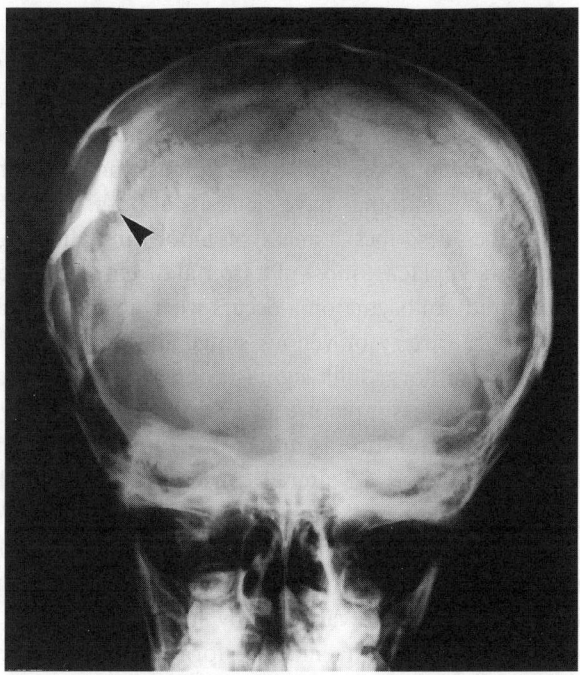

Fig. 3. Depressed fracture of the skull vault.

Table 4. *Types of intracranial pathology seen on CT*

Haematoma
  Extradural
  Intradural
    Subdural
    Intracerebral
    Mixed (burst lobe)

Contusion
  Low/mixed-density area with swelling

Brain swelling
  Generalized
    Loss of cortical sulci and fissures
    Effacement of third ventricle
    Effacement of basal cisterns
  Focal
    Shift of brain and ventricles

Indirect evidence of primary brain damage
  Small haematomas in basal ganglia, corpus callosum, or brainstem

- Periorbital haematoma (unilateral or bilateral).
- Subconjunctival haemorrhage without visible posterior margin.
- Haematoma over mastoid process (Battle's sign)—after 48 h.
- Haemotympanum.

Stab, gunshot and blast wounds of the head are occasionally seen in UK civilian practice. Although the skull is invariably fractured the injury to the brain dominates the clinical picture in most cases.

CT scanning and intracranial lesions

A CT scan can show haematoma, brain contusion, or focal or generalized swelling of the brain, and the appearances can be used for classification and prognosis (Tables 4 and 5) (Marshall *et al.*, 1991). Knowing what intracranial lesions the patient has is crucial for management. Current UK guidelines for referral to a neurosurgeon are based largely on which patients need a CT scan, but nowadays a scan has often been done before referral. Those involved in early care should know when to do a scan (Table 6), how to interpret what it shows, and what to do next.

Patients who fulfil any of the first three criteria need immediate referral to a neurosurgeon, whatever the hour.

Table 5. *CT scan classification of intracranial pathology*

Diffuse injury

I	No visible intracranial pathology seen on CT scan
II	Basal cisterns are visible, with or without: Midline shift of 0–5 mm; Visible lesions and/or bone fragments or foreign bodies; No high- or mixed-density lesion >25 ml
III (swelling)	Basal cisterns compressed or absent: Midline shift 0–5 mm; No high- or mixed-density lesion >25 ml
IV (shift)	Basal cisterns compressed or absent: Midline shift >5 mm; No high- or mixed-density lesion >25 ml

Non-evacuated high- or mixed-density mass lesion >25 ml

Any evacuated mass lesion, whatever its size

Time is of the essence, especially if the patient proves to have a haematoma, as outcome will be closely related to how long the brain has been allowed to remain compressed (Mendelow *et al.*, 1979; Seelig *et al.*, 1981).

Table 6. *Criteria for arranging a CT scan*

From the A&E department or resuscitation room (only after initial assessment and resuscitation)

- Fractured skull with:
  —confusion or worse impairment of consciousness
  —focal neurological signs
  —seizures
  —any other neurological symptoms or signs
- Coma continuing after resuscitation, even if no fracture
- Deteriorating conscious level or developing focal neurological signs

After admission to hospital

- Confusion or other neurological disturbance persisting after 6–8 h (even without a skull fracture)
- Neurologically well patient with CSF leak or other penetrating injury
- Worsening headache or vomiting, especially in a child

Haematomas

Acute haematomas appear as high-attenuation lesions on a CT scan. They are either extradural (20%) or intradural (80%), and the latter can be subdivided into subdural and intracerebral haematomas, though many intradural haematomas have elements of both. The term 'burst lobe' describes a mass of blood and disrupted brain tissue replacing most of a frontal or temporal lobe.

An extradural haematoma occurs when a skull fracture tears a dural artery or venous sinus, and appears on a scan as a lentiform high-signal lesion within the skull (Fig. 4). The classic picture of an initial lucid interval with later deterioration is in fact quite uncommon, and most patients have an altered conscious level from the start because of associated primary brain injury. An extradural haematoma enlarges quickly, compressing the brain and causing neurological deterioration and death unless it is promptly evacuated by surgery.

An acute subdural haematoma forms when a cerebral vein bridging the subdural space is torn, and forms a

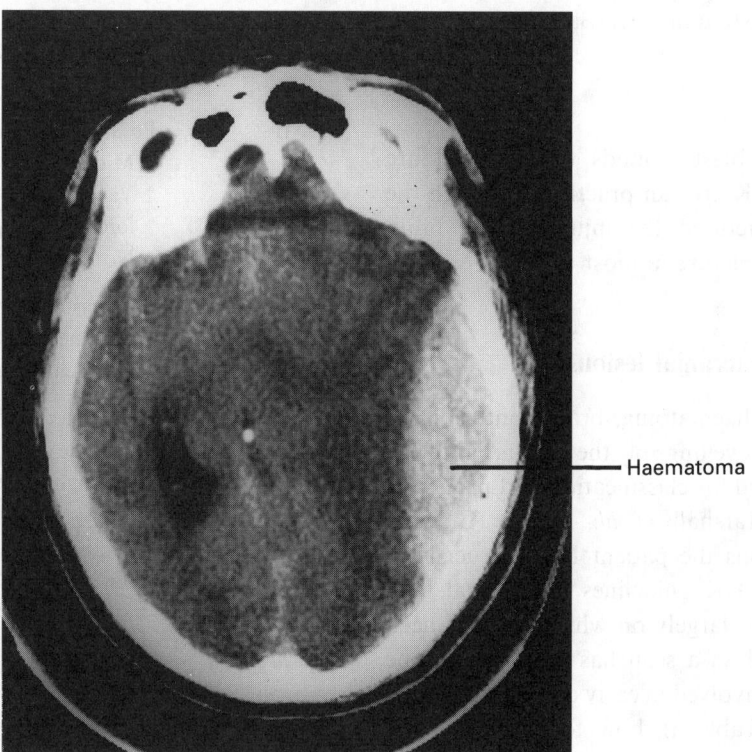

Fig. 4. Left extradural haematoma, causing brain compression, ventricular distortion, and midline shift.

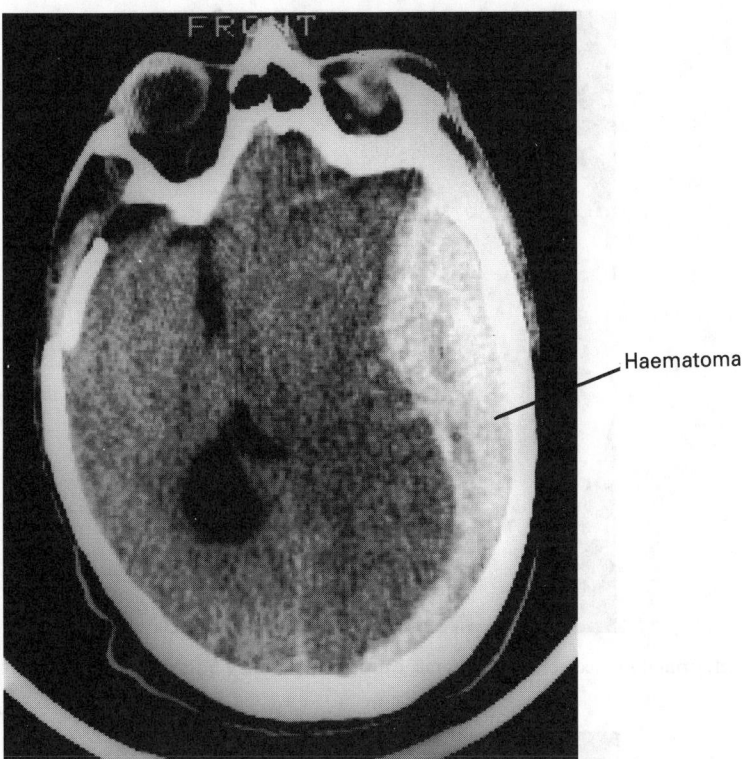

Fig. 5. Left acute subdural haematoma, causing brain compression, ventricular distortion and midline shift.

high-signal extracerebral collection following the contour of one cerebral hemisphere (Fig. 5). An intracerebral haematoma results from torn vessels within the brain parenchyma, usually in a frontal or temporal lobe. These patients usually have an altered conscious level from the time of injury because of associated primary brain damage. Some subdural and intracerebral haematomas are small and can be left alone, but larger ones distort and compress the adjacent brain, raise ICP, and cause progressive neurological deterioration if not surgically evacuated (Fig. 6). Monitoring ICP by an implanted intracranial transducer can help decision-making with borderline haematomas (Galbraith & Teasdale, 1981).

Some subdural haematomas start small but grow over weeks or months by a variety of mechanisms. This is particularly common in alcoholics and the elderly. The chronic subdural haematoma eventually presents with the features of a slowly expanding intracranial mass (headache, confusion, drowsiness, focal deficits), and appears as a mixed- or low-attenuation lesion on a CT scan (Fig. 7). Treatment is by burrhole evacuation of the old liquefied blood, and the prognosis is excellent.

Brain contusions

These appear on a scan as low- or mixed-attenuation lesions (often with mass effect) in one or more lobes of the brain (Fig. 8). They vary greatly in size, and if large can act as focal mass lesions and cause progressive neurological deterioration similar to that seen with a haematoma. Substantial haemorrhage within a large area of contused brain results in a burst lobe.

Diffuse axonal injury

Most primary brain damage is invisible on a CT scan, but in severe cases small haemorrhages are seen in the corpus callosum, brain stem, or basal ganglia. These do not need surgical evacuation, but are markers of the severity of primary brain injury, and carry a poor prognosis. MRI shows diffuse axonal injury more clearly because of signal change caused by focally raised brain water content (Jenkins et al., 1986) (Fig. 9). This can persist for some weeks after injury.

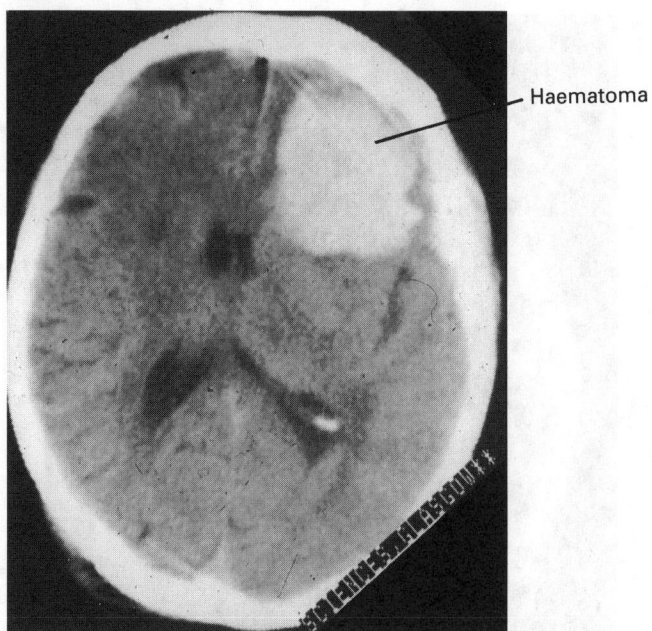

Fig. 6. Left frontal intracerebral haematoma, causing surprisingly little distortion and shift of brain.

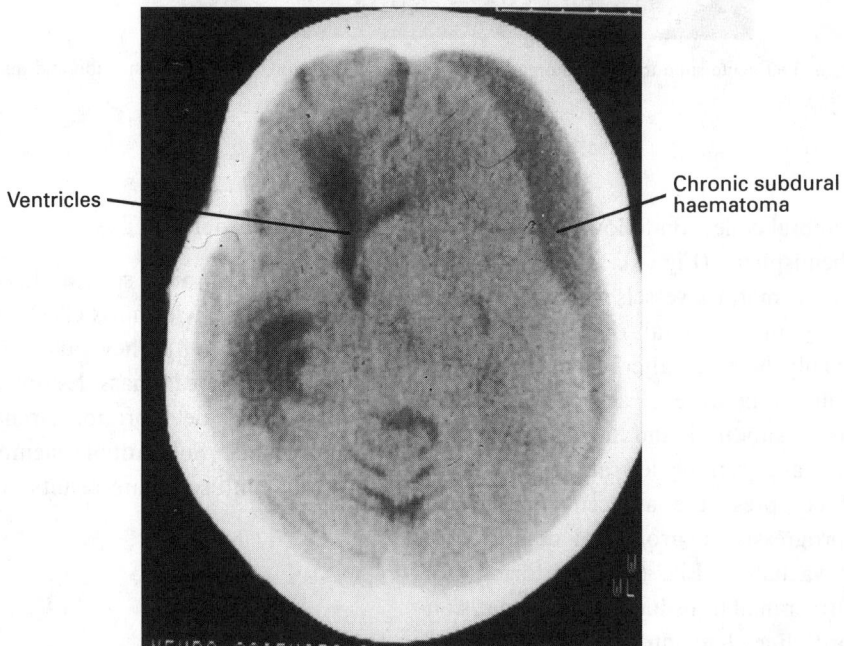

Fig. 7. Left chronic subdural haematoma, causing considerable distortion and shift.

Brain swelling

Generalized brain swelling can follow cerebral hypoxia or ischaemia from systemic or intracranial complications of injury. On a CT scan it causes loss of definition of the third ventricle and the CSF cisterns at the base of the brain (Fig. 10). Localized brain swelling is associated with a haematoma or contusion.

DECIDING ON A PLAN OF MANAGEMENT

The current guidelines give advice which is centred on estimating the risk of the patient having (or developing) a haematoma or other complication needing neurosurgical treatment. Nowadays those who manage seriously head-injured patients in the resuscitation room are

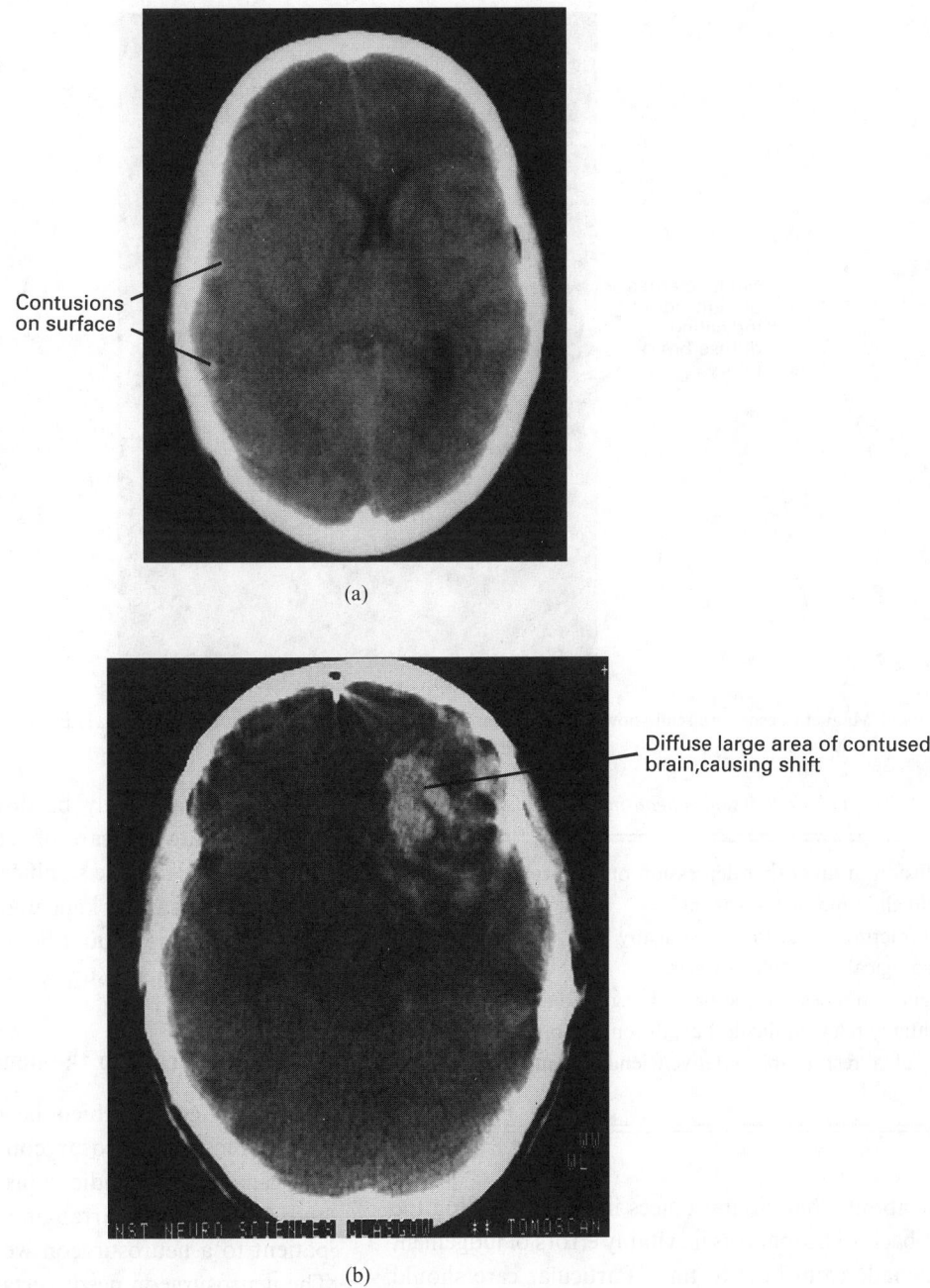

Fig. 8. Two films showing (a) small surface contusions; (b) large frontal contusion with shift, amounting to a 'burst lobe'.

likely to have access to considerable information, including a CT scan, to guide the action they need to take.

Patients with minor head injuries

The great majority of head-injured patients can safely be sent home from the A&E department after assessment and first aid treatment. The decision to discharge at this stage requires experience and should never be taken lightly, as the consequences of missing a serious complication can be catastrophic. Discharge should be reserved for patients whose conscious level is normal by the Glasgow Coma Scale, who have normal findings on neurological examination, have no skull fracture clinically or radiologically (or no good reason to look for one), and have a relative or friend willing to accept responsibility for looking after them at home. It is essential that clear, written instructions are given to the patient and the

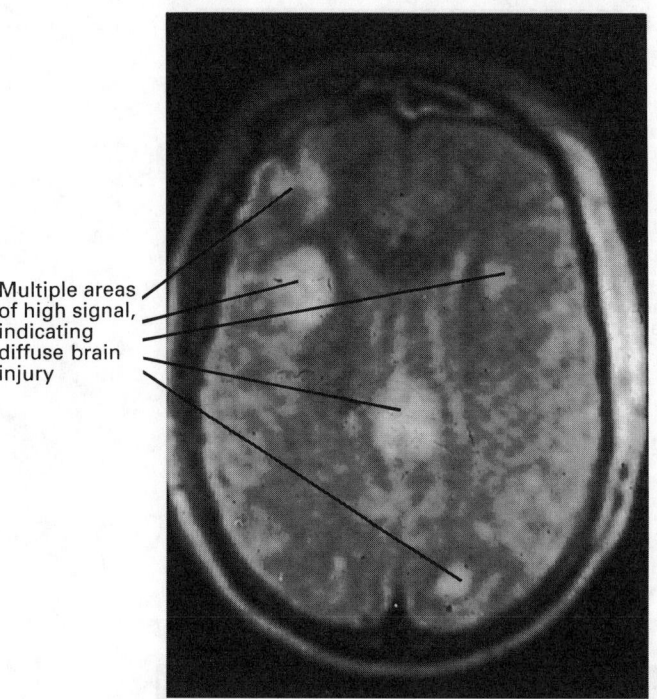

Multiple areas
of high signal,
indicating
diffuse brain
injury

Fig. 9. Magnetic resonance scan showing multiple areas of high signal (white) within the brain, indicating widespread diffuse injury.

Table 7. *Criteria for admission of head-injured adults to hospital*

- Confusion or any other depression of the level of consciousness at the time of assessment
- Skull fracture, on X-ray or clinically
- Neurological symptoms or signs
- Difficulty in assessing the patient, e.g. intoxication, epilepsy
- Potentially relevant medical condition, e.g. bleeding tendency
- Lack of a responsible relative/friend for supervision after discharge

relative about what circumstances in which to bring the patient back to hospital, as inevitably errors of judgement will be made from time to time. Particular care should be exercised with drunks (including those who will be going into police custody), and the very young and very old. If in any doubt, err on the side of caution and admit the patient to hospital.

Patients admitted to hospital

Guidelines for admitting head-injured patients to hospital for a period of neurological observation are given in Table 7. A few patients deteriorate neurologically during this period and should be referred promptly to a neurosurgeon. Most will improve or remain well during obser-

vation and can safely be discharged after about 24 h, preferably into the care of relatives or friends. Patients who continue to have significant neurological symptoms at that stage can be kept under further observation for longer, but there should be a low threshold for seeking advice from a neurosurgeon at this stage.

Patients referred to the neurosurgeon

Table 8 suggests which head-injured patients should be referred to a neurosurgeon. These referral criteria are very similar to the indications for performing a CT scan, and until recently arranging a scan and referring the patient to a neurosurgeon were often the same process. The neurosurgeon needs certain information at the time of referral (Table 9) in order to make an informed decision about the need for transfer and its timing.

EMERGENCY MANAGEMENT BEFORE TRANSFER

The importance of thorough assessment, resuscitation and continuing reassessment before transfer to the neurosurgical unit has already been made clear. Any cardiorespiratory or neurological deterioration is likely to be due to an extracranial complication like airway compromise or a pneumothorax. However, some intracranial

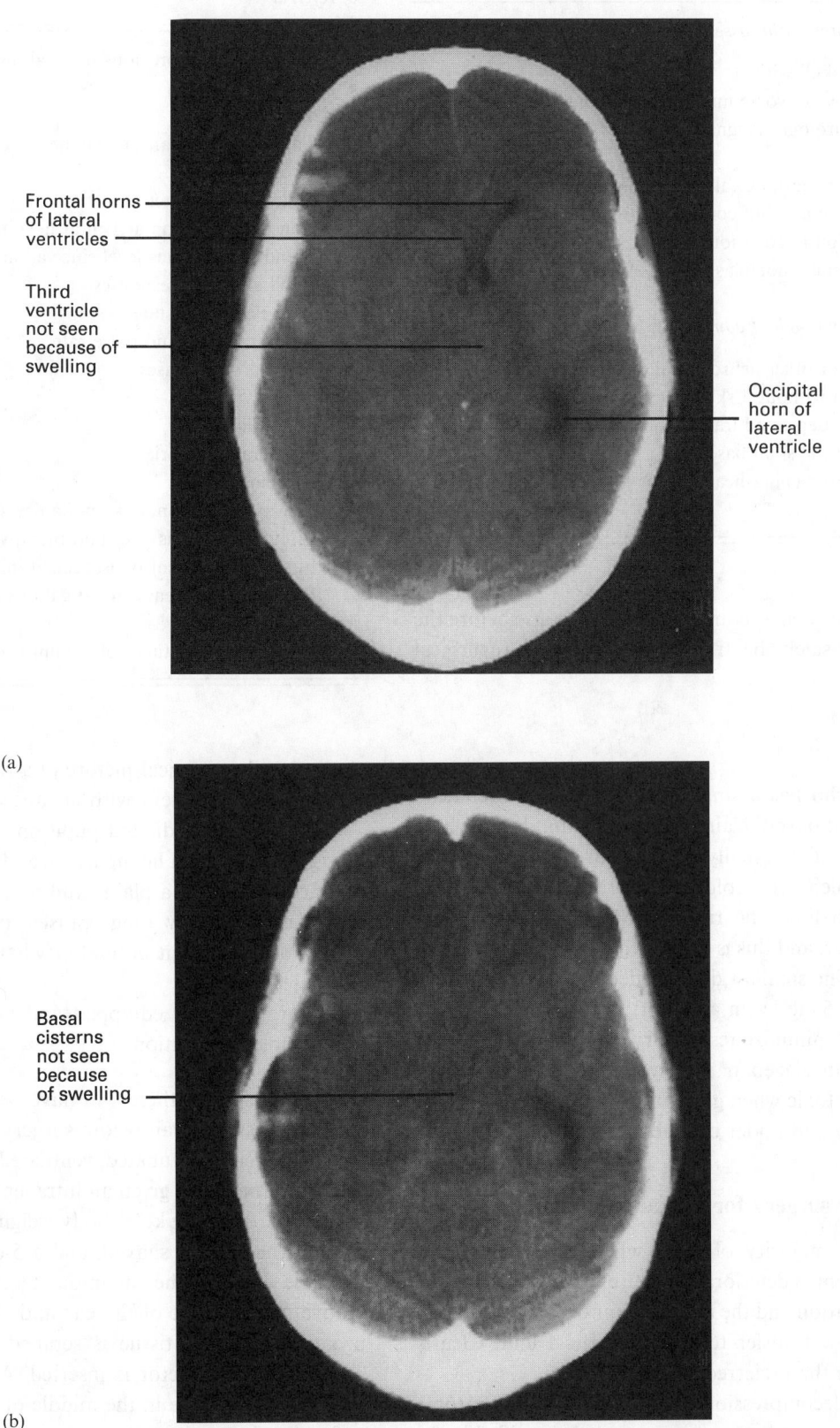

Frontal horns of lateral ventricles

Third ventricle not seen because of swelling

Occipital horn of lateral ventricle

(a)

Basal cisterns not seen because of swelling

(b)

Fig. 10. Swelling has obliterated the third ventricle (a) and the basal cisterns (b). (N.B. This is the same patient as in Fig. 8(a).)

Table 8. *Criteria for referral to the neurosurgeon*

Immediate (after initial assessment and resuscitation)

- Fractured skull with:
  —Confusion or worse impairment of consciousness
  —focal neurological signs
  —seizures
  —any other neurological symptoms or signs
- No skull fracture, but coma continuing after resuscitation
- Deterioration in conscious level or other neurological signs
- Suspected stab/shot/blast injury of head

Urgent (within 6–8 h of admission)

- Confusion or other neurological disturbance persisting after 6–8 h (even without a skull fracture)
- Compound depressed fracture of the skull vault
- Fracture of the skull base
- Persistent/worsening headache or vomiting, especially in a child

Table 9. *What the neurosurgeon needs to know at the time of referral*

- Patient's age and previous medical history (if known)
- History of injury
  Time of injury
  Cause and mechanism (e.g. height of fall)
- Neurological state
  Talked or not after injury
  Conscious level on arrival at hospital
  Trend in conscious level since admission
  Pupil and limb responses
- Cardiorespiratory state
  Blood pressure and pulse rate
  Arterial blood gases
- Injuries
  Skull fracture
  Extracranial injuries
- Management so far
  Airway protection and ventilatory status
  Circulatory status and fluid therapy
  First aid treatment of associated injuries
  Proposed emergency investigations/surgery
  Monitoring
  Drug doses and times of administration

complications demand an immediate response before the patient can safely be transferred to the neurosurgical unit.

Seizures

A patient who has a single epileptic seizure after head injury should have the airway protected until the seizure has stopped, as it usually does within a minute or two. Seizures which are prolonged or repeated need to be abolished to limit the rise in $CMRO_2$ and secondary brain damage, and this is done with intravenous or rectal diazepam. The smallest dose needed to stop the seizures is used (e.g. 5 mg IV in an adult), repeated if necessary, and this will minimize respiratory depression. Phenytoin is better than diazepam for preventing further seizures, but is cardiotoxic when given intravenously and must be given slowly and under cardiac monitoring.

Emergency surgery for extradural haematoma

In the vast majority of cases when a severely head-injured patient is deteriorating neurologically, intubation, hyperventilation and the use of mannitol can buy enough time to allow transfer to a neurosurgical unit. Clearly this is much the preferred course of action.

Surgical decompression of an extradural haematoma other than by a neurosurgeon can only be justified in the rare circumstances when certain factors coincide:

- A very clear clinical picture of a rapidly deteriorating unconscious patient with advanced and clear localizing signs (e.g. a dilated pupil on the left, then on the right, with a right hemiparesis) and perhaps a temporal fracture seen on a plain skull film.
- An unacceptably long transfer time to the nearest neurosurgical unit no matter what mode of transport is used.
- A surgical team equipped and willing to carry out burrhole exploration.

It is unlikely that there will have been time to confirm the diagnosis by scan before surgery.

The patient is intubated, ventilated to lower the PCO_2 below normal, and given an intravenous loading dose of mannitol ($0.3–0.7$ g kg^{-1} body weight). The appropriate side of the head is shaved, and a 5-cm vertical incision is made down to the squamous temporal bone, slightly above and in front of the ear and almost down to the zygoma. The soft tissue is scraped back, and a small self-retaining retractor is inserted. A perforator is used to make a burrhole in the middle of the incision (where a fracture is usually seen) and once through both tables of the skull a burr is used to ream out the hole. A large-bore sucker is used to aspirate as much haematoma as possible from the extradural space (the haematoma has the appearance and consistency of blackcurrant jam). Bone nibblers can be used to enlarge the burrhole to form a small craniectomy, exposing and coagulating any bleeding point (almost always an artery anterior and inferior to the burrhole). The wound is closed quickly around a vacuum drain and the patient transferred speedily to a neurosurgical unit, still ventilated.

If an extradural haematoma is not found, no attempt should be made to open the dura to deal with any other presumed haematoma, unless the surgeon has previous experience of operative neurosurgery. The patient should be transferred as soon as possible to the neurosurgical unit.

SAFE TRANSFER TO THE NEUROSURGICAL UNIT

Information on the risks of transfer and how to minimize them has accumulated in recent years (Gentleman & Jennett, 1990; Gentleman, 1992; Andrews *et al.*, 1990) and guidelines and standards for safe transfer have been published (Gentleman *et al.*, 1993; Munro & Laycock, 1993). The first step is to recognize the potential for avoidable secondary brain damage from unsuspected hypoxia or shock, during even a short transfer. The second step is to organize the service so as to minimize this risk. Table 10 summarizes what is needed.

Once the decision has been made to transfer the patient, unnecessary delay should be minimized. In the UK, transport by helicopter or aeroplane is useful in special circumstances (remoteness or traffic), but a land ambulance is the usual transport to the neurosurgical unit. Modern ambulances are less cramped and bumpy than their predecessors, but still provide an isolated and potentially hostile environment for a seriously head-injured patient and escort. This must be remembered by those responsible for the standard of care during the journey.

Before transfer the patient must be fully resuscitated. All life-threatening injuries are dealt with first. The airway must be secure before the journey starts. Even if the patient's condition has not until then demanded intubation and ventilation with sedative and paralysing drugs, this should be considered before transfer in a patient with an abnormal conscious level or who has deteriorated. Care must continue to be taken with the cervical spine during intubation. Reliable venous access is essential throughout the journey, the patient should

Table 10. *What is needed for a safe transfer*

- Trained escort (medical and nursing/paramedic)
- Ambulance
- Trolley which can be taken in and out of ambulance
- Functioning monitors with an adequate power supply
- Intubation equipment
- Intravenous lines
- Adequate oxygen supply
- Drugs
  —To institute and maintain ventilation
    —Depolarizing and non-depolarizing muscle relaxants
    —Short-acting analgesics
    —Intravenous sedatives
  —For cardiac resuscitation
  —Anticonvulsants
  —Mannitol

have a urinary catheter, and blood for transfusion should be sent in the ambulance, not in a taxi. Monitoring should be to the same standard as in an operating theatre: blood pressure, ECG and pulse oximetry. During transfer the patient must be accompanied by an experienced doctor (an anaesthetist if intubated) and a nurse or paramedic. They must have the equipment and drugs needed to deal with any crisis en route: tubes or lines can block or fall out, the patient can have a respiratory arrest or a fit, or can develop a fixed dilated pupil. All notes and films should be sent with the patient, as part of good communication between referring and receiving teams.

MANAGEMENT AT THE NEUROSURGICAL UNIT

The neurosurgical team should begin by reassessing the patient, using the ATLS system. Just because a complication was not present before the journey does not mean one has not developed by the time of arrival at the neurosurgical unit.

If a CT scan has not been done before transfer it is done soon after arrival at the neurosurgical unit, while continuing to monitor the patient. What the scan shows dictates what happens next. Some patients need an emergency operation to remove an intracranial haematoma, to deal with a penetrating injury, or so that other surgeons can deal with important extracranial injuries whose priority could only be determined after the CT scan. Other patients do not need surgery but admission to an intensive therapy unit for sophisticated monitoring and ventilation. A third group can safely be admitted to a ward for observation, as their injuries prove to be less serious.

Surgery

The details of operative management of haematomas and penetrating injuries are beyond the scope of this book, but the principles should be clearly understood by all in the chain of management after head surgery.

An acute haematoma forms a clot and so cannot be properly evacuated through a burrhole, only through a more substantial opening in the skull. The standard operation is a craniotomy, reflecting a scalp flap and cutting a window in the skull to expose the dura. Unless the problem is an extradural haematoma, the dura is opened to reveal the brain and any haematoma or contusion. Blood clot is sucked and washed away, bleeding points are identified and coagulated, and the wound is closed: dura, skull flap and scalp.

A depressed fracture or other penetrating brain wound is managed by gently mobilizing and removing in-driven bone fragments, sucking away non-viable brain tissue, suturing or patching torn dura, and replacing the bone fragments unless they are heavily contaminated. A key point is the debridement of the overlying traumatic wound to remove dirt, hair, foreign bodies and devital-ized tissue before the wound is sutured. Many neuro-surgeons recommend a broad-spectrum antibiotic with antistaphylococcal action (e.g. a cephalosporin) for a few days afterwards, and the patient's protection against tetanus should be checked.

The great majority of CSF leaks from the nose or ear stop spontaneously. Many neurosurgeons give a short course of an antibiotic active against pneumococci (e.g. benzylpenicillin), but the value of this is controversial. A minority of leaks persist beyond a few days, and in these cases the fistula is located using modern scanning tech-niques, surgically explored, and repaired with a bio-logical or synthetic graft to reduce the risk of penetrat-ing brain infection. Occasionally a patient injured some time previously presents with post-traumatic meningitis because of an unsuspected CSF leak, and requires surgi-cal closure of the fistula.

Management of patients with severe diffuse brain injury in an intensive therapy unit

Many patients with severe head injuries have no surgi-cally treatable lesion on the CT scan, and are managed on a general or neurosurgical intensive therapy unit. This involves increasingly extensive and sophisticated neuro-logical and cardiorespiratory monitoring (and often intervention) over a period of days or weeks, with neurosurgeon and anaesthetist sharing responsibility for management decisions.

Some UK neurosurgeons do not regard patients with diffuse brain injuries as their legitimate concern—a view often coloured by the limited beds and resources available in some units. The contrary view is that a neurosurgical unit is the most appropriate place to monitor and treat patients with severe diffuse brain injury. The Edinburgh unit has led the way by showing how often these patients suffer from hypoxic/ischaemic insults during the hours and days following injury, and how even short-lived insults can adversely influence outcome unless they are promptly recognized and treated (Jones *et al.*, 1994). Few drugs are yet of direct use in treating diffuse brain injury, but more effective therapies are likely to become available soon with the advent of novel neuroprotective drugs (Fadden & Salzman, 1992; Scatton *et al.*, 1991). A further argument for neurosurgical involvement in the care of these patients is that some will develop problems which need later neurosurgical intervention, such as enlargement of haematomas or contusions to cause critical elevations of ICP. What is quite clear is that more neurosurgical facilities (especially intensive therapy unit beds) are needed to improve patient care.

The technology available for ICP monitoring is now sophisticated yet easy to apply, even in a non-specialist intensive therapy unit. The practice of indi-vidual consultants regarding ICP monitoring is very variable, reflecting continuing controversy about the exact place of this technique in clinical practice. Most neurosurgeons would advocate monitoring of patients with 'borderline' haematomas which might require evacu-ation if the ICP is shown to be high or to rise during monitoring. Many would also monitor ICP in patients whose initial scan shows no focal lesion but evidence of generalized raised ICP, and who are treated by venti-lation and drugs to improve brain perfusion and oxygen-ation. Some neurosurgeons would extend ICP monitoring to all patients in coma with a conscious level below an arbitrary level (e.g. GCS 6), irrespective of what the scan shows.

What is clear is that the value of ICP monitoring is greatly enhanced when the data obtained is linked to other information—e.g. MAP, cerebral blood flow velocity, cerebral oxygen extraction (Chan *et al.*, 1992, 1993).

Neuroprotection

Neurosurgeons have unwittingly used neuroprotective drugs for many years to manage head-injured patients. For example, mannitol is an effective scavenger of free radicals from traumatized brain tissue. Recently, molecules have been synthesized which have a variety of protective effects on the structure and function of injured or ischaemic neurones *in vitro* and in animal experiments: neurotransmitter blockade, free radical scavenging, membrane stabilization, ionic channel effects and probably other mechanisms as yet undiscovered. Much excitement has been generated by the possibility that drugs could be used to protect damaged neurones after a head injury (or indeed after a spinal injury, a stroke, or a subarachnoid haemorrhage) (Fadden & Salzman, 1992; Scatton *et al.*, 1991; Bracken *et al.*, 1990; Argentino *et al.*, 1989; Gorio, 1988), and several pharmaceutical companies are now active in this field. Perhaps in years to come the doctor in the A&E department or the paramedic in the field will begin the treatment of the head-injured patient not just by applying an oxygen mask but by giving an intravenous injection of a neuroprotective drug.

CONCLUSION

Those who provide early care to head-injured patients carry great responsibility. Their actions and omissions in the A&E department, the resuscitation room, or the ambulance can profoundly affect both survival and the quality of survival. Fortunately there is now a good deal of information and advice available to guide good practice, and diagnostic facilities in most general hospitals are excellent.

The most important step is always to identify and correct potential causes of secondary brain damage, so that the initial injury is not compounded by a later insult. Organization, education, and practice must all be geared to this end.

Bibliography

AMERICAN COLLEGE OF SURGEONS COMMITTEE ON TRAUMA (1993). *ATLS Course Manual.* Chicago: American College of Surgeons.

ANDREWS, P.J.D., PIPER, I.R., DEARDEN, N.R. *et al.* (1990). Secondary insults during intrahospital transfer of head injured patients. *Lancet*, **i**, 327–30.

ARGENTINO, C., SACCHETTI, M., TONI, D. *et al.* (1989). GM1 ganglioside therapy in acute ischaemic stroke. *Stroke*, **20**, 1143.

BRACKEN, M.B., SHEPARD, M.J., COLLINS, W.F. *et al.* (1990). A randomised controlled trial of methylprednisolone or naloxone in the treatment of acute spinal cord injury: results of the Second National Acute Spinal Cord Injury Study. *N. Engl. J. Med.*, **332**, 1405.

BRIGGS, M., CLARKE, P., CROCKARD, A. *et al.* (1984). Guidelines for initial management after head injury in adults: suggestions from a group of neurosurgeons. *Br. Med. J.*, **288**, 983–985.

CHAN, P.H., YURKO, M. & FISHMAN, R.A. (1982). Phospholipid degeneration and cellular edema induced by free radicals in brain cortical slices. *J. Neurochem.*, **38**, 525–31.

CHAN, K.H., MILLER, J.D., DEARDEN, N.M. *et al.* (1992). The effect of changes in cerebral perfusion pressure upon middle cerebral artery blood flow velocity and jugular venous oxygen saturation after severe brain injury. *J. Neurosurg.*, **77**, 55–61.

CHAN, K.H., DEARDEN, N.M., MILLER, J.D. *et al.* (1993). Multimodality monitoring as a guide to treatment of intracranial hypertension after severe brain injury. *Neurosurgery*, **32**, 547–52.

FADEN, A.I. & SALZMAN, S. (1992). Pharmacological strategies in CNS trauma. *Trends Pharmacol. Sci.*, **13**, 29–35.

FADEN, A.I., DEMEDIUK, P., PANTER, S.S. *et al.* (1989). The role of excitatory amino acids and NMDA receptors in traumatic brain injury. *Science*, **244**, 798–800.

GALBRAITH, S. & TEASDALE, G.M. (1981). Predicting the need for operation in the patient with an occult traumatic intracranial haematoma. *J. Neurosurg.*, **55**, 75–81.

GENTLEMAN, D. (1990). Preventing secondary brain damage after head injury: a multidisciplinary challenge. *Injury*, **21**, 305–8.

GENTLEMAN, D. (1992). Causes and effects of systemic complications among severely head injured patients transferred to a neurosurgical unit. *Int. Surg.*, **77**, 297–302.

GENTLEMAN, D. & JENNETT, B. (1990). Audit of unconscious head injured patients transferred to a neurosurgical unit. *Lancet*, **i**, 327–30.

GENTLEMAN, D., DEARDEN, M., MIDGLEY, S. *et al.* (1993). Guidelines for resuscitation and transfer of patients with serious head injury. *Br. Med. J.*, **307**, 547–52.

GOLDSTEIN, M. (1990). Traumatic brain injury: a silent epidemic. *Ann. Neurol.*, **27**, 327.

GORIO, A. (1988). Gangliosides as a possible treatment affecting neuronal repair processes. *Adv. Neurol.*, **47**, 523.

JENKINS, A., TEASDALE, G., HADLEY, M.D.M. *et al.* (1986). Brain lesions detected by magnetic resonance imaging in mild and severe brain injuries. *Lancet*, **ii**, 445–6.

JENKINS, L.W., MOSZYNSKI, K., LYETH, B.G. *et al.* (1989). Increased vulnerability of the mildly traumatised rat brain to cerebral ischemia: the use of controlled secondary ischaemia as a research tool to identify common or different mechanisms contributing to mechanical and ischaemic brain injury. *Brain Res.*, **447**, 211–24.

JENNETT, B. & CARLIN, J. (1978). Preventable mortality and morbidity after head injury. *Injury*, **10**, 31–9.

JONES, P.A., ANDREWS, P.J., MIDGLEY, S. *et al.* (1994). Measuring the burden of secondary insults in head injured patients during intensive care. *J. Neurosurg. Anesthesiol.*, **6**, 4–14.

KRAUS, J.F. (1987). Epidemiology of head injury. In *Head Injury*, 2nd edn., ed. P. R. Cooper. pp. 1–19. Baltimore: Williams & Wilkins.

MARSHALL, L.F., MARSHALL, S.B., KLAUBER, M.R. *et al.* (1991). A new classification of head injury based on computed tomography. *J. Neurosurg.*, **75**, S14–S20.

MENDELOW, A.D., KARMI, M.Z., PAUL, K.S. *et al.* (1979). Extradural haematoma: effect of delayed treatment. *Br. Med. J.*, **1**, 1240–2.

MENDELOW, A.D., TEASDALE, G., JENNETT, B. *et al.* (1983). Risks of intracranial haematomas in head-injured adults. *Br. Med. J.*, **287**, 1173–6.

MILLER, J.D. & BECKER, D.P. (1982). Secondary insults to the injured brain. *J. R. Coll. Surg. Edinb.*, **27**, 292–8.

MILLER, J., MURRAY, L. & TEASDALE, G. (1990). Development of traumatic intracranial haematoma after 'mild' head injury. *Neurosurgery*, **27**, 669–73.

MUNRO, H.M. & LAYCOCK, J.R.D. (1993). Inter-hospital transfer: standards for ventilated neurosurgical emergencies. *Br. J. Intensive Care*, **3**, 210–14.

REILLY, P.L., ADAMS, J.H., GRAHAM, D.I. *et al.* (1975). Patients with head injury who talk and die. *Lancet*, **ii**, 375–7.

ROSE, J., VALTONEN, S. & JENNETT, B. (1977). Avoidable factors contributing to death after head injury. *Br. Med. J.*, **2**, 615–18.

SCATTON, B., CARTER, C., BENAVIDES, J. *et al.* (1991). *N*-Methyl-D-aspartate receptor antagonists: a novel therapeutic perspective for the treatment of ischaemic brain injury. *Cerebrovasc. Dis.*, **1**, 121–35.

SEELIG, J.M., BECKER, D.P., MILLER, J.D. *et al.* (1981). Traumatic acute subdural haematoma: major mortality reduction in comatose patients treated within four hours. *N. Engl. J. Med.*, **304**, 1511–18.

SERVADEI, F., FACCANI, G., ROCCELLA, P. *et al.* (1989). Asymptomatic extradural haematomas: results of a multicenter study of 158 cases in minor head injury. *Acta Neurochir. (Wien)*, **96**, 39–45.

SERVADEI, F., VERGONI, G., NASI, M. *et al.* (1993). Management of low-risk head injuries in an entire area: results of an 18 months survey. *Surg. Neurol.*, **39**, 269–75.

STEIN, S. & ROSS, S. (1992). Mild head injury: a plea for routine early CT scanning. *J. Trauma*, **33**, 11–13.

TEASDALE, G. & JENNETT, B. (1974). Assessment of coma and impaired consciousness. *Lancet*, **ii**, 81–4.

TEASDALE, G., GALBRAITH, S., MURRAY, L. *et al.* (1982). Management of traumatic intracranial haematoma. *Br. Med. J.*, **285**, 1695–7.

TEASDALE, G., MURRAY, G., ANDERSON, E. *et al.* (1990). Risks of acute traumatic intracranial haematoma in children and adults: implications for managing head injuries. *Br. Med. J.*, **300**, 363–7.

19 Faciomaxillary and dental emergencies

I. HUTCHISON (A: Faciomaxillary and dental trauma; B: Oral and maxillofacial diseases)

Chapter plan

A: Faciomaxillary and dental trauma

Introduction
Aetiology
Pathophysiology
Management in A&E
Timing of treatment
Examination of soft tissues and bones
Fractured facial bones and their management in A&E
Complications
Radiology
Suturing in the face
Conclusion

B: Oral and maxillofacial diseases

Introduction
Symptomatology
History, examination and investigations
Normal flora and pathogenic microorganisms
Decreased host defence mechanisms
Specific organ systems and their infections
Specific organisms

A: Faciomaxillary and dental trauma

I. HUTCHISON

*Department of Oral and Maxillofacial Surgery,
St Bartholomew's Hospital, London, UK*

INTRODUCTION

Injuries to the face are common but rarely life-threatening. The importance of these injuries lies not only in their disturbance of the functions of this region such as vision, smell, taste, eating and speech, but also in their cosmetic aspects. Facial appearance is important in all societies. Even the most minor injury may cause psychological distress if a satisfactory cosmetic result is not achieved.

Facial injuries provoke inordinate anxiety in staff because they destroy the patient's usual appearance. This anxiety may be exacerbated by the profuse initial bleeding associated with these injuries.

The unique anatomical properties of the face enable more conservative approaches in trauma management. Firstly, there is an excellent blood supply to the soft tissues and bones so that even the most parlous soft tissue pedicle and isolated bone fragment will survive. No tissue should be discarded before consultation with a maxillofacial expert. Secondly, the facial bones have been rendered light by pneumatization of the maxilla, frontal bone and ethmoids. This allows inspired air to be warmed and imparts resonance to speech. It also means that humans do not have to support a heavy head. These light facial bones have buttresses to transmit the strong vertical forces of mastication up to the base of the skull. These buttresses include the zygomatic bones, the lateral orbital margin and the lateral wall of the nose.

However, the facial bones are weak in the horizontal plane and are therefore susceptible to blows delivered anteriorly or laterally.

The bones of the face articulate with each other at various suture lines and these constitute important points of weakness where fractures commonly occur. The middle facial bones—the zygoma, maxilla, nose and ethmoids—articulate with the base of the skull on an inclined plane. Fractures separating the facial bones from the base of the skull often cause downward and backward impaction. This obstructs the pharynx and the upper airway.

The two most commonly injured facial bones are the prominent nose and zygoma (malar or cheekbone). Blows to the mandible are also relatively common. The mandible's condylar neck is weak and frequently fractures as a result of indirect trauma to the point of the chin. There is only a thin membrane of bone between the condylar fossa of the mandible and the middle cranial fossa. If the mandibular condyle did not readily fracture, this force would push it into the middle cranial fossa with consequent neurological damage.

The thin bony walls of the orbit are weak and this weakness may have a protective function. Blows to the globe will result in blow-out fractures of the orbital walls before the globe itself is ruptured.

The mandible is of prime importance in mastication and swallowing and therefore has many muscles gaining origin or inserting into its surface. These muscles tend to distract mandibular fractures in different directions depending on the site of the fracture.

AETIOLOGY

Alcohol consumption has an important role in facial trauma (Brook & Wood, 1983).

Road traffic accidents

Thirty-nine per cent of road traffic accident victims suffer facial injuries (Grattan & Hobbs, 1985). The incidence of facial injuries has reduced remarkably following legislation governing the compulsory wearing of car seat belts (Perkins & Layton, 1988; Pye & Waters, 1984) and helmets for motorcyclists, limitations on alcohol consumption, the introduction of motorway speed limits and, more recently, airbags for front seat passengers (Rogers et al., 1992). Furthermore, windscreen injuries have been reduced by the advent of toughened safety glass.

Motorway accidents are associated with severe trauma.

However, motorways may well have reduced the rate of road traffic accidents.

For the car passenger, common sources of injury are the windscreen, windscreen pillars, dashboard, steering wheel, other passengers acting as secondary missiles within the car, the bonnet and the mirror, and the front seats for back seat passengers. Motorcyclists are most frequently injured by other vehicles' bonnets, bumpers and windscreens, the road itself, their helmets and their motorbikes. Cyclists and pedestrians are injured by motor vehicles.

The nature of these injuries depends on the speed of impact and the amount of protection, and varies from the simplest of lacerations, through multiple glass puncture wounds, to severe complex trauma affecting the whole body.

Assault

Victims and protagonists have often consumed large amounts of alcohol prior to an assault (Hill et al., 1984). The assault may be perpetrated using fists, elbows, knees or feet, or blunt implements such as baseball bats, or sharp instruments such as knives. It may occur in the domestic environment and involve regular battering of wives (Shepherd et al., 1988; Zachariades et al., 1990) or children (Needleman, 1986). It may also occur at work (Brook & Wood, 1983; Iizuka et al., 1990) or during sports or leisure activities (Linn et al., 1986). Increasingly, though, in the inner cities, the assault may be perpetrated by an unknown assailant with minimal provoking factors (Adi et al., 1990; Telfer et al., 1991).

The incidence of human and other animal bites has also increased.

Industrial accidents

Legislation governing health and safety at work was designed to reduce industrial accidents, but workers in the construction industry are particularly prone to facial injuries. Other industries affected are those of mining, fishing and oil exploration (Brook & Wood, 1983; Iizuka et al., 1990). Historically, soldiers on guard duty fainted as a result of poor venous return to the heart and low cardiac output when they failed to use their calf muscle pump. They sustained parasymphyseal and bilateral condylar neck mandibular fractures (Bradley, 1985).

Accidents in the home

These are commonly associated with falls.

Medically compromised patients

Alcoholics and epileptics are particularly prone to falls and often sustain severe mandibular fractures.

Gunshot and bomb blast injuries

These injuries carry a higher risk of infection and are associated with significant tissue loss requiring specific reconstructive procedures (Shuker, 1986; Marshall, 1986; Rowe, 1985).

PATHOPHYSIOLOGY

Facial injuries usually occur in isolation. However, in cases of severe trauma, skull, cervical spine and chest injuries frequently occur concomitantly. In the patient with severe facial injuries one should always assume a cervical spine injury until proven otherwise and take the appropriate precautions with the use of a neck collar and 'log rolling' if the patient has to be turned (Haugh *et al.*, 1991).

Airway problems

The mouth and nose constitute the upper airway and, as such, any damage to these sites may result in airway compromise. Fragments of tooth, bone, blood, vomit or dentures may block the upper airway or be inhaled into the lung, blocking a main bronchus. The tongue is attached to the mandible just behind the lower incisor teeth. Therefore, when this site suffers comminuted fractures, the tongue may drop back obstructing the airway. The maxilla may slip backwards and downwards obstructing the upper airway in Le Fort I, II or III injuries. Finally, there may be associated injuries to the larynx and trachea further compromising the airway (Smith & Bradley, 1986).

It is therefore vital that the airway should be secured in all facial injury patients prior to their visiting the radiography department for radiographic examination.

Blood supply

The main blood supply to the face comes from the external carotid artery via the lingual, facial, maxillary

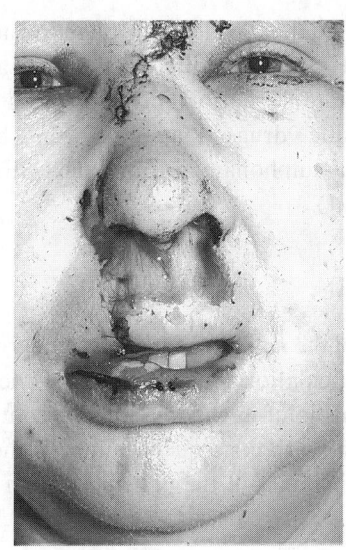

Fig. 1. This patient demonstrates cerebrospinal fluid, mixed with blood, leaking from the nose. She sustained a Le Fort II fracture with disruption of the cribriform plate of the ethmoid bone.

and superficial temporal arteries. The internal carotid artery makes a small contribution via the anterior ethmoidal arteries. There is a further blood supply to the base of the skull through the vertebrobasilar system which may occasionally be injured in this type of trauma.

Lacerations usually bleed profusely and then stop without significant blood loss. Conversely, puncture wounds may bleed significantly before the blood loss is recognized by cardiovascular collapse. This usually occurs when instruments such as sharp glass edges lacerate medium-sized arteries such as the facial artery. In these situations, the puncture wound needs to be opened widely and the artery clamped. The patient should be resuscitated simultaneously with intravenous fluid replacement.

The mandible receives its blood supply from the inferior dental artery travelling within the bone and from periosteal plexuses which gain a blood supply from branches of the facial and lingual arteries. The maxilla, nose and zygoma are supplied by branches of the maxillary artery such as the greater palatine artery and infraorbital arteries and by the anterior ethmoidal artery from the internal carotid artery.

Cerebrospinal fluid

The disruption of the skull base at the cribriform plate or around the petrous temporal bone may result in cerebrospinal fluid (CSF) leaks through the nose and ear respectively (Fig. 1). The patient is therefore at risk from meningitis. Suitable antibiotic prophylaxis should be instituted using drugs that cross the blood/brain barrier, such as sulphonamides, until the CSF leak ceases (Leopard, 1971).

Growth centres

The condyle of the mandible functions as a growth centre and as an articulation for movement of the mandible. Damage to this joint in children may be complicated by bony ankylosis with consequent failure of the mandible to grow and inability of the patient to open the mouth (Rowe, 1982).

Sensory and motor nerves

Branches of the trigeminal nerve run through the facial bones to supply the overlying skin with sensation. Fractures of these bones frequently result in neuropraxia or neurotmesis with classically distributed alteration in sensation. The facial or seventh cranial nerve exits from the base of the skull at the stylomastoid foramen and arborizes within the parotid gland to supply the muscles of facial expression. It may be damaged within the petrous temporal bone or when lacerations involve the parotid region.

Occlusion

Fractures of the facial bones result in derangement of the occlusion of the teeth. If this is left untreated, the malocclusion may cause permanent discomfort and secondary temporomandibular joint problems. Conversely, the teeth may be used to site the facial bones in their correct relationship when the facial swelling obscures accurate, direct visual assessment.

Limited mouth opening

Several different facial injuries may limit mandibular movement:
1. The commonest cause is muscle spasm and pain due to mandibular fracture.
2. Fractured zygomatic arches can impact on the temporalis muscle or the coronoid process of the mandible preventing mouth opening.
3. Damage to the mandibular condylar head or its condylar neck may be responsible.
4. Whiplash injuries may damage the intra-articular

fibrocartilaginous meniscus within the temporomandibular joint, resulting in its anterior displacement (Weinberg & LaPointe, 1987).

Eyelids and eye

The orbicularis oculi muscles of the eyelids gain attachment to the facial skeleton through the medial canthal ligaments which in turn surround the lacrimal sac. Damage to the medial canthal region causes alteration in shape of the eyelids and may be associated with lacrimal drainage problems.

The globe of the eye is protected by the supraorbital bar, lateral orbital wall, prominence of the zygoma and infraorbital rim. It occupies only a quarter of the orbital volume and sits suspended in periorbital fat. Damage to any of the orbital walls may result in alteration of level of the eye and entrapment of the periorbital tissues, resulting in double vision and limitation in eye movement. The superior orbital fissure may rarely be compressed in severe craniofacial trauma, resulting in damage to the lacrimal, frontal, trochlear, oculomotor, nasociliary and abducens nerves (Bowerman, 1969).

Infection

Fractures of the facial bones frequently open into the sinuses and mouth. This is not usually a problem if the fractures are dealt with rapidly. If fractures are left untreated for several days then infection and non-union may ensue.

Salivary glands

The parotid gland and its duct may be injured in facial lacerations. Saliva containing amylase then leaks into the facial soft tissues producing either a sialocele (a collection of saliva within the tissues) or a parotid fistula (Landau & Stewart, 1985).

MANAGEMENT IN A&E

Resuscitation always takes precedence.

TECHNIQUES

Airway

Several aspects of the upper airway require specific attention in facial injuries:
- The mouth should be opened, examined with a reasonable light and debris aspirated with a sucker.

The mouth can also be cleared by inserting the right index finger inside the cheek as far back as it will go and then hooking it forwards bringing all the debris to the front of the mouth.

- If possible the patient should be sat with the head up or nursed on one side. This, however, may be contraindicated if there is a suspected spinal injury.
- A nasopharyngeal airway may help secure the airway in maxillary fractures but this must be aspirated regularly to ensure it does not block.
- If the lower jaw is fractured and there is anxiety over the tongue dropping back then the midline of the lower jaw may be pulled forward. Alternatively, in the A&E department, a 2/0 black silk suture should be placed through the dorsum of the tongue and this suture taped to the side of the face, holding the tongue forward (Hutchison *et al.*, 1990).
- Upper jaw fractures may be disimpacted by inserting the left index finger behind the soft palate and the right index finger and thumb around the premaxillary region then pulling the maxilla forward whilst the forehead is supported by an assistant (Hutchison *et al.*, 1990).
- Dexamethasone 8 mg given intravenously will reduce post-traumatic pharyngeal oedema if this develops.
- The neck should be examined for surgical emphysema and if there is suggestion of a laryngeal or tracheal fracture then X-rays of the neck should be arranged.
- Unconscious patients or those with potential airway compromise must not be sent to the radiology department in the supine position with an unprotected airway.
- Endotracheal intubation is usually relatively easy when the facial bones are disrupted providing a good light and suction are available. Failing this, cricothyroid puncture may be appropriate. Emergency tracheostomy is rarely indicated.
- Chest X-rays are mandatory if inhaled foreign bodies are suspected. They may not show the foreign body but will show collapsed lobes and other direct chest injuries such as flail segments, pneumothoraces and ruptured diaphragms.
- Bronchoscopy should be arranged if there is a suspicion of inhaled debris in the lungs.

Haemorrhage

Outside the A&E department
- Haemorrhage from the face and neck is dramatic but usually stops spontaneously.
- First aid measures include manual compression of bleeding points rather than diffuse packing.
- If the injury is severe enough, blood should be taken for cross-match and intravenous fluid commenced.
- If there is an obvious bleeding point and artery clips are available, these may be applied to the vessel in question.

In A&E
- If the patient is bleeding significantly from a facial injury then venous access must be assured with two cannulae in central or large peripheral veins.
- Blood should be cross-matched and an infusion started.
- The patient's cardiovascular status should be monitored every few minutes.
- If possible, artery clips should be applied to any obvious bleeding vessels. Failing this, local compression with packs may be necessary.
- If the patient is bleeding profusely from the nose then anterior and posterior nasal packs should be used (Hutchison *et al.*, 1990).
- In certain instances it may be necessary to under-run a bleeding vessel with a suture but this carries significant risks.
- Vessels exiting from bony foramina may be plugged with bone wax or oxidized cellulose.
- In extremis, the external carotid artery or anterior ethmoidal arteries may need to be ligated (Dimitroulis & Steidler, 1992; Thaller & Beal, 1991).
- If it has been necessary to transfuse more than 4 units of blood to maintain the patient's blood pressure, a coagulopathy may develop. Clotting studies and fibrin degradation products aid in diagnosis but are often relatively normal. If the patient bleeds continuously from all sites despite local measures, consider this possibility. Treatment is with clotting factor concentrates, platelet infusions, and 10 ml of 10% calcium gluconate in conjunction with local measures.
- If the patient has circulatory collapse suggestive of significant blood loss, then injuries to the abdomen, chest, and limbs must be considered.

Pain control
- Surprisingly, there is very little pain associated with fractures of the middle third of the facial skeleton or with soft tissue lacerations. However, mandibular fractures are associated with significant pain. In the first instance, simple analgesia alone should be employed.

Prevention of complications
- This is usually linked to the recognition of all injuries. Having averted life-threatening problems, other injuries should be identified, and treatment should be instituted with the aim of restoring normal function.
- Specific complications are listed in Table 3 (see section on complications, below).

TIMING OF TREATMENT

All life-threatening problems such as chest, abdominal and neurological injuries should be controlled, and ischaemic limbs and nerve injuries should be dealt with prior to definitive management of the facial injury.

Ideally, facial soft tissue injuries should be sutured within 24 h. Most simple facial lacerations may be closed under local anaesthesia, but careful debridement, examination and meticulous closure should be achieved. In children, local anaesthesia may be supplemented with a sedative. If the soft tissue injury is severe or involves deep tissues such as the parotid gland or nasolacrimal apparatus, then the suturing should be performed under general anaesthesia. The local anaesthetic solutions that are currently used contain 0.5–2% lignocaine with a vasoconstrictor such as adrenaline at concentrations varying from 1 in 200 000 to 1 in 80 000. Alternatives include prilocaine hydrohloride with felypressin. Fine needles should be used to administer the local anaesthetic to minimize pain.

Bony injuries of the facial skeleton can wait for longer periods for definitive treatment, but pain, the risk of infection and failure to feed effectively all militate in favour of early surgery.

If the patient is being taken to theatre for other injuries, then the maxillofacial surgeon should be involved. More detailed assessment and interim or definitive treatment for the maxillofacial injuries may then be performed at the same operating theatre visit. This is particularly relevant in combined neurological and maxillofacial trauma (Jensen et al., 1992). If there is a complex maxillofacial injury in isolation, then treatment should be delayed for a few days until all the diagnostic information is available.

It is wise to obtain photographs of all patients prior to treatment as they may be helpful in later legal actions.

EXAMINATION OF SOFT TISSUES AND BONES

Prior to examination the source of trauma should be identified. This may help in identifying the site and type of injury; also, it is important statistically and legally and may uncover domestic violence.

The face should be examined systematically (Table 1) from the top of the skull to the bottom of the mandible and from the front of the face to the occipital region (Fig. 2). The two sides of the face should be compared. All orifices should be examined. Injuries are best recorded on a simple line drawing of the face. Measurements of injuries such as facial lacerations are helpful. The examination may be subdivided into inspection and palpation. The patient is inspected for lacerations, bruises, swellings and hollows, and the possibility of underlying damage

should be considered in these instances. Limitation of movement of the soft tissues such as the muscles of facial expression and the globe of the eye, and hard tissues such as the mandible, should be noted. The presence of blood or other fluid exuding from the nose or ear must be recorded. The function of the facial nerve should be assessed in detail. The patient should be palpated for abnormal movement of the facial bones, pain, crepitus and altered sensation of the facial skin.

FRACTURED FACIAL BONES AND THEIR MANAGEMENT IN A&E

The nasal bones

This fracture is the commonest injury of the facial bones and is usually caused by a direct blow to the nose. The injury may affect the nasal bones or the septum alone but more commonly involves both.

The patient complains of epistaxis and difficulty in breathing through the nose and may have noticed deformity.

Palpation over the nasal bones and over the nasal tip will elicit tenderness at the site of the fracture and may cause discomfort at the nasal spine.

Lateral radiographs of the nasal bones should be requested and an occipitofrontal 25° view may show the disposition of the septum and uncover damage to the lamina papyracea of the ethmoid bone in the more complex nasoethmoid fracture (Ellis, 1993).

Although there is no urgency to treat these fractures, early referral allows treatment to be instituted before post-traumatic swelling develops.

The zygoma

This is the second most common facial bone fracture and results from a blow to the side of the face. The zygomatic prominence probably protects the globe of the eye. The zygoma usually separates at its sutures with other bones. Patients present with depression of the cheek prominence, anaesthesia of the cheek, ipsilateral epistaxis and limitation in jaw opening (Fig. 3a). They may also have double vision and limitation of eye movements because the zygoma contributes to the orbital floor.

Examination demonstrates lateral subconjunctival ecchymosis where the posterior extent is not visible (Fig. 3b). There is tenderness and separation at the frontozygomatic, and/or zygomaticomaxillary sutures, and/or over the zygomatic arch. If the nose has been blown, there may be surgical emphysema of the periorbital tissues.

Table 1. *Examination of soft tissues and bones from top of head to bottom of mandible*

Inspection	Palpation (bilaterally simultaneously)
Forehead and temple	
• Laceration and swelling, bruising, depression, flattening and deformity	• Palpate skull gently • Feel for anaesthesia over forehead • Feel superior and lateral orbital margins, zygomatic arches and frontonasal region for steps and tenderness
Nose	
• Swelling • Deviation • Laceration • Depression • Epistaxis • CSF leak • Septal haematoma • Signs of nasoethmoid injury • Flat naso-orbital valley	• Fracture lines • Depression • Tenderness • Blocked nostrils • Measure intercanthal distance: > 36 mm abnormal • Palpate medial canthal ligaments
Eyes	

• Globe
  —Eye movements
  —Ex/enophthalmos
  —Subconjunctival ecchymosis
  —Visual acuity
  —Diplopia
  —Pupillary levels
  —Fundi
• Eyelids
  —Change of shape and angle
  —Swelling
  —Lacerations or ptosis
• Lacrimal apparatus
  —Tears down cheek
• Medial canthus
  —Signs of traumatic telecanthus
	• Feel inferior orbital margins for steps and tenderness
	• Anaesthesia: feel cheek, nose and upper lip for anaesthesia in distribution of infraorbital nerve
	• Tenseness of globe
	• Feel for surgical emphysema around eyes and on face. This may be caused by fracture of:
	  —zygoma
	  —nasoethmoid complex
	  —orbits

Face	

• Look for movement of muscles of facial expression
• Parotid duct injuries
  —Leaks
  —Sialoceles	

Ear	
• Lacerations • CSF leak • Subperichondrial haematoma • Bleeding from ear —Examine external auditory meatus for site of bleeding a. Anterior wall = fractured mandibular condyle b. Posterior wall or blue bulging tympanic membrane = fractured middle cranial fossa	

Table 1. *Continued*

Inspection	Palpation (bilaterally simultaneously)
Mastoid	
● Bruising of skin (Battle's sign) = fractured middle cranial fossa	
Mandible	
● Movement	● Feel inside ear for temporomandibular joint tenderness
● Deviation	● Feel lower border of jaw for steps and tenderness
● Retrusion	● Feel lower lip for anaesthesia
● Anterior open bite	
● Preauricular hollow	
● Deviation of chin point	
Mouth	
● Bloody saliva	● Mobile teeth
● Limited opening	● Independent movement of parts of mandible
● Bruising, especially sublingual	● Feel zygomatic buttress for tenderness
● Gingival and mucosal lacerations	● Feel mobility of maxilla on face
● Misplaced teeth	● Feel mobility of mandible as a whole
● Loose teeth	
● Steps in occlusion	
● Malocclusion	
● Fractured teeth in the premolar and molar regions: these are often vertical due to indirect trauma	
● Fractured teeth in the incisor region: these are horizontal due to direct trauma	
● Fetor	
● Drooling	
● Gagging	
● Anterior open bite	

Fractured zygomas invariably result in lateral orbital wall and floor fractures. If there is severe disruption of these orbital walls, there may be compression of the lateral rectus muscle, or the muscle cone around the optic nerve, and entrapment or herniation of the periorbital fat with consequent visual symptoms, or alteration in pupillary level, enophthalmos, and an antimongoloid slant of the palpebral fissure. Fortunately, although fractured zygomas are common, significant damage to the intraorbital contents is rare with this injury.

Occipitomental radiographs taken with a 0° and a 30° tilt of the X-ray tube will show separation at the frontozygomatic, zygomaticomaxillary and zygomaticotemporal sutures on the zygomatic arch (Fig. 4). The affected maxillary sinus may have a fluid level or be completely opaque and there will be disruption of the lateral sinus wall on this view.

Immediate referral is advisable because of the rare but definite risk of retrobulbar haemorrhage which may lead to blindness. Also, when the patient is referred early, it may be possible to institute immediate treatment for the fracture within the first 24 h before post-traumatic oedema develops. Failing this, treatment of the injury may be deferred for up to 1 week.

The mandible

Mandibular fractures are usually caused by direct blows over the mandible. There are several distinct fracture sites with their own characteristics. Two or more sites are frequently fractured simultaneously. For example, condylar neck fractures are often associated with contralateral body or angle fractures.

The temporomandibular joint

Condylar neck fractures

These are commonly caused by an indirect blow on the chin. It is the commonest site of mandibular fracture as

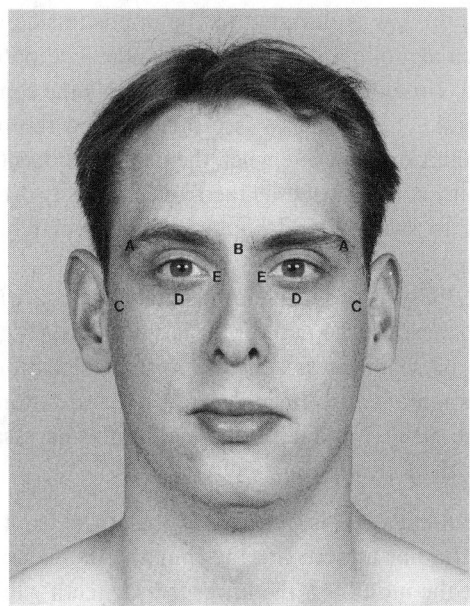

Fig. 2. If a facial fracture is suspected the following sites should be palpated for tenderness, depression or separation: A, frontozygomatic suture; B, frontonasal suture; C, zygomatic arch; D, zygomaticomaxillary suture; E, medial canthal ligament.

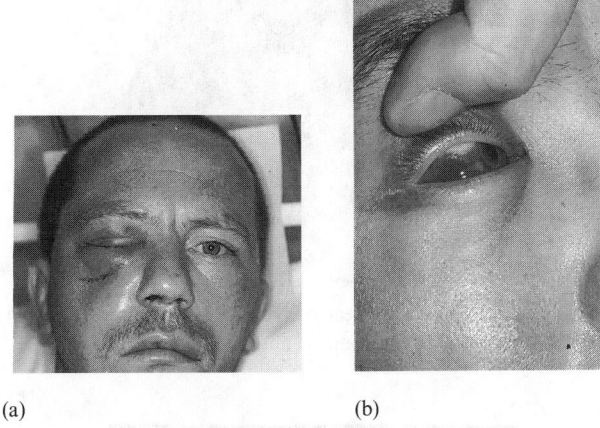

(a)　　　　　　　　　　　　(b)

Fig. 3. This man has a displaced fractured right zygoma. (a) Note the depressed cheek bone, periorbital haematoma and oedema, and the unilateral right-sided epistaxis. He also has numbness of his right cheek and is unable to fully open his mouth. (b) There is a lateral subconjunctival ecchymosis which extends beyond the right lateral conjunctival reflection.

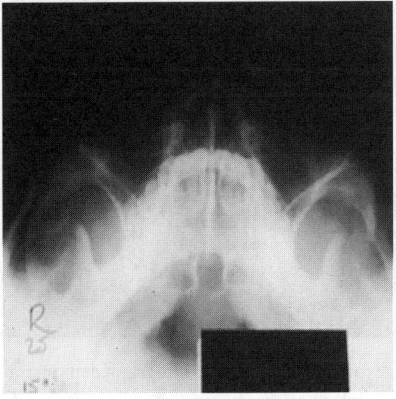

Fig. 4. Rotated occipitomental radiograph (40°) showing fractured left zygoma with depression of the zygomatic arch.

the condylar neck is weak. If this is the only mandibular injury the patient may have minimal symptoms and overlook the injury for several days.

The common presenting symptoms are pain and swelling over the affected joint with limited jaw opening. Occasionally, associated muscle spasm causes a malocclusion. If the anterior wall of the external auditory meatus has been damaged then blood leaks from the external auditory meatus (Loh et al., 1991) (Fig. 5). Examination in these cases will reveal a small tear just inside the anterior wall of the meatus. Very rarely, the head of the condyle may be forced into the external auditory meatus resulting in deafness (Antoniades et al., 1992). Even more rarely, the head of the condyle may be forced into the middle cranial fossa (Musgrove, 1986).

Posteroanterior views of the jaws, a Towne's view (Fig. 6), an orthopantomogram (OPG) or a posterior lateral oblique view of the jaws on the affected side will all demonstrate the fracture and its displacement.

With isolated condylar neck fractures, conservative measures usually suffice. The patient is maintained on a soft diet for 3 weeks. Occasionally, the patient may require indirect fixation of the jaws to rest the joint or, rarely, open surgery to reduce and fix a severe fracture dislocation of the condyle. It is not essential that the patient is referred immediately to the maxillofacial sur-

geon but this is advisable so that diagnosis and relief of symptoms is instituted as rapidly as possible.

Intracapsular condylar head fracture and haemarthrosis

This is much rarer but may be complicated by serious sequelae. It commonly occurs in children following an indirect blow such as a fall on their chin. They present with pain and swelling and limitation of jaw movement. OPG, Towne's views and lateral obliques should be arranged, but it may be that the fractures will only be demonstrated by tomography of the joint itself.

Untreated, this fracture may result in bony or fibrous

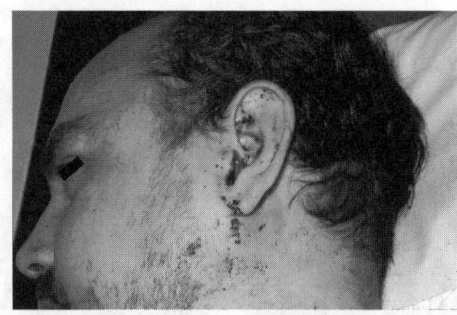

Fig. 5. Bleeding from the left ear was caused by a fractured condylar neck of the mandible. This patient did not have a fractured skull base.

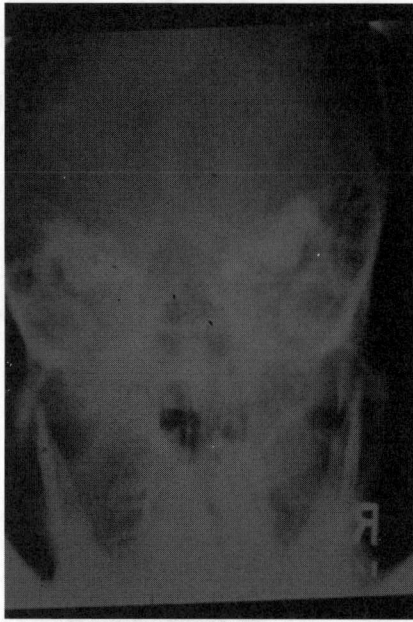

Fig. 6. Reverse (modified) Towne's radiograph demonstrating bilateral mandibular condylar neck fractures.

ankylosis of the joint and failure of the affected side of the jaw to grow (Rowe, 1982).

If this injury is suspected, the patient should be seen by a maxillofacial surgeon on the same day. The immediate management is usually conservative but aspiration of the joint may be indicated. The patient should be kept under constant review to ensure that ankylosis does not develop.

Dislocated temporomandibular joint

This occurs spontaneously but may be found more frequently in patients who are on phenothiazine medication or in patients who have suffered previous trauma to the joint and have lax joint capsules. If one joint is affected, the jaw is deviated to the opposite side with a preauricular hollow on the affected side. The patient is unable to close the mouth. More commonly the condition is bilateral. The lower jaw is protruded and the patient has an anterior open bite when the back teeth meet while the mouth is open wide at the front. There is drooling, inability to swallow and bilateral preauricular hollows are present.

The OPG will show an empty condylar fossa with the condylar head of the mandible placed anteriorly.

If the presentation is acute, then the dislocation may reduce spontaneously using intravenous sedation with an agent such as midazolam. Usually it is necessary to perform the following manoeuvre:

- The patient's jaw is pulled forward at the front using both thumbs underneath the chin and the index finger inside the mouth on the lower incisor teeth whilst the middle and ring fingers press down on the lower molars.
- This disimpacts the condyles from the temporal fossa and the jaw usually falls back into the condylar fossa.

The patient is then instructed to rest the jaw for the next few days by taking a soft diet.

If the patient suffers with recurrent dislocation then the jaw may dislocate again immediately. If the dislocation is associated with the extrapyramidal effects of drugs, then an appropriate antidote can be administered. A barrel bandage placed under the chin and over the top of the head to prevent mouth opening may temporarily prevent further dislocation. The patient should be referred immediately to the maxillofacial surgeon for observation and surgical treatment.

If the dislocation has lasted more than a few hours, then a maxillofacial opinion should be sought as it will not respond to reduction in the A&E department. General anaesthesia may be necessary to reduce the dislocation. If the dislocation is of several weeks duration then open surgical exploration and reduction of the articular eminence is necessary.

Dislocated temporomandibular joint meniscus

The temporomandibular joint consists of two compartments separated by a fibrocartilaginous meniscus. If the posterior attachment of this meniscus is torn, anterior dislocation of the meniscus results. This may occur in whiplash injuries. The patient has symptoms of pain in the joint and limitation of jaw movement but may not have any swelling.

Radiology is unhelpful and the patient should be referred to the next maxillofacial out-patient clinic if no fracture is seen on plain radiology.

If the injury is not recognized the patient may develop chronic symptoms of clicking with jaw movement, limitation of mouth opening, and painful temporomandibular joints.

Coronoid process fractures

These are usually caused by an indirect blow, are uncommon and no active treatment is indicated. It is wise to refer patients with these fractures for an opinion on the same day as they often have other mandibular fracture sites which may not be readily diagnosed (Rapidis *et al.*, 1985).

Angle, body and symphyseal

These usually occur at the site of direct trauma and pass through a tooth socket. Surprisingly, they rarely cause fracture of the tooth root and although the tooth involved appears mobile it is often fixed to one or other fragment of the mandible. The patient presents with pain and swelling at the affected site, bloody saliva, malocclusion and difficulty with jaw movements (Fig. 7). There is numbness in the distribution of the affected inferior dental nerve (i.e. the ipsilateral lower lip) and often an associated sublingual haematoma due to tearing of the medial (lingual) periosteum of the mandible (Fig. 8).

Posteroanterior radiographs (Fig. 9) with either lateral oblique views of the jaws (Fig. 10) or an OPG will demonstrate most fractures. Superimposition of the fractures may obscure the fracture line itself. Occasionally intraoral radiographs, such as periapical or occlusal, of the fracture site are required (Fig. 11).

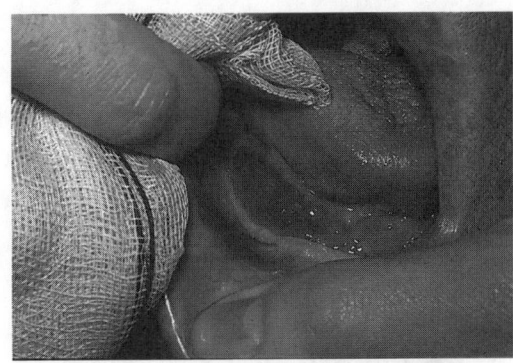

Fig. 8. This haematoma, situated medial to the mandible, strongly suggests a fractured mandible

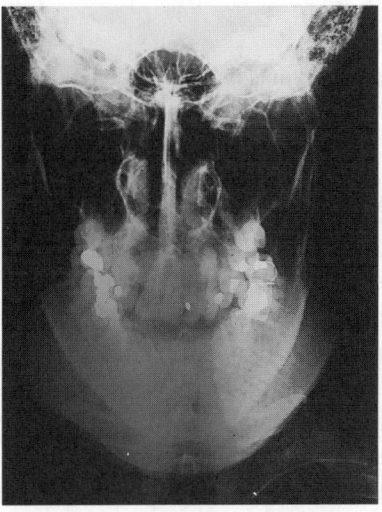

Fig. 9. Posteroanterior jaw radiograph showing right mandibular angle fracture.

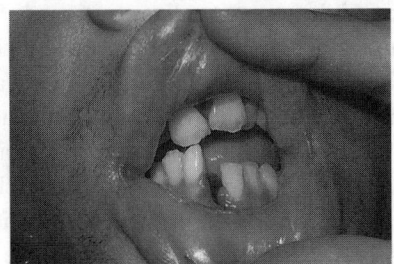

Fig. 7. The step in this man's occlusion between the lower central incisors clearly demonstrates a mandibular fracture.

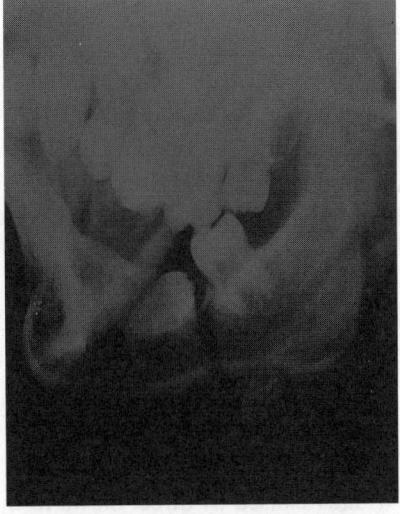

Fig. 10. Lateral oblique radiograph showing mandibular body fracture.

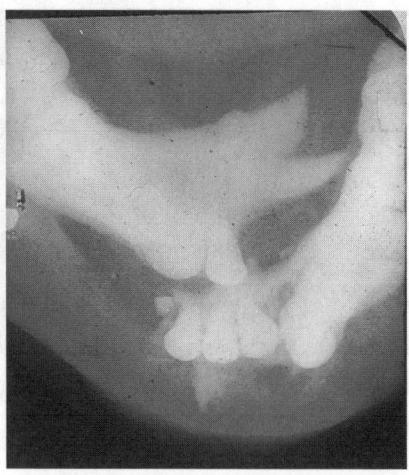

Fig. 11. Intraoral occlusal radiograph showing midline mandibular fracture.

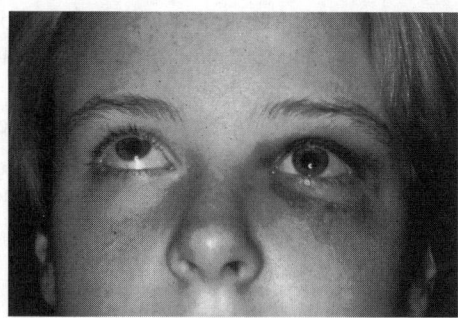

Fig. 12. This young girl with a blow-out fracture of her left orbital floor cannot elevate her left eye 4 days following a blow. She also has altered sensation of her left cheek.

If a spinal injury has been excluded, the patient should be nursed sitting up, or on the side if unconscious, and the mouth should be cleared of any loose debris such as vomit, blood and tooth fragments. There is no specific first aid treatment but antibiotics and simple non-steroidal analgesics should be given. These patients should see a maxillofacial surgeon immediately. Their definitive treatment should be instituted within the first 2 days to minimize the patient's discomfort and reduce the possibility of later complications such as infection, malunion and non-union. When the fracture involves the symphyseal region, tongue control may be lost, particularly in the unconscious patient. A tongue suture should be placed and taped to the side of the face (Hutchison *et al.*, 1990).

Guardsman's fracture

This is a tripartite fracture of the parasymphyseal region and both condylar necks (Bradley, 1985). It results in an anterior open bite and is particularly difficult to treat. It is also associated with marked discomfort as the patient has very little tongue control and cannot close the mouth effectively to contain the saliva.

It is commonly caused by a fall on the chin and was particularly associated with guardsmen fainting on parade.

Isolated orbital wall injuries

These are usually caused by direct blows to the globe of the eye.

The globe of the eye is supported in the orbital cavity by periorbital fat and is surrounded by four orbital walls. These are all thin plates of bone. The floor and medial wall are adjacent to the maxillary air sinus and ethmoid air sinuses, respectively. The lateral wall is supported outside the orbit by the temporalis muscle. The roof is inferior to the frontal lobe of the brain and the frontal sinus.

In isolated orbital wall fractures, the orbital rim remains intact. The orbital floor is the most commonly affected in isolation, followed by the medial orbital wall.

The orbital floor injury frequently lies over the infra-orbital nerve canal. The nerve is compressed by orbital fat herniating into the maxillary sinus. This results in altered sensation of the ipsilateral cheek. Entrapment of periorbital tissues causes limitations in eye movements, particularly upward gaze, and diplopia (Fig. 12). Surgical emphysema in the eyelids may develop after nose blowing. The patient may have alteration in position of the globe in the vertical or anteroposterior planes. Globe rupture fortunately occurs rarely.

The patient with a large orbital floor defect often has minimal symptoms initially. The defect is so large that there is no entrapment of periorbital tissues and post-traumatic oedema masks the loss of intraorbital contents so that the globe is normally positioned. It is wise to maintain a high index of suspicion. Radiology with occipitomental radiographs often shows a teardrop shaped radio-opacity in the roof of the maxillary antrum (Fig. 13). This represents herniated periorbital fat or haematoma at the site of the injury. An orbital floor fracture must be considered in the patient who presents with infraorbital paraesthesia and fluid in the maxillary sinus in the absence of any other fracture of the sinus walls.

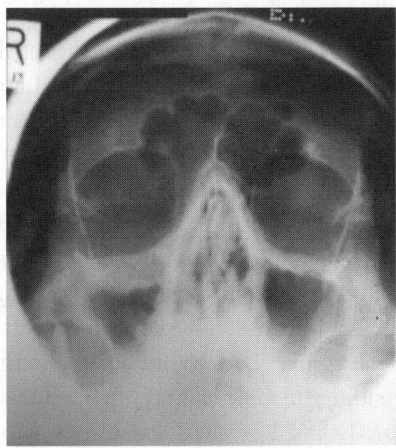

Fig. 13. Occipitomental radiograph showing hanging drop effect in superior aspect of right maxillary sinus pathognomonic of orbital floor blow-out fracture.

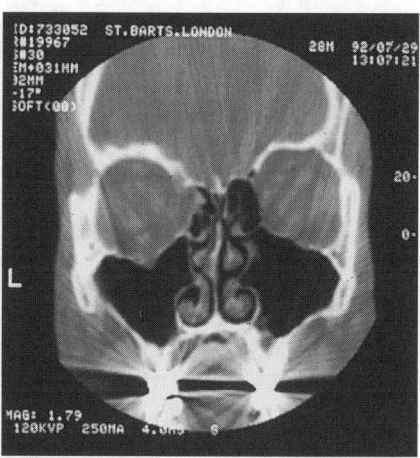

Fig. 14. CT scan with fine cuts in the coronal plane demonstrates a left orbital floor and medial wall fracture with herniation of periorbital fat into the maxillary and ethmoid sinuses respectively.

Significant lateral orbital wall damage is rare and occurs in association with marked depression of the zygoma, temporal bone fractures or fractures of the sphenoid wing. The patient may have pain on abduction of the affected eye and may also have progressive deterioration of vision due to compression of the optic nerve in the muscle cone and optic canal.

Orbital roof injuries are even rarer (Penfold *et al.*, 1992). They are always associated with injuries involving the frontal bone or frontal sinus or anterior cranial fossa floor. They present with proptosis, dropping of the pupillary level on the affected side, a mongoloid slant to the palpebral fissure and surgical emphysema if the frontal sinus is involved. The superior orbital fissure may be involved if the fracture line extends posteriorly in which case there is ptosis of the upper eyelid and failure of the affected eye to move. The eye has a fixed dilated pupil.E

Occipitomental and posteroanterior facial views will frequently reveal lateral orbital wall and orbital roof fractures.

All these cases of orbital wall fractures should be referred immediately for maxillofacial assessment. They will require CT (computed tomography) scanning in the coronal and sagittal planes and possibly three-dimensional formatting and volume measurements prior to reconstruction of the orbital walls (Fig. 14). In the case of orbital floors and medial walls, scans taken within 1 week of the injury overestimate the magnitude of the injury because haematoma mimics orbital fat. Scans should ideally be arranged at least 1 week after the injury and surgery should be performed, where indicated, within 2 weeks of the injury.

Dentoalveolar fractures

These injuries are caused by direct blows to teeth or blows on the mandible which then impacts upwards causing vertical fractures of the molar and premolar teeth. The vertical fractures may be particularly difficult to see unless the fractured segment of tooth is moved, when pain will be elicited.

Incisor teeth are commonly fractured in children. These fractures may be through the outer layer of enamel alone, or through dentine when pain on consuming hot and cold drinks is produced, or into the pulp chamber when there is usually continuous pain. The crown of the tooth may remain intact but there may be a root fracture of the tooth in which case the crown of the tooth appears mobile. Alternatively, the tooth itself may be avulsed completely, or subluxed and malpositioned in the mouth.

Alveolar bone segments containing one or more teeth may be fractured, in which case the whole fragment is mobile. The adjacent gum margin is torn and bleeds.

Patients present with pain, malocclusion, bloody saliva and malpositioned, painful or avulsed teeth.

Ideally, intraoral radiographs should be obtained, but this may prove difficult because of lack of facilities or lack of cooperation on the part of the children. In these instances OPGs may suffice.

All avulsed teeth must be kept in milk until reimplantation. It is essential to ensure that the tooth is reimplanted the correct way around and the tooth root should not be scrubbed clean as this will only induce rapid resorption of the root. Subluxed teeth should be repositioned under local anaesthesia when radiographs have confirmed that there is no root fracture.

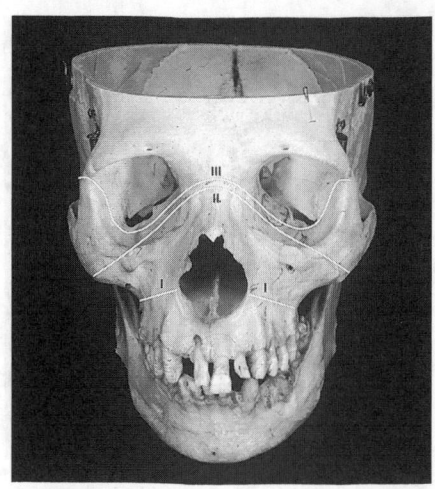

Fig. 15. The Le Fort I, II and III fractures are marked by their respective lines on the skull. The Le Fort I separates the tooth-bearing upper jaw from the rest of the maxilla. The Le Fort II separates at the frontonasal and zygomaticomaxillary sutures and the pterygoid plates. The Le Fort III fracture separates at the frontonasal, frontozygomatic and zygomaticotemporal (zygomatic arch) sutures as well as through the orbital floor and pterygoid plates. These fractures can coexist in any combination.

All children with these fractures should be referred for an urgent maxillofacial opinion because of the pain and distress associated with the injury.

Maxillary fractures

Since the advent of seat belt legislation and the reduction in road traffic accidents as a cause of facial trauma, these severe facial injuries have reduced in incidence. They have been subdivided into Le Fort I, II and III fractures and are usually caused by heavy direct blows over the maxilla, nose or zygomaticomaxillary complex. They may result in bilateral symmetrical fractures of the facial skeleton or a variety of fractures on different sides. Le Fort fractures are more frequently associated with penetrating injuries to the globe of the eye, neurosurgical injuries and severe trauma to the rest of the body. The face may split in the midline or the bones may be united across the middle of the face but separated in a horizontal manner. The Le Fort I, II and III fractures are illustrated in Fig. 15.

The Le Fort I injury involves the maxillary alveolus and floor of the nose so that the patient presents with bilateral epistaxis, a malocclusion in which the teeth of the upper jaw lie behind the teeth of the lower jaw, submucosal haemorrhage in the upper buccal sulcus, and lengthening of the middle third of the face. The upper jaw containing the teeth is mobile on the rest of the face.

This sign can be elicited by holding the upper jaw with the right hand and the forehead with the left hand then gently producing differential movement. Lateral facial views often show a fracture line passing through the lower part of the maxilla and the pterygoid plates posteriorly. The OPG may also be helpful.

The Le Fort II fracture is pyramidal in shape, passing through the pterygoid plates at the back and separating the maxilla and nose from the zygoma and frontal bone at the relevant sutures. The cribriform plate of the ethmoid bone is likely to be involved, so there is the distinct possibility of CSF leaking through the nose with both Le Fort II and Le Fort III fractures. Movement of the lower face on the upper face can be detected by holding the upper jaw and moving it backwards and forwards whilst keeping a finger on the frontonasal or zygomaticomaxillary sutures. The patient presents with similar symptoms to the Le Fort I injury. They often complain that they are unable to open their mouth when in fact their upper jaw has dropped onto their lower jaw and their mouth is already fully open.

The radiographs of choice are occipitomental views, lateral facial views, and a brow-up lateral to show fluid in the sinuses.

The Le Fort III fracture involves dysjunction of the face from the base of the skull at the cribriform plate, medial and lateral orbital walls (Fig. 16a and b). The zygoma, maxilla and nose are mobile on the skull. The patient presents with the same symptoms as before but mobility can be detected at the frontozygomatic suture in addition to the frontonasal suture. The same radiographs should be used.

It is also possible to have an isolated anterior maxillary wall fracture due to a direct blow from a small object. This is rare and may present with numbness over the affected cheek, surgical emphysema around the eye, tenderness and hollowing of the affected area and possible orbital floor, medial canthal, or lacrimal apparatus symptoms.

In all these fractures the patient should ideally be nursed sitting up with no nasal packs unless there is severe haemorrhage from the nose. Prophylactic sulphonamides are used in Le Fort II and Le Fort III fractures because of the risks of meningitis and the patients are advised not to blow their nose (Leopard, 1971). They should be referred immediately for a maxillofacial opinion.

Nasoethmoid complex

This more complex nasal bone injury is often overlooked and treated as a simple nasal fracture, unsuccessfully. It

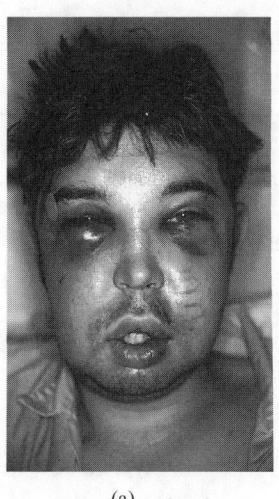 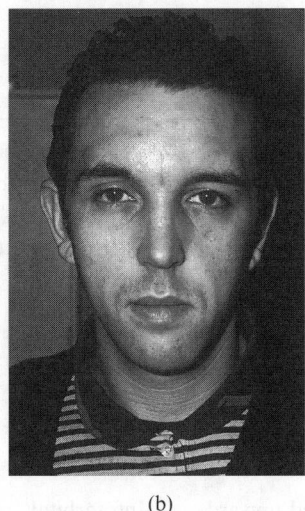

(a)   (b)

Fig. 16. (a) This young man presented with marked lengthening of his face and bilateral black eyes. He had a Le Fort III fracture. (b) Post-treatment view of the same patient.

is usually caused by a blow with a heavy object over the bridge of the nose. The nose is forced back through the ethmoids and the ethmoid complex is splayed laterally.

The key to recognition is the presentation. The patient has a very depressed nose and increased distance between the medial canthi of greater than 36 mm. There is flattening and loss of the normal naso-orbital valley, loss of palpable medial canthal ligaments and an alteration in the palpebral fissure's shape and angulation (Fig. 17). This changes to an almond-shaped rather lax-looking palpebral fissure with a mongoloid slant (Ellis, 1993). If the lacrimal canaliculi or lacrimal sacs have been disrupted then the patient will have epiphora.

Occipitofrontal radiographs at a 25° angulation show

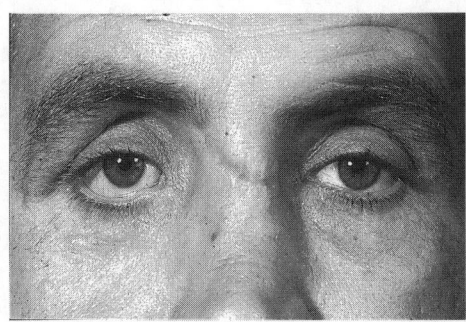

Fig. 17. This man sustained a fracture involving his left nasoethmoid region. Note the widening of the distance between the left medial canthus and the midline, the alteration in eyelid shape (loss of acute medial angle between the upper and lower eyelids) and flattening of the gap between the nose and eye. It is not possible to palpate the left medial canthal ligament.

fractures through the lamina papyracea of the ethmoid bones. The patient should be immediately referred for a maxillofacial opinion so that treatment can be instituted as soon as possible. This fracture is particularly difficult to treat effectively. It is advisable to institute treatment as early as possible, ideally within the first 2 days.

Frontal bones

High frontal bone injuries are caused by severe trauma and are associated with intracranial injury. In the glabella region of the frontal bone in the low midline there is an area of weakness because of the presence of the frontal sinus. Less powerful blows to this region may cause fracture of the anterior wall of the frontal sinus, or of the anterior and posterior walls. The patient presents with depression of the glabella and may also have surgical emphysema and hypoaesthesia of the frontal region. Lateral skull radiographs demonstrate these fractures.

In all frontal bone injuries, a maxillofacial opinion should be sought, even if there is an associated intracranial injury, because it may be appropriate to perform surgery to prevent later cosmetic problems.

COMPLICATIONS

Early complications relate to problems such as airway obstruction or pain control. Later complications may be physical or non-physical. Non-physical complications include failure to recognize child abuse or wife battering. It is frequently difficult to diagnose domestic violence. Women in fear of their partners will often disguise the source of their or their children's injuries. Sympathetic questioning can sometimes elicit the true facts. Even if the patient does not wish to report the incident to the legal authorities it is worthwhile recording the event in hospital notes. Unfortunately, there is a tendency for violence to escalate with each subsequent assault in abusive relationships.

Failure to deal with the psychosocial trauma produced by the cause of injury, such as assault, or the ensuing cosmetic deficit, will prevent the patient returning to normal life after the injury (Shepherd, 1992).

The late physical complications are almost universally associated with failure to diagnose and treat the injuries effectively, Classical examples that are frequently overlooked are the isolated orbital floor and medial orbital wall injuries. Nasoethmoid injuries are frequently misdiagnosed as simple nasal bone fractures.

The late complications are listed in Table 3.

Table 2. *Summary of maxillofacial fractures*

Injury	Cause	Symptoms	Inspection	Palpation	X-ray and findings

Zygoma	—Blow over cheekbone (e.g. punch)	—Flat cheek
		—Unilateral nose bleed
		—Limited mouth opening
		—Cheek numbness
		—Double vision
			—Flattening of cheekbone
			—Subconjunctival ecchymosis
			—Periorbital swelling
				—Tenderness and separation of bony sutures and zygomatic buttress intraorally
				—Infraorbital paraesthesia
					1. Occipitomental (OM):
					  a. Fluid level in antrum
					  b. Separation at zygomatic sutures with maxilla, frontal bone, lateral antral wall and zygomatic arch

Orbital floor	—Blow over globe (e.g. squash ball)	—Pain on eye movement —Double vision —Sunken in eye —Limited upward gaze —Surgical emphysema with nose blowing	—Limited upward gaze —Enophthalmos or exophthalmos —Alteration in pupillary level	—Infraorbital paraesthesia	1. OMs Tear drop from orbital floor in antral roof 2. CT (in sagittal and coronal planes) After 1 week
Mandible	—Blow on jaw	—Mandibular fractures are often paired			
A. Condylar neck		—Limited mouth opening —Malocclusion —Bleeding from ear —Swelling over joint —Pain over joint	—Swelling over joint	—Tender joint —Malocclusion —Tear in anterior wall of external auditory meatus	—OPG (orthopantomogram) —Lateral oblique (LO) jaws —Posteroanterior (PA) jaws —Towne's view
B. Body		—Loose teeth —Pain —Swelling over fracture —Malocclusion —Drooling of saliva —Bleeding from gums	—Swelling of face —Intraoral step in occlusion —Tear in gingiva —Bloody saliva —Sublingual haematoma	—Abnormal mobility and tenderness at fracture site —Anaesthesia of lower lip	1. OPG 2. PA jaws 3. LO jaws

Dentoalveolar	—Direct blow on teeth
	—Blow on lower jaw smashing lower teeth against upper teeth
		—Pain over tooth
		—Mobility of tooth/teeth
			—Torn gingiva
			—Gagged occlusion
			—Tooth out of place
			—Bloody saliva
			—Broken teeth
				—Vertical fractures of teeth
				—Mobility of teeth
					1. Intraoral
					  a. Occlusal
					  b. Periapical
					2. OPG
					  —Tooth out of socket
					  —Fractured tooth root

Table 2. *Continued*

Injury	Cause	Symptoms	Inspection	Palpation	X-ray and findings
Le Fort I	—Heavy diffuse anterior blow over upper jaw	—Gagging of occlusion —Cannot open mouth —Nose bleed	—Long face —Bruising in upper buccal sulcus —Bruising of palate —Midline tear of palate	—Mobility of upper jaw on nose	1. OPG 2. Lateral face (fracture line through pterygoid plates)
Le Fort II & III	—Heavy anterior blow to nose and face	—Gagging of occlusion —Cannot open mouth —Nose bleed	—Panda eyes —Long middle third of face —Swelling of face	—Mobility of face on skull palpable at zygomaticomaxillary or zygomaticofrontal sutures	1. OM 2. PA face 3. Lateral face
Nasoethmoid	—Small heavy blow to bridge of nose	—Flat nose —Epistaxis —Pain —Tears running down cheek	—Epiphora —Wide intercanthal distance —Flat nasal bridge —Nostrils pointing forwards —Flat naso-orbital valley —Almond-shaped palpebral fissure	—Absent medial canthal ridge	—Occipitofrontal (OF) 25° (fracture of lamina papyracea of ethmoids)

Table 3. *Late complications of facial injury*

Injury	Complication
Le Fort II and III and nasoethmoid injuries	CSF rhinorrhoea, meningitis
Overlooked orbital fractures	Enophthalmos, diplopia and tethering of the globe of the eye
Nasoethmoid injuries	Traumatic telecanthus, alteration in shape of the eyelids and nose, and epiphora (Fig. 18)
Lacrimal apparatus damage	Epiphora (Fig. 19)
Parotid gland damage	Parotid fistula and sialocele
Zygomatic fractures	Infraorbital anaesthesia dolorosa and cosmetic flattening
Mandibular fractures	Malocclusion and cosmetic problems
Dislocated mandible	Trismus, drooling and inability to eat properly
Temporomandibular joint intracapsular fracture	Ankylosis and failure of the jaw to grow
Tooth fractures	Discoloration of the tooth and abscess in the underlying bone
Tooth subluxation	Tooth becomes fixed in an abnormal position
Soft tissue wounds	Failure of tetanus and rabies prophylasix when necessary may lead to life-threatening infections
Failure to place appropriate transition lines when suturing	Unsightly scars
Dirty skin wounds not cleaned effectively	Tattooing of wounds
Inhaled teeth and debris	Lobar collapse of the lung
Through and through wounds from the face to mouth or nose	If the mouth or nasal mucosa is not closed then fistulae may occur

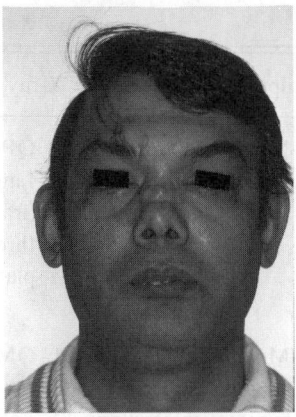

Fig. 18. This man sustained a nasoethmoid fracture which was misdiagnosed and treated only as a simple nasal fracture. He has been left with marked depression of the nasal bridge and nostrils pointing forward.

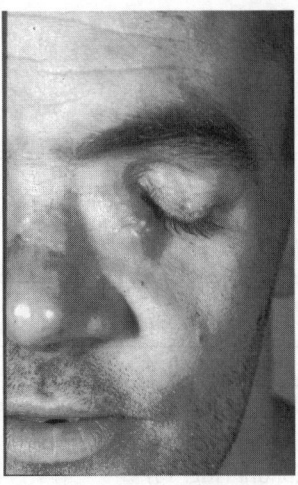

Fig. 19. Untreated damage to this man's left lacrimal drainage system resulted in a chronic dacrocystocele treated successfully with a dacrocystorhinostomy.

RADIOLOGY

With soft tissue injuries it is often necessary to arrange radiographs to ensure that no foreign bodies remain in the soft tissues. In severe complicated trauma, it is mandatory to arrange cervical spine views and a chest X-ray.

The most important specific view of the facial bones is the occipitomental (Fig. 20). This is taken with X-ray tube tilts of 0°, 15°, 30° and 45° (OM 0°, 15°, 30°, 45°). Lateral views of the face and an occipitofrontal view at 25° (OF 25°) tube tilt are supplementary. Wherever

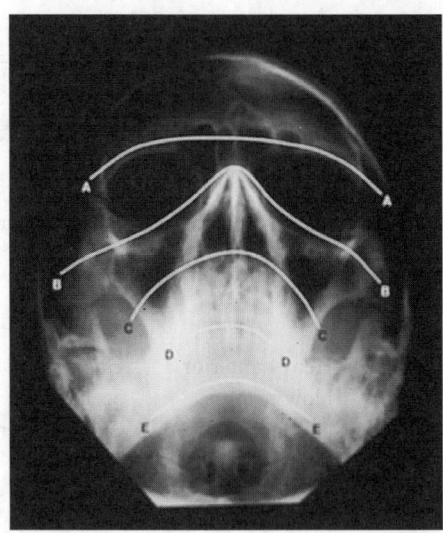

Fig. 20. The occipitomental radiograph should be analysed along five horizontal lines:
- Line A passing across the superior orbital margin will show separation at the frontozygomatic and frontonasal sutures and the supraorbital bar itself.
- Line B passes through the zygomatic arch and shows separation along the arch, body of zygoma, zygomaticomaxillary suture and nasal bones.
- Line C shows fractures in the lateral antral wall, fluid in the maxillary sinus and the 'hanging drop' effect from a fractured orbital floor.
- Line D shows the upper teeth.
- Line E shows the lower border of the mandible.

possible these views should be taken with the X-ray beam passing from the back to the front of the face. This reduces radiation to the eyes and produces clearer pictures of the facial bones. However, in the severely injured patient it may be necessary to take views using an X-ray beam passing from the front of the face to the back of the head. In these cases it is not worthwhile taking many views as the results are never perfect.

If the patient has Le Fort II or Le Fort III fractures then a brow-up lateral of the face should be taken to look for fluid levels in the sphenoid and other air sinuses.

The views of the mandible include posteroanterior views of the jaws, the OPG (Fig. 21) and lateral oblique views of the jaws. The lateral oblique radiographs can be taken to show the anterior or posterior aspect around the temporomandibular joint. In some situations and in some departments it is possible to arrange for intraoral radiographs and tomograms of the temporomandibular joints. CT scans of the facial bones are not usually necessary in the immediate phase, but if the patient is having CT scans for neurological trauma then it would be advisable to include the face and generate good-quality coronal pictures for treatment planning.

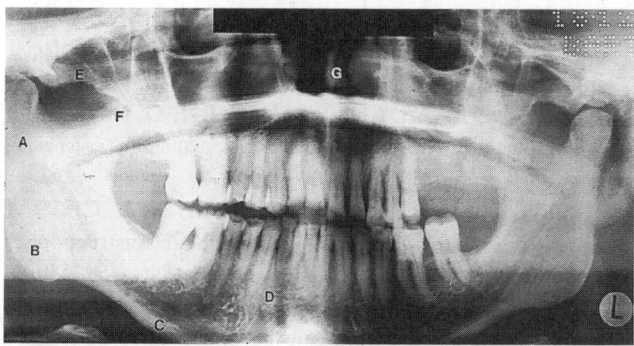

Fig. 21. This orthopantomogram (OPG) shows common mandibular fracture sites: A, condylar neck; B, angle; C, body; D, parasymphyseal. Other features can be seen: E, zygomatic arch; F, pterygoid plates; G, nasal septum.

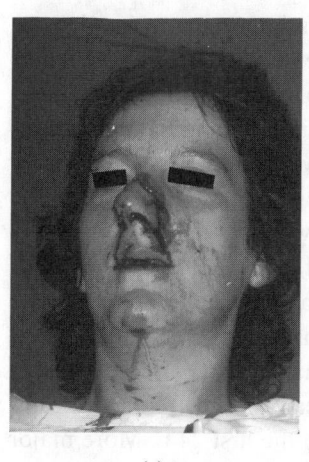
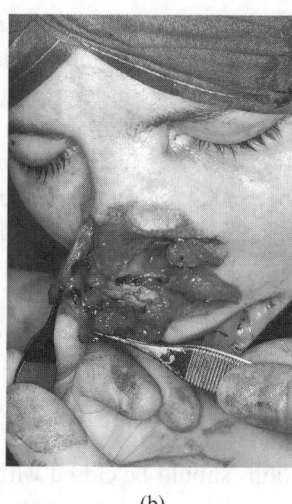

(a)   (b)

Fig. 22. (a) All facial lacerations must be thoroughly explored and cleaned. (b) Opening this laceration reveals extensive disruption of the underlying nasal architecture including the septum and alar cartilages.

SUTURING THE FACE

There are several points of distinction between the face and other parts of the body when suturing is undertaken.

TECHNIQUE

- The wound should be cleaned thoroughly. In most cases this can be done with soapy solutions such as aqueous chlorhexidine. If there is any dirt in the wound then this should be cleaned off with a toothbrush or nail brush to prevent later tattooing of the wound. If there is oil in the wound then acetone or xylol should be used. The wound should be explored thoroughly and all foreign bodies removed (Fig. 22a and b). If foreign bodies are suspected, soft tissue radiographs must be ordered prior to or after exploring the wound.
- Avoid shaving around the wound unless absolutely necessary. The eyebrows and edge of the hairline should not be shaved and the eyelids not cut as these help in correct apposition of wounds at these transition points.
- No soft or hard tissue should be discarded in the facial region.
- The deep tissue injuries should be repaired as accurately as those placed superficially. For example, the nasal septum and oral mucosa must be repaired accurately.
- Haemostasis should be ensured and deep tissues closed to eliminate dead space and prevent wound infection.
- There should be minimal tension on skin wounds.
- Margins of skin lacerations should only be debrided if they are shelved or ragged or contused. The edges should be made perpendicular if they are shelved.
- All fragments of tissue which have been avulsed should be retained. For example, if the ear is no longer attached then it can be de-epithelialized and implanted subcutaneously with a drain in anticipation of later uncovering at the correct site. Skin that has been separated from the body may be defatted and used as a skin graft.

- All haematomas should be drained to prevent fibrosis or even later ossification.
- Subperichondrial haematomas of the ear and nasal septum should be aspirated to prevent later cauliflower ears or nasal collapse, respectively.
- Parotid duct injuries should be recognized and referred for repair by maxillofacial surgeons.
- Facial nerve injuries that are involved in soft tissue lacerations proximal to the midpupillary line should be referred for immediate repair under general anaesthetic.
- It is vital to approximate the soft tissues accurately in transition zones such as the vermilion border of the lip, the alar region of the nose and the eyelids to prevent later cosmetic deficits.
- Antirabies and antitetanus prophylaxis should be instituted where necessary.
- War wounds should be closed loosely in the first instance.
- Bites from humans, dogs, cats, rodents or other wild animals should be referred for a senior opinion. Any tissue that has been bitten off completely should be retained but may have to be discarded after expert advice has been sought. The wound should be cleaned thoroughly with a soapy solution and then with quaternary ammonium compounds. The wound itself should be excised and sutured. Puncture wounds should be left open.

CONCLUSION

Facial injuries are common. They are rarely life-threatening and it is therefore technically possible to delay referral for a maxillofacial opinion. However, for the patient's convenience, it is preferable to arrange an immediate maxillofacial opinion to enable early diagnosis and treatment planning. Where the patient has suffered multiple injuries it is important to involve the maxillofacial surgeon at the outset so that they participate in the treatment planning and early operations. Delays in the treatment of mandibular fractures beyond 4 or 5 days usually produce less satisfactory results. It is possible to delay treatment of zygomatic and nasal fractures for a week. It is wise to delay treatment of complex facial trauma for 1 or 2 days until all the investigations are available and accurate treatment planning can be instituted.

Facial lacerations can usually be repaired effectively under local anaesthesia. Ideally, all soft tissue lacerations should be closed within the first 24 h. More major soft tissue injuries involving deeper structures such as the major vessels, the lacrimal apparatus, seventh cranial nerve, and parotid gland and duct are best sutured under general anaesthesia.

Bibliography

ADI, M., OGDEN, R.G. & CHISHOLM, D.M. (1990). An analysis of mandibular fractures in Dundee, Scotland (1977 to 1985). *Br. J. Oral Maxillofac. Surg.*, **28**, 194–9.

ANTONIADES, K., KARAKASIS, D. & DAGGILAS, A. (1992). Posterior dislocation of mandibular condyle into external auditory canal. A case report. *Int. J. Oral Maxillofac. Surg.*, **21**, 212–14.

BOWERMAN, J.E. (1969). The superior orbital fissure syndrome complicating fractures of the facial skeleton. *Br. J. Oral Surg.*, **7**, 1–6.

BRADLEY, P. (1985). Injuries of the condylar and coronoid process. In *Maxillofacial Injuries*, ed. N.L. Rowe & J.Ll. Williams. p. 339. Edinburgh: Churchill Livingstone.

BROOK, I.M. & WOOD, N. (1983). Aetiology and incidence of facial fractures in adults. *Int. J. Oral Surg.*, **12**, 293–8.

DIMITROULIS, G. & STEIDLER, N. (1992). Massive bleeding following maxillofacial trauma. Case report. *Aust. Dent. J.*, **37**, 185–8.

ELLIS, E. (1993). Sequencing treatment for naso-orbito-ethmoid fractures. *J. Oral Maxillofac. Surg.*, **51**, 543–58.

GRATTAN, E. & HOBBS, J.A. (1985). Mechanisms of injury to the face in road-traffic accidents. In *Maxillofacial Injuries*, ed. N.L. Rowe & J.Ll. Williams. pp. 37–41. Edinburgh: Churchill Livingstone.

HAUGH, R.H., WIBLE, R.T., LIKAVEC, M.J. *et al.* (1991). Cervical spine fractures and maxillofacial trauma. *J. Oral Maxillofac. Surg.*, **49**, 725–9.

HILL, C.M., CROSHER, R.F., CARROLL, M.J. *et al.* (1984). Facial fractures—the results of a prospective four-year study. *J. Maxillo-Fac. Surg.*, **12**, 267–70.

HUTCHISON, I.L., LAWLOR, M.G. & SKINNER, D.V. (1990). ABC of major trauma: major maxillofacial injuries. *BMJ*, **301**, 595–9.

IIZUKA, T., RANDELL, T., GUVEN, O. *et al.* (1990). Maxillofacial fractures related to work accidents. *J. Cranio-Maxillo-Fac. Surg.*, **18**, 255–9.

JENSEN, J., SINDET-PEDERSEN, S. & CHRISTENSEN, L. (1992). Rigid fixation in reconstruction of craniofacial fractures. *J. Oral Maxillofac. Surg.*, **50**, 550–4.

LANDAU, R. & STEWART, M. (1985). Conservative management of post-traumatic parotid fistulae and sialoceles: a prospective study. *Br. J. Surg.*, **72**, 42–4.

LEOPARD, P.J. (1971). Dural tears in maxillofacial injuries. *Br. J. Oral Surg.*, **8**, 222–30.

LINN, E.W., VRIJHOEF, M.M.A., DE WIJN, J.R. *et al.* (1986). Facial injuries sustained during sports and games. *J. Maxillo-Fac. Surg.*, **14**, 83–8.

LOH, F., TAN, K.B.C. & TAN, K. (1991). Auditory canal haemorrhage following mandibular condylar fracture. *Br. J. Oral Maxillofac. Surg.*, **29**, 12–13.

MARSHALL, W.G. (1986). An analysis of firearm injuries to the head and face in Belfast 1969–1977. *Br. J. Oral Maxillofac. Surg.*, **24**, 233–43.

MUSGROVE, B.T. (1986). Dislocation of the mandibular condyle into the middle cranial fossa. *Br. J. Oral Maxillofac. Surg.*, **24**, 22–7.

NEEDLEMAN, H.L. (1986). Orofacial trauma in child abuse: types, prevalence, management and the dental profession's involvement. *Pediatr. Dent.*, **8**, 71–80.

PENFOLD, C.N., LANG, D. & EVANS, B.T. (1992). The management of orbital roof fractures. *Br. J. Oral Maxillofac. Surg.*, **30**, 97–103.

PERKINS, C.S. & LAYTON, S.A. (1988). The aetiology of maxillofacial injuries and the seat belt law. *Br. J. Oral Maxillofac. Surg.*, **26**, 353–63.

PYE, G. & WATERS, E.A. (1984). Effect of seat belt legislation on injuries in road traffic accidents in Nottingham. *BMJ*, **288**, 756–7.

RAPIDIS, A.D., PAPAVASSILIOU, D., PAPADIMITRIOU, J. *et al.* (1985). Fractures of the coronoid process of the mandible. An analysis of 52 cases. *Int. J. Oral Surg.*, **14**, 126–30.

ROGERS, S., HILL, J.R. & MACKAY, G.M. (1992). Maxillofacial injuries following steering wheel contact by drivers using seat belts. *Br. J. Oral Maxillofac. Surg.*, **30**, 24–30.

ROWE, N.L. (1982). Ankylosis of the temporomandibular joint. Parts 1 and 2. *J. R. Coll. Surg. Edinb.*, **27**, 67–79, 167–173.

ROWE, N.L. (1985). Maxillofacial injuries—current trends and techniques. *Injury*, **16**, 513–25.

SHEPHERD, J.P. (1992). Strategies for the study of long-term sequelae of oral and facial injuries. *J. Oral Maxillofac. Surg.*, **50**, 390–9.

SHEPHERD, J.P., GAYFORD, J.J., LESLIE, I. J. *et al.* (1988). Female victims of assault: a study of hospital attenders. *J. Cranio-Maxillofac. Surg.*, **16**, 233–7.

SHUKER, S.T. (1986). Prevention of tongue prolapse by immediate stabilization in severely avulsed mandibular war injuries. *J. Maxillo-fac. Surg.*, **14**, 317–20.

SMITH, A.C. & BRADLEY, P.J. (1986). Progressive dyspnoea following facial injury. *Br. J Oral Maxillofac. Surg.*, **24**, 28–30.

TELFER, M.R., JONES, G.M. & SHEPHERD, J.P. (1991). Trends in the aetiology of maxillofacial fractures in the United Kingdom (1977–1987). *Br. J. Oral Maxillofac. Surg.*, **29**, 250–5.

THALLER, S.R. & BEAL, S.L. (1991). Maxillofacial trauma: a potentially fatal injury. *Ann. Plast. Surg.*, **27**, 281–3.

WEINBERG, S. & LAPOINTE, H. (1987). Cervical extension-flexion injury (whiplash) and internal derangement of the TMJ. *J. Oral Maxillofac. Surg.*, **45**, 653–6.

ZACHARIADES, N., KOUMOURA, F. & KONSO-LAKI-AGOURIDAKI, E. (1990). Facial trauma in women resulting from violence by men. *J. Oral Maxillofac. Surg.*, **48**, 1250–3.

Further reading

BANKS, P., ed. (1987). *Killey's Fracture of the Middle Third of the Facial Skeleton.* London: Wright

BANKS, P., ed. (1991). *Killey's Fracture of the Mandible*, 4th edn. London: Wright

ROWE, N.L. & WILLIAMS, J.Ll., eds (1985). *Maxillofacial Injuries*, Vols 1 & 2. Edinburgh: Churchill Livingstone.

B: Oral and maxillofacial diseases

I. HUTCHISON

Department of Oral and Maxillofacial Surgery, St. Bartholomew's Hospital, London, UK

INTRODUCTION

Infections of the head and neck are common. The three major sources of infection in the region are the upper respiratory tract, the teeth and their supporting structures, and the skin. Although diseases of these tissues occur frequently, they are rarely serious. However, the proximity of the brain, eye and airway, and the presence of potential spaces leading to the thorax, allow some of these relatively innocuous diseases to progress to life-threatening complications. Examples include Ludwig's angina and parapharyngeal abscesses which can be complicated by mediastinitis, pleural effusions, pericarditis, and sinus infections leading to cavernous sinus thrombosis. These patients will usually attend their doctor or dentist initially, but may also present direct to Accident and Emergency (A&E). Whenever a patient is experiencing severe symptoms, an urgent maxillofacial opinion should be sought.

Patients presenting to A&E have one or more of the following symptoms:

- Pain
- Swelling
- Ulceration
- Lymph node enlargement
- A blocked or discharging nose
- Redness of the skin of the face or neck
- Sore throat or pain on swallowing
- Gum swelling or bleeding
- Rarely, in extremis, symptoms of upper airway obstruction

SYMPTOMATOLOGY

Pain

Facial pain

Pain from the face is often severe. This may be because the face has a large cerebral cortical representation. The major contribution to facial sensation is from the three divisions of the fifth cranial nerve, the trigeminal. Briefly, the mandibular, maxillary and ophthalmic divisions enter the skull through the foramen ovale, rotundum and superior orbital fissure, respectively. The cell bodies of these nerves lie in the trigeminal ganglion situated in the middle cranial fossa. The nerve then follows a route into the posterior cranial fossa to enter the brainstem at the cerebellopontine angle. Relays occur in the spinal nucleus of the trigeminal nerve before pain fibres transmit to the thalamus and sensory representation fibres pass to the cerebral cortex.

Sensory receptors in the skin of the face overlying the angle of the jaw and the ear transmit in the great auricular nerve travelling around the posterior edge of the sternomastoid muscle to enter the spinal column at C2–C3 and relay here. The back of the head is supplied by sensory fibres from the occipital nerves which are posterior primary rami of C1 and C2. Deep somatic pain fibres from the tongue travel in the chorda tympani to the facial nerve and from the pharynx in the glossopharyngeal nerve.

Central pain

Pain is usually a manifestation of peripheral pathology. However, it may also represent pathology anywhere along the path of the affected nerve. For example, trigeminal neuralgia is thought to be caused by demyelination of the nerve, particularly by compression from adjacent arteries at the cerebellopontine angle (Jannetta, 1967). Pain mimicking trigeminal neuralgia can be caused by tumours compressing the trigeminal nerve at the cerebellopontine angle (Fig. 1), or other sites along its

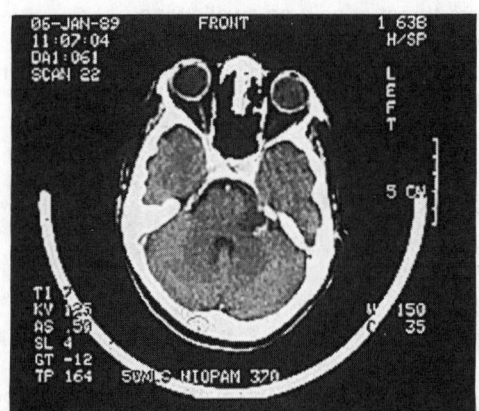

Fig. 1. This patient with an acoustic neuroma at the cerebellopontine angle presented with left facial pain and numbness in the distribution of the infraorbital nerve.

path such as the infratemporal fossa (Schnetler & Hopper, 1989). Tumours at these sites frequently present with the unusual combination of reduced sensation and pain affecting one or more divisions of the trigeminal nerve. Paraesthesia is an ominous symptom which should be investigated fully.

Referred pain

Classically, the pain radiates to sites served by the same division of the trigeminal nerve. For example, pain from the maxilla radiates to the eye, whilst pain from the mandible radiates to the ear. Pain from a single site does not radiate across the midline. Conversely, periodontal (gum) disease and pain affects the whole mouth, and atypical stress-related pains do cross the midline.

Dental pain

The pain caused by dental decay (caries) is initially precipitated by hot, cold and sweet stimuli around the affected tooth. It is sharp and lasts for a few moments. When the dental pulp is involved, the pain is severe, continuous, throbbing and radiates to the cheek and eye for upper teeth and to the ear for mandibular teeth. The patient is unable to sleep with the pain and simple analgesia does not control it. The pain lasts for a few days until the pulp dies, when it resolves spontaneously. Some months later, when an abscess develops, the same pain recurs and may be associated with a swelling adjacent to the affected tooth (Fig. 2a and b). The pain of pulpitis and abscess is exacerbated by biting on or tapping the affected tooth.

Jaw joint pain

Jaw joint pain is usually associated with decreased jaw opening and noises from the joint. The masticatory muscles may also be stiff and painful.

Swellings

These may be single or multiple. They may be a direct result of infections such as an abscess, secondary to infection such as lymph node enlargement in the drainage area, or not infective at all, such as a tumour. Pyrexia and pain usually denote an infective cause.

When the swelling is localized it often points to the diagnosis. Examples include dental abscesses and cysts. Diffuse swellings can be confusing. For example,

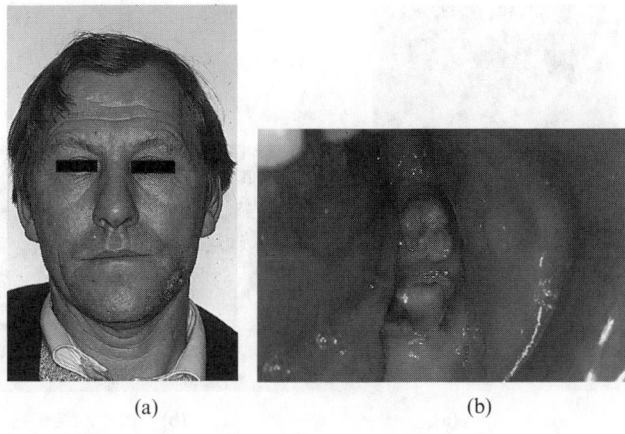

Fig. 2. (a) Left facial swelling and sinus secondary to (b) infected left molar teeth.

generalized enlargement of the jaws may be a manifestation of systemic disease processes such as myeloma, Paget's disease, acromegaly or cherubism.

Salivary gland swellings

These occur at the classic sites in the parotid, submandibular and sublingual regions. There are many minor salivary glands within the oral cavity which can also be affected by disease. Salivary glands may enlarge with meals, subsiding afterwards when a bad taste is noted. This is usually caused by sialadenitis secondary to obstruction by calculi. Salivary swellings which persist usually represent salivary gland neoplasms.

Ulceration

Ulcers are either primary, when oral mucosa or facial skin breaks down, or secondary to the rupture of an abscess or bulla. They can occur singly or at several sites simultaneously. They may be associated with fever or lymphadenopathy. In conditions such as herpes zoster they have a characteristic distribution involving one dermatome.

The commonest causes of mouth ulcers are trauma and aphthous ulceration (recurrent periodic attacks of crops of ulcers of unknown aetiology). Herpes simplex, herpes zoster and other viral infections, carcinoma, syphilis, tuberculosis and rare vesiculobullous lesions such as pemphigus may all present with ulcers on the face or in the mouth.

Cervical lymphadenopathy

Enlargement of the cervical lymph nodes occurs frequently in head and neck infection. Usually, the lymph nodes enlarge shortly after the onset of illness and disappear within a week or two of resolution of the infection. Any persistently enlarged lymph nodes should be treated with suspicion and investigated fully.

Acute bacterial infections of the teeth, jaws, gums and throat usually cause single lymph node enlargement in the drainage area. Cancers at these sites also produce cervical lymph node metastases which may be indistinguishable from infective nodes when examined.

Viral infections are more frequently associated with multiple cervical lymph node enlargement. Lymphoma and tuberculosis may present with single or multiple cervical lymphadenopathy.

Gingival swelling, redness and bleeding

Gingival and periodontal (gum) disease is very common and is due to plaque deposits accumulating around the cervical margins of teeth. If this plaque is not removed by careful toothbrushing it calcifies and becomes calculus (tartar). The toxins released by bacteria in the plaque cause inflammation in the gums which are then tender, red, oedematous and bleed readily when touched. If left untreated, the disease will involve the bone around the teeth with progressive bone loss and loosening of the teeth.

This gum swelling may be localized to one or two teeth or generalized. Classically, the patient complains of pain and gum discomfort which is relieved by simple analgesics and clenching their teeth. It does not keep them awake at night. They usually have fetor oris.

Systemic diseases such as leukaemia may also present with swollen, red, bleeding gums.

Sore throat and dysphagia

Sore throat is a common symptom and is usually due to an upper respiratory viral or bacterial infection. Pain from the throat may radiate to the ear, and pain from the mandible may radiate to the throat, thus confusing the unwary clinician. Persistent unilateral sore throats may represent sinister pathology such as carcinomas of the base of tongue or tonsillar fossa. A history of the site, duration and any associated symptoms are therefore important clues as to the likely cause of the sore throat.

Pain with swallowing always accompanies a sore throat, but difficulty with swallowing or dysphagia is a more significant symptom. Painless dysphagia not associated with any orofacial symptoms is usually a manifestation of pathology in the lower part of the pharynx and the oesophagus. Often the patient may be able to point to the site at which they feel the obstruction.

When the dysphagia is associated with infections of the mouth and face then parapharyngeal abscesses or Ludwig's angina should be considered.

Respiratory symptoms

Orofacial infections may lead to life-threatening airway obstruction with parapharyngeal abscesses and Ludwig's angina. In Ludwig's angina the tongue is elevated on to the roof of the mouth, the patient is unable to open the mandible and develops brawny bilateral neck swelling (Fig. 3a and b). The voice also becomes hoarse and the patient develops tachycardia, tachypnoea and drooling of saliva which they are unable to swallow.

Epiglottitis is another complication of upper respiratory tract infections which may cause acute airway obstruction, particularly in children (see Chapter 60).

Nasal symptoms

The commonest nasal symptoms are blocked nasal passages and epistaxis. Again, the duration of the nasal blockage, its occurrence at particular periods of the year such as spring and summer, and other associated symptoms will be important in defining the cause.

Unilateral recurrent nose bleeds may be caused by infection, prominent vessels at Little's area, systemic diseases, coagulopathies and rare entities such as Osler–Weber–Rendu (Fig. 4). When there is an associated infraorbital nerve paraesthesia, the possibility of maxillary sinus neoplasms should be considered.

HISTORY, EXAMINATION AND INVESTIGATIONS

Most diagnoses are made following accurate history-taking. Examination and special investigations usually serve to confirm a diagnosis already made from the history.

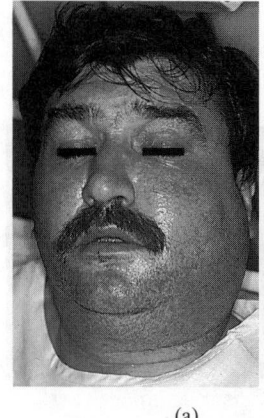
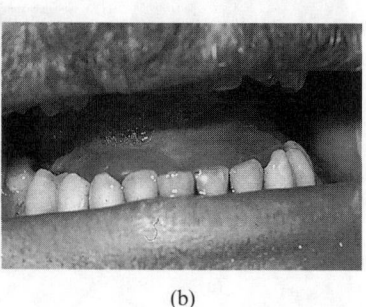

(a)   (b)

Fig. 3. (a) Ludwig's angina with bilateral neck swelling, respiratory difficulty; (b) difficulty opening the mouth and floor of mouth oedema forcing the tongue onto the plate.

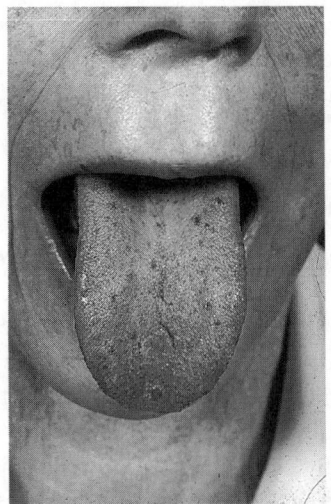

Fig. 4. Hereditary haemorrhagic telangiectasia.

History

Pain

When the patient presents with pain, the character of the pain, its site, duration, radiation, and precipitating, exacerbating and relieving factors should all be distinguished. For example, dental pain is deep-seated, aching, not relieved by analgesics, and keeps the patient awake at night. Sinus pain is similar in character, but is relieved by analgesics and does not keep the patient awake.

Swellings

Swellings may remain static in size, steadily increase or decrease, or fluctuate with certain events. Their site, duration and any factors associated with the swelling should be noted.

Ulcers

Ulcers may be single or multiple, regular and recurrent, shortlived for only a few days, or persistent. A careful note should be made of the history of the ulcer and any precipitating factors such as trauma. In recurrent ulcers, their duration, lengths of period of remission and frequency should be recorded.

Lymphadenopathy

The duration of lymph node enlargement and any association with pain and symptoms from the drainage area should be recorded. There may be generalized body symptoms such as malaise, weight loss and night sweats, and the patient may also have noted lymph node swellings elsewhere in the body.

Gingival swelling

Generalized gingival swelling, discomfort and bleeding is common. It is usually caused by chronic periodontal or gum disease. The patients are infrequent dental attendees and have poor oral hygiene. Their discomfort is classically relieved by clenching their teeth. In contrast, when the gingival swelling is caused by an abscess, it is localized to the affected tooth and there is severe dull throbbing pain which is exacerbated by biting on the affected tooth. Gingival swelling may also be caused by infiltrative processes such as leukaemia. These patients are often frequent dental attendees and have a sudden onset of gum symptoms. They may have associated symptoms of tiredness, easy bruising and frequent infections elsewhere.

Airway symptoms

Sore throats are also common. They are usually due to viral infection in which there are associated bodily symptoms such as muscle pain and headaches. The patient may have laryngeal and tracheal symptoms of voice alteration and cough. These symptoms should all settle over a few days. If the sore throat is persistent and unilateral then this may signify more sinister pathology such as neoplasia. The patient may be able to point to the site of soreness and there may be associated difficulty or pain with swallowing. Similarly, persistent hoarseness or cough merit further investigation. Patients

with Ludwig's angina or parapharyngeal abscesses present with swallowing problems which rapidly progress to respiratory difficulties. There is associated bilateral neck and sublingual swelling.

Nasal discharge

Mucopurulent nasal discharge occurs in upper respiratory tract infections. This resolves over a period of a few days. Continual mucous discharge associated with nasal blockage is found in allergic rhinitis. Upper respiratory tract infections may progress from simple nasal discharge to sinusitis when the patient complains of pain over the affected sinus exacerbated by jolting the head or bending. They have a sensation of blockage and headache.

Epistaxis

Epistaxis is common and is often associated with a small haemorrhagic area in the anterior caudal region of the nasal septal mucoperiosteum (Little's area). Unexplained unilateral epistaxis associated with infraorbital anaesthesia and maxillary sinus swelling on the face or in the palate is suggestive of maxillary sinus neoplasia.

Examination

The site of the patient's symptoms will be the main focus for the examination. However, confusion can occur when the patient's pain symptoms are at the site of radiation. For example, a patient may present with ear pain when the pathology is in the throat or lower jaw. It is therefore wise to rapidly examine the face, neck, mouth, throat and ears with most facial pains. In addition where no local pathology is found, it may be appropriate to perform a brief neurological examination. The format of inspection, palpation and percussion should be followed. Auscultation is rarely indicated.

The face

The face should be inspected for swellings and redness. In cavernous sinus thrombosis the eye may be proptosed and pulsating. Cellulitis and lymphangitis will manifest with diffuse areas of erythema. Swellings should be palpated for tenderness and fluctuation. If there is emphysema, sometimes found in association with a perforated sinus wall, the examining finger will detect crepitus. In sinusitis, there will be tenderness over the affected sinus, and when the patient bends the head down between the knees or shakes it from side to side the pain will worsen.

Dental decay

When the history is suggestive of dental pathology then the teeth should be examined for obvious breakdown and decay (brown/black discoloration and loss of tooth contour). More subtle caries will impart a chalky white appearance to undermined enamel. The tooth affected is often tender to pressure or percussion. There will be swelling adjacent to the affected tooth if an abscess or cyst penetrates one of the cortical plates of the jaws. Pus may discharge from the swelling or from the gum margin around the affected tooth.

Salivary glands

If the salivary glands are swollen or painful, their ducts should be milked toward the mouth to assess whether there is any salivary flow (none in obstructive saliadenitis) or discharge of pus (in acute infection). The parotid duct opens inside the cheek opposite the upper second molar; the submandibular duct opens in the midline floor of the mouth behind the lower central incisors.

Gums

The gums should be examined for swelling, redness and bleeding and the throat for inflammation and abnormal swellings. The oral mucosal surface of the tongue, floor of the mouth, soft palate and cheek are the likely sites of ulceration. The site of any ulcers should be recorded. Their size, surface, colour, depth of invasion and whether the margins are smooth or irregular, flat or raised should be noted.

Lymph nodes

When an enlarged lymph node is discovered, the drainage area of that node should be examined thoroughly. This would include the scalp, facial skin, ears, nose, sinuses and the oral cavity. If no obvious cause is found for the lymph node enlargement, then the rest of the lymphoreticular system, including the axilla, groins, liver and spleen, and para-aortic nodes should be assessed.

A record should be made of the site of lymph node enlargement, whether this is single or multiple, the size and texture of the lymph nodes, and whether there is any associated pain. The duration of lymph node enlargement should be noted and the texture and mobility of the lymph node should be assessed.

The site, size, fluctuance, mobility, tenderness and fixation to superficial and deep tissues of all swellings should be recorded. The status of the overlying skin including erythema and any sinuses should be assessed.

Respiratory difficulty

Impending respiratory obstruction in head and neck infections may be heralded by agitation, alteration in head posture and use of the accessory muscles. Examination should focus on the patient's mouth opening, and note whether there is any swelling of the floor of the mouth lifting up the tongue, or of the pharynx. The thyroid cartilage and trachea should be palpated for deviation, and the pulse rate, respiratory rate and pattern, and voice quality should be noted.

Investigations

In principle, clinicians should always start with the simplest, cheapest and least invasive investigations that will yield a diagnosis. Urine should therefore be tested for glucose.

Blood tests

Haematological investigations routinely include full blood count and sometimes erythrocyte sedimentation rate (ESR). Urea and electrolytes and liver function tests may be appropriate in certain circumstances. Patients with evidence of septicaemia should have blood taken for culture. Serum amylase is helpful in the rapid diagnosis of acute parotitis. Sarcoidosis can cause swellings in the head and neck region and serum angiotensin converting enzyme will usually yield the diagnosis. Sjögren's syndrome presents with bilateral parotid and sometimes lacrimal and submandibular swelling (Fig. 5). The patient may have a history of connective tissue disease, and autoimmune studies often demonstrate positive rheumatoid factor or antinuclear antibodies. Wegener's disease is a rare problem but the antineutrophil cytoplasmic antibody will be positive in many of these cases. The monospot or Paul–Bunnell test, cytomegalovirus antibody titres and the toxoplasma dye test should be done in cases of infectious mononucleosis. Serum antibody titres may be measured for specific viral infections, although these investigations do not provide rapid results.

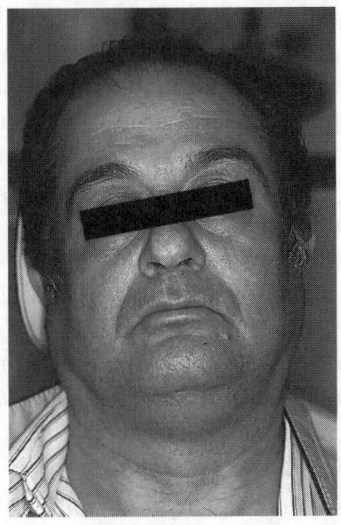

Fig. 5. Bilateral parotid enlargement in Sjögren's syndrome.

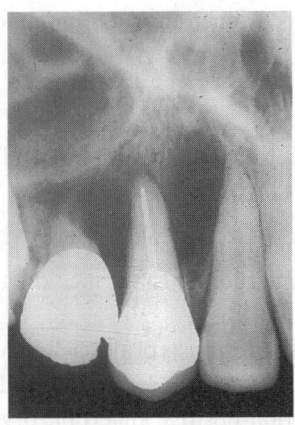

Fig. 6. Cyst causing bone destruction around an upper premolar tooth.

Radiology

Plain radiology of teeth, such as the orthopantomogram (OPG) and periapical radiographs, can show periapical radiolucencies or decay in the affected teeth (Fig. 6). In gum infections, bone loss may be visible around certain teeth. Occipitomental radiographs of the sinuses demonstrate fluid levels or mucosal thickening in sinusitis. (Fig. 7) Lateral radiographs of the neck can show soft tissue swelling affecting the airway in conditions such as epiglottitis and air–fluid levels in laryngoceles. Calcified masses in tuberculosis or opaque salivary calculi will also be detected on plain radiographs.

Contrast radiology, such as sialography, is usually only safe when the acute symptoms have resolved. CT scanning or Magnetic Resonance Imaging is occasionally useful in the acute situation for conditions such as parapharyngeal abscesses. Ultrasound is very useful in determining whether there is any fluid present which can be drained or aspirated.

Microbiology

Microbiology results are obviously vital in diagnosis and therapy. In oral candidiasis and herpetic infections, skin or mucosal swabs obtained from surface scrapings may be adequate for culture. Deep-seated abscesses may be aspirated in the first instance to obtain specimens for culture and sensitivity. Alternatively, surgical drainage will be therapeutic as well as providing specimens.

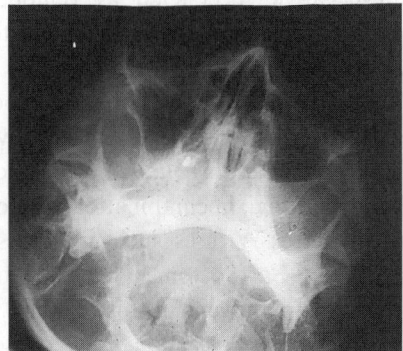

Fig. 7. Left maxillary sinus fluid level in sinusitis.

Cytology

Lymph nodes may be aspirated with 21 gauge needles for cytological specimens to ascertain whether their enlargement is caused by infection or neoplasia. Tuberculosis can also sometimes be diagnosed cytologically if epithelioid and Langerhans giant cells are present or acid/alcohol-fast bacilli are found. However, in suspected tuberculosis open or 'trucut' biopsy may be necessary for diagnosis.

Flexible fibre-optic endoscopy extends the possibility of examination to include the whole of the upper aerodigestive tract. It can also aid in the placement of an endotracheal airway in patients with impending airway obstruction. Nuclear medicine scans with radio-labelled diphosphonates are occasionally indicated to confirm the presence of chronic osteomyelitis. Similarly, radiolabelled white cells can locate sources of infection.

Intradermal tests (type IV immunology reactions) are important in the diagnosis of tuberculosis (Mantoux or Heaf) and sarcoidosis (Kveim).

If there is a suggestion of immunodeficiency, blood

glucose, white cell function tests, immunoglobin levels, bone marrow aspirates and HIV studies may be indicated.

NORMAL FLORA AND PATHOGENIC MICROORGANISMS

Cultures from head and neck infections frequently grow a mixture of microorganisms, including normal oral flora.

Normal oral flora consists of alpha- and non-haemolytic streptococci, *Staphylococcus epidermidis* and *aureus*, peptostreptococci (Gram-positive anaerobic organisms), diphtheroids, *Lactobacillus* and *Actinomyces* species, Gram-negative anaerobic rods such as fusobacteria and bacteroides, Gram-negative cocci such as veillonellae and neisseriae, and spirochaetes and yeasts (Schuster, 1987).

Specific pathogenic bacteria, notably the tubercle bacillus, *Treponema pallidum* and the gonococcus, can cause head and neck infections. Gram-negative enteric bacteria such as *Escherischia coli*, *Klebsiella* and *Pseudomonas* are often cultured, in combination with oral flora, from dental abscesses. Viruses such as herpes simplex and zoster, Epstein–Barr, cytomegalovirus, mumps and measles may act as pathogens in this region.

The fungi *Mucor*, *Rhizopus* and *Absidia* cause the rare but life-threatening cephalic phycomycosis in immunosuppressed patients. *Aspergillus* can affect a similar population.

Protozoa such as *Toxoplasma gondii* may cause an infectious mononucleosis-like syndrome in young adults.

In general terms, staphylococci cause soft tissue abscesses, osteomyelitis, and superficial soft tissue infections such as furuncles. Streptococci are associated with odontogenic infections, pharyngitis, tonsillitis, epiglottitis, Ludwig's angina, erysipelas, impetigo, scarlet fever, and subacute bacterial endocarditis.

DECREASED HOST DEFENCE MECHANISMS

Patients with impaired defence mechanisms may have inherited these or acquired them as a result of disease or therapy. Inherited disorders such as sickle cell disease may predispose to unusual forms of osteomyelitis caused by *Salmonella*. Subtle abnormalities in phagocyte activity or complement activation are sometimes found in patients with chronic infections. Alternatively, the patient's B or T lymphocytes may not function perfectly.

Diabetics, patients with chronic renal and liver disease, rheumatoid arthritics and patients with leukaemia may all have an increased susceptibility to infection. The use of immunosuppressants in transplant patients or corticosteroids may predispose to infection. The chemotherapeutic agents used in oncology often suppress the bone marrow production of white cells, resulting in infections. Patients with AIDS and malnourished patients are also susceptible to rare and life-threatening infections.

Candida species, *Aspergillus* and *Mucor* are associated with these debilitating states. *Pneumocystis* and *Clostridium* species can cause problems in these patients.

A further group of patients, such as those with prosthetic heart valves, may develop persistent infection after simple bacteraemias when bacteria settle on the prosthetic material. The prosthetic heart valve must usually be replaced to resolve this.

SPECIFIC ORGAN SYSTEMS AND THEIR INFECTIONS

In this section the symptoms, signs, investigations and management of diseases in organ systems of the head and neck will be described. A further section will deal with specific disease processes such as syphilis.

Upper respiratory tract infections

These infections are usually caused by viruses. They may be complicated by sinusitis, tonsillitis, orbital cellulitis and abscesses, and cavernous sinus thrombosis, and can progress to bronchitis and pneumonia. When acute sinusitis occurs, *Streptococcus pneumoniae* or *Haemophilus influenzae* are implicated. In chronic sinusitis, the organisms may change to bacteroides, peptostreptococci and corynebacteria. In debilitated patients, such as diabetics and patients on immunosuppressants, fungal sinus infections with *Aspergillus* and phycomycosis may occur, although these are exceedingly rare.

Streptococcus pyogenes (group A beta-haemolytic streptococci) sore throats can be complicated by immune complex diseases such as rheumatic fever and glomerulonephritis. Other rarer causes of sore throat include *Candida albicans*, *Neisseria gonococcus*, herpes simplex, *Corynebacterium diphtheriae* and Epstein–Barr virus. Tonsillitis may be complicated by peritonsillar abscesses or parapharyngeal abscesses. Upper respiratory tract infections often cause mucosal oedema around the eustachian tube opening, resulting in eustachian dysfunction and middle ear effusions.

Presentation

Patients present with sore throats, coughs and runny noses. The cough and runny nose usually produce clear mucus, but as secondary bacterial infection occurs this changes to a purulent discharge. Examination of the pharynx reveals inflammation in the fauces. The patient often has cervical lymphadenopathy. These nodes are mobile and usually less than 1 cm in diameter.

Sinusitis

If sinusitis develops, the patient has continuous, dull, aching pain in the region of the affected sinus with a sensation of blockage. This pain is exacerbated by bending or jolting the head. It is usually relieved by simple analgesics and does not keep the patient awake. The patient may develop erythema and oedema of the facial skin and periorbital oedema.

If the eustachian tube is affected then the patient may have severe earache and decreased hearing on the affected side. Tonsillitis, peritonsillar and parapharyngeal abscesses are accompanied by difficulty and pain with swallowing and discomfort on the affected side. The patient may also have difficulty breathing.

Investigations

There are no specific haematological investigations that will aid in diagnosis. All pus obtained should be sent for culture and sensitivity. If sinusitis is suspected, occipitomental X-rays will reveal fluid levels or mucosal thickening in the affected sinuses (Fig. 7). Lateral soft tissue views of the neck may reveal obstruction of the airway and swelling of such structures as the epiglottis. In the rare condition of laryngocele, the patient presents with a neck swelling, hoarseness of the voice and difficulty swallowing and breathing. Soft tissue X-rays of the neck often reveal an air–fluid level.

Treatment

Any underlying predisposing medical condition such as diabetes should be treated. Simple upper respiratory tract viral infections should be treated symptomatically, but secondary bacterial infections are treated with antibiotics.

Sinusitis

If sinusitis occurs, then decongestants such as ephedrine nasal drops should be used at a dosage of 0.5–1% to encourage drainage down the affected nostril. Steam inhalations also help as a temporary decongestant. Systemic antibiotics such as the penicillins, cephalosporins, tetracyclines or erythromycin may be used empirically until cultures are available. If the patient shows signs of developing orbital complications, they should be admitted to hospital and treated with intravenous antibiotics in high dosage, and surgical drainage. In cases of phycomycosis of the sinuses, immediate referral is necessary followed by systemic amphotericin and resection of the affected sinus (MacArthur et al., 1992).

When simple sore throats progress to parapharyngeal or peritonsillar abscesses or epiglottitis, then control of the airway is paramount (Andreassen et al., 1992). Senior A&E staff, anaesthetists and specialist surgeons should therefore be called in urgently. High-dose intravenous ampicillin or cephalosporins should be commenced immediately. The use of steroids in high dosage may reduce accompanying oedema, thereby improving the airway for a sufficient length of time whilst expert advice is awaited. In extremis, cricothyroidotomy may be required. The ideal treatment is drainage of the abscess after intubation.

Dental infections

Tooth decay associated with a diet high in refined sugar is endemic. The carious process of tooth decay starts with a lesion in the tooth enamel and, if left untreated over months or years, proceeds to involve the more deeply situated dentine and ultimately the pulpal tissues. The pulp dies and an abscess develops in the bone around the apex of the root. The abscess may initially be contained within the bone or may perforate one of the cortical plates of the jaws to present in the adjacent soft tissues. If the condition becomes chronic then cysts occasionally develop around the root apices. These enlarge slowly, expanding and sometimes perforating bone to cause a hard swelling opposite the affected tooth.

When abscesses penetrate the soft tissues they can cause facial swellings overlying the maxilla and mandible, or swellings in the submandibular or parotid regions. The abscess can develop between the masseter muscle and ramus of the mandible (submasseteric) in which case the patient has profound limitation of jaw opening associated with a diffuse swelling in the parotid region. Abscesses may also present in the floor of the mouth or progress to involve the parapharyngeal region.

Ludwig's angina

Occasionally, particularly in patients with chronic disease or a poor nutritional state such as alcoholics, the infection may become the bilateral sublingual, submandibular and parapharyngeal cellulitis known as Ludwig's angina. In this case the patient develops progressive difficulty in opening the mouth, swallowing and, finally, breathing. The tongue is forced up onto the palate and the initial submental and submandibular swelling progresses to involve the whole neck (Fig. 3a and b). This condition can also occur several days after the offending tooth has been extracted, and occasionally may not be related to tooth infection at all (pseudo-Ludwig's angina).

Rarely, dental infection may permeate the mandible or maxilla creating osteomyelitis. This may develop *de novo* or follow inadequately treated abscesses. In malnourished patients, dental infection may be complicated by an aggressive erosive destruction of large volumes of soft tissue of the face. This condition is known as cancrum oris and is particularly prevalent in the African continent.

The organisms causing dental bony and soft tissue infections are usually mixtures of alpha- and non-haemolytic streptococci with bacteroides, fusiforms, spirochaetes, propionobacteria and veillonellae.

Presentation

Dental caries

In early dental decay, the patient may have no pain whatsoever. When the dentine is involved, the patient experiences sharp pain lasting a few seconds on hot, cold and sweet stimuli. The tooth itself will not be tender unless the cavity is probed.

Pulpitis, when the pulp of the tooth becomes hyperaemic as the decay process approaches it, is associated with severe throbbing pain which is not controlled by simple analgesics. The pain keeps the patient awake and the tooth affected is exquisitely tender. The pulp then dies over the course of 2 or 3 days, after which the patient may not experience any pain from the tooth until bacterial toxins from the necrotic pulp cause acute inflammation of the bone at the apex of the tooth. This

pain-free interval may last many months or years. The patient then experiences pain similar to that of pulpitis.

Dental abscesses

If an abscess ensues, the patient is pyrexial and the pain does not resolve spontaneously. Alternatively, the bacterial toxins may stimulate chronic inflammation at the root apex. In this case, the tooth is persistently uncomfortable when touched or used for biting but the patient does not experience severe pain. This condition may be associated with a discharging sinus on the gum opposite the tooth. Cysts may develop around the root apex in response to the chronic inflammation. These grow steadily, causing expansion of the bony cortical plate, and they may destroy large volumes of jaw bone by simple expansion. These cysts usually become infected at some stage, when the patient presents with swelling, acute pain and fever. Soft tissue abscesses present with hot, red, tender swellings at the affected site. There may be associated oedema of the surrounding tissues and occasionally the swelling may be fluctuant. The mouth should be examined and the offending tooth is usually obvious as a blackened broken-down stump. If there is any doubt, then the teeth may be tapped with a wooden spatula when the affected tooth will be exquisitely sensitive.

In Ludwig's angina, the respiratory rate is not always increased, but the respiratory pattern is altered with no pauses between inspiration and expiration and the respiratory accessory muscles, such as sternomastoid, are often in use. The patient is tachycardic and frequently drools saliva from the mouth.

Investigations

With infection rather than simple decay, the patient will have a neutrophilia and a raised ESR. Radiology of the teeth and underlying bone will demonstrate radiolucency at the site of an abscess, granuloma or cyst. Ultrasound will be helpful in determining whether there is any fluid present in the abscess and therefore whether it is worthwhile draining. Fine-needle aspiration may achieve a similar effect and will also provide material for culture and sensitivity.

Pulse oximetry is advisable when respiratory embarrassment is suspected, but the patient may maintain normal oxygen saturation and blood gases until respiratory collapse occurs.

Treatment

Ludwing's angina

Any suspicion about impending airway obstruction should result in an immediate call to senior A&E staff, maxillofacial surgeons and anaesthetists. A nasopharyngeal airway may be helpful as a temporary measure.

In Ludwig's angina, treatment with high-dose steroids improves the airway, rapidly reducing oedema and improving mouth opening. The regimen recommended in adults is 8 mg of dexamethasone intravenously, repeated at 15-min intervals for half an hour, then at half-hourly intervals for intervals for 2 h. At this stage, there should have been a dramatic improvement. The dexamethasone frequency can then be adjusted according to requirements, but in general it continues at 2-h intervals for 8 h, and 4-hourly thereafter for the next 24 h. Alternatively, after an initial loading dose of 8 mg, an intravenous infusion of 1 mg of dexamethasone hourly can be started (Hutchison & James, 1989). The steroids should gradually be reduced to zero over the next 3 days. This treatment is combined with high-dose intravenous antibiotic therapy—for example gentamicin, cephalosporins and metronidazole in combination. Often over the course of the next 2 days, an abscess localizes which can be drained with ease. If the steroid therapy is successful it may not be necessary to intubate the patient in the emergency situation. However, should the airway still be compromised, awake intubation, using the flexible fibreoptic laryngoscope, is the safest treatment. Cricothyroidotomy is often impossible because of massive cellulitis in the neck. Occasionally, emergency tracheostomy is necessary.

Dental caries

In A&E, the pain of dental decay is best treated using simple analgesics. The only permanent remedy is to remove the decay and fill the tooth. When pulpitis develops simple analgesics do not control the pain completely and antibiotics have no immediate effect. The tooth should either be extracted or the pulp opened and drained using dental drills. With abscesses, the aim is drainage as soon as possible in combination with antibiotic therapy. The penicillins, cephalosporins, erythromycin and tetracyclines are all effective when used in combination with metronidazole. The maxillofacial surgeon should be informed immediately so that these measures can be instituted.

When patients present with chronic symptoms such as discharging sinuses on the face or neck, or unexplained facial swellings, it is still wise to inform the maxillofacial surgeon immediately so that appropriate investigation and treatment can be started before the patient is seen in out-patients.

Periodontal and gingival (gum) infections

The periodontium consists of the gingiva (gums), the alveolar bone supporting the teeth and the periodontal ligament holding the tooth roots in the bone. Diseases of these tissues have a different pathogenesis and behaviour to infections arising from tooth decay.

Presentation

Chronic marginal periodontility

The commonest condition is chronic marginal gingivitis where plaque builds up at the necks of teeth. Toxins from the bacteria within plaque cause sore gums with a line of erythema extending 2–5 mm below the necks of the teeth (Fig. 8). The gums bleed easily on brushing and touching but may not be particularly sore. Acute symptoms can develop if there is a particular area of food trapping (acute marginal gingivitis).

The supporting bone of the teeth is gradually destroyed by this process when the condition is called chronic marginal periodontitis. Here, in addition to the other symptoms, the teeth may be loose and the gums feel sore and congested. The discomfort is often relieved by clenching the teeth. Acute periodontal abscesses may develop which have similar features to those caused by dental decay.

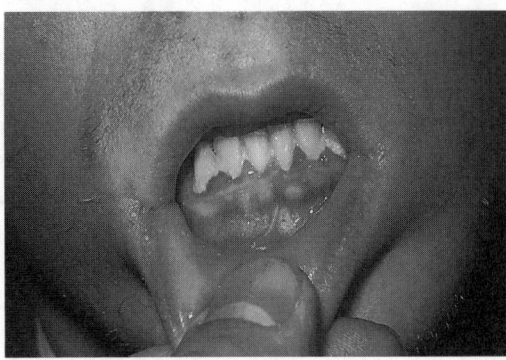

Fig. 8. Plaque around the teeth with red gum margins in marginal gingivitis.

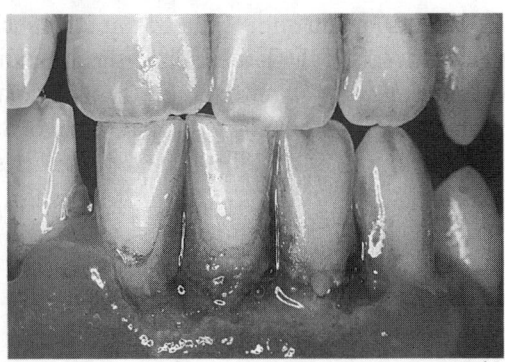

Fig. 9. Loss of gum margins in acute ulcerative gingivitis.

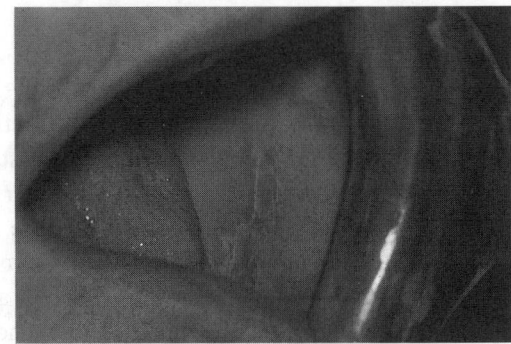

Fig. 10. White lacy pattern of lichen planus.

Acute ulcerative gingivitis

Acute ulcerative gingivitis (trench mouth, Vincent's angina) is found in malnourished or debilitated patients. Here, the interdental papilla becomes ulcerated and destroyed (Fig. 9). The bacteria implicated are *Fusiformis fusiformis* (= *Fusobacterium nucleatum*) and *Borrelia vincentii*.

Pericoronitis

Pericoronitis is the periodontitis that occurs around erupting teeth, especially impacted wisdom teeth. The patient has dull throbbing pain, especially on biting, and infection may track into the submasseteric or parapharyngeal spaces or the floor of the mouth.

White patches

Patients may notice white patches in their mouths and consider that these have an infective origin. Oral candidiasis presents with white curds overlying an erythematous, sore, diffusely inflamed oral mucosa. Oral lichen planus is marked by white striae in a lacework pattern (Fig. 10). The patient does not have any soreness unless there are erosive, red changes in the underlying mucosa. Unexplained white patches (leukoplakia) must be considered to be premalignant (Fig. 11).

The commonest causes of mouth ulcers are chemical and mechanical trauma and recurrent aphthous stomatitis when the patient suffers regular attacks of one or more ulcers which last 5–7 days. Squamous carcinoma (Fig. 12), vesiculobullous disorders such as pemphigus, tuberculosis and syphilis may all cause indolent or atypical ulcers which fail to heal within 2 weeks.

Gingival lumps

Benign polyps (Fig. 13), extravasations of saliva outside minor salivary glands (mucoceles) (Fig. 14), minor

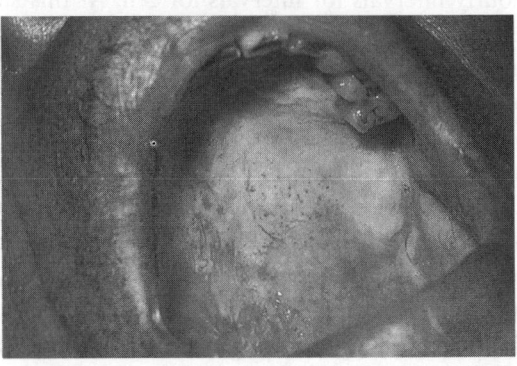

Fig. 11. Smoker's keratosis of the hard palate with a premalignant white and red path on the right soft palate.

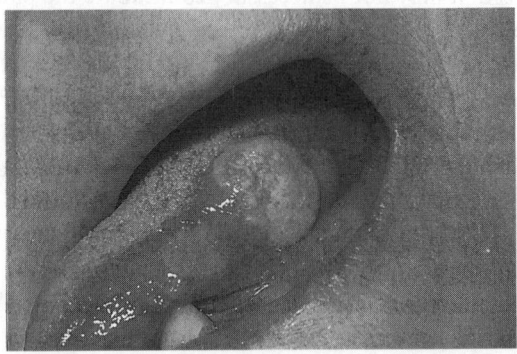

Fig. 12. Squamous cell carcinoma on left side of tongue: Irregular central ulcer with raised firm rolled margins. Note the premalignant white patch anteriorly.

salivary gland tumours, sarcoidosis and Crohn's disease may all cause oral mucosal swellings which are usually painless.

Investigations

It is always wise to take a full blood count and ESR in gingivitis or periodontitis as the rare case of leukaemia may be discovered. Where pus can be obtained, it should

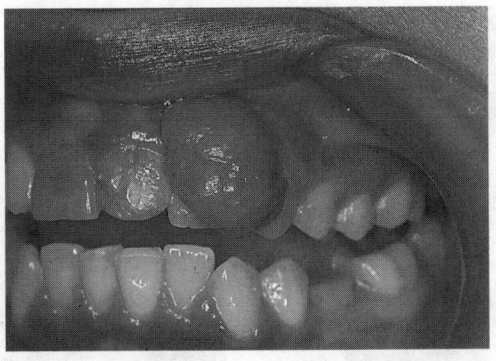

Fig. 13. Benign pedunculated pregnancy epulis attached to gum margin. Surgical removal with tooth scaling is curative.

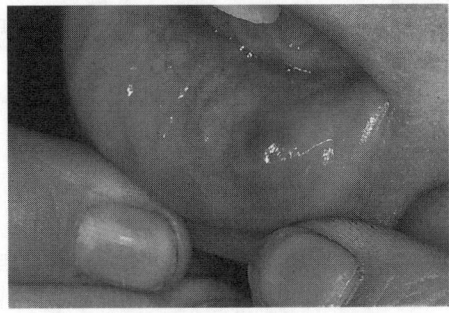

Fig. 14. Mucous extravasation cyst of the lower lip.

be cultured and tested for sensitivities. In cases of oral candidiasis or suspected herpetic ulceration, surface scrapings should be sent for fungal and viral culture.

With recurrent aphthous ulceration, blood should be taken for serum iron, total iron-binding capacity, vitamin B_{12} and folic acid, as deficiencies of these elements and vitamins may cause recurrent aphthous stomatitis.

Radiographs of the teeth and bone, such as the OPG, are helpful with periodontitis and acute abscesses.

If ulcers fail to heal, investigative biopsy should be performed by the maxillofacial surgeon.

Treatment

In gingivitis and periodontitis, the patient is best referred to their general dental practitioner for cleaning of the teeth and oral hygiene instruction. With acute ulcerative gingivitis, periodontal abscesses and pericoronitis, the patient should be treated with penicillin and metronidazole and referred for a maxillofacial opinion. In oral candidiasis, nystatin pastilles or amphotericin mouthwash are curative. However, the patient's blood sugar should be tested to exclude diabetes.

With unexplained mouth ulcers, white patches or swellings, a maxillofacial opinion should be sought for further investigation and treatment.

Jaw infections

Presentation and investigation

Osteomyelitis

Osteomyelitis of the jaws is not common. In the neonate, a haematogenous osteomyelitis can develop. The child does not take food, and is pyrexial and unwell with facial swelling. The patient has a neutrophilia and raised ESR. Radiographs are not helpful in the acute situation but a radionuclide white cell scan or bone scan can be diagnostic. Blood or bone cultures may distinguish the causative organism, usually *Staphylococcus aureus*. Other acute forms of facial bone osteomyelitis are rare.

Chronic osteomyelitis usually complicates dental infection or follows unsuccessfully treated facial bone trauma, but may also arise *de novo*. The patient has jaw pain, tenderness and a firm swelling of the affected site. There may be numbness of the ipsilateral lip (inferior dental nerve) or cheek (infraorbital nerve) in mandibular and maxillary osteomyelitis, respectively. There is a neutrophilia and raised ESR. Radiographs, such as the OPG, show thickening with patchy sclerosis and rarefaction of the affected bone. Once again, the radionuclide white cell and bone scans may be helpful in diagnosis. The patient with no antecedent cause for chronic osteomyelitis should be thoroughly investigated for subtle defects in their immune status, including white cell, lymphocyte and complement function.

Patients with sickle cell disease are prone to osteomyelitis. This can sometimes be caused by *Salmonella*. Rarer causes of osteomyelitis include the tubercle bacillus, *Actinomyces israelii* and syphilis.

Other jaw swellings

Benign conditions such as cysts and fibrous dysplasia also cause persistent jaw swellings. Tumours such as ameloblastoma (Fig. 15), lymphoma, histiocytosis X, osteosarcoma and Ewing's sarcoma present with enlarging jaw swellings which are often mildly painful and can be associated with paraesthesia in the lower lip (mandibular tumours) or cheek (maxillary tumours). They are often mistaken for jaw infections such as osteomyelitis. Paget's disease, acromegaly and cherubism cause generalized jaw bone enlargement which is usually painless.

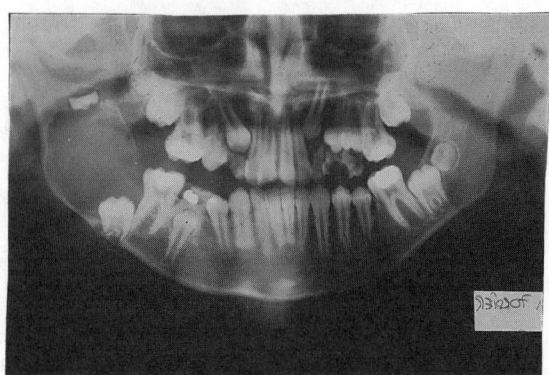

Fig. 15. OPG showing right mandibular radiolucency caused by an ameloblastoma. The patient presented with swelling in the parotid region.

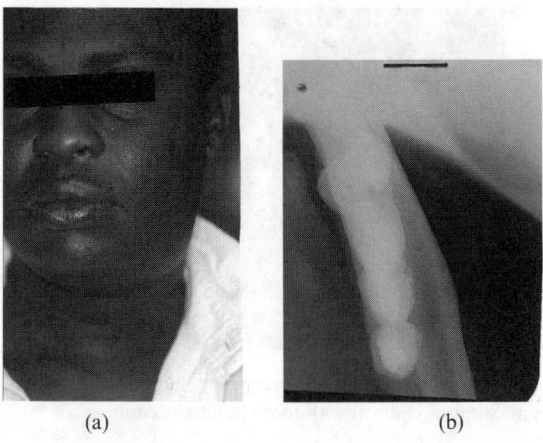

(a)   (b)

Fig. 16. (a) Left submandibular salivary swelling caused by (b) calculi blocking the salivary duct shown on this occlusal radiograph.

Once the diagnosis is reached, bone specimens should be cultured, and serum should be studied for raised antibody titres to specific organisms. Even then, there may not be unequivocal evidence for the causative organism. Bone biopsy will be diagnostic in the case of bone tumours, and calcium studies including alkaline phosphatase will identify generalized conditions such as Paget's disease.

Treatment

Acute osteomyelitis responds well to antibiotic therapy augmented occasionally by surgical decortication. In chronic osteomyelitis, even prolonged courses of antibiotics, augmented by physical techniques such as hyperbaric oxygen, may sometimes be unsuccessful (Hudson, 1993).

Aggressive surgical debridement and high-dose local antibiotic therapy using antibiotic beads or closed circulating systems can sometimes cure the condition. If this fails, then resection of the affected bone with well-vascularized reconstruction may be the only alternative.

Salivary gland infections

Presentation

Salivary gland diseases mainly present either as acute diffuse painful glandular enlargement, or chronic solitary painless nodules.

Sialadenitis

Obstructive sialadenitis of the major salivary glands is usually caused by radio-opaque calculi blocking the main duct, although radiolucent mucous plugs and debris can have a similar effect (Fig. 16). If the stone does not occlude the duct completely, the patient complains of periprandial pain and swelling of the affected gland which subsides after meals. The patient may give a long history of this problem or describe recurrent episodes. If the duct becomes completely occluded, the gland is permanently swollen and painful. Infection develops and the overlying skin becomes hot and tender and the patient is pyrexial. The patient presents within a few hours of developing these symptoms. The submandibular gland is more frequently affected.

In partial occlusion, it may be possible to milk saliva from the duct. Often, small flakes of debris are visible in this. In acute sialadenitis, pus may exude from the duct orifice (Fig. 17). Alternatively, it may not be possible to produce any secretions from the duct. The stone may be palpable in the mouth floor (submandibular gland) or cheek (parotid gland).

Trauma to the duct orifice and dehydration in hot weather, or after surgery, may also result in acute sialadenitis. The parotid gland is particularly prone to this.

If the patient suffers chronic damage to the acinar structure of the gland, they may have recurrent episodes of acute sialadenitis not related to calculus disease.

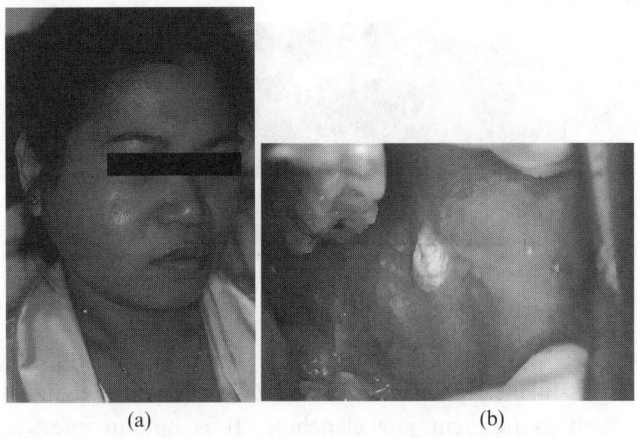

Fig. 17. (a) Acute parotitis with (b) pus exuding from the duct orifice opposite the upper second molar.

Mumps

Mumps classically causes fever, malaise and bilateral parotid swelling and pain. The submandibular glands can also be involved. The disease may not affect all glands symmetrically.

Sjögren's syndrome

Sjögren's syndrome—the autoimmune disease complex of a connective tissue disorder (e.g. rheumatoid arthritis) associated with dry mouth and dry eyes—presents as bilateral painless symmetrical parotid and/or submandibular gland enlargement (Fig. 5). However, acute sialadenitis can develop in the damaged gland, and the patient may also present with an enlarging solitary painless nodule in an affected gland if a MALT (mucosa-associated lymphoid tissue)-type lymphoma occurs.

Alcoholics, the malnourished, and diabetics can develop persistent diffuse enlargement of the parotids which is either painless or mildly uncomfortable.

Salivary tumours

Solitary painless salivary gland nodules are usually tumours. Normal saliva can be milked from the ducts. The parotid gland is most frequently affected but the submandibular and intraoral salivary glands can also develop tumours. The most common tumour is the benign pleomorphic adenoma (Fig. 18). Lymphomas, mucoepidermoid tumours (of intermediate status) and the malignant adenoid cystic and adenocarcinoma can also occur. If the patient has pain or facial nerve weakness in association with the lump, the tumour is likely to be

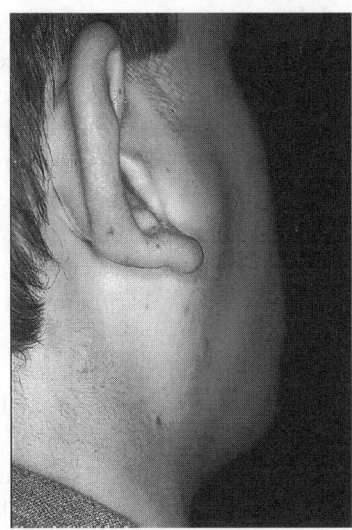

Fig. 18. Pleomorphic adenoma of the parotid—the earlobe is pushed out by the tumour.

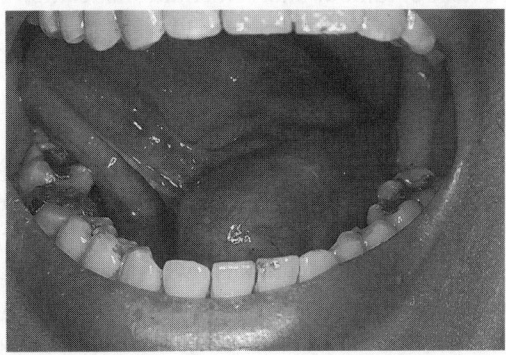

Fig. 19. Swelling left mouth floor caused by a blocked sublingual gland—the ranula.

malignant. Malignant tumours are also more likely to invade skin and infiltrate, producing induration and sinuses. Tuberculosis and actinomycosis of the parotid can produce a similar effect but do not cause facial nerve weakness.

Blockage of the sublingual gland and intraoral minor salivary glands cause persistent mucus-filled vesicles, the ranula (Fig. 19) and mucocele, respectively.

Investigation

Serum amylase is elevated in acute salivary gland infection. This can be helpful when there is uncertainty over diagnosis. When mumps is suspected, viral titres should be measured, but there is a long delay before these results are available.

Plain radiology (lateral oblique of the jaws and intraoral lower occlusal radiographs) will show submandibular calculi, but parotid calculi (lateral face radiograph with open mouth, and intraoral periapical radiograph of the cheek) are more radiolucent and rarely visualized. Contrast sialography can be used when the acute symptoms have settled and will show damage to the ducts (dilatation or ectasia) and acini (sialectasis) and filling defects at the site of radiolucent calculi.

Ultrasound can show duct dilatation and fluid collections, but is rarely diagnostic.

All pus collected should be sent for culture and sensitivity testing. If tuberculosis is suspected, a Mantoux or Heaf test should be arranged.

In solitary nodules, fine-needle aspiration cytology is the investigation of choice, but this should be left to the specialist surgeon. Sialography has no role in tumour assessment, but MRI (magnetic resonance imaging) and CT (computed tomography) scanning will define the exact extent of tumour and, sometimes, its relation to the facial nerve.

Treatment

In most cases, there are few options for emergency treatment, and definitive investigation and treatment is best left to the maxillofacial surgeon. Urgent referral is indicated in acute conditions, whilst an out-patient appointment is appropriate for a chronic condition.

With acute sialadenitis, the patient often requires admission for intravenous fluid replacement, antibiotics, and glandular rest with a nil by mouth regime. Calculi can often be removed by an intraoral approach. Surgical removal of the gland is indicated for tumours, calculi situated in the hilum of the gland, and symptomatic glands which are diffusely damaged.

Temporomandibular joint diseases

Temporomandibular joint pain dysfunction syndrome (i.e. jaw joint or masticatory muscle pain, clicking, or difficulty opening the mouth) is common, affecting as much as 70% of the population at some point in their lives (Rugh & Solberg, 1985). Radiographs show no abnormality as the pathological process involves the soft tissues of the joint (the disc and capsule). Arthrography and arthroscopy will define these soft tissue changes. The syndrome usually resolves spontaneously. However, treatment with mouth appliances, low-dose tricyclic antidepressants, or even joint surgery may be necessary in about 20% of cases. It frequently occurs around

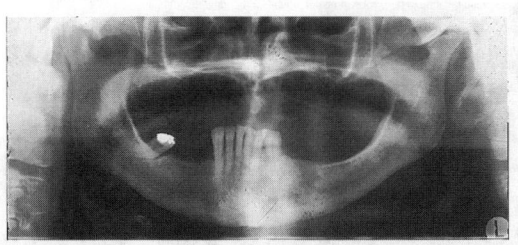

Fig. 20. OPG radiograph showing osteoarthritic change with flattening of the left mandibular condyle.

stressful life events and is associated with abnormal habits such as frequent jaw clenching. It is not an infective process. Referral for a maxillofacial surgery out-patient opinion is indicated.

Jaw joint infections are rare. They may be caused by:

- Direct extension from ear, mastoid or meningeal infections.
- Haematogenous spread.
- Direct instrumentation of the joint.
- Laceration of the overlying skin.

The patient has pain over the affected joint which is exacerbated by moving the jaw. The overlying skin may be red and is tender. Staphylococci, streptococci and gonococci are the common causative organisms. Plain radiology of the joint is unhelpful, but radionuclide scans with radiolabelled diphosphonates will show increased uptake (hot spots). The joint is aspirated for culture and, in haematogenous cases, blood cultures should be taken. High-dose intravenous antibiotic therapy and absolute jaw rest is instituted rapidly. In young children, whom this condition particularly affects, failure to provide effective early treatment can result in destruction of the growth potential of the joint and bony ankylosis (Guralnick, 1992).

Osteoarthritis (Fig. 20), rheumatoid arthritis and gout can all affect the temporomandibular joint and generate symptoms of joint pain, stiffness and grating sounds. The OPG will often show irregularity, erosions and osteophytes of the mandibular condyle.

Skin conditions

Skin lumps

All dermatological conditions can affect the face. Acne, folliculitis, furuncles, carbuncles and infected epidermoid (sebaceous) cysts are common in the head and neck. They present as white/yellow spots varying in size from 1 mm to greater than 2 cm. They are tender when infected, and fixed to surrounding skin. Staphylococci are usually implicated. In acute infection, surgical drainage, collection of material for culture and cytology, and antibiotic therapy may be necessary. Rarely, metastatic carcinoma in lymph glands can erode into the skin producing a similar clinical picture, but with more marked induration and fixation. If in doubt, a maxillofacial opinion should be sought before any drainage is attempted. Fine-needle aspiration cytology will usually differentiate.

Skin rashes

Redness of the facial skin can be caused by rashes in scarlet fever, measles and other childhood viral diseases, systemic lupus erythematosus, contact allergic reactions, eczema and erysipelas. In erysipelas, there may be blistering and the patient is unwell with a fever. The causative organism is a group A beta-haemolytic streptococcus and the patient should be treated with high-dose antibiotics. Redness of the skin can also be caused by infection in the underlying tissues, such as sinusitis or dental abscesses. The key to recognition lies in the associated symptoms.

Skin blisters

Crusting of the skin is caused by impetigo (*Staphylococcus* or *Streptococcus*), herpes simplex and herpes zoster. The vesiculobullous disorders of pemphigus and bullous pemphigoid can also cause blistering of the skin and mouth. The blisters rapidly burst to form ulcers or crusts.

Necrotizing fasciitis

Necrotizing fasciitis occurs rarely. It is caused by group A beta-haemolytic streptococci or *Staphylococcus aureus*. The initial presentation is of red, cellulitic skin which over the course of a few days becomes purple and necroses. The condition is treated with aggressive antibiotic therapy combined with surgical debridement and later reconstruction. An urgent opinion should be sought if this condition is suspected.

Skin tumours

The skin tumours of basal cell carcinoma (raised, rolled, pearly edge with overlying telangiectasia and central pit or ulcer) (Fig. 21), squamous cell carcinoma (initially scaly lesion, enlarging, deepening and ulcerating

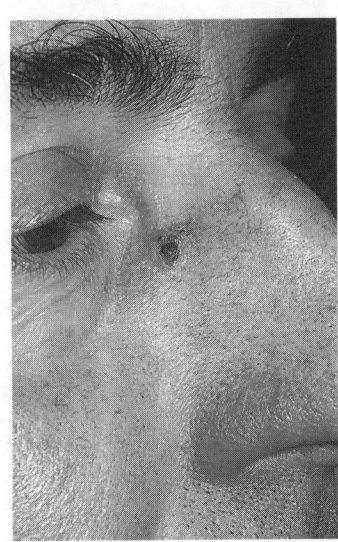

Fig. 21. Basal cell carcinoma of the right side of the nose.

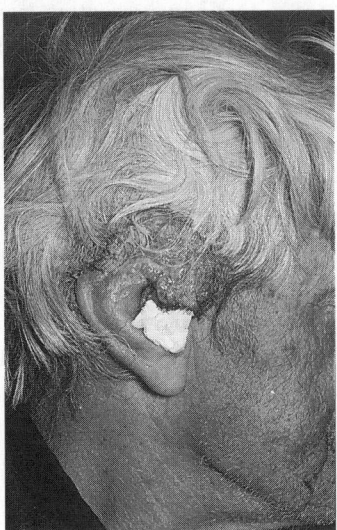

Fig. 22. Squamous cell carcinoma of the ear with actinic skin change on the face.

to form an irregular indurated persistent ulcer) (Fig. 22), and melanoma (irregularly pigmented lesion with uneven borders, which itches, continues to grow, has surrounding erythema and occasionally bleeds or crusts) are usually readily recognized and should be referred for an urgent out-patient appointment for biopsy and definitive surgical treatment.

Temporal or giant cell arteritis presents with linear, tender, swollen, red skin overlying the affected artery in patients over 50 years of age. The ESR is markedly raised to values around $100\ \text{mm}\,h^{-1}$. Treatment is with high-dose steroids after biopsy of the affected artery.

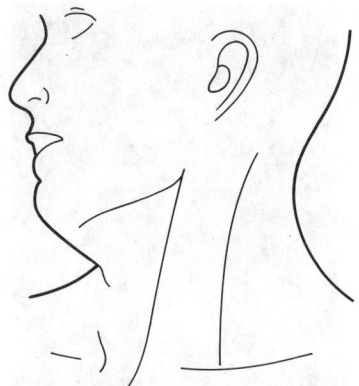

Fig. 23. The anterior and posterior triangles of the neck are separated by the sternomastoid muscle.

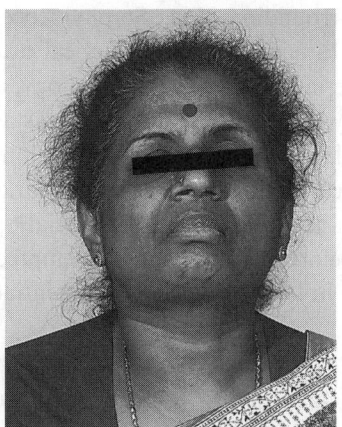

Fig. 24. Submandibular lymph node enlargement in sarcoidosis.

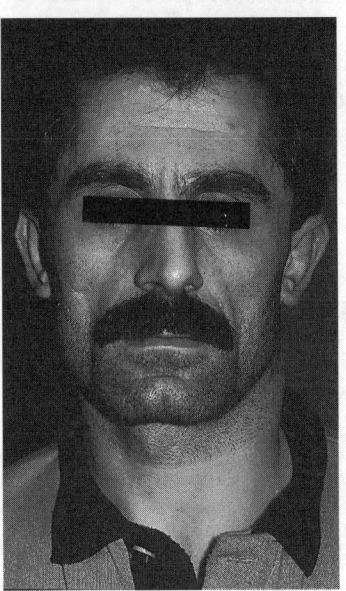

Fig. 25. Left posterior triangle lymphadenopathy in tuberculosis.

Neck lumps

Presentation

Neck lumps are a common presenting symptom. They are usually enlarged lymph glands or soft tissue abscesses secondary to primary pathology in the drainage area. However, there are many other sources of pathology in this region. The easiest method of recognition is to classify lumps anatomically: those lumps that are only found in the anterior triangle, and those that can be found in both anterior and posterior triangles. Pathological lesions common to both include lymph nodes, skin lesions, lipomas, vascular and nerve lesions. The anterior and posterior triangles are divided by the sternomastoid muscle (Fig. 23).

Structures found in the anterior triangle only, include the salivary glands (parotid tail and submandibular), second branchial arch remnants, the thyroid gland and the carotid artery and jugular vein.

Investigations

Investigations for the drainage area of lymph nodes and abscesses have been listed in the sections above. The neck lumps themselves can be investigated by ultrasound to determine whether they are cystic or solid, and plain radiology for air–fluid levels or calcification. Fine-needle aspiration is used to obtain culture and cytological material, and for distinguishing between solid and fluid-filled lesions.

Cervical lymphadenopathy

When the patient has persistent cervical lymph node enlargement and is generally unwell, blood should be taken for full blood count, Paul–Bunnell or monospot, cytomegalovirus titres and toxoplasma dye test to exclude infectious mononucleosis. Liver function tests and immunoelectrophoresis may be abnormal in lymphoma although the diagnosis is best made with fine-needle cytology followed up by open biopsy. Serum angiotensin converting enzyme, the Kveim test and a chest radiograph should be arranged when sarcoidosis is suspected (Fig. 24). In tuberculosis, intradermal Heaf or Mantoux tests supplement cytology of the nodes in suggesting the diagnosis (Fig. 25). Plain radiology of the neck rarely shows calcification (Fig. 26). A chest radiograph may show opacities suggestive of tuberculosis, and daily sputum and early morning urine specimens for 3 days sometimes yield positive tubercle bacillus cultures. However, open biopsy of the affected node is often

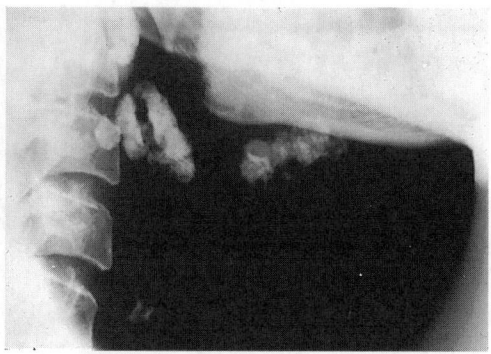

Fig. 26. Lateral neck radiograph showing calcified tuberculous lymph nodes.

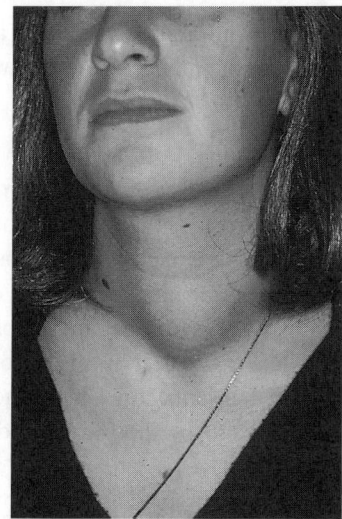

Fig. 27. Left solitary thyroid nodule.

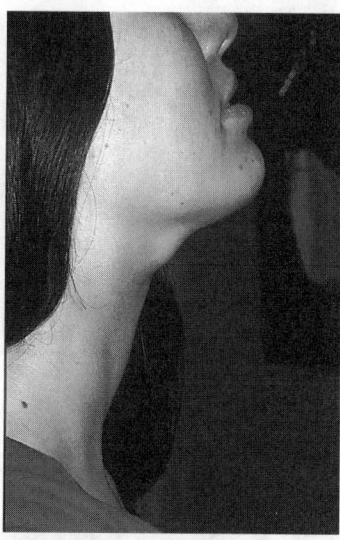

Fig. 28. Midline thyroglossal duct cyst overlying the hyoid bone.

necessary to confirm the diagnosis. In open lymph node biopsies, wherever indicated and when possible, one specimen should be sent to histopathology and one to microbiology. Both specimens should be sent fresh and not in fixative.

Thyroid swellings

With diffuse thyroid enlargement, blood is sent for thyroid function tests and autoantibodies, and an ultrasound is arranged to exclude any potentially neoplastic nodules. If the patient presents with a solitary thyroid nodule (Fig. 27), then fine-needle cytology and nuclear medicine (technetium or radioiodine) scans are added to the previous investigations.

Thyroglossal duct cysts

Thyroglossal duct cysts may be recognized by their position in the midline of the neck between the thyroid gland and hyoid bone (Fig. 28). They usually move with swallowing but rarely move with tongue protrusion. Fine-needle cytology and ultrasound confirm the diagnosis.

Carotid body tumours

The carotid body tumour is rare but can mislead the unwary. It occurs at the site of one of the most commonly enlarged lymph nodes in the jugulodigastric region and can therefore be mistakenly diagnosed as simple cervical lymphadenopathy. However, the carotid body tumour can usually be compressed and will return to full size with three arterial pulsations. Also, it is often visible, expanding the ipsilateral lateral oropharyngeal wall (Fig. 29a) (Dickinson *et al.*, 1986). If there is any doubt, angiography will confirm the diagnosis (Fig. 29b). Carotid body tumours may rarely secrete catecholamines. Therefore, when the carotid body tumour has been diagnosed, urinary vanillylmandelic acid levels should be measured.

CT and MRI have a distinct role in surgical planning for neck lumps and in staging of lymphoma (Fig. 30), along with bone marrow aspirates. However, they are usually not important in diagnosis.

Treatment

With most isolated neck lumps not caused by primary pathology elsewhere, there is no necessity for treatment

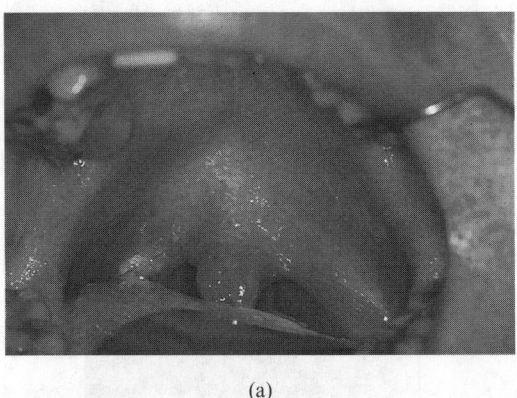

(a)

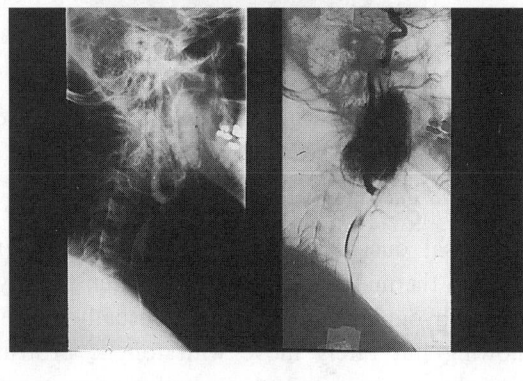

(b)

Fig. 29. This patient presented with a neck mass. (a) Intraoral examination revealed that the mass extended into the pharynx. (b) Arteriography confirmed the diagnosis of carotid body tumour.

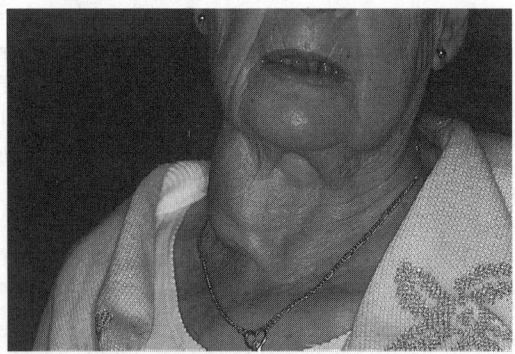

Fig. 30. Non-Hodgkin's lymphoma infiltrating and enlarging the cervical lymph nodes.

in the A&E department and the patient should simply be referred to the oral and maxillofacial surgeons for definitive management. The two most useful, cheap and rapidly available investigations in neck lumps are ultrasound and fine-needle aspiration cytology.

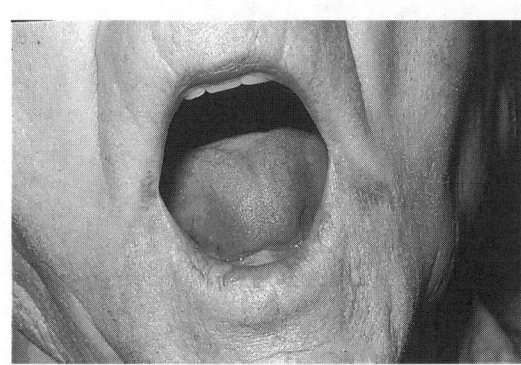

Fig. 31. Sores at the mouth angles associated with iron deficiency and colonised by *Candida albicans* (angular cheilitis).

SPECIFIC ORGANISMS

This section does not comprehensively cover all organisms affecting the face, mouth and neck but deals with the most significant.

Candida albicans

This organism is part of the normal oral flora. It overgrows in stagnant areas such as the mucosa underlying dentures when patients do not leave their dentures out overnight, and in creases at the angles of the mouth (angular cheilitis) (Fig. 31). It is also troublesome in immunosuppressed patients on chemotherapy, those receiving radiotherapy to the head and neck, and diabetics.

It presents in the mouth as white curds overlying raw, red mucosa. Scrapings sent for culture yield the diagnosis. The patient is treated with topical antifungal agents such as nystatin and amphotericin B administered as pastilles, creams or mouthwashes. Any underlying medical condition, such as uncontrolled diabetes, should be corrected. Edentulous patients should be instructed to leave their dentures in dilute hypochlorite solutions overnight.

Herpes simplex

This organism is endemic. Most people do not suffer a significant disease on first exposure. However, acute herpetic gingivostomatitis can occur at first exposure or occasionally as a recurrence in debilitated or immunosuppressed patients. In this, the patient has widespread mouth and throat ulcers, a pronounced fever and is usually unable to take any fluid or food by mouth because of the severe pain (Fig. 32). Viral cultures from swabs of ulcers are diagnostic but supportive treatment is instituted immediately. The patient frequently requires admission

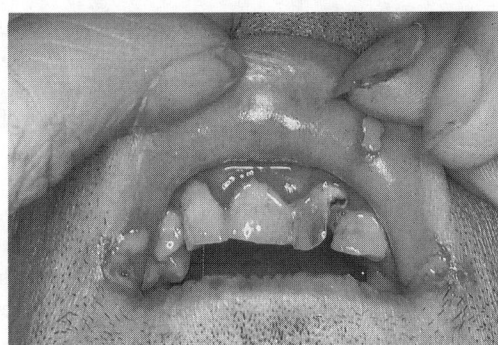

Fig. 32. Multiple lip and mouth ulcers in acute herpetic gingivosto-matitis.

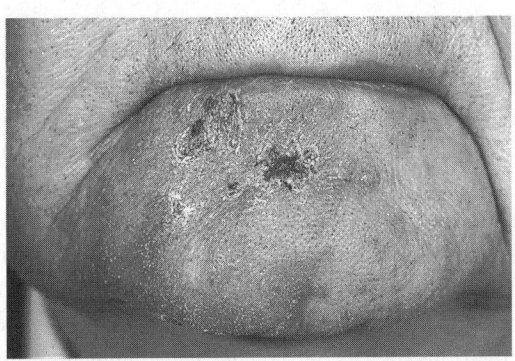

Fig. 33. Involvement of the mandibular division of the trigeminal nerve by herpes zoster with crusting of the affected side of the lower lip.

for intravenous fluid replacement. Topical analgesics such as benzydamine, or anaesthetic gels such as ligno-caine, are used to control pain, and aspirin or paracetamol are used to reduce the fever. Specific antiviral agents (e.g. acyclovir) are used systemically to shorten the duration of the acute attack and minimize the the possibility of complications such as corneal ulceration and herpetic encephalitis.

Recurrent herpes simplex infections usually present as 'cold sores' at mucocutaneous junctions such as the lip and nose. Small blisters form which rapidly burst leaving the classic crusted appearance. The patient has an initial tingling sensation at the site followed by mild pain and discomfort when the blisters burst and before the crust forms. Viral cultures confirm the diagnosis. The patient may be treated with barrier ointments such as petroleum jelly, or topical acyclovir.

Herpes zoster

Chicken pox affects most children as a short-lived, self-limiting disease with blistering followed by crusting of the trunk and face associated with fever and malaise. Shingles usually affects adults and the immunosuppressed. Any division of the trigeminal nerve can be involved (Fig. 33). The patient presents with vesicles along the distribution of the nerve; for example, if the maxillary division is affected, then half the palate is covered with vesicles and ulcers. In the Ramsay Hunt syndrome the facial nerve is affected. There may be some crusting around the ear and the patient has a facial nerve palsy. The patient usually experiences a prodrome of pain in the area served by the nerve prior to the development of blisters.

Treatment is with a systemic course of acyclovir. Some authorities supplement this in Ramsay Hunt

syndrome with a short course of steroids (Stafford & Welch, 1986).

Mycobacterium tuberculosis

The commonest presentation of tuberculosis in the head is as a persistently enlarged cervical swelling (Fig. 25). The patient is often unwell and may have a fever, night sweats and have lost weight. The patient with cervical tuberculosis does not usually have pronounced chest symptoms. Lower socioeconomic groups, diabetics and the debilitated are more frequently affected.

The 'cold' or 'collar-stud' abscess occurs much less frequently. In this, the patient is often constitutionally well but has a neck sinus which discharges intermittently. Radiographs may reveal calcification in this case (Fig. 26).

Finally, tuberculosis may present with a punched-out indolent mouth ulcer which is not particularly indurated.

The patient is investigated with fine-needle aspiration of lumps for cytology and culture, chest and cervical radiographs, sputum and urine culture, and intradermal Heaf or Mantoux tests. Ulcers should be biopsied and neck nodes may have to be biopsied for definitive diagnosis.

Treatment is with antituberculous medication.

HIV and AIDS

Patients infected with HIV can present with unexplained cervical lymphadenopathy, intraoral Kaposi's sarcoma, hairy leukoplakia, destructive acute ulcerative gingivitis, persistent oral candidiasis, or recurrent herpetic infections.

The patient should be referred immediately for counselling and investigation with their consent.

Syphilis

All stages of syphilis may manifest in the head and neck. Chancres can develop on the lips with cervical lymph node enlargement. In the second stage, snail track ulcers may occur on the oral mucosa, whilst gummata can present as deep eroding ulcers in the oral cavity in the tertiary stage. Oral cancer was thought to occur more frequently in syphilitics when syphilis was more prevalent.

The patient should have blood taken for specific investigations such as the *Treponema pallidum* immobilization test from the second stage onwards. Smears should be obtained from chancres for examination under dark ground illumination for the treponeme in the primary stage. Treatment is with penicillin.

Bibliography

ANDREASSEN, U.K., BAER, S. NIELSEN, T.G. *et al.* (1992). Acute epiglottitis—25 years experience with nasotracheal intubation, current management policy and future trends. *J. Laryngol. Otol.*, **106**, 1072–5.

DICKINSON, P.H., GRIFFIN, S.M., GUY, A.J. *et al.* (1986). Carotid body tumour: 30 years experience. *Br. J. Surg.*, **73**, 14–16.

GURALNICK, W.C. (1992). Ankylosis. In *Surgery of the Temporomandibular Joint*, 2nd edn, D.A. Keith. pp. 119–37. Boston, Blackwell Scientific.

HUDSON, J.W. (1993). Osteomyelitis of the jaws: a 50 year perspective. *J. Oral Maxillofac. Surg.*, **51**, 1294–301.

HUTCHISON, I.L. & JAMES, D.R. (1989). New treatment for Ludwig's angina. *Br. J. Oral Maxillofac. Surg.*, **27**, 83–4.

JANNETTA, P.J. (1967). Arterial compression of the trigeminal nerve at the pons in patients with trigeminal neuralgia. *J. Neurosurg. Suppl.*, **26**, 159–62.

MACARTHUR, C.J., LINDBECK, E. & JONES, D.T. (1992). Paranasal phycomycosis in the immunocompetent host. *Otolaryngol. Head Neck Surg.*, **107**, 460–2.

RUGH, J.D. & SOLBERG, W.K. (1989). Oral health status in the United States: temporomandibular disorders. *J. Dent. Educ.*, **49**, 398–405.

SCHNETLER, J. & HOPPER, C. (1989). Intracranial tumours presenting with facial pain. *Br. Dent. J.*, **166**, 80–3.

SCHUSTER, G.S. (1987). The microbiology of oral and maxillofacial infections. In *Oral and Maxillofacial Infections*, ed. R.G. Topazian & M.H. Goldberg. Philadelphia: W.B. Saunders.

STAFFORD, F.W. & WELCH, A.R. (1986). The use of acyclovir in Ramsay Hunt syndrome. *J. Laryngol. Otol.*, **100**, 337–40.

20 Ear, nose and throat emergencies

V.J. LUND and D.J. HOWARD

Institute of Laryngology & Otology, London, UK

Chapter plan

Trauma to the ear
Trauma to the nose
Trauma to the throat
Non-traumatic emergencies of the ear
Non-traumatic emergencies of the nose
Non-traumatic emergencies of the throat

Signs of ENT involvement in head injuries

- Fresh blood or cerebrospinal fluid coming from the ear, nose or nasopharynx
- Facial paralysis
- Haemotympanum or perforated tympanic membrane
- Hearing loss
- Dizziness and nystagmus

TRAUMA TO THE EAR

Auricle and external meatus

The auricle may suffer lacerations, avulsion, thermal injury, and blunt trauma resulting in haematoma. The external meatus is frequently injured by objects such as hairpins and cotton-buds used for wax removal.

History, examination and diagnosis

The cause of the problem is usually self-evident. In the case of haematoma, there is painful swelling and displacement of the auricle (Fig. 1). Otoscopic examination of the canal may reveal an injury. Specialist examination using a microscope may be required.

Management

Lacerations of the pinna should be cleaned and repaired under local anaesthesia (lignocaine 1%) and foreign

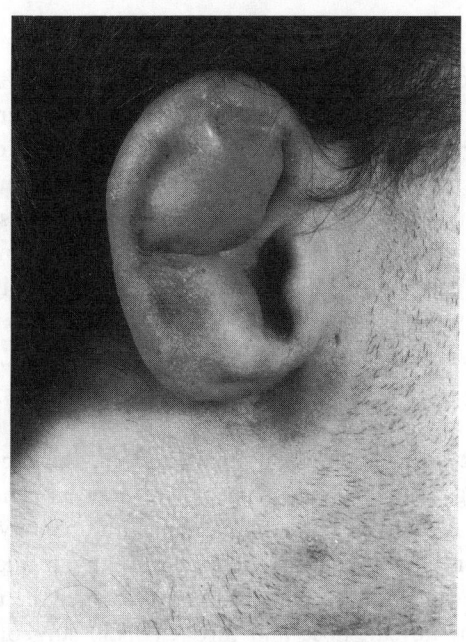

Fig. 1. A haematoma of the pinna.

debris and any obviously devitalized tissue removed. Skin sutures should be placed avoiding the underlying cartilage. Loss of up to 2 cm of the helical rim may be accepted for primary closure, though this will often require additional wedge resection of the pinna and should be referred for repair. However, if the tissue is available, even quite large portions of the ear may be reattached using appropriate reconstructive techniques if the time between injury and repair is short. In the canal, superficial abrasions will heal spontaneously but circumferential injuries may produce stenosis and require referral for suction cleaning, topical antibiotic drops and packing.

Haematoma formation between the perichondrium and pinna cartilage can lead to significant cosmetic

481

deformity due to cartilage destruction – the 'cauliflower ear' (English, 1976). The haematoma should be incised at the anterolateral aspect of the concha, drained under broad-spectrum antibiotic cover (against *Staphylococcus aureus*) and a supportive pressure dressing applied, contoured to the external ear. This should be removed daily for inspection.

Thermal injuries, such as frostbite and burns, vary in degree and can result in deep necrosis and stenosis of the external auditory meatus (Dowling *et al*, 1968; Sessions *et al*, 1971). They require the same management as elsewhere in the body, which may include skin grafting.

Middle ear

The middle ear may be damaged by penetrating injuries with sharp objects, flying debris as encountered in welding or steel mills or by blunt/barotrauma during water sports, flying, blast injuries or overzealous ear syringing (Kerr & Smyth, 1987). These can result in perforation of the eardrum, ossicular disruption or a haemotympanum. More severe injuries will involve the inner ear and base of skull.

History and examination

The patient will complain of pain and may have noticed bleeding following the injury. There may be a hearing loss; examination of the tympanic membrane may show a perforation, though blood can prevent an adequate view and necessitate suction clearance under the microscope by an ear, nose and throat (ENT) surgeon. The anterior inferior quadrant of the drum is the commonest site for injury. Alternatively the drum may be intact but the middle ear is filled with blood, giving the drum a purple appearance. If the appearances are those of a 'serous' otitis media or there is clear watery otorrhoea, the possibility of cerebrospinal fluid (CSF) leak should be considered. Similarly the presence of vertigo, nystagmus and facial paralysis is more indicative of damage to the inner ear.

Under these circumstances syringing and other manipulations in the external canal should not be performed.

Investigation

Any significant injury to the ear requires specialist assessment to determine the degree of damage and the

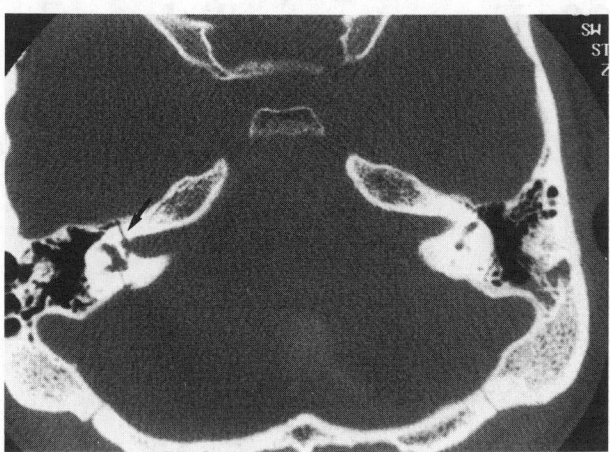

Fig. 2. Axial CT scan of petrous temporal bone showing a transverse fracture.

need for urgent surgical intervention. These investigations will include adequate examination under the microscope, audiometry and imaging to exclude fractures of the base of skull and disruption of the ossicular chain. The hearing loss may be conductive, sensorineural or mixed, depending upon the type of injury.

Management

The majority of cases will require an ENT opinion. Most perforations of the drum will heal spontaneously and require only simple cleaning under the microscope and short-term administration of topical antibiotic drops. However, it is always necessary to exclude the possibility of ossicular disruption even in the presence of an intact drum as this usually requires surgical reconstruction. Incudostapedial joint disruption is the commonest ossicular injury. A haemotympanum will generally resolve spontaneously, though occasionally myringotomy is required to relieve pain and improve hearing.

Inner ear and fractures of temporal bone

Forty-five per cent of fractures of the base of skull extend to the temporal bone and may affect the middle and inner ear. Thus in any head injury the ears should be examined at the earliest opportunity (Hough, 1970). Damage to the temporal bone may result from direct penetrating injuries such as gunshot wounds or blunt external trauma as in road traffic accidents. Fractures are divided into longitudinal, extending along the pyramidal axis to the middle ear, or transverse, crossing the axis into the bony labyrinth and internal auditory meatus (Fig. 2). Combinations of these may occur and in all cases there is the potential for direct intracranial communication and spread of infection via dural tears.

History and examination

Longitudinal fractures These present with a haemotympanum, tympanic perforation, bleeding from the external auditory canal, possible change in contour of the canal walls and hearing loss. Facial paralysis occurs in about 20% of cases.

Transverse fractures The drum and contours of the canal are intact though a haemotympanum may be found. Hearing loss and vertigo are evident, with spontaneous nystagmus beating towards the healthy ear. Facial paralysis is more common, occurring in at least half of patients, and CSF leak may occur down the eustachian tube, though this can be difficult to detect.

Sometimes facial paralysis may be delayed (>6 h), resulting from oedema of the nerve sheath and compression. It should also be noted that, even in the absence of any otological and radiological abnormalities, patients may experience hearing loss and vertigo due to labyrinthine concussion.

Diagnosis

Otoscopic examination, specialized imaging and evaluation of facial nerve function are required.

Management

The most important factor in the accident and emergency (A&E) department is to recognize the potential of the situation and obtain specialist advice. Prophylactic antibiotics are mandatory when any suspicion exists of a base of skull fracture. They are given parenterally, in high doses to avoid otogenic meningitis.

Barotrauma and acute acoustic trauma

Sudden changes in air pressure during flying or diving can cause bleeding in the middle ear cavity and tympanic perforation (Head, 1976). In severe cases disruption of the round window and ossicles may occur. The ear may also be injured by the gas emboli occurring in decompression sickness. Exposure to loud noise can specifically injure the cochlea.

Diagnosis and management

Depending upon the predominant site of injury, the patient experiences acute otalgia, pulsating tinnitus, deafness and vertigo. All require specialist management.

TRAUMA TO THE NOSE

Because of its prominent position, the nose is frequently injured and the commonest facial fracture is that of the nasal bones. The nose may sustain a circumscribed injury such as a punch or be involved in more severe midfacial trauma as in a road traffic accident.

Fractures may be linear (lateral, frontal or frontolateral) or severely comminuted 'smash' fractures involving frontal and lacrimal bones, orbital rim and ethmoid including the cribriform plate (Maran & Lund, 1990). A C-shaped fracture of the nasal septum frequently accompanies injuries to the nasal bones and the upper lateral cartilages are often displaced. Sometimes only the septum is affected, though this may still affect the external appearance of the tip and columella.

The injury is usually closed, though open fractures can occur with facial abrasions exposing the underlying nasal skeleton.

History and examination

The nature and timing of the injury should be elicited with information regarding any pre-existing nasal deformity. If the nasal bones are fractured, the injury will be rapidly followed by a change in shape, due to lateral dislocation or depression of the nasal bridge with soft tissue swelling and bruising.

The patient will complain of pain, nasal obstruction and epistaxis and will experience pain on pressure applied to the nasal pyramid. Crepitation of the bony fragments and even abnormal mobility of the external nose may be evident. The degree of internal swelling may be determined using a large aural speculum on an otoscope (with the glass eye-piece removed) placed in the nasal vestibule and this should be performed to exclude the presence of a septal haematoma.

Investigation and diagnosis

Deformity can be masked by the degree of soft tissue swelling which rapidly develops. Radiography of the nasal pyramid is often unhelpful and requires experienced interpretation. Lateral soft tissue (with dental film) and

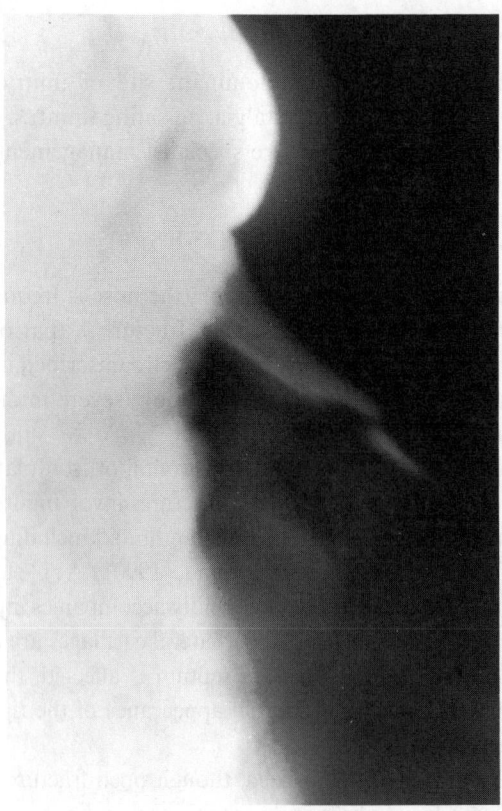

Fig. 3. Lateral X-ray showing fractured nasal bones. (Courtesy of T.R. Bull & G.A.S. Lloyd.

superoinferior (occlusal) views are the preferred method, but X-rays are generally performed to exclude the presence of impacted foreign bodies, to demonstrate more major trauma to the facial skeleton and for medicolegal reasons (Fig. 3).

Management

In the A&E department any abrasions should be cleaned and the edges of any lacerations approximated once the presence of foreign material has been excluded. Broad-spectrum antibiotics should be given in the case of open fractures.

If the patient is seen within 1–2 h of the injury it may be possible to easily reduce the fracture under sedation, but most cases present with significant swelling preventing a clear assessment of the deformity and they are consequently referred to an ENT surgeon for manipulation under general anaesthesia. This should ideally be performed within 10 days of the injury at which time the nasal septum can also be dealt with.

If a septal haematoma is suspected, this should be referred immediately for drainage under antibiotic cover

to avoid necrosis of septal cartilage and resultant saddling of the nasal bridge and retraction of the columella. More complex comminuted injuries may require soft tissue debridement and fixation of the bony fragments.

In young patients in whom a greenstick fracture may prove difficult to detect and can have serious long-term effects on midfacial development, specialist referral is recommended.

Complications

Serious cosmetic and functional problems can result from nasal trauma due to inadequate management or secondary infection, so an ENT opinion is advisable in most circumstances. Anosmia may result from the shearing effect at the cribriform plate and this may be accompanied by a CSF leak. Unilateral watery discharge increased or provoked by bending the head forwards requires treatment with antibiotics and referral for investigation.

TRAUMA TO THE THROAT

The mouth

The soft tissues of the mouth may be injured accidentally by small children with sharp objects such as wire coat hangers, or by falling whilst sucking a pencil, ice lolly or similar object. In adults the tongue may be bitten during fights and in accidents.

History and examination

The cause is usually self-evident but assessment of the extent of the injury may be difficult if the patient is uncooperative. It is important to ensure that no foreign material is left impacted in the tissues. Quite severe bleeding can occur from the tongue and tonsil region and this combined with oedema of the soft tissues may compromise the airway.

Management

The primary objectives are to protect the airway, stop haemorrhage and repair the damage. In severe cases, intubation will be difficult in a sea of blood so if there is concern for the airway a cricothyroidotomy or tracheostomy is preferable and will allow immediate assessment and intervention. However, in the majority of cases the injury requires no action as small lacerations will heal and one only needs to ensure that subsequent oedema and infection do not pose problems by administration of antibiotics and steroids. Small children are usually admitted overnight to observe their airway.

TECHNIQUES

Tracheostomy and cricothyroidotomy

Tracheostomy may be performed under a number of circumstances: as an emergency for immediate resuscitation, under local anaesthesia or as an elective procedure. Only the first is strictly relevant to the A&E department. Cricothyroidotomy can also be employed when immediate establishment of the airway is needed and endotracheal intubation is not possible (Howard, 1991). It has the advantage of speed and ease and requires little surgical experience. However, it should be regarded only as a temporary holding measure until more formal access to the airway can be achieved. It may be of use when other injuries prevent or contraindicate extension of the neck.

Objective
● To secure and maintain the airway.

Indications
● Mechanical obstruction:

  – Congenital anomalies, e.g. subglottic stenosis.
  – Infection/inflammation of upper aerodigestive tract.
  – Trauma.
  – Inhaled foreign bodies.
  – Obstructive tumours.
  – Bilateral paralysis of vocal cords.

● Retained secretions in lower respiratory tract.
● Prophylactically in major head and neck surgery.

Contraindications
● There are no specific contraindications to tracheostomy, assuming the necessary expertise of the operator.
● Cricothyroidotomy is inappropriate if there is subglottic pathology, and in children. It may be associated with an increased incidence of subglottic stenosis.

Preoperative investigations
● If time allows:

  – Inspection and palpation of the neck.
  – Indirect and/or direct laryngoscopy.
  – Laryngeal tomography.
  – Assessment of pulmonary function.

Emergency tracheostomy (Figs 4 and 5)

The patient lies supine with the neck extended and some padding under the shoulders unless this position is contraindicated.
● The head is kept in the midline and the landmarks of the neck palpated.

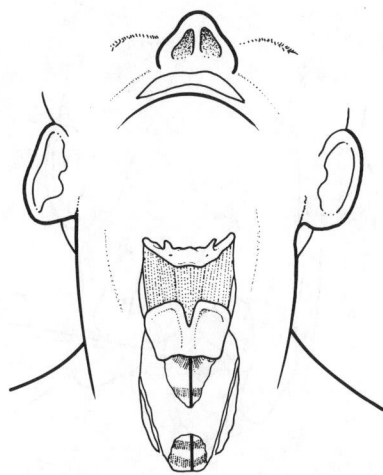

Fig. 4. Schematic drawing showing landmarks, position of patient and site of skin incision for emergency tracheostomy. (Reproduced with permission, from Howard, D.J. (1991). Emergency and elective airway procedures: tracheostomy, cricothyroidotomy and their variants. In *Rob & Smith's Operative Surgery. Head & Neck*, Part 1, ed. I.A. Mcgregor & D.J. Howard pp. 27–44. London: Butterworth-Heinemann.)

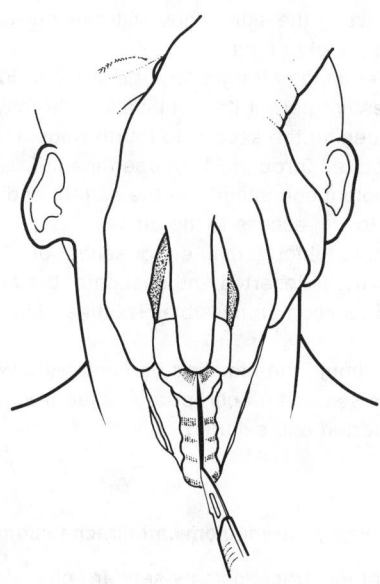

Fig. 5. Schematic drawing showing vertical incision in trachea following vertical skin incision. (Reproduced with permission, from Howard, D.J. (1991). Emergency and elective airway procedures: tracheostomy, cricothyroidotomy and their variants. In *Rob & Smith's Operative Surgery. Head & Neck*, Part 1, ed. I.A. Mcgregor & D.J. Howard pp. 27–44 London: Butterworth-Heinemann.)

● A vertical midline incision is made from the inferior aspect of the thyroid cartilage to the suprasternal notch straight down through the muscles.
Considerable haemorrhage will occur but other than suction, no attempt should be made to stop it.

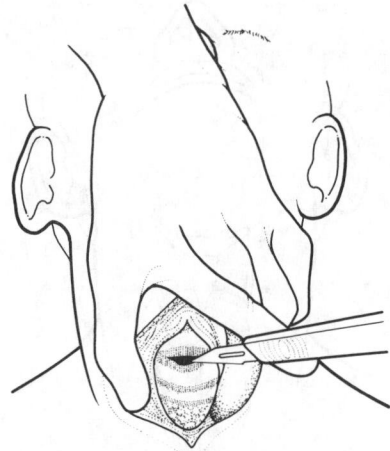

Fig. 6. Schematic drawing showing position of incision in cricothyroid membrane for cricothyroidotomy. (Reproduced with permission, from Howard, D.J. (1991). Emergency and elective airway procedures: tracheostomy, cricothyroidotomy and their variants. In *Rob & Smith's Operative Surgery. Head & Neck*, Part 1, ed. I.A. Mcgregor & D.J. Howard pp. 27–44 London: Butterworth-Heinemann.)

- The cricoid cartilage is found with the index finger whilst retracting the skin edges with pressure from the thumb and middle finger.
- A cut is then made straight through the thyroid isthmus, if time does not permit its mobilization, directly into the trachea, opening the second to fourth rings and the blade is rotated through 90° to open the cut. This will provoke violent coughing from the patient and there is a danger of losing access to the airway.
- Any available tubing (small endotracheal or tracheostomy) is inserted and suction of the airway performed as soon as possible. Tracheal dilators can be useful.
- Only then should the bleeding be dealt with. When the situation is stable, an appropriate cuffed tracheostomy tube is inserted and secured.

Cricothyroidotomy (laryngotomy,minitracheostomy) (Fig. 6)

- A variety of minitracheostomy sets are now available but in extremis this procedure can be performed with a scapel alone plus a pair of curved artery forceps and small tube.
- The neck is extended if possible and the area between the prominence of the thyroid and cricoid cartilages palpated with the index finger of the free hand.
- A vertical incision is made straight down to the cricothyroid membrane and a 1 cm transverse cut made in it.
- The blade is turned through 90° and the tube inserted. A tracheal hook or dilators will aid this manoeuvre.
- In an elective situation a transverse skin incision is preferable and attention can be paid to haemostasis.

- Once the airway is secured, direct laryngoscopy may enable intubation or it may be necessary to proceed to a tracheostomy.

Complications

The postoperative care and complications of tracheostomy are beyond the scope of this book. Intraoperative and early problems include:

- *Haemorrhage.* This should be carefully controlled as soon as the airway is secured.
- *Injury to paratracheal structures.* Dissection lateral to the trachea should be avoided as damage to the carotid vessels and recurrent laryngeal nerves may result. Hyperextension of the neck, particularly in children, renders the pleural domes and left brachiocephalic veins vulnerable.
- *Unnessary injury to the trachea.*
- *Apnoea.* This may occur in patients with prolonged respiratory difficulty due to a sudden fall in carbon dioxide. Administration of 5% carbon dioxide may be required with monitoring of blood gases.
- *Subcutaneous emphysema, pneumothorax.* If the tracheostomy or trachea becomes obstructed, or the skin edges of the wound are closed tightly, massive surgical emphysema, pneumothorax and pneumomediastinum can occur.
- *Accidental extubation or anterior placement of the tube.* The greatest care must be taken in placement and securing of any tube, however temporary.

Larynx and trachea

Trauma of the larynx and trachea is frequently life-threatening and may leave the patient with permanent airway problems and dysphonia (Maran *et al.*, 1981). The injury may be blunt from impaction on dashboard or steering wheel, from a fist or foot, by running into a stretched wire, or from attempted hanging or strangulation. Penetrating injuries can also occur (e.g. from gunshot wounds). Thus the injury may be open or closed and may involve other structures.

Varying degrees of damage to the laryngeal skeleton may occur, from a simple contusion to complete laryngo-tracheal separation. The cricoarytenoid joint may be dislocated and the hyoid, thyroid and cricoid cartilages may fracture.

History and examination

The degree of pain, hoarseness and dyspnoea will vary with the extent of the injury. In a simple contusion these symptoms will be slight with some tenderness over the larynx. However, depending upon the urgency of the situation, any laryngeal injury should be examined by an

ENT surgeon as soon as practicable to determine oedema, haematoma formation and loss of vocal cord mobility. This can be done by indirect laryngoscopy or preferably by flexible fibreoptic nasendoscopy.

Dislocation of the cricoarytenoid joint may also be associated with dysphagia, and aspiration and examination of the larynx will reveal the abnormal arytenoid and vocal cord position. Fractures of the laryngeal skeleton produce severe pain, dyspnoea, hoarseness or aphonia, stridor, swelling and surgical emphysema. Indeed, few survive a fracture of the cricoid due to the rapid development of a circumferential haematoma within the solid cartilage ring. The fracture contour may be evident though it is often obscured by oedema. There may be ecchymosis of the skin, dysphagia and haemoptysis.

Serious disruption of the laryngeal skeleton and laryngotracheal separation lead rapidly to respiratory obstruction.

Investigations

Securing the airway must take precedence over all else in the acute situation, but if time permits soft tissue X-rays (posteroanterior and lateral) including high-kilovolt films of the neck, may show obvious disruption of the laryngeal skeleton, which is usually partially calcified, and/or free air within the soft tissues.

A chest X-ray is mandatory to check for mediastinal emphysema or a pneumothorax.

Once the situation is stable, direct laryngoscopy under general anaesthetic and a CT (computed tomography) scan of the larynx will determine the extent of the injury.

Management

In the case of mild contusions, a combination of observation, steroids and oxygen/helium mixtures will often suffice. However, if the airway is compromised, the course of action lies between intubation, tracheostomy or cricothyroidotomy. In the presence of a distorted and oedematous larynx, an external approach is advised and the choice will then be determined by the experience of the operator and the urgency of the situation. Ancillary treatment includes antibiotics and steroids.

Formal repair will be required once the situation is stabilized.

Pharynx and oesophagus

The upper digestive tract can be injured in similar ways to and in combination with the larynx and trachea.

History and examination

Pain and dysphagia result with haemoptysis and/or haematemesis depending on the site of bleeding. Crepitus from subcutaneous emphysema may be palpable though sometimes such injuries are silent or obscured by accompanying problems and may present later as a retropharyngeal abscess or mediastinitis.

Investigations

Soft tissue (posteroanterior and lateral) X-rays may show air in the oesophagus or expansion of the retropharyngeal tissues. An ENT opinion should be requested if in any doubt, and direct pharyngo-oesophagoscopy performed.

Management

Whilst the nature of the injury is being established, the patient should be kept nil by mouth, receive fluid replacement and, if appropriate, antibiotics. The patient is usually admitted, at least overnight, and an ENT opinion sought.

Fortunately most perforations will heal spontaneously without major sequelae if the patient is fed via a nasogastric tube and given intravenous antibiotics, but the possibility of abscess formation and mediastinal infection should always be kept in mind (Drakeley, 1987). Retro- or parapharyngeal abscesses require formal drainage which should never be attempted in the A&E department.

NON-TRAUMATIC EMERGENCIES OF THE EAR

Wax and foreign bodies

Wax is naturally carried out of the external canal by the movement of the squamous epithelium. Unfortunately many patients prefer to assist nature, leading to impaction of wax, loss of cotton-bud ends in the ear canal and trauma. Other individuals, particularly small children, place a variety of objects in the external auditory meatus and often present to the A&E officer.

History and examination

It is often possible to see the object with an otoscope though infection and bleeding may obscure the view. An obstructed canal will produce symptoms of deafness, and occasionally pain.

Management

If the object is visible and the individual cooperative, it may be possible to remove it without assistance. However, attempts with a simple pair of forceps tend to push the foreign body further in. It is much easier to extract it with a wax hook placed beyond the object. If in doubt, refer to an ENT colleague as there is little point in unsucessfully traumatizing the ear and the patient.

Some foreign bodies and wax can often be sucessfully syringed out using gentle irrigation with water at 37°C. However, this should only be done if there is no possibilty of a tympanic perforation; if the wax is hard and impacted, specialist referral is recommended. In children a short general anaesthetic is often required.

Infection

Otitis externa and furuncle

Non-specific infection of the external auditory canal can be caused by trauma or excessive water exposure and it may simply represent a form of eczema caused by irritation, although *Proteus*, *Staphylococcus*, *Pseudomonas* and anaerobes may be found (Peterkin, 1974). Localized infection of a hair follicle produces a circumscribed furuncle.

Viral infections such as herpes zoster and influenza can also affect the ear as can certain fungal agents.

History and examination

In diffuse otitis externa the canal is swollen and obstructed with debris. The pinna may also be affected in severe cases. There is offensive discharge and the ear may be itchy but rarely very painful. A furuncle by contrast is characterized by a circumscribed exquisitely painful swelling in the outer canal, with pain increased by pressure on the tragus. There may be enlargement of preauricular nodes. As furunculosis and an aggressive 'malignant' form of otitis externa can occur in diabetics, the urine always should be tested.

Herpetic vesicles can sometimes be found on the pinna, in the canal and on the drum. In severe cases, the hearing, balance and facial nerve function may be affected. A bullous myringitis which can be extremely painful can also occur in flu.

A fungal infection should be suspected if mycelial masses varying in colour from whitish yellow to black are seen in the canal.

Management

Thorough regular suction cleaning of the external canal under the microscope combined with the insertion of wicks soaked in various topical agents are the mainstay of treatment for most cases of otitis externa so referral to an ENT clinic is recommended. In addition to oral antibiotics and adequate analgesia, a furuncle may require drainage if it does not burst spontaneously.

Acute otitis media

Acute infection of the middle ear cleft is extremely common, especially in children, and is generally associated with an effusion. This may persist and is then referred to variously as serous or secretory otitis media or glue ear. Viruses such as respiratory syncytial virus or influenza virus may be the initiating pathogen, but in suppurative otitis the common upper respiratory tract organisms are *Streptococcus pneumoniae* and *Haemophilus influenzae*, though a range of others have been found.

History and examination

The patient initially experiences severe otalgia, which may dissipate if the drum perforates. This is then accompanied by some bleeding and a purulent discharge. Hearing is affected to some degree. In young children the symptoms may be more generalized, with pyrexia, irritability, general malaise and gastrointestinal disturbance as the only clues. Thus it is important to routinely examine the ears in all young children who are unwell (Howie *et al*, 1970).

Normally the pinna appears normal and there is no tenderness or swelling of the mastoid. Similarly, unless the external canal is involved, tragal pressure is not painful. The drum, if intact, will appear red and inflamed, and may bulge. There may be purulent discharge and a visible perforation. Examination of the ear, particularly in a small distressed child, can be a difficult exercise.

Management

Broad-spectrum antibiotics such as amoxycillin, erythromycin or cefaclor will cover most common upper respiratory pathogens. If the patient has already received an adequate course without resolution it is worth considering one of the agents able to overcome beta-lactamase production. Antipyretics and nasal decongestants can produce symptomatic relief.

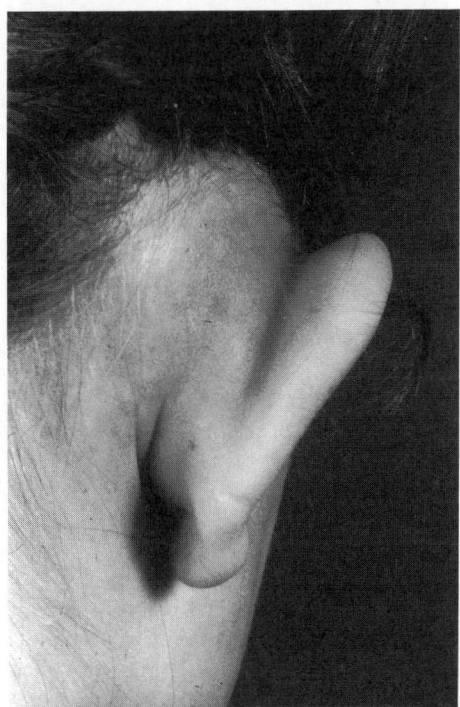

Fig. 7. Clinical photograph of patient with acute mastoiditis showing displacement of auricle with swelling over mastoid bone.

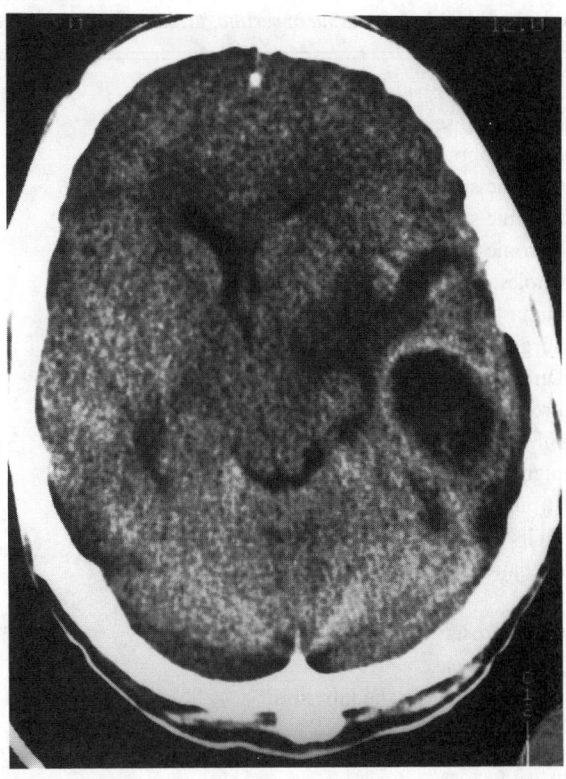

Fig. 8. Axial CT scan of brain showing temporal lobe abscess.

Myringotomy in the acute phase prior to spontaneous perforation can be helpful in reducing pain but is not as popular in the UK as in the USA.

If there is any suggestion of mastoid tenderness or swelling, or inappropriate malaise, headache or drowsiness, an ENT opinion should be sought to exclude local or intracranial complications (Fig. 7). Infection of the middle ear is still one of the commonest causes of intracranial sepsis (Fig. 8) (Gower & McGuirt, 1983).

Any adult with a persistent unilateral middle ear effusion must be referred for further investigation to exclude nasopharyngeal malignancy.

Cochleovestibular emergencies

Sudden sensorineural hearing loss

This condition is often not recognized as a medical emergency and, although it is not always possible to improve matters, the list of causes includes some for which early intervention may be worthwhile (Booth, 1987). Many cases are probably caused by viral infections but fistulae of the round and oval windows may also present in this way, as may conditions such as acoustic neuroma.

History and examination

The patient may wake with hearing loss or find that it suddenly appears after a popping sensation. This can be accompanied by loud tinnitus and vertigo but is rarely painful.

There may be few clinical signs other than the deafness. Tuning fork tests and an audiogram will clarify the sensorineural nature of the loss and a range of specialized audiological tests and imaging are usually performed to establish the diagnosis. This is obviously beyond the remit of the A&E department so specialist referral should be made.

Acute vertigo

Vertigo specifically refers to the hallucination of movement as opposed to feeling unsteady or light-headed. It is a complex problem and may result from a plethora of causes, some related to the inner ear such Menière's disease, others to more diffuse disorders of the central nervous system such as multiple sclerosis (Wright, 1988) (Table 1).

Table 1. *Conditions resulting in vertigo, dizziness or unsteadiness*

Ear conditions resulting in vertigo
Middle ear disease
    Acute suppurative otitis
    Chronic suppurative otitis media
    Chronic serous labyrinthitis
    Chronic suppurative labyrinthitis
    Cholesteatoma
Trauma to the inner ear
    Surgical
    Direct trauma to the head
    Pressure-induced damage
Menière's disease and syndrome
Benign paroxysmal positional vertigo
Vestibular neuronitis and the Ramsay Hunt syndrome
Syphilis
Miscellaneous ear conditions
    Wax
    Otosclerosis
    Paget's disease
    Drugs damaging the labyrinth

Peripheral neuropathies likely to result in unsteadiness –
caustive factors
Alcohol
Diabetes
Chronic uraemia
Drugs
    Isoniazid
    Nitrofurantoin
    Vincristine
    Gold
    Allopurinol
Organic chemicals and solvents
Heavy metals – arsenic
Vitamin deficiencies
    B complex
    B_{12}
Non-metastatic effects of carcinoma
Hypothyroidism
Spinal cord – stretching compression or disease

Central causes
Inflammation
    Meningitis
    Meningoencephalitis
    Cerebellar abscess
Trauma
    Cerebral concussion and confusion
Space-occupying processes
    Infratentorial tumours
    Cerebellopontine angle tumours
    Glomus tumours
    Arachnoid cysts

Vascular processes
    Vertebrobasilar insufficiency
    Basilar artery migraine
    Arteriovenous anomalies
Intoxication
    Barbiturates
    Alcohol
Degenerative diseases of the central nervous system
    Multiple sclerosis
    Syringobulbia
    Cerebellar degeneration

Drugs
Narcotic analgesics
    Morphine
    Dextropropoxyphene
    Codeine
    Dihydrocodeine
    Paracetamol
    Pentazocine
Psychotropics
    Tricyclic antidepressants
    Phenothiazines, e.g. chlorpromazine
    Benzodiazepines, e.g. diazepam
Anticonvulsants
    Carbamazepine
    Clonazepam
    Primidone
    Phenytoin
Antiparkinsonians
    Benzhexol
    L-Dopa

History and examination

A careful history regarding the character, duration, severity and precipitating factors of the dizziness will often point strongly towards the diagnosis. A full ENT and neurological examination is required followed by a number of audiological, vestibular and radiological investigations.

Management

In the A&E department the primary objective should be symptomatic control of the vertigo and accompanying nausea and vomiting whilst arrangements are made for further investigation and possible admission. Intravenous diazepam (5–10 mg) given slowly over 3–5 min or vestibular sedatives such as prochlorperazine by intramuscular injection or suppository may be effective.

Acute facial nerve paralysis

In the absence of obvious trauma or middle ear pathology, patients may present with sudden onset of partial or complete hemifacial paralysis, often referred to as Bell's palsy.

It is possible that a viral infection is responsible. As a proportion of cases recover spontaneously, there is some controversy as to whether medical or surgical intervention helps but it is advisable to obtain an ENT opinion if only to exclude other causes such as middle ear pathology.

NON-TRAUMATIC EMERGENCIES OF THE NOSE

Foreign bodies

An interesting variety of objects find their way into the noses of young children and the mentally retarded.

History and examination

The most important feature is a unilateral foul-smelling purulent discharge. This has often been present for some time. Soft tissue swelling and pus may obscure any view of the nasal cavity and X-rays are of limited value unless the object is known to be radio-opaque. If the history is strong enough, the individual must be referred for an ENT opinion and examination under anaesthesia.

Epistaxis

Nose bleeds can result from many conditions, both local and systemic, but the commonest cause is trauma in its many forms (Table 2). The majority of bleeds probably emanate from the front of the nasal septum (Little's area) which is the area most readily traumatized, but they can arise from any part of the nose.

History and examination

The severity of the problem will again dictate the immediate response to this condition but pertinent points in the history will include relevant medical conditions and medication, precipitating factors and previous episodes. With a profuse haemorrhage, general examination must relate primarily to establishing the vital signs and general condition of the patient as much as the precise source of the bleeding.

Table 2. *Causes of epistaxis*

Local
Idiopathic
Trauma
  Self-inflicted
  Facial fractures
  Iatrogenic – surgery
  Septal deviation
  Foreign bodies
  Septal perforation
Inflammatory – atrophic rhinitis
Infective
Tumours
  Benign, e.g. angiofibroma
  Malignant

General
Atherosclerosis
Bleeding dyscrasia
  Coagulation disorders
  – Congenital
    Haemophilia
    Christmas disease
    Von Willebrand's
  – Acquired
    Renal and liver failure
    Massive transfusion
    Vitamin deficiency
    Anticoagulants
    Myelosuppressive drugs
  Haemopoetic
    Leukaemia
    Aplastic anaemia
    Lymphoma
    Widespread metastases
Hereditary haemorrhagic telangiectasia
Endocrine
  Vicarious menstruation
  Pregnancy

Management

Adequate preparation is important in dealing with a severe nose bleed. The patient should be seated comfortably, draped with a plastic cover and given a bowl to collect the blood. The doctor should also be suitably gowned and gloved, with mask and glasses to avoid contamination. A suction device and good illumination should be to hand. If the patient has already lost a significant amount of blood, start an intravenous infusion and arrange for cross-match, full blood count, and other haematological tests such as a clotting screen if appropriate.

It may be impossible to examine the nose adequately if bleeding is profuse and bilateral, in which case simply pack the nose in the first instance with a reasonable length of 2 cm wide plain ribbon gauze (1 m or less) soaked in a vasoconstrictor and topical anaesthetic. Also, ask the patient to firmly squeeze the front of the nose for 10 min whilst leaning forwards over the bowl. This will often stop the bleeding. If it continues then a more permanent pack is required, preferably using 2 cm wide vaseline gauze. It is rarely realized that the nasal cavity can accommodate at least 2 m of packing on each side if inserted in a systematic way (Fig. 9a). In a severe bleed it is usually necessary to pack both sides of the nose and even then bleeding may continue into the nasopharynx. Under these circumstances a postnasal pack is required and is best inserted by an ENT surgeon. Alternatively a Foley catheter (18FG) can be placed in the postnasal space on each side and the balloons inflated with air or cold water, though care should be taken not to overfill them and cause swelling of the soft palate (Fig. 9b). The nose can then be repacked. The placing of ice packs on the forehead or nape of the neck to produce reflex vasoconstriction is of doubtful value.

Once the nose has been packed, the patient should be admitted for observation. Many elderly patients' respiratory reflexes are considerably compromised by occluding the nose and this, combined with the loss of blood, renders these patients vulnerable to respiratory problems. Consequently they must be monitored, preferably using an oximeter, and the temptation to oversedate or depress the respiratory drive with strong analgesics must be resisted. Similarly, hypertension will often settle with bed rest and should not be lowered therapeutically. The packs must be secured by taping them to the side of the face and must not rub on the columella which is easily traumatized. Antibiotics should be given whilst the packs are in place. If Foley catheters have been inserted, the balloons should be deflated the following day and the catheters left in place for a few hours to ensure bleeding does not restart into the nasopharynx.

On removing the packing it may be possible to see an obvious source of the bleeding on the anterior septum which is amenable to cautery, but this and subsequent follow-up should be arranged with ENT colleagues.

More modest bleeding may respond to simple pressure, followed by application of vaseline to the anterior septum twice a day for several weeks. This is frequently the case in children.

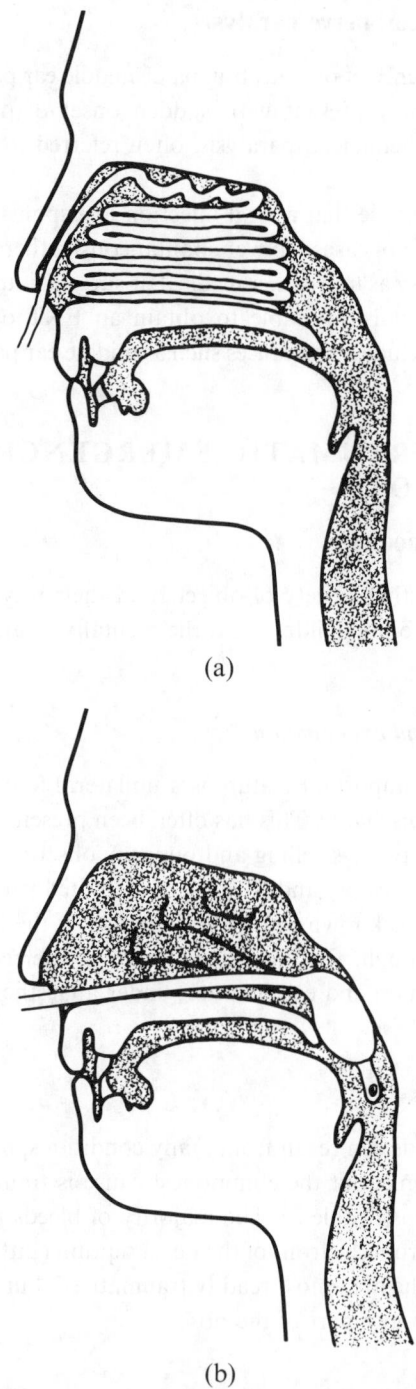

(a)

(b)

Fig. 9(a) Diagram showing placement of anterior nasal packing for epistaxis, (b) diagram showing the placement of Foley urinary catheter to control posterior nasal bleeding.

Acute sinusitis

Viral infections of the nose and sinuses are common conditions. However, viral damage to the respiratory epithelium may allow invasion by common respiratory pathogens responsible for bacterial sinusitis and otitis media such as *Streptococcus pneumoniae* and *Haemophilus influenzae* (Gwaltney & Hayden, 1982). Most infections (except those of dental origin) affect all the sinuses to a greater or lesser degree. The majority of these attacks are self-limiting or require one course of antibiotics. Occasionally they may persist in the acute form, progress to a serious complication or become chronic, when they fall into the realm of the ENT surgeon. The complications may be broadly divided into orbital, intracranial and bony. Orbital complications range from cellulitis to a localized abscess which may be extraperiosteal, intraperiosteal or simply in the anterior upper lid. As with otitis media, intracranial complications include all forms of abscess (extradural, subdural, intracerebral), cavernous sinus thrombosis, and disseminated infection (meningitis and encephalitis). It should be remembered that complications are multiple in 30% of cases and the mortality from intracranial complications, once they occur, has not changed significantly in 20 years.

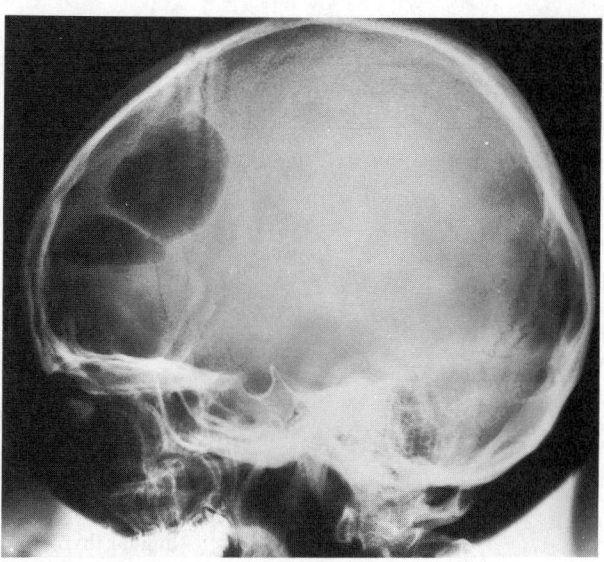

Fig. 10. Plain lateral skull X-ray showing large air-containing abscess cavity in frontal lobes in a child with orbital cellulitis secondary to acute ethmoiditis.

History, examination and investigation

In an uncomplicated case, the patient will complain of nasal obstruction, purulent discharge if the sinus is draining, facial pain, headache, general malaise and pyrexia. There may be visible pus in the nose or postnasal space. Significant swelling or tenderness over the sinuses suggest either a complication or, in the case of the maxilla, a dental abscess.

Orbital problems manifest themselves with swelling around the eye which may make it difficult to determine whether any genuine proptosis, limitation of movement or visual change has occurred. Nevertheless, it is mandatory that the eye is properly examined, however uncomfortable, as vision rarely returns once lost. The first sign is the inability to distinguish red from brown or blue from black. It can be difficult at this stage to determine whether an ophthalmic or ENT opinion is required. A plain sinus X-ray, although not completely reliable, will usually show gross change within the sinuses and may make the choice easier. However, the patient must *not* be allowed to languish in the A&E or X-ray department for several hours as the window of opportunity to decompress the eye and save vision may be lost (see Chapter 21).

The symptoms of intracranial involvement may be overlooked if the patient is complaining primarily of sinus symptoms with headache, malaise and pyrexia but signs of meningism, focal neurological signs and drowsiness should alert one to the possibility (Fig. 10).

Management

In uncomplicated cases of sinusitis, a broad-spectrum antibiotic may be given orally. If the patient has already had an adequate course of one of these, it is worth adding metronidazole as anaerobes can sometimes be present, an agent (flucloxacillin) effective against staphylococci which can be responsible for some aggressive sinus infections, or changing to a drug with beta-lactamase stability (e.g. cefuroxime axetil). Intranasal decongestants can be helpful for a few days to encourage drainage of the sinuses but should not be used long term.

If there is any doubt, an ENT opinion should be sought. It is now possible with rigid and flexible endoscopes to easily examine the nose and obtain accurate microbiology without resort to antral lavage which is less popular than in the past.

NON-TRAUMATIC EMERGENCIES OF THE THROAT

Foreign bodies

Oropharynx and hypopharynx

Foreign bodies can become lodged in any part of the upper aerodigestive tract. Sharp objects such as fish bones, pins and pen caps can be caught in the palatine or lingual tonsils and, during a road traffic accident, teeth and dental prostheses may be displaced and overlooked as attention is focused on other injuries.

Table 3. *Causes of inspiratory stridor*

Site of obstruction	Disease

Oro- and hypopharynx	Infection – diphtheria
	 – Ludwig's angina
	 – abscess
	     retropharyngeal
	     peritonsillar
	     base of tongue
	Inflammatory – angioneurotic
	     oedema
	Mechanical – posterior displace-
	     ment of tongue
	     in the uncon-
	     scious
	     –lingual thyroid
	Tumours – benign and malignant

Larynx	Congenital – laryngomalacia Infection – diphtheria – epiglottitis – croup Inflammatory – glottic oedema Laryngeal spasm Bilateral vocal cord paralysis Mechanical – foreign body Cysts and laryngocoele Tumours – benign and malignant Trauma
Trachea and bronchus	Congenital – tracheomalacia Infection – tracheitis and bronchitis Mechanical – foreign body Tumours Trauma – tracheal subluxation – tracheal stenosis

History, examination and investigations

In small children, it may be difficult to elicit a history as the initial episode may have been missed. Usually a history of pain and difficulty swallowing is given and there may be drooling. Frequently the sensation of 'something in the throat' may persist for some time after the object has been swallowed due to scratching of the mucosa, but it must never be assumed that this is the case without adequate examination. With large objects there may be associated dyspnoea and inspiratory stridor (Table 3). If there is significant airway obstruction there may be obvious intercostal and suprasternal retraction and use of accessory respiratory muscles.

Careful examination of the mouth may show a foreign body in the mouth and oropharynx though fish bones and pins can often be quite difficult to see. Indirect laryngoscopy or flexible nasendoscopy may be needed.

Plain X-rays may show a foreign body but many are not radio-opaque and a failure to show one does not exclude its presence. Occasionally the X-ray will confirm the presence of surgical emphysema from pharyngeal perforation.

Management

In a cooperative patient, with good illumination and angled forceps it may be possible to remove the object and this can sometimes be made easier with a little topical anaesthetic sprayed in the throat. However, in all but the easiest cases, ENT assistance is advisable and in children, or when the object is not readily accessible, a general anaesthetic is needed. This must be done with care as the object may move and obstruct the airway once muscle relaxation occurs.

Complete obstruction of the airway is obviously an acute emergency and only immediate action can prevent death. If aspiration of a foreign body is suspected, the Heimlich manoeuvre may displace it. This is performed by standing behind the patient, clasping the hands around them, with one hand in a fist under the diaphragm and applying a sudden upward and inward thrust over the epigastrium. If the patient is supine, apply epigastric pressure from the front. If this is unsuccessful, an emergency tracheostomy or cricothyroidotomy should be performed to secure the airway until removal of the foreign body can be performed.

Fine sharp objects may pass through the walls of the pharynx, leading to retro- and parapharyngeal abscesses which may present at a later time with dysphagia, airway obstruction, pain and prevertebral swelling on X-ray.

Oesophagus

History and examination

Foreign objects may lodge lower down the digestive tract, though many such as coins will pass through without mishap. In the elderly a large bolus of unchewed meat may stick at the cricopharyngeal sphincter. A history of problems following eating chicken, duck or lamb must be taken very seriously as long thin bones may perforate the oesophagus, causing mediastinitis and even death. Symptoms range from nothing to severe dysphagia, drooling and stridor (Drakeley, 1987). After a time the adjacent trachea becomes oedmatous, affecting the airway. The crepitus of surgical emphysema may be felt in the supraclavicular fossae.

Investigation and management

Plain X-rays of the neck and chest (posteroanterior and lateral) may show soft tissue swelling, free air or a radio-opaque object. Contrast studies with Omnipaque rather than barium (which may obscure future visualization) may aid diagnosis but, irrespective of these findings, a patient should undergo formal rigid oesophagoscopy by the ENT surgeon on the basis of a good history alone.

A large meat bolus may pass unaided if the patient is kept in overnight, but referral for further investigation is recommended to exclude the possibility of a malignant stricture.

Larynx and trachea

It is unusual for foreign bodies to lodge in the larynx, though occasionally this can occur whilst laughing and eating (e.g. throwing a whole pickled onion into the mouth). In the acute situation, a Heimlich manoeuvre and/or emergency tracheostomy or cricothyroidotomy may be required to avert disaster. Otherwise, specialized examination by indirect or flexible laryngoscopy followed by direct laryngoscopy under general anaesthesia will be needed.

Bronchi

It is extremely important to treat seriously all patients claiming to have inhaled foreign material. In children the initial episode may have been missed and the only complaint is a cough, stridor, or pyrexia due to localized infection. Unilateral chest symptoms, such as wheeze and decreased or absent breath sounds are suspicious and there may be evidence of mediastinal shift.

The chest X-ray may occasionally show a radio-opaque object but more often evidence of obstructive emphysema, segmental collapse or mediastinal shift (Fig. 11). Posteroanterior and lateral views, including inspiratory and expiratory films, should be obtained and right and left lateral decubitus views may show absence of volume loss on the dependent side with partially obstructing objects.

The extent of collapse will depend upon the position of the foreign body. Objects commonly, but not exclus-

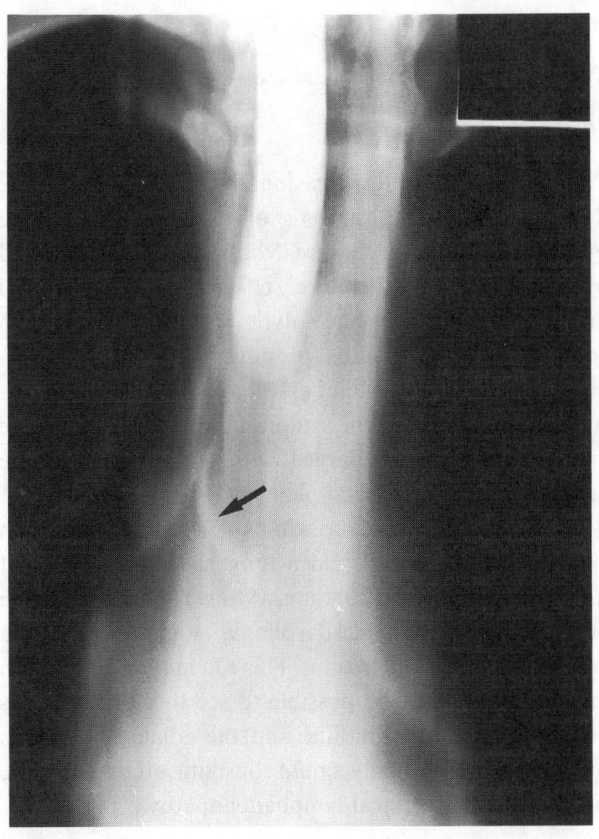

(a)

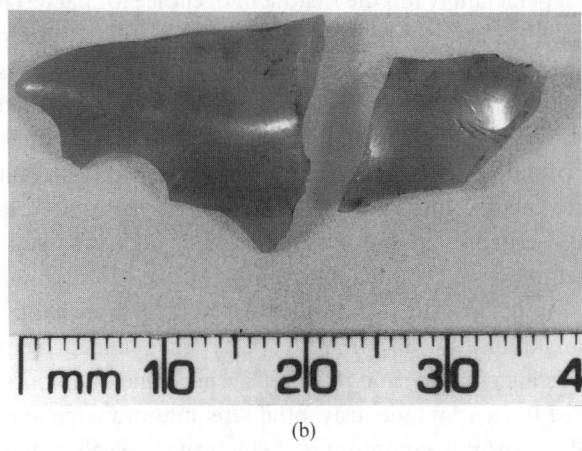

(b)

Fig. 11(a) Hilar tomogram showing foreign body at carina. (b) Piece of denture aspirated during a road traffic accident, found overlying the carina at bronchoscopy.

ively, lodge in the right main bronchus. It should be remembered that vegetable material such as peanuts create a considerable local reaction after a short time.

Referral for bronchoscopy is mandatory in all such cases.

Infections

Tonsillitis and peritonsillar abscess

History and examination

Patients with tonsillitis occasionally present to the A&E department if the symptoms of pain, dysphagia and pyrexia are sufficiently severe. Many episodes are caused by viruses and are, therefore, self-limiting, but bacterial infection with a beta-haemolytic streptococcus is also common. Viral tonsillitis produces little obvious abnormality other than slight erythema of the oropharynx. In bacterial tonsillitis, the symptoms are somewhat worse and the tonsils are enlarged with a purulent exudate and a generalized marked pharyngitis.

A peritonsillar abscess or quinsy most often occurs in a patient who has not had a long history of recurrent tonsillitis (Herbild & Bonding, 1981). The pain is severe and there is significant dysphagia, sometimes with a drooling of saliva and trismus. This can make examination difficult, but it may be possible to see that one tonsil is pushed towards the midline and the adjacent palate is bulging. There is usually a mild tonsillitis on the opposite side and tender cervical lymphadenopathy.

Management

Oral penicillin is still the treatment of choice for bacterial tonsillitis but dysphagia can be sufficiently bad to require admission for rehydration and systemic antibiotics. As infectious mononucleosis can also produce a marked tonsillitis, ampicillin should not be used as it may precipitate a rash. It should also be remembered that occasionally blood dyscrasias (leukaemia, aplastic anaemia) may present in this way, as can the odd rarity such as diphtheria. A unilateral lesion of the tonsil must always be investigated further to exclude malignancy. Many quinsies will settle with conservative management consisting of intravenous fluid replacement and antibiotics. Some burst spontaneously, others require drainage and, if the airway is compromised, emergency tonsillectomy is sometimes performed. More usually the patient is offered tonsillectomy at a later date if more than one peritonsillar abscess develops.

Ludwig's angina

History and examination

Cellulitis or a localized abscess of the floor of the mouth may arise following trauma or dental infection. It can produce significant pain, drooling, dysphagia and airway obstruction, together with obvious swelling of the intraoral tissues.

Management

These patients normally require hospitalization, intravenous fluid, antibiotics and careful observation of the airway. Localized collections of pus may require drainage and breathing may be improved by use of a nasopharyngeal airway, Occasionally intubation or even tracheostomy/cricothyroidotomy is necessary.

Epiglottitis

This infection is caused mainly by *Haemophilus influenzae* type B and is commonest in children between 3 and 6 years old, although adults may be affected.

History and examination

Dysphagia, drooling and pyrexia develop rapidly. Food and fluid are refused and the patient sits upright with the neck thrown forward and obvious inspiratory stridor. The speech is thick – the so-called 'hot potato' voice of supraglottic swelling (Baxter, 1967).

It is important to realize that attempts to examine the mouth and larynx may precipitate respiratory collapse so preparations for intubation or tracheostomy should be made in advance of examination. Oximetry can be very useful.

Management

If such a diagnosis is suspected, obtain the assistance of an experienced anaesthetist and otolaryngologist immediately (Fearon & Cinnamond, 1977; Oh & Motoyama, 1977; Kinnefors & Oloffson, 1983). Do not attempt to move or upset the child in any way without adequate resuscitation equipment to hand. Which method is adopted to maintain the airway will depend upon the facilities and experience of the unit but this must be a first priority combined with intravenous fluid replacement, appropriate broad-spectrum parental antibiotics and steroids. With care the majority of children can be successfully intubated and will rapidly recover. The diagnosis should be confirmed by direct examination of the larynx, culture of secretions and blood, chest X-rays and lateral X-rays of the neck.

The differential diagnosis includes impacted foreign bodies, infected epiglottic cysts, angioneurotic oedema and tumours, though these are obviously more common in adults.

Bibliography

BAXTER, J.D. (1967). Acute epiglottitis in children. *Laryngoscope*, **77**, 1358–61.

BOOTH, J.B. (1987). Sudden and fluctuant sensorineural hearing loss. In *Scott-Browne's Otolaryngology*, Vol. 3, *Otology*, ed. J.B. Booth, pp. 387–434. London: Butterworths.

DOWLING, J.A., FOLEY, F.D. & MONCRIEF, J.A. (1968). Chrondritis in the burned ear. *Plast. Reconstr. Surg.*, **42**, 161–5.

DRAKELEY, M.J. (1987). The oesophagus in otolaryngology. In *Scott-Browne's Otolaryngology*, Vol. 5, *Laryngology*, ed. P. M. Stell, pp. 392–402. London: Butterworths.

ENGLISH, G.M. (1976). Common injuries to the ear. *Prim. Care*, **3**, 507–9.

FEARON, B. & CINNAMOND, M. (1977). Tracheotomy in acute supraglottis: the treatment of choice. *Laryngoscope*, **87**, 879–83.

GOWER, D. & McGUIRT, W.F. (1983). Intracranial complications of acute and chronic infectious ear disease: a problem still with us. *Laryngoscope*, **93**, 1028–33.

GWALTNEY, J.M. & HAYDEN, F.G. (1982). The nose and infection. In *The Nose; Upper Airway Physiology and the Atmospheric Environment*, ed. D.F. Proctor & I. Anderson, pp. 399–422. Amsterdam: Elsevier.

HEAD, P.W. (1976). Otitic barotrauma. *Br. J. Audiol.*, **10**, 91–8.

HERBILD, O. & BONDING, O. (1981). Peritonsillar abscess. *Arch. Otolaryngol.*, **107**, 540–6.

HOUGH, J.V.D. (1970). Fractures of the temporal bone and associated middle and inner ear trauma. *Proc. R. Soc. Med.*, **63**, 245–52.

HOWARD, D.J. (1991). Emergency and elective airway procedures: tracheostomy, cricothyroidotomy and their variants. In *Rob & Smith's Operative Surgery. Head and Neck*, Part 1, ed. I.A. McGregor & D.J. Howard, pp. 27–44. London: Butterworth-Heinemann.

HOWIE, V.M., PLOUSSARD, J.H. & LESTER, R.C. (1970). Otitis media: a clinical and bacteriological correlation. *Pediatrics*, **45**, 29–35.

KERR, A.G. & SMYTH, G.D.L. (1987). Ear trauma. In *Scott-Browne's Otolaryngology*, Vol. 3, *Otology*, ed. J.B. Booth, pp. 172–184. London: Butterworths.

KINNEFORS, A. & OLOFFSON, J. (1983). Acute epiglottitis in children. *Clin. Otolaryngol.*, **8**, 25–30.

MARAN, A.G.D. & LUND, V.J. (1990). Trauma to the nose and sinuses. In *Clinical Rhinology*, pp. 110–139. Stuttgart: Georg Thieme.

MARAN, A.G.D., STELL, P.M., MURRAY, J.A.M. *et al.* (1981). Early management of laryngeal injuries. *J. R. Soc. Med.*, **74**, 656–60.

OH, T. H. & MOTOYAMA, E. K. (1977). Comparison of nasotracheal intubation and tracheostomy in the management of acute epiglottitis. *Anesthesiology*, **46**, 214–18.

PETERKIN, G.A.G. (1974). Otitis externa. *J. Laryngol. Otol.*, **88**, 15–21.

SESSIONS, D.G., STALLINGS, J.O., MILLS, W.J. Jr *et al.* (1971). Frostbite of the ear. *Laryngoscope*, **81**, 1223–32.

WRIGHT, T. (1988). *Dizziness. A Guide to Disorders of Balance*. London: Croom Helm.

Further reading

BECKER, W., NAUMANN, H.H. & PFALTZ,C.R. (1989). *Ear, Nose and Throat Diseases. A Pocket Reference.* Stuttgart: Georg Thieme.

LUCENTE, F.E. & SOBOL, S.M. (1988). *Essentials of Otolaryngology*, 2nd edn. New York: Raven Press.

SUEN, J.Y. & WETMORE, S.J. (1986). *Emergencies in Otolaryngology*. Edinburgh: Churchill Livingstone.

21 Ocular trauma and emergencies

R.J. COOLING

Moorfields Eye Hospital NHS Trust, London, UK

Chapter plan

Introduction
Superficial injuries
Non-penetrating ocular injuries
Penetrating ocular injuries
Chemical and thermal burns
Ocular effects of remote injury
Inflammatory disorders
Acute visual loss
Acute diplopia

INTRODUCTION

In a large survey of a district general hospital accident and emergency (A&E) department, 6.1% of all new attendances presented with ophthalmic complaints. The majority of ophthalmic emergencies were either self-referred minor injuries or external inflammatory eye disorders. Referral for specialist advice was deemed necessary in one-third of cases and, by implication, most presenting emergencies could be handled satisfactorily by the non-specialist (Edwards, 1987).

Clearly many patients presenting with acute ocular problems perceive the general A&E department as offering a service appropriate to their needs. Competence to deal with this workload should fall within the capabilities of A&E medical staff. It is therefore important that appropriate training is received, including practical instruction. This can be achieved through a comprehensive induction programme for new staff and may usefully include attachment to an ophthalmic casualty department or primary care clinic. Furthermore, there is the need for close cooperation with an ophthalmic unit, not only to provide ready access to specialist advice but for the regular updating of clinical guidelines.

In order to meet this service requirement, it is essential that an appropriate range of equipment is immediately to hand. Accurate diagnosis depends upon the availability of proper examination facilities including a slit-lamp microscope which will also be required for on-site specialist opinion.

Essential equipment

- Visual acuity charts (distance and reading)
- Pin-hole occluder
- Pen-torch and magnifying loupe
- Slit-lamp microscope
- Direct ophthalmoscope
- Lid retractors
- Flourescein-impregnated strips
- Universal indicator paper
- Topical anaesthetic agents – amethocaine 1%
- Topical mydriatic agents – tropicamide 0.5%

The only genuine ophthalmic emergencies are acute chemical burns and central retinal artery occlusion. In addition to the many patients presenting as emergencies with either minor trauma or superficial inflammatory conditions, there may be others with sight-threatening disorders that warrent urgent treatment and which can easily be overlooked or misinterpreted. Attention given to a detailed history of the onset of the complaint or the precise circumstances of injury together with a systematic ophthalmic examination will go a long way towards avoiding such diagnostic pitfalls. The importance of complete documentation – including recording visual acuity in both eyes – should not require emphasizing but regrettably is often omitted. Frequently, inappropriate immediate management or delayed recognition compromises the outcome of secondary care and can result in irrevocable loss of vision. Unfortunately the penalties for the clinician may prove high and the situation indefensible.

Although many ocular injuries occur in isolation, it is particularly important to exclude ophthalmic injury in the comatose patient or in the presence of serious multiple injuries including head injury or faciomaxillary trauma (Holt & Holt, 1983). It is not uncommon in this situation for the ophthalmic component to form a significant element of the residual disability. Vigilance is also required when dealing with the injured child where the history is often unreliable or there is no adult witness to the event and detailed examination is notoriously difficult.

SUPERFICIAL INJURIES

Abrasions or lacerations of the conjunctiva are often associated with subconjunctival bleeding. This may conceal a penetrating wound of the underlying sclera. Injury caused by a sharp pointed object should raise the possibility of more extensive injury, and ophthalmoscopy of the fundus with the pupil fully dilated may reveal damage to deeper tissues. Fortunately, the majority of conjunctival lacerations are uncomplicated and do not require suturing. If the extent of the injury is in doubt, referral for wound exploration is advisable. If the conjunctival defect is extensive or there is gaping of the wound, the edges are best apposed using 7/0 absorbable material.

Conjunctival and corneal abrasions

An abrasion of the corneal epithelium is a frequent minor injury. The circumstances are often trivial and typically involve the intruding finger of a child, the glancing blow of a branch or in association with the wearing of contact lenses. Pain is often intense, with profuse lacrimation and severe lid spasm. Topical anaesthesia may be necessary before detailed examination is possible when the area of epithelial loss is readily defined by fluorescein staining. Corneal epithelial defects are quickly resurfaced and even extensive abrasions are healed within 2–3 days. Foreign debris or loose epithelium should be removed with a sterile cotton bud and a short-acting cycloplegic (cyclopentolate 1%) is used together with antibiotic ointment. Traditionally an eyepad or pressure bandage is recommended, but this appears to confer little or no benefit and may in fact compromise epithelial regeneration (Kirkpatrick et al., 1993; Easty, 1993).

Superimposed infection of a corneal abrasion is fortunately rare but is suggested by a history of increasing pain, discharge and the appearance of a greyish opacity of the stroma underlying the epithelial defect. Urgent referral for diagnostic microbiology and intense topical and systemic antibiotic therapy is essential.

A recurrent corneal abrasion or erosion within weeks or months of injury is not an uncommon event. This typically develops on waking and sometimes the severity of the attack is worse than the original episode. Liberal use of simple eye ointment at night for at least 3 months will often prevent or at least reduce the number of further episodes.

Foreign bodies

Airborne foreign bodies, if not ejected from the conjunctival sac by reflex tear secretion, tend to lodge beneath the upper lid. The foreign body is likely to escape detection unless the lid is everted. Discomfort occurs on blinking with telltale vertical linear abrasions of the cornea. Alternatively, the foreign body adheres to the exposed conjunctiva or cornea. Hot metallic fragments (e.g. during grinding) may become embedded within the corneal epithelium. The immediate foreign body sensation disappears only to be followed by a painful, red and watering eye for some hours later. Such embedded or adherent foreign bodies are best removed with a hypodermic needle mounted on a syringe and under slit-lamp observation. Accompanying rust deposit in the bed of the foreign body should be removed to facilitate healing but is more easily achieved after a delay of 24 h. Where the foreign body is located in the visual axis, utmost care is necessary during removal to minimize corneal scarring. If buried within the stroma, referral for specialist management is recommended. Again, prophylactic use of a broad-spectrum topical antibiotic (e.g. chloramphenicol) is required and if the eye is inflamed a short-acting mydriatic such as tropicamide 0.5% is indicated. Many of these injuries continue to occur in the workplace and the opportunity should be taken to advise on the need for protective eyewear (MacEwen, 1989).

Ultraviolet keratoconjunctivitis (arc eye)

Unshielded exposure to a welding arc or sunlamp causes intense discomfort, watering and light sensitivity within 6–10 h. Ultraviolet photochemical damage is confined to the surface epithelium, the cornea showing punctate staining with fluorescein. Topical anaesthesia provides temporary relief but should not be repeated. The condition is self-limiting but discomfort is reduced by instilling a short-acting cycloplegic and steroid/antibiotic ointment together with systemic analgesics.

Lid lacerations

Superficial lid wounds in general need little more than simple taping but if there is gaping of the wound, closure with a continuous subcuticular or interrupted 6/0 nylon suture is required. Vertical lacerations of the lid, however, are often full-thickness and involve the lid margin, requiring meticulous, layered repair to avoid permanent deformity. The excellent vascular supply of the lids allows conservation of all tissues even when there is extensive disruption including avulsion. All ingrained foreign material should be vigorously removed. Upper lid lacerations may involve the levator complex and primary repair should always be attempted, although later ptosis repair is often necessary (Collin, 1989). Lacerations of the medial aspect of the lid may include the lacrimal canaliculae, the medial canthal tendon or lacrimal sac. Accurate apposition is required with possible marsupialization of the divided distal end of the lower canaliculus (Welham, 1987).

Lacerations of the lid or brow may extend to involve the underlying globe and this merits careful exclusion. Puncture wounds of the lid also require careful assessment as the orbital septum will have been breached, with the risk of secondary orbital cellulitis. Such wounds may harbour foreign material sometimes deep within the orbital tissues. In addition, the orbital roof may be penetrated with the risk of intracranial complications. Detailed radiological studies, including CT (computed tomography) scans, should be considered to determine the possible extent of the injury (Bedrossian, 1987).

NON-PENETRATING OCULAR INJURIES

Non-penetrating eye trauma resulting from blunt force is a common pattern of injury and accounts for the majority of serious eye injuries. Many occur during domestic or leisure activities, especially in the young and as a consequence of assault. Contusion injury may be confined to the globe (e.g. from a direct blow), but damage may also occur in association with facial or closed head injury. The prevalence of ocular involvement in faciomaxillary injuries has been highlighted in a number of reports, impaired visual acuity and defective ocular movement being the most sensitive predictors (Dutton et al., 1992).

Contusion damage characteristically affects multiple intraocular structures and often at sites of inherent weakness such as the iris root, drainage angle, lens zonule

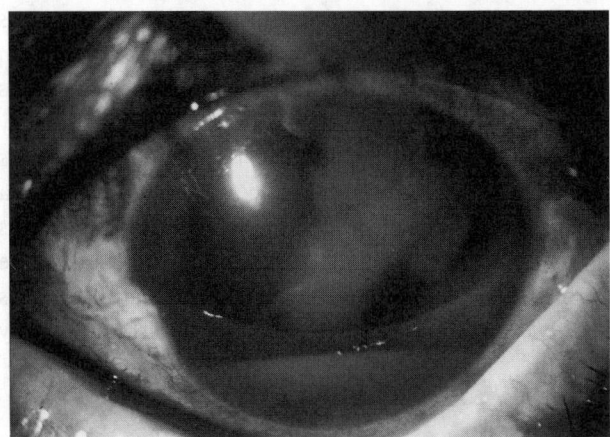

Fig. 1. Traumatic hyphaema. Fluid level and clotted hyphaema and paresed pupil following concussional injury.

and vitreous base. Accompanying swelling or haematoma of the lids or damage to the orbital contents may conceal underlying and potentially serious ocular injury and must be carefully excluded.

Contusion injury predominantly affects structures in the anterior segment but often the recovery of vision is good. Where tissue damage involves the posterior compartment, the visual outcome is less favourable. In the immediate stages, clouding of the media by haemorrhage or breakdown of the blood/ocular barriers is a common sequel and precludes complete assessment of internal damage. Similarly, visual acuity on presentation is often severely reduced and although vision may rapidly improve complete recovery may take weeks or months.

Hyphaema

Bleeding into the anterior chamber originating from the iris or ciliary body is a common manifestation of serious blunt injury (Fig. 1). At first diffused, blood rapidly settles to form a fluid level and will usually reabsorb over several days to allow identification of associated structural damage. About 10% of cases rebleed within 7 days of injury and this may cause elevated intraocular pressure, bloodstaining of the cornea or optic nerve damage. The presence of hyphaema always warrants referral to exclude permanent or sight-threatening damage. Out-patient supervision is now more commonly adopted and does not appear to increase the risk of secondary haemorrhage (Williams et al., 1993). Some authorities advocate the use of systemic antifibrinolytic agents to reduce the incidence of rebleeding (Kutner et al., 1987) but this has not been routinely adopted. Surgical intervention to remove clotted blood is rarely necessary unless raised intraocular pressure cannot be controlled by medical means.

Iris and pupil damage

Damage to the iris may cause haemorrhage, pigment release or secondary inflammation. Tears of the iris usually affect the pupil margin and involve the iris sphincter muscle with permanent deformity of the pupil (traumatic mydriasis). Sphincter tears may be single or multiple and appear as triangular notches of the pupil margin. Mydriasis may also result from concussional damage, normal pupil size and reactivity returning over several weeks. Tears may also involve the iris root at the junction with the ciliary body and, if large, such iridodialyses produce a characteristic D-shaped pupil. Damage is likely to be sustained by adjacent structures including the aqueous drainage angle or lens zonule. Persistent double vision or photophobia may necessitate surgical repair of an iridodialysis at a later date once the full extent of injury is established.

Lens opacity and displacement

The lens and its supporting ligament or zonule are especially vulnerable to the effects of blunt injury. Immediate or delayed cataract is usually located beneath the anterior or posterior capsule and appears as a rosette opacity against the red reflex. Sometimes the cataract is reversible, particularly in the young, or may show little progression and preservation of good vision. Disruption of the supporting zonule may cause partial or complete displacement of the lens with herniation of vitreous gel into the anterior chamber. The iris often appears tremulous and the edge of the displaced lens may be visible within the pupil. Definitive surgical treatment is usually deferred and is largely governed by the visual potential allied to the nature and extent of associated damage. Rarely, and usually in the elderly, the lens becomes displaced into the anterior chamber to cause raised intraocular pressure and corneal endothelial damage necessitating urgent lens removal.

Retinal oedema

Concussional damage takes the form of reversible opacity affecting the central or peripheral retina (commotio retinae). This results in immediate and often profound visual loss. There may be accompanying intraretinal or subretinal haemorrhage. The milky opacity resolves in a matter of days but the level of visual recovery is unpredictable and determined by the severity of damage to the underlying tissues and disruption of the blood/ocular barriers.

Retinal breaks and detachment

Retinal breaks may develop in the posterior or central retina but more commonly occur in the periphery or vitreous base region (Cooling, 1986). The detection of peripheral retinal breaks requires referral for specialist examination. Although breaks occur at the moment of injury, identification may be hampered by opacities in the media. If identified early, prophylactic sealing with cryotherapy or laser photocoagulation prevents the development of retinal detachment. Full-thickness breaks located at the macula give rise to severe and permanent visual loss and at present are not amenable to treatment.

Choroidal tears

Ruptures of the choroid occur peripherally at the point of impact or remotely beneath the central retina. Initially they may be obscured by associated retinal or choroidal haemorrhage. Single or multiple, indirect choroidal ruptures appear as crescentic defects and are usually disposed concentrically with the optic disc. The overlying retina is intact and bare sclera is visible in the bed of the tear. Recovery of vision is likely unless the tear is located beneath the macula. Delayed visual loss may occur following the development of secondary choroidal neovascular ingrowth and may require focal laser treatment (Wood & Richardson, 1990).

Optic nerve injury

Direct injury to the globe may induce partial or complete avulsion of the optic nerve with immediate and irreversible visual loss. More often, indirect force from a blow to the brow or frontal region inflicts damage to the optic nerve within the optic canal from the effects of skeletal distortion (Lessell, 1989). Usually there are minimal external signs of injury and the fundus appears normal, but poor visual acuity is accompanied by an obvious relative afferent pupil defect. High-dose systemic steroids may help to reduce neuronal oedema (Spoor et al., 1990) and in selected cases vision may be restored by surgical decompression of the roof of the optic canal.

Orbital fractures

Diffuse blunt impact may induce orbital haemorrhage and, if severe, necessitate emergency decompression by incision of the orbital septum. More commonly the impact of an object larger than the orbital aperture results in a blow-out fracture usually affecting the floor or medial wall. There may be coexisting ocular damage or merely displacement of the globe backwards (enophthalmos) or downwards. The ocular movements are restricted with variable diplopia and surgical emphysema of the lids may be detected. Plain X-ray examination usually shows an opaque antrum or ethmoid sinus, but CT scans may demonstrate the fracture site and associated tissue incarceration. There is now much greater emphasis on a conservative approach unless there is significant enophthalmos or persistent diplopia in the straight ahead position 10–14 days following injury (Koornneef, 1982).

PENETRATING OCULAR INJURIES

The exclusion of a penetrating wound of the eye is likely to be the prime objective in the evaluation of most ocular injuries. A disturbingly high proportion of these injuries occur in childhood and an increasing number result from urban assault. In addition, accidents in the workplace, often involving machine tools, continue to take their toll. Damage may be inflicted by a variety of sharp objects, high-velocity missiles, or airgun pellets. Severe blunt force may rupture the globe.

Corneoscleral lacerations

Lacerating wounds usually affect the exposed cornea and may extend across the limbus or corneal margin to involve the anterior sclera. Isolated scleral wounds are far less common. In most instances evidence of serious injury is all too apparent with the findings of a collapsed globe, extensive bleeding or pigmented tissue on opening the lids. With shallowing or loss of the anterior chamber, there may be prolapse or incarceration of the iris within the wound resulting in obvious distortion of the pupil (Fig. 2). Hyphaema may be present and damage to the lens may be evident.

Ruptured globe

Ruptures of the globe from severe blunt force are usually located at the limbus with obvious disruption of internal structures and major intraocular haemorrhage. On occasions the rupture affects the more posterior sclera, often beneath the extraocular muscles, producing no visible wound. Differentiation from a blunt non-penetrating injury may be difficult. Although CT scans and ultrasonic imaging techniques may demonstrate the rupture, surgical

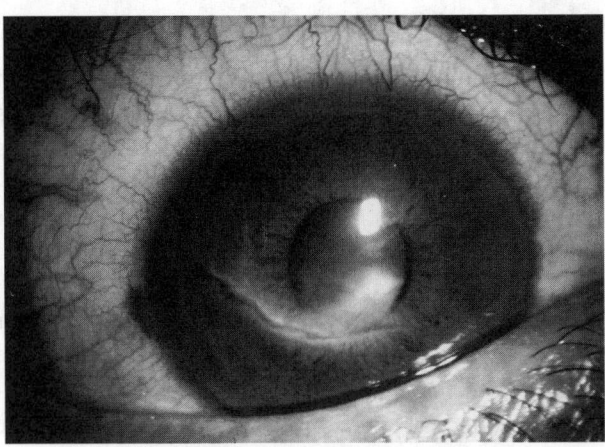

Fig. 2. Corneal laceration with shallowing of the anterior chamber, iris incarceration and distortion of pupil and early cataract.

exploration of the globe may be necessary to exclude an open wound.

Puncture wounds caused by darts, wire, or small metallic fragments can be difficult to identify, as they show few if any of the usual hallmarks of a penetrating injury. Without the benefit of a detailed slit-lamp examination, such wounds are easily overlooked and often misinterpreted as superficial corneal abrasions.

Inevitably, all penetrating ocular injuries carry the risk of intraocular infection or endophthalmitis. This represents the most serious consequence of failure to promptly identify a penetrating ocular injury. Infection is highest in the presence of an intraocular foreign body, or where injury occurs in rural surroundings, and may complicate up to 10% of cases. The results of treatment remain poor, although modern therapeutic regimens – including the use of intraocular antibiotics – have improved the prognosis, provided there is no significant delay.

The possible retention of foreign material within the eye should be considered in all penetrating ocular injuries. Foreign debris is often found to contaminate the wound but is frequently of an inert nature (e.g. glass).

If a penetrating wound is identified or suspected, further examination should be curtailed to limit extrusion of intraocular contents. The eye should be covered by a protective shield and the patient referred immediately. Systemic antibiotic treatment is commenced (e.g. intravenous ciprofloxacin) and antitetanus measures are taken if appropriate.

The majority of penetrating wounds require accurate microsurgical repair using atraumatic monofilament nylon materials. Incarcerated uveal tissue is cleared from the wound by repositioning or, if devitalized, by excision. If disrupted, the opaque lens is aspirated and extruding

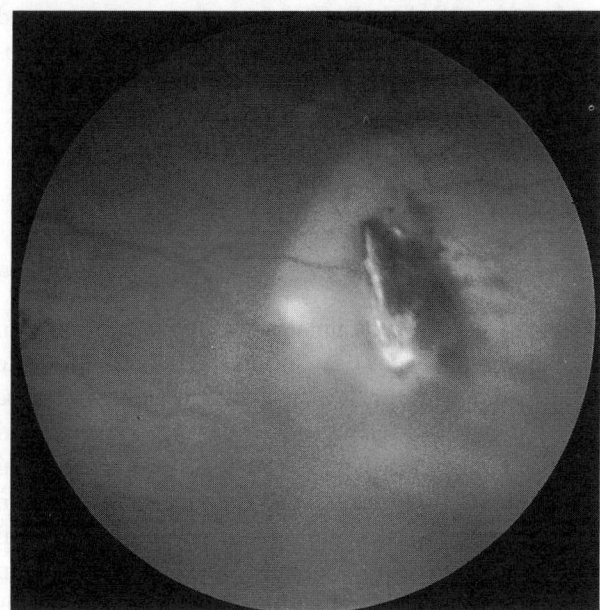

Fig. 3. Fundus photograph showing metallic foreign body impacted in the retina with surrounding oedema and haemorrhage.

vitreous cleared from the wound. All ocular compartments are reformed to restore normal ocular contours.

Intraocular foreign bodies

The archetypal intraocular foreign body (IOFB) is a small metallic fragment measuring 2–3 mm at most and ferromagnetic in composition. The foreign body usually penetrates the cornea to leave a self-sealing wound and creates a small transilluminating defect in the adjacent iris easily identified against the red reflex. The momentum of the foreign body is such that it continues along its trajectory through the lens or zonule, coming to rest in the vitreous cavity or becoming impacted in the retina (Fig. 3).

The recognition of an IOFB can be very elusive as the presenting clinical appearances so often suggest a relatively innocuous injury. Typically there is little discomfort and minimal impairment of vision. A complaint of floaters will accompany vitreous haemorrhage resulting from retinal impact damage. Dilatation of the pupil may reveal a track of opacity through the lens, and if the media are clear the foreign body is visible in a high proportion of cases.

The single most important and possibly the only pointer is provided by a detailed history of the circumstances of injury, which characteristically involves the use of a hammer. Once such a history is elicited, plain X-ray

examination is imperative. Only rarely is a metallic foreign body not detectable radiologically (McElvanney & Fielder, 1993). The possibility of an IOFB should also be entertained in accidents involving the use of industrial power tools, explosions or gunshot injuries.

If the typical IOFB injury goes unrecognized, the patient is likely to present several months later with insidious loss of vision due to the effects of chemotoxic damage (siderosis). The metabolic damage which ensues affects most intraocular structures but particularly the photoreceptors, causing irrevocable loss of sight (Hope-Ross et al., 1993).

Once the presence of an IOFB has been detected, accurate localization is necessary prior to removal. Axial and coronal CT scans are performed if the foreign body is obscured by cataract or vitreous haemorrhage. Gone are the days of 'blind' extraction with an electromagnet, although removal using a magnet is still applicable to uncomplicated IOFBs. Increasingly, modern vitreoretinal surgery allows controlled removal of the foreign body with intraocular microforceps at an early stage as well as the repair of intraocular tissue damage, producing marked improvement in visual outcome (Williams et al., 1988). Furthermore, these techniques have transformed the management of non-magnetic IOFBs, including copper-containing fragments and organic materials which are frequently associated with progressive intraocular inflammation.

CHEMICAL AND THERMAL BURNS

Chemical injuries of the eye involve a wide range of noxious agents which may rapidly inflict extensive tissue damage with devastating consequences for vision. Such injuries arise from accidents within the home or workplace, or from malicious assault (Morgan, 1987). The severity of injury is determined by the volume, concentration and precise composition of the agent but, most importantly, by the duration of contact. Alkalis (and strong acids) rapidly penetrate the surface layers of the eye by disrupting epithelial barriers and saponification of cell membranes to gain access to the anterior chamber and deeper structures (Pfister, 1983). These effects are enhanced by additives including ionic detergents present in many domestic chemicals. In contrast, most acid radicals are confined to surface structures by immediate tissue fixation. Antipersonnel agents are often confused with ammonia but their effects are fortunately transient.

On presentation, the precise nature of the chemical is often in doubt as well as the efficacy of immediate first aid measures. Universal indicator paper should be used to determine the conjunctival pH and guide irrigation. Sterile physiological fluid is best delivered using a standard intravenous infusion line but care must be taken to remove particulate chemical from the conjunctival fornices.

The initial clinical appearance offers a guide to the severity of injury, but may be deceptive. Superficial burns show conjuctival injection and oedema, with areas of epithelial loss demonstrated by fluorescein staining. Treatment is limited to topical anti-inflammatory and antibiotic therapy. Moderate or severe burns show blanching or ischaemia of the conjunctiva and corneal opacification. Ischaemia of the limbal zone is a particularly adverse prognostic factor. Severe burns are characterized by progressive inflammatory destruction of the anterior segment with the risk of corneal perforation. Topical (10%) and systemic ascorbate are used together with steroids and may be combined with proteolytic enzyme inhibitors (L-cysteine). Extensive ischaemic damage to the conjunctiva and lids is likely to result in a severe dry eye, conjunctival adhesions (symblepharon) and deformity of the lids.

Thermal burns predominantly affect the lids, but splashes of molten metal can cause extensive damage to ocular surface tissues. The greatest need is to secure protection of the globe, prevent corneal exposure, and prevent infection.

OCULAR EFFECTS OF REMOTE INJURY

Generalized disturbance of the posterior ocular circulation affecting one or both eyes may develop in association with serious head injury, crush injuries of the chest or multiple limb fractures. This vascular change is associated with the name of Purtscher, who first documented the retinal changes. Various aetiological factors have been incriminated, including raised intravenous pressure, arteriolar spasm and lipid emboli (Roden et al., 1989). The predominant features may suggest a venous origin with extensive intraretinal haemorrhages or arterial with micro-infarction of the retina and accumulation of axoplasmic debris (cotton-wool spots), but these features are often combined (Archer, 1986). Visual recovery is unpredictable but systemic steroids may be beneficial. Similar but less extensive changes of inner retinal ischaemia may result from chest compression by seat belts often accompanied by whiplash injuries of the neck (Archer et al., 1988). Symptoms, including variable blurring of vision, develop within 48 h of injury. Good visual recovery is the rule

but is often delayed. Defective colour perception and paracentral field loss usually remain and persistent abnormalities are identifiable with electrodiagnostic studies or by fluorescein angiography.

INFLAMMATORY DISORDERS

Lids

The focus of acute inflammation of the lid is usually an infected lash follicle or its associated glands (stye). Acute inflammation of a tarsal or meibomian gland gives rise to a tender deep swelling with overlying erythema and oedema. Application of local heat combined with topical antibiotics will usually suffice and once acute inflammation has resolved, incision and curettage of any residual granuloma (chalazion) is undertaken. There is often an associated chronic inflammation of the lids or blepharitis manifested by marginal crusting and hyperaemia. Bicarbonate lid scrubs with topical antibiotic/steroid ointment applied sparingly to the lid margins is usually all that is required, but a course of systemic tetracycline is worth considering in recalcitrant blepharitis.

Lacrimal

Acute inflammation of the lacrimal gland (dacryoadenitis) is characterized by tenderness and swelling in the upper outer quadrant of the orbit. This rare condition may be bacterial in origin but is most often associated with infectious mononucleosis.

Acute inflammation of the lacrimal outflow system usually complicates atresia or acquired obstruction of the nasolacrimal duct with a history of constant epiphora. A distended, inflamed lacrimal sac (dacryocystitis) presents as an obvious tender swelling at the medial canthus with surrounding cellulitis. Dacryocystitis is usually streptococcal in origin and responds to appropriate systemic antibiotic therapy without the need for incision and drainage. Following resolution of acute infection, elective lacrimal bypass surgery (dacryocystorhinostomy) is required to prevent further episodes.

Orbital

Orbital cellulitis usually results from the spread of infection from the adjacent paranasal sinuses. Early diagnosis is essential if serious complications including blindness, cavernous sinus thrombosis and intracranial infection are to be avoided (Martin-Hirsch, 1992). Lid

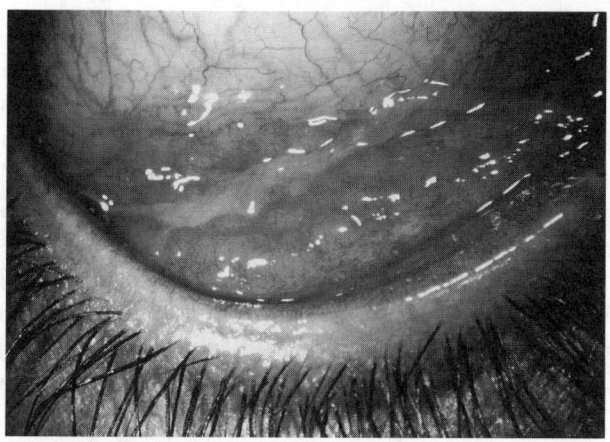

Fig. 4. Adenovirus conjunctivitis showing follicular changes affecting the inferior conjunctiva.

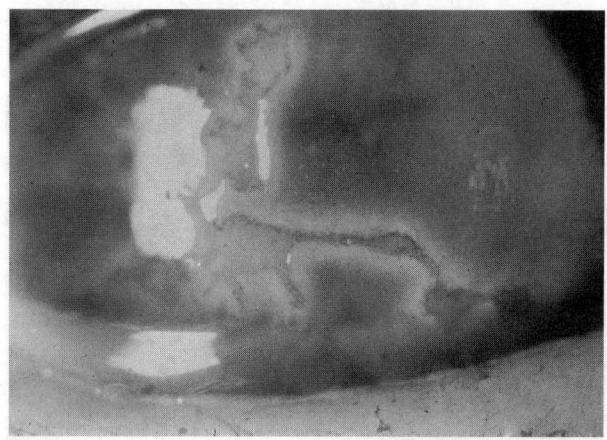

Fig. 5. Slit-lamp photograph of herpes simplex dendritic corneal ulceration stained with fluorescein

swelling is accompanied by variable proptosis and limitation of ocular movements. Urgent investigations should include blood cultures and CT scans. Immediate intravenous antibiotic therapy is essential as well as prompt referral for ophthalmic and ear, nose and throat opinions.

Conjunctiva

Acute conjunctivitis is the most common presenting inflammatory eye condition and may be bacterial, viral, or allergic in origin. One eye, or more often both eyes, are affected by a foreign body or gritty sensation with a watery or sticky discharge. Generalized congestion of the conjunctiva is evident with a clear corneal reflex and vision is unimpaired. In acute allergic conjunctivitis, oedema or chemosis of the conjunctiva is evident accompanied by lid swelling. In cases of bacterial origin, rapid resolution follows topical broad-spectrum antibiotic treatment.

Viral conjunctivitis and particularly adenovirus infection occurs in epidemics. Being highly contagious, there is considerable risk of cross-infection within hospital services and hand washing after examination of a suspected case is essential. The disorder is characterized by a follicular conjunctival reaction (Fig. 4) composed of subepithelial collections of lymphocytes and may be accompanied by preauricular lymphadenopathy. Corneal involvement is suggested by the development of photophobia with superficial punctate infiltrates visible on slit-lamp microscopy. There may be an associated upper respiratory tract infection or abdominal upset. There is no specific antiviral therapy but symptoms may be ameliorated by frequent topical chloramphenicol 0.5%. Follicular conjunc-

tivitis may also occur in primary herpes simplex infection and in response to chlamydial oculogenital infection.

Cornea

Infected corneal ulceration or suppurative keratitis is an urgent sight-threatening condition and almost always implies compromised ocular surface defences. Infection may supervene following traumatic abrasion or complicate lid or tear film disorders. Case-control studies have demonstrated that contact lens wear is now the major risk factor in microbial keratitis (Dart, 1993). Bacterial organisms, including pneumococci, staphylococci and pseudomonas species prevail but fungi, herpes simplex infection and rarely acanthamoeba (Bacon et al., 1993) may be responsible. Reduced vision is accompanied by pain, photophobia and watering. In the area of ulceration the corneal light reflex is disturbed and an underlying greyish infiltrate is observed. Although the clinical appearances may suggest the likely organism, urgent microbiological studies are imperative. Early identification and prompt therapy is often successful in the prevention of endophthalmitis, corneal perforation and loss of the eye.

Acute corneal ulceration resulting from recurrent herpes simplex infection shows a characteristic branching or dendritic pattern enhanced by fluorscein staining (Fig. 5). Topical acyclovir is the treatment of choice and is highly specific with minimal toxicity. Topical steroid therapy without antiviral cover must be avoided as this will induce progressive ulceration and permanent corneal scarring.

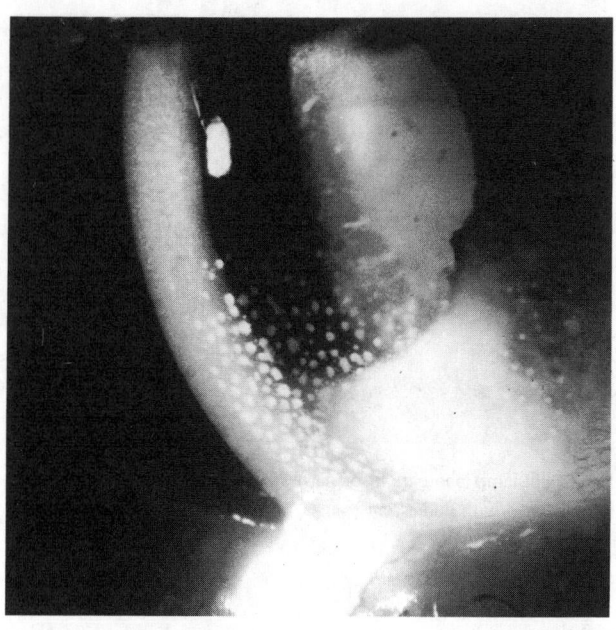

Fig. 6. Slit-lamp photograph of acute iritis with endothelial precipitates.

Marginal corneal ulceration is a benign condition attributable to staphylococcal sensitivity. A linear area of paralimbal infiltration is seen with adjacent conjunctival injection. This is a self-limiting disorder but topical steroids provide symptomatic relief and shorten the duration of the condition.

Uvea

Acute anterior uveitis (iritis), commonly misinterpreted as conjunctivitis, is distinguished by a short history of pain in the eye and light sensitivity. Vision is often maintained. Conjunctival vascular congestion surrounds the cornea but may be generalized. Breakdown of the blood/ocular barriers causes flare, and cells in the anterior chamber and inflammatory deposits may be visible on the corneal endothelium (Fig. 6). In severe or neglected cases, accumulation of inflammatory cells in the anterior chamber (hypopyon) occurs. The pupil is usually small and irregular from adhesions to the anterior lens capsule. In most instances there is no associated systemic disorder but acute uveitis may accompany ankylosing spondylitis, sarcoidosis or Reiter's syndrome. Recurrences are common and the condition may independently affect the other eye. Prompt treatment is required comprising intensive dilatation of the pupil and hourly topical steroids. In severe or recalcitrant cases, steroids are given by periocular injection.

Herpes zoster

Herpes zoster affecting the ophthalmic division of the trigeminal nerve may give rise to anterior uveitis even in the early stages. Vasculitic damage to the iris is not uncommon, causing irregularity of the pupil and impaired reactivity. Severe ocular pain precedes the rash and can cause diagnostic confusion. Other inflammatory changes include conjunctivitis or keratitis as well as corneal anaesthesia with the risk of trophic ulceration. Topical steroids and mydriatics are used but the influence of systemic acyclovir on the ocular sequelae is unproven (Marsh & Cooper, 1993).

Acute glaucoma

Acute angle closure glaucoma is a rare condition which develops in the anatomically predisposed eye with a shallow anterior chamber. The patient is usually elderly or middle-aged and hypermetropic (long-sighted). Occlusion of most of the drainage angle by the iris root arrests the outflow of aqueous leading to an abrupt rise of intraocular pressure. Angle closure may be brought on by physical or mental stress and often arises under conditions of dim illumination. Sudden onset of ocular pain or unilateral headache is accompanied by visual loss and haloes from corneal oedema. A history suggestive of previous aborted episodes of angle closure may be elicited. On occasions, nausea or vomiting may be the predominant complaint. Examination reveals a congested eye with diffuse corneal oedema and a semidilated, oval and non-reactive pupil. The globe is tender and digitally firm.

The essential aim of treatment is to immediately reduce the intraocular pressure by intravenous acetazolamide (500 mg), where necessary supplemented by oral glycerol. The pupil is constricted by pilocarpine drops 3–4 hourly. Topical steroids are added to combat the inflammatory effects of the accompanying ischaemia. Once the acute effects have subsided and permanent damage to the drainage angle is assesed, laser (neodymium-YAG) or surgical iridotomy is undertaken to prevent further attacks. In addition, prophylactic laser iridotomy is performed on the predisposed fellow eye. The recovery of vision is related to the duration of the attack, but in some cases sight is lost at an early stage due to ischaemic optic nerve damage.

Episclera

Episcleritis is a benign disorder prone to recurrence. A localized area of brick-red superficial vascular injection is seen. There is no discharge, and soreness rather than pain is experienced. Frequent topical steroids will relieve the discomfort and shorten the episode.

Sclera

Scleritis may be nodular or diffuse and is often associated with serious disorders, particularly autoimmune disorders. Unlike episcleritis, there is constant severe pain and the vascular congestion takes on a violaceous hue best appreciated in daylight. There may be signs of intraocular inflammation with flare and cells in the anterior chamber. The condition may respond to non-steroidal anti-inflammatory agents but often systemic steroids are necessary and essential if there is scleral necrosis (Tuft & Watson, 1991).

ACUTE VISUAL LOSS

Reference has already been made to sudden painful loss of vision accompanying certain inflammatory ocular disorders and acute angle closure glaucoma. The causes of acute loss of vision in the absence of pain can usually be differentiated on the basis of the pupillary responses, confrontation fields and the findings on ophthalmoscopy.

Transient visual loss

An episode of transient visual loss may be the forerunner of a cerebrovascular accident and always merits further investigation. The majority of these ischaemic episodes are due to platelet or cholesterol emboli most commonly derived from the carotid artery or an abnormal heart valve.

Transient obscuration of vision may also occur in patients with impending retinal vascular occlusion, elevated intraocular pressure or papilloedema.

Vitreous haemorrhage

Major vitreous haemorrhage causes severe loss of sight and abolition of the red reflex on ophthalmoscopy. Minor bleeds appear to the patient as a shower of floaters, and streaks of blood or floating debris may be identified on ophthalmoscopy. It is essential to establish the cause as early as possible and, although the possibilities are legion, diabetic or hypertensive retinal vascular disease is the most likely. Alternatively, sudden onset of floaters may be due to an acute posterior vitreous detachment. Although this is usually an innocent phen-

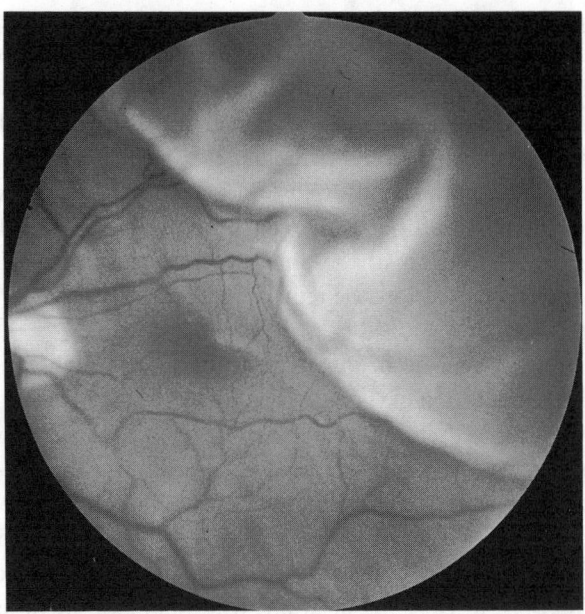

Fig. 7. Fundus photograph of superotemporal bullous retinal detachment with macula attached.

omenon, vitreous separation may induce retinal breaks which should be treated without delay to prevent retinal detachment.

Retinal detachment

Premonitory symptoms of retinal detachment include flashes of light indicative of vitreous traction or floaters of sudden onset due to vitreous separation or haemorrhage. As retinal detachment evolves, a field defect may be observed or central vision becomes blurred or distorted following macular involvement. With direct ophthalmoscopy, the detached retina appears as a greyish membrane with darkened vessels (Fig. 7). Most retinal detachments develop as a result of one or more breaks in the peripheral retina of the myopic eye but may be secondary to other retinal or choroidal disorders (e.g. choroidal melanoma). In all cases the status of the macula should be assessed and if still attached prompt surgical intervention is necessary to preserve central vision.

Retinal vascular occlusion

This is a common cause of sudden visual loss in the elderly or hypertensive patient. Central or branch retinal artery occlusions are usually embolic in nature but may be due to local thrombosis. Central retinal artery occlusion presents an unmistakable picture of almost complete visual loss with attenuation of the retinal arterioles and no apparent flow. Ischaemic swelling of the retina produces central pallor with sparing of the macula or the so-called cherry red spot. In branch occlusions, pallor is confined to a sector of the retina and sometimes the responsible calcific or cholesterol embolus can be observed. In central retinal arterial occlusion, lowering of the intra-ocular pressure by massage, intravenous acetazolamide or decompression of the anterior chamber by corneal puncture may restore the retinal circulation with recovery of vision.

Retinal vein occlusions tend to occur overnight and the deterioration of vision is generally less than in arterial obstructions. Central retinal vein occlusion or thrombosis causes widespread intraretinal haemorrhages, engorged tortuous retinal veins and optic disc swelling. In branch retinal vein occlusions, vision is reduced if the macula is involved, or alternatively a sector field defect is observed. There is a close association with diabetes mellitus, systemic hypertension and open angle glaucoma. There is no immediate treatment, but if there is prominent retinal ischaemia panretinal laser treatment is indicated to prevent painful rubeotic glaucoma.

Optic neuritis

Sudden loss of central vision in a young patient accompanied by pain on ocular movement is highly characteristic of optic neuritis. The fundus appearances are usually normal and pupil testing reveals a relative afferent pupil defect. Most cases are due to demyelination and there may be a history of previous episodes of transient visual loss or diplopia. Systemic steroids may expedite visual recovery but do not appear to influence the ultimate level of vision.

Ischaemic optic neuropathy

This condition causes sudden visual loss in middle-aged or elderly patients. Again there is a relative afferent pupil defect and the optic disc shows pallid swelling. Ischaemic optic neuropathy caused by temporal arteritis must be excluded by erythrocyte sedimentation rate and temporal artery biopsy. Urgent treatment with high-dose systemic steroids may reverse visual loss and protect the fellow eye. Systemic steroids are of no value in non-arteritic cases, but surgical fenestration of the optic nerve sheath may be beneficial (Flaharty *et al.*, 1993). The condition often affects both eyes and anatomical factors appear significant (disc at risk).

ACUTE DIPLOPIA

Sudden onset of double vision may be the presenting symptom of a number of serious neurological or systemic disorders. Paresis may affect one or more of the extraocular muscles resulting in defective ocular movement in the direction of the affected muscle. Examination should include assessment of the relative position of the eyes, testing of the ocular movements in all directions of gaze, pupil responses and a complete neurological examination. Closed head injury may result in bilateral sixth or fourth nerve palsies, the latter producing disabling torsional diplopia (Lee, 1983). Third nerve paresis may result from a posterior communicating artery aneurysm with ocular pain, ptosis and pupil involvement. Pupil-sparing third nerve palsy is most often seen in the diabetic patient and carries a favourable prognosis.

Bibliography

ARCHER, D.B. (1986). Traumatic retinal vasculopathy. *Trans. Opthalmol. Soc. UK*, **105**, 361–84.

ARCHER, D.B. *et al.* (1988). Traumatic retinal angiopathy associated with wearing of car seat belts. *Eye*, **2**, 650–9.

BACON, A.S. *et al.* (1993). A review of 72 consecutive cases of acanthamoeba keratitis, 1984–1992. *Eye*, **7**, 719–25.

BEDROSSIAN, Jr., E.H. (1987). Evaluation of orbital injuries. *Adv. Ophthalmic. Plast. Reconstr. Surg.*, **6**, 37–49.

COLLIN, J.R.O. (1989). *A Manual of Systematic Eyelid surgery*, 2nd edn. Edinburgh: Churchill Livingstone.

COOLING, R.J. (1986). Traumatic retinal detachment – mechanisms and management. *Trans. Ophthalmol. Soc. UK*, **105**, 575–9.

DART, J.K.G. (1993). Disease and risks associated with contact lenses. *Br. J. Ophthalmol.*, **77**, 490–503.

DUTTON, G.N. *et al.* (1992). Ophthalmic consequences of mid-facial trauma. *Eye*, **6**, 86–9.

EASTY, D.L. (1993). Is an eyepad needed in cases of corneal abrasion? *Br. Med. J.*, **307**, 1022.

EDWARDS, R.S. (1987). Ophthalmic emergencies in a District General Hospital Casualty Dept. *Br. J. Ophthalmol.*, **71**, 938–42.

FLAHARTY, P.M. *et al.* (1993). Optic nerve sheath decompression may improve blood flow in anterior ischaemic optic neuropathy. *Ophthalmology*, **100**, 297–305.

HOLT, G.R. & HOLT, J.E. (1983). Incidence of eye injuries in facial fractures: an analysis of 727 cases. *Otolaryngol. Head Neck Surg.*, **91**, 276–9.

HOPE-ROSS, M., MAHON, G.J. & JOHNSTON, P.B. (1993). Ocular siderosis. *Eye*, **7**, 419–25.

KIRKPATRICK, J.N.P., HOH, H.B. & COOK, S.D. (1993). No eyepad for corneal abrasion. *Eye*, **7**, 468–71.

KOORNNEEF, L. (1982). Current concepts on the management of orbital blow-out fractures. *Ann. Plast. Surg.*, **9**, 185–200.

KUTNER, B. *et al.* (1987). Aminocaproic acid reduces the risk of secondary haemorrhage in patients with traumatic hyphema. *Arch. Ophthalmol.*, **105**, 206–8.

LEE, J. (1983). Ocular motility consequences of trauma and their management. *Br. Orthop. J.*, **40**, 26–33.

LESSELL, S. (1989). Indirect optic nerve trauma. *Arch. Ophthalmol.*, **107**, 382–6.

MacEWEN, C.J. (1989). Eye injuries: a prospective study of 5671 cases. *Br. J. Ophthalmol.*, **73**, 888–94.

MARSH, R.J. & COOPER, M. (1993). Ophthalmic herpes zoster. *Eye*, **7**, 350–70.

MARTIN-HIRSCH, D.P. (1992). Orbital cellulitis. *Arch. Emerg. Med.*, **9**, 143–8.

McELVANNEY, A.M. & FIELDER, A.R. (1993). Intraocular foreign body missed by radiography. *Br. Med. J.*, **306**, 1060–1.

MORGAN, S.J. (1987). Chemical burns of the eye: causes and management. *Br. J. Ophthalmol.*, **71**, 854–7.

PFISTER, R. (1983). The effects of chemical injury on the ocular surface. Ophthalmology, **90**, 601–9.

RODEN, D. *et al.* (1989). Purtscher's retinopathy in fat embolism. *Br. J. Ophthalmol.*, **73**, 677–9.

SPOOR, T.C. *et al.* (1990). Treatment of traumatic optic neuropathy with corticosteroids. *Am. J. Ophthalmol.*, **110**, 665–9.

TUFT, S.J. & WATSON, P.G. (1991). Progression of scleral disease. *Ophthalmology*, **98**, 467–71.

WELHAM, R.A.N. (1987). The lacrimal drainage apparatus. In *Clinical Ophthalmology*, ed. S. Miller pp. 408–9. Bristol: Wright.

WILLIAMS, C. *et al.* (1993). Outpatient management of small traumatic hyphemas: is it safe? *Eye*, **7**, 155–7.

WILLIAMS, D.F. *et al.* (1988). Results and prognostic factors in penetrating ocular injuries with retained intraocular foreign bodies. *Ophthalmology*, **95**, 911–16.

WOOD, C.M. & RICHARDSON, J. (1990). Chorioretinal neovascular membranes complicating contusional eye injuries with indirect choroidal ruptures. *Br. J. Opthalmol.*, **74**, 93–6.

22 Trauma to the spine and spinal cord

A. SWAIN

Accident and Emergency Department, General Hospital, Weston-super-Mare, UK

Chapter plan

Introduction
Unstable spinal injuries
Clinical management
Stable injuries
Conclusion

INTRODUCTION

Man's susceptibility to spinal injury was appreciated by early civilisations and the first reference to it is contained in the Edwin Smith Papyrus which dates from about 3000 BC (Bennett, 1964). In this text, an early Egyptian physician used the following description of a cervical dislocation.

> "If thou examinest a man having a dislocation in a vertebra of his neck, shouldst thou find him unconscious of his two arms and his two legs on account of it, while his phallus is erected on account of it and urine drops from his member without his knowing it ... it is a dislocation of a vertebra of his neck ... an ailment not to be treated."

The precise incidence of spinal injury in the UK is unrecorded. Of all complications the most serious is spinal cord involvement which occurs each year in 10–15 cases per million of the population (Swain & Grundy, 1993). As 50% of patients admitted to one spinal injury unit suffered neurological deterioration at the receiving district hospital (Toscano, 1988), the prevention of secondary injury to the spinal cord is vitally important in accident and emergency (A&E) departments.

Neurological complications are usually associated with unstable injuries of the spine and an appreciation of the causes, nature and management of such injuries is important.

UNSTABLE SPINAL INJURIES

Definition

Stability may be defined as the ability of the spine to limit its displacement under physiological loads so as not to damage or irritate the spinal cord or nerve roots (White *et al.*, 1975). Unstable injuries, therefore, are those in which normal movement places the spinal cord at risk. Holdsworth (1970) emphasized the importance of intact posterior ligaments in maintaining stability. The supraspinous and interspinous ligaments, the ligamentum flavum and the capsules of the facet (apophysial) joints form a tetrad he referred to as the posterior ligament complex (Fig. 1). Their integrity is largely responsible for spinal stability.

More recently, a three-column concept has been proposed in which the posterior column of neural arch

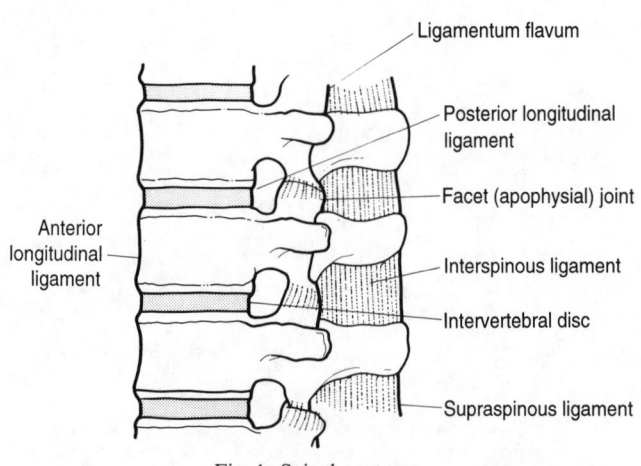

Fig. 1. Spinal anatomy.

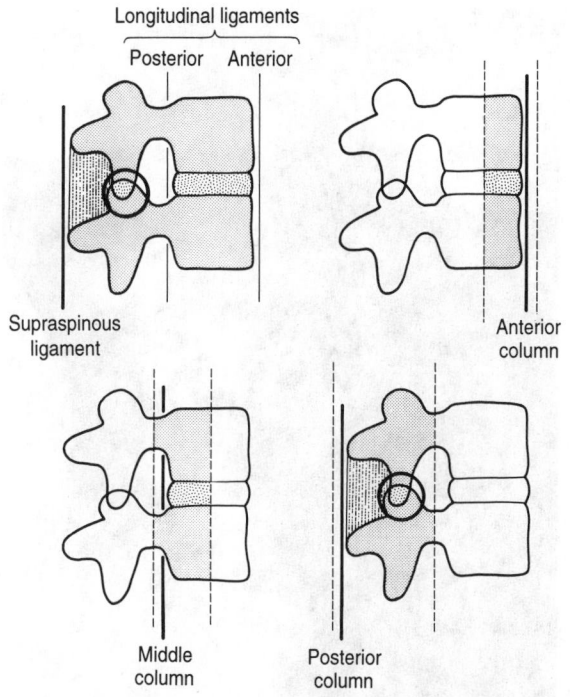

Fig. 2. The three spinal columns. (Reproduced, with permission, from Denis, F. (1983). *Spine*, **8**, 817–31.)

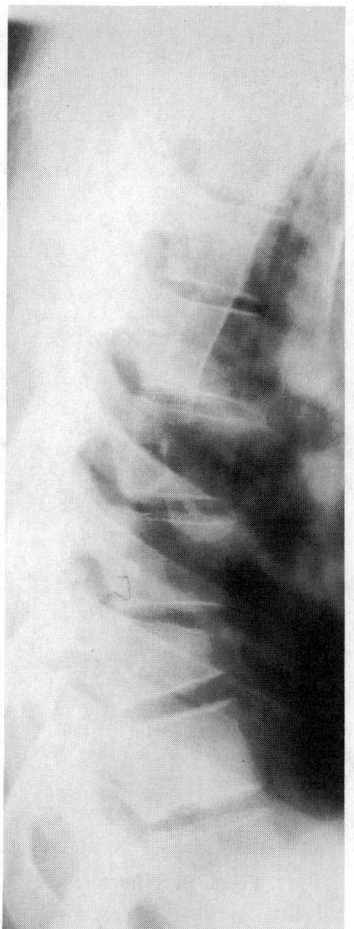

Fig. 3. Stable wedge fracture.

structures and ligaments described by Holdsworth is supplemented by middle and anterior columns (Denis, 1988). The middle column consists of the posterior halves of the vertebral bodies and discs with the adjacent posterior longitudinal ligament whilst the anterior portions of the bodies and discs joined by the anterior longitudinal ligament constitute the anterior column (Fig. 2). Instability is now known to result from simultaneous disruption of the posterior and middle columns (particularly the posterior longitudinal ligament and the adjacent disc).

This three-column model may be used to determine the degree of instability in different types of injury. For example, it explains why isolated fractures of the anterior and central parts of the vertebral bodies are normally stable and also why severe ligament injuries can produce instability without any associated fracture or dislocation. The system is less easily applied to atypical vertebrae such as the atlas or axis. Radiological signs of an unstable ligament injury will be described later.

Classification

Compression fractures

These are of two main types. When only the anterior column is affected, a wedge fracture (Fig. 3) results and

the injury remains stable unless the degree of collapse causes the posterior column to fail under tension. The second type of compression injury is associated with axial loading and failure of the anterior and middle columns which produces a burst fracture (Fig. 4). Although this is a stable injury because the posterior column remains intact, retropulsion of the posterior vertebral wall or disc into the neural canal places the spinal cord at risk and this fracture is often associated with neurological injury.

Flexion Injuries

Posterior distraction may be a more potent component of this injury than anterior compression and the posterior and middle columns can rupture under tension whilst the anterior column remains intact (Fig. 5). This is clearly an unstable injury which is usually associated with a posterior vertebral fracture.

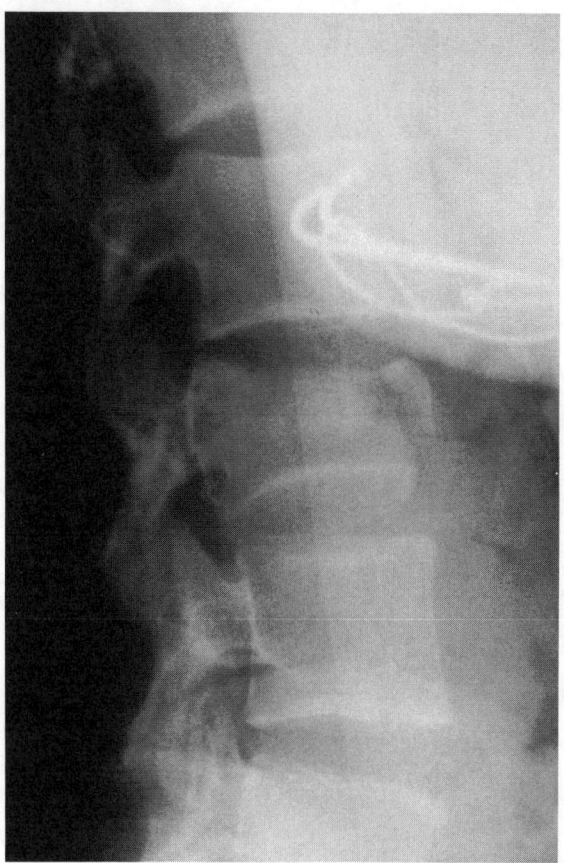

Fig. 4. Burst fracture.

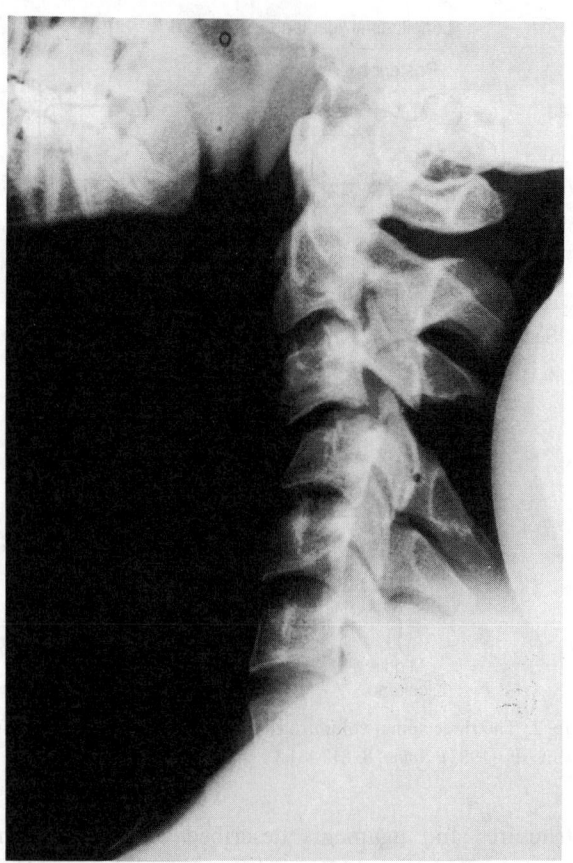

Fig. 5. Rupture of posterior ligamentous complex and forward displacement of C3 on C4.

Fracture-dislocations result from combinations of compression, tension, rotation and shearing. They disrupt all three columns, are the most dangerous of injuries and are commonly associated with trauma to the spinal cord. Dislocation may be regarded as a horizontal shearing injury without an associated fracture.

Extension injuries

These are more commonly encountered in the cervical region. Forced extension may produce a fracture which tends to reduce spontaneously in the neutral position and may not be evident on X-rays. However, the anterior longitudinal ligament can avulse a small fracture from the front of the vertebral body (Holdsworth, 1970) and this marker normally persists (Fig. 6).

The practical significance of instability in spinal injury is its potential for neurological disability or death. For this reason, all patients with suspected spinal injuries must be placed and splinted in the anatomical position until investigations confirm or refute the diagnosis.

Causation and incidence of spine and spinal cord injury

There is said to be a 5–10% coincidence of unstable cervical injury with significant head trauma (Irving & Irving, 1967; Evans, 1971; ATLS, 1993). This figure has been contested by others and sometimes patients with relatively minor head injuries have been included in the calculations (O'Malley & Ross, 1988; Bayless & Ray, 1989). Facial trauma is also said to be associated with cervical spine injury (ATLS, 1993) but some studies do not bear this out (Luce et al., 1979; Andrew et al., 1992).

Approximately 14% of all spinal injuries implicate the cord (Riggins & Kraus, 1977) and these patients are usually admitted to a spinal centre. Half have been involved in road traffic accidents, 30% have been injured at work or home and 20% at sport (Peach & Grundy, 1991). Diving carries particular risks (Peach & Grundy, 1991) and casualties removed from water should always be suspected of having a spinal injury (Morgan & Winter, 1986; Grundy et al., 1991). Sadly, many accidents responsible for spinal cord injury are associated with

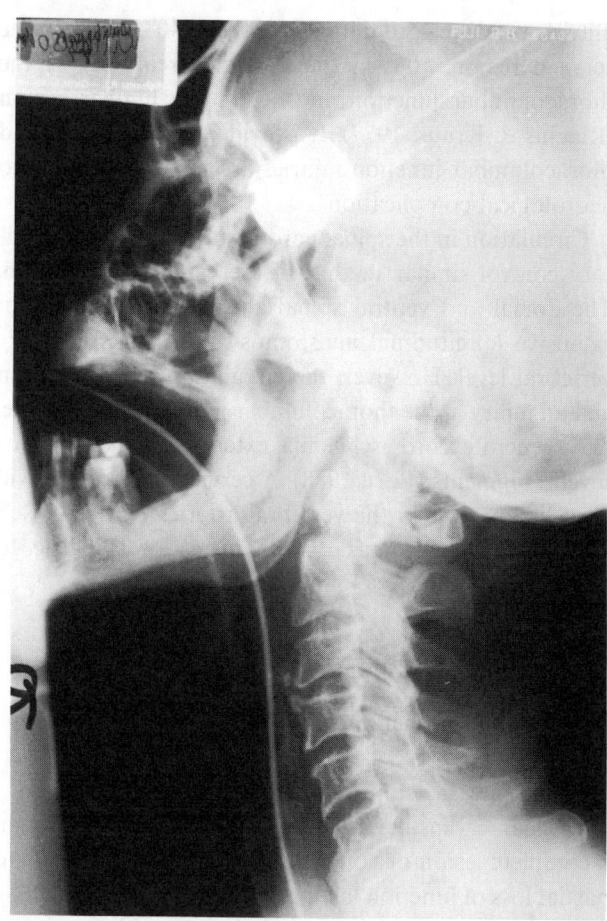

Fig. 6. Extension avulsion fracture of body of C4, fracture of posterior arch of C1 and type II fracture of the odontoid process.

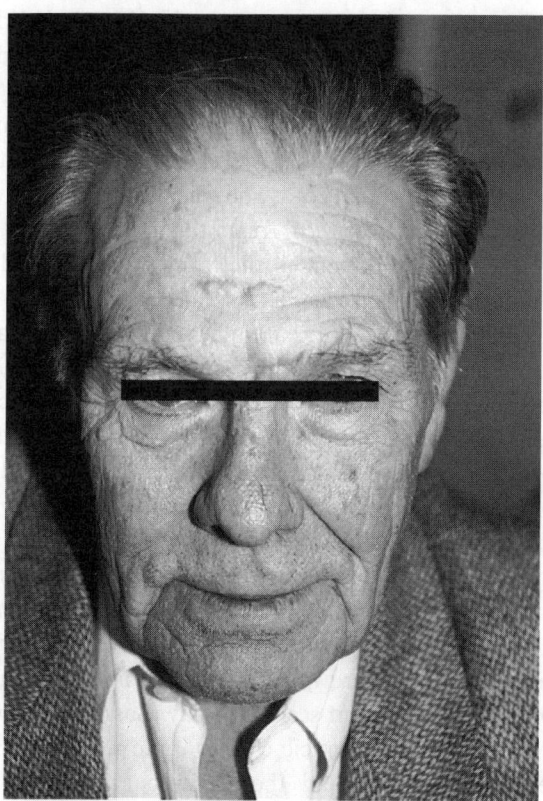

Fig. 7. Minor forehead wound associated with an odontoid fracture.

alcohol consumption and are potentially preventable (Peach & Grundy, 1991).

Although neck sprains are often seen in restrained car drivers and passengers, one study showed that 80% of serious neck injuries occurred in unrestrained car occupants compared with only 5% of those who wore a seatbelt (Huelke *et al.*, 1981). The same study revealed that one in 14 casualties ejected from a vehicle suffered a serious neck injury compared with one in 483 of those who remained in a vehicle which was sufficiently damaged to be towed away. When ejection does not occur, the greatest threat to the neck is posed by the vehicle turning over (Wigglesworth, 1992).

Although the efficacy of seat belts for protection against serious cervical injury is well established (Cadoux *et al.*, 1987), a pattern of visceral and lumbar injury associated with pressure from the lap belt has been described in adults (Williams & Ratliff, 1993) and children (Newman *et al.*, 1990).

Clinical anatomy and pathogenesis of injury

Any force may injure the spine and excessive flexion, extension, rotation, lateral tilt, axial distraction or impaction are all detrimental. Flexion with rotation or vertical impaction is the commonest mechanism but extension injuries are seen in the cervical spine, often in association with a relatively minor forehead wound (Fig. 7).

A number of anatomical factors influence the patterns of injury in the four segments of the spine: cervical, thoracic, lumbar and sacral.

The cervical spine commences superiorly with two atypical vertebrae – the atlas and axis. The atlas has no body as this fused during evolution with that of the axis to form the odontoid process (dens). The 1st cervical vertebra (C1) therefore consists of a ring which articulates with the anterior surface of the odontoid and the lateral masses of the axis. The main structure responsible for stabilizing their anatomical relationship is the cruciate ligament which holds the odontoid peg forwards allowing the spinal cord to pass through a relatively wide spinal canal behind. Between the spinal cord and the odontoid process lies areolar tissue so that the anterior third of the cavity of C1 is occupied by the odontoid, the middle third by areolar tissue and the posterior third by the spinal cord (Steel, 1968). Significant displacement must therefore occur at the C1/2 level before the odontoid impinges on the spinal cord. The spinal canal is relatively capacious in the cervical region compared with the thoracic, and movement in the former is facilitated by obliquely orientated facet joints.

The thoracic vertebrae have more coronally orientated apophysial (facet) joints which allow rotation but limit other movements which are also restricted by the rib cage and sternum. The chest wall serves to splint the thoracic spine and a severe impact is therefore required to produce a thoracic fracture-dislocation. Because the spinal canal in this region is less capacious, unstable and displaced injuries are more often associated with partial or complete cord transection, particularly when sternal or multiple rib fractures are present. However, exceptions are recorded and cord transection must not be assumed from the displacement seen on X-ray (Sasson & Mozes, 1987). Whilst the thoracic cord is quite well protected, the cervicothoracic and thoracolumbar junctions are sites of stress where the more mobile cervical and lumbar vertebrae articulate with the relatively immobile thoracic spine and survivable cord injury most commonly occurs (Riggins & Kraus, 1977; Green *et al.*, 1981). In fatal accidents there is a high incidence of injury to the upper cervical spine (Bucholz *et al.*, 1979; Alker *et al.*, 1975).

In the lumbar spine the facet joints are orientated sagittally and the main movements are therefore flexion, extension and lateral tilt. In the adult, the spinal cord terminates as the conus medullaris at the lower border of the 1st lumbar vertebra. Injuries at the thoracolumbar junction may therefore damage the lowest (sacral) segments of the cord, or inferior to this the cauda equina, interfering with bladder and bowel function. As the nerve roots of the cauda equina only partially fill the lumbar canal, neurological injuries in this area tend to be incomplete and less disabling.

It should be emphasized that, in at least 5% of cases, injuries coexist in two or more non-contiguous areas of the spine and the identification of one injury must not preclude the search for another (Calenoff *et al.*, 1978; Korres *et al.*, 1981). A displaced fracture or dislocation should be evident on X-rays but a central disc prolapse can compress the cord in the absence of any obvious radiological abnormality (Young *et al.*, 1986).

Whatever the mechanism of trauma, 14% of all spinal injuries produce cord damage; of these, 40% occur in the cervical region, 10% in the thoracic area, 35% at the thoracolumbar junction and 3% in the lumbar region (Riggins & Kraus, 1977). It is evident that cervical and thoracolumbar junction injuries are most susceptible to neurological complications.

Circulation in the spinal cord is subject to autoregulatory control similar to that of the cerebral circulation. The dorsal and ventral spinal arteries form part of an extensive longitudinal anastomosis with links at every vertebral level. However, the circulation is not uniform and an injury at the thoracolumbar junction, for example, may generate cord ischaemia extending superiorly for several segments (Burt, 1988). A cervical dislocation will also disrupt flow in the vertebral arteries.

There are three basic mechanisms of spinal cord impairment:

1. Mechanical.
2. Hypoxic.
3. Ischaemic or haemorrhagic.

Oedema may develop as a secondary event.

Mechanical insults may transect the cord, produce an incomplete lesion or concuss it generating transient and partial loss of function lasting several days (Benes, 1968). More subtle compression may be produced by an extradural haematoma or prolapsed disc. In some cases, such as those with delayed neurological deterioration, local vascular obstruction may be an important factor in the pathogenesis of the cord injury. Hypoxia and hypotension are as deleterious to the spinal cord as they are to other neural tissues (Sonntag & Douglas, 1992) and resuscitation of vital functions is therefore just as important for a patient with spinal injury as it is for any other trauma casualty. The patient must be laid supine, not only to relieve spinal deformity and cord compression, but also because the head of hydrostatic pressure within the circulation may fall in the sitting or standing position and infarct the cord at a site of incomplete injury. Nowadays, incomplete injuries are more common, but whether this results from improved safety or better care before or after arrival at hospital is not known.

The possibility of a brachial plexus injury should be considered in the differential diagnosis of patients with post-traumatic neurological symptoms or signs in the upper limb (Grundy & Silver, 1981). Avulsion of the roots of the brachial plexus can damage the spinal cord at the level of detachment (Flannery & Birch, 1990).

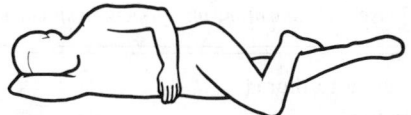

Fig. 8. Lateral position. (Reproduced from *ABC of Spinal Cord Injury*, with permission of BMJ publishing group.)

CLINICAL MANAGEMENT

Casualty positioning

At the earliest opportunity, the patient should be placed in the anatomical position by gently correcting any flexion, extension, rotation or lateral tilt of the spine. This will reduce displacement at any level of injury and help to relieve compression of the spinal cord or arteries. The anatomical position is best achieved by carefully placing the patient supine and this position facilitates resuscitation and the rapid assessment of immediately life-threatening injuries. However, unconscious supine patients are susceptible to silent gastric regurgitation and aspiration unless intubated. If tracheal intubation cannot be performed, the patient should be 'log-rolled' carefully into the lateral position with the upper shoulder tilted slightly forward and the head supported in neutral on the underlying arm (Fig. 8). This position allows secretions to drain freely from the mouth.

The patient with known or suspected spinal injury should be turned ideally by four people in a coordinated manner, one person being responsible for the head and neck, one for the shoulders and chest, one for the hips and abdomen, and one for the legs (Fig. 9). The person holding the head and neck directs movement. In turning the patient to the lateral or supine position, it is essential that unnecessary movement of any part of the spine is avoided. It is not acceptable for the injured spine to be splinted in a position of deformity; definitive treatment seeks to achieve normal alignment which should be restored at an early stage by gentle movement and avoidance of traction until the nature of any injury is known. The only contraindication to neutral alignment is precipitation or aggravation of neurological symptoms during attempts to straighten the spine. Patients with suspected spinal injury must be placed and transported in the horizontal position to avoid orthostatic hypotension in the spinal arteries.

Spinal immobilization

Nowadays, unconscious casualties and those with suspected spinal injury are usually positioned and splinted correctly by ambulance personnel. Soft collars are totally inadequate for cervical splintage and one of the semirigid types which cup the chin is essential (Johnson *et al.*, 1981; Podolsky *et al.*, 1983). In the supine position, the collar should be supplemented by sand bags each side of the head and forehead tape crossing the sand bags to the stretcher or trolley on each side. Proprietary head immobilizers serve the same function. In the uncooperative or active patient, the head should not be taped down as movement of the trunk can manipulate the cervical spine from below. Similarly, a semirigid collar alone is appropriate if the patient has to be nursed in the lateral position. It should be emphasized that, in the event of any difficulty, the most secure way to immobilize the neck is to grasp each side of the head without occluding the ears. However, splintage does release the doctor to attend to other duties.

A short backboard (Cline *et al.*, 1985) or equivalent lightweight splint such as the Kendrick or Russell extrication device (Fig. 10) will effectively immobilize the whole of the spine from head to pelvis if used in conjunction with a semirigid collar. Similar splints for children incorporate padding to support the thoracolumbar spine and counteract the effect of the prominent

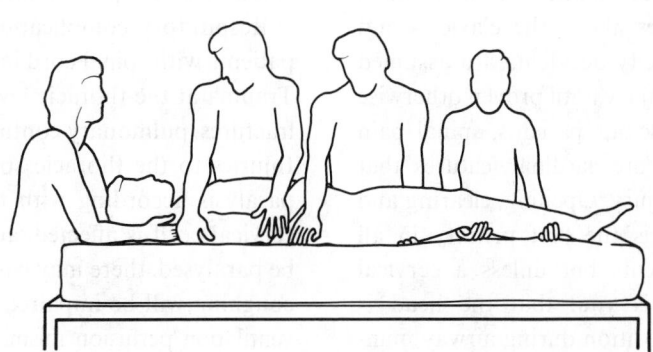

Fig. 9. Log-roll. (Reproduced from *ABC of Spinal Cord Injuries*, with permission of BMJ publishing group)

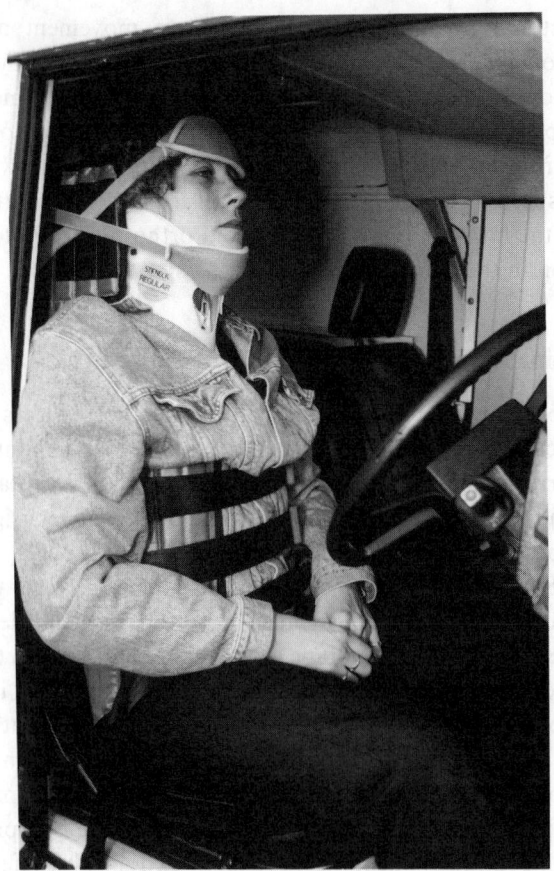

Fig. 10. Spine immobilizer (Kendrick extrication device).

occiput by allowing the neck to extend into the neutral position. Conversely, elderly and kyphotic patients need occipital padding to prevent cervical hyperextension.

Spinal splints are being used increasingly by ambulance services in the UK. On arrival in the A&E department, the patient may also be placed on a long spinal board for complete immobilization.

Primary survey

It is essential that patients unconscious from trauma, those with significant injuries above the clavicles and those who survive high-velocity accidents are assumed to have an unstable cervical injury until proven otherwise by adequate X-rays. In conscious patients, spinal pain and neurological symptoms are cardinal features that help to localize the level of injury. Opening, clearing and maintenance of the airway is the first priority in all seriously ill or injured patients but unless a cervical injury can be excluded it is vital that the head is immobilized in the neutral position during airway manoeuvres. As a first approach, the head may be held firmly

Table 1. *Causes of respiratory impairment in spinal cord injury*

- Direct trauma to thorax
  - Rib fractures
  - Pulmonary contusion
  - Haemopneumothorax
- Spinal cord lesions
  - Intercostal muscle paralysis
  - Partial phrenic nerve involvement: immediate/delayed
- In either case
  - Impaired cough
  - Ventilation/perfusion mismatch

with a hand on each side whilst the fingers open the airway with a jaw thrust. Once the head is immobilized as described above, the hands are free to manage the airway.

When the patient is unconscious and the head is splinted, the risk of aspiration may be reduced by tipping the casualty head down and applying suction, but it is best prevented by tracheal intubation. In skilled hands this manoeuvre may be performed blindly by the naso-tracheal route without moving the neck (Aprahamian *et al.*, 1984). However, there is no evidence that orotracheal intubation carries any risk as long as movement of the head is minimized by an assistant (Majernick *et al.*, 1986; Rhee *et al.*, 1990; Bivins *et al.*, 1988). Flexible fibreoptic nasotracheal intubation is probably the ideal technique (Delaney & Hessler, 1988) but it is rarely available in an emergency, such as airway occlusion by a large prevertebral haematoma (McLauchlan *et al.*, 1991).

Vigorous suction must be avoided in the presence of a high spinal cord lesion because unopposed vagal stimulation can precipitate cardiac arrest (Baker & Silver, 1984). A nasogastric or orogastric tube should be passed to reduce the likelihood of aspiration since ileus is common after spinal injury.

Respiratory complications (Table 1) are common in patients with spinal cord injury (Grundy & Swain, 1993). Trauma at the thoracic level is often associated with rib fractures, pulmonary contusion or haemopneumothorax. Injuries to the thoracic spinal cord produce intercostal paralysis according with the level of injury. When the cervical cord is affected, all the intercostal muscles may be paralysed, there may be a partial phrenic nerve injury, coughing will be impaired and hypoxia will result from ventilation/perfusion mismatch. Ascending post-traumatic cord oedema may develop within 24 h and precipitate respiratory failure. It is therefore important that clinical assessment of respiratory function is combined with pulse oximetry and monitoring of blood gas tensions. The splinting effect of the ribs and sternum on unstable thoracic injuries will be lost if these bones are also fractured.

Circulatory assessment may reveal shock which should be attributed to hypovolaemia unless haemorrhage can be excluded. Cardiogenic shock may occasionally develop and electrocardiographic monitoring is mandatory, but injuries to the cervical or thoracic cord above T5 are more frequently associated with neurogenic shock (Burt, 1988; Sonntag & Douglas, 1992). Neurogenic shock is produced by high cord lesions which interrupt the sympathetic outflow between the 1st thoracic and 2nd lumbar segments causing bradycardia and peripheral vasodilatation. The bradycardia may not be profound but it should certainly be treated with atropine if the pulse rate drops below $50 \, min^{-1}$. When the systolic blood pressure is less than 80 mmHg and unresponsive to elevation of the legs or a fluid challenge, inotropic support should be considered, usually with dopamine (Grundy & Swain, 1993). Other causes of bradycardia must be considered in the differential diagnosis (e.g. drugs). The response to treatment should be assessed by measuring central venous pressure and the hourly urine output.

An additional cardiovascular risk to patients with spinal cord injury is the use of suxamethonium for tracheal intubation. This drug is contraindicated between 3 days and 9 months after injury as it may precipitate hyperkalaemic cardiac arrest which can be avoided by using a non-depolarizing muscle relaxant (John *et al.*, 1976).

At the end of the primary survey, the patient must be fully undressed to permit a full examination of the back and other areas. Administration of oxygen at high concentration, intravenous fluid volume replacement and other therapeutic interventions during the primary survey will help to improve spinal cord nutrition. However, care should be taken not to overinfuse patients whose shocked state is exclusively neurogenic in origin (Meyer *et al.*, 1971). By performing a rectal examination before passing a urinary catheter, an opportunity is provided to check for anal sphincter tone and perianal sensation.

The fully conscious and orientated patient with spinal injury will be able to provide a history during the primary survey but may not always complain of neck or back pain (Maull & Satchatello, 1977; Bresler & Rich,

Table 2. *Factors responsible for failure to identify spinal cord injury*

- Distraction of patient and/or doctor by more painful, obvious or multiple injuries
- Any impairment of consciousness
  - Head injury
  - Shock
  - Alcohol
  - Drugs
- Atypical neurological picture, e.g. partial cord injury
- Assumed longstanding neurological defect, e.g. stroke
- Patient thought to be feigning symptoms or hysterical

1982). Consciousness is often impaired by head injury, alcohol, drugs or shock, and sometimes more overt and painful injuries distract the patient and doctor alike. These factors (Table 2) are responsible for the failure to promptly diagnose spinal cord injury in a significant number of patients (Bohlman, 1979; Ravichandran & Silver, 1984; Ravichandran, 1989). Spinal cord involvement in conscious patients produces sensory and/or motor impairment below a neurological level and these symptoms are normally accompanied by spinal pain which often radiates along nerve roots at the level of injury. Complete spinal cord lesions should not be difficult to diagnose in orientated patients but the spectrum of incomplete cord injury means that sensory and motor symptoms must never be disregarded, even if they do not fit a typical pattern (Maroon, 1977).

Partial cord lesions are those associated with some preservation of distal neurological function. Their diagnosis is important as they carry a better prognosis for recovery and are now more common. However, they would not normally be diagnosed until the end of the secondary survey and even then the diagnosis is often missed (Bicknell & Fielder, 1992).

Secondary survey

At this stage in the assessment of a traumatized patient, the treatment of life-threatening injuries should have commenced. The secondary survey is a top-to-toe examination which commences at the head. This is important as 5–10% of significant head injuries are associated with trauma to the cervical spine (Irving & Irving, 1967; Evans, 1971). With the head properly immobilized, examination of the neck in the supine patient is difficult but with the head held and the collar released for a few moments, only the back of the neck is concealed from view and this area can be palpated without moving the patient.

In the chest, injury to the thoracic spine may be associated with fractures of the sternum or ribs, haemopneumothorax or pulmonary contusion. Although this part of the spine cannot be palpated in the supine patient, the anteroposterior chest X-ray must be examined carefully as it may reveal alterations in vertebral contour, a paravertebral haematoma or fractures of the upper three ribs resulting from a severe deceleration or acceleration force at the base of the neck. Cervical and high thoracic cord injuries cause paralysis of the intercostal muscles and paradoxical (diaphragmatic) respiration (Sandor, 1966).

In the abdomen, spinal cord injury produces further physiological changes as the abdominal wall becomes anaesthetic, flaccid and areflexic. Signs of peritonism such as rigidity and rebound tenderness are absent in such cases but referred pain at the tip of the shoulder is a useful sign, particularly if it is aggravated by abdominal palpation. When spinal cord and abdominal trauma are thought to coexist, peritoneal lavage is a particularly important and helpful investigation as abdominal emergencies in these patients are responsible for 10% of deaths (Tibbs *et al.*, 1979). Upward movement of the umbilicus when the abdomen tenses is associated with spinal cord injury at the 10th thoracic level (Beevor's sign) but this is an uncommon sign. Priapism is more obvious and is pathognomonic of cord injury.

In the arms, a flexed posture may indicate paralysis of extensors and other muscle groups supplied by nerve roots distal to the 5th cervical. After examination of the limbs, the patient should be log-rolled ideally by four people (as previously described) but with the semirigid collar still in place. The doctor in charge is responsible for examining the back and must not therefore take part in the log-roll which is coordinated by the person at the head end. During the turn, which should be performed only as far as is necessary to expose the back, it is important that movement is synchronous and that the head is moved carefully through an arc, as well as rotated. In the tilted position, the spine and the posterior ribs can be inspected and palpated. Bruising, swelling and tenderness over the spine are all significant, as is widening of the interspinous gap (White *et al.*, 1975). The collar should be removed briefly to permit a proper examination of the back of the head and neck. Only patients with an established diagnosis of unstable injury or with symptoms or signs of spinal cord trauma should

have their log-roll deferred until they have been assessed by a senior doctor. Occasionally, casualties are transported to hospital in the lateral position and the back can then be examined before the patient is turned supine.

The secondary survey ends with an examination of the nervous system which should be more detailed when spinal or spinal cord injury is suspected or confirmed.

Neurological examination

In the conscious patient, all the major neurological modalities should be tested including fine touch (posterior columns), pin-prick (spinothalamic tracts), proprioception (posterior columns), power (corticospinal tracts), tone and reflexes (including abdominal and sacral). The response to pain must be tested in all four limbs and above the clavicles as a tetraplegic patient is likely to respond only to the latter. The root values of dermatomes and muscle groups must be known if the neurological examination is to be interpreted correctly. A search should be made for sacral sparing by checking the bulbocavernosus (S3–4) and anal reflexes (S5). The anal reflex consists of a visible contraction of the external sphincter in response to perianal pin-prick. The bulbocavernosus reflex is a similar response felt by the examiner's finger in the anal canal when the glans penis (or clitoris) is squeezed. If these reflexes are preserved in an incomplete cord injury throughout the phase of spinal shock, bladder and bowel control will probably return. However, the absence of a bulbocavernosus reflex is not necessarily significant and the plantar response is also an unreliable sign in the diagnosis of acute spinal cord injury.

Spinal shock is a shutdown of spinal cord function associated with flaccidity and areflexia below the level of injury. It may last for hours, days or weeks but ultimately resolves producing upper motor neurone signs (hyperreflexia and hypertonicity) below the level of cord injury. Spinal shock is therefore responsible for flaccid areflexia.

Diagnosis of spinal cord injury

This may be obvious in a conscious patient with sensory and motor impairment distal to a neurological level. However, be wary of neurological symptoms and signs which do not fit a classical pattern: a partial cord lesion may be present. The majority of these injuries conform to one of several patterns. If the zone of cord injury lies centrally (Fig. 11) and encroaches on the cervical axons

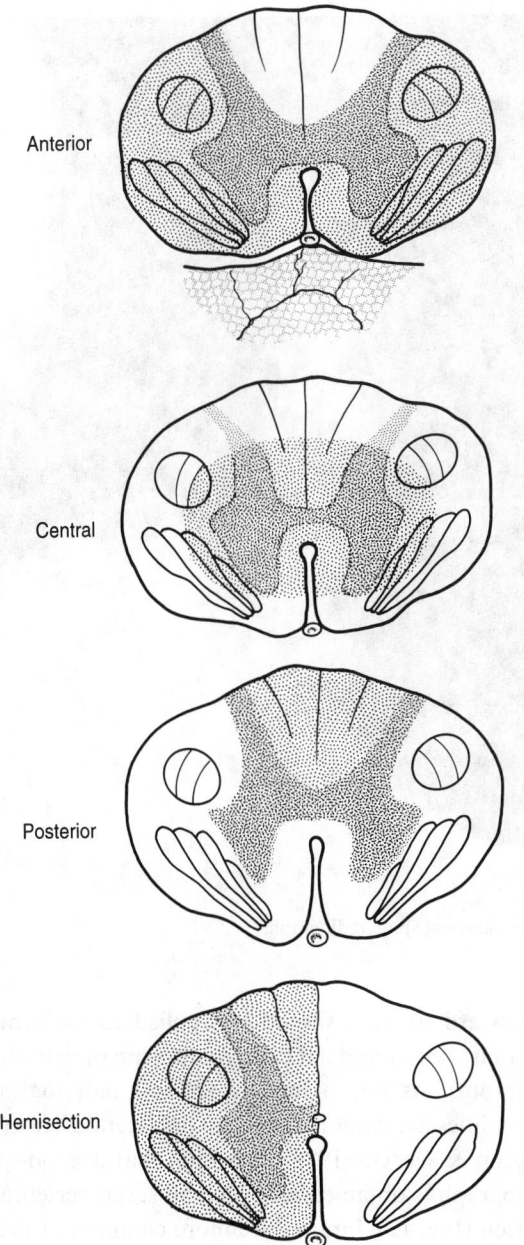

Anterior

Central

Posterior

Hemisection

Fig. 11. Partial cord injuries. (Reproduced from *ABC of Spinal Cord Injuries*, with permission of BMJ publishing group.)

Table 3. *Signs of spinal cord injury in the unconscious*

- Flaccid areflexia (spinal shock)
- Diaphragmatic breathing
- Flexed posture of the upper limbs
- Priapism
- Neurogenic shock
- Pain response above clavicles only

1989). In the anterior cord syndrome, contusion affects the spinothalamic and corticospinal tracts producing weakness and impaired pain and temperature sensation. The anterior spinal artery is often injured at the same time. The posterior cord syndrome affects proprioception and may cause ataxia, whilst lateral injuries to the spinal cord from penetrating trauma or lateral fractures of the vertebrae can produce a Brown-Séquard lesion in which the ipsilateral corticospinal tract and the crossed spino-thalamic tract are injured. Ipsilateral weakness and contralateral loss of pain and temperature sensation result. Incomplete cord injury may manifest a range of neurological symptoms.

In the unconscious patient, diagnosis of spinal cord injury is much more difficult but important signs (Table 3) are flaccid areflexia, diaphragmatic breathing, flexed posturing of the upper limbs, priapism and neurogenic shock. Trauma to the spinal cord must not be discounted until the return of consciousness allows a more accurate clinical assessment.

If the diagnosis of spinal cord injury is confirmed, it should be classified according to its completeness and the neurological and skeletal level of injury. Examples are: incomplete paraplegia below the 9th thoracic segment (T9I) caused by a fracture of the 8th thoracic vertebra; or complete tetraplegia below the 6th cervical vertebra (C6C) resulting from a fracture of the 6th cervical vertebra.

Radiological investigations

The spinal cord may be injured in the absence of any fracture, dislocation or extensive ligament injury. Spinal cord injury without radiological abnormality is common in children (Burke, 1974) in whom the articular facets are flatter and soft tissues more elastic (Sherk *et al.*, 1976) and in elderly patients with cervical spondylosis (Johnston, 1989) when a prolapsed disc may be responsible (Young *et al.*, 1986). The aim of obtaining X-rays is

of the long tracts, there will be flaccid weakness in the arms, spasticity in the lower limbs, and usually urinary retention. This central cord syndrome (Schneider *et al.*, 1954) is more common in older patients in whom the spinal canal is narrowed by the changes of cervical spondylosis. There is often no fracture or dislocation but the cord is compressed between the sclerotic ligamentum flavum posteriorly and a degenerate disc or osteophytes anteriorly, usually during an extension injury (Johnston,

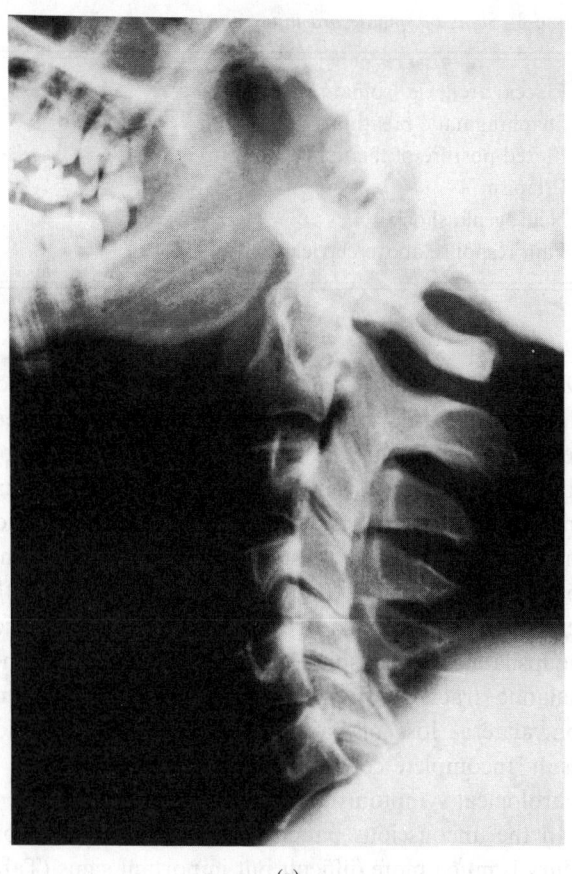

(a)

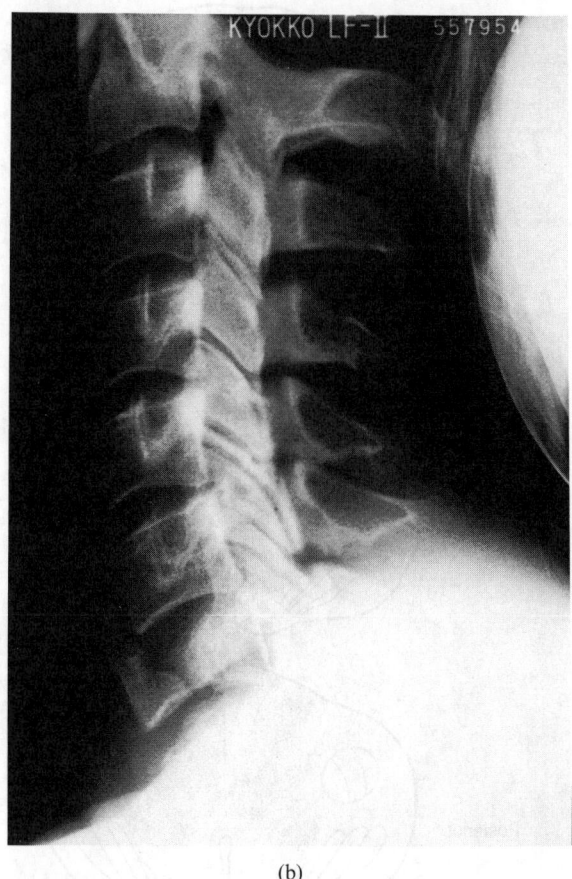

(b)

Fig. 12. Inadequate (a) and adequate (b) lateral cervical spine radiographs.

to identify unstable injuries requiring reduction, immobilization or surgery to restore stability.

Many workers have attempted to establish criteria for requesting X-rays of the cervical spine in casualties suffering serious or potentially serious trauma. Patients who are fully alert with no cervical symptoms or signs do not need cervical spine films, but care must be taken that they are fully orientated and not distracted by the pain of other more obvious injuries. X-rays of the cervical spine should be obtained on trauma patients who manifest any reduction in conscious level, impairment from drugs or alcohol, spinal pain or tenderness, or neurological symptoms or signs (Jacobs & Schwartz, 1986; Bachulis *et al.*, 1986; Roberge *et al.*, 1988).

Cervical spine

Lateral views of the cervical vertebrae are obscured by the shoulders, and the lower jaw and incisor teeth encroach on the anteroposterior and open-mouth views. To expose the lower cervical spine on the lateral X-ray,

downward traction should be applied to the arms but this must be reduced if it exacerbates pain or neurological symptoms. As approximately 85% of radiological abnormalities are demonstrated on the lateral X-ray (Dunnington & Gervin, 1983), it is vital that a good-quality radiograph is obtained on which all seven vertebrae can be seen (Fig. 12). Injuries are more common at the base of the neck and, if this is not well demonstrated, a swimmer's view should be requested (Fig. 13).

The swimmer's view (so named because of its resemblance to the 'crawl' position) may be taken with the patient supine by fully abducting one arm (Fig. 14). The risk associated with any slight movement of the spine is theoretical rather than actual and the head and neck can remain splinted during the procedure. In the UK it is standard practice to put the X-ray plate on the side of the abducted arm whilst the X-ray source is situated adjacent to the opposite shoulder. Staff unfamiliar with this radiograph often find it difficult to interpret, but the first rib and vertebra prominens are helpful landmarks. Chip fractures and minor abnormalities may not

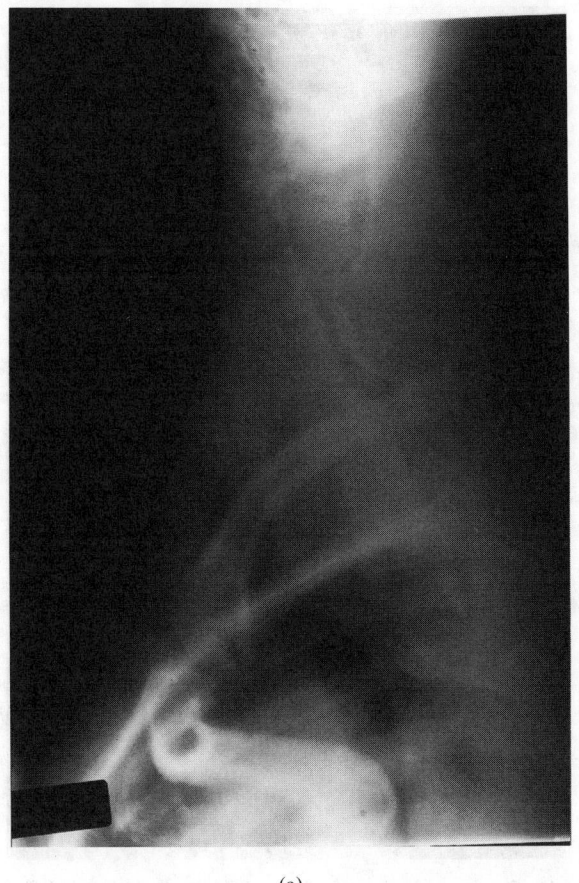
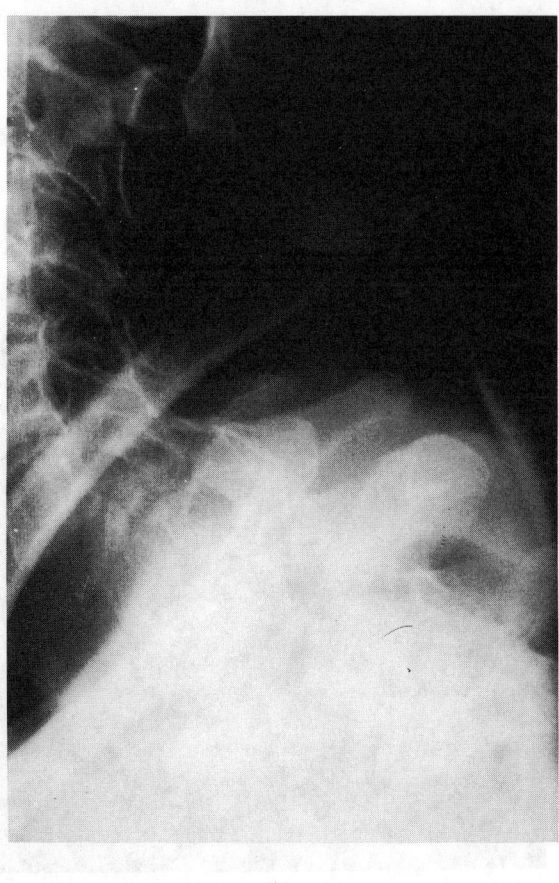

(a)   (b)

Fig. 13. Swimmer's radiographs demonstrating subluxation (a) and dislocation (b) at C6/7.

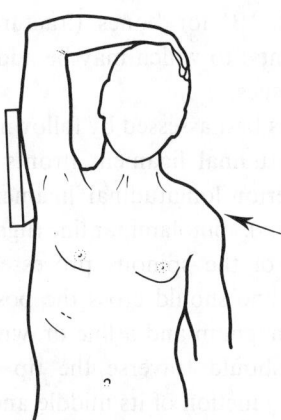

Fig. 14. Technique for obtaining swimmer's view. (Reproduced from *ABC of Spinal Cord Injury*, with permission of BMJ publishing group.)

be detected but vertebral alignment is normally shown.

The anteroposterior cervical spine X-ray is usually less informative than the lateral view. However, attention should be given to the alignment of spinous processes which may change abruptly at the level of a rotatory deformity (Fig. 15). Fractures of the 1st, 2nd and even 3rd ribs are occasionally seen on the anteroposterior view and indicate that the base of the neck has been subjected to a severe force. A prevertebral haematoma at the thoracic inlet may produce tracheal shift (Langford et al., 1989). On the anteroposterior film the upper cervical spine is obscured by the chin and teeth and for this reason an additional open-mouth odontoid view (Fig. 16) is required to complete the standard series of three X-rays required in all patients with known or suspected injury to the cervical spine. To obtain a clear view of the odontoid process, the head and/or X-ray beam often have to be tilted and this investigation should therefore be deferred until the lateral X-ray has been scrutinized.

Some authors have recommended a five-view series of the cervical spine which includes right and left lateral oblique X-rays (Doris & Wilson, 1985). These oblique films sometimes reveal abnormalities at the base of the cervical spine that are not demonstrated on standard

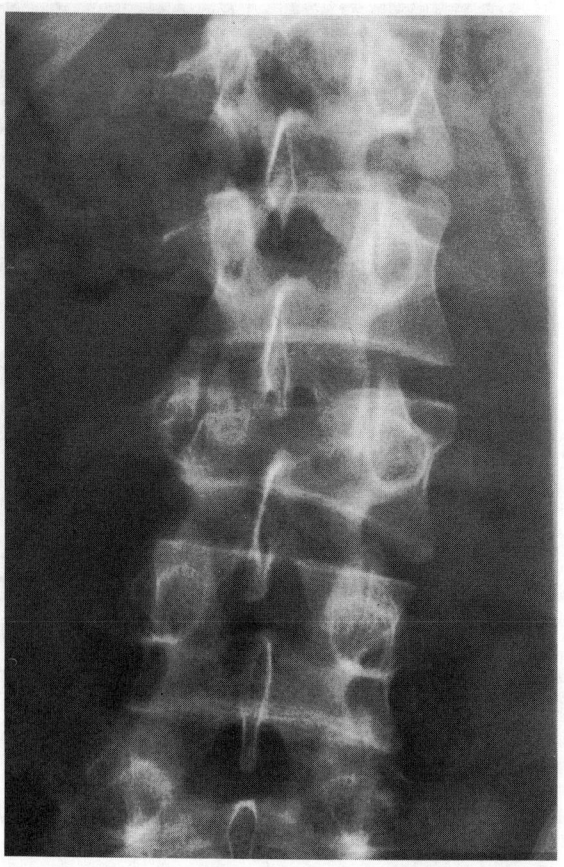

Fig. 15. Anteroposterior view of lumbar spine demonstrating altered alignment of spinous processes (rotatory deformity) at level of L3 fracture.

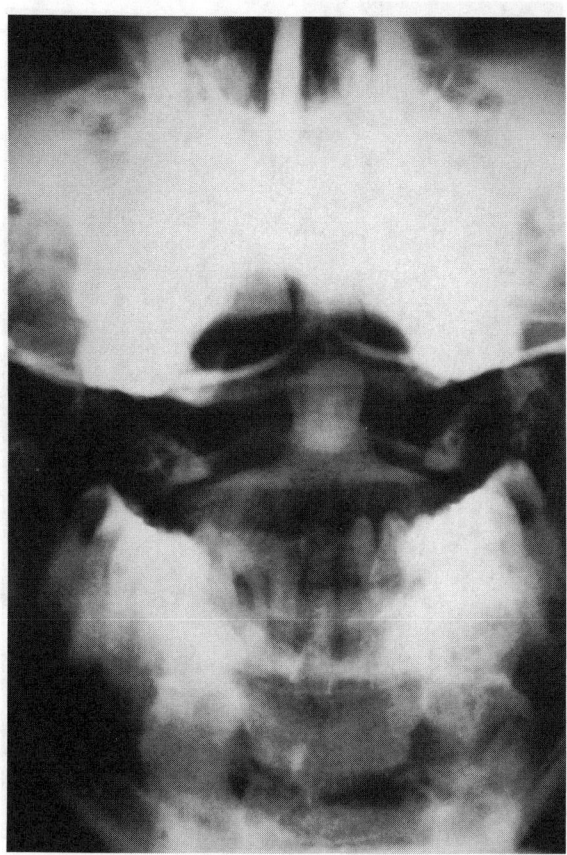

Fig. 16. Open-mouth view of odontoid process revealing a Jefferson fracture of C1.

views (Fig. 17). However, alternative investigations such as tomography, computed tomography (CT) or magnetic resonance imaging (MRI) may also be considered according to circumstances.

Lateral views of the cervical spine taken in flexion and extension under medical supervision may help to elucidate an unstable ligamentous injury with no associated fracture or radiological evidence of instability (see below). The main indication for this investigation is severe neck pain persisting from the moment of impact in a patient whose X-rays reveal no convincing post-traumatic abnormality (Plunkett et al., 1987). Flexion and extension views must not be undertaken in the presence of neurological symptoms or signs or impaired consciousness and the patient should only flex and extend the neck as far as symptoms will allow. Investigations of this type are best left to experienced doctors.

The interpretation of cervical spine radiographs may pose problems for the inexperienced. A recommended system (Williams et al., 1981) follows the sequence 'A'

for alignment, 'B' for bones (fractures), and 'C' for cartilages (joints) to which may be added 'D' for dense connective tissues.

Alignment is best assessed by following the lines of the anterior longitudinal ligament (fronts of the vertebral bodies), posterior longitudinal ligament (backs of the vertebral bodies), spinolaminar line (ligamentum flavum) and the tips of the spinous processes (Fig. 18). The spinolaminar line should cross the posterior margin of the foramen magnum and a line drawn along the clivus of the skull should traverse the tip of the odontoid process at the junction of its middle and anterior thirds. The anterior arch of the atlas (C1) passes in front of the odontoid peg of the axis (C2) and lies anterior to the first line described. When it does not, an odontoid fracture is likely (Fig. 19). Traumatic rupture of the transverse part of the cruciate ligament allows the anterior arch of C1 to displace forwards producing an abnormally large atlanto-odontoid gap (Fig. 20) exceeding 2.5 mm in adults (Jackson, 1950; Hinck & Hopkins, 1960; De Beer et al., 1988) or 5 mm in children (Locke et al., 1966).

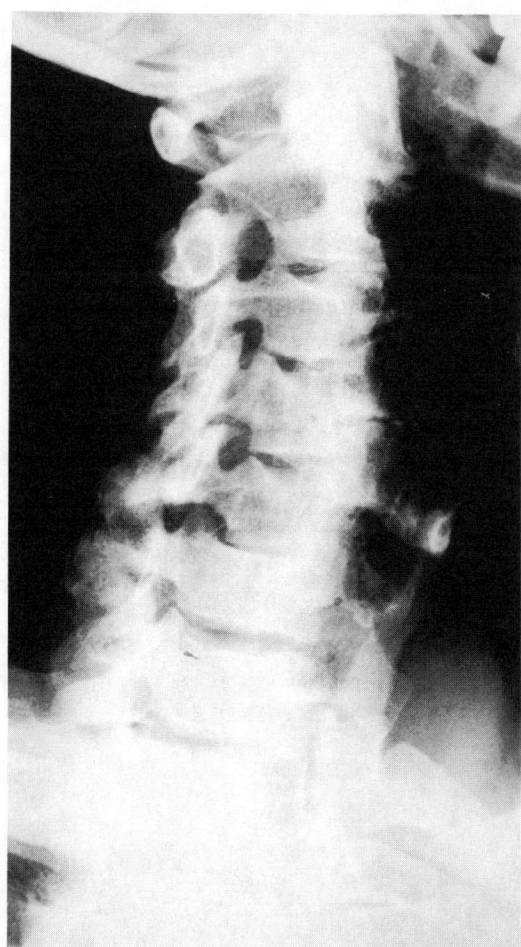

Fig. 17. Unilateral facet dislocation and associated malrotation at C5/6.

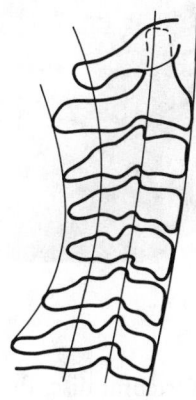

Fig. 18. Lines of alignment.

Other deviations in alignment include subluxation of one vertebra on another which is permitted to a maximum of 3.5 mm (White *et al.*, 1975). Attention should be focused on any abrupt alteration in the spinal contour. Loss of the normal lordotic curvature is noteworthy (Webb *et al.*, 1976) but is often attributable to muscle spasm. Subluxation equivalent to less than half the width of the vertebral body usually denotes a unilateral facet joint dislocation (Fig. 21) which is associated with rotational deformity seen on the anteroposterior or lateral views. Forward displacement greater than this normally indicates bilateral facet dislocation (Fig. 22) which is an unstable injury. In an A&E department, the degree of stability of spinal injuries is academic and the simplest approach is to regard all as being unstable or potentially so.

Turning to the bones ('B'), fractures may be demonstrated on any of the three standard X-rays. C1 fractures involve the anterior or posterior arches (Fig. 6) or the lateral masses (Fig. 16). In some cases of axial compression, the fracture is a burst type with separation of the ring into several fragments and outward displacement of the lateral masses (Fig. 16). This is the Jefferson fracture (Jefferson, 1920). In 50% of cases, fractures of the posterior arch of C1 are accompanied by fractures of C2 (Fig. 6) or another cervical vertebra (Levine & Edwards, 1989). Odontoid fractures are classified into three types (Anderson & D'Alonzo, 1974): an oblique type I fracture passing through the attachment of the alar ligament, a type II injury across the base of the peg (Fig. 26) and a type III extending down into cancellous bone (Fig. 23). The type II fracture is unstable and prone to non-union. Another common fracture of C2 (Fig. 24) is traumatic spondylolysis through the pedicles – the hangman's fracture (Wood-Jones, 1913; Schneider *et al.*, 1965). In this injury, C1 together with the body and odontoid peg of C2 are separated from the posterior part of C2 and the remainder of the cervical spine.

Fixed rotatory subluxation of the atlas on the axis is an unusual injury which usually develops spontaneously or from minor rather than major trauma (Fielding & Hawkins, 1977). Diagnosis is difficult and falls within the province of an orthopaedic surgeon but is based on the presence of a persistent torticollis in young patients and fixed rotation of C1 on C2. The open-mouth odontoid view reveals on one side a wider and medially displaced lateral mass of C1 whilst the opposite lateral mass appears narrow and laterally situated.

The 3rd to 7th vertebrae may fracture through the body, neural arch or spinous process and each part of the vertebra should be examined carefully on the X-ray. Chip fractures commonly detach from the anterosuperior corner of the vertebral body (usually in extension injuries) or anteroinferior angle (during forced flexion). The former may be avulsed by the anterior longitudinal ligament

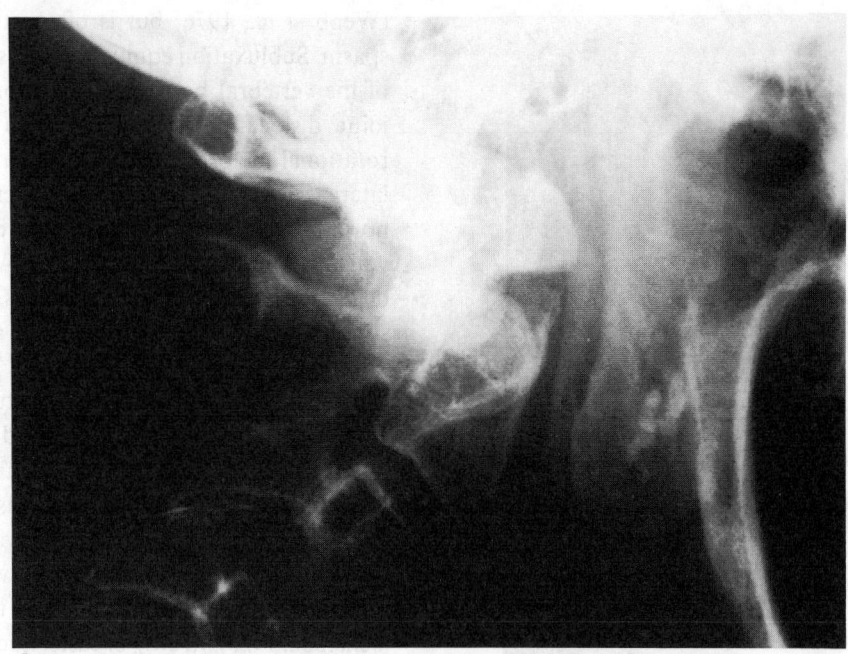

Fig. 19. Posteriorly displaced odontoid fracture in an elderly patient..

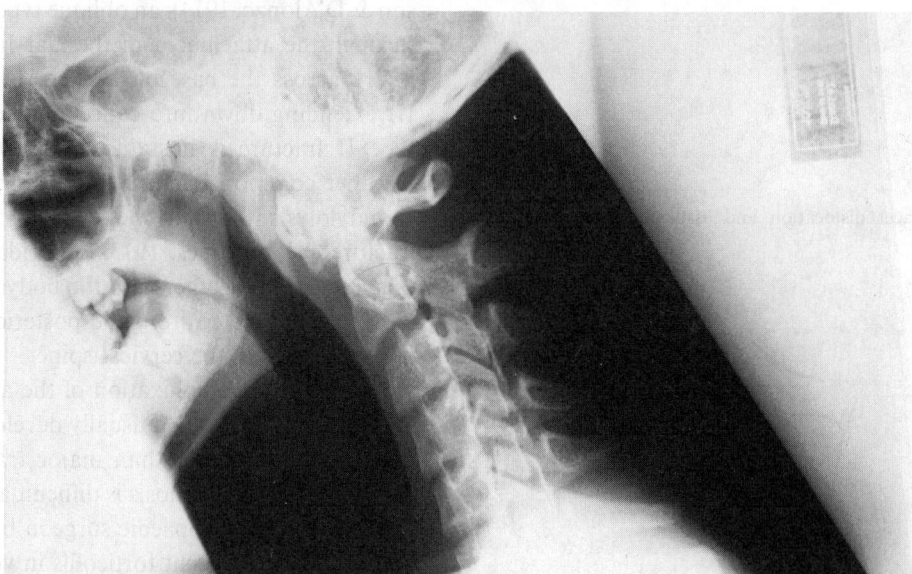

Fig. 20. Increased atlanto-odontoid gap.

(Fig. 6) but the latter is produced by impingement between adjacent vertebrae. The anteroinferior fragments are referred to as 'tear drop' fractures (Fig. 25) and are often associated with intervertebral disc rupture, posterior displacement of the vertebral body and instability (Schneider, 1956). They must therefore be treated with respect.

Cartilage ('C') is a component of the joints of the spine

which are the intervertebral disc, the facet (apophysial) joints and the small uncovertebral synovial joints situated on the posterolateral aspect of the cervical vertebral bodies. These joints are all subject to degenerative changes. The intervertebral disc may undergo traumatic rupture and in facet joint dislocations forward displacement of one vertebra on another is seen.

Abnormalities of the dense connective tissues ('D')

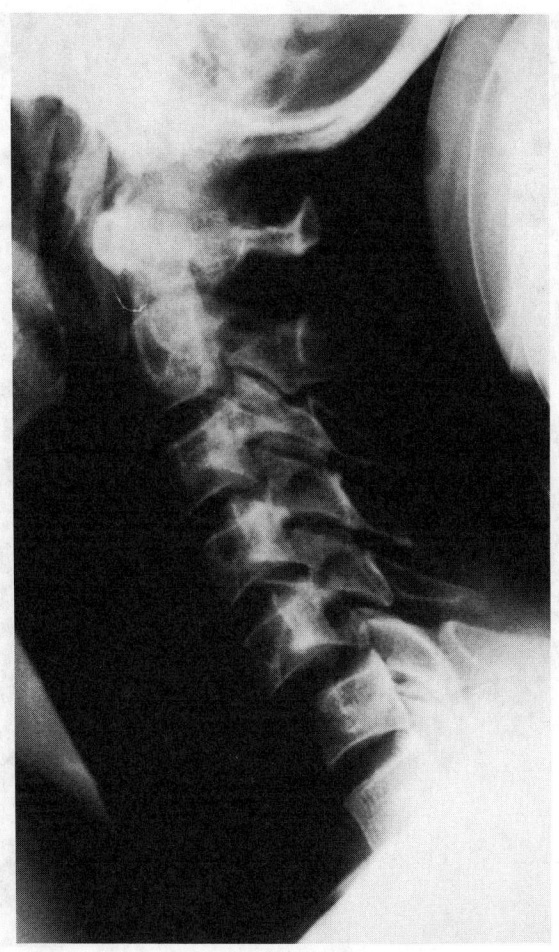

Fig. 21. Unilateral facet dislocation at C5/6.

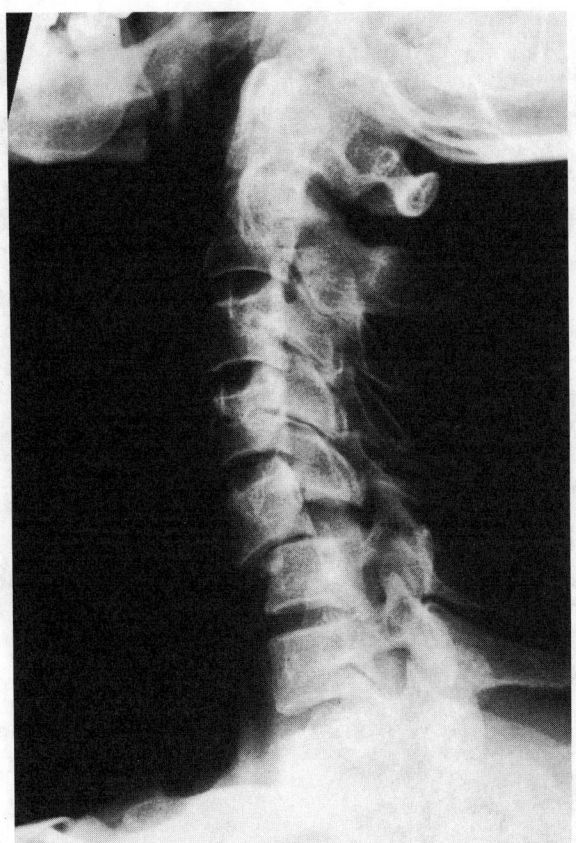

Fig. 22. Bilateral facet dislocation at C5/6.

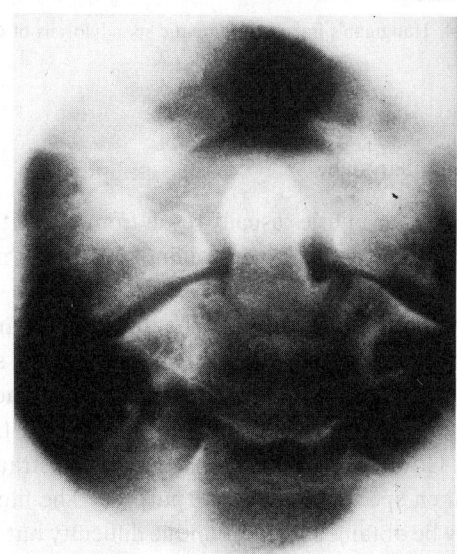

Fig. 23. Odontoid fracture type III.

may portend unstable injury in the absence of any fracture. Anterior ligamentous injuries often produce a prevertebral haematoma which may be diagnosed by displacement of the prevertebral fat-stripe or an increase in the size of the retropharyngeal or retrotracheal space (Webb *et al.*, 1976). The retropharyngeal space (at the level of C2) should not exceed 6 mm in adults or children, whereas the retrotracheal space at C6 should not exceed 22 mm in adults or 14 mm in children (Timberlake, 1989). (A distance of 22 mm in adults approximates to the anteroposterior width of the vertebral body.) However, it is more important to look for a bulge or alteration in soft tissue contour (Fig. 26) than adhere to precise measurements which may be influenced by crying, respiratory distress or swallowing (Martinez *et al.*, 1988), especially in children. Posterior ligamentous injury (Fig. 5) may produce an increased interspinous gap (Webb *et al.*, 1976), and divergent angulation of 11° or more is evidence of instability (White *et al.*, 1975). Prevertebral

swelling, tear-drop fractures, subluxation and widening of the interspinous gap are all radiological signs of potential instability in the cervical spine (Webb *et al.*, 1976).

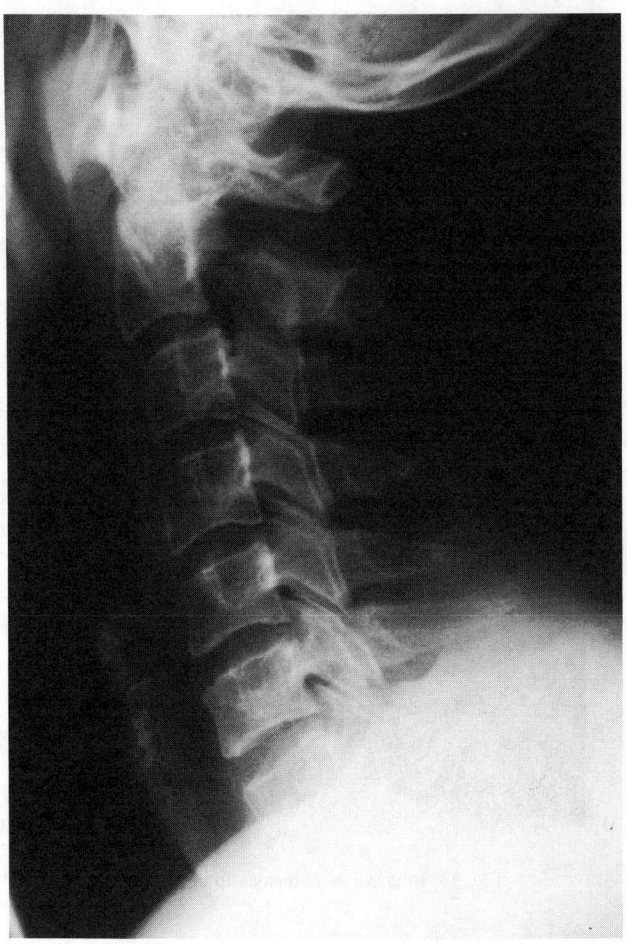

Fig. 24. Hangman's fracture (traumatic spondylolysis of C2).

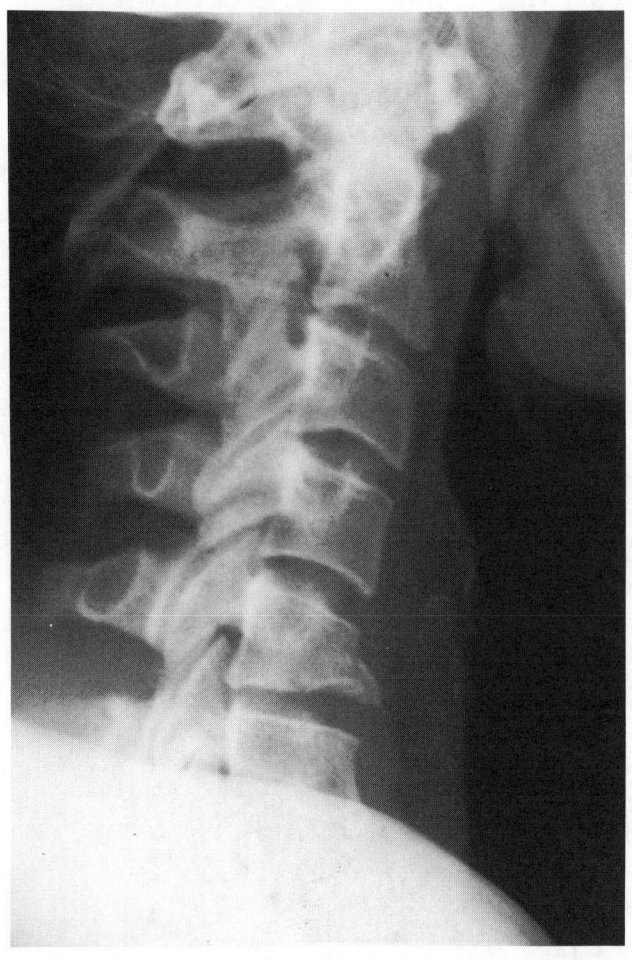

Fig. 25. 'Tear-drop' fracture of C5.

Thoracolumbar spine

Thoracolumbar injuries usually result from severe trauma and it is vital that the spine is maintained in the neutral position.

The standard radiographs of the thoracolumbar spine are the anteroposterior and lateral views. Care should always be taken to try and discern the vertebrae on a chest X-ray taken during the investigation of a trauma patient. However, the spine is best demonstrated on views taken specifically for that purpose. The films can normally be obtained without undue difficulty but lateral X-rays of the upper thoracic spine are often obscured by the ribs and scapulae. Tomography or CT may be required to visualize the vertebrae in this area where fractures can go undetected. In the thoracolumbar region, prevertebral haematomata are best seen on the anteroposterior film.

X-rays may be interpreted according to the ABCD sequence, but the degree of stability is often difficult to assess from the films and is influenced by the integrity of the ribcage and sternum. Anterior compression fractures (Fig. 3) produce wedging of the vertebral bodies but the posterior body and neural canal remain intact. Burst fractures are compression injuries of the anterior and middle columns which are characterized by increased separation of the pedicles on the anteroposterior X-ray and retropulsion of bone into the neural canal on the lateral film (Fig. 4). The posterior ligament complex in the thoracolumbar region may also rupture under tension, but this injury is usually accompanied by a fracture. Fracture dislocations normally result from combined injuries to the anterior, middle and posterior columns and are therefore manifestly unstable. However, an orthopaedic or radiological opinion must be obtained immediately if there is any uncertainty about the radiological diagnosis.

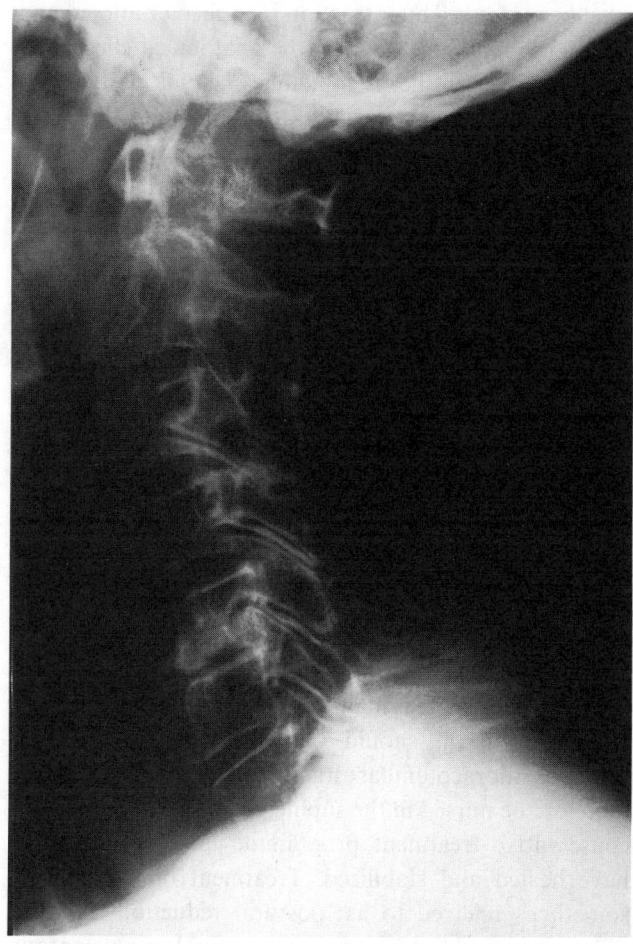

Fig. 26. Prevertebral swelling at level of C6.

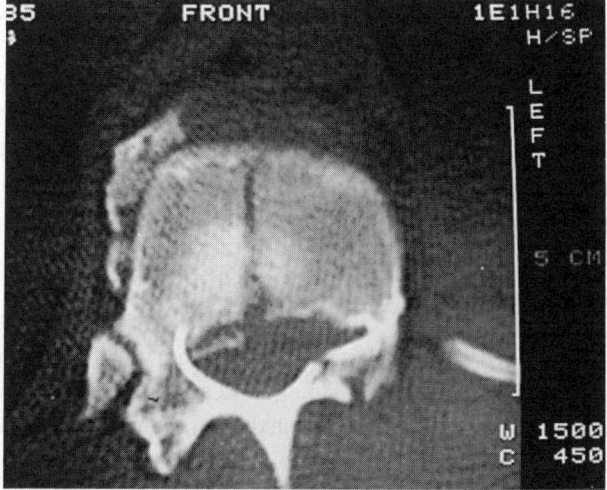

Fig. 27. Computed tomogram of fractured vertebra.

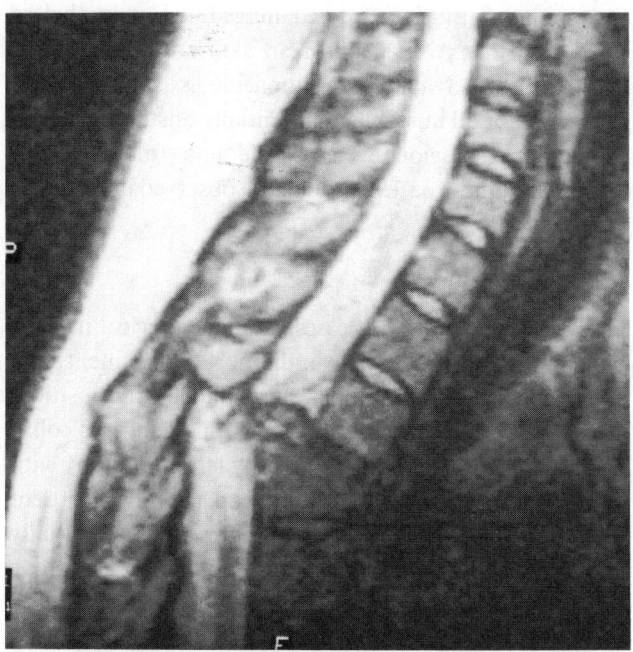

Fig. 28. Magnetic resonance image of spinal cord transection.

Other imaging techniques

CT is at present the most readily available second-line investigation for spinal trauma. Its strength is the effectiveness with which it delineates bony structures, disc material and dense tissues in difficult areas such as the lower cervical and upper thoracic spine (Fig. 27). However, it normally provides views in one plane and should always be used in conjunction with a standard series of X-rays for which it is no substitute (Cacayorin & Kieffer, 1982; Donovan Post et al., 1982). The contents of the neural canal are not well demonstrated on CT images, and spinal curvature – normal or abnormal – interferes with interpretation.

MRI is now the investigation of choice for visualizing the spinal cord and adjacent soft tissues (Fig. 28). The vertebrae are demonstrated but with less bony detail than on CT scans. MRI can distinguish pathological conditions in and around the traumatized cord such as haemorrhage, oedema, contusion, transection or central disc prolapse, and these features assist in determining the prognosis (Kulkarni et al., 1987; Silberstein et al., 1992; Harris et al., 1992). Some lesions in the extradural space are amenable to surgery.

Principles of treatment

Definitive treatment of spinal injury will be undertaken by orthopaedic or neurological surgeons, or consultants in a spinal unit if the cord is damaged. It is nevertheless important that A&E department staff are familiar with the treatments available. Orthopaedic assistance should be sought for all unstable or potentially unstable injuries. In the lumbar region, even a stable injury may give rise to ileus and these patients should be observed in hospital.

Cervical injuries

In by far the majority of cases, unstable cervical injuries can be nursed satisfactorily in the A&E department with the head and neck immobilized in the neutral position. This may be achieved as described with a semirigid collar of appropriate size supplemented by lateral support with sand bags or cushions and forehead tape. The patient should be fully resuscitated and have any potentially life-threatening conditions addressed before definitive treatment of the spinal injury is initiated. Patients with anaesthetic areas resulting from spinal cord injury should be turned regularly and receive skin care if their transfer from the A&E department is delayed.

Splintage in a semirigid collar is adequate treatment for some cervical injuries but, for others, skull traction may be applied in the emergency room by an appropriately trained doctor. Care must be taken not to overdistract the vertebrae at the level of injury. This is more likely to occur in the upper cervical spine where traction requirements are less (Fried, 1974), and is a particular risk with the hangman's fracture where excess traction is borne directly by the spinal cord. Most unstable cervical injuries are treated by skull traction because it helps to correct alignment, reduce fractures and dislocations, provide stability and decompress the cord, spinal arteries and nerve roots. Various skull calipers are available but those with spring-loaded points, such as the Gardner–Wells (Gardner, 1973) or University of Virginia types, embed more securely in the outer table of the skull without drilling and they are less likely to penetrate the skull if properly applied. In recent years, traction through a halo has been more popular because the device can be connected to a spinal brace to permit earlier mobilization.

Traction, manipulation or surgery becomes more urgent when there are signs of deteriorating spinal cord function. Surgery has not been shown to improve the neurological outcome when the patient's condition is stable (Young & Dexter, 1978). As a guide, 1–2 kg of traction are usually adequate for injuries of the upper cervical spine, whilst 3–5 kg are required for injuries in the lower part of the neck. However, the patient's neurological state must be reassessed after traction is applied or altered and X-rays are required to assess the anatomical effect. Use of an image intensifier is sometimes helpful, particularly if any attempt is being made to manipulate the neck. Manipulation is fraught with risk but, in experienced hands, neurological recovery has been reported (Duke & Spreadbury, 1981; Kleyn, 1984). To restore normal spinal curvature, patients on skull traction should have a neck roll placed posteriorly.

In the UK, penetrating injuries to the neck from stabbing or gunshot injuries are rare but open wounds require surgical exploration. Surgery may also be appropriate for non-union and persistent instability. Minimal intervention is appropriate for children and the elderly when spinal cord injury is sustained in the absence of radiological abnormality. These patients do not necessarily require anything more than a firm collar.

Thoracolumbar injuries

As long as the spine is maintained in the neutral position, no further harm should befall the patient with an unstable thoracolumbar fracture. These patients can therefore be nursed in the supine position as part of their conservative treatment programme until the fractures have healed and stabilized. Treatment of this type is sometimes referred to as 'postural reduction' because pillows are used to try and restore normal spinal contour during the period of bed rest.

Many centres now prefer to accelerate mobilization and ease the nursing burden by internal fixation of the spine with rods and other devices normally used in conjunction with a bone graft. However, there is no evidence that such treatment ameliorates the spinal cord injury and the only strong indication for emergency surgery is neurological deterioration (Gaines & Humphreys, 1988). Surgery also has a part to play in the relief of spondylitic cord compression, the correction of post-traumatic spinal deformity and the treatment of complications of spinal cord injury (e.g. syringomyelia).

Spinal cord injury

The majority of patients with spinal injury will be taken to the nearest A&E department and admitted to hospital under the care of the orthopaedic surgeon or occasionally a neurosurgeon. When spinal cord injury is present, the patient is best cared for in one of the 11 spinal injury units in the UK. Advice should be sought from the staff at the nearest spinal injury unit as soon as the diagnosis is made as many complications can develop in these patients who are best treated in specialist units (Carvell & Grundy, 1989). However, the patient must be stabilized before transfer, which may be delayed by prolonged resuscitation or emergency surgery at the receiving hospital.

Patients with cord injury may be transferred to a spinal unit by ambulance which should proceed at a modest but not a crawling pace. Patients with cervical or upper thoracic cord lesions should be accompanied by an anaesthetist who can intubate with minimal neck movement if respiratory failure develops. If a long distance is to be covered or the patient's condition is poor, helicopter transport minimizes the transfer time and has improved survival in the emergency situation (Hachen, 1977). The maintenance of steady skull traction during the journey may pose problems. The RAF pattern turning frame overcomes this by incorporating a constant tension device which can be linked by cable to the skull calipers. Traction, however, is not a prerequisite for the safe transfer of patients with unstable cervical injuries; effective splintage is adequate (Burney et al., 1989).

Many drugs have been tested experimentally and clinically on patients with spinal cord injury in the hope that some improvement in neurological outcome might be achieved (Anderson et al., 1985). Mannitol and naloxone have no proven benefit and the first American multicentre study of steroid therapy (NASCIS-1) was inconclusive. In 1990, NASCIS-2 appeared to show that high-dose methylprednisolone given during the first 24 h after spinal cord injury (30 mg kg^{-1} as an initial bolus followed by 5.4 mg kg^{-1} h^{-1} for 23 h) improved neurological function significantly in comparison with a control group (Bracken et al., 1990). The structure of the study has been criticized (Young, 1992; Hanigan & Anderson, 1992) but most centres now recommend that methylprednisolone should be given in accordance with the NASCIS-2 protocol as soon as spinal cord injury is diagnosed and certainly within 8 h.

It should be emphasized that the prognosis for recovery from spinal cord injury is very uncertain immediately after injury but becomes more predictable as the days go by. Spinal shock in particular mimics a complete cord lesion and may take days or weeks to resolve. It is therefore vital that A&E staff are non-committal about the prospects of neurological recovery and that relatives are advised not to make any premature assumptions. The most accurate prognosis will be given by the consultant in the spinal centre.

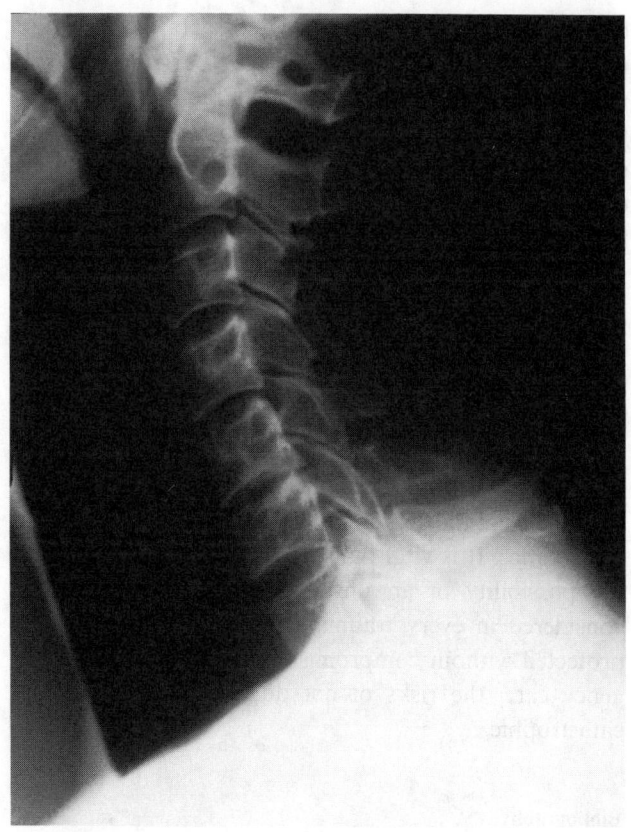

Fig. 29. Clay shoveller's fracture of spinous process of C7.

STABLE INJURIES

These are fractures and incomplete ligament injuries which do not materially affect the integrity of the spine. Common stable fractures are those of the transverse and spinous processes (e.g. the clay shoveller's fracture of C7; Fig. 29) and anterior wedge fractures which leave the neural arch intact and undisplaced. Transverse process fractures are most common in the lumbar region where they may be associated with renal tract injury. Wedge compression fractures can occur at any level but are most frequently seen at the apex of the thoracic kyphosis or lumbar lordosis.

Fractures of the transverse and spinous processes require symptomatic treatment only, and hospital admission is necessary only if symptoms are severe, mobility is lost or there is an associated visceral injury. Patients with isolated cervical and thoracic wedge fractures need not be admitted, but lumbar fractures may be associated with ileus or visceral trauma and patients with these complications must be observed in hospital.

Sacral fractures, particularly those involving the sacro-iliac joint or ala of the sacrum, often form one component of a pelvic ring disruption. Isolated sacral fractures do not impair pelvic stability but require bed rest and pain relief until mobility can be regained. Fractures or dislocations of the coccyx are also treated to relieve symptoms: sitting should be avoided, the tender area should be cushioned and a high-fibre diet will help to soften the faeces. Persistent pain from a coccygeal injury (coccydynia) may respond to local physiotherapy or steroid injection but sometimes the coccyx has to be excised.

CONCLUSION

Spinal injuries present with a broad spectrum of severity from insignificant to lethal. Between these extremes there is variation in the degree and nature of any physiological disturbance. It is vital that no further harm is done and the possibility of an unstable spinal injury must be considered in every trauma patient. The spine can be protected without compromising other aspects of emergency care; the risks of not doing so are potentially catastrophic.

Bibliography

ALKER, G.J., YOUNG, S.O., LESLIE, E.V. et al. (1975). Postmortem radiology of head and neck injuries in fatal traffic accidents. *Radiology*, **114**, 611–17.

ANDERSON, L.D. & D'ALONZO, R.T. (1974). Fractures of the odontoid process of the axis. *J. Bone Joint Surg.*, **56-A**, 1663–74.

ANDERSON, D.K., DEMEDIUK, P., SAUNDERS, R.D. et al. (1985). Spinal cord injury and protection. *Ann. Emerg. Med.*, **14**, 816–21.

ANDREW, C.T., GALLUCCI, J.G., BROWN, A.S. et al. (1992). Is routine cervical spine radiographic evaluation indicated in patients with mandibular fractures? *Am. Surg.*, **58**, 369–71.

APRAHAMIAN, C., THOMPSON, B.M., FINGER, W.A. et al. (1984). Experimental cervical spine injury model: evaluation of airway management and splinting techniques. *Ann. Emerg. Med.*, **13**, 21–4.

ATLS (1993). Trauma to the spine and spinal cord. In *Advanced Trauma Life Support for Physicians*. Chicago: American College of Surgeons.

BACHULIS, B.L., LONG, W.B., HYNES, G.D. et al. (1986). Clinical indication for cervical spine radiographs in the traumatized patient. *Am. Surg.*, **153**, 473–7.

BAKER, J.H.E. & SILVER, J.R. (1984). Atropine toxicity in acute cervical spinal injury. *Paraplegia*, **22**, 379–82.

BAYLESS, P. & RAY, V.G. (1989). Incidence of cervical spine injuries in association with blunt head trauma. *Am. J. Emerg. Med.*, **7**, 139–42.

BENES, V. (1968). *Spinal Cord Injury*, pp. 41–2. London: Baillière, Tindall & Cassell.

BENNETT, G. (1964). History. In *Injuries of the Spine*, ed. M.B. Howorth & J.G. Petrie, pp. 2–3. London: Baillière, Tindall and Cox.

BICKNELL, J.M. & FIELDER, K. (1992). Unrecognised incomplete cervical spinal cord injury. *Am. J. Emerg. Med.*, **10**, 336–43.

BIVINS, H.G., FORD, S., BEZMANILOVIC, Z. et al. (1988). The effect of axial traction during orotracheal intubation of the trauma victim with an unstable cervical spine. *Ann. Emerg. Med.*, **17**, 25–9.

BOHLMAN, A.H. (1979). Acute fractures and dislocations of the cervical spine. *J. Bone Joint Surg.*, **61-A**, 1119–41.

BRACKEN, M.B., SHEPPARD, M.J., COLLINS, W.F. et al. (1990). A randomised controlled trial of methylprednisolone or naloxone in the treatment of acute spinal cord injury. *N. Engl. J. Med.*, **322**, 1405–11.

BRESLER, N.J. & RICH, G.H. (1982). Occult cervical spine fracture in an ambulatory patient. *Ann. Emerg. Med.*, **11**, 440–2.

BUCHOLZ, R.W., BURKAGAD, W.Z., GRAHAM, W. et al. (1979). Occult cervical spine injuries in fatal traffic accidents. *J. Trauma*, **19**, 768–71.

BURKE, D.C. (1974). Traumatic spinal paralysis in children. *Paraplegia*, **11**, 268–76.

BURNEY, R.E., WAGGONER, R. & MAYNARD, F.M. (1989). Stabilisation of spinal injury for early transfer. *J. Trauma*, **29**, 1497–9.

BURT, A.A. (1988). Thoracolumbar spinal injuries: clinical assessment of the spinal cord injured patient. *Current Orthop.*, **2**, 210–13.

CACAYORIN, E.D. & KIEFFER, S.A. (1982). Applications and limitations of computed tomography of the spine. *Radiol. Clin. North Am.*, **20**, 185–205.

CADOUX, C.G., WHITE, J.D. & HEDBURG, K.C. (1987). High-yield roentgenographic criteria for cervical injuries. *Ann. Emerg. Med.*, **16**, 738–42.

CALENOFF, L., CHESSARE, J.W. & ROGERS, L.F. (1978). Multiple level spinal injuries: importance of early recognition. *Am. J. Roentgenol.*, **130**, 665–9.

CARVELL, J. & GRUNDY, D.J. (1989). Patients with spinal injuries. *Br. Med. J.*, **229**, 1353–4.

CLINE, J.R., SCHEIDEL, E. & BIGSKY, E.F. (1985). A comparison of methods of cervical immobilisation used in patient extrication and transport. *J. Trauma*, **25**, 649–53.

DE BEER, J. DE V., THOMAS, M., WALTER, J. et al. (1988). Traumatic atlanto-axial subluxation. *J. Bone Joint Surg.*, **70-B**, 652–5.

DELANEY, K.A. & HESSLER, R. (1988). Emergency flexible fibreoptic nasotracheal intubation: a report of 60 cases. *Ann. Emerg. Med.*, **17**, 919–25.

DENIS, F. (1988). Thoracolumbar spinal injuries: classification. *Curr. Orthop.*, **2**, 214–17.

DONOVAN POST, K.J., GREEN, B.A., QUENCER, R.M. *et al.* (1982). The value of computed tomography in spinal trauma. *Spine*, **7**, 417–31.

DORIS, P.E. & WILSON, R.A. (1985). The five view trauma series. *J. Emerg. Med.*, **3**, 371.

DUKE, R.F.N. & SPREADBURY, T.H. (1981). Closed manipulation leading to immediate recovery from cervical spine dislocation with paraplegia. *Lancet*, **i**, 577–8.

DUNNINGTON, G.L. & GERVIN, A.S. (1983). Cervical spine trauma: A review of 107 fractures in 90 patients. *J. Trauma*, **23**, 634.

EVANS, J.P. (1971). The International Symposium on Head Injuries. *J. Neurosurg.*, **35**, 367–70.

FIELDING, J.W. & HAWKINS, R.J. (1977). Atlanto-axial rotatory fixation. *J. Bone Joint Surg.*, **59A**, 37–44.

FLANNERY, M.C. & BIRCH, R. (1990). Acute compression of the cervical spinal cord: a complication of pre-ganglionic injury to the brachial plexus. *Injury*, **21**, 247–8.

FRIED, L.C. (1974). Cervical spinal cord injury during skeletal traction. *J. Am. Med. Assoc.*, **229**, 181–3.

GAINES, R.W. & HUMPHREYS, W.G. (1988). Thora-columbar spinal injuries: role of operative treatment. *Curr. Orthop.*, **2**, 231–5.

GARDNER, W.J. (1973). The principle of spring-loaded points for cervical traction. *J. Neurol.*, **39**, 543–4.

GREEN, B.A., CALLAHAN, R.A., KLOSE, K.J. *et al.* (1981). Acute spinal cord injury: current concepts. *Clin. Orthop.*, **154**, 125–35.

GRUNDY, D.J. & SILVER, J.R. (1981). Problems in the management of combined brachial plexus and spinal cord injuries. *Int. Rehab. Med.*, **3**, 57–70.

GRUNDY, D.J. & SWAIN, A.H. (1993). Early management and complications. In *ABC of Spinal Cord Injury*. London: BMJ Publications Group.

GRUNDY, D.J., PENNY, P. & GRAHAM, L. (1991). Diving into the unknown. *Br. Med. J.*, **302**, 670–1.

HACHEN, H.J. (1977). Idealised care of the acutely injured spinal cord in Switzerland. *J. Trauma*, **17**, 931–6.

HANIGAN, W.C. & ANDERSON, R.J. (1992). Commentary on NASCIS-2. *J. Spinal Disord.*, **5**, 125–31.

HARRIS, J.H., KRAMAR, L.A. & YEAKLEY, J.W. (1992). Magnetic resonance imaging of acute spinal injury. *Instr. Couse Lect.*, **41**, 265–73.

HINCK, V.C. & HOPKINS, C.E. (1960). Measurement of the atlanto-dental interval in the adult. *Am. J. Roentgenol.*, **84**, 945–51.

HOLDSWORTH, F. (1970). Fractures, dislocations and fracture-dislocations of the spine. *J. Bone Joint Surg.*, **52A**, 1534–51.

HUELKE, D.F., O'DAY, J. & MENDELSOHN, R.A. (1981). Cervical injuries suffered in automobile crashes. *J. Neurosurg.*, **54**, 316–21.

IRVING, M.H. & IRVING, P.M. (1967). Associated injuries in head injured patients. *J. Trauma*, **7**, 500–11.

JACKSON, H. (1950). The diagnosis of minimal atlanto-axial subluxation. *Br. J. Radiol.*, **23**, 672.

JACOBS, L.M. & SCHWARTZ, R. (1986). Prospective analysis of acute cervical spine injury: a methodology to predict injury. *Ann. Emerg. Med.*, **15**, 44–9.

JEFFERSON, G. (1920). Fracture of the atlas vertebra. *Br. J. Surg.*, **7**, 407–21.

JOHN, D.A., TOBEY, R.E., HOMER, L.D. *et al.* (1976). Onset of succinylcholine-induced hyperkalaemia following denervation. *Anaesthesiology*, **45**, 294–9.

JOHNSON, R.M., OWEN, J.R., HART, D.L. *et al.* (1981). Cervical orthoses. *Clin. Orthop.*, **154**, 34–43.

JOHNSTON, R.A. (1989). Management of old people with neck trauma. *Br. Med. J.*, **299**, 633–4.

KLEYN, P.J. (1984). Dislocations of the cervical spine: closed reduction under anaesthesia. *Paraplegia*, **22**, 271–81.

KORRES, D.S., KATSAROS, A., PANTAZOPOU-LOS, T. *et al.* (1981). Double or multiple level fractures of the spine. *Injury*, **13**, 147–52.

KULKARNI, M.B., McARDLE, C.B., KOPAN-ICKY, D. *et al.* (1987). Acute spinal cord injury: MR imaging at 1.5 T. *Neuroradiology*, **164**, 837–43.

LANGFORD, R.M., FERRIS, D.D. & WALKER, C.R. (1989). Tracheal shift in cervicothoracic dislocation. *Injury*, **20**, 237–8.

LEVINE, A.M. & EDWARDS, C.C. (1989). Traumatic lesions of the occipitoatlantoaxial complex. *Clin. Orthop.*, **239**, 53–68.

LOCKE, G.R., GARDINER, J.I. & VAN HEPPS, E.F. (1966). Atlas–dens interval in children. *Am. J. Roentgenol.*, **97**, 135–40.

LUCE, E.A., TUBB, T.D. & MOORE, A.M. (1979). Review of 1,000 major facial fractures and associated injuries. *J. Plast. Reconstr. Surg.*, **63**, 26–30.

MAJERNICK, T.G., BIENIEK, R., HOUSTON, J.B. *et al.* (1986). Cervical spine movement during orotracheal intubation. *Ann. Emerg. Med.*, **15**, 59–62.

MAROON, J.C. (1977). Burning hands in football spinal cord injuries. *J. Am. Med. Assoc.*, **238**, 2049–51.

MARTINEZ, J.A., TIMBERLAKE, G.A., JONES, J.C. *et al.* (1988). Factors affecting the cervical prevertebral space in the trauma patient. *Am. J. Emerg. Med.*, **6**, 268–72.

MAULL, K.I. & SACHATELLO, C.R. (1977). Avoiding a pitfall in resuscitation: the painless cervical fracture. *South. Med. J.*, **70**, 477–8.

McLAUCHLAN, C.A.J., PIDSLEY, R. & VANDEN-BERK, P.J.M. (1991). Minor trauma – major problem. Neck injuries, retropharyngeal haematoma and emergency airway management. *Arch. Emerg. Med.*, **8**, 135–9.

MEYER, G.A., BERMAN, I.R., DOTTY, D.B. *et al.* (1971). Haemodynamic responses to acute quadriplegia with or without chest trauma. *J. Neurosurg.*, **34**, 168–77.

MORGAN, G.A.R. & WINTER, R.J. (1986). Drowning and near drowning. *Br. Med. J.*, **293**, 395.

NEWMAN, K. D., BOWMAN, L.M., EICHELBER-GER, M.R. et al. (1990). The lapbelt complex: intestinal and lumbar spine injury in children. *J. Trauma*, **30**, 1133–8.

O'MALLEY, K.F. & ROSS, S.E. (1988). The incidence of injury to the cervical spine in patients with craniocerebral injury. *J. Trauma*, **28**, 1476–8.

PEACH, F. & GRUNDY, D. (1991). How preventable are spinal cord injuries? *Health Trends*, **23**, 62–6.

PLUNKETT, P.K., REDMOND, A.D. & BILLS-BOROUGH, S.H. (1987). Cervical subluxation: a deceptive soft tissue injury. *J. R. Soc. Med.*, **80**, 46–7.

PODOLSKY, S., BARAFF, L.J., SIMON, R.R. et al. (1983). Efficacy of cervical spine immobilisation methods. *J. Trauma*, **23**, 461–4.

RAVICHANDRAN, G. (1989). Errors and omissions in the acute management of spinal cord injury. *J. Med. Def. Union*, 14–16.

RAVICHANDRAN, G. & SILVER, J.R. (1984). Recognition of spinal cord injury. *Hosp. Update*, January, 77–86.

RHEE, K.J., GREEN, W., HOLDCROFT, J.W. et al. (1990). Oral intubation in the multiply injured patient: the risk of exacerbating spinal cord damage. *Ann. Emerg. Med.*, **19**, 511–14.

RIGGINS, R.S. & KRAUS, J.F. (1977). The risk of neurologic damage with fractures of the vertebrae. *J. Trauma*, **17**, 126–33.

ROBERGE, R.J., WEARS, R.C., KELLY, M. et al. (1988). Selective application of cervical spine radiography in alert victims of blunt trauma: a prospective study. *J. Trauma*, **28**, 784–8.

SANDOR, F. (1966). Diaphragmatic respiration: a sign of cervical cord lesion in the unconscious patient. *Br. Med. J.*, **1**, 465–6.

SASSON, A. & MOZES, G. (1987). Complete fracture-dislocation of the thoracic spine without neurologic deficit. *Spine*, **12**, 67–70.

SCHNEIDER, R.C. (1956). Chronic neurological sequelae of acute trauma to the spine and spinal cord. *J. Bone Joint Surg.*, **38A**, 985–97.

SCHNEIDER, R.C., CHERRY, G. & PANTEK, H. (1954). The syndrome of acute central cervical cord injury. *J. Neurosurg.*, **11**, 54–77.

SCHNEIDER, R.C., LIVINGSTON, K.E., CAVE, A.J.E. et al. (1965). Hangman's fracture of the cervical spine. *J. Neurosurg.*, **22**, 141–54.

SHERK, H.H., SHUT, L. & LANE, J.M. (1976). Frac-tures and dislocation of the cervical spine in children. *Orthop. Clin. North. Am.*, **7**, 593–604.

SILBERSTEIN, M., TRESS, B.M. & HENNESSY, O. (1992). Prediction of neurological outcome in acute spinal cord injury: the role of CT and MRI. *Am. J. Neuroradiol.*, **13**, 1597–608.

SONNTAG, V.K.H. & DOUGLAS, R.A. (1992). Management of cervical spinal cord trauma. *J. Neurotrauma*, **9**, S385–S394.

STEEL, H.H. (1968). Anatomical and mechanical considerations of the atlanto-axial articulations. *J. Bone Joint Surg.*, **50-A**, 1481–2.

SWAIN, A.H. & GRUNDY, D. (1993). At the accident. In *ABC of Spinal Cord Injury*, p. 1. London: BMJ Publications Group.

TIBBS, P.A., BIVINS, B.A. & YOUNG, A.B. (1979). The problem of acute abdominal disease during spinal shock. *Am. Surg.*, **45**, 366–8.

TIMBERLAKE, G.A. (1989). In *Cervical Spine Trauma*, ed. N.E. McSwain, J.A. Martinez & G.A. Timberlake, pp. 52–53. New York: Thieme.

TOSCANO, J. (1988). Prevention of neurological deterioration before admission to a spinal cord injury unit. *Paraplegia*, **26**, 143–50.

WEBB, J.K., BROUGHTON, R.B.K., McSWEE-NEY, T. et al. (1976). Hidden flexion injury of the cervical spine. *J. Bone Joint Surg.*, **58-B**, 322–7.

WHITE, A.A., JOHNSON, R.M., PANJABY, M.M. et al. (1975). Biomechanical analysis of clinical stability in the cervical spine. *Clin. Orthop.*, **109**, 85–95.

WIGGLESWORTH, E.C. (1992). Motor vehicle crashes and spinal injury. *Paraplegia*, **30**, 543–9.

WILLIAMS, N. & RATLIFF, D.A. (1993). Gastrointestinal disruption and vertebral fracture associated with the use of seatbelts. *Ann. R. Coll. Surg. Engl.*, **75**, 129–32.

WILLIAMS, C.F., BERNSTEIN, T.W. & JELENKO, C. (1981). Essentiality of the lateral spine radiograph. *Ann. Emerg. Med.*, **10**, 198–204.

WOOD-JONES, F. (1913). The ideal lesion produced by judicial hanging. *Lancet*, **i**, 53.

YOUNG, W. (1992). Medical treatment of acute spinal cord injury. *J. Neurol. Neurosurg. Psychiatry*, **55**, 635–9.

YOUNG, J.S. & DEXTER, W.R. (1978). Neurological recovery distal to the zone of injury in 172 cases of closed, traumatic spinal cord injury. *Paraplegia*, **16**, 39–49.

YOUNG, S., TAMAS, L. & O'LAOIRE, S.A. (1986). Prolapse of a cervical disc in elderly patients with cervical spondylosis. *Br. Med. J.*, **293**, 749–50.

23 Chest and cardiac trauma

P.A. DRISCOLL[a], C.L. GWINNUTT[b] and T.R. GRAHAM[c]

[a]*Department of Emergency Medicine, Hope Hospital, Salford, UK*
[b]*Department of Anaesthesia, Hope Hospital, Salford, UK*
[c]*Department of Cardiothoracic Surgery, Queen Elizabeth Hospital, Birmingham, UK*

Chapter plan

Objectives
Introduction
Mechanism of injury
Applied anatomy
Respiratory pathophysiology
Primary survey and resuscitation
Secondary survey
Definitive care
Transfer
Summary

OBJECTIVES

This chapter starts by outlining the mechanism of chest trauma and the relevant applied anatomy and physiology of the thoracic region. This will help the reader understand the reasons behind the medical management of the thoracic conditions subsequently described. Finally, the principles of transferring patients with thoracic trauma are discussed.

INTRODUCTION

Injuries to the thorax are responsible for 25% of all trauma deaths, mainly as a result of hypoxia or hypo-volaemia. Nevertheless 85% of them may be treated without the immediate need of a thoracic surgeon (Committee on Trauma of the American College of Surgeons, 1993; Ross, 1990). It is therefore extremely important that the clinician develop the expertise to recognize and manage these injuries, as well as being aware of those problems which require expert help.

MECHANISM OF INJURY

Injuries can be divided into 'blunt' or 'penetrating' depending on their cause. These can occur separately or in combination (e.g. following a blast injury). In all cases, however, the severity of the injury is dependent upon the site of the impact and the energy transferred to the tissues from the causative agent (Ross, 1990).

Blunt trauma

In blunt trauma, the force can be spread over a wide area. This minimizes the energy transfer at any one spot and so reduces tissue damage. After low-energy impacts, damage is usually localized to the superficial structures. In contrast following high-energy transfer, considerable tissue disruption can be produced with the clinical consequences being dependent upon the organs involved. Injuries resulting from baton rounds (i.e. plastic and rubber bullets) represent an intermediate state (Richie, 1992).

Penetrating trauma

The significance of the local damage following this type of injury is dependent upon both its site and the depth of penetration. However, it is also affected by the amount of energy transferred to surrounding tissues. This, in turn, depends upon several factors:

- The kinetic energy of the missile on impact.
- The mean presenting area of the missile.
- The missile's tendency to deform and fragment.
- Mechanical characteristics of the tissues.
- Length of the track.

The kinetic energy of the missile on impact with the patient is the product of half its mass and the square of its velocity at the moment of contact. As a result, objects with a high velocity (e.g. a rifle bullet or bomb casing) possess a large amount of kinetic energy. In contrast, a knife has a low level of kinetic energy even though its mass is large. It is important to remember that low-energy transfer can still produce significant clinical problems, a good example being a stab wound to the heart.

There is both functional and mechanical disruption of the neighbouring tissues following impact with the missile. The extent of this damage is dependent upon the amount of energy transferred and the tissue characteristics. For example, low-density organs, such as the lungs, sustain less damage than solid organs because their greater elastic properties enable them to 'ride the punch' created by the shift in energy.

(For further details on ballistic injuries, the reader is referred to Chapter 40.)

Blast injuries

Following an explosion, there is a sudden release of considerable energy which leads to an instantaneous rise in pressure in the surrounding air. This band of very high pressure is known as the *shock front* (or *blast wave*) and it spreads out in all directions faster than the speed of sound. However, it gets weaker as the distance from the edge of the band to the epicentre of the explosion increases.

Behind the shock front comes a movement of air which is called the *blast wind*. As this spreads out from the epicentre, it carries with it fragments from the bomb or surrounding debris. Close to the explosion, this material will be travelling at high velocity and can produce 'high-energy transfer' wounds.

It follows that a variety of injuries may be seen after bomb blasts and these are described below.

Primary effects

When the shock front hits the surface of the patient's body, a wave of deformation spreads through all the air/tissue interfaces because of their relative freedom of movement. The extent of the resulting tissue damage is directly dependent on both the magnitude and rate of onset of this deformation. The higher the rate, the bigger the pressure wave traversing the body.

As the deformation mainly affects air-containing organs, the lungs and gut are at particular risk. It is these waves which produce the damage of the lung's air/tissue interface which leads to the syndrome known as 'blast lung':

- Haemorrhage into alveolar spaces.
- Damage to alveolar septa.
- Stripping of bronchial epithelium.
- Emphysematous blebs produced on the pleural surface.

If this disruption is extensive, ventilation/perfusion (V/Q) mismatch develops and the patient becomes hypoxic (see below). High blast pressures can also lead to air emboli which may precipitate sudden death if they obstruct the cerebral or coronary arteries.

Secondary effects

These result from the direct impact on patients of fragments carried in the blast wind. High-energy transfer wounds are more likely to be sustained by those who were originally close to the explosion. However, as the distance from the explosion increases, the velocity of the fragments declines and the lesions become more superficial. Consequently, victims may sustain grossly contaminated multiple wound of varying depth depending upon their location in relation to the bomb.

It is important to note that the lethal environment for these secondary effects is usually much greater than that of the shock front and, in civilian explosions, most injuries are caused in this manner.

Tertiary effects

These result from the dynamic force of the blast wind itself giving rise to impact (deceleration) injuries and, in extreme cases, avulsion amputation. In civilian explosions, the latter is usually only seen in those victims close to the detonation. As these people will also be subjected to both primary and secondary effects of the explosion, they usually die at the scene.

In addition to these effects, patients may also sustain injuries as a result of damage caused to surrounding structures by the explosion (e.g. falling masonry).

(For a fuller description of blast injuries the reader is referred to Chapter 40.)

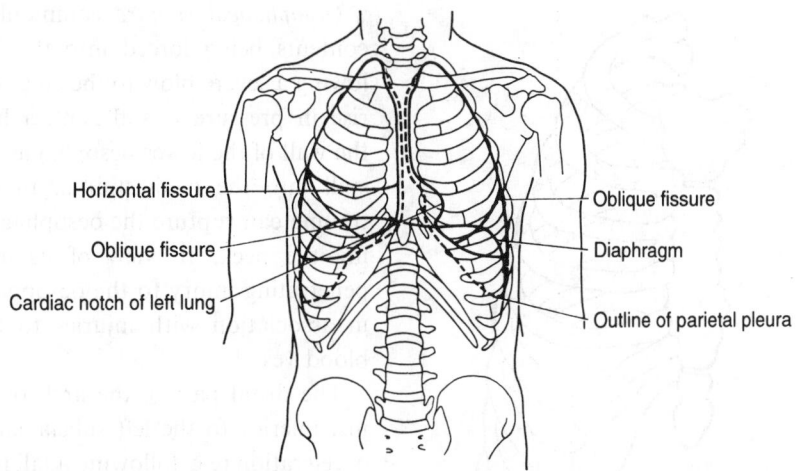

Fig. 1. Diagram of the chest wall with thoracic contents and diaphragm. (Reproduced, with permission, from Romanes, 1969.)

APPLIED ANATOMY

Fig. 1 demonstrates anatomical features which are clinically important.

Chest wall

Lung injuries, or air in the pleural space (pneumothorax), most commonly occur following chest trauma. However, they can also result from penetrating injuries to the lower neck. This is because the pleural cavity and the lung apices both project above the clavicles. Consequently, a pneumothorax can be caused by a misplaced needle during the insertion of a central venous cannula.

A potentially fatal type of pneumothorax is a *tension pneumothorax*. This can result from trauma to the lung surface creating a one-way valve. Consequently, with successive respiratory cycles, air accumulates within the pleural cavity and pressure within it increases. Eventually the ipsilateral lung collapses and profound hypoxia ensues. Furthermore, the mediastinum is displaced towards the opposite hemithorax, with the result that venous return is impeded and cardiac output falls (Fig. 2).

When a rib is fractured in two places the middle section can move independently from the relatively fixed end pieces. A *flail segment* is produced when two or more ribs are fractured in two or more places (Fig. 3). This also applies when both the clavicle and 1st rib are similarly affected. In the early stages, spasm of the chest wall musculature often splints these fractures. However, this leads to an increased energy expenditure for breathing and, over time, the muscles fatigue. At this point, abnormal or paradoxical movement of the injured part of the chest may be visible as the flail segment is drawn in

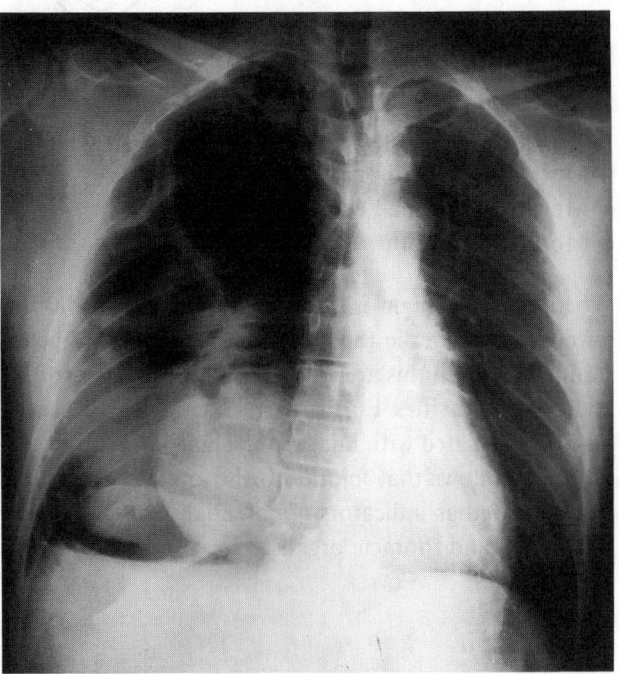

Fig. 2. Radiograph showing compression of the right lung and displacement of the heart due to a right tension pneumothorax.

during inspiration and pushed out with expiration. This results in impairment of ventilation and the development of hypoxia.

A flail segment can be life-threatening, particularly if there is underlying pulmonary contusion. The reason for this is that both conditions impair ventilation and lead to hypoxia. This is demonstrated in the increase in mortality rates if these two conditions coexist (Clark *et al.*, 1988).

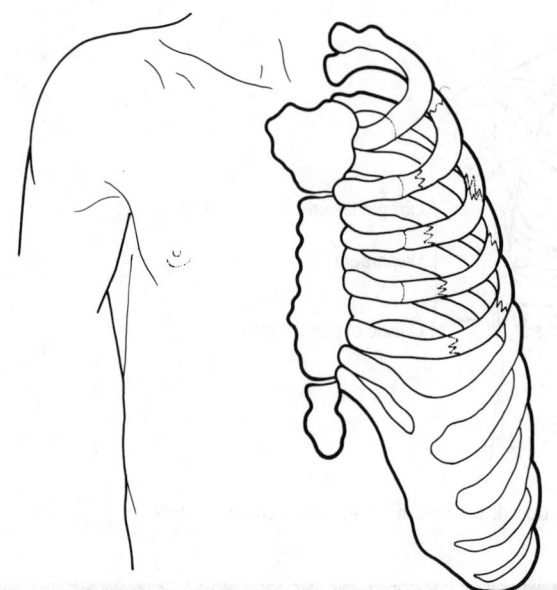

Fig. 3. Line diagram of a flail chest. (Redrawn from Landon *et al.*, 1993.)

- Mortality for pulmonary contusion   16%
- Mortality for a flail chest   16%
- Mortality for both   42%

When the diaphragm is elevated during expiration, the lower six ribs overlie the abdominal cavity and a penetrating wound in this area may enter both the peritoneal and thoracic cavities. Furthermore, fractures of these ribs may be associated with injury to the underlying liver and spleen. It follows that injuries to the lower chest should be considered as indicators of potential damage to both abdominal and thoracic organs.

Mediastinum

In the chest the trachea, oesophagus and major blood vessels lie in close proximity and are contained along with the heart in the mediastinum. The surface landmarks of the mediastinal margins are the nipple lines anteriorly and the medial edges of the scapulae posteriorly. Consequently, a penetrating injury in this area may damage one or more of these structures.

As the bronchi are more firmly anchored than the trachea, injuries to the former commonly result from rapid deceleration. *Bronchial tears* usually occur within 1 inch of the carina (80%) and can be either partial or complete with both sides equally affected. Of those who reach hospital alive, up to 30% will die of associated injuries.

Oesophageal rupture commonly results from gastric contents being forced into the lower oesophagus following a severe blow to the epigastrium. When the acute rise in pressure is sufficient, a linear tear develops in the wall of the lower oesophagus and intestinal contents spill into the mediastinum. In contrast, penetrating trauma can rupture the oesophagus at any level, including the neck. In view of its anatomical position, a penetrating injury to the oesophagus is at risk of being in association with injuries to the trachea and main blood vessels.

The distal part of the arch of the aorta is anchored just inferior to the left subclavian artery. During rapid deceleration (e.g. following a fall from a great height) the unanchored section of the aortic arch moves freely with the forward momentum. This can lead to tearing of the inner two layers of the descending aorta just distal to the left subclavian artery with the result that blood escapes into the wall of the aorta. In 90% of cases a complete disruption occurs because the outer (adventitial) layer of the aorta is also breached. This injury is invariably fatal because of rapid exsanguination. However, in 10% of cases the blood is contained, for a variable time, by the adventitial layer.

The heart is covered with tough, fibrous pericardium. Consequently, a small collection of blood within the pericardium can compromise ventricular filling, contraction and hence cardiac output in the healthy state. This condition is *cardiac tamponade* and it may follow penetrating trauma of the heart.

Cardiac contusion commonly follows blunt trauma to the chest causing bleeding into the myocardium or its subepicardial surface. It results from, and can lead to, coronary artery occlusion due to spasm, neighbouring tissue oedema and intimal tearing. The end result in all cases is further myocardial damage due to ischaemia.

Usually it is the arrhythmias produced by cardiac contusion which compromise the cardiac output. However, in severe cases the contusion can lead to a reduction in myocardial contractility. Further impairment may also occur as a result of the catecholamine response to trauma which can increase the myocardial oxygen demand above that which can be delivered. When a significant amount of the left ventricular myocardium has been severely damaged, cardiogenic shock will ensue.

The clinician should remember that antiarrhythmic drugs being taken by the patient prior to the injury, or administered acutely, may further reduce cardiac contractility and output.

Table 1. *Normal arterial blood gas values on air*

• H^+	35–45 nmol l^{-1} (pH 7.35–7.45)
• $PaCO_2$	4.7–6.0 kPa (35–45 mmHg)
• PaO_2	11.8–13.0 kPa (90–100 mmHg)
• Standard bicarbonate	24–32 mmol l^{-1}
• Base excess	± 2 mmol l^{-1}

RESPIRATORY PATHOPHYSIOLOGY
(West, 1987, 1990)

The main functions of the lungs are oxygen uptake and carbon dioxide elimination. To do this air has to get to the alveoli (ventilation, V), blood has to reach the pulmonary capillaries (perfusion, Q), and oxygen and carbon dioxide have to cross the gas/blood interface (diffusion). Finally, the balance between ventilation and perfusion (V/Q ratio) has to be correct. Impairment of any of these processes can lead to hypoxaemia and hypercapnia (Table 1).

Lung structure is ideally suited for diffusion as the surface area of the alveoli is approximately 50 m² and the gas/blood barrier is only 0.0005 mm thick. A reduction in the former when a lung collapses (e.g. pneumothorax) or an increase in the latter (e.g. interstitial pulmonary oedema) will reduce gas exchange, in particular oxygen uptake.

The partial pressure of oxygen in arterial blood (PaO_2) is dependent upon the inspired partial pressure of oxygen, alveolar ventilation and pulmonary perfusion. However, it is the ratio of ventilation to perfusion which is probably the most important factor in determining the PaO_2.

The reason why the V/Q ratio has such a profound effect on PaO_2 can be understood if the following points are borne in mind:

- Blood leaving an area of lung with a low V/Q ratio (perfusion in excess of ventilation) will not be fully saturated with oxygen and therefore will have a reduced oxygen content.
- The small increase in the oxygen content in blood coming from the high V/Q areas (ventilation in excess of perfusion) is due primarily to extra oxygen dissolved in the plasma, as the haemoglobin is virtually 100% saturated.
- The oxygen deficit from the low V/Q ratio areas is much larger than the very small increase in the oxygen content of blood that occurs in the areas with a high V/Q ratio.

Therefore most of the excess oxygen delivered to the high V/Q area is 'wasted' and cannot offset the reduced oxygen content of blood from areas of lung with a low V/Q ratio.

The reason why carbon dioxide is not affected by the V/Q mismatching is because there is an almost linear relationship between the partial pressure of carbon dioxide and the carbon dioxide content of blood. Consequently, an area of high ventilation can compensate for areas of low ventilation to eliminate carbon dioxide. Furthermore, if the partial pressure of carbon dioxide in arterial blood ($PaCO_2$) rises above a particular level the respiratory rate increases and the elimination of carbon dioxide is again increased.

An example of diffusion, ventilation and perfusion pathology is seen in patients with a *pulmonary contusion* (Repine, 1992). This is one of the commonest causes of death following thoracic trauma and usually follows blunt injury in which energy is transmitted to the underlying lung tissue. It results in an increase in permeability of the small pulmonary capillaries leading to interstitial and alveolar oedema. This leads to a reduction in lung compliance (the lungs become 'stiffer') and less air is drawn into the lungs with each breath. Therefore a greater volume of lung is being perfused but not ventilated (i.e. there is a low V/Q ratio) and hypoxia follows. Consequently, further damage to the epithelial barrier occurs. In addition, as the compliance falls, the work needed to inflate the lungs increases and ventilation decreases. The respiratory rate also increases to try and compensate and maintain alveolar ventilation but as the patient becomes exhausted alveolar ventilation falls, the hypoxia worsens and the process becomes self-perpetuating. If the patient survives, infection in the contused area may develop at a later stage, particularly in those patients who are elderly or have coexistent lung disease.

In contrast to oxygen, carbon dioxide can diffuse across the damaged alveolar/pulmonary capillary barrier, at least in the early stages. Consequently, as the respiratory rate increases due to hypoxia more carbon dioxide is expired and the $PaCO_2$ falls. However, as the patient tires and the ventilatory rate falls, $PaCO_2$ rises.

PRIMARY SURVEY AND RESUSCITATION

The aim of the primary survey for chest injuries is to detect and correct the six immediately life-threatening conditions (Committee on Trauma of the American College of Surgeons, 1993). These will be covered in the order that they are most likely to be discovered.

Immediately life-threatening thoracic conditions

A	Airway obstruction
T	Tension pneumothorax
C	Cardiac tamponade
O	Open chest wound
M	Massive haemothorax
F	Flail chest

A mnemonic for this list is: **A**ll **T**rauma **C**linicians **O**ccasionally **M**iss **F**ractures.

Airway and cervical spine

Airway obstruction has been dealt with in detail in Chapter 2. The personnel responsible must assess, clear and secure the airway whilst maintaining in-line cervical stabilization. All trauma patients have an increased oxygen demand and therefore require a high inspired oxygen concentration.

Before the cervical collar is applied, the neck should be examined for any visible injuries, distended veins and the position of the trachea noted. If a collar is already in place it may be removed to allow examination of the neck but the cervical spine must be stabilized manually whilst this is carried out.

Breathing

The patient's chest must be exposed and inspected for bruising, penetrating wounds, intercostal or supraclavicular indrawing, lack of movement or abnormal movement and surgical emphysema. The rate and depth of breathing should be noted because rapid, shallow respiration suggests a chest injury or developing hypoxia. The axillae can then be auscultated to determine if the air entry is equal over both sides of the thorax and, finally, both sides are percussed and compared to elicit hyper-resonance or dullness.

Tension pneumothorax

This is commonly due to rupture of an emphysematous bulla as a result of blunt trauma, but it can also result from penetrating trauma. Classically the patient will be tachypnoeic (and tachycardic) and the chest may appear overinflated and immobile (Table 2). Hyper-resonance may be detected over the hemithorax on the affected side and, if there is no coexisting hypovolaemia, the neck

Table 2. *Signs of a tension pneumothorax*

- Tachypnoea
- Shocked
- Hyper-resonant hemithorax
- Splinted hemithorax
- Decreased air entry to the hemithorax
- Deviated trachea (late)
- Raised JVP (if no hypovolaemia)
- Cyanosis (very late)

JVP, jugular venous pressure.

will be deviated to the contralateral side (Fig. 2). Cyanosis is a very late sign which depends on there being more than 5 g of deoxygenated (reduced) haemoglobin in the circulation.

Patients with a tension pneumothorax rapidly become shocked and ventilation becomes more difficult as the intrapleural pressure increases and the contralateral lung becomes compressed. This may become apparent in ventilated patients either as increasing resistance to manual ventilation or raised inflation pressures on a ventilator.

Following trauma, a tension pneumothorax can be easily missed so a high index of suspicion is required by the clinician. It may also occur at any point during resuscitation, especially after insertion of a central line or during manual or mechanical ventilation when there are rib fractures.

Patients with this condition rapidly deteriorate and can die in the time it takes to obtain and process a chest X-ray. Therefore, if a tension pneumothorax is suspected, a needle thoracostomy should be performed as an emergency measure (Fig. 4).

A tension pneumothorax should be a clinical and not a radiological diagnosis.

TECHNIQUE

Needle thoracostomy

Objective
- Rapid decompression of a tension pneumothorax, resulting in a simple pneumothorax.

Indication
- Suspected tension pneumothorax.

Contraindications
- None.

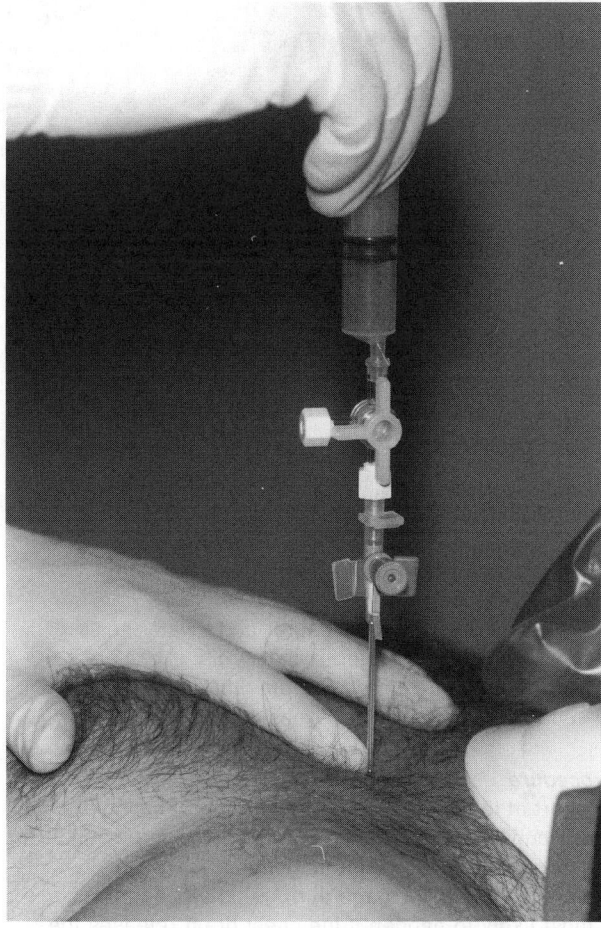

Fig. 4. Needle thoracostomy.

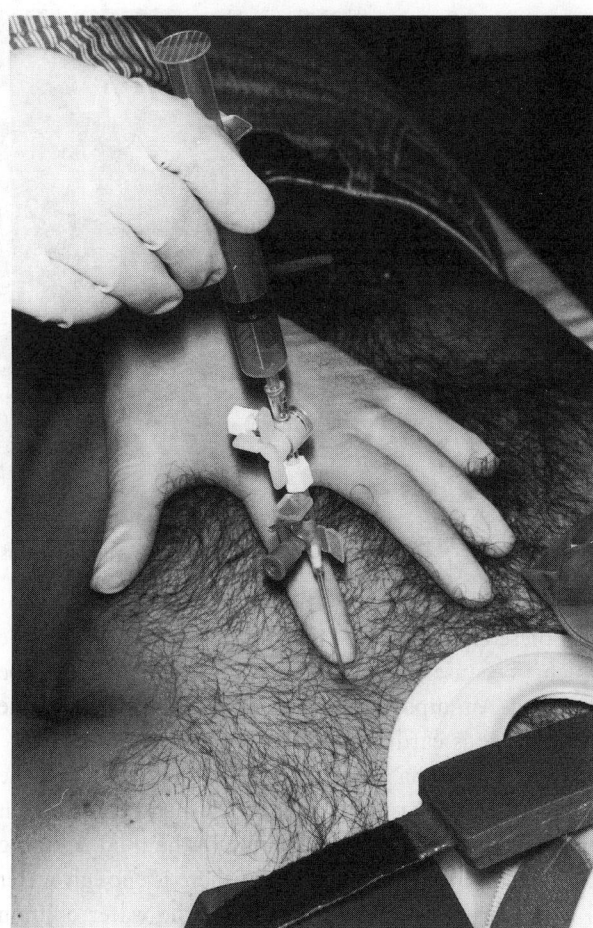

Fig. 5. Needle thoracostomy.

Technique

- Ensure the patient is receiving 12–15 litres of oxygen min^{-1} by the most appropriate means available.
- A 16G cannula is connected to a 10 ml syringe by a three-way tap. This is inserted into the 2nd intercostal space just above the third rib, perpendicular to the chest wall, in the midclavicular line (Fig. 5). Do not be surprised if the cannula has to be inserted almost fully due to the amount of overlying soft tissues.
- A rapid release of air confirms the diagnosis. The cannula can then be slid over the needle into the pleural cavity, and the syringe and needle removed. Aspirate as much air as possible.

Potential complications

- Creation of a pneumothorax if one did not exist initially.
- Soft tissue haematoma and infection.

Postprocedure checks

- Reassess the chest by inspection and auscultation. Remember there will still be no breath sounds.
- Reassess the adequacy of ventilation by arterial blood gas analysis and pulse oximetry.

- Check that the cannula does not kink as this will allow the tension pneumothorax to redevelop.

Aftercare

- Tube thoracostomy.
- Chest radiograph must be taken after the drain is inserted.

A needle thoracostomy gives enough time for the clinician to definitively treat the condition by inserting an underwater seal chest drain (see below).

If insertion of the cannula is followed only by a slow release of air and froth, then the diagnosis remains in doubt. Furthermore, there is now the possibility that a pneumothorax has been created as a result of the needle puncturing the lung. As this can be transformed into a tension pneumothorax if the patient is being ventilated, an urgent chest X-ray is required. However, if this is not possible, it is safer to insert a chest drain prophylactically.

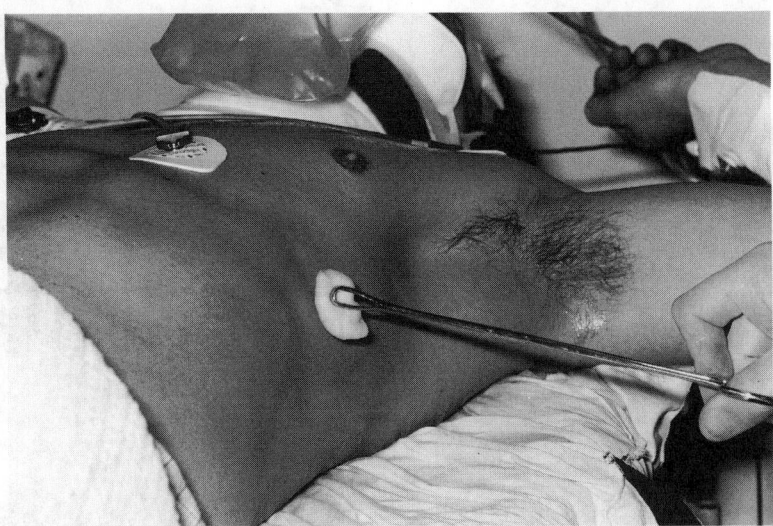

Fig. 6. Tube thoracostomy: chest wall preparation.

In these circumstances, the clinician must reassess the patient because the cause of shock still has to be identified. An important diagnosis to confirm or exclude at this stage is cardiac tamponade (see later).

If a chest tube has been inserted prior to arrival in the accident and emergency (A&E) department, the clinician must check the nature and volume of the fluid draining into the container and ensure that there is enough water to form an underwater seal and that the water column swings with respiration.

TECHNIQUE

Tube thoracostomy

Objective
- Decompression of a pneumo- or haemothorax.

Indication
- Pneumothorax, haemothorax and open chest wound.

Contraindications
- None.

Investigations prior to thoracostomy
- In most situations a chest radiograph will be performed to confirm the diagnosis.

Technique
Make sure all the required equipment is available:
- Skin preparation solution.
- Swabs.
- Sterile sheets.
- Sterile gowns and gloves for the doctor and nurse.
- Local anaesthetic (10 ml of 1% lignocaine).
- Syringe and needle.
- Scalpel and blade.
- Suture (at least O in thickness) and sterile scissors.
- 36G silastic chest drain with trocar removed.

- A closed chest drainage bag or underwater seal containing 200 ml of sterile water.
- 1 large straight clamp (for drain tubing).
- 1 curved clamp (Spencer Wells).

Procedure
- Insert at least one large-bore peripheral cannula in the antecubital fossa. This is to make sure intravenous access is available if the patient suddenly develops significant haemorrhage during this procedure. This is most likely to happen if the chest drain releases the tamponade effect of a massive haemothorax.
- The patient's arm is abducted and the 5th intercostal space palpated, usually at the level of the nipple in males. If there is an underlying rib fracture then an intercostal space immediately above or below is chosen.
- Using an aseptic technique, the patient's chest is cleaned and draped (Fig. 6). Local anaesthetic is injected into the skin and then deeper structures in the 5th intercostal space just anterior to the midaxillary line (Fig. 7). Finally, the needle is then directed down onto the 6th rib and local anaesthetic is injected onto its periosteum and over its superior surface into the underlying pleura. This approach is important because the intercostal vessels lie under the inferior surface of the ribs.
- It is important to draw back frequently on the syringe to make sure the needle has not entered a blood vessel. A 3 cm transverse incision is then made down to the 6th rib, through the anaesthetized area (Fig. 8).
- Using the curved clamp, the intercostal muscle layers are opened in a cruciate fashion, the pleura above the rib is breached and a track is formed *perpendicular* to the skin (Fig. 9). If the tract runs obliquely to the skin then it will collapse once the clamp is removed and it will be difficult to find.
- The operator must then insert a finger through the

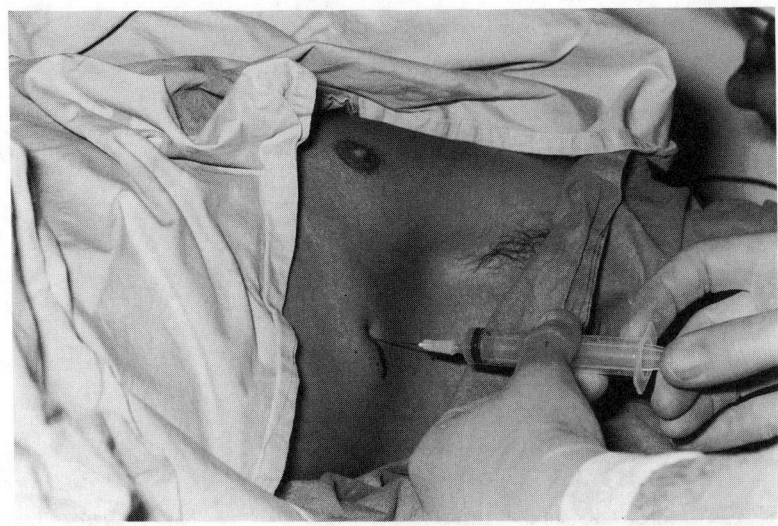

Fig. 7. Tube thoracostomy: local anaesthetic infiltration.

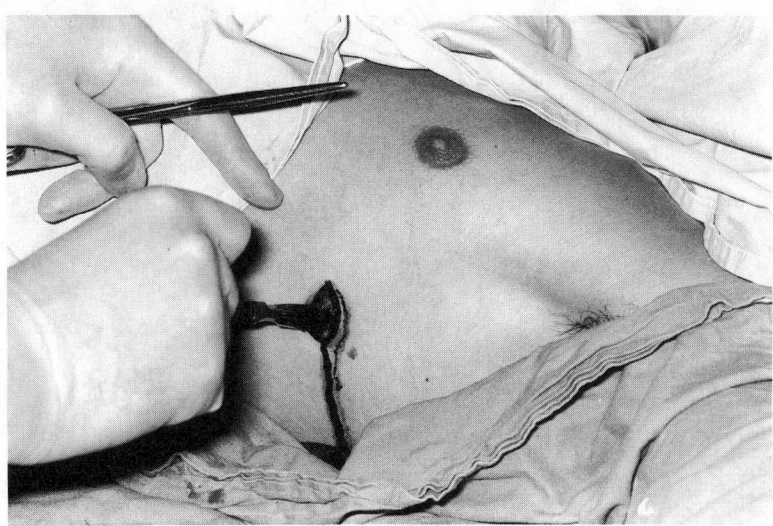

Fig. 8. Tube thoracostomy: incision.

incision and sweep around the intrapleural space to detect the presence of a ruptured diaphragm or lung adhesions (Fig. 10). If adhesions prevent the passage of a finger, then a fresh incision should be made in the 4th or 6th intercostal space, just anterior to the midaxillary line.

- The chest tube inserted into the incision is directed with the curved clamp (Fig. 11). Condensation of water vapour in air escaping from the pleural cavity causes fogging of the tube once it is in the intrapleural space. It is then connected to an appropriate drainage set. If the underwater set is used, there is initially a rush of air into the container as demonstrated by a mass of bubbles. Later, this settles and the fluid level is noted to rise and fall with the respiratory cycle.
- The chest drain must then be secured. This is done with both suture (Fig. 12) and tape. The incision is then covered with gauze and tape (Fig. 13).

- Although trocars are usually supplied in chest drains, they should never be used as they can seriously injure the patient's lung, mediastinum and abdominal viscera due to inappropriate placement.

Potential complications

The insertion of a chest drain should be carried out by trained staff because it can give rise to several complications if it is performed incorrectly. The main ones are:

- Bleeding.
- Damage to the intercostal vessels and nerves.
- Lung and mediastinal injury.
- Damage to abdominal organs and vessels.
- Infection.
- Allergic reactions.

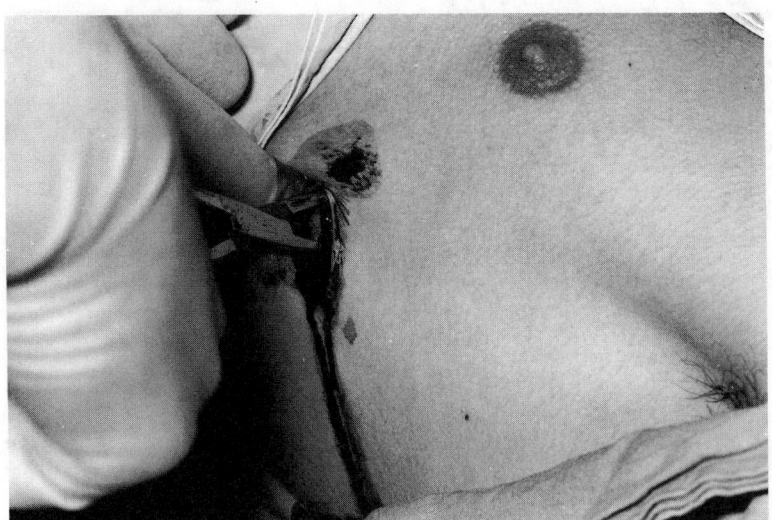

Fig. 9. Tube thoracostomy: breaching the pleura.

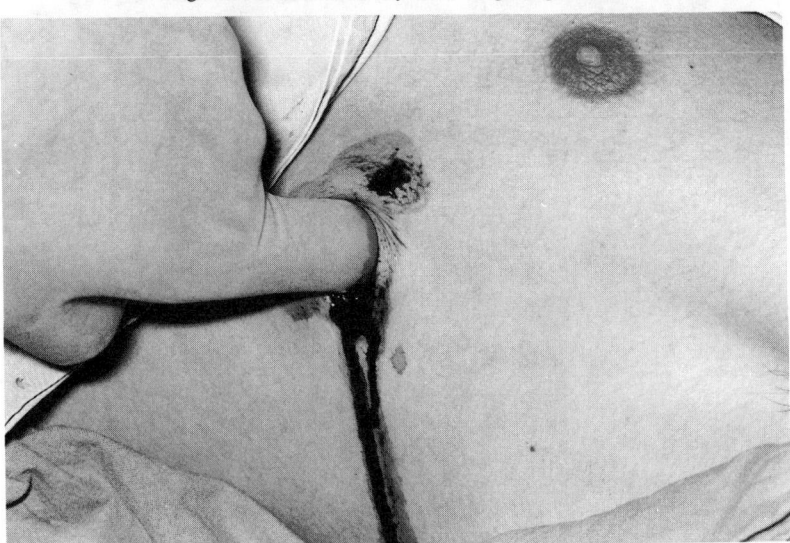

Fig. 10. Tube thoracostomy: finger exploration.

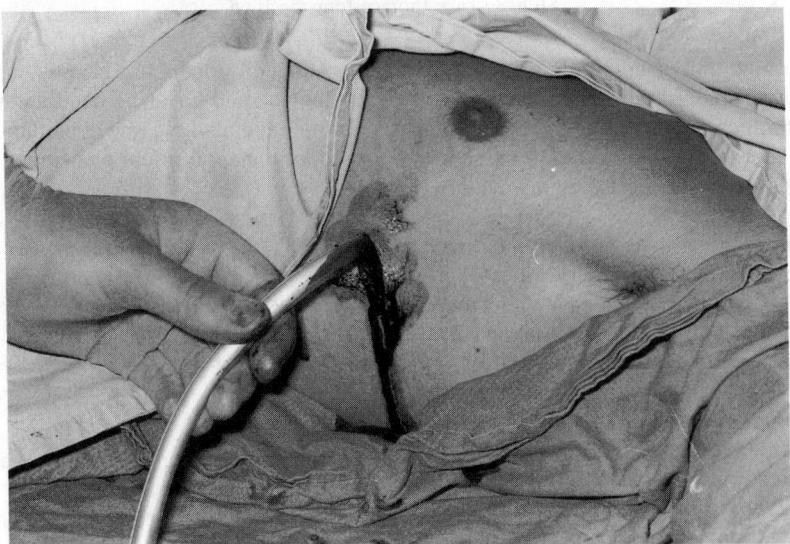

Fig. 11. Tube thoracostomy: inserting the chest drain.

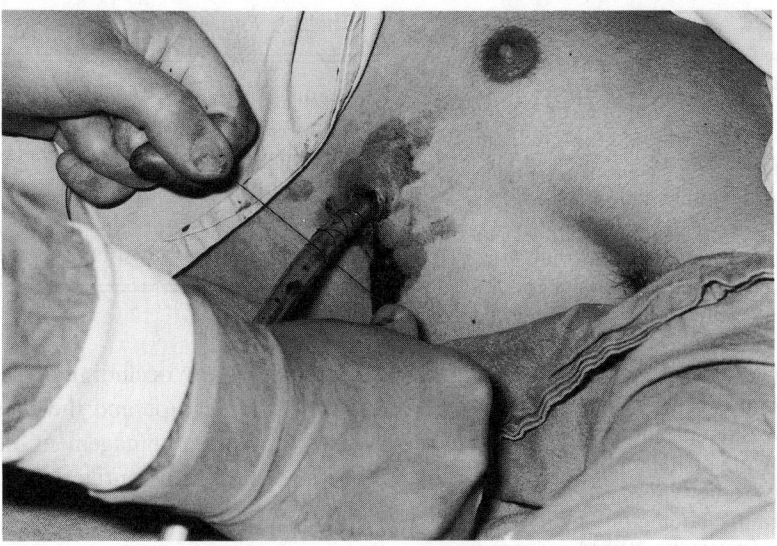

Fig. 12. Tube thoracostomy: securing the chest drain.

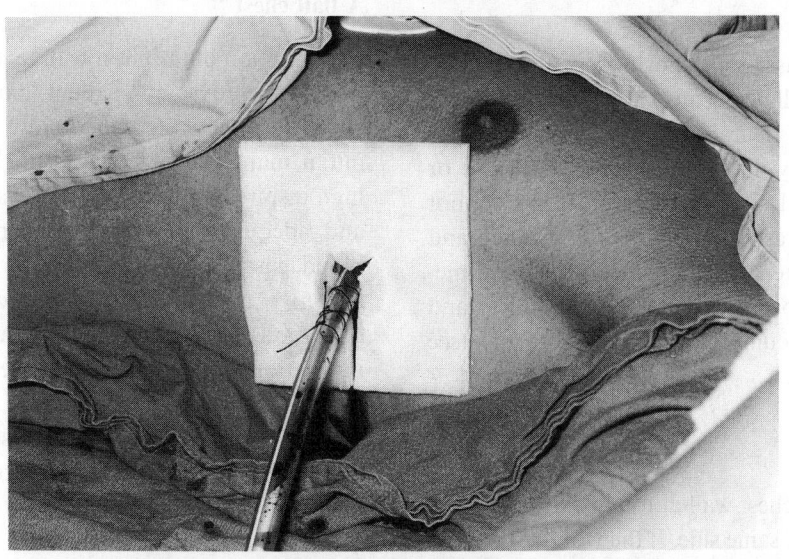

(a)

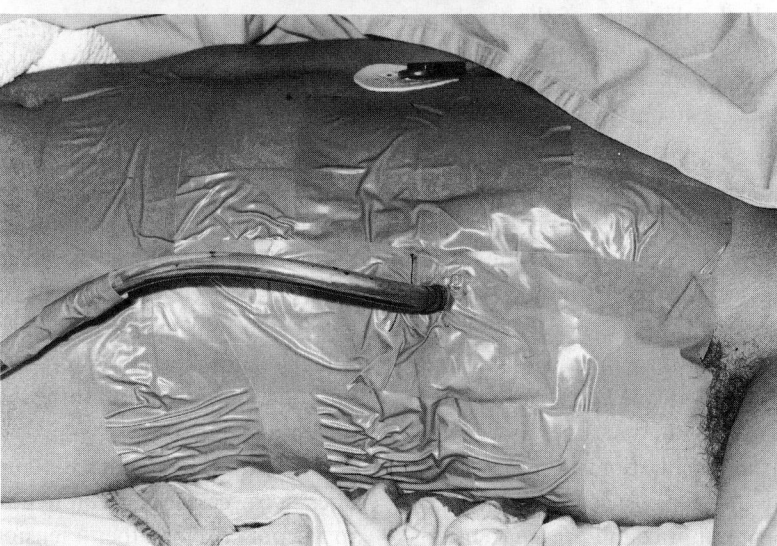

(b)

Fig. 13a, b. Tube thoracostomy: covering the incision.

Postprocedure checks

- Once a chest drain has been inserted, the patient's chest needs to be re-examined to ensure the lung is now ventilating, and a chest X-ray should be taken to ascertain the position of the drain and the presence of residual lung pathology.
- If an underwater seal drainage system is used, it is important to remember:
  - The container must not be lifted higher than the patient, as fluid will drain back into the chest.
  - The chest drain should only be clamped when bottles are being changed.
  - Connections between the intercostal drain and the drainage tube is reinforced with zinc oxide adhesive tape to prevent inadvertent disconnections.
- Reassess the adequacy of ventilation by arterial blood gas analysis and pulse oximetry.
- Kinking of the chest drain, clogging of the chest drain with blood, or displacement of the chestdrain may cause a recurrence of the initial problem.

The clinician must assess the position of the drain if the water does not oscillate because it implies that either the tube is not in the pleural cavity, or it has become blocked. This is usually due to kinking of the drain or obstruction from blood clots. If these problems cannot be corrected easily, a fresh drain should be inserted and a chest radiograph taken. The presence of a non-functioning chest drain imparts a false sense of security and may allow a tension pneumothorax or haemothorax (see later) to go undiagnosed.

Open chest wound

An open defect on the chest wall automatically produces a pneumothorax on the same side. If the wound diameter is greater than two-thirds the diameter of the trachea, then air preferentially enters the chest through this hole during inspiration. This leads to failure of ventilation of the lung which will collapse. A particularly dangerous situation is when a tension pneumothorax develops because a one-way valve has been created which allows air to enter the pleural cavity but not escape. This can be due either to the configuration of the wound (a condition known as the 'sucking chest wound'), or the application of an occlusive dressing.

The immediate management of an open chest wound is to apply a sterile cover, sealed on *three* sides so that air can escape during expiration but does not enter through the defect during inspiration. A chest tube should then be urgently inserted, via a freshly created incision, to drain the pneumothorax and prevent tension developing. In the event of a tension pneumothorax

Table 3. *Patients with a flail chest requiring artificial ventilation*

- Falling PaO_2 or <6.6 kPa (50 mmHg) on air
- PaO_2 <10.4 (80 mmHg) with supplemental oxygen
- Rising $PaCO_2$ or >6.0 kPa (45 mmHg)
- Exhaustion
- Respiratory rate >30 min^{-1}
- Significant associated injuries of the abdomen and head

developing, any occluding dressing must be removed so that air can escape and the chest can be decompressed. The long-term management of the majority of these patients is definitive surgical closure, utilizing the expertise of a thoracic surgeon.

A flail chest

Examination of the chest wall reveals crepitus, instability and, in the conscious patient, pain.

As these patients can rapidly become hypoxic, their initial management consists of the administration of a high inspired concentration of warm, humidified oxygen and adequate fluid resuscitation. In all cases arterial blood gases need to be monitored frequently to allow objective assessment of the progress of the patient's condition. A selected group of patients will require early intubation and ventilation (Table 3). Analgesia, by intercostal or epidural block, may be given during the definitive management phase (see Chapter 10) but it requires expert advice and monitoring in an appropriate intensive care area.

Circulation

A rapid assessment is made of the patient's pulse for rate, volume, regularity and (if time) the presence of paradox. This is followed by noting the time for capillary return and the blood pressure. If the neck veins have not been examined by this stage it must be done now. Two large peripheral intravenous cannulae (14G or 16G) should then be inserted with 20 ml of blood being withdrawn before the infusions are connected. This blood sample will enable routine laboratory investigations to be carried out and, more importantly, allow typing and cross-matching of blood.

It must be remembered that a poor cardiac output does not necessarily mean hypovolaemia. It may be due to the presence of either a tension pneumothorax (which should already have been treated) or cardiac tamponade.

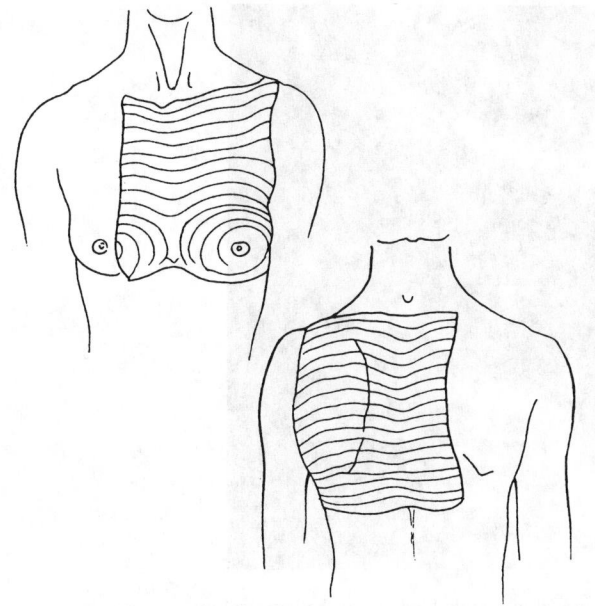

Fig. 14. Sites of wounds which are associated with cardiac tamponade. (Redrawn from Landon *et al.*, 1993.)

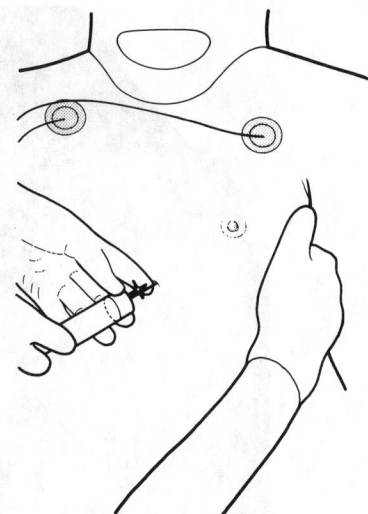

Fig. 15. Pericardiocentesis. (Redrawn from Landon *et al.*, 1993.)

Cardiac tamponade

This condition must be suspected if there is a wound within the area indicated in Fig. 14. Only a third of trauma patients will have the classic presentation of Beck's triad, pulsus paradoxus and Kussmaul's sign:

- Beck's triad
  - Arterial hypotension.
  - Raised jugular venous pressure (JVP).
  - Decrease in heart sounds.
- Pulsus paradoxus
  - A decrease in systolic blood pressure of >10 mmHg during inspiration.
- Kussmaul's sign
  - Raised JVP on inspiration.

The central venous pressure is elevated due to the obstructed venous return to the right ventricle. However, distension of the neck veins and a raised jugular venous pressure (JVP) will only be seen if the patient is normovolaemic. Furthermore, muffled heart sounds, due to blood in the pericardium, are always difficult to ascertain in the resuscitation room.

In contrast to these manifestations, the patient usually demonstrates signs of hypovolaemic shock because of impaired ventricular filling.

Temporary relief of the symptoms of cardiac tamponade can be achieved initially by increasing the rate of intravenous infusions to optimize venous return while

preparations are made for pericardiocentesis (Fig. 15). This procedure has significant risks and can be falsely negative in up to 25% of cases because the blood within the pericardium clots easily. In those cases where aspiration has been successful, the cannula must be left in the pericardial space and allowed to drain freely because this will delay the development of any recollection. However, irrespective of the success or failure of the initial aspiration, the assistance of a thoracic surgeon must be sought for the definitive care of these patients. Furthermore, once the initial treatment has been carried out, continuous assessment of these patients is essential because of the high chance of tamponade recurring either in the resuscitation room or during transfer.

TECHNIQUE

Pericardiocentesis

Objective
- Rapid decompression of a cardiac tamponade.

Indication
- Suspected cardiac tamponade.

Contraindications
- None.

Technique
Make sure all the required equipment is available:

- A skin preparation solution.
- Swabs.
- Sterile sheets.

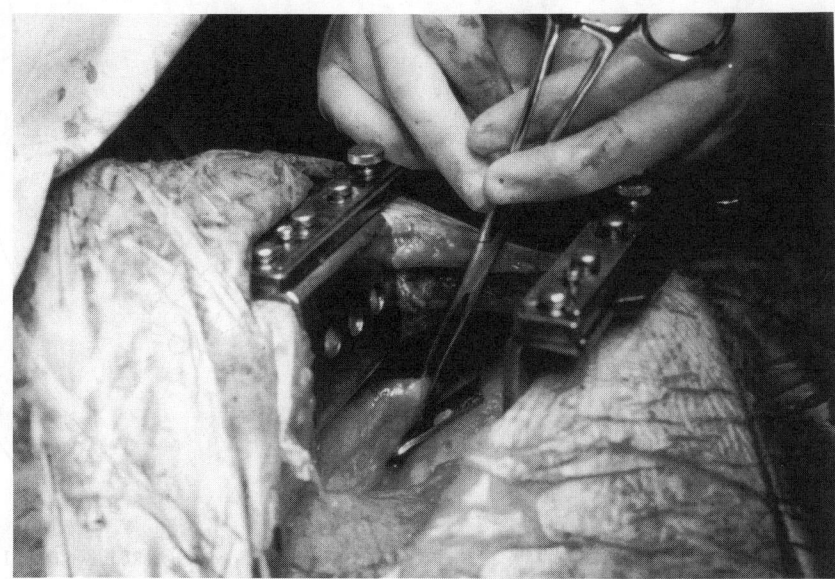

Fig. 16. Emergency room thoracotomy showing the removal of a knife blade from the pericardium.

- Sterile gowns and gloves for the doctor.
- A 15 cm, 16G or 18G cannula connected to a 10 ml syringe.
- A three-way tap.
- ECG monitor.

Procedure
- The presence of any significant mediastinal shift is determined and the position of the xiphisternum noted. The patient must be connected to an ECG monitor with the screen visible to the clinician.
- If there is time, aseptic precautions are taken and the patient's subxiphoid area is cleaned, draped and anaesthetized.
- The cannula is connected to a 10 ml syringe by a three-way tap. The skin is then punctured, 1–2 cm inferior and to the left of the xiphochondral junction at a 45° angle. Whilst aspirating continually, the needle is advanced towards the tip of the left scapula. Simultaneously, the ECG monitor must be constantly checked for injury patterns (ST elevation or depression) and arrhythmias (ventricular ectopics). Their appearance indicates that the needle has advanced too far and is now touching the myocardium. It should therefore be withdrawn slowly until a normal ECG is achieved.
- Once the needle enters the pericardium as much blood as possible should be aspirated. As the cardiac tamponade is drained, ventricular filling will increase and the myocardium will move towards the needle and the ECG may change as described previously. Once again, slowly withdrawing the needle should result in a normal ECG. Following removal of the needle, the cannula is left in place and connected to the three-way

tap. The tap and cannula is then secured in place with gauze and tape.

Potential complications
- Pneumothorax.
- Damage to the coronary arteries and veins.
- Damage to the myocardium.
- Damage to lung.
- Infection of the skin, mediastinum and peritoneum.

Postprocedure checks
- Once the cannula has been inserted, the patient's chest needs to be re-examined to ensure the lung is still ventilating.
- Should the symptoms of a cardiac tamponade recur, the pericardium can be reaspirated.

Aftercare
- Once haemodynamic stability has been restored, the patient must be considered for transfer to theatre, where definitive surgery can be carried out.

The patient must be transferred to an operating theatre immediately so that a thoracotomy can be carried out under more ideal conditions if (Selficiano, 1992):

- The systolic blood pressure is over 70 mmHg.
- Appropriate personnel and equipment are available to transfer and receive the patient (see later).
- The transfer time will be less than 5 min.

Thoracotomy in the resuscitation room is reserved for patients who have a penetrating injury to the chest and are in electromechanical dissociation (EMD); i.e. have electrical activity but no cardiac output (Bodai *et al.*, 1983; Champion *et al.*, 1986; Jones *et al.*, 1987; Jurkovic *et al.*, 1992; Lorenz *et al.*, 1992).

As delays in performing this procedure significantly decrease the patient's chances of survival, it should be carried out sooner rather than later once the diagnosis has been made (Fig. 16). In all cases it must be performed by a clinician who is both familiar with the equipment and the procedure.

TECHNIQUE

Emergency room thoracotomy and median sternotomy

Objective
- Rapid decompression of a cardiac tamponade, internal cardiac massage, control of a penetrating cardiac injury, major vascular haemorrhage or a bronchial tear.

Indication
- Penetrating thoracic trauma with EMD.
- Massive haemorrhage into the tracheobronchial tree such that the airway cannot be cleared and secured by any other method.
- Drain over 1000 ml of blood from the chest and have a systolic blood pressure under 70 mmHg despite rapid fluid replacement.

It must only be performed by a trained clinician who is familiar with the equipment and procedure.

Contraindications
- Lack of appropriate skill.
- Blunt trauma with EMD.

Technique
Ensure all required equipment is available, which is the same as that used for chest drain insertion plus:

- Thoracotomy/sternotomy retractor.
- Bone saw (Gigli/oscillating).
- Bone cutters.
- Satinsky vascular clamp.
- Metzenbaum scissors.
- Vascular clamps.
- Long forceps (toothed and non-toothed).
- Needle holder.
- Teflon pledgets.
- 2-O double-armed Ethibond.

Procedure
- Ensure that the patient is intubated (preferably with a double lumen tube) and that a chest drain is in position on the opposite side of the patient from the thoracotomy.
- *Median sternotomy approach*. This should be considered for anterior wounds between the nipples and posterior wounds between the medial borders of the

scapula causing cardiac tamponade and/or life-threatening haemorrhage. It is performed by incising the skin and soft tissues from the jugular notch of the manubrium to 2 cm below the xiphisternum onto the periosteum of the sternum. A bone or Gigli saw is then used to divide the sternum. The thymus is then divided so that the pericardium can be exposed. If access to the lungs or hila are required then the appropriate pleura can be breached.

- *Lateral thoracotomy approach*. Barring those cases mentioned previously, this approach is used in all cases of thoracic trauma when a thoracotomy is indicated. Start by internally rotating the patient's left arm and tucking the left hand under the patient's waist. This provides better access to the chest wall. The approach to the chest is through an anterolateral incision in the interspace immediately below the nipple. This is usually carried out on the left side as this provides access to the heart and descending aorta. The operator should avoid the internal mammary artery by starting the incision approximately 5 cm lateral to the sternum. Further access can be achieved by extending the incision posteriorly and having the patient partially turned. The latter manoeuvre is dependent on the team leader's suspicion of potential spinal injury. Another option is to extend the incision anteriorly through the sternoxiphoid junction, after the internal mammary arteries have been clamped. This provides a good approach to the pericardium.

- Irrespective of the approach used, once the incision has been opened with the retractor, the trained surgeon can deal with most emergency problems inside the chest. After a rapid inspection the emergency procedures which may be carried out are:
  - Compressing the aorta just above or below the left subclavian artery to selectively shunt the available blood into the central circulation. It is important that a covered Satinsky vascular clamp is used. Periodic assessment of the patient's volume status is needed once the aorta is compressed to prevent ventricular distension and other problems of aortic occlusion such as spinal ischaemia.
  - Opening the pericardium fully to release any cardiac tamponade and allow the source of the bleeding to be controlled by direct pressure or suture. The phrenic nerve may be at risk during this procedure; consequently, the operator must identify this structure and must cut anteriorly to it.
  - External cardiac compression in a patient with a normal blood volume only produces 10% of the normal cardiac output. However, it can be increased to 50 % with internal cardiac massage. This is carried out by placing a hand inside the pericardial sac and squeezing the heart at a rate of approximately $60\ min^{-1}$. It is preferable to use the palm of the hand as finger tips can traumatize the heart wall. Internal cardiac massage is an exhausting activity because the operator needs to squeeze hard and then abruptly relax to facilitate ventricular filling. Barring

defibrillation, this must be continued without interruption until spontaneous cardiac output is established or the patient is pronounced dead by the clinician in charge.

– Internal defibrillation is necessary if VF (ventricular fibrillation) develops. However, the paddles should be covered with wet saline gauze to prevent burning the myocardium. One paddle needs to be placed over the base of the right atrium and another over the cardiac apex. Lesser energies must be used compared with external defibrillation (10–60 J as opposed to 200–360 J).

– Significant bleeding can usually be controlled by direct pressure from either finger compression or laparotomy packs. Occasionally, a bleeding organ, such as the hilum of the lung, will require the direct application of a non-crushing clamp of the vascular paddle.

Potential complications

An emergency room thoracotomy should only be carried out by trained staff because it can give rise to many complications if it is performed incorrectly. The main ones are:

- As for tube thorocostomy.
- Major haemorrhage.
- Significant damage to mediastinal and pulmonary structures.

Postprocedure checks

- Check the patient ventilation and cardiovascular status.

Aftercare

- Once haemodynamic stability has been restored, the patient must be transferred to theatre, where definitive surgery can be carried out.

Massive haemothorax

This is defined as the loss of more than 1.5 litres of blood into the chest cavity (Fig. 17) or the drainage of greater than 200 ml h^{-1} for 4 h. It is usually the result of either a torn intercostal vessel or lacerated internal mammary artery, but occasionally is secondary to a torn hilum. Bleeding from any of these vessels tends to continue unabated as there is no tamponading effect from the thoracic contents. Conversely, bleeding from the lung parenchyma usually stops once the lung has re-expanded because of the low pulmonary perfusion pressure.

The physical signs of a massive haemothorax are:

- Decreased air entry to the hemithorax.
- Dull percussion note over the hemithorax.
- Shocked, grade 2–3.
- Raised JVP (variable).

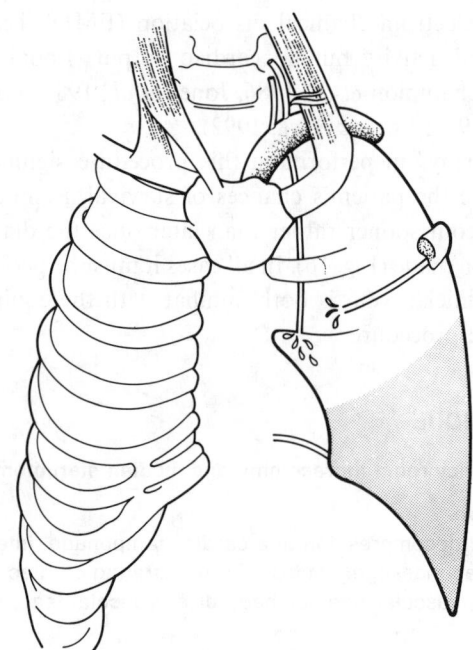

Fig. 17. Line diagram showing a massive haemothorax. (Redrawn from Landon *et al.*, 1993.)

It should be noted, however, that the JVP may be high or low depending on coexisting problems.

Patients with a massive haemothorax usually require a formal thoracotomy to correct the condition. Therefore, the appropriate surgeon should be informed and in the meantime resuscitation should be continued with type-specific blood.

Monitoring and reassessment

At the end of the primary survey and resuscitation phase it is essential that the life-threatening problems involving the airway, breathing and circulation have been identified and managed appropriately. A policy of continual vigilance is essential in patients with thoracic trauma because the above problems may not only be present on arrival in the A&E department but may also develop at any time during resuscitation. Therefore a reassessment must be carried out if a patient's condition deteriorates. This should start with the airway in the manner described above.

In addition to the continuous observation of the patient's pulse, blood pressure, respiratory rate, skin perfusion and level of consciousness, an electrocardiographic (ECG) monitor should be attached and a chest X-ray ordered. An arterial blood sample must be sent to assess adequacy of ventilation and acid–base status; if

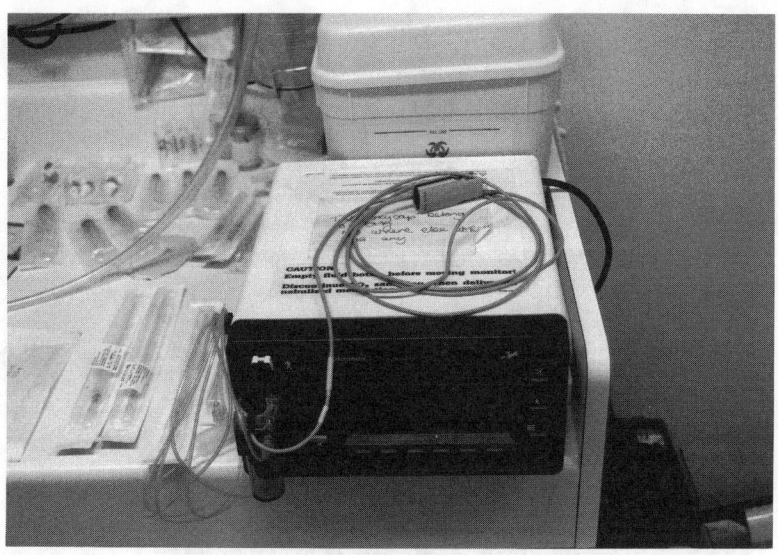

Fig. 18. Pulse oximeter.

there are any signs suggesting cardiac injury, a 12-lead ECG is required.

Pulse oximeters (Fig. 18)

The adequacy of oxygenation can be assessed using a pulse oximeter. This device measures the absorption of red and infrared light by oxyhaemoglobin during the pulsatile phase of blood flow through tissues. The result is then used to calculate the arterial haemoglobin saturation with oxygen (SaO_2) (Tremper & Barker, 1989).

Although reliable and accurate under normal circumstances, there can be an underestimation of the saturation or the loss of the signal altogether when the pulsatile phase is reduced. This typically occurs in patients who are severely vasoconstricted from either a low cardiac output or hypothermia (West, 1990). Pulse oximeters are also very susceptible to motion artefact and patient shivering, and both of these conditions may occur and present problems during resuscitation. Finally, if a patient has a high circulating carboxyhaemoglobin level, this will artificially elevate the reading. Clearly results from these devices must be interpreted in light of these facts.

PaO_2 (and hence SaO_2) can be maintained by increasing the inspired oxygen concentration (FiO_2). Consequently, patients who are hypoventilating with a high FiO_2 can have a normal SaO_2 but a raised $PaCO_2$ (Hutton & Clutton-Brock, 1993).

Capnography (Fig. 19)

Under normal circumstances, the partial pressure of carbon dioxide in the gas at the end of expiration (end-tidal carbon dioxide) is very close to that in pulmonary capillary blood and hence arterial blood ($PaCO_2$). The latter is a good indicator of the efficacy of ventilation, to which it is inversely related. Consequently end-tidal carbon dioxide can also be used as an indicator of ventilation. However, in patients who develop ventilation/perfusion mismatch, end-tidal carbon dioxide will underestimate $PaCO_2$ as carbon dioxide is not being delivered to ventilated alveoli and so does not appear in the gas at the end of expiration. In these circumstances, end-tidal carbon dioxide cannot be used to assess ventilation and an arterial blood sample must be analysed for a true $PaCO_2$ reading.

SECONDARY SURVEY

The secondary survey of the chest involves a detailed physical examination to detect any potentially life-threatening conditions as well as other minor chest conditions (Committee on Trauma of the American College of Surgeons, 1993). In this way, a definitive management plan for the patient can be devised.

The front and sides of the chest should be fully examined in detail by looking, listening and percussing. Subsequently each rib must be palpated for tenderness and crepitus and the thoracic cage squeezed in two

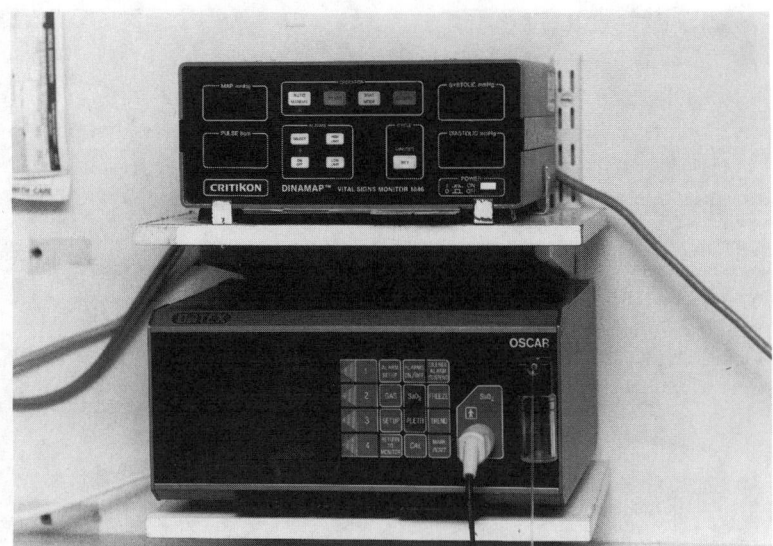

Fig. 19. Capnograph.

planes to determine rib stability if no obvious fractures have been identified. The presence of surgical emphysema must also be noted.

Examination of the back of the chest is very important but it will require sufficient people to enable the patient to be log-rolled onto their side safely. Consequently this part of the examination is usually left until the whole of the back is inspected. However, if the clinician is suspicious of a posterior penetrating injury, then the patient's back must be inspected at the earliest opportunity.

There are six potentially life-threatening conditions which need to be ruled out during the secondary survey.

Potentially life-threatening thoracic conditions

P   Pulmonary contusion
C   Cardiac contusion
R   Ruptured diaphragm
D   Disruption of the thoracic aorta
O   Oesophageal rupture
A   Airway rupture

A mnemonic for this list is: **P**hysicians **C**annot **R**esuscitate **D**ead **O**n **A**rrivals.

Unfortunately, these conditions result in subtle changes which require a high index of suspicion and can lead, if they are missed, to a significant increase in mortality. Knowledge of the mechanism of the injury and a detailed physical examination are therefore essential for their early detection.

Pulmonary contusion

Often the only initial indicators of this condition are tenderness or marks on the chest wall from the original injury along with rapid shallow respiration. Fractured ribs can be present, but in the young the natural elasticity of the chest wall may prevent this. Auscultation can also be normal. However, as the disease process develops, respiratory distress increases as ventilation becomes progressively more difficult (Macnaughton & Evans, 1992; Martin, 1993; Murphy & Jones, 1991).

A plain chest radiograph will commonly show hazy shadowing after a few hours (Fig. 20) and serial arterial blood gases will reveal a gradual fall in the PaO_2 as the ventilation/perfusion mismatch develops. As the patient becomes exhausted by the work of ventilation, there will also be a rise in the $PaCO_2$.

These patients require a high inspired oxygen concentration, careful fluid administration and close observation, preferably in a high-dependency/intensive care unit. This will also facilitate the use of analgesic techniques to allow physiotherapy so that infection can be prevented. A selective approach to mechanical ventilation is undertaken in most hospitals:

- Elderly.
- Decreased level of consciousness.
- Associated long bone fractures.
- Progressive rise in $PaCO_2$.
- Progressive fall in PaO_2.
- Requiring a general anaesthetic for surgery.
- Requiring transfer.

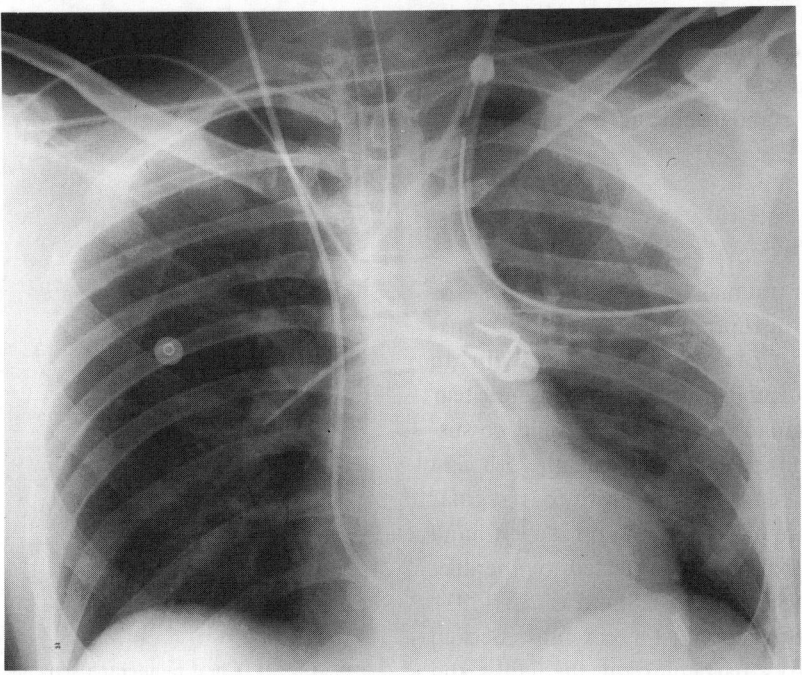

Fig. 20. Chest radiograph taken on a multiply injured patient 4 h after the injury. Pulmonary contusion and multiple fracture ribs are visible. Note that the patient is intubated, a pulmonary artery catheter and nasogastric tube are in place and that the chest drain is inserted too far on the left.

- Renal failure.
- Pre-existing lung disease.

The actual criteria for starting this form of treatment will vary between hospitals, and the clinician must therefore be aware of the local policy.

The potential for an increase in pulmonary oedema as a result of overtransfusion in these patients is well recognized. Nevertheless, significant injury can also result from undertransfusion leading to a fall in cardiac output, pulmonary perfusion and, in turn, areas of high V/Q ratios. The development of a high V/Q ratio results in further hypoxia and additional leakage through the alveolar membrane. It follows that invasive monitoring is the only safe way of determining the appropriate fluid requirements for these patients and this is a further reason why they should be managed in a high-dependency/intensive care unit.

Cardiac contusion

In the reported cases of thoracoabdominal trauma, cardiac contusion has an incidence of 16–76%. Should the contusion be significant then the patient may develop arrhythmias, heart failure or hypotension which will not respond to fluid resuscitation. The incidence of ar-

rhythmias also increases if there is any associated hypoxia or acidosis. However, in the majority of cases it is often missed because the patient is asymptomatic.

Clearly, any patient who on examination has sternal bruising and tenderness from a blow to the front of the chest, a fracture of the sternum or wedge fractures of the thoracic vertebrae, must be considered to be at a high risk of having a cardiac contusion.

The principle investigations are a 12-lead ECG and a plasma assay of the cardiac creatine phosphokinase isoenzyme (CPK-MB). Although an elevation of greater than 30% in the enzyme assay is diagnostic of myocardial damage, there are few hospitals which can do this biochemical investigation whilst the patient is in the resuscitation room. Therefore its value tends to be as a retrospective confirmatory test. During the definitive phase, information on the ventricular wall motion can be obtained by performing either a transoesophageal or transthoracic echocardiogram (Hiatt et al., 1988). Isotope studies performed later may be confirmatory.

A variety of arrhythmias may be present, particularly premature ventricular contractions, atrial fibrillation, sinus tachycardia and ST elevation or depression. A right bundle branch block pattern may also be seen. Patients with suspected cardiac contusion with arrhythmias require the facilities of a high-dependency unit for their long-term management. It is therefore important to make sure the appropriate doctor is informed. Heart failure and arrhythmias producing haemodynamic instability should be treated by standard medical protocols (see Chapter 45B).

Ruptured diaphragm

Blunt or penetrating trauma to either the chest or abdomen can result in a ruptured diaphragm. In penetrating trauma, 75% of cases are associated with an intra-abdominal injury and there is usually a discrete tear in either hemidiaphragm. This condition should be suspected if a wound is found lying between the 5th and 12th ribs. In contrast, blunt trauma produces irregular multiple tears, which are more common on the left-hand side (79% of cases) as the right is 'protected' by the liver (Demetriades *et al.*, 1988; Kaulesar Sukul *et al.*, 1991).

On examination, the patient must be carefully checked for any wounds or marks, particularly in the flanks and on the back. Breath sounds may be decreased over the inferior aspect of the affected hemithorax and occasionally bowel sound can be heard on auscultation of the chest. Unfortunately these physical signs are not always present and the first suspicion usually comes from the plain chest radiograph (Maddox *et al.*, 1991). The affected hemidiaphragm is elevated, and occasionally bowel is seen herniating through it into the pleural space (Fig. 21). These features are best seen on an erect chest X-ray but this should only be obtained once spinal injury has been eliminated. If a naso- or orogastric tube has been inserted it may be seen coiled up above the left hemidiaphragm. Occasionally, peritoneal lavage fluid will leak out of a chest drain if the diaphragm is ruptured, thereby confirming the diagnosis. However, the diagnostic peritoneal lavage itself may be negative (free of blood).

Once the diagnosis has been made or is suspected, surgical advice is required to deal with any associated intrathoracic or abdominal injury. Operative repair of the diaphragm prevents bowel herniation and possible obstruction.

Disruption of the thoracic aorta

Of the 10% of patients who reach hospital alive with this condition, 50% will die each day if the diagnosis is missed and surgery is not performed. The clinician therefore needs to have a high index of suspicion of this injury and request early advice from a thoracic surgeon.

It is important to note that as usually only a relatively

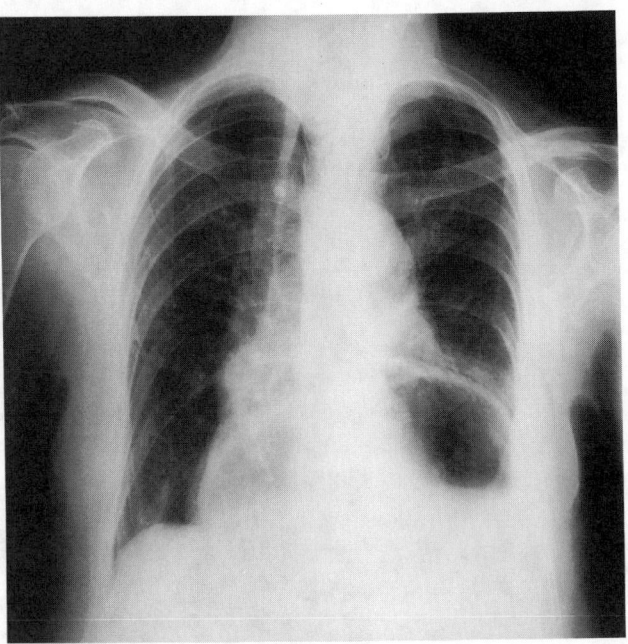

Fig. 21. Chest radiograph showing a ruptured diaphragm.

small volume of blood (approximately 500 ml) is lost from the systemic circulation, these patients do not demonstrate the classical signs of shock providing there are no other sources of haemorrhage. A variety of other signs may be present, including hoarseness, pulse differences between upper and lower limbs, and upper limb hypertension due to an inappropriate baroreceptor response. Hypertension will need pharmacological control both prior to theatre and during transport to reduce the risk of haemorrhage. A common recommendation consists of labetalol infusion to achieve central hypotension and 2–5 µg of dopamine kg^{-1} to optimize renal perfusion.

An erect plain chest radiograph is an important preliminary investigation as it can demonstrate several signs of a disrupted thoracic aorta, of which a widened mediastinum is the most important:

- Widened mediastinum.
- Fractured first two ribs.
- Trachea displaced to the right.
- Oesophagus displaced to the right.
- Pleural capping.
- Blurring of the aortic notch.
- Elevation of the right mainstem bronchus.
- Depression of the left mainstem bronchus.
- Decrease in space between the pulmonary artery and aorta.

The definitive investigation is either angiography, a CT (computed tomography) scan of the aortic arch or transoesophageal echocardiography. The choice depends on the policy of the local thoracic surgeons (Treasure & Raphael, 1991).

If these patients are to survive then the aorta needs to be surgically repaired before the adventitial layer ruptures. If there is no thoracic surgical team in the receiving hospital, advice must be sought on which investigation to perform because of the risk of deterioration during transfer.

Oesophageal rupture

The patient with this condition has a degree of shock and pain greater than that normally expected from the apparent injury. Suspicions should be raised if a left-sided pneumothorax or pleural effusion is seen on the chest radiograph, without there being any history of left-sided chest trauma. Occasionally, a pneumomediastinum or a fluid level may be present behind the heart shadow. Surgical emphysema in the neck and upper chest may also develop with time. If a chest drain has been inserted the fluid swing should be observed. Normally this is maximal during expiration, but with an air leak from the oesophagus the swing is equal in both stages of the ventilatory cycle. Very occasionally bowel contents are extruded through the chest drain, indicating that a viscus has been ruptured.

These patients require further investigations and in almost all cases surgical repair. Therefore the appropriate surgical team should be involved once the secondary survey is finished.

Airway rupture

This can occur at three different anatomical levels.

Larynx

Impacts with dashboards, steering wheels, clothes lines, fists or feet can fracture this cartilaginous structure causing pharyngeal haematomas and oedema which may eventually cause respiratory obstruction.

On examination the three classical signs may be present. These are:

- Hoarseness.
- Crepitus.
- Surgical emphysema.

Any haemoptysis, tenderness, bruising around the larynx, reduced prominence of the thyroid notch, dyspnoea or stridor should also be noted.

The first priority in these patients is to ensure they have a patent airway. This must be secured by an experienced anaesthetist because the distorted anatomy can make this procedure very difficult. To avoid rendering a patient with a compromised airway apnoeic by injecting a muscle relaxant, the anaesthetist may choose to perform inhalational induction of anaesthesia to allow direct laryngoscopy. In this way the airway can be inspected without paralysing the patient.

Whatever technique is used, an experienced surgeon should be immediately available to perform an emergency tracheostomy in case intubation fails. A cricothyroidotomy is contraindicated in these patients because the distorted anatomy and the risk of significant haemorrhage would make the procedure extremely difficult (see Chapter 2). Once the airway has been cleared and secured, a CT scan can then be performed (Myers & Iko, 1987).

The patient will require skilled ENT (ear, nose and throat) advice during the definitive treatment phase.

Tracheal tears

The causes of blunt trauma to the trachea are similar to those fracturing the larynx, with tears usually occurring at the cricotracheal junction. Conversely, penetrating trauma can occur at any level. The latter is frequently associated with injuries to adjacent structures, especially when the lesion is in the neck. Coexisting injuries to the carotid arteries, jugular veins, oesophagus and laryngeal and phrenic nerves must be excluded or treated.

Apart from external evidence of injury, the only finding of tracheal injury may be noisy breathing as a result of partial airway obstruction from the presence of a haematoma, oedema or blood clot. If obstruction is complete, ventilation will be absent, causing extreme respiratory distress in the conscious patient. In the deeply unconscious patient this may present a diagnostic dilemma, as the cause of apnoea may not be recognized.

If penetrating trauma has exposed the lumen of the trachea, blood and bubbles may be seen escaping from the base of the wound. The clinician must immediately clear and secure the airway, either by orotracheal intubation or, in some instances, by directly inserting a tracheal tube into the trachea through the wound.

In cases of complete obstruction just proximal to the carina, it may be necessary to deliberately pass a tracheal tube into one main bronchus relying on one-lung ventilation with 100% oxygen as an emergency measure. If the defect is only small then basic airway control may be all that is required until a detailed examination of the trachea can be performed.

Once the patient with a tracheal injury has been adequately resuscitated the clinician must remember to examine and investigate the trauma victim for injuries to the closely aligned structures.

Bronchial tears

On examination the only finding may be haemoptysis with overt signs of a chest injury. Mediastinal or surgical emphysema suggests a tear proximal to the pleural reflection, whilst a pneumothorax (simple or tension) indicates a tear between the parietal and visceral pleura. Often the diagnosis is made after a chest drain has been inserted as the initial rush of air does not settle. Instead many bubbles are produced with each expiration, indicating a large, persistent leak. If this is large enough, a second chest drain may have to be inserted.

If an oral intubation is attempted (for whatever reason), it may be technically difficult or impossible to perform because of distorted anatomy. Therefore expert anaesthetic assistance is crucial. The expertise of a thoracic surgeon will be necessary for definitive management. Some patients will require surgery whilst others will be managed conservatively. However, all will require a bronchoscopy to determine the extent of the injury and to remove clots and debris.

DEFINITIVE CARE

The thoracic surgical team will be required to help in the management of approximately 15% of cases of chest trauma. The receiving trauma team must therefore make sure they are aware which cases the surgeons will need to be involved with and, if the surgeons are not on site, what the local protocols are for dealing effectively with these problems.

The management of the following conditions should fall within the capability of any clinician involved in the care of trauma patients.

Pneumothorax

All traumatic pneumothoraces need to be evacuated with an appropriately sized chest drain, inserted using the open technique, in the correct location. If the lung becomes fully inflated and the pleural space dry, then there is less than a 1% chance of side-effects such as infection and adhesions (Fig. 22).

Haemothorax

Bleeding into the pleural cavity usually follows lung or vessel injury and is often self-limiting. The treatment required is drainage of the blood through a large chest tube to stop the formation of clots which would prevent full expansion of the lung. In addition, an adequate circulating volume must be maintained using cross-matched blood as appropriate.

Occasionally, the bleeding does not stop. To ensure that this is detected it is important to monitor closely the amount of blood draining via the chest drains. Surgical intervention may be required to arrest the haemorrhage (see above).

Surgical emphysema

This does not need treating unless it is severe enough to interfere with respiration when a chest drain may be required. However, it should be viewed as an indicator of more serious underlying injuries and a detailed examination is required to identify the cause, which will require definitive treatment:

- Laryngeal, tracheal or bronchial tears.
- Oesophageal tear.
- Sucking chest wound.
- Blast injury.
- Lung injuries.

Fractured sternum

Isolated sternal fractures, in the absence of clinical evidence of cardiac or respiratory complications and with a normal 12-lead ECG and chest radiograph, require no further investigations. Following observation for 24 h, these patients may be discharged without follow-up (Heyes & Vincent, 1993). In contrast, if cardiac or pulmonary contusions are suspected from the clinical presentation or from these initial tests, then the specialist investigations discussed previously are necessary. The management of these patients depends on their clinical state.

Fractured ribs

Ribs usually fracture at their point of maximum curvature laterally. Young people, especially children, have very pliable bones which do not break, even when subjected

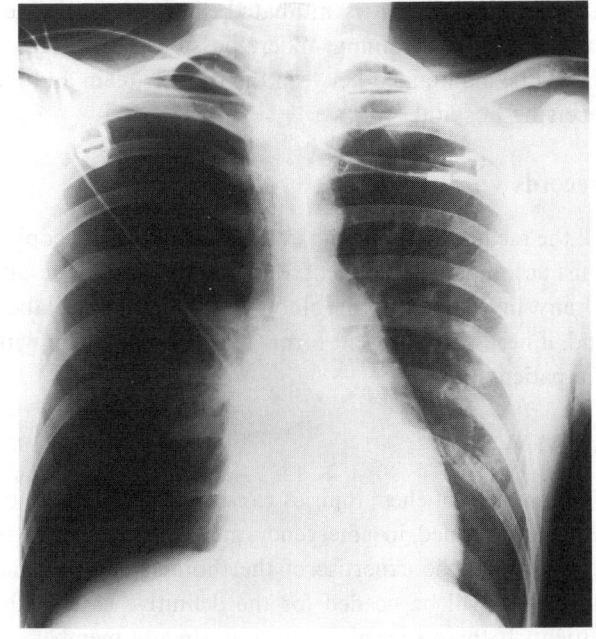

(a)

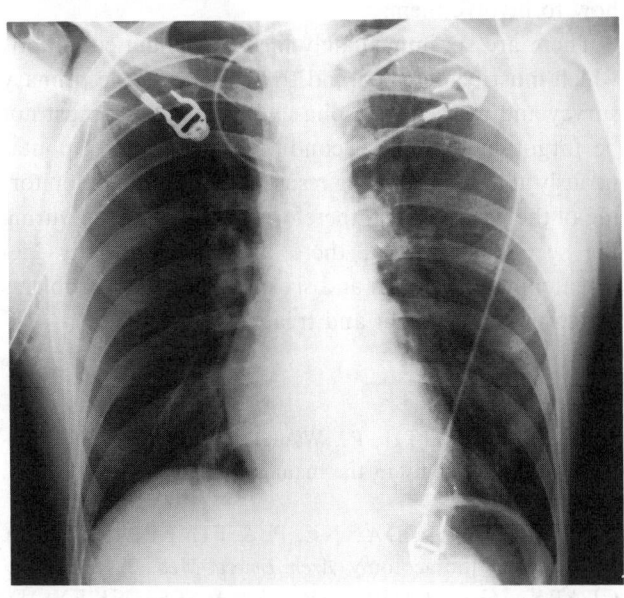

(b)

Fig. 22. Chest radiographs showing a right pneumothorax before (a) and after (b) the chest drain has been inserted. Note that the mediastinum returns to its normal position following insertion of the drain, indicating a degree of tension was present in the initial radiograph.

to considerable forces. Consequently, in these cases, there can be significant internal thoracic injuries without overlying rib fractures. These fractures are often not visible on the initial radiograph unless there is significant displacement, but as muscle spasm relaxes the fractures open out and they can be clearly seen (Fig. 20).

Great force is required to produce fractures of the upper three ribs which are protected by the overlying muscles and clavicle. These fractures are therefore associated with severe intrathoracic pathology and a mortality of 50%. Their presence should alert the clinician to the potential for severe underlying conditions which must be identified or excluded.

Ribs 4–9 may be broken in the axillary region from either a direct blow or an anteroposterior compression force. The former will push the broken ends of the bone into the chest cavity, causing an increased risk of lung damage.

The lower ribs also cover the abdominal cavity. Therefore, when fractured, there may be associated intra-abdominal visceral injury and blood loss into the peritoneal cavity. Both of these complications need to be excluded.

Rib fractures are painful, especially when multiple. In spontaneously breathing patients, severe pain will restrict expansion of the lungs and coughing, leading ultimately to retention of secretions, consolidation and infection. Therefore, once any underlying pathology has been ruled out, analgesia should be provided so that intensive chest physiotherapy can be started. Pain can be relieved by a variety of techniques (e.g. local or regional block), depending upon the expertise available (see Chapter 10).

Chest compression (traumatic asphyxia)

If severe, this can obstruct venous return causing raised intrathoracic and intracranial pressure. Patients are plethoric and cyanotic with engorged faces, upper limbs and chests. They may be confused or unconscious. Associated signs are petechial and scleral haemorrhages and respiratory distress. Once the compression force has been relieved, the raised pressures abate and mortality is related to associated injuries.

TRANSFER

This is a particularly dangerous time for the patient. Great care must be taken to anticipate and minimize any potential problems (Ridley *et al.*, 1990).

Communication

To facilitate a smooth transfer, it is important to ensure that the receiving facility and personnel have been contacted directly by the clinician in charge of the patient. If an interhospital transfer is envisaged, the clinician must also decide on the most suitable method of transportation and how the patient should be prepared for the journey (see below). Air transport should be avoided if possible in patients with thoracic trauma. However, if this mode of transport is necessary, it is best to replace any underwater seal drains with a Heimlich-type flutter valve or closed chest drainage system.

Irrespective of the mode of transport never clamp the chest drain!

Assessment

All aspects of the primary survey must be reassessed before the patient leaves and appropriate adjustments made. Ideally the patient should be stable in terms of their respiratory and cardiovascular systems. The patient who tolerates an oropharyngeal airway should be intubated and ventilated so that the airway can be protected and hypoxia and hypercarbia prevented. All cannulae, catheters, tubes and drains must be secured with the knowledge that, if they can fall out, they will fall out! Adequate supplies of oxygen, intravenous fluids and drugs must be taken, particularly if the oxygen is driving a ventilator.

Monitoring

This ensures that ventilation and tissue perfusion remain adequate. If a parameter needs to be monitored before transfer, it will also need to be monitored during transfer. As a minimum, an ECG monitor, automatic blood pressure recorder and pulse oximeter are essential. All of these devices must be fully charged with adequate battery supplies for long journeys.

Equipment and drugs

The trolley carrying the patient during an interhospital transfer must also transport the suction system, oxygen supply, ventilator, blood pressure monitor, syringe pumps and defibrillator-monitor. Smaller items, such as airway adjuncts, needles and drugs are usually carried separately in a prepared box by one of the medical team.

Transfer personnel

During transit, the patient needs to be accompanied by appropriately skilled staff who are able to monitor and intervene with any potential problems which may arise.

If the trauma victim is intubated, the personnel must have anaesthetic training. Where possible, radio contact should be maintained between the transfer team and the receiving hospital.

Records

All the medical and nursing notes, or high-quality copies, must accompany the patient. Radiographs and the results of any investigations or blood tests, identifying labels and, if necessary, consent forms must also be taken with the patient.

SUMMARY

The majority of chest injuries can be treated initially by clinicians trained in emergency medicine. However, in certain cases the expertise of the thoracic surgeon and intensivist will be needed for the definitive care of the patient. If these specialists are not already members of the resuscitation team, the clinician must know when and how to involve them.

There are six immediately life-threatening conditions which must be detected and treated during the primary survey and resuscitation phase. Nevertheless it must not be forgotten that these conditions may occur spontaneously at any time during resuscitation. Careful monitoring of the patient must, therefore, be maintained. During the secondary survey, there are six potentially life-threatening conditions and six minor thoracic problems which must be sought and treated.

Bibliography

BODAI, B., SMITH, P., WARD, R. *et al.* (1983). Emergency thoracotomy in the management of trauma. *JAMA*, **249**, 1891–6.

CHAMPION, H., DANNE, P. & FINELLI, F. (1986). Emergency thoracotomy. *Arch. Emerg. Med.*, **3**, 95–9.

CLARK, G., SCHECTER, W. & TRUNKEY, D. (1988). Variables affecting outcome in blunt chest traums: flail chest vs. pulmonary contusion. *J. Trauma*, **28**, 298–304.

COMMITTEE ON TRAUMA OF THE AMERICAN COLLEGE OF SURGEONS (1993). *ATLS Program*, pp. 111–41. Chicago: American College of Surgeons.

DEMETRIADES, D., KAKOYIANNIS, S., PAREKH, D. *et al.* (1988). Penetrating injuries of the diaphragm. *Br. J. Surg.*, **75**, 824–6.

HEYES, F. & VINCENT, R. (1993). Sternal fracture: what investigations are indicated? *Injury*, **24**, 113–5.

HIATT, J., YEATMAN, L. & CHILD, J. (1988). The value of echocardiography in blunt chest trauma. *J. Trauma*, **28**, 914–22.

HUTTON, P. & CLUTTON-BROCK, T. (1993). The benefit and pitfalls of pulse oximetry. *Br. Med. J.*, **307**, 457–8.

JONES, T., BARNHART, G. & GREENFIELD, L. (1987). Cardiopulmonary arrest following penetrating trauma: guidelines for emergency hospital management of presumed exsanguination. *J. Trauma*, **27**, 24–31.

JURKOVICH, G., ESPOSITO, T. & MAIER, R. (1992). Resuscitation thoracotomy performed in the operating room. *Am. J. Surg.*, **163**, 463–8.

KAULESAR SUKUL, D., KATS, E. & JOHANNES, E. (1991). Sixty three cases of traumatic injury to the diaphragm. *Injury*, **22**, 303–6.

LANDON, B., DRISCOLL, P. & GOODALL, J. (1993). *An Atlas of Trauma Care: The First Hour*. Carnforth: Parthenon Publishing.

LORENZ, H., STEINMETZ, B., LIEBERMAN, J. *et al.* (1992). Emergency thoracotomy: survival correlates with physiological status. *J. Trauma*, **32**, 780–8.

MACNAUGHTON, P. & EVANS, T. (1992). Management of adult respiratory distress syndrome. *Lancet*, **339**, 469–72.

MADDOX, P., MANSEL, R. & BUTCHART, E. (1991). Traumatic rupture of the diaphragm: a difficult diagnosis. *Injury*, **22**, 299–302.

MARTIN, L. (1993). Crush injuries of the chest: an historical perspective in a single unit. *J. R. Coll. Surg. Edinb.*, **38**, 4–8.

MURPHY, P. & JONES, J. (1991). Acute lung injury. *Br. J. Intens. Care*, **12**, 110–14.

MYERS, E. & IKO, B. (1987). The management of acute laryngeal trauma. *J. Trauma*, **27**, 448–52.

REPINE, J. (1992). Scientific perspectives on adult respiratory distress syndrome. *Lancet*, **339**, 466–9.

RICHIE, A. (1992). Plastic bullets: significant risk or serious injury above the diaphragm. *Injury*, **23**, 265–6.

RIDLEY, S., WRIGHT, I. & ROGERS- P. (1990). Secondary transport of critically ill patients. *Hosp. Update*, **16**, 289–98.

ROMANES, G., ed. (1969). *Cunningham's Manual of Practical Anatomy*, Vol. 2, *Thorax and Abdomen*, 13th edn. Oxford: Oxford University Press.

ROSS, S. (1990). Epidemiology of thoracic injuries: mechanisms of injury and pathophysiology. *Top. Emerg. Med.*, **12**, 1–9.

SELFELICIANO, D. (1992). The diagnostic therapeutic approach to chest trauma. *Semin. Thor. Cardiovasc. Surg.*, **4**, 156–75.

TREASURE, T. & RAPHAEL, M. (1991). Investigation of suspected dissection of the thoracic aorta. *Lancet*, **338**, 490–5.

TREMPER, K.K. & BARKER, S.J. (1989). Pulse oximetry. *Anaesthesiology*, **70**, 98–106.

WEST, J. (1987). *Pulmonary Pathophysiology – The Essentials*. Baltimore: Williams & Wilkins.

WEST, J. (1990). *Respiratory Physiology – The Essentials*. Baltimore: Williams & Wilkins.

24 Abdominal trauma

B. J. ROWLANDS

Department of Surgery, The Queen's University of Belfast, Belfast, Northern Ireland

Chapter plan

Introduction
Pathophysiology of injury
Initial assessment and resuscitation
Surgical intervention in abdominal injury
Summary

INTRODUCTION

Intra-abdominal trauma is a contributing factor to approximately 20% of fatalities. In the Report of the Royal College of Surgeons of England on Major Trauma, published in 1988, it was identified as a significant cause of preventable deaths. Both blunt and penetrating abdominal injury may cause damage to solid and hollow viscera within the peritoneal cavity or to their associated blood vessels within the mesentery or retroperitoneal tissues. Blunt abdominal trauma is often associated with multisystem injury which may include head, thoracic or limb injury. The most common cause of demise following penetrating trauma is major intra-abdominal vascular trauma leading to hypovolaemic shock. Septic complications may follow disruption of solid organs and injury to the bowel. They are a significant cause of late mortality and morbidity.

This chapter will review the mechanisms of intra-abdominal injury and the recognition of important diagnostic features that suggest significant life-threatening injury. The principles underlying the optimal management of selected injuries to individual organs will also be discussed. Application of sound surgical principles to the management of abdominal trauma should decrease the incidence of unnecessary death when major lesions remain undiagnosed or untreated. Immediate appropriate resuscitation, diagnosis and definitive management should also reduce the incidence of postinjury septicaemia, pulmonary insufficiency, renal failure and malnutrition.

PATHOPHYSIOLOGY OF INJURY

Some trauma patients may suffer injuries that are rapidly fatal. Other injuries produce remarkably little tissue destruction or haemodynamic instability. The former group have injuries that are not amenable to treatment and death is inevitable within minutes. The latter group require careful assessment and observation and may require minimal attention to soft tissue injuries. Usually, if they remain stable, they may be discharged from hospital within several hours. In between these two extremes, which account respectively for 5% and 80% of all trauma admissions, are a group of potentially salvageable unstable victims whose injuries may be life-threatening if not given urgent medical attention. These patients benefit most from rapid transportation to a hospital that provides facilities and personnel to cope with a spectrum of injuries. As one-fifth of postinjury deaths are due to abdominal injuries associated with blunt and penetrating trauma, it is particularly important to suspect abdominal injury in this group of unstable patients.

Factors requiring a high degree of suspicion for intra-abdominal injury

- Revised Trauma Score of less than 12
- Glasgow Coma Scale of less than 13
- Rapid deceleration injury
- High-velocity penetrating injury
- Falls from more than 4.5 m

} Highest correlation with multiple injury

- Massive blunt soft tissue injury
- Combination of blunt and penetrating trauma, e.g. bomb blast
- Crush injury, e.g. burial alive
- Penetrating trauma between nipples and midthigh
- Traumatic amputation of arm or leg
- Limb paralysis – partial or complete
- Road traffic accidents involving:
  - prolonged extraction
  - passenger compartment 'invaded' by 30 cm or more
  - vehicle roll-over
  - backward displacement of the front axle
  - ejection or death of another occupant
  - pedestrians struck at more than 20 m.p.h.

Table 1. *Incidence of injuries in blunt and penetrating abdominal injury*

	Blunt (%)	Penetrating (%)
Spleen	25	6
Liver	15	16
Retroperitoneal haematoma	13	1
Kidney	12	5
Small bowel	9	30
Bladder/ureter	6	2
Mesentery/omentum	5	18
Large bowel	4	9
Pancreas	3	3
Urethra	2	–
Diaphragm	2	8
Vascular	2	4
Stomach	1	7
Duodenum	1	2
Biliary	–	1

Blunt trauma

In Britain, blunt trauma is the more common cause of abdominal injury and is usually associated with multiple system injury. This makes initial assessment difficult and may present conflicts concerning the priorities of treatment. The causes of blunt trauma are motor vehicle, auto/pedestrian and industrial accidents as well as sporting injuries. Blunt injury produces damage by direct impact, rapid deceleration or by shearing and rotational forces. In motorvehicle and auto/pedestrian accidents, all these mechanisms may be operative, resulting in ejection from the vehicle or violent contact with the fabric of the car. In deceleration injury (e.g. head-on collisions or falls from a height) the vessels and tissue of solid and hollow organs are torn from their attachments. Rotational forces cause similar injuries at the juxtaposition of relatively fixed and mobile structures. Shearing and crushing forces may compromise blood supply to organs and cause massive soft tissue injury to the anterior and posterior abdominal wall. Bursting of the bowel may occur when intraluminal and intra-abdominal pressure rises rapidly at the moment of impact. The abdominal organs most commonly involved in blunt trauma are the spleen, liver and kidney, and the most common manifestation of solid organ injury is bleeding into the peritoneal cavity or retroperitoneal tissue (Table 1).

Penetrating trauma

Penetrating trauma occurs less frequently, but stab wounds and penetrating injuries from urban violence are now common in large cities. Gunshot wounds are seen more frequently than in the past, especially in large cities. Knife wounds are relatively clean, rarely life-threatening and rarely require urgent exploration. Exceptions include injuries to major abdominal vessels or when the injury occurs between the nipples and costal margins so that the mediastinum and pleural cavities are traversed in addition to the peritoneal cavity. Gunshot wounds are more serious and produce varying degrees of injury and tissue destruction depending on the type of weapon, the velocity of the bullet and the distance between assailant and victim (Barach *et al.*, 1986a, b) Handguns fire bullets at a low velocity and produce less injury to tissue than magnum weapons, paramilitary firearms and shotguns, which use high-velocity ammunition and whose energy is dissipated over a wider area producing cavitation and destruction. Injuries may involve several organs and massive soft tissue necrosis. Whereas a selective policy of operative management may be appropriate for knife wounds that penetrate the peritoneal cavity, all gunshot wounds should be explored.

Extensive injuries due to bombs and explosive devices may cause a combination of penetrating and blunt injury resulting in massive soft tissue injury, blast effects and loss of life and limb (see Chapter 40). Survivors all need exploration of the peritoneal cavity and extensive debridement of necrotic tissue and removal of foreign bodies. The pattern of organ injury in penetrating trauma is different from blunt trauma, as bowel injury is more common than solid organ injury and major vessel injury is more likely to occur (Table 1).

INITIAL ASSESSMENT AND RESUSCITATION

The patient should be admitted to the trauma receiving area in the accident and emergency (A&E) department, equipped with ventilator support, monitoring, venous access and diagnostic evaluation, as well as with resuscitation fluids (Yates, 1984). Physical examination and resuscitation should proceed simultaneously and external evidence of trauma such as penetrating wounds, soft tissue injury, limb deformity, haematoma formation and bruising noted. The initial examination should include rapid assessment of the airway, chest, abdomen and neurological status together with pulse and blood pressure, and should take less than 60 sec. The immediate priority in management should be to establish and maintain an adequate airway and respiratory effort. In the conscious, spontaneously breathing patient oxygen may be given by mask but the unconscious patient may require an oropharyngeal airway or tracheal intubation and mechanical ventilation using a bag and mask or ventilator. The airway should be cleared of blood, saliva and foreign bodies. The air entry into each lung should be checked by auscultation.

The next priority is the cardiovascular system, the blood pressure and pulse being noted along with the presence of peripheral vasoconstriction and skin temperature. Signs of hypovolaemic shock should be treated by immediate insertion of large-bore intravenous cannulae into uninjured limbs either percutaneously or by venous cut-down into the cubital fossa, ankle or groin. Isotonic saline should be infused rapidly (up to 2 litres) followed by colloid infusion of blood, plasma, albumin, dextrans or gelatin solutions (Rowlands, 1988).

Intra-abdominal injury should be suspected in any patient who is unconscious, has respiratory difficulty and evidence of hypovolaemia.

Physical examination

After initial airway clearance and fluid resuscitation, a more thorough examination may be carried out, particularly of the chest and abdomen. The chest wall is examined for movement, evidence of fractured ribs, bruising and penetrating injury. A chest X-ray should be taken and pneumothorax or haemothorax treated with tube thoracostomy to the affected side. The abdomen should be examined carefully and the patient 'log-rolled' to examine the back and flanks. Palpation may reveal abdominal distension and voluntary guarding in the conscious patient. Evidence of penetration, bruising and haematoma formation on the anterior abdominal wall and flanks is noted. The pelvis is compressed to assess pelvic stability and possible fracture and the external genitalia and rectum are examined for blood and a pelvic haematoma. Penetrating injuries require little in the way of diagnostic skills and all injuries between the nipple and costal margins should be suspected of entering the abdominal cavity. Blunt injury may require further diagnostic tests, if the patient is stable, to ascertain the extent and nature of the injuries; 20% of head-injured patients have associated abdominal trauma, so hypotension in this group of patients should arouse a high index of suspicion of unrevealed haemorrhage in the abdominal or thoracic cavities.

Diagnostic tests

Initial laboratory evaluation should include blood for typing and cross-matching, haematocrit, white blood cell count, electrolytes and urea, amylase, toxicology and arterial blood gases. Abdominal X-rays give little information apart from location of bullet fragments in gunshot wounds and bony injury to the spine and sacrum. Pelvic films document fractures of the pelvic ring. Urinalysis may reveal haematuria and an intravenous pyelogram should be performed when haematuria is present to assess excretion from both kidneys and ureters. This is also essential in any penetrating injury that may involve the urinary tract. A urinary catheter should be inserted, provided urethral injury is not suspected, to monitor urinary output and assess effectiveness of resuscitation.

Diagnostic peritoneal lavage

The most useful diagnostic procedure for suspected intra-abdominal visceral injury is diagnostic peritoneal lavage (Fischer et al., 1978). It is particularly useful in the assessment of blunt trauma but may also be beneficial in the assessment of penetrating abdominal trauma due to stab wound where local exploration suggests no violation of the peritoneal cavity. Diagnostic peritoneal lavage is contraindicated in certain circumstances when intra-abdominal injury is obvious and mandatory laparotomy is indicated. The 'open' technique involves the introduction of a peritoneal dialysis catheter under direct vision into the peritoneal cavity through a midline subumbilical incision after evacuation of the bladder. One litre of warm normal saline is infused into the peritoneal

Diagnostic peritoneal lavage

Indications

- Head injury or impaired level of consciousness when abdominal injury cannot be excluded
- Unexplained hypotension – particularly in association with head injuries
- Suspicion of abdominal trauma, e.g. bruising pattern, guarding, tenderness, no bowel sounds
- Wounds that penetrate the peritoneum (except gunshot wounds)
  - Suspect all anterior plus lateral abdominal wounds and anterior plus lateral chest wounds below the level of the nipple
  - Do not probe chest wounds in the A & E department

Contraindications – mandatory laparotomy required

- Abdominal gunshot wound
- Bomb blast to the abdomen
- Subphrenic air on chest radiograph
- Unable to resuscitate patient due to persistent hypotension, unstable patient, gross abdominal distension

Beware!

- Previous abdominal operations – adhesions prevent free passage of the cannula
- Patients with large pelvic fractures – the pelvic haematoma causes false positives

Complications

- Instillation of fluid into extraperitoneal tissues.
- Bowel perforation.
- Trauma to the iliac vessels.
- Bladder perforation.

Table 2. *Objective criteria for assessing diagnostic peritoneal lavage*

Positive criteria – laparotomy

- Lavage fluid appears in chest drain or bladder catheter
- Gross blood on entering abdominal cavity or in lavage fluid (>10 ml)
- RBC count $>100\,000\ \mu l^{-1}$ (in penetrating trauma: RBC count $>50\,000\ \mu l^{-1}$)
- WBC count $>500\ \mu l^{-1}$
- Amylase >175 U ml^{-1}
- Obvious faeces or bile

Equivocal criteria – reassess clinically/other diagnostic tests

- Dialysis catheter tube fills with blood
- RBC count $>50\,000$ but $<100\,000\ \mu l^{-1}$ (in penetrating trauma: RBC count $>25\,000$ but $<50\,000\ \mu l^{-1}$)
- WBC count >100 but $<500\ \mu l^{-1}$
- Amylase >75 but <175 U ml^{-1}

Negative criteria – observe

- RBC count $<50\,000\ \mu l^{-1}$ (in penetrating trauma: RBC count $<25\,000\ \mu l^{-1}$)
- WBC count $<100\ \mu l^{-1}$
- Amylase <75 U ml^{-1}

RBC, red blood cells: WBC, white blood cells.

cavity and allowed to 'equilibrate' for several minutes. The fluid is then allowed to run back into the infusion bag and a 50 ml sample is sent for analysis of red blood cell count, white blood cell count and amylase. The 'closed' technique uses the Seldinger principle and has no advantages but a higher incidence of complications (4.8% compared to 2.2% with the open technique).

TECHNIQUE

Principles of performing peritoneal lavage

Open technique

- Full aseptic technique.
- Catheterize urinary bladder.
- Insert nasogastric tube.
- Local anaesthetic with 0.5% lignocaine plus 1:100 000 adrenaline.
- Subumbilical midline incision; when pelvic fracture is present, supraumbilical incision should be used.
- Dissect down to peritoneum and insert cannula under direct vision and pointing towards pelvis.
- Infuse 1000 ml of warm saline (15 ml kg^{-1} in children); tilt patient to redistribute fluid; wait 10 min; position bag below level of patient and observe lavage fluid; send sample to laboratory for quantitative analysis (full blood 'picture', amylase).

A number of objective criteria are used to assess diagnostic peritoneal lavage and a positive result for any one value, or the aspiration of frank blood from the peritoneal cavity, requires mandatory exploratory laparotomy (Table 2). An equivocal result requires reassessment clinically, help from a more senior colleague, repeat lavage after 2–3 h or the use of other diagnostic tests, (e.g. ultrasound or CT (computed tomography) scan).

Following a negative result the patient should be admitted for observation and the test repeated or other investigations performed in the event of development of new physical signs or deterioration in the patient's general condition. The lavage catheter may be left in place pending repeat lavage.

Diagnostic peritoneal lavage has good sensitivity and specificity in both blunt and penetrating trauma (blunt: false negative 1.2%, false positive 0.2%; penetrating: false negative 3.8%, false positive 1.0%).

Other diagnostic tests

Other diagnostic modalities may give useful information which indicates whether surgical intervention is required or continued medical support and observations are more appropriate.

Plain abdominal radiographs

These are of limited use in blunt trauma. Free gas may be seen in some cases of bowel perforation and the retroperitoneal gas bubble associated with duodenal perforation is characteristic. Blurring of the psoas shadow suggests retroperitoneal blood or fluid. The plain radiograph should include the pelvis to exclude fracture. In penetrating injury due to gunshot wound, abdominal X-ray is useful in detecting bullets, bullet fragments and associated bony injury.

CT (computed tomography) scanning

This should be performed when abdominal injury is suspected in an unconscious patient undergoing CT evaluation of head injury and where diagnostic peritoneal lavage gives equivocal results. It has similar diagnostic accuracy to diagnostic peritoneal lavage, ultrasound and minilaparoscopy provided the films are interpreted immediately by an expert radiologist. Its drawbacks are that, to obtain good-quality films, it is operator-dependent, expensive and is not widely available, especially in developing countries. Injuries to solid viscera are easily seen whereas rupture of a hollow viscus is easily missed. Patients undergoing CT scan must be haemodynamically stable. It is particularly useful in evaluation of combined head and torso injury, retroperitoneal injuries (e.g. duodenum, pancreas and kidneys) and abdominal injury associated with pelvic fracture. Contrast-enhanced CT scan gives useful anatomical and functional information about several organs.

Ultrasound

This can detect free fluid and solid organ injury (especially liver, kidney and spleen) and associated haematomas. It may also be useful in detecting rupture of the hemidiaphragm.

Contrast studies of the gastrointestinal tract (see also Chapter 25)

These are rarely used but will delineate rupture of the oesophagus, duodenum and rectum. The *intravenous* urogram (*IVU*) and *cystogram* are the main methods of assessing the urinary tract. The possibility of urethral injury must be considered if blood is present at the urethral meatus and may be excluded by a normal urethrogram. *Cystography* should be performed by distending the bladder with up to 400 ml of water-soluble contrast. A *limited IVU* (films at 5 min and 20 min after injection of contrast) should be performed to look for normal renal function and extravasation of dye. The incidence of adverse dye reactions is low and the inability to obtain an allergic history should not delay the examination. Angiography is rarely used (probably underused) in the initial assessment of abdominal injuries but is essential for investigating previously documented abnormalities such as a non-functioning kidney on IVU in a haemodynamically stable patient.

Radionuclide scanning, endoscopy and minilaparoscopy

These techniques have little place in the assessment of abdominal injuries although advocates of the latter technique claim that its use lowers the rate of exploratory laparotomy with negative findings, because stable bleeding injuries can be identified directly and conservative management instituted.

Assessment of severity of injury

The final phase of patient evaluation, which should be carried out during initial resuscitation and evaluation, is an estimate of the severity of injury using one of the trauma scoring systems which readily identify the patient who has fatal injuries, those at the greatest risk of dying or developing complications and those most likely to make an uneventful and full recovery (Champion et al., 1983). The Glasgow Coma Scale (Teasdale & Jennett, 1974) gives an assessment of the level of consciousness, motor and verbal response and, when combined with the systolic blood pressure and respiratory rate, can be used to generate the Revised Trauma Score. These simple observations, together with consideration of mechanism of injury, environmental factors and the anatomical features of the injury, readily identify the most seriously injured and provide guidelines for triage and management priorities. Other scoring systems such as the Injury Severity Score (Baker et al., 1974) and the Penetrating Abdominal Trauma Index (Moore et al., 1981) require full assessment of the anatomical disruption or physiological derangements (APACHE II; Knaus et al., 1985) caused by injury and are, therefore, not useful in the initial assessment. They do, however, correlate well with survival and development of complications and so are useful in audit of trauma management (Rowlands & Blair, 1992).

SURGICAL INTERVENTION IN ABDOMINAL INJURY

The principles of management should be to stop haemorrhage, debride devitalized tissue, repair wounds to the bowel by suture or resection and eliminate all foreign bodies, haematoma and intestinal contents to reduce postoperative infective complications. The management of injuries to individual organs is considered briefly below, but the surgeon should quickly identify the full extent of intra-abdominal injury and plan his operative strategy so that injuries are dealt with in an orderly fashion, with speed and safety.

Blunt trauma

About 20% of patients with blunt trauma have sufficient physical signs – continuing hypovolaemia despite adequate resuscitation and progressive abdominal distension – to warrant immediate laparotomy. In stable patients following initial resuscitation, the results of peritoneal lavage, together with the results of X-ray and other invasive investigations, should guide surgical intervention. A chest X-ray that indicates free peritoneal air and diaphragmatic rupture, intravenous urogram that shows intraperitoneal bladder rupture or major kidney injury, or arteriogram indicating major vessel damage should lead to urgent surgical exploration. Soft tissue injury to the anterior abdominal wall or flank indicates sufficient force to cause visceral injury. A negative peritoneal lavage or a decision to pursue nonoperative therapy should be followed by frequent re-examination and further investigation when clinically indicated.

Stab wound

In penetrating trauma due to stab wounds, immediate laparotomy is indicated for evisceration, unexplained blood loss and signs of peritonitis – absent bowel sounds, diffuse tenderness and guarding. If the patient is stable, local exploration of the wound can be used to determine if the peritoneal cavity has been entered. Superficial wounds require no further treatment, but if peritoneal penetration is confirmed the patient should undergo laparotomy or diagnostic peritoneal lavage to confirm the need for laparotomy, depending on the experience of the physician supervising management. A policy of exploration of all stab wounds that penetrate the peritoneal cavity is recommended for surgeons with little experience of these injuries. Less than half the patients will have significant intraperitoneal injuries but negative laparotomy has a low morbidity. A selective policy based on peritoneal lavage will save a significant number of unnecessary laparotomies and will miss fewer than 5% of important injuries, but this policy is best practised by units with a large experience of penetrating abdominal trauma.

Gunshot wound

Following gunshot wound, irrespective of bullet velocity, exploration of the abdomen is mandatory as visceral injury is present in the majority of cases in which the peritoneal cavity is violated. Penetrating wounds between the nipple and costal margin should all be treated with placement of tube thoracostomy on the affected side followed by laparotomy because injuries to the upper abdominal viscera are common and the diaphragmatic laceration must be repaired. Entrance or exit wounds involving the buttocks, perineum, groins, genitalia or upper thigh should all be suspected of associated intra-abdominal injuries unless definite evidence is obtained that the peritoneal cavity and pelvic viscera have not been violated. Again, it should be remembered that negative laparotomy has a low morbidity and mortality.

Infection

Sepsis is a major cause of morbidity and mortality following blunt and penetrating abdominal trauma. Therefore broad-spectrum prophylactic antibiotics against enteric microorganisms (both aerobic and anaerobic) should be given to these patients as soon as possible after injury and prior to surgical exploration (Rowlands & Ericsson, 1984; Rowlands et al., 1987). A combination of metronidazole plus an aminoglycoside or a second/third generation cephalosporin gives an adequate spectrum of antimicrobial cover and the duration of therapy should be decided on the basis of intraoperative findings.

All injuries should be regarded as 'low' risk for infective complications unless there is:

- Bowel perforation.
- Major injury to solid viscera (especially liver and pancreas).

- Incomplete haemostasis at operation.
- Residual tissue of doubtful viability.
- Repair of major splenic injury.
- Close-range gunshot wound.
- High-velocity wound.
- Preoperative haemodynamic instability.
- Foreign body contamination.
- Blast injuries.

'Risk' is fully assessed at operation. 'Low'-risk cases should receive antibiotic cover for 12 h (one preoperative and two postoperative doses) and 'high'-risk cases receive cover for 72 h postoperatively. At that time, if the 'high'-risk patient is apyrexial and making good progress antibiotic therapy should be discontinued. If, however, ongoing sepsis is suspected, therapy should be reviewed and changed if appropriate.

Management of injuries to individual intra-abdominal organs

Diaphragm

Injuries to the diaphragm are more common following penetrating trauma than blunt trauma and should be repaired at initial laparotomy to avoid the late complication of diaphragmatic hernia, which is more common if injuries of the left hemidiaphragm are missed. The undersurface of the diaphragm should be carefully palpated and inspected by inferior retraction of the stomach, liver and spleen. Lacerations should be repaired with interrupted, non-absorbable, mattress sutures. Large diaphragmatic defects due to blast injuries require the use of Marlex mesh to bridge them. Following repair, abdominal drainage is not required and tube thoracostomy of the affected side should be performed to drain intrathoracic fluid and to obtain full re-expansion of the lung.

Stomach

The stomach is rarely injured in blunt trauma but injury is common in penetrating trauma of the upper abdomen between the xiphisternum and umbilicus that punctures the rectus muscle. The anterior and posterior walls of the stomach should be carefully inspected by taking down the greater curvature to gain access to the lesser sac. Injuries may be missed in the least accessible parts of the stomach – the fundus, gastro-oesophageal junction posteriorly and intra-abdominal oesophagus. Entrance and exit wounds must be identified. The stomach has an excellent blood supply and most simple lacerations or penetrating wounds can be closed primarily in two layers following debridement of contaminated or devitalized tissue. The stomach contents should be emptied and decompressed postoperatively with a nasogastric tube. More severe trauma may require resection of the stomach wall, body or antrum. Re-establishment of continuity of the bowel will depend on the site and extent of injury, but injuries to the antrum and pyloric region are best managed by closure of the duodenal stump distal to the pylorus, and gastroenterostomy away from the visceral injury.

Duodenum

Duodenal injuries, although uncommon, are associated with a high morbidity and mortality which usually relates to delay in diagnosis and management after blunt trauma. Factors associated with an increase in complications include a delay in definitive operative management of greater than 24 h, defects larger than 75% of the circumference, injuries to the first and second parts of the duodenum, and associated pancreatic, major vessel (portal vein, inferior vena cava) or bile duct injury (Synder et al., 1980). The duodenum must be carefully inspected by incision of the lateral peritoneum and mobilization together with the head of the pancreas (Kocher's manoeuvre). Simple lacerations may be sutured in two layers. More extensive injuries may be managed using a variety of techniques including closure of the injury with tube duodenostomy, decompression through a separate incision proximal to the injury, omental or serosal patch, gastroenterostomy and/or duodenal 'diverticulization' (Stone & Fabian, 1979; Berne et al., 1974). The most common complications are duodenal fistula, dehiscence of the repair and intra-abdominal sepsis which have a high mortality; postoperative drainage of the right subhepatic region and right paracolic gutter is therefore advocated. Injuries to the duodenum may tax the most experienced surgeons and operative management should never be left to surgical trainees.

Small bowel

The small bowel should be inspected at laparotomy from the ligament of Treitz to the ileocaecal valve. Injuries may consist of single or multiple perforations, lacerations of the bowel and mesentery, haematoma formation, maceration of the bowel or ischaemia due to crush, blast or vascular injury. Simple injuries are closed in two layers making sure that all entrance and exit wounds are identified. Multiple perforations or lacerations to the bowel and mesentery are best treated with resection and primary anastomosis. Non-viable bowel must be excised. If there is massive intraperitoneal contamination with bowel contents or multiple associated injuries, it may be safer to defunction the bowel by constructing an ileostomy and mucous fistula than risk subsequent dehiscence of an anastomosis performed in unfavourable circumstances. Mesenteric haematomas are sometimes associated with perforation of the mesenteric border of the bowel. Small bowel injuries due to blunt trauma have a greater morbidity and mortality than penetrating trauma due to the complications of associated injuries (Donohue *et al.*, 1985).

Colon

Injuries to the colon are usually due to penetrating trauma and are associated with a mortality of approximately 10%. The incidence of complications and death is related to the presence of shock, the amount of intraperitoneal contamination with bowel contents, the number and type of associated injuries and the age of the patient (Burch *et al.*, 1986). Controversy exists concerning the initial management of these injuries between primary closure of the colonic wound, defunctioning colostomy and exteriorization of the repair. Most civilian injuries of the colon are due to knife wounds or low-velocity bullets, and many of these injuries can be treated with primary repair provided there is little or no faecal contamination, hypotension or major associated injuries. Centres with a large experience of penetrating trauma now advocate primary repair as the mainstay of treatment for colonic injury, indicating that mortality is not related to type of repair and that colostomy requires a subsequent operation which may also give rise to complications (Burch *et al.*, 1986). Where experience is less, a different approach is advocated; several contraindications to primary closure of colonic wounds have been identified and include delay between injury and operation, extensive peritonitis or contamination, high-velocity missile wounds, blast injuries, blunt trauma producing massive body trauma, and associated pancreatic and duodenal injuries (Parks, 1981). If resection of the right colon is necessary, primary anastomosis may be effected between the ileum and transverse colon, but injuries to the distal transverse, descending and sigmoid colon requiring resection of the injury should probably be managed by construction of

a colostomy and mucous fistula, with bowel continuity being restored when the patient has recovered. Exteriorization of a colonic repair appears to have few advocates at present and is associated with similar morbidity to colostomy and subsequent reanastomosis. The repair may break down if the exteriorized segment is not managed meticulously to avoid further tissue damage.

Rectum

All injuries of the rectum must be treated with diversion of the faecal stream, repair of the injury, drainage of the presacral space and irrigation of the distal segment of the bowel to remove all faecal material. These injuries are associated with a high incidence of septic complications. An end colostomy should be constructed in the left iliac fossa and a mucous fistula brought separately on to the abdominal wall to achieve complete diversion. The rectum is repaired with interrupted sutures. Presacral Penrose drains are placed via an incision posterior to the anus and by further blunt dissection between the rectum and coccyx through the levator ani. The continuity of the bowel should be restored several months after the injury when all sepsis is resolved and after radiological and functional assessment of the rectum and anal sphincters.

Spleen

The spleen is the most common solid organ to be injured in blunt trauma. It has important immunological and reticuloendothelial functions and, therefore, if damage is only minor, efforts should be made to preserve the spleen in children, adolescents and young adults. The extent of injury can only be judged by mobilization of the spleen to the midline and elevation into the wound by division of the lateral peritoneal reflection and gentle blunt dissection away from the posterior abdominal wall. The surfaces can easily be inspected following mobilization, and haemostasis obtained by occluding the splenic pedicle. Superficial capsular and parenchymal lacerations may be controlled with pressure, electrocautery or suture. Deeper laceration may be treated with partial or hemisplenectomy. When parenchymal injury is more severe or haemorrhage is not easily and quickly controlled, and if there is haemodynamic instability or other associated major injury, splenectomy is the favoured treatment. Care should be taken to ligate the splenic artery and vein separately, and damage to the tail of the pancreas or avulsion of the short splenic vessels to the greater curvature of the stomach should be avoided during removal of the spleen. Following splenectomy, patients should be treated with antibiotics during convalescence and should be given polyvalent pneumococcal vaccine and haemophilus influenza vaccine prior to discharge. Splenorrhaphy is possible in about half the patients undergoing laparotomy for splenic trauma, and splenic reimplantation may be a viable method of control of immediate haemorrhage without the long-term sequelae of postsplenectomy sepsis (Moore *et al.*, 1984). Non-operative management of splenic trauma should only be pursued if there is absolute haemodynamic stability, minimal abdominal physical indication, negative peritoneal lavage, and a blood transfusion requirement of less than 2 units (Mucha *et al.*, 1986). However, laparotomy and splenorrhaphy or splenectomy can be carried out with minimal morbidity and may return the patient to full activity sooner.

Liver

The liver is the most commonly injured organ following civilian trauma, and presents a spectrum of injury ranging from simple capsular avulsion or tear which requires little operative management to retrohepatic caval injury associated with bilobular parenchymal disruption which is often rapidly fatal. The basic principles in the management of hepatic trauma are the control of haemorrhage, removal of devitalized tissue and perihepatic drainage (Moore, 1984). Laparotomy should be performed through a generous midline incision and, if haemoperitoneum is present and liver injury suspected, the right upper quadrant should be rapidly evacuated of blood and packed while the rest of the abdominal contents are assessed for life-threatening injury. Haemostasis may be aided by use of the Pringle manoeuvre to occlude the vessels in the porta hepatis, and hypotension may respond to aortic occlusion at the hiatus. The majority of injuries can be controlled with suture of the liver capsule, individual ligation of vessels and biliary radicals following exploration of lacerations extending into the liver parenchyma, or ligation of a branch of either the portal vein or hepatic artery supplying a segment of injured liver tissue. In less than 5% of cases will a more major procedure such as resection of a segment or hepatic lobectomy be required. Injuries to the vena cava and hepatic veins are unusual and have a high mortality. These procedures should not be undertaken by inexperienced surgeons. Temporary packing of the liver injury and immediate transfer to a surgeon with experience of hepatic surgery is advocated. Access to the liver may be improved by extending the abdominal incision into the right chest through the right costal margin and diaphragm. Devitalized and macerated liver parenchyma should be removed. Minimal liver injuries should not require postoperative drainage, but if there is significant parenchymal destruction or resection is carried out leaving a raw parenchymal surface then closed suction drainage should be used postoperatively for approximately 48 h. Mortality from hepatic injury is about 10% and the most common cause of death is shock and transfusion coagulopathy in the perioperative period (Feliciano *et al.*, 1986). Sepsis due to intra-abdominal abscess is the most common late complication.

Pancreas

Pancreatic injury has a high associated morbidity. It may be particularly difficult to manage when penetrating injuries cause associated injury to major vessels (vena cava, portal vein, superior mesenteric vessels), the extra-hepatic biliary system, and the duodenum. Important determinants of the outcome are the magnitude of associated injuries and the presence or absence of injury to the pancreatic duct or duodenum (Jones, 1985). Injuries to the parenchyma of the pancreas should be assessed by opening the lesser sac and reflecting the hepatic flexure of the colon inferiorly to expose the head, body and tail of the pancreas. Injuries to the left of the mesenteric vessels (distal pancreas) should be treated by drainage of the lesser sac using sump or closed suction drains provided there is no associated ductal injury. Severe injuries to the body and tail as well as ductal injuries may be managed by distal pancreatectomy in a stable patient. Injuries to the head of the pancreas that do not involve the duct, or adjacent vessels, ducts or organs may also be managed by appropriate surgical drainage. More complex injuries need an individualized approach by an experienced surgeon to assess the possibility of repair of the injury, and the use of techniques to limit complications due to anastomotic breakdown or leakage in the postoperative period (Feliciano *et al.*, 1987). Major complications in patients who survive more than 48 h are intra-abdominal sepsis, and pancreatic and duodenal fistula. Rarely is pancreaticoduodenal resection necessary, the indications being proximal pancreatic duct, ampullary or distal bile duct injuries that preclude reconstruction and combined devascularizing injuries to the pancreas and duodenum (Oreskovich & Carrico, 1984).

Kidney and bladder

Haematuria should be investigated with an IVU to exclude renal trauma or bladder rupture. If either kidney is not visualized, elective angiography should be carried out to assess the renal vessels and their function. The kidneys should be approached through a standard laparotomy with reflection of the right or left colon, but access to the aorta for control of renal vessels can be obtained through the base of the transverse mesocolon provided there is no extensive retroperitoneal haematoma. Renal salvage is possible in the majority of blunt and penetrating injuries. Injuries to the renal pedicle carry the greatest morbidity (Sagalowski et al., 1983). Renal and ureteral injuries should usually be drained following repair. Intraperitoneal bladder ruptures can be treated with formal closure of the bladder wound and either suprapubic or urethral drainage with little or no mobidity, whereas extraperitoneal rupture may be treated effectively with bladder drainage alone (Corriere & Sandler, 1986).

Vascular injuries (see also Chapter 46)

Major haemorrhage from intra-abdominal arteries and veins is the main cause of immediate death following blunt and penetrating injury. The principles of management are as for elective vascular surgery in that proximal and distal control of the vessel is required on either side of the injury. The abdominal aorta and its branches should be approached by medial mobilization of the viscera and not by dissection through a retroperitoneal haematoma. Initial control of the aorta may be achieved by a transthoracic approach to the descending thoracic aorta or by encircling the abdominal aorta as it passes through the hiatus. Penetrating injury may cause entrance and exit wounds in major vessels or tangential injury. With arterial injury, when control is obtained, the vessel should be debrided to remove damaged intima and repaired by primary suture, venous patch, venous on-lay graft or the use of autogenous artery (Holcroft, 1982). Venous injuries may, in general, be treated by suture repair or ligation of the vessel; exceptions are injuries to the superior mesenteric vein and suprarenal vena cava. Penetrating injuries of the infrarenal vena cava should be treated by repair of both the posterior and anterior wall, the former being accomplished by suture inside the vessel. Attempts to mobilize or encircle the vena cava may cause damage to major lumbar veins resulting in further haemorrhage which is difficult to control. Control of inferior venacaval haemorrhage may be achieved with direct pressure on the vein above and below the injury. The use of Dacron grafts to replace arteries or veins should be avoided in the presence of significant contamination.

Pelvic fractures

Massive blunt trauma may cause unstable pelvic fractures with a large loss of blood into the pelvis and retroperitoneal tissues. Because the force involved in producing a pelvic fracture is considerable, abdominal and pelvic organs may be injured by blunt trauma or from penetration by pieces of pelvic bone. Resuscitation with large volumes of fluid and blood may be necessary. Angiography may be indicated if haemodynamic instability persists despite resuscitation. Embolization and external fixation to reduce the fracture may be necessary to achieve adequate resuscitation. The rectum, urethra and bladder are particularly susceptible to injury and should be carefully assessed. Injury to major vessels may require operative repair.

SUMMARY

Blunt and penetrating abdominal injury may affect several intra-abdominal organs and are often associated with injuries to other regions of the body. Prompt resuscitation and definitive treatment of all injuries provide the best chance of successful and complete recovery and of avoiding the complications of sepsis and multiple organ dysfunction syndrome.

Bibliography

BAKER, S. P., O'NEILL, B., HADDON, W. et al. (1974). The injury severity score: a method of describing patients with multiple injuries and evaluating emergency care. J. Trauma, 14, 187–96.

BARACH, E., TOMLANOVICH, M. & NOWAK, R. (1986a). Ballistics: a pathophysiologic examination of the wounding mechanisms of firearms. Part I. J. Trauma, 26, 225–35.

BARACH, E., TOMLANOVICH, M. & NOWAK, R. (1986b). Ballistics: a pathophysiologic examination of the wounding mechanisms of firearms. Part II. J. Trauma, 26, 374–83.

BERNE, C. J., DONOVAN, A. J., WHITE, E. J. et al. (1974). Duodenal 'diverticulization' for duodenal pancreatic injury. Am. J. Surg., 127, 503–7.

BURCH, J. M., BROCK, J. C., GEVIRTZMAN, L. et al. (1986). The injured colon. Ann. Surg., 203, 701–11.

CHAMPION, H. R., SACCO, W. J. & HUNT, T. K. (1983). Trauma severity scoring to predict mortality. *World J. Surg.*, **7**, 4–11.

CORRIERE, J. N., & SANDLER, C. M. (1986). Management of ruptured bladder; seven years of experience with 111 cases. *J. Trauma*, **26**, 830–3.

DONOHUE, J. H., CRASS, R. A. & TRUNKEY, D. D. (1985). The management of duodenal and other small intestinal trauma. *World J. Surg.*, **9**, 904–13.

FELICIANO, D. V., MATTOX, K. L., & JORDAN, G. L. *et al.* (1986). Management of 1000 consecutive cases of hepatic trauma (1979–1984). *Ann. Surg.*, **204**, 438–45.

FELICIANO, D. V., MARTIN, T. D., CRUSE, P. A. *et al.* (1987). Management of combined pancreatico-duodenal injuries. *Ann. Surg.*, **205**, 673–9.

FISCHER, R. P., BEVERLIN, B. C., ENGRAV, L. H. *et al.* (1978). Diagnostic peritoneal lavage, fourteen years and 2,586 patients later. *Am. J. Surg.*, **136**, 701–4.

HOLCROFT, J. W. (1982). Abdominal arterial trauma. In *Trauma Management*, Vol. I, *Abdominal Trauma*, ed. W. Blaisdell & D. Trunkey. pp. 226–51. New York: Thieme Stratton.

JONES, R. C. (1985). Management of pancreatic trauma. *Am. J. Surg.*, **150**, 698–704.

KNAUS, W. A., DRAPER, E. A., WAGNER, D. P. *et al.* (1985). APACHE II: a severity of disease classification system. *Crit. Care Med.*, **13**, 818–29.

MOORE, E. E. (1984). Critical decisions in the management of hepatic trauma. *Am. J. Surg.*, **148**, 712–16.

MOORE, E. E., DUNN, E. L. & MOORE, J. B. (1981). Penetrating abdominal trauma index. *J. Trauma*, **21**, 439–45.

MOORE, F. A., MOORE, E. E., MOORE, G. E. *et al.* (1984). Risk of splenic salvage after trauma, analysis of 200 adults. *Am. J. Surg.*, **148**, 800–5.

MUCHA, P., DALY, R. C. & FARNELL, M. B. (1986). Selective management of blunt splenic trauma. *J. Trauma*, **26**, 970–9.

ORESKOVICH, M. R. & CARRICO, C. J. (1984). Pancreatico duodenectomy for trauma, a viable option. *Am. J. Surg.*, **147**, 618–23.

PARKS, T. G. (1981). Surgical management of injuries to the large intestine. *Br. J. Surg.*, **68**, 725–8.

ROWLANDS, B. J. (1988). Management of major trauma. In *Recent Advances in Surgery*, vol. 13, ed. R. C. G. Russell, pp. 1–17. London: Churchill Livingstone.

ROWLANDS, B. J. & BLAIR, P. H. B. (1992). Infection scoring systems. In *Infection in Surgical Practice*, ed E. W. Taylor. pp. 101–8. Oxford: Oxford University Press.

ROWLANDS, B. J. & ERICCSON, C. D. (1984). Comparative studies of antibiotic therapy following penetrating abdominal trauma. *Am. J. Surg.*, **148**, 791–5.

ROWLANDS, B. J., ERICSSON, C. D. & FISCHER, R. P. (1987). Penetrating abdominal trauma: the use of operative findings to determine length of antibiotic therapy. *J. Trauma*, **27**, 250–5.

SAGALOWSKI, A. I., McCONNELL, J. D. & PETERS, P. C. (1983). Renal trauma requiring surgery, an analysis of 185 cases. *J. Trauma*, **23**, 128–31.

SNYDER, W. H., WEIGELT, J. A., WATKINS, W. L. *et al.* (1980). The surgical management of duodenal trauma, precepts based on a review of 247 cases. *Arch. Surg.*, **115**, 422–9.

STONE, H. H. & FABIAN, T. C. (1979). Management of duodenal wounds. *J. Trauma*, **19**, 334–9.

TEASDALE, G. JENNETT, B. (1974). Assessment of coma and impaired consciousness. *Lancet* **ii**, 81–4.

YATES, D. W. (1984). Emergencies and catastrophies. In *Surgical Management*, ed. S. Taylor, G. D. Chrisholm, N. O'Higgins *et al.* pp. 707–39. London: Heinemann.

25 Urological trauma

R.S. KIRBY and S.A.V. HOLMES

Department of Urology, St Bartholomew's Hospital, London, UK

Chapter plan

Introduction
Pathophysiology and classification of urological injuries
Diagnosis and investigations
Management in the A&E department
Criteria for consultation with a urologist and/or transfer
  to a specialist urological service
Summary

INTRODUCTION

By virtue of its retroperitoneal and pelvic location, the urinary tract is mainly protected from injury in minor trauma. However, in more major blunt and especially penetrating injuries of the chest, abdomen or pelvis the urinary tract may become involved. Because the urinary tract is highly vascularized, the kidneys in particular receiving 20% of cardiac output (1200 ml min^{-1}), and the body is constantly producing urine, damage to the urinary tract carries the danger not only of considerable haemorrhage but also of extensive urinary extravasation. This can in turn lead to intense tissue inflammation and subsequent wound infection. The key to the correct management of urological injuries therefore lies in the early and accurate recognition of the nature and extent of trauma and urgent institution of the appropriate corrective management. Coexisting injuries to other systems must also be promptly recognized and the correct intervention employed.

PATHOPHYSIOLOGY AND CLASSIFICATION OF UROLOGICAL INJURIES

Trauma to the urinary tract may be conveniently divided into blunt and penetrating injuries. It is also appropriate to divide them according to the structures damaged as follows:

- Renal injuries.
- Ureteric injuries.
- Bladder trauma.
- Urethral trauma.
- Injury to the external genitalia.

Each of these will be considered in turn.

Renal trauma

Prompt recognition and accurate characterization of renal injuries are necessary to obtain maximal renal salvage and minimize morbidity. Delayed or misdiagnosis of renal injury may exacerbate the original trauma.

The kidneys are located high in the retroperitoneum and are protected posteriorly by the large psoas and quadratus lumborum muscles and anteriorly by the peritoneum and abdominal viscera. In addition, the kidneys are surrounded by cushioning perinephric fat inside Gerota's fascia. The lower ribcage (ribs 10–12) provides an outer defence to the kidney but it must be remembered that, in terms of surface anatomy, one must consider the kidneys as potentially susceptible to intrathoracic injuries as well as to retroperitoneal trauma. Traditionally, discussions of renal trauma have dealt separately with blunt and penetrating injuries but the distinction between these causes is more important in terms of the associated injuries than in terms of the different degrees of renal damage itself. For example, penetrating wounds more commonly involve intrathoracic or intraperitoneal structures. With modern diagnostic modalities the extent of renal injury can be estimated quite accurately and this is an important factor in determining the appropriate therapy (Federle *et al.*, 1987).

Penetrating renal trauma is usually the result of an assault and is most frequently due to either stab wounds or gunshot injuries. The trauma clinician must be aware that penetrating renal trauma will almost certainly be accompanied by intra-abdominal and/or intrathoracic injury, involving the liver, small bowel, stomach and colon. Combined renal and ureteric injuries in such cases are not uncommon.

The most difficult problems to deal with are gunshot wounds to the kidney from high-velocity missiles (greater than 1100 ft sec^{-1}). The majority of the tissue damage is caused by the *cavitation* effects of the missile. This widespread damage can cause bleeding and fistula formation in areas that may appear viable at the time of injury. If a kidney is directly involved, the entire organ tends to be disrupted to produce a 'shattered kidney', which is usually irreparable.

Blunt renal trauma is often associated with sudden deceleration of the body. Motor vehicle accidents of all types and in particular injuries from seat belts, falls from a considerable height, or blunt physical contact are the most common causes of this type of renal injury. Rib or upper lumbar vertebral transverse process fractures may lacerate or contuse the renal parenchyma. Deceleration or crush injuries may thrust the kidneys internally against the ribcage or vertebra, or externally against the steering wheel or dashboard of the vehicle, resulting in contusion, laceration or avulsion of renal parenchyma. A direct blow to the abdomen or flank is possibly the most common cause of blunt renal injury. Renal arterial intimal tear with subsequent thrombosis and disruption of the ureteropelvic junction are two renal injuries particularly associated with deceleration (Cass, 1989). Children are more prone to the latter injury owing to the greater mobility of the longitudinal spinal ligaments which permit hyperextension injuries in the young. Pre-existing renal abnormalities such as hydronephrosis, renal tumour, vascular malformation or cystic/polycystic disease may also make the kidney more susceptible to injury. One should always suspect such predisposing factors when the renal injury appears disproportionate to the trauma induced.

Renal injuries may be classified as minor or major. The most commonly employed nomenclature separates renal trauma into three subdivisions:

1. Minor parenchymal laceration or contusion.
2. Major parenchymal laceration usually through the corticomedullary junction and often involving the collecting system.

3. Shattered kidney or renal pedicle injury.

In general, about 70% of renal injuries are minor, 10–15% are major and the remainder are shattered kidneys or renal pedicle injuries that may be irreparable (McAninch *et al.*, 1991).

In fact, the greatest determinant of mortality in patients with renal trauma is usually the nature and extent of associated non-renal injuries. Renal pedicle injury has a high association with other non-renal events such as major thoracic trauma.

Ureteric injury

A simple classification of ureteric injury which also helps determine the optimum form of management is as follows:

- *Site*: upper, middle or lower third of ureter.
- *Time of recognition*: immediate or delayed.
- *Nature of the injury*: blunt trauma with laceration or avulsion, penetrating trauma from knife wounds or low- or high-velocity missiles.
- *The presence of concomitant injuries.*

Ureteric injuries secondary to trauma are often associated with knife or bullet wounds. Although rare, they are the most common ureteric injuries seen in the emergency unit. Late presentation of iatrogenic injury is occasionally seen; for example, ureteric avulsion may occur during endoscopic stone extraction. However, probably the most common form of iatrogenic injury to the ureter occurs at the time of abdominal hysterectomy (Daly & Higgins, 1988), caesarean section or colonic or ovarian surgery for extensive pelvic malignancy.

Bladder injuries

Owing to its location deep within the pelvis where it is protected by bony structures laterally, the urogenital diaphragm inferiorly, and the rectum posteriorly, the bladder is infrequently injured. Its shape varies with the amount of urine contained and the type of injury that may occur depends on the volume of the bladder at the time of injury. Bladder injuries secondary to blunt trauma may be classified as:

- Contusion.
- Extraperitoneal rupture.
- Intraperitoneal rupture.

Penetrating injuries may also involve the bladder, especially when it is full (Fig. 1). Bladder contusions

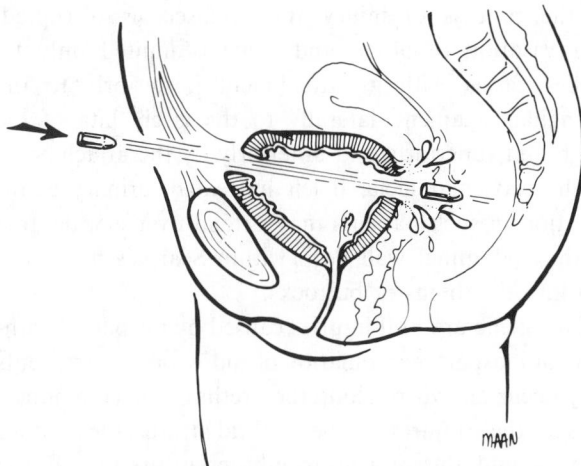

Fig. 1. Example of penetrating injury to the bladder.

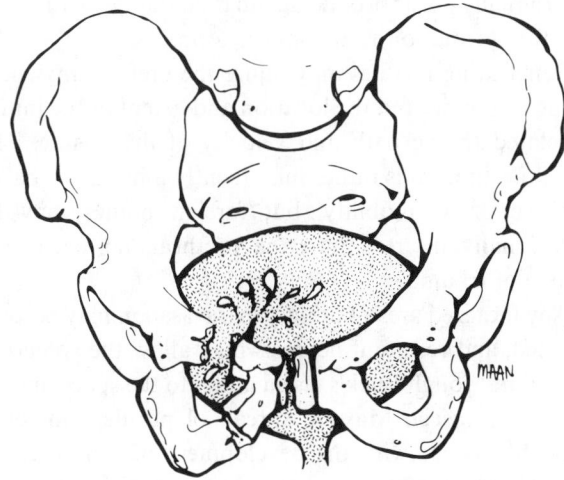

Fig. 2. Extraperitoneal rupture of the bladder by a fragment of fractured pelvis.

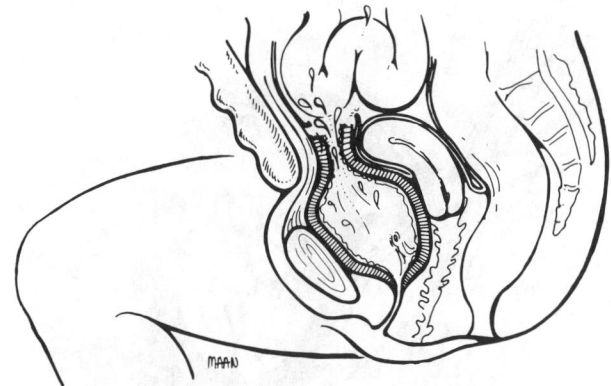

Fig. 3. Intraperitoneal rupture of the bladder following blunt trauma to the lower abdomen.

secondary to blunt or penetrating trauma may be associated with gross haematuria carrying a risk of clot retention but this does not usually require surgical intervention. By contrast, extraperitoneal rupture of the bladder occurs secondary to penetration of the bladder wall by a bone fragment when the pelvis is fractured (Fig. 2). In such circumstances there is considerable extravasation into the perivesical space and open surgical repair is usually necessary (Robards *et al.*, 1976).

Intraperitoneal rupture of the urinary bladder may have a different cause. This injury usually occurs in a patient who sustains a blow to the lower abdomen whilst the bladder is distended with urine. The force of the blow is therefore transmitted equally to all surfaces of the bladder wall which will usually rupture at its weakest point, generally the dome (Fig. 3). The bladder contents are then lost into the peritoneal cavity and free intraperitoneal flow of urine continues and may present as ascites if unrecognized. It must be borne in mind that in children the bladder is more intra-abdominally than intrapelvically located and such trauma in young patients is more likely to result in intraperitoneal rather than extraperitoneal leakage.

Urethral injuries

Rupture to the urethra is much more common in men than women and is an unusual but serious injury. In the male, the urethra is divided into four portions (Carroll & Dixon, 1992):

1. Prostatic urethra.
2. Membranous urethra.
3. Bulbous urethra.
4. Penile or penulous urethra.

Most urethral injuries occur as a result of blunt forces in motor vehicle accidents or crush injuries. Penetrating injuries such as gunshot wounds and stab wounds are rarely a cause of urethral damage. Iatrogenic factors from urethral instrumentation may cause urethral trauma and very rarely there may be spontaneous urethral rupture associated with urethral stricture; either of these may result in urinary extravasation and periurethral abscess formation.

In considering the classification of urethral injuries, it is convenient to group them into those occurring above the urogenital diaphragm and those occurring below it. Urethral rupture superior to the urogenital diaphragm is most commonly the result of a violent external force. The prostate may be separated from its attachments to the urogenital diaphragm and the puboprostatic

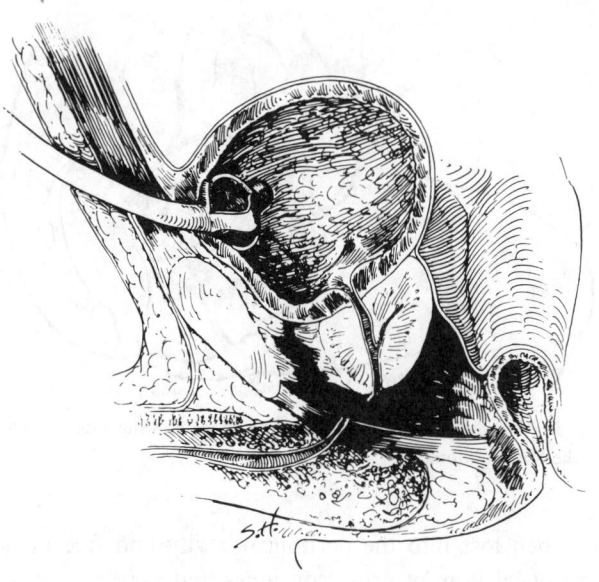

Fig. 4. Position of urethral rupture following pelvic fracture.

ligaments may or may not be ruptured. The urethra is consequently torn at the level of the pelvic diaphragm and this injury is almost invariably associated with a fracture of the pelvis. Tears of the urethra superior to the urogenital diaphragm may be either complete or incomplete. In the patient with complete disruption of the urethra above the urogenital diaphragm, the bladder and prostate may ascend above the normal anatomical position and the defect will fill with haematoma and urine (Fig. 4). If the tear is incomplete and the puboprostatic ligaments are only partially severed, there may be only a minimal degree of prostatic and bladder displacement. The distinction between a complete and an incomplete tear is important and its significance in the management of this injury will be discussed later. At the time of injury the bladder neck frequently remains competent and thus urinary extravasation may be minimal (Turner-Warwick, 1989). In such circumstances the bladder itself may be palpable or visualized by means of ultrasonography.

Urethral injuries inferior to the urogenital diaphragm usually result from a straddle-type injury or other direct blow to the perineum along the path of the urethra. This may produce complete or partial severance of the urethra as well as extensive extravasation of blood and urine which is usually confined to the fascial plane of the perineum (McAninch, 1981). If the superficial fascia remains intact, extravasation of blood and urine will be limited to the space between the tunica albuginea and the corpus spongiosum, essentially a sleeve of the penis, and discoloration is confined to the penis. If, however,

in the process of injury Buck's fascia is disrupted, extravasation of blood and urine is limited only by Colles' fascia with its attachment posteriorly to the triangular ligament, laterally to the fascia lata of the thigh and superiorly and anteriorly by the attachments of the clavicular facia. If left untreated, urinary extravasation in such patients may extend over a wide area of the abdominal wall deep within Scarpa's fascia but not into the thighs or buttocks.

Iatrogenic urethral injuries caused by misplaced catheters or inexpert manipulation of endoscopic instruments may occur anywhere along the urethra. The commonest sites for these injures are the urethral meatus, the bulbous urethra and the prostatomembranous urethra. If too large an instrument is forced through the urethra, ischaemic necrosis at the meatus or bulbar region may occasionally occur producing inflammation, scarring and stricture formation in the longer term.

Penetrating missiles may injure the urethra anywhere along its course and the location and extent of the injury is related to the path and velocity of the missile. The penulous urethra is rather infrequently injured, probably because of its mobility, but foreign bodies may be occasionally inserted into the urethra and become a source of trauma.

Any localized area of urinary extravasation may become infected, and resultant necrosis may allow the spread of infection through Buck's fascia and into the space limited by Colles' fascia. Massive spread of purulent material may then occur with the development of a necrotizing fasciitis, which when involving the scrotum is known as Fournier's gangrene and is a surgical emergency.

Injury to the external genitalia

Injury to the penis and scrotum occur from penetrating missiles such as gunshot wounds, land mine explosions or stab injuries, or from blunt trauma. Burn injuries may involve the penis, the scrotum and its contents. The main structures that form the penis are the two corpora cavernosa and the corpus spongiosum with the enclosed urethra. The corpora cavernosa are thick bodies of vascular erectile tissue surrounded by the sturdy tunica albuginea. Trauma involving the penis may affect one or all of its structural components. Strangulation of the penis with ischaemia and distal necrosis may be caused by various constricting devices. In addition, blunt injury to the erect penis may occur during intercourse and result in corporal (Pryor et al., 1981) and, very occasionally, urethral rupture.

DIAGNOSIS AND INVESTIGATIONS

Renal trauma

Physical examination will often suggest renal trauma. Flank or upper abdominal tenderness, contusion or a palpable mass and tenderness over the lower ribcage or lumbar vertebra are all associated with renal injury and require evaluation. It must be remembered, however, that absence of these findings does not rule out major, or even life-threatening, renal trauma in a patient with a suggestive history. Examination of the urine is a useful diagnostic aid. Renal injury must be excluded in every patient with gross or microscopic haematuria following trauma, but the degree of haematuria may bear no relationship to the severity of the renal injury. Generally, however, severe renal injuries are associated with considerable haematuria and sometimes clot retention.

Sometimes patients with blunt or more often penetrating renal trauma are too unstable from the cardiovascular viewpoint for preoperative studies. However, the following investigations are desirable when circumstances allow. Chest and abdominal X-rays should be performed as patterns of calcification over the kidney may suggest pre-existing pathology. Ground-glass density in the flank suggests urinary extravasation and/or haematoma. Absence of the psoas muscle shadow is non-specific but suggests renal trauma.

Evaluation of the upper urinary tract then proceeds with a high-dose pyelogram (Cass et al., 1987). Standard low-dose pyelography has a false negative rate of around 30% in renal trauma, and double the normal dose for intravenous urography is necessary to identify with certainty more than 80% of renal injuries.

TECHNIQUE

Intravenous urography

Objective
- To provide anatomical imaging of the urological tract, as far as the bladder.

Indications
- Suspected trauma to kidneys or ureter.

Contraindications
- History of allergic reaction to intravenous contrast material.

Investigations
- Access to emergency drugs should always be available in the event of an anaphylactic reaction.

- In the absence of a detailed history of allergies, a non-ionic contrast medium should be selected.

Practical technique
- Intravenous access is obtained with a cannula.
- A plain X-ray film is obtained.
- Intravenous contrast, approx. 1.5 ml kg^{-1}, is injected.
- Films are obtained at 5 min to look at the kidneys, at 10 min to look at the ureters and at 20 min to look at the bladder.

Potential complications
- Anaphylaxis to contrast.

Interpretation of results
Comparison between the speed of concentration and excretion of contrast on the two sides should be made. Depending on the degree of damage the affected side will show delay and the level of damage can sometimes be determined by visible extravasation.

The pyelogram has two important functions in the evaluation of renal trauma. First, the presence and function of a contralateral kidney can be documented in unilateral renal injuries. Second, the extent of the injury to the affected renal unit is classified (Elkin et al., 1966). Renal injury is suggested by:

- Decreased excretion of contrast.
- Obliteration of the psoas shadow by extravasation of blood or urine.
- Spinal scoliosis away from the injury as a result of ipsilateral psoas muscle spasm.
- Extravasation of contrast from the kidney, renal pelvis or ureter.

A normal intravenous urogram (IVU) in a traumatized patient with haematuria suggests minor renal or bladder contusion and rules out major injury. Incomplete or poor visualization of a portion of the kidney on intravenous pyelography suggests major renal trauma, including a laceration, avulsion or vascular injury. Further delineation of the injury should be sought with a selective angiogram whenever possible. Angiography may reveal complete parenchymal fracture with preserved vascularity to all of the kidney. It also allows identification of areas of renal devascularization; these may be important because necrosis and abscess formation, or hypertension, may follow.

Failure to visualize one or both kidneys on pyelography, assuming adequate contrast dosage has been given, requires immediate arteriography whenever possible. Although severe contusion and renal artery spasm

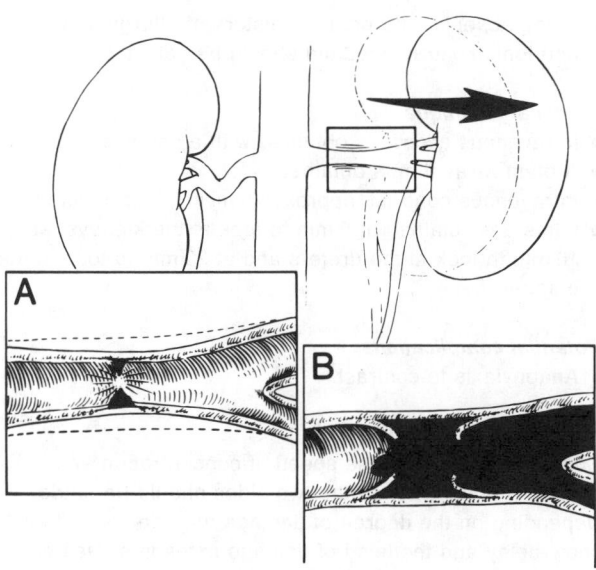

Fig. 5. Mechanism of intimal tear of renal artery and subsequent thrombosis.

may occasionally be responsible, a renal artery intimal tear with thrombosis is the most common cause (Figs 5 and 6) and the only prospect of satisfactory repair is very early diagnosis and urgent operative intervention. Arteriography may also be useful to assess areas of renal damage or infarction (Fig. 7) and associated aortic, hepatic or splenic injuries with extravasation.

Urgent computed tomography (CT) scanning is an-

other way of evaluating abdominal and renal trauma; in the USA particularly this has assumed a dominant role. Unfortunately, in UK centres, urgent CT scanning is not always available. CT is capable of identifying urinary extravasation more often than pyelography and it more precisely defines the extent of the injury. In particular, perinephric haematomata and renal lacerations are well shown on CT films taken after injection of intravenous contrast. Segmental devascularization or arterial spasm reveals a sharp demarcation on CT unlike a contusion or an intrarenal haematoma.

Retrograde pyelography is rarely useful in the diagnosis of renal parenchymal injury and ultrasonography has also rather limited value. Radionuclide scanning accurately depicts renal blood flow. However, parenchymal defects are less precisely imaged with isotope scans than with CT scans or arteriography, although radionuclide scanning is often useful in the follow-up of these lesions.

Ureteric injury

The presence or absence of haematuria is of little value in diagnosing ureteric injury (Carlton, 1978). Damage to the ureters from penetrating wounds is usually suspected by the presence of extravasation on the IVU together with some degree of hold up on the same side. Ureteric injury must be suspected in all abdominal gunshot

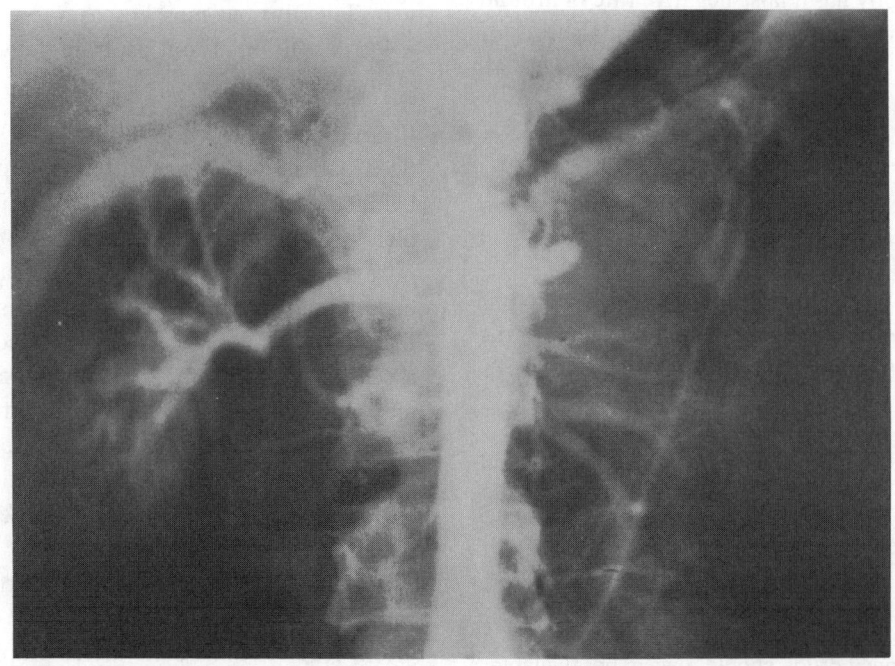

Fig. 6. Angiogram of renal artery thrombosis following trauma.

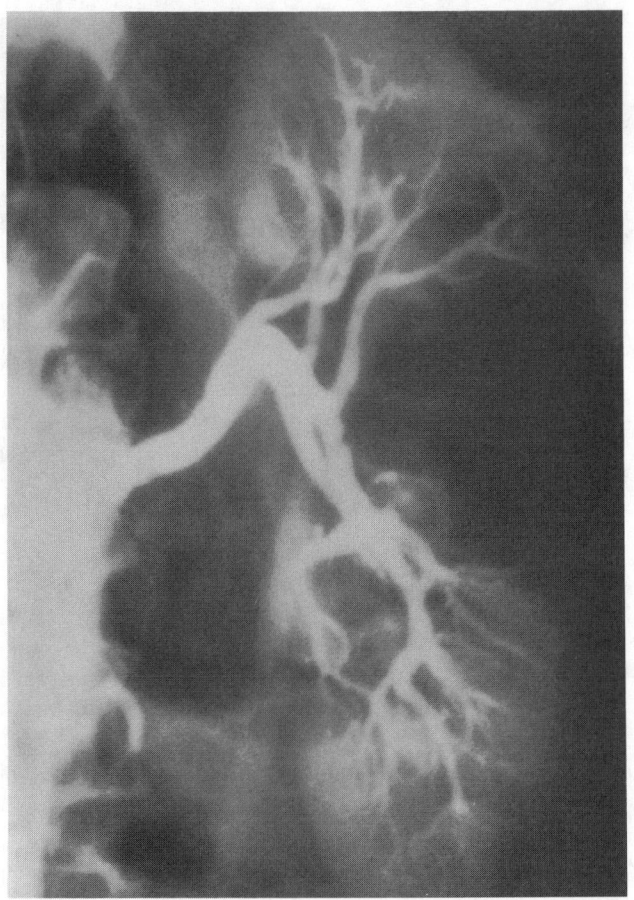

Fig. 7. Angiogram of renal vasculature demonstrating area of lack of perfusion in middle pole of the kidney following blunt renal trauma.

wounds, and the normal intravenous urogram does not exclude ischaemic damage to a ureter from the cavitation effect of a high-velocity missile. Computed axial tomography scanning is an alternative way of diagnosing extravasation preoperatively, although it is more commonly employed in trauma patients with blunt injury rather than those with penetrating injuries. Patients with penetrating injuries usually have associated trauma and shock and their injuries tend to be explored promptly.

An alternative way of assessing ureteric continuity and the presence or absence of extravasation is to perform retrograde pyelography prior to exploration of the abdomen. Obviously this can only be done if there is no urgency about opening the abdomen to deal with concomitant injuries.

Since percutaneous techniques can be performed under local anaesthesia, the urologist may prefer this approach in the patient who is gravely ill and is not a candidate for general anaesthesia, especially if there is considerable hydronephrosis present which will facilitate the puncture of the collecting system. Once drainage of the kidney has been achieved, subsequent antegrade ureterograms can be performed to more closely evaluate the degree of ureteric trauma and if necessary, antegrade placing of a stent can be accomplished.

Bladder injuries

On presentation to the A&E department, the patient with a bladder injury usually complains of suprapubic pain associated with absence of micturition since the injury. They may also give a history of a sharp blow to the lower abdomen. Physical examination may reveal suprapubic and inguinal swelling but usually the only clinical sign is suprapubic tenderness without any muscular rigidity or indications of peritoneal irritation, unless associated visceral injuries are present. Bowel sounds may be normal. Only 3% or so of patients present in shock when they have an isolated bladder injury; when shock is present other causes of hypotension such as splenic or hepatic bleeding should be meticulously excluded.

After the patient has undergone initial assessment the evaluation of the urinary tract should be accomplished as follows. A plain abdominal film is arranged and fractures sought, especially those of the ribs, transverse processes and pelvis that may be associated with urinary tract injuries. Calcifications and foreign bodies, including missile fragments, should be noted. Urethral trauma should be excluded by the history and physical examination of the pelvis and perineum. If any doubt remains, urethrography should be performed by means of gentle retrograde infusion of a water-soluble contrast medium. If urethrography is normal, a catheter can be gently passed and through this a cystogram is performed with up to 300 ml of sterile water and soluble X-ray contrast material. An anteroposterior film is then taken and the shape and size of the bladder is noted, as well as irregularity, trabeculation or signs of extravasation (Fig. 8).

TECHNIQUE

Urethral catheterization

Objective
● To provide drainage of urine from the lower urinary tract.

Indications
● Both diagnostic, as for cystography, and therapeutic to empty bladder or overcome outflow obstruction.

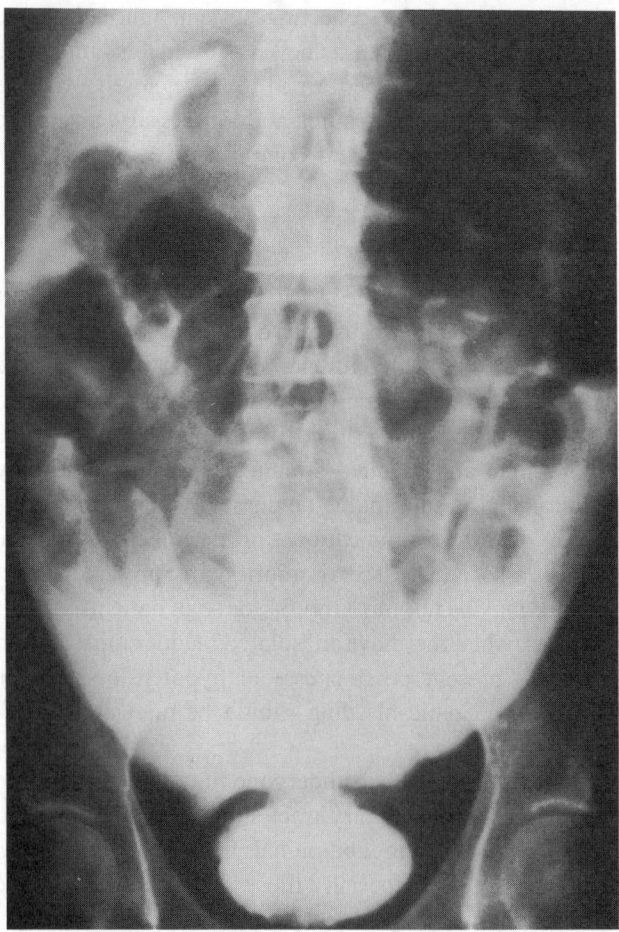

Fig. 8. Cystogram demonstrating intraperitoneal rupture of bladder.

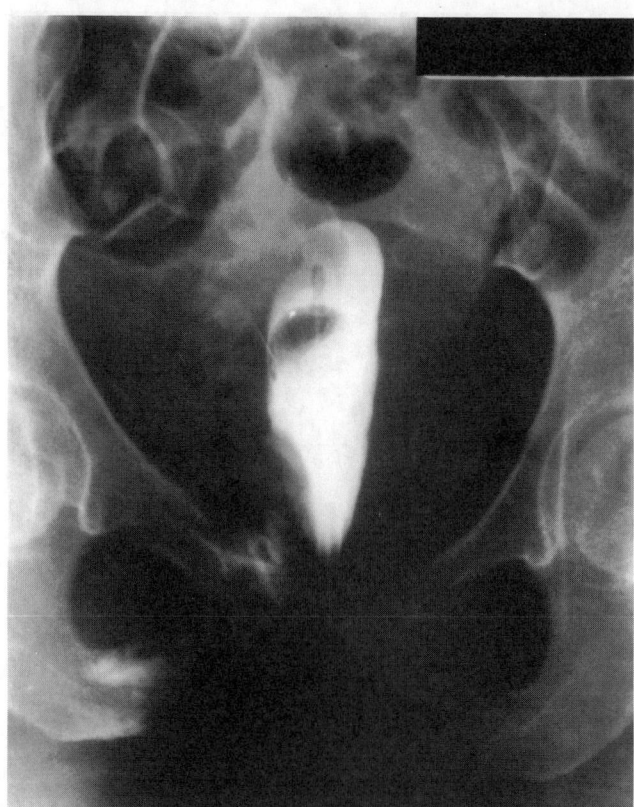

Fig. 9. Cystogram of bladder following pelvic fracture demonstrating 'tear drop' appearance of bladder due to surrounding haematoma.

Contraindications
- Blood at the urethral meatus in the presence of a pelvic fracture.

Practical technique
Male catheterization:

- Clean penis with sterile fluid, always keeping one hand sterile.
- Insert anaesthetic/lubricant jelly into urethral meatus.
- Keep urethra straight with slight traction on the penis and introduce catheter.

Potential complications
- *Development of a false passage.* This occurs in the presence of a urethral stricture. If the catheter does not pass with ease, DO NOT PUSH.
- *Sphincter damage.* This can occur when the balloon is blown up in the prostatic urethra/sphincter mechanism and is prevented by never blowing up the balloon until urine is flowing out of the catheter.

Aftercare
- The system is a closed drainage system and so the catheter bag should be attached immediately and should not be removed unless really necessary.
- Undue tension on the catheter should be avoided.

In the patient with a severe pelvic fracture there may be massive blood loss into the surrounding tissues and the bladder can be compressed into the so-called 'tear drop' deformity (Fig. 9). In patients with extraperitoneal rupture, flame-like wisps of urinary extravasation are noted on the film of the full bladder (Fig. 10). Next the bladder is allowed to drain and a further film is taken as this may reveal subtle areas of urinary extravasation that may not have been obvious when the bladder was filled. Once a satisfactory cystogram has been accomplished, evaluation of the upper urinary tracts should be performed as described above (Sandler *et al.*, 1981).

Urethral injury

In the patient with a history of trauma to the perineum or pelvis a urethral injury must always be suspected.

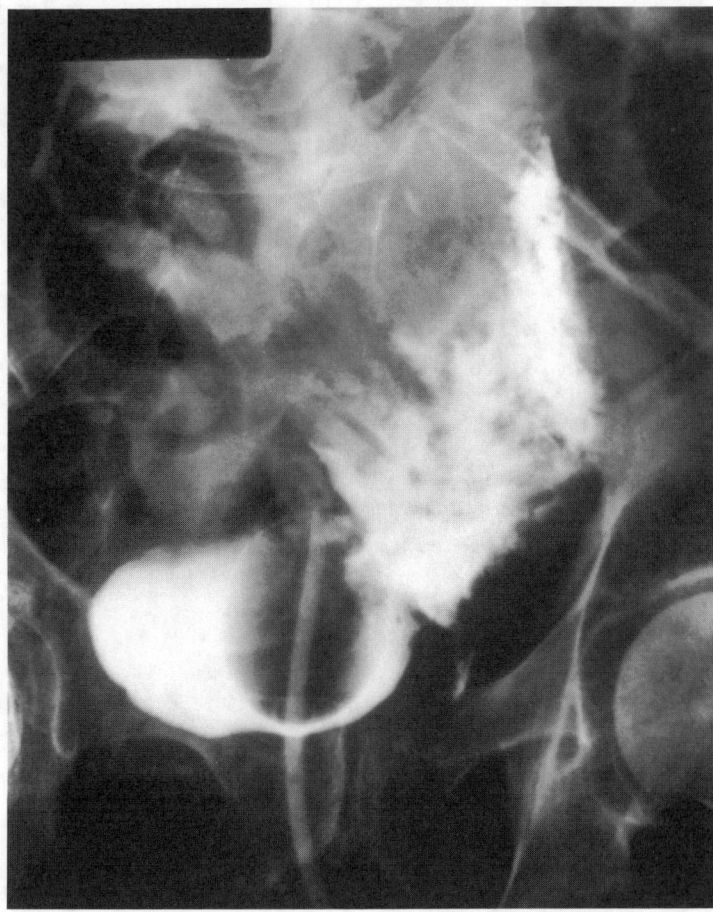

Fig. 10. Cystogram showing extraperitoneal rupture of bladder.

Careful questioning may reveal that the patient has noticed bleeding at the meatus even though there may not be any visible by the time that he arrives in the A&E department. He may also have noticed swelling in the perineum during or after voiding which may represent extravasation of urine. Physical examination may reveal swelling or discoloration of the genitalia suggesting the presence of a urethral injury.

Rectal examination is essential in a patient with lower abdominal or perineal injury. Not only may the prostate be elevated above its normal position by a supradiaphragmatic urethral rupture, but concomitant injuries to the rectum itself may be detected and will need urgent management, usually by defunctioning colostomy. If, on the basis of history and physical examination, a urethral injury is suspected, catheterization should not be attempted but an oblique retrograde urethrogram should be performed immediately using water-soluble contrast. An anteroposterior film of the pelvis is taken first and any calcification or pelvic fracture is noted. Then with the patient in the oblique position,

between 20 and 30 ml of diluted water-soluble contrast material is gently introduced through a syringe into the urethral meatus (Fig. 11). An X-ray is taken during the injection to ensure that the urethra is full and distended with contrast material. If for some reason a urethral catheter has already been placed and the urine is draining well, then injection of water-soluble contrast material alongside the catheter may sometimes be worthwhile. An adequate urethrogram can be obtained and serious urethral injury excluded without the removal of the catheter.

TECHNIQUE

Retrograde urethrogram

Objective

- To obtain anatomical definition of the urethra.

Indications

- Whenever a urethral injury is suspected. For example when blood is seen at the meatus in the presence of a

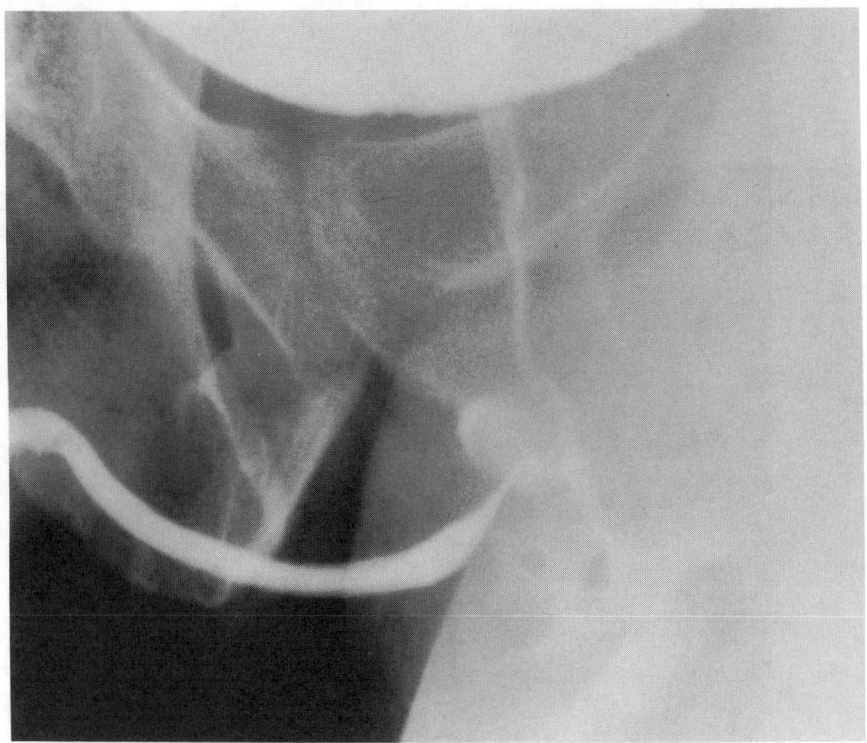

Fig. 11. Urethrogram demonstrating contrast extravasation due to a urethral rupture.

fractured pelvis or the patient is unable to void after such an injury.

Practical technique
- If possible patient should be placed in the oblique position.
- 20–30 ml of dilute water-soluble contrast are injected into the urethra with a catheter-tip syringe.
- Screen urethra during filling to look for adequate urethral distention and any injury.

Potential complications
- Injection of contrast up the urethra followed by extravasation through a urethral rupture can invite sepsis and the procedure should be covered with a systemic broad-spectrum antibiotic.

Injury to the external genitalia

Although the mechanism of injury is important, physical examination of the external genitalia will usually reveal the type and extent of the injury. The entrance of a penetrating missile will usually be obvious. The extent of extravasation of blood and urine in blunt penile trauma is determined by the integrity of Buck's fascia. If this layer remains intact then all bleeding from a ruptured corpus cavernosum and/or urethra will be limited to

Buck's fascia. On the other hand, if Buck's fascia has been damaged then the extravasation will extend to Colles' fascial attachments.

MANAGEMENT IN THE A&E DEPARTMENT

As previously mentioned, urological injuries are frequently associated with other major injuries and attention to these may take priority over the urological injuries. Hypoxia, haemorrhage and shock are the immediate threats to life. The immediate priorities are airway patency and the mechanics of ventilation and circulation. The next priority is restoration of intravascular volume and control of any external bleeding.

The management of blunt renal trauma depends on the degree of injury. The great majority of patients have minor parenchymal injury and are best treated by observation. Approximately 10% of patients with blunt renal trauma have severe injuries and these patients usually require exploration to control haemorrhage and to have any chance of renal salvage. However, these injuries frequently require nephrectomy owing to extensive renal parenchymal trauma and other life-threatening non-renal injuries.

When a ureteric injury is suspected on the excretory

intravenous urogram, the next step is to arrange an ascending ureterogram and the gentle passage of a guidewire up the ureter in an attempt to locate a double J stent passed from the renal pelvis down to the bladder. Ureterography may more precisely localize the area of ureteric injury and in patients in whom there is not complete disruption of ureteric continuity, the passage of a double J stent and a bladder catheter may be all that is necessary.

When the bladder is the site of injury then the principles of management include adequate urinary diversion from the area of injury, usually by catheterization, and prompt and adequate drainage of the perivesical area, or other areas of extravasation. Closure of the defect in the vesical wall is usually employed unless laceration and extravasation are very minor. In the patient with penetrating trauma, surgical exploration should always be promptly performed, not only to evaluate the bladder injury but also to assess the integrity of the surrounding abdominal viscera and vasculature.

When a urethral injury has occurred either above or below the urogenital diaphragm, a plan of management should be made for the initial phase and for any subsequent reconstructive procedure. Initial management of the urethra that has been ruptured above the urogenital diaphragm may be accomplished by several methods. Because of associated injuries, the usual treatment is insertion of a suprapubic catheter and delayed repair of the prostatobulbous urethra. The suprapubic catheter can be put in under ultrasound control. More commonly, the patient will be transferred to the operating theatre for open insertion of a suprapubic catheter and inspection of other abdominal viscera for associated injuries. As described above, if a urethral tear is suspected then a urethrogram with water-soluble contrast should be undertaken prior to attempted insertion of the urethral catheter. If the urethra appears intact, a urethral catheter is not only valuable for performing a cystogram to exclude bladder injury but it also provides an invaluable means of measuring urinary output to assess the success of other resuscitation manoeuvres.

Management of injuries to the penis, scrotum and scrotal contents depends on their nature and severity. Injuries to the corpora cavernosa usually require operative repair to prevent the development of erectile impotence and/or curvature of the penis. Scrotal injuries will often be contaminated and thorough debridement is necessary together with antibiotic prophylaxis to prevent the complication of Fournier's gangrene. At the time of surgical exploration, the viability of the testes and associated structures should be assessed. If the tunica albuginea of the testis has been violated, seminiferous tubules will extrude from the wound. Necrotic and devitalized tubules should be debrided and the tunica albuginea closed primarily with absorbable sutures. This is best done in the operating theatre under general anaesthesia rather than in the A&E unit.

Blunt trauma of the scrotum requires individualized treatment. The differential diagnosis of testicular torsion and epididymitis must always be considered. Patients often attribute the swelling and pain of testicular torsion to an episode of minor trauma. The clinician can often make a clear differential diagnosis by means of urine analysis, scrotal examination and rectal palpation but if doubt persists surgical exploration is mandatory. It must be remembered that a ruptured testis may result from blunt trauma and any chance of salvage of the testis will be lost with conservative treatment. Prompt exploration in the operating room in cases of blunt scrotal trauma decreases not only the chances of testicular loss, but also the morbidity to the patient. A large haematoma may take months to resolve and if it becomes secondarily infected an abscess may result.

CRITERIA FOR CONSULTATION WITH A UROLOGIST AND/OR TRANSFER TO A SPECIALIST UROLOGICAL SERVICE

The criteria for consultation and/or transfer in urological injury depends on the individual patient. Other injuries may take priority, but when urological injury does occur it is important that a urologist is consulted because delayed or inappropriate management may result in long-term loss of function and morbidity for the patient. The majority of renal injuries are managed conservatively, but a urologist should be consulted at an early stage when the decision between conservative and operative management has to be made. Ureteric injuries will need intervention and this is best undertaken by a urologist since ureteric reanastomosis and reimplantations have a tendency to stenose if inexpertly performed. Bladder ruptures are relatively simple to repair but again this is best carried out by a urologist who will be well versed in pelvic anatomy and the surgical techniques. Urethral injuries provide the most complex problems associated with urological trauma and are best managed in specialist units by those with experience in urological reconstruction. The initial management is urinary diversion by means of a suprapubic catheter. Generally the patients will have other injuries that may require immediate treatment and after a period of 12 weeks or so they should be transferred to a specialist unit for reconstruction of the urethra. In experienced hands, success rates approach 100% but the injury itself and the surgery necessary to correct it may produce erectile impotence in a proportion of cases.

SUMMARY

- The greatest determinant of mortality of patients with urological trauma is the extent of associated non-urological injuries.
- 70% of renal injuries are minor, 15% are major and 15% are irreparable.
- The degree of haematuria may bear no relationship to the severity of renal injury.
- Pelvic fracture injuries involve the membranous urethra and occur when the prostate, which is attached to the pubis by the puboprostatic ligaments, moves with the pubic bone fragments.
- Bulbar urethral injuries occur as a result of perineal blunt trauma or iatrogenic urethral instrumentation.

In the severely traumatized patient with a pelvic fracture and blood at the urethral meatus the following should be performed:

- Retrograde urethrography to look for injury to the urethra.

  If normal:

- Cystography following passage of urethral catheter.

  If normal:

- Intravenous urography to look for upper tract or ureteric damage.

If renal or ureteric injury is suspected, intravenous urography should be performed at the earliest opportunity. If bladder or urethral trauma is suspected, retrograde cystourethrography is the investigation of choice.

The principle of managing serious lower urinary tract injuries involves diversion of urine away from the site of injury.

Bibliography

CARLTON, C.E. (1978). Injuries of the kidney and ureter. In *Campbells Urology*, 4th edn, ed. J.H. Harrison, R.F. Gittes, A.D. Perlmutter, T.A. Stamey & P.C. Walsh. Philadelphia: W.B. Saunders.

CARROLL, P.R. & DIXON, C.M. (1992). Surgical anatomy of the male and female urethra. *Urol. Clin. North. Am.*, **19**, 339–46.

CASS, A.S. (1989). Renovascular injuries from external trauma. *Urol. Clin. North Am.*, **16**, 213–20.

CASS, A.S., LUXENBURG, H. & GLEINCH, P. (1987). Clinical indications for radiographic evaluation of blunt renal trauma. *J. Urol.*, **136**, 370–3.

DALY, J.W. & HIGGINS, K.A. (1988). Injury to the ureter during gynaecological surgical procedures. *Surg. Gynecol. Obstet.*, **167**, 19–23.

ELKIN, M., MENCH, C.H. & DE PANEDES, R.G. (1966). Correlation of intravenous urography and renal angiography in kidney injury. *Radiology*, **86**, 496–8.

FEDERLE, M.P., BROWN, T.R. & McANINCH, J.W. (1987). Penetrating renal trauma: CT evaluation. *J. Comput. Assist. Tomogr.*, **11**, 1026–30.

McANINCH, J.W. (1981). Traumatic injuries to the urethra. *J. Trauma*, **21**, 4–7.

McANINCH, J.W., CARROLL, P.R., KLOSTERMAN, P.W. *et al.* (1991). Renal reconstruction after injury. *J. Urol.*, **145**, 932–7.

PRYOR, J.P., HILL, J.T. & PACKHAM, W.A. *et al.* (1981). Penile injuries with particular reference to injury to the erectile tissue. *Br. J. Urol.*, **53**, 42–6.

ROBARDS, V.L., HAGLUND, R.V., LUBIN, E.N. *et al.* (1976). Treatment of rupture of the bladder. *J. Urol.*, **116**, 178–9.

SANDLER, C.M., PHILLIPS, J.M., HARRIS, J.D. *et al.* (1981). Radiology of the bladder and urethra in blunt pelvic trauma. *Radiol. Clin. North Am.*, **19**, 195–204.

TURNER-WARWICK, R.T. (1989). Prevention of complications resulting from pelvic fracture urethral injuries and from their surgical management. *Urol. Clin. North Am.*, **16**, 335–52.

26 Management of open fractures

A.J. FORESTER and S.P.F. HUGHES

Department of Orthopaedic Surgery, Hammersmith Hospital, London, UK

Chapter plan

Historical perspective
Consequences of open fracture
Aetiology
Classification
Prehospital care
Emergency treatment
Examination and debridement of the wound
Fracture stabilization
Wound coverage
Limb salvage or amputation
Postoperative care

Definition

- An open fracture is one in which the skin and soft tissues overlying the fracture have been broken and communicate directly with the fracture or its haematoma

---

HISTORICAL PERSPECTIVE

The importance of open fractures has long been recognized. Hippocratic physicians (Lloyd, 1978) demonstrated that wound size, fracture stability and associated proximity of neurovascular structures influenced the outcome of these injuries. They recommended removal of protruding fragments, use of antiseptic dressings and stable fracture fixation. Free drainage of pus was thought desirable also.

Until 150 years ago an open fracture usually meant death from sepsis within a month and amputation was frequently indicated. Amputation carried a high mortality rate from sepsis. Traditional methods of treatment involved cauterization of the wound, often inducing tissue necrosis and sepsis.

Ambroise Paré, a French Army surgeon, described in 1538 the ligation of bleeding vessels following amputation (Paré, 1634). He advocated removal of dead tissue and foreign material from the wound and enlargement of the wound to allow free drainage of pus. Desault at the end of the eighteenth century developed the concept of debridement (Wangensteen & Wangensteen, 1978). This has come to mean the removal of all foreign and dead material from a wound, but is derived from the French *débrider*, 'to unbridle'. Larrey in 1829 used the term to include splitting of the deep fascia in order to ligate bleeding vessels, explore the wound and allow for swelling to occur. This lesson has been learnt and forgotten by successive generations of surgeons. As each new advance became established then debridement was neglected, usually with catastrophic effects.

CONSEQUENCES OF OPEN FRACTURE

These depend on the extent of soft tissue injury but include:

- Contamination of the injury by bacteria.
- Crushing or devitalisation of soft tissues such that they are susceptible to infection.
- Limitation of treatment options due to loss of bone or soft tissue.

Prognosis

This is determined by the degree of bacterial contamination and the amount of dead and devitalized soft tissue.

> **Aims of treatment**
>
> - To prevent infection.
> - To achieve bone and soft tissue healing.
> - Early rehabilitation to restore function.

AETIOLOGY

Open fractures are high-energy injuries. Over the last 100 years there has been a steady rise in such injuries. Fractures occurring in two, three or four limbs are not uncommon and are frequently associated with trauma elsewhere, particularly cerebral lesions, chest and abdominal injuries. Knowledge of the mechanism of injury is useful since it may influence treatment. Kinetic energy (KE) transferred to the body at injury is described by the equation

$$KE = \tfrac{1}{2}mv^2$$

where m is the mass and v the velocity of the wounding force. Doubling the mass of the object will double the kinetic energy, but doubling the velocity quadruples the energy available for injury.

Extent of injury

This will depend on how much energy is absorbed by the soft tissues prior to injury occurring and the ability of the tissues to resist or dissipate the energy. Typically, open fractures are associated with soft tissue loss, compartment syndromes, neurovascular injuries, displacement and comminution of the bone and, in severe injuries, bone loss.

CLASSIFICATION

This 'tool' allows surgeons to communicate with each other concerning an open fracture. Treatment and prognosis is dependent on more factors than injury alone. Most classifications concentrate on the size and extent of the skin defect and soft tissue damage. Of these the classification of Gustilo & Anderson (Table 1) is the most widely used and understood. This system concentrates on the degree of soft tissue injury and the degree of contamination, with particular emphasis on wound size. In addition, gunshot wounds and farmyard injuries are automatically considered to be grade III severity. Other classifications in use include that of Tscherne &

Table 1. *Gustilo & Anderson classification* (Gustilo & Anderson, 1976; Gustilo *et al.*, 1984)

Grade I	Low-energy wound Skin wound <1 cm Minimal contamination Minimal soft tissue damage Simple fractures with minimal comminution
Grade II	Skin wound >1 cm Moderate contamination Moderate soft tissue injury Minimal/moderate crushing component Moderate comminution of bone
Grade III	High-energy injuries Skin wound >10 cm Gross contamination Extensive soft tissue damage with crushing IIIA: Extensive soft tissue laceration, with adequate bone coverage IIIB: Extensive soft tissue injury with periosteal stripping and bone exposure; soft tissue reconstruction required IIIC: Severe loss of coverage plus vascular injury requiring repair

Oestern (1982), which has four severity grades dependent on the extent of skin injury, soft tissue injury, degree of contamination and severity of the fracture. In the UK the CEPOD (Confidential Enquiry into Peri-Operative Deaths) classification grades open fractures as 'urgent', i.e. they should be operated on within the first 6 h following injury.

PREHOSPITAL CARE

At the accident scene the rescue crew will either 'scoop and run' or resuscitate the patient prior to transporting them to the accident unit. Following stabilization of vital functions, the wounds will be covered with sterile dressings and the fracture splinted. Haemorrhage is best controlled by direct pressure. There is no indication for the use of tourniquets, particularly in the prehospital phase.

EMERGENCY TREATMENT

Immediate assessment and treatment is required for all patients presenting with open fractures. Attention should be drawn to treatable life-threatening conditions and not to the fracture *per se*.

Resuscitation

Management priorities are to establish an airway, evaluate breathing and to control haemorrhage. Immediate venous access should be obtained with two 14G cannulae inserted into large veins, by cut-down, if necessary. Any evidence that there is inadequate circulation requires immediate fluid resuscitation. Neurological function must be assessed, and reassessed frequently. Following adequate resuscitation a thorough physical examination should be carried out unless life-threatening conditions demand surgery. If this is the case, then the secondary survey must be completed postoperatively.

It must be assumed that in the multiply injured patient the cervical spine is injured until proven otherwise. A hard cervical collar must be applied until X-rays of the cervical spine from the occiput to the C7/T1 junction are obtained which reveal no abnormality. However, it is vital to realize that the lateral cross-table cervical spine film may appear normal in 10% of cases that have a significant structural abnormality. Neck symptoms indicate that further radiological evaluation of the cervical spine is necessary.

Initial wound care

The wound should ideally be photographed with a polaroid camera prior to a sterile dressing being applied and then left undisturbed until the patient reaches the operating theatre (Fig 1). If it is not possible to photograph the wound then a sketch should be drawn. Reinspecting wounds raises the infection rate by a factor of 3 to 4 (Tscherne, 1984) and must be avoided.

Antibiotic prophylaxis

Strictly speaking the administration of antibiotics in cases of open fracture is therapeutic, not prophylactic. Intravenous antibiotics should be commenced. A suitable regimen for an adult would be: 1.5 g cefuroxime IV plus 2 mega-units of benzylpenicillin stat.

Antibiotics should be continued intravenously for the next 48–72 h (Patzakis, 1982) and thereafter if there is microbiological evidence of infection. Cefuroxime is used since it is effective against *Staphylococcus* and benzyl-

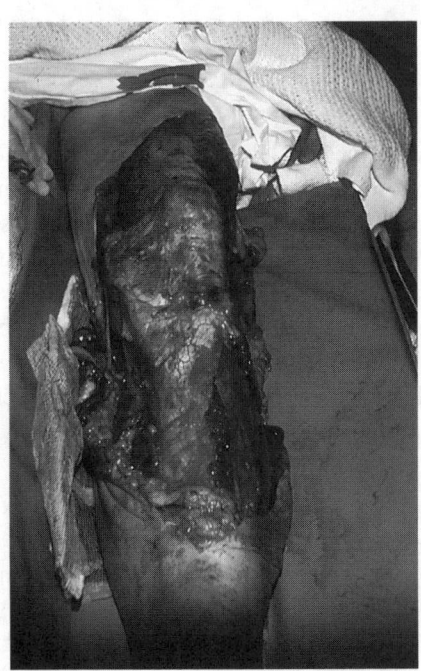

Fig. 1. Initial presentation of grade IIIA open tibial fracture at accident unit

penicillin is effective against *Clostridium* and *Streptococcus*. A suitable alternative would be metronidazole.

Tetanus prophylaxis

In fully immunized patients who have sustained an open fracture tetanus toxoid should be administered. Unimmunized patients, or in cases where there is uncertainty, should receive tetanus immunoglobulin.

Investigations

Blood is taken for full blood count, urea and electrolytes, group and cross-match and blood arterial gases (if indicated). A wound swab should be taken.

Radiological examination

X-rays of the cervical spine, chest and pelvis should be taken in the polytraumatized patient. This is in addition to X-rays of the injured extremity which will depict fracture patterns allowing selection of an appropriate method of fracture stabilization. If there is suspicion that there is vascular compromise in a limb then urgent angiography or exploration in the operating theatre is required.

EXAMINATION AND DEBRIDEMENT OF THE WOUND

This should be carried out in the operating theatre under general anaesthesia. The dressing should be removed, and further photographs taken if possible. The skin around the wound should be inspected and the findings carefully noted. Wound swabs should be obtained and sent for culture and sensitivity. Large foreign bodies can be removed from the wound. A tourniquet should be applied to the limb but *not* inflated unless massive bleeding occurs. The wound should then be scrubbed clean with a brush and a scrub solution.

Irrigation

This is probably one of the most important manoeuvers of the debridement process. Copious irrigation should be used; this will remove loose foreign material, necrotic tissue and reduce the bacterial load. There is no consensus on what 'copious' means but it is generally taken to mean 10 litres. Ideally this irrigation fluid should be a sterile isotonic solution; however, in the absence of this tap water is preferable to not performing irrigation at all. Pulsatile irrigation with a sprinkler head appears to the most effective method of delivery of the irrigation fluid. Antibiotics may be added to the fluid for final irrigation, although there is no evidence that this is beneficial.

Debridement

There is no more critical aspect in the treatment of open fractures than the removal of all dead and devitalized tissue (Wangensteen & Wangensteen, 1978). In particular, dead muscle is an ideal pabulum for infection and incomplete debridement is the commonest cause of subsequent infection. If the skin wound is small the underlying muscle injury may be misjudged.

Extending the skin wound

Judging severity of injury by the skin wound may be misleading. The wound must be extended to allow access to all damaged tissue. The skin edge should be trimmed approximately 1–2 mm removing contaminated and non-viable skin. Contaminated fat should be freely debrided since it has a poor blood supply. Skin from amputated parts or from non-viable flaps may be harvested with a dermatome for subsequent use.

Fascia

Devitalized or contaminated fascia should be freely resected. Open fractures do not always decompress fascial compartments and complete fasciotomy of all muscle compartments may well be indicated.

Muscle and tendons

It is traditionally taught that the 'four Cs' allow identification of dead or devitalized muscle. These are Consistency, Contractility, Colour and Capacity to bleed. Dead muscle is said to be plum-coloured, mushy in consistency, does not bleed when cut and does not contract when pinched. Of these signs the colour is the least reliable sign. During debridement each muscle compartment must be examined and all dead muscle excised. Occasionally this will mean the removal of a complete muscle group.

Contaminated tendons should be carefully cleaned by irrigation but may be left intact for debridement at a later point. However, if skin cover is not possible in an open wound then a moist dressing will be required to prevent desiccation.

Bone and joints

Bone fragments should be adequately irrigated, and obviously contaminated small fragments with no soft tissue attachments should be removed. Problems arise with a large bony fragment with no soft tissue attachments which may be necessary for bony reconstruction. If the surgeon is not sure how contaminated the fragment is then it is wise to *remove* it rather than risk an infected non-union.

If the wound has entered a joint it must be explored and any foreign material removed. Following adequate irrigation the synovium should be closed although the tissues overlying it may be left open.

Neurovascular structures

Small blood vessels identified at wound exploration may be ligated. Extensive use of diathermy should be avoided since it increases the non-viable tissue load. Any major vessels that require reconstruction are usually identified prior to surgery. Early stabilization of the fracture is necessary if vascular repair is indicated.

Major nerves found to be divided at surgery require repair. Should facilities not be available at the time of

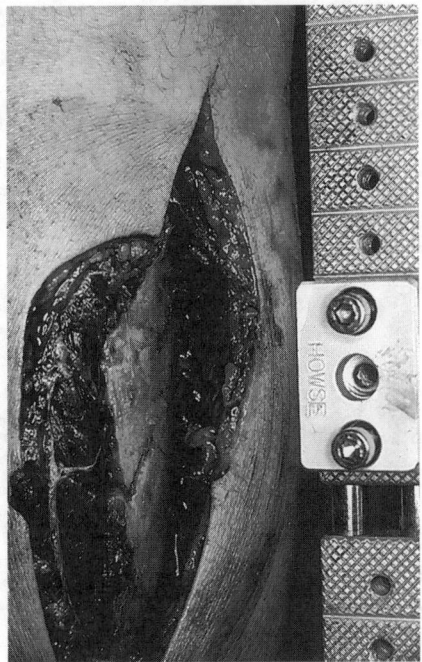

Fig. 2. Postdebridement of grade IIIA open tibial fracture

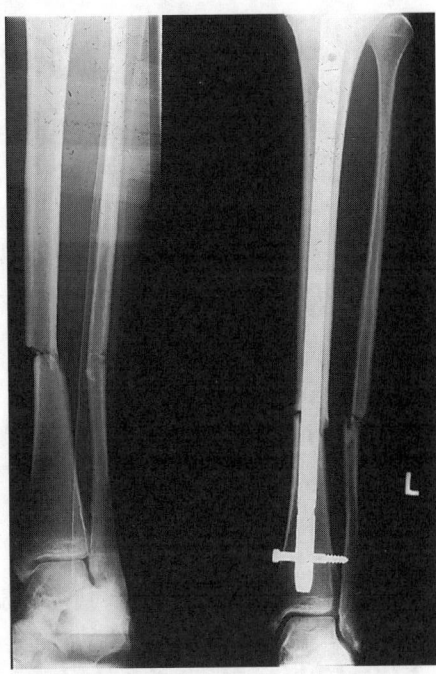

Fig. 3. Intramedullary nailing fixation of open tibial fracture

surgery then the ends of the nerve trunks should be marked with a non-absorbable suture such that they will be easily identified at a future date.

Foreign bodies

All obvious foreign bodies should be removed during the debridement; however, a protracted search for small fragments may cause more damage to the soft tissues than leaving them *in situ*.

Reappraisal

At the end of wound exploration it is important to re-examine the wound and any further obviously non-viable tissue should be removed. The skin should NOT be closed (Fig. 2).

FRACTURE STABILIZATION

Stabilization of the fracture is necessary for bone and soft tissue healing. It prevents further damage occurring, decreases pain and simplifies nursing care. The definitive treatment for an open fracture depends on its location, the facilities available, the expertise of the surgeon, and also the quality of the rehabilitation services. In general terms the methods available include the following.

(a) Non-operative treatment

Use of plaster casts or splints, and traction are suitable for open fractures but are intensive of nursing care and require long hospital admissions. They are used for some grade I and II fractures and as temporary immobilization for grade III injuries.

(b) Internal fixation

Although considered contraindicated until relatively recently, internal fixation allows early stabilization of fractures. Plate fixation may be indicated for the upper extremity and for fractures around joints. Intramedullary nails are now the treatment of choice for grade I, II and IIIA open femoral and tibial fractures (Klemm & Börner, 1986; Llowe & Hansen, 1988) (Fig. 3).

(c) External fixation

External fixation was considered to be the treatment of choice for open fractures particularly of the lower extremity (Fig. 4). Recent advances in intramedullary nailing in these fractures have meant that grade IIIB and IIIC injuries that are severely contaminated are the only indication for the application of an external fixator (Edwards et al., 1988; Klemm & Börner, 1986; Llowe and Hansen, 1988) (Fig. 5).

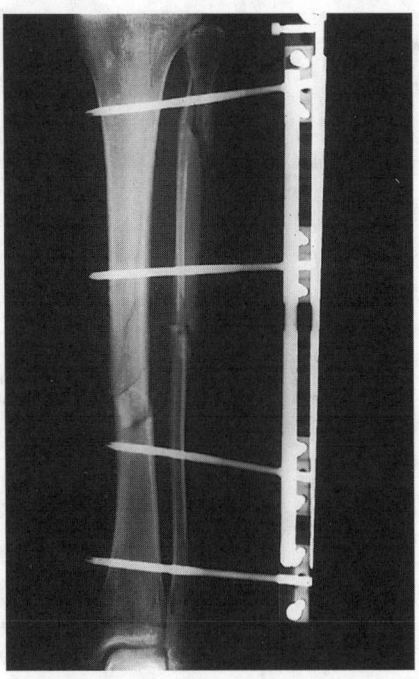

Fig. 4. Hughes fixator on open tibial fracture

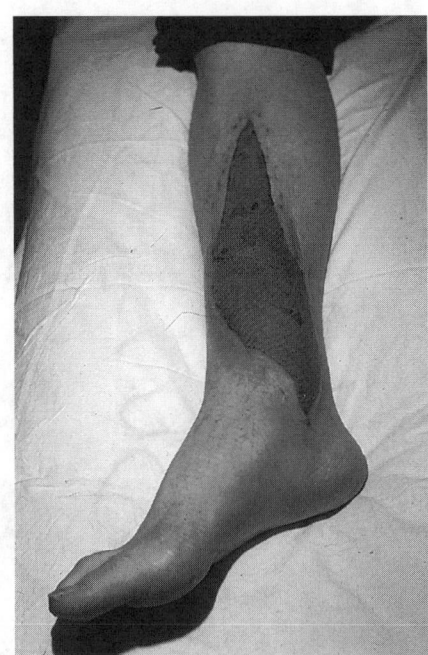

Fig. 6. Split skin graft following open fractures can cover most defects

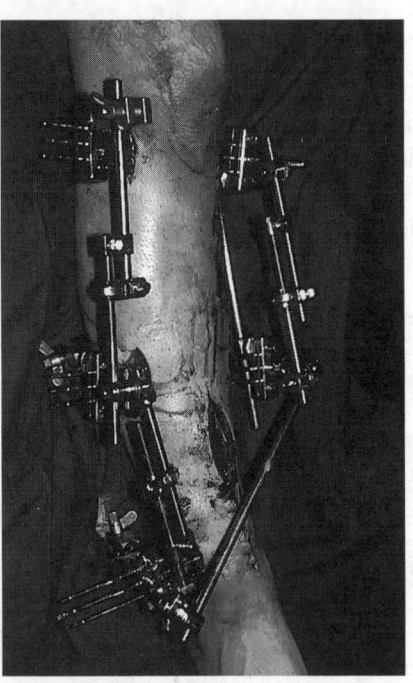

Fig. 5. Double bar fixation, double configuration and cross-connections may aid stability and be configured to manage most fracture patterns

WOUND COVERAGE

Primary closure is rarely indicated. It is safer to perform delayed primary closure at 3–5 days than to risk infection with anaerobic organisms. Wounds should be dressed with fluffed gauze laid over the wound but never packed into it. If there is a lack of bone or tendon coverage a moist dressing should be used. The wound should not be reinspected until the time of delayed primary closure, unless clinical evidence in the form of pyrexia or a raised white blood cell count indicates that early further inspection is warranted. At delayed primary closure further wound inspection and debridement should be performed to remove any remaining non-viable tissue. If, at second look, skin closure is not possible then a local or free flap will be necessary although a split-thickness skin graft is suitable if the wound bed is well vascularized (Yaremchuk et al., 1987) (Fig. 6).

LIMB SALVAGE OR AMPUTATION

In severe open fractures where there is loss of bone with severe comminution, extensive crushing of muscle, neurovascular damage, extensive skin loss with contamination, then primary amputation may be considered. This is more likely if there has been prolonged limb ischaemia (> 8 h). Although amputation should not be considered without the advice of at least one other surgeon, and only if the limb is non-salvageable, it is important to take a decision early. Multiple surgical procedures and prolonged hospital stays over a long period are detrimental to both patient and society especially if the final outcome is amputation. In deciding on appropriate treatment for a case the Mangled Extremity Severity Score (Johansen *et al.*, 1988) may be helpful. A score of greater than 7 is considered a reliable guide for the need to amputate. The factors and their scoring are as follows:

Mangled Extremity Severity Score (Johansen *et al.*, 1988)

(*a*) *Skeletal/soft tissue injury*
- Low-energy injury (stab wound; closed fracture; low-energy transfer gunshot wound) 1
- Medium-energy injury (open fracture; multiple fractures; dislocation) 2
- High-energy injury (shotgun wound; high-energy transfer gunshot wound; crush injury) 3
- Very high-energy wounds (as above but with gross contamination, soft tissue avulsion) 4

(*b*) *Limb ischaemia*
- Pulse reduced or absent, normal perfusion:
  <6 h 1
  >6 h 2
- Pulseless, paraesthesiae; decreased capillary refill:
  <6 h 2
  >6 h 4
- Cool, paralysed, insensate limb:
  <6 h 3
  >6 h 6

(*c*) *Shock*
- Systolic blood pressure >90 mmHg 0
- Transient hypotension 1
- Persistent hypotension 2

(*d*) *Age*
- <30 years 0
- 30–50 years 1
- >50 years 2

POSTOPERATIVE CARE

Following surgery the most important factor in controlling swelling is elevation of the limb. Swelling may prevent delayed primary closure, increase the risk of infection and may cause loss of the position of the fracture if a plaster cast has to be split.

Systemic complications

Hypovolaemic shock

This can be defined as inadequate tissue perfusion with tissue hypoxia which may threaten vital organ function. A closed fracture of a long bone such as the femur may result in the loss of 2–3 units of blood such that transfusion may be required. Open fractures may have bled much more and for a longer period in the absence of any tamponade. Repeated transfusion can lead to problems with haemostasis and may cause disseminated intravascular coagulation.

Fat embolism

This is the occurrence of hypoxia, confusion and multiple petechiae a few days following long-bone fracture. Fat embolism is an important cause of acute respiratory distress syndrome. The only specific treatment of fat embolism is to reduce the hypoxaemia by administering oxygen. Failure to maintain oxygenation by mask is an indication for intermittent positive pressure ventilation with positive end-expiratory pressure.

Thromboembolic disorders

Deep venous thrombosis and pulmonary embolism are dangerous complications of musculoskeletal injury, especially in the lower extremity. Physical and pharmacological prophylaxis are valuable especially if there is a history of risk factors.

Local complications

Soft tissue and vascular problems

Failure to obtain skin coverage with subsequent soft tissue necrosis may necessitate multiple reconstructive procedures. Vascular injuries may produce haematomata or false aneurysms and require exploration. Limbs that require revascularization may ultimately come to amputation.

Osteomyelitis

Infection is a significant risk in open fractures (Fig. 7). This may range from an infected fracture haematoma to chronic osteomyelitis. Infection in bone may lead to great morbidity because inflammation causes pressure necrosis and occlusion of the blood supply. This in turn causes

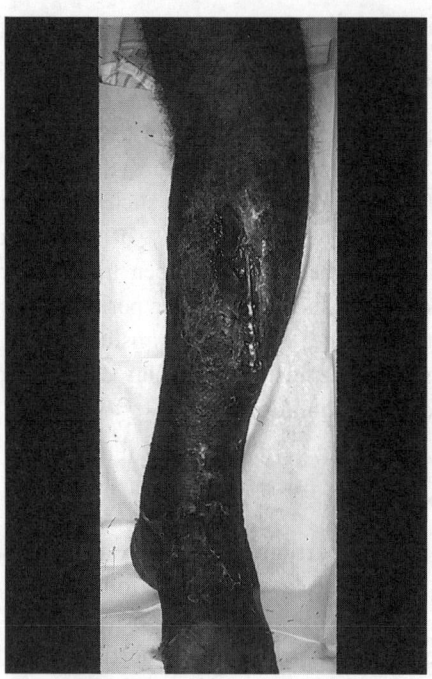

Fig. 7. Infected tibia following internal fixation for an open fracture

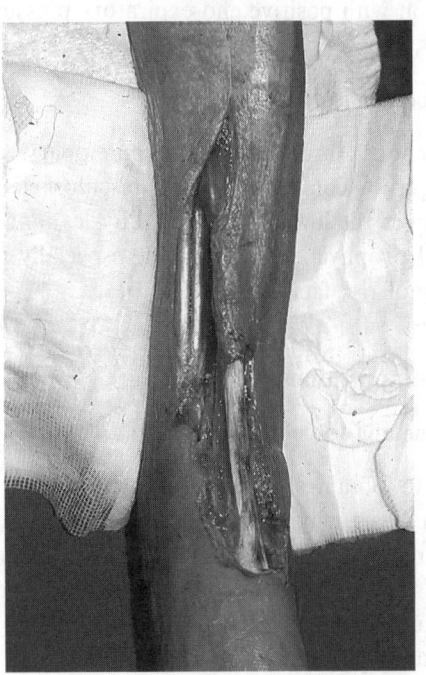

Fig. 8. Chronic osteomyelitis following an open fracture

bone necrosis with dead fragments of bone acting as foreign material and therefore a nidus for further infection (Weiss, 1989). Treatment of chronic osteomyelitis may be prolonged and complex (Fig. 8) and is beyond the scope of this chapter. However, prompt treatment with

intravenous antibiotics on arrival at the accident department reduces the incidence of this complication.

Tetanus

This is one of the most serious complications of wounds, but it is rare.

Bibliography

EDWARDS, C. C., SIMMONS, S. C., BROWNER, B. D. *et al.* (1988). Severe open tibial fractures: results treating 202 injuries with external fixation. *Clin. Orthop.*, **230**, 98–115.

GUSTILLO, R. B. & ANDERSON, J. T. (1976). Prevention of infection in the treatment of one thousand and twenty five open fractures of the long bones. *J. Bone Joint Surg.*, **58A**, 453.

GUSTILLO, R. B., MENDOZA, R. M. & WILLIAMS, D. N. (1984). Problems in the management of type III (severe) open fractures: a new classification of type III open fractures. *J. Trauma*, **24**, 742–6.

JOHANSEN, K., DAINES, M., HOWIE, T. *et al.* (1988). Objective criteria for amputation after lower extremity trauma. Paper presented at OTA Annual Meeting, Dallas, 27–29 October 1988.

KLEMM, K. W. & BÖRNER, M. (1986). Interlocking nailing of complex fractures of the femur and tibia. *Clin. Orthop.*, **212**, 89–100.

LLOWE, D. W. & HANSEN, S. T. (1988). Immediate nailing of open fractures of the femoral shaft. *J. Bone Joint Surg.*, **70A**, 812–19.

LLOYD, G. E. R., ed. (1978). In *Hippocratic Writings*, pp. 277–314. New York: Pelican Books.

PARÉ, A. (1634). In *The Workes of That Famous Chirurgion Ambrose Parey*, translated by Thomas Johnson, London.

PATZAKIS, M. F. (1982). Management of open fractures. *AAOS Instr. Course Lect.*, **31**, 62–4.

TSCHERNE, H. (1984). The management of open fractures. In *Fractures With Soft Tissue Injuries*, pp. 10–32. Eds. Tscherne, H. & Gotzen, L. Berlin: Springer-Verlag.

TSCHERNE, H. & OESTERN, H.-J. (1982). Die Klassifizierung des Weichteilschadens bei offenen und geschlossenen Frakturen. *Unfallheilkunde*, **85**, 111–15.

WANGENSTEEN, O. H. & WANGENSTEEN, S. D. (1978). In *The Rise of Surgery from Empiric Craft to Scientific Discipline*, pp. 3–64, 301–325, 407–452, 479–525. Minneapolis: University of Minnesota Press.

WEISS, S. J. (1989). Tissue destruction by neutrophils. *N. Engl. J. Med.*, **320**, 365–76.

YAREMCHUK, M. J., BRUMBACK, R. J., MANSON, P. N. *et al.* (1987). Acute and definitive management of traumatic osteocutaneous defects of the lower extremity. *Plast. Reconstr. Surg.*, **80**, 1–12.

27 Hand injury

I.W.R. ANDERSON and A. SEN

Department of Accident and Emergency Medicine, Victoria Infirmary, Glasgow, UK

Chapter plan

Introduction
Anatomy
Clinical examination
Investigations
Soft tissue injuries
Fractures and dislocations
Infections of the hand
Burns and cold injuries
Anaesthesia in hand injury
Wound care in hand injury
Specialist referral

INTRODUCTION

There have been few human achievements that have not depended on the ability of the hand to perform with versatility, ranging from movements of great intricacy to feats of great strength, each embodying that remarkable human capacity to create and also to destroy.

The hand is a highly sensitive organ in keeping with its role in searching out an environment which is frequently hostile and it is thus prone to injury. Large sections of the population, both in the developing and the developed world, depend on manual skills for their economic well-being and even survival. Injury leading to impairment in the use of the hand can condemn a person to a life of dependency.

In the UK, some 20% of all patients attending an accident and emergency (A&E) department have an injury distal to the wrist. Thus some 1.4 million patients seek hospital treatment for a hand injury each year.

The role of the clinician involved in treating these patients is to prevent further harm and arrange for the appropriate investigations, treatment and rehabilitation.

The aim should be to return the injured patient to as close a level of preinjury activity as possible, as soon as possible.

Only 5% of hand-injured patients require the skill of the 'expert' in diagnosis and treatment. The challenge is to blend a high index of suspicion for underlying injury with a low threshold of appropriate level of referral to a hand surgeon.

Pitfalls in hand injury

- Inadequate prevention
- Inadequate diagnosis
- Inadequate treatment
- Inadequate follow-up

ANATOMY

A working knowledge of hand anatomy is essential for accurate clinical diagnosis of injury.

Skin

Palmar skin is thick and tethered to the underlying palmar aponeurosis. Dorsal skin is lax and contains the veins and lymphatics in the loose areolar tissue plane. Hence swelling and oedema from whatever cause always involves the dorsum of the hand.

Bones

Three sets of bones constitute the skeleton of the hand. Eight carpal bones are arranged in two rows, proximal ones articulating with the distal radius to form the wrist joint. Distally they articulate with the five metacarpals. The thumb metacarpal articulates with the trapezium on a plane at right-angles to the rest. Hence the plane of abduction for the thumb is at 90° to the rest of the palm. The phalanges are short bones that articulate axially to form proximal and distal interphalangeal joints (PIPJ and DIPJ).

Muscles

In the *volar compartment*, the four fingers have a slip each of a long flexor, the flexor digitorum profundus (FDP), and a short flexor, the superficialis (FDS), inserted into the base of the distal and the middle phalanges, respectively. The thumb bears a separate long flexor tendon, flexor pollicis longus (FPL), attached to the base of the distal phalanx. The fibrous flexor sheath forms an osteofascial tunnel for these tendons in relation to the phalangeal bones and possesses intermittent thickenings known as pulleys.

The *intrinsic muscles* that make up the thenar eminence are abductor pollicis brevis (APB), opponens pollicis (OP), flexor pollicis brevis (FPB) and adductor pollicis (AP). The hypothenar eminence does not contain an adductor for the little finger metacarpophalangeal joint (MCPJ). The four lumbrical muscles are each attached to a long flexor tendon. There are three palmar and four dorsal interossei filling up the web spaces, of which the first dorsal alone constitutes the bulk of the first web space. The intrinsic muscles are responsible for intricate finger movements of the hand.

In the *dorsal compartment*, there are three long tendons of the thumb – extensor pollicis longus (EPL), extensor pollicis brevis (EPB) and abductor pollicis longus (APL) attached to the distal phalanx, proximal phalanx and the metacarpal, respectively. The four fingers have one extensor tendon, the extensor digitorum (ED), except for the index and the little finger which have an additional slip from extensor indicis and extensor digiti minimi respectively.

Tests

FDP should be tested by asking the patient to flex the terminal phalanx while holding the middle phalanx steady. FDS is tested by flexing one finger at the PIPJ while the others are held in extension. This is pure FDS action as FDP is a mass action muscle.

Function

The muscles act on various joints (Table 1).
- **P**almar interossei **AD**duct at finger MCPJ: **PAD**.
- **D**orsal interossei **AB**duct at finger MCPJ: **DAB**.

Table 1. *Joints of the hand*

Joint	Extension	Flexion	Range
DIPJ	Interossei	FDP	0–65°
PIPJ	Interossei	FDS	0–110°
MCPJ	ED	Lumbricals	0–85°
IPJ (thumb)	EPL	FPL	0–90°
MCPJ (thumb)	EPB	FPB	0–45°

See text for abbreviations.

- Opposition of thumb (thumb touching little finger tip) is a combined action of OP, APB and AP.
- The axis of finger abduction and adduction runs along the middle finger.

Nerve supply

The motor supply of the extrinsic and intrinsic muscles and the sensory supply is shared by the median, ulnar and radial nerves.

Motor nerves

All the long flexor tendons to the hand are supplied by the *median nerve* (C5–8, T1) except flexor carpi ulnaris and the medial (ulnar) two slips of flexor profundus to the little and ring fingers. These are supplied by the ulnar nerve. The median nerve enters the wrist under the flexor retinaculum deep and to the ulnar side of the flexor carpi radialis tendon. By asking the patient to hold the thumb in an abducted position (APB), the examiner can test the integrity of the motor division of the median nerve.

The *ulnar nerve* (C8, T1) lies superficial to the retinaculum in relation to the tendon of flexor carpi ulnaris, passes through the short canal of Guyon and supplies all the intrinsic muscles of the hand except some of the muscles of the thenar eminence, and the lumbricals to the index and middle fingers. Finger adduction (Card test) and adduction of the extended thumb (Froment's sign) are the means of testing ulnar nerve function.

The radial nerve (C5–8, T1), after supplying all the long muscles of the extensor compartment in the forearm, is purely sensory in the hand.

Sensory nerves

On the volar surface, the median nerve supplies the thenar eminence and the area including the thumb, index, middle and the radial half of the ring finger. The ulnar nerve supplies the hypothenar eminence and the area including the little finger and the ulnar side of ring finger. There can be variations in the overlap between the median and ulnar nerve in the hand.

The digital nerves originate in the palm under the palmar aponeurosis and lie close to the volar skin in their whole course along the side of the respective digit. Note that the volar nerves also supply the extensor surface of all the digits distal to the DIPJ crease.

On the dorsal surface, the radial nerve supplies the first web space and adjacent area, while the rest is supplied by the ulnar nerve.

Blood supply

The radial and ulnar arteries both enter the hand through the volar compartment. There is an extensive collateral supply to all parts of the hand from the superficial and deep palmar arches formed by these two vessels. The distal and proximal palmar creases correspond to these arches.

Lymphatic drainage

The lymph vessels start in the dorsum and travel along either side of the hand. The ulnar lymphatics reach the epitrochlear nodes first (these vessels are often visible in cases of lymphangitis) and terminate in the axilla.

CLINICAL EXAMINATION

The patient with hand trauma may present with multiple injuries. In such cases, life-threatening problems take priority and initial assessment and resuscitation should proceed according to the basic principles (ABC) of trauma management (see Chapter 17). The hand injury may be limb-threatening, but in only one circumstance (an incomplete division of a major vessel) can it be life-threatening. The hand is thus assessed during the secondary survey in a patient who has already been adequately resuscitated and stabilized.

The initial examination in the A&E department is the best opportunity for accurate diagnosis of any hand problem. The hand should be perceived as part of the whole patient and treated accordingly. An apparently 'minor' injury may cause much pain and apprehension.

The patient should be placed on a couch and the hand elevated. The examination should be conducted under good light and in a gentle, reassuring manner. Control of bleeding is important to allow proper inspection. This should be achieved by elevation and gentle direct pressure with a sterile dressing. The urge to 'clamp the bleeder' should be strongly resisted. The examination should follow a routine of LOOK – FEEL – MOVE – X-RAY (if necessary). The aim should be to identify all anatomical deficits.

It is important to note the normal hand posture at rest. When the hand is fully supinated, the wrist lies in 30° of extension and the MCPJs progressively flexed from 40° at the index to 70° at the little finger. This 'cascade effect' is lost in the presence of flexor tendon injuries. With the hand fully prone, loss of extension through tendon injury may cause drooping of the affected finger. In the presence of an open wound, more information is gained by covering the wound and examining the whole anatomy with the 'eye of a scanner'. The mechanism of injury is a useful guide to diagnosis as clinical signs may be misleading in certain injuries. A high index of suspicion is always necessary.

Injuries sustained by high-pressure injection, crushing in roller machines, etc., are associated with significant tissue damage and yet clinical signs are sparse. The integrity of structures should be tested individually, especially tendons. Nerves should be examined for motor and sensory deficit, often the first sign of injury being the absence of sweating over the cutaneous distribution of that nerve. Clinical diagnosis is frequently made all the more difficult by factors like alcohol or drug intoxication, alteration in conscious level, extremes of age and apprehension on the part of the patient.

Clinical findings are best documented according to tissue types (e.g. skin, tendon, nerve, etc). A sketch is of great help as part of clinical note-keeping.

INVESTIGATIONS

X-ray is the mainstay of diagnosis following clinical examination. Specific views should be requested rather than including the whole hand. Sophisticated imaging techniques like MRI (magnetic resonance imaging) are likely to play an increasingly major role in the future.

SOFT TISSUE INJURIES

These are the commonest form of hand injury. Rapid healing and complete return of function depend on precise diagnosis at the time of presentation. Failure to appreciate the nature of a wound may mean avoidable

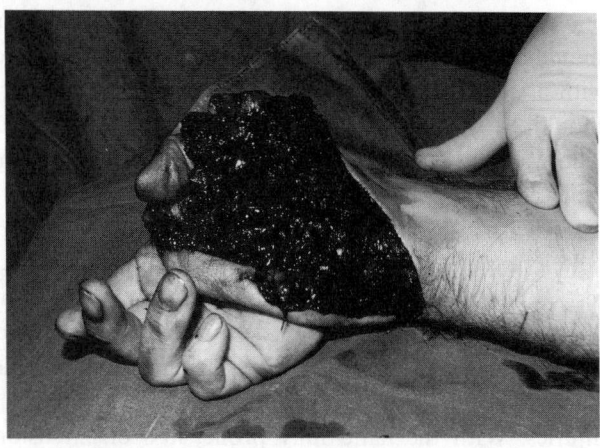

Fig. 1. Crush injury.

disability. Sound surgical principles of wound management apply to all hand wounds.

The mechanism of injury may be blunt, penetrating or a combination. Post-traumatic swelling of the hand is a constant finding and should be treated by high elevation. Following a period of rest, early mobilization helps prevent stiffness.

Blunt injury

This is universally painful. Tissue damage beneath the skin must be excluded clinically and radiologically. In the absence of deep injury, elevation and analgesia are all that are required.

Crush injury

This is usually caused by accidents involving industrial processes which may result in considerable energy transfer. The tissue damage may not be immediately obvious, yet in-patient treatment is almost always necessary to guard against compartment syndrome and to assess for nerve or vascular damage (Fig. 1).

Finger tip injuries

These are common and often occur in children. The wounds normally heal satisfactorily with conservative treatment. Examination may be difficult in the presence of pain which may be relived by a ring block at the outset. An associated terminal phalangeal fracture should not alter soft tissue management.

Subungual haematoma should be drained by trephining the nail, even in late presenters.

Partial avulsion of nail should be completed under a ring block. Any damage to the nail bed must be repaired by precision suturing with fine suture material (e.g. 6/0 nylon). Temporary replacement of the nail helps to splint the healing bed and prevent adhesions.

Pulp avulsion, when partial, is similarly repaired with care to appose the nail bed. Flap viability should be monitored.

Pulp loss is common in blunt injuries. Any loss smaller than 1 cm^2 in an adult may be treated conservatively if the terminal phalanx is not exposed. Even larger pulp defects involving exposed bone have been treated on a similar regime. All dressings should be non-adherent and changed at weekly intervals. Frequent changes are counter-productive. More complex tissue losses should be referred to a specialist for reconstruction.

Penetrating injury

According to the mechanism of injury, these wounds may be clean, lightly contaminated or contaminated. A meticulous clinical examination of the whole hand must be carried out to establish the extent of tissue damage. Gentle pressure with elevation should be used to control bleeding. The degree of contamination has an important bearing on any treatment plan. The possibility of a foreign body in the wound should be borne in mind and appropriate X-rays requested. Deeper penetration may not be apparent and, if suspected, can only be excluded by formal surgical exploration. Therefore referral to a hand surgeon should be early rather than late.

Incised wounds and lacerations

Clean, incised wounds and tidy lacerations of the skin and subcutaneous tissue may be sutured without tension using fine sutures (e.g. 5/0 nylon). Any contaminated wound should be thoroughly irrigated with sterile normal saline solution. All contaminated wounds and wounds with doubtful tissue viability should be left open for delayed primary closure. Antibiotics are only needed for spreading infection and gross contamination. Tetanus prophylaxis is relevant for all wounds.

Foreign bodies

Foreign bodies that are lodged in hand wounds are usually wooden splinters or glass. All glass will be shown on X-ray provided appropriate exposures are used. An X-ray or ultrasound scan may be helpful for localization.

A foreign body that is readily visible may be removed under a local anaesthetic. Attempts to remove deeply embedded foreign bodies should never be made in the A&E department under poor light and in a bloody operative field. Specialist referral is essential under these circumstances.

Tendon injuries

These should be suspected in all penetrating wounds overlying the route of a tendon. Division of a tendon should be identified by careful clinical examination of each. Early referral is essential for the best operative results.

Mallet finger

Mallet finger is a closed rupture of the insertion of terminal extensor slip into the distal phalanx. This may be associated with an avulsion fracture of the phalanx. The patient is unable to extend the flexed DIPJ – mallet deformity. The fracture may be confirmed by X-ray which is also essential to exclude a dislocation. Treatment consists of splintage of the DIPJ in extension for 6 weeks full time and a further 2 weeks at night only, even for late presentations. The mallet splint must allow free movement of the PIPJ.

Nerve injury

Injury to nerves is another possibility to be considered in all penetrating hand wounds. The median and ulnar nerves at the wrist and the volar digital nerves in the fingers are particularly susceptible. A high index of suspicion is needed to identify nerve damage which may not be evident initially because of temporary conduction of impulses across the extracellular gap. The initial presentation may be deceptive or misleading even in the most cooperative patient. Distal motor and sensory loss should be clearly documented and the patient referred for formal exploration and primary repair.

Other soft tissue injuries

Carpal tunnel syndrome

This results from compression of the median nerve under the flexor retinaculum. Blunt trauma, carpal fractures, rheumatoid arthritis, pregnancy, oedema etc., are the usual causes. The presenting features are wrist pain that is worse in the night and neurological deficit (sensory and later motor) in the median nerve distribution. Tinel's test and Phalen's test (exacerbation of sensory symptoms by passive wrist flexion) may be helpful. Specialist referral is needed for confirmation of the diagnosis and decompression.

Ring avulsion injuries

These injuries may produce simple contusion or major tissue avulsion requiring replantation. Assessment of circulatory impairment is often difficult. Local dressing and elevation is adequate for the simple injury. Most others need to be discussed with a specialist who may consider a microvascular surgical procedure. This injury frequently occurs in the ring finger of a young female patient and every effort should be made to refer such a patient to an appropriate specialist to salvage the finger (Figs 2 and 3).

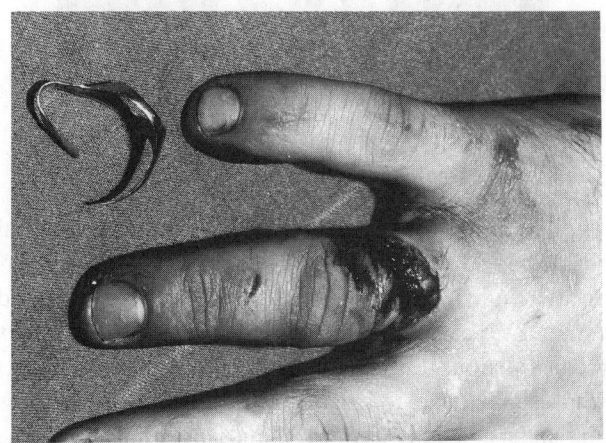

Fig. 2. Ring degloving injury.

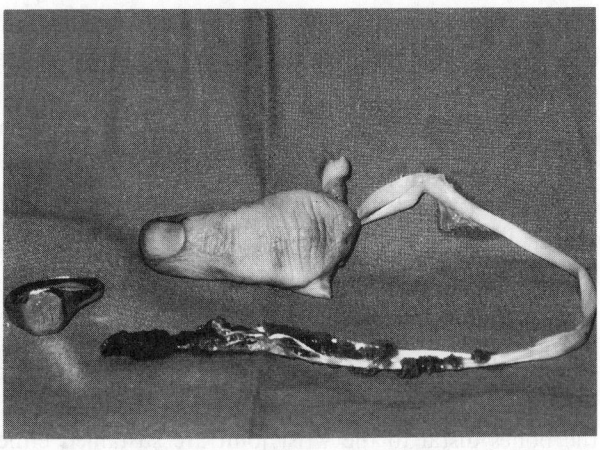

Fig. 3. Ring degloving injury.

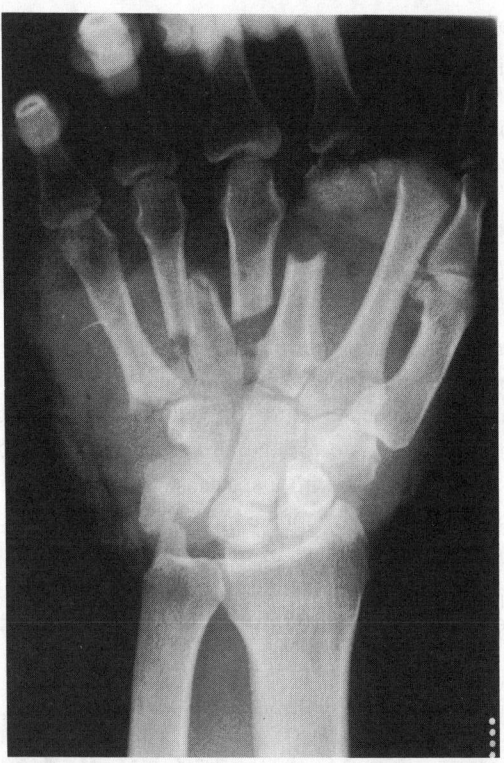

Fig. 4. Mutilating hand injury caused by roller machine.

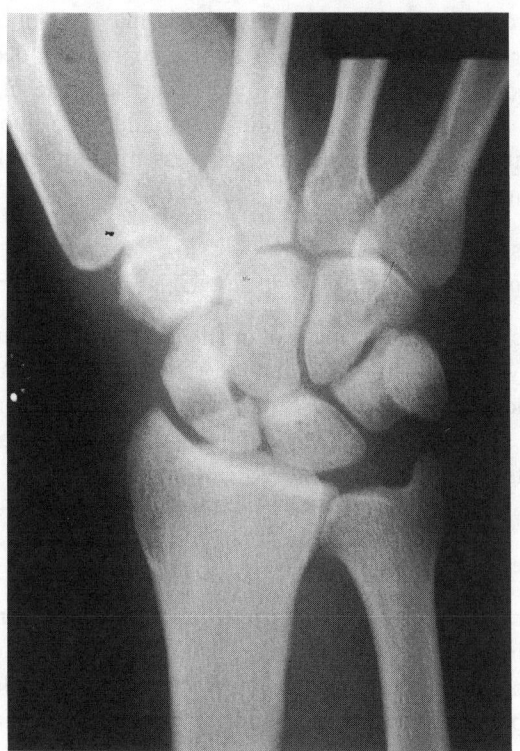

Fig. 5. Scaphoid fracture – non-union.

The mutilated hand

Mutilation usually results from blast injuries, industrial accidents and severe ripping forces. The external appearances are obvious and distressing. The services of a hand expert are necessary for limb salvage and complex reconstruction. It is important to reassure these patients who usually have an isolated injury, are fully conscious and understandably terrified. Clinical assessment of tissue viability may be misleading in these situations. The patient should receive adequate intravenous analgesia. The wound should be covered with a sterile dressing and not be exposed repeatedly for inspection. The limb should be elevated prior to X-ray and specialist referral (Fig. 4).

Extensive degloving injuries should be treated in the same manner. These commonly involve distally based flaps, characteristically do not bleed briskly and will require extensive reconstructive surgery.

FRACTURES AND DISLOCATIONS

Fractures around the wrist involving forearm bones are discussed in Chapter 28. Fractures and dislocations of the bones distal to the wrist joint are sustained either by direct blows or falls on the outstretched hand.

The mechanism of injury and clinical localization of bony tenderness help determine the relevant part to be X-rayed. Although manipulation is not a common requirement in these injuries, follow-up and physiotherapy play a vital role.

Open bone and joint injuries need early debridement under an anaesthetic and operative fixation by a specialist.

Scaphoid fracture

These are usually caused by a fall on the outstretched hand or occasionally from a blow. Tenderness is localized to the anatomical snuffbox and also the dorsal and volar aspects of the scaphoid. This injury should be suspected, even in the present of minimal signs, and proper 'scaphoid views' requested. A normal X-ray does not rule out a fracture, although most are evident with hindsight (Fig. 5). These patients should be referred for follow-up so that further X-rays or a bone scan may be considered. A temporary wrist support should be applied.

Lunate and perilunate dislocation

This may easily be missed in cases of 'wrist sprain'. The important clue is pain out of proportion to the clinical findings. The lateral wrist radiograph is diagnostic and should be examined carefully. Delayed diagnosis may be associated with median nerve compression in the carpal tunnel. Prompt referral is needed for open reduction under anaesthesia. There is sometimes an associated scaphoid fracture.

Carpal bone fractures other than simple avulsions

These are uncommon and can usually be treated in a neutral Colles-type plaster. Complex carpal fractures and dislocations can occur and should be referred to a specialist.

Metacarpal fractures

These are usually caused by punching, and the neck of the little finger metacarpal is the commonest site of injury. Most of these fractures are stable and should be rested (e.g. in a volar splint) for 2 weeks. Any malrotation must be corrected. Operative fixation is required for unstable fractures. Open metacarpal fractures have an evil reputation for infective complications and long-term problems. Aggressive surgical treatment of these injuries is required.

Metacarpophalangeal dislocations

These result from a hyperextension force and should be reduced under metacarpal block. The hand should be rested in a volar splint (in the rest position) for a short time before mobilizing.

Phalangeal fractures

These are caused by either direct trauma or a twisting force. Distal phalangeal fractures are treated for the associated soft tissue injury. A ring block offers good analgesia in these patients. Both middle and proximal phalangeal fractures are potentially unstable and carry risks of rotatory or angulatory malunion. Specialist referral is advisable.

Interphalangeal dislocations

These are usually obvious at presentation and should be reduced by traction under a ring block. Rest in neighbour strapping followed by mobilization is all that is required. If the volar plate is disrupted in PIPJ dislocation, reduction may be difficult. One attempt at reduction is permissible and, if unsuccessful, these injuries must be referred directly to a specialist.

Thumb metacarpal fractures

These may involve the shaft or the base, including the carpometacarpal joint (Bennett fracture). They are potentially unstable and need manipulation and plastering or internal fixation under regional or general anaesthesia. Specialist advice must be sought.

Thumb metacarpophalangeal injuries

These usually involve an abduction force which disrupts the ulnar collateral ligament of the MCPJ with or without a small avulsion fracture of the base of proximal phalanx. The MCPJ is unstable on abduction stress and the patient should be referred for either splintage or operative repair of the ligament.

Phalangeal fractures (thumb)

These are treated in the same way as other phalangeal injuries.

Traumatic amputations

These are not common. Amputations through the middle of the distal phalanx (base of nail) or those that are excessively mutilated may not be suitable for replantation. Specialist referral is necessary for advice and early skin cover. The amputated part and the hand must be X-rayed prior to referral. Factors influencing the need for replantation are occupation, dominance, type of amputation, complexity of fractures, etc. Clean-cut amputations fare better. The patient should be transported to the nearest microvascular facility with the amputated digit in saline-moistened gauze in a plastic bag maintained at 4°C on ice. The patient must be discussed on a 'doctor to doctor' basis prior to referral.

INFECTIONS OF THE HAND

Fluctuation is a late sign.

Most hand infections resolve completely with adequate treatment. Many start as trivial infections, but have the potential to cause major disability if improperly diagnosed and treated. Foreign bodies, penetrating injuries and neglected wounds are the usual cause. Early diagnosis of a collection of pus is essential. Important principles of treatment are adequate drainage, rest in a splint and timely mobilization.

All procedures should be carried out under effective local, regional or general anaesthesia. Antibiotics are infrequently necessary and should be reserved for cases of cellulitis or lymphangitis and systemic infection. The predominant organism is *Staphylococcus aureus*, which is susceptible to penicillinase-resistant antibiotics.

Paronychia

This is infection of the nail fold and surrounding tissues and is common in nail biters. In advanced cases, pus may cause the nail to float. Under a ring block, the pus should be drained through a narrow 1 cm ellipse. The nail usually needs removal for effective drainage. The hand should be elevated. Antibiotics are not required in the absence of ascending infection or systemic upset.

Pulp space infection

This is extremely painful as pus accumulates in the compact interstices of the terminal pulp space between the fibrous septa. The pus should be drained under a ring block through an adequate pulp incision. Antibiotics are not required for local infection. If neglected, these infections may cause troublesome osteitis of the terminal phalanx (Fig. 6).

Web space infection

This usually results from a penetrating wound and may spread to the palm unless drained early. It causes separation of the web space and dorsal oedema. It is best drained by a specialist under anaesthetic and tourniquet.

Palmar infections

These are fortunately rare and result from direct penetrating injury or spread from distal sites. There is extensive dorsal oedema and pain. The patient is often toxic and should be referred to the specialist urgently.

Tendon sheath infections

These are rare nowadays but cause serious problems of disability if the diagnosis is delayed. The causative penetrating injury on the volar aspect of the fingers

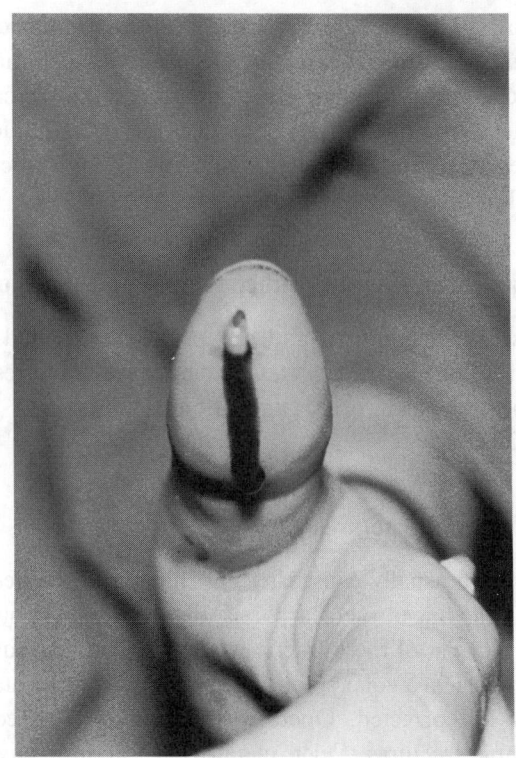

Fig. 6. Pulp space infection.

may easily be overlooked. Suppuration in the synovial sheath causes pain and swelling over the whole finger, which is held in a flexed posture. Passive finger extension is extremely painful. Tenderness may be present proximally in the palm with involvement of the whole sheath (Kanavel's sign). Immediate specialist referral is required for drainage and irrigation of the tendon sheath (Fig. 7).

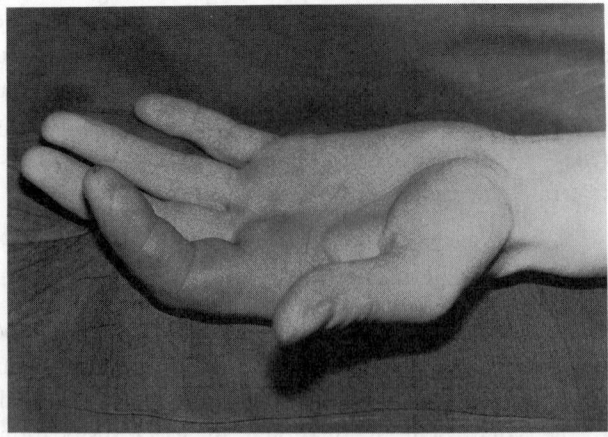

Fig. 7. Flexor sheath infection. Note passive flexed position of finger.

INADEQUATE INCISION

under

INADEQUATE ANAESTHESIA

produces

INADEQUATE DRAINAGE

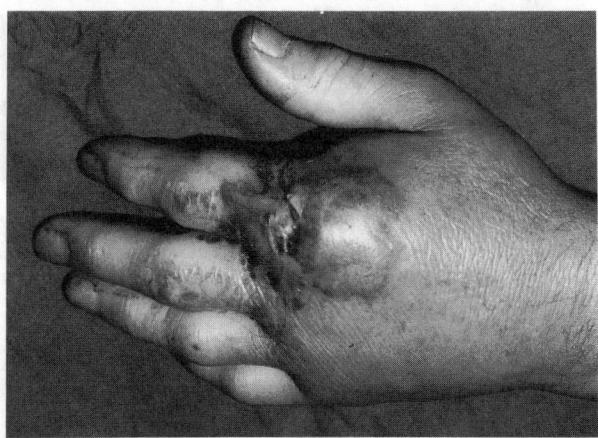

Fig. 9. Neglected human bite over knuckle of index finger.

High-pressure injection

This injury is caused by hydraulic or air-pressured devices commonly used in industry. The patient should be asked about the nature of the industrial process and the pressure under which the air or the hydraulic fluid operates.

Initial symptoms may be very few and the wound may look innocuous. However, extensive tissue damage and infection will follow if the injury is not identified and treated by early surgical exploration and rigorous debridement. An X-ray may reveal radio-opaque material in the tissue planes. All cases must be referred to the specialist urgently (Fig. 8).

Bites

Human bites are usually sustained on the knuckles following a punch injury. The patient may be circumspect about the mechanism of injury. The wound is usually inoculated with *Bacteroides* and carries a high risk of cellulitis or septic arthritis of the MCPJ. Treatment should include thorough wound debridement under

anaesthetic and a course of prophylactic broad-spectrum antibiotics including metronidazole. Suturing such wounds is contraindicated. These injuries must be referred to the specialist (Fig. 9). Penetrating wounds sustained by simple mechanisms such as falls also pose a risk of septic arthritis.

Animal bites involve deeper tissues and should be treated on similar lines. The likely organism is *Pasteurella multocida*, so the choice of antibiotic is penicillin. Butchers and fishmongers are at risk of developing serious hand infections in relatively trivial wounds due to contamination from carcasses and delay in seeking treatment. The principles of wound management are the same and these cases will require appropriate antibiotics guided by the results of wound swab culture.

Cellulitis and lymphangitis

These complications should be identified early from findings of erythema, tenderness and red streaks. There is usually a wound of entry. Treatment includes rest in a volar splint with the MCPJs flexed and the IPJs extended, elevation and appropriate antibiotics. These cases are best treated in hospital.

Pyogenic granuloma

These arise from exuberant granulation in a chronic wound. They cause contact bleeding and pain. Treatment is silver nitrate cautery or excision under local anaesthetic if possible. The diagnosis must be confirmed histologically and the possibility of squamous cell carcinoma or melanoma ruled out (Fig. 10).

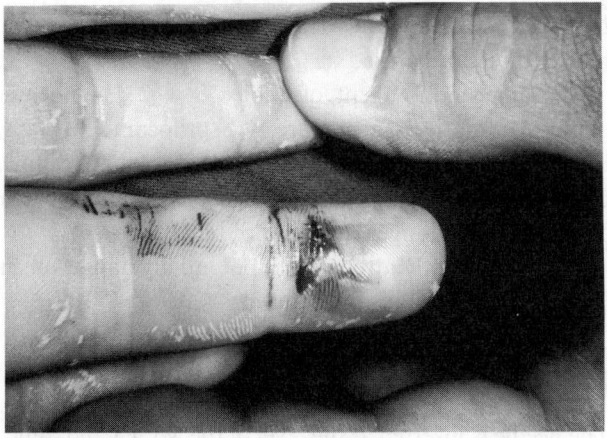

Fig. 8. Innocuous entry wound of high-pressure injection injury.

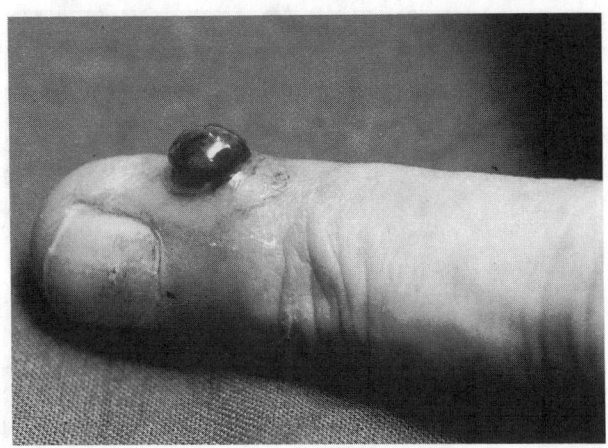

Fig. 10. Pyogenic granuloma.

BURNS AND COLD INJURIES (see also Chapter 34)

Its very function makes the hand prone to thermal injury. Treatment is aimed at pain relief and early return of function. The usual causative agents are hot water (scald), cooking fat or flame, and these may cause either partial or full-thickness burns. The need for specialist referral lies in the assessment of depth, tissue viability and rehabilitation. Immediate cooling with water provides good analgesia and reduces damage. Small areas of superficial burn may be treated by non-adherent dressing (e.g. paraffin gauze) and elevation. Early mobilization is vitally important (particularly with volar injuries) and antiseptic bags facilitate this. Most hand burns should be referred to a specialist for evaluation and possible in-patient treatment (Fig. 11).

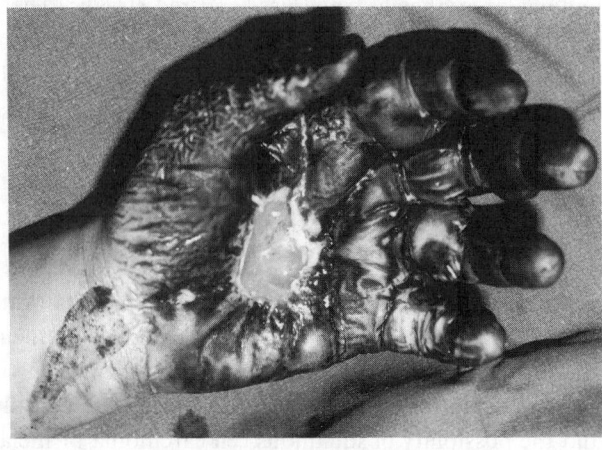

Fig. 11. 'Flash burn'.

Chemical burns

These usually result from industrial accidents with corrosive substances. The hand should be copiously irrigated with water and antidotes are best avoided. Prediction of depth may be difficult at the initial presentation, particularly with alkali which binds to tissues and continues to act. Specialist advice should be sought as the patients usually required hospital admission.

Electrical burns

These may be caused by direct passage of the current or the flash. The former causes more damage and the entry and exit points are most susceptible. Every structure in the path of the current may be damaged. High-voltage (>1000 V) injuries inflict extensive tissue coagulation. Muscle damage can give rise to myoglobinuria. Specialist referral is essential for contact burns (see also Chapter 36).

Frostbite

This causes intracellular crystallization and microvascular thrombosis leading to gangrene. Less severe cold injuries cause pain, swelling and blistering of the skin. The extent of tissue damage caused by cold is similar to that caused by heat. Tissues of apparently doubtful viability can sometimes survive and dumbfound the gloomiest of pundits. Extensive frostbite injuries require specialist care (see also Chapter 38).

ANAESTHESIA IN HAND INJURY

Most of the procedures required for hand injuries and infection presenting to the A&E department may adequately be carried out under local anaesthesia. It is useful to have a working knowledge of some of the regional blocks that can be used.

The anaesthetic agent of choice is 1–2% lignocaine plain. Alternative agents are 4% prilocaine or 0.5% bupivacaine. A combination agent using equal volumes of 1% lignocaine and 0.5% bupivacaine is quite useful and provides a longer duration of block.

Lignocaine with adrenaline is potentially dangerous in the hand and should not be used.

Ring block

The needle is inserted at the level of the MCPJ and aimed towards the volar surface at a 45° angle. The anaesthetic

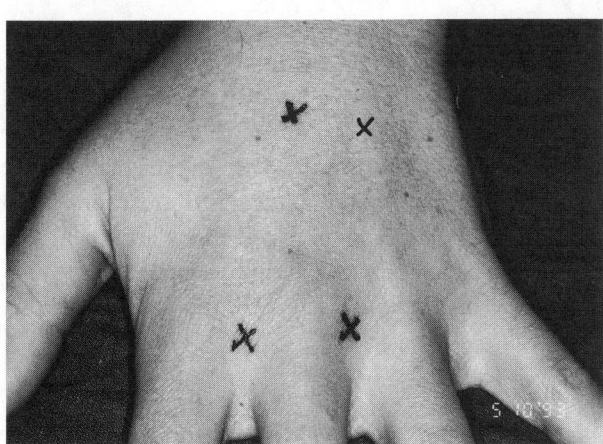

Fig. 12. Surface marking for digital and metacarpal block.

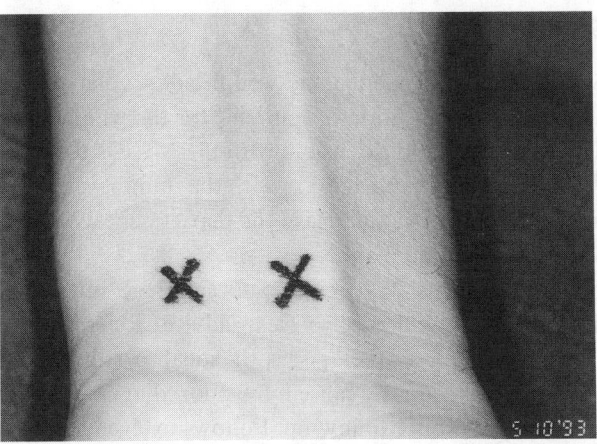

Fig. 13. Surface marking for wrist block (median and ulnar nerves).

agent is deposited nearer the volar aspect to block the digital nerve along with some dorsal infiltration. This provides good anaesthesia from the MCPJ distally. The volume required is about 3 ml.

Metacarpal block

This provides more proximal anaesthesia for procedures on the web spaces. The needle is introduced at the apex of each web space vertically from dorsal surface. The anaesthetic is injected as close to the volar surface as possible with some dorsal infiltration. The average volume of anaesthetic required is about 6 ml (Fig. 12).

Wrist block

This anaesthetizes virtually the whole hand distal to the wrist and is aimed at the three nerves at this level.

Median nerve

The needle is aimed at the gap between the two tendons of flexor carpi radialis and palmaris longus on the proximal wrist crease. The anaesthetic should be injected when paraesthesia is elicited in the median nerve distribution. Intraneuronal injection causes nerve damage.

Ulnar nerve

The needle is inserted in the gap between the ulnar artery and the flexor carpi ulnaris tendon and should evoke a similar paraesthesia when in contact with the nerve (Fig 13).

Radial nerve

The nerve is blocked over a wide area on the dorsum of the wrist extending from the radial styloid process in an ulnar direction.

Axillary and supraclavicular brachial plexus

These blocks are best carried out in theatre by a specialist.

WOUND CARE IN HAND INJURY

Examination of the injured hand and all procedures should be gentle and unhurried. Adequate analgesia must be provided during and after all treatment and this may involve using various regional blocks. Normal saline should be used copiously for irrigation of wounds. This can be delivered in a jet from a needle mounted on a syringe, taking care to irrigate and not to infiltrate tissue. Use of hydrogen peroxide should be restricted to contaminated wounds of small surface area.

Suturing should be done without tension and follow skin creases where possible. Delicate instruments and fine suture material (e.g. 5/0 nylon) should be used. Sutures should not invert skin edges. Contaminated wounds or those containing tissue of doubtful viability must not be sutured but should be left open for delayed closure. More harm is often done by injudicious attempts to close wounds. Dressings should have a non-adherent layer of tulle-gras or silicone-impregnated tulle in contact with the wound, covered with absorbent gauze. Bandages should not cause circumferential compression.

Splintage

Splints should be padded and well-fitted. A volar plaster slab offers the best form of splintage for the whole hand. The wrist is held in extension, with the MCPJs flexed to 90°, the IPJs in near extension with the thumb web space open. No patient should leave the department without a sling to elevate the hand.

Those patients who require no splintage but active movements should receive clear advice. Referral to a trained hand physiotherapist is the ideal. A stiff hand is an iatrogenic disease caused by poor diagnosis, poor treatment and poor follow-up. Follow-up, even for what might appear to be a minor problem, should be supervised in every case by a competent clinician. Most hand morbidity is caused by factors other than the severity of the initial injury.

The need for antibiotics, tetanus toxoid and hepatitis B prophylaxis should be considered in every patient and not be overlooked.

SPECIALIST REFERRAL

Hand surgery has become a speciality in its own right. Every A&E department should have access to a local or regional hand service. Despite the fact that a small number of hand injuries require the services of a hand specialist, any hand problem presenting to an A&E department should receive the best possible treatment.

Clinicians in any A&E department should avail themselves of that advice and assistance by adopting a low threshold of referral. Discussion over the phone should paint a clear picture of the injury to the specialist. The required information from the A&E doctor includes the mechanism of injury, the patient's occupation, hand dominance, clinical and X-ray findings together with details of the preliminary treatment. Full functional recovery is often the outcome of early and appropriate referral.

Bibliography

AMERICAN SOCIETY FOR SURGERY OF THE HAND (1983). *The Hand – Examination and Diagnosis*, 2nd edn. New York: Churchill Livingstone.

BURKE, F.D., McGROUTHER, D.A. & SMITH, P.J. (1990). *Principles of Hand Surgery*. Edinburgh: Churchill Livingstone.

GREEN, D.P. & HOTCHKISS, R.N. (1993). *Operative Hand Surgery*, 3rd edn. New York: Churchill Livingstone.

LISTER, G. (1984). *The Hand – Diagnosis and Indication*, 2nd edn. Edinburgh: Churchill Livingstone.

McMINN, R.M.H., HUTCHINGS, R.T., PEGINGTON, J. *et al.* (1993). *A Colour Atlas of Human Anatomy*, 3rd edn. London: Wolfe Publishing.

MENNEN, U. & WIESE, A. (1993). Fingertip injuries: management with semi-occlusive dressing. *J. Hand Surg.*, **18B**, 416–22.

WARDROPE, J. & SMITH, J.A.R. (1992). *The Management of Wounds and Burns*. Oxford: Oxford University Press.

28 Upper limb injuries

K.M. WILLETT

Trauma Service, John Radcliffe Hospital, Oxford, UK

Chapter plan

Scapular injuries

Sternoclavicular joint injuries

Fractures of the clavicle

Acromioclavicular dislocations and fractures at the lateral
   end of the clavicle

Scapulothoracic dissociation

Fractures of the proximal humerus

Dislocations of the shoulder

Fractures of the humeral shaft

Fractures of the distal humerus

Elbow dislocation

Fractures of the radius and ulna at the elbow

Fractures of the forearm bones

Fractures of the distal radius

Conclusions

SCAPULAR FRACTURES

Fracture of the scapula is an uncommon injury and represents less than 1% of all fractures. The body of the scapula is embedded in a large muscle mass and is relatively protected. Fractures of the body of the scapula are seen after high-energy vehicular trauma or crushing injuries. They are frequently associated with injuries of the cervical spine, ipsilateral limb, thorax and hips and may be overlooked in a seriously injured patient. Fracture displacement, despite the force, is usually minimal because of the soft tissue envelope and accordingly healing is usually uncomplicated. Fractures of the acromion may occur following a direct blow. The coracoid process may fracture across its base or be avulsed at the tip. Occasionally traumatic dislocation of the shoulder may be associated with a glenoid rim fracture and, if large, the rim fragment may require internal fixation to restore stability following reduction of the dislocation.

Treatment

For most scapular fractures, simple support of the upper limb in a broad arm sling and appropriate analgesia is appropriate initially. As soon as pain and swelling permit (after 3–5 days), pendulum exercises and then active assisted movement should be encouraged. Hand, wrist and elbow exercises should be promoted from the outset. Fracture healing is achieved by 6–8 weeks and maximum function can be expected by 3–4 months. Many patients require admission because of associated injuries. Surgical stabilization is only necessary when soft tissue damage is severe or there are displaced fractures of the glenoid fossa, anatomical neck or spine of the scapula such that function will not be restored by conservative measures.

STERNOCLAVICULAR JOINT INJURIES

Injuries to the sternoclavicular joint are very uncommon and usually occur as a result of direct violence to the clavicle or a blow to the point of the shoulder. The patient frequently presents with intense local pain and tenderness but deformity may not be obvious. The commonest injury is a mild anterior subluxation of the clavicle presenting as a tender prominence at the sternoclavicular joint and asymmetry of the medial ends of the clavicles. The diagnosis is a clinical one as plain radiographs are not helpful, and either tomography or CT (computed tomography) scanning is necessary to determine the extent of displacement. Rare, but potentially more serious, is the posterior dislocation where the medial end of the clavicle passes behind the sternum and may impinge on the subjacent structures occupying the thoracic inlet. This injury may present with dyspnoea, dysphagia or signs of vascular compression.

Treatment

The common mild anterior subluxation requires no immediate intervention and may be adequately managed conservatively; the displacement and prominence are accepted and no attempt at reduction is necessary. Simple support with a broad arm sling and body bandage for 3 weeks followed by a graduated programme of mobilization and avoidance of heavy lifting for 8 weeks, usually results in a return to full function. Gross posterior displacement with compression symptoms in the thoracic inlet may require immediate reduction and this should be performed under general anaesthesia. The patient should be positioned supine with a large sand bag placed between the scapulae and traction is applied to both shoulders with the arm abducted and extended. The use of pointed bone forceps carefully applied percutaneously to the medial end of the clavicle will obtain good purchase and facilitate a reduction. Irreducible dislocations are rare and open reduction by an experienced surgeon will then be necessary.

FRACTURES OF THE CLAVICLE

Most clavicle fractures result from a fall on the outstretched hand. Less commonly the mechanism may be direct trauma. The force transmitted up the arm usually results in a fracture of the clavicle and displacement of the fracture ends; the proximal fragment is held up by the pull of the sternocleidomastoid muscle while the distal fragment is depressed by the weight of the upper limb. Overlap of the fragments is normal with shortening of the anterior strut of the shoulder girdle. With greater violence the fracture pattern may be more complex and penetration of the overlying muscle, fascia and occasionally skin may occur.

Diagnosis

The pain is localized to the fracture site where there is marked tenderness at presentation. There may be obvious deformity with local swelling and the patient usually supports the ipsilateral elbow with the opposite arm.

Neurovascular complications are surprisingly rare considering the proximity of the subclavian bundle but rarity should not distance the recognized association with brachial plexus injuries and scapulothoracic dissociation (see later).

Radiographs

A simple anteroposterior radiograph is usually adequate to confirm most fractures. Fractures of the distal end of the clavicle will be discussed with injuries to the acromioclavicular joint.

Treatment

Simple support of the arm to relieve its weight on the disrupted shoulder girdle affords considerable pain relief in this injury. This is best achieved with a broad arm sling which may be supplemented by a body bandage or stocking. Union is usually rapid and the functional recovery and remodelling potential even in adults make exhaustive efforts at maintaining reduction unnecessary. There is no indication for surgical stabilization of isolated closed fractures of the clavicle. Historically, numerous methods have been described to try to restore clavicle length and correct the scapular protraction. Figure-of-eight bandaging, axillary loops and strapping have been tried. These methods, however, are ineffective in achieving a reduction and require such frequent adjustment and attention to maintain alignment as to make them impractical. Despite careful padding, these methods involve application of local pressure and may compromise axillary structures and cause skin breakdown. They are poorly tolerated by patients, particularly the elderly. The excellent functional results in most patients after simple supporting measures question the need for more aggressive treatment. The administration of simple analgesia and the use of a broad arm sling for 3 weeks followed by gentle mobilization within the limits of comfort is standard treatment. Clavicle fractures are seen frequently in the elderly and the duration of arm immobilization should then be minimized to 1 week or less in order to prevent glenohumeral joint stiffness.

Fracture union may be anticipated in 6–10 weeks. The non-union rate for this fracture has been estimated at 1–5% with a greater incidence in the high-energy fracture group. Acceptance of the fracture overlap means that malunion is normal and the patient should be warned from the outset of a prominence at the fracture site. Anxiety to obtain a better cosmetic result should not be seen as an indication for surgical treatment. A broad surgical scar is far more unsightly.

Indications for surgery

Open reduction and internal fixation is only indicated for an open fracture of the clavicle, or when an associated vascular repair is necessary. Occasionally a bone spike or fracture fragment may threaten to breach the overlying skin. Support of the weight of the limb in a broad arm sling and immobilization with a body bandage is usually sufficient to maintain skin integrity. Rarely an imminent breach of the skin will require reduction of the fracture and stabilization.

ACROMIOCLAVICULAR DISLOCATIONS AND FRACTURES AT THE LATERAL END OF THE CLAVICLE

A discussion of the management of acute injury to the acromioclavicular joint must be considered in the light of anatomical and biomechanical factors.

Disruption of the acromioclavicular joint usually occurs as a result of a direct blow to the point of the shoulder. This frequently follows an unrestrained fall from a bicycle or in sport. The force depresses the acromion (scapula) and the clavicle by way of the acromioclavicular joint and the coracoclavicular ligaments. The integrity of the joint will be maintained until the clavicle strikes the first rib impeding any further descent. Depending on the continued application of force, the acromioclavicular joint will disrupt, followed by the conoid and trapezoid (coracoclavicular) ligaments.

Diagnosis

The patient usually has a clear recollection of the mechanism of injury and can accurately localize the injury. However, pain and disability may be such that all shoulder movement is inhibited and the patient's awareness of something displaced is misinterpreted as a glenohumeral dislocation by the unwary. The patient is best examined standing or sitting with the arms dependent. There may be obvious deformity with prominence of the outer end of the clavicle. This deformity may be masked by muscle spasm and swelling in the acute phase. Tenderness is usually localized to the acromioclavicular joint and to the anterior part of the shoulder. Shoulder movements are painful and there is usually a restriction of active movement, particularly in abduction. In the event of a fracture in the lateral third of the clavicle, crepitus may be palpable on movement.

Within the spectrum of joint disruption, the most minor is that of acromioclavicular sprain. In this circumstance, the damage is confined to the acromioclavicular ligaments, the clavicle remains in contact with the acromion and the coracoclavicular ligaments are intact. There may be no significant deformity and the only finding is of tenderness along the joint line. Subluxation of the joint may accompany acromioclavicular ligament disruption, even in the presence of intact coracoclavicular ligaments. This subluxation may be confirmed by downward pressure on the clavicle while the examiner's opposite hand supports the ipsilateral elbow. The joint deformity will be felt to reduce and then recur when the arm is left dependent.

Complete disruption of the scapuloclavicular structures with tearing of the acromioclavicular and coracoclavicular ligaments results in marked and persistent displacement. There is a clinically palpable and usually visible deformity with an apparent loss of shoulder height and prominence of the distal third of the clavicle. Confirmation of dislocation of the acromioclavicular joint can be made by flexing and extending the shoulder with the arm abducted to 90°. Careful palpation of the acromioclavicular joint during this manoeuvre will confirm that the distal clavicle does not follow the excursion of the acromion. Other patterns of anatomical distortion such as loss of the prominence of the lateral clavicle or more obvious posterior displacement suggests one of the rarer acromioclavicular disolocations (see below).

Radiographs

Accurate diagnosis of injuries to the acromioclavicular joint requires specific instructions for the radiographer. An anteroposterior projection should be centred on the joint and in the majority of cases radiographic evidence of displacement is obvious. Confirmation of minor subluxation may be obtained on the same projection by including both shoulders with a weight attached to each hand. The weight will exaggerate any deformity; the information obtained is unlikely to change management and is therefore of dubious value. This investigation should not be ordered routinely as it is extremely painful for a patient who has a clinically obvious joint disruption. Oblique and lateral projections will be necessary to confirm the rare posterior or inferolateral dislocations of the lateral end of the clavicle.

Fractures of the lateral end of the clavicle

Identification on a radiograph of a fracture of the lateral third of the clavicle should be interpreted as part of the spectrum of acromioclavicular joint complex injury. The distal clavicle is normally under a balanced load between the inferior pull of the coracoclavicular ligament complex and the acriomoclavicular joint capsule. In opposition, elevating the clavicle are the stronger upward forces of the trapezius and sternocleidomastoid muscles. The location of the fracture and its relative displacement forms the basis of its classification. Fractures lateral to the coracoclavicular ligament complex are stable, displace little and usually heal without complication. A more complex injury pattern occurs when the fracture (usually oblique) separates the lateral third of the clavicle with an intact acromioclavicular joint from the coracoclavicular ligament complex. For management purposes these should be considered as the complete (type III) acromioclavicular joint disruption.

Treatment of acute acromioclavicular injuries

Immediate care of the injury requires careful assessment to exclude associated neurovascular injuries and the application of a supportive broad arm sling. It is essential that the weight of the arm is relieved for pain relief.

There are few areas in orthopaedic trauma that are more contentious than the definitive management of acromioclavicular joint dislocation. The controversy has resulted from two distinct management philosophies but neither demonstrates convincing evidence of a better outcome. For acromioclavicular joint strain (type I) and the acromioclavicular joint subluxation with intact coracoclavicular ligaments (type II), there is general agreement that they should be treated conservatively. A supporting sling should be worn for 3–6 weeks depending on the severity of the injury, preferably under clothing as this will increase compliance and shoulder immobilization. Symptoms rapidly settle. Joint stiffness is rare (except in the elderly) and physiotherapy is rarely necessary. Numerous modifications of the simple sling have been developed, many with a shoulder strap which crosses the involved clavicle in an attempt to apply counter-pressure to reduce the subluxation. This is an improvement on the historical adhesive tape bandage applied in a similar fashion which nearly always resulted in skin maceration. However, there is little evidence to suggest that any functional or cosmetic improvement is achieved with the use of these modified slings, braces or harnesses. The more sophisticated the immobilization the greater is the requirement for regular supervision and adjustment, and both skin and nerve compression symptoms have been recorded. Usually, a good restoration of movement and shoulder strength is achieved provided that the muscle envelope of deltoid and trapezius remains intact. The fibrous union which occurs across the unreduced joint inevitably interferes with the normal biomechanics of shoulder function and may account for persisting pain in a small proportion of patients. The deformity may be obvious but is usually tolerated well in the presence of good function.

Many types of surgical treatment have been described in the orthopaedic literature. Open techniques are either directed at transfixing the acromioclavicular joint with wires or pins, or indirect reduction by fixation of the clavicle to the coracoid process using screws or implanted materials such as ligament substitutes. Many of these surgical procedures require a long period of immobilization equal to or longer than conservative management. Frequently, a second procedure to remove implanted metal is necessary. On current knowledge, operative management is difficult to support except for rare inferior or posterior clavicular dislocations.

For the minority of patients with untreated acromioclavicular joint dislocations who have persisting disability, successful late surgical procedures involving resection of the lateral end of the clavicle are available.

SCAPULOTHORACIC DISSOCIATION

Scapulothoracic dissociation is a rare injury resulting from very severe high-energy trauma. Previously unrecognized, this injury may be missed or underestimated. It represents a closed forequarter amputation and is the result of a severe traction injury to the shoulder girdle with partial or complete separation of the limb and scapula from the torso.

The diagnosis should be prompted by the massive soft tissue swelling that develops around the shoulder girdle, frequently coupled with a brachial plexus lesion and vascular injury. It is a complex injury and the neurovascular disruptions are frequently concealed. The initial chest X-ray may reveal lateral displacement of the scapula (commonly associated with disruption of the acromioclavicular joint or sternoclavicular joint, or clavicle fracture). In most cases there is unusually wide displacement at these sites. Life-threatening haemorrhage may occur and immediate arteriography is recommended followed by appropriate vascular repair. Amputation may prove necessary.

Even less frequent is the intrathoracic dislocation of the scapula in which the inferior angle of the scapula becomes impaled between two ribs. Direct manipulation of the scapula is necessary under general anaesthesia.

FRACTURES OF THE PROXIMAL HUMERUS

Anatomy and biomechanics of the shoulder joint

To understand the pathology that results from fracture and dislocation in the proximal humerus and shoulder joint, the normal shoulder anatomy and function must be understood. The glenohumeral joint has the greatest range of movement of any joint in the human skeleton. The maintenance of stability in such a joint is therefore complex and is achieved by a combination of the encompassing rotator cuff muscles (subscapularis, supraspinatus, infraspinatus and teres minor) and the glenohumeral ligaments. The latter represent condensations in the capsule of the shoulder joint passing as restricting bands from the humeral neck to the glenoid rim and labrum. It has been estimated that only 25% of the articular surface of the relatively large humeral head is in contact with the glenoid at any one time. The rotator cuff stretches over the large spherical head and is inserted beyond its equator. This anatomical arrangement produces the biomechanical advantage necessary to produce the wide range of movement. In combination with the deltoid muscle and a stabilized shoulder girdle, the arm may also be used powerfully in the abducted or overhead position. The line of muscle tension, its point of insertion and the relative position of the centre of rotation of the humeral head are critical for normal shoulder biomechanics. Disruption of any of these positions or disturbance of this intricate mechanism will result in a disproportionate loss of function, coordination, stability and strength.

In fractures of the proximal humerus, the fragments usually represent the insertions of the components of the rotator cuff (lesser and greater tuberosities), a capital articular fragment and the humeral shaft. Residual displacement of only a few millimetres after healing of these bony components is sufficient, particularly in association in adhesions formed during the repair process, to produce marked permanent loss of movement. Derangement of the architectural relationships of the humeral head or tuberosities, or disruption of the rotator cuff, leads to destabilization of the shoulder, superior subluxation on attempted elevation, and loss of movement range.

Diagnosis

Proximal humeral fractures account for 5% of all fractures. There is an increased frequency in elderly people with osteoporosis. The mechanism of injury is usually a direct blow to the anterior or lateral part of the arm, or a fall on to the pronated forearm. Similar fracture patterns in young adults represent high-energy injuries, frequently as a result of heavy falls, motor vehicle accidents and contact sports. The patient should be examined with full anterior and posterior exposure of both shoulders. This is best achieved by sitting the patient on an examination couch, allowing observation from in front and behind. Careful inspection for swelling, deformity, preservation of the normal shoulder profile and the attitude of the limb is required. Simultaneous comparative palpation of both shoulders is useful proceeding sequentially from the sternoclavicular joint across the clavicle to the acromioclavicular joint and then around the anterior and posterior glenohumeral joint lines. Depressions are as important as bony prominences in determining joint dislocations and may be subtle in the presence of muscle bulk and swelling. Pain frequently restricts the ability to palpate deeply and radiographs are essential. The patient should be invited initially to demonstrate active motion in the shoulder and then this range should be reproduced passively, carefully assessing for pain, fixed deformity and any further excursion. In the presence of an obvious fracture, passive joint movement should not be pursued. In late presentations, extensive bruising will be visible in the arm and chest. A full examination of the shoulder includes testing the important muscle groups. Because of pain, it is frequently only possible to assess these isometrically by asking the patient to attempt the movement actively while the examiner resists. A momentary push is all that is necessary to ascertain muscle innervation and tendon integrity.

The axillary neurovascular bundle is immediately anteromedial to the glenoid and may be compromised by fractures and dislocations of the shoulder. The cords of the brachial plexus and axillary artery are similarly at risk when the mechanism of injury produces a fracture of the neck of the humerus with medial displacement of the humeral shaft. The shaft may be driven superiorly and medially into the axilla at the moment of impact and this fracture pattern should raise considerable suspicion concerning neurovascular injury. It is essential, therefore, that muscle group testing includes the following: deltoid, biceps, supraspinatus, infraspinatus and latissimus dorsi muscles and the forearm and hand muscles that indicate radial, median and ulnar nerve functional integrity. Dermatomal sensation should also be carefully assessed with particular reference to the lateral aspect of the upper arm which is the dedicated dermatome for the axillary nerve. The preservation of sensation in this territory is not, however, a reliable indicator of axillary nerve motor function.

Vascular injuries are reported to occur in approximately 5% of the more complex proximal humeral fractures. The extensive collateral circulation of the shoulder may mask the immediate effect of the vascular deficit. The diagnosis must therefore be pursued based on suspicion and the presence of a reduced pulse volume or impalpable radial pulse, limb paraesthesia and the presence of an expanding haematoma. Urgent vascular repair is necessary as late deterioration with secondary thrombosis is recognized.

The radiographic classification of proximal humeral fractures

Much confusion has existed over the description of complex fractures of the proximal humerus. The usefulness of any classification is dependent on its ability to identify the fracture patterns associated with complications that may be modified by specific treatment regimes. Compounding elements in proximal humeral fractures are the number of major fragments, the degree of displacement, the involvement of the capital segment, dislocation of the glenohumeral joint and the integrity of the rotator cuff. As previously mentioned, the biomechanics of the shoulder are complex and the correct orientation and position of the rotator muscle insertions (tuberosities) and the fulcrum (humeral head) are essential. The blood supply to the humeral head and its articular surface is derived from the circumflex humeral arteries which enter the head predominantly via the tuberosities. Displacement of a capital segment or combined tuberosity fractures may interrupt nutrition. Avascular necrosis of the humeral head may become evident over a 1–2 year period. This is the main complication seen in four-part fractures but it may also occur in three-part or two-part fractures.

The pattern of fractures seen about the proximal humerus in adults may be classified into:

1. Avulsion fractures of the tuberosities.

2. Impacted fractures of the surgical or anatomical neck.
3. Displaced combined fractures of the neck and tuberosities (two-, three-, or four-part fractures).
4. Fracture dislocations.

Immediate treatment

Simple immobilization of the shoulder is best achieved by supporting the arm in a sling bandaged to the side of the body. For impacted stable fractures, a broad arm sling alone is appropriate but in those fractures in which there is displacement between the humeral head and shaft, traction produced by the weight of the limb supported in a collar and cuff may be more beneficial. If glenohumeral dislocation is considered likely, radiographs should be obtained prior to any attempted reduction. Consultation with an orthopaedic surgeon is necessary for these injuries which frequently require more sophisticated reduction manoeuvres or open procedures.

For undisplaced or impacted fractures the arm should be placed in a sling for comfort and early gentle passive pendulum exercises may be commenced after a few days. Active assisted movement may rapidly follow but strenuous, passive movement should be avoided until the fracture is healed.

In fractures treated conservatively in which the fragments are angulated or unimpacted, immobilization may be necessary for 2–3 weeks prior to commencing physiotherapy.

Patients with proximal humeral fractures should be made aware from the outset that a long period of recovery can be expected lasting between 4 and 6 months. Some permanent limitation of movement is common but, as a result of adaptation, functional impairment is not usually great. The presence of an axillary nerve palsy will significantly compromise rehabilitation. Although the majority of these recover spontaneously, the persistence of deltoid paralysis into the rehabilitation phase is frequently accompanied by marked long term joint stiffness. Reflex sympathetic dystrophy is occasionally associated with proximal humeral fractures and may produce considerably more stiffness and disability.

Avulsion fractures of the tuberosities

These fractures most commonly occur as a result of glenohumeral dislocation and have the same mechanism of injury. The greater tuberosity fragment is displaced by the resisted pull of supraspinatus. In up to 10% of anterior dislocations, there is an avulsion fracture of the greater tuberosity which usually remains attached to the rotator cuff complex. Following relocation of the glenohumeral joint, anatomical reduction of the tuberosity is frequently seen. It is accepted practice, therefore, that these injuries should be managed as if they were uncomplicated anterior dislocations of the shoulder (see later). If the tuberosity fragment remains displaced superiorly or posteriorly after relocation of the joint, this suggests there is either a rotator cuff tear. Surgical cuff repair and reattachment of the tuberosity is then essential if shoulder function is to be restored, and an orthopaedic surgical opinion should be requested. Avulsion of the lesser tuberosity is rare and represents a resisted external rotation force injury. These may be treated conservatively unless displacement is marked.

Immediate treatment

Tuberosity avulsion fractures if undisplaced should be treated in a broad arm sling for comfort and early gentle passive pendulum exercises begun after a few days. If the injury is part of a fracture-dislocation then a period of immobilization is necessary prior to movement. Exercises may proceed as fracture and soft tissue healing occurs with passive range being superseded by active assisted, isometric and ultimately full active movement at 6 weeks.

Definitive treatment of complex proximal humeral fractures

With recognition that reconstruction of the bony and soft tissue anatomy is essential for the restoration of shoulder function, more sophisticated management is now frequently selected. The options include:

1. Closed reduction.
2. Percutaneous wiring.
3. Open reduction and internal fixation with wires, rods, plates or screws.
4. Immediate prosthetic arthroplasty.

The selection of a particular management protocol depends on the patient's age, mental state, medical condition, degree of osteoporosis, the fracture pattern and the presence of nerve palsy. Two-part impacted fractures may be treated with a sling and early movement. Displaced fractures of the surgical neck may be similarly treated with the anticipation of a reasonable functional result. However, complex fractures involving the tuberosi-

ties may produce a poor result. Open reduction and internal fixation is advocated for displaced fractures and fracture-dislocations in which closed reductions are unsuccessful. Surgery is not without complications and there is a significant risk of avascular necrosis in three- and four-part fractures treated with open reduction and internal fixation. Prosthetic replacement of the humeral head is increasingly preferred in three- and four-part fractures, particularly in the elderly and certainly for those fractures in which there is splitting of the capital fragment.

DISLOCATIONS OF THE SHOULDER

Diagnosis

Dislocation of the shoulder is a common disorder. It should be differentiated from the inferior subluxation frequently seen as a result of muscle hypotonia. The latter condition is often an incidental finding in the elderly, accompanies chronic shoulder conditions, previous injury or neuromuscular disorders but should always raise the suspicion of a deltoid muscle palsy.

True shoulder dislocation follows a traumatic event, usually a fall on the hand with the shoulder abducted and externally rotated. The force of the humeral head against the anterior capsule results in tearing of the capsule or avulsion of the labrum from the glenoid rim. The vast majority of dislocations are anterior as the applied forces are directed by anteversion of the humeral head. The injury is most commonly seen in the young adult athlete or elderly patient. The humeral head comes to lie anteromedially in front of the scapula (subcoracoid) and the patient is seen to support the arm at waist level with the arm internally rotated and slightly abducted at the shoulder. The classic feature of an an angular deformity at the shoulder is produced by a residual prominence of the acromion after flattening of the normal curvature (created by the deltoid muscle). No shoulder movement is tolerated. Neurovascular evaluation must be carried out. The axillary nerve is at particular risk as it follows a short fixed course around the medial side of the neck of the humerus, having arisen from the posterior aspect of the brachial plexus. Vascular compromise (e.g. absent pulses or a cold blue hand) dictates immediate reduction of the joint dislocation. In the absence of neurovascular compromise a radiograph should be obtained prior to attempted reduction to confirm the type of dislocation and identify coexisting fractures.

Posterior dislocation

This rare injury is renowned for its frequency as a missed injury. The mechanism of injury is usually a direct blow to the front of the shoulder or forced internal rotation. It may be associated with an avulsion fracture of the lesser tuberosity and should be suspected after an epileptic fit or electrocution. The diagnosis is 'missed' because of a failure to examine. There is always a loss of external rotation at the shoulder, the arm being held by the side, locked in internal rotation. The loss of shoulder profile is less apparent seen from in front but inspection from above reveals a posterior humeral head prominence and residual prominence of the coracoid process anteriorly. A reliance on radiographs compounds the error as the humeral head may still be seen to apparently oppose the glenoid on the anteroposterior projection but is never congruent on the axillary view. The axillary view requires some shoulder abduction and this may not be possible. The alternative lateral view in the scapular plane may be more difficult to interpret. There is no substitute for a thorough examination.

Subglenoid dislocation (luxatio erecta)

Inferior dislocation of the shoulder is a very rare injury occurring when the arm is strongly adducted at the time of trauma. The humeral head dislocates inferiorly and becomes jammed beneath the glenoid. The diagnosis is clinically obvious with the arm held in wide abduction or vertically at the side of the head.

Immediate care of dislocations of the shoulder

In the absence of neurovascular compromise, radiographs should be performed, including an anteroposterior projection in the scapular plane and a lateral axillary view. Prompt reduction of the shoulder dislocation is mandatory and several methods are available. Intravenous sedation and analgesia usually produce satisfactory muscle relaxation to facilitate a gentle reduction and should always be employed unless there is a specific contraindication. If pain or spasm prevents efficient traction or arm movement, general anaesthesia will be necessary. Reduction is possible without anaesthesia but often fails and is frequently unacceptably painful. The key to reduction is to overcome the restraining muscle spasm and the application of traction for several minutes (by the clock) with the shoulder in 45° of abduction is often sufficient. This may be supplemented by placing the doctor's stockinged foot in the axilla to act as a fulcrum to guide the humeral head into the joint as the arm is adducted (Hippocrates' manipulation). Forceful counter-traction in the axilla should be avoided as it may produce neurovascular injury.

In Kocher's method, the doctor first applies traction to the flexed elbow for several minutes and then gently maximally externally rotates the humerus. With the arm maximally externally rotated, the elbow is then brought across the chest, adducting the shoulder and finally internally rotating the arm.

Each method is useful and has its advocates but all depend on adequate traction and sufficient muscle relaxation. Failure to reduce the joint is an indication for greater muscle relaxation and therefore for a general anaesthetic with a short-acting muscle relaxant rather than a more forceful second attempt!

The 'hanging arm technique' has been popularized as a method of reduction without anaesthesia. The patient is given sufficient parenteral analgesia and lies prone on the examination couch with the affected arm hanging vertically down, the shoulder being supported by a sand bag. Spontaneous reduction may be achieved by the traction effect of the arm's weight but many patients find this position uncomfortable and it should not be persisted with if reduction is not achieved within 30 min.

Following reduction a re-evaluation of the neurological and vascular status must be performed with specific reference to axillary nerve sensory and motor function. Radiographs must be taken to confirm reduction and exclude associated fractures of the tuberosities or glenoid rim. The arm should be immobilized in a sling and body bandage with a wool pad in the axilla to absorb perspiration. Hand and elbow movements are commenced immediately but shoulder movement should be restricted (especially external rotation) for a minimum of 3 weeks. Aftercare in the elderly should be modified to prevent stiffness; a sling for 1 week is sufficient and may be followed by physiotherapy.

In the presence of a greater tuberosity fracture, the shoulder reduction should be performed in the usual manner. In most instances the fracture fragment reduces after glenohumeral reduction. These cases may then be managed similarly except that active abduction will be inhibited by pain and should not be strenuously pursued until early fracture healing (3–4 weeks). Occasionally after reduction, persisting displacement of a lesser or greater tuberosity fracture signifies a rotator cuff injury which dictates early surgical exploration, fixation and repair.

Posterior dislocation of the shoulder is reduced under general anaesthesia by traction in 90° of abduction with external rotation of the arm and the humeral head is pushed forwards. An orthopaedic consultation should be arranged as residual instability may be present. Subglenoid dislocation (luxatio erecta) should be reduced by traction applied in the axis of the limb in the position of deformity. Reduction is usually easily achieved and the arm is then brought to the side and supported in a sling.

Recurrent dislocation

Frequently, despite adequate initial treatment, shoulder dislocations recur, particularly in the young muscular male. Recurrent dislocation typically follows progressively less traumatic episodes and may ultimately occur during normal activities. Patients may effect their own reductions or may present with the shoulder dislocated. Standard reduction manoeuvres are effective but there is no requirement for a period of immobilization after the initial pain has settled. Surgical reconstruction is necessary to produce long-term stability, although symptoms may be reduced by physiotherapy, avoidance behaviour and restricting shoulder braces. In recurrent anterior dislocation, radiographs will frequently identify a compression defect (Hill–Sachs lesion) on the posterolateral aspect of the humeral head seen on the lateral axillary projection. This is caused by repetitive impaction on the glenoid margin.

Beware – recurrent dislocation or its symptoms, and habitual voluntary dislocation, are common presenting ploys of patients seeking to deceive healthcare workers and obtain drugs of dependence.

Late unreduced dislocations

This is a formidable challenge which should be referred to an orthopaedic surgeon at the outset. Closed reduction is frequently unsuccessful and open reduction may be necessary. Forceful attempts at reduction should not be made, particularly in the elderly.

FRACTURES OF THE HUMERAL SHAFT

Most humeral shaft fractures are sustained as a result of twisting falls on the arm, direct blows and as a component of multiple injuries.

A flail arm without voluntary movement at the elbow and shoulder and with detectable mobility at the fracture site usually makes diagnosis easy. The commonest complication of this injury is radial nerve palsy and this must be sought while completing a full neurological and vascular assessment of the distal limb. Radial nerve palsy occurs in 10–15% of closed humeral shaft fractures but 90% recover spontaneously within 6 months. Radial nerve palsy is detected by identifying wrist drop or weakness of wrist extension and sensory impairment over the dorsum of the hand in the region of the first web space.

Radiographs in two projections confirm the diagnosis. Fracture displacement is dictated by the local muscle action and the force of the injury.

Immediate treatment

For the uncomplicated midshaft fracture, a collar and cuff and body bandage will afford considerable pain relief. The traction effect of the arm's weight may be increased by the addition of an above elbow cast with the elbow at 90° of flexion (hanging arm technique). Swelling and pain predominate in the first few days and splintage is difficult, but the U-slab plaster method has some advantages. The plaster is applied to include the point of the shoulder and the elbow. Shoulder immobilization is not achieved but the parallel splint is beneficial for pain relief. Significant displacement of the fracture necessitates reduction under general anaesthesia and the application of a U-slab plaster. Definitive management consists of a humeral functional brace after pain and swelling have subsided in approximately 2 weeks. Fracture union can be anticipated in 8–12 weeks.

Surgical stabilization is mandatory in open fractures, fractures associated with vascular injury, fractures associated with penetrating wounds and in those fractures in which early management has precipitated a radial nerve palsy. In this latter case it must be assumed that the nerve has become trapped in the fracture gap or impaled on a bone spike. The Holstein–Lewis fracture (the spiral or oblique fracture at the junction of the distal and middle third of the humerus) has a high incidence of radial nerve damage, and the presence of a radial nerve palsy is a further indication for surgical exploration, fracture fixation and nerve repair as appropriate. Patients with multiple injuries and those with concurrent chest injuries should have their humeral fractures treated by surgical fixation as casting techniques demand an upright posture.

The traditional non-operative treatment of the humeral shaft fracture which yielded 90% union rates is now being questioned in certain circumstances. With the advent of the locked intramedullary humeral nail, patients who have segmental fractures, ipsilateral forearm fractures and transverse or short oblique diaphyseal fractures (recognized to carry a risk of delayed or non-union) are now frequently treated operatively. Early referral to an orthopaedic surgeon in these circumstances is advised.

FRACTURES OF THE DISTAL HUMERUS

Adult injuries of the distal humerus are uncommon and usually result from a direct blow to the elbow or olecranon. The complexity of the epiphyseal arrangement of the elbow in children produces important fracture patterns which are considered separately (see Chapter 29). The distal humerus may be considered to have a two-column construction supporting the trochlear articulation for the elbow joint between its limbs. Adult fractures involve one or both columns and are differentiated by their articular involvement. A direct blow to the point of the elbow with the elbow flexed beyond 90° may drive the olecranon upwards, splitting the condyles (columns) or creating a shear fracture of one condyle and its articular component. Bicondylar fractures are the most common and represent a severe high-energy injury in the young and a complex fracture in the elderly making it one of the most difficult to treat. Neurovascular injury is surprisingly uncommon.

Diagnosis

The elbow becomes rapidly swollen and deformity is common. The subcutaneous position of the bone makes a careful inspection for open wounds imperative. Distal neurological and vascular function must be assessed. Standard anteroposterior and lateral radiographs are frequently of poor quality because of positioning problems and the inability to extend the elbow. High-quality radiographs are essential for preoperative planning and further attempts to obtain radiographs are best deferred until the patient is in the operating room and anaesthetized.

Immediate treatment

The arm should be placed in a supporting plaster slab in 90° of flexion, or the position of ease for the patient where there is neurovascular compromise. Traditional treatment has been temporary casting for 3 weeks followed by early active movement. This produces variable results with a high incidence of long-term stiffness. More complex fractures have also been treated by olecranon traction with some effect. Recent studies have supported improved outcomes, even in the elderly, by open reduction and internal fixation with the aim of restoring the column structure and reconstituting the articular surface. Surgery may be demanding and lengthy but should be performed as soon as possible before swelling becomes established. Refer directly to an experienced orthopaedic trauma surgeon for assessment.

Fractures of the capitellum

The capitellar surface may suffer a shear fracture in the coronal plane, the fragment migrating proximally to lie anterior to the radial head. These fractures are extremely rare and are the source of considerable debate. The clinical presentation is very similar to a radial head fracture and may occur in association with this injury. It is also a recognized element of a fracture dislocation of the elbow and a careful examination for evidence of medial ligament complex injury would support the latter diagnosis. The immediate management is to achieve pain relief which can be accomplished by aspiration of the haemarthrosis. This is a sterile technique with the needle inserted immediately posteriorly to the radio-capitellar joint line. The arm should be rested in a broad sling after aspiration. If the displaced fragment is large, closed reduction under general anaesthesia may be successful but is often difficult and stability is difficult to assess; late displacement is common. The presence of a large displaced capitellar fragment therefore demands a surgical orthopaedic opinion and internal fixation is frequently performed. A less common fracture pattern is seen with a shearing of just the articular surface. This may later block elbow flexion; fixation is often not possible and excision of this bone fragment may be beneficial.

ELBOW DISLOCATION

Dislocation of the elbow joint is the second most common major dislocation after the shoulder joint. The injury may follow a fall onto the outstretched hand with the elbow slightly flexed or hyperextended. The radius and ulna usually dislocate together and in the majority of cases lie posteriorly and laterally in relation to the distal humerus. Medial, anterior or direct posterior displacement is also recognized. In every case major ligament and capsule disruption and muscle damage is inherent. The clinical diagnosis may be made by the loss of the three-point anatomical arrangement of the medial and lateral humeral epicondyles and the olecranon. Rapid swelling frequently precludes accurate palpation, and the differential diagnosis of a complex distal humeral fracture makes radiographic examination essential prior to attempted reduction. The exception to this rule is in the case of major forearm ischaemia. As with all major joint dislocations, a high incidence of neurovascular injuries can be expected and should be sought. Radiographs should be scrutinized for associated fractures commonly involving the radial head, coronoid process, capitellum or the humeral epicondyles.

Immediate treatment

Reduction of the elbow dislocation should be performed under anaesthesia or sedation and the minimum of force should be applied to produce a gentle relocation, avoiding further articular damage. Prolonged traction is again a prerequisite of any manipulation and may often alone be sufficient. A good guide for manipulation is to aim to restore the three-point relationship of the humeral epicondyles and the olecranon process. A palpable clunk is usually evident if successful.

It is often forgotten, but vital, to put the reduced elbow through a full range of motion to exclude a block to movement and assess persisting instability. This will serve as an important guide for subsequent management by determining the safe range of movement which can be allowed initially. The elbow should also be assessed for varus and valgus instability. The identification of associated fractures, particularly the presence of instability, demands a surgical opinion as the outcome in these patients is considerably worse.

After reduction, the elbow should be supported in a well-padded posterior splint in 90° of flexion and the neurovascular state is re-evaluated. Careful monitoring for the development of forearm compartment syndromes following this injury is essential because of the extensive swelling and potential for vascular compromise.

FRACTURE OF THE RADIUS AND ULNA AT THE ELBOW

Fracture of the olecranon

This common fracture is usually produced by a blow on the point of the elbow; the olecranon is subcutaneous and vulnerable to direct trauma. More complex fracture patterns may follow a fall onto the outstretched hand or high-velocity injuries. An open fracture is surprisingly rare. This fracture is articular and the goals are therefore anatomical reduction and restoration of the elbow extension mechanism. Articular comminution is an important factor in determining treatment and outcome.

Clinical examination will identify local tenderness and swelling and will frequently detect the 'gap' created by the pull of triceps on the proximal fragment. Radiographs in two projections will usually demonstrate the fracture pattern, but the lateral must be a true projection to judge articular involvement. Immediate treatment involves a neurovascular assessment of the arm with careful examination of the wrist and shoulder for coexisting injuries. The arm should be supported in a broad arm sling or splinted with the elbow flexed at 90°. Optimal function will only be restored by operative treatment of displaced fractures and this should be pursued within 1 or 2 days of injury. Surprisingly good functional results are occasionally seen in neglected cases in the elderly although weakness and limitation of movement are the rule.

Fracture of the radial head

Compression of the radial head against the capitellum may produce fracture of the radial head or neck. Such a valgus compression force may be generated by a fall on the abducted outstretched pronated forearm.

Diagnosis

After the initial injury there is frequently little pain and reasonable elbow movement; this is replaced over several hours by severe pain and loss of function as a tense haemarthrosis develops. Passive movements are restricted and pain is felt in the region of the radial head. Localized tenderness is frequently diagnostic and a tense swelling immediately posterior to the radial head indicates a haemarthrosis. Care must always be taken to palpate the medial ligament complex; tenderness in this site indicates a more major injury and suggests a fracture dislocation pattern that has reduced spontaneously. The distal radioulnar joint and wrist should also be carefully examined. Routine radiographs usually demonstrate the fracture or a fat-pad sign (haemarthrosis), but radial (tangential) head views may be helpful.

Immediate treatment

Aspiration of the radiocapitellar joint confirms the presence of a haemarthrosis and is most effective in relieving pain, particularly if supplemented by the instillation of a few millilitres of a local anaesthetic agent. This procedure must be performed as a sterile technique and the site of puncture is immediate posterior and proximal to the radiocapitellar joint at the point of maximum capsular distension. Isolated fractures with minimal angulation or displacement involving less than a third of the joint surface are quite reasonably treated in a broad arm sling for 5 days and then actively mobilized anticipating discomfort and stiffness for 6 weeks. Isolated displaced radial head fractures that exhibit a block to either forearm rotation or elbow flexion should be considered for open reduction and internal fixation. If the fracture is part of a more serious ligamentous or fracture dislocation injury, the argument for surgical fixation is strengthened.

FRACTURES OF THE FOREARM BONES

To be effective, the prehensile forelimb in the human demands exceptional versatility in its articulations and mechanical advantage. The more proximal a limb injury the greater is the adaptation available to overcome residual deformity. Conversely the more distal the injury the less tolerant one can be of suboptimal healing and function if dexterity is to be preserved. The difficulties in the treatment of forearm fractures have long been recognized. The unique rotatory movement of the forearm bones requires exact restoration of both alignment and length and this goal must dominate the treatment of adult forearm fractures. Diaphyseal (shaft) fractures of the radius and ulna are commonly caused by a twisting force (a fall onto the hand) or a direct blow producing spiral or transverse fractures respectively.

Diagnosis

Deformity, local tenderness and loss of function are usual. The pulses must be felt and the hand examined for neurological deficit. Signs of raised muscle compartment pressure must be specifically looked for if this complication is to be avoided (see later).

Radiographs

When requesting X-ray examination of the forearm, the final radiographs must show the full length of both radius and ulna and the radiocarpal and elbow joints in both projections. The radius and ulna are bound together by the strong interosseous membrane, the annular ligament, radioulnar ligaments and the triangular cartilage. They are one functional unit. By necessity, if one forearm bone is fractured with shortening or angulation there must be at least one other injury, usually a dislocation of the radial head (Monteggia injury) or ulnar head (Galeazzi fracture-dislocation). An isolated fracture of radius or ulna alone is uncommon and usually follows a direct blow. A single forearm fracture must never be accepted until Monteggia or Galeazzi fracture-dislocation patterns have been excluded.

Immediate treatment

Baseline assessment of vascular and neurological function is essential. Gross deformity with vascular compromise dictates immediate correction. Open fractures are common, particularly in the distal third of the forearm where the bone has a less bulky muscular envelope. In these cases, a sterile dressing should be applied, broad-spectrum antibiotics and tetanus prophylaxis administered and a surgical consultation obtained promptly (see Chapter 26).

Compartment syndrome in the forearm

The unyielding investing fascia is responsible for the high incidence of compartment syndromes complicating forearm and elbow injuries. This complication may be evident acutely in severe fractures and crush injuries or may develop during the first few hours in hospital. Injuries more proximal in the limb associated with vascular compromise must also be considered likely to precipitate a forearm compartment syndrome. This risk is particularly high after perfusion is restored when the damaged basement membrane of the capillaries is overwhelmed. Morbidity, and rarely mortality, from delayed treatment or missed compartment syndromes remains a major cause of avoidable disability and successful negligence claims. The under appreciation of risk, poor understanding of the mechanism and tardy response to clinical signs are the main causes. Local haemorrhage, swelling and altered capillary permeability cause a rise in tissue pressures within the closed spaced. At a pressure greater than the arteriolar perfusion pressure, shunting occurs within the compartment, and muscle and nerve perfusion ceases. A period of ischaemia commences and further swelling develops as a result of cell damage and anaerobic metabolism.

The symptoms of an impending compartment syndrome are:

1. Unrelenting pain dispropionate to the injury, especially if the pain is progressive.
2. The muscle compartment is tensely swollen and tender to palpation.
3. Attempted passive stretching of the muscle within the compartment causes severe pain and is a very reliable sign.
4. Nerve tissue is most sensitive to hypoxia and there will be early sensory impairment or hyperaesthesia in the sensory dermatome of any nerve passing through the involved compartment.

Palpable pulses are present. Capillary refill remains normal and the hand remains pink and warm. Pressure will rarely rise to a level which occludes the main arteries traversing the compartment yet tissue within the compartment may be profoundly ischaemic. The presence of pulses and normal capillary filling in the hand must not distract from the diagnosis of compartment syndrome. In the unconscious patient, compartment pressure monitoring may be necessary. Commercial systems are now available employing a slit catheter and pressure transducer.

It is imperative to respond rapidly to symptoms and signs of an incipient compartment syndrome. Dressings should be removed, any cast should be bivalved and orthopaedic wadding must be divided along the whole length of the cast. The limb should be elevated to the level of the heart to promote arterial inflow. Failure to rapidly reverse the pain, swelling and neurological dysfunction by means of these simple approaches, and the presence of an established compartment syndrome, are indications for surgical decompression. Surgery is urgent and decompressions must be extensive involving division of the skin and investing fascia in both the volar and dorsal compartments of the forearm, extending from the elbow to wrist. It must also be appreciated that within the volar compartment there are fascial divisions which require separate decompression. Fasciotomy wounds are left open and frequently require indirect closure and split skin grafts.

Definitive treatment of forearm fractures

Undisplaced forearm fractures are rare except for the occasional isolated distal ulna or radial fracture. These may be treated in a cast for 6–8 weeks. Displaced fractures of the forearm are best treated by early operation and excellent results have been achieved with plate fixation and early functional rehabilitation (Anderson *et al.*, 1975).

Monteggia lesion

Fractures of the ulna associated with disruption of the radiohumeral joint may be considered within this description. A relatively rare injury pattern, it has generated a substantial volume of literature and discussion, not least because of problems persisting after inadequate treatment or failure to recognize the radial head dislocation on initial radiographs. In adults, the radial head dislocation is usually posterior but anterior and lateral dislocations are recognized.

The injury presents as a painful elbow and the ulna bone deformity is usually obvious. The patient will allow no forearm rotation or movement of the elbow. Posterior and anterior interosseous and ulnar nerve lesions may be present. The wrist and elbow joint must be visualized on radiographs, and the head of the radius (which normally points directly at the capitellum in any position on any projection) is dislocated or subluxed.

Immediate treatment

The forearm and elbow should be supported in a splint in a position of comfort and pain relief administered. Regular observations of the neurological, vascular and compartment function are essential. Unlike the Monteggia fracture in childhood, open reduction and internal fixation in the adult is the absolute rule. Stable anatomical reduction of the ulna fracture is essential to relocate the radial head. Occasionally, open reduction of the radial head is also necessary because of the interposition of the annular ligament.

Galeazzi fracture-dislocation

More common in adults than the Monteggia lesion, this fracture of the radius associated with subluxation or dislocation of the distal radioulnar joint has been termed the reverse Monteggia lesion. The diagnosis is confirmed by X-rays having recognized the deformity and tenderness of the distal radioulnar joint. The radial fracture is usually in the distal third, is oblique with shortening and may be comminuted. Disruption of the distal radioulnar joint is best seen on the true lateral projection.

This fracture pattern is inherently unstable and closed treatment and casting yield unsatisfactory results. Acceptable outcomes are only achievable with operative treatment.

FRACTURES OF THE DISTAL RADIUS

Fractures of the distal radius are the most common; the majority occur in elderly osteoporotic females and are the result of low-energy trauma. The low demands of this patient group, the acceptance of deformity and the reasonable function usually achieved by manipulation and cast treatment has unfortunately produced complacency in the treament of these injuries. The wide spectrum of fracture patterns must be appreciated, together with an understanding of the greater severity of the injury in the younger patient. Individual fractures should be analysed and treated taking account of the patient's age, energy of injury, bone strength, premorbid function and demands of the patient. For the purpose of discussion, distal radial fracture will be considered according to the presence or absence of radiocarpal articular involvement and the patient's age.

Extra-articular fractures

In the elderly patient, the commonest injury is that which presents with the deformity described by Abraham Colles in 1814. This pattern of injury occurs after a fall on the outstretched hand and produces a fracture in the distal radial metaphysis. The bone is frequently osteoporotic and the clinical deformity is both striking and typical, resembling the curvature of a 'dinner fork' viewed from the side. Examination will demonstrate many of the features of this injury which is a fracture of the radius with dislocation or subluxation of the radio-ulnar joint. Local tenderness and shortening of the radius may be identified by comparative palpation of the radial and ulnar styloids, together with a step deformity of dorsal displacement. Radial displacement and lateral rotation are also common elements of the injury. Impaction is common so the presence of distal radial tenderness after a fall warrants radiographic examination. A note of caution: the frequency of this fracture in the elderly must be borne in mind as patients with healed malunions of previous fractures may present with new injuries. Assessment of the neurovascular status of the hand is essential; the median nerve is the structure most likely to be compromised by fracture displacement. Occasionally the distal ulnar fracture may be open.

Radiographs

Good-quality anteroposterior and lateral radiographs should be taken. In the majority of cases the fracture is easily located, but careful tracing of the cortical outline in both views may be necessary in impacted fractures. A useful indicator on the lateral view is the loss of the normal 10° of anterior angulation of the distal end of the radius. Articular extensions of the fracture, comminution and distal radioulnar joint involvement should all be noted.

Immediate treatment

The limb is best supported on pillows or in a sling with a temporary splint extending from the forearm to the metacarpals. It is undesirable to leave reductions for more than a few hours, but logistics and the frequency of the condition may demand designated resources in a busy accident unit. Anaesthesia is essential and for the primary reduction attempt a regional anaesthetic block (i.e., Bier's block) is satisfactory. General anaesthesia carries greater risks in the elderly unprepared patient and should be reserved for difficult or delayed cases (see Chapter 10). Direct injection of the fracture haematoma ('haematoma block') has its advocates and offers some advantages when dealing with large numbers of these injuries. It may be performed rapidly, by one doctor, requires a minimum of readily available equipment and local anaesthetic agent. However, the pain relief is less predictable, muscle relaxation is not achieved and the closed fracture haematoma is, in theory, violated, presenting a risk of infection. With articular extension of the fracture, joint distension pain may be a problem. Reduction of the fracture must address the known displacements. With the patient supine, the shoulder abducted and the elbow flexed, traction is applied along the line of the forearm by grasping the hand. Counter-traction is applied above the elbow by an assistant without force or violence: the elderly are often frail and have poor skin which is easily damaged. Traction for 2–3 min disimpacts the fracture; an attempt to manipulate before this is achieved may be unsuccessful and is the single commonest reason for poor or failed reductions. Radial length, lateral displacement and lateral angulation are usually corrected by simple traction. Firm pressure over the dorsal radius will effect reduction of the dorsal displacement and angulation. The forearm and wrist should be left in a pronated position with 10° of wrist flexion and ulnar deviation. A radial plaster slab is then applied over adequate padding extending from the metacarpal necks to the proximal third of the forearm. The thumb metacarpal should be excluded. The aim of casting is to maintain flexion and ulnar angulation and the reduction may be further secured by moulding over the dorsal radius as the plaster sets. Orthopaedic surgeons should agree local management protocols for these fractures. Postreduction radiographs are essential and should be carefully scrutinized for displacement. In particular, residual dorsal angulation, lateral angulation and radial shift are known to impair long-term function. Persisting radial shortening after reduction implies insufficient traction and may account for failure to correct other displacements. Remanipulation should be considered before anaesthesia is lost.

The presence of dorsal cortical comminution indicates an unstable fracture pattern and the patient should be warned of redisplacement. Involvement of the distal radioulnar joint, intra-articular extensions and articular impaction are all known to adversely influence outcome. With the exception of open fractures, all extra-articular fractures of the distal radial metaphysis in the elderly warrant closed manipulation. Local arrangements must be established for early review and intervention in cases that remain unsatisfactory or are unstable. Contemporary management of more difficult fractures involves the use of percutaneous Kirschner wires, the application of external fixator frames from radius to metacarpals and limited open reduction and internal fixation.

Following application of a cast the patient should be given specific instructions regarding elevation of the hand and the promotion of finger, elbow and shoulder exercises. The patient should also be warned to return immediately if symptoms and signs of vascular or neurological compromise develop. A plaster check and examination by trained staff is mandatory within 24 h of cast application. Completion of the cast should be delayed until no further acute swelling is anticipated. In the elderly, a Colles' forearm cast will be necessary for 3–6 weeks depending on the individual surgeon.

The equivalent extra-articular fracture in the young patient is a different beast and should be approached in a more critical manner. Neurovascular compromise is more likely to be present and fracture displacement is usually marked. These features are to be expected from the mechanism of injury which usually involved a much greater force. These injuries are typically seen following motorcycle injuries, falls from a height and in sporting accidents. Reduction may be more difficult and anatomical restoration is critical. Late displacement cannot be accepted and there should be a low threshold for supplementary fixation with percutaneous wires, or external fixation. Prompt orthopaedic consultation is advised.

A reverse deformity to that described by Colles, in which there is palmar displacement of the distal radial fragment with a dislocation of the inferior radioulnar joint, was described by Smith in 1847. His name has been given to the fracture of this pattern caused by a fall on the dorsum of the flexed wrist. This injury is considerably less common than the dorsally displaced fracture and represents a greater challenge in management because of inherent instability. Traditional treatment was closed manipulation under regional anaesthesia and immobilization in an above elbow plaster case with the elbow flexed, the forearm supinated and the wrist dorsiflexed. Closed manipulation may be unsuccessful or, more frequently, reduction cannot be maintained conservatively for the 6 weeks necessary. Many orthopaedic surgeons perform open reduction and internal fixation on these fractures using a volar buttress plate.

Intra-articular fractures

Involvement of the radiocarpal joint is common with distal radial fractures. In the absence of major joint incongruity, management need not differ from the extra-articular fracture, but increased joint stiffness should be anticipated and early mobilization favoured. The use of haematoma block anaesthesia may be less effective and produce discomfort as a result of joint capsule distension.

Two important articular fracture patterns do, however, need to be specifically addressed to ensure restoration of hand and wrist function and to limit the rise of post-traumatic osteoarthritis. First, the radiocarpal two-part dislocation must be considered. This is a high-energy shearing injury in which the carpus displaces with the distal radial fragment. The displacement (first described by Barton in 1838) may be dorsal or palmar and includes subluxation of both radiocarpal and radioulnar joints. Initial management, reduction and casting techniques are as for dorsal and palmar extra-articular fractures, respectively, but the incidence of instability is very high, frequently necessitating early open reduction and internal fixation.

Perhaps the fracture with the poorest outcome from closed manipulation and casting is the high-energy complex articular fracture seen in young people. The radial metaphysis explodes, disrupting the radiocarpal and radioulnar joints. Rapid gross swelling often masks the bony deformity. Neurological and vascular injuries are more common and compartment syndromes may develop. The ulnar and median nerves are frequently injured. This injury pattern is commonly seen in the multiply injured patient and may also be associated with other injuries in the ipsilateral limb, including carpal instability.

Plain radiographs illustrate the degree of comminution, displacement and joint damage and the inevitable fracture instability. In particular, the lunate and scaphoid facets of the distal radial articular surface may be separated and impacted. Oblique radiographs, tomography and CT scanning may be necessary to evaluate the fracture, but perhaps the most useful and expeditious investigation is a traction film under general anaesthesia. These fractures are now known to require more aggressive reconstructive surgery and the modern orthopaedic trauma surgeon will utilize a combination of percutaneous wires, limited open reduction and internal fixation, ligamentotaxis and external fixation to effect and maintain a reduction. Except in gross deformity or vascular compromise there is no requirement for provisional manipulation of these fractures in the emergency room. The forearm and hand should be splinted, cold dressings applied intermittently and the hand monitored prior to surgical stabilization.

CONCLUSIONS

Fractures of the upper limb and pectoral girdle are amongst the most common injuries seen in A&E departments. The priorities of management are the rapid identification of limb-threatening injuries, usually resulting from vascular compromise, open fractures or the development of compartment syndromes. In these circumstances, prompt surgical intervention must be established. It is essential that the complete neurological and vascular status of the limb distal to any recognized injury is documented prior to radiographic studies or treatment. The key to diagnosis in limb injuries is careful observation and palpation of the limb bones and assessment of joint function. Careful examination will ensure that appropriate radiological examinations are requested and accurate diagnoses made. Treatment must be individually assigned, based on the characteristics of the patient (including functional demand and age), as well as the energy of injury, fracture pattern, quality of bone and patient compliance.

Significant progress in many areas of orthopaedic trauma management has now established standards and goals unobtainable by traditional conservative treatment. Close cooperation and consultation at a local level and the facility for early evaluation by experienced orthopaedic surgeons are essential. There is no substitute for meticulous attention to detail and critical patient review in the management of upper limb injuries.

Further Reading

ADA, J.R. & MILLER, M.E. (1991). Scapular fractures: Analysis of 113 cases. *Clin. Orthop.*, **269**, 174–80.

ANDERSON, L.D., SISK, T.D., TOOMS, R.E. *et al.* (1975). Compression plate fixation in acute diaphyseal fractures of the radius and ulna. *J. Bone. Joint Surg.*, **57A**, 287–97.

AXELROD, T.J., McMURTRY, R.Y. (1990). Open reduction and internal fixation of comminuted intra-articular fractures of the distal radius. *J. Hand Surg.*, **15A**, 1–11.

AXELROD, T.J., PALEY, D., GREEN, J. *et al.* (1988). Limited open reduction of the lunate facet in comminuted intra-articular fractures of the distal radius. *J. Hand Surg.*, **13A**, 372–77.

BADO, J.L. (1967). The Monteggia lesion. *Clin. Orthop.*, **50**, 71–6.

BRADWAY, J., AMADIO, P.C. & COONEY, W.P. (1989). Open reduction and internal fixation of displaced, comminuted intra-articular fractures of the distal end of the radius *J. Bone Joint Surg.*, **71A**, 839–47.

GABEL, G.T., HENSON, G., BENNETT, J.B., *et al.* (1987). Intra-articular fractures of the distal humerus in the adult. *Clin. Orthop.*, **216**, 99–107.

HARDEGGER, F.H. & SIMPSON, L.A. (1984). *J. Bone Joint Surg.*, **66B**, 315–24, 725.

HOWARD, P.W., STUART, H.D., HIND, R.E. *et al.*, (1989). External fixation or plaster for severely displaced comminuted Colles fractures. *J. Bone Joint Surg.*, **71B**, 68–73.

JENKIN, N.H., JONES, D.G., JOHNSON, S.R. *et al.* (1987). External rotation of Colles fracture: an anatomic study. *J. Bone Joint Surg.*, **69B**, 207–11.

JUPITER, J.B., NEFF, U., HOLZACH, P. *et al.* (1985). Intercondylar fracture of the humerus. *J. Bone Joint Surg.*, **67A**, 226–39.

MEHNE, D.K., & JUPITER, J.B., (1992). Fractures of the distal humerus. *Skeletal Trauma*, Vol. II, ed. B.D. Browner, J.B. Jupiter, A.M. Levene & P.G. Trafton, pp. 1146–76. Phildelphia: W.B. Saunders.

MOORE, T.M., KLEIN, J.P., PATZAKIS, M.J. *et al.* (1985). Results of compression plating of closed Galleazzi fractures. *J. Bone Joint Surg.*, **67A**, 1015–21.

NEER, C.S. (1960). Nonunion of the clavicle. *J. Am. Med. Assoc.*, **172**, 1006–11.

NEER, C.S. (1984). Injuries to the acromio-clavicular joint. In *Fractures in Adults*, ed. C.A. Rockwood Jr. & D.P. Green, p. 895. Philadelphia: J.B. Lippincott.

ORECK, S.L., BURGESS, A. & LEVENE, A. (1984). Traumatic lateral displacement of the scapula: a radiographic sign of neurovascular disruption. *J. Bone Joint Surg.*, **66A**, 758–63.

POLLOCK, S.H., DRAKE, D., BOVILL, E.G. *et al.*

(1981). Treatment of radial neuropathy associated with fractures of the humerus. *J. Bone Joint Surg.*, **63A**, 239–43.

PORTER, M. & STOCKLEY, I. (1987), Fractures of the distal radius: intermediate and end results in relation to radiologic parameters. *Clin. Orthop.*, **220**, 241–51.

RUBENSTEIN, J.D., EBRAHEIM, N.A. & KELLAM, J.F. (1985). Traumatic scapulo-thoracic dissociation. *Radiology*, **157**, 297–8.

VAN DE LINDEN. W. & ERICKSON, R. (1981). Colles fracture: how should displacement be measured and how should it be immobilised? *J. Bone Joint Surg.*, **63A**, 1285–91.

WEAVER, J.K. & DUNN, H.K. (1972). Treatment of acromio-clavicular injuries, especially complete acromio-clavicular separation. *J. Bone Joint Surg.*, **54A**, 1187–94.

ZENNI, E.J. Jr, KRIEG, J.K. & ROSEN, M.J. (1981). Open reduction and internal fixation of clavicular fractures. *J. Bone Joint Surg.*, **63A**, 147–51.

29 Paediatric orthopaedics

M. BELL

Orthopaedic Department, Royal Hallamshire Hospital, Sheffield, UK

Chapter plan

Why children's fractures are different
Upper limb
Spinal injuries
Pelvic fractures
Acetabular fractures
Hip fractures
Lower limb

WHY CHILDREN'S FRACTURES ARE DIFFERENT

The aim of the treatment of children's fractures is exactly the same as that for adults: identification of an injury and treatment of that injury such that full function is restored. However, there are a number of differences in children's fractures compared to those of adults. These include the bone structure itself, the presence of growth plates and the capacity for remodelling. Because bone structure varies with age, the pattern of injury in children also varies.

Pattern of injury

Fractures under the age of 1 year are very uncommon. If they do occur, pathological fracture of the bone should be considered (e.g. osteogenesis imperfecta or other brittle bond conditions).

Fractures under the age of 2 years are rare and child abuse must be considered.

At certain ages specific injuries tend to occur. Spiral fractures of the tibia are frequent in children between the ages of 2 and 5 years and supracondylar fractures of the elbow between the age of 5 and 10 years.

Ligament injuries and dislocations become more frequent as the child becomes older.

In children the bone still has the capacity for growth. Any injury to the physis (growth plate) can affect future development of the bone. A diffuse injury to the growth plate may arrest growth and local damage may result in an angular deformity.

Bony elasticity

In children the bones are more elastic than they are in adults. As a result, when force is applied, the bones may bend without obvious fracture. This is called plastic deformation.

The elasticity of the bone is responsible for greenstick fractures which are unique to children.

Types of fractures

Greenstick fracture (Fig. 1)

This is a tension and compression fracture. The fracture occurs on the tension side; on the compression side the periosteum is intact. As bone stiffness increases with age greenstick fractures become less common.

Torus fractures (buckle fractures) (Fig. 2)

These fractures occur when the bone buckles under compression. The fracture is rarely displaced.

Pathological fractures

These fractures are uncommon. They can occur in neuromuscular conditions and in children suffering from metabolic bone disease, benign bone tumours and bone cysts.

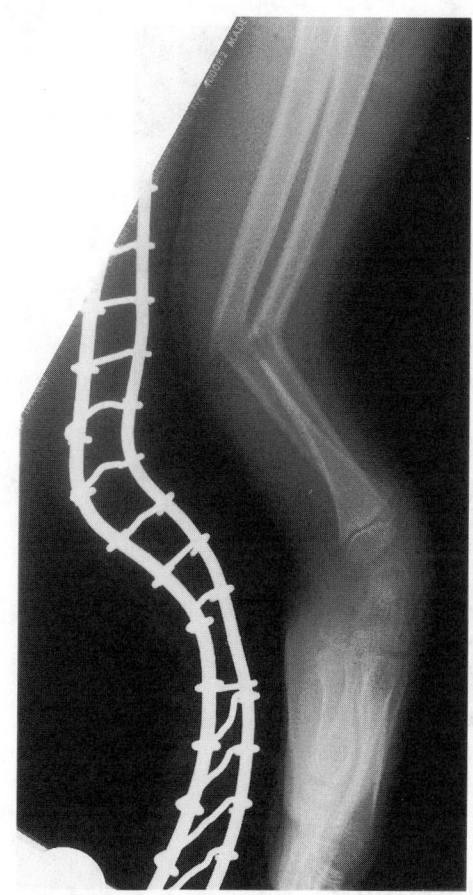

Fig. 1. A greenstick fracture of both bones of the forearm.

Remodelling

A specific feature in the young child is the ability of the bones to remodel. As a consequence, some deformity that occurs following fracture may be corrected by the body as growth continues. Remodelling has its greatest potential in the younger child with an injury which is close to the physis. Fractures remodel in the plane of the joint and rotational injuries do not. Remodelling takes place at the ankle, the knee and the wrist and, perhaps best of all, at the shoulder. Significant displacement of shoulder fractures can correct completely over 1–2 years.

Increased growth

Long bone fractures can stimulate increased growth. There may be two reasons:

1. An increase on the blood supply to the epiphysis as a result of the hyperaemia which follows fracture.
2. A tearing of the periostial tether allowing the bone to increase in length.

These factors must be considered with femoral fractures as anatomical reduction can lead to a significant overgrowth in bone length.

Healing rate

Children's fractures heal very quickly and physeal injuries even faster – approximately half the time taken by metaphyseal fractures. Non-unions are very rare.

Periosteum

This is a very thick layer which lifts off easily from the bone. Identification of some undisplaced fractures of the tibia is difficult in the early stages and may only be apparent from the new bone laid down subperiosteally 1 week to 10 days after the injury. The periosteum itself is firmly attached to the epiphysis and the zone of Ranvier. It is a very important structure in the healing of fractures and the laying down of new bone.

What's normal?

A number of difficulties in the management of children's fractures surround the identification of what is normal and what is a fracture. The presence of physeal lines and the absence of secondary centres of ossification make interpretation of X-rays difficult. A high index of suspicion is needed in dealing with children's injuries. An area where significant problems do occur is around the elbow in the younger child.

Physeal injuries

Physeal disruptions represents 15% of all children's fractures and can be classified according to Salter and Harris (Fig. 3).

Physeal injuries of the Salter–Harris type I tend to occur in the younger infant. Types II, III and IV increase in incidence as the secondary centre of ossification enlarges. Physeal injuries are more common in the upper limb and in males as opposed to females. It is suggested that distal radial fractures represent 30% of physeal injuries and the average age of these injuries is 11 years in girls and 12 years in boys.

Some 97% of physeal injuries can be treated by closed methods. Salter–Harris type II fractures account for 73% of the injuries. Salter–Harris type I for 8.5%, type III for 6.5% and type IV for 12%. Type V injuries are very rare,

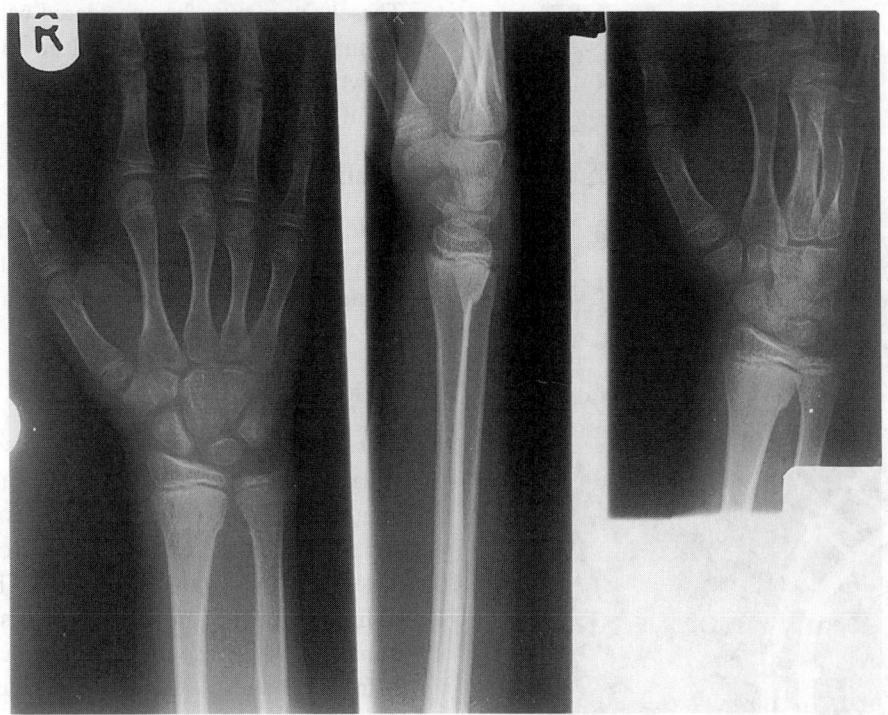

Fig. 2. A buckle fracture of the distal radius with no displacement.

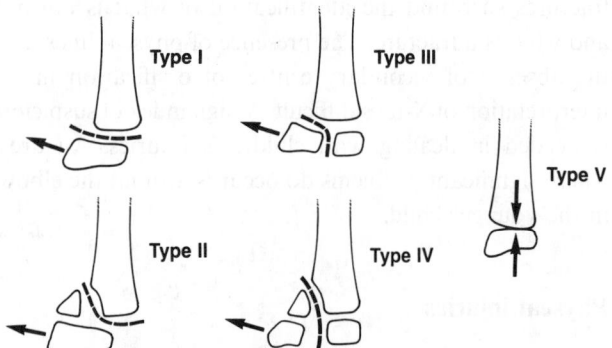

Fig. 3. Illustration of Salter–Harris classification of physeal injuries: Type I, a fracture is through the growth plate; Type II, a fracture through the growth plate and takes a small fragment of the metaphysis; Type III, a fracture of the epiphysis and then through the growth plate; Type IV, a fracture through the epiphysis across the growth plate and into the metaphysis; Type V, a crush of the epiphysis.

occurring in only 1% of the patients. Type III and IV have a significant risk of localized growth arrest. Type III fractures of the ankle have a very high risk of angular deformity.

Questions have been raised as to whether Salter–Harris type V truly exists. Petersen has suggested that it may occur as a vascular phenomenon.

UPPER LIMB

The hand

Hand fractures in children are less common than in adults. They account for 7% of children's injuries; 34% of the fractures are physeal injuries. All types of fracture can occur as a direct result of violence to the hand.

Young children do not tolerate regional anaesthesia well. Under these circumstances consideration must be given to the use of general anaesthesia to reduce any fracture.

The principles of management are identical to those in adults. Reduction of any intra-articular fracture must be anatomical and rotational deformities must be identified and corrected.

Finger tip injuries may need help from plastic surgeons, especially if there is significant skin or pulp loss.

Salter–Harris type II fracture of the proximal phalanx is the most common injury in children. In the majority of cases these injuries need no specific treatment other than the use of neighbour strapping. If there is angulation of more than 15°, consideration must be given to manipulation under anaesthetic.

Common injuries are fractures of the neck of the fifth metacarpal. This may be a Salter–Harris type II injury or a fracture of the metaphysis. They occur as a resul of fighting. Up to 40° of angulation can be accepted. When treating hand fractures the 'safe' position for immobilization must be used to prevent the development of joint contractures.

Carpal injuries

Carpal injuries in children are exceptionally rare. Scaphoid fractures are very infrequent in any child under the age of 10 years. Above this age they are not common until the child had reached skeletal maturity at around 15 years of age in girls and 17 years in boys. Fractures before this age are most likely to involve the scaphoid tubercle rather than the waist or proximal pole.

Carpal dislocations do occur and are written up as case reports in journals. As with adults, they can occur in association with fractures of the distal radius. It is essential in any child who presents with a distal radial fracture that the carpus is scrutinized to ensure that there is no associated injury.

Distal radial fractures

Distal radial fractures can be divided into four types:

1. Physeal injuries.
2. Torus fractures.
3. Greenstick fractures.
4. Complete fractures.

Of distal radial injuries physeal fractures are the most frequent between the ages of 6 and 12 years. The commonest are type I and type II; the others are exceptionally rare. Fractures of the distal radial physis are often associated with fractures of the distal ulna.

Associated injuries of the carpus do occur and must be looked for but they are exceptionally rare.

Physeal injuries

Salter–Harris type II fractures of the distal radius are very common. The mechanism of injury is a fall on the outstretched hand. Treatment depends on the degree of displacement and some fractures may require manipulation. It has been reported that remodelling of physeal injuries takes place up to the age of 12 or 13 years.

Usually the fractures are dorsally displaced by the distal radial physis; however, a volar displacement has been reported.

Torus fracture

This is a compression fracture of the distal radius which buckles the bone. The vast majority of these fractures have little in the way of angulation. The only treatment required is that of pain relief. A short period in a below elbow cast is sufficient. A full range of motion and return of full function is the expected outcome.

Greenstick fracture

These are less common than epiphyseal injuries to the distal radius. Whether manipulation is required depends on the degree of displacement. If manipulation is advised then the decision has to be made whether or nor to break the periostial hinge. The intact periostial hinge may increase the risk of the fracture displacing when in a plaster cast.

The overall outcome of these fractures is excellent and full restoration of normal function should be expected.

Complete fractures

Complete fractures occur in the slightly older child and are more common between the ages of 10 and 14 years. Decisions regarding manipulation are made on the degree of displacement and angulation. Some degree of overlap can be accepted as long as there is no angular rotation deformity.

In these fractures it is important to assess the distal neurovascular status. Median nerve injury can occur as a result of these injuries and compartment syndromes have been reported.

If a reduction is obtained with only slight rotatory angular displacement and overlap, the overall outcome is excellent.

Both bones of forearm (Fig. 4)

Fractures of both bones of the forearm occur distally in 75% of cases, in the midshaft in 18% and proximally only in 7%.

If an isolated fracture of the radius is identified, close examination of the distal radial joint must be made. An isolated fracture of the radius with a dislocation of the distal radial ulnar joint is known as a Galleazzi fracture. Isolated fractures of the ulna do occur but in some cases, they are associated with dislocation of the proximal radial ulnar joint. This injury is known as a Monteggia fracture. Therefore it is essential in all injuries to the

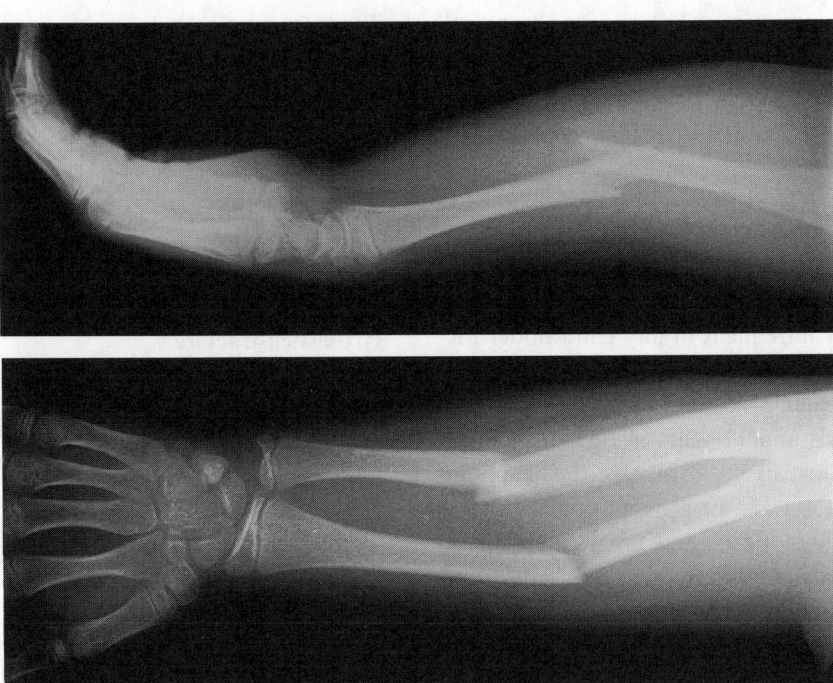

Fig. 4. A complete fracture of both bones of the forearm.

forearm that X-rays of the joint above and below the level of the fracture are taken to ensure that dislocations are not missed.

Some degree of angulation can be accepted, especially in the younger child, but this is a matter of judgement. Midshaft fractures of the radius and ulna will not completely remodel after the age of 8 years. The vast majority can be treated conservatively in plaster, with or without a manipulation. Distal fractures should be held in an above elbow cast in pronation, midshaft fractures in neutral rotation and upper shaft fractures in supination.

It is important to try to obtain anatomical alignment, but as long as the fractures are hitched and there is no angular or rotational deformity an incomplete reduction can be accepted because of the ability of the bones to remodel.

It is essential that the possibility of associated nerve damage is considered in any forearm fracture. This must be sought prior to any treatment being instituted.

Monteggia fractures

These are fractures of the proximal ulna associated with dislocations of the radial head. They have been classified into four types depending on the displacement of the radial head:

- Type 1 – anterior dislocation.
- Type 2 – posterior dislocation.
- Type 3 – lateral dislocation of the radial head.
- Type 4 – dislocation of the radial head associated with a fracture of the radius.

The most important part of the treatment of this injury is identification so that appropriate treatment can be instituted to reduce the dislocated radial head.

Elbow injuries

These account for approximately 9% of children's injuries. This is an area where the greatest problems lie for the accident and emergency (A&E) physician. Fractures in this region may be difficult to identify radiologically because of the late appearance of secondary centres of ossification and the possibility of injuries through the physeal plate and cartilaginous portions of the epiphysis. A high index of suspicion must be levelled at any child who has a history of significant injury to the elbow associated with soft tissue swelling.

The radiographic appearances of the elbow alter as the child matures and it is essential that the A&E department carries a book depicting the normal X-ray appearances of the elbow at different ages. This will help the unwary to identify some of these difficult fractures.

Pulled elbow

This occurs between the ages of 2 and 5 years and is caused by a pull on the outstretched arm. The radial head subluxes beneath the annular ligament. The child screams and is reluctant to move the arm. However, on pronation and supination in flexion the radial head reduces. The child should be observed for a few minutes and if the manipulation fails to correct the condition and X-rays taken at this stage are normal, no treatment is indicated as the radial head will relocate spontaneously in a collar and cuff within 1 or 2 days. If this does not occur the injury must be reassessed.

Distal humerus

Supracondylar fractures occur between the ages of 5 and 10 years. They account for 70% of injuries around the elbow, with lateral condylar fractures 17% and medial epicondylar fractures around 12%. 'T' intercondylar fractures are very uncommon.

Appearance of secondary centres of ossification

Ossification of the capitellum is present at and around a year. It appears slightly sooner in girls than in boys. The next secondary centres appears in the medial epicondyle between the ages of 5 and 6 years. The secondary centre of ossification in the radial head appears at the same age. The trochlea ossification centre appears between the ages of 9 and 10 years when one would expect the lateral epicondylar centre also to be present. Ossification in the olecranon appears between the ages of 7 and 8 years. All the secondary centres of ossification fuse together in the early teens.

On clinical examination of the normal elbow at full extension, there is a carrying angle of approximately 18°. It is not significantly different in boys or girls. When the elbow is fully flexed the long axis of the forearm lies parallel to the long axis of the humerus. These factors are important when considering whether deformity is present.

Supracondylar fractures

These occur between the ages of 5 and 10 years as a result of a fall onto the outstretched hand. They should be classified into three groups:

1. Extension fractures.
2. Flexion fractures.
3. Distal metaphyseal fractures.

The extension and flexion fractures can be classified further as to whether they are undisplaced, displaced, displaced with the posterior cortex intact, flexion fractures with the anterior cortex intact, or completely displaced. Completely displaced fractures are then subdivided as to whether displacement is medial or lateral.

Following identification of a supracondylar fracture careful examination of the distal nervous system and vascular tree must be carried out. Commonly associated are injuries to the anterior interosseous or radial nerves. Vascular injuries occur but a true Volkmann's ischaemic contracture is uncommon. Careful examination of the arm is necessary to prevent the development of compartment syndromes and subsequent Volkmann's ischaemic contracture. The presence of a radial pulse is no guarantee that the deep flexor compartment of the arm is being adequately perfused and the absence of a radial pulse does not necessarily mean the deep compartment is inadequately perfused. Clinical examination must exclude the presence of pain on extension of the fingers.

The patient should be asked if he/she can:

1. Make the sign of an 'O' which ensures that the anterior interosseous nerve is intact.
2. Make the hand into the form of a star indicating the ulnar nerve is intact.
3. Extend the thumb like a hitch-hiker to make sure the radial nerve is intact.
4. Make a fist indicating the median nerve is intact.

When assessing the limb be careful to ensure that associated injuries are not missed. Forearm fractures and distal radial fractures can accompany injuries to the elbow.

Treatment

Undisplaced fractures
Collar and cuff. These will heal, depending on the age of the child, within 3 weeks.

Minimally displaced fractures
Depending on the degree of displacement there may be a need for manipulation by elbow flexion which, in the majority of cases, will restore normal alignment. Treatment is then with a collar and cuff for a period of 3 weeks before mobilization.

Displaced fractures (Fig. 5)
These always need realignment. The surgeon must be aware of all treatment modalities. The principles are that:

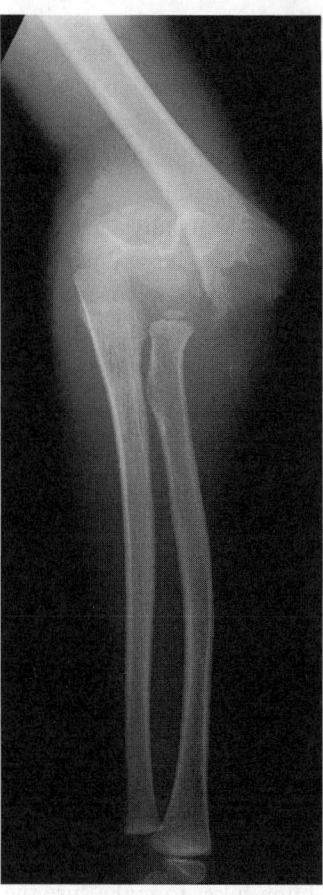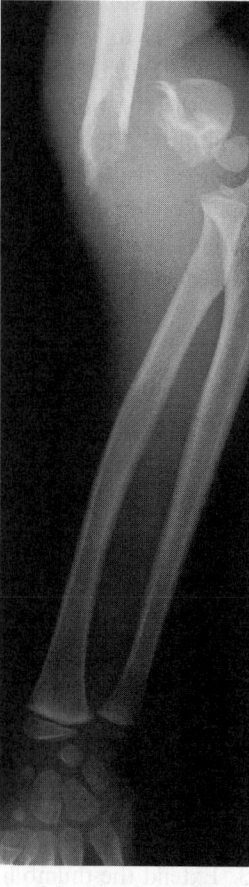

Fig. 5. An extension supracondylar fracture of the distal humerus with gross displacement. Assessment of the neurovascular status of the forearm and hand is essential.

1. Reduction must be obtained.
2. The reduction must be adequate.
3. The reduction must be maintained.

The failure of any of these criteria is an indication that other treatment modalities including percutaneous pinning or open reduction and fixation must be employed. Another option is traction. Dunlop traction and straight lateral traction have their advocates but recently the use of a screw in the olecranon for overhead traction has become more popular.

Reduction must be carried out under general anaesthesia and the surgeon performing the reduction must be prepared to proceed to other treatment modalities. If he cannot, senior help should be called. Once the reduction has been obtained it is important to determine the adequacy of this reduction and exclude rotary malalignment of the distal fragment.

There are few indications for open reduction: these are the presence of an open fracture, vascular com-

promise, or an irreducible fracture. If the fracture can be reduced but is unstable, traction is a reliable alternative.

The best quality reduction obtains the best long-term results. Vascular complications are said to occur in 5% of cases and the incidence of Volkmann's ischaemic contracture is 1%.

The significant complication of supracondylar fracture is cubitus varus deformity. This is reported to occur in 3% of cases which have been treated by closed percutaneous pinning and 14% following a simple closed reduction. The deformity results from rotatory malalignment of the distal fragment. To reduce the incidence of this, close evaluation of post-operative reduction films is essential. The fracture must be stabilized to prevent this deformity occurring.

Physeal injuries of the elbow

Lateral condyle physeal injuries account for approximately 17% of elbow fractures. The most common age of presentation is 6 years. These injuries have a bad reputation as the fracture pattern is difficult to identify. They can be divided into two types depending on the line of the fracture.

The fracture usually begins in the metaphysis and crosses the epiphysis. However, it may go across the epiphysis in one of two places: the ossification centre of the lateral condyle or between the ossification centres of the capitellum and trochlea. The second type of injury could be treated as a Salter Type II but the first is a Salter Harris type IV injury. As a consequence there is a significant incidence of abnormal growth following these injuries. Non-unions of children's fractures are rare but a number occur associated with lateral condylar fractures.

To avoid missing injuries of the lateral condyle of elbow a high index of suspicion is essential. They are associated with significant soft tissue swelling. If in doubt as to the severity of the injury or whether the fracture line enters the elbow joint, an arthrogram is helpful. Anatomical reduction of any fracture which enters the joint must be achieved and therefore an open reduction may be indicated.

Capitellar fractures

These are very rare in children.

Medial condyle fractures

These are uncommon but occur after the trochlea ossification centre has appeared. They can be of either type 1 or type 2 patterns as previously described for lateral condylar fracture. All the problems associated with lateral condylar fractures pertain to this injury.

Medial epicondylar fractures

These injuries occur between the ages of 9 and 12 years and they are more common in boys than girls; 30% are associated with dislocation of the elbow joint, and in 14% the medial epicondylar fragment is incarcerated into the elbow joint. A classification has been proposed:

- Type 1 – undisplaced fracture.
- Type 2 – minimally displaced fracture.
- Type 3 – displaced.

The type 3 is subdivided as to whether it is associated with an elbow dislocation or whether the fragment is trapped in the joint.

The medial epicondyle should be present on X-rays between the ages of 5 and 6 years. It is essential to check its position. Incarceration into the joint can occur even if the elbow reduces spontaneously in the A&E department.

Undisplaced fractures can be treated conservatively but any fracture with significant displacement should be treated by open reduction and internal fixation to ensure that the stability of the elbow is maintained.

Lateral epicondylar fractures

These are uncommon. Avulsion fractures can occur, or isolated fragmentation as a result of direct injury.

Radial head fractures

Fracture of the radial head in a child is a serious injury accounting for approximately 1% of fractures in children. The presenting age is usually between 9 and 10 years and the cause is a fall on the outstretched hand.

The three types of injury which can produce this are a Salter II, Salter IV and fracture of the proximal metaphysis. These may be associated with fractures of the proximal ulna. It is important to determine whether there is angulation, rotation, translocation or complete separation of the fragments.

Better results are obtained under the age of 10 years.

Poor results occur if there is an associated injury, greater than 30° of angulation or 3 mm of translocation. Without associated injury an angulation of 40° can be accepted.

The first line of treatment for translocation and angulation is closed reduction. If this fails to achieve an acceptable reduction, percutaneous manipulation using a small Steinmann pin should be recommended. Open reduction is associated with a poor outcome because of devascularization, stiffness or arrested growth.

Elbow dislocations

These occur in the older child, usually between the ages of 13 and 14 years. They are often associated with other injuries, especially avulsion of the medial epicondyle. Dislocation is usually posterolateral. Associated nerve injuries are uncommon.

Humeral fractures

Humeral shaft fractures are much less common than fractures at the proximal or distal end of the bone. They usually occur as a result of direct violence and represent only 10% of humeral fractures and 2% of children's fractures. Certain injury patterns should be looked for. Any child with a spiral fracture of the humerus under the age of 2 years should be considered as suffering abuse from wrenching until proven otherwise.

Humeral shaft fractures can occur with delivery but the most common mechanism over the age of 3 years is direct violence which usually produces a transverse or a short spiral fracture. In this type of injury there is a greater incidence of radial nerve damage.

Fractures of the upper shaft of the humerus can occur through pathological bone, a simple or aneurysmal bone cyst, enchondroma or deposits of eosinophilic granuloma.

Fractures of the shaft of the humerus in children should be treated by strapping the arm to the side. Occasionally splintage may be required.

Neonates to 3-year-olds

These tend to be incomplete greenstick fractures which can usually be treated by strapping the arm to the chest in a collar and cuff. Any angulation should remodel within the course of 1–2 years.

5 years to 12-year-olds

These children may be treated with a collar and cuff and a body bandage but occasionally some form of external splintage may be required to control angulation.

Adolescents

These fractures should be treated like those of an adult. Reduction is rarely required.

The prognosis is excellent. Up to 40° of angulation often remodels without difficulty. In some cases overgrowth does occur by as much as 2 cm.

Radial nerve lesions are less common in children than in adults.

SPINAL INJURIES

Cervical spine

Children's spinal injuries do present a problem in interpretation of radiographs. Epiphyseal lines can mimic fractures. In addition there are occasional congenital absences of bony structures or ligaments which can lead to significant injuries in 'at risk' groups.

The incidence in children is rare but is said to account for approximately 3% of all spinal injuries. In contrast to adult fractures, the vast majority of spinal injuries in children occur above the level of C3. It is stated that there is a lower incidence of neurological abnormalities and if neurological damage does occur the outcome is better.

Radiological features

The distance between the anterior arch of the atlas and the dens should measure less than 4.5 mm. Any increase suggests there is some degree of instability at this level. Soft tissue swellings at the level of C2 should measure less than 4 mm and at C6 less than 8 mm but this is variable, especially in children that cry. There is hypermobility in children's spines. This is prevalent at C2 and C3, and can give the impression of subluxation but may well be a normal variant (Fig. 6). Care must be taken in interpreting subluxation at this level and if there is any doubt a series of flexion/extension views may be taken under medical supervision.

Injuries

A whiplash/shaken infant syndrome occurs in children under the age of 3 months. This is a recognized pattern of child abuse (see Chapter 61).

Occiput/C1 fractures

In children, dislocation of the occiput on C1 does occur but is usually fatal.

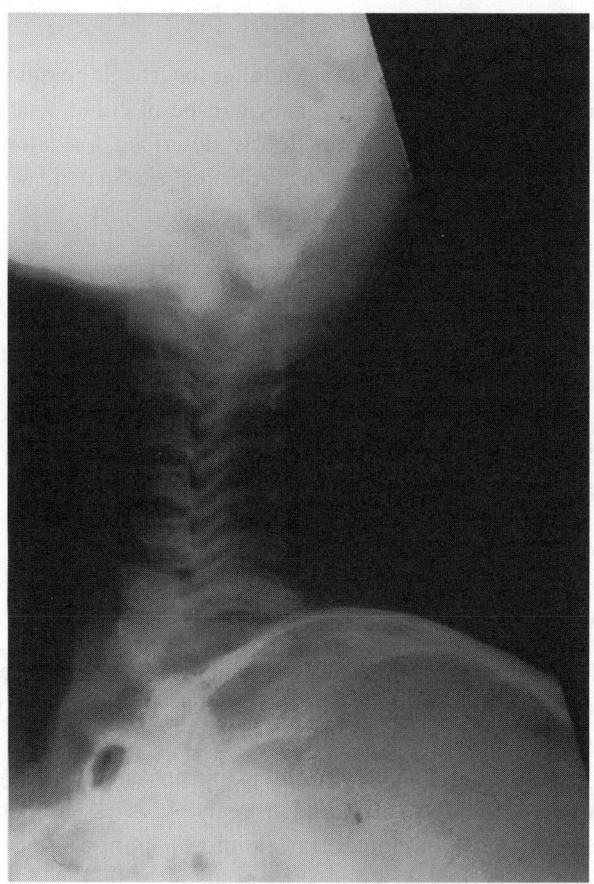

Fig. 6. Pseudo-subluxation of the cervical spine.

Atlas fractures

Compression injuries are uncommon and they occur much less frequently in children than in adults.

Atlanto/axial injuries

Atlantoaxial instability

Atlantoxial instability due to ligamentous disruption is exceptionally rare. However, it is a chronic problem in a number of disorders including Down's syndrome, juvenile rheumatoid arthritis, Larsen's syndrome and mucopolysaccharidosis. The presence of chronic instability at this level can lead to significant neurological dysfunction following minimal trauma. Care must be taken when evaluating any children with unusual syndromes who have had a fall.

Atlantorotary displacement

This is perhaps the best term used to describe rotary subluxation of C1 and C2. It is a cause of acute torticollis and is thought to be due to excessive mobility and forward subluxation of C1 on C2. The overall outcome is excellent. However, there are four types of increasing significance.

- Type 1 – rotary displacement with no anterior shift of C1 on C2.
- Type 2 – rotary displacement with anterior shift less than 5 mm.
- Type 3 – rotary displacement with anterior shift greater than 5 mm.
- Type 4 – rotary displacement with posterior shift.

Types 3 and 4 are associated with a significant risk of neurological impairment.

The most important X-ray to take is the open mouth view which demonstrates the subluxation of C1 on C2. A lateral view is also indicated to see if there is any evidence of anterior displacement of C1 on C2.

Odontoid fracture

This is a frequent injury associated with hyperextension. The highest incidence is at the age of 4 years. It is not really a fracture but a slip of the synchondrosis. The outlook is excellent.

In children over the age of 10 years, adult injury patterns may occur. Facet dislocations, either unilateral or bilateral, may occur and these are often related to diving accidents.

Thoracolumbar spine

The incidence of injury is much lower than that of the cervical spine. Again, skeletal development makes the interpretation of X-rays difficult. At least two-thirds of the fractures are stable. Compression fractures or Chance fractures can occur.

However, there is an increased incidence of spinal cord damage with no radiological abnormality so care must be taken in the evaluation of all children who are suspected of having a thoracolumbar injury.

Traumatic spondylolysis

Spondylolysis does not occur congenitally. It is thought to be a stress fracture of the pars interarticularis. The peak incidence is between the ages of 7 and 8 years. However, the symptoms may not appear until much later in life. If plain lateral X-rays are taken 20% of cases will be missed. Either oblique films or a bone scan must be performed. The presenting feature is back pain, particularly on lateral stress. It is said to be more common in athletic children, particularly those participating in gymnastics. It is unusual for any neurological signs to be present in these children.

PELVIC FRACTURES

Pelvic fractures in children have a high mortality because, as in adults, a high degree of violence is required. There is also a high incidence of associated injuries. The mortality rate is reported as being between 9% and 18%.

The overall outlook for pelvic fractures in children is excellent. They usually heal without complications which tend to arise from associated injuries.

It is best to use the adult classification of pelvic injuries. However, some features differ (e.g. avulsion fractures). It is possible to avulse any of the apophyses around the pelvis, such as the anterior superior iliac spine, anterior inferior iliac spine, ischial tuberosity and the lesser trochanter. These result from strenuous activity in athletes. The peak incidence is between the ages of 12 and 14 years.

ACETABULAR FRACTURES

Acetabular fractures are exceptionally rare. However, they have a similar pattern in children as in adults. One complication is growth arrest due to damage to the acetabular growth plate.

HIP FRACTURES

Hip fractures are unusual in children and their prognosis is worse than in adults because the blood supply to the hip is precarious and fractures of the femoral neck have a high incidence of avascular necrosis. A considerable degree of violence is required to cause fractures of the femoral neck which result from road traffic accidents or falls from a significant height.

Classification

Transepiphyseal fractures

- With dislocation of the capital epiphysis.
- Without dislocation of the capital epiphysis.

The outcome of both these injuries is poor. The incidence

of avascular necrosis is at least 50%. Aggressive treatment is needed to obtain as good a reduction as possible.

Transcervical fractures

- Undisplaced.
- Displaced.

Again the outlook is poor. The average incidence of avascular necrosis is 42% and it appears that displaced fractures carry a greater risk than those which are undisplaced. Aggressive treatment should be instituted with decompression of the haematoma within the capsule of the hip joint and internal fixation to stabilise the fracture.

Cervicotrochanteric fractures

- Undisplaced.
- Displaced.

This group corresponds to basal cervical fractures in adults. In children there is a 30–35% risk of avascular necrosis according to the displacement of the fracture. Internal fixation is strongly recommended.

Peritrochanteric fractures

These usually unite without complication and they account for approximately 70% of all femoral neck fractures.

Dislocation of the hip

This is more common than a fracture. There are two peaks:

1. In early childhood.
2. In adolescence.

Fifty per cent are said to occur between the ages of 12 and 15 years. The vast majority are posterior dislocations. Avascular necrosis is reported in 8–10%. The longer the hip is out of joint the greater the risk of avascular necrosis. Early reduction is essential.

LOWER LIMB

Femoral fractures

This is a common injury in childhood. There are two peaks:

1. At the age of 2 years.
2. At 14 years.

The former usually result from falls. The layer peak results from road traffic accidents and recreational activities. Seventy per cent fractures of the femur involve the midshaft. The overall outlook for these fractures is excellent and non-union is unusual. Malunion can occur as a result of inappropriate treatment.

Most fractures are either transverse or spiral. Open fractures and comminution are uncommon in children.

Birth injuries involving the femur

In difficult births, transverse midshaft fractures of the femur can occur. Any condition in which the knees are in fixed extension predisposes to birth fractures.

Sixty per cent of fractures that occur in children under the age of 1 year have been attributed to child abuse. The remainder must be considered pathological or due to bone dysplasia.

Fractures and dislocations of the knee

Separation of distal femoral epiphysis

This accounts for between 1% and 6% of all epiphyseal injuries. The separations are usually either of a Salter I or Salter II type with some compression and there is significant risk of growth arrest with these injuries.

The injuries can be classified in two different ways:

1. According to the direction of displacement: for displacement type 1 anterior, type 2 posterior, type 3 medial or lateral.
2. By the Salter–Harris classification on I to V.

Anterior separation is due to hyperextension injury and as a result there is a significant risk of neurovascular damage. This is often a Salter–Harris type I injury. It can occur in the newborn, especially in breach delivery. It has also been identified in child abuse. There is a significant risk of growth arrest.

Posterior displacement is very rare.

Medial and lateral displacement is the most common of the distal femoral epiphysis separations. They are usually Salter–Harris type II with compression and a significant risk of growth arrest. An anatomical reduction should be obtained.

These injuries can be associated with significant trauma to the anterior cruciate and the collateral ligaments.

Careful evaluation of these structures must be made before treatment is instituted.

Some injuries to the epiphyseal plate are undisplaced. Stress views may be of value in determining the degree of instability. All should be evaluated for neurovascular injury.

Proximal tibial epiphysis separation

This is a very rare injury. However, there is a high risk of associated neurovascular damage and growth arrest.

The majority of injuries are Salter I or Salter II caused by direct or indirect violence. The displacement is usually posterior which can compress the vessels at the trifurcation. It can occur in breach delivery. Sometimes the fibula is also fractured and there is damage to the lateral popliteal nerve.

Undisplaced fractures do occur and stress views may be of value. Anatomical reduction should be obtained and most patients can be managed satisfactorily in plaster. The major complications are growth arrest with deformity, recurrent instability because of associated ligamentous injury and neurovascular compromise.

Tibial tubercle avulsion

This is a rare injury. The diagnosis is complicated because of Osgood–Schlatter's disorder which is common in childhood and presents with pain and tenderness over the tibial tuberosity. In some series, Osgood–Schlatter's disorder and tibial tuberosity avulsions have been grouped together.

Patellar injuries

The patella is a sesamoid bone in the quadriceps tendon. The thick cartilaginous mass of the patella in childhood protects the ossific centre against injury and therefore fracture is unusual. However, a number of unusual injuries occur specifically in children.

Avulsion injuries can affect the inferior pole. This is known as Sinding–Larsen–Johansson syndrome. It is said to be more common in athletes, especially in people involved in sports which require sudden take-off and jumping.

Osteochondral fractures

Osteochondral fractures are quite common following patellar dislocation. However, they are often difficult to diagnose because of the small ossific component and large chondral fragment. It is important to be aware of this injury and X-rays are mandatory.

Sleeve fracture

This occurs between the ages of 8 and 12 years. It is an avulsion of a small chondral fragment with an extensive sleeve of articular cartilage. The retinaculum is also pulled off the bony patella. There is displacement of the fracture with disruption of the extensor mechanism so the patient is unable to straight leg raise. Awareness of the severity of the injury is essential to ensure that it is accurately diagnosed.

Transverse fractures

As in adults and in adolescence, transverse fractures can occur as a result of direct violence. It is essential to ensure that the extensor mechanism is intact as this will affect treatment.

Knee injuries

Ligamentous injuries around the knee itself are uncommon. The ligament's attachment to bone is stronger than are the epiphyseal plates around the knee and this usually results in epiphyseal separations rather than ligamentous injuries.

Injuries specific to children are osteochondral fractures and tibial spine injuries.

Osteochondral fractures

These can arise from the patella in lateral dislocation or from the femoral condyle. There is some difficulty making a diagnosis because of the small osseous component. Injuries to the femoral condyle can occur as a result of direct trauma and produce a significant haemarthrosis. The fracture should if at all possible be reduced.

Tibial spine injuries

Rupture of the anterior cruciate in children is very unusual. The bony attachment is very much weaker than the ligament itself and fractures of the anterior tibial spine are more common. The injury is associated with accidents on bicycles and motorized off-road vehicles. The classification is:

1. Minimal displacement.
2. Displacement with a posterior hinge.
3. Complete separation.

The mechanism is thought to be forced hyperextension. It is a severe injury and other ligaments within the
knee joint may be affected.

The treatment is reduction which usually takes place
in extension. However, type III injuries require open
reduction and stabilization.

Ligamentous injuries

Ligamentous injuries in children become progressively
more common as the child approaches skeletal maturity.
The treatment is as for adults. Anterior cruciate injuries
are uncommon but their outlook is poor.

Treatment is designed to prevent meniscal injuries
until the epiphyses have fused and a formal anterior
cruciate reconstruction can be performed.

Meniscal lesions

Again these are uncommon injuries in children which
occur as they approach skeletal maturity and are known
to be associated with discoid menisci. Peripheral detachments are frequent and, instead of excision, meniscal
repair should be considered. MRI (magnetic resonance
imaging) is advisable in children to exclude meniscal
injury which should be referred to the appropriate
surgeon.

Tibial fractures (Fig. 7)

This is the most common lower limb injury in children.
The causes are sport or road traffic accidents.

The toddler's fracture

This is a spiral fracture of the tibia which occurs in
children under the age of 2 years and results from a fall.
Children often present to the A&E department with a
reluctance to bear weight. There is often no significant
bruising or swelling over the tibia but some localized
tenderness. The injury is best treated by a long leg cast.
X-rays taken 10 days later will show callus beneath the
raised periosteum.

This fracture should not make the casualty officer
particularly suspicious of non-accidental injury.

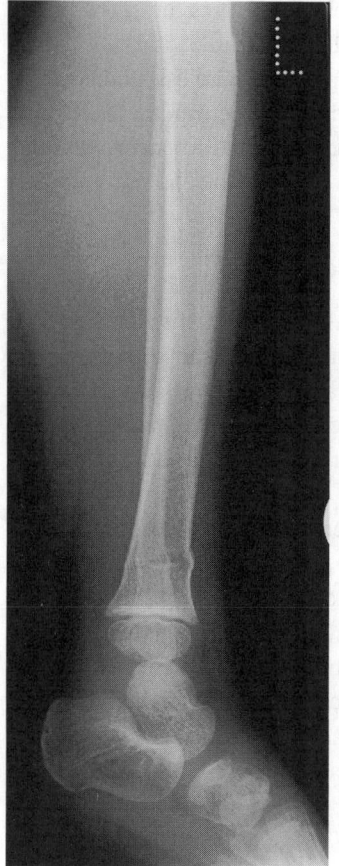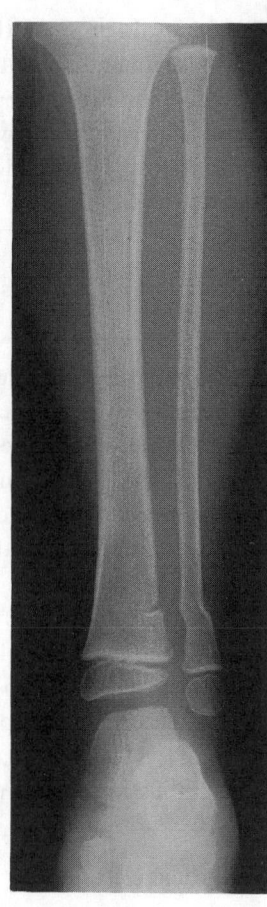

Fig. 7. A fracture of the distal tibial compression type, with also a
fracture of the fibula with some angulation and no displacement. The
cortex appears to be intact.

Spiral fracture

Spiral fractures occur in children as do short oblique
fractures with an intact fibula. In some instances the
fibula has undergone plastic deformation producing
varus deformity at the fracture site and some difficulty
obtaining a reduction.

Stress fracture

These do occur in children and present with pain in the
tibia on bearing weight. X-rays show some thickening of
the cortex posteriorly and the bone scan reveals a hot
area. Treatment is by immobilization.

The surgeon must be aware that all tibial injuries may
be associated with neurovascular trauma.

Injuries to the foot

Significant injuries to the foot are exceptionally rare in
children.

Talar fractures

These do occur as a consequence of forced dorsiflexion. The risk of avascular necrosis is increased in children. Identification of this injury depends on awareness. The cause is usually a road traffic accident. The physical signs are swelling and localized tenderness.

Calcaneal fractures

These are often difficult to diagnose, are benign, usually involve slight depression and heal without complication. They occur, as in adults, following a fall from a height and awareness of associated injuries is essential in patient management. The patient should be carefully examined for injuries to the hips and to the back. Fractures can be divided into three major groups:

1. Extra-articular.
2. Intra-articular.
3. Fractures with bone loss and damage to the achilles tendon.

Groups 1 and 2 have been further subdivided.

Metatarsal fractures

These are very common injuries resulting from direct violence. The fracture is usually transverse involving the neck of the metatarsal. They heal without complication. Aggressive treatment is indicated if more than one metatarsal is fractured.

Fracture of the base of the fifth metatarsal is a frequent injury seen in the A&E department. It is caused by inversion and the pull of peroneus brevis which produces an avulsion fracture.

This injury is often in doubt as the apophysis is often confused with a fracture. The apophysis lies parallel to the shaft of the fracture, is not present below the age of 8 years and fuses after the age of 12 years in girls and 15 years in boys. Failure to identify this as an apophysis often leads to unnecessary immobilization.

Jones fracture

Fracture of the shaft of the metatarsal distal to the tuberosity is known as a Jones fracture. It presents at the age of 15–21 years. People involved are usually athletic.

Ankle injuries

Injuries around the ankle produce a significant workload for all A&E departments. The injuries range from a minor sprain of the anterior talofibular ligament to a significant fracture of the physeal plate of the distal tibia. Any child presenting with a history of ankle injury who cannot bear weight and has significant swelling must be treated as having a potentially serious injury.

Radiographs can be confusing because of a number of accessory ossicles and physeal lines which mimic avulsion fractures.

A number of classifications of ankle injury have been published. These help the surgeon to determine how the force was applied and how the fractures can be reduced. However, they do not accurately describe the prognosis which depends on the degree of physeal injury.

Twenty-five per cent of all physeal injuries occur at and around the ankle. Some are exceptionally serious. Damage includes growth arrest, producing shortening or asymmetrical development and deformity. Careful evaluation of the X-rays is essential to identify the fracture plane as the same fracture patterns do not occur in an adult and become more complex if part of the physis has closed. Examples are the juvenile Tillaux fracture (Fig. 8) which is a Salter–Harris type III fracture of the lateral part of the tibial epiphysis. The other injury unique to children is the triplane fracture consisting of three fragments (Fig. 9). The first involves the anterolateral portion of the distal tibial physis – a Salter–Harris type III injury. The second is made up of the remainder of the physis anterolaterally, and a posterior portion with an attached posterolateral spike of the distal tibial metaphysis and is again a Salter–Harris type III injury. The third is the remainder of the distal tibial metaphysis. Care must be taken evaluating the lateral radiograph as the oblique fracture can be thought to be a fracture of the fibula. These fractures need anatomical reduction.

The Salter–Harris type I epiphyseal separation of the distal fibular presents with significant swelling over the lateral aspect of the ankle following an inversion injury. The vast majority are undisplaced and just need to be immobilized.

Other fracture patterns which occur as a result of injuries to the ankle are Salter–Harris type III fractures of the distal tibial epiphysis on the medial side. The medial malleolus fractures but there is also a significant crush injury which will lead to growth disturbance and a poor outlook.

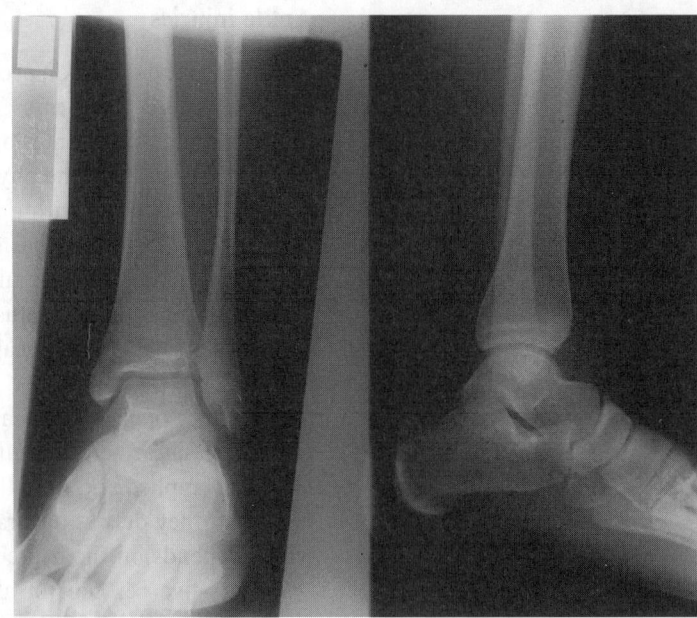

Fig. 8. A Tillaux fracture of the ankle.

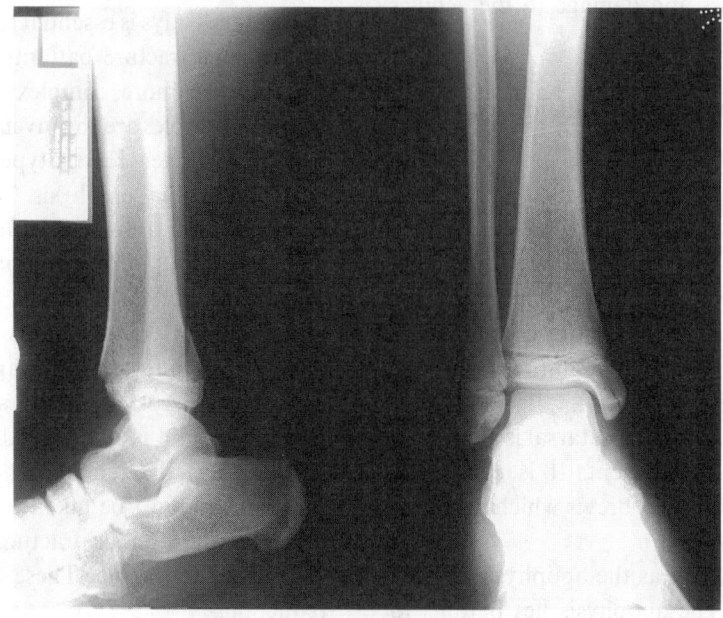

Fig. 9. A complex triplane fracture with a fracture extending into the metaphysis through the epiphysis through the medial malleolus. Note there is posterior displacement of the fracture.

Salter–Harris type II and type IV injuries occur; anatomical reduction produces the best result.

Selected further reading

BENSON, M. K. D. *et al.* (1994). *Children's Orthopaedics and Fractures*, Edinburgh: Churchill Livingstone.

RANG, M. (ed.) (1983). *Children's Fractures* 2nd edn, Philadelphia, PA: Lippincott.

SHARRARD, W. J. W., *Paediatric Orthopaedics and Fractures*, Oxford: Blackwell Scientific.

WILKINS, K. *et al. Rockwood and Green Fractures in Children.*

30 Injuries of the lower limb

M. PEARSE[a] and M. JACKSON[b]

[a]Department of Orthopaedic Surgery, Charing Cross Hospital, London, UK
[b]Department of Orthopaedic Surgery, Bristol Royal Infirmary, Bristol, UK

Chapter plan

Femoral shaft fractures
Fractures around the knee
Fractures of the tibial shaft
Fractures and dislocations of the hindfoot
Acute compartment syndromes
Fractures of the ankle

FEMORAL SHAFT FRACTURES

Fractures of the strongest bone in the body occur as a consequence of high-energy injuries such as road traffic accidents (vehicular and pedestrian), gunshot injuries, falls from a height, horse riding accidents and plane crashes. Most series show a male preponderance with an average age of 25–30 years. However, there is an increasing incidence of femoral shaft fractures in the elderly (Moran *et al.*, 1990). These fractures are typically the result of low- to moderate-energy trauma.

The femoral shaft fracture is probably the commonest orthopaedic injury in a multiply injured patient and virtually all major traumatic injuries can occur in association with this fracture. Associated injuries to the head, chest, spine and abdomen are common (Bone *et al.*, 1989). Several musculoskeletal injury patterns are frequently seen in association with a femoral shaft fracture. Coexisting ipsilateral proximal femoral and femoral shaft fractures are not uncommon, particularly in the multiply injured patient. However, some series have reported a failure to diagnose a proximal femoral fracture in up to 30% of cases (Swiontkowski, 1987). Failure to diagnose a femoral neck fracture may increase the risk of avascular necrosis or non-union of the femoral neck. Therefore all patients with a femoral shaft fracture must have an anteroposterior pelvic radiograph and care must be taken not to obscure the femoral neck with the ring of a Thomas splint or other traction device. A significant knee ligament injury may occur in association with femoral shaft fractures in up to 15% of cases (Swiontkowski, 1987). Once fracture stability has been achieved by surgical treatment, the knee must be evaluated for ligament injury, preferably immediately following shaft stabilization while the patient is still anaesthetized.

Ipsilateral fracture of the tibia, the 'floating knee', occurs relatively commonly in conjunction with femoral shaft fracture. Multiply injured patients with long-bone fractures have approximately a 50% incidence of ipsilateral femoral shaft and tibial fractures (Karlstrom & Olerud, 1977). All patients with this injury pattern should be regarded as polytraumatized because of the high frequency of injury to other body regions. Stabilization of both femoral and tibial fractures is required to optimize the functional outcome and prevent loss of knee motion.

Open femoral shaft fractures are relatively common. In one study of 520 shaft fractures, 16.5% were open injuries (Winquist *et al.*, 1984); the majority were type I (88.4%) or type II (9.3%). Therefore, the extent of open injury tends to be reduced because of the large soft tissue envelope surrounding the femur.

The clinical diagnosis of a femoral shaft fracture is usually simple. The patient is in severe pain and the limb is swollen and shortened. Angulation tends to be anterior and lateral. Associated injuries to other systems must be recognized and hypovolaemic shock treated. A femoral shaft fracture can result in the loss of approximately 2 units of blood and all patients with this injury must have an intravenous infusion. Pain in the hip or pelvic region may indicate a hip dislocation or fracture. Knee effusion is not uncommon and may indicate a significant ligament injury. A careful evaluation of the nerve status of the

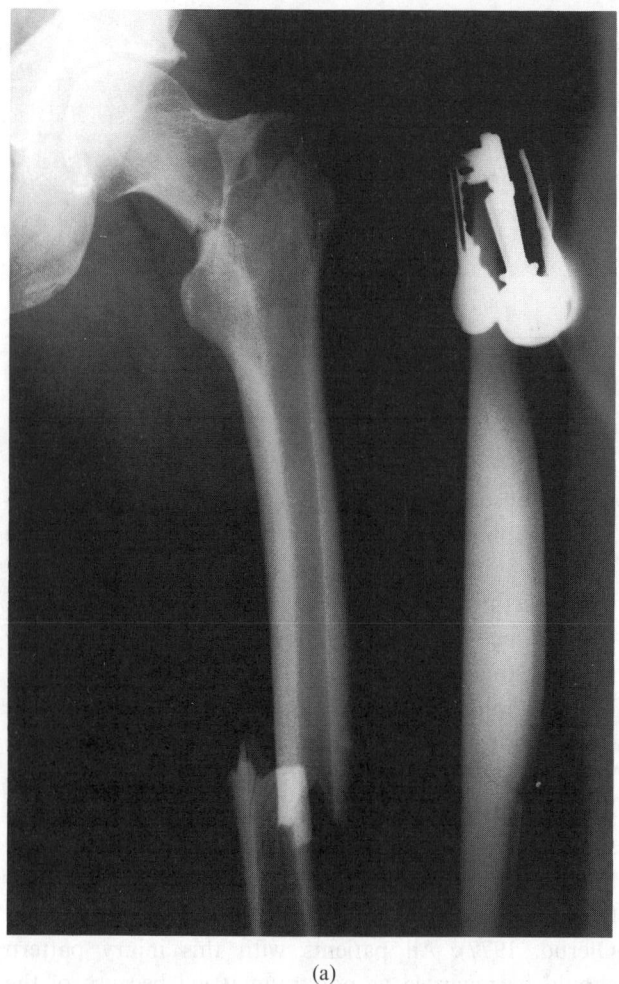

(a)

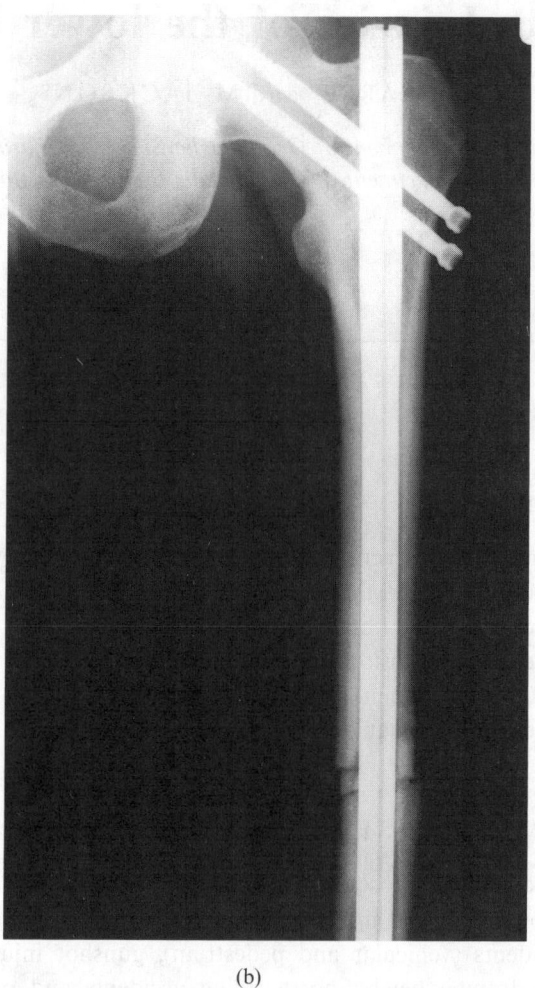

(b)

Fig. 1. Radiographs showing ipsilateral femoral shaft and neck fracture (a) treated by intramedullary reconstruction nailing (b).

injured limb must be recorded at presentation and the extent of all soft tissue injuries evaluated and documented. The fracture should then be gently splinted by the application of a Thomas splint or other traction device. Immediately after splinting the leg, the neurovascular examination is repeated.

All patients require anteroposterior and lateral radiographs of the whole femur and an anteroposterior radiograph of the pelvis. Multiply injured patients should also have a chest radiograph and a lateral radiograph of the cervical spine unless the patient is alert and completely asymptomatic.

The femur is a common site for metastases, particularly the proximal metaphysis. A patient who presents with a fractured femur without a history of significant trauma must be investigated for a pathological fracture. Patients with symptomatic lesions (pain on weight bearing), or with lesions greater than 50% of the circumfer-

ence of the bone, should be considered for prophylactic stabilization.

Prior to 1940, femoral shaft fractures were treated by closed reduction and immobilization with skeletal traction utilizing the Thomas splint or a modification thereof. Following the introduction of intramedullary femoral nails by Gerhardt Küntscher in 1939 (Johnson, 1992), the treatment of femoral shaft fractures changed dramatically. Closed locked intramedullary nailing is now the treatment of choice for virtually all femoral shaft fractures (Fig. 1) (Johnson, 1992). However, the immediate management of a femoral shaft fracture still involves immobilization of the fracture by splinting and the application of traction—either skin or skeletal traction. Doctors involved in the immediate care of trauma patients must be able to quickly apply a traction splint following resuscitation and evaluation of the patient. This is particularly important if the patient is to be transferred to another hospital or if intramedullary nailing is delayed beyond the first 24 h. If the patient is to be admitted to the presenting hospital, skin or skeletal traction applied over a pulley at the foot of the bed is acceptable for a short period prior to surgery. Skeletal traction in a Thomas splint with modification to allow early knee motion can be used as a definitive treatment if surgical expertise is not available.

TECHNIQUE

Application of a Thomas splint

- The aim is to immobilize a fractured femur and thereby reduce pain and bleeding at the fracture site.
- Check distal neurovascular status first.
- Photograph and dress any wounds as necessary.
- Measure the circumference of the proximal thigh on the uninjured side if possible, allowing some room for further swelling of the thigh when selecting the appropriate ring size.

Skin traction

- Shave the skin, then apply adhesive tape starting at the medial malleolus and proceeding proximally.
- Apply tape to the lateral side and, with an assistant applying traction, secure the adhesive tape with encircling crepe bandage.

Skeletal traction

- Alternatively, a Steinmann pin placed though the tibia (behind the tibial tuberosity) or distal femur (at the level of the adductor tubercle) may be used, particularly in an older patient with inelastic skin and where heavy traction is required.
- A metal loop (e.g. Tulloch–Brown) is then attached to each end of the Steinmann pin.
- Slings to bridge the splint side irons are applied. A circular bandage (e.g. tubigrip) or calico and canvas slings may be used.
- A large pad (e.g. wool dressing) should be placed directly beneath the fracture to act as a fulcrum.
- Traction is applied to the leg by pulling on the traction cords connected to the spreader pad of the adhesive tapes, or to the metal loop if skeletal traction is being used.
- The Thomas splint is then pushed up the leg, while an assistant is maintaining traction, until the ring reaches the ischial tuberosity.
- The traction cords are then tied to the end of the splint. A Chinese windlass (e.g. spatula or metal rod) may be used to take up the slack.
- Following the fitting of a Thomas splint and the application of traction, the neurovascular status of the limb must be re-evaluated. If a distal pulse is not palpable immediately after applying traction, the traction should be released and the leg re-examined.

Aftercare

- Check regularly for thigh swelling which may render the ring tight around its circumference.
- Ensure all pressure areas are well padded, particularly around the ring, over the malleoli and in the region of the Achilles tendon.

In the multiply injured patient (injury severity score, ISS > 15), stabilization of the fracture within 24 h holds many advantages. Early stabilization decreases the incidence of pulmonary complications (Bone et al., 1989), systemic infection and mortality rate in multiply injured patients (Border et al., 1975). A study by Johnson et al. (1985) has shown that the benefits of early fracture stabilization are greatest in the severely injured. An isolated femoral shaft fracture should be stabilized as a planned procedure.

FRACTURES AROUND THE KNEE

Supracondylar and intercondylar fractures of the femur

The supracondylar area of the femur extends from the junction of the metaphysis with the diaphysis to the femoral articular surface of the knee. The mechanism of injury in most supracondylar fractures is an axial loading force combined with a varus/valgus or rotational force. These fractures are relatively common in elderly patients following a fall onto the flexed knee, leading to a comminuted fracture through osteoporotic bone. Similar fractures in younger patients are associated with high-energy trauma and there may be significant fracture displacement with open wounds and associated injuries. Clinically the limb is shortened and angulated at the fracture site and the deformity is usually varus. The distal neurovascular status must be checked. When the distal fragment is intact the pull of gastrocnemius may flex it, endangering the popliteal artery.

Radiographs should be carefully studied for fracture comminution, displacement and intra-articular extension. The AO classification (Muller et al., 1991b) divides these injuries into three types, each with three subtypes (Fig. 2).

Displaced comminuted fractures of the distal femur, particularly fractures with intra-articular involvement, present considerable challenges in management. The management of supracondylar fractures, however, is controversial (Wiss, 1991). Early reports comparing internal fixation and closed methods noted a high incidence of surgical complications, and numerous authors concluded that closed methods were preferable (Neer et al., 1967).

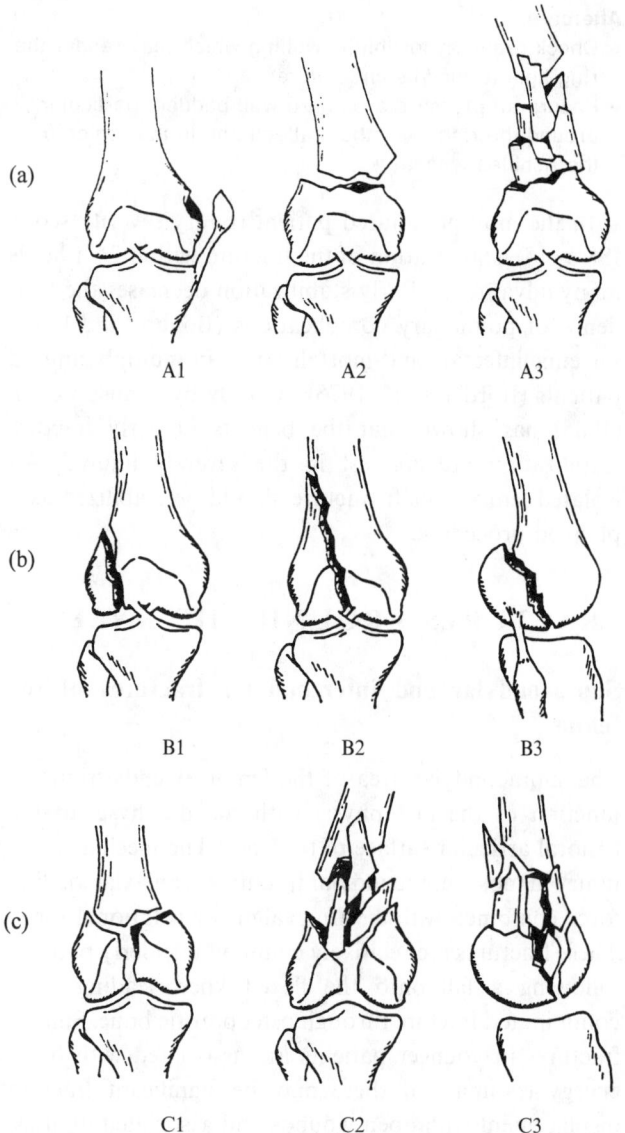

Fig. 2. AO classification of distal femoral fractures (after Muller *et al.*, 1991b). (a) Type A1, A2, A3. (b) Type B1, B2, B3. (c) Type C1, C2, C3.

Over the past two decades, surgical techniques and implants have improved considerably. More recent studies comparing the results of surgical and non-surgical methods have favoured open reduction and internal fixation (Schatzker & Lambert, 1979).

Indications for closed management include undisplaced or impacted stable fractures, severe osteoporosis, concomitant medical conditions precluding anaesthesia and spinal cord injury with fracture. To minimize the complications of closed treatment (e.g. long periods confined to bed and knee stiffness) most authorities combine skeletal traction with early cast-bracing. The fracture is reduced by traction through a distal femoral or proximal tibial Steinmann pin. The patient is placed in a cast-brace when there is minimal tenderness at the fracture site and radiographic signs of callus formation, usually between 3 and 6 weeks postinjury. Careful clinical and radiographic follow-up is required to monitor for loss of fracture reduction. The brace will be required until the fracture has healed, which is usally by 16 weeks.

Rigid internal fixation with anatomical alignment allows early mobilization and provides the best chance of an excellent result (Wiss, 1991). However, operative management of these complex fractures is difficult and surgical complications may produce the poorest results.

Careful preoperative planning is essential (Mast *et al.*, 1989). Surgeons attempting operative management of these injuries must be fully trained and have the complete instrumentation available and be supported by experienced theatre staff. Indications for surgery include:

- Displaced intra-articular fractures.
- Open fractures.
- Associated vascular injuries.
- Ipsilateral limb injuries.
- Associated knee ligament injuries.
- Pathological fracture.
- Failed closed treatment.

The most commonly used implant is the dynamic condylar screw; the 95° condylar blade plate is now indicated for the most distal fractures only. Bone grafting is recommended for comminuted fractures. If rigid fixation is achieved at surgery, postoperative continuous passive motion should be instituted.

Fractures of the patella

The patella is the largest sesamoid bone and lies within the quadriceps tendon. The function of the patella is to increase the efficiency of the quadriceps muscle. The patella elevates the extensor mechanism from the knee joint axis and increases the leverage of the quadriceps muscle by making it act over a greater angle. Recognition of the importance of the patella has led to a shift towards reconstruction and preservation of patellar function following fracture (Einola *et al.*, 1976).

Patellar fractures may result from direct or indirect forces. The majority are a result of direct trauma—a fall on the knee or a direct blow as in vehicular trauma. An ipsilateral femoral shaft fracture or posterior hip dislocation may occur in association with direct injuries. Fractures resulting from direct trauma may be incomplete, stellate or comminuted. If the quadriceps expansion is not torn there may be active extension against gravity and little separation of the fragments.

Indirect forces tend to cause a transverse fracture. The pull of the quadriceps muscle tears the medial and lateral expansions and the fracture fragments become widely separated. This injury typically follows a stumble or partial fall and active knee extension is usually lost.

The patella is subcutaneous and clinical suspicion of a fracture may be confirmed by palpation of its margin, away from any wound. It is important to assess the continuity of the extensor mechanism. Full active extension against gravity indicates an intact extensor mechanism. An injection of local anaesthetic may aid the clinical examination.

Operative treatment is not indicated for undisplaced fractures where the extensor mechanism is intact. Aspiration of the haemarthrosis, if present, and cylinder casting for 4–6 weeks are all that is necessary.

Displaced (>2 mm) articular fractures of the patella with loss of the extensor mechanism usually require operative repair. The fracture is exposed through a longitudinal midline or lazy 'S' incision. Following irrigation of the joint, the fracture is reduced and held with two Kirschner wires and an anterior tension band (Muller et al., 1991a).

It is important to preserve the patella whenever possible and thereby maintain quadriceps function. Severely comminuted fractures may be reduced and held by 'indirect reduction' utilizing two anterior wire loops and two Kirschner wires (Johnson, 1991). Total patellectomy may be indicated in a small subgroup with very comminuted fractures. Whichever technique is employed, the injury to the medial and lateral quadriceps expansion must be identified and repaired.

Tibial plateau fractures

Fractures of the tibial plateau are caused by axial loading combined with a valgus/varus force. The tibial condyle is crushed or split by the opposing femoral condyle which usually remains intact. The collateral ligament may act like a hinge with the fracture occurring on the opposite side (Kennedy & Bailey, 1968). Approximately half of all tibial plateau fractures are due to vehicular trauma and they account for 8% of fractures in the elderly (Hohl, 1991).

Patients may present with a swollen, painful knee and a varus or valgus deformity may be obvious. However, symptoms and signs are often more subtle and condylar tenderness should always be sought. Difficulty weight-bearing is an important symptom. The leg and foot must be examined for any neurovascular injury or signs of a compartment syndrome. Careful examination (a general anaesthetic may be required) may demonstrate instability if the collateral ligaments are injured. If a tense haemarthrosis is present the joint should be aspirated under aseptic conditions. Fat globules in the aspirate are highly suggestive of an intra-articular fracture.

Anteroposterior, lateral and occasionally oblique X-rays usually show the fracture, but further imaging is required to assess the degree of comminution or plateau depression. Tomograms, CT (computed tomography) scanning or MRI (magnetic resonance imaging) are all available in this respect. Schatzker (1987) has described six types of tibial plateau fractures (Fig. 3).

The treatment of tibial plateau fractures is controversial. A sensible management plan can, however, be made according to the degree of fracture comminution and/or plateau displacement and the age and medical status of the patient. Minimally displaced fractures (<2–3 mm) can be treated conservatively. Full assessment of the knee requires an examination under anaesthesia to assess any ligament damage. Any doubt regarding the extent of fracture displacement can be resolved by an arthroscopic washout and inspection of the fracture. A hinged cast brace can then be applied allowing early movement. Full weight-bearing should be delayed until there are signs of healing radiographically.

Displaced type 1 fractures usually require open or arthroscopically assisted reduction and internal fixation. Type 2 fractures with <4 mm depression in the elderly may be treated conservatively. Skeletal traction via a tibial pin, allowing early mobilization, is employed for 3 weeks before the application of a cast-brace (Apley, 1979). Open reduction with elevation of the fracture and bone grafting is usually preferred in younger patients. Similar principles apply to type 3 and type 4 fractures. Type 5 and type 6 fractures are very severe injuries and are often associated with neurovascular damage and compartment syndromes. The operative treatment of these fractures is difficult and the surgical complication rate is high. Therefore closed treatment with skeletal traction is generally the preferred option (Hohl, 1991). Complications of tibial plateau fractures include joint stiffness and residual deformity. Post-traumatic osteoarthritis is not a particularly common sequela (Lansinger et al., 1986).

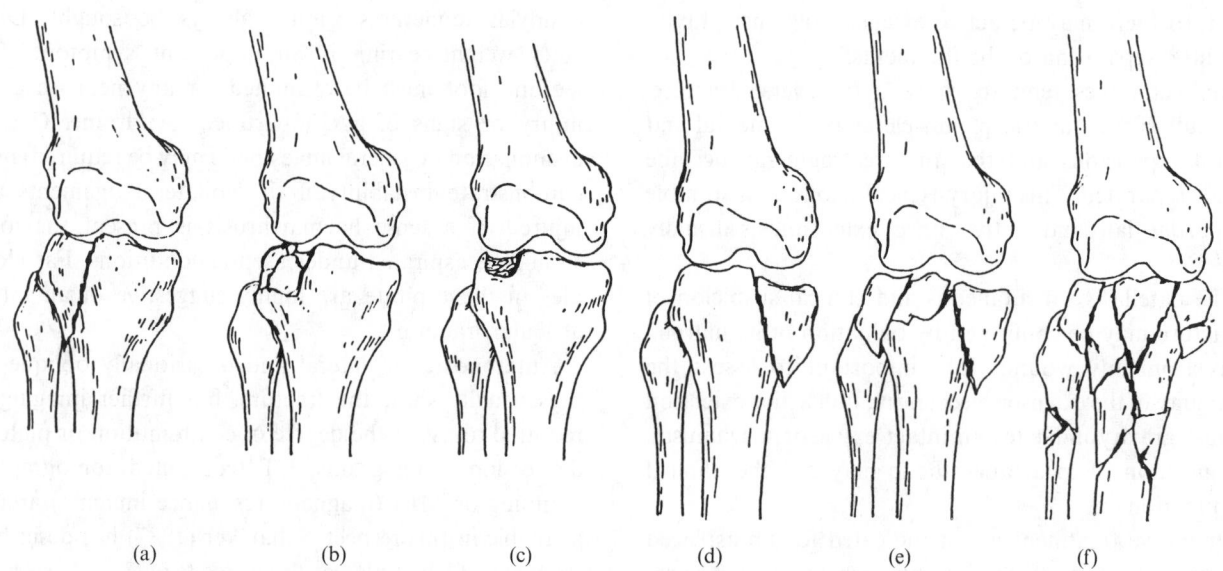

Fig. 3. Classification of tibial plateau fractures (after Schatzker, 1987). (a) Type 1 – shear fracture of lateral condyle. (b) Type 2 – combined joint depression and shear fracture of lateral condyle. (c) Type 3 – joint depression fracture of lateral condyle. (d) Type 4 – fracture medial tibial condyle. (e) Type 5 – bicondylar fracture. (f) Type 6 – plateau fracture with associated metaphyseal fracture.

FRACTURES OF THE TIBIAL SHAFT

The tibia is the most common lower limb long-bone fracture. In children, healing is rapid and complications such as non-union, malunion and infection are rare. In adult fractures complications frequently occur, the most serious of which is osteomyelitis, particularly as a result of open fractures. These comprise 10–20% of all tibial fractures and are amongst the most challenging problems facing the modern orthopaedic trauma surgeon. The most important steps in the prevention of osteo-myelitis rest on the management in the first 24 h. Tibial fractures are amongst the leading causes of temporary and permanent disability in young adults in the Western world.

An increasing proportion of tibial fractures result from direct violence as the subcutaneous location of the bone affords little protection from this type of injury. Many of these occur as a result of sports injuries or road accidents. Gunshot and rifle bullet wounds, although rare in the UK, are relatively common in the USA and may result in an associated severe and contaminated soft tissue injury. Indirect violence may occur as a result of a twisting force applied to the limb whilst the foot is held in a fixed position.

In virtually all instances tibial shaft fracture precludes weight-bearing and, if the fracture is displaced, pain may be severe. Signs of tibial fracture include angular and rotational deformity of the limb, swelling and bruising over the subcutaneous border as well as in the calf muscles. Tenderness will be maximal at the fracture site(s).

The distal circulation and sensation must be care-fully assessed, including signs of impending and early compartment syndrome (see below). Evidence of skin damage should be sought, including non-viable areas of degloving as well as open wounds.

Good-quality standard anteroposterior and lateral views to include the knee and ankle joints are usually the only radiographs necessary.

Tibial shaft fractures are frequently associated with ligamentous injuries of the knee. In one study (Temple-man & Marder, 1989), 22% of patients with closed fractures had significant instability. The medial collateral ligament was involved in all cases and the posterior cruciate ligament in 6%.

Management of closed tibial fractures

Many tibial fractures can be adequately treated by manipulation under anaesthetic and application of a moulded long-leg cast. This may be reduced to a below knee patellar bearing cast after 4 – 6 weeks until union. Patients require hospital admission for observation and elevation after reduction and application of a cast.

Operative fixation is increasingly considered if rapid functional recovery is required or the fracture pattern is complex and unstable. Those fractures considered

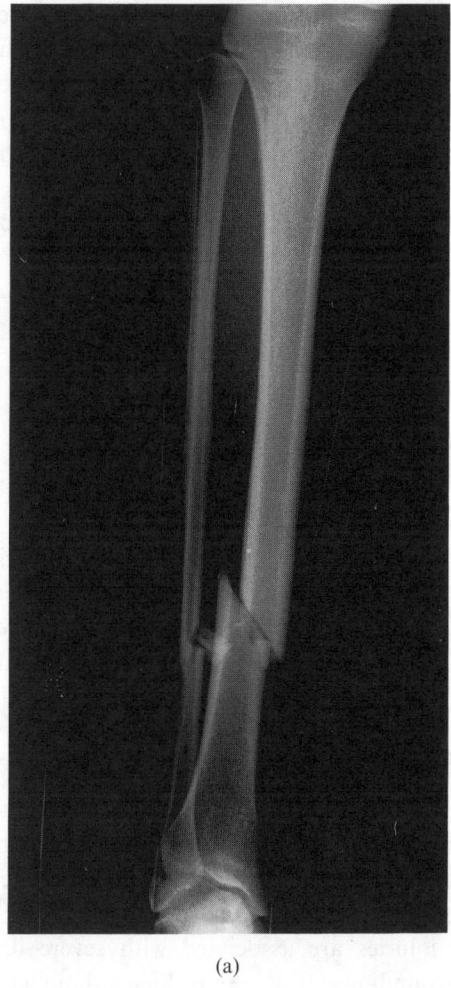
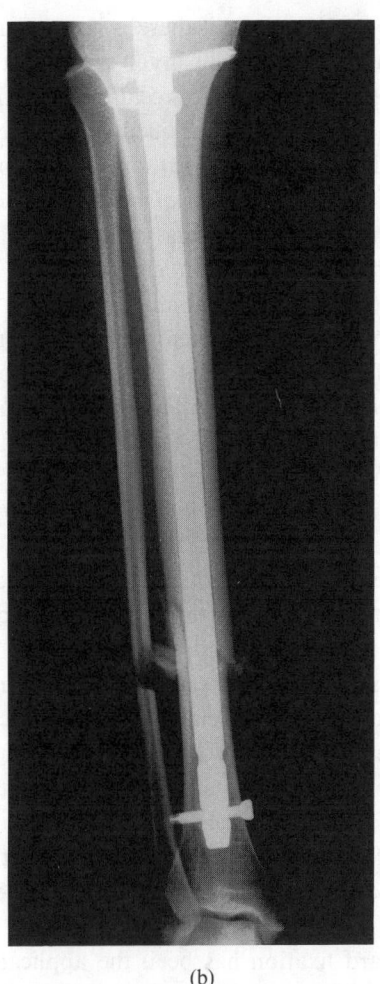

(a)   (b)

Fig. 4. Radiographs of tibial shaft fracture (a) treated by locked intramedullary nailing (b).

unsuitable for non-operative treatment are those where the fracture is segmental, multifragmented or where the initial displacement is greater than 50% of the shaft diameter.

The current fixation of choice for fractures of the tibial diaphysis is a closed interlocked intramedullary nail (see Fig. 4). Clinical results are superior to compression plating or external fixation, with fewer complications (Court-Brown *et al.*, 1990).

Management of open tibial fractures

The early management of open fractures of the tibia is of paramount importance if the functional outcome is to be satisfactory. The major complication of open tibial fracture is infection, which may lead to osteomyelitis.

The fundamental aim of management should be early restoration of the soft tissue envelope, allied to stable fixation of the fracture itself. The early use of rotational and free flap grafts has been a major advance. The immediate involvement of a plastic surgeon is now recognized to be an important step in improving the outcome of these injuries.

Accurate assessment of the degree of soft tissue injury using a standard classification system is essential, particularly in deciding on a management plan (see below).

Inevitably in an open fracture, there is a considerable degree of soft tissue injury and contamination and therefore urgent removal of all non-viable tissue and treatment of incipient infection is mandatory.

As soon as the injury is noted, the wound should be photographed on Polaroid film, then covered temporarily with dressings soaked in antiseptic. These must not be disturbed again until the patient reaches the operating theatre. Antibiotic therapy is commenced. This should be effective against *Staphylococcus aureus*, *Streptococcus* and *Clostridia*, particularly if there is heavy contamination. Standard protocols will involve use of a second-generation cephalosporin, such as cefuroxime, with benzylpenicillin. These should be continued until skin cover has been restored. Recently some authorities have noted the emergence of *Pseudomonas aeruginosa* as a cause of deep infection after open fractures and hence have advocated the use of a third-generation cephalosporin such as ceftazidime to cover this eventuality.

The patient should be taken to theatre for wound excision, preferably within 6 h of injury to avoid significant bacterial colonization. All non-viable tissue should be removed; this includes skin, fascia, muscle and devascularized cortical bone. The wound should then be irrigated with copious quantities (about 5 litres) of either normal saline or, preferably, a 0.05% solution of aqueous chlorhexidine. This should produce a clean field. Under *no* circumstances should primary closure be undertaken.

Stable fixation of the fracture is then carried out, but it must be emphasized that cast immobilization has no part in the current management of these fractures. It restricts access to the limb for plastic procedures and does not bestow adequate stability to prevent the development of infection. Recent experimental studies have shown that fracture instability is a potent aetiological factor in the development of infection (Worlock *et al.*, 1994).

The standard fixation has been the application of a uniaxial external fixator. The use of these devices leads to simple, safe and rapid stabilization of tibial fractures, although access to the limb is inevitably restricted. Union is also slow and may require bone grafting. Any subsequent conversion to intramedullary fixation is subject to an increased risk of infection.

For these reasons, there has been much recent interest in primary locked nailing of these fractures, particularly using small diameter solid nails which can be inserted without reaming. Initial clinical results with both reamed and unreamed intramedullary nails appear promising and are comparable with or superior to external fixation (Court-Brown *et al.*, 1991). However, proponents of these techniques rightly emphasize the importance of the restoration of soft tissue cover within 48–72 h of injury.

The role of amputation in the management of severe tibial fractures

In cases where extremely severe soft tissue injury accompanies a tibial fracture, particularly where there is neuro-

vascular damage, reconstruction may not be feasible or can only be expected to provide a very poor functional outcome. Primary amputation should then be considered. Until recently this was a subjective judgement based on the experience of the surgeon treating the case. However, an objective scoring system has been developed, validated by both retrospective and prospective data, to indicate when amputation should be performed. The Mangled Extremity Survival Score (MESS) (Johansen *et al.*, 1990), predicts amputation with 100% accuracy where scores are 7 or greater. It comprises four elements:

- The mechanism and energy of injury.
- Systemic hypotension.
- Limb ischaemia.
- The age of the patient.

The system is undoubtedly useful in the evaluation of the injury, leading to the inevitably difficult decision to amputate the limb; it does not follow, however, that a MESS score of less than 7 will predict a satisfactory clinical outcome.

Fractures of the tibial plafond

These injuries result from a vertical compression force applied to the hindfoot with the talus impacting on the distal tibia creating a fracture which involves the articular surface and the distal metaphysis of the tibia.

The injuries are associated with severe damage to the surrounding soft tissue envelope although damage to major neurovascular structures is rare. As a result, compartment syndrome may accompany this fracture.

Management should be directed towards the initial reduction of the swelling by elevation and ice. The injured limb should be supported by a plaster shell to prevent the development of an equinus deformity.

Standard radiographs, while showing the extent of the injury, are inadequate for management purposes. CT scanning is necessary for accurate imaging of the articular surface to permit anatomical reduction.

Definitive management of the bony injury must be achieved operatively, by internal fixation, usually with bone graft to restore the articular surface. This will enable good function in fractures where displacement is minimal or moderate. In cases where comminution is severe, results are poor leading to deep infection (13%), malunion (25%), non-union (25%) and degenerative arthritis (53%) (Bourne, 1989). Recent innovations include the concept of minimal internal fixation with axial stabilization using fine wire circular fixators. Preliminary reports have yielded encouraging results.

Ruptures of the Achilles tendon

The Achilles tendon is susceptible to inflammation as a result of overuse, and to acute partial or complete rupture.

Achilles tendonitis usually produces pain localized to the tendon itself and is caused by a recent increase in use. The tendon is tender but intact, and is treated with anti-inflammatory medication, rest and alteration of footwear.

Complete rupture presents with the typical sudden onset of pain, often likened to a sharp blow to the back of the calf. Under these circumstances, clinical examination will demonstrate a palpable defect in the tendon and the squeeze test will be negative. This is performed with the patient kneeling on a chair. Absence of plantar flexion when the calf muscles are squeezed indicates that the tendon is ruptured.

The management of this injury is controversial, both operative and non-operative methods having been shown to be effective. Conservative management consists of the application of a full below knee cast for a period of 4 weeks in full equinus, semiequinus for a further 4 weeks and then a heel raise for a further period of 4 weeks. If treatment is commenced within 48 h of injury, results are equivalent to surgery, in terms of both strength of plantar flexion and duration of disability (Carden et al., 1987). However, the rate of complications is much lower (19% vs 4%) for those treated in plaster. For those patients presenting more than 7 days after injury, the rate of rerupture becomes significant, as does calf weakness, and non-operative management is not appropriate.

There has been recent interest in percutaneous surgery for this condition; however, this seems to be associated with a high incidence of sural nerve complications, and reports of clinical results show little advantage over non-operative treatment.

FRACTURES AND DISLOCATIONS OF THE HINDFOOT

Fractures of the talus

The talus has a complex morphology and forms an intercalated segment, without muscle insertion, of the articulations of ankle, subtalar and transverse tarsal joints. It is therefore extensively (60%) covered by articular cartilage. Fractures may involve the dome, the neck, the body or the smaller processes of the talus. There are significant differences in the mechanism of injury, and the management of these types, and they are therefore considered separately.

Fracture of the talar neck

Fractures of the talar neck result from a direct high-energy impact force applied to the plantar flexed foot and are seen following car accidents. The injury has been classified by Hawkins (1970). The vascular supply of the proximal part of the talus may be compromised by displacement of the fragments; this may lead to non-union and to avascular necrosis of the dome. Management consists of prompt anatomical reduction of displaced fractures and compression screw fixation in an attempt to reduce the incidence of complications.

Fracture of the talar dome and lateral and medial processes

These are osteochondral fractures caused by inversion injuries of the ankle. They frequently present following persistent ankle pain on exercise. Although diagnosed by plain radiographs, management decisions require accurate imaging, preferably with CT or MRI, to delineate the injury exactly. Small displaced fragments from the lateral or medial dome are treated by excision; those from the lateral process involve the articular surface of the talocalcaneal joint and if significantly displaced require reduction and fixation.

Fractures of the calcaneum

These are caused by vertical compression forces applied to the hindfoot, usually as a result of a fall from a height. Clinically this injury is associated with marked soft tissue swelling and a varus deformity of the hindfoot leading to a short heel. The fracture is diagnosed by plain lateral and axial radiographs of the heel (Fig. 5a). These are usually adequate to identify whether the fracture line involves the subtalar joint. If subtalar joint involvement is suspected, further imaging using CT is necessary to assess the degree of displacement of the articular surface (Fig. 5b).

Minor extra-articular fractures require only ice, elevation and early mobilization of the hindfoot and ankle with the aid of physiotherapy.

Fractures causing displacement of the articular surface of the joint are best managed by operative reduction and

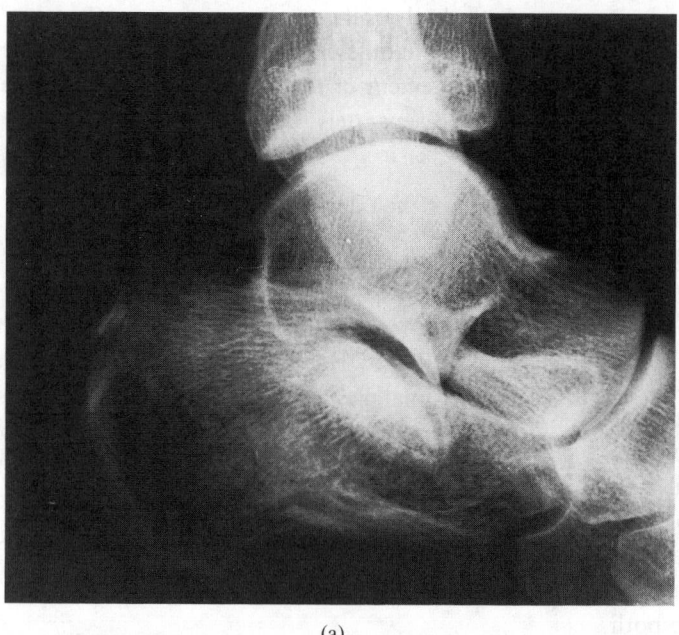 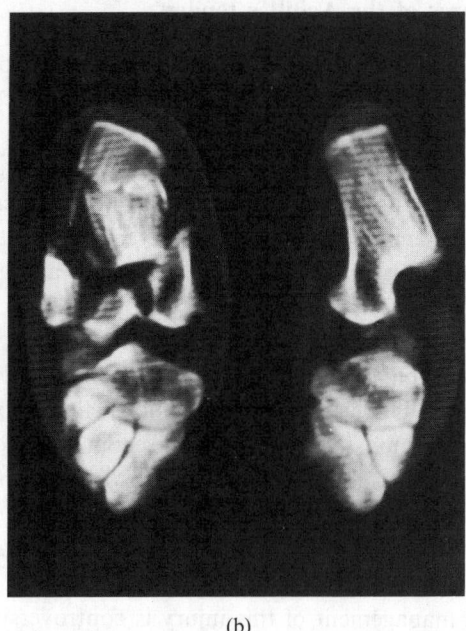

(a)   (b)

Fig. 5. (a) Plain lateral radiographs of intra-articular fracture of the calcaneum, (b) CT scans of the same fracture showing displacement of the fracture.

internal fixation via an extended lateral approach in order to restore congruity (Eastwood *et al.*, 1993). Treatment by non-operative means leads to significant and disabling symptoms and deformity.

Fractures of the cuboid

This fracture occurs as a result of lateral subluxation of the midtarsal joint with subsequent longitudinal compression of the cuboid. This rarely causes significant displacement and treatment of the injury is by casting and initial elevation. If there is significant loss of length, the deformity will cause abduction of the forefoot and subsequent disability. Under these circumstances, open reduction and bone grafting of the cuboid supplemented with external fixation are required to restore the lateral column of the foot.

Fractures of the navicular

These may involve the tuberosity, the body or the dorsal lip.

The tuberosity is avulsed by the tibialis posterior tendon if the foot is forcibly everted. It may be associated with a fracture of the cuboid and the lateral side of the tarsus should be visualized on the radiographs. The fracture is rarely displaced but may be confused with an accessory navicular bone. This is distinguished by smooth rounded borders and is commonly bilateral. Treatment, where the tuberosity is displaced, is by reattachment using a small fragment screw; otherwise, cast immobilization is sufficient.

Fractures of the body of the navicular are often associated with injuries involving the talonavicular and navicular cuneiform articulations of the midtarsal joint occurring as a result of high-energy trauma. Operative reduction of the involved joint is necessary although post-traumatic midfoot stiffness and pain are common.

Avulsion fractures of the dorsal cortex are caused by forced eversion of the foot. Simple cast immobilization from between 4 and 6 weeks is all that is necessary unless the fragment exceeds 25% of the articular surface, in which case screw fixation is indicated.

Fractures of the shaft and necks of the metatarsal bones

These fractures generally result from a heavy object falling onto the foot. Often more than one lateral metatarsal bone may be injured and there may be significant soft tissue trauma. Fracture displacement is rare, and ice, elevation and casting are all that is necessary. In cases where there are multiple displaced fractures, reduction and fixation using Kirschner wires is indicated and should be supplemented by cast immobilization.

Fracture of the fifth metatarsal base

This fracture is often referred to as the 'Jones' fracture as it was first described in 1903 by Sir Robert Jones with a radiograph of his own foot. The base of the metatarsal is avulsed by the tendon of peroneus brevis during forced inversion of the foot. The injury is now subdivided into those fractures of the peroneal tuberosity alone (type I) and those of the junction of proximal metaphysis and diaphysis (type II) – the true 'Jones' fracture. Each injury type should be immobilized in a below knee walking cast or strapped. It should be recognized that type II injuries have a significant rate of non-union and refracture.

Dislocation or fracture-dislocation of the tarsometatarsal (Lisfranc's) joint of the foot

This rare but important injury is frequently overlooked at first presentation. Failure to treat it may lead to significant disability, even after minimal displacement. Severe displacement is associated with entrapment or tear of the dorsalis pedis artery and consequent forefoot ischaemia if not reduced.

The injury is caused by direct crush, an indirect twisting force or an axial load applied to the trapped foot. The foot will appear swollen and pain will be elicited by supination/pronation while the subtalar joint is held. Distal perfusion may be reduced. Radiographic signs may be subtle, requiring a high degree of clinical suspicion. Anteroposterior, oblique and, importantly, true lateral projections are required. Four signs may be present:

- Diastasis between the first and second metatarsal shafts.
- Small fracture fragments of the bones comprising the midtarsal joint.
- Residual subluxation of the metatarsal bases seen on the lateral projection.
- Note the alignment of the medial side of the base of the second metatarsal with the medial cuneiform; these should normally form an unbroken line.

Treatment requires anatomical reduction under anaesthesia. This is achieved by toe traps and traction. The stability of the reduction should then be tested, with stress radiographs if necessary. Persisting instability should be treated with percutaneous Kirschner wires or screws, one placed from the fifth metatarsal base into the

cuboid with a second wire or screw passing through the first metatarsal base into the medial cuneiform. Cast immobilization should be used to supplement this fixation.

ACUTE COMPARTMENT SYNDROMES

A compartment syndrome can be defined as the occurrence, within a myofascial compartment, of a sufficiently high pressure to impair function and viability of the tissue in that space. The absolute values of intracompartmental pressure that lead to this syndrome are not clear. Several variables may be relevant, including systemic perfusion pressures, the degree of primary muscle damage and the period during which raised pressures have persisted. Severe and irreversible damage to limb function may occur if the compartment is not rapidly decompressed. Diagnosis is based on symptoms and signs, and can be confirmed by direct measurement of the compartment pressure.

Clinical evidence of compartment syndrome should be sought in all injuries of the lower limb, although it most commonly complicates fractures of the tibia and crush injuries of the foot. An early and sensitive test is to perform passive, vigorous stretching of the muscles within the compartment; this will elicit pain, indicating an impending compartment syndrome. Persisting, severe pain despite adequate analgesia and immobilization, and distal parasthesia, indicate an established compartment syndrome. Accompanying signs in the late case include absent distal pulses, paralysis and pallor of the limb. At this stage irreversible muscle necrosis will have taken place.

The clinical appearance alone is usually sufficient grounds for decompressive fasciotomy, but in equivocal cases direct measurement of pressure may be helpful. This must be related to the diastolic blood pressure, compartment perfusion requiring a 30 mmHg gradient to maintain normal metabolic function. However, a single pressure reading of greater than 45 mmHg indicates that fasciotomy should be performed. If facilities for continuous monitoring are available, it may be permissible to delay decompression at this stage provided that the trend is downward. Fasciotomy should release all affected myofascial compartments with division of the fascia over the length of the muscle compartment; the wound should never be closed, allowing delayed primary closure or grafting once the swelling has resolved.

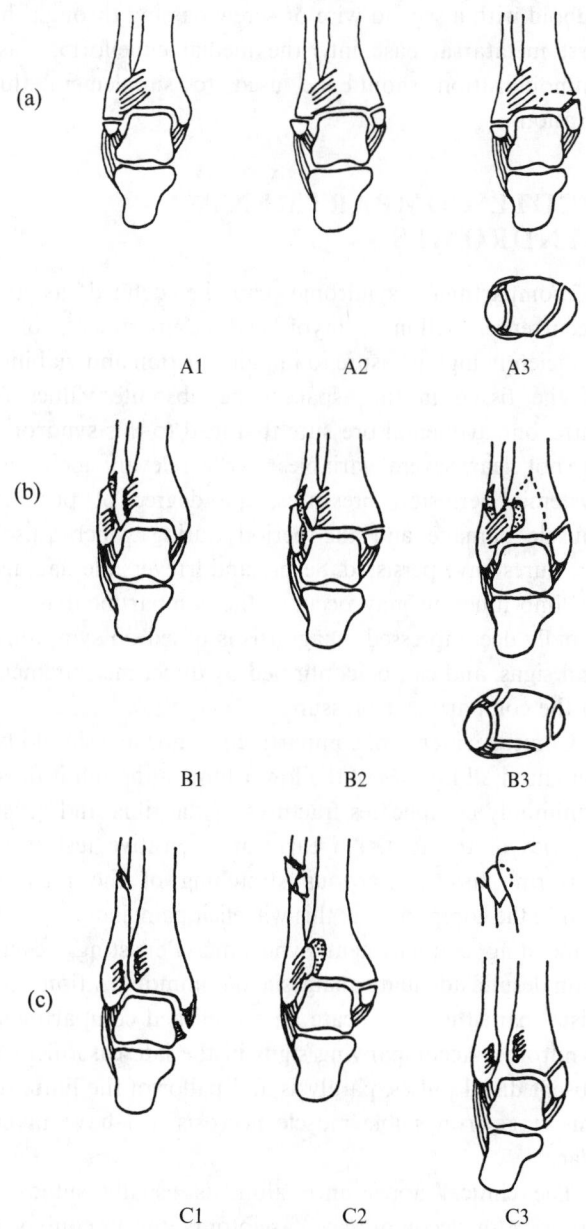

Fig. 6. AO classification (modified Danis – Weber) of ankle fractures. (a) Type A: fibula fracture below syndesmosis (infrasyndesmotic). A1, isolated; A2, with fracture of medial malleolus: A3, with a postero-medial fracture. (b) Type B: fibula fracture at the level of syndesmosis (trans-syndesmotic). B1, isolated; B2, with medial lesion (malleolus or ligament); B3, with posteromedial tibial fracture. (c) Type C: fibula fracture above syndesmosis (suprasyndesmotic). C1, simple fibular fracture; C2, complex fibular fracture; C3, proximal fibular fracture.

FRACTURES OF THE ANKLE

Fractures of the ankle are common injuries. Normally the square talus or 'tenon' fits snugly into the square 'mortise' formed by the distal tibia and fibula – an arrangement offering rigidity and stability. This stability is reinforced by the ankle joint capsule and ligaments. If the talus tilts excessively in the mortise either the ligaments may rupture or the malleoli fracture. If a malleolus is pushed off, it usually fractures obliquely; if it is pulled off (by intact ligaments), it fractures transversely. A spectrum of instability exists, depending on the degree of soft tissue and bony injury (Lauge-Hansen, 1950). The pattern of injury depends on many factors and in particular the position of the foot at the time of injury (supinated or pronated) and the direction and magnitude of the loading forces. The most important forces are external rotation, abduction and adduction. Usually the foot is anchored to the ground while the momentum of the body continues forward.

The AO-modified Danis – Weber system is a simple classification of ankle fractures (Fig. 6) which is useful in planning treatment. This system is based on the level of the fibular fracture: the more proximal the fracture of the fibula, the greater the risk of injury to the syndesmosis and the more likely the joint will be unstable. Type A is a supination injury with a fracture of the fibula below the syndesmosis. Further force results in a fracture of the medial side. Type B involves a fibular fracture at the level of the syndesmosis. The more severe type C injury involves a fibular fracture above the syndesmosis with disruption of the syndesmosis and an associated injury on the medial side. The fibular fracture may involve the fibular diaphysis or the more proximal fibula (Maisonneuve type).

Clinically an injured ankle is swollen and any deformity is obvious. The site of tenderness is important; if tenderness is present medially and laterally an unstable injury must be suspected. A clinically dislocated or subluxed joint must be promptly reduced and placed into a padded cast.

Appreciation of the ankle joint axis is important in interpreting ankle radiographs (Fig. 7). This axis is externally rotated about 15° from the frontal plane. The true mortise view is taken with the foot internally rotated 15° and will clearly show the entire joint space and the presence of any talar shift.

Ankle fractures are intra-articular injuries and the aim of treatment is to obtain an anatomical reduction and maintain the reduction until the fracture has healed (Vander Griend et al., 1991). Closed reduction may be indicated for displaced fractures if an anatomical reduction can be obtained and held without repeated manipulations, if operative treatment is contraindicated because of the general condition of the patient or the fractured limb, and for undisplaced or stable fractures.

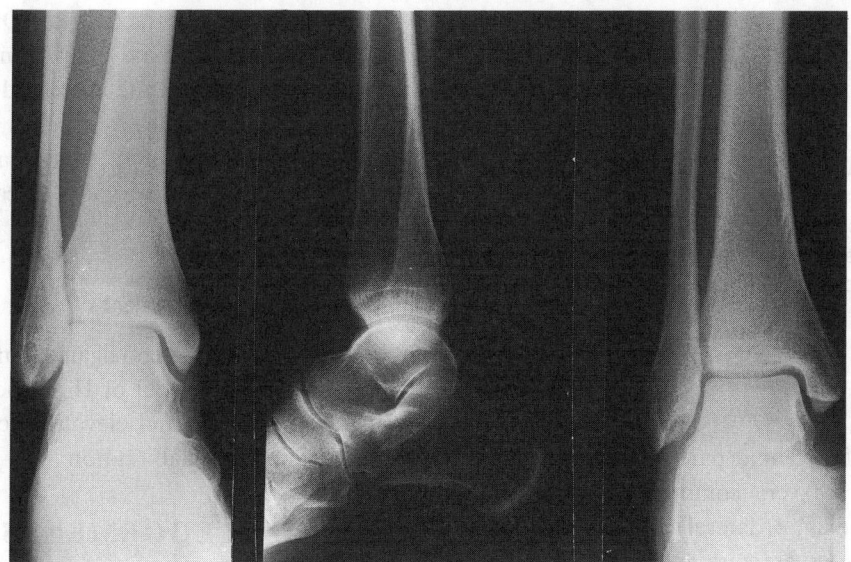

Fig. 7. Left—Anteroposterior radiograph of the ankle along the axis of the foot. The entire fibula should be included if there is any lateral tenderness above the joint line. Centre—Lateral view. The talar dome is centred under the tibia and the fibula lies posterior to the tibia. Right—True mortise view with the foot internally rotated 15°. The joint space is clearly shown and should be equal in width at all parts of the joint.

A closed reduction is obtained by reversing the mechanism of injury by manipulation under anaesthesia and holding the reduction in a well-padded, moulded plaster cast. Accurate X-rays are essential in interpreting a fracture reduction.

A reduction is satisfactory only if all of the following radiographic criteria are met:

1. Fibular length is restored
2. Talus sits squarely in the mortise with parallel tibiotalar articular surfaces
3. The ankle joint space is equal at all points
4. There is no tibiofibular diastasis (widening between the tibia and fibula)

Some fracture patterns may be difficult or unsuitable for treatment by closed means: for example, type C injuries, which are usually unstable. Furthermore, loss of position is common following closed reduction, and repeated manipulations may be required.

Operative treatment is indicated:

- For failure of closed methods.
- If closed reduction requires abnormal positioning of the foot.
- For unstable fractures, particularly of both malleoli with talar shift or widening of the mortise and type C injuries.
- For open fractures.

The timing of surgery is crucial and is best done before the onset of any soft tissue swelling or after the swelling has resolved. In practice, operative fixation should either be within 8 h of the injury or after at least 4 days, during which time the limb is elevated.

The internal fixation technique depends on the fracture type (Muller *et al.*, 1991); the most common is the Weber type B. The fibula fracture is fixed with one or two interfragmentary compression screws placed perpendicular to the fracture line. A one-third tubular plate is also commonly used to neutralize the rotational and axial forces on the fibula. If a medial malleolar fracture is present it is usually fixed after the lateral side.

Fractures of the posterior distal tibia, commonly referred to as the posterior malleolus, require fixation if the fragment contains 25% or more of the articular surface of the distal tibia.

The treatment of a disrupted syndesmosis (Weber type C injury) is controversial. The indication for syndesmotic fixation is based on an intraoperative assessment of stability after fixation of the fibular fracture and any medial malleolar fracture if present. A hook is placed around the fibula at the level of the syndesmosis and lateral traction is applied. Lateral movement of the fibular or widening of the mortise on intraoperative X-rays are indications for a syndesmotic screw.

Complications of ankle fractures
● Non-union
● Malunion
● Poor wound healing
● Infection
● Post-traumatic osteoarthritis
● Reflex sympathetic dystrophy
● Tibiofibular synostosis

Ligament injuries

Ligament injuries of the ankle, particularly of the lateral ligament complex, are very common and are usually classified by site (medial or lateral) and by grade (Kay, 1985). Grade I injuries are sprains, grade II involve a partial tear but no instability, and grade III are complete tears of the ligament.

Lateral collateral ligament

Injuries to the lateral ligament complex account for more than 85% of all ankle ligament injuries. The majority are produced by an inversion force on the supinated foot which injures the anterolateral capsule, the anterior talofibular ligament and the anterior tibiofibular ligament. Finally, if the force continues, the calcaneofibular ligament is injured. Although these injuries are very common, their treatment is controversial. Many authors, however, agree that non-operative treatment provides satisfactory results for most patients. Immediate use of ice, elevation and compression along with splinting of the injured ankle are helpful. Grade I and II injuries are then best managed either by protected mobilization with strapping or immobilization in a walking cast.

Patients with mild sprains may be allowed to weight-bear as tolerated and rehabilitation is commenced as soon as pain and swelling allow, with emphasis on peroneal strengthening exercises. Patients with more severe sprains may require a 2 – 3-week period of immobilization and non-weight-bearing prior to rehabilitation. Surgical repair is reserved for the occasional patient with a severe grade III injury who is involved in high-stress activities (e.g. athletics).

Chronic lateral ligament instability

Patients with chronic lateral instability complain that the ankle gives out or that they have recurrent lateral pain after athletic activities. On examination, increased inversion may be present and stress radiographs will demonstrate increased talar tilt compared with the normal side. A number of operative repairs can be performed and these have been shown to give good results in over 90% of cases (St. Pierre et al., 1982).

Medial collateral ligament

Isolated medial collateral ligament injuries are uncommon and are usually grade I or II injuries. Treatment is non-operative with ice and elevation followed by strapping or bracing and rehabilitation.

ACKNOWLEDGEMENTS

We thank Mrs M. van der Lem for help with typing and Mr J. Kitson FRCS for help with the illustrations.

Bibliography

Femoral shaft fractures

BONE, L.B., JOHNSON, K.D., WEIGETT, J. et al. (1989). Early versus delayed stabilisation of femoral fractures: a prospective randomised study. *J. Bone Joint Surg.*, **71A**, 336–40

BORDER, J.R., LaDUCA, J. & SEIDEL, R. (1975). Priorities in the management of patients with polytrauma. *Prog. Surg.*, **14**, 84–120.

JOHNSON, K.D. (1992). Femoral shaft fractures. In *Skeletal Trauma*, eds. B.D. Browner, J.B. Jupiter, A.M. Levine & P.G. Trafton, pp. 1525–641. Philadelphia: W.B. Saunders

JOHNSON, K.D., CADAMBI, A. & SEIBERT, G.B. (1985). Incidence of adult respiratory distress syndrome in patients with multiple musculoskeletal injuries: effect of early operative stabilisation of fractures. *J. Trauma*, **25**, 375–84.

KARLSTROM, G. & OLERUD, S. (1977). Ipsilateral fractures of the femur and tibia. *J. Bone Joint Surg.*, **59A**, 240–3.

MORAN, C.G., GIBSON, M.J. & CROSS, A.T. (1990). Intramedullary locking nails for femoral shaft fractures in elderly patients. *J. Bone Joint Surg.*, **72B**, 19–22.

SWIONTKOWSKI, M.F. (1987). Ipsilateral femoral shaft and hip traction. *Orthop. Clin. North Am.*, **18**, 73–84.

WINQUIST, R.A., HANSEN, S.T. & CLAWSON, D.K. (1984). Closed intramedullary nailing of femoral fractures: a report of five hundred and twenty cases. *J. Bone Joint Surg.*, **66A**, 529–39.

Fractures around the knee

APLEY, A.G. (1979). Fractures of the tibial plateau. *Orthop. Clin. North Am.*, **10**, 61–74.

EINOLA, S., AHO, A.J. & KALLIO, P. (1976). Patellectomy after fracture: long-term follow-up results with special reference to functional disability. *Acta Orthop. Scand.*, **47**, 441–7.

HOHL, M. (1991). Fractures of the proximal tibia and fibula. In *Fractures in Adults*, ed. C.A. Rockwood, D.P. Green & R.W. Bucholz. pp. 1725–62. Philadelphia: J.B. Lippincott.

JOHNSON, E.A. (1991). Fractures of the patella. In *Fractures in Adults*, ed. C.A. Rockwood, D.P. Green & R.W. Bucholz, pp. 1726–77. Philadelphia: J.B. Lippincott.

KENNEDY, J.C. & BAILEY, W.H. (1968). Experimental tibial plateau fractures. *J. Bone Joint Surg.*, **50A**, 1522–34.

LANSINGER, O., BERGMAN, B., KORNER, L. *et al.* (1986). Tibial condylar fractures. *J. Bone Joint Surg.*, **68A**, 13–19.

MAST, J., JAKOB, R. & GANZ, R. (1989). Planning and reduction technique. In *Fracture Surgery*. pp. 100–14. New York: Springer-Verlag.

MULLER, M.E., ALLGOWER, M., SCHNEIDER, R. *et al.* (1991a). Patella and tibia. In *Manual of Internal Fixation Techniques. Recommended by the AO-ASIF Group*, 3rd edn. pp. 564–7. Berlin: Springer-Verlag.

MULLER, M.E., ALLGOWER, M., SCHNEIDER, R. *et al.* (1991b). The comprehensive classification of long bone fractures. In *Manual of Internal Fixation Techniques Recommended by the AO-ASIF Group*, 3rd edn. pp. 140–1. Berlin: Springer-Verlag.

NEER, C.S., GRUTHAM, S.A. & SHELTON, M.L. (1967). Supracondylar fractures of the adult femur. *J. Bone Joint Surg.*, **49A**, 593–613.

SCHATZKER, J. (1987). Fractures of the tibial plateau. In *The Rationale of Operative Care*, eds. M. Tile & J. Schatzker, pp. 279–96. Berlin: Springer-Verlag.

SCHATZKER, J. & LAMBERT, D.C. (1979). Supracondylar fracture of the femur. *Clin. Orthop.*, **138**, 77–83.

WISS, D.A. (1991). Supracondylar and intercondylar fractures of the Femur. In *Fractures in Adults*, ed. C.A. Rockwood, D.P. Green & R.W. Bincholz, pp. 1778–97. Philadelphia: J.B. Lippincott.

Fractures of the tibial shaft

BOURNE, R.B. (1989). Pilon fractures of the distal tibia. *Clin. Orthop.*, **240**, 42–46.

CARDEN, D.G., NOBLE, J., CHALMERS, J. *et al.* (1987). Rupture of the calcaneal tendon. *J. Bone Joint Surg.*, **69B**, 416–20.

COURT-BROWN, C., CHRISTIE, J. & McQUEEN, M.M. (1990). Closed intramedullary tibial nailing. *J. Bone Joint Surg.*, **72B**, 605–11.

COURT-BROWN, C., McQUEEN, M.M., QUABA, A.A. *et al.* (1991). Locked intramedullary nailing of open tibial fractures. *J. Bone Joint Surg.*, **73B**, 959–64.

JOHANSEN, K., DAINES, M. & HOWEY, T. (1980). Objective criteria accurately predict amputation following lower extremity trauma. *J. Trauma*, **30**, 568–72.

TEMPLEMAN, D.C. & MARDER, R.A. (1989). Injuries of the knee associated with fractures of the tibial shaft. *J. Bone Joint Surg.*, **71A**, 1392–5.

WORLOCK, P., SLACK, R., HARVEY, L. *et al.* (1994). The prevention of infection in open fractures: an experimental study of the effect of fracture stability. *Injury*, **25**, 31–8.

Fractures and dislocations of the hindfoot

EASTWOOD, D.M., LANGKAMER, V.G. & ATKINS, R.M. (1993). Intra-articular fractures of the calcaneum. *J. Bone Joint Surg.*, **75B**, 189–94.

HAWKINS, L.G. (1970). Fractures of the neck of the talus. *J. Bone Joint Surg.*, **52A**, 991–1002.

Fractures of the ankle

KAY, D.B. (1985). The sprained ankle: current therapy. *Foot Ankle*, **6**, 22–8.

LAUGE-HANSEN, N. (1950). Fractures of the ankle. Combined experimental-surgical and experimental-roentgenologic investigations. *Arch. Surg.*, **60**, 957–85.

MULLER, M.E., ALLGOWER, M., SCHNEIDER, R. *et al.* (1991). *Manual of Internal Fixation Techniques Recommended by the AO-ASIF Group*. 3rd edn, pp. 595–612. Berlin: Springer-Verlag.

ST. PIERRE, R., ALLMAN, F. & BASSETT, F.H. (1982). A review of lateral ankle ligamentous reconstruction. *Foot Ankle*, 3, 114–23.

VANDER GRIEND, R.A., SAVOIE, F.H. & HUGHES, J.L. (1991). Fractures of the ankle. In *Rockwood and Green's Fractures in Adults*, Vol. 2, 3rd ed. pp. 1983–2039. Philadelphia; J.B. Lippincott.

31 Injury to the pelvis and proximal femur

M. BIRCHER

Department of Orthopaedics, St George's Hospital, London, UK

Chapter plan

Introduction

Pelvic injury

Dislocation of the hip, acetabular fracture and fracture dislocation, fracture of the femoral head

Fractures of the proximal femur

INTRODUCTION

Injuries to the pelvis and proximal femur in the young are usually associated with high-energy trauma. In the elderly they are most often caused by minor falls. For very different reasons both groups have a significant mortality. The high-energy injuries are complicated by severe haemorrhage. The elderly usually sustain less severe fractures but recovery is hampered by coexisting medical problems.

A subgroup of pelvic injury – hip dislocation and acetabular fracture – has a lower mortality rate but high morbidity associated with later post-traumatic osteo-arthritis. A mismanaged pelvic fracture can lead to early death from haemorrhage whereas complications arising from acetabular fractures are associated with premature articular cartilage degeneration.

PELVIC INJURY

Within the group sustaining high-energy blunt trauma, there is a very significant incidence of associated injury to the head, chest and abdomen. Reported mortality rates run as high as 50% in open pelvic fractures with an average in the whole group approaching 10%. These unstable pelvic fractures are rare. An average district general hospital serving a population of 200 000 patients will probably only see two to three such fractures a year. The rarity of these injuries inevitably leads to an under-estimation of the injury. The major problem is bleeding and there is unfortunately a tendency to undertransfuse. An efficient trauma team and the early involvement of senior help using practised and tested management protocols will reduce this tendency (Advanced Trauma Life Support, Royal College of Surgeons).

Pelvic fractures in the elderly are usually associated with fairly minor trauma. Haemorrhage, although not usually marked can again be problematical as hypo-volaemia is poorly tolerated. Early mobilization and discharge from hospital is delayed by coexisting medical problems and inadequate social support.

At present in the UK we have not developed a particularly sophisticated and rapid transfer system from the accident site to A&E departments. We likewise have very few true 'trauma centres'. There is, therefore, a theoretical risk that some patients with multiple injuries may die before reaching hospital who might otherwise have survived.

Anatomical considerations

The bones of the pelvis form a ring, stabilized by strong posterior ligaments. The pelvic floor is a dense weave of tendon, ligament and muscle which provides further stability. Different amounts of force will produce differing degrees of pelvic instability depending upon the extent of pelvic floor and posterior ligament damage (Fig. 1). If the pelvis is broken in one place, search for a second disruption elsewhere in the ring. More often than not the anterior pelvic fracture is obvious on the trauma film, but the second (and usually more significant) posterior injury is often hidden by a combination of faeces and gas shadows.

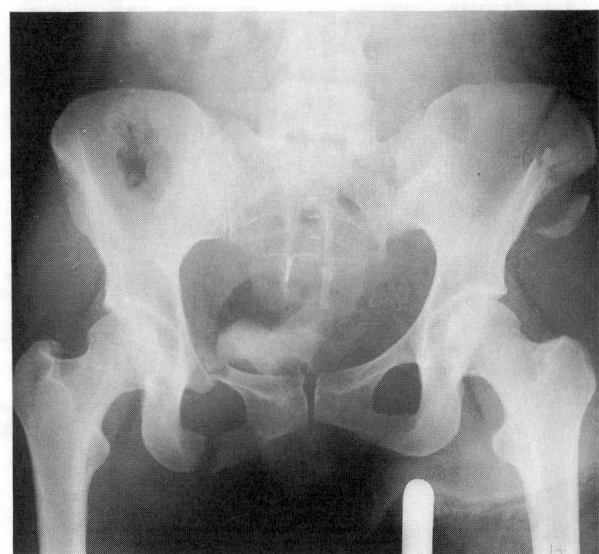

Fig. 1. Anteroposterior X-ray of unstable pelvic fracture. There is a left-sided sacroiliac dislocation, fracture of the iliac blade, and contralateral fracturing of the superior and inferior pubic rami.

The pelvic basin contains the bladder, rectum and uterus. The pelvic floor is pierced by the rectum, vagina and urethra. Significant pelvic injury can damage some or all of these structures. Fixed to the inner wall of the pelvis is a complex network of blood vessels. The pelvic fracture combined with shearing of the pelvic floor will produce significant haemorrhage. If the pelvic floor is torn, vast amounts of blood can leak into the upper thigh, perineum and retroperitoneal space. The skeleton must be stabilized at an early stage. This allows clots to form and remain *in situ*. Temporary fracture reduction will reduce pelvic volume and improve the tamponade effect. If this is not undertaken, haemorrhage will continue, diffuse intravascular coagulation may develop and death is possible.

Classification

Classification into unstable and stable injuries is still the most useful. However, it is sometimes extremely difficult to decide from an antero-posterior pelvic X-ray whether an injury is stable or unstable. It is thus essential to be cautious and treat all pelvic fractures aggressively. Tile (1988) considers pelvic instability as being rotational or vertical. Rotational instability can occur in either an internal or an external direction. The most common example of this type of pelvic fracture is the lateral compression injury. This may be produced by side-impact road traffic accidents or falls from a height onto

the greater trochanter. If there is no associated acetabular fracture, the hemipelvis is driven inwards and rotated upwards. Spontaneous reduction is common, as is urethral damage. External rotation of the pelvis is produced by anteroposterior trauma. As force is applied to the hemi-pelvis, the pubic symphysis or rami are disrupted and the anterior pelvic floor is torn. If the force is continued the sacroiliac joint opens. If further violence is applied, posterior ligamentous structures are ruptured and the fracture moves from being rotationally unstable to being vertically unstable. The most extreme variety of this injury is a traumatic hemipelvectomy.

Vertical instability is always associated with posterior ligamentous disruption in association with a fracture or fracture dislocation. These are extremely violent injuries associated with shearing forces and involve sacroiliac dislocation, sacral fracture, iliac fracture or combinations. There is a high incidence of lumbosacral nerve damage, urethral and bladder rupture. Posterior degloving injuries are also common.

Pelvic fractures – The high-energy injury

History, management and early treatment

Before the patient arrives in the accident and emergency (A&E) department the paramedics may report a fall from a height or a high-speed road traffic accident. This should alert the physician to the strong likelihood of pelvic injury. It is possible to predict the injury pattern from the accident report. For example, a 30-year-old male falling 35 feet onto his right side should be suspected as having the following injuries: right-sided head injury, right-sided rib fracture plus lung contusion, liver laceration and lateral compression pelvic injury

Group O negative blood should be available in the A&E department at all times.

All patients with unstable pelvic fractures are shocked and invariably require blood.

Assessment and resuscitation along Advanced Trauma Life Support guidelines should be undertaken. As conditions are identified in the primary survey they require prompt treatment. Once the airway is secured (with cervical spine control) and chest injuries are dealt with, the circulation requires special attention. Two large-bore intravenous cannulae need to be set up and 8 units of type-specific blood ordered. The abdomen, perineum and urethral meatus must be inspected. At this stage, the diagnosis of a serious pelvic fracture is purely a clinical one. However, treatment must not be delayed. Sometimes it is necessary to stabilize the pelvis before any X-rays are taken. The lower limbs are often externally rotated with extensive bruising and swelling over the flanks, upper thighs and suprapubic perineal region. There is usually a scrotal haematoma and occasionally blood at the external urethral meatus. Rectal examination needs to be performed early. The iliac blades can be compressed and quite often crepitus or abnormal rotation and vertical movement can be felt. This manoeuvre should only be performed once for fear of clot dislodgement. A nasogastric tube and urinary catheter should be inserted (if not contraindicated). Towards the end of the primary survey, lateral cervical spine, chest and pelvic X-rays should be obtained.

The management of persistent shock – the external fixator

Despite vigorous resuscitation the patient may still remain hypovolaemic and unstable. All other bleeding sources need to be excluded. The possibility of pericardial tamponade or myocardial dysfunction needs to be considered. Sources of bleeding may be the abdomen, the pelvis or the retroperitoneal space. Diagnostic peritoneal lavage, ultrasound and/or laparotomy may be indicated. However, prior to these investigations it is strongly recommended that an unstable pelvic fracture is stabilized with an external fixator. Immediate laparotomy in the presence of an unstable pelvic fracture is an extremely dangerous undertaking. Tamponade will be released and can lead to a catastrophic terminal bleed. A simple external fixator needs to be available to the trauma room at all times. A&E staff should be familiar with its indications and use.

Two types of external fixator are now available. The first is a frame constructed of standard fixator equipment. Two or three 5 mm pins are inserted into both hemipelvises behind and above the anterior superior iliac spine. Significant pelvic injury will distort the hemipelvises and make pin insertion difficult. Orientation of the iliac blades must be judged by palpation and the use of two thin spinal needles slid either side of the iliac blades will provide vital information to assist pin placement. The superior surface of the iliac bone can be opened with a drill and the pins inserted using a T-handle. They should be screwed in gently to find their way between two bony cortices. Three pins are usually necessary as at least one pin will have a poor hold. The lower route utilizing the bone above the acetabulum in

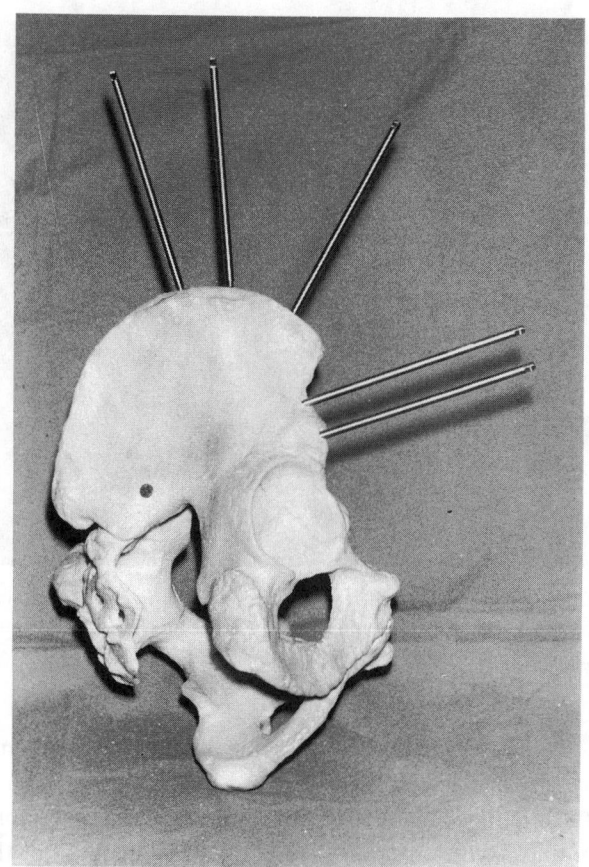

Fig. 2. Lateral view of pelvis showing upper and lower routes of pin insertion. Note the proximity of the pins to the acetabulum in the lower routes. Image intensifier should always be used if this technique is being used.

the region of the anterior inferior iliac spine is not recommended in a trauma situation. This method requires an image intensifier to reduce the possibility of acetabular penetration. The orientations of the pins is illustrated in Fig. 2.

After pin insertion, two cross-connecting rods are constructed superiorly and inferiorly. They can be moved up and down to allow access to the abdomen and perineum. Should laparotomy be required the fixator will not prevent access. Before the frame is finally tightened a 'clinical reduction' needs to be made. Pressure should be applied posteriorly, external to the sacroiliac joint, combined with pressure anteriorly over the iliac blades and longitudinal traction on the affected limb. Once satisfactory closure of the pelvis has been achieved the frame is tightened.

A new type of external fixator – the Ganz Pelvic Anti-Shock Clamp (Fig. 3) – has been developed. Single pins are applied percutaneously external to the sacroiliac

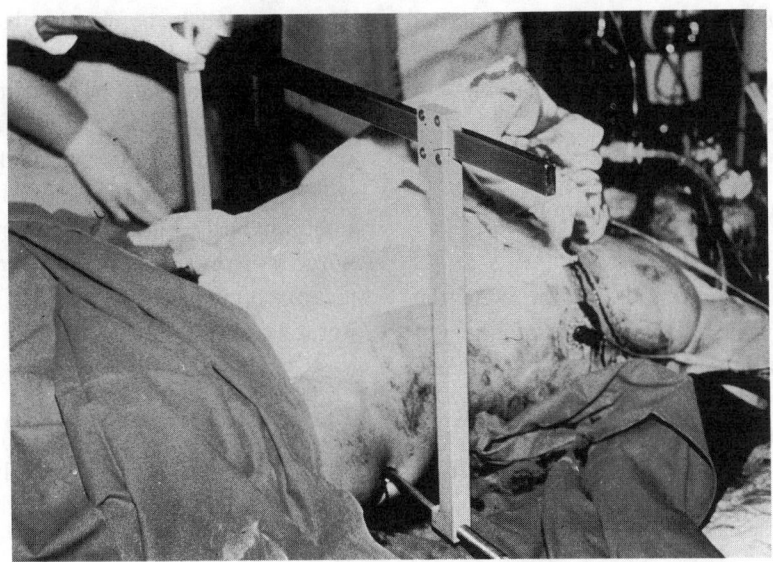

Fig. 3. The Ganz Pelvic Anti-Shock Clamp.

joint. A single anterior bar is constructed over the front of the patient resembling a carpenter's clamp.

The cross-bar can be moved superiorly and inferiorly to allow access to the abdomen. The pelvic antishock clamp applies pressure more posteriorly, theoretically affords a better reduction and with practice may be easier to apply.

The use of a pneumatic antishock garment has largely been abandoned due to difficulties encountered with patient access once applied. In very rare circumstances one or both iliac blades may be severely disrupted and in these patients it may be impossible to apply an anterior frame. This is where the Ganz clamp seems to have a clear advantage. However, if this piece of apparatus is not available, pelvic bandaging may as a last resort improve tamponade and assist in stabilizing the patient. In Germany, patients are transferred onto bean bags which support the fractured pelvis both during transport and during the initial resuscitation.

Diagnostic peritoneal lavage

The results of diagnostic peritoneal lavage and the presence of a pelvic fracture must be viewed with caution. As previously stated, indiscriminate laparotomy can prove fatal. Diagnostic peritoneal lavage often needs to be performed and the usual indications must be observed. In the presence of a pelvic fracture, a supraumbilical route should be employed. The aspiration of 8–10 ml of fresh blood is positive and laparotomy indicated. Ideally an external fixator should be applied before or while the

laparotomy is performed. Close liaison between the orthopaedic and general surgeons must be maintained. If the cell count in the lavage fluid is lower than 100 000 red cells per mm^3 then laparotomy is not indicated but close observation must be maintained. A count above 100 000 red cells in a patient without pelvic fracture requires laparotomy. However, in the presence of a serious pelvic fracture an expectant policy may be adopted. This depends very much on the clinical picture (including the results of CT (computed tomography) and ultrasound scanning, if time permits) and the views of the surgical team.

Ultrasound

In many European centres members of the trauma team are trained in the use of ultrasound. In such units this technique is used to decide if there is free blood in the abdomen. The advantages are that it is non-invasive and can be repeated a number of times. However, there are disadvantages, the main problem being that it is very 'user dependent' and it will not easily detect a damaged or ruptured viscus. Ultrasound is not widely used in UK accident centres.

Open pelvic fractures

Severe open pelvic fractures involve pelvic floor disruption with bone spicules entering the rectum and/or vagina. Fractures with faecal contamination carry the highest mortality. Once the diagnosis has been made, early skeletal stabilization and longitudinal skeletal traction combined with colostomy need to be undertaken. Large amounts of blood are required. The genitourinary system requires special attention.

The management of bladder and urethral rupture (See Chapter 25)

Urinary output is one of the major indicators of the effectiveness of patient resuscitation. In the presence of a pelvic fracture, urethral and bladder injury should be assumed until proved otherwise. Early involvement of an experienced urologist is ideal. The clinical diagnosis of urethral rupture is based on the presence of scrotal haematoma and blood at the urethral meatus. A high-riding prostate is said to be a classical feature but is difficult to detect.

One gentle attempt, by the senior responsible surgeon, at passing a small-gauge catheter is permissible in the trauma room. If clear urine is produced the management of the patient as a whole is simplified. However, it is possible to catheterize a patient who has had a severe urethral disruption. A patient who has sustained a pelvic fracture and is haemodynamically stable should have a urethrogram prior to catheterization. If this is normal then one should proceed to a cystogram. If either or both of these tests are abnormal, further management depends upon urological advice. In general terms, bladder rupture requires repair and urethral disruption is treated by splintage coupled with suprapubic drainage. It must be noted that insertion of a suprapubic catheter in the presence of a pelvic fracture can be extremely dificult. Patients are often shocked, urine output is reduced and the suprapubic swelling associated with the fracture makes identification of the bladder difficult. Bladder repair can often be coupled with anterior skeletal stabilization if there is no faecal contamination. In urethral rupture, early alignment is probably the treatment of choice.

Pelvic fracture not associated with hypotension

A large number of patients with pelvic injury are haemodynamically stable. These injuries are usually of a lateral compression type. The pelvic floor is intact and radiographic assessment often shows minimal displacement and minor malrotation of the hemipelvis. Anterior bony displacement may have been greater at the time of the accident and, although these injuries look innocuous, urethral and bladder damage is still a common finding.

Patients need to be closely observed. Hypovolaemia is often less of a problem, but associated injuries (e.g. lung contusion) can lead to later complications. Intravenous fluid is still required. Definitive treatment of the fracture can be less hurried and external fixation is rarely required as an emergency procedure. The pelvis often derotates spontaneously, but specific anterior injuries may require surgery involving plating or the application of an external fixator often used in 'reverse' with frames externally rotating the hemipelvis.

Pelvic fractures in the elderly

Elderly patients may be involved in high-speed road accidents. The prognosis with this type of injury is poor as severe hypovolaemia is poorly tolerated by this group. Most pelvic fractures in the elderly are caused by minor falls. Rami fractures can produce bleeding and there is often an associated sacral crush injury. Resuscitation needs to be undertaken. Patients must not be left on hard trolleys and pressure areas must be protected. It is essential not to miss the possibility of a second injury (e.g. an impacted subcapital fracture of the femur), which may be of more clinical signifcance in this age group.

Radiology of the pelvis

An anteroposterior X-ray of the pelvis needs to be taken towards the end of the primary survey. Further X-rays after stabilization of the patient include inlet and outlet views. Early CT scanning may be undertaken for other reasons, such as assessment of head or chest injury. CT scanning of the pelvis is said to be difficult in the presence of an external fixator but, if the gantry is angled and the frame is moved up and down, excellent 'cuts' of the posterior structures where the hidden injuries occur can be obtained (Fig. 4).

Definitive fracture management

Definitive management of the pelvic fracture depends upon the classification of the injury. Vertical instability needs to be controlled, often with early external fixation combined with longitudinal skeletal traction. Sophisticated forms of internal fixation may be instituted at a later date. Stabilization of the posterior structures is essential. Rotational instability often derotates spontaneously without any specific treatment. External rotation of the pelvis requires anterior external fixation, and marked internal rotation of the hemipelvis combined

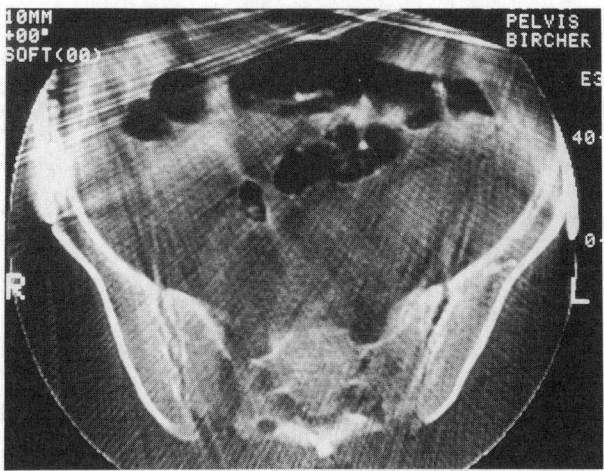

Fig. 4. CT scan of pelvis with external fixator in position. Note anterior interference but good visualization of posterior structures. Sacral facture is visible on the right side.

with upward migration may require complex internal fixation to prevent inequality of leg length and difficulty sitting.

Fractures of the pelvis in children

Teenage children often present with avulsion fractures of the pelvis. There is usually a history of sudden movement causing a sharp pain around the iliac crest or ischial area. X-rays will often reveal avulsion fractures of the iliac crest, anterior superior iliac spine, or the ischial tuberosities. These conditions are painful but rarely cause any significant disability and it is very unusual for them to require any specific treatment other than rest and analgesia.

Checklist for pelvic fracture management

- Do not miss associated injuries
- Do not underestimate hypovolaemia; large volumes of blood may be required
- Does the patient require emergency external fixation?
- Is the bleeding intra-abdominal or associated with the pelvic fracture?
- Complete bladder and urethral assessment

More serious unstable pelvic fractures in children are usually caused by road traffic accidents. Children are all too frequently run over, causing severe multisystem injuries. Management is as outlined for adults with rapid fluid replacement. The capacity for recovery even in the most desperate situations is excellent in this group. There is a high incidence of urethral and rectal damage requiring faecal and urinary diversions at an early stage.

External fixation with skeletal traction is often used for temporary and definitive management.

DISLOCATION OF THE HIP, ACETABULAR FRACTURE AND FRACTURE DISLOCATION, FRACTURE OF THE FEMORAL HEAD

To produce such injuries considerable force is required. However, in isolation, hypotension is unusual and is usually a result of other injuries. These are essentially intra-articular injuries and management is directed at prompt reduction and stable anatomical reconstruction.

Hip dislocation

Anatomical considerations and classification

The hip is a naturally stable joint. Considerable force and soft tissue damage must occur during the dislocation. The blood supply to the femoral head is precarious, with a high percentage coming via the capsule, particularly posteriorly. Dislocation will not only directly damage the capsule but the malpositioned head will cause stretching of undamaged areas of capsule and thus lead to a greater risk of avascular necrosis. The sooner the dislocation is reduced the quicker the blood supply will be improved and the lower the incidence of post-traumatic avascular necrosis. As the head dislocates, it is quite usual for small fragments of acetabular rim to be torn off. These may prevent relocation, as does buttonholing of the head through the capsule. The close proximity of the sciatic nerve to the posterior hip capsule should alert the physician to the possibility of direct nerve damage. Isolated hip dislocation is either anterior or posterior, the latter being much more frequent. 'Central dislocation' of the hip is always associated with some type of acetabular fracture.

Anterior dislocation

This injury accounts for approximately 10% of all dislocations. The hip will be shortened and held in some degree of external rotation. This is an extremely painful condition. After general assessment, a check on the circulation of the limb and the function of the femoral and sciatic nerve needs to be made. Diagnosis is confirmed by X-ray

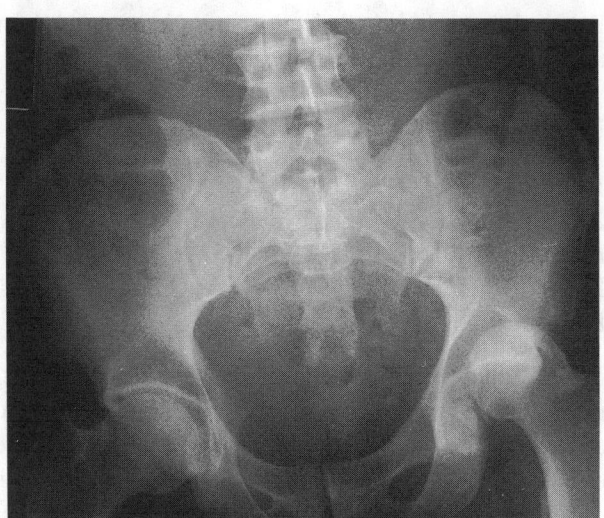

Fig. 5. Anteroposterior view showing posterior dislocation of hip; the head thus appears smaller. An associated lip fracture is visible.

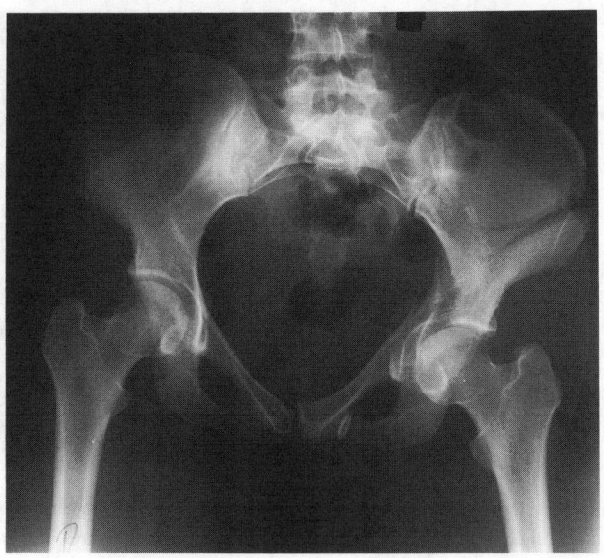

Fig. 6. Acetabular fracture. A left-sided complex fracture of both columns.

and urgent arrangements for relocation need to be made. If closed reduction fails, an open reduction is necessary. Postreduction X-rays and CT scan are mandatory.

Posterior dislocation

Posterior dislocation (Fig. 5) is a common injury usually produced as a result of head-on road traffic accidents. Other injuries must not be missed. There is association between posterior dislocation of the hip, ipsilateral posterior cruciate injury and fracture of the patella. The leg is shortened and the hip held in internal rotation. The diagnosis can be confirmed by X-ray. A careful inspection of the pelvic X-ray needs to be made to exclude acetabular or femoral neck fractures. Urgent arrangements must be made for relocation of the hip, which usually requires a general anaesthetic. If the hip is reduced in the A&E department, the doctor must assess postreduction stability. This is very important for future treatment planning. If the hip feels unstable there is usually an underlying posterior wall fracture. A small percentage of pure posterior dislocations will not reduce by closed methods under general anaesthesia. This is invariably due to buttonholing of the hip through the posterior capsule which requires open reduction. Postreduction X-ray and CT scanning are essential to check for entrapped bone fragments which will need surgical removal. The timing of reduction has a direct bearing on the overall avascular necrosis rate.

Acetabular fracture

Acetabular fractures (Fig. 6) should be managed as any other intra-articular fracture. The joint is deeply seated and thus clinical and radiographic assessment is awkward. Injuries are usually produced by falls from a height or from a side-impact road traffic accident. Right-sided acetabular fractures have a strong association with hepatic injury; likewise, left-sided acetabular fractures are often associated with splenic rupture.

Acetabular fractures in children are unusual but should be managed like any other intra-articular fracture. Three-dimensional CT and MRI (magnetic resonance imaging) may help define the injury as much of the acetabulum is cartilaginous. Growth arrest and malunion are potential long-term problems.

Anatomical considerations and classification

The acetabulum is a deep socket surrounded by a number of large muscles. Neurovascular structures run behind and in front of the joint and coincidental injury is common. The acetabulum itself it made up of posterior and anterior columns. A variety of classifications are used for acetabular fractures but, essentially, injuries involve the anterior column or posterior column or both (Letournel & Judet, 1994). A new alpha numeric classification has been recently developed. Acetabular fractures in the young are commonly associated with high-energy trauma but there is a second peak in the elderly usually associated with falls onto the greater trochanter.

Management

Associated injuries must not be missed. Distal circulation and neurology need to be assessed and traction applied to the hip. The leg itself may need support. An antero-posterior X-ray of the pelvis is all that is necessary at this stage.

Subsequent definitive treatment

Longitudinal tibial skeletal traction is applied and good quality Judet views need to be obtained, together with a CT scan. All displaced fractures should be considered for open reduction and stabilization.

Checklist for acetabular fractures and hip dislocations

- Associated injuries – general
- Associated injuries – local
- Circulation and neurology
- Urgent relocation – ? stability

Femoral head fractures

These are rare injuries that usually accompany hip dislocation and/or acetabular fracture. They are usually classified according to Pipkin (1957). Associated hip dislocation requires reduction as soon as possible. Small femoral head fractures usually require no specific treatment but larger fragments may need open reduction and internal fixation.

Acute upper femoral epiphyseal separation

Unlike classical slipped upper femoral epiphysis, these injuries are caused by direct violent trauma. Radiographically there is no evident of preslip or old bone formation. These injuries require prompt anatomical reduction and skeletal stabilization.

FRACTURES OF THE PROXIMAL FEMUR

Unlike fractures of the pelvis, most of these injuries are caused by trivial falls in the elderly. The numbers of fractures per year is on the increase with 43 220 being reported for the UK in 1985 (J. R. Coll. Physicians, 1989). They are approximately twice as common in females. Most of the fractures can be considered pathological, associated with severe osteoporosis in an ageing population. The injury itself is usually very minor. It is rare to sustain a proximal femoral fracture through normal bone without significant violence. Across the country, one quarter of all orthopaedic beds are occupied by patients with fractured femoral necks. Mortality rates are high because of the frail nature of the patients rather than the fracture itself. Associated injuries are rare in the elderly and not usually responsible for any immediate mortality. They include humeral neck fractures and distal radial fractures.

Clinical presentation

The typical patient is an elderly lady who reports a minor fall. In some cases it is thought that the fracture actually precipitates the fall, implying that many of these injuries are stress fractures in abnormal bone. The patient cannot bear weight on the leg and, if the fracture is displaced, the affected limb will be short and externally rotated. There is often a bruise over the greater trochanter.

A small number of patients will have either an inter-trochanteric crack or an undisplaced subcapital fracture and in either case the leg is orientated normally. X-rays may not be diagnostic but patients will be reluctant to bear weight. If this is the case they should not be sent home and need to be investigated further with better quality X-rays, oblique views or even an urgent bone scan. Other injuries must be excluded (e.g. rami fractures). In most cases, however, the fracture can be visualized on a good-quality anteroposterior X-ray of the pelvis or a true lateral view of the hip. Both are essential.

Treatment principles

Most orthopaedic units treat proximal femoral fractures operatively. This allows early mobilization and reduces complications. Early management in the A&E department involves swift diagnosis and assessment of suitability for operation. Patients have often been lying alone for some hours and may be in a poor general condition. Hypothermia needs special attention as do pressure areas. Patients must not be left on hard trolleys as sores will develop quickly and this greatly prolongs hospital stay and increases the overall mortality rate. Rapid referral to the orthopaedic team is essential. Routine blood tests including full blood count, urea and electrolytes and cross-match should be performed and an intravenous infusion instituted. A chest X-ray and ECG (electrocardiogram) are required to detect coexisting medical problems that may delay treatment.

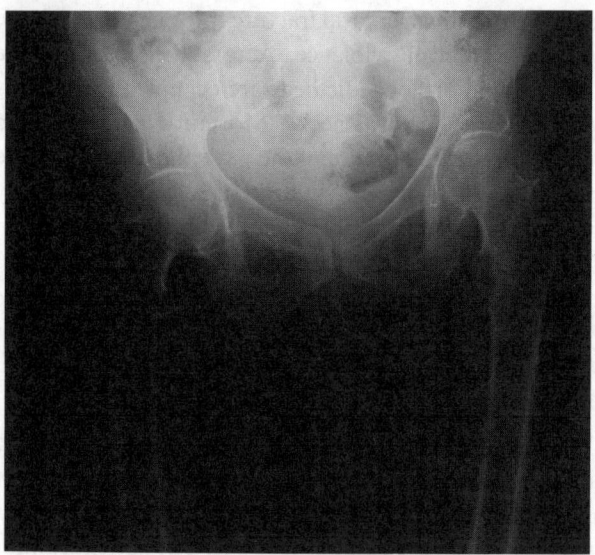

Fig. 7. Impacted minimally displaced transcervical fracture of neck of left femur.

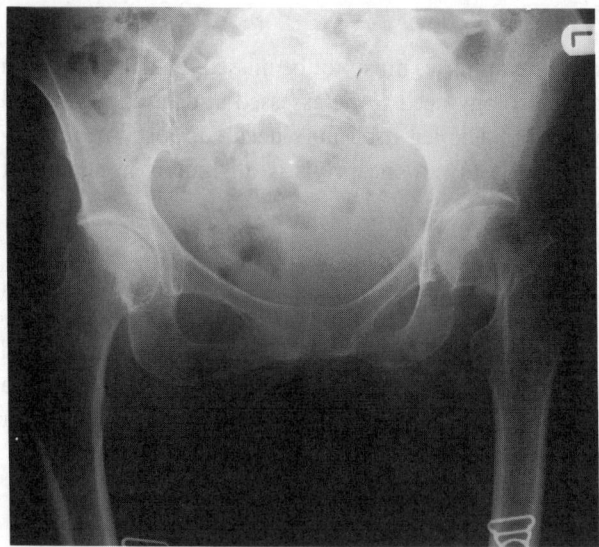

Fig. 8. Completely displaced transcervical fracture at neck of femur.

Anatomical considerations, classification and treatment

Proximal femoral fractures fall into two main groups: transcervical fractures and intertrochanteric fractures.

Transcervical fractures of the neck the femur (including basal fractures)

It is rare to see a transcervical fracture in a patient with osteoarthritis of the hip. The thickened calcar forms a protection against fracture. The femoral head has a poor blood supply, and a fracture through the neck inevitably interrupts the flow of blood to the head. The fracture haematoma increases intracapsular pressure and further jeoparidzes the circulation. Finally, fracture displacement impinging on the capsular vessels (particularly posterior) further complicates the circulatory problem. If the definitive management involves the preservation of the femoral head, rapid reduction and stabilization will afford better long-term results. In the elderly (70 plus) with a displaced fracture, the head is usually sacrificed as the avascular necrosis rate following reduction and internal fixation is usually unacceptably high.

Classification

The most widely used classification is that described by Garden. There are four grades of fracture which are classified according to appearances on an anteroposterior X-ray of the hip. A good-quality film is essential. Grades I and II are undisplaced or minimally displaced fractures that have a degree of impaction (Fig. 7). The real danger with this group is that they can be missed. Garden grades III and IV are significantly displaced fractures (Fig. 8). In this group of patients the blood supply to the femoral head is severely compromised.

Treatment

In children and young adults these fractures are often associated with high-energy injuries. They represent a surgical emergency as prompt reduction and internal fixation should be performed to preserve viability.

The 50–70 age group Defining a specific age group raises certain problems. More active elderly patients may be considered 'younger' within this group and treatment modified accordingly. Biological age is far more important than real age. Grade I and II fractures are treated with reduction and internal fixation. The management of displaced femoral neck fractures is more controversial in this age group. In younger patients with less displacement and comminution with good bone quality, open reduction and internal fixation is probably the best treatment. In the older patient with more displacement and comminution with poor bone stock, a hemiarthroplasty is probably the best treatment. In a small group of patients who are very active but who have suffered very severe displaced fractures (or in fractures that have presented late), total hip replacement is an option. If the

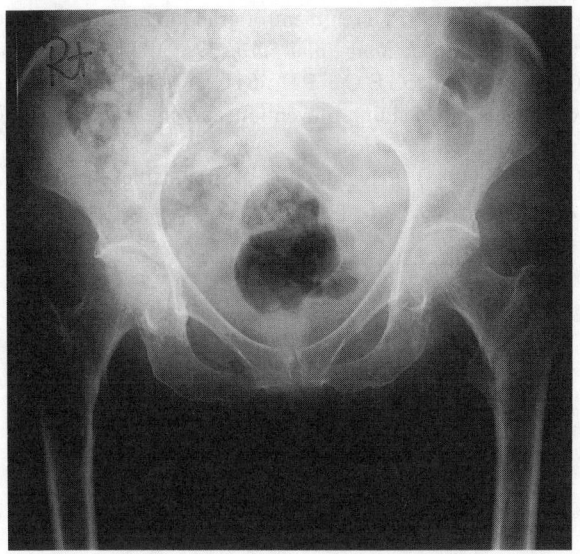

Fig. 9. Minimally displaced 'stable' intertrochanteric fracture of neck of the left femur.

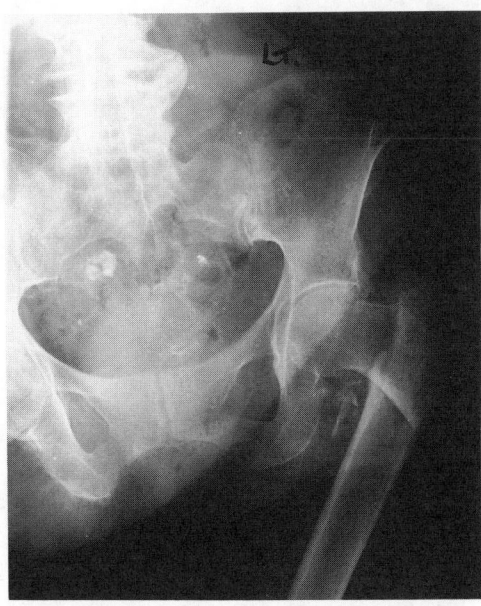

Fig. 10. Displaced 'unstable' intertrochanteric fracture of neck of left femur. Note displacement of lesser trochanter.

fracture has been left markedly displaced for over 24 h, the likelihood of avascular necrosis rises.

Patients over 80 If the fracture is at all displaced hemiarthroplasty is the best method of treatment and therefore emergency intervention is not essential. Patients need to be assessed and prepared for surgery on the next available daytime list which ideally should be within 24 h.

Intertrochanteric fractures

Intertrochanteric fractures do not interfere significantly with the femoral head blood supply and avascular necrosis is not a problem. Most of the fractures unite without operation, but patients will need to be in bed on traction for approximately 3 months. There is also likely to be a significant degree of malunion. The vast majority of these fractures are therefore internally fixed to allow early mobilization and discharge from hospital.

Classification

Essentially these fractures are either unstable or stable. They have been classified according to Evans (1949). Stable injuries have an intact medial buttress with the lesser trochanter in place. There is usually minimal displacement of the fracture (Fig. 9). More unstable injuries are those in which there is marked displacement, comminution, explosion of the medial buttress and displacement of the lesser trochanter (Fig. 10). Subtrochanteric extension needs to be noted and, if present, different methods of treatment considered.

Treatment

Conservative treatment of these fractures leads to a higher complication rate, malunion and longer hospital stay. Most units stabilize these fractures with some kind of sliding hip screw or intramedullary device. Anatomical reconstruction in the young is mandatory but some fracture collapse is accepted and indeed encouraged in the elderly. All operations on proximal femoral shaft fractures should be carried out within 24 h of hospital admission.

Proximal femoral fracture checklist

- Subcapital or intertrochanteric?
- Coexisting medical or social problems?
- Associated injury?
- Pressure areas
- Rapid assessment and referral to orthopaedic department

Bibliography

ADVANCED TRAUMA LIFE SUPPORT (1993). Programme for Physicians. London: Royal College of Surgeons of England.

EVANS, E. M. (1949). The treatment of trochanteric fractures of the femur. *J. Bone Joint Surg.*, **31B**, 190–203.

GARDEN, R.S. (1974). Reduction and fixation of subcapital fracture of the femur. *Orthop. Clin. North Am.*, **5**, 683–712.

LETOURNEL, E. & JUDET, R. (1994). *Fractures of the Acetabulum*, 2nd edn. Springer-Verlag.

PIPKIN, G. (1957). Treatment of grade IV fracture dislocation of the hip. *J. Bone Joint Surg.*, **39A**, 1027–42.

ROYAL COLLEGE OF PHYSICIANS. (1989) Fracture of the neck of femur—prevention and management. *J. R. Coll. Physicians London.*

TILE, M. (1988). Pelvic fractures. Should they be fixed? *J. Bone Joint Surg.*, **70B**, 1–12.

32 Sports injuries

N. TUBBS

Department of Trauma and Orthopaedic Surgery, University Hospital Birmingham, Birmingham, UK

Chapter plan

Introduction
Classification
Sports injury clinics
Principles of diagnosis and treatment
Prevention
Acute injuries
Chronic injuries
The foot
The ankle
The lower leg
The knee
The thigh
The pelvis and hips
The spine
The upper limb

INTRODUCTION

Patients with sports injuries form about 10% of those attending most accident departments although it is less easy to define what is meant by a sports injury. For statistical purposes most will define it as any injury occurring in a place of sport or recreation, and for comparative purposes this is a useful definition, albeit inaccurate if one has to define a road, for example, as a place of recreation for the marathon runner. Nonetheless most of us know what is meant by a sports injury and the grey areas occur where there is difficulty in knowing what is a sport (e.g. motor racing and chess). In this chapter it is taken to be an athletic pursuit.

CLASSIFICATION

Williams (1971) classified sports injuries into extrinsic and intrinsic injuries (Table 1), a classification which has

Table 1. *Classification of injury in sport*

Consequential injury
1. PRIMARY
A Extrinsic
(i) Human
(ii) Implemental
(a) incidental
(b) overuse
(iii) Vehicular
(iv) Environmental
B Intrinsic
(i) Incidental
(ii) Overuse
(a) acute
(b) chronic
2. SECONDARY
A Short term
B Long term
Non-consequential injury

served a purpose but would be more usefully replaced by a classification involving the mechanism of acquisition or rationale for treatment, as do many of the classifications of fractures. A practical division is into acute and chronic (sudden and overuse) injuries which implies a mechanism and frequently a form of treatment. Some would prefer a system which only included injuries specific to sport, but this would be inaccurate as most mechanisms of injury can be found in work or pastimes other than sport; for example, tennis elbow is most frequently *not* caused by tennis.

In this chapter, the common injuries occurring in sport will be described according to the region of the body as most will present as pain or dysfunction of a particular part. Fractures in general are described elsewhere and will only be mentioned if they tend to be sport-specific (such as stress fractures). The remainder are soft tissue injuries and, indeed, many sports injury clinics have been euphemistically called soft tissue clinics.

SPORTS INJURY CLINICS

In the UK the Sports Council has a slogan of 'Sport for All' which was welcomed by many. Lay people imagined that facilities would improve (which they have) and the medical profession imagined that sports clinics would be funded (which they have not). Sports clinics were founded and then floundered either through lack of enthusiasm or through lack of funds. Some of the issues are:

1. Whether it is justifiable to have a clinic for a limited section of the public.
2. Whether sports injuries are a specialty.
3. How to set up such a clinic.

Justifying a clinic is not easy unless sports injuries can be regarded as a specialty, although it would be just as justifiable as having an obesity or disordered pulmonary function clinic. On the whole, sports people are trying to keep themselves healthy and away from hospitals whereas the same cannot be said of overeaters and smokers.

Many injuries occurring in sport can occur during other pursuits; a plumber can just as easily sprain his ankle as a cross-country runner and indeed they may be one and the same person. Preferential treatment should be given to neither. However, it may be appropriate to give different treatment (not better treatment) to the elderly plumber and to the professional athlete. A more cogent argument for distinguishing the sports person from others is the different pathology. Fractures and sprains occur in both but some chronic overuse injuries tend to occur in the sports person; the iliotibial tract syndrome rarely occurs except in runners and is frequently not recognized by those without a specialist interest in sporting injuries. Such injuries have a different aetiology, require different recognition and need different (but not better) treatment.

Sports injuries have already become recognized as a specialty as evidenced by the number of sports clinics in existence, but their presence does nothing to justify their existence, nor does it add to their credibility. A specialty can be based on a disease process (oncology), a region of the body (thoracic surgery), the age of the patient (paediatrics), chronicity of the illness (accident and emergency medicine), a system of the body (endocrinology) or method of acquisition (aviation medicine). Should this be needed as a justification then sports injuries fall into at least two categories, being solely acquired through sport and affecting the musculoskeletal system. The practical side to this applies to all branches of medicine and surgery; conditions are treated by those who are interested and trained in that condition, i.e. those who are good at it. There is no shortage of those interested in sports injuries but there are few who have the training either through experience or by completing a formal course. In the future, such clinics should be run by someone who has obtained recognition in the subject by diploma, degree, etc.

Organizing a clinic is little different from organizing other specialty clinics. It is no longer sufficient to have one person interested in the subject – a back-up team is necessary. An orthopaedic surgeon with a diploma in sports medicine may well be the most appropriate person to lead the team particularly as that provides an outlet for all forms of treatment, but physiotherapists, nutritionists, physiologists, psychotherapists, etc. must all be readily available. An ideal set-up is for the physiotherapist and clinician to run the clinic and see the patients together. As in all branches of medicine, the labelling of the clinic is less important than the training and ability to perform the task required.

PRINCIPLES OF DIAGNOSIS AND TREATMENT

Musculoskeletal and most other tissue can only be damaged in a limited number of ways. Acute injuries result in bruising and partial or complete rupture of a structure. The injury may be extrinsic (from outside the body; e.g. from a cricket ball) or intrinsic (from within; e.g. a ruptured hamstring muscle). Chronic injury produces inflammation and is usually intrinsic (e.g. Achilles tendonitis). The simplicity of this is reflected in the nomenclature in which '-itis' (inflammation of) is added to the name of the tissue: tendonitis, fasciitis, synovitis, tenosynovitis, periostitis. Many will baulk at musculitis (chronic muscle strain) and ligamentitis (chronic ligament strain) even if these terms more accurately describe the pathology.

Diagnosis

Diagnosis relies heavily on understanding the mechanism of injury, particularly in chronic overuse injuries. Again, the body's local reaction to damage is limited; the early reaction is inflammation and this will be followed by repair and fibrosis. The symptoms will therefore be those of inflammation (pain, swelling and loss of function) followed by the effects of repair and fibrosis (e.g. nerve entrapment), or occasionally the failure of repair (e.g. non-union of a fracture).

Treatment

Treatment of the *acute injury* relies on either repairing the ruptured part or allowing it to repair itself. It may be kind to prescribe analgesia, it is sometimes sensible to splint and rest the part but it is illogical to give anti-inflammatory drugs; inflammation is part of the repair process and should not usually be diminished. Immediately after the injury the traditional treatment is ICE – Ice, Compression, Elevation – which may limit the painful effects of swelling.

Immediate treatment of acute injury	
I	Ice
C	Compression
E	Elevation

For the *chronic overuse injury* it is logical to reduce inflammation. Withdrawing the stimulus by rest or modifying the style of use, non-steroidal anti-inflammatory drugs, local injections of steroids and physiotherapy may all be used. Once fibrosis has occurred the treatment may need to be operative. In this group of injuries the treatment must be tailored to the needs of the athlete; rest is frequently anathema to the high-class athlete and instruction to this effect will be ignored; better to diminish the localized inflammation and allow that athlete to continue such that eventually the part will adapt to overuse. Supervision at this stage is all important. Wolff's Law (1892) applies:

'Every change in the form and the function of bones, or of their function alone, is followed by certain definite changes in their internal architecture, and equally definite secondary alterations in their external conformation, in accordance with mathematical laws.'

This can equally well be applied to other musculoskeletal tissue but is exemplified best by bones and gives a rationale for treatment of conditions such as stress fractures, tendonitis, tract syndromes, etc. In stress fractures, use of the bone sufficient to cause pain, indicates further trabecular fracturing and inflammation and is clearly counterproductive. It is equally senseless to enforce complete rest such that the bone returns to its previous state. It is better to allow some stress so that the repair process (callus) continues to build up and eventually strengthens the bone.

The following is a plan for treating chronic overuse injuries:

1. Modify training, e.g. run less.
2. Modify equipment, e.g. shoes.
3. Modify style, e.g. orthoses.
4. Non-steroidal anti-inflammatory drugs (NSAIDs).
5. Local steroids.
6. Physiotherapy.
7. Operation.

PREVENTION

Prevention is correctly a function of a sports injury clinic but not necessarily of an A&E department. Understanding the mechanisms involved and the methods used in sport will help in giving advice about preventing the occurrence or recurrence of an injury. To this extent it is easier but not essential if the adviser has been involved in sport. Even in the A&E department, appropriate advice about prevention can be given provided there has been audit of all injuries. A good example of this has been the introduction of helmets for cyclists.

ACUTE INJURIES

Muscle injury

This may be due to direct or indirect force which is usually obvious from the history. A hamstring muscle rupture can be diagnosed in a sprinter from the television screen. The ruptured part of the muscle will be tender and sometimes swollen if there is a large haematoma. The two ends of completely ruptured muscle may be palpated. There is a complete or partial loss of function. Practically, it does not matter whether the rupture is central or peripheral.

Suturing a partially torn muscle is rarely worthwhile. After initial treatment for the pain (analgesia, rest, elevation and occasionally strapping) physiotherapy is devoted to the prevention of shortening by fibrosis. Some fibrosis is inevitable, being the process of healing, but excessive contracture will predispose to further ruptures. It is rarely possible to aspirate a haematoma and should it be deemed harmful (e.g. by its size), surgical exploration is the answer. At this time the ruptured muscle ends should be apposed to obliterate the cavity. The need to repair a complete rupture will depend on which muscle is involved. It is rarely necessary to repair a complete rupture of the rectus femoris.

Tendons

These are usually ruptured, partially or completely, by an indirect force in sport. The athlete will give a history of a sudden force applied to the tendon, although occasionally the history may be misleading as in the classic rupture of the Achilles tendon in which almost invariably the story is that of being hit on the back of the calf. Partial ruptures are tender and swollen without loss of function, whereas complete ruptures may not be tender but are invariably accompanied by loss of function.

Partial ruptures do not need surgical intervention. Except in unimportant tendons, complete ruptures should be treated by apposition of the ruptured ends, most frequently by suturing.

Tendon avulsions are the adolescent equivalent of adult tendon ruptures. Most frequently the avulsions are accompanied by detachment of a small fragment of bone. Unless the separation is trivial the fragment should be replaced. The tendon sheath is rarely injured acutely in sport, other than as part of a more widespread injury involving the tendon. The desirability of closing the sheath is discussed elsewhere (hand injuries).

Ligaments

Like tendons, ligaments may be partially or completely ruptured – nearly always by indirect force. The rupture is often an avulsion with or without a fragment of bone. Ligament ruptures can be graded into three categories:

- Grade I – few torn fibres.
- Grade II – more than 50% of fibres torn.
- Grade III – all fibres torn.

The diagnosis and treatment is along the same lines as that of tendon injury. In a partial rupture, stressing the ligament will be painful but there will not be laxity unless the fibres of the ligament are extradigitated rather than completely ruptured in part of the tendon. In a complete rupture, stressing the ligament may not be painful as the pain fibres have all been ruptured and will not be stressed. However, there will be laxity.

Partial ruptures will not need operative intervention; in complete ruptures, the ends need to be apposed

although it is rare to find two neatly ruptured ends. In both, the patient will need proprioceptive re-education.

Fibrocartilage

This is most frequently injured by a compressive shearing force. The symptoms are mechanical. The vascular part is capable of repair and in many instances it should be repaired.

Acute injuries of articular cartilage, bone, skin, nerve and vessels are described elsewhere.

CHRONIC INJURIES

Overuse injuries are the true sports injuries in that they tend to occur only in sporting activities. Clearly it is not the sport itself which is to blame but the repetitive mechanism which may be exclusive to that sport. Overuse injuries are more common in the endurance sports of rowing, running, swimming and cross-country ski-ing, but they frequently occur in any sport involving excessive repetition. The body will adapt if progression is slow, but adaptation fails if progression is too quick and one or more parts will react to this failure by inflammation. A useful, but grammatically awful, way of describing the condition is to add the suffix '-itis' to the tissue involved (see above).

Muscle

Overuse without adaptation results in inflammation of the muscle whether one calls it musculitis, myositis or chronic muscle strain. Over a short period it results in stiff muscles well known to most athletes after the first outing of the year, while over a longer period a localized area of muscle may be involved such as the hamstrings in sprinters. A predisposing cause is shortening of the muscles which may be localized due to fibrosis from a previous rupture. Rest, anti-inflammatory drugs, massage and stretching all help.

Tendons

Tendons become inflamed from tension or friction. One of the commonest overuse injuries is Achilles tendonitis due to recurrent tension or jarring. Frequently this results from microruptures of individual fibres which sometimes form soft degenerate areas and cysts (Williams et al., 1976). Treatment is aimed at diminishing the

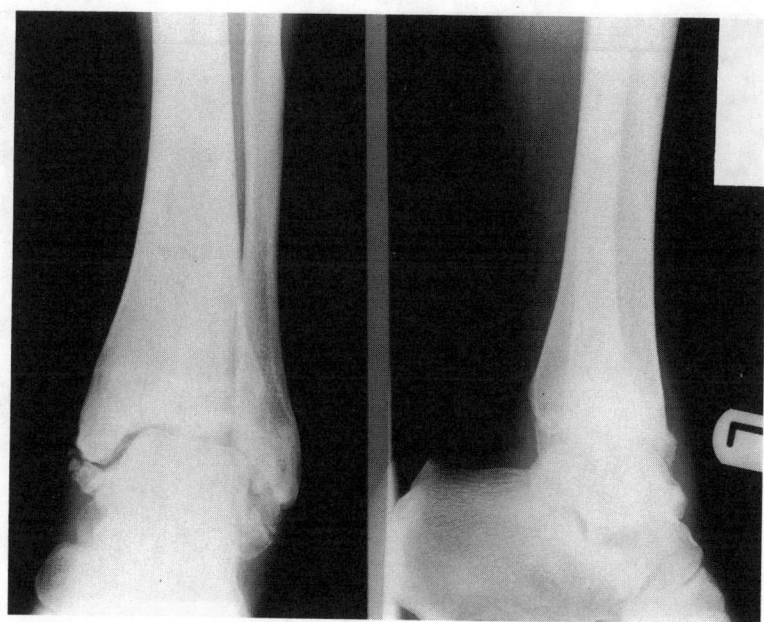

Fig. 1. Footballer's ankle.

jarring, decreasing the inflammation and, occasionally, decompression of the cyst. Similarly, friction as in the iliotibial tract syndrome (see below) causes inflammation which may be treated using the same principles.

The tendon insertion

This may also become inflamed; these are the enthesiopathies. Before the apophyses are fused the inflammatory change may be associated with radiographic fragmentation of the apophysis as in Osgood–Schlatter disease (tibial apophysitis) and Sever's disease (calcaneal apophysitis).

Tendon sheaths

These may become inflamed separately or in combination with tendonitis. Trigger finger, sometimes seen as part of a generalized disorder such as rheumatoid arthritis, is a common example of this combination. Tenosynovitis causes pain, swelling and crepitus.

Ligaments

Ligaments frequently undergo repeated strain resulting in chronic ligament injury which presents with pain and swelling. Ligamentitis would be a more accurate, but less euphonious, description of the condition which indicates

the pathology and hence the treatment. Over a long period, recurrent tearing and inflammation produce calcification and even ossification, as in the well-known footballer's ankle (Fig. 1).

Fibrocartilage

The menisci of the knee may react in a similar way; the force is more often shearing from rotation and results in repeated ruptures of the fibres, areas of degenerate change and small cysts.

Bones

Bones also respond to overuse with inflammatory change; microfractures are associated with inflammation and pain and may progress to more extensive fractures seen on a radiograph. Raised periosteum may be accompanied by a partial lucency (fracture) or density (callus). A contentious way of treating this is to keep exercising the limb without applying the causative force (e.g. swimming for runners) until the area is pain-free, and then maintaining a tolerable stimulus in order to strengthen the bone. The safe method of treatment is to rest the limb completely until the fracture has healed after about 8 weeks, and then gradually resume sport.

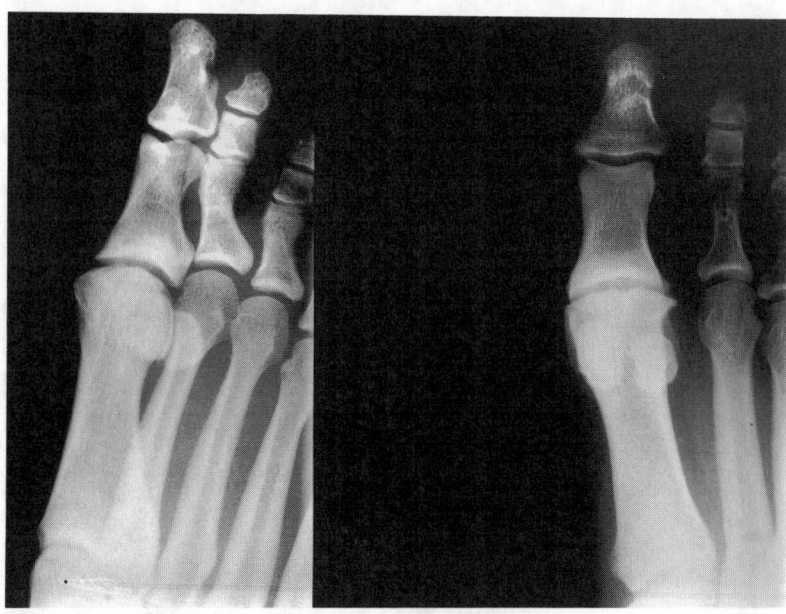

Fig. 2. Osteochondritis dissecans of head of first metatarsal.

THE FOOT

Acute injuries

These differ little from acute injuries in other walks of life. Tendon and ligament ruptures, tendon avulsions, dislocations and fractures all occur and are treated along standard lines. The tissues are replaced and held in their anatomical position either operatively or by manipulation. Avulsion of the base of the fifth metatarsal tends to be overdiagnosed; an avulsion fracture is usually transverse whereas the physis is always longitudinal. Crush injuries should always be taken seriously as soft tissue damage is almost always more extensive than the external appearance suggests.

Chronic overuse injuries

These are common, particularly in runners.

Subungual haematoma

This is an almost universal complaint of road-runners in which the nail of the toe, often the hallux, is rubbed off its bed resulting in bleeding beneath the nail. It is rarely worth trephining. The nail will eventually fall off and regrow. Rest is not necessary.

Blisters

These are common and may be dressed or deroofed.

Osteochondritis dissecans

This can affect the head of a metatarsal causing pain and swelling of the metatarsophalangeal joint. Recurrent tangential forces may cause a fragment of convex bone and cartilage to shear off, particularly during jumping sports such as netball. One option is to remove the bony fragment (Fig. 2). Osteochondritis dissecans, usually of the second metatarsal head (Freiberg's disease), may not be caused by trauma; the metatarsophalangeal joint is swollen and painful and a radiograph confirms the diagnosis. Severe symptoms are relieved by excision of the metatarsal head and this allows a rapid return to sport.

Stress fractures

These particularly affect the metatarsal shafts and navicular and have increased in incidence with the popularity of running. The second metatarsal stress fracture is the March fracture (Fig. 3). Pain and localized tenderness are characteristic and treatment is as described above. The sesamoid bones of the hallux may occasionally be congenitally bipartite or split by an acute or stress fracture.

Plantar fasciitis

This is frequently precipitated by overuse but sometimes occurs *de novo*. Pain and tenderness are felt at the origin

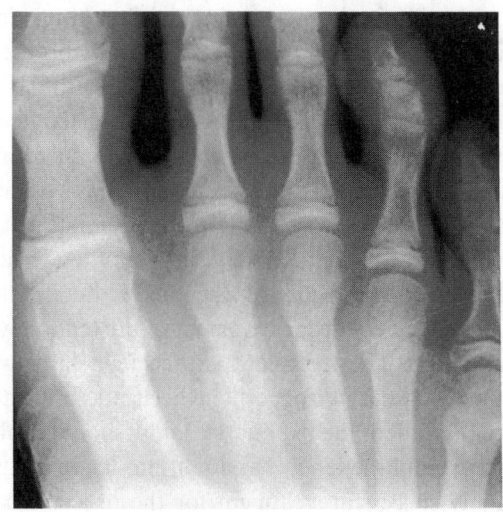

Fig. 3. March fracture.

of the fascia from the calcaneum. A calcaneal spur may be seen on the radiograph but the condition frequently occurs without. If standard anti-inflammatory methods fail, it is occasionally necessary to divide the origin of the fascia.

Bruised heel fat pad

This usually results from running on hard surfaces and gives much the same symptoms as plantar fasciitis but the tenderness is more posterior. It is a difficult condition to treat successfully without advising complete rest. A sorbothane heel pad helps to lessen the impact and a local steroid injection frequently reduces the pain but may damage the fat pad and render it more liable to further injury.

Traction apophysitis

This may occur at the base of the fifth metatarsal. An intractable case should be relieved with a steroid injection around the insertion of the peroneus brevis.

Interdigital (Morton's) neuroma

This may occur at any age and is especially common between the third and fourth metatarsals in runners and walkers, but may occur between any of the metatarsals. The digital nerve is compressed between the heads of adjacent metatarsals resulting in neuroma formation. The patient complains of pain or paraesthesia radiating into the adjacent toes. There is plantar tenderness at the site of the neuroma and pain is elicited by transverse compression of the metatarsals. Numbness may be present on the adjoining surfaces of the two toes. Non-operative treatment includes orthoses to alter the load-bearing area and local injections of steroids, but excision of the neuroma and sometimes of an associated bursa is often needed, in which case the patient should be warned about permanent but harmless numbness.

THE ANKLE

Ankle injuries are some of the commonest conditions seen in an A&E department. Morbidity, however, is not as common as might be expected.

Acute injuries

Acute ligament injuries

These are often referred to as sprains whatever the grading and are caused by inversion or eversion forces which rupture the lateral or medial ligaments, respectively. If a crack is heard, a ligament has ruptured completely or there is an associated fracture. Indeed, the anterolateral ligament is frequently avulsed distally and the small bony fragment may be seen on the lateral radiograph. There is localized swelling and tenderness but laxity is not always demonstrable in the acute phase. However, laxity should always be tested for; anterior laxity demonstrated by the drawer test indicates rupture of the anterolateral ligament and is most frequently associated with later instability. Most sprains can be satisfactorily treated by elevation and early restoration of movements but the more serious ruptures may need splinting. Repair of the ligament should be considered for a grade III rupture in an ardent athlete. Proprioceptive re-education (physiotherapy) should be given to all.

A trap for the unwary is the extensive rupture of the interosseous membrane and anteroinferior tibiofibular ligament associated with a high spiral fibular fracture (the Maisonneuve fracture). The ankle is extremely swollen and the wary physician will have detected the tenderness of the fibula before the fracture and diastasis have been revealed by the radiograph. Morbidity will result unless the diastasis is corrected operatively.

The peroneal tendons

These occasionally rupture singly or in pairs due to sudden resisted active eversion. This is a difficult diagnosis, especially if only one tendon has ruptured. There will be weakness of eversion but this is easily put down to pain from lateral ligament rupture. Surgical exploration may be the best option if there is doubt.

The tendo Achillis

This frequently ruptures and the diagnosis is missed. Almost invariably there is a classic history and it is difficult to understand why the injury is missed. The middle-aged athlete believes there was a sudden blow on the calf which, on a squash court, is mistaken for a blow from the opponent's racket. Pain, weakness and swelling may only be moderate. Initially the gap between the two ends of the tendon may be palpated. Active plantar flexion will be intact due to the action of other posterior tendons. Simmonds' squeeze test will almost invariably give the answer: the patient kneels on a padded chair with the feet hanging over the edge and the calves are squeezed in their bulky part. On the normal side, the foot plantar-flexes and on the ruptured side there is no movement. Partial ruptures can occur and in these cases the squeeze test may be negative.

Complete ruptures should always be treated by apposition of the tendon ends until they unite at 6–9 weeks. Splinting the leg, initially with the ankle plantar-flexed and the knee slightly flexed, gives satisfactory results. The splint can be brought below the knee at 3 weeks and the ankle can be brought up to a neutral position at 6 weeks. More certain apposition is achieved by suturing which may be strong enough to allow mobilization and is probably the treatment of choice in the quality athlete.

Chronic overuse injuries

These are common and often result from a previous acute injury.

Achilles tendonitis and paratendonitis

This is the commonest single entity in a sports injury clinic. The tendo Achillis and its paratenon (there is no anatomical sheath) become inflamed due to repeated jarring. It is most often seen in runners, particularly long-distance runners. The condition probably starts as microrupture of individual fibres which initiate an inflammatory response and may progress to form foci of ruptured or degenerate fibres and sometimes cyst formation.

The history is almost always that of excessive running.

Pain and stiffness is most common first thing in the morning and when beginning a run. Examination reveals tenderness at the junction of the mid-third with the distal third of the tendon. In the more advanced chronic condition there is a fusiform swelling and surrounding oedema. The whole length of the tendon may be affected. Some authors claim to be able to differentiate between tendonitis and peritendonitis by the site of tenderness in plantar and dorsiflexion of the ankle, but operative findings reveal very little movement of the tendon within the paratenon. The treatment is the same. Jarring may be limited by wearing sorbothane heels and anti-inflammatory treatment helps but steroids should only be injected around the tendon and not into it. An irrational but highly successful treatment for the resistant case is paratenon stripping with decompression (longitudinal splitting) of the tendon. The author favours operating on both tendons as it so frequently becomes bilateral.

Achilles insertional tendonitis

This is caused by recurrent jarring at the insertion of the tendon, usually in the younger patient. Before the apophysis is fused there is often radiographic fragmentation and increased density of the apophysis. Clinically there is localized tenderness which responds to anti-inflammatory treatment (rest, NSAIDs, physiotherapy and localized steroid injection around the insertion).

Achilles bursitis

This gives a similar clinical picture to the two conditions above. A bursa may enlarge and become inflamed anterior or posterior to the tendon, just superior to the insertion. The tender cyst may be felt separate from the tendon. Aspiration and injection of a little steroid will relieve the condition.

Os trigonitis

This may be confused with an anterior Achilles bursitis. The os trigonum is an anatomical variant. It is a small bone situated immediately posterior to the talus although occasionally the bony prolongation is just part of the talus. In hyperflexion of the ankle, often seen in hurdlers and footballers, the os trigonum is repeatedly squeezed between the posterior lip of the tibia and the calcaneum, like a nut in a nut cracker, causing an inflammatory reaction. The athlete complains of pain on plantar flexion. Examination reveals deep tenderness posterior to the

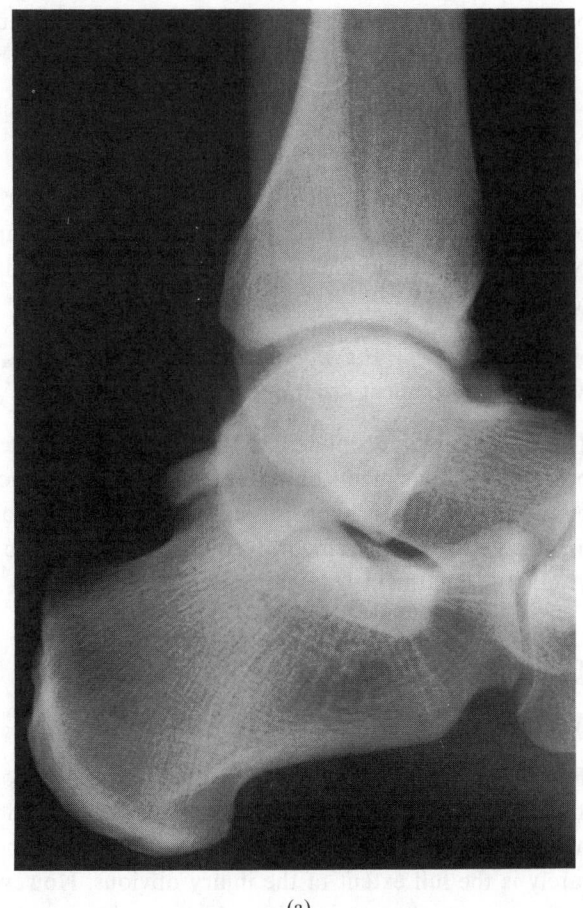

(a)

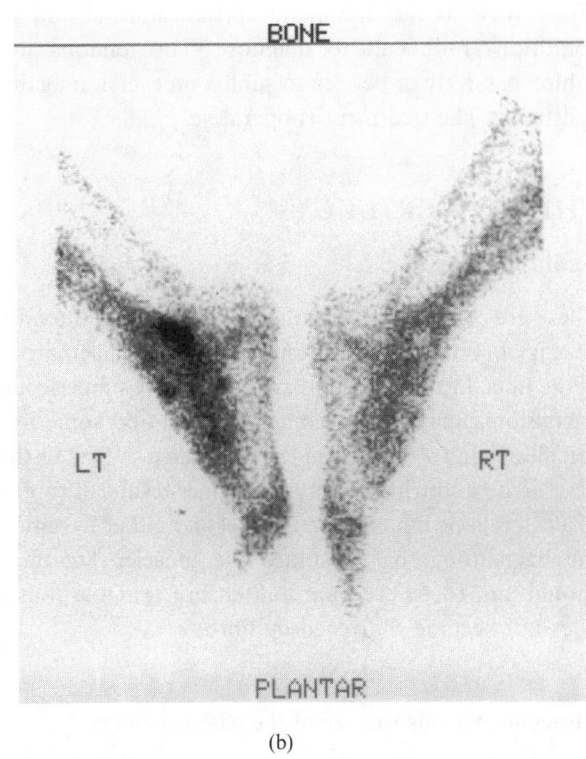

(b)

Fig. 4. (a) Os trigonum. (b) Technetium bone scan of os trigonitis.

ankle and radiographs show the bone (Fig. 4a). Anti-inflammatory measures usually settle the condition but the recalcitrant case needs excision of the bone (Fig. 4b).

The anterior impingement syndrome

This is a similar condition occurring on the front of the ankle. The anterior lip of the tibia, often enlarged by an osteophyte, impinges on the talus in dorsiflexion, pinches the synovium and causes inflammation and pain. If anti-inflammatory treatment fails, the redundant synovium and osteophyte may be excised arthroscopically or at open operation.

Osteochondritis dissecans

This affects the angles of the dome of the talus. If the fragment becomes loose it should be removed.

Tenosynovitis

This occurs in all three muscle groups (anterior, lateral and posterior). Crepitus is frequently heard and felt. In the more acute form, rest is sufficient; in the chronic form, a steroid injection may be necessary.

Tarsal coalition

This is most frequently calcaneonavicular. It alters the mechanics of the foot and predisposes to peroneal teno-synovitis. In children, it presents as painful spasmodic flat foot. Excision of the bony bar should cure the condition.

Footballer's ankle

This term is sometimes given to the stiff calcified ligaments which result from repeated sprains (Fig. 1). Treatment is symptomatic.

Peroneal tendon subluxation

This may occur primarily, or secondary to lateral ligament and retinacular rupture. The tendons sublux superficial to the lateral malleolus creating pain, snapping and giving way. At rest the ankle appears normal and the condition is difficult to diagnose. The tendons may sublux passively or be seen to sublux on eversion against resistance. The treatment is operative.

THE LOWER LEG

Acute injuries

These are commonplace in the calf and shin and tend to be trivial. With the exception of periosteal haematoma of the tibia, bruising is rarely bothersome. A subperiosteal haematoma may be exceedingly painful and sometimes calcifies giving a radiographic appearance similar to that of a sarcoma. Intrinsic injury sometimes results in rupture of a calf muscle but is is rarely necessary either to remove the haematoma or to suture the muscle. Treatment should aim to relieve pain and ensure that the muscle does not become shortened by fibrosis.

Musculotendinous rupture of the gastrocnemius

This most frequently affects the medial head and gives very similar symptoms to rupture of the Achilles tendon. Repair is only indicated in the good athlete with major disruption and wide separation of the muscle and aponeurosis. Rest in equinus is usually sufficient.

Chronic overuse injuries

These usually present with shin pain, often called 'shin splints', and it may be difficult to differentiate stress fracture, insertional fasciitis and compartment syndrome. Pronation of the foot predisposes to all of these conditions so that occasionally an antipronation orthosis in the shoe is the only treatment necessary.

Stress fractures

These are diagnosed clinically from the history, localized swelling and transverse tenderness of the bone in the early stages as there are no radiographic changes. The most frequent site is the junction of the mid-third with the distal third of the tibia. Later, periosteal elevation (Fig. 5a) is seen and, in the well-established case, there are obvious radiographic changes (Fig. 5b). A technetium bone scan will confirm the diagnosis.

Insertional fasciitis

This produces pain and tenderness along the anterior or posterior borders of the tibia. Relative rest, physiotherapy, NSAIDs and steroid injections help; fasciotomy is a last resort.

Muscle compartment syndromes

These are mainly confined to the anterior and deep posterior compartments of the leg. Shin pain is produced by running and the diagnosis is confirmed with compartment pressure measurement during exercise (Matsen *et al.*, 1980). Treatment is fasciotomy.

THE KNEE

Acute injuries

The knee is the most frequently injured part of the body in sport and the commonest sports injury seen in most A&E departments. Often the problem is one of diagnosis; rarely is the full extent of the injury obvious. However, there are some acute injuries which are important to diagnose early such as ligament and tendon avulsions, and the task is made easier and more successful by taking a full history and making an appropriate examination, even in the rushed atmosphere of the A&E department.

In the history only six questions need to be asked regarding:

1. Type of injury.
2. Crack at time of injury.
3. Swelling.
4. Locking.
5. Stability.
6. Pain.

Most athletes will be able to talk through the circumstances of the injury. It should become clear whether the limb was bearing weight, if the force was angular and/or rotational and if there was hyperflexion or hyperextension. The direction of the force gives the clue as to which ligament may be injured and weight-bearing is necessary to cause a longitudinal tear of the meniscus.

If a crack, often likened to the sound of a rifle shot, is heard at the time of the injury, this indicates that a major structure such as a ligament or meniscus has ruptured.

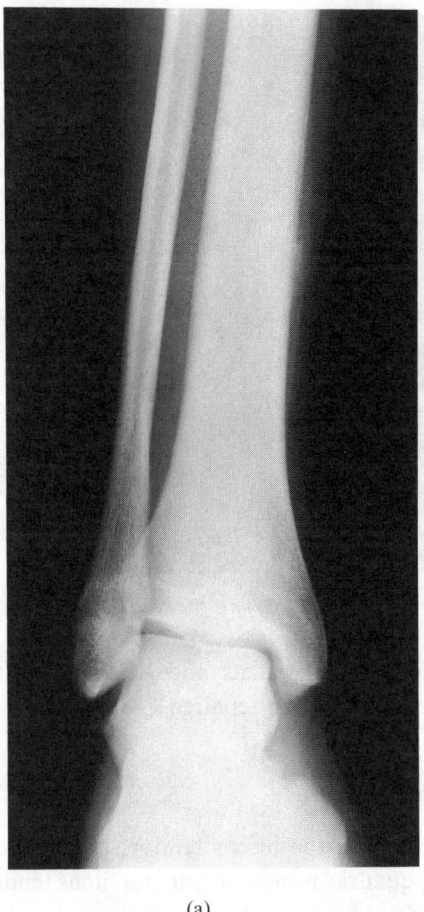 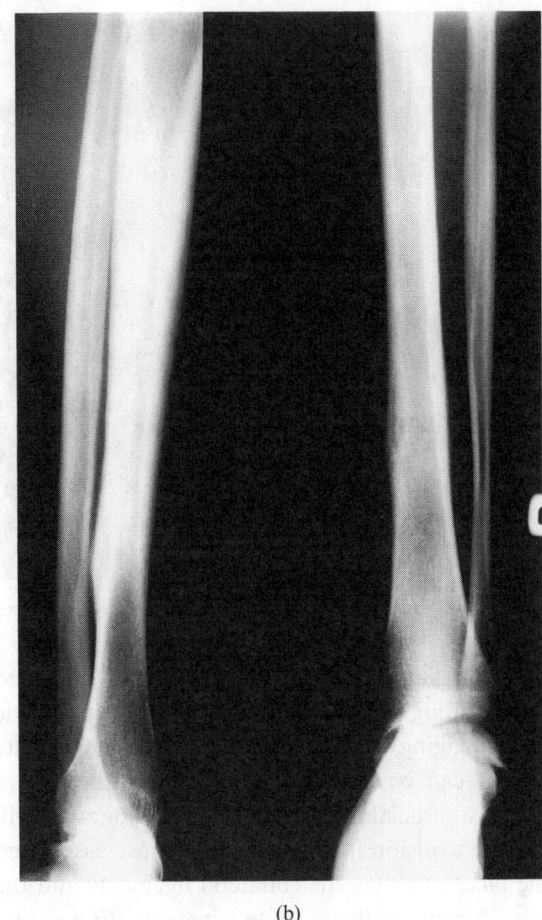

(a) (b)

Fig. 5. (a) Tibial stress fracture with periosteal elevation. (b) Healing tibial stress fracture.

Early swelling within an hour of the injury indicates a haemarthrosis due to rupture of a well-vascularized structure, most often the anterior cruciate ligament.

Surgical locking is the sudden inability to extend the knee but some flexion is possible. Blocking would be a better term as it does not imply the same mechanism as locking a door in which there is no movement either way. Surgical locking is caused by a loose intra-articular body which may be meniscal, cartilaginous or bony.

Early instability of the knee may indicate ligament rupture or a loose intra-articular structure, but it may just be a reflection of pain.

The site of the pain is a crude indication of the site of the injury.

Examination is often less helpful than the history. Tenderness may localize the rupture of a ligament or tendon, the tearing of a meniscus or the site of a fracture. An effusion is easily distinguished from soft tissue swelling by its distribution and, in the author's opinion, should only be aspirated for diagnosis (e.g. of haemarthrosis,

gout, infection) or to relieve pain in a tense effusion.

A loss of extension may be caused by true locking or pain from an injured posterior structure. Laxity of the knee is one of the most difficult and contentious subjects in knee surgery, from the point of view both of demonstrating the laxity and of interpreting the findings. In the A&E department it is sufficient to elicit whether there is anterior, posterior, medial or lateral laxity. The definitive diagnosis can wait for the operating theatre. It is by no means easy to distinguish between anterior and posterior laxity, and between medial and lateral laxity. If there is doubt, stress radiographs are helpful. Anterior laxity is tested with the knee at 90° (the drawer test) and 20° (Lachman's test). The latter is more likely to be accurate in the acutely injured knee due to the lack of hamstring action. Medial and lateral laxity should also be tested at 20° of flexion to negate the action of the anterior cruciate ligament. In the acutely injured knee it is rarely possible to obtain sufficient muscle relaxation to allow the important pivot shift test.

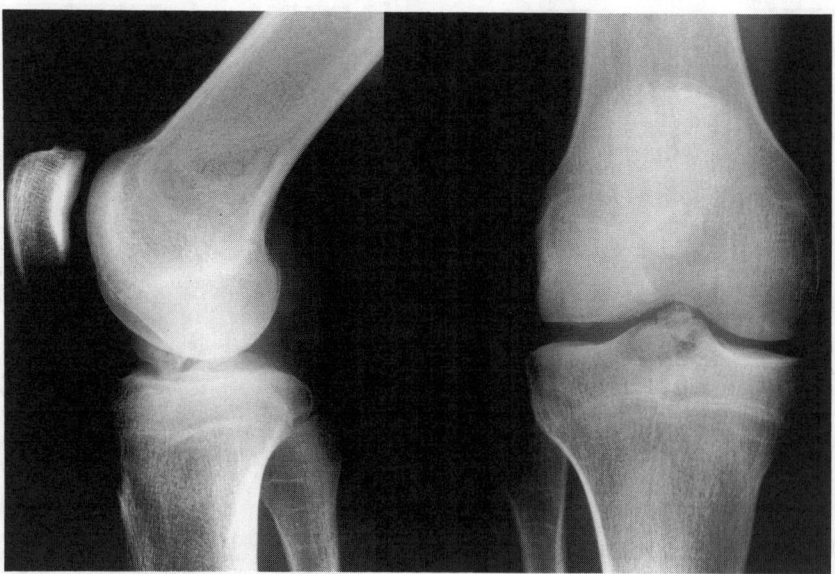

Fig. 6. Avulsion of tibial attachment of anterior cruciate ligament.

The history and examination will have indicated whether a radiograph is necessary. A MRI (magnetic resonance imaging) scan is not needed for most acute injuries but can be helpful in determining the site of rupture of a cruciate ligament. The radiograph will demonstrate avulsion fractures such as those associated with the biceps tendon, the collateral ligaments and the tibial attachments of the cruciate ligaments (Fig. 6) and the Segond fracture (from the anterolateral lip of the tibia) which almost invariably accompanies a ruptured anterior cruciate ligament (Fig. 7a, b).

A tentative diagnosis should be made. If this is delayed by advising the patient to come back in 2 weeks when things have had time to settle down, it may be too late to reattach an avulsed cruciate ligament. A haemarthrosis is an indication for further investigation, usually examination under anaesthetic and arthroscopy. A reliable MRI scan is less invasive but no use as therapy. A locked knee needs rapid operative intervention.

Indications for early operation

- A haemarthrosis
- A locked knee
- An osteochondral fracture
- A displaced intra-articular fracture
- grade III ligament laxity

Ligament ruptures

These are diagnosed and graded under anaesthesia and by direct vision at arthroscopy. Grade III ruptures of the collateral ligaments and avulsions of the cruciate ligaments should be repaired.

Tendon avulsions

These involve the biceps tendon, patellar tendon (ligament), quadriceps tendon and popliteus tendon. Rupture of the quadriceps mechanism is frequently misdiagnosed by mistaking an inability to raise the straight leg as being due to pain. Electrical stimulation will usually demonstrate whether the mechanism is intact, but if there is doubt it should be explored surgically. Avulsion of the tibial tuberosity tends to occur in children and teenagers and it should be replaced.

Meniscal tears

These are usually longitudinal from an acute injury and may convert into a complete bucket handle by anterior extension, or to a flap tear by radial extension. Both can cause locking by displacing and jamming in the anterior segment of the joint. If the tear is in the peripheral vascular third of the meniscus which is otherwise undamaged, it may be sutured; otherwise it is best removed.

Chondral fractures, osteochondral fractures

These also cause locking when the fragment jams anteriorly. A chondral fracture cannot be seen on a radiograph and should be removed if it causes symptoms. There is frequently only a sliver of bone attached to an osteo-

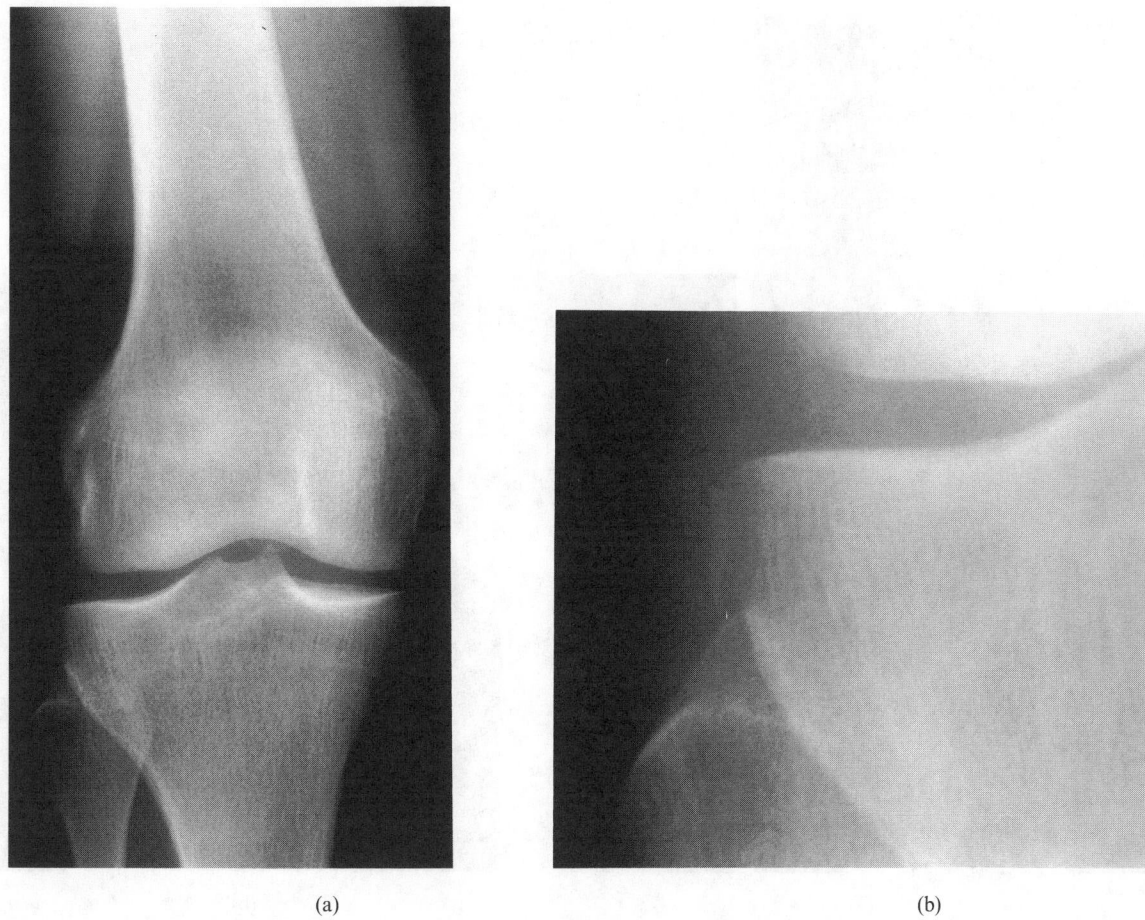

(a)   (b)

Fig. 7. (a) & (b) Segond fracture.

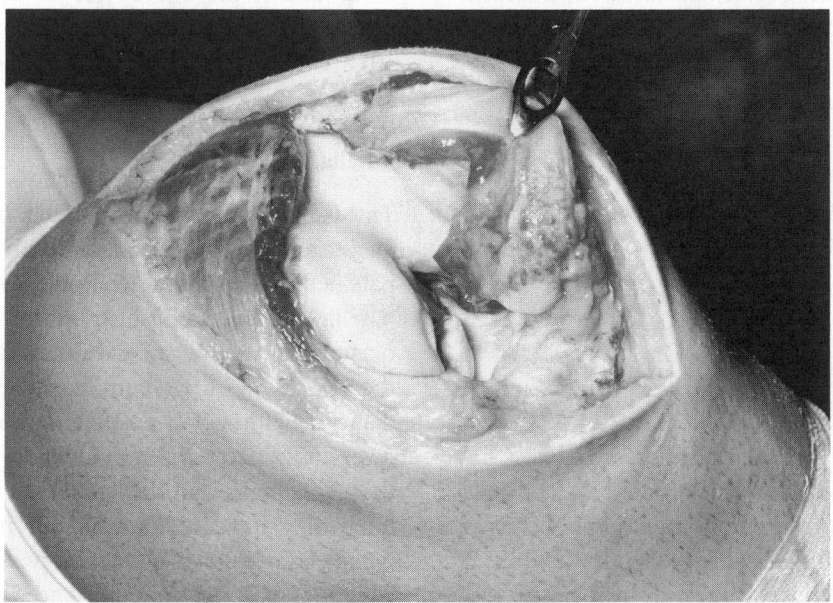

Fig. 8. Osteochondritis dissecans of medial femoral condyle.

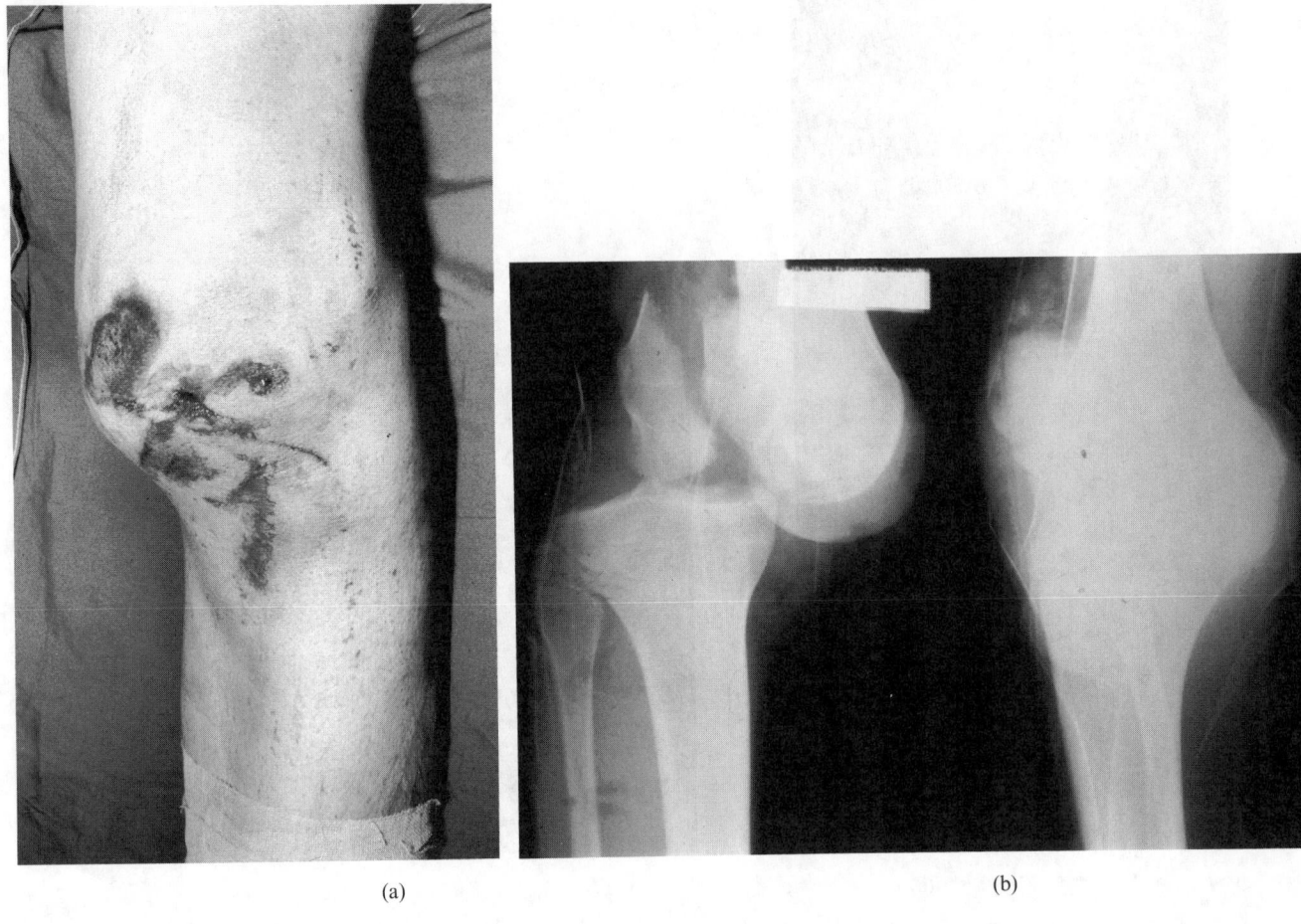

(a)   (b)

Fig. 9. (a) & (b) Fracture-dislocation of knee.

chondral fracture which is therefore difficult to see on a radiograph, but there will be haemarthosis. The fragment should be replaced surgically (Fig. 8) unless very small.

Articular fractures

These sometimes release sufficient fat as well as blood to give a lipohaemarthrosis seen as a fluid level on a radiograph. Displacement of more than a millimetre or two is best corrected to produce a smooth articular surface.

Tibiofemoral dislocations

These are caused by considerable force and are uncommon in sport. Fracture-dislocations (Fig. 9a, b) are associated with speedway riding or road traffic accidents. Rarely is there difficulty in diagnosing the condition but the frequency with which they are associated with popliteal nerve and vascular damage is not so well appreciated. A full neurovascular examination must be made and if there is doubt an angiogram should be performed. Urgent relocation and surgical repair (Fig. 10) are needed.

Patellar dislocation

This is invariably lateral. A high patella, an increased Q angle, a deficient lateral femoral condyle and a flat patella all predispose to dislocation, but even the normal patella is subject to dislocation from either a direct blow or sudden twisting on an almost straight leg. Usually the patella relocates spontaneously causing difficulty in diagnosis although a positive patellar apprehension test gives the answer. If the patella was avulsed from the vastus medialis and medial retinaculum, a fragment of bone may have been pulled off its medial border (a Goodfellow lesion) which makes repair worthwhile. Otherwise it is best to keep the knee moving and perform vastus medialis exercises.

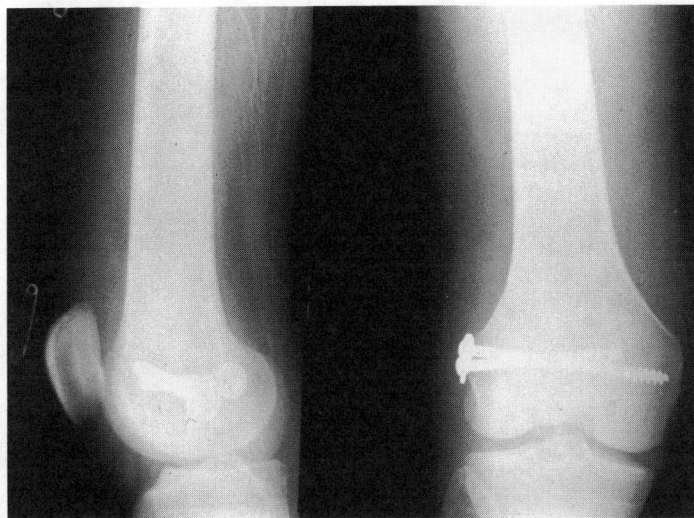

Fig. 10. Relocation of fracture-dislocation of knee.

Superior tibiofibular dislocation

This is rare and persisting dislocation is even rarer. It is caused either by landing badly from a jump or from a direct blow. Pain and swelling are limited to the joint and the knee mechanism is not involved. It should be relocated.

Chronic overuse injuries of the knee

Fathoming the multitudinous causes of chronic knee pain is akin to unravelling the Gordian knot. Nonetheless many athletes come to the A&E department with pain and expect help. An incomplete list of some of the causes of chronic knee pain (mostly due to overuse) is given in Table 2. Many of these can be differentiated by the site of pain and tenderness. Irrespective of the causation, patellar pain is frequently helped by vastus medialis exercises in an attempt to alter the alignment of the patella.

Chronic meniscal tears are probably caused by repeated shearing forces resulting in localized pain and occasionally instability. Treatment is excision of the torn part of the meniscus. Cysts of the lateral meniscus are associated with this type of tear and are felt as a smooth tender hard swelling at the centre of the lateral joint line, most prominent at 70° of flexion. These cysts can be decompressed arthroscopically at the same time as partial meniscectomy.

A medial synovial plica sometimes becomes inflamed and can be felt as a thin tender band just superior to the medial joint line; it usually responds to non-operative measures.

Table 2. *Some causes of chronic knee pain*

- Patellar
  - Recurrent dislocation/subluxation
  - Chrondromalacia
  - Excessive lateral pressure syndrome
  - Bipartite patella (occasionally)
  - Stress fracture
  - Osteochondritis dissecans
- Meniscal
  - Horizontal cleavage tears
  - Radial tears
  - Cysts
- Femoral
  - Osteochondritis dissecans
- Synovial
  - Plicae
  - Fat pad syndrome (Hoffa's)
- Tendonitis
  - Patellar (ligament)
  - Popliteus
  - Biceps
  - Iliotibial tract
- Insertional tendonitis
  - Quadriceps
  - Patellar tendon (ligament)
- Traction apophysitis
  - Osgood–Schlatter disease
  - Sinding–Larsen–Johansen syndrome
- Bursitis
  - Pes anserinus
  - Semimembranosus
  - Biceps

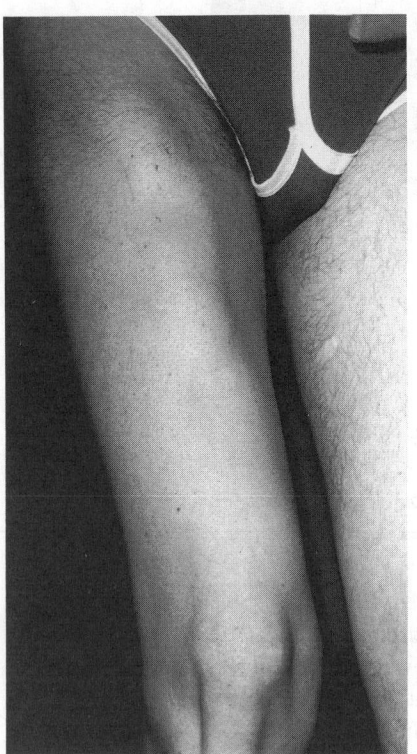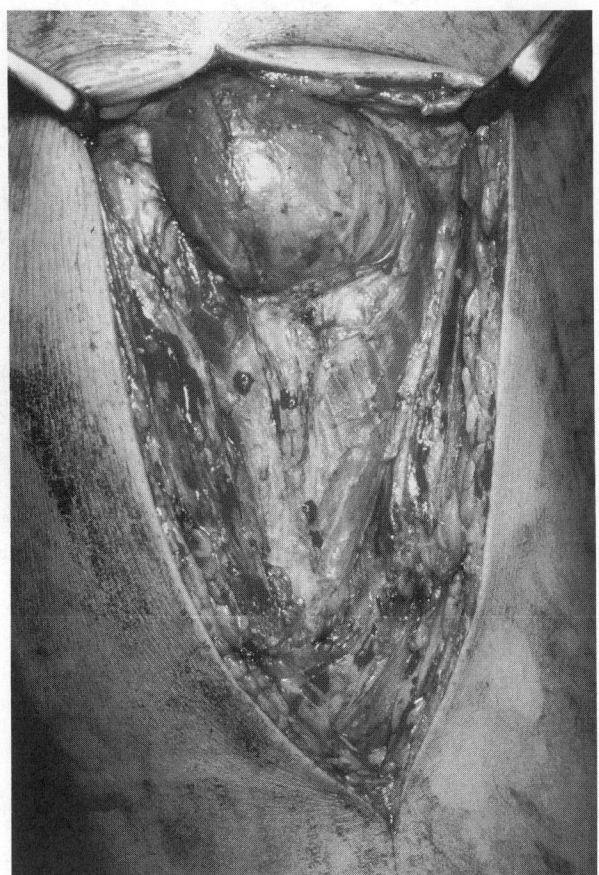

Fig. 11. (a) & (b) Rupture of rectus femoris.

The fat pad occasionally becomes nipped between the femoral condyle and tibia in hyperextension running downhill; the resulting inflammation gives rise to anterior pain and tenderness which also responds to non-operative treatment. The iliotibial tract syndrome (Noble, 1980) presents with pain and tenderness at the point where the iliotibial tract rubs over the lateral femoral condyle. It is a long-distance runner's complaint. Physiotherapy, including stretching the tract, and local injections help.

Osgood–Schlatter's pain is the well-known tibial tubercle apophysitis characterized by pain, swelling and radiographic fragmentation of the tibial tubercle mainly in active children. It usually resolves with or without treatment. Splinting is not necessary as exercise will do no harm but will hurt. The Sinding–Larsen–Johansen syndrome is a similar condition at the lower pole of the patella. Insertional tendonitis is the adult equivalent of these conditions and responds to physiotherapy or local injections around the insertion.

Patellar tendonitis is similar to Achilles tendonitis and responds to the same treatment.

THE THIGH

Acute injuries

A dead leg or Charley Horse injury

Recovery is rapid unless there is an intramuscular haematoma.

A rectus femoris rupture (Fig. 11a, b)

This is caused by kicking an immovable object. It does not need repair in the average athlete.

Hamstring rupture

This is common in sprinters. Treatment is aimed at avoiding recurrence by lengthening the hamstrings and preventing contracture from fibrosis.

Chronic injuries

The superior iliotibial tract syndrome

This is caused by friction of the iliotibial tract on the greater trochanter. Diagnosis and treatment are the same as for the inferior variant. Trochanteric bursitis may occur separately or in association with the syndrome.

THE PELVIS AND HIPS

Acute injuries

Avulsion injuries of tendons

These occur with or without the bony apophysis in the adductor tendons, both heads of the biceps femoris and the hamstrings. The latter is particularly common in long-jumpers in whom the ischial apophysis is pulled off and unites with a mass of callus which may be mistaken for an osteosarcoma (Fig. 12a, b). The iliac apophysis may also be pulled off in cricketers.

A snapping hip

This is commonly seen in young female athletes. Usually it arises from the iliotibial tract on the greater trochanter or the iliopsoas tendon over the hip joint. Surgical lengthening is rarely needed.

Chronic overuse injuries

These are seen in a variety of athletic pursuits and often give rise to 'groin pain' (a symptom found in adductor tendonitis, iliopsoas tendonitis, pubic symphysitis, stress fractures, sports hernias, conjoint tendonitis and others). Tenderness is usually confined to the structure affected. The instability of pubic symphysitis can be demonstrated on radiographic stork views. The sports hernia and conjoint tendonitis are hotly debated subjects, but it is undoubted that many of the sufferers, mainly footballers, are cured by an operation akin to a herniorrhaphy. Stress fractures are seen in the pubic or ischial rami of runners (Fig. 13).

THE SPINE

Acute injuries

These are rarely sports-specific.

Chronic overuse injuries

A few are particularly common in athletes.

Road-runner's back

This is nothing more than back pain from recurrent jarring in which the clinical and radiographic findings may be normal.

Spondylolytic stress fractures

These occur in the twisting sports of cricket and tennis and are treated in a standard manner.

Osteochondritis dissecans of the vertebral ring epiphyses (Scheuermann's disease)

This is frequently seen in young gymnasts. Rest is needed.

THE CHEST

A few chest wall injuries are seen in athletes.

Costochondritis

This usually involves the second costochondral junction. Tietze's disease is seen in rowers and swimmers. Physiotherapy and steroid injections may help.

Costotransverse subluxation

This is also seen in rowers and may be cured by manipulation without anaesthetic.

Jogger's nipple

This affects males and females and is often not recognized for what it is – a sore nipple from the rubbing of the runner's vest.

Distal avulsion of the pectoralis major (Fig. 14)

This is seen in weight-lifters, swimmers and runners. It may be sutured back in place, but if left it causes surprisingly little deficit. Occasionally the track calcifies (Fig. 15).

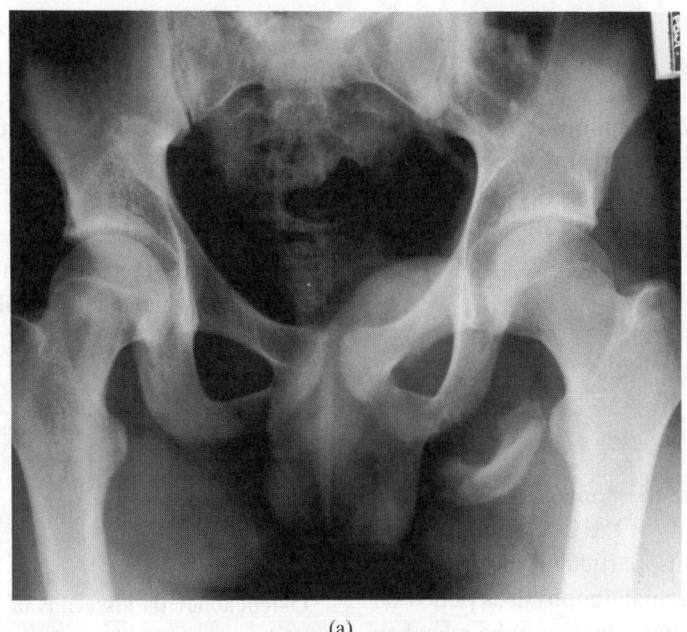

(a)

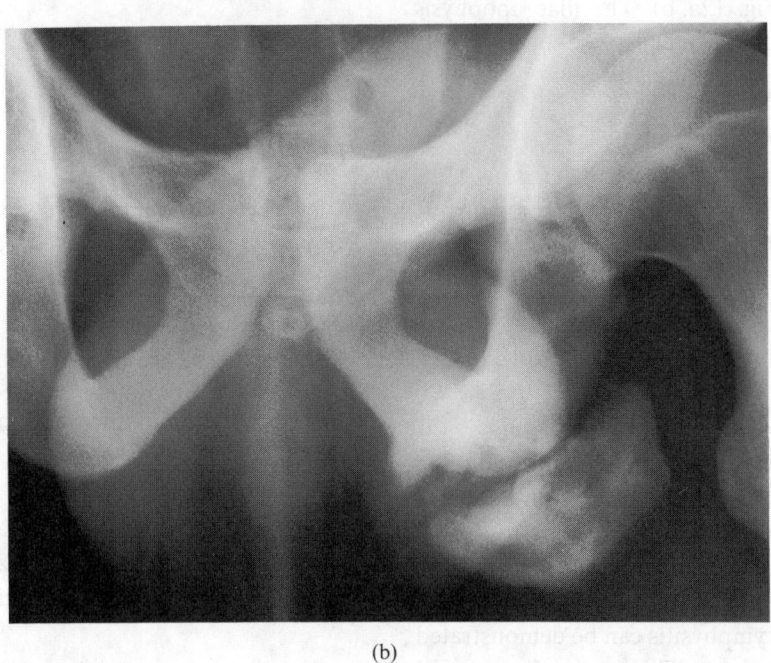

(b)

Fig. 12. (a) Avulsion of ischial tuberosity. (b) Healing avulsion of ischial tuberosity.

THE UPPER LIMB

There are few true sports injuries of the upper limb and many are diagnosed and treated along the standard lines described at the beginning of the chapter.

Acute injuries

These are mainly muscle and tendon ruptures. The supraspinatus tendon, and the tendons of the biceps (Fig.

16a, b) may rupture with sudden intrinsic force as in weight-lifting. In the acute phase, these injuries are best sutured in athletes.

Glenohumeral dislocation

This injury is common in rugby. After reduction of an anterior dislocation, external rotation and abduction should be prevented for 6 weeks. Even then recurrent

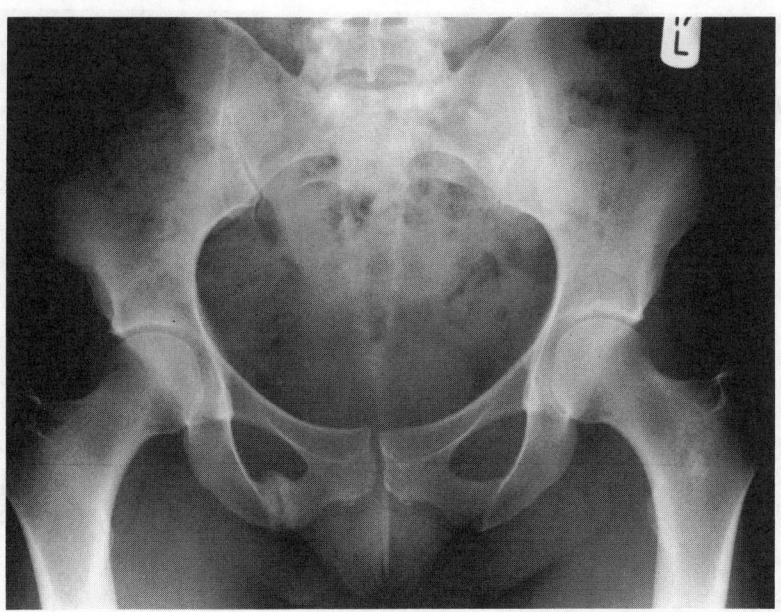

Fig. 13. Stress fracture of ischial ramus of 400 metre runner.

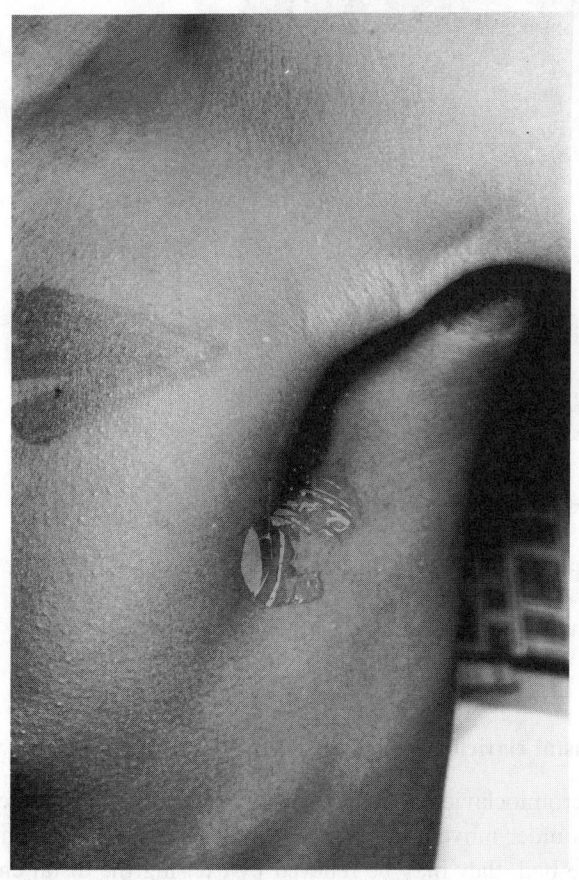

Fig. 14. Avulsion of pectoralis major.

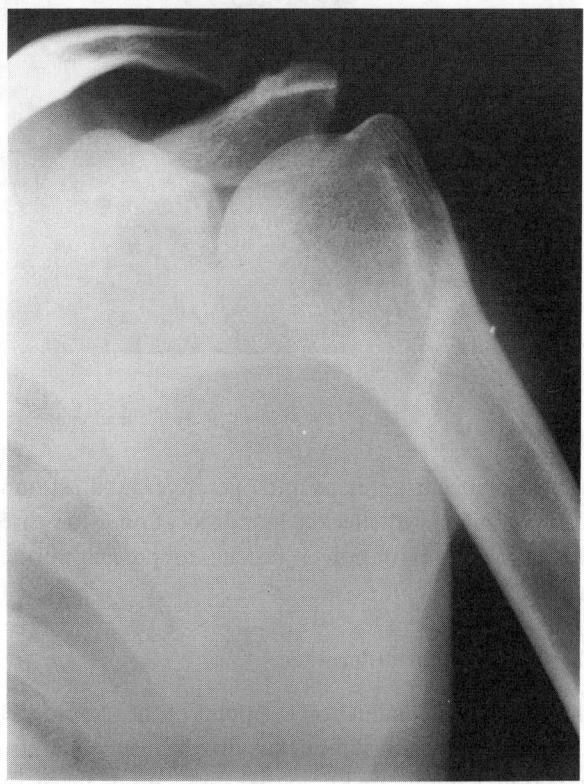

Fig. 15. Calcification in tract of pectoralis major.

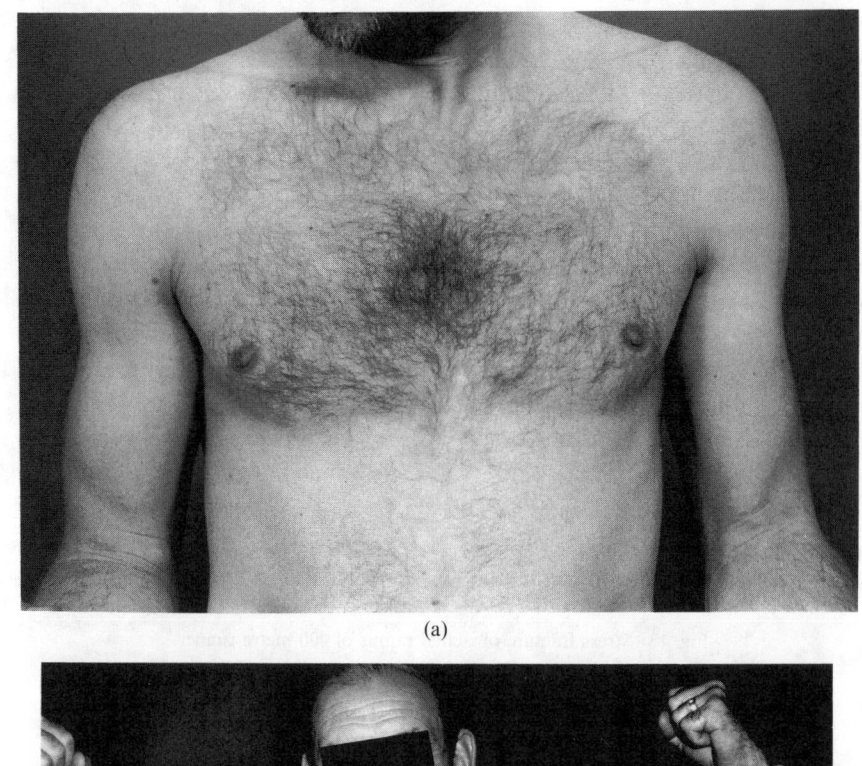

(a)

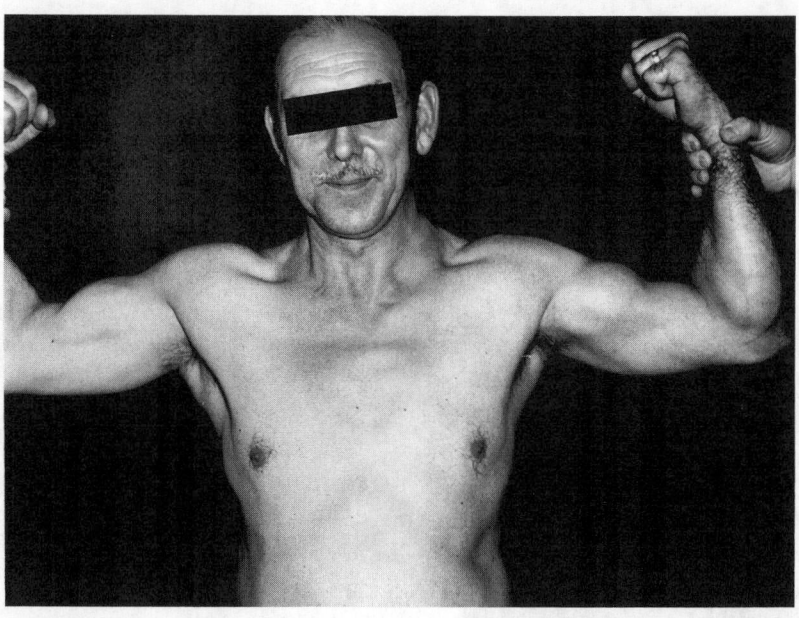

(b)

Fig. 16. (a) Avulsed left biceps tendon at rest. (b) Abulsed left biceps tendon with muscle contraction.

dislocation occurs in many and operative stabilization is often recommended after the first dislocation. After three dislocations stabilization is needed to prevent further damage to the joint.

Acromioclavicular dislocation

This is caused by falling on the point of the shoulder. It does not usually give sufficient trouble to justify operative reduction. Complicated grade III dislocations merit fixation.

Chronic overuse injuries

These occur particularly in throwing sports.

Distal clavicular osteolysis

Acromioclavicular joint pain may occur with repeated shoulder movements such as canoeing. If the symptoms are bad, they may be relieved by excising the distal end of the clavicle.

Subacromial impingements

These may require subacromial decompression.

Bicipital tendonitis

This occurs most frequently in the long head of biceps but also in the distal conjoint tendon. It is not a cause of rupture which is due to sudden excessive force.

Epicondylitis

This affects the medial (golfer's elbow) and lateral (tennis elbow) humeral epicondyles spontaneously or after excessive use. The tenderness tends to be very localized. A deep injection of steroid into the tender spot and down to bone will often relieve the pain.

Epiphysitis

This occurs at the distal humerus (little leaguer's elbow) and is caused by repeated throwing in children. Throwing should be forbidden to prevent growth disturbance.

Olecranon impingement and coronoid impingement

These occur from repeated sudden extension (or flexion) of the elbow which causes the bony point to impact into the humerus. Inflammation is treated in the usual way but occasionally bony excision is needed. In javelin throwers especially, loose bodies form. They should be removed arthroscopically.

Tenosynovitis

Tenosynovitis around the wrist is extremely common in all sports which use wrist action. A sports-specific tenosynovitis is found in rowers and canoeists who develop the condition in the extensor pollicis brevis and abductor pollicis longus tendons. Rapid relief is achieved following surgical decompression.

Skier's thumb

Rupture of the ulnar collateral ligament of the thumb results from hyperextension when the thumb is caught in the straps of the ski pole or the holes of an artificial ski slope. This injury should be explored surgically and sutured as necessary.

Bibliography

MATSEN, F. A., WINGUIST, R. A. & KRUGMIRE, R. B. (1980). Diagnosis and management of compartment syndromes. *J. Bone Joint Surg.*, **62A**, 286.

NOBLE, C. A. (1980). Illio-tibial band friction syndrome in runners. *Amer. J. Sports Med.*, **8**, 232.

WILLIAMS, J. G. P. (1971). Aetiological classification of injuries in sportsmen. *Brit. J. Sports Med.*, **5**, 228.

WILLIAMS, J. G. P. & SPERRYN, P. N. (1976). *Achilles Tendon Lesions in Sports Injuries*, p. 475. London: Arnold.

WOLFF, J. (1982). *Das Gesetz der Transformation de Knocken*. Berlin: Hitschwald.

33 Special trauma cases

T. D. BELL and B. L. ENDERSON (A: Paediatric trauma)

P. NASH (B: Trauma in pregnancy)

G. HUGHES (C: Trauma in the elderly)

P. NASH (D: Rape, sexual assault and female genital injuries)

Chapter plan

A: Paediatric trauma

Introduction
Incidence and consequence
Prevention
'Not just little adults'
Triage, trauma team and transport
Management of minor injuries
Management of serious injuries
Organ system injuries
Summary

B: Trauma in pregnancy

Introduction
Causes of trauma in pregnancy
The effects of anatomical changes of pregnancy on the response to trauma
The effects of physiological changes of pregnancy on the response to trauma
Assessment of the mother
Assessment of the fetus
Blunt trauma
Penetrating trauma
Burns
Surgical intervention in trauma in pregnancy

C: Trauma in the elderly

Introduction
Epidemiology
Spectrum of injury
Specific injury patterns
Age-related complications and their prevention in the A&E department
Intercurrent drugs
Metabolism
Nutrition
Circulatory insufficiency
Respiratory insufficiency
Anaesthetic problems
Ethical aspects

D: Rape, sexual assault and female genital injuries

Rape and sexual assault
Genital trauma

A: Paediatric trauma

T.D. BELL and B.L. ENDERSON

Department of Surgery, University of Tennessee Memorial Hospital, Knoxville, Tennessee, USA

INTRODUCTION

Caring for traumatic injury in the child is a particularly poignant experience. Juggling the need for objective assessment with the need to be sensitive to the child can be difficult, especially since the child is likely to have additional pain during the course of his examination and treatment. Unfortunately, trauma is the leading cause of paediatric mortality in the industrialized world, responsible in some countries for 40% or more of deaths in children under 15 years of age. It far outweighs any other cause of death in children.

INCIDENCE AND CONSEQUENCE

In the USA there are approximately 19.3 traumatic deaths per 100 000 children (Waller *et al.*, 1989); rates

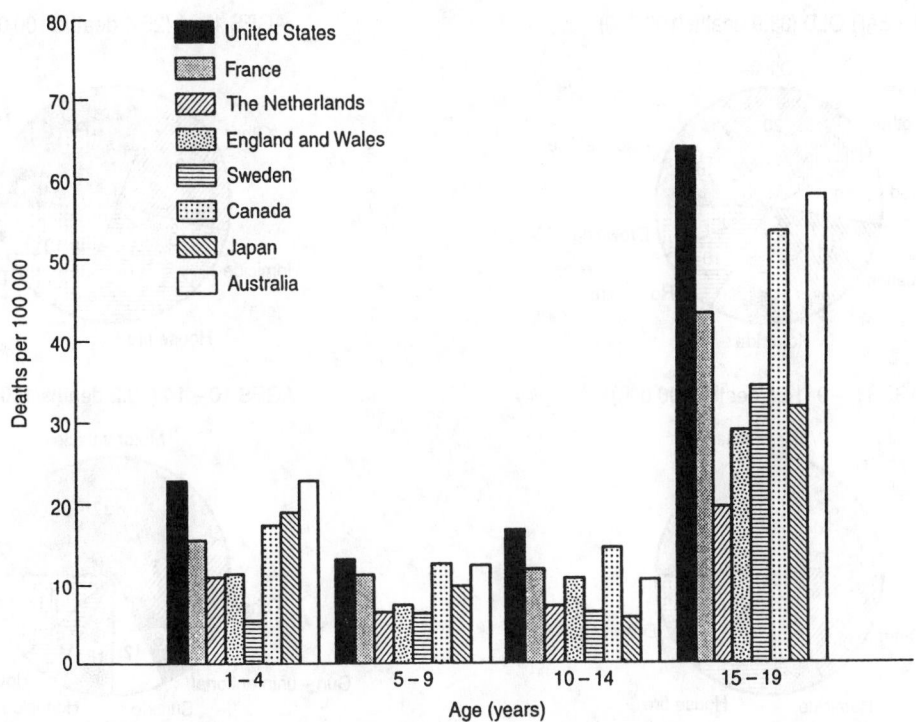

Fig. 1. International death rates from injuries and violence, 1985. (Reprinted, with permission, from Centers for Disease Control (1990). Childhood injuries in the United States. *Am. J. Dis. Child.*, **144**, 627–46.)

are somewhat lower in other industrialized countries (Fig. 1) (Division of Injury Control, Centers for Disease Control, 1990). In 1985, emergency department visits by children were most frequently associated with falls (3.6 million), followed by sports injuries (2.6 million) and motor vehicle related injuries (1.1 million); the leading cause of death, however, in 0–15-year-olds was motor vehicles (31%), followed by drownings (13%) and burns (12.5%) (Guyer & Ellers, 1990). Motor vehicle crashes are responsible for 7.2 deaths per 100 000 children, while drownings cause 2.8/100 000, pedestrian injuries 2.4/100 000, fires 2.3/100 000, and homicide (mostly child abuse) 1.9/100 000 (Waller *et al.*, 1989). The rate for each type of injury changes with different age ranges. The rate of drowning deaths in under 5-year-olds (5.2/100 000) is twice that of 5–10-year-olds or 11–14-year-olds, with similar hospitalization rates (Wintemute, 1990). Pedestrian injury death rates are almost twice as high in both under 5-year-olds and 5–10-year-olds than they are in 11–14-year-olds, even though the hospitalization rate is highest (by a factor of two) in the 5–9-year-olds. Fire deaths (burns and smoke inhalation) at 5.2/100 000 in under 5-year-olds, are two times the rate for older children, but the hospitalization rate is nearly four times that of older children (Centers for Disease Control, 1990)

(Fig. 2). These rates are a reflection of the activities a child is likely to engage in at different ages, the child's physiological adaptability to injury, and the types of injury he is likely to sustain (i.e. fall with isolated extremity injury versus cyclist struck by a car causing multisystem injury). Peak hours for injury are in the afternoon and evening when children are out of school and not yet home for the night.

Mortality differs by mechanism, location and severity of injury, as well as by age and sex. In one study (Peclet *et al.*, 1990a), motor vehicle crashes caused 28.5% of admissions, with 9.7% being motor vehicle occupants (mortality rate of 4.4%) and 18.8% being struck by a motor vehicle (mortality rate of 2.8%). Child abuse cases were only 2.2% of admissions but accounted for 20% of deaths in the series because the mortality rate was 15.8%. Conversely, motor vehicle crashes were the most frequent cause of deaths – even though mortality rates were low – because the number of motor vehicle crashes was high.

As expected, mortality rates also vary according to the severity of injury. For instance, closed head injury (CHI) is very common, present in 70–80% of injured children admitted to hospital (Pascucci, 1988). Most are due to falls, resulting in 82% mild CHI, 14% moderate to severe CHI and 5% overall mortality (Krause *et al.*, 1990).

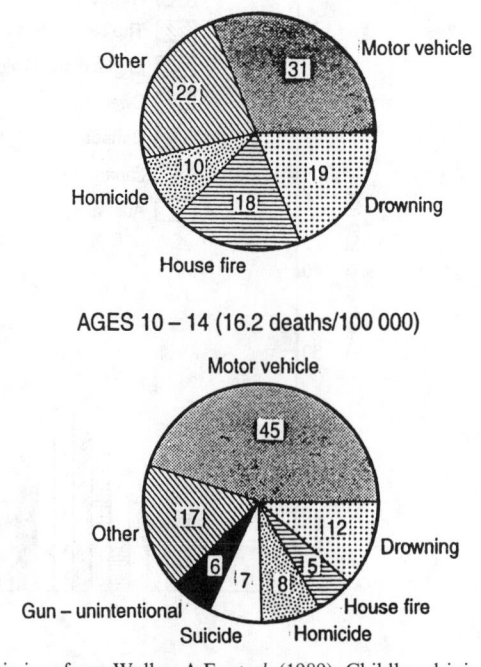

Fig. 2. Childhood injury deaths by cause, USA, 1980–1985. (Reprinted, with permission, from Waller, A.E. *et al.* (1989). Childhood injury deaths: national analysis and geographic variations, *Amer. J. Public Health*, **79**, 311. Copyright American Public Health Association.)

Another study showed a severe CHI (Glasgow Coma Scale <8) rate of 5.6% with overall mortality 2.5% (Luerssen *et al.*, 1988). Looking only at the population of children with severe CHI, however, reveals a 30% mortality (Luerssen *et al.*, 1988; Berger *et al.*, 1985). It is also worth noting that, of children who die after trauma, 75–90% will have a CHI as the primary cause of death (Breaux *et al.*, 1990; Chan *et al.*, 1989; Barlow *et al.*, 1983; Fischer *et al.*, 1988), which is only true for 38–48% of adults (Shackford *et al.*, 1989; Fischer *et al.*, 1988). Abdominal injury causes about 15% of childhood injury deaths (Breaux *et al.*, 1990; Fischer *et al.*, 1988). In large studies, the overall mortality rate in adults hospitalized for trauma is 6.6% (Shackford *et al.*, 1989), while for children it is 2.4% (Peclet *et al.*, 1990a). The rate of death from CHI is 10.4% in adults, 2.5% in children. Adult mortality rate for severe CHI is greater than 45% (Luerssen *et al.*, 1988). Multiple studies have shown that survival is poorest in cases of an abused child 2 years of age or less (Michaud *et al.*, 1992; Waller *et al.*, 1989; Peclet *et al.*, 1990a); they have less mass absorbing the force of a blow and are physiologically less compensated on arrival. Finally, multiple studies have shown both the injury and the death rates for boys to be twice that for girls.

Although childhood death rates due to trauma are alarming, the resulting disability and the economic losses are equally staggering. Trauma is second only to infection as a cause of childhood morbidity. In a study of 34 multiply injured children, over one-third had residual abnormalities when examined an average of 2.4 years after discharge (Klein & Marcus, 1986). A study of children surviving severe CHI (GCS <8) found only 33% with good recovery, though another 19% were functional (Berger *et al.*, 1985). Another study looking specifically at predictors of good or moderate recovery found that a 72-h postinjury score of 4–6 on the motor component of the GCS correlated well, as did an arterial Po_2 of 350 mmHg or more in the emergency department (Michaud *et al.*, 1992). Even in cases of isolated mild CHI or multiple injury without CHI, there are frequently behavioural disturbances resulting in dysfunction and/or use of special school programmes (Michaud *et al.*, 1993; Basson *et al.*, 1991). The effects of childhood trauma can be devastating to families; marital discord increases, the financial burden is significant and siblings are at risk of developing behavioural problems (Harris *et al.* 1989). Economic losses are difficult to estimate since the hospital bill is just the tip of the iceberg. The loss of future earning potential due to fatalities amounts to billions of dollars.

Falls – which have a very low mortality – cause $810 million a year in direct and indirect costs due to the high number of occurrences resulting in emergency department visits and hospitalizations (CDC, 1990). Economic losses are compounded by parents leaving work temporarily or permanently to care for the child.

PREVENTION

Improvement in childhood mortality has been seen with the development of paediatric trauma systems and paediatric intensive care units. However, improving the delivery and effectiveness of trauma care to injured children is not enough. As discussed above, these children do not return to their preinjury status. The dictum from the American College of Surgeons is 'trauma is no accident'. Paediatric trauma events are indeed highly predictable and should be amenable to preventive measures.

Prevention of childhood injury has three arms:

1. Improvement of product design.
2. Regulation of product use and enforcement of these regulations.
3. Education of parents and children about risks and risk-control measure including 1 and 2.

Improved product measures include seat belts and airbags in cars, window bars in apartments above the second story (Barlow et al., 1983) and fencing directly around pools and other bodies of water (Wintemute, 1990). Regulatory changes include enforcement of laws for the above measures, as well as against drunk driving and for helmet use when engaging in sport and recreational activities. Education consists of both public education campaigns and use of every interaction between healthcare providers and the public to reinforce safety issues. These measures can be very effective. The 'Children Can't Fly' programme in New York City, consisting of public education and an ordinance requiring window bars, dramatically reduced the hospital admissions for falls (Barlow et al., 1983). A campaign in Seattle, Washington, has increased bicycle helmet use in school-age children from 5% to 38% (Diguiseppi et al., 1989).

'NOT JUST LITTLE ADULTS'

There are several important differences between adults and children which make it essential that paediatric trauma patients be managed by trauma care providers familiar with children. The most obvious difference is the smaller size of the child, but there are many other structural differences of more significance. Differences in metabolism and psychology related to the normal growth and development of a child also have an impact on injury response and treatment.

Structure

Differences in structure mean differences in both patterns of injury and the mechanics of caring for injured children when compared to adults. The wide range of sizes in paediatric patients requires that a wide range of sizes in catheters, endotracheal tubes, intravenous catheters and immobilization devices be immediately available (Table 5). Appropriate sizes can usually be estimated based on the child's age and/or approximate weight, and multiple formulae have been developed to aid in these estimations. One particularly useful device is the Broselow Pediatric Resuscitation Tape. It is printed on one side with length-based average weight as well as size recommendations for endotracheal tubes, nasogastric and urinary catheters, and laryngoscope blades. The other side has weight-based drug dosages. Any estimations may need modifications for individual variations.

Although the child's *head* is smaller than an adult's, in relation to the rest of his body a child's head is large and heavy. This makes it very susceptible to trauma since there is relatively more of it. The head is often the first point of impact – arresting the flight of a child in motion – especially in falls, motor vehicle crashes and recreational injuries. There is a theoretical advantage for infants in whom the cranial sutures have not yet closed because they will not have the build-up of intracranial pressure, but mortality data in traumatic brain injury actually shows the highest death rate in children less than 2 years of age (Luerssen et al., 1988; Michaud et al., 1992). This may be a reflection of injury mechanisms rather than an indicator of physiological tolerance.

The relatively large weight of the head also contributes to the vulnerability of the paediatric *cervical spine* to injury as the cervical spine tethers the head to the body. Additionally, the neck muscles are weak, the ligaments are lax and the bones are immature in both strength and architecture (Bonadio, 1993a). This contributes to an injury seen more commonly in children than in adults, in which cervical cord injuries are sustained without any cervical spine fractures. Fortunately, cervical cord and spine injuries are not common in children who arrive alive in the emergency department; the incidence of cervical spine injury taken from the trauma registry at our level I trauma centre over a 5-year period is 1.2% (13/118) in children under 16 years versus 4.4% (377/8653) in adults.

Until late childhood the *airway* of the paediatric patient is significantly different from the adult airway. The tongue is relatively larger and more likely to obstruct the airway of a supine patient by falling backwards into the oropharynx. The epiglottis viewed end-on is markedly curved. In tends to 'flop' posteriorly into the pharynx; this is due to the softness of the cartilage and to the short distance between the thyroid cartilage and hyoid bone, resulting in less soft tissue tension to hold the epiglottis erect. The larynx is relatively shorter, and lies more anterior and more cephalad than in adults. In the newborn, the larynx from glottic opening to inferior border of the cricoid ring spans the length of one cervical vertebral body, with the glottis at the C3/4 interspace. In the adult the larynx spans the length of just over two vertebral bodies, with the glottis at the bottom of C4. The cricoid ring is the narrowest part of the airway of a child up until about 8 years of age, unlike the adult where the glottic opening is the narrow point. Fig. 3 demonstrates these differences. In addition, the infant or young child has a very soft and compliant airway which can be occluded by flexion or extension of the neck (an action to be avoided in the trauma victim with a potential cervical spine injury). The cricoid ring is the primary point of support in these small airways and is easily injured during emergency cricothyroidotomy. Long-term airway complications due to iatrogenic cricoid injury can be severe and cricothyroidotomy should not be performed in children less than 8 years of age. The carina is at T4 in adulthood but in the infant it is only at T2, increasing the risk of mainstem bronchus intubation. Finally, the mucosa and submucosal soft tissues below the glottis are loose and subject to oedema. This is a concern with direct or inhalational airway injury or with resuscitation since a small amount of oedema in paediatric air passages has much more impact on resistance to air flow (due to

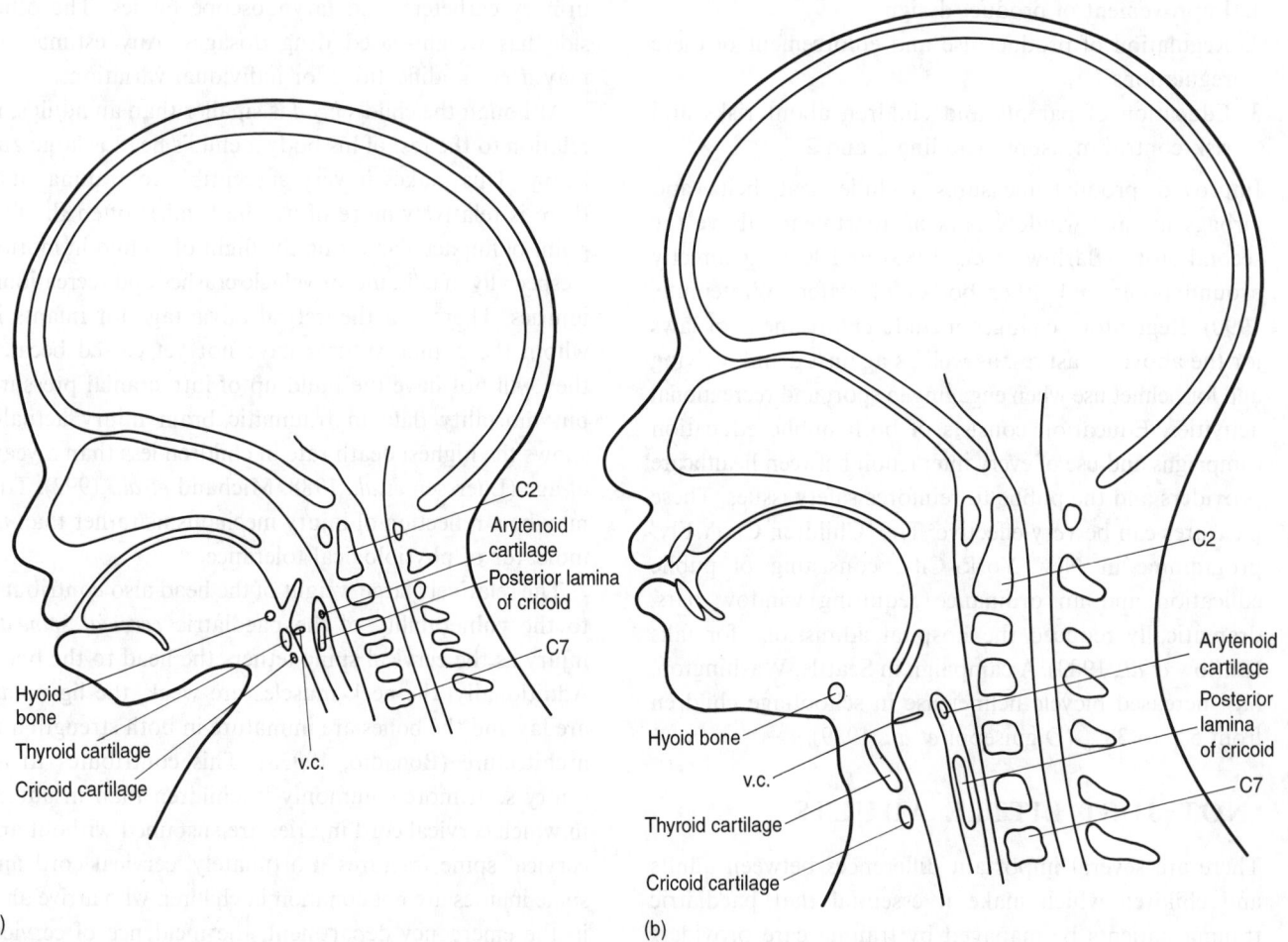

(a)   (b)

Fig. 3. The larynx in a newborn (a) and adult (b). Note the cephalad placement and short length of the newborn larynx in comparison to the adult. Note also the angulation of the posterior lamina of the cricoid cartilage in the neonate and the narrowness of the airway at the level of the cricoid. v.c., vocal cords (glottic opening); C2, second cervical vertebral body; C7, seventh cervical vertebral body.

decreased airway cross-sectional area) than oedema in the large adult air passages.

The *thorax* in children is also different. Like other bones the ribs are porous and relatively compliant, with a large cartilaginous component. Both of these facts contribute to the marked flexibility of the paediatric rib cage. As a result, rib fractures in children are less frequent than in adults. Pulmonary or cardiac contusions can occur without rib fractures and must therefore be suspected in any child with chest wall contusions or abrasions or with a significant mechanism of injury (i.e. a motor vehicle occupant striking the dashboard or a pedestrian struck by a motor vehicle). Although significant chest injury is not common in children it contributes significantly to mortality; in one series the mortality rate in injured children with a thoracic component was 26% vs 1.5% in those without chest injury (Peclet *et al.*, 1990b). Chest injury also greatly increases the mortality rate for paediatric patients with head injury (Michaud *et al.*, 1992). Children with thoracic injury are much more likely to have multisystem injury (69–97%, most commonly a CHI; Peclet *et al.*, 1990b; Nakayama *et al.*, 1989; Roux & Fischer, 1992) which contributes to mortality. Chest trauma is the only area where paediatric mortality is probably greater than adult mortality (Eichelberger, 1993) due to the facts that the soft tissues absorb the force and multisystem injury is common.

Other differences exist in the paediatric chest in infants and young children. The heart makes up a greater percentage of the anterior chest contents than in adults. The lungs are small and immature; few alveoli are mature at birth and alveoli continue to develop in form and number until the child reaches 8 years of age, with the greatest increase in numbers from birth to 3 years. This means that a young child has less pulmonary reserve than an older child or young adult. The mediastinum in a child is more mobile than in an adult. Therefore, even though pneumothorax is relatively uncommon in children (only 33% of children with blunt trauma injuries to the chest; Roux & Fisher, 1992), if the child develops a tension pneumothorax the circulatory effects can rapidly be profound as the inferior vena cava (two-thirds of normal venous return) is essentially pinched off by angulation at the diaphragm. This can occur even if intrathoracic pressure by itself is not high enough to significantly impair blood return.

Organs in the child's *abdomen* are structurally at increased risk of injury. The rib case is not only softer than in an adult but covers less of the abdominal cavity and flanks, leaving upper abdominal viscera and kidneys vulnerable. The spleen and liver are at additional risk because they are large in relation to the size of the child. The kidneys are also relatively larger than in adults, lie more anteriorly and in less perinephric fat. Therefore, they are susceptible to blows from the front as well as from the back or side of the child. Not surprisingly, the liver is the most commonly injured intra-abdominal organ followed by the spleen and the kidneys. In addition to relatively larger solid organs, the child's abdominal wall is thinner with less subcutaneous tissue and less well-developed musculature, affording less protection to abdominal contents. Due to the shape of the pelvis, young children do not have a true pelvic cavity and the bladder and female reproductive organs are essentially intra-abdominal.

Intra-abdominal injury has been noted in 4.1–5.7% of all children admitted with blunt trauma (Fischer *et al.*, 1988; Peclet & Murphy, 1993) and in 33% of 'seriously' injured children (injury severity score > 16) (Chan *et al.*, 1989). Paediatric trauma deaths in these series are overwhelmingly associated with severe head injury; however, a significant number of *preventable* deaths are from missed intra-abdominal injury (Dykes *et al.*, 1989; McKoy & Bell, 1983). Although overall mortality from childhood injury is 2.4% (Peclet *et al.*, 1990a), the mortality rate in children with abdominal injury is given at 14% (Peclet & Murphy, 1993). Abdominal examination in a frightened, uncooperative or obtunded child is difficult, but the mortality data associated with abdominal injury make it clear that aggressive evaluation of the abdomen in the injured child is imperative.

The *bones* of children are relatively soft and compliant, both weaker and more resilient than mature bone. This is due to the porosity of the cortex, a high cartilage content (including growth plates) and a thicker periosteum. Additionally, children have strong ligamentous tissue, such that the strength of the ligaments is greater than that of the bone, which is greater than that of the physes. This means that children are prone to fractures at the growth plates and that joint dislocations are rare without concomitant fracture. Children are also prone to greenstick and buckle fractures, which are unusual in adults. Fractures and dislocations in children are dealt with more fully in Chapter 29.

Physiology

As a general rule children tolerate severe degrees of injury better than do adults (with limitations). This is most remarkable in the cardiovascular system but is true also of the central nervous system and kidneys.

The infant *heart* has marked microstructural and physiological differences in comparison to the heart of an adult or even a 5-year-old child. Contractile proteins make up only 30% of myocardial cell volume (as opposed to 60% in adults) and are more disorganized in arrangement. This results in less ventricular compliance and relative inability of the infant heart to alter stroke volumes in response to hypovolaemia; cardiac output is essentially heart rate dependent. Sympathetic innervation is also immature, with parasympathetic innervation being more completely developed. As a result the infant has poor ability to peripherally vasoconstrict in response to volume losses, and may actually become bradycardic in response to stress-induced high autonomic output, due to the relative dominance of the parasympathetic system (see Ludwig & Liselle, 1993, for additional discussion). Therefore, a pink infant with a history or suspicion of trauma and heart rate of 100 (normal 110–170) must be assumed to be hypovolaemic and offered a volume challenge, especially if the infant is exhibiting any signs of cerebral compromise. The relative non-compliance of the ventricle in an infant means that the ventricle is less tolerant of excessive preload. Consequently, the immature heart is very sensitive to volume overload and can be pushed into failure without much effort. Because of this, care of an injured or otherwise potentially hypovolaemic infant or small child mandates use of volumetric intravenous fluid tubing which should never contain more than 20 ml of fluid per kg of the child's weight in the reservoir.

By the time a child is 5 years old, the cardiovascular system is essentially more mature although resting heart rate remains high, decreasing through adolescence. The older child has tremendous physiological reserve and can compensate for hypoxia by increasing cardiac output with an increase in stroke volume and only a slight increase in heart rate, or for hypovolaemia with intense vasoconstriction and slight to moderate increase in heart rate. Because of this reserve, children's vital signs do not show evidence of haemodynamic decompensation until dangerously late in the course of their deterioration. A more sensitive measure of compromise is frequently repeated evaluation of perfusion by physical examination. Although less precise, indicators such as mental status (cerebral perfusion), skin colour, turgor and temperature, pulse quality and capillary refill (peripheral perfusion), and urinary output (renal perfusion) are better monitors of volume status. Haemodynamic decompensation or

cardiac arrest due to hypovolaemia in a traumatized child is a grave prognostic indicator.

Immature *renal* function is manifested as inability to concentrate urine. As a result, especially in infants, some urinary output will continue even in the face of pronounced degrees of hypovolaemia. Volume resuscitation should continue until normal amounts of urine are produced. Urinary output should be maintained at $2\,\mathrm{ml\,kg^{-1}\,h^{-1}}$ in the infant and $1\,\mathrm{ml\,kg^{-1}\,h^{-1}}$ in the child.

The paediatric *brain* is less tolerant of injury than other paediatric organs but seems to be much more so than the adult brain. This is especially true in children less than 10 years old, approximately half of whom exhibit good functional recoveries after severe head injury (Berger *et al.*, 1985). As shown in Fig. 4, in children between 2 and 15 years of age the mortality also is markedly less than it is in adults (Luerssen *et al.*, 1988; Michaud *et al.*, 1992). This is a consequence of the plasticity of the very young nervous system, of both its ability to learn and the ability of uninjured neural tissue to assume some of the roles of dead or injured cells. This plasticity diminishes with age. There is growing evidence, however, that even though there is usually full functional recovery after head injury, these children are at a much increased risk of severe behavioural disturbances, especially if they are injured in the preschool years (Michaud *et al.*, 1993). If injured when less than 2 years of age, not only does the mortality for head injury in children approach that for adults (Luerssen *et al.*, 1988) but intelligence quotient testing shows a 17–20 point drop in children who had any head injury for which medical

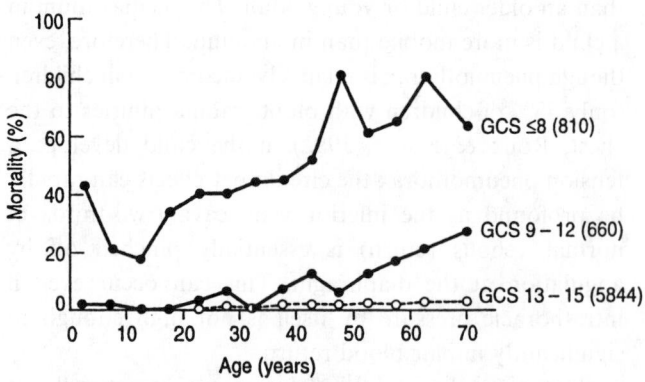

Fig. 4. Mortality, by age and Glasgow Coma Scale (GCS) score on admission. (Reprinted, with permission, from Luerssen, T.G. *et al.* (1988). Outcome from head injury related to patient's age. *J. Neurosurg.*, **68**, 409–16.)

treatment was sought (Michaud et al., 1993). So even though children tolerate head injuries better than adults there are definite sequelae.

In children with severe head injuries who do die there is a high correlation with increased intracranial pressure (ICP) (Magnuson & Maier, 1993; Ghajar & Hariri, 1992; Muizelaar et al., 1989a). This increase in ICP can result from an increase in volume of any of the contents of the cranium – brain, blood, CSF (cerebrospinal fluid) or a combination. The addition of other components – intra-cerebral, subdural or extradural haematoma – to the intracranial space will also increase ICP. More than adults (Muizelaar et al., 1989a), children with severe head injuries are likely to develop a reactive cerebral hyper-aemia 24 h postinjury (Ghajar & Hariri, 1992; Bruce et al., 1981), which correlates well with a lower GCS. The above study (Muizelaar et al., 1989a) shows that after 24 h there was an uncoupling of cerebral blood flow and cerebral oxygen consumption such that, in the hyper-aemic, high-flow state, oxygen consumption was low. A related study showed that cerebrovascular autoregula-tion was intact 59% of the time in severely head injured children, only failing when cerebral blood flow was greatly increased or decreased (>2 standard deviations from normal); when blood pressure was low cerebral vessels dilated, increasing cerebral blood volume and increasing ICP (Muizelaar et al., 1989b). Studies have shown that patients whose intracranial hypertension can be controlled have better survival rates and no increase in the rates of vegetative outcome (Marshall et al., 1979; Kumar et al., 1991). This indicates that aggressive measures to control ICP by decreasing the volume of intracranial contents is worthwhile. The aim of these measures is to prevent secondary brain injury due to conversion of injured and dysfunctional but potentially viable neurones to dead neurones by further insult from oedema and/or hypoxia.

First and foremost the child must have good mean arterial pressure and oxygenation to maintain adequate perfusion and prevent cerebral hypoxia; hypotension and prolonged resuscitation have been shown to have a very bad influence on head injury outcome (Marshall et al., 1979; Luerssen et al., 1988). In the presence of intact autoregulation, good blood pressure acts to decrease cerebral blood volume by vasoconstriction. Keeping the patient's P_{CO_2} at 25–30 mmHg does the same, but patients whose P_{CO_2} is kept below 25 mmHg run the risk of cerebral ischaemia from excessive vasoconstriction. Brain volume can also be reduced by minimizing oedema and haemorrhage into cerebral contusions. Large hae-matomas obviously need to be promptly evaluated for evacuation by a neurosurgeon.

Psychosocial development

In addition to structural and physiological differences, children have unique developmental and psychosocial vulnerabilities. The developmental stage of the child has an impact on both the type of trauma sustained and the optimum approach to care in the emergency room (Table 1).

The child 0–1 year old is almost completely dependent. He is a receiver of trauma either by abuse or neglect. In the emergency room this child needs comforting, sooth-ing and pain control.

Between 1 and 3 years of age the child is learning to distinguish self from others. Between 9 months and 2 years separation anxiety is paramount and having a parent and/or 'security object' (the child's favourite blanket or teddy bear) present early or continuously can ease fears. Two-year-olds go through a period of defiant individuation ('terrible two's') that can actually contribute to caregiver-inflicted trauma, but they still benefit from a comforting presence. There are occasions when a parent is unable to be comforting in a post-traumatic situation, in which case it may be wise to delay their access to the child. Throughout the toddler years injuries stem primarily from exploration: poisonings, burns, drownings and falls, with a certain incidence of child abuse. Although their verbal skills are poor, receptive language ability is quite good. They will benefit from verbal reassurance and explanations even if they cannot respond in kind.

The 3–6-year-old child has a grasp of permanence and can therefore tolerate separations, but thinking is con-crete and egocentric and ability to judge danger is poor. These children continue to explore and begin to imitate the behaviour of adults. In addition to injuries that 1–3-year-olds are subject to, 3–6-year-olds are prone to 'tool-using' injuries such as lawnmower injuries and bicycle spills. Imitative behaviour can be used to facilitate medical care, as in wearing an oxygen mask 'like a fighter pilot' or 'an astronaut', or getting a cast applied 'like Uncle Jack'. Because they are egocentric they may perceive the trauma and the additional assault of medical care as punishment. Frequency reassurances as well as explanations of medical examinations and the need for them (before they are done!) can be used in alleviating some of the child's anxiety. Explanations should be kept very basic in accordance with the concrete thinking of this age group. Pain control remains important.

Table 1. *Effects of growth and development on aetiology and management of injury* (Ludwig & Loiselle, 1993)

Age (years)	Period	Trauma type	Communication pattern	Management concepts
Birth–1	Dependency	Abuse Neglect MVC – passenger	Tactile Preverbal	Meet needs
1–2	Individuation	Exploration injury Abuse	Receptive language good Expression language poor	Use parental contact
2–4	Imitative	MVC – pedestrian Fires Falls	Expressive language excellent Fantasy life rich	Use fantasy and make-believe
5–9	Competence	MVC – pedestrian Sports injury	Mature language Understanding of concepts, including death	Describe mechanics Project outcome
10–14	Peer-oriented	MVC – pedestrian, passenger Inflicted trauma Suicide	Mature language 'Slang'	Use adult communication Childlike reassurance
15–19	Young adult	MVC – driver, passenger Inflicted trauma Suicide	'Adult' interaction	Use informed consent Decision-making

MVC, motor vehicle crash.

The school-age child is approaching adult mentation and coping skills. The *6–10-year-old* child has reasonable motor competence and has become aware of his vulnerability. This age group in fact has the lowest incidence of traumatic events (Peclet *et al.*, 1990a; Gallager *et al.*, 1984). They are most commonly pedestrian or bicycling victims who are struck by motor vehicles after school. Because of their relatively mature information-processing ability they do well with explanations of injury, disease and treatments needed. They also do well if allowed to control some aspects of their treatment and if recognition for their ability to handle pain and stress is expressed. Because they are aware of vulnerability and have active imaginations, early reassurance on the subject of death and loss of body parts is important; even a very brief explanation and reassurance given on the way to radiology or the operating room is worthwhile.

Young *adolescents* focus primarily on peer groups and assertion of independence, and seem to lose any sense of vulnerability. This results in risk-taking behaviour. In addition, this age group starts experimenting with alcohol and drugs and spends more time in adolescent-driven automobiles. The incidence of motor vehicle crashes – and in the USA homicides and suicides – goes way up, as does the mortality rate (CDC, 1990; Peclet *et al.*, 1990a). Because of their preoccupation with autonomy and their emotional immaturity, young adolescents are frequently hostile and uncooperative in the emergency department even though they are cognitively capable of understanding what is going on. They need communication at an adult level with reassurances offered as for a younger child, including reassurances about peer-group acceptability. The physician needs to be alert for possible self-inflicted injuries in this age group. Modesty is an important issue at all the school ages as gender identification is firmly in place.

As is true for adults, at times of stress or injury all children have a tendency to regress and may behave in ways consistent with earlier developmental stages. This is normal and will usually resolve as the injury resolves but can be disconcerting or even alarming to parents and other caretakers. Parents themselves have differing and unpredictable reactions to their child's trauma which can impair the child's full recovery (Walsh, 1993). Severe head injuries are well-recognized as highly correlated with behavioural changes such as increased aggressiveness, irritability and poor control, hyperactivity and social withdrawal. There is now evidence that milder degrees of head trauma may also predispose to behavioural problems (Michaud *et al.*, 1993), as may trauma without any head injury (Basson *et al.*, 1991). These changes can persist for months or years.

There is no question that major trauma is economically devastating to society (Michaud *et al.*, 1993; CDC, 1990).

Table 2. *Paediatric Trauma Score (PTS) and mortality data*

A. Paediatric Trauma Score (PTS)

Component	Component score		
	+2	+1	−1
Size (kg)	>20	10–20	<10
Airway	Normal	Maintainable	Unmaintainable
Systolic blood pressure (mmHg)	>90	50–90	<50
If no BP cuff, pulse palpable at:	Wrist	Groin	None
Central nervous system	Awake	Obtunded/unconscious	Comatose
Open wounds	None	Minor	Major/penetrating
Fractures	None	Single closed	Open or multiple

B. Mortality data (13,162) patients

PTS	< −2	−1 to 2	1–2	3–4	5–6	7–8	9–10	11–12
Mortality	96.6%	70.9%	39.3%	28.1%	11.7%	0.9%	0.1%	0.0%
Distribution	0.21%	0.8%	1.45%	2.54%	5.45%	14.6%	30.6%	44.3%

Score is assessed by assigning the patient +2, +1 or −1 for each of the six components, then adding the numbers. PTS can thus range from −6 to 12. Mortality data are from the National Pediatric Trauma Registry based on PTS. (Reprinted, with permission from Ramenofsky, M.I. (1993) Early Assessment and Management of Trauma. In *Pediatric Surgery*, ed. K.W. Ashcraft & T.M. Holder, p. 112. W.B. Saunders.).

It can also be devastating to the family both economically and functionally. A final risk to be aware of is creation of a 'vulnerable child syndrome' in which a child who has returned to good health remains overprotected (Walsh, 1993). Education of parents and/or other caretakers about these issues prior to the child's discharge from the emergency department or the hospital should be undertaken to minimize dysfunction in the child, the family and the school. Families should be encouraged to seek out and take advantage of community resources if appropriate. They should be advised to seek assessment and counselling early if behavioural problems emerge, before maladaptive patterns become ingrained.

TRIAGE, TRAUMA TEAM AND TRANSPORT

The need to rapidly assess the severity of a child's injury in terms of mortality risk is apparent. Injury severity plays a major role in decision-making about the speed, location and type of interventions performed. Multiple scoring systems have been proposed: the injury severity score (ISS); the trauma score/ISS (TRISS) (Chan *et al.*, 1989; Eichelberger *et al.*, 1988); modified ISS (MISS) (Mayer *et al.*, 1980, 1984) and the paediatric trauma score (PTS) (Tepas *et al.*, 1987, 1988). Most of these scoring systems, though good predictors of mortality, are too unwieldy to be used for triage. The PTS, however, is quickly and easily done and highly correlated to ISS and mortality risk. The marked increase in mortality risk for the very small child and the child who has progressed to the point of circulatory collapse is built into the score, as is the absolute priority of maintaining an airway (Table 2). The survival of patients with a PTS of 9–12 is nearly 100%, while the survival of patients with a PTS of −2 to 0 is rare (Ramenofsky, 1993) and was initially thought to be 0% (Tepas *et al.*, 1988). Therefore it is possible to decide at the scene of injury if a child can be treated in a community centre or needs to go to a resource-intensive centre specializing in trauma care. Specialized paediatric trauma care centres will have the biggest impact on the population of patients with a PTS of 0–8, though those with a PTS of −2 to 0 may also benefit.

Centres that specialize in paediatric care need to have certain facilities and personnel immediately available. Since the majority of injured children are not severely injured and go home from the emergency department, it is not reasonable to expect all emergency departments to have these resources. Any facility which sees children, however, should ideally have written protocols to define serious injury and transfer criteria (Table 3), personnel

Table 3. *Criteria for activation of full trauma team response, or for transfer to a trauma centre*

I. Mechanism of trauma
  A. Falls from third floor or from 40 feet or more
  B. Motor vehicle crash occupant
    1. High-speed crash or significant (20 inches) vehicle deformity
    2. Vehicle rolled over
    3. Patient ejected
    4. Death of another vehicle occupant
  C. Pedestrian (or cyclist) struck by motor vehicle

II. Physiology
  A. Pediatric trauma score of 8 or less
  B. Unstable or deteriorating vital signs
  C. Compromise of airway, breathing, or circulation
  D. Severely compromised neurological status (GCS 8 or less)

III. Injuries
  A. Multiple system injury
  B. Open penetrating injury below subcutaneous tissue of neck, chest, abdomen, or groin
  C. Evidence of spinal cord injury
  D. Pelvic fracture with unstable pelvic ring
  E. Flail chest
  F. Complete or near-complete extremity amputation

GCS, Glasgow Coma Scale.

skilled in initial trauma management who can safely control the airway and establish intravenous access, and appropriately sized and designed equipment for children (Table 5).

A hospital centre for the care of the seriously injured child should have a designated team and immediate access to the radiology department, an operating room, paediatric intensive care and a designated and fully-stocked resuscitation room in the emergency department. Necessary personnel for an optimal paediatric trauma response are:

- Ambulance crews and emergency medical technicians who have some training in paediatric care and can communicate directly with the hospital.
- Immediately available hospital personnel, including physicians, nurses and radiographers who may respond on demand from other parts of the hospital.
- Readily accessible acute care specialists such as anaesthetists, orthopaedic surgeons and neuro-surgeons.

Team leadership – responsibility for overall care of the patient – alters as the child is transported from the scene of injury to the hospital and additional personnel become available, but for the seriously injured child should culminate in the attendance of a paediatric surgeon. The trauma team leader must be aware of the child's status at all times, directed care given by other team members and deciding which procedures, diagnostic tests or operations have the highest priority. The surgeon should be present from the start of emergency department assessment and resuscitation to facilitate immediately the necessary surgical procedures (venous cut-down, tracheotomy, chest tube, diagnostic peritoneal lavage, thoracotomy) and to provide coordination and continuity of care as the patient moves from the emergency department to other hospital areas, from acute care to critical care to routine care. All physician members of the trauma response team should have completed the Advanced Trauma Life Support (ATLS) Provider Course and nurse members should be familiar with ATLS principles.

Issues during transport of children are similar to those for adults. The first priority is assessment of the airway and control of both airway and breathing if needed. Intubation of an infant or small child should be part of the training of transport personnel. In the child with blunt injury, cervical spine immobilization must be maintained. In a child less than 8 years old this means using specialized collars which are smaller and relatively shorter. Due to the relatively greater size of a child's head, the standard spine board must be modified to prevent flexion of the cervical spine (Fig. 5). The external auditory meatus should line up with the shoulders (Herzenberg *et al.*, 1989). Circulation is less of a priority than airway and breathing. Obvious bleeding should be controlled by direct pressure on the bleeding site. Intravenous lines can be attempted en route. One must remember that vital signs in small children consist of a higher heart rate and lower systolic blood pressure than is acceptable in an adult; a heart rate of 80 in a toddler is bradycardia, and a systolic blood pressure of 80 is normal. If intravenous lines are established, volumetric tubing should be used since children can easily be volume overloaded. Obvious fractures should be immobilized to reduce both pain and blood loss into a fracture. Finally, if not precluded by other issues, parents should be allowed to ride in the ambulance with the child, especially a very young child. This and a gentle caring manner may help to minimize the psychological impact of the trauma experience on the young child.

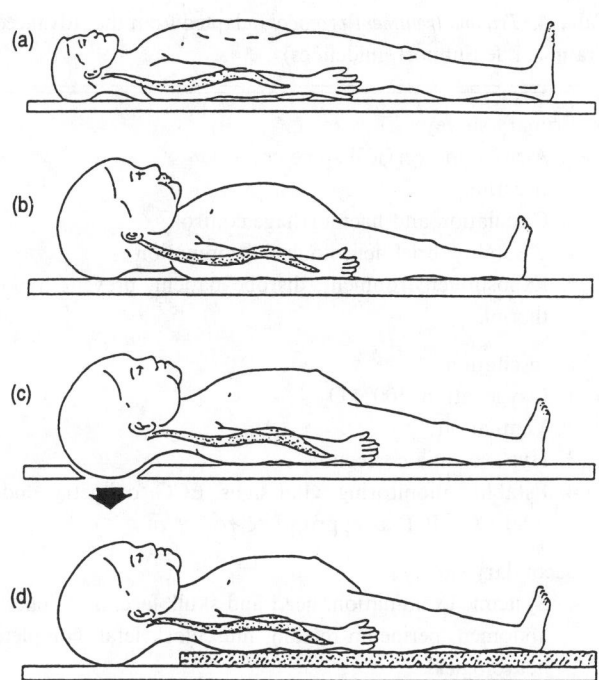

Fig. 5. Immobilization on backboard. (a) Adult. (b) Young child; note flexion at the cervical spine due to the large relative head size. (c & d) Backboard modifications for transport of young children allowing proper cervical spine alignment. (Reprinted, with permission, from Herzenberg, J.E. *et al.* (1989). Emergency transport and positioning of young children who have an injury of the cervical spine. *J. Bone Joint Surg.*, **71A**, 15–22.)

MANAGEMENT OF MINOR INJURIES

The majority of children presenting to the emergency department have minor injuries: contusions, lacerations or an isolated extremity fracture. These are the result of low-energy events such as blows, short falls or misuse of a sharp object. These patients can usually be treated and released if history and physical examination give no indication of serious injury. Careful judgement of congruency between injury and history is required to detect abuse or neglect. Parents should be educated about the expected course of recovery and any necessary follow-up. They need to be warned that children frequently regress to a previous developmental stage or become fearful and dependent after trauma, and may need additional nurturing. They should be encouraged to seek assistance early if the child manifests behaviour problems, especially after head injury.

Wound care is detailed in Chapter 12, but a few points relating to children will be made here. Caring for a child's wound means caring for the wound, the child and the

child's parent(s). The sight of blood is upsetting to both child and parent so, as soon as an initial assessment reveals stability, efforts should be made to clean up blood around the wound and in the treatment area. A calm and confident manner on the part of physician and nurse is reassuring to both patient and parent, as is direct verbal reassurance. Active bleeding can almost always be controlled by direct pressure over the wound with a gauze pad, which also removes a bloody wound from sight. A saline-soaked dressing should be applied to wounds that are not actively bleeding to prevent desiccation. A more thorough examination can now be done to assess neurovascular function distal to a wound and to evaluate the child for other injuries. Anaesthetics should not be infiltrated until after the neurological examination is completed. Assessment for nerve and tendon injury in a very young child can be difficult and the resting posture of the extremity or face should be examined. An older child can frequently be talked into cooperating if he is made a part of the examination rather than the object of it ('can you do this?' or 'show me this' rather than 'do this'). The time spent in this way can be used to build rapport with the child through eye contacts, verbal interactions and reassurances. The older child will often tolerate instillation of lignocaine if he understands that the increased pain will be brief and then most of the pain will go away. Very young children can occasionally be handled in the same way but usually will need to be restrained for local anaesthetic, wound exploration and wound repair. In this instance, consideration should be given to both sedation and to sending the parent to the waiting room until repair is complete. A child over 3 years of age is aware of body integrity, so a hurried and insensitive examination – especially of the genitoanal area – adds to the psychological damage of the original injury. An explanation of procedures and examinations is in order prior to performance. Consideration should be given to closing lacerations with subcuticular suture and/or tape strips to avoid later suture removal. The multiple small, shallow triangular lacerations from automobile glass are best closed with carefully applied benzoin and tape strips (Templeton, 1993b). Never shave an eyebrow to close a laceration as they don't always grow back. Abrasions should be thoroughly scrubbed to prevent 'tattooing' from embedded particles, and then treated like burns. Contusions and sprains can be treated with elevation and ice for 24 h, then gentle motion and warm soaks or heat. Tetanus prophylaxis or immunization must be given when indicated.

MANAGEMENT OF SERIOUS INJURIES

Management of a child who is potentially seriously injured follows the same guidelines as for adults, but one must keep in mind the structural and metabolic differences of children and their developmental stages in order to minimize the potential for iatrogenic injury. Obviously life-, limb- or organ-threatening injuries have first priority but treatment of the child as a whole cannot be neglected. In an alert child who has triggered a full trauma team response it may be appropriate to ask a team member to hold the child's hand, explain procedures and offer reassurance while the rest of the team proceeds with medical care.

The team leader must continuously reassess the patient to make sure all priority issues are receiving attention in appropriate order. This includes prevention of hypothermia, a potentially devastating problem to which children are particularly prone because of their high surface area/volume ratio. The child should be covered as much as possible with a warm blanket, all resuscitation fluids and inspired gases should be warmed and the latter humidified. Finally, the vast majority of injuries to children are due to blunt forces. This means that the energy is dissipated over a broad area, not confined to a missile track or stab wound. Multiple system injuries and injury complexes must be anticipated. In this section, the protocol for initial evaluation of a seriously injured child will be reviewed, followed by a discussion of injury to particular organ systems.

Initial assessment

The initial assessment is a continuous process of prioritization and treatment, not a rigid routine. The outline below is a hierarchy of priorities, not a timetable (Table 4). Many of these issues can and should be addressed simultaneously. If a patient deteriorates one should go back to the top of the list and reassess the airway, breathing and circulation.

Primary survey

The primary survey consists of the ABCs, plus D and E: Airway, Breathing, Circulation, Disability (brief neurological examination) and Exposure. The *airway* is the first priority: death from an obstructed airway occurs in 3–4 min, from hypovolemic shock in 10+ min (Ramenofsky, 1993). The alert child will usually maintain his own

Table 4. *Trauma treatment protocol* (adapted from the Advanced Trauma Life Support guidelines)

A. Primary survey
  1. Airway and cervical spine control
  2. Breathing
  3. Circulation and haemorrhage control
  4. Disability: brief neurological examination
  5. Exposure/environment: disrobe patient, prevent hypothermia

B. Resuscitation
  1. Oxygenation: 100% O_2
  2. Ventilation
  3. Hypovolemia correction
  4. Establish monitoring: vital signs, ECG, oximetry, end-tidal CO_2, ICP as appropriate

C. Secondary survey
  1. Systemic examination: head and skull, face, neck, chest, abdomen, perineum/rectum, musculoskeletal, complete neurological
  2. Diagnostic studies
  3. Treatment: temporizing or definitive

ECG, electrocardiography; ICP, intracranial pressure.

airway, at least initially. Airway maintenance in the obtunded child may be as simple as removing obstructing blood or vomitus, or performing a jaw thrust followed by a naso- or oropharyngeal airway to displace the relatively large tongue. Appropriate size airways should be used (Table 5). In a child less than 8 years of age, the oral airway should be inserted following the curve of the tongue to avoid lacerating the soft palate and pharynx. An awake child will tolerate a nasal but not an oral airway. If these measures do not secure the airway, tracheal intubation is indicated. Remember that the infant pharynx is small and soft, and the larynx is located relatively higher and more anterior than in the pre-adolescent or adult. Intubation of the very young child is accomplished by inserting the appropriate size straight laryngoscope blade perpendicularly into the mouth until the tip is at the uvula; the laryngoscope is then pushed directly towards the child's feet lifting slightly when the epiglottis is seen. This should bring the vocal cords into view. Nasotracheal tubes are difficult or impossible to place and are not indicated for trauma. An uncuffed endotracheal tube which passes very freely through the cords should be used in a child less than 8–10 years old; the cricoid ring will give a sufficiently snug seal and absence of a cuff means a larger diameter endotracheal

Table 5. Guidelines for paediatric vital signs and equipment in acute trauma care

	Estimation guidelines	Premature	Newborn	6 months	12 months	18 months	3 years	5 years	8 years	12 years	15 years
Weight (kg)	2 (age in years) + 8	3	3.5	7	10	11	15	18	25	35	50
Vitals											
HR[a]		120–170	110–170		100–160			80–130			
SBP[a]	2 (age) + 70	>70	>70		>80			>90		>90	<90
RR[a]		<50	<50	<40	<40			<30		<20	<20
Hb/Hc[b]		14.5/45	16.5/51	12.36/36		12.0/36	12.5/37		13.5/40		14/40 m 14.5/43 f
Airway[c]											
Cervical collar size		Sandbags, rolled towel[d]	Sandbags, rolled towel	Sm	Sm	Sm	Sm	Sm	Sm/med	Med	Med
O₂ mask		Prem/tent[e]	NB/tent	Paed/tent	Paed/tent	Paed/tent	Paed	Paed	Paed/adult	Adult	Adult
Oral airway	Corner of mouth to earlobe	Infant	Infant	Infant/sm	Sm	Sm	Sm	Med	Med	Large	Large
Bag–valve–mask		Infant	Infant	Infant	Paed	Paed	Paed	Paed	Paed	Paed/adult	Adult
ETT[a]	ID: 1/4 (age) + 4 / ED: distal phalanx of 5th finger	2.5–3.0	3.0	3.5		4.0	4.5	5.0	6.0	6.5	7.0–8.0
		Uncuffed	Uncuffed	Uncuffed	Uncuffed	Uncuffed	Uncuffed	Uncuffed	Cuffed or uncuffed	Cuffed	Cuffed
Laryngoscope[f]		0, st	0–1, str	1, st	1, st	1–2, st	2, st	2, st	2, st or curv	2–3, st or curv	3, curv or st
Breathing[f]											
Tidal volume (ml)	10–15 ml kg⁻¹	40	50	80	120	150	200	250	320	450	650
Rate		40–50	40	40	30	30	30	20	20	15	15
Circulation											
Blood volume (ml)	80 ml kg⁻¹	240	280	560	800	880	1200	1.44 l	2.0 l	2.8 l	4 l
Bolus size (ml)	20 ml kg⁻¹	60	70	150	200	220	300	360	500	700	1 l
Catheters											
Intravenous (G)		22	22	22	22–20	20	20	20	18	18–16	16
NG Nasogastric (F)		12	12	12	12	12	12	14	14	16	18
Urinary (F)		5 (f.t.)	5–8 (f.t.)	8 (f.t.)	8	10	10	10–12	12	12–14	16
Chest tube (F)		10–14	12–16	14–18	14–20	16–20	18–24	20–30	24–32	28–36	32–40

[a] Burg, J.M. & Fleischer, G.R. (1993). Prehospital care of the injured child. In: *Pediatria Trauma: Prevention, Acute Care, Rehabilitation*, ed. M.R. Eichelburger. St Louis: Mosby Year Book.

[b] *The Harriet Lane Handbook*, 13th edn, 1993. St Louis: Mosby Year Book.

[c] *Advanced Trauma Life Support Manual*, 5th edn, 1993. Chicago: American College of Surgeons.

[d] A hand towel can be rolled up and snugly wrapped around the neck.

[e] An oxygen tent can be used if the child will not tolerate a face mask, but inspired oxygen concentration is less.

[f] These values are for mechanical ventilation and are biased toward hyperventilation; arterial blood gases should be checked.

HR, heart rate; SBP, systolic blood pressure; RR, respiratory rate; Hb/Hc, haemoglobin (g dl⁻¹)/haematocrit (%); ETT, endotracheal tube; ID, internal diameter; ED, external diameter; m, male; f, female; st, straight; curv, curved; NB, newborn; sm, small; med, medium; paed, paediatric; f.t., feeding tube; G, gauge; F, french.

tube can be used. An endotracheal tube which is snug at the cords will be too big at the cricoid and cause pressure necrosis and subglottic stenosis, either acutely from oedema or chronically due to scarring. Consistent with the child's normal pattern, small tidal volumes at a rate near 40 should be given. Surgical cricothyroidotomy should not be done in a child less than 8 years of age because of the risk of injury to the cricoid. A needle cricothyroidotomy using a 14 G catheter is a good temporizing measure while an emergency surgical tracheotomy is organized. The child can be ventilated using intermittent occlusion of a three-way adapter with 100% oxygen going through the third port. Throughout airway manipulation, cervical spine immobilization must be maintained until a spinal injury is excluded.

Once a secure airway is assured, attention is turned toward *breathing*. If the airway is opened the child may breathe on his own. Conversely, his airway may be intact and breathing impaired by decreased excursion, loss of respiratory drive (as in a head injury), or injured lung. Decreased excursion is immediately life-threatening in cases of tension pneumothorax, but it can be quickly and easily relieved by placing a 14 G intravenous catheter just above the third rib in the midclavicular line, followed by a chest tube. Other causes of decreased excursion are haemo- or pneumothorax, chest wall injury and diaphragmatic compromise due to laceration or gastric distension. These conditions can be temporized or definitively treated by a chest tube in the first two instances and a nasogastric tube in the last two. Respiratory insufficiency due to head injury or pulmonary contusion must be treated with intubation and mechanical ventilation. A distinction should be made between a child intubated for airway control and for respiratory compromise as extubation criteria are different.

Circulation in a trauma patient is compromised by loss of cardiovascular function or loss of volume. As discussed, hypotension from hypovolaemia occurs late in children and early signs are more reliable (see Table 6 and discussion in section on physiology). If signs of poor circulation are present, intravascular fluid should be given and sources of blood loss sought. Acute external bleeding (which may not be readily apparent before volume resuscitation is begun) must be controlled. This is best done by direct pressure: haemostats placed blindly into a bleeding wound can crush nerves or other vital structures previously uninjured, and a circumferentially wrapped 'pressure' dressing acts as a tourniquet. Large scalp wounds can be quickly controlled with a skin stapling device though the closure must be redone if the galea is not closed or the wound is incompletely cleaned. Little or transient response to volume loading should trigger a search for occult blood loss. Rarely, circulatory failure in the child is due to cardiac tamponade or to cardiac contusion, treated by pericardiocentesis and supportive measures, respectively. Finally, spinal cord injury may be the cause of persistent circulatory compromise but without signs of vasoconstriction. In this case, occult sources of bleeding must be ruled out; low-dose vasoconstrictors can be used to support vasomotor tone.

Disability is assessed by a brief neurological examination evaluating level of consciousness, presence and vigour of extremity movement, and pupillary reactivity. The Glasgow Coma Scale (adapted for children) (Table 7) is a quantitative measure of level of consciousness and should be recorded if possible. If a patient must be paralysed for intubation, this examination should be done beforehand and the results noted.

Table 6. *Paediatric organ system responses to blood loss* (adapted from the ATLS Manual)

	Early <25% blood volume loss	Prehypotensive ≥25% blood volume loss	Hypotensive ≥40% blood volume loss
Cardiac	Weak, thready pulse, increase heart rate	Increased heart rate	Hypotension, tachycardia to bradycardia
CNS	Lethargic, irritable, confused, combative	Depressed level of consciousness, dulled response to pain	Very depressed level of consciousness or comatose
Skin	Cool, clammy	Cyanotic, decreased capillary refill, cold extremities	Pale, cold
Kidneys	Decreased urinary output	Decreased urinary output	Decreased or no urinary output

Table 7. *Glasgow Coma Scale, paediatric modifications*

Score	Eye opening		
4	Spontaneous		
3	To speech		
2	To pain		
1	None		

Score	Best 'verbal' response		
	Adult/adolescent	Child	Young child
5	Oriented	Appropriate	Smiles, fixes and follows
4	Confused	Inappropriate	Cries but consolable
3	Inappropriate	Moaning	Inconsolable, irritable
2	Incomprehensible	Restless, agitated	Restless, agitated
1	None	None	None

Score	Best motor response
6	Follows commands or spontaneous appropriate movement
5	Localizes to pain
4	Withdraws to pain
3	Decorticate (flexor) posturing
2	Decerebrate (extensor) posturing
1	None

E is for *exposure* – which is required to fully assess the patient – and also for *environment*. The patient should be fully disrobed but immediately covered up and placed in proximity to a heat source to prevent hypothermia.

In an unstable patient, cervical spine, chest and pelvic radiographs should be done in the resuscitation room during the primary survey. A 'one-shot' IVP (intravenous pyelogram) should be obtained as part of the primary survey if possible when the patient is going directly to the operating room for abdominal exploration.

Resuscitation

Resuscitative measures are begun as soon as the patient arrives, if not started during transportation. Every seriously injured child should have two large-bore intravenous (in an infant, 20 or 22 G) catheters, supplemental oxygen and a nasogastric catheter. Intravenous access can be difficult to obtain in a child, especially in the face of the intense vasoconstriction children have in response to hypovolemia. Alternatives are intraosseous infusion, venous cut-down and central venous lines. Intraosseous infusion can be established in the proximal tibia of a young child or just above the medial malleolus of an older child (Driggers *et al.*, 1991) (see Fig. 6 for technique). Blood products, fluids and medications can be infused, but there should be no proximal fracture.

Venous cut-down should be done using the saphenous vein at the ankle or the groin, depending on the size of the child and the skill of the operator. Central access via the subclavian or internal jugular approach is discouraged except in the hands of a skilled operator or in a large older child. Femoral access is probably safe but the line should be removed in 24–48 h to decrease the risk of line sepsis. Blood should be drawn in paediatric tubes at the time of intravenous line placement and sent for blood count, electrolytes, amylase and blood typing. Coagulation studies and blood alcohol or other analyses should be considered. A urinary catheter should be placed to monitor urine output and a urinalysis undertaken for red blood cells.

As the above measures are proceeding, the child with signs of circulatory compromise should receive a 20 ml kg^{-1} bolus of crystalloid infused at a rapid rate. A second bolus should be given if there is no improvement in signs of perfusion. During the second bolus the child should be rapidly assessed for possible non-hypovolaemic causes of hypoperfusion: spinal shock, tension pneumothorax and cardiac injury or tamponade. A third bolus, this time of blood (10 ml kg^{-1}) should be given and repeated as needed if signs of shock persist. Blood should be given as the second bolus if there is obvious large blood loss or the patient is frankly hypotensive. The possible locations of occult blood loss are limited:

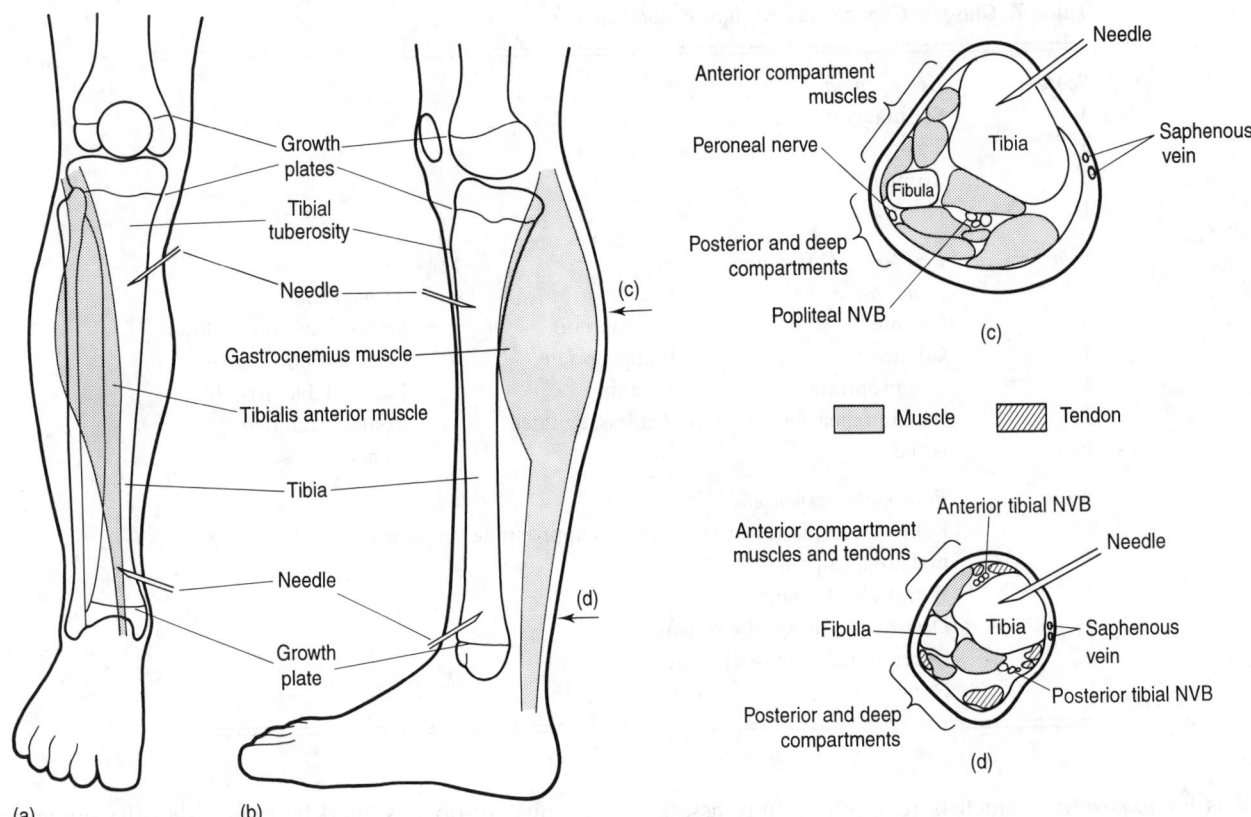

Fig. 6. (a) & (b) Anterior and medial views of the right lower leg showing levels of needle placement. (c) & (d) Cross-sectional views at the levels of needle placement. NVB, neurovascular bundle.

TECHNIQUE

- A heavy-gauge needle (16 g hypodermic, bone-marrow needle or designated intraosseous needle) is introduced with a twisting motion 2–4 cm below the tibial tuberosity or above the medial malleolus.
- Resistance will decrease when the cortex is penetrated.
- The needle is adequately positioned when it feels 'solid' in the bone, marrow can be aspirated easily and fluid flows freely.
- Care should be taken to avoid the growth plates; the needle can be angulated away from the metaphysis but this increases the chance of it bending when introduced.
- Careful sterile technique is necessary to avoid osteomyelitis.

abdomen, chest, badly fractured pelvis, retroperitoneum. If the child remains unstable he must be rapidly assessed for emergency operative intervention by diagnostic peritoneal lavage, chest and pelvis radiographs, and/or a one-shot IVP. External bleeding is controlled initially by direct pressure on the bleeding point, followed by definitive control when the patient is more stable.

Secondary survey

After the ABCs are assured, attention is turned to a systematic examination of the patient from head to toe, including log-roll to assess the patient's back for wounds and deformity. This is a careful examination aimed at defining all serious injuries. If not already done, chest tubes and urinary and nasogastric catheters should be placed. Pelvic stability should be assessed and a rectal examination done to screen for urethral injury prior to placement of a urinary catheter. If significant facial or basilar skull fractures are suspected, the nasogastric tube should be inserted as an orogastric tube to avoid the possibility of passage into the cranium. Fractures should be splinted and wounds covered with saline-soaked gauze, or dry gauze if the patient is hypothermic. The secondary survey is a good point at which to obtain further history. Transport personnel are an excellent source of information. After completing the secondary survey, a medical history (allergies, past hospitalizations, etc.) can be obtained from the parents who are allowed to visit if the child is stable. Frequent vital signs and perfusion evaluations should continue, with any abnormalities or changes prompting a return to the primary survey.

Diagnostic procedure are also part of the secondary survey. These include plain radiographs, special radiological studies and invasive procedures. Plain films are taken of any area exhibiting signs of injury. A complete series of spinal radiographs is obtained in patients with any known spine fracture, ejection from a vehicle, a history of significant axial loading, or pedestrian/cyclist struck by a vehicle. A computed tomography (CT) scan of the head should be requested in every unconscious or obtunded child. If immediate laparotomy is required, CT scan of the head and the remainder of the secondary survey must be completed afterwards. A CT scan of the abdomen is now the gold standard for diagnosis of abdominal and retroperitoneal injury in children because much information can be obtained (degree of solid organ disruption, renal function, amount of intra- or retroperitoneal blood) and there is now a bias towards non-operative management of paediatric solid organ injury. DPL (diagnostic peritoneal lavage) is arguably more sensitive to pancreatic injury (high amylase; Rothenberg et al., 1987) and bowel injury (bile or food fibers) but it gives no information on renal functions. DPL is indicated as part of the primary survey in an unstable child, as part of the secondary survey if the child is going directly to the operating room for another injury (i.e. extradural haematoma, major arterial injury), where the abdomen cannot be monitored, or if CT scan is delayed. The technique of DPL is the same for children as for adults, using lavage volumes of 10 ml kg^{-1} and the same criteria for 'positive' lavage. The abdomen must be investigated if there is any suspicion of intra-abdominal injury from the examination or mechanism of injury, failure of resuscitation, or spinal cord injury. Other diagnostic studies include angiography, urethrography and cystography, duodenography, oesophagoscopy and bronchoscopy as indicated.

If a child has sustained a penetrating injury, the wounding force will be localized to that point, but one must keep in mind the possibility of additional blunt injury such as a concomitant fall or beating. In the far more common case of blunt injury, the wounding force is dissipated over a large surface area and injuries may not be readily apparent. Injury may result from differential deceleration of soft tissue and bone as well as from the direct blow (i.e. 'coup' and 'contre-coup' cerebral injuries). Multiple injuries are common and certain injury complexes well-recognized (Table 8). Keeping this in mind, a search must be made for any associated injuries.

Continuing assessment

Once the early flurry of diagnosis and treatment settles down, the child should be reassessed from head to toe as injuries are frequently missed during the initial assessment. Daily reassessments should be made until the patient is discharged from the hospital. Although missed injuries are not usually life-threatening they can affect function and limb viability and need to be addressed.

ORGAN SYSTEM INJURIES

Since other chapters have been devoted to organ system injuries, only those more or less unique to children will be addressed here.

Head

As discussed, children are particularly susceptible to reactive cerebral hyperaemia after trauma. In this situation the most important issue is preventing secondary brain injury by maintaining a good systemic blood pressure, monitoring and controlling intracranial pressure, correcting coagulopathy, and ensuring adequate or excessive oxygen delivery. Although not widely practised, there are institutions in the USA where ICP monitors are inserted in the emergency department. As in adults, intracranial bleeding will not cause hypovolaemia, but in the very young child a scalp haematoma or cephalhaematoma can cause loss of volume sufficient to produce symptoms. Symptoms should correct with one or two fluid boluses, however, as these haematomas do not cause persistent haemodynamic instability unless there are open wounds which continue to bleed.

An infant with CHI and inconsistent history should be checked for retinal haemorrhages, which are virtually diagnostic of the 'shaken-baby syndrome'. If severely compromised, 'shaken' babies need intubation and hyperventilation; if the fontanelle is tight and there is abnormal posturing or pupillary dilation they should have a fontanelle tap. This is performed 2 cm from the midline (to avoid the sagittal sinus) bilaterally through the anterior fontalle as an emergency to release raised ICP (Bruce, 1993).

Lastly, small children are also subject to 'ping-pong' skull fractures. These are small circular depressed fractures resulting from low-energy impacts and are usually not significant; neurological symptoms should prompt CT evaluation.

Table 8. *Injury complexes*

Sentinel injury	Associated injuries	Mechanism
Head injury or facial fractures	Cervical spine fracture	Hyperflexion, hyperextension or axial loading of cervical spine
Chin laceration	Mandible fracture	Direct blow, or transmitted force to mandibular condules
Facial injury	Closed head injury (usually mild)	Direct to face, with coup and contre-coup to brain
Spine fracture	Other remote spine fracture	Axial loading
Chest wall injury	Pulmonary contusion	Direct blow
Sternal injury	Cardiac contusion	Direct blow
Ribs 1–3 fractured	Aortic rupture	Both result from massive force
Lower ribs fractured	Liver, spleen, diaphragmatic lacerations	Direct blow, or injury from intrusion of the broken rib
Chance (transverse) lumbar spine fracture	Small bowel injury, pancreatic injury	'Lap belt complex': acute flexion around an abdominal restraint
Upper abdominal abrasion or tenderness	Pancreatic injury, duodenal injury	Blow to upper abdomen, compressing organs against spine
Pelvic fracture	Sacral fracture, bladder rupture, urethral injury	Disruption of ring, laceration by sharp bone, overdistension of (full) bladder
Sacral or sacroiliac fracture	Pelvic vascular injury	Laceration and/or stretch of vessels (consider angiographic embolization if exsanguinating)
Femoral shaft fracture	Acetabulum or femoral neck fracture	Translated force
Knee laceration or severe lower leg injury	Acetabulum or femoral neck fracture, hip dislocation	Axial loading through femoral shaft
Calcaneus fracture	Lumbar spine fracture, hip fracture/dislocation	Axial loading (classically from a fall landing feet first)
Knee dislocation or fracture distal third of humerus	Arterial injury (femoral or popliteal artery)	Direct laceration or stretching injury of intima
Humeral shaft fracture	Radial nerve injury	Direct laceration or stretch of nerve
Distal radius fracture	Scaphoid fracture	Direct blow to extended wrist

Face

Facial fractures are much less common in children than adults. This is due to the relatively large size of the cranium, the undeveloped sinuses and thick soft tissues (Hunter, 1992). However, lacerations due to falls and play injuries are common and frequently extend down to the bone. They need to be carefully explored and meticulously reapproximated to avoid significant deformity as the child's face grows and develops. Primary hyphaemia is more common in children than adults, who usually have a late, secondary haemorrhage (Hiatt, 1991; Bloom, 1990). The eye should be covered and the child kept quiet for several days to avoid secondary bleeding.

The eye must be carefully examined for concomitant retinal injury.

Nasal and mandibular fractures are the most common fractures in children. Nasal septal haematomas must be promptly evacuated and the nasal cavity packed (ensuring close approximation of mucosa to cartilage) to prevent septal necrosis and a saddle nose deformity. Injury to the mandibular condyle can cause growth disturbances and deformity. An injury peculiar to childhood is that sustained as a result of running around with an object such as a pencil or toothbrush in the mouth with subsequent impalement in the oral cavity. If this affects the lateral palate, there is some risk of injury to the internal carotid artery which runs posterior to the tonsillar fossa. A neurological deficit may result.

Neck

Soft tissue injuries of the neck are uncommon in children since the neck is short and the chest and face relatively protuberant; but they can occur, for instance in a fall onto bicycle handlebars. In these instances vigilant attention to the airway is necessary with a bias towards early intubation before oedema completely obstructs the small-diameter airway.

Spinal cord injury without radiographic abnormality (SCIWORA) has been reported in 30–67% of children who have spinal cord trauma. The traumatic event may be trivial and cord injury symptoms may have a delayed onset (Riviello et al., 1990). When cervical spine injuries occur, they tend to be high in the neck (C1, C2, C3) rather than low as in adults. There are several reports of atlanto-occipital disruption. Death at the scene of injury is the rule in these cases, or quadriplegia in most who make it to the emergency department, but there are at least two cases of full neurological function (Harmanli & Koyfman, 1993; Papadopoulos et al., 1991). Bonadio (1993a, b) and Woodward (1993) have written comprehensively on neck injury and the interpretation of paediatric cervical spine films. Unless the child is alert and cooperative, with a normal neurological examination, the paediatric cervical spine cannot be considered normal on the basis of the standard three views (anteroposterior, lateral, odontoid). Ligamentous laxity and bony immaturity cause spinal hypermobility which renders the cords susceptible to injury. If the child is obtunded or there is suspicion of spinal injury, work-up should continue with CT or MRI (magnetic resonance imaging), or both.

Chest

Because of the compliant chest wall the most common chest injury in children is pulmonary contusion, accounting for over half of all chest injuries, frequently without rib fracture (Roux & Fisher, 1992; Templeton, 1993a; Nakayama et al., 1989). Respiratory function must be monitored closely after blunt chest trauma as decompensation may take 24–48 h to manifest. Next in frequency is rib fractures, followed by pneumo- and haemothorax. One-quarter of pneumothoraxes in one series were under tension (Nakayama et al., 1989). As previously discussed, children are particularly susceptible to the haemodynamic effects of tension pneumothorax and need prompt correction of this condition. Ruptured diaphragm, flail chest, aortic transection, tracheobron-chial rupture and cardiac injury are rare. They do, however, occur and a high index of suspicions must be maintained as these are highly morbid or fatal missed injuries.

Abdomen

A child's *solid organs* are susceptible to injury but injury is usually well-tolerated. They don't require operative intervention, even if initially symptomatic from hypovolaemia, as long as the child stabilizes with resuscitation and requires less than 50% (40 ml kg^{-1}) of blood volume in transfusions over the next 24 h. The child should be admitted to hospital for several days and activity restricted for 6–8 weeks after injury. Children with renal trauma should be evaluated for hypertension and have urinalysis 1 year after injury. Pancreatic injuries are probably more common in children than adults. Although consisting primarily of pancreatitis, disruption of a major duct may occur. An increase in serum amylase 24 h after admission heralds this and other major pancreatic injury and laparotomy and/or endoscopic retrograde pancreatography (Smith et al., 1988) should be considered.

Hollow viscus injury is much less common in children than in adults and accounts for only about 10% of laparotomies for blunt trauma (Brown et al., 1992; Fischer et al., 1988). As in adults, surgery is indicated. Three points about bowel injury should be made:

1. There is no good means of early diagnosis; frequent serial examinations and signs of peritonitis are most reliable.
2. Missing an injury leads to significant morbidity and a high index of suspicions is imperative.
3. Bowel injury is more common in child abuse and in these cases can present distressingly late, or after death.

Duodenal haematomata are probably more common in injured children than injured adults, although still very infrequent. They are usually managed conservatively with nasogastric suction and parenteral nutrition.

The bladder in children is more susceptible to injury without pelvic fracture due to its intra-abdominal location. Young boys may sustain disruption of the anterior urethra from a straddle injury in which the urethra is compressed against the pubis. Genital trauma in boys or girls should always arouse suspicion of child abuse.

Extremities

Fractures are an indication of significant soft tissue damage in children, who have relatively flexible bones. Neurovascular function must be carefully assessed, especially with a known or suspected joint dislocation, and the patient needs to be monitored closely for development of compartment syndrome. Early immobilization of fractures, particularly operative fixation or cast application, significantly reduces pain and allows early mobilization

SUMMARY

Management of paediatric trauma patients consists of the same priorities as for adults but most incorporate the special needs and vulnerabilities, both physical and psychosocial, of children and their carers. Children with minor injuries can be managed in the emergency department and discharged with appropriate follow-up instructions. Treating children with major injuries is more complex and involves training prehospital and hospital personnel, an adequate transport system, and designation of facilities offering an immediate and appropriate response. Control of airway, breathing and haemorrhage followed by resuscitation and treatment or triage are the priorities in the emergency department. Trauma remains by far the biggest contributor to paediatric morbidity and mortality. Although treatment has improved survival, the biggest impact on reducing these numbers will be from improvements in preventing childhood injury.

Bibliography

BARLOW, B., NIEMIRSKA, M., GANDHI, R. P. *et al.* (1983). Ten years of experience with falls from a height in children. *J. Pediatr. Surg.*, **18**, 509–11.

BASSON, M.D., GUINN, J.E., McELLIGOTT, J. *et al.* (1991). Behavioral disturbances in children after trauma. *J. Trauma*, **31**, 1363–8.

BERGER, M.S., PITTS, L.H., LOVELY, M. *et al.* (1985). Outcome from severe head injury in children and adolescents. *J. Neurosurg.*, **62**, 194–9.

BLOOM, J.N. (1990). Traumatic hyphema in children. *Pediatr. Ann.*, **19**, 368–75.

BONADIO, W.A. (1993a). Cervical spine trauma in children: Part I. General concepts, normal anatomy, radiographic evaluation. *Am. J. Emerg. Med.*, **11**, 158–65.

BONADIO, W.A. (1993b). Cervical spine trauma in children: Part II. Mechanisms and manifestations of injury, therapeutic considerations. *Am. J. Emerg. Med.*, **11**, 256–78.

BREAUX, C.W., SMITH, G. & GEORGESON, K.E. (1990). The first two years experience with major trauma at a pediatric trauma center. *J. Trauma*, **30**, 37–43.

BROWN, R.A., BASS, D.H., RODE, H. *et al.* (1992). Gastrointestinal tract perforation in children due to blunt abdominal trauma. *Br. J. Surg.*, **79**, 522–4.

BRUCE, D.A. (1993). Head trauma. In *Textbook of Pediatric Emergency Medicine*, 3rd edn., ed. G.R. Fleischer & S. Ludwig, pp. 1102–12. Baltimore, MD: Williams & Wilkins.

BRUCE, D.A., ALAVI, A., BILANIUK, L. *et al.* (1981). Diffuse cerebral swelling following head injuries in children: the syndrome of 'Malignant Brain Edema', *J. Neurosurg.*, **54**, 170–8.

CENTERS FOR DISEASE CONTROL, DIVISION OF INJURY CONTROL, CENTER FOR ENVIRONMENTAL HEALTH AND INJURY CONTROL (1990). Childhood injuries in the United States. *Am. J. Dis. Child.*, **144**, 627–46.

CHAN, B.S.H., WALKER, P.J. & CASS, D.T. (1989). Urban trauma: an analysis of 1,116 paediatric cases. *J. Trauma*, **29**, 1540–7.

DIGUISEPPI, C.G., RIVARA, F.P., KOEPSELL, T.D. *et al.* (1989). Bicycle helmet use by children: evaluation of a community-wide helmet campaign. *J. Am. Med. Assoc.*, **262**, 2256–61.

DRIGGERS, D.A., JOHNSON, R., STEINER, J.S. *et al.* (1991). Emergency resuscitation in children: the role of intraosseous infusion. *Postgrad. Med.*, **89**, 129–37.

DYKES, E.H., SPENCE, L.J., YOUNG, J.G. *et al.* (1989). Preventable pediatric trauma deaths in a metropolitan region. *J. Pediatr. Surg.*, **24**, 107–11.

EICHELBERGER, M. (1993). Thoracic trauma. In *Pediatr. Surgery*, 2nd edn., ed. K.W. Ashcraft & T.M. Holder, pp. 122–32. Philadelphia, PA: W.B. Saunders.

EICHELBERGER, M.R., MANGUBAT, E.A., SACCO, W.S. *et al.* (1988). Comparative outcomes of children and adults suffering blunt trauma. *J. Trauma*, **28**, 430–4.

FISCHER, R.P., MILLER-CROTCHETT, P. & REED, R.L. (1988). Gastrointestinal disruption: the hazard of nonoperative management in adults with blunt abdominal injury. *J. Trauma*, **28**, 1445–9.

FLEISHER, G.R. (1991). Controversies in pediatric emergency medicine: prehospital intravenous access in pediatric trauma. *Pediatr. Emerg. Care*, **7**, 117–19.

GALLAGER, S.S., FINISON, K. *et al.* (1984). The incidence of injuries among 87,000 Massachusetts children and adolescents: results of the 1980–81 statewide injury prevention program surveillance system. *Am. J. Public Health*, **74**, 1340–7.

GHAJAR, J. & HARIRI, R.J. (1992). Management of pediatric head injury. *Pediatr. Clin. North Am.*, **39**, 1093–125.

GUYER, B. & ELLERS, B. (1990). Childhood injuries in the United States. *Am. J. Dis. Child.*, **144**, 649–52.

HARMANLI, O.T., KOYFMAN, Y. (1993). Traumatic atlanto-occipital dislocation with survival: a case report and review of the literature. *Surg. Neurol.*, **39**, 324–30.

HARRIS, B.H., SCHWAITZBERG, S.D., SEMAN, T.M. *et al.* (1989). The hidden morbidity of pediatric trauma. *J. Pediatr. Surg.*, **24**, 103–6.

HERZENBERG, J.E., HENSINGER, R.N., DEDRICK, D.K. *et al.* (1989). Emergency transport and positioning of young children who have an injury of the cervical spine. *J. Bone Joint Surg.*, **71A**, 15–22.

HIATT, R.L. (1991). Eye trauma in children. *South. Med. J.*, **84**, 747–50.

HUNTER, J.H. (1992). Pediatric maxillofacial trauma. *Pediatr. Clin. North Am.*, **39**, 1127–43.

KLEIN, L. & MARCUS, R.E. (1986). Trauma in children: management, prognosis, and metabolism. In *Trauma in Children*, ed. R.E. Marcus, pp. 1–10. Rockville, MD: Aspen Publishers.

KRAUSE, J.F. ROCK, A. & HEMYARI, P. (1990). The causes, impact and preventability of childhood injuries in the United States: brain injuries among infants, children, adolescents and young adults in the United States. *Am. J. Dis. Child.*, **144**, 684–91.

KUMAR, R., WEST, C., QUIRKE, C. *et al.* (1991). Do children with severe head injury benefit from intensive care? *Childs Nerv. Syst.*, **7**, 299.

LUDWIG, S. & LOISELLE, J. (1993). Anatomy, growth and development: impact on injury. In *Pediatric Trauma: Prevention, Acute Care, Rehabilitation*, ed. M.R. Eichelberger. pp. 39–58. St Louis, MO: Mosby Year Book.

LUERSSEN, T.G., KLAUBER, M.R. & MARSHALL, L.F. (1988). Outcome from head injury related to patients' age. *J. Neurosurg.*, **68**, 409–16.

MAGNUSON, D.K. & MAIER, R.V. (1993). Pathophysiology of injury. In *Pediatric Trauma: Prevention, Acute Care, Rehabilitation*, ed. M.R. Eichelberger, pp. 59–83. St Louis, MO: Mosby Year Book.

MARSHALL, L.F., SMITH, R.W. & SHAPIRO, H.M. (1979). The outcome with aggressive treatment in severe head injuries. Part I: The significance of intracranial pressure monitoring. *J. Neurosurg.*, **50**, 20–5.

MAYER, T., MATLAK, M.E., JOHNSON, D.G. *et al.* (1980). The modified injury severity scale in pediatric multiple trauma patients. *J. Pediatr. Surg.*, **15**, 719–26.

MAYER, T., WALKER, M.L. & CLARK, P. (1984). Further experience with the modified abbreviated injury severity scale. *J. Trauma*, **24**, 31–4.

McKOY, C. & BELL, M.J. (1983). Preventable traumatic deaths in children. *J. Pediatr. Surg.*, **18**, 505–8.

MICHAUD, L.J., RIVARA, F.P., GRADY, M.S. *et al.* (1992). Predictors of survival and severity of disability after severe brain injury in children. *Neurosurgery*, **31**, 254–64.

MICHAUD, L.J., RIVARA, F.R., JAFFE, K.M. *et al.* (1993). Traumatic brain injury as a risk factor for behavioural

disorders in children. *Arch. Phys. Med. Rehab.*, **74**, 368–75.

MUIZELAAR, J.P., MARMAROU, A., DeSALLES, A.A.F. *et al.* (1989a). Cerebral blood flow and metabolism in severely head-injured children, Part I: Relationship with GCS Score, outcome, ICP and PVI. *J. Neurosurg.*, **71**, 63–71.

MUIZELAAR, J.P., WARD, J.D., MARMAROU, A. *et al.* (1989b). Cerebral blood flow and metabolism in severely head-injured children, Part II: Autoregulation. *J. Neurosurg.*, **71**, 72–6.

NAKAYAMA, D.K., RAMENOFSKY, M.L. & ROWE, M.I. (1989). Chest injuries in childhood. *Ann. Surg.*, **210**, 770–5.

PAPADOPOULOS, S.M., DICKMAN, C.A., SONNTAG, V.K.H. *et al.* (1991). Traumatic atlantooccipital dislocation with survival. *Neurosurgery*, **28**, 574–9.

PASCUCCI, R.C. (1988). Head trauma in the child. *Intensive Care Med.*, **14**, 185–95.

PECLET, M. & MURPHY, J.P. (1993). Abdominal and urinary tract trauma. In *Pediatric Surgery*, 2nd edn., ed. K.W. Ashcraft & T.M. Holder. pp. 133–40. Philadelphia, PA: W.B. Saunders.

PLECET, M.H., NEWMAN, K.D., EICHELBERGER, M.R. *et al.* (1990a). Patterns of injury in children. *J. Pediatr. Surg.*, **25**, 85–91.

PECLET, M.H., NEWMAN, K.D., EICHELBERGER, M.R., *et al.* (1990b). Thoracic trauma in children: an indicator of increased mortality. *J. Pediatr. Surg.*, **25**, 961–6.

RAMENOFSKY, M.L. (1993). Early assessment and management of trauma. In *Pediatric Surgery*, 2nd edn., ed. K.W. Ashcraft & T.M. Holder. pp. 110–21.

RIVIELLO, J.J., MARKS, H.G., FAERBER, E.N. *et al.* (1990). Delayed cervical central cord syndrome after trivial trauma. *Pediatr. Emerg. Care*, **6**, 113–17.

ROTHENBERG, S., MOORE, E.E., MARX, J.A. *et al.* (1987). Selective management of blunt abdominal trauma in children – the triage role of peritoneal lavage. *J. Trauma*, **27**, 1101–6.

ROUX, P. & Fisher, R.M. (1992). Chest injuries in children: an analysis of 100 cases of blunt chest trauma from motor vehicle accidents. *J. Pediatr. Surg.*, **27**, 551–5.

SHACKFORD, S.R., MACKERSIE, R.C., DAVIS, J.W. *et al.* (1989). Epidemiology and pathology of traumatic deaths occurring at a Level I Trauma Center in a regionalized system: the importance of secondary brain injury. *J. Trauma*, **29**, 1392–7.

SMITH, S.D., NAKAYAMA, D.K., GANTT, N. *et al.* (1988). Pancreatic injuries in childhood due to blunt trauma. *J. Pediatr. Surg.*, **23**, 610–14.

TEMPLETON, J.M. (1993a). Thoracic trauma. In *Textbook of Pediatric Emergency Medicine*, 3rd edn., ed. G.R. Fleischer & S. Ludwig, pp. 1143–66. Baltimore, MD: Williams & Wilkins.

TEMPLETON, J.M. (1993b). Minor trauma. In *Textbook of Pediatric Emergency Medicine*, ed. G.R. Fleischer & S. Ludwig, pp. 1288–97. Baltimore, MD: Williams & Wilkins.

TEPAS, J.J., MOLLITT, D.L., TALBERT, J.L. & BRYANT, M. (1987). The pediatric trauma score as a predictor of injury severity in the injured child. *J. Pediatr. Surg.*, **22**, 14–18.

TEPAS, J.J., RAMENOFSKY, M.L., MOLLITT, D.L *et al.* (1988). The pediatric trauma score as a predictor of injury severity: an objective assessment. *J. Trauma*, **28**, 425–9.

WALLER, A.E., BAKER, S.P. & SZOCKA, A. (1989). Childhood injury deaths: national analysis and geographic variations. *Am. J. Public Health*, **79**, 310–15.

WALSH, T. (1993). Psychosocial aspects of care. In *Pediatric Trauma: Prevention, Acute Care, Rehabilitation*, ed. M.R. Eichelberger. pp. 84–8. St Louis, MO: Mosby Year Book.

WINTEMUTE, G.J. (1990). Childhood drowning and near-drowning in the United States. *Am. J. Dis. Childr.*, **144**, 663–9.

WOODWARD, G.A. (1993). Neck trauma. In *Textbook of Pediatric Emergency Medicine*, 2nd edn., ed. G.R. Fleischer & S. Ludwig. pp. 1113–42. Baltimore, MD: Williams & Wilkins.

B: Trauma in pregnancy

P. NASH

Accident and Emergency Department, Neath General Hospital, Neath, UK

INTRODUCTION

Trauma in pregnancy is the commonest cause of non-obstetric maternal death. Data from the USA suggest that the degree of trauma is sufficiently severe to necessitate hospital admission of 3–4 expectant mothers per 1000 deliveries (Lavin & Scott Polsky, 1983).

When dealing with the pregnant trauma patient it is essential to remember that two lives are at risk. The fetus may die unless the mother is adequately resuscitated. Treatment priorities are the same as for the non-pregnant patient but resuscitation and stabilization need modification to take account of the anatomical and physiological changes of pregnancy. Early involvement of an obstetrician is advocated.

The pregnant patient who sustains trauma is usually extremely anxious about herself and her baby. Allocation of a nurse to establish rapport and give reassurance assists the trauma team.

CAUSES OF TRAUMA IN PREGNANCY

Road traffic accidents are the commonest reason for hospital admission following trauma in pregnancy. Other causes include blunt trauma as a result of assault or falls, penetrating trauma due to stabbing or gunshot wound, and burns (Drost *et al.*, 1990; Timberlake & McSwain, 1989).

THE EFFECTS OF ANATOMICAL CHANGES OF PREGNANCY ON THE RESPONSE TO TRAUMA

During the first trimester the fetus lies within the thick-walled uterus and is protected against injury by the bony pelvis. As pregnancy progresses beyond the 12th week of gestation the uterus becomes an intra-abdominal organ and is therefore more vulnerable to direct injury (Fig. 1). During the second trimester the fetus is cushioned by a large volume of amniotic fluid, but by the end of the third trimester the uterus is thin-walled, offering little protection to the fetus (Nash & Driscoll, 1990).

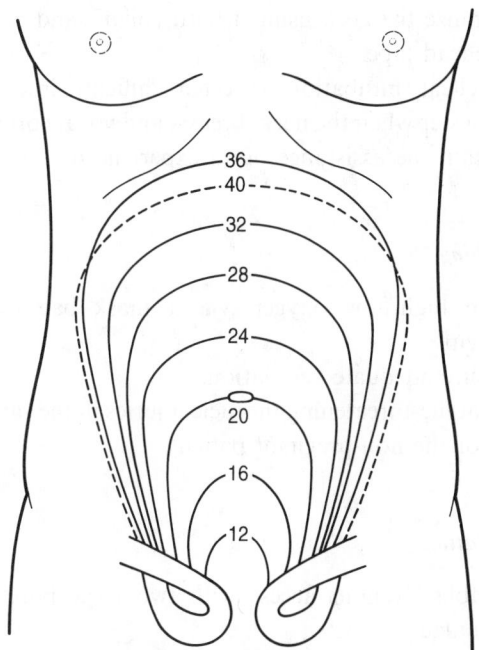

Fig. 1. Fundal height by gestation in weeks.

Enlargement of the uterus displaces the intestines to the upper abdomen.

Compared to the uterine wall the placenta lacks elastic tissue. When shearing forces are applied to the abdomen the difference in elasticity may result in placental abruption.

The anatomical changes of pregnancy make the uterus and its contents more susceptible to penetration, uterine rupture, placental abruption and rupture of the membranes. Myometrial injury can destabilize decidual lysosomes, releasing arachidonic acid which can cause uterine contractions.

THE EFFECTS OF PHYSIOLOGICAL CHANGES OF PREGNANCY ON THE RESPONSE OF TRAUMA

Respiration

The respiratory rate in pregnancy is unchanged, but tidal volume increases by 40% and residual capacity falls by 25%. This causes a 'physiological hyperventilation' of pregnancy which produces a Pco_2 of 4.0 kPa (30 mmHg). An apparently normal Pco_2 of 5.3 kPa in a pregnant trauma patient reflects both maternal and fetal acidosis.

Circulation

During pregnancy the cardiac output increases by 1.0–1.5 litres min^{-1}. However, in the supine position, the pressure of the uterus on the great vessels (aortocaval compression) may decrease cardiac output by 30–40%. The resting pulse rate increases by 15–20 beats min^{-1} in the third trimester. Both systolic and diastolic blood pressures fall by 15 mmHg in the second trimester, returning to normal by term. Blood volume increases by 50% at 34 weeks of gestation (Pearlman et al., 1990).

Damage to the placental bed may result in massive haemorrhage because of its vascularity. Similarly, fractures of the pelvis are often associated with exsanguinating haemorrhage from dilated pelvic veins.

Circulatory assessment in the injured pregnant patient can be difficult. Because of the increased circulating volume the pregnant patient can lose 50% more blood than her non-pregnant counterpart before signs of hypotension occur. The placental circulation is sensitive to catecholamines and vasoconstriction of the placental vessels may preserve the maternal circulation at the expense of fetal perfusion. The fetus may therefore be shocked before signs of maternal shock develop. If the patient is nursed in the supine position, aortocaval compression may cause hypotension which can be corrected by positioning the patient.

Although the resting central venous pressure in pregnant patients is variable, the response to fluid challenge is the same as for the non-pregnant patient so this is a useful means of monitoring the circulatory volume.

Gastrointestinal tract

The pregnant trauma victim is at increased risk of aspiration of gastric contents into the lungs because of a rise in intragastric pressure without concomitant increase in gastro-oesophageal sphincter tone. Stretching of the peritoneum and abdominal musculature by the gravid uterus diminishes rebound tenderness and guarding as signs of abdominal injury.

Urinary tract

The glomerular filtration rate and renal plasma blood flow increase during pregnancy causing falls in blood urea and creatinine. Glycosuria is common in pregnancy when the renal threshold is reduced. The renal calyces, pelvices and ureters are dilated. The bladder is displaced upwards and anteriorly by the enlarging uterus becoming an intra-abdominal organ after the 12th week and more susceptible to direct injury.

Endocrine system

During pregnancy the mass of the pituitary gland increases by up to 50%. Haemorrhagic shock can cause necrosis and insufficiency of the anterior pituitary.

Musculoskeletal system

Ligamentous laxity results in widening of the symphysis pubis by up to 8 mm and relaxation of the sacroiliac joints.

Nervous system

Eclampsia is a complication of pregnancy which may mimic head injury. Eclampsia should be considered in the pregnant patient who has a convulsion and is likely if proteinuria, oedema and hyper-reflexia are present. Hypertension may be absent if shock coexists.

Blood composition

Dilutional anaemia occurs because of a smaller increase in red cell mass than circulatory volume. The white cell count is increased. Serum fibrinogen and clotting factors are increased and prothrombin time and partial thromboplastin time may be shortened. In response to injury the myometrium releases high concentration of placental thromboplastin or plasminogen activator which reverse the normal haemostatic mechanisms of pregnancy and can result in disseminated intravascular coagulation.

ASSESSMENT OF THE MOTHER

Primary survey

When a severely injured pregnant patient presents to the accident and emergency (A&E) department the priorities for her care are the same as for a non-pregnant patient. The Advanced Trauma Life Support protocol provides a suitable framework for assessment and resuscitation of the patient (American College of Surgeons, 1988). The important modifications required in the pregnant patient are detailed below.

Airway and neck

- Ensure that the airway is patent and be alert to the high risk of regurgitation and aspiration of gastric contents.

- Stabilize the neck using a hard collar, sand bags and forehead tape.
- Tracheal intubation is often difficult in the last trimester when the neck, breasts and vocal cords swell. Obtain the assistance of an experienced anaesthetist.

Breathing

- Give high-flow oxygen via a mask–bag–reservoir system.
- Ensure adequate ventilation.
- Treat life-threatening thoracic injuries in the same way as for the non-pregnant patient.

Circulation

- Establish venous access with two large bore (14 G) cannulae.
- Take blood for Kleihauer test (see assessment of the fetus), group and cross-match in addition to routine tests.
- Commence vigorous fluid therapy with crystalloid and blood. In the UK the synthetic colloid gelatin preparations can be used before blood is available.
- To avoid aortocaval compression and resultant hypotension, the patient should be nursed in the left lateral position once spinal injury has been excluded. Alternatively, the right hip can be elevated using a sand bag and the uterus can be displaced manually to the left.
- If pneumatic antishock garments are used, only the leg compartments should be inflated (Stauffer, 1986).
- Vasopressors are particularly contraindicated in the pregnant patient because they restore maternal blood pressure at the expense of uterine blood flow producing fetal hypoxia.

Secondary survey

During the secondary survey the mother should be examined from head to toe for evidence of injury. Assessment of the fetus also forms part of the secondary survey (see below).

X-rays should not be withheld because the patient is pregnant: the small risk to the fetus is outweighed by the need to detect life-threatening maternal injury. Use of abdominal shields when peripheral films are being taken minimizes fetal irradiation. The greater risk to the fetus is at 8–15 weeks of gestation, a time when the mother does not look obviously pregnant. A teratogenic risk

Table 1. *Absorbed radiation dose to the unshielded gravid uterus during radiological investigation*

X-ray investigation	Uterine dose range (rad)
Cervical spine	No detectable contribution
Chest	0.0003–0.0043
Pelvis (anteroposterior)	0.142–0.486
Intravenous pyelogram	0.202–0.815
Full spine	0.154–0.527
CT head	<0.05
CT upper abdomen	<3.0

CT, computed tomography.

has been established at 5–10 rad of radiation, and a risk of childhood cancer at slightly lower doses (Drost *et al.*, 1990). The absorbed radiation dose of some commonly performed X-rays is shown in Table 1.

If abdominal surgery is required to treat maternal injuries this should not be delayed because of pregnancy. Peritoneal lavage can be performed in the pregnant patient, but the site of incision should be displaced cranially. When the pregnant uterus reaches the umbilicus a vertical midline incision should be made above it. When the uterus is at term the incision should be made over its dome taking care not to damage the uterus or fetus (Higgins, 1988).

ASSESSMENT OF THE FETUS

This should be performed as part of the secondary survey of the mother, preferably by an obstetrician, Three key questions need to be addressed:

1. Is the fetus potentially viable (over 24–25 weeks gestation)?
2. Has there been damage to the fetal environment?
3. Are there signs of fetal distress?

Gestation can be estimated by fundal height (Fig. 1) and/or the date of the last menstrual period. Many pregnant women carry their obstetric records with them and if available these are a useful source of information.

Abdominal palpation will reveal the presence of uterine contractions. The onset of labour is likely when moderate intensity contractions occur regularly (e.g. every 5 min) lasting 45–80 sec (Bojanowski *et al.*, 1988). Tetanic contractions accompanied by vaginal bleeding imply placental abruption. Palpation of fetal parts separate from the uterus is diagnostic of uterine rupture. The presence of normal movements is reassuring to both mother and doctor.

Vaginal examination should be performed by the obstetrician to check for vaginal bleeding, suggestive of placental abruption or placenta praevia. Facilities for urgent surgical intervention should be available.

Leakage of amniotic fluid suggests rupture of the chorioamniotic membranes. Dilatation and effacement of the cervix and fetal presentation should also be assessed at the time of vaginal examination.

The normal fetal heart rate is 120–160 beats min^{-1} and can be assessed using doppler ultrasound from 12–14 weeks. Bradycardia of less than 100 beats min^{-1} and loss of beat-to-beat variation are signs of fetal distress. Later in pregnancy a cardiotocogram can be used to monitor heart rate and uterine contractions while the conscious mother records fetal movements. Signs of fetal distress include late decelerations in response to uterine contractions and inadequate accelerations in response to fetal movement. Continuous monitoring is advocated for between 4 h (Pearlman *et al.*, 1990) and 48 h (Esposito *et al.*, 1989) for all patients carrying a viable fetus following blunt abdominal trauma.

Gestational age and viability can be confirmed using pelvic ultrasound. The heart beat is visible from 7 weeks of gestation. Ultrasound also provides information on placental position, abruption and the presence of intra-amniotic haemorrhage.

The Kleihauer test detects fetal blood cells in the maternal circulation indicating fetomaternal haemorrhage, which is associated with anaemia and a poor prognosis for the fetus (Rose *et al.*, 1985).

Anti-D immunoglobulin should be given to all rhesus negative women with fetomaternal haemorrhage to prevent rhesus isoimmunization.

BLUNT TRAUMA

In a study of 208 pregnant patients injured in road traffic accidents, overall maternal mortality was 7.5% and fetal mortality was 13.5% (Crosby & Costiloe, 1971). Head injury and intra-abdominal injury were the commonest causes of maternal death. Maternal death was the commonest cause of fetal death, with placental abruption the second most common cause. Injury to maternal abdominal organs including liver, spleen, kidney and intestines occurs in 15.6–26.2% of pregnant patients with blunt abdominal trauma (Lavin & Scott Polsky, 1983). Pelvic fractures are also common following blunt trauma and are often associated with massive retroperitoneal haemorrhage from dilated pelvic veins (see also Chapter 33D). Coexistent injury to the lower urinary tract occurs in 10–15% of cases of pelvic fracture. Stable fractures rarely interfere with delivery but unstable fractures may be further displaced at the time of vaginal delivery causing damage to the bladder and urethra.

Direct injury to the fetus is rare following blunt trauma but when it does occur head injury and long bone fractures are most common (Lavin & Scott Polsky, 1983).

In a study of 40 pregnant patients with blunt abdominal trauma, three required immediate laparotomy for fetal distress, accompanied by maternal haemodynamic instability in one case (Esposito et al., 1989). Pregnant patients with minor injuries (mean injury severity score 5.9) including blunt abdominal trauma were safely observed. Those with major injuries, shock, altered mental status or neurological deficit required further studies including diagnostic peritoneal lavage, CT (computed tomography) scanning and ultrasound to rule out intra-abdominal injury.

The use of seat belts by pregnant car occupants reduces both maternal and fetal mortality by preventing ejection from the vehicle in the majority of accidents (Crosby & Costiloe, 1971). Three-point harnesses give the best protection and should be worn with the lap belt across the upper thighs and the diagonal belt between the breasts, i.e. above the bump (Pearce, 1992). This minimizes the risk of placental abruption.

Placental abruption

The reported incidence of placental abruption in traumatized pregnant patients ranges from 6.6% to 66% (Higgins & Garite, 1984). The majority of abruptions occur within 48 h of abdominal trauma. Placental abruption can also be precipitated by shock from other causes and may be seen following the rise in venous pressure that occurs distal to compressiom of the inferior vena cava in the supine position. Clinical signs of placental abruption include vaginal bleeding, uterine tenderness, uterine irritability, tetanic contractions and rising fundal height, with or without maternal shock. There are also signs of fetal distress. In equivocal cases the diagnosis can be confirmed by ultrasound. If less than 25% of the placenta is involved, external vaginal bleeding and labour ensue. Greater involvement threatens maternal and fetal survival with fetal death likely if there is greater than 50% separation. Large abruptions are associated with disseminated intravascular coagulation in the mother.

Any urgent decision concerning an emergency caesarean section should be made by an obstetrician.

Uterine rupture

Uterine rupture, although rare, has a higher incidence in those with a previous uterine scar (e.g. previous caesarean section). It is usually associated with damage to another major organ (Stauffer, 1986). Symptoms of uterine rupture include a sudden onset of sharp, lower abdominal pain and cessation of contractions. Physical examination reveals loss of fetal movements and heart sounds, separately palpable fetus and uterus, vaginal bleeding and profound maternal shock. Plain abdominal X-rays show a uterus and separate fetus, usually with extended extremities. There may also be free intraperitoneal air (Auerbach, 1979). Immediate surgical intervention is indicated because fetal mortality approaches 100% and maternal exsanguination is likely if surgery is delayed. The uterus can sometimes be repaired but if damage is extensive or if the laceration has extended into the parametrial vessels, caesarean hysterectomy may be required.

PENETRATING TRAUMA

Stab and gunshot wounds are common forms of penetrating trauma in pregnancy. The pattern of injury is altered by the presence of the pregnant uterus which by virtue of its size is commonly injured. It may afford protection to other intra-abdominal organs.

In gunshot wounds to the abdomen, bullets tend to strike the uterus because of its large size, and much of their energy is dissipated in this muscular organ. Injury to other abdominal organs occurs in less than 20% of cases (Lavin & Scott Polsky, 1983), but should always be suspected because of the unpredictable trajectory. Because the uterus is a non-vital organ, maternal death following abdominal gunshot wounds is rare. However, the fetus, umbilical cord and/or placenta are commonly injured resulting in high fetal mortality.

Abdominal stab wounds carry a better prognosis for mother and fetus than do gunshot wounds. As with gunshot wounds the uterus shields other abdominal organs but loops of bowel may be injured in the upper abdomen. Many fetal, placental and umbilical cord injuries have been reported.

Exploration should be considered in all cases of penetrating injury (Higgins, 1988). In cases of less than 28 weeks' gestation every attempt should be made to preserve the pregnancy if the fetus is alive and there is a minor penetrating injury to the uterus. Beyond 28 weeks with no uterine penetration at laparotomy and no evidence of fetal distress, Higgins suggests preserving the pregnancy and close postoperative fetal monitoring. Where uterine penetration is evident, he advocates delivery because the risk of fetal death from injury greatly exceeds the risk of perinatal death through prematurity.

BURNS

In a review of 50 pregnant patients admitted to a burns unit, mother and fetus survived in 23 (Matthews, 1982). All except two had burns of less than 50%. The patients with burns greater than 50% were in the first trimester of pregnancy. Of the 27 patients whose pregnancy ended in hospital, only two of the 14 mothers with greater than 50% burns survived. Their survival was attributed to delivery within 14 h of the burn, with loss of the physiological load of pregnancy. As a result of this work Matthews concluded that survival is optimal in the first trimester but that for patients with greater than 50% burns in the second or third timester of pregnancy immediate fetal delivery is indicated because maternal death is otherwise certain and fetal survival is not improved by waiting.

SURGICAL INTERVENTION IN TRAUMA IN PREGNANCY

The main indication for surgical intervention following trauma in pregnancy is the need to treat maternal injuries, especially those associated with internal haemorrhage and penetrating abdominal trauma. Uterine rupture necessitates urgent laparotomy. Emergency caesarean section is indicated for fetal distress, placental abruption and for those with burns of greater than 50% in the second or third trimester. On occasion the enlarged uterus limits surgical exposure and for the treament of life-threatening injuries the fetus should be delivered regardless of gestation.

Postmortem caesarean section may be required to deliver a viable fetus after cardiopulmonary arrest. The fetal prognosis is then based on the time interval between maternal death and delivery. It is optimal if delivery is achieved within 5 min but if there is a delay of greater than 20 min, survival is unlikely (Higgins, 1988). Prior to postmortem caesarean section fetal viability must be ascertained and maternal cardiopulmonary resuscitation (CPR) must be continued throughout. A vertical midline incision is made through the abdominal wall into the uterus, then the fetus is removed, the cord is clamped and the baby is resuscitated by the paediatrician. The placenta is removed. There have been occasional reports in which the mother revived following delivery of the fetus so it is worthwhile continuing CPR and assessing the mother for signs of life.

Bibliography

AMERICAN COLLEGE OF SURGEONS (1988). *Advanced Trauma Life Support Manual Provider Manual.* Washington, DC: American College of Surgeons.

AUERBACH, P.S. (1979). Trauma in the pregnant patient. *Topics Emerg. Med.,* **1**, 133–47.

BOJANOWSKI, C., HILL, K. & MARTIN, D. (1988). Assessment of the pregnant trauma patient. *Dimens. Crit. Care Nurs.,* **7**, 356–62.

CROSBY, W.M. & COSTILOE, J.P. (1971). Safety of lap-belt restraint for pregnant victims of automobile collisions. *N. Engl. J. Med.,* **284**, 632–6.

DROST, T.F., ROSEMURGY, A.S., SHERMAN, H.F *et al.* (1990). Major trauma in pregnant women: maternal/fetal outcome. *J. Trauma,* **30**, 574–8.

ESPOSITO, T.J., GENS, D.R., GERBER SMITH, L. *et al.* (1989). Evaluation of blunt abdominal trauma occurring during pregnancy. *J. Trauma,* **29**, 1628–32.

HIGGINS, S.D. (1988). Trauma in pregnancy. *J. Perinatol.,* **8**, 288–92.

HIGGINS, S.D., & GARITE, T.J. (1984). Late abruptio placenta in trauma patients: implications for monitoring. *Obstet. Gynecol.,* **63**, 10S–12S.

LAVIN, J.P. SCOTT POLSKY. S. (1983). Abdominal trauma during pregnancy. *Clin. Perinatol.,* **10**(2), 423–37.

MATTHEWS, R.N. (1982). Obstetric implications of burns in pregnancy. *Br. J. Obstet. Gynaecol.,* **89**, 603–9.

NASH, P.E. & DRISCOLL, P. (1990). ABC of major trauma: trauma in pregnancy. *Br. Med. J.,* **301**, 974–6.

PEARCE, M. (1992). Selt belts in pregnancy. *Br. Med. J.,* **304**, 586–7.

PEARLMAN, M.D., TINTINALL, J.E. & LORENZ R.P. (1990). Blunt trauma during pregnancy. *N. Eng. J. Med.,* **323**, 1609–13.

ROSE, P.G., STROHM, M.T. & ZUSPAN, F.P. (1985). Fetomaternal haemorrhage following trauma. *Am. J. Obstet. Gynecol.,* **153**, 844–7.

STAUFFER, D.M. (1986). The trauma patient who is pregnant. *J. Emerg. Nurs.,* **12**, 89–93.

TIMBERLAKE, G.A. & McSWAIN, N.E. (1989). Trauma in pregnancy. A ten year perspective. *Am. Surg.,* **55**, 151–3.

C: Trauma in the elderly

G. HUGHES

Department of Accident and Emergency Medicine, Bristol
Royal Infirmary, Bristol, UK

INTRODUCTION

By the year 2000 one-fifth of the population of Europe
and North America will be over 60 years of age (Rabbitt,
1992). Compared to younger populations this age group
has a higher mortality from any given injury and is more
likely to sustain more serious injuries in any given
accident. Elderly patients with equivalent injury severity
scores (ISS) have higher admission rates, spend longer
in hospital and have a significantly increased mortality
(McCoy *et al.*, 1989). Appropriately aggressive management in these people is rewarding and leads to increased
survival without loss of quality of life or independence
(DeMaria *et al.*, 1987).

EPIDEMIOLOGY

People aged over 65 years are less likely than persons in
other age groups to be injured at all, but they are more
likely to have fatal outcomes from the injuries that do
occur and they represent 25% of injury fatalities in all
age groups. Falls, fire and road traffic accidents account
for three-quarters of injury deaths (Oreskovich *et al.*,
1984). Road traffic accident deaths occur in all types of
road user but the elderly pedestrian is the most common
category (McCoy *et al.*, 1989). As many as 96% of elderly
accident victims were mobile and independent prior
to the accident; the immobile are low-risk individuals
(Oreskovich *et al.*, 1984).

General characteristics of injury in the elderly

- Elderly represent 25% of all injury fatalities
- Majority are independently mobile prior to injury
- Compared to younger age groups, the elderly:
  - sustain more serious injuries
  - have higher admission rates
  - spend longer in hospital
  - have deeper burns and higher mortality from them
- Road traffic accident related deaths are commonest
  in pedestrians

Although 75% of all home accidents go unreported to
the medical services, more than 300 000 people aged over
65 years attend accident and emergency (A&E) departments in England and Wales each year following a
domestic accident. The incidence increases with age from
6% in the 65–74 age group to 11% in the over-85s
(Livesley, 1992).

The true incidence of accidental hypothermia (defined
as core body temperature of less than 35 °C) is unknown.
However, nearly half of all hypothermic admissions are
in patients over 65 years and the mortality ranges from
40% to 80% (Mills, 1973).

Although the incidence of burns is lower than in the
young, the elderly have a higher mortality rate following
thermal injury.

SPECTRUM OF INJURY

The elderly are most likely to be injured in road traffic
accidents as pedestrians, sustaining injuries to the pelvis,
lower limbs and head. They walk directly into the path
of an oncoming vehicle and respond slowly, if at all, to
the danger (McCoy *et al.*, 1989). As drivers they have
impaired skills and may also suffer acute medical conditions while at the wheel. As vehicle occupants they have
a similar distribution of injuries to the young but their
injuries are generally more severe. Fracture of the sternum
when wearing a seat belt is seen six times more frequently
than in the young (McCoy *et al.*, 1989).

As in all age groups, the majority of older patients
who die have a serious head injury. Non-survivors have
twice the incidence of central nervous system injury
compared to survivors; one-third of elderly road traffic
accident victims with major injuries require thoracic or
abdominal surgery (Oreskovich *et al.*, 1984).

The elderly may come to injury as a result of a
pre-existing chronic medical condition and these patients
have significantly longer periods in hospital. The effect
of a pre-existing medical condition on length of hospital
stay is more noticeable in patients with less severe
injuries (MacKenzie *et al.*, 1989).

Precipitating factors for home accidents include adverse
environmental conditions (poor lighting, loose rugs,
etc.), poor mobility and slow response times to danger,
multiple pathology, and drug-induced side-effects
(Livesley, 1992).

Accidental hypothermia results from a combination of
cold exposure, impaired responses (thermoregulation,
shivering and temperature perception) and the effects of
systemic disease (e.g. hypothyroidism) and medication.

Burns in the elderly tend to be deeper because of a

combination of poor reaction times, impaired mobility and age-related atrophic changes in the skin (Anous & Heimbach, 1986).

SPECIFIC INJURY PATTERNS

Head injury

Although less common than in the young, head injury is a cause of significant morbidity and mortality in the elderly (Table 1). As many as one in seven patients admitted to neurosurgical units are over 65; intracranial haematoma is three times more common than in the under-65s. Elderly patients with minor head injury are more likely to be admitted to non-specialist units than younger people, primarily because of social factors. As many as half live alone at the time of injury.

In younger populations head injury is at least three times as common in males as females but in the elderly the sex incidence is equal and the cause is more likely to be a fall than road traffic accident. Alcohol is an associated factor in half of elderly men (Pentland et al., 1986).

Doctors tend to be less critical in assessing the elderly head-injured patient. Obtaining a good history can be difficult and physical signs such as confusion may be attributed to non-traumatic causes. Although coexisting medical disorders may be obscured by a head injury, patients with head injuries may be misdiagnosed as suffering from a medical condition. For example, head injury may not be considered in patients with a hemiplegia but no skull fracture. Prompt and appropriate use of X-rays and CT (computed tomography) scanning is essential and should not be withheld on grounds of age.

Table 1. *Characteristics of head injury in the elderly*

- Equal sex incidence
- Alcohol is an associated factor in 50% of males
- Injury is more likely to result from a fall than road traffic accident
- Intracranial haematomata are three times more common than in the young
- Admission rates are higher than in the young following minor injury
- Medical conditions may obscure a head injury
- Head injury may be misdiagnosed as a medical condition (e.g. cerebrovascular accident)

The reduced cerebral reserve of the elderly means they are less likely to tolerate a minor head injury. The resulting impairment (particularly of cognitive function) may lead to loss of independence, and average hospital stays are nearly three times longer than for younger age groups. It is likely that more community support will be needed after discharge.

Age is an important consideration in certain types of head injury. A 75-year-old in coma for longer than 6 h (after resuscitation) has an almost 100% chance of dying or persisting in a vegetative state. Despite this depressing figure initial treatment and resuscitation, including prompt neurosurgical intervention, should not be withheld simply because a patient is old (Galbraith, 1987).

Cervical spine injury

Although cervical spine injury is predominantly a disease of young males, it does occur in the elderly and is easily missed; a particularly difficult problem is cord damage in hyperextension injuries. Complete and incomplete cord lesions, in addition to causing permanent disability, hasten the early death of an elderly patient.

Initial management and assessment of cervical spine injuries is similar to that in younger age groups: immobilization, resuscitation and radiological investigation are followed by fracture/dislocation reduction and stabilization according to standard guidelines.

Respiratory failure may develop from spinal cord injury alone but is more likely to occur in combination with pre-existing respiratory disease or coexistent thoracic trauma. Post-traumatic autonomic dysfunction may complicate pre-existing cardiovascular disease, manifesting as arrhythmia, myocardial ischaemia or systemic hypertension (Johnston, 1989).

A particularly common syndrome in the elderly is acute injury to the central cervical cord. It is misdiagnosed because complex neurological signs are not recognized (poor 'pattern recognition') and X-rays of the cervical spine rarely show any acute injury. It is commonly caused by a fall with hyperextension of the cervical spine; the spinal canal is reduced in size by degenerative disease and the cord is compressed between anterior cervical osteophytes and the inward buckling of the posterior ligamentum flavum or a disc. Lesions to anterior horn cells, adjacent lateral corticospinal and spinothalamic tracts and central grey matter occur. The legs are spared because their axons are situated more peripherally in the spinal cord. Clinically, the patient has a greater weakness of the arms than the legs, a variable and inconsistent sensory loss in the upper limbs and often evidence of an injury to the forehead such as a bruise or abrasion (Johnston, 1989). Cervical spine X-rays show only degenerative disease. Half the patients recover function with conservative treatment, the legs improving more than the arms. Mobilization and walking may be compromised by an inability to use a stick or walking frame.

Central cord lesions in younger age groups are sometimes associated with cervical disc prolapse. The relevance of this to the elderly is unknown, but as better imaging techniques (such as MRI – magnetic resonance imaging) develop, it may become clearer (Johnston, 1989).

Chest injury

Although mechanisms and patterns of injury from blunt chest trauma are similar in all age groups, the elderly have a higher morbidity and mortality; elderly patients with isolated chest injury have a death rate three times that of young patients (Shorr et al., 1989).

Despite evidence that the elderly are more likely to present with shock or cardiorespiratory arrest, a high index of suspicion is needed in assessment of chest injuries, and aggressive diagnosis and treatment should not be withheld.

Fractures of the bony thorax are the most common injury in major trauma, followed by haemopneumothorax, pulmonary contusion and ruptured aorta. Osteoporotic changes occur in ribs as well as long bones and the decreased elasticity of the chest wall more readily produced rib fractures. Sternal fractures in seat belt users are six times more common in the elderly than in the young. Even in the absence of respiratory or cardiac disease, chest wall injuries which are often benign in younger people may be dangerous in the elderly as the respiratory system has marginal reserve. Parameters such as peak flow and vital capacity are reduced and accessory and intercostal muscles tire more easily. Simple rib fractures therefore necessitate admission for observation, monitoring of coexistent medical conditions or pain relief management. Although the elderly are more likely to need mechanical ventilation, it is the functional rather than just the anatomical consequences of injury which determine the need for ventilation, as in younger patients.

The heart and great vessels are less resilient in the elderly. Baseline coronary flow is reduced as is the cardiovascular response to physiological demand. The myocardium is more sensitive to hyposia and acidosis but less sensitive to circulating catecholamines. Arrhythmias resulting from conduction system disturbance are more common. Aortic inelasticity associated with ageing and atherosclerosis makes the vessel more vulnerable to transection or traumatic aneurysm formation.

Secondary complications seen in the postresuscitation phase include atelectasis, pneumonia, adult respiratory distress syndrome, pleural effusion and pulmonary embolus.

Penetrating chest injuries, rare in the elderly, are managed as they are in the young.

Abdominal injury

Blunt abdominal trauma severe enough to cause intra-abdominal injury is easily misdiagnosed in the elderly and has a mortality rate nearly five times greater than in the young (Finelli et al., 1989).

The elderly are more vulnerable to hypovolaemic shock after relatively minor injury; when elderly patients do show evidence of hypovolaemic shock the aetiology is less likely to be intra-abdominal than in the young (Pedowitz & Sjackford, 1989). Additionally, peritonitis is more difficult to detect.

Although the elderly tolerate surgery less well and are more prone to postoperative complications, an aggressive surgical approach is needed; of necessity there will be a higher incidence of negative laparotomies than in the young (Sutherland et al., 1989).

Penetrating abdominal injuries, rare in the elderly, are managed as they are in the young.

Pelvic injury

Pelvic injuries represent 3% of all fractures and are the third most common cause of road traffic accident deaths. The incidence of pelvic fractures, of all grades, rises with age to 446 per 100 000 in women aged 85 or over (Mucha & Farnell, 1984).

Pelvic fractures represent a spectrum ranging from minor injuries which do not require hospital admission to complex injuries with haemodynamic instability that prove fatal. In the elderly the former usually result from a fall, and the latter from road traffic accident.

Pubic rami fractures are common and easily overlooked, particularly by inexperienced doctors looking at an X-ray to exclude a fracture of the femoral neck. Fractures which cause haemodynamic instability contribute significantly to mortality, death being 12 times more common than in pelvic injuries without cardiovascular compromise (Mucha & Farnell, 1984). Major fractures require early reduction and stabilization with angiography and embolization if necessary to control haemorrhage; age is not a contraindication to such treatment.

Soft tissue and major organ injury from pelvic fractures are managed according to standard techniques.

Skeletal limb injury

A combination of falls and osteoporosis account for the majority of upper and lower limb fractures in the elderly. Although osteoporosis is the most frequently documented predisposing cause, other types of metabolic bone disease (e.g. hyperparathyroidism and Paget's disease) and pathological fractures secondary to malignancy (including myeloma) should be considered in the differential diagnosis. In addition, cardiovascular syndromes and other conditions responsible for falls should be identified.

Temporary loss of function in a limb can rapidly lead to loss of independence and institutionalization in the elderly. Emergency management should include a social and nursing assessment to help coordinate and consolidate community support, promote early discharge and hopefully avoid inappropriate hospital admissions (Nankhonya et al., 1991; Williams et al., 1992).

Fractures in the elderly heal at the same rate as in young adults; the healing process itself does not require additional treatment (Pennig, 1992). Fracture reduction, stabilization and rapid mobilization to promote a return to functional and independence are ideal treatment goals. An isolated fracture of a long bone may well be the precipitating factor responsible for the death of the patient and it must be treated expeditiously. The type of operation or method of internal fixation must take into account the quality of the bone to be fixed.

Old people with skeletal injury *only* may suffer haemorrhage which is significant enough to increase mortality. Isolated long bone fractures may be the cause of death, particularly if the fracture is open and sepsis develops.

Upper limb

Shoulder girdle

Injuries to the clavicle, scapula and acromioclavicular joint are unusual in the elderly, but rotator cuff lesions are more common than in the young (Stableforth, 1992). The incidence of fractures of the proximal humerus rises progressively with age from the fifth to the eighth decades, accounting for 5–10% of all joint and bone injuries and 30% of all upper limb fractures. They are twice as common in elderly women as in men.

Acute glenohumeral dislocation is a common problem needing prompt reduction. The greater the delay the more difficult is the reduction and the more likely the development of persistent shoulder pain and stiffness. This injury is commoner in females and is associated with a high incidence of rotator cuff tears and fractures of the greater tuberosity which may well be responsible for persistent unsatisfactory results (Astley, 1986). Functional recovery normally occurs over a 4–6 month period and requires physiotherapy, which should commence as soon as the pain allows. Recurrent anterior dislocation, which is common in the young, is rare in the elderly.

Elbow

Fractures and dislocations in this area account for 15% of upper limb injuries, fracture of the radial head being particularly common. Fixed flexion deformities are more readily acceptable than in young patients unless they lead to loss of independence because of inability to use a walking aid. Slightly displaced fractures of the olecranon in the elderly and frail may be treated conservatively.

Wrist

Colles' fracture is common in the elderly. In females there is a sharp increase in incidence between the ages of 45 and 60 years, peaking at 95 per 100 000. As many as 75% of people with a Colles' fracture have osteoporosis (Dias, 1992). As these injuries tend to be caused by a fall onto the outstretched hand, the rest of the limb and shoulder girdle should be carefully examined to exclude injury.

Complications following wrist fractures in the elderly include deformity, stiffness, weakness and pain in the vicinity of the ulnar styloid. Median nerve compression, extensor pollicis longus rupture and reflex sympathetic dystrophy (Sudeck's atrophy) are more amenable to treatment (Cooney et al., 1980).

Maintenance of wrist function is more important than cosmetic perfection. One study has shown that 19% of patients have persistent moderate or severe pain at 6 years and 17% have persistent wrist stiffness at 6 years. One in four patients will have some wrist deformity and disability affecting their daily activities (Dias, 1992).

Lower limb

Fracture of the femoral neck is an age-related condition, the incidence rising from 1 in 1000 in both sexes at age 55, to 30 per 1000 in women and 15 per 1000 in men at age 85. Additionally there has been an increased incidence since the Second World War unrelated to age; in a 20-year period from 1955 to 1975 age-specific hip fracture incidence doubled in both sexes (Warnes, 1992). The reason for this is not known.

The injury is most commonly caused by a fall with axial compression loading and a medially directed force to the hip. Factors such as age, body weight and environment are also relevant. The majority (70%) occur indoors. Although osteoporosis is undoubtedly a factor which predisposes to injury, there is a debate as to its exact contribution; above the age of 75 years the increasing risk of sustaining a fracture because of reduced bone mass is small (Cooper et al., 1987). There is a negative association between fracture and osteoarthritis.

Avascular necrosis is a well-known complication of femoral neck fractures, occurring in at least 80% of subcapital fractures but in less than 1% of intertrochanteric fractures (Catto, 1965).

The specific details of each type of fracture (traditionally classified as extra- or intracapsular) and their operative management will not be discussed here. The differential diagnosis, which should be straightforward with examination and careful X-ray screening, includes pubic ramus fracture. The injured should undergo surgery within 24 h following appropriate resuscitation. Additional medical treatment such as rehydration and cardiovascular stabilization should be completed as quickly as is reasonable. A preoperative blood transfusion may be inappropriate as a 2–3-day delay is required to allow the donor blood to become an efficient oxygen carrier.

Mortality statistics for this injury should include figures at 6 and 12 months postinjury in addition to the immediate postoperative period. Death rates vary from 10% to 40% at 6 months. Recent evidence suggests that the most negatively discriminating features relating to 6-month survival are the presence of dementia, postoperative chest infection, neoplasia, increasing age and the development of wound infection (Stevens, 1992).

Isolated fractures of the long bones are best treated by surgical internal fixation rather than conservative methods. Management decisions should be aimed at early fracture stabilization and mobilization. Surgery to relieve pain and assist nursing may be appropriate in bedridden patients.

Spinal injury

Compression fractures of the thoracic and lumbar spine are the most common vertebral fractures in the elderly. Pain may arise spontaneously or after minimal trauma to an osteoporotic spine. Management of stable injuries involves good analgesia and early mobilization. Pathological fractures secondary to malignancy (including myeloma) must be considered in the differential diagnosis.

Fracture patterns after trauma are similar to those in younger age groups; cord injuries are most commonly seen in cervical injury followed by thoracolumbar and thoracic lesions. The nature of the body lesion can be elucidated with CT scanning.

Accidental hypothermia

In the elderly this is frequently associated with underlying illness or injury (e.g. thyroid disease or hip fracture). Protocols for rewarming are similar to those in the young. Resuscitation should continue until warming has failed to revive the patient or rewarming is not achieved. Ninety per cent of elderly patients are dead within 1 year of suffering an episode of accidental hypothermia (Gilbert 1992).

Burns

The mortality rate for a burn of any particular size is higher in the elderly than in the young. Baux's formula is well-known and predicts that the mortality rate is equal to age plus the percentage surface area of the burn.

Extensive and deeper burns in the elderly result from slow reaction times and poor mobility in response to danger; also age-related changes to the skin predispose to deeper burns.

Burn management protocols are similar to those applied to younger patients, but lower thresholds for admission to hospital are appropriate. Patients with 70% burns or greater do not survive and this should be considered during resuscitation (Anous & Heimbach, 1986).

AGE-RELATED COMPLICATIONS AND THEIR PREVENTION IN THE A&E DEPARTMENT

The elderly have impaired physiological, immunological and metabolic responses to trauma. Injury severity scores (ISS), when age-adjusted, are a good indicator of outcome; scores predicting 10% mortality for blunt trauma in the under 55s predict a 40% mortality in the over 55s (Boyd et al., 1987). In addition to this natural effect of ageing, the elderly are more likely than younger patients to have a pre-existing chronic medical condition (PEC). The presence of a PEC has a significant influence on outcome, leading to longer hospital stays because of increased susceptibility to complications, reduced physiological and immunological reserve, the need for complex multidisciplinary discharge planning and treatment of the PEC itself (Mackenzie et al., 1989).

Soft tissue

Elderly skin becomes atrophic with decreased vascularity, epidermal thinning and loss of elasticity and subcutaneous fat. These changes are associated with impaired wound healing and infection. Immobility and decreased soft tissue bulk encourage pressure sore development. Urinary and faecal incontinence, diabetes mellitus and peripheral vascular disease exacerbate these problems.

Pressure sores are most commonly seen over the sacrum, buttocks and heel. As many as 60% of patients with femoral neck fracture develop them within 5 days of admission (Versluysen, 1986) and prevention should begin in the A&E department. Prolonged periods on hard trolleys awaiting admission are sometimes unavoidable and appropriate turning and skin care should be part of the management of the patient in the A&E department. Proper care should reduce the incidence of pressures sores to less than 2% in high-risk patients.

Deep venous thrombosis in calf or thigh veins occurs in 40–50% of postoperative patients, and pulmonary embolism develops in 3% of such cases (Stevens, 1992). The role of prophylactic anticoagulation in trauma is limited; physiotherapy and early mobilization are the best prophylactics. Other complications include sepsis, particularly pneumonia and urinary tract infection and septicaemia secondary to wound infection. These may occur despite expeditious surgical treatment and mobilization.

INTERCURRENT DRUGS

Adverse drug reactions arise in the elderly for two main reasons:

1. Altered drug handling (e.g. decreased renal and hepatic elimination resulting in an extended half-life).
2. Iatrogenic polypharmacy because of lack of awareness of drug interactions and ignorance of the correct drug regimen.

Patients may be confused or forgetful of their daily drug requirements; indeed a drug-induced side-effect may have been the precipitating factor in a fall leading to the presenting injury. Age-related changes which affect drug handling include decreased body water and mass and increased body fat; hence water-soluble drugs have higher initial plasma levels because volumes for distribution are decreased. Lipid-soluble drugs tend to have longer elimination half-lives and larger volumes for drug distribution.

The correct dose and route of administration is important. It is prudent to commence treatment at a lower dosage in the elderly and increase it gradually according to response. When prescribing oral analgesics and anti-inflammatories for home use it is wise to remember that the elderly have difficulty swallowing tablets, opening bottles and reading labels and may not be compliant because of confusion or memory loss.

Elderly patients require prescriptions tailored to their needs. The doctor must ask the question 'Is the drug really necessary?'.

METABOLISM

The elderly have an altered metabolic response to injury. Inadequate nutritional reserve and coexistent disease means that the catabolic response to major trauma may be inadequate.

Post-traumatic hyperglycaemia, which resolves within 2–3 weeks in the young regardless of the severity of injury, is exaggerated and prolonged in the elderly (Desai et al., 1989). This is attributed to a slight increase in basal plasma glucose seen with age, decreased sensitivity to insulin and increased gluconeogenesis and glycogenolysis. Elevated circulating catecholamines may be partly responsible and prolonged immobility following injury or surgery may also be relevant (Frayn et al., 1983). Protracted insulin resistance is detrimental to nitrogen balance and tissue repair.

Although cortisol secretion and clearance decrease with age, serum cortisol levels in response to trauma are increased in the elderly according to the degree of injury. There is evidence of a prolonged and sustained increase following femoral neck fractures (Frayn et al., 1983), but this is not seen in patients who have severe multiple injuries, perhaps because the adrenal cortex is less responsive to ACTH (adrenocorticotropin) (Barton et al., 1987).

End organ sensitivity to circulating hormones is also

age-related, resulting in decreased heart rate and cardiac output responsiveness to circulating catecholamines.

NUTRITION

Although the elderly are particularly at risk, malnutrition is difficult to quantify as it may be subclinical. Protein calorie malnutrition will lead to increased sepsis, decreased muscle bulk and white cell function. Decreased plasma protein binding affects drug handling. Malnutrition impairs thermoregulation and predisposes to hypothermia, decreased muscle bulk, immobility and ataxia, increasing susceptibility to injury (Bastow et al., 1983). Vitamin C depletion is associated with pressure sore development in elderly patients with femoral neck fractures (Goode et al., 1992).

CIRCULATORY INSUFFICIENCY

Differentiating between the effects of disease and ageing on the cardiovascular system is difficult. Structural changes in the myocardium seen with increasing age cause a reduction in a stroke volume and a decrease in the force of ejection. Cardiac output during exercise probably decreases with age. Peripheral vascular resistance increased with age as does systemic blood pressure. The clinical assessment of cardiac output in the elderly patient with multiple injuries may be difficult and inaccurate. Apparent haemodynamic stability may conceal a dangerously low cardiac output which, if left untreated, will lead to cardiogenic shock and multiple organ failure (Scalea et al., 1988). Early invasive monitoring to measure haemodynamic parameters, including arterial blood pressure, is appropriate in the elderly and it increases survival.

RESPIRATORY INSUFFICIENCY

Many factors contribute to respiratory insufficiency. Chest wall and lung compliance decrease with age and this is compounded by the development of a kyphosis, barrel chest, airway narrowing, decreased tidal volume and vital capacity, increased closing volume and ventilation/perfusion mismatch. All predispose to arterial hypoxia. Weak accessory and intercostal muscles also contribute to respiratory failure. Decisions to ventilate patients with chest trauma and respiratory disease need to be based on pathophysiological considerations as well as on the anatomical injury.

ANAESTHETIC PROBLEMS

Airway control and maintenance may be hampered by lack of dentition and loss of facial muscle tone. Atrophic skin and fragile veins contribute to cannulation difficulties. The skin is easily torn by fraction or shearing in transferring patients from stretcher to X-ray or operating tables. Irritating substances or solvents injected intravenously (e.g. diazepam) are more likely to predispose to thrombophlebitis and caution is needed. Circulation times increase steadily with age and allowance must be made for this when using intravenous agents.

Hypotension is a difficult problem to deal with, especially if associated with spinal cord injury; invasive monitoring is appropriate and often essential.

Aspiration of gastric contents is a major problem in the elderly. Symptoms vary from tachypnoea and temporary bronchospasm to severe respiratory failure with pneumonitis. Prevention by aspiration of gastric contents through a nasogastric tube followed by rapid sequence induction with preoxygenation and endotracheal intubation is appropriate.

Experienced surgeons are required to decrease anaesthesia time and the problems associated with prolonged surgery in elderly patients.

Anaesthesia may cause suppression of the cough reflex and a fall in the functional residual capacity. Atelectasis in a dependent lung contributes to prolonged postoperative hypoxia which may be resistant to manipulation with positive and expiratory pressure ventilation and large tidal volumes. Early postoperative respiratory physiotherapy with appropriate analgesia to promote coughing helps to prevent atelectasis.

Confusion is common pre- and postoperatively in the elderly and is readily exacerbated by hypoxia and sedation.

ETHICAL ASPECTS

Ethical decisions in the A&E department are particularly challenging when dealing with the elderly. There is little opportunity to obtain a medical history or form a doctor/patient relationship and a patient's personal beliefs regarding resuscitation from trauma may be unknown. Many doctors have negative attitudes to treating the elderly. Patient care consists not only of making a diagnosis, prescribing medication and performing technical procedures. The indiscriminate application of modern technology, treatment and surgery is not always acceptable as they lead to a painful, prolonged, undignified and predictable death. Informed consent may be lacking, in which case common law may be applied when urgent intervention is required. If in doubt, resuscitate first and ask questions afterwards, although there are specific situations in which the prospect of survival is poor. For example, patients with 70% burns of whatever age are unlikely to survive, and patients aged 75 with a head injury who are in coma after 6 h are likely to die or persist in a vegetative state. Independent factors associated with poor long-term outcome include shock, sepsis and a Glasgow Coma Score $\leqslant 7$ (Van Aalst et al., 1991).

When assessing the need to treat an orthopaedic injury, the outcome sought and absolute necessity for a technically correct procedure should be considered. For example, anterior dislocation of the shoulder which has been present for several months in an elderly person may best be treated with physiotherapy rather than surgery. If the patient has a hemiplegia, an injury to the disabled side is unlikely to benefit from sophisticated treatment.

It is important to treat injuries which interfere with the use of a walking aid or appliance. In general, mobilization and maintenance of independence should be the over-riding goal. Prolonged and unnecessary immobility is particularly dangerous in the elderly and will lead to their demise.

Bibliography

ANOUS, M.M. & HAIMBACH, D.M. (1986). Causes of death and predictors in burned patients more than 60 years of age. J. Trauma, 26, 135–9.

ASTLEY, T.M. (1986). Dislocation of the shoulder in the elderly. J. Bone Joint Surg., 686, 676.

BARTON, R.N., STONER, H.B. & WATSON, S.M. (1987). Relationships among plasma control, adrenocorticotrophin, and severity of injury in recently injured patients. J. Trauma, 27, 384–92.

BASTOW, M.D., RAWLINGS, J. & ALLISON, S.P. (1983). Undernutrition, hypothermia and injury in elderly women with fractured femur: any injury response to altered metabolism? Lancet, i, 143–5.

BOYD, C.R., TOLSON, M.A. & COPES, W.S. (1987). Evaluating trauma care: the TRISS method. J. Trauma, 27, 370–8.

CATTO, M. (1965). The histological appearance of late segmented collapse of the femoral head after transcervical fracture. J. Bone Joint Surg., 47B, 777–91.

COONEY, III, W.P., DOBYNS, J.H. & LINSCHEID, R.L. (1980). Complications of Colles' fracture. J. Bone Joint Surg., 62A, 613–19.

COOPER, C., BARKER, D.J.P., MORRIS, J. et al.

(1987). Osteoporosis, falls, and age in fracture of the proximal femur. Br. Med. J., 295, 13–15.

DeMARIA, E.J., KENNEY, P.T., MERRIAM, M.A. et al. (1987). Aggressive trauma care benefits the elderly. J. Trauma, 27, 1200–6.

DESAI, D., MARCH, R. & WATTERS, J.M. (1989). Hyperglycemia after trauma increases with age. J. Trauma, 29, 719–23.

DIAS, J.J. (1992). Wrist fractures. In Orthogeriatrics: Comprehensive Orthopaedic Care for the Elderly Patient, ed. R.J. Newman, pp. 167–74. Oxford: Butterworth Heinemann.

FINELLI, F.C., JOHNSON, J., CHAMPION, H.R. et al. (1989). A case control study for major trauma. J. Trauma, 29, 541–8.

FRAYN, K.N., STONER, H.B. & HEATH, D.F. (1983). Persistence of high plasma glucose, insulin and cortisol concentrations in elderly patients with proximal femoral fractures. Age Ageing, 12, 70–6.

GALBRAITH, S. (1987). Head injuries in the elderly. Br. Med. J., 294, 325.

GILBERT, M. (1992). Lecture to Resuscitation 92 Conference, Brighton, UK.

GOODE, H.F., BURNS, E. & WALKER, B.E. (1992). Vitamin C depletion and pressure sores in elderly patients with femoral neck fracture. Br. Med. J., 305, 925–7.

JOHNSTON, R.A. (1989). Management of old people with neck trauma. Br. Med. J., 299, 633–4.

LIVESLEY, B. (1992). Reducing home accidents in elderly people. Br. Med. J., 305, 2–3.

MacKENZIE, E.J., MORRIS, J.A. & EDELSTEIN, S.L. (1989). Effect of pre-existing disease on length of hospital stay in trauma patients. J. Trauma, 29, 757–65.

McCOY, G.F., JOHNSTONE, R.A. & DUTHIE, R.B. (1989). Injury to the elderly in road traffic accidents. J. Trauma, 29, 494–7.

MILLS, G.L. (1973). Accidental hypothermia in the elderly. Br. J. Hosp. Med., 2, 691–699.

MUCHA, P. & FARNELL, M.B. (1984). Analysis of pelvic fracture management. J. Trauma, 24, 379–86.

NANKHONYA, J.M., TURNBULL, C.J. & NEWTON, J.T. (1991). Social and functional impact of minor fractures in elderly people. Br. Med. J., 303, 1514–15.

ORESKOVICH, M.R., HOWARD, J.D., COPASS, M.K. et al. (1984). Geriatric trauma: injury patterns and outcome. J. Trauma, 24, 565–9.

PEDOWITZ, R.A. & SHACKFORD, S.R. (1989). Non-cavitary hemorrhage producing shock in trauma patients: incidence and severity. J. Trauma, 29, 219–22.

PENNIG, D. (1992). Principles of fracture management in elderly patients. In Orthogeriatrics: Comprehensive Orthopaedic Care for the Elderly Patient, ed. R. J. Newman. pp. 120–4. Oxford: Butterworth Heinemann.

PENTLAND, B., JONES, P.A., ROY, C.W. et al. (1986). Head injury in the elderly. Age Ageing, 15, 193–202.

RABBITT, P. (1992). Ageing gracefully. *Lancet.* **339**, 1157–8.

SCALEA, T., DUNCAN, A., ATWEH, N. *et al.* (1988). Geriatric blunt multiple trauma: improved survival with early invasive monitoring. *J. Trauma*, **28**, 1096.

SHORR, R.M., RODRIGUEZ, A., INDECK, M.C. *et al.* (1989). Blunt chest trauma in the elderly. *J. Trauma*, **29**, 234–6.

STABLEFORTH, P.G., (1992). Shoulder injuries in the elderly. In *Orthogeriatrics: Comprehensive Orthopaedic Care for the Elderly Patient*, ed. R.J. Newman. pp. 159–66. Oxford: Butterworth Heinemann.

STEVENS, J. (1992). Fractures of the femoral neck. In *Orthogeriatrics: Comprehensive Orthopaedic Care for the Elderly Patient*, ed. R.J. Newman. pp. 138–58. Oxford: Butterworth Heinemann.

SUTHERLAND, F.R., TEMPLE, W.J., SNODGRASS, T. *et al.* (1989). Predicting the outcome of exploratory laparotomy in ICU patients with sepsis or organ failure. *J. Trauma*, **29**, 152–7.

VAN AALST, J.A., MORRIS, J.A., YATES, H.K. *et al.* (1991). Severely injured geriatric patients return to independent living: a study of factors influencing function and independence. *J. Trauma*, **31**, 1096–102.

VERSLUYSEN, M. (1986). How elderly patients with femoral neck fractures develop pressure sores. *Br. Med. J.*, **292**, 1311–13.

WARNES, A.M. (1992). Demographic processes and health forecasts. In *Orthogeriatrics: Comprehensive Orthopaedic Care for the Elderly Patient*, ed. R.J. Newman. pp. 1–12. Oxford: Butterworth Heinemann.

WILLIAMS, M., LAMBERT, M., MILLINGTON, H. *et al.* (1992). Social and functional impact on minor fractures in elderly people. *Br. Med. J.*, **304**, 447.

D: Rape, sexual assault and female genital injuries

P. NASH

Accident and Emergency Department, Neath General Hospital, Neath, UK

RAPE AND SEXUAL ASSAULT

Introduction

Rape is a violent crime characterized by intercourse with vaginal penetration, with or without ejaculation, without the woman's consent. Consent to intercourse can be negated by force, fear or fraud. The legal criteria for rape are shown in Table 1. Violation of a man or woman by buggery or fellatio are tried as different forms of sexual assault (The Sexual Offence Act (Amendment) 1976). A recent legal precedent has allowed the crime of rape within marriage to be recognized.

The true incidence of rape is unknown. Crime statistics represent only the tip of the iceberg as many women do not report the crime of rape to the police. However, a woman who has been raped may present to a hospital or to her general practitioner immediately after the assault, or at any time up to several years later. Medical personnel must therefore have an understanding of the medical, legal and psychological aspects of care of the woman who has been raped. She may require treatment of injuries sustained at the time of the assault, screening for sexually transmitted diseases, contraception or counselling and psychological support. A multidisciplinary approach to the rape patient in specially planned sexual assault centres has been advocated (Duddle, 1985).

Contrary to the myth that rape occurs to 'other

Table 1. *Legal criteria for rape*

A man commits rape if:	he has unlawful sexual intercourse with a woman who at the time of that intercourse does not consent to it
	and at that time he knows that she does not consent to the intercourse or he is reckless as to whether she consents to it

people', in a dark alley and at the hands of a stranger, sexual assault crosses all boundaries of class and culture. Rape was perpetrated by an acquaintance in 21 of 51 cases in one study from Belfast (Bownes *et al.*, 1991). Acquaintance rapes were associated with significantly more prior contact in a social setting, verbal abuse during the rape and verbal interaction following the rape than stranger assaults. By comparison, significantly more of the stranger rapists initially encountered their victim in an outdoor setting and displayed a weapon. As a result, proportionately more of the stranger-rape victims had serious injuries.

Clinical assessment

Because rape is a violent crime the woman may have life-threatening injuries. The first priority is therefore to resuscitate the woman and save her life. Non-genital injuries occur in 20–50% of rapes (Geist, 1988). Fortunately, the majority are minor injuries such as abrasions, contusions, haematomas or lacerations. The commonest anatomical sites for injury are the face, head and neck (50%), extremities (33%) and trunk (15%). Less than 1% of rape patients have injuries for which they require hospital admission. Such injuries include multiple trauma, major fractures, major lacerations and stab wounds.

If there is no serious physical injury the woman should be assessed in privacy, preferably by a female doctor. She should be offered the opportunity to report her case to the police, but medical confidentiality must be respected if she does not wish police involvement. The collection of forensic samples must only be undertaken by a doctor who is a trained forensic medical examiner (police surgeon). Some hospital doctors are trained as forensic medical examiners and have facilities to deal with rape patients within their hospital. If the woman is initially reluctant to report to the police, forensic evidence can be taken with her consent by such a doctor and stored for several weeks while she considers police involvement. Medical personnel should be aware that valuable forensic evidence may be lost if the patient is allowed to wash, clean her teeth, eat, drink or undress while she is waiting to be seen by the police surgeon.

Before commencing forensic medical examination the police surgeon must obtain the patient's consent, stressing that any information given may be made available to the police.

History

The aims of taking the history from the patient are to establish rapport, to clarify details of the attack which help in finding physical signs consistent with the mechanisms of injury, and to guide the examining police surgeon in the collection of forensic samples.

The history of the alleged assault starts with events leading up to the attack including whether the patient has taken any drugs or alcohol. Details of the attack should include when and where it took place, and whether weapons, force or physical restraints (gags, ligatures) were used. Note should be made of whether the patient's clothing was damaged or stained by the assailant's body fluids. It is important to ascertain whether vaginal, anal or oral intercourse occurred, and whether the assailant(s) ejaculated or wore a condom. The assailant may have left saliva on the patient's skin if she was licked, bitten or sucked. If the woman was menstruating, her sanitary towel or tampon may be contaminated with semen. She may have inflicted injury on the assailant or contaminated his clothing if she was bleeding.

Following the attack it is important to note whether the woman washed herself or changed her clothes. She may have cleaned her teeth or taken oral fluids including alcohol. She may also have had subsequent intercourse.

In addition to the history of the attack, the woman's recent sexual, menstrual and contraceptive history should be noted.

Examination

Ordinarily a female police officer assists the police surgeon during the forensic medical examination.

- The patient is asked to undress whilst standing on a large piece of paper which collects any trace evidence which may fall from her clothes (Lacey, 1991). The clothes are retained for forensic examination, each item being individually bagged and labelled by the accompanying female police officer.
- General physical examination includes identification of wounds, bruises and other evidence of physical injury. The assistance of a police photographer is useful in the documentation of any such injuries. Loose fibres or debris relating to the scene of the crime found on the patient's skin should be preserved as evidence.
- If there is a history of oral penetration there may be signs of petechial bruising inside the mouth. Swabs

should be taken from the outer and inner aspects of the lips and gums.

- Examination with a Wood's light may show fluorescence at the site of saliva and semen stains. Any such stains should be swabbed.
- The perineum should be examined for signs of external injury and bleeding. Genital injury occurs in 5–25% of rape cases, being most common in young girls and older women (Geist, 1988). If there is matting of the pubic hair, combings are taken. Swabs of the external genitalia are taken and speculum examination is performed to enable high vaginal or cervical swabs to be taken. Anal intercourse should be suspected and anal swabs taken if there is anal spasm, perianal erythema or haematoma.
- Fingernail clippings are taken if circumstances suggest that blood or fibres are present.
- Control samples of blood and saliva are taken from the patient. If pubic hair samples were taken as evidence, control specimens are plucked from the head and pubic regions. Blood and urine samples may be taken for estimation of drug and alcohol levels.

Table 2 shows a check list of samples which can be taken for forensic examination.

Interpretation of forensic samples

When interpreting the results of forensic swabs for spermatozoa it is important to know both the time after the assault and the site from which the swabs have been taken. Following oral intercourse spermatozoa persist in the mouth for only 16 h (Keating, 1988a). If the woman has eaten, had oral fluids, cleaned her teeth

Table 2. *Forensic sample checklist*

- Patient's clothing
- Sheet of paper on which she undresses
- Loose debris found on skin
- Swabs of skin contaminated with assailant's body fluids
- Oral swabs
- Anal swab (if history of anal intercourse)
- Perineal swab
- External vaginal swab
- High vaginal swab (cervical swab if >48 h since assault)
- Hair combings
- Nail clippings
- Patient controls – blood, saliva and hair

or used a mouth wash, spermatozoa may be lost. Spermatozoa can be found on swabs taken up to 46 h after anal intercourse. By comparison, spermatozoa persist for up to 6 days in the high vagina and have been found up to 10 days postassault on cervical swabs. The patient's clothing is extremely useful as forensic evidence because spermatozoa can be identified on contaminated clothing until the item is washed, which may be weeks or months after the assault.

Specimens of semen, seminal fluid and saliva are subject to DNA fingerprinting and ABO secretor status, the former providing an almost unique marker of the assailant (Honma *et al.*, 1989). In addition to being used as evidence in individual cases, the results of such investigations, together with the modus operandi and details of the persons involved, are held on a computerized Sexual Assault Index which facilitates identification of serial rapes by the same assailant.

Hairs are considered of little value as evidence by forensic scientists because discrimination of samples is often difficult. Hair evidence is most likely to be of value when victim and assailant are of different races or where hair dyes have been used (Keating, 1988b). Fibres can prove useful in linking the victim or assailant with the scene of the crime.

Contraception

If the woman is of child-bearing age she may require postcoital contraception (see Chapter 59). If intercourse occurred within 72 h previously and there are no contraindications, a postcoital pill (e.g. Eugyon-50 two tablets stat followed by two tablets 12 h later) may be given. Alternatively, an intrauterine contraceptive device may be inserted up to 5 days after the assault. The patient should be followed up by her general practitioner to ensure that pregnancy has not ensued. On occasion it may be necessary for the patient to be referred for termination of pregnancy. The fetus may provide useful genetic evidence concerning the assailant.

Screening for sexually transmitted diseases

Women who are raped are at risk of contracting sexually transmitted diseases (STD), although some women may already be infected at the time of the rape. Police surgeons do not screen for STD immediately following the assault as evidence of infection may be used in court to discredit the victim. The women should be referred to the genitourinary medicine clinic for screening

Table 3. *Sexually transmitted disease screen checklist*

- Gram stain of genital discharge
- Cultures for *Neisseria gonorrhoeae* and *Chlamydia trachomatis* (oral, vaginal, anal and urethral)
- Wet preparation for *Trichomonas*
- Culture of lesions for Herpes simplex
- Syphilis serology
- Frozen serum

approximately 1 week after the attack to allow incubation of infection. Table 3 shows a list of samples that should be taken for STD screening (Glaser, 1986). Antibiotic prophylaxis is not recommended prior to screening, but a suitable regimen after samples have been taken would be ciprofloxacin 500 mg orally followed by a 1-week course of either oxytetracycline or erythromycin 500 mg four times daily (Lacey, 1991). The reported prevalence rates for STD following rape range from 3.9% to 56%. *Trichomonas* is found in 6–18% of women, *Chlamydia* in 5–13% and *Neisseria gonorrhoeae* in 2.2–13.3%. By contrast, positive syphilis serology is uncommon, occurring in less than 3% of cases (Forster, 1992).

Many women who have been raped are concerned about contracting HIV (human immunodeficiency virus) infection. Although the risks are low, four patients were found to be HIV positive following rape (Clayton *et al.*, 1991). It is therefore appropriate that women who have been raped are counselled about HIV infection and offered screening at the time of initial assessment, and 3 months after the assault for seroconversion.

Psychological aspects

Following rape, women experience profound psychological reactions characterized by the rape trauma syndrome (Burgess & Holstrom, 1974). In the first 6 weeks there is an immediate reaction with initial shock, disbelief and denial, followed by guilt and self-blame. Some victims express intense feelings of anger, fear, anxiety, humiliation and helplessness; others remain calm and composed with little outward display of emotion. Physical symptoms including headaches, nausea, abdominal and genital pain may occur. Some patients experience dissociation, during which they feel as though they are outside their body watching the assault. The subsequent reorganization phase lasts from 6 weeks to 6 months after the assault. During this period the patient may make changes in lifestyle, may experience mood swings, may

develop phobias and experience sleep disturbance in addition to numerous somatic complaints.

There are some individuals who never resolve the rape trauma syndrome and go on to develop post-traumatic stress disorder.

Psychological support for the patient should begin at her initial presentation. An unbiased, non-judgemental approach to the patient minimizes her feelings of self-blame (Beebe, 1991). The doctor should discuss the common psychological sequelae of rape and offer referral for counselling, either to hospital psychologists or to other agencies such as the local victim support scheme or rape crisis centre.

GENITAL TRAUMA

Vulval trauma

Vulval trauma may occur as a result of sexual assault, including the insertion of foreign bodies (e.g. bottles) into the vagina with resultant perineal tears. Falls astride hard objects such as bicycle crossbars also cause perineal trauma (Sill, 1987). Initial management of vulval haematomas includes bed rest, application of cold packs and hot sitz baths to reduce oedema. Indications for surgical evacuation of a haematoma and ligation of bleeding vessels include increasing size of the haematoma with extension into the perineum or lower abdomen, and urethral obstruction by the haematoma.

Vaginal trauma

Vaginal lacerations may result from normal coital activity, especially at the time of first intercourse and during the months following childbirth, or may occur as a result of rape or instrumentation with foreign bodies (Geist, 1988). Lower vaginal lacerations are more common in virgin women. Tears to the hymen tend to be posterior and associated with only minor bleeding and pain. Occasionally the hymeneal laceration extends into the perineal body and rectum producing significant haemorrhage and necessitating surgical repair. Upper vaginal lacerations are caused by penile thrust or foreign bodies. The posterior fornix is most commonly affected. Eighty per cent of patients present with vaginal bleeding and 10% experience pain. Profuse vaginal bleeding occurs in half of these patients. Occasionally vaginal lacerations extend into the peritoneum. Treatment consists of temporary control of haemorrhage with moist vaginal packs followed by surgical repair. Transfusion may be required.

Because patients may conceal a history of trauma, the diagnosis should be considered in any woman with unexplained vaginal bleeding, and excluded only after thorough speculum examination.

Uterine trauma

Because the uterus comprises a thick muscular wall and is well protected by the pelvis, blunt trauma to the non-pregnant uterus is unusual, but it may accompany pelvic fractures. Uterine perforation may occur following instrumentation (e.g. 'back-street' abortion). Patients present with vaginal haemorrhage and may have signs of peritonitis. Resuscitation followed by gynaecological referral for laparotomy is indicated.

Bibliography

BEEBE, D. K. (1991). Initial assessment of the rape victim. *J. Miss. State Med. Assoc.*, **32**, 403–6.

BOWNES, I.T., O'GORMAN, E. & SAYERS, A. (1991). Rape – a comparison of stranger and acquaintance assaults. *Med. Sci. Law*, **31**, 102–9.

BURGESS, A.W. & HOLMSTROM, L.L. (1974). Rape trauma syndrome. *Am. J. Psychiatry*, **131**, 981–6.

CLAYDON, E., MURPHY, S., OSBORNE, E.M. *et al.* (1991). Rape and HIV. *Int. J. STD, AIDS*, **2**, 200–1.

DUDDLE, M. (1985). The need for sexual assault centres in the United Kingdom. *Br. Med. J.*, **290**, 771–3.

FORSTER, G. (1992). Rape and sexually transmitted disease. *Br. J. Hosp. Med.*, **47**, 94–5.

GEIST, R.F. (1988). Sexually related trauma. *Emerg. Med. Clin. North Am.*, **6**, 439–66.

GLASER, J.B. (1986). Sexually transmitted diseases in victims of sexual assault. *N. Engl. J. Med.*, **315**, 625–7.

HONMA, M., YOSHI, T., ISHIYAMA, I. *et al.* (1989). Individual identification from semen by the deoxyribonucleic acid (DNA) fingerprint technique. *J. Forensic. Sci.*, **34**, 222–7.

KEATING, S.M. (1988a). The laboratory's approach to sexual assault cases. Part 1: Sources of information and acts of intercourse. *J. Forensic. Sci. Soc.*, **28**, 35–47.

KEATING, S.M. (1988b). The laboratory's approach to sexual assault cases. Part 2: Demonstration of the potential offender. *J. Forens. Sci. Soc.*, **28**, 99–110.

LACEY, H. (1991). Rape, the law and medical practitioners. *Br. J. Sexual Med.*, **18**, 89–91.

SILL, P.R. (1987). Non-obstetric genital tract trauma in Port Moresby, Papua New Guinea. *Aust. N.Z. J. Obstet. Gynaecol.*, **27**, 164–5.

34 Burns and Scalds

J. M. RYAN

Accident and Emergency Directorate, University College Hospital, London, UK

Chapter plan

Introduction
Mechanisms
Pathophysiology
Management

INTRODUCTION

Burn and scald injury is common and management often less than adequate. This is particularly true of early management where care is usually undertaken by inexperienced and often fatigued medical staff working in the accident and emergency (A&E) room. The objective in this chapter is to provide a guide and reference source for those whose are likely to be involved in the early management of a burn or scald victim.

The exact incidence of burn injury in the UK is not known. It is probable that the majority are treated in the home, the workplace and by the general practitioner or practice nurse. However, burns and scalds result in over 10 000 hospital admissions each year, and over 600 patients die. A larger number are managed in the A&E department on an out-patient basis.

Two groups are particularly at risk:

- Children under the age of 5 years, typically presenting with scald injury.
- The elderly, presenting with burns of mixed aetiology.

The possibility of non-accidental injury should be considered in children under the age of 3 years. Scalds involving the buttocks or lower limbs where the history is indifferent or inconsistent should arouse particular suspicion. In young adults who are less at risk (see Chapter 61), flame burns predominate. Susceptible groups are patients with epilepsy, drug addicts and alcoholics.

These factors should be considered in all unconscious burn or scald victims.

MECHANISMS

Injury is nearly always accidental and preventable, and in civilian practice it usually involves an individual or small group. In war, terrorist incidents and natural disasters, casualties may present in large numbers.

Clearly defined mechanisms may be described, including flame, liquid, flash, electrical or chemical injury. This chapter is concerned with flame and liquid injury; others deal with flash, electrical and chemical injury (see Chapters 35 and 36).

Flame

Flame burn results from the ignition of clothing or items in the environment (e.g. furniture) and may occur in domestic or industrial settings. Injury is usually accidental but may be associated with a suicide or murder attempt. Recent legislation concerning inflammable materials in night attire and domestic furniture has had some effect in reducing the incidence and severity of injury.

Flame injury taking place in a closed environment (house or factory) is usually complicated by inhalation of smoke or toxic gases and mortality is considerably increased. The injury is usually patchy with wide variations in extent and depth.

Liquid

Scald injuries are associated with spillage or immersion. Injury due to spillage varies in extent and depth and is usually accidental. Immersion injury is commonly seen in young children and may be deliberate – a high index of suspicion is warranted. In general, injury is severe, resulting in areas of deep dermal and full thickness scald. Deliberate immersion is associated with high morbidity and significant mortality.

Steam

A specialized and potentially disastrous form of scald injury results from exposure in a closed space to superheated steam – a boiler room explosion, for example. Inhalation of superheated steam is particularly dangerous and may result in tracheobronchial burns and disruption of respiratory epithelium.

PATHOPHYSIOLOGY

Local features

Burn and scald injury results in coagulative necrosis of variable depth involving tissues in immediate contact with the flame or hot liquid. A zone of stasis lies lateral and deep to the area of necrosis and outside this is an area of hyperaemia. Changes in capillary permeability occur immediately resulting in a shift from plasma to interstitial fluid; severe oedema is therefore a very early clinical sign.

Tissues damaged by flame or hot liquid are notoriously unstable – the zone of stasis is particularly vulnerable in the early hours following injury. In the presence of tissue hypoxia and/or infection, it may become necrotic. Thus a deep dermal burn (see below) may readily change to a full thickness burn if management is inadequate in the immediate postinjury period.

Burn classification

Burns and scalds are classified according to the depth of the zone of coagulative necrosis. They may be described as partial or full thickness. Partial thickness burns and scalds are further subdivided into two groups: superficial or deep dermal.

- Superficial dermal (or superficial partial thickness) injuries are red, warm, tender, oedematous and wet. Blistering of the skin is characteristic and the blisters are readily disrupted (Fig. 1). Pain and hypersensitivity to touch and pinprick are marked features.
- Deep dermal (or deep partial thickness) injuries exhibit a necrotic superficial epidermis but deeper structures such as hair follicles and sweat glands remain viable (Fig. 2). Deep pressure sensation and a blunted

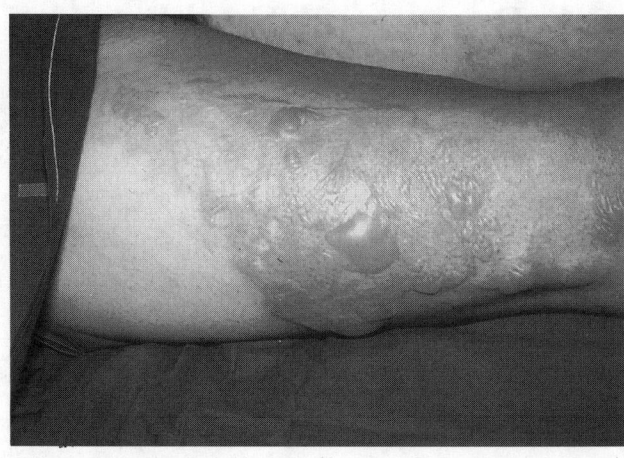

Fig. 1. Superficial burn exhibiting areas of redness and blistering. (Courtesy of Department of Military Surgery, RAM College.)

awareness of pin-prick is usually retained. Recovery without grafting is possible provided early measures to combat hypovolaemic shock and wound infection are adequate.

- Full thickness injuries are typically charred or pearly white. Thrombosed vessels may be evident and the wound is totally anaesthetic (Fig. 3). Pain is not a feature but acute anxiety is invariable.

Careful examination (see below) will reveal superficial, deep dermal and full thickness areas to a variable extent in most victims. It is important to distinguish them.

General Features

Burn or scald injury results in a systemic illness with notable clinical features and consequences.

Airway and breathing

Injury due to flame or liquid, including steam, may result in marked oedema of the upper airway of rapid onset. The possibility of such injury must always be borne in mind – the mouth and oropharynx should be carefully and repeatedly examined.

Injury to the lower airway or chest wall may result in respiratory failure. Mechanisms include direct burns of the respiratory mucosa, inhalation of smoke or other noxious agents, or splinting of the chest by a full thickness circumferential burn. Respiratory failure may also supervene early as a result of poorly managed hypovolaemic shock, or it may arise later secondary to infection or multiple organ failure. The cardinal clinical feature is an altered conscious level.

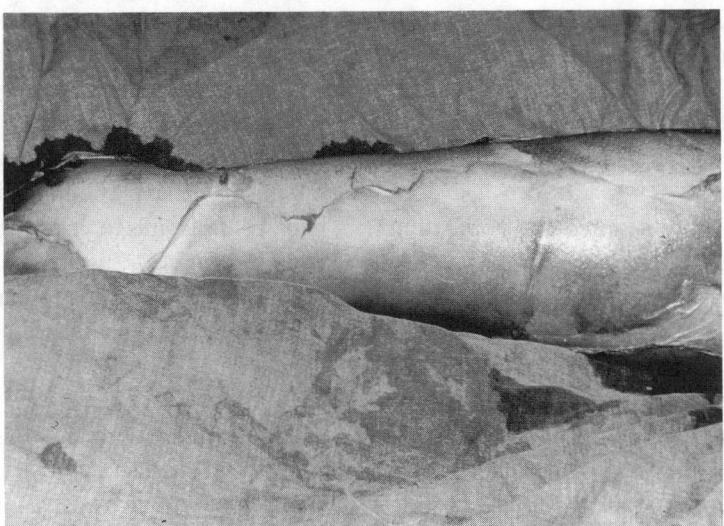

Fig. 2. Deep dermal burn exhibiting areas of necrosis interspersed with areas of redness and blistering. (Courtesy of Department of Military Surgery, RAM College.)

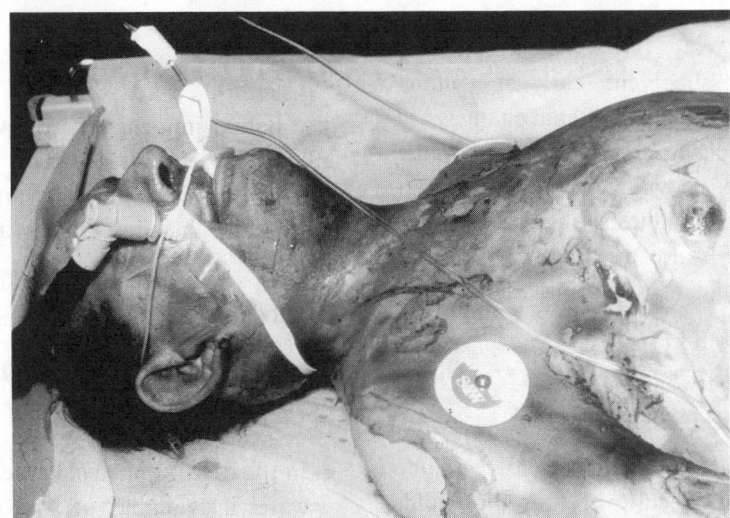

Fig. 3. Typical appearance of a full thickness burn. (Courtesy of Department of Military Surgery, RAM College.)

Careful attention must be paid to the history, physical examination and selective investigations. A chest X-ray and serial arterial blood gas analysis are required early in the resuscitation phase. Respiratory failure is characterized by a persistently low PO_2 (<8.0 kPa despite adequate oxygen therapy) and high PCO_2 (>5.5 kPa). Other features of impending respiratory failure are:

- Stridor.
- Inability to speak.
- Obvious respiratory distress.
- Respiratory rate greater than 40 (adult).
- Tachycardia.

Circulation

The pathophysiological event of importance is shock which is a state of inadequate tissue/organ perfusion. The concept of shock has already been discussed (Chapter 6). Although hypovolaemic shock is characteristic, burn and scald victims may have other shock-inducing injuries (e.g. myocardial contusion/tamponade or spinal injury) and these should be considered. The onset and severity of burn/scald hypovolaemia will be determined by site, extent and depth of the wound, the delay before instituting treatment, and the adequacy of such treatment.

Hypovolaemic shock resulting from burns or scalds has unique features:

- Immediate and generalized capillary leakage of molecules up to a molecular weight of 250 000 results in a plasma to interstitial fluid shift; leakage is maximal during the first 8 h and lasts for about 48 h.
- Haemolysis of red cells in the injured area as a result of direct thermal injury.
- Generalized fragility of the entire red cell population with a reduced lifespan.
- Changes in the osmotic gradient and obstruction of lymphatics by coagulated proteins, resulting in loss of utilizable proteins and water.
- Impaired tissue perfusion and direct thermal injury to cells leads to tissue hypoxia, impairment of the sodium pump, metabolic acidosis and a sodium deficit.

All of the above lead to a progressive fall in plasma volume which, if untreated, results in circulatory collapse and renal shutdown.

Renal sequelae

Acute renal failure will supervene early if volume replacement is delayed or inadequate. Renal changes are initially reversible but tubular necrosis follows if volume replacement continues to be withheld. The principal indicator of impending renal failure is oliguria.

Late-onset renal failure is also a feature of burn and scald injury and may result from systemic infection or disseminated intravascular coagulopathy.

Nutritional and metabolic consequences

A burn or scald is a catabolic insult. Extensive injury may raise the basal metabolic rate two- or three-fold. Glycogen stores are mobilized. Energy requirements are great and daily calorific needs in excess of 2000 kcal per m^2 are typical. Oral or enteral administration of a high-carbohydrate, high-protein and high-fat diet is indicated. Parenteral nutrition via a centrally placed long venous catheter imposes an unacceptable risk of septicaemia and is best avoided. Clinical signs of increased basal metabolic rate include a rise in core temperature and an increased cardiac output.

Wound and systemic infection

The exposed surface of a partial or full thickness burn is a perfect pabulum for bacterial contamination and subsequent wound infection. Research by Pruitt and others has shown that when the bacterial density of a burn exceeds 10^5 organisms per gram of tissue, systemic invasion takes place leading to septicaemia. Growth and invasion is further enhanced by immune deficiency. White cell function is impaired, IgC and complement levels fall and T cell function is diminished. A wide range of organisms behave as opportunistic pathogens and many may be resistant to local and systemic antibacterials. Colonization by multiresistant nosocomial organisms may result from early and inappropriate use of systemic broad-spectrum agents (see below).

Gastrointestinal features

Stress-related erosive gastritis and frank duodenal ulceration are seen increasingly in burn centres. Distal small bowel and colonic ulceration with haemorrhage and perforation have also been reported, typically in late or neglected burns. Ileus, cholecystitis and pancreatitis occur late in association with infection.

MANAGEMENT

The period immediately following burn or scald injury is critical; measures taken during this period will profoundly affect outcome and are determined by the setting and the equipment available.

Prehospital setting

Stop the burning / scalding process – send for assistance.

- In the case of *flame injury*, extinguish by dousing with water if available, or by rolling or wrapping in any material to hand.
- In the case of *scald injury*, removal of clothing soaked in hot liquid may have some effect on the extent and depth of injury.
- In *both instances*, the aim is to halt injury.
- Time is critical – an early call for skilled help is vital and is easily forgotten.
- Commence immediate assessment using a system – the ATLS approach is particularly recommended (see Chapter 5).

Airway

The absence of advanced equipment in the prehospital setting does not preclude adequate airway maintenance. Speak to the victim – a clear, articulate response is evidence *at that moment* of a clear airway, reasonable ventilation and the presence of at least 50% of circulating blood volume. Failure to respond demands immediate airway attention. Open the airway using the chin lift or jaw thrust manoeuvres. Check inside the mouth – look for burn swelling/oedema, blood or mucus, vomitus or loose teeth. Note particularly any evidence of upper airway burn.

Breathing

Burn or scald victims may have other injuries. Check neck veins and the position of the trachea to rule out a tension pneumothorax, for example. Assess ventilation – check rate and depth. Expired air resuscitation will be required if the patient is not breathing spontaneously. Remember, a full thickness circumferential burn of the chest will impede respiration and result in progressive hypoxia. Early transfer to hospital for escharotomy is essential (see early hospital phase, below).

Circulation

Assess again the level of consciousness. Note the colour in an uninjured area and check capillary refill if possible. Note the rate and quality of a central arterial pulse. Such observations may be critical in later management.

Assess rapidly for other sites of volume loss – in particular, the abdomen, pelvis and limbs.

Establish intravenous lines.

Disability (neurological)

A rapid qualitative assessment of the neurological state can be carried out by assessing pupils and level of consciousness using the AVPU method.

The AVPU method of characterizing level of consciousness

A   Alert
V   Responds to voice
P   Responds to pain
U   Unresponsive

Exposure – environment and history

Depending on environment (location/season/ambient temperature) the victim should ideally be undressed in preparation for a full assessment. In most instances this is best left until arrival in the hospital setting.

The injury environment should be noted and a history obtained. The time and place of injury must be noted. The location may be critical – indoors or outdoors, domestic or industrial? Such information may increase the likelihood of additional injury (e.g. jumping from a building to escape flames) or may point to a risk of inhalation or chemical injury.

Transfer to hospital

The medical attendant should ideally accompany the victim. If this is not possible, paramedics should be fully briefed on all prehospital measures taken and the relevant history. In general, a burn/scald victim is best served by an early, supervised transfer to hospital.

Early hospital phase – primary survey and resuscitation

The sequence is similar to that in the prehospital setting. The steps taken should be repeated and any changes noted, particularly in the vital signs. Start with the primary survey and resuscitate concurrently. Use the A, B, C, D, E system to identify immediately life-threatening injuries.

The A, B, C, D, E system

A   Airway (with cervical spine protection)
B   Breathing
C   Circulation and volume replacement
D   Disability (neurological assessment)
E   Exposure

TECHNIQUES

- Start by stopping the burning process if this has not already been done.

Airway [A]

- The upper airway is very susceptible.
- With good light, check the inside of the mouth for evidence of direct injury.
- Look for mucosal burns, blistering or carbon deposits.
- Listen for stridor or hoarseness.
- Check for facial burns, singeing of eyebrows/lashes or nasal hairs (Fig. 4).

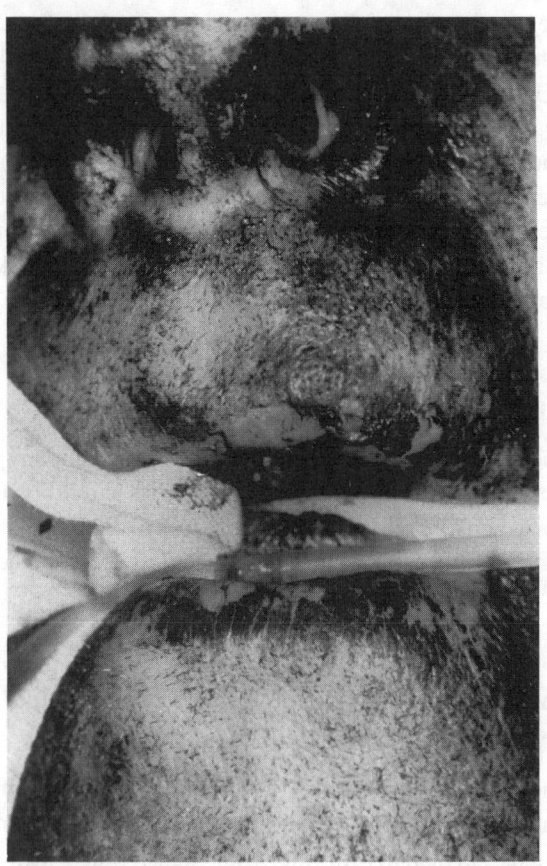

Fig. 4. Carbon deposits around the mouth and nose indicating burn injury to the airway. (Courtesy of Department of Military Surgery, RAM College.)

- Note the history – if it points to the likelihood of airway burn or inhalation, assume this is present even in the absence of clinical signs.
- If the airway is thought to be jeopardized, secure it.
- Consider the need for early endotracheal intubation.
- Establish an oropharyngeal or nasopharyngeal airway and call for skilled anaesthetic assistance.
- Using a mask with a reservoir device, give high concentrations of oxygen (10–12 litres min^{-1}).
- Remember – an intact airway does not guarantee adequate ventilation.

Breathing [B]

- Check the neck veins and tracheal position.
- Expose the chest fully, back and front.
- Look for full thickness, circumferential burns as these will impede respiration.
- If present, immediate escharotomy is required (see below) (Fig. 5).
- Assess chest movement and note the rate and depth of respirations.

- Listen to all areas of chest – take particular note of crepitations which may indicate pulmonary injury.

Circulation and volume replacement [C]

- Assessment of the circulation can be difficult in the severely burned or scalded patient.
- The principal tasks are to gain access to the circulation and to obtain a crude assessment of burn size.
- Children with burns/scalds of more than 10% and adults with injuries exceeding 15% of body surface area *must* be resuscitated with intravenous fluids.
- Oral resuscitation is usually appropriate for smaller, superficial burns.
- Two large bore cannulae are sited percutaneously or by cutting down onto a peripheral vessel – do not hesitate to cut through injured areas.
- Central access should be avoided because of the risk of sepsis.
- Blood is withdrawn for baseline investigations and fluid replacement commenced with Hartmann's solution.
- Carry out a rapid assessment of burn size; use the 'rule of nines' or a paediatric modification for children (Fig. 6) This is an initial assessment only – during the secondary survey a more comprehensive method is used to accurately estimate extent and depth.
- For significant burns or scalds in the adult (>15%), 2 litres of crystalloid should be infused rapidly.
- For significant burns/scalds in the child (>10%), the initial fluid challenge is calculated from the formula: 20 ml kg^{-1} body weight.
- The concern in this phase is to *commence* fluid resuscitation pending full assessment and estimation of the exact volumes required.

Disability (neurological assessment) [D]

- A rapid assessment of pupil size and conscious level is all that is required now.
- Use the AVPU method.

Exposure [E]

- Fully undress the casualty in appropriate surroundings.

Resuscitation measures

It is axiomatic that life-threatening conditions are treated as they are found. Therefore, the primary survey and resuscitation phases run concurrently.

Supplemental high-flow oxygen is instituted via a mask–reservoir device. If inhalation/lung injury was noted during the primary survey, tracheal intubation

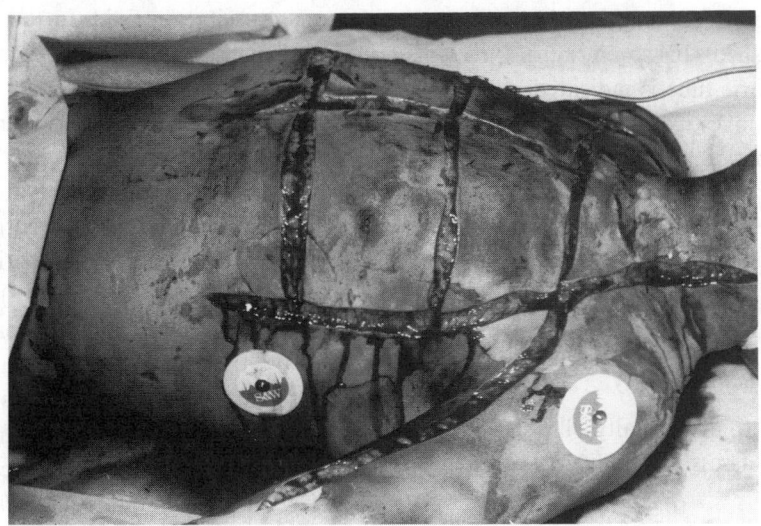

Fig. 5. Circumferential full thickness burn of chest. The appearance following escharotomy. (Courtesy of Department of Military Surgery, RAM College.)

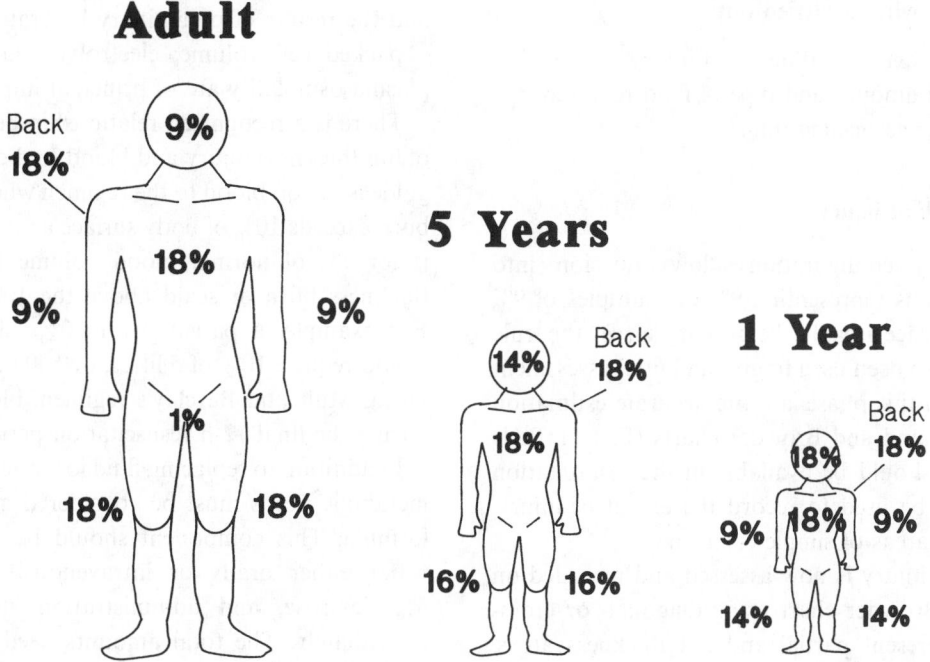

Fig. 6. The 'rule of nines' for adults and its modification for infants and children. Note that the surface area of the head decreases with age and the surface area of the lower limbs increases.

and assisted ventilation should have been established. If not, a surgical airway (i.e. surgical cricothyrotomy) may be needed.

Emergency escharotomy may also be performed as a resuscitation measure. Initial circulatory support should consist of warmed Hartmann's solution infused rapidly pending the institution of a planned regimen.

Quantitative assessments of vital signs are started as soon as possible and include pulse, respiratory rate, pulse pressure, blood pressure and level of consciousness. Values should be recorded, timed and dated.

A urinary catheter should be sited and hourly measurements commenced. The aim is to achieve a urinary output of $50 \, \text{ml h}^{-1}$ in the adult and older child, and $1 \, \text{ml kg}^{-1} \text{h}^{-1}$ in children under 30 kg. Urinary output is one of the best early indicators of the efficiency of fluid resuscitation after injury. Core temperature monitoring should also be established. In severe burns, ileus is common and a nasogastric tube is indicated.

Important baseline investigations should also be performed during this period. These include:

- Haemoglobin.
- Packed cell volume.
- Grouping and saving serum for later cross-match.
- Arterial blood gases, electrolytes and carboxyhaemoglobin estimation. These tests will be repeated later. An early chest X-ray is mandatory.

The immediate threat to the casualty's life should now be over. A more detailed assessment may now commence.

Secondary survey

This is a phase of detailed burn/scald assessment and continuing stabilization and monitoring.

The following will be carried out:

- Assessment of extent and depth of injury.
- Assessment of amount and type of fluid required.
- Assessment for associated injuries.

Extent and depth of injury

The adult body configuration allows division into anatomical regions representing 9% or multiples of 9% of total body surface area. In the primary survey the 'rule of nines' will have been used to give an initial assessment of injury size. In this phase, a more accurate estimation is made using Lund and Browder charts (Fig. 7). Pads of these charts should be available in the resuscitation room and may be used to record the extent of injury. Do not include areas of simple erythema.

The depth of injury is now assessed and recorded on the Lund and Browder chart using diagonal- or cross-hatching to represent partial and full thickness areas. When tested with a pin, wet, blistered and sensitive areas are partial thickness injuries; white areas are deep dermal if sensation is present or full thickness if not.

All charts *must* be named, timed and dated. This is vital if dealing with more than one victim.

Calculation of fluid loss and replacement needs

There is still no consensus on the ideal fluid for burn/scald resuscitation. The essential requirements are electrolyte, colloid and water. A myriad of regimens exist. In the USA, considerable reliance is placed on electrolyte alone

as a resuscitation fluid. In the UK, most centres advise a regimen with a colloid component. The colloid in widespread use is human plasma protein fraction solution. This solution contains 4.5% human albumin and about 150 mmol $Na^+ l^{-1}$.

To calculate requirements, use a formula dictated by the local regional burns centre or a widely accepted formula. The most popular British formula is that devised by Muir and Barclay (Fig. 8). This predicts the total volume of plasma required over a 36-h period. However, unlike other formulae, the fluid requirements are calculated for short, successive resuscitation periods of 4, 4, 4, 6, 6 and 12 h, which allows frequent reassessment and fine-tuning of the volumes required. The whole 36-h period begins *at the time of injury*, not at the time of admission or commencement of the regimen. Thus, in the first 4 h considerable catching up may be necessary. At the end of each resuscitation period, progress is assessed by reviewing the patient's clinical state, urinary output and the results of preliminary laboratory investigations – packed cell volume, electrolyte status, urinary and plasma osmolality are of principal importance.

There is a recognized relationship between the extent of full thickness injury and blood (red cell) loss. A useful guide is to add blood to the regimen when a full thickness burn exceeds 10% of body surface area. The requirement is for 1% of normal blood volume for each 1% full thickness burn or scald above the 10% starting point. For example, a patient with 20% full thickness burn would require 10% of 5 litres, or 500 ml of whole blood. Using Muir and Barclay's regimen, blood is best given during the final 12-h resuscitation period.

In addition to replacing fluid loss due to injury, normal metabolic needs must be considered and added to any formula. This component should be given as salt-free water either orally or intravenously in the form of 5% dextrose, and administration should commence immediately. The total amounts need to be calculated carefully and there will probably be a catching-up period. Urine output and insensible losses must be replaced – typical volumes will be of the order of 2–3 litres per day.

Finally, it must be emphasized that all formulae are, at best, guides to the actual volumes required. There is no substitute for close and frequent reassessments with adjustment in rate of infusion as clinically indicated.

Associated injury

Most patients with significant burns or scalds will be transferred to a regional burns centre once stabilized. It

CHART FOR ESTIMATING SEVERITY OF BURN WOUND

NAME_____WARD_____NUMBER_____DATE_____
AGE_____ ADMISSION WEIGHT_____

LUND AND BROWDER CHARTS

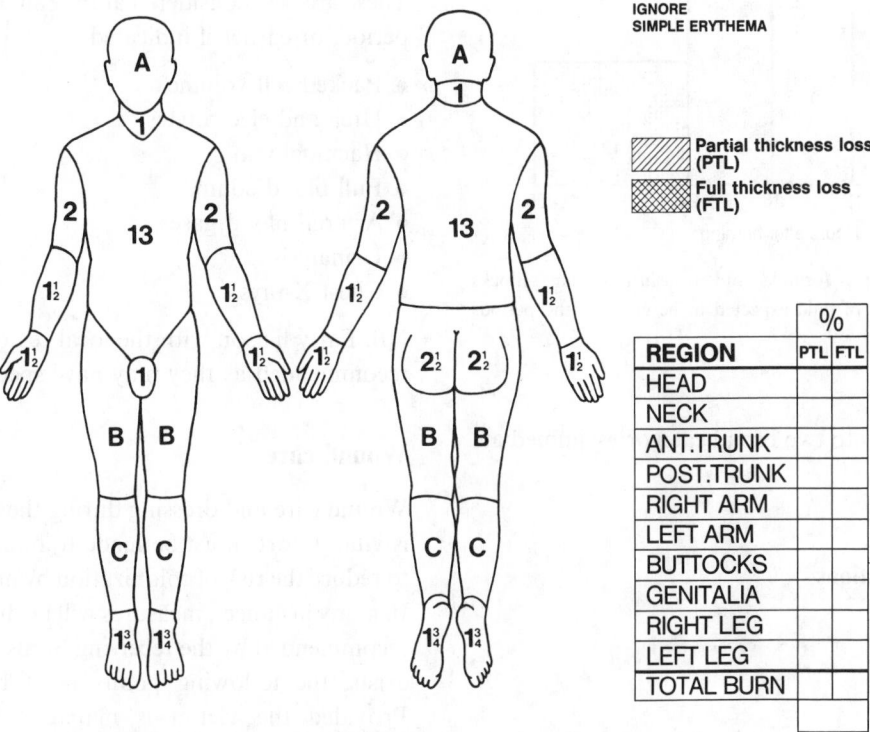

IGNORE
SIMPLE ERYTHEMA

Partial thickness loss (PTL)

Full thickness loss (FTL)

REGION	%	
	PTL	FTL
HEAD		
NECK		
ANT.TRUNK		
POST.TRUNK		
RIGHT ARM		
LEFT ARM		
BUTTOCKS		
GENITALIA		
RIGHT LEG		
LEFT LEG		
TOTAL BURN		

RELATIVE PERCENTAGE OF BODY SURFACE AREA AFFECTED BY GROWTH

AREA	AGE 0	1	5	10	15	ADULT
A=½ OF HEAD	9½	8½	6½	5½	4½	3½
B=½ OF ONE THIGH	2¾	3¼	4	4½	4½	4¾
C=½ OF ONE LEG	2½	2½	2¾	3	3¼	3½

Fig. 7. Lund and Browder charts. (Courtesy of Smith and Nephew Pharmaceuticals Ltd.)

is of particular importance that they are not transferred with an occult injury which may manifest itself during transfer or in the burns unit. A burn casualty with a quietly bleeding spleen will not, as a rule, do well in a regional burns centre!

In excluding additional injury, the history is vital – a victim who has jumped from a first or second floor window to escape flames will have additional injury until proven otherwise. If no history is available, the secondary survey must be a particularly thorough 'head-to-toe' examination of the fully undressed patient.

Finally, a burn or scald victim, no matter how severe the injury, must not be transferred until fully stabilized and should ideally be transferred with a medical escort (see below).

Investigation

This chapter deals with the resuscitation phase only; investigations more appropriate to definitive care are not included. Preliminary investigations have already been

Total percentage area of burn × weight in kg/2 = ml of fluid required by end of first four hour period
i.e. 0.5 ml/kg/% burn

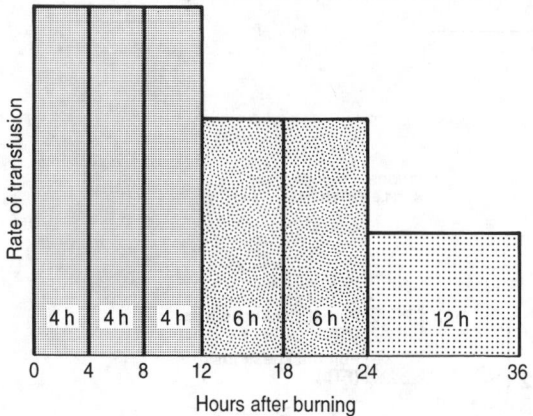

Fig. 8. Muir and Barclay formula and transfusion plan. Blocks represent equal volumes of fluid expected to be given in the periods shown.

mentioned and fall into two broad categories: immediate and periodic.

Immediate investigations

Blood

- Haemoglobin.
- Full blood count.
- Packed cell volume.
- Platelets.
- Urea and electrolytes.
- Glucose.
- Liver function tests.
- Clotting profile.
- Group and save serum for cross-match.
- Serum Ca^{2+}.
- Blood culture (neglected burn).
- Arterial blood gases and carboxyhaemoglobin (if smoke inhalation suspected).

Microbiology

- Culture swabs in nutrient medium from:
  - Burn area (multiple).
  - Throat.
  - Groins/axillae.
  - Perineum.
- Catheter specimen of urine for culture and sensitivity.

Radiology

- Chest X-ray.
- Other X-rays as appropriate if additional injury suspected.

Periodic investigations

These are best considered at the end of each resuscitation period, or earlier if indicated:

- Packed cell volume.
- Urea and electrolytes.
- Haemoglobin.
- Full blood count.
- Arterial blood gases.
- Urinalysis.
- Chest X-rays.

NB: Early liaison with the local regional burns centre is recommended as they may have special requirements.

Wound care

Wound care and dressing during the resuscitation phase is vital. Efforts must be made to minimize heat loss and to reduce the risk of colonization by microbial pathogens. In many instances, measures will be dictated by protocols recommended by the receiving burns unit. If no protocol exists, the following points must be borne in mind. Provided the victim is managed in a warm, clean environment it is best to leave the burn/scald exposed during the phase of initial assessment and resuscitation. If protection is considered necessary, sterile towels or cling film may be applied as these do not preclude later assessment or access by burns unit medical staff.

Definitive dressings or topical creams should not be applied in the resuscitation phase unless specifically recommended by burns unit medical staff. However, there are usually no contraindications to the use of sterile polythene bags for the hands and feet. These reduce pain, permit early movement and function and are in widespread use (Fig. 9).

There are no indications for deroofing burn blisters during the resuscitation phase – it is unnecessary, painful and increases the likelihood of microbial colonization and infection.

Antibiotic policy

Early use of systemic or local antimicrobial agents is controversial and should be avoided. Liaison with the

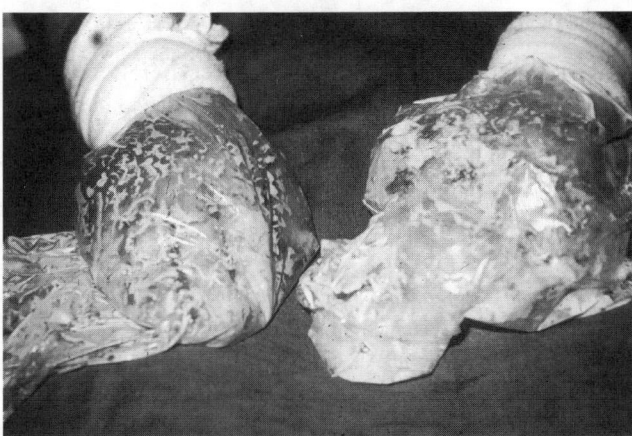

Fig. 9. 'Burn bag' in use for a hand injury. (Courtesy of Department of Military Surgery, RAM College.)

local regional burns centre to ascertain their antibiotic policy is recommended. There is no doubt that broad-spectrum systemic antibiotics, given indiscriminately, encourage colonization of the victim and the local environment by antibiotic-resistant opportunistic organisms including yeasts and fungi. However, there is a caveat. Early colonization of a burn with beta-haemolytic streptococci is life-threatening, particularly in a child. If a burn victim has a known or suspected sore throat, immediate microbiological examination is mandatory and if beta-haemolytic streptococcus is isolated, systemic benzylpenicillin or erythromycin should be administered.

There is also concern over the widespread use of topical antibiotics, particularly the use of 1% silver sulphadiazine cream in association with polythene hand and foot bags. Again, the regional centre should be contacted for advice.

There is no controversy concerning tetanus prophylaxis. The patient's status should be determined; if it is not known, prophylaxis should be commenced.

Monitoring

Most hospitals will have differing transfer criteria for burned patients and the amount of time spent in the A&E department or resuscitation room will vary. Medical staff in the A&E department have a responsibility to continue monitoring the victim until the patient arrives at the burns centre.

Non-invasive

Continuing assessment of the following is important:

- Airway patency.
- Respiratory rate and depth.

- Pulse.
- Blood pressure.
- Pulse pressure.
- Capillary refill.
- ECG (electrocardiogram).
- Urinary output (hourly).
- Level of consciousness (Glasgow Coma Scale/AVPU).
- Core and peripheral temperature.
- Radiological investigations as listed earlier.

Invasive

Assessment of the following may be considered:

- Central venous pressure line – risk of sepsis.
- Pulmonary wedge pressure – risk of sepsis.

Surgical intervention (injury to special sites)

Surgical intervention may be indicated;

- Immediately to save the casualty's life and limbs.
- *Early* to prevent life-, limb- or sight-threatening complications.
- *Late and planned.*

Medical staff in the A&E department are principally concerned with life- and limb-saving interventions. These include surgical access to the airway and escharotomy for circumferential burns to the torso or limbs. Early interventions (12 h onwards) may be indicated for burns to eyelids, hands, feet or genitalia, or following certain chemical burns. Although not carried out in the A&E department, resuscitation staff should be aware of indications for early intervention and should seek specialist help.

Admission to hospital – burns unit consultation and transfer

A&E personnel should, if possible, have protocols for admission to general wards and for transfer to specialized centres.

In the absence of firm protocols, the following guidelines are recommended:

- Admit the very young and the very old, even with small surface area injury (<10%). Both are vulnerable and prone to complications. Toxic shock syndrome in children may supervene after very modest burns and it carries a significant mortality.

- Admit all facial injuries, however minor – the risk of airway burn and inhalation injury is considerable.
- Admit all victims with burns or scalds to hands, feet, genitalia and perineum. Seek immediate consultation – many will be discharged quickly but this should be a specialist decision.
- Admit and get urgent specialist opinion on all eye and eyelid injuries – contractures can develop in under 24 hrs.
- Admit all full thickness burns or scalds of surface area greater than 3 cm^2.
- Children with burns/scalds greater than 10% and adults with greater than 15% require urgent intravenous fluid resuscitation and therefore hospital admission. If deep dermal or full thickness, liaise with burns unit and transfer depending on the extent or local policy.
- Admit pregnant patients, even those with apparently trivial injuries. Although the aetiology is unclear, burns and scalds in pregnancy are associated with an increased incidence of abortion or premature onset of labour.

Bibliography

AMERICAN COLLEGE OF SURGEONS COMMITTEE on TRAUMA (1993). Injuries due to burns and cold. *Advanced Trauma Life Support Manual*. pp. 245–59. Chicago: American College of Surgeons.

FRAME, J. D. & KELLY, D. A. (1992). Early management of burns. *Surgery*, **10**(5), 109–16.

HACKETT, M. E. J. (1989). Management of burns. In *Trauma – Pathogenesis and Treatment*, ed. S. Westaby, pp. 296–311. Oxford: Heinemann Medical.

MUIR, I. F. K., BARCLAY, T. L. & SETTLE, J. A. D. (1987). *Burns and Their Treatment*, 3rd edn. London: Butterworths.

PRUITT, B. A. (1982). Burns and soft tissues. In *Clinical Surgery International*, Vol. 4, *ed*. H. C. Polk. pp. 113–31. London: Churchill Livingstone.

PRUITT, B. A. (1984). Biopsy diagnosis of surgical infections. *N Engl. J. Med.*, **310**, 1737–8.

WIENER, S. L. & BARRETT, J. (1986). Burn injury and management. In *Trauma Management for Civilian and Military physicians*, ed. S. L. Wiener & J. Barrett. pp. 53–76. Philadelphia: W. B. Saunders.

35 Chemical and radiation injuries

T. DAYNES and A. D. REDMOND

Accident and Emergency Department, North Staffordshire Hospital, Stoke on Trent, UK

Chapter plan

Chemical emergencies
Radiation accidents

CHEMICAL EMERGENCIES

Introduction

Chemical incidents are rare in the UK. It is therefore essential that local authorities, chemical plants and emergency services have a well-rehearsed strategy in place. Following the Flixborough disaster in 1974, the Advisory Committee on Major Hazards produced the Notification of Installations Handling Hazardous Substances Regulations. This requires users of hazardous chemicals to register with the Health and Safety Executive. In 1984, in response to European guidelines, the Control of Industrial Major Accident Hazard Regulations (CIMAH) were introduced. These involve regular inspection and updating of on- and offsite plans for dealing with a major disaster, and require copies of the plans to be held by the manufacturer, the emergency services, and the planning officer, district council, and health authority.

Identification of the chemical hazard

Fire services play a central role in the identification of the chemical or chemicals involved. They have access to CHEMDATA, a computerized record of chemicals and treatment, as well as the information for interpreting the hazard warnings and codes displayed on vehicles and storage tanks. They also have a team of personnel and equipment that can perform on- or offsite analysis of substances released.

Warnings are displayed on the UKHIS board (Fig. 1)

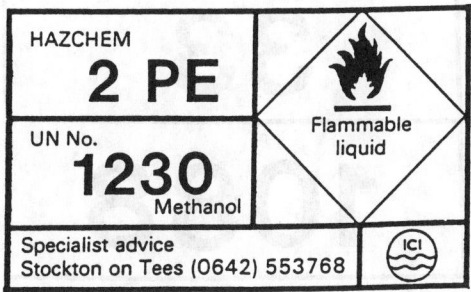

Black lettering on orange background.
Black symbol and letters in red diamond on white square background.

Fig. 1. Example of signs displayed on vehicles carrying hazardous chemicals in the UK.

and the ECE-ADR KEMLER board (Fig. 2). The UKHIS Board is standard in the UK, and contains the HAZCHEM code (see Fig. 3), the United Nations (UN) diamond which shows the physical properties of the chemical (e.g. inflammability, toxicity, etc.), the UN number specific to that chemical, and a contact for further information. The KEMLER board is standard throughout the European Community, and gives the UN number and a hazard code.

All emergency services must be familiar with the HAZCHEM code, and a copy must be available in all emergency departments. It gives the form of the chemical, the type of protective clothing and breathing apparatus required, the risk of explosion, and whether it should be diluted or prevented from entering the local water supply or drains. It also tells you if local evacuation may be necessary. As well as hazard warnings, each vehicle will carry transport emergency cards which provide information on appropriate first aid, fire-fighting methods and protection.

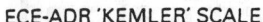

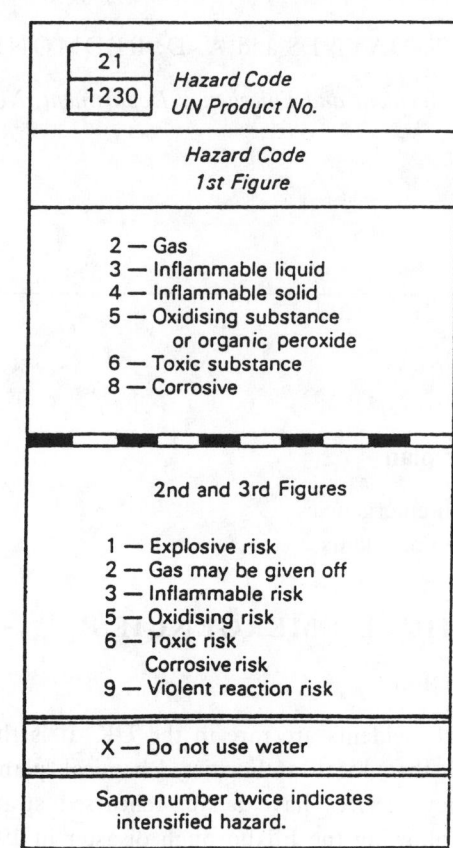

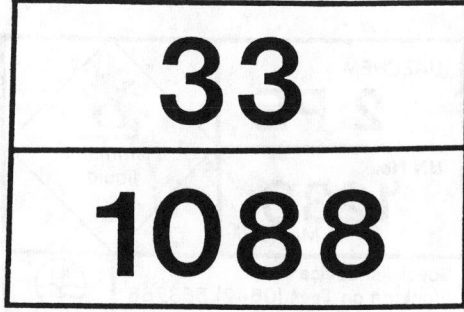

Fig. 2. (a) Example of signs displayed on vehicles carrying hazardous chemicals in the European Community. (b) The KEMLER scale.

Decontamination

At the scene of a chemical spillage the fire service is responsible for decontaminating the area and personnel. They will attempt to limit the spread and prevent contamination of local water supplies. In the case of an explosion or leakage of toxic gas, limiting spread is far more difficult. The fire brigade uses protective suits but also has mobile decontamination vehicles and equipment, and high-pressure jet showers. Decontamination does not take precedence over basic life support, and when the airway, breathing, or circulation is compromised this is dealt with first. Decontamination involves removing all clothing, which must be bagged and left at the scene, and performing one of the following:

1. Wet, containment: water spray with all water retained for safe disposal later.
2. Wet, non-containment: water spray with diluted chemical washed into local drainage.
3. Dry: for powders, using vacuum cleaners.

Decontamination is not without hazard and wet patients may become hypothermic. Scrubbing should not be used as it will create abrasions through which systemic absorption will be increased. Particular care should be taken to wash eyes and mucous membranes from where chemicals are rapidly absorbed. Water should not be used for lime (use brushing instead) or heavy metals such as sodium, potassium and lithium because an exothermic reaction occurs with these. Phosphorus should be immersed in water, as it ignites in air, and then scraped off carefully under water.

Containment

A planned approach will minimize casualties and ensure that rescuers and hospital staff do not become contaminated. Contaminated clothing and equipment should be left at the scene and only where life is threatened should decontamination take place elsewhere. The police will be responsible for keeping the public and press at a safe

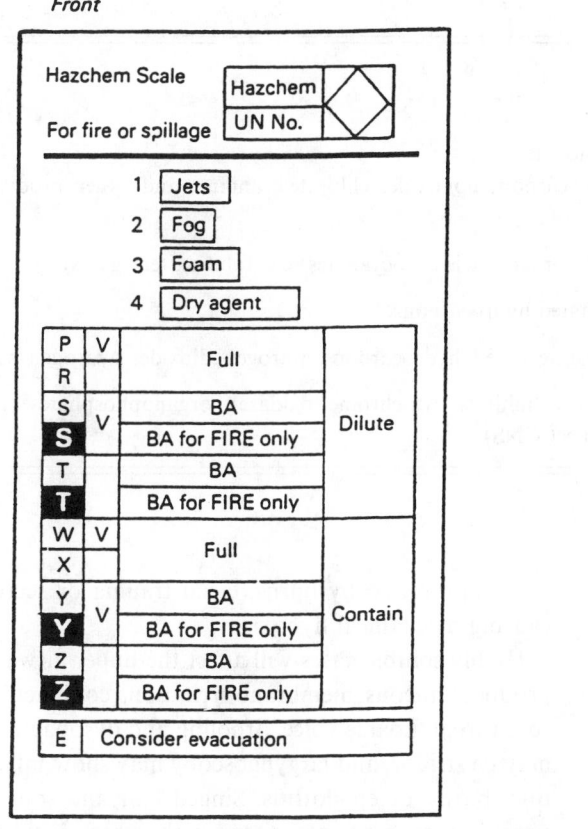

Front

Hazchem Scale

For fire or spillage

Hazchem

UN No.

1	Jets	
2	Fog	
3	Foam	
4	Dry agent	

P R	V	Full	Dilute
S	V	BA	
S		BA for FIRE only	
T		BA	
T		BA for FIRE only	
W X	V	Full	Contain
Y	V	BA	
Y		BA for FIRE only	
Z		BA	
Z		BA for FIRE only	

E	Consider evacuation

(a)

Back

Notes for Guidance

Fog
In the absence of fog equipment a
fine spray may be used.

Dry agent
Water must not be allowed to come
into contact with the substance at risk.

V
Can be violently or even explosively
reactive.

Full
Full body protective clothing with BA.

BA
Breathing apparatus plus protective
gloves.

Dilute
May be washed to drain with large
quantities of water.

Contain
Prevent by any means available, spillage
from entering drains or water course.

(b)

Fig. 3. The HAZCHEM code: (a) front; (b) back.

distance and accurate details should be released to the media by a designated person. The police will also coordinate any evacuation of local communities. Long-term effects on local water supplies, arable land and livestock may require monitoring by local authorities.

A full debriefing with psychological support for staff and public should follow any major incident.

A&E management

Most casualties arriving in the A&E department will have already undergone decontamination, but should still be isolated from the rest of the hospital staff and patients. Those who for medical reasons have been evacuated first, should be transferred to a decontamination area. This ideally should be a suite based on the guidelines in Table 1 and the DHSS building notes produced in 1986, or advice obtained from the Health and Safety Executive.

All hospitals likely to receive casualties from a chemical incident should have plans for isolation, decontamination and appropriate protective clothing for staff.

Table 1. *Requirements for a decontamination suite*

1. Air lines for breathing apparatus
2. Standing showers, and irrigation for supine casualties
3. Separate drainage
4. Separate entrance
5. Easily isolated
6. Protective suits
7. High-flow ventilation
8. Trolley facilities
9. Separate disposal facilities
10. Oxygen and resuscitation equipment

Triage and assessment

Patients should be triaged on the basis of airway, breathing and circulation. Contamination, like cervical spine control, should be considered in parallel. It should be remembered that a patient from a chemical incident may have sustained physical trauma (e.g. from the blast) and primary and secondary surveys must be carried out.

The history should include details of time and length of exposure, type of chemical, enclosed or open space,

Table 2. *Respiratory effects of inhalation of chemicals*

Early 0–6 h	Chemicals most likely to be the cause
Asphyxia	
Simple	Nitrogen, methane, propane, carbon dioxide
Chemical	Nitrites, cyanides, hydrogen sulphide, carbon monoxide, chlorates, aniline, and other producers of methaemoglobinaemia
Bronchoconstriction	Oxides of sulphur, oxides of nitrogen, inorganic acids, isocyanates (e.g. toluene, tear gases)
Acute laryngeal oedema	Chlorine, ammonia, phosgene, halogenated hydrocarbons
Pulmonary oedema	All the above, especially phosgene, halogenated hydrocarbons, nitrogen dioxide, hydrogen sulphide
Systemic toxicity	Arsine (haemolysis), hydrogen sulphide (inhibits cytochrome oxidase), organophosphates (inhibits acetylcholinesterase), hydrocarbons (affect CNS)

explosion or spillage, the extent of injury to other victims, and the condition of the patient at the scene. Particular note must be made of respiratory symptoms, collapse, loss of consciousness, or confusion, suggesting significant toxic inhalation, or hypoxia, and previous respiratory or cardiovascular conditions.

Physical examination should be directed towards the mental state, the chest, the face, nose and mouth for singed hair, burns or soot.

Baseline investigations must include arterial blood gases, carboxyhaemoglobin, chest X-ray, peak expiratory flow rate, ECG (electrocardiogram) monitoring, full blood count, urea and electrolytes. Blood and urine should be saved for a toxicology screen.

Symptomatic patients should be admitted for at least 24 h observation. Normal investigations do not exclude pathology and life-threatening bronchospasm may occur up to 24 h after exposure, although the risk is less after 8 h. All patients should be told to reattend if symptoms develop in the next 48 h. Pulmonary oedema and systemic organophosphate poisoning present less acutely but are equally life-threatening.

Airway and breathing (Table 2)

The most immediate life-threatening problem is asphyxia due to displacement of oxygen in the air by released gases. This is more likely in enclosed spaces, resulting in loss of consciousness and inability to rescue oneself. It may be worsened by chemical asphyxia (e.g. cyanide combining with ferric ion of mitochondrial cytochrome oxidase, causing intracellular hypoxia and lactic acidosis). It should be remembered that the patient's airway may be compromised by burns, facial trauma or secretions, causing mechanical hypoxia.

Highly soluble gases will affect the upper airways and produce mucous membrane irritation, conjunctivitis, a sore throat, hoarse voice, drooling and dysphagia. There may be stridor, and largyngoscopy may show inflammation, burns, or epiglottitis. Singed hair and soot in the nose or mouth are associated with a high incidence of largyngeal burns and inhalation injury (see Chapter 34). Lower airway injury is suggested by cough, carbonaceous sputum, wheeze, chest pain and signs of atelectasis. The peak flow may be reduced, and lung collapse may be visible on the chest X-ray. Oedema, sloughing of the bronchial mucosa and bronchorrhoea in combination are referred to as bronchiolitis obliterans.

Pulmonary parenchymal injury is seen with less soluble gases such as phosgene. It may present with acute breathlessness and hyperventilation, or more insidiously. Fine crackles in the lung field are accompanied by hypoxia. The chest X-ray appearance may vary from normal to signs of patchy or diffuse infiltration. Mild pneumonitis produces pulmonary oedema with a high protein exudate and alveolar wall damage, which may heal with fibrosis.

Immediate care should include clearing and control of the airway, administration of 100% oxygen, and removal from the scene. Decontamination should be performed at the same time as advanced life support when possible. Intubation should be considered in the following circumstances and performed by the most senior person available:

- No spontaneous respiration after basic life support.
- Cyanosis or hypoxia (PO_2 below 8 kPa) not improving with 100% oxygen.

- Coma.
- Respiratory distress, with stridor or drooling.
- Full-thickness face or neck (circumferential) burns.
- Laryngeal, pharyngeal or pulmonary oedema.
- Respiratory failure, with rising PCO_2.
- NB: Early intubation is better than late and difficult intubation.

  Anaesthetic drugs may be needed.

Intubated patients should be fully decontaminated before transfer to intensive care. This must include the oropharynx. Care should be taken not to precipitate hypothermia.

Bronchodilators should be administered when there is bronchospasm, wheeze, or a reduced peak flow. These must be administered with 100% oxygen even when chronic airway disease is present, as severe hypoxia may follow subsequent pulmonary vasodilation.

Steroids remain controversial and are not indicated for pneumonitis or pulmonary oedema and may increase mortality from infection. Some advocate a single large dose on initial presentation. Pulmonary oedema should be treated with intravenous diuretics, and close monitoring of the central venous pressure and cardiac output. Overenthusiastic administration of intravenous fluids will worsen the patient's condition. Positive end expiratory pressure ventilation should be considered for those who do not respond. Prophylactic antibiotics are of no benefit and treatment should be based on isolation of an organism in a patient with persisting fever and leucocytosis.

Respiratory function, peak flow, and arterial blood gases must be monitored. A chest X-ray should be repeated after 24 h. Adult respiratory distress syndrome is a late complication requiring ventilation and close monitoring of fluid balance and cardiac output. Severely affected patients may eventually develop lung fibrosis.

Skin contamination

The skin can be affected directly, or be the route of systemic absorption. Strong acids tend to cause necrosis by coagulation, which forms a layer limiting further caustic damage. Strong alkalis liquefy tissue and therefore cause deeper necrosis. Organophosphates, arsenic, mercurial compounds and phenol cause severe blistering followed by systemic effects. Hot gases or liquids will cause thermal burns.

Skin contamination is a hazard for unprotected hospital staff. Decontamination, as outlined above, with copious amounts of water is the first line of treatment after life support and removal of non-adherent clothing. This may need to be repeated on arrival at the receiving hospital.

Phenol may be identified by its smell. It causes painless burns. Its systemic effects are coma, convulsions, haemolysis, shock and renal failure. These can be limited by swabbing with polyethylene glycol after washing.

Hydrofluoric acid is used in the electronics industry, glass manufacture and horticulture. It causes severe necrosis and painful burns, which may be limited by intralesional injection of calcium gluconate (0.5 ml per cm^2 of burn).

Phosphorus ignites in air. Burns should be kept moist and particles removed. Phosphorescence or copper sulphate solution can be used to reveal small particles.

Lime or quicklime reacts with water, producing heat. Small amounts of water may cause more damage. Cement burns are alkaline; they tend to progress and may be deceptive. Like other alkali burns they should be assessed by more experienced staff.

Treatment of the burn should follow that for thermal burns, and involves dressings, analgesia, fluids and possible referral to a plastic surgeon.

Chemical burns of the eyes

The eyes are affected by gases, liquid or sprays. Solids may get under the eyelid. The eyes will become red, watery and sore. Vision may be blurred or reduced. Examination may show conjunctivitis, with or without corneal abrasion or oedema. Limbal ischaemia, an opaque cornea, dilated pupil and signs of raised intraocular pressure with a risk of optic nerve damage are signs of more severe injury. Cataracts may develop over the first 24 h. Healing with corneal vascularization will cause long-term visual impairment. Alkalis penetrate more deeply than acids and therefore cause more damage. Volatile chemicals and detergents cause conjunctivitis, but rarely any permanent damage.

Treatment requires immediate copious irrigation with a litre of normal saline. Amethocaine drops should be used to make this procedure more comfortable. Irrigation should be continued in the case of acids and alkalis until litmus paper shows a neutral pH. Mydriatic drops such as cyclopentolate or homatropine will relieve pain, and if there is epithelial damage shown by fluorescein staining a topical antibiotic such as chloramphenicol should be used. The eyelids must be everted and particles removed

Table 3. *Use of antidotes*

Poison	Target organ	Antidote and dose
Carbon monoxide	CNS toxicity	Hyperbaric oxygen
Organophosphates and carbamates	Acetylcholinesterase	Atropine 2–4 mg repeated at 15-min intervals until fully atropinized
Organophosphates only		Pralidoxime 30 mg kg^{-1} in 250 ml of normal saline over 60 min
Hydrogen sulphide	Cytochrome oxidase	Sodium nitrate 10 ml of a 3% solution IV
Cyanides	Cytochrome oxidase	Dicobalt edetate 300–600 mg IV
Mercurials and arsenics	CNS, kidney	Dimercaprol 3 mg kg^{-1} IM 4-hourly for 2 days, then 12-hourly for 8 days
		D-Penicillamine for inorganic compounds

CNS, central nervous system.

followed by irrigation. The patient should be referred to an ophthalmologist for intraocular pressure measurement and further treatment. The use of topical steroids is controversial: they are beneficial in the acute stage but prolonged use may delay healing.

The use of antidotes

An antidote may be used in cases of moderate and severe poisoning (see also Chapter 11). The use of antidotes is limited to the listing in Table 3 and relies on identification of the chemical, recognition of the clinical risk of contamination and measurement of the appropriate blood level. Before the use of an antidote the local poisons unit should be contacted for advice.

Common chemical poisons

Carbon monoxide

This is a colourless gas released by combustion of natural gas and found in smoke fumes and car exhausts. It produces headache, dizziness, nausea and agitation. In severe cases there may be coma with cerebral oedema, papilloedema, hyper-reflexia, arrhythmias and cardiovascular collapse.

Measurement of the arterial carboxyhaemoglobin level and the use of a standard nomogram (see Clark *et al.*, 1986) will give an estimate of the original concentration at exposure. A smoker will have an average level of about 8% and levels below 10% are not associated with symptoms. Levels above 20% suggest significant exposure. For levels above 40%, hyperbaric oxygen should be considered

as part of the following indications:

- Carboxyhaemoglobin level >40%.
- History of unconsciousness.
- Cardiac complications.
- Persistent neurological deficit or coma.
- Pregnancy.

Immediate treatment should be management of the airway, breathing and circulation, and high-flow oxygen through a reservoir bag. Hyberbaric oxygen at 3 atmospheres will increase the elimination of carbon monoxide and may reduce long-term neurological damage.

Cyanide

This is widely used in the chemical industry and hydrogen cyanide is released by burning plastic. It should be suspected when there are neurological signs associated with respiratory symptoms, an odour of bitter almonds on the patient's breath, and a metabolic acidosis. As the antidote is potentially toxic in the absence of cyanide ions, plasma levels should be confirmed where possible. A conscious patent is unlikely to require treatment with antidote, which should be reserved for severe poisoning associated with coma, convulsions, or cardiovascular collapse, and when other causes have been excluded.

Organophosphates

These are found mainly as insecticides and inhibit cholinesterase, causing peripheral and central nervous overstimulation. Muscarinic effects are salivation, lacrimation, urination, diarrhoea, gastrointestinal cramps and emesis (SLUDGE). Pupillary constriction, bronchospasm and

---

Muscarinic effects of organophosphates (SLUDGE)

S   Salivation
L   Lacrimation
U   Urination
D   Diarrhoea
G   Gastrointestinal cramps
E   Emesis

---

bradycardia may also occur. Nicotinic effects are hypertension, hyperglycaemia, muscle fasciculation and paralysis. Central effects are headache, slurred speech, ataxia, seizures and coma.

Diagnosis can be confirmed by cholinesterase activity. Activity less than 50% is significant, activity less than 10% indicates severe poisoning. Treatment includes oxygen and decontamination, particularly of skin burns to reduce systemic absorption. Atropine will reverse the muscarinic effects and should be given every 15–30 min until a dry mouth, dilated pupils, flushed skin and a pulse of 80 min^{-1} are achieved. Pralidoxime will reverse the nicotinic effects and, if clinical improvement is noted after two initial doses, an infusion of 0.5 mg h^{-1} is indicated for 24 h. Seizures and muscle fasciculation can be controlled with diazepam.

RADIATION ACCIDENTS

The sources of radiation that may generate casualties include radioactive material used in industry, medicine and research, and any originating from a nuclear reactor or released during transport. The source can be particulate or involve electromagnetic radiation. There are five types of ionizing radiation which differ in the amount of penetration, and therefore the amount of damage produced:

- *Alpha-particles.* Do not penetrate skin; damage results from ingestion or entry via wounds.
- *Beta-particles.* Penetrate skin but no further; may cause burns.
- *Gamma-rays.* Penetrating electromagnetic radiation; the main cause of acute radiation syndrome.
- *X-rays.* Same as gamma-rays.
- *Neutron particles.* Penetrating radiation causing both skin burns and the radiation syndrome.

The measure of the amount of radioactive material is the Becquerel (Bq), which is equivalent to the number of atoms which distintegrate per second. The unit of absorbed dose is the Gray (Gy), measured in joules per kilogram. The same dose may have a different biological effect. Therefore a more useful unit is the dose equivalent, or Sievert (Sv), which measures the number of joules per kilogram causing the same effect as 1 Gy of low-energy radiation such as X-rays.

There are two types of exposure. If the casualties are exposed to an external source (e.g. gamma-rays, X-rays or neutrons) the whole body will be affected. They can be removed from the source and are therefore irradiated but not contaminated. These patients are not a risk to emergency staff and can be managed as any other patient. Exposure to radioactive solids, dust or liquid spillage results in contamination of clothes, skin and wounds. There is a risk of ingestion, and full precautions should be taken to limit exposure of others. These patients may also receive high doses over small areas, resulting in localized burns.

The effects of radiation exposure

Ionizing radiation mainly affects cells undergoing high rates of division in the gastrointestinal tract, the haemopoietic system and the skin. The time to onset of symptoms and their severity depend on the dose of radiation:

- *Early effects.* Immediate symptoms are anorexia, nausea, vomiting, diarrhoea, headache, fever and malaise. If the dose is greater than 4 Sv then symptoms will develop within 2 h; if they have not developed by 6 h then the dose is less than 0.5 Sv. After exposure to over 6 Sv, symptoms may continue for up to 2 weeks. A massive dose will cause central nervous symptoms of severe vomiting, delirium, ataxia, seizures and coma; death may occur in the following 2 days, and may be immediate if the dose is over 100 Sv. The changes in the lymphocyte count over the first 48 h give an idea of the prognosis: if the count is less than 0.5, the prognosis is poor.
- *Intermediate effects.* There may be a latent period of 2–3 weeks followed by acute watery diarrhoea, vomiting and dehydration. Bone marrow suppression results in thrombocytopenia and neutropenia. Overwhelming sepsis or mucosal haemorrhage leads to death in the next 6 weeks.
- *Late effects.* If the patient survives the acute illness he has an increased risk of malignancy, leukaemia and infertility.

Skin

The effect of exposure to less than 2 Sv is erythema in the first 24 h. Above this erythema will last longer, there will be hair loss and blistering will occur. Third-degree burns are likely if the dose is above 8 Sv, but these burns are still painful because nerve endings are preserved.

Management of the contaminated casualty

At the scene

Protective clothing must be worn and the scene must be safe from other hazards. Life support takes priority, followed by decontamination if facilities are available. When life support is not required, transfer to a hospital that is fully prepared to receive casualties and has been notified of the details is appropriate. Plastic sheeting is used at the scene to reduce the spread of contamination. Clothes should not be removed over the head because this will spread contamination to the face and hair. If burns are extensive or there are signs of shock, intravenous fluids should be started.

Preparation of the receiving hospital

A designated area should be isolated and covered with plastic sheeting. The requirements for decontamination are the same as those outlined for chemical incidents. Specified personnel only should be allowed into the area; they should have full protective clothing and ideally a personal dosimeter as used in most X-ray departments. Equipment to monitor radioactivity must be available as well as access to expert advice.

Decontamination

When possible, casualties should be surveyed with a Geiger-Müller counter and areas of activity mapped in the same way that burns are charted. Solid and dust particles must be lightly brushed off the skin, avoiding abrasion, and swabs taken from the ears, mouth and nose. Wounds should be irrigated until clear of activity, and debrided if they remain contaminated. Irrigation of eyes, ears and nose should be done with warm water and the mouth cleaned with mouth wash and a soft toothbrush, taking care that water is not swallowed. When wounds have been cleaned and dressed, the casualty is washed all over with soapy water or cetrimide, taking care over areas previously identified. Contaminated hair should be cut, not shaved, and upright showering avoided because this will spread contamination to other parts. Nails must be clipped and cleaned. Urine and faeces should be kept for analysis and routine blood count, electrolytes and blood grouping performed. Blood must be saved for tissue typing in the event that a bone marrow transplant is required.

Internal decontamination for inhaled or swallowed material requires specialist advice because the methods include gastric or bowel lavage and bronchoalveolar lavage. Activated charcoal may be recommended to reduce absorption.

Radioiodine

This is released into the atmosphere with other radioisotopes and after absorption is taken up by the thyroid. Potassium iodide (100 mg) should be distributed to all members of the public as well as to hospital casualties within 1 h of exposure; this will block uptake of radioiodine by the thyroid.

Prognosis

This is directly related to the dose received. It is generally agreed that below 2 Sv the chance of survival is good; above 6 Sv more than 90% of cases will have received a fatal dose. Other indicators are:

- Nausea, vomiting and diarrhoea within minutes, or ataxia, coma and shock within hours when a fatal dose has been received.
- Bloody diarrhoea within 4 days, lymphocytes less than 0.5 within 3 days, or other evidence of severe bone marrow suppression within a week means that a fatal dose is likely in over 80% of cases.
- The extent of skin burns.

Bibliography

ABBUHL, S.B. (1991). Acetylcholinesterase inhibitor poisoning. In *Clinical Practice of Emergency Medicine*, ed. A. Harwood-Nuss, C. Linden, R.C. Luten, G. Sternbach & A.B. Wolfson. Ch. 169. Philadelphia: J.B. Lippincott.

CLARK, C.J., CAMPBELL, E. & REID, W.H. (1986). Blood carboxyhaemoglobin and cyanide levels in fire victims. *Lancet*, i, 1332–5.

EDELMAN, P.A. (1991). Irritant gas inhalation. In *Clinical Practice of Emergency Medicine*, ed. A. Harwood-Nuss, C. Linden, R.C.Luten, G. Sternbach, & A.B. Wolfson. Ch. 159. Philadelphia: J.B. Lippincott.

HALL, A.H. & RUMACK, B.H. (1991). Cyanide poisoning. In *Clinical Practice of Emergency Medicine*, ed. A.

Harwood-Nuss, C. Linden, R.C. Luten, G. Sternbach & A.B. Wolfson. Ch. 170. Phildelphia: J.B. Lippincott.

HEIFETZ, I.N. (1991). Radiation accidents. In *Clinical Practice of Emergency Medicine*, ed. A. Harwood-Nuss, C. Linden, R.C. Luten, G. Sternbach & A.B. Wolfson. Ch. 212. Phildelphia: J.B. Lippincott.

HINES, K. *et al.* (1988). Chemical accidents. In *Medicine for Disasters*, ed. P. Baskett & R. Weller. Ch. 27. Bristol: Wright.

LINDEN, C.H. (1991). Smoke inhalation. In *Clinical Practice of Emergency Medicine*, ed. A. Harwood-Nuss, C. Linden, R.C. Luten, G. Sternbach & A.B. Wolfson. Ch. 209. Philadelphia: J.B. Lippincott.

MURRAY, V.S.G. (1989). *Major Chemical Disasters – Medical Aspects of Management*. London: Royal Society of Medicine Services Ltd.

OLSON, K.R. (1991). Carbon monoxide poisoning. In *Clinical Practice of Emergency Medicine*, ed. A. Harwood-Nuss, C. Linden, R.C. Luten, G. Sternbach & A.B. Wolfson. Ch. 157. Philadelphia: J.B. Lippincott.

ORGANISATION FOR ECONOMIC CO-OPERATION AND DEVELOPMENT. (1994). Health aspects of chemical accidents – guidance on chemical accident awareness, preparedness and response for health professionals and emergency responders. Paris: OECD.

WELLER, R. (1988). Nuclear accidents. In *Medicine for Disasters*, ed. P. Baskett & R. Weller. Ch. 30. Bristol: Wright.

36 Electrical and lightning injuries

J. WARDROPE

Department of Accident and Emergency Medicine, Northern General Hospital NHS Trust, Sheffield, UK

Chapter plan

Physical characteristics and biological effects of electricity
Epidemiology
Pathophysiology
Prehospital care
A&E department care

PHYSICAL CHARACTERISTICS AND BIOLOGICAL EFFECTS OF ELECTRICITY

Electricity is the flow of electrons from an area of high electrical potential to that of low potential. Modern life is highly dependent on a continuous supply of this form of energy and almost every household will have a large number of electrical appliances, each with the ability to kill if not properly installed and operated. Prevention of electrical injury is the best strategy to reduce the morbidity and mortality from accidents. However this can only be achieved by continuing programmes of industrial health and safety, design standards, product quality control, building regulations and public education.

The *energy* released by an electrical contact with the human body is dependent on three variables: voltage, current and contact time.

Amount of energy released depends on three variables

- Voltage – the measure of the difference in the electrical potential between the entry and exit points.
- Current – the amount of electricity flowing through the body
- Contact time – the duration of current flow

Energy = *Voltage × Current × Contact time*

Voltage

Examples of the voltages of electrical sources are illustrated in Fig. 1. Some authorities define low voltage as less than 50 V but for clinical purposes any voltage below 1000 V may be regarded as low voltage. Domestic supply voltage of 240 V is therefore low voltage.

Current

The current will depend on the *resistance* of the body pathway to earth. For very low voltage the main resistance is in the skin. At high voltage the skin resistance is negligible and the total body resistance is 500–1500 ohm.

Contact time

The longer the current flows through the body the greater the damage and also the greater the possibility of ventricular fibrillation (VF) and loss of consciousness.

Alternating current (AC) is induced by moving a magnet in and out of a conducting coil. This is the basis for almost all domestic and industrial electrical supplies which cause most injury and death.

Direct current (DC) is produced by electrochemical sources such as batteries, AC that has been processed (rectified) to produce DC, or by static electricity as in lightning. AC produces tetanic spasm of major muscle groups and the victim may be unable to let go of the source. AC is also much more likely to produce VF than DC.

EPIDEMIOLOGY

Electrical injury

Electrical current causes on average 200 deaths per annum in England and Wales. Young men are the most

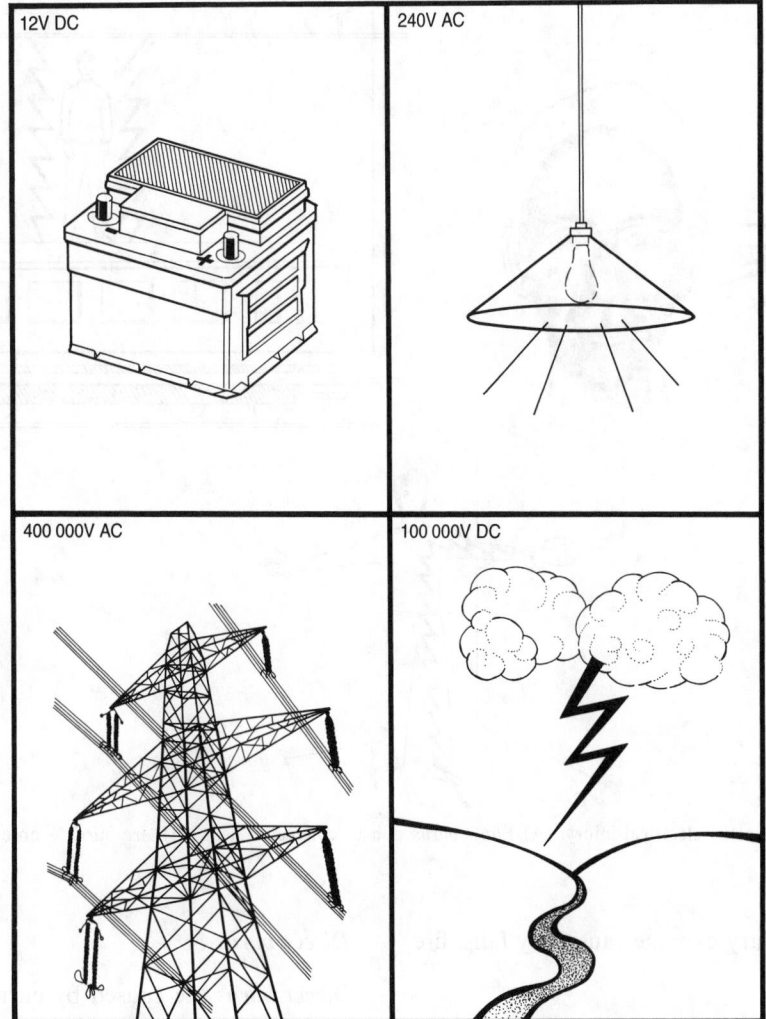

Fig 1. Examples of the voltages typically associated with different types of electrical source.

commonly killed (male/female 6:1) (OPCS, 1993, personal communication).

There are over 1000 deaths every year in the USA from electrical accidents.

Lightning

Lightning is the leading cause of death from a natural phenomenon in the USA with 600 deaths per year on average (Fulde & Marsden, 1990). The incidence of death from lightning varies from country to country depending on climatic conditions. Death rates vary from 0.7 deaths per million in the USA to 0.2 per million in Scandinavia. In England and Wales the yearly average of deaths due to lightning is two to three. There are distinct seasonal variations in death rates, again dependent on the weather.

Most of the deaths occur in young people engaging in outdoor activity.

PATHOPHYSIOLOGY

General mechanisms

Electrical current will flow from an area of high potential to that of low potential – usually the zero potential of earth. It will follow the path of least resistance.

The degree and pattern of injury will depend on the amount of energy (voltage × current × contact time), the path taken by the current and the type and frequency of the current.

The major pathological mechanisms causing injury are burns, dysfunction of conducting tissue within the body, cell damage by large transmembrane potentials induced

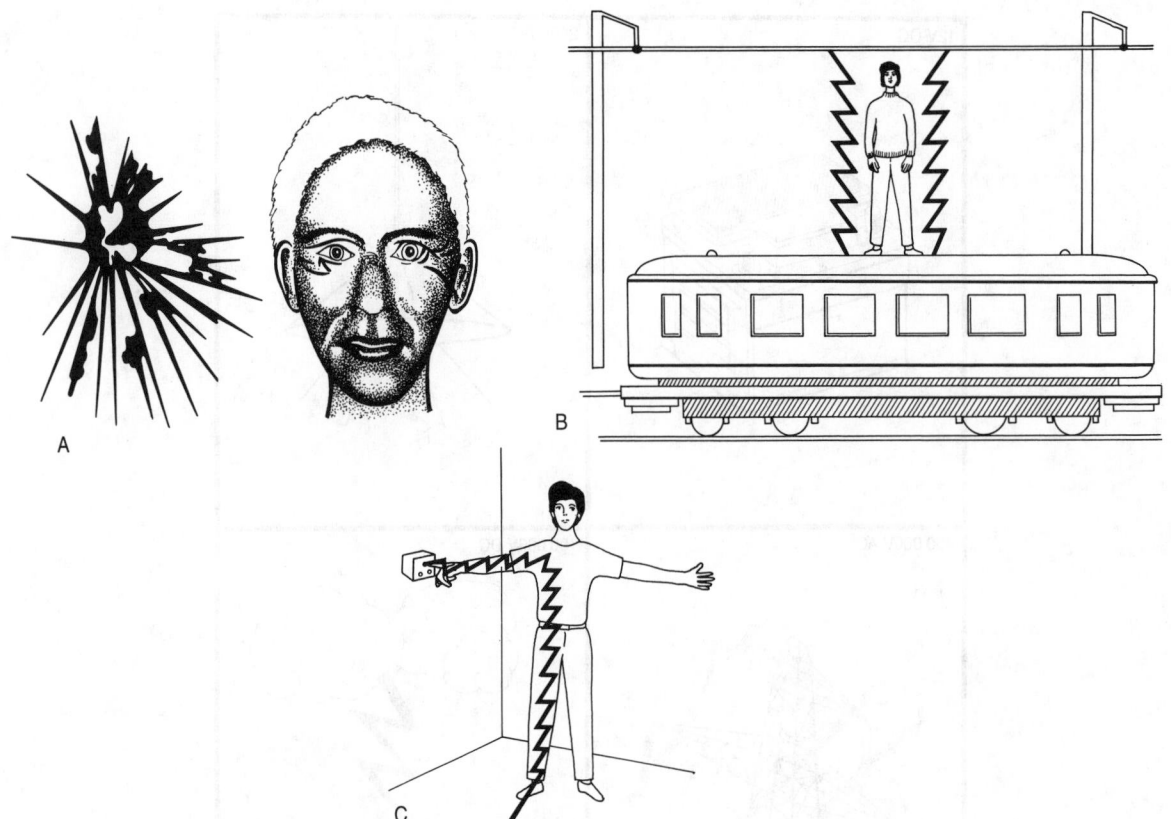

Fig. 2. Mechanisms of burns in the electrical injury. (A) *Flash burns* due to convected heat. (B) *Arc burns* – note the current flows around the body. (C) *Direct burns.*

by currents, and secondary damage caused by falls, fire and blast injury.

Burns

Flash burns

Flash burns are probably caused by *convected heat* (Barnes & Mercer, 1989). No current flows through or around the body but a remote electrical flash causes a wave of heat. Typical flash burns involve the face and exposed parts of the body (Fig. 2A). The burns tend to be superficial but the heat may cause ignition of clothing leading to more extensive and serious burns.

Arc burns

Arc burns are caused by high-voltage electrical currents, short-circuiting *external* to the body, often generating temperatures in the range 3000–20 000°C. In high-voltage arc injury the victim does not have to touch the source: the arc will cross 2–3 cm for every 1000 V (Fig. 2B). Victims are often thrown some distance by the arc and secondary injury is common (Koller, 1991).

Direct burns

Direct burns are caused by current flowing through the body (Fig. 2C). The degree of the damage is proportional to the intensity and duration of current flow. The maximum current will flow through structures with least electrical resistance and highest cross-sectional area. Thus in the limbs the muscle groups will carry the largest electrical load (see Fig. 4).

Early interruption in cellular function

Those structures and cells with specialized electrical functions are susceptible to electrical shock. A current flowing across the heart may cause VF. Current flow through the brain may cause unconsciousness or respiratory arrest. Often this interruption in function is short-lived and, if immediate treatment is given, full recovery is expected in most cases. Where there has been a prolonged period of hypoxia, lasting cerebral or myocardial damage may be seen. If a very large current flows through the brian, for example in some lightning strikes, there will be major direct structural damage. This is relatively rare.

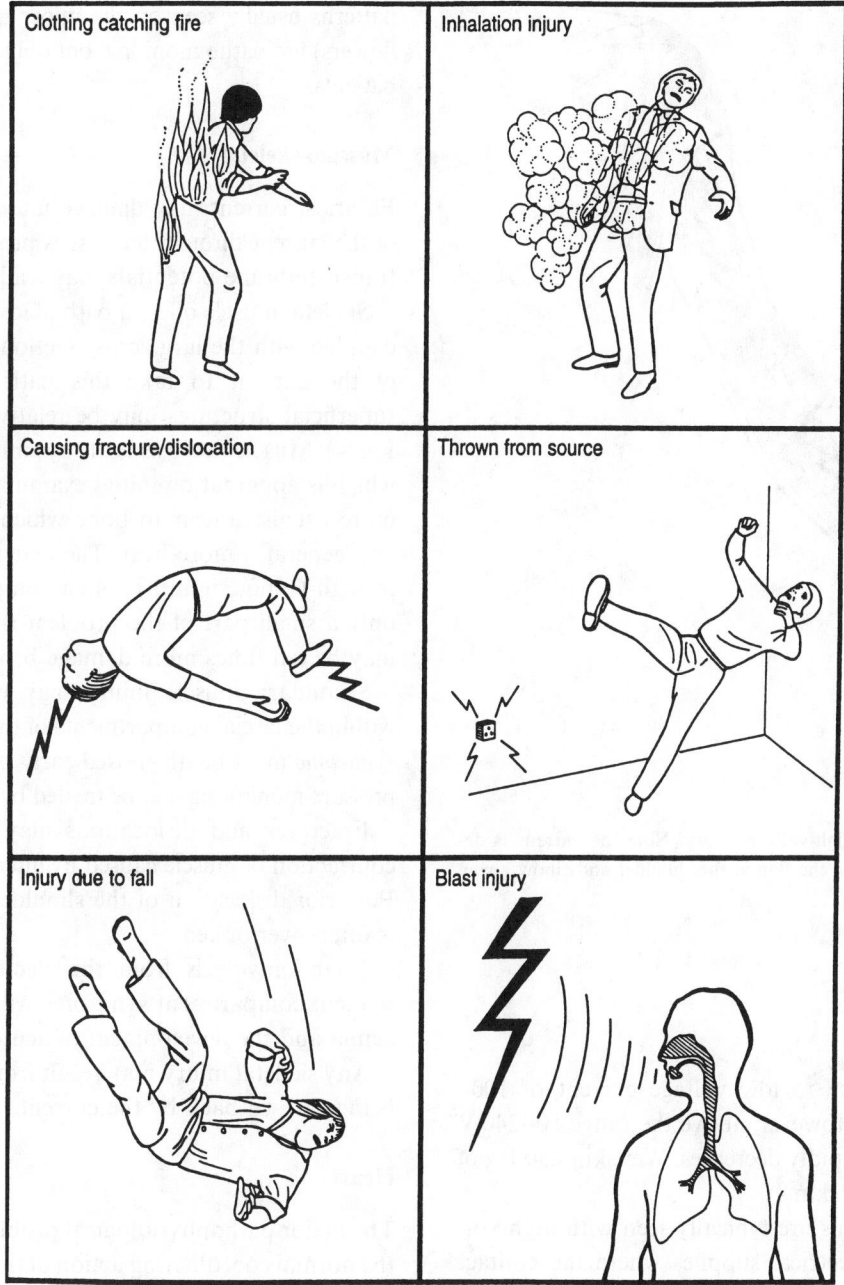

Fig. 3. Mechanisms of secondary injury following electrical contacts.

Transmembrane potential injury

The flow of electricity produces electromagnetic fields. Living cells are very dependent on the maintenance of electrical gradients and may be damaged by the induction of large transmembrane potentials. This causes water to enter the lipid layer of the cell membrane creating large pores, a process known as *electroporation* (Lee, *et al.*, 1992). If these pores are large enough the cell will rupture. These effects are most marked in large cells such as neurones and muscle cells. This may explain neurological damage in patients with high-voltage arc burns where there has been no direct passage of electricity through the body (Gaylor *et al.*, 1988).

Secondary injury

Falls from a height, exposure to fire and smoke, and blast injury may all occur in addition to the electrical injury and such injuries should be excluded in these patients (Fig. 3).

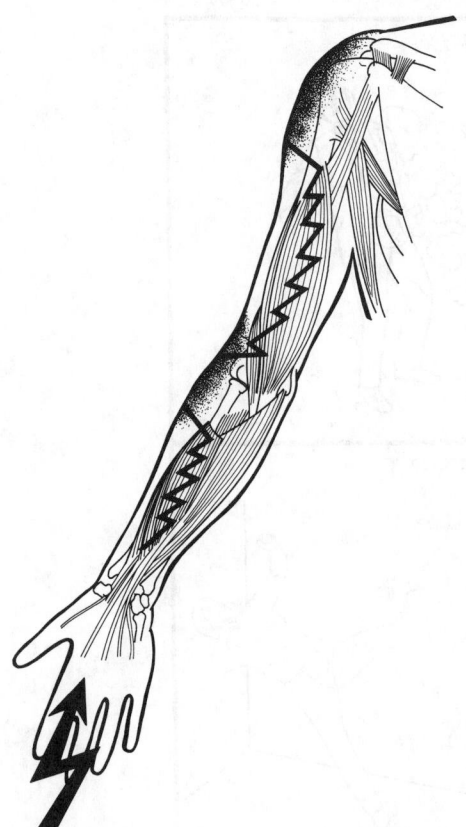

Fig. 4. Current flow in high-voltage injury. Note the current is deflected from the muscles to the skin at the shoulder and elbow giving 'skip' burns.

Individual tissues

Skin

Skin has a resistance to low voltage current of 100–300 kohm per cm^2. However, above the range 50–240 V the skin resistance rapidly decreases. Wet skin has 1% of the resistance of dry skin.

Full-thickness burns are typically seen with high voltage or domestic electrical supplies where the contact area is small. The burns may not be confluent and 'skip lesions' are observed. In this phenomenon the skin at the wrist, elbow and shoulder may be burnt as current is deflected to the surface because of poor muscle bulk over these ares (Fig. 4) (Daniel et al., 1988).

Arcing of the current in high-voltage injuries or lightning strikes may result in very high temperatures. Burns may be extensive (25–75% of body surface area), although not always full-thickness. The burns are more severe if the clothing catches fire.

In lightning injury, superficial burns and hair scorching are common findings, usually on the head and lower limbs (Eriksson & Ornehult, 1988). Feather-like branching patterns usually seen on the upper thorax (Lichtenburg's flowers) are pathognomonic but only seen in a minority of patients.

Musculo-skeletal

Electrical current may damage muscle by direct passage of the current through the tissues producing heat. Induced transmembrane potentials may lead to cell rupture.

Skeletal muscle offers a path of low resistance and this, coupled with the large cross-sectional area, causes most of the current to take this pathway. The skin and superficial structures may be relatively undamaged (see Fig. 4). Muscle necrosis is always much greater than that which is apparent on initial examination. The damage is more extensive near to bone which has high resistance and generates more heat. The extent of muscle damage in high-voltage injury is often compared to an iceberg: only a small part of the problem is apparent and there may be ten times more damage beneath the surface.

Secondary muscle injury may occur from swelling within the fascial compartments of the limb. *Compartment syndrome* must be diagnosed early by intracompartment pressure monitoring and be treated by extensive fasciotomy.

Fractures and dislocations may occur from tetanic contraction of muscle caused by alternating current (AC). Posterior dislocation of the shoulder is an injury which is often overlooked.

Rhabdomyolysis from the electrical injury or subsequent compartment syndrome will lead to myoglobin-aemia and the development of acute renal failure.

Any skeletal injury may result from falls or the patient being thrown back by the current.

Heart

The major pathophysiological problem is interruption of the normal coordinating action of the cardiac conduction system leading to arrhythmias.

VF is the commonest fatal arrhythmia. The magnitude of the current that may cause VF is designated the *fibrillation threshold*. This is dependent on:

- The intensity of current (see Table 1).
- The contact time.
- The current path (a path from left hand to foot is 2.5 times more likely to produce VF than foot to foot).
- The frequency of the AC current (the higher the frequency the greater the current required to produce VF).

Electric stun guns use a combination of low contact

Table 1. *Fibrillation thresholds for 240 V AC at 50 Hz, current path left hand to foot* (British Standards Institution, 1981)

Contact time	Minimum current to cause VF	Current producing VF in 50% of victims
10 msec	500 mA	1000 mA
0.1 sec	400 mA	700 mA
1 sec	50 mA	70 mA
3 sec	40 mA	50 mA

VF, ventricular fibrillation.

times and high-frequency current to minimize the risk of VF (Robinson *et al.*, 1990).

Many supraventricular arrhythmias may be triggered by electrical injury, the commonest being supraventricular tachycardia and atrial fibrillation. These usually revert to sinus rhythm spontaneously but if persistent may be managed along conventional lines.

In most large reported series it is found that significant arrhythmias seldom develop if the initial 12-lead electrocardiogram (ECG) is normal (Cunningham, 1991; Purdue & Hunt, 1986). Two cases of late arrhythmias have been reported following otherwise uncomplicated low-voltage shocks but in neither case was an ECG carried out immediately after the injury (Jensen *et al.*, 1987).

Disturbances in ventricular function have been noted on ultrasound but such abnormalities have been found after cardiac arrest and the exact aetiology of the problem is not clear. Myocardial ischaemia during the cardiac arrest is the probable mechanism. Acute myocardial infarction may occur but this is most likely the result of ischaemic damage at cardiac arrest and not the direct effect of the shock on cardiac muscle (Homma *et al.*, 1990).

Cases of acute pulmonary oedema have been reported following electrical shock or lightning injury. These may have been caused by a blast injury effect on the lungs (Lutalo & Pratt, 1989) or myocardial damage (Schein *et al.*, 1990).

Nervous system

Central nervous system – immediate effects

Loss of conciousness is the commonest complication. This may occur in up to 20% of the victims of low-voltage injury and in up to 50% of cases of high-voltage injury (Grube *et al.*, 1990). In low-voltage injury, transient loss of conciousness causes no long-term problems. Uncon-

ciousness may result from direct brain injury or secondary hypoxic damage from cardiorespiratory arrest. If the patient is still unconcious at the time of arrival in the accident and emergency (A&E) department then there is a 50% mortality. In lightning injury direct neural damage is the second most common cause of death.

Peripheral nervous system – immediate effects

Acute peripheral neural dysfunction may occur in low-voltage injury and up to 50% of cases of high-voltage injury. Nerve compression syndromes (especially at the wrist), compartment syndrome or spinal cord injury may all cause neurological deficit after electrical injury and potentially treatable complications should be excluded (Kanitkar & Roberts, 1988).

In low-voltage injury over 80% of patients make a complete recovery. In high-voltage injury over 50% of acute neurological problems result in permanent disability.

Nervous system – delayed effects

Delayed neuropathy is well described in high-voltage electrical injury. The neuropathy may affect the spinal cord or the peripheral nervous system. The cause of this damage has not been explained satisfactorily. The induction of transmembrane potentials is most marked in large cells, which may explain the selective damage to motor neurones (Koller & Osagh, 1989). The reported incidence varies from 0% to 27% and the median incidence is around 6%. The onset of symptoms may be within a few hours but is typically in the range 4–30 days.

Motor deficits are the most common but there is usually no interruption of bladder function. Most recover, at least partially. Delayed peripheral neuropathy has also been described but tends not to be severe and most cases resolve (Grube *et al.*, 1990). There is also an association between electrical injury and the onset of motor neurone disease (Gallagher & Talbert, 1990).

Post-traumatic stress disorders are well described following high-voltage or lightning injury (Silva *et al.*, 1991).

Eyes

The major effect is that of delayed cataract formation. This is most common when one of the contact points is the head. It is uncommon with low-voltage injury but 5–10% of high-voltage cases or lightning victims may have these problems (Boozalis *et al.*, 1991). Retinal injury, iritis and corneal injury have also been reported.

Ears

Perforation of the tympanic membrane may occur in lightning strike victims. This is especially common when the injury occurs whilst using a telephone (Andrews & Darveniza, 1989).

Renal

The extensive muscle damage caused by high-voltage injury leads to myoglobinuria. This, coupled with renal hypoperfusion from shock, may lead to acute tubular necrosis and renal failure. Fluid replacement should be rigorous in the victims of high-voltage injury to try and prevent this complication.

PREHOSPITAL CARE

The rescue of a victim of electrical injury places the rescuer at high risk. A collapsed patient may still be attached to a live electrical source and there may be no warning of this. If attempts are made to move the victim before turning off the current there is a great risk that the rescuer will suffer the same effects as the victim.

Always turn off the electrical source before treating the victim of electrical injury.

Even greater care is needed with victims of high voltage, which can jump significant distances. In dry air a spark can leap 3 cm per 10 kV, but once the arc is established it may propagate several metres. Before entering such areas ensure the current has been switched off. For example, for overhead railway power lines a distance of 2.7 m (8 ft) is recommended.

In lightning injury there are special risks to prehospital personnel. Lightning can strike twice in the same location. Many of these injuries occur in the open where there is little shelter. Spend as little time as possible in the open and evacuate early to a vehicle or building. Trees are dangerous, as is electrical equipment, especially radios with aerials (Duclos & Sanderson, 1990).

Cardiac arrest is managed according to conventional protocols. In lightning injury there have been reports of survival after prolonged periods of cardiac arrest, perhaps due to arrested cerebral metabolism caused by the lightning strike. In most most cases the heart will have been previously healthy.

Always consider the possibility of coexistent injury and open the airway by chin lift or jaw thrust with adequate spinal immobilization. Give high-flow oxygen. If possible establish venous access and commence fluid resuscitation. Burns should be covered with dry sterile sheets.

A&E DEPARTMENT CARE

The clinical presentations of electrical injury are varied but two common patterns are encountered in A&E departments: contact with domestic supply (low voltage) and contact with high-voltage power lines. Lightning will be dealt with separately.

Domestic supply injury

In the UK the mains supply is 240 V AC. If the body acts as a mass conductor with a resistance of 1000 ohm, a current of 0.25 amps is generated. If the limb in contact with the source is thrown back from the current then the contact times are small and the tissue damage is limited. Full-thickness skin burns may be seen at the entry site but deep damage does not occur.

AC may cause tetanic spasm leading to longer contact times and greater damage. The life-threatening problem is that of VF.

Cardiac arrest is managed according to conventional protocols (see Chapter 3). The arrest rhythm is usually VF.

The conscious patient

Procedure

- Assess to ensure that there are no immediately life-threatening problems.
- Carry out a full history and examination and arrange appropriate investigations.
- Elucidate the exact source of the shock. If there is suspicion that high voltage may have been involved then have a low threshold for admitting the patient. Ask if the patient was thrown back from the source or if the source made it difficult to let go.
- Enquire about tetanus status, allergy and any concurrent medical illness or medications.
- Examine the whole body. Record the Glasgow Coma Score, the pulse rate, blood pressure and respiratory rate.
- Note the size and depth of the burn at the entry site. Look for burns at possible exit sites such as the contralateral limb or the feet.
- Examine for signs of cardiac failure.

- A 12 lead ECG should be recorded in all cases.
- If there is a significant area of full-thickness burning $>1\,cm^2$ on the hands), then referral to the appropriate surgical in-patient team will be required.
- Tetanus toxoid is given if indicated.

Aftercare

Most patients who have no signs or symptoms following minor contact with domestic electricity may be discharged home. If there are no cardiac abnormalities on examination or on the initial ECG then it is unlikely that they will occur subsequently. However, note the indications in Table 2 for a senior opinion or admission to hospital.

Table 2. *Indications for admission to hospital following contact with domestic electricity.*

- Loss of conciousness at any time
- Significant burn, especially full-thickness
- New abnormalities on cardiovascular examination or on the ECG
- Doubt whether the source was high voltage
- Any neurological signs or symptoms
- Established cardiorespiratory disease

High-voltage burns

These are critical injuries and the patient must be managed in the resuscitation room with early and aggressive support of the airway breathing and circulation. If there is any indication of upper airway burns then early endotracheal intubation is essential.

Procedure

- Fluid replacement in line with local burns protocols should aim to obtain a urine output of $50-100\,ml\,h^{-1}$ to prevent renal tubular damage from myoglobinuria.
- If full-thickness burns interfere with circulation to a limb or digit or inhibit chest expansion, then early escharotomy is required. The burnt tissue is incised for the whole length of the injured area and the incision must be deep enough to allow the constricted tissue to spread apart.
- Examination to reveal the full extent of the burns and exclude other injuries which may have been sustained in falls.
- Compartment pressures in the injured limb should be monitored and fasciotomy performed if they are found to be above 30 mmHg (Hammond & Ward, 1988).

- Neurological examination is especially important in view of the high incidence of subsequent neurological problems.

Investigations

Early investigations should include cross-matching of blood, and estimation of urea and electrolytes, haematocrit, osmolality and blood gas tensions. Urine is tested repeatedly for free haemoglobin and myoglobin. If the patient has been exposed to fire in a confined space check carboxyhaemoglobin levels.

X-rays of the chest, cervical spine and pelvis should be obtained routinely because of the risk of serious injury. Damaged limbs must also be X-rayed together with other areas as necessary. Have a low threshold for ordering X-rays of the whole spine and shoulders. Fractures and dislocations resulting from tetanic muscle contraction may be difficult to diagnose.

Detailed investigation is outwith the scope of most A&E departments but technetium isotope scanning is a useful technique for imaging the extent of muscle damage in high-voltage injury (Chang & Yang, 1991; Delpassand *et al.*, 1990). Early and radical debridement of dead tissue is required and amputation is often necessary. Mortality rates are dependent on the degree of damage, but in the best centres high-voltage injury has survival rates of 90–95%.

Discuss such injuries early with the regional burns centre but do not transfer patients until they have been fully resuscitated, other injuries defined and treated, and the patient is stable.

Lightning injury

Lightning may strike directly causing all the current to flow through the body resulting in major tissue damage. The current may also arc around the body producing more widespread burns. Bolts may be deflected from a nearby object (side-flash), or if the bolt strikes the ground near the victim there may be such a large potential difference between one foot and the other that the current may travel up one leg and down the other (Fulde & Marsden, 1990). Blast injury may damage the lungs or bowel.

Cardiac arrest is managed according to conventional guidelines. Respiratory arrest and asystole are common causes of arrest. Prolonged cardiac massage is indicated since good survival and recoveries have been reported.

Presenting complaints are varied and at first may seem bizarre. Always take any symptoms seriously.

If the patient is stable, perform a full head-to-toe examination looking for evidence of burns, neurological injury and musculo-skeletal trauma.

Detailed examination of the eyes and ears is necessary to establish a baseline; these examinations will need to be repeated following admission.

Investigations should be carried out as detailed above for high-voltage injury. Computerized tomography (CT) may be required in cases of impaired consciousness. Radiographs of the chest and ECG recording should be routine.

All patients should be admitted for monitoring of cardiovascular and lung function and repeated neurological assessment.

Bibliography

General and biological effects of electricity

BRITISH STANDARDS INSTITUTION (1988). *Effects of Current Passing Through the Human Body*. Part 1. *General aspects*. London: British Standards Institution.

DANIEL, R.K., BALLARD, P.A., HEROUX, P. *et al.* (1988). High voltage electrical injury: acute pathophysiology. *J. Hand Surg.*, **13A**, 44–9.

GAYLOR, D.C., PRAKAH-ASANTE, K. & LEE, R.C. (1988). Significance of cell size and tissue structure in electrical trauma. *J. Theor. Biol.*, **133**, 223–37.

KOLLER, J. (1991). High tension electrical arc induced thermal burns caused by railway overhead cables. *Burns*, **17**, 411–4.

LEE, R.C., CRAVALHO, E.G. & BURKE, J.F. (1992). *Electrical Trauma: The Pathophysiology, Manifestations and Clinical Management*. Cambridge: Cambridge University Press.

ROBINSON, M.N., BROOKS, G.A. & RENSHAW, G.D. (1990). Electric shock devices and their effects on the human body. *Med. Sci. Law*, **30**, 285–300.

Complications and treatment

Nervous system

BOOZALIS, G.T., PURDUE, G.F., HUNT, J.L. *et al.* (1991). Ocular changes from electrical burns, a literature review and report of cases. *J. Burn Care Rehab.*, **12**, 458–62.

GALLAGHER, J.P. & TALBERT, O.R. (1990) Motor neurone syndrome after electric shock. *Acta Neurol. Scand.*, **83**, 79–82.

GRUBE, B.J., HEIMBACH, D.M., ENGRAV, L.H. *et al.* (1990). Neurological consequences of electrical burns. *J. Trauma*, **30**, 254–8.

KANITKAR, S. & ROBERTS, A.H.N. (1988). Paraplegia in an electrical burn. *Burns*, **14**, 49–50.

KOLLER, J. & OSAGH, I. (1989). Delayed neurological sequelae of high tension elecrical burns. *Burns*, **15**, 175–8.

LEHMAN, L.B. (1991). Successful management of an adult lightning strike victim using intracranial pressure monitoring. *Neurosurgery*, **28**, 907–10.

SILVA, J.A., LEONG, G.B. & FERRARI, M.M. (1991). Posttraumatic stress disorder in burn patients. *South. Med. J.*, **84**, 530–1.

Burn injury

BARNES, S.J. & MERCER, D.M. (1989). Flash burns to the face. *Burns*, **15**, 250–1.

CHANG, L.Y. & YANG, J.Y. (1991). The role of bone scans in elecrical burns. *Burns*, **17**, 250–3.

DELPASSAND, E.S., DHEKNE, R.D., BARRON, B.J. *et al.* (1990). Evaluation of soft tissue injury by Tc-99m bone agent scintigraphy. *Clin. Nucl. Med.* **16**, 314–9.

HAMMOND, J.S. & WARD, C.G. (1988). High voltage electrical injuries: management and outcome of 60 cases. *South. Med. J.*, **81**, 1351–2.

Cardiac

CUNNINGHAM, P.A. (1991). The need for cardiac monitoring after electrical injury. *Med. J. Aust.*, **154**, 765–6.

HOMMA, S., GILLAM, L.D. & WEYMAN, A.E. (1990). Echocardiographic observations in survivors of acute electrical injury. *Chest*, **97**, 103–5.

JENSEN, P.J., THOMSEN, P.E.B., BAGGER, J.P. *et al.* (1987). Electrical injury causing ventricular arrhythmias. *Br. Heart J.*, **57**, 279–83.

PURDUE, G.F. & HUNT, J.L. (1986). Electrocardiographic monitoring after electrical injury: necessity or luxury. *J. Trauma*, **26**, 166–8.

SCHEIN, R.M.H., KETT, D.H., DE MARCHENA, E.J. *et al.* (1990). Pulmonary oedema associated with electrical injury. *Chest*, **97**, 1248–50.

Lightning

ANDREWS, C.J. & DARVENIZA, M. (1989). Telephone mediated lightning injury: an Australian survey. *J. Trauma*, **29**, 665–71.

DUCLOS, P.J. & SANDERSON, L.M. (1990). An epidemiological description of lightning related deaths in the United States. *Int. J. Epidemiol.*, **19**, 673–9.

ERIKSSON, A. & ORNEHULT, L. (1988). Death by lightning. *Am. J. Forensic Med. Pathol.*, **9**, 295–300.

FULDE, G.W.O. & MARSDEN, ST J. (1990). Lightning strikes. *Med. J. Aust.*, **15**, 496–8.

LUTALO, S.K. & PRATT, G.P. (1989). Acute pulmonary oedema caused by lightning. *Cent. Afr. J. Med.*, **35**, 534–7.

37 Near drowning and diving injuries

D. STEEDMAN

Department of Accident and Emergency Medicine, Royal Infirmary, Edinburgh, UK

Chapter plan

Near drowning
Diving injuries
Appendix: Where to get help

NEAR DROWNING

Introduction

Drowning is defined as death by suffocation following submersion in a liquid and near drowning is the term used when there is at least temporary survival from this. There are on average 700 deaths from drowning per annum in the UK and the victims are predominantly children and young adults. Drowning is the third commonest cause of accidental death in children in Britain after road traffic accidents and burns (Office of Population Census and Surveys (OPCS), 1988). In 1988 and 1989, 149 children aged between 0 and 14 years drowned giving an incidence of 0.7 per 100 000 (Kemp & Sibert, 1992) but the incidence of drowning is considerably higher in the USA (2.7); (Wintemute, 1990) and Australia (5.2); Pearn *et al.*, 1976). Much of this difference can be attributed to warmer climates and the prevalence of domestic swimming pools in these two countries.

These mortality figures probably underestimate the size of the problem. There are no data available on the numbers of victims of submersion incidents seen in accident and emergency (A&E) departments. However, up to 90% of near drowning victims may not reach hospital with further morbidity being prevented by prompt local action (Geddis, 1984).

Most accidents occur in fresh water. Coastal waters are usually associated with better surveillance and rescue systems, but a survey conducted by the Royal Life Saving Society of 51 British beaches judged over half to have inadequate provisions for beach safety (Holiday Which?, 1991). The majority of drowning and near drowning incidents in children under 5 years take place at home. Bath drownings occur mainly in babies and young toddlers. Garden pools and domestic swimming pools continue to be a significant problem (Barry *et al.*, 1982). There is a strong correlation between lack of adult supervision and drowning deaths in children. Most children admitted to hospital after nearly drowning in public baths have been effectively resuscitated at the poolside and the mortality is remarkably low (Kemp & Sibert, 1992). Mortality is higher in submersion accidents associated with unsupervised swimming or falls into open waterways such as lakes, rivers, canals or flooded quarries. Incidents in farmyards involving sheep dips, animal drinking troughs, slurry pits and septic tanks are sporadically reported. Thirty per cent of adult drownings occur because of boating accidents.

The specific cause of a submersion accident may be difficult to determine. Certain factors are, however, associated with drowning and near drowning which may alter management and outcome. The single most important precipitating factor in adult drownings is the recent consumption of alcohol (Mackie, 1979)

Factors associated with drowning and near drowning

- Cervical spine and cord injury (especially in diving accidents)
- Head or other injury (due to falls or boating accidents)
- Alcohol or drug intoxication
- Hypoglycaemia (diabetics or alcohol intoxication)
- Epilepsy
- Cerebral air embolism (Scuba divers)
- Non-accidental drowning (suicide, homicide, child abuse)

Pathophysiology

Involuntary submersion typically results in a period of intense struggling and breath-holding before a breakpoint is reached and involuntary inspiration occurs. The breath-holding capacity of an average individual in water colder than 15°C is in the region of 15–25 sec, which is approximately one-third of normal and increases the risk of drowning. In about 15% of cases intense laryngospasm is precipitated by fluid contacting the larynx and asphyxiation occurs without fluid entering the lungs ('dry drowning'). More commonly, however, water enters the tracheobronchial tree either initially upon submersion or as the laryngospasm abates when loss of consciousness supervenes.

Pulmonary injury

Aspiration of water results in pulmonary injury. The mechanisms involved will depend on whether salt or fresh water is aspirated and on the presence of contaminants such as mud, sand, sewage and bacteria. The culmination of these effects is profound hypoxia. Inhalation of water results in vagally mediated pulmonary vasoconstriction and pulmonary hypertension. Intrapulmonary shunting may increase from the normal level of 10% to as much as 75%. Fresh water is a particularly effective trigger of this response which can occur following aspiration of very small (1 ml kg^{-1}) quantities of fluid. Both fresh water and salt water aspiration produce diffuse alveolar capillary membrane damage. Sea water, which has an osmolality three to four times that of plasma, results in a rapid exudation of protein-rich fluid into the alveoli and interstitium of the lung. In fresh water aspiration fluid moves across the alveolar capillary membrane into the circulation. These rapid fluid fluxes cause severe destruction of pulmonary ultrastructure. Endothelial changes consist of microvesicle formation, swelling, detachment from the basement membrane and disruption of both type 1 and type 2 pneumocytes (Nopanitanya *et al.*, 1974). Loss of surfactant in both salt water and fresh water aspiration by a wash-out effect or denaturation result in atelectasis and stiff non-compliant lungs. The presence of chlorine in 1–2 parts per million, such as occurs in swimming pools, does not influence the degree of pulmonary injury. Large amounts of water can be swallowed during involuntary submersion which may lead to vomiting and contribute to pulmonary injury from aspiration of gastric contents.

About 5% of submersion victims who respond well to initial resuscitation subsequently deteriorate from a respiratory distress syndrome (Pearn, 1980). The syndrome has been observed after both salt water and fresh water near drowning and is commonly referred to as 'secondary drowning'. The phenomenon is thought to be due to loss of surfactant from chemical, anoxic and osmotic damage to the pneumocytes that line the alveoli. Other respiratory causes of post-rescue respiratory deterioration which must be considered include bacterial pneumonia, foreign body or chemical pneumonitis, and pulmonary barotrauma.

Central nervous system effects

The cause of death in acute drowning is irreversible cerebral anoxia (Colebatch & Halmagyi, 1961). There is, however, a period of reversibility before the cerebral hypoxic insult produces permanent damage to neurones (Safar, 1993). Cerebral hypoxia and ischaemia result in a breakdown in the blood/brain barrier and intracellular and extracellular increases in osmotic pressure develop as vascular and cell wall integrity are lost. Cerebral oedema may consequently develop in survivors but several reports suggest that an increase in intracranial pressure is not a common complication of global anoxia in near drowning at least in the first 24 h. Central nervous system (CNS) damage may continue after restoration of cerebral blood flow. During complete cerebral ischaemic anoxia, calcium shifts, brain tissue lactic acidosis, and increases in brain free fatty acids, osmolality and extracellular concentrations of excitatory amino acids set the stage for reperfusion injury (Safar, 1993). Neurones demonstrate selective vulnerability and skills which require visual–motor coordination have been reported to be particularly affected in survivors of submersion accidents (Pearn, 1977).

Cardiovascular effects

Cardiac arrhythmias and depression of myocardial function may result from hypoxia caused by the pulmonary injury and can be compounded by a metabolic acidosis. Increased catecholamine release secondary to the stress of the submersion incident has also been implicated (Karch, 1985).

Salt water versus fresh water aspiration

The effect of aspiration of hypertonic sea water and the rapid shift of plasma into the alveoli and interstitium should produce a reduction in circulating blood volume and a rise in serum electrolytes. Shifts from the alveoli to the intravascular compartment in fresh water aspiration should result in expansion of blood volume, haemolysis and a decrease in serum electrolyte concentrations. Despite these theoretical changes, however, few near drowning victims presenting to the A&E department have blood electrolyte abnormalities requiring treatment. Modell and colleages have demonstrated that electrolyte abnormalities do not occur if less than 22 ml kg^{-1} is aspirated (Modell & Davis, 1969). Autopsy studies have demonstrated that only 15% of those who die in the water aspirate more than this quantity (Modell *et al.*, 1976).

Immersion hypothermia

Immersion in cold water may rapidly lead to hypothermia due to surface heat loss. In addition, core cooling can occur after swallowing and aspirating cold water (Orlowski, 1987; Hayward *et al.*, 1984). Thermal conductivity of cold water is up to 25 times that of air; the average sea temperature around Britain is 11°C in summer. The rate of fall of temperature after immersion is dependent on multiple variables including surface area/mass ratio, volume of water aspirated or swallowed, body/water temperature gradient, thickness of subcutaneous fat and type of clothing worn. Children have less subcutaneous fat and relatively greater body surface area compared to adults.

Cases of drowning and near drowning are often the consequence of the hypothermic victim losing consciousness. Coordinated motor activity becomes progressively more difficult as hypothermia supervenes. Increased peripheral blood flow during exercise increases the conductive loss from uninsulated extremities and movement will increase convective losses. Associated exhaustion may hasten eventual collapse and subsequent drowning in cold water. Scuba divers are usually in negative thermal balance despite wearing a wet suit or dry suit for thermal protection. If a life jacket is worn it will keep the airway clear of water and will in most instances prevent drowning. Although a life jacket will also delay the onset of hypothermia by reducing the need for limb movement, hypothermia will eventually develop. A life jacket is not always a guarantee against drowning or near drowning in rough seas especially when consciousness becomes impaired as a result of hypothermia.

On immersion in cold water (<15°C) sympathetic increase in heart rate and precipitous elevation in blood pressure may result in myocardial infarction or cerebro-vascular accident. Sudden cardiac arrest may follow catecholamine-induced arrhythmias (Keatinge & Hayward, 1981).

During prolonged cold water immersion, peripheral vasoconstriction and hydrostatic squeeze on tissues below the surface shunts blood into the deep capacitance vessels. The relative excess volume is removed by a diuresis. Cold exposure also results in fluid shifts from the extracellular to the intracellular compartment. Significant volume depletion can precipitate cardiovascular collapse during rescue and resuscitation.

There have been reports of children surviving with restoration of normal neurological function after being rescued following prolonged submersion (40–60 mins) in very cold water (Siebke *et al.*, 1975). Submersion in cold water and the development of hypothermia decrease metabolic demands. Brain temperatures fall at up to 1°C min^{-1} during agonal respirations of drowning animals submerged in fresh water at 20–22°C. The rapid onset of hypothermia during fresh water drowning is due to the rapid absorption of cold water with significant cooling taking place prior to cessation of circulation (Conn & Barker, 1984). When the temperature falls to below 28°C ventricular fibrillation (VF) or asystole can occur.

The diving reflex

One explanation for survival following long periods of submersion in very cold water has focused on the possibility that the diving reflex present in aquatic mammals may operate in humans. Although apnoeic submersion of humans elicits the oxygen-conserving 'dive reflex', evidence suggests that this is insignificant in potentiating the protective effects of hypothermia (Ramey *et al.*, 1987). The dive reflex in humans is very weak compared to aquatic mammals and is only present whilst breath-holding occurs. In addition, cold water further weakens the reflex by diminishing breath-holding duration. Consequently, for humans submerged in cold water the reflex peripheral and splanchnic vasoconstriction and associated bradycardia stimulated by trigeminal afferents following facial submersion is only a transient phenomenon and would not be able to conserve sufficient oxygen to provide neurological sparing. Any bradycardia beyond the period of involuntary breath-holding and consciousness is a pathological loss of autonomic control or directly related to hypothermia rather than the centrally regulated bradycardia of the dive reflex (Hayward *et al.*, 1984). Circulatory arrest resulting from VF occurs in children at a lower temperature than in adults, thus permitting more profound central cooling (Harries, 1986). This has been attributed to blunting of catecholamine release during rapid cooling (Orlowski, 1987).

Prehospital care

The initial management of fresh and sea water submersion accidents is identical. At the scene, resuscitation should follow basic first aid principles. Expired air resuscitation can be started while the victim is still in the water but external cardiac compressions cannot be adequately delivered until the victim has been rescued. In near drowning accidents associated with sport diving, scuba regulators have been used to assist ventilation. The pressure required to inflate the lungs may be considerable.

During rescue from prolonged cold water immersion, impairment of baroreceptor response together with sudden release of the 'hydrostatic squeeze' applied to tissues below the surface may precipitate severe hypotension and cardiac arrest. If possible the casualty should be removed horizontally. It is often more important, however, to get the casualty out of the water quickly. If horizontal rescue is not practicable the victim should be placed in a level position as quickly as possible after removal from the cold water. If the rescue is performed on a steeply sloping beach the patient should be placed parallel to the water's edge.

Adequate cervical spine immobilization should be maintained during rescue and resuscitation following submersion accidents from surfing or diving into water, in those patients with signs of injury, and in unconscious casualties. The risk of further aspiration secondary to regurgitation of large volumes of water and stomach contents is high. Therefore the unconsious self-ventilating patient should be placed and transported in the recovery position. A modified position avoiding flexion or rotation of the neck must be used if cervical spine injury is suspected.

If the victim is breathing spontaneously, high-flow oxygen (12–15 litres min^{-1}) should be given via a mask. Frequent suctioning to maintain a patent airway is necessary in most unconscious submersion victims. If ventilation is inadequate or the patient is apnoeic, assisted ventilation will be required by bag–mask or mouth-to-mask techniques. Skilled tracheal intubation will greatly assist ventilation and clearing of secretions. Attempts to drain fluid from the lungs are unhelpful and will delay ventilation and external chest compression. Gastric drainage may be required in patients who have swallowed large volumes of water since gastric distension can interfere with ventilation. This can be achieved by abdominal compression or gravity drainage with adequate suction immediately available. Attempts to empty the stomach should not precede initial attempts at ventilation and when deemed necessary should be performed with minimal delay in the basic life support sequence.

The casualty should be insulated from the environment to prevent further heat loss and to allow spontaneous rewarming. It is important when applying insulation to remember the head, since up to 70% of total heat production can be lost from this site depending on ambient temperature. Conduction losses will continue if a patient is simply covered with a blanket and no insulation is provided between the body and the ground. Using polythene sheeting or bags for insulation is as effective and cheaper than commercially available metallized plastic sheeting and space blankets. A thick fibre pile 'casualty bag' covered by a waterproof layer is even better.

In profound hypothermia there is significant respiratory depression and the patient may appear apnoeic. If the patient is found in respiratory arrest, assisted ventilation should be commenced. Palpation of peripheral pulses is difficult in vasoconstricted hypothermic patients when the cardiac rate is extremely slow. Careful palpation of the carotid or femoral pulse for at least 1 min may be necessary. The low cardiac output may be sufficient to meet the demands in these patients and ventricular fibrillation can be precipitated by unnecessary external chest compressions. In hypothermic victims chest compressions should be performed at the same rate as in normothermic patients. If a monitor is available the cardiac rhythm should be determined. DC countershock at 2 J kg^{-1} should be given if indicated. Attempts at defibrillation are usually unsuccessful until the core temperature is above 28–30°C. Most drugs are ineffective in hypothermic patients or are dangerous to use because of increased cardiac irritability.

All victims of submersion, including those patients who are asymptomatic, should be taken to the A&E department. Estimates of duration of submersion are notoriously inaccurate when made by bystanders, patients or even trained rescuers. Death should not be diagnosed in the field but hazardous conditions may render prolonged attempts at resuscitation or evacuation to hospital impossible.

Management in the A&E department

Investigations

Patients may be triaged according to an ABC classification system popularized by Modell & Conn (1980) for prognosis: patients who are fully alert and orientated (**A** for 'awake'); patients who are not fully conscious but are rousable and demonstrate purposeful responses to painful stimuli (**B** for 'blunted'); patients who are comatose (**C**). Patients in groups A and B require a chest radiograph and arterial blood gas determinations. Those in group B may also require baseline biochemical and respiratory function studies. Careful clinical monitoring of these two groups should prevent overinvestigation (Pearn, 1985).

Victims who are comatose (group C), and all others who are not improving clinically, required further investigation for immediate diagnosis and to establish baselines for monitoring progress.

Investigations in near drowning

- Chest radiographs
- Skull and cervical spine radiographs
- Skeletal survey (suspected non-accidental injury)
- Serial blood gas determinations
- Urea and electrolytes
- Blood glucose
- Full blood count
- Coagulation screen
- Anticonvulsant levels (if appropriate)
- Drug screen (if indicated)
- Electrocardiogram.
- Core temperature
- Sputum culture
- Respiratory function studies

In cases of aspiration, the typical radiographic pattern on chest X-ray is generalized pulmonary oedema with patchy shadowing. The radiograph may be normal despite a pulmonary insult and the initial appearances often underestimate the extent of the pulmonary injury.

There should be a high index of suspicion for cervical spine injury. Whenever there is uncertainty surrounding the incident and especially if the casualty's conscious level is depressed, it should be assumed that the patient has an unstable cervical spine injury. Cervical spine radiographs must be performed in these circumstances. Physical examination may reveal associated injuries

which will require appropriate radiological investigation. A full skeletal survey will be required in cases of suspected non-accidental injury. A CT (computed tomography) scan may be necessary in comatose patients not responding to treatment in whom head injury is suspected.

Initial treatment

The complete recovery of apparently lifeless individuals justifies aggressive resuscitation and support of all victims of near drowning brought to the A&E department.

High-flow oxygen (12–15 litres min^{-1}) should be administered via a face mask to conscious patients while awaiting the results of arterial blood gas analysis.

Clearing the airway of regurgitated fluid and debris by suctioning is of primary importance in unconscious casualties. If the gag reflex is significantly impaired or the patient is not breathing, the airway should be protected by skilled tracheal intubation. If aspiration of particulate matter is suspected, bronchoscopy is required. Intermittent positive pressure ventilation should be commenced if necessary and, in near drowning patients, high inflation pressures are often required. Maintaining positive end expiratory pressure (PEEP) typically results in marked improvement in the patient's oxygenation. PEEP increases functional residual capacity, reduces ventilation/ perfusion mismatch and prevents atelectasis following surfactant loss. In cooperative patients able to tolerate a tight fitting mask, continuous positive airway pressure (CPAP) ventilation may avoid the need for tracheal intubation and assisted ventilation. After obtaining adequate levels of oxygenation, PEEP or CPAP should be maintained for at least 24 h to allow the regeneration of sufficient surfactant.

Mechanical ventilation is required when a patient cannot maintain satisfactory arterial oxygen and carbon dioxide concentrations: a PaO_2 of 8.0 kPa (60 mmHg) or less breathing air, a PaO_2 of 10.0 kPa (75 mmHg) or less on 50% oxygen, or a $PaCO_2$ of 7.5 kPa (50 mmHg) or more.

Expansion of plasma volume may be required if a satisfactory circulating volume cannot be maintained, especially if hypovolaemia is unmasked by PEEP. A Swan–Ganz catheter is advised in patients who develop haemodynamic instability or who require high levels of CPAP or PEEP.

If cardiac arrest occurs, advanced life support measures should be initiated and cardiac arrhythmias treated according to standard protocols. In patients with reduced core temperatures the guidelines for the management of hypothermic victims presented in Chapter 38 should be followed. Cardiopulmonary resuscitation should not be abandoned until the core temperature exceeds 33°C and drugs have been excluded as far as is possible as a cause of the arrest. When metabolic and thermal imbalances have been corrected and resuscitation has continued for a further 30 min in the presence of asystole without response, it is usually reasonable to stop.

Acidosis is the commonest and most serious metabolic abnormality encountered in submersion victims. Initial management is directed towards restoration of adequate ventilation. In prolonged resuscitation and/or known arterial pH levels $\leqslant 7.1$ ($H^+ > 80$ nmol l^{-1}), sodium bicarbonate 1 mmol kg^{-1} may be given, but further aliquots should be guided by arterial blood gas values. Clinically important serum electrolyte disturbances are not common and if present usually resolve following adequate resuscitation and rewarming.

Substantial volumes of water may be absorbed from the stomach, especially in infants, and pulmonary aspiration causes severe complications. A nasogastric tube should therefore be passed. Patients with facial injury or in whom there is suspicion of a cribriform plate or basal skull fracture, should have an orogastric rather than a nasogastric tube inserted to avoid inadvertent intracranial placement.

Prophylactic antibiotics need not be administered to all submersion victims. Antibiotic treatment is usually restricted to patients with confirmed sepsis on sputum or blood culture. Although still controversial, antibiotic therapy to cover a broad spectrum of Gram-negative organisms should probably be started early if contaminated water is implicated. Sea water incidents are much less likely to be associated with aspiration of infective organisms.

Steroids have not been shown clearly to improve the outcome from cerebral oedema or pulmonary injury associated with near drowning and are not recommended (Calderwood et al., 1975).

Following resuscitation and stabilization of the cardiovascular system, comatose patients should be admitted to an appropriate intensive therapy unit.

Signs of secondary drowning usually develop within 4 h of the submersion accident. Asymptomatic patients with normal serial blood gas results while breathing air and a normal chest radiograph after 6 h are unlikely to develop problems and can be safely discharged.

Cerebral resuscitation in near drowning

Appropriate use of muscle relaxants, sedation and analgesia, and gentle handling of the patient should minimize potential increases in intracranial pressure (ICP). Cerebral oedema is not easily detected or controlled using basic clinical measurements and some units advocate ICP monitoring by an extradural or intraventricular pressure transducer. Sudden increases in ICP can be controlled by hyperventilation but reduction in Pa_{CO_2} can cause differential cerebral blood flow to non-ischaemic areas of the brain (the steal phenomenon) as well as causing systemic hypotension; a Pa_{CO_2} of 4.0–4.5 kPa (30–34 mmHg) offers an optimal compromise. Mannitol 0.5–1.0 g kg^{-1} as an intravenous bolus can also be used to reduce cerebral oedema.

Empirical regimes used in 'cerebral resuscitation' of near drowning victims have been advocated, and include hypothermia, barbiturates and aggressive treatment of raised ICP. While hypothermia during immersion may be protective, the use of therapeutic hypothermia to treat the secondary effects of cerebral hypoxia is more controversial. Usually, if the core temperature is above 30°C, the aim should be to rewarm the patient over 6–8 h following rescue. Some units advocate inducing hypothermia (30 ± 1°C) when the ICP cannot be controlled by other means. However, hypothermia is associated with a reduction in neutrophil count and activity and may lead to a higher incidence of sepsis. Barbiturates reduce cerebral metabolic rate, decrease membrane permeability and reduce cerebral oxygen demand. The use of barbiturates such as thiopentone in paralysed and ventilated victims of submersion, however, remains inconclusive and may even compromise cerebral perfusion by lowering cardiac output (Nussbaum & Maggi, 1988).

Intensive therapy should be directed at optimal cardiorespiratory support with full monitoring so that the potentially damaging effects of hypoxia, hypercarbia and inadequate cerebral perfusion pressure will not contribute to further brain damage. Although raised ICP is associated with a poor outcome (Dean & McComb, 1981), aggressive treatment has not been convincingly demonstrated to improve outcome and there are reports that it may lead to a rise in the number of patients surviving in a persisting vegetative state (Biggart & Bohn, 1990). Cerebral resuscitation should therefore not be employed routinely and only after careful consideration.

Prognosis

The management of near drowning includes giving a prognosis to parents and relatives. The initial clinical history is almost always incomplete. Although prolonged submersion times are associated with an unfavourable prognosis, reports on the duration of submersion are usually unreliable when the patient is admitted to the A&E department (Kemp & Sibert, 1991). The history has to be built up following admission and help is required from bystanders, rescuers, police and ambulance personnel.

The skill of basic life support provided at the scene is recognized as one of the most important factors influencing ultimate survival. A delay in instituting effective cardiopulmonary resuscitation of more than 10 min following rescue is associated with an unfavourable prognosis (Orlowski, 1979). One of the best prognostic indicators is the time to the first respiratory gasp which if made within 20 min of the rescue is associated with an excellent outcome (Pearn, 1985). Respiratory effort on admission to the A&E department is usually associated with a good recovery.

Although a third of children in the British Isles admitted unconscious after near drowning either die or have subsequent severe neurological deficit, most children admitted unconscious with reactive pupils survive normally after submersion incidents and a third of children admitted to hospital unconscious with fixed dilated pupils also do well (Kemp & Sibert, 1991). This contrasts with studies in the USA referring largely to incidents involving warm swimming pools, which have shown that fixed dilated pupils and coma predict those patients who will die or have neurological deficit. Most outdoor drownings in the UK are in water temperatures of less than 20°C and all the children in the British Isles study previously mentioned were hypothermic with a mean core temperature of 31°C.

In child victims, pupils remaining fixed and dilated 6 h after admission or fits continuing 24 h after admission predict a poor outcome (Kemp & Sibert, 1991). Of all children who survive only about 3% will exist in a persistent vegetative state. The incidence of severe handicap such as spastic quadriplegia varies between 5% and 20% in children admitted to hospital unconscious. Following recovery of children who appear to function normally, approximately one-third have minimal cerebral dysfunction revealed on formal psychometric testing (Pearn, 1977).

DIVING INJURIES

Introduction

It is estimated that there are 50 000 sport divers in the United Kingdom performing 1–2 million dives every year (Douglas, 1985). In addition 1500 commercial divers operate in the North Sea. The medical care of these professional divers is strictly controlled by law, supervised by trained personnel and accidents are now uncommon. Although there is no legislation controlling recreational diving, national subaqua clubs promote high standards of training and safety. Despite this 10–12 deaths and 200 serious diving accidents are reported every year (Sykes, 1990). Doctors and paramedics may have to start resuscitation of a diving casualty at the scene and arrange evacuation to a specialist diving medical facility. Furthermore, divers may present to A&E departments far removed from the dive site with vague symptoms which may herald serious illness.

This section is concerned with problems which affect recreational divers. Such divers use self-contained underwater breathing apparatus (SCUBA) at pressures associated with depths down to 50 m. SCUBA uses a compressed air cylinder carried on the back; the pressure is reduced with a demand valve so that the pressure of the air breathed by the diver is exactly equal to the surrounding water pressure.

Pathophysiology

Pressure and volume

The pressure exerted by air contained in the atmosphere at sea level is about 100 kPa (1 atmosphere). This is called the atmospheric pressure. When a diver descends under water the ambient pressure increases. Water is much denser than air and the pressure exerted by 10 m of sea water is the same as that exerted by the entire atmosphere above sea level. Pressure is measured from one of two reference points. It can be expressed with reference to a vacuum, i.e. zero pressure. This reading is called the *absolute pressure*. The second method measures pressure above local pressure and these readings are called *gauge pressures*. Thus at sea level the absolute pressure is 1 atmosphere and the gauge pressure is zero. With descent in water the gauge pressure remains 1 atmosphere less than the absolute pressure. For example, at 50 m the gauge pressure reads 5 atmospheres (ATG) and is equivalent to 6 atmospheres absolute

(ATA). Sport diving is performed at a pressure of up to 6 ATA.

The tissues of the body are composed mostly of water which is not compressible and not significantly affected by pressure changes. However, gases are compressible and consequently gas-containing spaces and organs are directly affected by changes in ambient pressure. The gases in these spaces obey Boyle's Law. This states that, if the absolute temperature remains constant, the volume (V) of a given mass of gas is inversely proportional to the absolute pressure (P) ($V \propto 1/P$). Thus if 10 litres of gas at sea level (1 ATA) is compressed to 2 ATA it will occupy 5 litres, and 2 litres at 5 ATA. The greatest changes in pressure ratio and consequently volume occur near the surface.

If a person fills their lungs at the surface and then dives to 10 m, the lung volume will decrease by 50%. On returning to the surface the gas will re-expand to its original volume. When SCUBA is used during a dive the pressure in the gas-filled spaces of the body is normally in equilibrium with the ambient pressure. If the volumes of the gas-filled spaces in the diver's body are to remain constant during a descent air has to be added as the ambient pressure increases. Should obstruction occur in the various portals of gas exchange a pressure disequilibrium develops and tissue damage can result. During the ascent phase ambient pressure decreases. Consequently, gas in the body spaces expands in volume. If a scuba diver ascends rapidly to the surface from 30 m without exhaling, the volume of gas will increase four-fold. Unless gas is vented as it expands it will exert pressure on the surrounding tissues. Injury caused by direct tissue damage following volume changes of gas consequent on pressure is called *barotrauma* and can occur during descent or ascent. Barotrauma can occur during rapid ascent from a shallow dive, even from the bottom of a swimming pool.

Partial pressures in gas mixtures

Increase in depth and associated pressures also affect the partial pressure of the respiratory gases. Air consists of approximately 21% oxygen, 79% nitrogen, 0.03% carbon dioxide and traces of other gases. The total pressure of this mixture of gases is equal to the sum of their partial pressures (Dalton's Law). The biological effects of each gas depends on its partial pressure which changes in proportion to the ambient pressure. The significance of partial pressure in diving concerns the toxic effects with which various gases have on the body at elevated

pressure; 100% oxygen cannot be used in diving because of the associated toxicity when breathed at a partial pressure in excess of 2 ATA.

The partial pressure of nitrogen in air increases with increasing depth, and below 30 m begins to exert a narcotic effect (*nitrogen narcosis*) which increases with increasing depth. Nitrogen is very soluble and dissolves in the lipid component of nerve cell membranes slowing impulse conduction. At depths below 30 m, euphoria, overconfidence and confusion develop and the decreasing level of consciousness below 50 m renders air diving unsafe. In commercial diving at greater depths helium is used to dilute the oxygen as helium has no narcotic effects. Although the narcotic effects are rapidly and entirely reversed as the diver ascends, nitrogen narcosis can be a precipitating factor in diving accidents.

Undesirable effects can also occur if the compressed air used in SCUBA contains contaminants. The air used is prepared by compressing and filtering normal atmospheric air. There are many potential contaminants in air especially if the compression process has occurred in an industrial area. Carbon monoxide and nitrogen oxides are toxic components of polluted city air and contamination may also occur if the compressor is operated near an engine exhaust. With pressurization even small concentrations of carbon monoxide can produce significant poisoning.

Solution of gases in liquids

As depth and therefore pressure increase during a dive, more gas will dissolve in body tissues (Henry's Law). While the excess oxygen acquired is capable of being used in metabolism producing carbon dioxide which is highly water-soluble, this is not the case with nitrogen. At sea level a diver's body tissues contain about 1 litre of nitrogen in solution. At a depth of 10 m breathing air at 2 ATA a diver will eventually reach equilibrium again and have twice as much nitrogen dissolved in his tissues. When he then ascends to the surface the extra nitrogen load must be expelled in a controlled manner. This is facilitated by an orderly ascent which may incorporate holding stages known as stops during which 'off-gassing' can occur. If insufficient time is allowed, desaturation of dissolved nitrogen forms bubbles in tissues and blood resulting in *decompression sickness*. These bubbles may cause tissue damage either at the sites of formation or at locations to which they have been delivered by the blood. The bubbles exert mechanical effects causing vascular or lymphatic occlusion and pressure on surrounding tissues. Bubbles also incite an inflammatory response due to a blood–bubble surface interaction. Activation of intrinsic clotting, kinin and complement systems result in cellular clumping, lipid embolization, increased vascular permeability, interstitial oedema and microvascular sludging (Kizer, 1983).

Barotrauma

Barotrauma of descent

Barotrauma of descent – or 'squeeze' as it is referred to by divers – results from compression of gases in enclosed spaces as ambient pressure increases. Equalization of middle ear pressure can be facilitated during a diver's descent by swallowing or performing a valsalva man-oeuvre. Mucosal congestion may obstruct the eustachian tube and as the pressure differential increases the diver will experience discomfort. As expected from the way in which gas volume changes with depth, most middle ear squeezes occur near the surface. If the diver continues to descend the pressure differential increases, mucosal oedema and haemorrhage occur and inward bulging of the tympanic membrane may eventually lead to rupture. Cold water then enters the middle ear causing vertigo and disorientation which can precipitate a diving acci-dent. Clinical examination will show erythema, haemor-rhage or perforation of the tympanic membrane with a conductive hearing loss.

External ear squeeze results if the external auditory canal is occluded (e.g. by cerumen plugs). Compression of the enclosed air will result in outward bulging of the tympanic membrane.

Rupture of the round or oval window (inner ear squeeze) can result if sudden and marked pressure changes occur between the middle and inner ear. A perilymphatic fistula results and classically the patient complains of tinnitus, vertigo and deafness. The typical features of middle ear barotrauma – sensorineural hear-ing deficit and vestibular dysfunction – are found on examination.

If tympanic rupture does not occur, middle ear squeeze can be managed with a decongestant which usually results in resolution of symptoms within 2 weeks. Anti-biotics should be prescribed when there is tympanic membrane rupture, previous infection or following a dive in polluted water. The diver must refrain from diving until the symptoms resolve and the rupture has completely healed. Specialized otolaryngological opinion is urgently required if a perilymphatic fistula is suspected.

Paranasal sinuses may also be affected by the develop-ment of pressure differentials. Precipitating factors include upper respiratory tract infections, nasal polyps and sinusitis. If a diver fails to exhale via his nose into his mask periodically during descent, a face mask squeeze can result with erythema, ecchymosis and petechial haemorrhages of the enclosed skin. Areas of skin tightly enclosed by part of the diver's suit can give similar appearances. These injuries appear dramatic but normally no treatment is required.

Barotrauma of ascent

Barotrauma of ascent is the reverse process of squeeze. It is unusual for the ears or sinuses to be affected by barotrauma with ascent since obstruction of gas exchange is unlikely if pressure equilibrium can be achieved during descent. 'Reverse squeeze' of the middle ear may result if the diver treats upper respiratory congestion with a short-acting topical vasoconstrictor and the effect wears off during a dive. Divers are strongly advised against diving with concurrent nasal or sinus congestion.

If the diver does not exhale adequately during ascent, alveoli may rupture allowing air to escape through the visceral and mediastinal pleura or alternatively into the pulmonary capillaries. *Pulmonary barotrauma* may be precipitated by breath-holding during rapid and uncon-trolled ascent or by air trapping which occurs in people with asthma or congenital bullae.

Pulmonary barotrauma may be asymptomatic or may present within minutes of surfacing with chest pain or dyspnoea. There may be a cough perhaps with the production of frothy bright red sputum usually in small amounts. Mediastinal emphysema is the commonest sequela of 'burst lung' and may develop several hours later either with gradually increasing hoarseness, neck fullness or with surgical emphysema in the neck or upper chest. Symptoms usually resolve spontaneously or fol-lowing treatment with high-flow oxygen.

Development of a pneumothorax following pulmonary barotrauma is unusual although it is a potentially serious complication if it develops during a dive. The intrapleural gas cannot be vented and will progress to a tension pneumothorax as the diver ascends. All patients suspected of pulmonary barotrauma should have a chest X-ray to exclude a pneumothorax. Treatment by needle thoraco-centesis or insertion of a chest drain is usually required. If recompression is necessary the chest drain must be clamped on compression and subjected to continuous suction at depth and during decompression.

The most dangerous complication of pulmonary baro-trauma is arterial air embolism. Cerebral air embolism causes symptoms immediately the diver surfaces. Classically the onset is dramatic with loss of consciousness, convulsions and cardiovascular collapse. Motor and sensory deficits tend to be unimodal and unilateral in contrast to the signs of decompression sickness which are usually bilateral and bimodal. Symptoms and signs attributed to brainstem involvement may be seen and subtle cognitive or personality changes also occur. A diagnosis of cerebral air embolism does not need to be substantiated by evidence of pulmonary barotrauma or of its other sequelae.

Decompression sickness

Decompression sickness is more likely to occur in cold water and in divers who exercise excessively during diving. Fifty per cent of divers who develop decompression sickness will become symptomatic in the first 10 min following diving, with 85% developing symptoms within 1 h (Francis *et al.*, 1989). However, divers may still present to the A&E department with symptoms 48 h after a dive.

Decompression sickness may be provoked by the reduction in barometric pressure experienced during air travel. This is liable to occur if there is insufficient time between diving and flying for residual inert gases to leave the body tissues in a controlled fashion. An interval of 12–48 h, depending on the depth and duration of dives performed, should be allowed between the last dive and flying (Sheffield, 1989).

Musculoskeletal manifestations

The colloquial term 'the bends' refers to acute peri-articular joint pain and is the commonest presenting symptom of decompression sickness. The shoulders and the elbows are most commonly affected in air diving decompression sickness. Symptoms are usually exacerbated by limb movement but are rarely associated with localized tenderness. Inflation of a blood pressure cuff around the joint may temporarily relieve the pain and assist with the diagnosis.

Cutaneous manifestations

Cutaneous manifestations may present as transient localized pruritic rashes which may be erythematous. A more important manifestation begins with itching which is usually situated over the trunk. Subsequently an erythematous rash appears which may be accentuated by coughing (Mellinghoff's sign). This is replaced by an area of cyanotic marbling known as cutis marmorata which may blanch on pressure. The affected skin may be warm to the touch and the area may become tender within a few hours even after treatment has successfully resolved other manifestations (Murrison & Francis, 1991). Local swelling or a peau d'orange effect can occur if lymphatic obstruction is present. Skin complications other than a transient itch indicate the need for recompression and a search for the other manifestations of decompression sickness should be made.

Neurological manifestations

Spinal decompression sickness may result from bubbles (venous, air embolic or autochthonous) pressing on the cord or obstructing venous drainage in the vertebral venous plexus (Hallenbeck *et al.*, 1975). The lower thoracic, lumbar and sacral segments are most commonly affected. Backache, girdle-type abdominal pain, lower limb weakness and paraesthesiae or urinary retention signify spinal decompression injury. Other manifestations of CNS involvement include coma and seizures, visual disturbance, dysphasia, and patchy motor and sensory deficits. Constitutional complaints such as lethargy or a general, non-specific feeling of ill-health may be noted. There may be impaired balance, vertigo and vomiting due to cerebellar involvement ('the staggers'). Increasingly subtle disturbance of higher cerebral function is being recognized as a manifestation with memory impairment and personality and mood changes.

Inner ear manifestations

Bubble formation within the confines of the inner ear can cause disruption of the vestibulocochlear apparatus. Although vestibular decompression sickness is not common and is predominantly seen in deep professional diving, it represents another cause of acute post-dive vertigo. It is important to differentiate between vestibular decompression sickness and inner ear barotrauma as recompression therapy is mandatory in the former and undesirable in the latter.

Pulmonary manifestations

Generalized liberation of nitrogen bubbles in the circulation can result in diffuse pulmonary embolization ('the chokes'). This rare manifestation presents with chest pain particularly on inspiration, cough and dyspnoea and may progress rapidly to cardiovascular collapse. It is commonly accompanied by other manifestations of decompression sickness. Cardiopulmonary decompression sickness demands urgent recompression and therefore needs to be clearly differentiated from pulmonary barotrauma which in the absence of cerebral arterial embolism does not. Cardiopulmonary decompression sickness is unlikely from a shallow short dive that has incorporated adequate provision for off-gassing.

Terminology

Decompression sickness has traditionally been subdivided according to the presumed site of injury and perceived clinical significance into type I or mild (limb bends and cutaneous changes) and type II or serious decompression sickness (Golding et al., 1960). It has been recommended that these arbitrary divisions should be abandoned (Murrison & Francis, 1991). The distinction between cerebral arterial air embolism and neurological decompression sickness, and between cerebral and spinal decompression sickness is clinically often very difficult to make. In addition, it is increasingly apparent that decompression insults tend to be multifocal rather than discrete (Adkisson et al., 1989). Furthermore, an artificial distinction between the conditions is not required for therapeutic purposes as the principles of treatment are the same. The Undersea and Hyperbaric Medical Society in 1990 (Francis & Smith, 1991) recommended the adoption of the generic term *decompression illness* to cover the various conditions associated with decompression.

Management of serious decompression illness

Prehospital management

- Serious diving casualties may require resuscitation prior to transfer to a unit with a hyperbaric chamber. However, recompression is the definitive treatment for decompression sickness and cerebral air embolism and any delay will reduce the efficacy of treatment.
- All divers developing manifestations of serious dysbaric illness should be given 100% oxygen. This promotes a maximum gradient for nitrogen gas excretion and improves oxygenation of ischaemic tissues.
- The left Trendelenberg position, previously recommended on theoretical grounds for use in patients

suspected of cerebral air embolism has now been identified firmly as of no benefit. Additionally, this position makes management procedures technically more difficult and the head down position may result in an increase in ICP and exacerbate cerebral oedema.
- Analgesics will mask the response to pressure and create difficulties for the recompression staff to monitor response to treatment. Their use is contraindicated. Development of pain following a recent dive is an absolute contraindication to Entonox (50% oxygen, 50% nitrous oxide) administration. If Entonox is breathed by a diver with decompression sickness a reverse gradient is created and nitrous oxide will diffuse into and enlarge nitrogen bubbles. Entonox is also contraindicated in divers injured following a road traffic accident shortly after a dive.
- The pain arising in a joint can often be improved by applying pressure around the joint. Inflating a sphygmomanometer cuff to 150–250 mmHg may immediately relieve pain of the bends. The pressure must be released periodically to prevent any neurovascular deficit. This symptomatic treatment is not an alternative to recompression.
- Attempts by a symptomatic diver to re-enter the water to perform recompression by descending to the depth of his original dive should be resisted. In UK waters the risk of developing hypothermia during the time required for such a procedure is considerable and is generally very hazardous.
- The history which can be ascertained at the scene and relayed to the hyperbaric unit staff should if possible include details of the depth and duration of the last two dives, problems experienced during ascent or descent phases, presence of undue exertion or cold during the dive, omission of any decompression procedures and any details of non-dive-related illness or medications.
- Divers usually dive in pairs and if one diver has symptoms of decompression sickness or pulmomary barotrauma his 'buddy' may also be at risk of developing serious dysbaric illness. Although recompression may not be required, he should be transferred along with the affected diver. Diving equipment should accompany divers for the hyperbaric staff to inspect.
- Diving is frequently carried out in situations remote from recompression chambers. If evacuation by aircraft is required it is critical that the cabin is maintained at sea level pressurization (1 atmosphere) during flight. Most aircraft are pressurized to approximately 2000 m above sea level (0.8 atmospheres) and therefore air

transport may result in deterioration in the clinical state. Examples of aircraft which can be pressurized to that of sea level include the C-130 Hercules, Lear jet and Cessna Citation. If the patient is to be moved by helicopter the crew must maintain the lowest possible flight altitude but never higher than 300 m above the take-off elevation.

A&E department management

With the increase in popularity of recreational diving and diversity of popular dive sites including inland waters, divers may be brought to A&E departments for their initial assessment and treatment. There has been a recent increase in the number of divers presenting with neurological features (Sykes, 1989). This may be due to a greater awareness of the potential of relatively minor neurological complaints to progress to more serious illness or to recreational divers undertaking deeper and longer dives made possible by improvements in equipment.

The only definitive treatment for severe dysbaric illness is recompression breathing 100% oxygen. If recompression is delayed, the risk of permanent damage to the brain and spinal cord is greatly increased.

The safest approach is to assume that any symptoms in a diver presenting to the A&E department within 48 h after a dive are dysbaric in origin.

Often the diagnosis of decompression sickness may only be confirmed following the response of the symptoms and signs to recompression.

Although the majority of patients presenting to the A&E department with dysbaric air embolism will have clinical evidence of CNS involvement, some patients experience marked resolution of their signs during transfer from the scene. Nevertheless these patients should be transferred to a diving medical centre and recompressed.

The seriously ill diver will require resuscitation prior to transfer to the recompression unit but there should be minimal delay in arranging transfer. High-flow oxygen (12–15 litres min⁻¹) should be administered to all patients with serious dysbaric illness if this has not already been commenced in the field. If tracheal intubation is required the cuff should be inflated with sterile water not air since during recompression an air-filled cuff will deflate.

Intravenous infusion is advocated in decompression sickness or air embolism. Normal saline (or a polygeline) may be used. Adequate circulating volume assists with oxygenation of the ischaemic tissues and facilitates the discharge of excess tissue nitrogen load into the venous system. The infusion should be sufficient to maintain the urine output at 60–100 ml hr⁻¹. Dextrans have received much attention and slight differences of opinion still prevail. Dextran 40 and Dextran 70 have both been used in an attempt to prevent capillary sludging.

An indwelling urinary catheter should be inserted in severe decompression sickness or spinal air embolism because of sacral nerve root dysfunction and to monitor urine output.

High-dose parenteral corticosteroids have been advocated to decrease cerebral or spinal cord oedema (Kizer, 1981) and oral aspirin may be given for its antiplatelet activity, but these adjuvant therapies should also be administered after discussion with the receiving recompression team.

Despite wearing a dry or wet suit for thermal protection, diving-related illness is often accompanied by hypothermia. Appropriate passive or active rewarming of the victim should be commenced.

Recompression therapy

Current management of decompression illness is based on the clinical experience of Workman (1968). The patient is compressed initially to a simulated depth of 18 m of sea water. During treatment 100% oxygen is breathed, interspersed with periods of air breathing to reduce the risk of oxygen toxicity. If relief is prompt the patient is then decompressed according to a standard treatment protocol modified as necessary. Rarely more complex hyperbaric therapies are required.

Early recompression is often effective in reversing even profound neurological disturbances and should be applied as soon as possible. It is estimated that 200 divers per year suffer from decompression sickness of whom 150 are treated in specialist centres. About 70% of these exhibit neurological symptoms and signs. Current treatment regimens result in clinical recovery in 95% of cases and in the remaining few only minor neurological abnormalities persist. About two patients per year in the UK become permanently paraplegic.

APPENDIX: Where to get help

- HM Coastguard (999) will provide a useful communication link for a doctor in a remote location faced with a seriously ill diver.

- The Royal Navy Duty Diving Medical Specialist may be contacted at HMS *Vernon* in Portsmouth (01705 818888). State that you have a diving emergency. Less urgent enquiries should be directed to the Institute of Naval Medicine (01705 822351).
- A similar service is provided by the Diving Diseases Centre at Fort Bovisand, Plymouth. In an emergency the duty doctor may be contacted via a 24-h air call bleeper (01752 261910), or for routine enquiries (01752 408093).
- In Northern Ireland the Regional Recompression Unit at Craigavon Hospital is available for consultation (01762 336711).
- In Scotland contact the Hyperbaric Medicine Unit at Aberdeen Royal Infirmary (01224 681818). State that you have a diving emergency and give your name and telephone number. Contact will then be made with the duty hyperbaric physician.

Bibliography

Near drowning

BARRY, W., LITTLE, T.M. & SIBERT, J.R. (1982). Childhood drownings in private swimming pools: an avoidable cause of death. *Br. Med. J.*, **285**, 542–3.

BIGGART, M.J. & BOHN, D.J. (1990). Effect of hypothermia and cardiac arrest on outcome of near-drowning accidents in children. *J. Paediatr.*, **117**, 179–83.

CALDERWOOD, H. W., MODELL, J.H. & RUIZ, B.C. (1975). The ineffectiveness of steroid therapy for treatment of fresh water near drowning. *Anesthesiology*, **43**, 642–50.

COLEBATCH, H.J.H. & HALMAGYI, F.J. (1961). Lung mechanics and resuscitation after fluid aspiration. *J. Appl. Physiol.*, **16**, 684–96.

CONN, A.W. & BARKER, G.A. (1984). Freshwater drowning and near drowning: an update. *Can. Anaesth. Soc. J.*, **31**, S38–S44.

DEAN, J.M. & McCOMB, J.G. (1981). Intracranial pressure monitoring in severe paediatric near drowning. *Neurosurgery*, **9**, 627–9.

GEDDIS, D.C. (1984). The exposure of pre-school children to water hazards and the incidence of potential drowning accidents. *N.Z. Med. J.*, **87**, 223–6.

HARRIES, M. (1986). Drowning and near drowning. *Br. Med. J.*, **293**, 122–4.

HAYWARD, J. S., HAY, C., MATTHEWS, B.R. *et al.* (1984). Temperature effects on the human dive response in relation to cold water near drowning. *J. Appl. Physiol.*, **56**, 202–6.

HOLIDAY WHICH? (1991). Beach safety. *Holiday Which?* January 8, 30–3.

KARCH, S.B. (1985). Pathophysiology of the heart in near drowning. *Arch. Pathol. Lab. Med.*, **109**, 176–8.

KEATINGE, W.R. & HAYWARD, M.G. (1981). Sudden death in cold water and ventricular arrhythmias. *J. Forens. Sci.*, **26**, 459–61.

KEMP, A.M. & SIBERT, J.R. (1991). Outcome for children who nearly drown: a British Isles study. *Br. Med. J.*, **302**, 921–3.

KEMP, A.M. & SIBERT, J.R. (1992). Drowning and near drowning in children in the United Kingdom: lessons for prevention. *Br. Med. J.*, **304**, 1143–5.

MACKIE, I. (1979). Alcohol and aquatic disasters. *Practitioner*, **222**, 662–5.

MODELL, J. H. & CONN, A.W. (1980). Current neurological considerations in near drowning. *Can. Anaesth. Soc. J.*, **27**, 197–8.

MODELL, J.H. & DAVIS, J.H. (1969). Electrolyte changes in human drowning victims. *Anesthesiology*, **30**, 414–20.

MODELL, J.H., GRAVES, S.A. & KETOVER, A. (1976). Clinical course of 91 consecutive near drowning victims. *Chest*, 7, 231–8

NOPANITANYA, W., GAMBILL, T.G. & BRANK-HOUSE, K.M. (1974). Fresh water drowning: pulmonary ultrastructure and systemic fibrinolysis. *Arch. Pathol.*, **98**, 361–6.

NUSSBAUM, E. & MAGGI, J.C. (1988). Pentobarbital therapy does not improve neurologic outcome in nearly drowned, flaccid comatose children. *Pediatrics*, **81**, 630–4.

OFFICE OF POPULATION CENSUSES AND SURVEYS (1988). *Mortality Statistics: Accidents and Violence*. London: OPCS.

ORLOWSKI, J.P. (1979). Prognostic factors in paediatric cases of near drowning. *J. Am. Coll. Emerg. Physicians*, **8**, 176–9.

ORLOWSKI, J.P. (1987). Drowning, near drowning and ice water submersions. *Pediatr. Clin. North Am.*, **34**, 75–92.

PEARN, J.H. (1977). Neurologic and psychometric studies in children surviving childhood fresh water immersion accidents. *Lancet*, i, 7–9.

PEARN, J.H. (1980). Secondary drowning in children. *Br. Med. J.*, **281**, 1103–5.

PEARN, J. (1985). The management of near drowning. *Br. Med. J.*, **292**, 1447–52.

PEARN, J., NIXON, J. & WILKEY, I. (1976). Fresh water drowning and near drowning accidents involving children. A five year total population study. *Med. J. Aust.*, **2**, 942–6.

RAMEY, C.A., RAMEY, D.N. & HAYWARD, J.S. (1987). The dive response of children in relation to cold water near drowning. *J. Appl. Physiol.*, **63**, 665–8.

SAFAR, P. (1993). Cerebral resuscitation after cardiac arrest: research initiatives and future directions. *Ann. Emerg. Med.*, **22**, 324–49.

SIEBKE, H., ROD, Y., BREIVIK, H. *et al.* (1975).

Survival after 40 minutes' submersion without cerebral sequelae. *Lancet*, **i**, 1275–7.

WINTEMUTE, G.J., (1990). Childhood drowning and near drowning in the United States. *Am. J. Dis. Child.*, **144**, 663–9.

Diving injuries

ADKISSON, G.H., HODGESON, M., SMITH, F. *et al.* (1989). Cerebral perfusion deficits in dysbaric illness. *Lancet*, **ii**, 119–21.

DOUGLAS, J.D.M. (1985). Medical problems of sport diving. *Br. Med. J.*, **291**, 1224–6.

FRANCIS, T.J.R., PEARSON, R.R., ROBERTSON, A.G. *et al.* (1989). Central nervous system decompression sickness: latency of 1070 human cases. *Undersea Biomed. Res.*, **15**, 403–17.

FRANCIS, T.J.R. & SMITH, D.C. ed. (1991). *A Workshop to Develop a Classification for Neurological Dysbarism*. Undersea and Hyperbaric Medical Society, Bethesda, Publication No. (DECO) 5/15/91.

GOLDING, F.C., GRIFFITHS, P., HEMPLEMAN, H.V. *et al.* (1960). Decompression sickness during construction of the Dartford Tunnel. *Br. J. Ind. Med.*, **17**, 167–80.

HALLENBECK, J.M., BOVE, A.A. & ELLIOT, D.H. (1975). Mechanisms underlying spinal cord damage in decompression sickness. *Neurology*, **25**, 308–16.

KIZER, K.W. (1981). Corticosteroids in the treatment of serious decompression sickness. *Ann. Emerg. Med.*, **10**, 485–8.

KIZER, K.W. (1983). Management of dysbaric diving casualties. *Emerg. Med. Clin. North Am.*, **1**, 659–70.

MURRISON, A.W. & FRANCIS, T.J.R. (1991). An introduction to decompression illness. *Br. J. Hosp. Med.*, **46**, 107–10.

SHEFFIELD, P.J., ed. (1989). *Flying after Diving*. Undersea and Hyperbaric Medical Society, Bethesda, Publication Number 77 (FLYDIV) 12/1/89.

SYKES, J.J.W. (1989). Is the pattern of acute decompression sickness changing? *J. R. Nav. Med. Serv.*, **75**, 69–73.

SYKES, J.J.W. (1990). The harzards of sport diving. *J. R. Coll. Physicians Edinb.*, **20**, 318–22.

WORKMAN, R.D. (1968). Treatment of the bends with oxygen at high pressure. *Aerospace Med.*, **39**, 1076–83.

38 Hypothermia and cold injury

E.L. LLOYD

Department of Anaesthesia, Western General Hospital NHS Trust, Edinburgh, UK

Chapter plan

Introduction
Hypothermia
Direct local cold injury
Other conditions and effects of cold

INTRODUCTION

Cold can kill. Man has known this since prehistory but appears to have forgotten with the development of high-tech civilization. Since cold is a feature of the environment which every human being experiences, its contribution to injury, illness and death is often overlooked.

Cold risk (Lloyd, 1986)

In the timber industry, and on building sites and farms, workers are exposed to all weathers. Because of cold, fishing is a particularly hazardous occupation, the accident rate being five times greater than the most dangerous land-based transport industry. Cold is also a hazard for divers, with the water temperature below 100 m depth being a constant 4°C dropping to −2°C in the Arctic. Deep-freeze stores are installed in large depots, individual shops (e.g. butchers), lorries and in medical facilities (e.g. blood transfusion), and workers are exposed to temperatures of −20°C to −40°C, sometimes with an additional fan-produced wind-chill. People can also be exposed to potentially dangerous levels of cold at home, in poor-quality houses, during travel and following an accident.

Man is also exposed to cold during sport and recreation. Any person in the hills, whether a climber, skier, or recreation walker, is at risk, especially if there is an injury or a sudden change in weather. The temperature drops 1°C per 150 m rise in altitude and at high altitude hypoxia compounds the problem. Sports people in winter are vulnerable whether participating in team sports, cross-country running or so-called winter sports. Water sports participants experience cold (e.g. scuba divers and swimmers are immersed in cold water), and sailors suffer wind-chill and wetting from spray and unexpected immersion. Cold can cause problems and injuries at any time of year; for example, muscle tears can occur in 'cold' muscles even in a heatwave.

Hypothermia is a risk of trauma, usually as a result of a combination of exposure, tissue hypoperfusion and infusion of inadequately warmed fluids. In trauma, hypothermia has a deleterious effect on survival producing 40% mortality if the core temperature is below 34°C compared with 7% if the core temperature is above 34°C. Hypothermia also contributes to the coagulopathy which accompanies massive transfusion (Nolan, 1993).

Cold stress

Cold stress applies to any degree of environmental cold which causes the physiological thermoregulatory mechanisms to be activated. The severity of cold stress is not related to the absolute temperature alone but is also affected by air movement (wind or draughts) (Table 1) and moisture (humidity, rain or damp).

The sensation of cold is related to the lowered average skin temperature, but man is more sensitive to change, and rate of change in temperature than to any absolute value. Cold applied to the skin is pleasant if the core temperature is raised but unpleasant if the core temperature is lowered.

Routes of heat loss

Human beings are constantly losing heat through convection, radiation, conduction and evaporation, and the

Table 1. *Wind-chill chart showing the effect of wind on increasing the degree of cooling at any particular temperature and wind speed*

Wind speed (m.p.h)	Equivalent chill temperature (°C)									
0	4	−1	−7	−12	−18	−23	−29	−34	−40	−46
5	2	−4	−9	−15	−21	−26	−32	−37	−43	−48
10	−1	−9	−15	−23	−29	−37	−34	−51	−57	−62
15	−4	−12	−21	−29	−34	−43	−51	−57	−65	−73
20	−7	−15	−23	−32	−37	−46	−54	−62	−71	−79
25	−9	−18	−26	−34	−43	−51	−59	−68	−76	−84
30	−12	−18	−29	−34	−46	−54	−62	−71	−79	−87
35	−12	−21	−29	−37	−46	−54	−62	−73	−82	−90
40	−12	−21	−29	−37	−48	−57	−65	−73	−82	−90
	Little danger			Increasing danger. Flesh may freeze within 1 min			Great danger. Flesh may freeze within 30 sec			

10 m.p.h = 16.1 km h$^{-1.}$

standard laws of physics apply. Radiation loss is maximal when the body is unclothed and erect, and least when curled up and insulated. The amount lost by conduction depends on the temperature difference between two surfaces in direct contact. Conduction is the major route for heat loss during immersion in very cold water, and even on land wet clothing increases conductive loss. Evaporative loss occurs from the skin through insensible moisture loss and active sweating, through evaporation from wet clothing, and from the respiratory tract during warming and humidifying the inspired air. Large quantities of heat are required to convert a liquid into its gaseous phase (latent heat of evaporation). Convective heat loss is increased by limb movement and shivering because the currents produced by the pendulum effect remove the warmed layer of air or water next to the skin, and this is aggravated by a bellows effect of clothing. Both convective and evaporative heat losses are increased in windy conditions – the 'wind-chill'.

Regulation of body temperature

Body temperature is controlled through a central mechanism in the hypothalamus which, while it acts in a manner similar to a thermostat, is not a simple on/off drive but is more akin to a 'black box' with a complex system of neurones cross-linking sensory input and effector output (Bligh, 1984). The thermostat is activated by impulses from central receptors, which respond to changes in the temperature of the blood, and from peripheral receptors mainly in the skin. There are also spinal thermostatic reflexes, though these alone are insufficient to control body temperature. The thermostat regulates the temperature of the body by adjusting heat production and heat loss, but the setting of the thermostat itself may be altered (Maclean & Emslie-Smith, 1977).

The body responds to cold by constriction of the peripheral vessels, mainly via the sympathetic nervous system but also through direct action on the blood vessels. Vasoconstriction is very effective in reducing heat loss by limiting blood flow to the periphery, thus increasing the depth of shell insulation and reducing the temperature differential between the skin and the environment. In fact, vasoconstriction can result in the outer 1 inch of the body having a thermal conductivity equivalent to that of cork (Maclean & Emslie-Smith, 1977). This, however, increases the risk of local cold injury. There is also a countercurrent exchange of heat between the arteries and veins in the distal half of the limbs. Below a temperature of 10–12°C the peripheral vasoconstriction fails and alternating vasodilation and vasoconstriction occur, although there may actually be very little increase in the volume of blood circulating in the skin during vasodilation (Pozos & Wittmers, 1983), and therefore the insulating effect of the vasoconstriction is preserved. The head has minimal vasoconstrictor activity, and the rate of heat loss through the head increases in a linear manner between +32°C and −20°C; indeed, at rest in −4°C the heat loss from the head may equal half the total heat production (Lloyd, 1986).

Heat production rises by increased muscle metabolism

and tone, leading to shivering, but any increase in heat production is always accompanied by a rise in oxygen consumption, and shivering may double or treble oxygen consumption. Deliberate activity also increases heat production 10–15-fold during hard physical exercise but, in the cold, additional heat may be needed to maintain normothermia. Therefore, for any level of exercise, the oxygen consumption is higher in a cold environment than in a warm one (Horvath, 1981). This is seen clinically when angina develops during a particular level of activity in the cold but not at normal temperatures. Activity and shivering are not economical in thermo-regulation because they are accompanied by an increased blood supply to the muscles and this increases heat loss. In fact, only 48% of the extra heat generated is retained in the body.

If hypoxia is present, as at high altitude, there will be a decrease in the total possible heat production and shivering may be inhibited (Alexander, 1979). Similarly, there is a limit to the maximum oxygen uptake and, in conditions of very severe cold, the maximal oxygen uptake may be insufficient to provide for the high demand of both the exercise and the severe cold stress. A person can develop unexpected and unsuspected hypo-thermia despite vigorous muscular exercise. Finally, if the person is exhausted or suffering from malnutrition, he cannot increase heat production because of the lack of substrate (fuel) for metabolism (Lloyd, 1986).

Even at complete rest at a comfortable temperature, the vital functions of the body continue and this generates heat. Reduced to a minimum this is called basal metabolic heat. This basal heat production is raised if the body temperature rises, and falls in hypothermia.

There are racial variations in the response to cold and at the extremes of age there is an increased risk of hypothermia. Many medical disorders predispose to hypothermia (Maclean & Emslie-Smith, 1977) and a range of drugs, including anaesthetics, increase the risk through impairing vasoconstriction or depressing metab-olism. Mental stress even of as mild a degree as mental arithmetic increases the heat loss as also do nausea, vomiting, fainting, trauma and haemorrhage (Lloyd, 1986).

During sleep the cerebral thermostat is reset to a new low level, vasoconstriction is reduced with an immediate rise in skin temperature and the metabolic rate is reduced (Lloyd, 1986). Although alcohol produces a number of effects which increase the risk of hypothermia, the greatest danger is because it decreases the awareness of cold and increases bravado while impairing the ability to assess risks (Lloyd, 1986). Improving fitness results in an increase in the maximum oxygen uptake and fit people work and sleep better and are more comfortable in the cold than unfit people (Horvath, 1981).

HYPOTHERMIA

Definition and classification

Hypothermia is subnormal body temperature, but therm-ally the body can be divided into zones. The 'core' consists of the deeper tissues of the body including all the vital organs (e.g. heart and brain) and the temperature of this core is kept stable over a surprising range of environmental thermal stresses. The 'shell' is superficial, and its size and temperature varies considerably according to the external environment, the degree of protection and the activity of the individual; however, in extremis, the tissues in the shell are thermally expendable. To allow for the diurnal variation of 1–2°C, it has now been agreed that a person is considered to be in a state of hypothermia if the core temperature is below 35°C (Royal College of Physicians, 1966).

It is no longer acceptable to consider hypothermia and its treatment purely on the measurement of core tempera-ture. (This is akin to classifying and deciding the treatment of anaemia purely on the measurement of the haemoglobin level). Among the many physiological effects of exposure to cold there are three which are of particular relevance to the safe management of cases of hypothermia (Lloyd, 1986, 1992).

1. *Energy reserves.* The body responds to cold by increasing heat output and therefore the energy reserves are utilized. With rapid cooling (e.g. in cold water) the energy reserves are relatively undepleted and, once removed from the cold, the person will rewarm. With less severe cold, the body temperature will only fall when the energy reserves are exhausted. With their reduced heat-generating capacity these people may continue to cool, and die, even in a mildly cold environment.

2. *Fluid balance.* Cold-induced vasoconstriction shunts blood into the deep capacitance vessels and the relative excess of volume is removed by a diuresis. Respiratory moisture loss is increased by exercise especially in dry air (e.g. in the polar regions and at high altitude). Cold air is dry, evaporation is rapid and even sweat loss of 1–2 litres per day may be unnoticed. However, even with total body dehy-dration, exercise causes an increase in the intravascular

fluid volume, thus increasing the cold diuresis and worsening any dehydration.

During exposure to cold, fluid also shifts from the intravascular space into the extravascular space and then into the intracellular space. During rewarming these fluid shifts reverse and the circulating blood volume increases (up to 130% of the value prior to cooling), depending on the potential volume of fluid available, which in turn is related to the duration of cold exposure.

The fluid status of any hypothermic individual will depend on the relative importance of these responses.

3. *Vascular responses.* When a subject is in the cold, there is a continuous stream of impulses from the cold receptors in the skin reinforcing vasoconstriction. But when the cold stress on the skin is removed, the cutaneous cold impulses are reduced, the vasoconstrictor tone is therefore also reduced, and the active volume of the vascular bed is increased. If there is insufficient available fluid (e.g. through dehydration due to diuresis and/or fluid shifts), the central venous pressure will fall and then the blood pressure (producing collapse due to relative hypovolaemia). Removal of a body from water will also increase the active vascular bed by removal of the hydrostatic squeeze.

In very prolonged exposure to mild cold, vasoconstriction, and therefore fluid loss from cold-induced diuresis, will be minimal. Loss of fluid from the vascular space due to fluid shifts will have been replaced by fluid intake, and any rapid return of fluid to the intravascular space during rewarming may result in fluid overload and pulmonary and/or cerebral oedema.

Using these physiological parameters, it is possible to describe different types of hypothermia (Lloyd, 1986).

In *acute* or 'immersion' hypothermia, the core temperature is forced down despite maximal heat production. Hypothermia occurs before the body becomes exhausted, and the person will have very little difficulty in rewarming once he has been removed from the severe environment. Because of the timescale the shifts of body fluid will be minimal. The commonest cause of accidental hypothermia. is falling into cold water (the average summer sea temperature in Britain is 11°C). Drowning, the commonest cause of death in water, may follow loss of consciousness due to hypothermia. Hypothermia has been implicated in 20% of scuba diving fatalities, and hypothermia in cavers often involves immersion in cold water. Deep diving (below 150 m) with the use of oxyhelium gas breathing mixtures may also cause 'immersion' hypo-

thermia because of the tremendous respiratory heat loss which occurs under these conditions and the heat transfer capacity of the compressed gas.

In *subacute* or 'exhaustion' hypothermia the heat production can maintain body temperature until exhaustion occurs, i.e. the supply of heat fails. Thermal protection must therefore counter every avenue of heat loss because even small quantities of additional heat may make the difference between life and death. There is also likely to be dehydration due to fluid loss as well as intercompartmental fluid shifts. This type of hypothermia is most commonly found in mountaineers or hill walkers. In Scottish hills between 1967 and 1977, 15% of surviving casualties were hypothermic, 10% of the fatalities were attributed to hypothermia and in many of the deaths due to physical injury the effects of cold exposure probably contributed to the fatal outcome. Runners and cyclists training or competing in long distance events are at risk, and not only in winter. Exhaustion hypothermia may occur during the event or after stopping.

In *subchronic* or 'urban' hypothermia, the cold is relatively mild but has been prolonged. The core temperature remains normal (35°C or above), possibly for weeks, before drifting or being precipitated into hypothermia (e.g. by a fall). The energy reserves will be very variable and there will be large intercompartmental fluid shifts. If rewarming is too rapid, even if spontaneous, the volume of fluid returning to the circulation may cause an overload and result in cerebral and/or pulmonary oedema. This is the most usual type of hypothermia found in the elderly or in association with malnutrition.

The different types of hypothermia can only be distinguished by the case history. For example, a climber in a snowstorm disabled by a broken leg will probably cool as rapidly as if immersed. The shock of the injury will increase the rate of heat loss and the fracture will prevent the person generating heat to his full capacity and may therefore prevent exhaustion. Similarly, a diver may suffer 'immersion' hypothermia even in a dry pressure chamber. On the other hand, a swimmer lost overboard in relatively warm water is a candidate for 'exhaustion' hypothermia. A child with severe malnutrition is likely to develop 'urban' hypothermia whereas a fit 70-year-old out walking in the hills probably has 'exhaustion' hypothermia.

The importance of making the correct diagnosis is that inappropriate treatment may result in death during rewarming. Collapse is almost unknown during rewarming from 'immersion' hypothermia whereas it is common with 'exhaustion' hypothermia.

Table 2. *Signs and symptoms at different levels of hypothermia*

37.6°C	'Normal' rectal temperature
37°C	'Normal' oral temperature
36°C	Increased metabolic rate to attempt to balance heat loss
35°C	Shivering maximum at this temperature; hyper-reflexia, dysarthria, delayed cerebration
34°C	Patients usually responsive and with normal blood pressure; lower limit compatible with continued exercise
33–31°C	Retrograde amnesia, consciousness clouded, blood pressure difficult to obtain, pupils dilated, most shivering ceases
30–28°C	Progressive loss of consciousness, increased muscular rigidity, slow pulse and respiration, cardiac arrhythmia develops, ventricular fibrillation may develop if heart irritated
27°C	Voluntary motion lost along with pupillary light reflex, deep tendon and skin reflexes; appears dead
26°C	Victims seldom conscious
25°C	Ventricular fibrillation may appear spontaneously
24–21°C	Pulmonary oedema develops (100% mortality in shipwreck victims in Second World War)
20°C	Heart standstill
18°C	Lowest adult *accidental* hypothermic patient with recovery
17°C	Isoelectric EEG
15.2°C	Lowest infant *accidental* hypothermic patient with recovery
9°C	Lowest artificially cooled hypothermic patient with recovery
4°C	Monkeys revived successfully
1°C to −7°C	Rats and hamsters revived successfully

Symptoms and signs

One of the earliest signs of hypothermia is a change in personality or behaviour, but unfortunately not only can similar changes be caused by other factors (e.g. hypoglycaemia, exhaustion or heat stroke), but the person involved is likely to be the last to notice the change. A variety of signs and symptoms have been described (Table 2) in an attempt to give a clinical guide to the level of hypothermia, but this is only a general guide since individuals show a great range of responses; for example loss of consciousness may occur at 33°C but in one case consciousness was still present at a rectal temperature of 24.3°C. Similarly, shivering is considered

to cease at 30°C but it has been recorded at a core temperature of 24°C. At the other extreme, some experimental subjects can cool without shivering, many mountain rescue cases never shiver, and one immersion victim did not start shivering during rewarming until the core temperature reached 37°C (Lloyd, 1986).

Despite the fact that hypothermia protects the brain from the effects of anoxia, in clinical practice survival in hypothermia is almost totally dependent on there being sufficient cardiac output to adequately perfuse the heart and brain. Therefore cardiac function has more relevance to ultimate survival than brain temperature.

Diagnosis

Hypothermia can only be diagnosed by recording the core temperature. The rectum is the usual site used, but when the core temperature is changing rectal recordings lag behind the rest of the core and the rectal temperature may still be falling when the temperature of the rest of the core is rising. The inner ear or tympanic membrane temperature is accurate but requires special equipment. The oesophagus is also accurate and sensitive but there is a remote risk of triggering ventricular fibrillation (VF), and inserting the probe may be difficult if the jaw is clenched with the cold. Using a low-reading thermometer, the mouth is the simplest site for an initial check of temperature in a conscious person since, unless the person has just drunk something hot, the mouth reading will never be higher than the core (Lloyd, 1986). In the situations where casualties occur, low-reading thermometers are unlikely to be available. For practical purposes, therefore, a casualty should be treated as 'cold' if the body feels 'as cold as marble' and, in particular, if the armpit is profoundly cold (Handley *et al.*, 1992). Probably the most important factor in making the diagnosis is suspicion that hypothermia may be present.

In hypothermia the diagnosis of other conditions is difficult because the features of hypothermia mask the signs of other disorders (Lloyd, 1986). In hypothermia the reflexes are affected and there is a general increase in rigidity which makes accurate neurological diagnosis impossible; slurred speech, ataxia and the development of incoordination or a change in personality may be due to hypothermia and not neurological damage. The changes in the electrical and mechanical functions of the heart cause problems for cardiologists. Gastrointestinal motility slows and may cease during cooling and as a result gastric dilatation and decreased or absent bowel sounds are common. The lungs may show clinical and X-ray

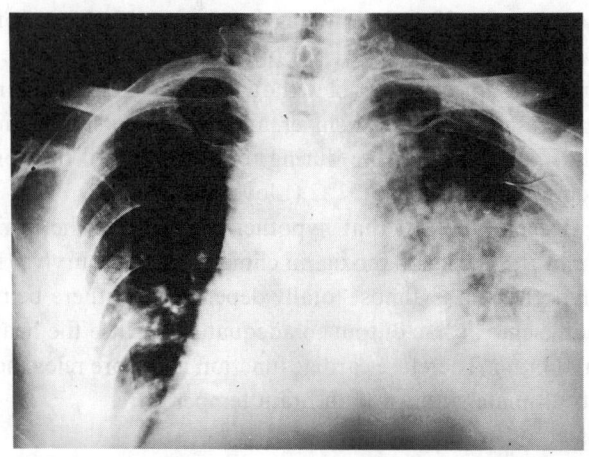

Fig. 1. X-ray of chest on admission showing pneumonic changes at a core temperature of 32.5°C.

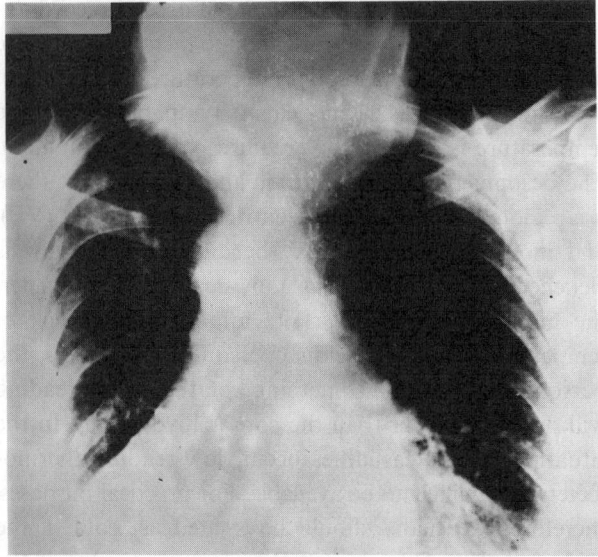

Fig. 2. X-ray of chest of same patient as Fig. 1 showing marked improvement on reaching normothermia after 12 h of airway warming treatment.

features similar to pneumonia (Fig. 1), although these clear on rewarming (Fig. 2). It is therefore important that the patient be normothermic before any diagnosis is made or any irrevocable treatment started.

Rescue

At all times it is vital that the safety of the rescuer as well as of the casualty is ensured. This is particularly important if the casualty is in a hostile environment (e.g. in water or on a hillside). As well as being aware of the dangers of falling rocks, unstable snow or unsafe ice, the rescuer must ensure that he does not also become hypothermic through exhaustion or donating his own clothing to the casualty.

If possible the casualty should be rescued horizontally, especially from water, but it is often more important to reach safety quickly than to delay for a horizontal rescue (Handley *et al.*, 1992).

Cause of death after a rescue (Lloyd, 1986, 1992)

There is a false assumption that, once a person has been removed from cold stress, he/she is safe: deaths still occur after rescue. During early experiments (Alexander, 1945) it was noticed that, after the person had been removed from cold water, the core temperature continued to drop for a while before rising. Because death often occurred at about the time this 'afterdrop' was at its lowest, it was assumed that the afterdrop caused the death. Subsequently, because VF was sometimes recorded during rewarming, it was postulated that death was due to VF caused by continued cooling. However, it is difficult to accept that a temperature reached at the nadir of the afterdrop is more dangerous than a similar temperature recorded while the body is continuing to cool.

The original explanation for the afterdrop was the return of cold blood from the periphery but, due to peripheral vasoconstriction, there is unlikely to be a large volume of blood sequestered in the periphery. Also, returning cold blood would cause the cardiac temperature to fall more than the rectal temperature, whereas the afterdrop is less at the heart than in the rectum. Furthermore, although the peripheral temperatures start to rise immediately on removal from the cold, there is no increase in limb or extremity flow during the afterdrop even during surface rewarming (Pozos & Wittmers, 1983). There is therefore no evidence of a peripheral pool of blood. If a small volume with high temperature is expanded to include an additional volume which is at a lower temperature, equilibration will result in a lower average temperature of the whole. The afterdrop is therefore the result of the normal physical laws of heat flow and reflects temperature equilibration and the re-establishment of the normal body temperature gradients. The ogre of the afterdrop should now be relegated to history.

Death following rescue (Lloyd, 1992) may result from:

1. An imbalance between the active vascular capacity and the effective circulating fluid volume. As discussed earlier, the different types of hypothermia have different physiological changes and inappropriate rewarming

may result in death if the vascular bed becomes too large for the actual circulating blood volume (relative hypovolaemic shock) or if the reversal of the fluid shifts is too great, thus overloading the circulation and resulting in cerebral and/or pulmonary oedema. This matches clinical and experimental observations and is the commonest cause of death during rewarming.

2. Ventricular fibrillation (VF). The risk rises as the core temperature falls, but VF is usually triggered by mechanical irritation, which may be as mild as the heart having its position changed by rolling a patient for bedmaking. Other triggers are hypoxia of the heart muscle and rapid changes in pH or electrolytes in the blood, or temperature gradients within the heart muscle. As the heart cools it becomes more susceptible to VF but, left undisturbed, the cooling heart usually stops in asystole. Occasional case reports have implicated tracheal intubation in hypothermia as being the event which triggered VF. However, in three large series, tracheal intubation was performed on many patients (lowest core temperature 24.3°C) and no cases of VF were recorded (Lloyd, 1986). All patients were preoxygenated before intubation. Defibrillation with DC countershock is usually unsuccessful until the core temperature is above 28–30°C.

3. Continued cooling.

Death in hypothermia (Lloyd, 1986)

The clinical picture in profound accidental hypothermia is very difficult to distinguish from death, with a pulse that is very slow and undetectable because of vasoconstriction, and such profound respiratory depression that the patient appears apnoeic. Temperature is no guide to survival: a 23-day-old infant has been revived from a core temperature of 15.2°C with no sequelae (Nozaki *et al.*, 1986). Neither is the total absence of cardiorespiratory activity, nor a flat EEG (electroencephalogram) a certain indicator of death in hypothermia. Failure to appreciate this has almost certainly meant that some autopsies have been carried out before the person is dead. It is now generally agreed that the only certain diagnosis of death in hypothermia is failure to recover on rewarming. This statement has to be tempered with commonsense for rescuers, since the victim can be accepted as dead if the core temperature is equal to or lower than the air temperature, or if the mouth and nose are filled with snow or ice.

Hypothermia is only one possible cause of death in water and is a major cause when the water is cold but not very cold (5°C or less). Drowning is the commonest cause of death in water.

Sudden entry into very cold water produces marked cardiorespiratory responses which may cause death, unconsciousness or incapacity and therefore drowning may occur from a stroke, a myocardial infarction, or because of uncontrollable hyperventilation. Anaphylaxis may occur in those with unsuspected allergy to cold. Swimming is impossible in very cold water and even Olympic class swimmers become incapacitated, probably because of the effect of cold on nerve and muscle function. Water in the ears and/or nose may cause a vagal reflex with instantaneous cardiac and respiratory arrest. In warm water, drowning will occur following exhaustion.

Casualties totally submerged in very cold water can recover after periods of up to 1 h, especially the young (normal submersion survival is about 3 min) (Lloyd, 1986). The diagnosis of death should only be made in hospital but survival depends on resuscitation being started immediately. One young woman was revived with expired air resuscitation after being buried for 20 min in a wet-snow avalanche (Gray, 1987).

Resuscitation

In hypothermia the heart may still be working even if clinically undetectable, and the mechanical irritation of chest compression may trigger VF with subsequent total loss of cardiac function. It is unsafe, however, to assume that hypothermia is present in isolation. Many patients are injured or have some illness, possibly cold-related, and drowning may precede or follow cooling. If the heart has stopped through drowning or heart attack, resuscitation with mouth-to-mouth respiration and chest compression must be started at once if there is to be any hope of the person surviving. This dilemma for the rescuers causes controversy, but the widest consensus (Handley *et al.*, 1992; Lloyd, 1986; Steinman, 1986) is that:

1. If breathing is absent, becomes obstructed or stops, standard airway management should be started including expired air resuscitation if appropriate.
2. Chest compression should be started *only* if:
   a. there is no carotid pulse detectable after feeling in the correct place for at least 1 min
   and
   b. Cardiac arrest is observed, i.e. a pulse which was present previously has disappeared, or there is a

reasonable chance that a cardiac arrest occurred within the previous 2 h

and

c. There is a reasonable expectation that effective cardiopulmonary resuscitation (CPR) can be provided with only brief periods of interruption for movement until the casualty can be transported to hospital where full advanced life support can be provided. There is the danger that if the rescuers become exhausted by doing CPR they may themselves become casualties. Resuscitation has been successful after CPR for 4.5 h during transport and rewarming when cardiac arrest occurred at a rectal temperature of 23°C with the rhythm varying between asystole and VF (Stoneham & Squires, 1992). It was also achieved after 6.5 h of CPR, including air transfer, when asystole occurred at 23.2°C (Lexow, 1991).

3. The rates for expired air ventilation and chest compression should be the same as for normothermic casualties. Because of stiffness of the chest wall the aims should be to inflate with a volume of air sufficient to cause the chest to rise visibly, and to compress the sternum to a depth of 4–5 cm in an adult (2–3 cm in a child, 1–1.5 cm in an infant).

4. If at any time a pulse is detected, CPR must stop while the pulse is still present.

Methods of rewarming

These should be assessed on the following criteria (Lloyd, 1986):

● Heat gain, not only in terms of absolute quantities of heat added and heat loss prevented, but also where the heat gain occurs.
● Other effects on the body. These may be beneficial or adverse, and should include consideration of cardiovascular, cerebral, respiratory and renal function.
● Where the method can be used (practical potential). Each method has to be evaluated for safety and utility through the whole sequence from discovery of the victim, through first aid treatment, transport, treatment at base or hospital, to final recovery.
● Mortality rates, not warming rates, should ultimately dictate the choice of therapy.

It is important to remember that people die slowly in the cold but inappropriate aggressive treatment can kill in a hurry.

Rubbing the skin of the victim is absolutely contra-

indicated since it provides a sense of warmth to the skin without providing heat. This suppresses shivering and increases the risk of hypotensive collapse. It may also damage the cold skin. The practical rewarming methods currently available are:

1. Spontaneous rewarming, i.e. preventing further heat loss to the environment and allowing the body to rewarm without supplying any additional heat from an external source.
2. Active rewarming, i.e. supplying additional heat which may be through two main routes:
   a. Surface heating.
   b. Central rewarming.
3. Combinations of a number of different methods.

Patients who are young and/or suffering from immersion or exhaustion hypothermia have a very low mortality whereas urban hypothermic patients tend to have a high mortality. However, where the treatment has been carried out in an intensive care unit (i.e. a unit with intensive monitoring of physiological and biochemical changes and facilities to make rapid corrections of any abnormality which may occur) there is a very low mortality in all types of hypothermia. In these circumstances, deaths are attributable to pre-existing medical conditions or others which develop after rewarming. It is probably true that, if a patient with hypothermia is in an intensive care unit, any method of rewarming can be safely applied.

Spontaneous rewarming

This technique is used automatically by the rescue services as soon as the victim is found. Insulating the body surface usually reduces the heat loss sufficiently to allow the patient to rewarm spontaneously from endogenous heat production. The insulation must include the head since up to 50% of total heat production can be lost by this route (Lloyd, 1986). Adequate insulation between the casualty and the ground must be ensured. A fine point of the technique is that the hands and feet should be kept cool (i.e. the hands should be down the side of the patient and not on the abdomen). Warm hands and feet reduce the stimulus for heat production and allow reduction of vasoconstrictor tone, thus increasing heat loss and the risk of vasomotor collapse. Any available material can be used, but the 'space blanket' made of metallized plastic sheeting was shown on theoretical grounds and in experiments to be no better than a similar thickness of polythene, which is much cheaper (Lloyd, 1986). Wet clothing should be removed when the victim is in a warm shelter out of the wind. If the shelter is not available, extra layers of clothing should be added, especially a layer that is impervious to wind and water (Handley *et al.*, 1992).

If the person is shivering, rewarming will be fairly rapid. However, shivering may be dangerous, especially in the presence of hypovolaemia (e.g. following trauma) because it requires an increase in peripheral blood flow and carries a risk of hypotension. Also shivering increases oxygen consumption (up to 400%), and the shift to the left in the oxyhaemoglobin dissociation curve in hypothermia will impair oxygen delivery, possibly leading to lactic acidosis. Shivering may therefore compound the lactic acidosis and decreased hepatic metabolic clearance of lactic acid which typically accompany hypovolaemia (Nolan, 1993).

In the field, part of the insulation is to provide shelter from the wind (e.g. a hut, lifeboat cabin, survival bag, snowhole or large boulder). However, if the environmental cold is very severe, if the insulation is poor or incomplete, or if the metabolism is depressed through drugs or low body temperature, heat production may be insufficient to compensate for the continued heat loss, and the patient may then fail to rewarm, or may in fact continue to cool.

In hospital, the rate of rewarming is very variable and depends on the metabolic rate. In urban hypothermia, if the rate exceeds $0.5°C\,h^{-1}$, covers should be removed to slow rewarming and avoid pulmonary or cerebral oedema.

Surface reheating

This is often used because rescuers feel that they must do something active.

The hot bath is the fastest method of rewarming a person, and it became standard therapy following early experiments (Alexander, 1945). It should only be used for casualities who are conscious, shivering and uninjured and can get into the bath with minimal assistance (Handley *et al.*, 1992). The temperature of the bath should approximate but not exceed 40°C (i.e. elbow comfort temperature). This temperature should be maintained by constantly stirring and adding hot water as necessary. This technique requires large quantities of hot water, too much for the ordinary domestic hot water supply. Heavy outer clothing should be gently removed before the casualty is immersed to the neck. Assistance should be given with removing the rest of the clothing once the casualty is comfortably settled in the bath. On

immersion, shivering will stop but this is not an indication for removing the casualty. He should be helped out of the bath when he feels comfortably warm, dried, covered with blankets and kept lying flat. He should not be allowed to stay in the bath if he feels hot or starts sweating.

Plumbed garments which circulate warm fluids, heating pads and hot water bottles placed at the neck, axilla and groin can also be used.

One method reputedly used by mountain rescue teams is body-to-body contact inside a sleeping bag. Unless three people can provide simultaneous body heat the method is dangerous and, in practice, the standard sleeping bag will only just admit one body – the victim.

Warmth on the skin will depress shivering and reduce vasoconstriction, and surface warming has been associated with rewarming collapse. The worst mortality occurs in casualties left exposed in a warm room (Pozos & Wittmers, 1983). However, radiant heat applied to the blush area of the head and neck will inhibit shivering and reduce oxygen consumption (Sharkey *et al.*, 1993) without markedly impairing vasoconstriction. In addition, cold tissues require less oxygen than warm tissues, but cold blood carries less oxygen than warm blood. In surface warming, the oxygen carried may be inadequate for the increased demand of the warmed superficial tissues, resulting in a dangerous metabolic acidosis (see also shivering in trauma above). Finally, if there is no circulation (or very little) through the skin, as may be the case with cardiac depression or arrest, surface warming is ineffective and may cause burning even at 'baby bath' temperatures.

Central rewarming

With central rewarming the heat is supplied to the 'core' first and rewarming proceeds from within out. The core organs, 8% of the total body weight, contribute 56% of the heat production in basal metabolism at normothermia and a higher percentage in hypothermia because the muscles and superficial tissues have cooled more than the core and are therefore producing a lower percentage of the total body heat production. As the temperature of a tissue rises, the heat generated also rises rapidly. Therefore, by concentrating the heat gain in the core, the thermal benefits will be significantly greater than calculations alone would suggest (Lloyd, 1986). The methods which have been used to date are:

- Extracorporeal blood warming, e.g. cardiopulmonary bypass, haemodialysis.

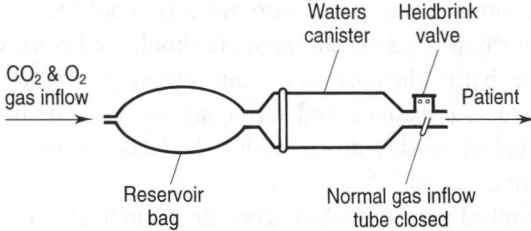

Fig. 3. Simple circuit for providing airway warming from an anaesthetic machine. The patient may be connected by face mask or endotracheal tube as appropriate, and ventilation assisted if required.

- Irrigation of body cavities, e.g. mediastinal irrigation, pleural irrigation, peritoneal dialysis.
- Other methods, e.g. intragastric, intraoesophageal and intracolonic balloons, intravenous infusion, diathermy.
- Airway warming.

All these methods of rewarming have been used successfully but all have disadvantages and problems. Some require expertise or equipment which is only available in a few large hospitals, and some that have been advocated for use by the emergency services (e.g. diathermy or peritonal dialysis) should only be used with medical supervision because of inherent dangers or risks.

Airway warming (Lloyd, 1986, 1990)

Even with perfect surface insulation the patient loses heat through breathing; airway warming provides a warmed, humidified atmosphere for the patient to breathe.

Airway warming is similar to spontaneous rewarming in that the main thermal input comes from the body's own metabolic heat production. It accelerates rewarming and should be used with surface insulation. It is effectively 'airway insulation' and should not be referred to as 'airway rewarming'. In the only studies which have compared airway warming with spontaneous rewarming during the same episode of hypothermia, airway warming produced a significant ($P < 0.001$) increase in the rate of rewarming.

Airway warming produces a marked improvement in cardiovascular function (a feature shared with peritoneal dialysis) and cerebral function, conscious level and cardiorespiratory control. With both airway warming and peritoneal dialysis there have been case reports of VF reverting spontaneously to sinus rhythm at a core temperature of about 28°C. Shivering is inhibited and, because of the reduction in oxygen demand, this can be very important if the patient has cardiovascular or

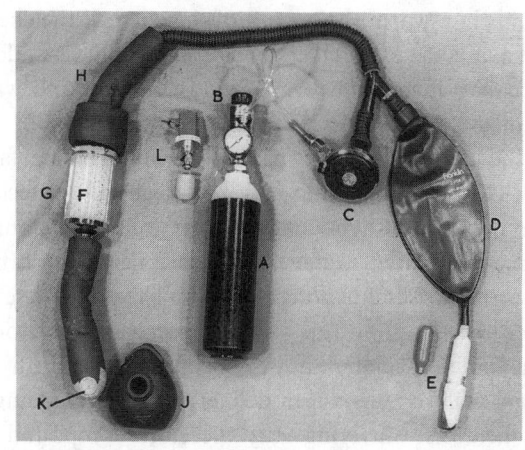

Fig. 4. Lightweight 'Lloyd' portable airway warming equipment. A, oxygen cylinder; B, first-stage reducing valve and gauge; C, demand reducing valve with manual over-ride; D, 2 l reservoir bag; E, Corkette (Sparklet corkmaster) with the distal portion of the needle removed and inserted into the tail of the reservoir bag (spare sparklet alongside); F, soda lime, G, paediatric Waters canister; H, insulation – neoprene foam tubing; J, facemask; K, thermometer registering mean air temperature at mask inflow; L, adaptor for refilling small oxygen cylinder from a large cylinder.

respiratory impairment, or trauma and hypovolaemia (Nolan, 1993). Despite the decreased oxygen consumption, rewarming is not slowed. Surface heat also inhibits shivering and reduces oxygen demand but at the expense of reduced heat production.

In young patients suffering from immersion or exhaustion hypothermia, airway warming has a lower mortality than spontaneous rewarming or hot bath rewarming (Miller *et al.*, 1980). However, in urban hypothermia airway warming should not be used without intensive care unit facilities because the accelerated rate of rewarming may precipitate cerebral and/or pulmonary oedema.

There is a variety of equipment (Lloyd, 1991a) which can produce warm moist air, which should not exceed 45°C to avoid thermal burns to the face and pharynx. These devices include electrically operated hospital humidifiers (not nebulizers), a design which utilizes the chemical reaction between soda lime and carbon dioxide (Fig. 3), a portable version weighing 3 kg (Fig. 4), and a condenser humidifier attached to a face mask (Fig. 5). Although the condenser humidifier is the least efficient, it is simple, light and cheap and could be carried as part of a first aid kit.

Airway warming has the advantage that it can be started in the field and continued in hospital. It is non-invasive and can be combined with other rewarming methods.

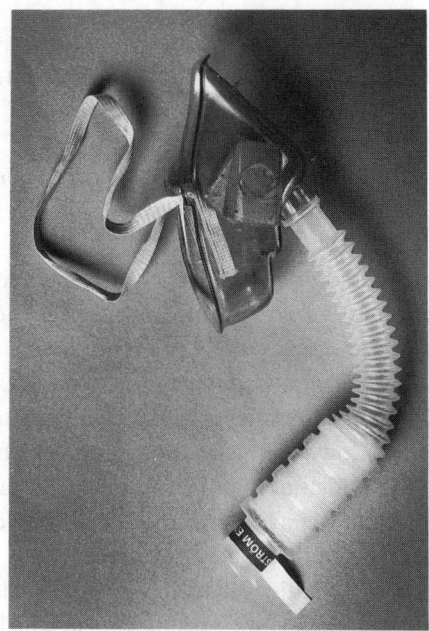

Fig. 5. Condenser humidifier with face mask attached. This can be used in the emergency treatment of accidental hypothermia. The end of the humidifier should be under the clothing next to the skin and the whole device, including mask, covered with a scarf.

Peritoneal dialysis

This does not require expensive equipment and can be set up in a few minutes. Normal (0·9%) saline at 45°C is run into the peritoneal cavity through an infusion set. After leaving the fluid for a few minutes to allow heat transfer, it is removed and replaced by a fresh warm supply. The operative technique and contraindications are as standard.

Rewarming the liver reactivates detoxifying and other enzymes. The heat warms the heart through the diaphragm and via blood returning in the inferior vena cava. This stabilizes cardiac conduction and VF has reverted spontaneously to sinus rhythm while the core temperature was below 27°C.

Intravenous fluids

All fluids, including blood, should be warmed during resuscitation in hypothermia. A level 1 fluid warmer warms all fluids from 10°C to 35°C at flow rates of 350–500 ml min^{-1} (Nolan, 1993). A microwave oven can also be used but the fluid must be mixed after heating and the system must be pretested with each oven. In the field, heat packs or body warming can reduce the risk of cold fluid. The addition of saline warmed to 70°C to an equal volume of cold (−4°C) packed red cells results in

a diluted unit of blood at 37°C with no adverse effect on red cell survival (Nolan, 1993). Unfortunately, the risk of fluid overload and cardiac arrhythmias reduces the value of this technique in pure hypothermia.

Extracorporeal warming

Cardiopulmonary bypass may be considered to be the ideal method of rewarming since the vital organs in the core are rewarmed first with well-oxygenated fluid and the circulation is artificially supported. It is certainly very effective when the heart is in asystole or VF. With the warmer set at 38–40°C femoral arterial flow rates of 2–3 litres min^{-1} can elevate core temperature by about 15°C h^{-1}. However, it is not always successful (Jui et al., 1988) and, in the few clinical case reports where it has been used, the patient's temperature has sometimes dropped back to hypothermic levels after treatment has stopped because only the core has been rewarmed. There have also been problems with cardiovascular stability, respiratory complications and renal failure (Lloyd, 1986). Cardiopulmonary bypass is only available in a few large hospitals, and even when the hospital has the equipment it may be in use. It requires an experienced team. In practice, it is usually adopted after other methods have been started.

Practical recommendations

In the prehospital situation, the choice of treatment is governed by many factors, including distance, local risk, weather, number and experience of rescuers, their physical condition, and the availability of equipment (Mills, 1992). The only methods of rewarming that can be considered practical are spontaneous rewarming, airway warming and surface heating, although the last is not first choice (Handley et al., 1992).

In the A&E department, spontaneous rewarming and airway warming can be used and peritoneal dialysis should also be available. These should be sufficient. Other measures require specialist expertise which is not always available.

Late effects

Most patients have no after-effects following rewarming, but some patients may develop intravascular coagulation which can produce thrombosis and stroke. This is more common following rapid rewarming from severe hypothermia, as are haemolysis and acute tubular necrosis. Post-rewarming pancreatitis also occurs from coagulopathy or a different mechanism.

Other treatment

In hypothermia, cardiac drugs are ineffective or dangerous because of increased cardiac irritability. The effects of other drugs are unpredictable and any medication should be given intravenously because of poor circulation in muscle and subcutaneous tissue.

The use of *oxygen* has been considered dangerous because of the suggestion that the respiratory centre in hypothermia may no longer respond to carbon dioxide and may only respong to the hypoxic drive. However, when measurements were made, patients required additional oxygen to avoid hypoxia while the carbon dioxide drive was normal. Oxygen can therefore be given, but if it is too cold (e.g. cylinder lying in the snow) changing from warm expired air resuscitation may cause cardiac arrest either through inhalation or through the vagal stimulation of cold on the face.

Measurements have shown that circulating *corticosteroid* levels are often above normal in hypothermic patients. However, these may have fallen from higher, stress-induced levels. While steroids cannot be recommended as routine treatment, they are worth considering *in extremis* in view of reports from the field where large doses, given as a last resort, have had almost miraculous effects.

Glucose levels are reported to be above normal in hypothermia because of failure of the metabolic capability of cold tissues. However, levels fall during rewarming and patients, particularly those with exhaustion hypothermia, may require glucose as a metabolic substrate. Also, hypothermia can be precipitated by hypoglycaemia and the symptoms of the two conditions are very similar. Glucagon will be ineffective in glycogen-depleted patients and therefore 50% dextrose should be considered.

Heated fluids should only be given by mouth if the victim is fully conscious. They do not provide much heat but give psychological comfort. Alcohol must not be given since it suppresses shivering, causes vasodilatation and induces drowsiness.

Intensive care is one of the most important measures in the hospital management of hypothermia. All patients should be transferred to intensive care after initial stabilization in the A&E department. If unnecessary deaths from urban hypothermia are to be avoided, rewarming should only be undertaken with intensive care monitoring.

Caution

Published papers on accidental hypothermia must be examined critically for the following reasons:

1. The morphology and thermoregulatory physiology of animals used in experiments may differ greatly from that of man.
2. The pharmacological effects of drugs, including anaesthetics, alter thermoregulation. Anaesthetic techniques may differ between experiments, and tracheal intubation alters the thermohydrodynamics of respiration.
3. With human experiments it is too dangerous to cool volunteers down to the body temperatures frequently found in accidental hypothermia; 34°C is the normal limit. At this temperature, the full physiological response to hypothermia is not present and shivering prevents some of the vasoconstriction associated with cold exposure. The only experiments in which humans were cooled to realistic temperatures were the unethical experiments carried out by the Nazis at Dachau (Alexander, 1945). However, recent work has suggested that the Dachau experiments contributed little to the general knowledge of hypothermia and they may have delayed progress.
4. Most experiments in hypothermia involve rapid cooling, usually in cold water, and the physiological changes are very different from hypothermia among climbers or the elderly.
5. In clinical cases of accidental hypothermia in man, there are many variables, even in a single study.
6. Many papers deal with very few patients and make claims that some particular method of rewarming is safe. However, the conclusions reached are often the authors' interpretation of the clinical observations and usually overlook important points such as treatment in an intensive care area.

DIRECT LOCAL COLD INJURY

Frostbite

Frostbite is a localized lesion caused by the direct effects of cold following moderate or long-term exposure to temperatures less than 0°C. Although most commonly associated with northern latitudes, it may also occur in unexpected parts of the world (e.g. in the Sahara desert at night) (Lloyd, 1986).

Pathophysiology

There are three elements which produce the 'frostbite lesion' (Foray, 1992; Mills, 1991).

1. Skin freezes at $-0.5°C$ but true frostbite occurs when there is sufficient heat loss in the local area to allow ice crystals to form in the extracellular fluid. The remaining hypertonic extracellular fluid causes intracellular dehydration as water runs down the osmotic gradient. This disturbs the enzyme mechanisms, pH and electrolyte imbalance, causing cell death. Cell survival is possible given appropriate treatment. Very rapid freezing over seconds or minutes causes ice crystals to form within the cells and immediate cell death occurs.
2. Blood hyperviscosity develops during cooling which is aggravated by dehydration and cold-induced fluid shifts.
3. Cold-induced vasoconstriction and stagnation increase cellular aggregation and sludging. Normally there is a decrease in local haematocrit and, on rewarming, vasodilatation occurs with immediate recovery of microvascular perfusion. However, if there is pathological local vasodilatation without rewarming, (e.g. because of histamine release) the part will be perfused with blood containing a high concentration of red cells. This will increase the risk of red cell aggregation and microvascular occlusion with complete stasis, and may result in gangrene and problems during rewarming.

These last two features produce microthombi, tissue anoxia and local metabolic acidosis which in turn damages the capillary endothelium (through bradykinin release) resulting in oedema and perpetuation of the vicious cycle.

Precipitating factors (Foray, 1992; Foray & Salon, 1985; Mills, 1983, 1991)

Frostbite affects the extremities preferentially – feet 57% (particularly the large toe), hands 46% (the thumb is frequently spared) – and open areas such as the face (ears, nose, cheeks) 7% (frostbite of the ears increases when short hairstyles are fashionable). The site of frostbite is influenced by physical immobility, position, pressure (e.g. on buttocks and perineum from sitting on a metal seat), lack of insulating fat, liability to wetting (including overflow incontinence), or by contact with cold metal (e.g. handling metal wrenches or penile frostbite from metal zips). Petrol or other organic solvents left outside in freezing weather become supercooled and cause in-

stantaneous freezing of tissues. Anything that restricts the circulation increases the risk of frostbite and worsens the outcome. For example, training shoes and similar shoes used for cross-country skiing are dangerous especially if too tightly laced, and snow boots have felt liners which shrink and freeze if they become wet. A similar compression can occur if neoprene boots are worn during ascent to altitude. Inadequate or tight clothing worn during skiing or running in extreme cold can also produce penile freezing. 'Snorting' cocaine causes vasoconstriction of the nasal mucous membrane and this has allowed the development of severe intranasal frostbite. The risk of frostbite of the hands is increased in the presence of the vibration white finger syndrome (Virokannas & Anttonen, 1993).

Negroid people are more susceptible than caucasians, and the risk is increased in smokers, in some medical disorders, including peripheral vascular disease and Raynaud's syndrome, and by a previous episode of frostbite. The risk is also increased by dehydration, which can often occur during exposure to cold, by alcohol, by excess tiredness and at altitude, where local haemoconcentration and dehydration are increased. Frostbite may occur in fully clothed individuals at extreme altitude and subzero temperatures if the oxygen uptake is insufficient for adequate heat production and mental function, such that proper preventive measures may be forgotten. If the body temperature is lowered, a small cold skin stimulus which normally has no effect will cause intense vasoconstriction in the fingers and feet.

Classification

Frostbite can be classified into a number of different grades of severity, but three divisions are enough for practical purposes (Ward *et al.*, 1989). In *frostnip* the exposed skin, which has been painful, blanches and loses sensation but remains pliable. In *superficial frostbite* the skin becomes white and frozen, with the deep underlying tissues remaining fairly pliable, although this may not be easy to determine. In *deep frostbite*, muscle, bone and tendons are involved as well as the skin and subcutaneous tissues. The part is insensitive, wooden and grey-purple or marble white. Because tendons are less sensitive to cold and the associated muscle groups are distant from the injury, the part can still be moved voluntarily.

Prognosis and investigations (Foray, 1992; Mills, 1991)

Even if the damage is only superficial (Fig. 6), the initial assessment of severity is often inaccurate (even by

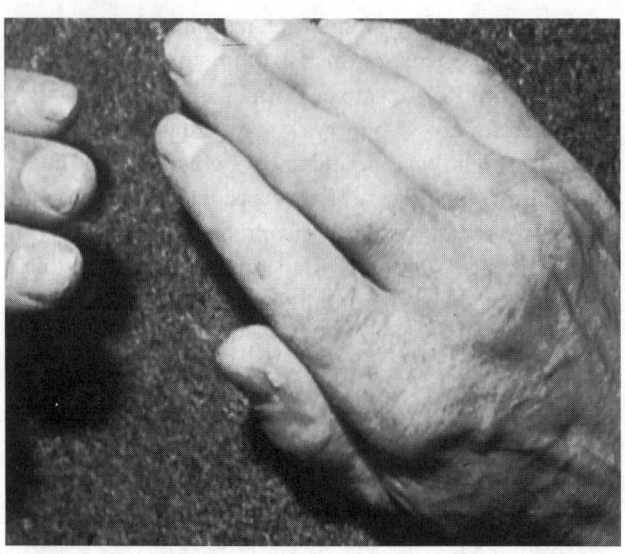

Fig. 6. A cold rigid hand without sensation or digital motion.

experienced practitioners) because the part is hard, cold, white and anaesthetic and appears solidly frozen through; 4–5 days are needed before it is possible to be sure whether the lesion involves superficial or deep freezing. There is no evidence that decisions about treatment are best determined by the severity of the damage, and in practice the extent of the final damage is determined by the changes occurring during rewarming as well as during freezing.

Because of arterial spasm, arteriography may be misleading and infra-red thermography is also of limited value. Other investigations are more useful.

Laser-doppler

The laser beam reflected by red blood cells gives an indication of flow velocity (Doppler effect). Laser-doppler testing is performed on presentation and on the third day. Unfortunately, on initial presentation, good doppler pulses in the extremities may not correlate with tissue perfusion – the distal digital vessels may remain patent for a short while even in the presence of total blockage of the deep capillary system.

Microwave thermography

This is a non-invasive means of measuring tissue temperature giving information on the vascularization and metabolism of the affected tissues.

Nuclear magnetic resonance: ^{31}P, H^+, ^{23}Na

This gives useful information about the state of the muscle masses and gives an early indication of the likelihood of a proximal amputation. It has limitations in the fingers and toes because there is so little muscular tissue.

Technetium-99 infusion

^{99}Tc isotopes are injected and the perfusion is examined radiologically. It is performed on the day of admission and appears of great value in deciding prognosis. Cold spots in the bones indicate deep frostbite and correspond to the areas of severe frostbite that will lead to subsequent amputation.

Treatment

This has to take into account the pathophysiology. With the provisos detailed below, the sooner treatment is begun the more complete it will be and the better the results.

Rewarming

The treatment of hypothermia, if present, takes precedence because it maintains vasoconstriction (Foray & Salon, 1985; Mills, 1983).

Only frostnip should be rewarmed in the field. This is done by placing the affected part in the armpit or under clothing. The part tingles and becomes hyperaemic. Within a few minutes sensation is restored and normal working can be resumed. There may be some skin desquamation several days later.

No attempt should be made to thaw frostbite if it is likely that the part will refreeze. Refreezing causes much more damage than continuous freezing (Mills, 1983). It is possible, and better, to walk to safety on frozen feet as has been achieved for up to 74 h. Before thawing, the frozen part should be protected to avoid trauma.

The currently recommended method is rapid rewarming (Foray, 1992; Foray & Salon, 1985; Mills, 1983, 1991; Ward *et al.*, 1989) by immersion of the part or the whole person in a whirlpool or bubble bath, or using warm wet packs (38–41°C) until the distal tip of the thawed part flushes or no further improvement occurs. The tissues will then be soft and pliable. Sensation returns after warming until blisters develop. If clear blebs develop over the next 48 h (Fig. 7) there is an optimal degree of tissue preservation and early function especially in deep injury

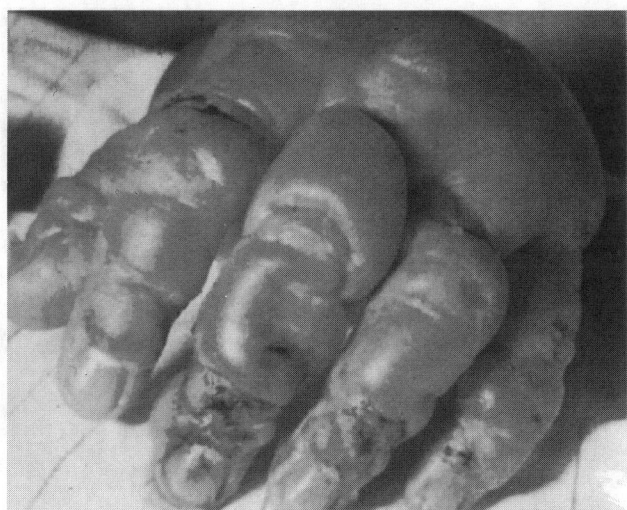

Fig. 7. 36 h post-thawing by rapid rewarming in warm water, showing clear blebs reaching to the ends of the fingers. Patient complained of severe pain.

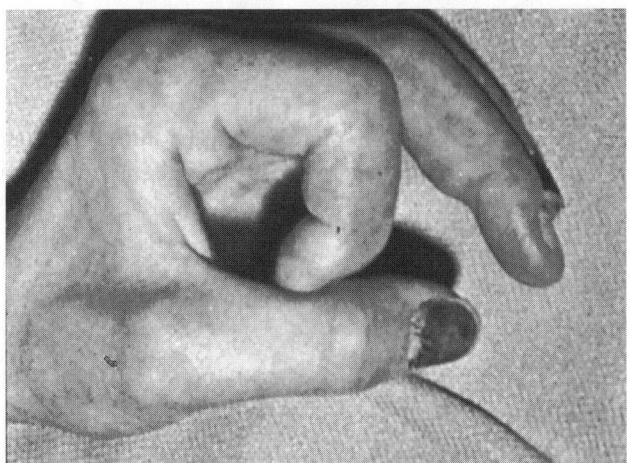

Fig. 8. Four months postinjury and rewarming in warm water. Epithelialization is complete and the anatomy has been preserved.

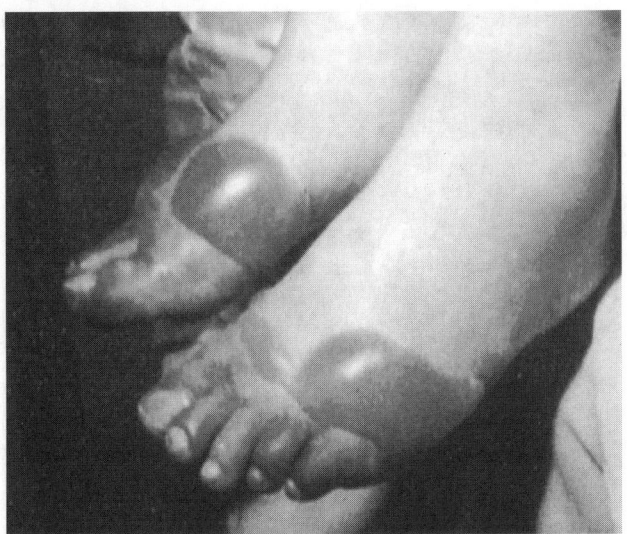

Fig. 9. The feet are approximately 5 days postfreezing and 48 h post-thawing after a freeze–thaw–refreeze injury. A very poor prognostic sign is evident. The blebs are all proximal and dark, while the toes and distal tissues are without blebs or blistering, and are dusky, oedematous, painless and insensitive. Phalangeal amputation is generally unavoidable with this pattern and may be predicted as early as 24 h post-thaw. See Fig. 10.

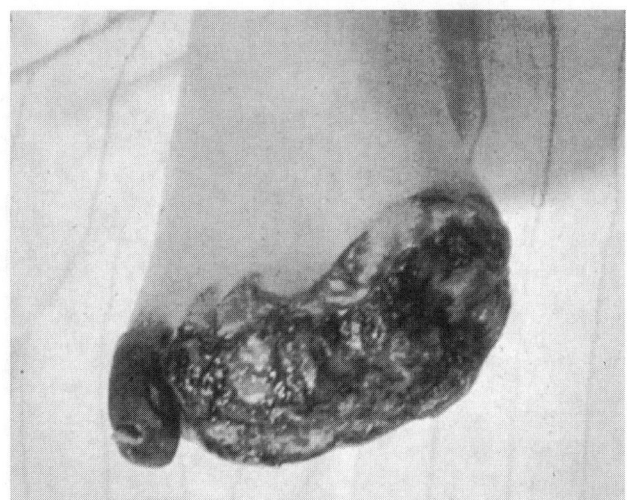

Fig. 10. Spontaneous amputation at the distal metatarsal level which was subsequently surgically trimmed and closed. Despite this the patient was back in the Arctic the following winter and continued trapping and hunting for many years.

(Fig. 8). If the part remains cyanotic and cold and small dark blisters appear late, it is ominous. If blebs do not develop (Fig. 9), there is no chance of tissue recovery (Fig. 10). (Rapid rewarming should not be used if the part has been thawed previously).

Gradual spontaneous thawing is satisfactory for superficial frostbite but not for deep injury. Beating, delayed thawing or using ice or snow rubbing often results in marked tissue loss. The worst results follow freeze–thaw–refreeze injury, 'Trench foot' followed by freezing (see later), or thawing with excessive heat (Figs 11–13) at or above 50°C (temperatures produced by diesel exhausts, stoves or wood fires, or scalding water) (Foray & Salon, 1985; Mills, 1991).

Rapid internal rewarming theoretically produces good results but these are no better than those achieved with the standard external method, and intra-arterial lines can cause severe damage (Mills, 1983).

After thawing there may be postfreezing injury with vasoconstriction, arteriovenous capillary thrombosis and/or severe cellular damage as a result of the freezing.

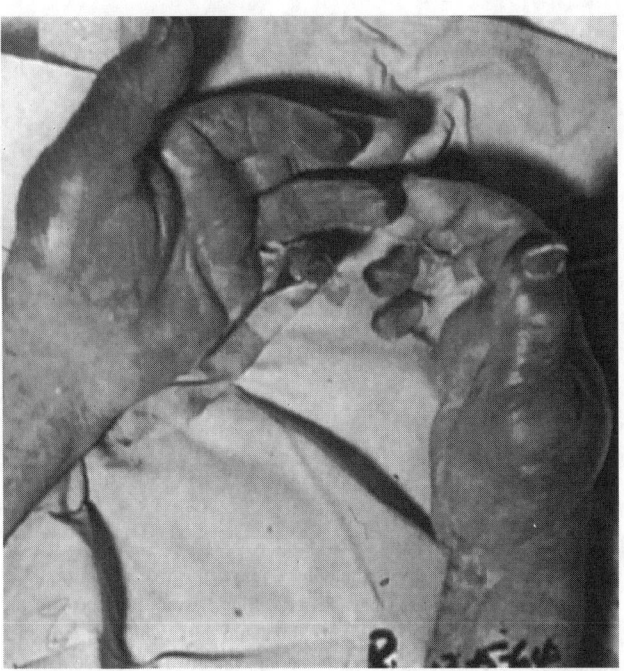

Fig. 11. The extremity less than 24 h after thawing frostbite by using excess heat (boiling water in this case). The hand is cyanotic, painful and foul-smelling and there are no blebs.

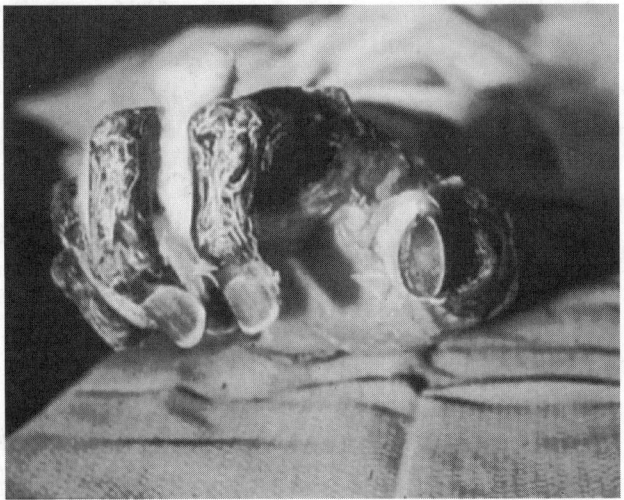

Fig. 12. At 3 weeks the digits show tissue death, being hard and rigid with the soft tissue completely mummified. There is evidence of infection, superficial only, at the area of tissue demarcation.

Hydration and haemodilution

Most patients with frostbite, and/or hypothermia, are dehydrated, and rehydration with warmed fluids is very important. Low molecular weight dextran may reduce the cellular aggregation and sludging and may be worth continuing for 10–12 days in the postrewarming phase (Foray & Salon, 1985).

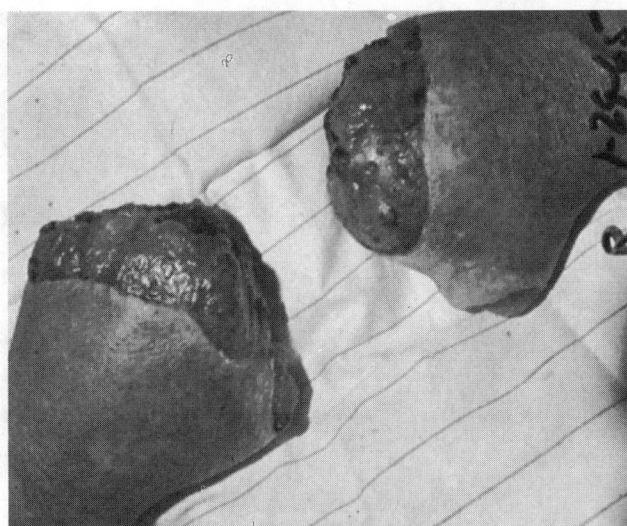

Fig. 13. Spontaneous amputation at the metacarpophalangeal junction at 6 weeks. This is typical of the extent of tissue loss and the hopelessness for recovery when gangrene is caused by 'cooking' frozen tissues with excessive dry or wet heat.

Pain relief

Narcotic analgesics are usually required during thawing but thereafter tranquillizers or aspirin is all that is needed in uncomplicated cases (Foray & Salon, 1985).

Measures to counter infection (Foray & Salon, 1985; Mills 1991)

After thawing the extremities should be elevated and exposed on sterile sheets with cradles to avoid damage. Sterile gauze or cotton-wool is placed between the digits. To remove necrotic and infected tissue without causing any damage to healthy tissue, treatment is continued with whirlpool or bubble baths (30–35°C) twice daily for 20 min with an antiseptic (e.g. hexachlorophene, 4% chlorhexidine gluconate or betadine) added to the water. After the whirlpool treatment 0.5% silver nitrate lavaged over the frostbitten area reduces pain and the incidence of infection, and also counteracts severe drying, splitting and separation of the eschar. Antibiotics are used only when there is a definite indication.

Sympathetic blockade and vasodilators

Sympathectomy reduces pain, decreases oedema, and lessens infection but, despite more rapid tissue demarcation, it does not result in increased tissue preservation (Mills, 1991). Sympathectomy is of value following fasciotomy. Continuous cervical or lumbar epidural infusion provides analgesia and sympathetic blockade. Current management includes alpha-adrenergic blockade using phenoxybenzamine hydrochloride 10 mg daily, increasing to 20–60 mg depending on effect and need. Naftidrofuryl oxalate (Praxilene) 100–200 mg three times daily has also been of value. The patient must be well hydrated if sympathetic blockade or vasodilators are used (Mills, 1983).

Smoking is prohibited because of its vasoconstrictor effect, but alcohol is permitted.

Other measures (Foray & Salon, 1985; Mills, 1991; Ward et al., 1989)

Prostaglandins and thromboxane are released from damaged epithelial cells and these promote vasoconstriction and clotting which is obviously hazardous in the post-thaw phase. These adverse effects can be countered by the use of non-steroidal anti-inflammatory drugs taken orally. Aspirin (1–2 tablets) should also be given while the part is still frozen and repeated every 6 h. Topical Aloe Vera cream every 6 h has also been shown to be of value.

Anti-tetanus prophylaxis must be given after rewarming.

Anticoagulants (low-dose heparin) prevent microthrombosis, and thrombolytic enzymes may be tried in the presence of deep thrombus. However, both are risky in the presence of associated trauma, especially if there is the possibility of a head injury. Hyperbaric oxygen and biofeedback training both appear to be of value in the post-thaw phase but are undergoing further evaluation.

The patient should be nursed in a pleasant environment and fed with a high-protein and high-calorie diet with vitamin supplements. Digital exercises are encouraged throughout the day and, for the lower limbs, Buerger's exercises four times daily.

Surgery

One study (Heggers et al., 1990) suggested that, after thawing, clear or white blisters/blebs should be debrided because the blister fluid contained prostaglandins and thromboxane which caused persistent vasospasm. Haemorrhagic blebs were left intact since they protected deep injury. The claim that this produced better results than standard treatment has been challenged on the grounds that the study was very badly designed (Richard & Butson, 1990). The consensus of opinion (Foray, 1992; Mills, 1991; Ward et al., 1989) is that blebs should be protected and kept intact to reduce infection but if they become infected they should be drained or debrided.

When the eschar is dry, escharotomy on the dorsal or lateral aspects of the digits releases splinting and allows exercises to continue.

After thawing, the formation of oedema may result in a compartment pressure syndrome; fasciotomy is then essential to avoid extensive tissue necrosis. Clinical judgement should not be over-ruled by sophisticated technology in deciding whether or not a fasciotomy is necessary.

Dislocations should be reduced immediately the part has been rewarmed but fractures are treated conservatively until the post-thaw oedema has settled.

Since the gangrene of frostbite is much more superficial than it appears, even in deep frostbite, debridement or amputation should be delayed up to 90 days till mummification and tissue demarcation is complete (Foray, 1992; Mills, 1991; Ward et al., 1989). After the blackened areas have separated, the underlying tissue is raw, shiny, tender and unduly sensitive, and there may be abnormal sweating. This should return to normal in 2–3 m (Ward et al., 1989).

Occasionally following freeze–thaw–refreeze or trauma plus freeze there is overwhelming local infection with systemic spread. This is the only situation in which immediate amputation is essential. A modified guillotine procedure should be used, with closed suction, irrigation of the wound with normal saline 100 ml h^{-1} and a flush of 50 ml of antibiotic solution every hour (Mills, 1991).

Skin grafting is performed late but, if the fasciotomy wound is extensive, immediate grafting reduces infection, morbidity and scarring. Late amputations should if necessary be closed with a skin flap and not with grafts.

In prehospital management, wounds should be sutured early since this results in less infection and tissue loss (Richard & Butson, 1990).

Trench foot (non-freezing cold injury)

Cold can also cause tissue damage without freezing: 'trench foot', 'paddy foot', 'immersion injury', 'non-freezing cold injury' (NFCI). There is sometimes confusion between frostbite and NFCI, though NFCI may be present proximal to areas of frostbite. NFCI may be followed by frostbite and this combination is usually disastrous. NFCI is certainly much more common than is usually recognized.

NFCI was frequent during the wars among soldiers living in wet trenches and among sailors after long periods spent in lifeboats. Even in the Falklands campaign in 1982, NFCI was present in 20% of the men received on the hospital ship Uganda. Prolonged trekking through boggy terrain in northern countries can result in NFCI.

Running barefoot on frozen ground, though painless during the run because of cold-induced neuropathy, has resulted in considerable loss of tissue on the soles of the feet.

Pathology and risk factors

NFCI requires longer exposure than frostbite does. It develops when the legs are exposed to the wet and cold above 0°C, but wet conditions are not absolutely necessary. If the part is wet, similar tissue damage may occur with skin temperatures above 16°C, even up to 29°C (Maclean & Emslie-Smith, 1977). There is a vicious pathogenic circle of cooling and vasoconstriction accompanied by a high level of sympathetic tone (Francis & Golden, 1985). The venous pressure rises causing sludging and thrombosis, and this results in tissue ischaemia and neurovascular damage without ice crystal formation (Schmid-Schonbein & Neumann, 1985). Failure of cellular calcium extrusion alters the intracellular ionic milieu. In NFCI there is muscle and nerve damage with the skin remaining intact – the reverse of frostbite.

As in frostbite (and hypothermia), predisposing factors include dehydration, inadequate nutrition, fatigue, stress, intercurrent illness or injury (Lloyd, 1986). Damage is more likely to occur and be more extensive if the limb is dependent, immobile or is constricted by footwear. If footwear has been soaked in sea water the incidence of NFCI is higher because the salt crystals attract water; in the mountains, NFCI can develop if the boots are impervious to water because the build-up of sweat inside the boot is the equivalent to immersion (Mills, 1983).

Signs and symptoms (Lloyd, 1986; Ward et al., 1989)

The feet are initially cold and numb. The loss of sensation gives the feeling of 'walking on cotton wool' and this combined with joint stiffness causes difficulty in walking, with the victims adopting a gait with their legs apart to maintain balance. When first examined the typical case has cold, swollen and blotchy pink-purple or blanched feet which feel heavy and numb. After rewarming this is succeeded by hyperaemia with hot, red, swollen feet, and paraesthesia and/or pain which may be severe. The pain is described by some as being like electric shock running up the legs from the toes, and it may be severe enough to prevent sleep. This phase lasts for days or weeks. There may be bleeding into the skin, ulceration and secondary infection. Severe injury is indicated by large blisters. The damage may progress to gangrene which tends to be deeper than in frostbite.

Treatment

This involves removing the person from the hostile environment, bed rest, and analgesics for the pain. The consensus is that NFCI should never be rewarmed actively. However, there is a view that, if the pulses are impalpable, rewarming the feet in a bath may be advisable. Whole-body warming and sympathectomy are controversial. Elevation reduces the oedema, and weight-bearing should be avoided because it causes very severe pain.

After-effects of local cold injury

There is a large overlap in the pathology and late sequelae of frostbite and NFCI. All nerves degenerate if kept below freezing for more than a few seconds. There is complete necrosis of all structures within the perineurium except the endothelial lining of the blood vessels. Even at temperatures above freezing, demyelination of nerves may occur. However, axon regeneration does occur and there may be full return of neurological function over 9 months or longer.

In freezing cold injury, the degree of muscle damage depends on the amount of exposure. There is coagulation necrosis in the superficial coldest layer, slow necrosis in the intermediate zone and muscle atrophy in the deepest layer. Repair is by fibrosis and wasting. Rhabdomyolysis with incipient renal failure has been reported after severe frostbite of both lower limbs and after NFCI of both feet in children.

After recovery, there may be persistent effects with vasomotor paralysis, analgesia and paraesthesia, which may be permanent; 61% report long-term burning sensations in their feet, and intractable pain has been known to last for 35 years (Mills, 1983; Ward et al., 1989). There may also be early anhidrosis or late hyperhidrosis.

Epiphyseal cartilage is more sensitive to cold than bone cells which are more sensitive than skin. Cartilage cells, epiphyseal growth plates and non-ossified carpal bones are irreversibly destroyed and the effect of cold on osteocytes may produce bone necrosis. In children this results in gross abnormalities during growth. After 6 months, X-rays may show typical changes with fine irregular lytic or cystic areas near articular surfaces. Even

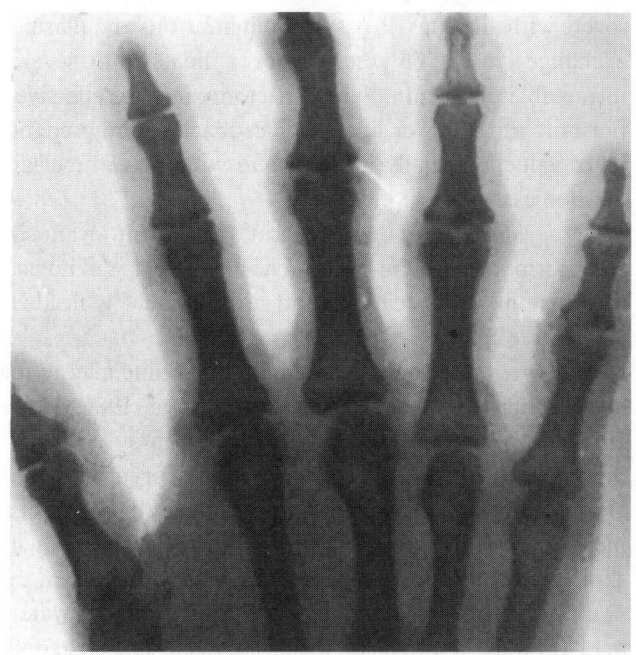

Fig. 14. X-ray showing fusiform enlargement of the proximal inter-phalangeal joints, and sub- and intra-articular lytic areas. Severe freezing 3 years previously.

following complete return of function, there is joint swelling, limited movement and pain (Fig. 14). Other late problems include toe rigidity, fallen arches and osteo-porosis, although new bone formation usually restores the normal X-ray appearance. Epiphyseal damage and eroded joints predispose to osteoarthritis (Mills, 1983; Ward *et al.*, 1989).

There may be hardening and atrophy of soft tissues. Some victims suffer permanently from intermittent ulcer-ation of the skin with fissuring and chronic infection. Fungating and ulcerating carcinoma of the heel occur occasionally and has been reported up to 40 years after frostbite. This is due to unstable scar tissue subjected to chronic irritation and pressure. The tumour is of low malignancy with little spread and treatment is by local excision and skin grafting (Ward *et al.*, 1989).

Obliterative endarteritis and Raynaud's syndrome may occur, with the feet in particular tending to develop a marked and persistent vasospasm when presented with cold stimuli. This cold hypersensitivity may persist for years or even be permanent, and re-exposure to cold is liable to cause relapse. Interestingly, 60% of 'normal' people are very susceptible to cold injury (Ahle *et al.*, 1990). Finally, there may be weakness and deformity because of muscle damage and/or amputation. Unfortu-nately, at present, there is no satisfactory treatment for the many late manifestations of NFCI.

Prevention of local cold injury

There should be adequate fluid intake to prevent dehy-dration. The disappearance of pain is an early warning of incipient cold injury and, where practicable, the feet and hands should be warmed at intervals, especially if there is total anaesthesia on attempting to move the fingers and toes. No existing boot or shoe will prevent NFCI or frostbite because the many functions shoes and boots have to perform cause conflict in design. The most useful preventive measures are:

1. To limit the time a person is exposed to the hazardous environment.
2. To take a hot drink whenever possible – of thermal and hydration benefits.
3. Maintain adequate foot care to keep the feet as dry and abrasion-free as possible.
4. 'Buddies' can keep a close watch on each other for early signs.

These measures were used in the Second World War by the British troops but not by the American troops, and the result was that, even under identical conditions, the US troops suffered ten times the incidence of cold injuries incurred by the British.

OTHER CONDITIONS AND EFFECTS OF COLD

Conjunctivitis due to cold, and cold injury or frostbite to the cornea, have been seen in downhill skiers, ice skaters and snowmobile drivers unprotected by goggles. In severe cases, a corneal transplant is the only treatment (Ward *et al.*, 1989).

Chilblains (pernio) are localized cold-induced inflam-matory lesions with erythema and swelling due to a vascular sympathetic hypersensitivity to cold (Lahti, 1982). Patients complain of intense pruritus and burning paraesthesia, the latter more common after rewarming. In severe cases, haemorrhagic vesicles or ulceration may occur. The underlying pathology is a dermal lymphocytic vasculitis associated with microvascular stasis, thrombosis and oedema. Chilblains usually occur on the dorsal surfaces of the hands and feet. They are most common in young women, in people with Raynaud's or other previous skin disease and in people who habitually work in cold, damp and wet conditions. Predisposing factors include injury, poor nutrition, sepsis, inadequate clothing and cold humid conditions. If severe, the affected areas should be elevated to reduce the oedema, cleaned and dressed. After rewarming, tender blue nodules appear which may persist for weeks leaving hyperpigmentation. Recurrence is common. Central heating reduces the incidence of chilblains but increases the problem of *winter itch* (asteototic eczema), because the low relative humidity causes water loss, decreased sweating and sebum secretion, the skin becomes dry, brittle and itchy, and cracks develop. Treatment involves humidification of the room, emulsifying skin ointments and the avoidance of too much washing (Lahti, 1982).

In *Raynaud's syndrome* (Belch, 1990; Lloyd, 1986) a cold stress, whose severity does not affect normal people, produces severe arterial vasoconstriction and the normal reactive hyperaemia following arterial occlusion is virtually absent. Even in the warm, there is an altered pulse contour. Raynaud's phenomenon is most marked in the fingers and toes, but the tips of the tongue, nose and ears may also be involved, and the vasospasm may affect internal organs. Raynaud's syndrome is more readily induced if the core temperature is below 36°C. Raynaud's phenomenon is associated with a large number of connective tissue disorders (such as rheumatoid arthritis, systemic lupus erythematosus, scleroderma) and arteriosclerosis, thoracic outlet syndrome and emboli. However, a large percentage of patients have detectable antinuclear antibodies without any other evidence of autoimmune disease. Those without antinuclear antibodies have lower noradrenaline levels than controls but higher cortisol levels which increase vasomotor reactivity.

Vasospastic attacks are precipitated by cold and/or emotional stress. Attacks may also be provoked by trauma, hormones and chemicals, including those in tobacco smoke, and by a number of drugs including beta-blockers, ergot and other antimigraine drugs, cytotoxic agents, bromocriptine and sulphasalazine. Exposure to arsenic in mining, to vinyl chloride and the hand vibration syndrome (e.g. from pneumatic drill usage, or by driving snowmobiles) all cause increased sensitivity to cold, as does previous cold injury.

Protection from cold exposure can be obtained through suitable clothing, shoes and gloves but, if attacks of digital ischaemia are incapacitating, chemical hand warmers or portable electrically heated gloves or socks should be considered. Smoking should be stopped.

In some cases, the condition is persistent, leading to digital ulceration and occasional loss of the tips of the digits. Drug treatment is possible and calcium channel blockers, prostaglandins and the anabolic steroid stanozolol are the most promising treatments. Unfortunately, side-effects and practical problems of administration are severe with all drugs. Prostaglandin infusions and plasma exchange should be reserved for patients with severe intractable ulceration. Sympathectomy may be effective, but only in the lower limbs. Biofeedback training might be of value, especially in the group without antinuclear antibodies.

Acrocyanosis is a symmetrical permanent cyanosis with normal peripheral pulses. The aetiology is unknown, there are no complications and no treatment is needed (Lahti, 1982).

Cold urticaria. Some people have a genuine allergy to cold (British Medical Journal, 1975; Lloyd, 1986; Ting, 1984), with exposure causing degranulation of sensitized mast cells in the skin. It is associated with cryoglobulins, cryofibrinogen or cold agglutinins. The local effects include redness, itching, wheals and oedema on exposed skin. Even cold drinks may produce lesions in the mouth and on the lips, and wading or swimming in cold water may produce a transient localized rash. The systemic features are malaise with shivering, tachycardia, aching joints and generalized urticaria, sometimes progressing to collapse, anaphylactic shock and death. The most common form is acquired and this is associated with histamine release. By contrast, the familial form is not associated with histamine release. The susceptibility is transmitted as a genetic dominant. The diagnosis of familial cold urticaria should not be missed since it may occur on any immersion, even in an indoor swimming pool. Proper counselling and prevention of exposure to cold may save the life of a susceptible person, since some deaths which occur within a few minutes of entering cold water may be due to anaphylaxis in a person with previously unsuspected cold urticaria. Treatment using an H1-receptor antagonist (e.g. cyproheptadine) may be of value.

Cold erythema is due to cryoglobulins which precipitate with chilling. Symptoms include purpura, severe pain, muscle spasm and sweating. Treatment is to remove the person from the cold, but unfortunately the signs and symptoms often become exacerbated during rewarming.

Paroxysmal cold haemoglobinuria (Gaunt et al., 1992) is a form of autoimmune haemolysis. On exposure, a cold-reactive antibody produces a complement-mediated massive haemolysis. It is more common in males. In children, the condition is acute and transient usually following a virus infection (e.g. measles, mumps or chickenpox). In adults it takes a more chronic form with episodes of haemoglobinuria, aching pains and cramps following exposure to cold. It may occasionally produce peripheral gangrene. In adults, it is associated with congenital and tertiary syphilis. There are signs of haemolysis (e.g. lowered haemoglobin with increased reticulocytes and raised bilirubin). The diagnostic test is to incubate the serum with red cells at 4°C and when these are then warmed to 37°C there is intense haemolysis due to Donath–Landsteiner antibody which acts at very low titres. Immediate treatment is bed rest and warmth; over the longer term the person should avoid cold following infection.

Oedema. Exposure to cold normally results in dehydration through diuresis and respiratory moisture loss. Exercise increases the loss through both routes. However, if the body cools very slowly, fluid shifts from the intravascular space to the intracellular space and this may produce oedema. Oedema may also occur within 12–24 h of rewarming due to plasma passing through cold damaged capillaries into the interstitial tissue. As has been seen in mountains, associated exercise may cause swelling of the feet.

Backache. The muscles of the back are very powerful, and heat production rises by increased muscle metabolism and tone. Therefore, in a cold environment, the back muscles may have to be constantly generating heat. Backache was found to be a symptom associated with cold housing (Platt *et al.*, 1989) and its mechanism may be similar to that of overuse injury.

*Systemic illness.*One of the disadvantages of the very precise definition of hypothermia is that people can be suffering from cold to a significant extent without ever becoming hypothermic. There are other adverse effects which cold may have on the body (Lloyd, 1986) which may lead to hospital admission or death. Hypothermia is not the most common cause of cold-related deaths, even among the elderly.

The effects of cold stress may cause heart attacks, strokes, ruptured aortic aneurysm (Lloyd, 1988) and heart failure, and cold may be implicated in the causation of ischaemic heart disease and high blood pressure (Lloyd, 1986, 1991b).

Breathing cold air triggers asthma and some people are very susceptible. The pulmonary responses to cold may explain some of the paradoxes in the transmission of the common cold, and if divers breathe cold oxyhelium under pressure they may drown in their own secretions. Cold, interacting with hypoxia, is probably a factor in the aetiology of high-altitude pulmonary oedema and high-altitude pulmonary hypertension. At lower altitudes, it is involved in the aetiology of chronic bronchitis and its acute exacerbations. Cold may be implicated in some 'cot deaths' and, even though some of the victims have had a raised core temperature (usually producing a diagnosis of hyperthermia), it could have been the end-result of vasoconstriction and an increased heat production in response to cold.

Cold affects nerves, muscles and joints, impairing manual performance (Enander, 1984) and increasing the risk of musculotendinous tears.There is impairment of the higher senses, slowing of reaction times, the development of incoordination and an increasing frequency of mistakes. There may be impairment of cerebration leading to misinterpretation or hallucinations. Some sufferers have even paradoxically undressed while exposed to the cold. The peripheral and central effects in various combinations make accidents more likely.

Bibliography

AHLE, N.W., BURONI, J.R., SHARP, M.W. *et al.*, (1990). Infrared thermographic measurement of circulatory compromise in trenchfoot-injured Argentinian soldiers. *Aviat. Space Environ. Med.*, **61**, 247–50.

ALEXANDER, L. (1945). The treatment of shock from prolonged exposure to cold, especially in water. *Combined Intelligence Objective Subcommittee, Item No.* 24, File No. 26-37.

ALEXANDER, G. (1979). Cold thermogenesis. In *Environmental Physiology III.* ed. D. Robertshaw pp 43–155. Baltimore: University Park Press.

BELCH, J.J.F. (1990). Management of Raynaud's phenomenon. *Hosp. Update*, **16**, 391–9.

BLIGH, J. (1984). Temperature regulation: a theoretical consideration incorporating Sherringtonian principles of central neurology. *J. Therm. Biol.*, **9**, 3–6.

BRITISH MEDICAL JOURNAL (1975). Cold hypersensitivity. *BMJ*, **1**, 643–4.

ENANDER, A. (1984). Performance and sensory aspects of work in cold environments – a review. *Ergonomics*, **27**, 365–78.

FORAY, J. (1992). Mountain frostbite. Current trends in prognosis and treatments (from results concerning 1261 cases). *Int. J. Sports Med.*, **13**, S193–6.

FORAY, J. & SALON, F. (1985). Casualties with cold injuries; primary treatment. In *High Altitude Deterioration*, ed. J. Rivolier, P. Ceretelli, J. Foray & P. Segantini. pp. 149–58. Basel: Karger.

FRANCIS, T.J.R. & GOLDEN, F.St.C. (1985). Nonfreezing cold injury; the pathogenesis. *J.R. Naval Med. Serv.*, **71**, 3–8.

GAUNT, M.E., CHAPMAN, C., LONDON, N. *et al.* (1992). Paroxysmal cold haemoglobinuria presenting as peripheral gangrene. *Hosp. Update*, **18**, 825–6.

GRAY, D. (1987). Survival after burial in an avalanche. *BMJ*, **1**, 611–2.

HANDLEY, A.J., GOLDEN, F.St.C., KEATINGE, W.R. *et al.* (1992). *Report of the Working Party on Out of Hospital Management of Hypothermia.* Medical Commission on Accident Prevention.

HEGGERS, J.P., PHILLIPS, L.G., MCCAULEY, R.L. *et al.*, (1990). Frostbite: experimental and clinical evaluation of treatment. *J. Wilderness Med.*, **1**, 27–32.

HORVATH, S.M. (1981). Exercise in a cold environment. *Exerc. Sport Sci. Rev.*, **9**, 221–63.

JUI, J., HAUTY, M. & HARDER, R. (1988). Hypothermia on Mt. Hood: 1986. *Wilderness Med. Newsl.*, **5**, 4–7.

LAHTI, A. (1982). *Cutaneous Reactions to Cold.* Nordic Council for Arctic Medical Research, Report No. 30, pp. 32–5.

LEXOW, K. (1991). Severe accidental hypothermia: survival after 6 hours 30 minutes of cardiopulmonary resuscitation. *Arctic Med. Res.*, **50** (Suppl. 6), 112–4.

LLOYD, E.L. (1986). *Hypothermia and Cold Stress.* London: Croom Helm.

LLOYD, E.L. (1988). Hypothermia in the elderly. *Med. Sci. Law*, **28**, 107–14.

LLOYD, E.L. (1990). Airway warming in the treatment of accidental hypothermia: a review. *J. Wilderness Med.*, **1**, 65–78.

LLOYD, E.L. (1991a). Equipment for airway warming. *J. Wilderness Med.*, **2**, 330–50.

LLOYD, E.L. (1991b). The role of cold in ischaemic heart disease: a review. *Publ. Health*, **105**, 205–15.

LLOYD, E.L. (1992). The cause of death after rescue. *Int. J. Sports Med.*, **13**, S196–9.

MACLEAN, D. & EMSLIE-SMITH, D. (1977). *Accidental Hypothermia.* Edinburgh: Blackwell Scientific.

MILLER, J.W., DANZL, D.F. & THOMAS, D.M. (1980). Urban accidental hypothermia: 135 cases. *Ann. Emerg. Med.*, **9**, 456–61.

MILLS, W.J. (1983). Frostbite. *Alaska Med.*, **25**, 33–8.

MILLS, W.J. (1991). Frostbite. In *A Colour Atlas of Mountain Medicine*, ed. F. Dubas & J. Vallotton. pp. 78–91. London: Wolfe Publishing.

MILLS, W.J. (1992). Field care of the hypothermic patient. *Int. J. Sports Med.*, **13**, S199–202.

NOLAN, J.P. (1993). Techniques for rapid fluid infusion. *Br. J. Intens. Care*, **3**, 98–105.

NOZAKI, R.N., ISHIBASHI, K., ADACHI, N. *et al.* (1986). Accidental profound hypothermia. *N. Engl. J. Med.*, **315**, 1680.

PLATT, S.D., MARTIN, C.J., HUNT, S.M. *et al.* (1989). Damp housing, mould growth and symptomatic health state. *Br. Med. J.*, **1**, 1673–8.

POZOS, R.S. & WITTMERS, L.E. ed. (1983). *The Nature and Treatment of Hypothermia.* London: Croom Helm.

RICHARD, A. & BUTSON, C. (1990). Notes on frostbite. *J. Wilderness Med.*, **1**, 33–5.

ROYAL COLLEGE OF PHYSICIANS (1966). *Report on Committee on Accidental Hypothermia.* London: Royal College of Physicians.

SCHMID-SCHONBEIN, H. & NEUMANN, F.J. (1985). Pathophysiology of cutaneous frost injury; disturbed microcirculation as a consequence of abnormal flow behaviour of the blood. Application of new concepts of blood rheology. In *High Altitude Deterioration*, ed. J. Rivolier, P. Ceretelli, J. Foray & P. Segantini. pp. 20–38. Basel: Karger.

SHARKEY, A., GULDEN, R.H., LIPTON, J.M. *et al.* (1993). Effect of radiant heat on the metabolic cost of postoperative shivering. *Br. J. Anaesth.*, **70**, 449–50.

STEINMAN, A.M. (1986). Cardiopulmonary resuscitation and hypothermia. *Circulation*, **74**, (Suppl. IV), IV-29–IV-32.

STONEHAM, M.D. & SQUIRES, S.J. (1992). Prolonged resuscitation in acute deep hypothermia. *Anaesthesia*, **47**, 784–8.

TING, S. (1984). Cold-induced urticaria in infancy. *Pediatrics*, **73**, 105–6.

WARD, M.P., MILLEDGE, J.S. & WEST, J.B. (1989). *High Altitude Medicine and Physiology.* London: Chapman and Hall.

39 Hyperthermia

M.T. ALI and J.H. COAKLEY

Intensive Care Unit, St. Bartholomew's Hospital, London, UK

Chapter plan

Introduction
Pathophysiology
Clinical features
Treatment

INTRODUCTION

Hyperthermia is not a disease but a complication which may arise from a variety of conditions. It is defined as elevation of core body temperature above normal. It is uncommon, but there has been an increase in the number of cases presenting to accident and emergency (A&E) departments over recent years. This is principally due to the popularity of long-distance running events such as city marathons and to the explosion in the availability and use of amphetamine-like drugs such as 'Ecstasy' at nightclubs, raves and parties.

This chapter will deal with conditions associated with failure of normal thermoregulatory mechanisms resulting in heat illness, but not with fevers of infective origin.

Hyperthermia develops when the body can no longer cope with excessive heat load and may arise from either excess heat production or from failure of heat dissipation, or a combination of both. It is a medical emergency that carries a high morbidity and mortality (Vicario *et al.*, 1986; Horowitz *et al.*, 1989; Khogali, 1983; Khogali & Weibner, 1980; Clowes & O'Donnell, 1974; Niroche & Marty, 1992) and requires prompt diagnosis and immediate management.

Definition and classification

Hyperthermia is defined as elevation of core body temperature above normal and severe hyperthermia or heat stroke produces a core temperature of 40.5°C or higher, sustained for at least 1 h (Rosenberg *et al.*, 1986). The more severe form is associated with neurological dysfunction ranging from confusion to seizures (Channa *et al.*, 1990; Bouchama *et al.*, 1991).

Mild hyperthermia includes the syndromes of heat cramps and heat exhaustion; *severe hyperthermia* encompasses the more serious heat stroke, malignant hyperthermia and neuroleptic malignant syndrome (Tek & Olshaker, 1992; Wagner, 1993).

Clinical features

Heat cramps occur in heavily exercised muscle, generally the calves, during unaccustomed exercise in the heat. The underlying disorder is a combination of dehydration and sodium loss and is more frequent in subjects who sweat profusely and replace lost fluids with water without added salt (Tek & Olshaker, 1992).

Heat exhaustion is characterized by headache, malaise, dizziness, nausea and vomiting. It is distinguished from the more serious heat stroke by a temperature of greater than 37°C but less than 39°C and by normal mental function (Tek & Olshaker, 1992). By the time a patient with heat stroke presents to the A&E department their temperature may have fallen from its peak; therefore any patient having a temperature above 38.5°C with mental changes must be assumed to have heat stroke.

Neither heat cramps nor heat exhaustion should lead to serious consequences and both respond rapidly to oral or intravenous rehydration, which will be discussed later.

Severe hyperthermia

Heat stroke is the most severe manifestation of thermal injury. It may develop from heat cramps and heat exhaustion.

Heat stroke has been divided into classic heat stroke, occurring in subjects with compromised homeostatic mechanisms (such as the elderly) in conditions of high ambient temperature, and exertional heat stroke which occurs in younger healthier patients usually associated with extreme physical exercise. Classic heat stroke has a slower onset and is often associated with absence of sweating whereas exertional heat stroke is of rapid onset and sweating may be present (Tek & Olshaker, 1992; Wagner, 1993).

The majority of cases of severe hyperthermia presenting to an A&E department are associated with the use of psychoactive drugs and accompanying severe exercise. The drug-related syndromes of malignant hyperthermia and neuroleptic malignant syndrome are both characterized by severe hyperthermia. Both are rare: malignant hyperthermia is a pharmacogenetic disorder which is triggered by drugs used mainly in anaesthetic practice; neuroleptic malignant syndrome is an idiosyncratic disorder associated with the administration of neuroleptic agents. Hyperthermia following drug abuse and exercise shares some of the features of both malignant hyperthermia and neuroleptic malignant syndrome. The causes of hyperthermia are summarized in Table 1.

Table 1. *Causes of hyperthermia*

Increased heat production
1. Increased muscular activity: exercise, seizures, agitation, rigidity
2. Uncoupling of oxidative phosphorylation: salicylates
3. Stimulation of hepatic metabolism: sympathomimetics
4. Alterations in brain chemistry

Increased heat production may be by central or peripheral mechanisms

Reduced heat dissipation
1. Behavioural dysfunction
2. High ambient temperature and humidity
3. Pre-existing disease
4. Drug-related

Specific syndromes
1. Malignant hyperthermia
2. Neuroleptic malignant syndrome

PATHOPHYSIOLOGY

Aetiology

Apart from a few specific syndromes, most cases of hyperthermia are due to a number of exogenous and endogenous factors which result in a multisystem disorder characterized by excess heat load, reduced heat dissipation, or a combination of both. The main factors are exertional, environmental and toxic. There are, however, many other causes of hyperthermia, which are summarized in Table 2.

Exertional

Most cases of severe hyperthermia presenting in an A&E department have followed exercise of some sort. It may occur in long-distance runners (Woolfe & Behrman,

Table 2. *Factors predisposing to hyperthermia*

Pre-existing disease
Cardiovascular disease
Endocrine disease
Autonomic dysfunction
Dehydration
Fever
Delirium tremens
Psychosis
Neonates/elderly
Malignant hyperthermia
Parkinsonism

Drugs
Anticholinergics
Phenothiazines
Tricyclic antidepressants
MAO inhibitors
Beta-blockers
Alpha-blockers
Alpha-agonists
Sympathomimetics
Hallucinogens
Salicylates
Diuretics
Alcohol

Behaviour
Overexertion
Inappropriate clothing
Poor fluid intake
Poor acclimatization

MAO, monoamine oxidase.

1981; Whitworth & Wolfman, 1983; Sutton & Bar-Or, 1980), armed forces recruits following training (Hopkins *et al.*, 1991) and drug abusers (Watson *et al.*, 1993; Henry, 1992) after prolonged dancing.

Environmental factors

The incidence of severe hyperthermia is increased in conditions of high ambient temperature and humidity. Many cases of severe hyperthermia have been documented during the Muslim Pilgrimage to Mecca in Saudi Arabia (Khogali & Weibner, 1980; Khogali, 1983; Sutton & Bar-Or, 1980) and these have allowed researchers to evaluate the most effective forms of treatment (Channa *et al.*, 1990; Bouchama *et al.*, 1991; Weiner & Khogali, 1980).

Humid atmospheric conditions reduce the ability of the body to dissipate heat by impeding evaporation of sweat. The Wet Globe Thermometer Index is an excellent measure of environmental heat stress, taking into account ambient temperature, humidity and wind speed. The American College of Sports Medicine (1975) has recommended that sporting events should be postponed if the temperature exceeds 28°C.

Toxic

Malignant hyperthermia and neuroleptic malignant syndrome are well-described conditions due solely to the effect of specific drugs.

Severe hyperthermia has been described following the use of many 'recreational drugs'. It is not always certain whether this is due to idiosyncratic reactions, overdose or because of associated overexertion and conditions of high ambient temperature. Drugs responsible include amphetamines (Baraie & Peppers, 1989; Kalant & Kalant, 1975; Ginsberg *et al.*, 1970), amphetamine derivatives (Henry *et al.*, 1992; Screaton *et al.*, 1992; Woods & Henry, 1992; Tehan *et al.*, 1993), cocaine (Rosenberg *et al.*, 1986; Wagner, 1993; Menashe & Gottlieb, 1988; Merigian & Roberts, 1987), lysergic acid diethylamide (LSD) (Wagner, 1993; Rosenberg *et al.*, 1986), mescaline (Wagner, 1993; Rosenberg *et al.*, 1986) and phencyclidine (PCP) (Wagner, 1993; Rosenberg *et al.*, 1986).

Drugs that reduce sweating (anticholinergic agents) such as tricyclic antidepressants (Rosenberg *et al.*, 1986; Vassallo & Delaney, 1989) and antihistamines, and those that increase metabolic rate such as salicylates (Rosenberg *et al.*, 1986; Vassallo & Delaney, 1989) have been implicated in severe hyperthermia. Additionally, the condition has been described following use of a variety of other agents (Vassallo & Delaney, 1989; Nimmo *et al.*, 1993; Parenti & Hoffmann, 1986; Perlman *et al.*, 1989; Litovitz & Trantman, 1983).

Mechanisms of increased heat production

Peripheral mechanisms

Increased heat production follows unremitting exercise which may be enhanced by the use of sympathomimetic agents such as amphetamines or derivatives. The rhabdomyolysis that often accompanies severe hyperthermia is probably due to overexertion and heat damage (Tek & Olshaker, 1992; Watson *et al.*, 1993) rather than a direct toxic effect of the agents themselves.

Similarly, drugs which cause seizures or rigidity such as tricyclic antidepressants or monoamine oxidase inhibitors may lead to excess heat production (Rosenberg *et al.*, 1986; Vassallo & Delaney, 1989). Muscular rigidity of the extrapyramidal type caused by dopamine antagonists such as haloperidol, chlorpromazine, fluphenazine or thioridazine may lead to the neuroleptic malignant syndrome (Nimmo *et al.*, 1993).

Sympathomimetic agents additionally increase heat production by increasing hepatic metabolism of glucose and fat.

Uncoupling of oxidative phosphorylation by salicylates causes cellular energy production to be released as heat rather than stored as ATP (adenosine triphosphate) (Vassallo & Delaney, 1989; Nimmo *et al.*, 1993).

Sweat gland activity is controlled via cholinergic pathways. Drugs that have anticholinergic effects such as tricyclic antidepressants (Rosenberg *et al.*, 1986; Nimmo *et al.*, 1993), antihistamines (Vassallo & Delaney, 1989) and atropine (Niroche & Marty, 1992) reduce sweat and block heat dissipation.

Similarly beta-blockers blunt the necessary increase in cardiac output to support maximal cutaneous vasodilatation, as do diuretics which diminish extracellular fluid volume.

Alpha-agonists such as phenylephrine or the appetite suppressor phenylpropranolamine promote cutaneous vasoconstriction and reduce heat loss (Kew *et al.*, 1982). Any drugs with sympathomimetic actions may reduce cutaneous vasodilation and have the same effect, as with amphetamine and its derivatives, cocaine and phenyclidine ('angel dust') or ketamine ('special K').

When temperature regulation is lost and core temperature exceeds 42°C, oxidative phosphorylation is uncoupled and enzymes cease to function. Simultaneously energy stores are depleted, membranes become more permeable and sodium influx increases. Cellular energy stores are depleted by increases in membrane depolarization and neurotransmitter activity, leading to further heat production.

Thus, as temperature control fails, hyperthermia is accelerated, proteins denature and widespread necrosis appears, leading to multiple system organ dysfunction and failure.

The tissues most at risk are vascular endothelium, nervous tissue and hepatocytes, but eventually all organs may be involved, producing the clinical picture of coma, liver failure, renal failure, acute respiratory distress syndrome, rhabdomyolysis and disseminated intravascular coagulation.

Central mechanisms

There appear to be two main reasons why drugs acting centrally may alter brain chemistry and cause increased heat production:

1. Dopamine hyperactivity results in thermogenesis (Nimmo et al., 1993) as well as causing extrapyramidal rigidity.
2. Excess serotonin is a trigger for centrally mediated thermogenesis (Sternbach, 1991) and is an additional mechanisms for hyperthermia associated with amphetamines and derivatives (Schmidt et al., 1990) as well as monoamine oxidase inhibitors and the antidepressant fluoxetine (Nimmo et al., 1993).

Whereas serotonin appears to be a thermogenic amine, noradrenaline appears to be thermolytic; hence drugs which inhibit noradrenaline such as alpha-blockers interfere with thermoregulation.

The primary methods of increasing heat dissipation are by increasing cutaneous blood flow and sweat gland activity. In hot conditions or during exercise the normal response is to remove excess clothing or to move to a cooler place. Failure to adapt to the conditions may occur with the mentally ill, small babies (e.g. being left in a car in hot weather, or well wrapped-up), the elderly, or in soldiers on exercise or in training (Niroche & Marty, 1992). Alcohol or drugs of abuse may contribute by inducing behavioural dysfunction.

High environmental temperature and humidity can lead to hyperthermia by inducing sweating, which leads to a reduction in extracellular fluid volume and reduced cardiac output, thus blunting the capacity to increase cutaneous blood flow which is essential for adequate heat dissipation. Additionally, exercise diverts blood to muscles which reduces cutaneous blood flow. Peripheral vasoconstriction combined with high metabolic heat output is a major factor in the pathogenesis of hyperthermia (Khogali & Weibner, 1980).

The ability to increase cardiac output is crucial to the dissipation of excess heat load and thus subjects with limited cardiac reserve such as the elderly, those with heart disease or the dehydrated with reduced extracellular fluid volume are at risk (Gold, 1960; El Sharif et al., 1970).

CLINICAL FEATURES

History

An adequate history may be difficult to take from an obtunded patient. The admitting doctor should question family, friends or bystanders. These individuals may be reluctant to give information, particularly if drug-taking is involved. Examination of clothes and personal belongings may be useful.

The important points to elicit are:

1. Whether there is a history of exposure to high heat loads.
2. The presence of risk factors such as drug abuse, intercurrent illness, medication or whether this has occurred before.
3. The presence of neurological symptoms such as syncope, convulsions, ataxia or irrational behaviour.

Neurological disability is the hallmark of severe hyperthermia.

Examination

In many cases the patient will appear severely ill with an altered mental state. The core temperature will be high (>40.5°C) although the patient may already have begun to cool by the time of presentation to the A&E department.

The patient may feel deceptively cool as late cutaneous vasoconstriction can occur and classically the skin feels dry, although profuse sweating may be present (Knochel, 1974).

Patients exhibit tachycardia and either normotension with a wide pulse pressure or hypotension. Tachypnoea is often present (Tek & Olshaker, 1992). The temperature should be monitored using a rectal or oesophageal probe. A high rectal temperature indicates a poor prognosis as the deep rectal compartment underestimates the central core temperature (Niroche & Marty, 1992). Temperature measurements should be continuous so as to avoid overshoot hypothermia or rebound hyperthermia.

Further examination should be directed to the central nervous system (CNS) and cardiorespiratory system.

The mental state is invariably altered and may vary from minor confusion to deep coma, including seizures, abnormal posturing and focal neurological signs. Coma may be profound and indicates a poor prognosis, but survival is possible in these circumstances.

The presence of neurological dysfunction means that the possibility of CNS infections or cerebrovascular accidents must be entertained in the differential diagnosis. The patient may have the flaccid muscles of exertional or environmental hyperthermia (Channa et al., 1990) or may exhibit the rigid or dystonic musculature of drug-induced hyperthermia.

The cardiovascular system is usually hyperdynamic (unless limited by pre-existing disease or dehydration) to meet the increased oxygen requirements and is characterized by a high cardiac output and peripheral vaso-dilatation, although late cutaneous vasoconstriction may supervene.

Laboratory investigations

In the severely hyperthermic patient, resuscitative measures should be instituted immediately and may include mechanical ventilatory support, intravenous fluids and empirical temperature reduction.

Tests allow the severity of the thermal injury to be gauged once empirical treatment has begun and the monitoring of complications.

Initial tests (see also Table 3)

- *Blood count.* Full blood count should be taken as a baseline and to monitor the platelet count which falls in disseminated intravascular coagulation. The white blood count is raised in hyperthermia but may also indicate an underlying infective process.
- *Clotting screen.* This should initially be measured as a baseline but thereafter to monitor coagulation abnormalities, which may develop with extraordinary rapidity.

Table 3. *Summary of useful tests in hyperthermia*

Blood tests	Urine tests
● Full blood count	● Myoglobin
● Clotting screen, fibrinogen	● Haemoglobin
● Liver function tests	
● Creatine kinase	**Others**
● Urea, creatinine, electrolytes	● Electrocardiogram
	● Chest radiograph

- *Liver function tests.* Liver enzyme activities are often raised, particularly in severe hyperthermia.
- *Creatine kinase.* This is raised in hyperthermia, helps confirm a non-infective origin and can be used to monitor the severity of rhabdomyolysis.
- *Urea and electrolytes.* Renal failure may complicate hyperthermia, and electrolyte abnormalities such as hypernatraemia, hypokalaemia, hypocalcaemia and hyper/hypophosphataemia may develop.
- *Arterial blood gas analysis.* This should be taken as a baseline, but may also reveal pulmonary complications such as hypoxaemic or ventilatory failure and metabolic acidosis.
- *Electrocardiogram (ECG).* This may show signs of ischaemia with ST depression and T wave inversion.
- *Chest X-ray.* This is usually normal initially, but may later reveal evidence of adult respiratory distress syndrome or focal infection. Rapidly progressive pulmonary haemorrhage may also occur.
- *Cerebrospinal fluid (CSF) analysis and culture and CT (computed tomography) scan.* These investigations may be required when there is a strong clinical suspicion of meningitis or other CNS infective or inflammatory process.

Differential diagnosis

The most important differential diagnosis in a hyperthermic patient with altered mental state is meningitis. If signs of meningeal irritation are present and the history is unclear, appropriate antibiotic treatment should commence immediately alongside cooling measures. Later lumbar puncture and/or CT scan may clarify the diagnosis.

Hyperthermia may be present in sepsis which may also be associated with altered mental status. It is important to ask about any recent history of foreign travel, of malaria or other tropical fevers.

Numerous agents (described earlier) are responsible for toxic hyperthermia and a history of drug intake should be elicited. It is essential to consider this if muscular rigidity is present.

Prolonged status epilepticus or other disorders of increased muscle tone such as discontinuation of anti-Parkinsonian treatment (Rosenberg et al., 1986; Nimmo et al., 1993), or some psychoses may occasionally present as hyperthermia.

Rarely, cerebrovascular accidents involving the hypothalamus or endocrine abnormalities such as thyroid storm (thyrotoxicosis) or phaeochromocytoma may present with severe hyperthermia and altered mental state (Tek & Olshaker, 1992).

Complications

After the initial resuscitation and treatment of the hyperthermic patient the continuing management of this condition can be difficult and challenging.

Severe hyperthermia is a multiple system insult and has repercussions in all organs of the body.

Central nervous system

Most neurological symptoms and signs resolve when treatment is instituted early; however, long-term sequelae may result and include cerebellar ataxia, paresis and personality changes. These are more likely if hyperthermia is prolonged and associated with cardiovascular failure. Petechial haemorrhages and cerebral oedema have been observed at autopsy (Bacon, 1983).

Cardiovascular system

The normal response to hyperthermia is to maximize heat dissipation via increased cardiac output and peripheral vasodilatation. Hypovolaemia is common due to a combination of sweating and transudation of fluid into interstitial and cellular spaces.

Fluid resuscitation should be cautious as cooling may redistribute the volume from the periphery to the core. Eventually cardiac failure may develop with a low cardiac output and normal or high peripheral vascular resistance. It is worth noting that myocardial contractility decreases when body temperature is greater than 40°C (Costrini et al., 1979).

Respiratory system

Pulmonary oedema, either cardiac or non-cardiac, is recognized following severe hyperthermia (El Kassini et al., 1986). The underlying mechanism is probably direct thermal injury to pulmonary vascular endothelium compounded by myocardial dysfunction. Additionally the return of large fluid volumes to the central circulation following cooling and aggressive fluid management may play a part.

Haematological system

Disseminated intravascular coagulation is a common and serious complication of hyperthermia, its presence increases mortality (Rosenberg et al., 1986; Tek & Olshaker, 1992) and is the usual mode of death in fatal cases (Chao et al., 1981).

Clotting factors are probably denatured by the heat and the clotting cascade is activated via vascular endothelial damage resulting in disseminated intravascular coagulation.

Renal

Renal failure is another well-recognized and common complication of severe hyperthermia (Vertel & Knochel, 1967). The causes of acute renal failure are complex, but direct heat injury coupled with hypovolaemia and hypotension are major factors. Rhabdomyolysis and haemolysis with consequent myoglobin and haemoglobin release compound the adverse effects on the kidney.

Muscle

Muscle damage and rhabdomyolysis are commonly seen in severe hyperthermia, particularly secondary to drug abuse or exercise. Muscles swell and become painful, serum muscle enzymes such as creatine kinase become grossly elevated and myoglobinuria occurs. Rhabdomyolysis rapidly impairs renal function and leads to acute renal failure.

Liver

Liver injury in hyperthermia is almost universal and is reflected in serum transaminase elevation and jaundice. The damage is either from direct thermal injury or from circulatory failure and hypoxia. Liver failure compounds any coagulopathy produced by the heat injury.

Acid–base balance and electrolytes

Excess production of lactate from overexercising, muscle rigidity, seizures or circulatory insufficiency leads to metabolic acidosis. Hypermetabolism and respiratory failure can also cause a respiratory acidosis (Niroche & Marty, 1992).

Hyperthermia may lead to alterations in serum electrolytes. Increased aldosterone secretion following dehydration and sodium loss may cause an initial hypokalaemia which may later be followed by a life-threatening hyperkalaemia secondary to rhabdomyolysis and acute renal failure. Hypocalcaemia is common but rarely requires intervention.

TREATMENT

Hyperthermia carries a high morbidity and mortality and the outcome is related to the peak temperature and the duration of its elevation. The success of treatment depends upon the speed at which treatment is instituted.

The primary goals of management of severe hyperthermia

1. Rapid and aggressive cooling of the patient. This should be simultaneous with:
   - Maintenance of the oxygen delivery mechanism
   - Rapid assessment and treatment of airway, breathing and circulation (ABC)
2. Specific therapy may be indicated depending on the aetiology of the hyperthermia
3. Continued support for vital organ function

Prehospital management

In the field, simple measures are all that may be required to prevent serious complications; the patient should be removed from the heat stress immediately. Clothing should be removed and cooling instituted by whatever means are at hand. The subject should be sprayed or splashed with water and a fan used to encourage evaporation. Alternatively, exposing the subject to a draught by keeping doors or windows open may help. The down-draught from helicopter blades has been used in the past!

If available, ice packs should be applied to the neck, axillae or groin.

If oxygen is available it should be administered together with a peripheral intravenous infusion of crystalloid.

Arrangements should be made for immediate transfer to hospital.

Hospital management

A&E department

In hospital, aggressive cooling measures should be instituted as soon as possible once the diagnosis is suspected and simultaneously with maintenance of airway, breathing and circulation.

Several alternatives exist for the rapid cooling of patients but often the simplest techniques are the most appropriate.

Immersion in ice baths has been advocated in the past but may promote cutaneous vasoconstriction, thus interfering with heat exchange and diminishing the capacity for heat loss. The difficulties of managing a patient in a bath of ice and water make this method unfeasible.

Evaporation of water consumes seven times as much heat as melting the same quantity of ice, and thus the most effective methods for cooling utilize evaporation combined with convection.

Splashing or sponging the patient with tepid (not cold) water and combining this with a continuous current of air is extremely effective.

The most effective method for cooling subjects was developed by Weiner & Khogali (1980) and involves the naked subject being sprayed with lukewarm (15°C) atomized water while warm air (40–45°C) is blown over the body keeping the skin temperature above 30°C to maintain cutaneous vasodilatation. The Mecca body-cooling unit (as it has been called) is unsurpassed in reducing body temperature and has been successfully employed on numerous occasions (Channa et al., 1990; Bouchama et al., 1991; Yaqub et al., 1986).

Other methods of cooling are of only minor significance: cold humidified oxygen and cold intravenous fluids contribute minimally to heat exchange, but iced gastric lavage may be used in combination with evaporative measures (Vicario et al., 1986; Kew et al., 1982; Syverud et al., 1985).

When cooling methods have failed to reduce core temperature below 40°C after 30 min, additional methods such as peritoneal lavage have been described (Horowitz, 1989); this involves instilling 2 litres of iced normal saline via open peritoneal lavage and draining after 30 min.

Extracorporeal cooling via cardiopulmonary bypass provides the most rapid technique for cooling concomitant with maintenance of oxygen delivery to tissues but is only of use if instituted early and will be of use mainly for cases of malignant hyperthermia occurring in the anaesthetic room.

Intensive care unit

Antipyretics such as aspirin and paracetamol have no place in the treatment of severe hyperthermia as they require a normally functioning hypothalamus, but other specific therapies may be indicated according to the aetiology of the condition.

Specific therapies

Dantrolene is a hydantoin derivative that inhibits the release of calcium from the sarcolemma of skeletal muscle as well as acting as a direct muscle relaxant. Its action prevents muscle contraction and thus reduces heat production.

Dantrolene is rapidly effective in reversing the clinical features of malignant hyperthermia (Kolb *et al.*, 1982) and also in preventing malignant hyperthermia when given prophylactically to susceptible patients undergoing anaesthesia.

Dantrolene may also be effective in neuroleptic malignant syndrome (Khan *et al.*, 1985; Coons *et al.*, 1982), exercise-induced hyperthermia (Larner, 1992; Lydiatt & Hill, 1981) and drug-induced hyperthermia (Singarajah & Lavies, 1992; Baraie & Peppers, 1989; Tehan *et al.*, 1993; Logan *et al.*, 1993; Woods & Henry, 1992; Padkin, 1994). Evidence from a large randomized double-blind trial suggests that it is of no benefit in exertional hyperthermia (Bouchama *et al.*, 1991). Although dantrolene has been advocated for use in severe hyperthermia secondary to toxicity from amphetamine sulphate and its derivatives such as Ecstasy and Eve (Singarajah & Lavies, 1992; Baraie & Peppers, 1989; Tehan *et al.*, 1993; Logan *et al.*, 1993; Woods & Henry, 1992; Padkin, 1994), there is as yet little evidence to support any additional efficacy beyond cooling measures and supportive therapy and its use as yet cannot be recommended (Watson *et al.*, 1993).

As some forms of drug-induced hyperthermia are thought to be due partly to altered neurotransmitter chemistry, then redressing any imbalance may play a part in specific therapy for severe hyperthermia. It appears that drugs such as fluoxetine, monoamine oxidase inhibitors and Ecstasy (3,4-methylenedioxymetamphetamine, MDMA) and Eve (3,4-methylenedioxyamphetamine, MDA) may exert some of their hyperthermic effect via increased serotinin levels (Tehan *et al.*, 1993; Padkin, 1994; Nimmo *et al.*, 1993). Blockage of $5-HT_2$ receptors antagonizes the hyperthermic effects of Ecstasy (MDMA) in rats (Schmidt *et al.*, 1990) and there may

be a place for specific serotonin antagonists (e.g. ketanserin) in the treatment of severe hyperthermia secondary to amphetamine sulphate and the related compounds Ecstasy and Eve. Additionally, the release of serotonin is calcium-dependent and animal studies suggest nimodipine may have a role in inhibiting its release (Azmita *et al.*, 1990).

Specific therapy to redress neurotransmitter imbalance is successful in neuroleptic malignant syndrome, with the use of bromocriptine, amantidine and levodopa leading to increased dopaminergic activity (Vassallo & Delaney, 1989; Rosenberg & Green, 1989; Zubenko & Pope, 1983; McCarron *et al.*, 1982). However, these agents have always been used in combination with other therapies and clear evidence of their efficacy (as with dantrolene and drug-induced hyperthermia) is lacking.

Supportive measures

Even after successful initial resuscitation and stabilization, further A&E department and intensive care unit management of a severely hyperthermic patient can be difficult and challenging.

Intubation and ventilation may be necessary in an unconscious patient to avoid hypoxia and hypercapnia. Paralysis with neuromuscular-blocking agents reduces muscular activity (thus reducing heat production) although it may not reduce the muscular rigidity seen secondary to drug toxicity.

Pulmonary oedema due to cardiac failure or acute respiratory distress syndrome may require a prolonged period of ventilation. Hypotension is common and, although it may resolve with aggressive cooling, intravenous fluid therapy may be necessary to restore circulating volume. Colloids should be used and guided with the aid of central venous pressure monitoring. Fluid therapy should be cautious to avoid volume overloading and pulmonary oedema. If hypotension or congestive cardiac failure are refractory, then a pulmonary artery flotation catheter should be used to guide inotropic therapy, bearing in mind that catecholamines increase thermogenesis.

Alpha-agonists such as noradrenaline and ephedrine should be avoided if possible as they cause peripheral vasoconstriction and impair heat loss. Agitation increases heat production, and sedation with benzodiazepines may be indicated. Seizures are common, often during cooling, and animal studies have shown that prevention of seizures reduces mortality in cases of amphetamine and cocaine toxicity (Rosenberg *et al.*, 1986).

Prophylaxis against convulsions with phenytoin should be considered in all cases of severe hyperthermia whilst recognizing the potential cardiovascular effects of this agent. If a patient requires muscle relaxant drugs a cerebral function monitor should be used to detect convulsions. Rhabdomyolysis is common, particularly with sympathomimetic toxicity (e.g. amphetamine sulphate, Ecstasy and Eve) and in exercise-induced hyperthermia. Patients should be well hydrated to maintain a high urine output (100 ml h^{-1}; Tek & Olshaker, 1992) and mannitol or frusemide may be indicated.

Alkalinization of urine is the usual recommended therapy for rhabdomyolysis, but it should be noted that alkaline urine reduces the renal clearance of amphetamine and its derivatives.

In cases of severe toxicity and rhabdomyolysis early use of haemofiltration should be considered to remove toxins and myoglobin and to correct acidosis and hypokalaemia. Disseminated intravascular coagulation is a common complication of severe hyperthermia and indicates a poor prognosis (Rosenberg et al., 1986; Tek & Olshaker, 1992; El Kassini et al., 1986; Chao et al., 1981; Jones et al., 1982). If complications of bleeding occur, treatment should proceed with blood products according to the pattern of the coagulopathy.

Liver injury following severe hyperthermia is almost universal and treatment should be supportive. Hypoglycaemia must not be missed and is treated with intravenous glucose.

In summary

Rapid institution of cooling and basic resuscitation are essential for the treatment of severe hyperthermia. The intensive care team should be involved from an early stage and in severe cases the use of cardiopulmonary bypass and early haemofiltration should be considered.

Prognosis

Morbidity and mortality are directly related to the peak temperature and the duration of its elevation (Channa et al., 1990; Bouchama et al., 1991; Tek & Olshaker, 1992). Mortality is greatly reduced if patients are rapidly cooled during the first hour of treatment (Vicario et al., 1986; Yaqub et al., 1986).

Although a core temperature of greater than 42°C is a poor prognostic factor, survival is possible if treatment is aggressive (Logan et al., 1993). Prolonged coma and disseminated intravascular coagulation are major indicators of poor prognosis but equally important is the premorbid health of the patient.

Bibliography

AMERICAN COLLEGE OF SPORTS MEDICINE (1975). Position statement on prevention of heat injuries during distance running. Med. Sci. Sport, 7, vii–ix.

AZMITA, E.C., MURPHY, R.B. & WHITAKER-AZNUITIA, P.M. (1990). MDMA (Ecstasy) effects on cultural serotonergic neurons: evidence for Ca^{2+} dependent toxicity linked to release. Brain Res., 510, 97–103.

BACON, C. (1983). Heatstroke and haemorrhagic shock and encephalopathy. Lancet, ii, 918–20.

BARAIE, J.A. & PEPPERS, M.P. (1989). Use of dantrolene in management of amphetamine induced hyperthermia. Clin. Pharm., 8, 326–7.

BOUCHAMA, A., CAFEGE, A., DEVOL, E.B. et al. (1991). Ineffectiveness of dantrolene sodium in the treatment of heatstroke. Crit. Care Med., 19, 176–80.

CHANNA, A.B., SERAJ, M.A., SADDIQUE, A.A. et al. (1990). Is dantrolene effective in heatstroke patients. Crit. Care Med., 18, 290–2.

CHAO, L.T.C., SIMMIAH, R. & PAKIA, J.F. (1981). Acute heatstroke deaths. Pathology, 13, 145.

CLOWES, G.H.A. & O'DONNELL, T.F. (1974). Heatstroke. N. Engl. J. Med., 291, 564.

COONS, D.J., HILLMAN, F.J. & MARSHALL, R.W. (1982). Treatment of neuroleptic malignant syndrome with dantrolene sodium: case report. Am. J. Psychiatry, 139, 944–5.

COSTRINI, A.M., PITT, H.A. & GUSTAFSON, A.B. (1979). Cardiovascular and metabolic manifestations of heatstroke and severe heat exhaustion. Am. J. Med., 66, 296–302.

EL KASSINI, F.A., AL-MASHADAMI, S.A. & AKHTAR, J. (1986). Adult respiratory distress syndrome and disseminated intravascular coagulation complicating heatstroke. Chest, 90, 571–4.

EL SHARIF, N., SHAHWARI, L. & SOROUR, A.H. (1970). The effects of acute thermal stress on general and pulmonary haemodynamics in the cardiac patient. Am. Heart J., 79, 305.

GINSBERG, M.D., HERTZMAN, M. & SCHMIDT-NOWARA, W.W. (1970). Amphetamine intoxication with coagulopathy, hyperthermia and reversible renal failure. A syndrome resembling heatstroke. Ann. Intern. Med., 73, 81–5.

GOLD, J. (1960). The development of heat pyrexia. J. Am. Med. Assoc., 173, 1175–82.

HENRY, J.A. (1992). Ecstasy and the dance of death. Br. Med. J., 305, 5–6.

HENRY, J.A., JEFFREYS, K.J. & SAWLING, S. (1992). Toxicity and deaths from 3,4 methylenedioxymethamphetamine (Ecstasy). Lancet, 340, 384–7.

HOPKINS, P.M., ELLIS, F.R. & HALSALL, P.J. (1991). Evidence for related myopathies in exertional heatstroke and malignant hyperthermia. *Lancet*, **338**, 1491–2.

HOROWITZ, B.Z. (1989). The golden hour of heatstroke: use of iced peritoneal lavage. *Am. J. Emerg. Med.*, **7**, 616–19.

JONES, T.S., LANG, A.P. & KILBOURNE, E.M. (1982). Morbidity and mortality associated with the July 1980 heat wave in St. Louis and Kansas City. *J. Am. Med. Assoc.*, **247**, 3328–31.

KALANT, H. & KALANT, O.J. (1975). Death in amphetamine users: cause and rates. *Can. Med. Assoc. J.*, **112**, 299–304.

KEW, M.C., HOPP, M. & ROTHBERY, A. (1982). Fatal heatstroke in a child taking appetite suppressant drugs. *S. Afr. Med. J.*, **62**, 905–6.

KHAN, A., JAFFE, J.H., NELSON, W.H. *et al.* (1985). Resolution of neuroleptic malignant syndrome with dantrolene sodium: case report. *J. Clin. Psychiatry*, **46**, 244–6.

KHOGALI, M. & WEIBNER, J.S. (1980). Heatstroke: report on 18 cases. *Lancet*, **ii**, 276–8.

KHOGALI, M. (1983). Epidemiology of heat illness during the Makkah pilgrimage in Saudi Arabia 1983. *Int. J. Epidemiol.*, **12**, 267.

KNOCHEL, J.P. (1974). Environmental heat illness: an eclectic review. *Arch. Intern. Med.*, **133**, 841–63.

KOLB, M.E., HORNE, M.L. & MARTZ, R. (1982). Dantrolene in human malignant hyperthermia: a multicenter study. *Anesthesiology*, **56**, 254–62.

LARNER, A.J. (1992). Dantrolene for exertional heatstroke. *Lancet*, **339**, 182.

LITOVITZ, T.L. & TRANTMAN, W.G. (1983). Amoxapine overdoses: seizures and fatalities. *J. Am. Med. Assoc.*, **250**, 1069–71.

LOGAN, A. ST. C., STICKLE, B., O'KEEFE, N. *et al.* (1993). Survival following 'Ecstasy' ingestion with a peak temperature of 42°C. *Anaesthesia*, **48**, 1017–18.

LYDIATT, J.S. & HILL, G.E. (1981). Treatment of heatstroke with dantrolene. *J. Am. Med. Assoc.*, **246**, 41–2.

McCARRON, M.M., BOETTGER, M.L. & PECK, J.J. (1982). A case of neuroleptic malignant syndrome successfully treated with amantadine. *J. Clin. Psychiatry*, **43**, 381–2.

MENASHE, P.I. & GOTTLIEB, J.E. (1988). Hyperthermia, rhabdomolysis and myoglobinuric renal failure after recreational use of cocaine. *South. Med. J.*, **81**, 379–81.

MERIGIAN, K.S. & ROBERTS, J.R. (1987). Cocaine intoxication hyperpyrexia, rhabdomyolysis and acute renal failure. *J. Toxicol.*, **25**, 135–48.

NIMMO, S.M., KENNEDY, B.W., TULLETT, W.M. *et al.* (1993). Drug induced hyperthermia. *Anaesthesia*, **48**, 892–5.

NIROCHE, Y. & MARTY, J. (1992). Hyperthermia. In *Care of the Critically Ill Patients*, 2nd edn., edn., J. Tinker & W.M. Zapol, pp. 1115–24. Berlin: Springer-Berlin.

PADKIN, A. (1994). Treating MDMA ('Ecstasy') toxicity. *Anaesthesia*, **49**, 259.

PARENTI, C.M. & HOFFMANN, J.E. (1986). Hyperpyrexia associated with intravenous cimetidine therapy. Report of a case. *Arch. Intern. Med.*, **146**, 1821–2.

PERLMAN, P.E., ADAMS, W.G. & RIDGEWAY, N.A. (1989). Extreme pyrexia during bretylium administration. *Postgrad. Med.*, **85**, 111–14.

ROSENBERG, M.R. & GREEN, M. (1989). Neuroleptic malignant syndrome. Review of response to therapy. *Arch. Intern. Med.*, **149**, 1927–31.

ROSENBERG, J., PENTEL, P., POND, S. *et al.* (1986). Hypothermia associated with drug intoxication. *Crit. Care Med.*, **14**, 964–9.

SCHMIDT, C.J., BLACK, C.K., ABBATE, G.M. *et al.* (1990). Methylenedioxymetamphetamine induced hyperthermia and neurotoxicity are independently mediated by $5HT_2$ receptors. *Brain Res.*, **529**, 85–90.

SCREATON, G.R., CAIRNS, H.S., SARNER, M. *et al.* (1992). Hyperpyrexia and rhabdomyolysis after MDMA abuse (ecstasy). *Lancet*, **339**, 677–8.

SINGARAJAH, C. & LAVIES, N.G. (1992). An overdose of ecstasy. A role for dantrolene. *Anaesthesia*, **47**, 686–7.

STERNBACH, H. (1991). The serotonin syndrome. *Am. J. Psychiatry*, **148**, 705–13.

SUTTON, J.R. & BAR-OR, O. (1980). Thermal illness in fun running. *Am. Heart J.*, **10**, 778–81.

SYVERUD, S.A., BARKER, W.J. & AMSTERDAM, J.T. (1985). Iced gastric lavage for the treatment of heatstroke: efficacy in a canine model. *Ann. Emerg. Med.*, **14**, 424–32.

TEHAN, B., HARDERN, R. & BODENHAM, A. (1993). Hyperthermia associated with 3,4-methylenedioxyamphetamine (Eve). *Anaesthesia*, **48**, 507–10.

TEK, D. & OLSHAKER, J.S. (1992). Heat illness. *Emerg. Med. Clin. North Am.*, **10**, 299–310.

VASSALLO, S.V. & DELANEY, K.A. (1989). Pharmacologic effects on thermoregulation: mechanism of drug related heatstroke. *Clin. Toxicol.*, **27**, 199–224.

VERTEL, R.M. & KNOCHEL, J.P. (1967). Acute renal failure due to heat injury. *Am. J. Med.*, **43**, 435–49.

VICARIO, S.J., OKUBAJRE, R. & HALTON, T. (1986). Rapid cooling in classic heatstroke: effect on mortality rates. *Am. J. Emerg. Med.*, **4**, 394–8.

WAGNER, M.B. (1993). Hyperthermia. In *Presenting Signs and Symptoms in the Emergency Department*, ed. G.C. Hamilton, pp. 259–65. Baltimore: Williams & Wilkins.

WATSON, J.D., FERGUSON, C., HINDS, C.J. *et al.* (1993). Exertional heat stroke induced by amphetamine analogues. *Anaesthesia*, **48**, 1057–60.

WEINER, J.S. & KHOGALI, M. (1980). A physiological body-cooling unit for treatment of heatstroke. *Lancet*, **ii**, 507–9.

WHITWORTH, J.A.G. & WOLFMAN, M.J. (1983).

Fatal heatstroke in a long distance runner. *Br. Med. J.*, **287**, 948.

WOODS, J.D. & HENRY, J.A. (1992). Hyperpyrexia induced by 3,4-methylenedioxyamphetamine (Eve). *Lancet*, **340**, 305.

WOOLFE, S.M. & BEHRMAN, N. (1981). Heatstroke and community runs. *Br. Med. J.*, **282**, 2060.

YAQUB, B.A., AL-HARTHI, S.S. & AL-ORAINEY, I.O. (1986). Heat stroke at the Mekkah pilgrimage: clinical characteristics and course of 30 patients. *Q. J. Med.*, **59**, 523–30.

ZUBENKO, G. & POPE, H.G. (1983). Management of a case of malignant neuroleptic syndrome with bromocriptine. *Am. J. Psychiatry*, **140**, 1619–20.

40 Ballistic injuries

J.W.R. PEYTON

Department of Surgery, South Tyrone Hospital, Dungannon, Northern Ireland

Chapter plan

Introduction
Types of weapon
Pathophysiology
Initial management of ballistic injuries
Conclusion

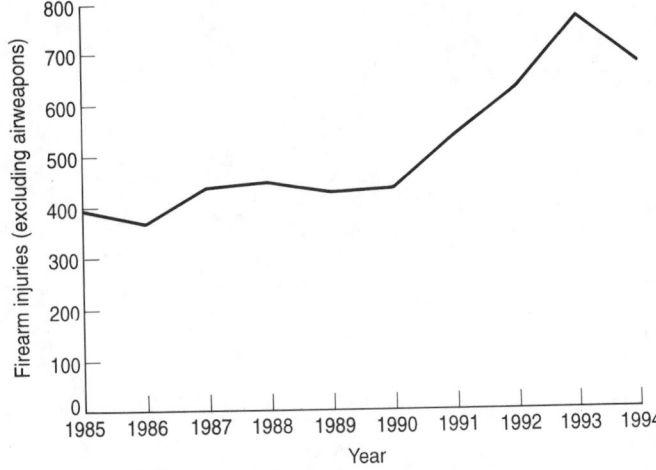

Fig. 1. Firearm injuries (excluding airweapons). Scotland, England and Wales 1985–1994 (Government Statistical Service, The Scottish Office, Edinburgh and Home Office, London).

INTRODUCTION

The term 'ballistics' comes from the latin 'ballista', which was a catapult used by the Romans to hurl heavy objects against fortified towns. The science of ballistic trauma is the study of missile injuries on animal tissue. The missiles are usually projected by an explosive force and they may be primary wounding agents (e.g. bullet or grenade fragments), or secondary agents in the form of objects displaced by the explosive force. The secondary agents may be external to the animal tissue (e.g. broken glass or pieces of masonry), or internal (e.g. teeth or shattered bone).

Generally, throughout the Western world the incidence of missile injuries has been rising in spite of a so-called peacetime environment. This is true not only in those areas subject to terrorist attack but also in the course of 'ordinary' criminal activities (Fig. 1).

This chapter will deal with the early management of missile injuries. Proper treatment of these casualties requires an understanding of some of the basic pathophysiology of missile injuries. Possibly the most vital principle to grasp is that all missile injuries have the potential to be multisystem in nature, no matter where the entrance or exit wounds are situated.

TYPES OF WEAPON

These can be grouped according to whether the missile was a primary or secondary feature; all may give rise to single or multiple wounds.

Primary missiles are very diverse, ranging from single bullets to small pieces of metal thrown out by the explosive force of a grenade. Military grenades usually produce uniform fragments varying in size down to the fleshettes designed to combat body armour (Fig. 2). The terrorist has improvised grenades containing various secondary objects packed around an explosive source (Fig. 3).

Secondary missiles also produce blast injuries. This may cause considerable trauma (e.g. to the ears or lungs; Fig. 4). Also, surrounding objects may be dislodged to form secondary missiles. The body itself may be turned into a secondary missile and be thrown into other objects

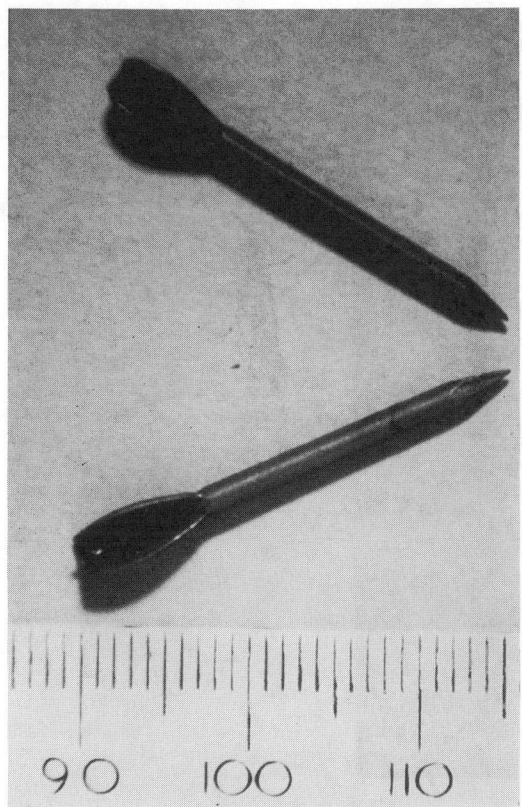

Fig. 2. Fleshettes. (Courtesy of Department of Military Surgery, RAM College.)

PATHOPHYSIOLOGY

While weapons may produce missiles of high or low velocity, speed alone is not the only determinant of the amount of tissue destruction. The damage depends on the amount of energy transferred to the tissue; in other words, the difference between the energy level of the missile when it penetrates the tissue and any residual energy it may have on leaving. The wounds may thus be divided into either high-energy transfer injuries or low-energy transfer injuries. The amount of energy transferred depends on two main features:

1. The characteristics of the missile.
2. The characteristics of the tissue.

Characteristics of the missile include its size, shape and especially its presenting surface both at the time of impact and throughout the duration of its passage through the tissues. Fragmentation of the missile within the tissues gives rise to multiple secondary missiles dispersing in all directions. Under the terms of the Hague Peace Conference (1899), attempts have been made to decrease the tendency for bullets to fragment by placing them in a shaped copper jacket. Therefore the leading edge encounters less resistance on its way through the tissues, thus limiting the amount of destruction around the track. Bullets used by criminals, terrorists or even certain police forces are not subject to the same regulations. Bullets may be partially jacketed or have their heads deliberately flattened to give greater retardation and so transmit more energy on impact (better 'stopping-power'). Consequently, this type of bullet is more deadly than those used routinely by the military.

causing blunt as opposed to penetrating trauma. The environment must also be taken into account, especially in industrial injuries where there may be chemicals or toxic gases (see Chapter 35).

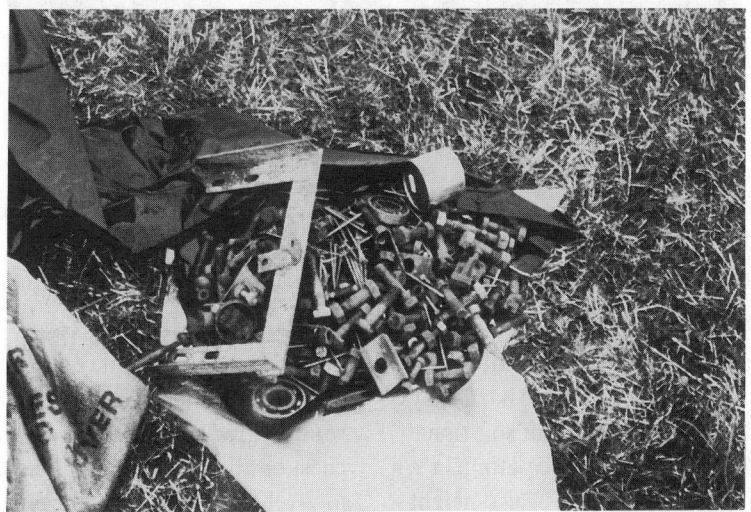

Fig. 3. Home-made terrorist device showing metal fragments packed round explosive.

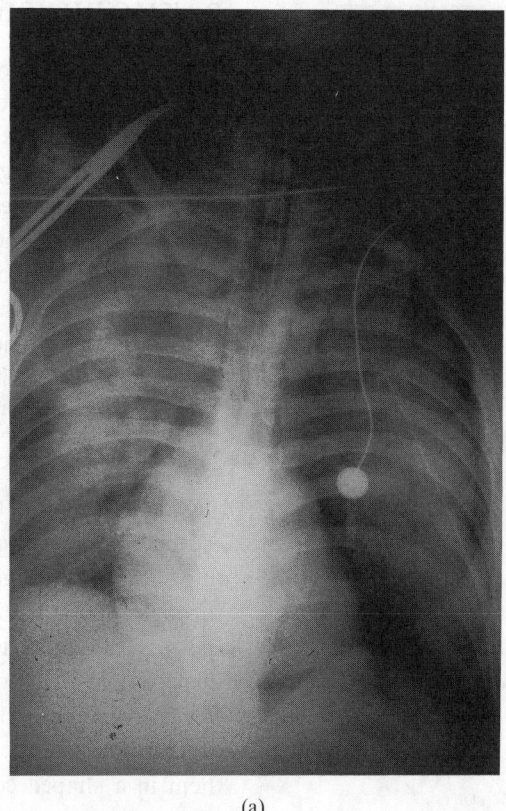

Fig. 4. Blast lung following a bus bombing. (a) X-ray appearance after one hour. (b) Lungs at post mortem.

The function of most missiles is to transmit their energy to the target, usually but not necessarily by penetration. Baton rounds deliver a significant soft tissue injury to discourage the victim from participating in a riot. They are meant to be aimed below waist height from outside a minimum range. Unfortunately waist height for an adult may well be face height for a child and severe injuries, even fatalities, have resulted from rounds fired at too short a range, or striking the head, chest or abdomen (Fig. 5). These are high-mass, relatively low-velocity missiles which are unstable in flight and usually present a large surface area on contact with the

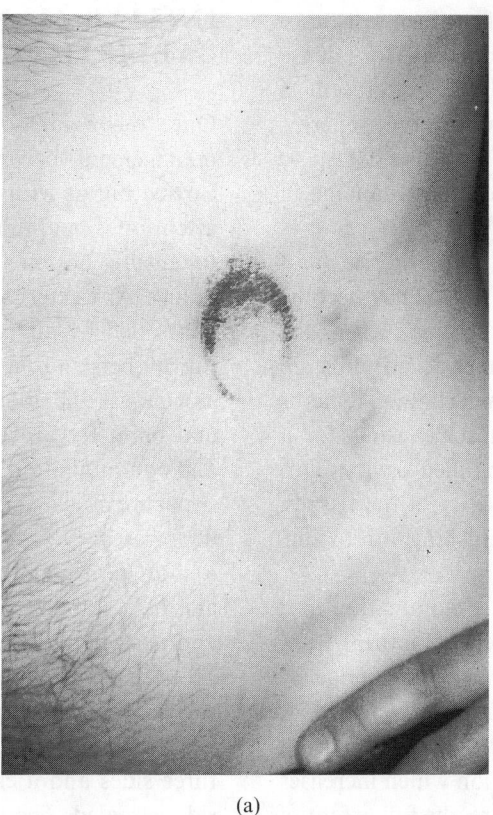

(a)

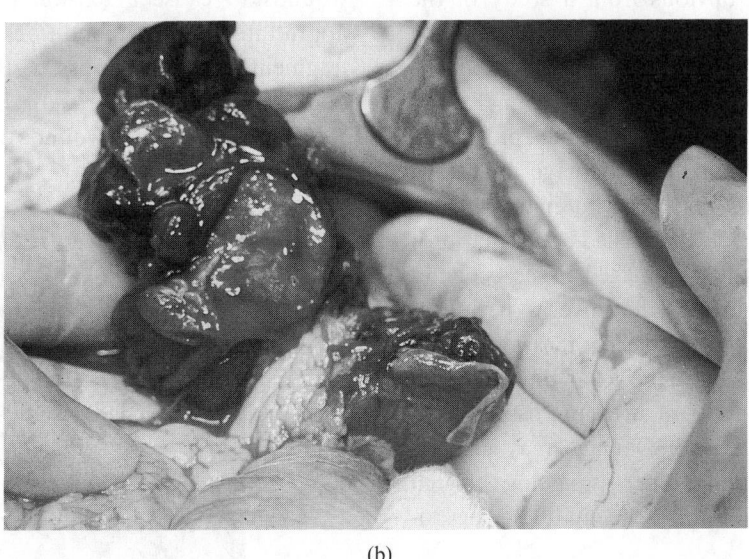

(b)

Fig. 5. Baton round injury to abdomen. (a) Skin marking; (b) ruptured spleen.

target. This ensures maximum transmission of energy without penetration.

The intrinsic energy of a missile at its time of impact is proportional to its mass times the square of the velocity ($E = MV^2$). If, however, the missile leaves the body without losing much of its mass (i.e. relatively intact) or

velocity, then the energy transmitted can be very small, producing less tissue disruption.

Apart from the characteristics of the bullet, the loss of energy to the tissues will depend on the amount of retardation afforded to the missile during its passage, which will in turn depend on the density of the tissue.

Elastic tissue such as lung does not offer much resistance and consequently may sustain less damage. More dense tissues such as liver, and especially bone, present a greater retarding force and therefore absorb more energy. Both are likely to shatter, and bone may also deflect or shatter the missile, causing gross secondary damage in tissues away from the main tract.

Wounding agents with low-energy transfer cause damage by pushing aside tissues in their path. They become lethal when they directly hit vital structures such as the heart and great vessels. High-energy transfer wounds are characterized by the process of cavitation. Tissue is accelerated away from the wound tract causing, for a fraction of a second, a large vacuum-filled cavity. This rapidly collapses because of the elasticity of the tissues. Considerable damage results from crushing, stretching, tearing and shearing forces.

Any penetrating missile can carry contamination into the tissues from the outside (e.g. cloth or buttons from items of clothing) and this effect may be compounded by the vacuum of the temporary cavity. The spread of damage outside the missile track and the contamination of tissue planes causes tissue destruction which increases with time. In the early stages, therefore, the full extent of the damage may not be obvious from a study of the entrance and exit wounds. Usually a high-energy missile will exit the body through a large tearing wound. On the other hand, it may completely dissipate its energy by being deflected and shattered within the body, producing no exit wound at all but maximum damage internally. Failure to appreciate this may lead to inappropriate surgery. If wounds are not widely opened or are inappropriately packed, the dead and damaged tissue becomes a potential culture medium. Swelling over a period of hours after injury leads to increased tension in the wound. This can severely limit the local blood supply leading to further anoxia and destruction of tissue which otherwise might have survived. Damage may also be caused by pressure on vessels and nerves passing through the area giving rise to distal ischaemia and neuropraxia.

The mass of dead and damaged tissue in the anoxic environment provides a perfect culture medium for the contamination brought into the wound by the missile and the negative pressure of cavitation. Intrinsic contamination may occur if the missile passes through tissues such as bowel. The effects of this contamination usually become clinically apparent after 6–8 h, but the whole process may be aborted by good initial management.

INITIAL MANAGEMENT OF BALLISTIC INJURIES

Once the nature of the missile wound is understood, management becomes logical. Initial resuscitation is carried out as with any other serious injury and specific attention is paid to the airway, breathing and circulation to ensure optimal perfusion and oxygenation of the tissues. Any external bleeding from the wound should be controlled by direct pressure, avoiding the use of clips, tourniquets and similar devices. At this stage X-rays such as views of the abdomen may add valuable information and point towards the potential for multisystem injury and contamination. Probing of such wounds in an A&E department is a very dangerous manoeuvre and is to be deprecated. Occasionally, wounds need to be packed as a short-term emergency procedure to stem blood flow and help stabilize the patient. Wounds around the head and neck may cause immediate or delayed airway compromise. Intubation may therefore be required at an early stage to secure the airway. Wounds to the chest should be covered with impervious dressing taped on three sides and a chest drain inserted before the fourth side is sealed. The potential for small entrance and exit wounds to cause a tension pneumothorax should be appreciated and the condition suspected (Fig. 6). Small fragments may also cross to the opposite chest cavity and cause pneumothorax or haemothorax there, even though there is no wound on the chest wall. It is

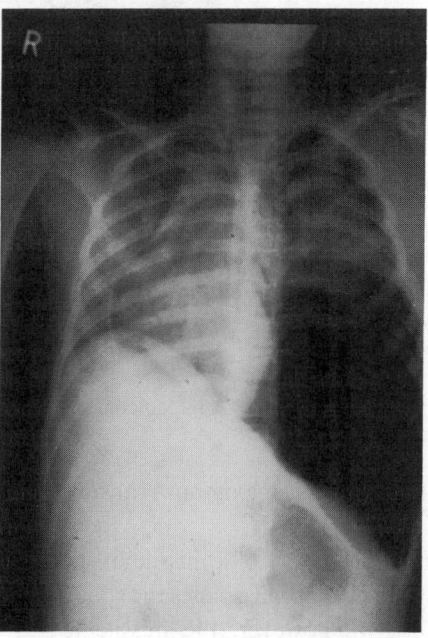

Fig. 6. Child with tension pneumothorax following shotgun injury.

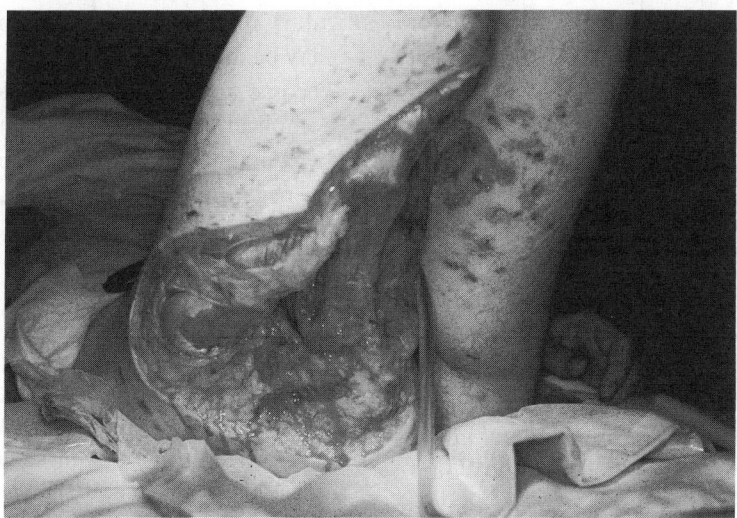

Fig. 7. Blast wound to buttock which penetrated the abdomen, requiring colostomy.

important to note that a tension pneumothorax may not develop until after the patient has been intubated and ventilated, positive pressure ventilation causing air to escape into the pleural cavity.

The use of dressings and insertion of a chest drain will treat up to 85% of all chest injuries. Approximately 10% will require emergency surgery if the initial blood loss is more than 1500 ml or if there is a continuing blood loss of more than 300 ml h^{-1}. Other indications for early surgery are large defects in the chest wall, continual air leak or potential mediastinal damage. Small missiles penetrating the pericardium and heart muscle can give rise to pericardial tamponade. For those surviving with this condition to an A&E department the initial management is pericardiocentesis (see Chapter 23).

Approximately 5% of patients with chest injury may require surgery at a later stage because of complications such as infection or a ruptured diaphragm. Surgery is not necessarily required for the presence of a foreign body in the chest cavity if there are no other complications.

In contrast to chest wounds, there is little place for conservatism in the management of abdominal wounds and all missile wounds in this area should be properly explored. The possibility of missiles entering the abdominal cavity through the chest, back, buttocks or even legs should be recognized (Fig. 7) and appropriate investigations carried out. In selected cases the use of peritoneal lavage, ultrasound or contrast radiography (e.g. intravenous urography or a urethrogram) may be required in the acute phase. A rectal examination may reveal bleeding into the alimentary tract. Perforation of

the bowel and the subsequent development of peritonitis may not be clinically obvious for several hours, especially with wounds around the duodenum or low colon and rectum.

Apart from direct damage to nervous tissue, indirect damage to the spinal cord and peripheral nerves may be caused by ischaemia following thrombosis of the arterial blood supply to these tissues. It may take several hours for the paralysis to develop. The best defence against this progressive tissue damage is adequate resuscitation with maintenance of high levels of oxygenation and perfusion, along with relief from local pressure effects associated with swelling of damaged tissue or haematoma formation. These problems become most obvious in areas with tight fascial compartments such as the limbs. The development of a compartment syndrome may be arrested by the early use of generous fasciotomies (see Chapter 30).

Cavitation effects may damage large blood vessels at an intimal level but this may not immediately affect the pulses. Bullet wounds near major vessels therefore demand early investigation with arteriography before thrombosis develops. Salvage of a limb requires repair of the vein as well as the artery to secure good venous drainage. Careful handling of the peripheral nerves is important to preserve or restore their blood supply whether interrupted by injury or by local pressure. Pressure can also damage the nerve bundles but these should recover well if the pressure is relieved at an early stage.

In summary, the overall aim in treating ballistic injuries is to prevent secondary tissue damage by maintaining tissue oxygenation. This requires early resuscitation involving airway maintenance, breathing and circulatory mechanisms, along with restoration of vascular continuity and the relief of pressure effects. Tissue damage is not always apparent in the very early phase and initial surgical management must recognize this. The biggest killer after the initial phase is infection and so all efforts must be directed towards diminishing this possibility. The factors giving rise to infection are the anoxic environment, ischaemic tissue and the presence of contamination. As well as the measures outlined above, the use of antibiotics is very important but only as an adjunct to adequate surgery. Intravenous third-generation cephalosporins are currently used for most peripheral injuries along with tetanus prophylaxis (see Chapter 12). Wounds involving the bowel require additional agents that are active against bowel organisms (e.g. metronidazole), and those involving the urinary tract, the addition of aminoglycosides.

CONCLUSION

The incidence of ballistic injuries is rising. Initial management should follow the same general principles as for any other trauma. Specific management of the missile injury requires an understanding from the outset that it may be multisystem in nature and that some effects only become apparent with the passage of time. These late complications may be compounded by infection caused by contamination. After resuscitation, attention is focused on negating these effects with timely, adequate surgery and the use of antibiotics.

Bibliography

BOWEN, T.E. & BELLAMY, R.F. (1988). *Emergency War Surgery*. Washington: US Government Printing Office.

COOPER, G.J. & RYAN, J.M. (1990). Interaction of penetrating missiles with tissues; some common misapprehensions and implications for wound management. *Br. J. Surg.*, **77**, 606–10.

HANSRAJ, K.K. & WEAVER, L.D. (Eds) (1995). Orthopaedic management of gunshot wounds. In *Orthopaedic Clinics of North America*, Vol. 26, No. 1. Philadelphia: WB Saunders.

HAYWOOD, I.R. (1989). Missile injury. *Problems in General Surgery*, **6** (2), 330–47.

HILKLE, J. & BETZ, S. (1995). Gunshort injuries. *AACN Clinical Issues* **6**(2), 175–86.

RYAN, J.M. & RICH, N. (Eds) (1996). *Ballistic Trauma*. London: Arnold.

41 Rehabilitation of soft tissue injuries

N.S.T. GENDI[a] and J. OUTHWAITE[b]

[a] Rheumatology Department, Basildon Hospital, UK
[b] The Nuffield Orthopaedic Centre, Oxford, UK

Chapter plan

Introduction
Neck sprain
Ankle sprain
Knee sprain

INTRODUCTION

A chapter on rehabilitation may superficially seem out of place in a textbook of emergency medicine. While rehabilitation is concerned with the long-term effects of injury, the accident and emergency (A&E) specialist is mainly interested in its acute management. The two aspects cannot, however, be completely separated. On the one hand, the A&E specialist needs to have an overview of the long-term aspects of injury in terms of course, prognosis, disability and management. This will enable him to provide a sound medicolegal opinion and information to patients, employers, insurance companies and compensation systems. On the other hand, prolonged disability could be prevented or minimized by sound acute management. The domain of injury rehabilitation is extensive. We will therefore limit our discussion to soft tissue injuries as these are the most common and are often followed-up in the A&E department. The following discussion will deal with neck sprain, ankle sprain and knee sprain. The physical aspects of acute management are covered in more detail in the chapter on physiotherapy.

NECK SPRAIN

The term 'whiplash' was first used by Crowe describing the effect of sudden acceleration–deceleration of the cervical spine (Crowe, 1928). Since then, neck sprain has become a major problem with the increasing use of cars and the introduction of seat belt legislation. The term is used to label soft tissue injuries of the cervical spine in the absence of bony or neurological involvement. The injury is most commonly encountered in car accidents and is a major source of litigation and claims to insurance companies. In a multicentre survey, conducted after the introduction of seat belt legislation in the UK, neck sprains were diagnosed in 18.5% of patients attending hospital within 12 h of road traffic accidents (Rutherford et al., 1985). Since the onset of neck symptoms is sometimes delayed beyond 12 h, the above figure is likely to be an underestimate.

Most frequently the victim is the driver or front-seat passenger in a rear-end collision, although neck sprains are also caused by collisions from other directions. In the absence of a well-positioned headrest, hyperextension of the cervical spine is only checked by the occiput hitting the posterior chest wall, far beyond the physiological range of movement. It is therefore believed that much of the damage involves the overstretched anterior neck structures. Pain arises from ligaments, facet joint capsules, annular fibres of intervertebral discs and cervical muscles. Interscapular pain arises from the anterior longitudinal ligament. Upper limb paraesthesia and pain may be explained by temporary thoracic outlet neurovascular compression. Headache arises from injury at the atlanto-axial articulation and subsequent irritation of the greater occipital nerve and less often from temporomandibular joint injury. Injury of the neck flexors accounts for the discomfort felt and swelling often noted at the front of the neck. Weakness of neck flexion results in difficulty in maintaining a correct posture. Protective muscle spasm leads to limitation of movements and later to contractures. It is postulated that injury to the sympathetic nerves as they emerge through the precervical fascia leads to such symptoms as dizziness, vertigo, blurred vision, light-headedness, dysphagia and the occasionally noted Horner's syndrome. Some of these symptoms could be accounted for by brain concussion or contusion and injury to the vestibular apparatus (Cailliet, 1991; Evans, 1992).

The development of disability

Various studies give different figures for the percentage of patients developing persistent symptoms or disability after neck sprain (Porter, 1989). This largely reflects different patient populations. The worst figures are reported in patients referred to specialized clinics, in contrast to a much better prognosis in those presenting to general practitioners (Livingston, 1992). Among patients presenting to the A&E department, 36% will have occasional symptoms and 6% will have constant pain persisting for more than a year after a whiplash injury (Deans et al., 1987). Very little recovery is likely to occur after a year (Gargan & Bannister, 1995).

We should try to understand the mechanisms and factors leading to disability if we are to prevent it. Both physical and psychosocial factors interact and contribute to the development of chronic disability. Physical factors are mainly related to immobilization and disuse. Prolonged immobilization using a collar leads to muscle and joint contractures and muscle weakness. This in turn leads to neck stiffness and pain on movement. The patient, interpreting further pain as further injury, will tend to reinforce immobility. This creates a vicious spiral with decreasing joint mobility, muscle strength and endurance and increasing pain. Symptoms are characteristically aggravated by exercise and the patient will therefore tend to reduce his or her activities with consequent loss of general fitness. This is sometimes referred to as the deconditioning syndrome (Gatchel et al., 1992). The use of sedating medications will aggravate the general feeling of tiredness and being unwell. A bad neck posture with the head lying forward to the centre of gravity will tend to increase lordosis and weight-bearing on the neck (Cailliet, 1991).

As the condition is often associated with a negative neurological examination and normal X-rays, it is often implicitly suggested to patients that their condition is mainly psychological. This attitude hardly helps the patient and is bound to lead to a loss of confidence in the medical profession. It is best to regard the syndrome as a real entity rather than behaviour (Hirsch et al., 1988). In a prospective study, psychosocial factors

assessed shortly after the accident were not found to influence the outcome at 3, 6 and 12 months (Radanov et al., 1991, 1994). There is no doubt, however, that psychosocial factors develop and interfere with recovery. Anger, anxiety and depression often complicate the picture and increase as the patient becomes unable to continue with work, domestic responsibilities and leisure activities. Loss of employment and income and dependence on benefits further complicate the picture. Litigation is disproportionately high after neck sprains. This may be related to insurance compensation systems and social copying (Livingston, 1992). It is tempting to consider that symptoms are exaggerated or prolonged for secondary gain. This probably plays a role only in a minority of patients. A proportion of patients who develop chronic symptoms are not involved in litigation and most of those whose litigation is settled are not cured by the verdict (Gargan & Bannister, 1995).

Rehabilitation of neck sprain

In the acute stage, accurate evaluation is mandatory. The aim is to detect those who require immediate referral for bony and neurological injuries, to establish an accurate record of the injury, to determine prognosis and to provide reassurance to the patient. In taking the history, it is important to determine the circumstances of the accident. The position of the patient's head, the direction and force of impact, the use of the seat-belt and properly adjusted headrest and the patient's awareness of the impending impact can all give clues to the anatomical structures injured and to the degree of damage (Cailliet, 1991).

Physical examination should include a thorough neurological assessment and a detailed examination of the neck looking for tenderness, swelling and weakness of the anterior neck muscles and recording the range of active and passive movements. X-rays reveal acute changes only in a minority of patients (MacNamara et al., 1988). Their use should therefore be limited to when symptoms are severe enough to suspect bony injury or if there are positive neurological signs. Poor prognostic factors include a severe injury, interscapular or upper back pain, occipital headache, multiple symptoms, upper limb pain or paraesthesia, neck stiffness, sleep disturbance, reduced speed of information processing, pre-existing degenerative changes, previous history of head trauma and headache and a relatively older age (Evans, 1992; Radanov et al., 1994).

The plan of initial treatment is a short period of rest, using a comfortable collar in slight neck flexion, followed within 2 days by gradual mobilization to restore movement and strength. The use of a collar should be limited in favour of early mobilization (Carroll, 1992). This aspect of treatment is discussed in Chapter 42. While simple analgesics and non-steroidal anti-inflammatory medications are useful for pain relief, sedating and addictive medications should be avoided. It is advisable to review the patient in 2 weeks, when a clearer idea of his/her progress and prognosis can be ascertained. At this stage counselling is appropriate.

Counselling is a vital component of treatment and is often greatly appreciated by the patient. This should be targeted at those with poor prognostic factors and persisting symptoms. The mechanism of injury and the origin of the patient's symptoms should be explained. The plan of treatment should be discussed, aiming to make the patient, at an early stage, an active participant rather than increasingly dependent on the medical profession. It is important for the patient to know that discomfort does not equate with injury and that he/she has to accept a certain degree of discomfort in order to regain a normal range of movement and muscle strength. He/she should be encouraged to resume work and other activities as early as possible.

The subacute stage begins within a few days, when the initial symptoms start to wane (Cailliet, 1991). A proportion of patients will need extended treatment during this stage to enable them to return to work and full function. Exercises are continued to strengthen and regain muscle length and range of movement. General exercises such as brisk walking and swimming should be encouraged to maintain fitness and promote a sense of well-being. Repeated counselling may be necessary to consolidate the issues discussed previously.

Special attention should be paid to the patient's psychological state as he is liable to develop depression or anxiety if his symptoms are slow to resolve. Sedative and habituating medications tend to increase patient tiredness, reduce motivation and increase dependence and should be avoided. Simple analgesics and non-steroidal anti-inflammatory medications can be a useful adjuvant to treatment. Amitriptyline in small doses, such as 25 mg at night, is beneficial in patients whose sleep is disturbed by pain. There are numerous other treatment modalities that are used to alleviate pain. A technique that deserves special mention is trigger point injection. Trigger points are tender points that give a radiating sensation when pressed upon. In a recent study (Byrn *et al.*, 1993), subcutaneous sterile water injection of tender and trigger points in the shoulder and neck regions was found to be beneficial in neck sprain patients.

Effort should be made to correct neck posture during walking, sitting and various daily activities. Ergonomic advice is valuable. Good posture during sleep can be achieved using special pillows that fit in the neck concavity. Surgery may have a small role to play in patients with persistent symptoms. In one study (MacNab, 1964), seven out of eight patients had complete relief of symptoms following cervical fusion. Avulsion of the intervertebral disc from the vertebral cartilaginous end-plate and stretching or tearing of the anterior longitudinal ligament were noted at surgery. Magnetic resonance imaging (MRI) can detect similar changes and may therefore have a role in defining patients suitable for surgery (Davis *et al.*, 1991).

In the chronic stage, efforts should be directed to disentangle and remedy the physical, psychological and social factors that contribute to persistence of symptoms and disability. An intensive multidisciplinary approach is needed. This is best undertaken by a team in a musculoskeletal rehabilitation unit. The emphasis in such treatment programmes is on function, hence the name 'functional restoration management' (Gatchel *et al.*, 1992).

ANKLE SPRAIN

Ankle sprains are frequent and are the most common sport injuries. They are particularly common in basketball, soccer and cross-country running. Although the general prognosis for ankle sprains is good, chronic disability in the form of functional instability can develop (Freeman *et al.*, 1965). Some degree of instability arises in 20–40% of lateral ankle sprains and, if longstanding, can lead to excessive loading of the medial joint space and degenerative arthritis (Harrington, 1979). In the chronic stage, the patient sustains recurrent sprains and complains of a feeling of instability on uneven surfaces, and later of persistent pain and swelling.

To understand the mechanism of ankle sprain, some knowledge of the functional anatomy of the ankle and its ligaments is necessary. The talus, articulating superiorly with the ankle mortise, allows plantar and dorsiflexion. The wider anterior portion of the talus fits snugly into the ankle mortise disallowing lateral or rotatory movements. In plantar flexion, the narrower posterior portion comes to lie between the lateral and medial malleoli, providing a relatively unstable position in which the ligaments contribute more towards ankle stability. The anterior talofibular, calcaneofibular and posterior talofibular ligaments provide lateral stability aided by the peroneal muscles. The anterior talofibular is the weakest and the first ligament to be torn in inversion injuries of the ankle (Dias, 1979). As it is adherent to the joint capsule, a tear in the capsule is usual and accounts for the swelling and bruising encountered. In more severe sprains, the calcaneofibular ligament can additionally be torn. The posterior talofibular ligament is only rarely torn causing complete ankle dislocation. Medially, the much stronger deltoid ligament is rarely ruptured without an associated fracture (Cox, 1985). Lateral ankle sprain is usually caused by an inversion injury when the foot lands on the ground in a position of plantar flexion (Lassiter et al., 1989).

Rehabilitation of ankle sprain

On initial evaluation, several issues are relevant to the process of rehabilitation. The severity of injury should be determined. Tenderness over both anterior talofibular and calcaneofibular ligaments, prominent soft tissue swelling, evidence of instability and inability to weight-bear, all point to a more severe injury (Lassiter et al., 1989). A history of recurrent ankle sprains indicates the need for more prolonged rehabilitation and for prevention. The high-level athlete needs a quicker return to full function compared to the sedentary patient. Other injuries such as malleolar, talar neck or fifth metatarsal fractures, osteochondral fractures, peroneal tendon subluxation and inferior tibiofibular diastasis should be excluded by appropriate clinical and radiological examination. Conditions such as diabetes, peripheral neuropathy and peripheral vascular disease can complicate recovery and should specifically be sought (Cass & Morrey, 1984).

The first principle of treatment is to reduce swelling. This helps to reduce ankle stiffness, and therefore the period of rehabilitation, and is achieved by a combination of ice, compression, elevation and a non-steroidal anti-inflammatory medication. Early mobilization, as opposed to plaster immobilization with or without surgery, gives the best results as regards to symptoms and return to full activities (Freeman, 1965; Brooks et al., 1981; Moller-Larsen et al., 1988). This is supported by experimental studies which show that ligament healing is enhanced by mobilization (Lassiter et al., 1989). Support is given by daily strapping using a non-elastic adhesive tape or, if the patient is unable to attend, a cast-brace that is easy

to apply. Special splints have also been developed and tested (Zwipp & Schievnik, 1992). Strapping should be applied in a position of eversion and dorsiflexion to approximate the torn ligament ends. Using crutches, progressive partial weight-bearing is allowed within the patient's tolerance. The crutches are discarded when the patient is able to walk without pain. Exercises progress from plantar and dorsiflexion to eversion–inversion exercises, and from range of movement to resisted active exercises. Strengthening exercises are applied to ankle dorsiflexors and evertors to protect against further inversion injuries. Stretching exercises, using a tilt board, are aimed at calf muscles and tendons in the belief that short calf musculature predisposes to further injury. Exercises on a balance board are used to regain proprioception.

In relation to sport, the patient progresses from walking through jogging, running straight lines, running with progressive cutting and specific sport-related exercises to full activity. In the active athlete, prevention of reinjury is achieved by protective strapping or the use of ankle braces (Fig. 1) and high-top shoes. These may have to be used for several months or longer after a severe ankle sprain (Cox, 1985).

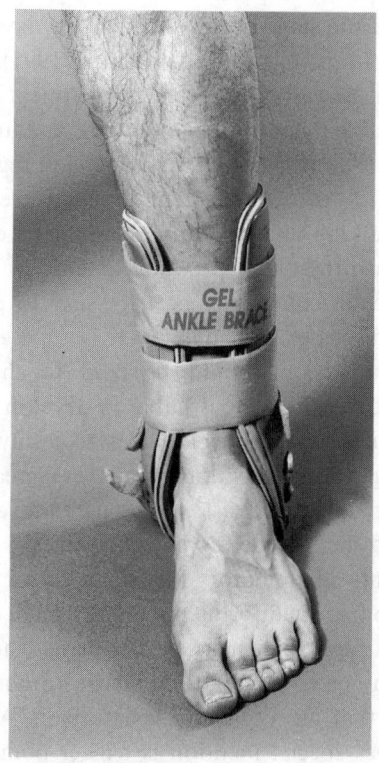

Fig. 1. The air/gel therapeutic ankle support system can be worn with a laced shoe after lateral ankle sprains.

Surgery is not generally indicated in the acute stage of isolated lateral ankle sprain. Although it offers more stability, there are risks of stiffness, reduced ankle agility, longer rehabilitation and infection. In addition, there is no significant difference between the results of primary and delayed reconstruction (Cass *et al.*, 1985). The role of surgery is therefore limited to those with recurrent ankle sprains and instability and to the high-level athlete for whom stability is very important. Reconstruction is usually done using the peroneus brevis or a free tendon graft from the extensor digitorum longus (Lassiter *et al.*, 1989). Surgical reconstruction can be beneficial even after the development of degenerative changes (Harrington, 1979). Persistent pain should alert the physician to the possibility of a missed additional injury, the development of reflex sympathetic dystrophy or traumatic synovitis which could respond to a local corticosteroid injection.

KNEE SPRAIN

The knee is the most complex and also the largest joint in the body. The articulating surfaces, which allow multidirectional motion, contribute little to joint stability. The latter depends on the joint capsule, ligaments, menisci and dynamic musculotendinous support. The term knee sprain is used here to cover ligamentous injuries; namely, that of the cruciate and collateral ligaments. Such injuries are the most frequent cause of sport-related disability (Leffers, 1992). They are especially common in contact sports and those associated with sudden twisting and deceleration such as soccer, rugby, basketball, wrestling and ski-ing. Another mechanism is dashboard injury in car accidents.

Medial collateral ligament sprain is the most common ligamentous injury of the knee. This ligament is the primary medial stabilizer for the knee and is injured by trauma to the lateral aspect of the knee with the foot fixed on the ground. The deeper portion of the ligament is closely related to the medial meniscus, which can therefore be simultaneously injured. Although complete tears can produce clinical instability, isolated injuries to the medial collateral ligament rarely produce functional disability.

Isolated injury to the lateral collateral ligament is unusual but the resultant lateral instability often causes a functional deficit.

Anterior cruciate ligament injury is much more serious and is a frequent cause of long-term disability which is mainly caused by the resultant anterior and rotatory instability. The anterior cruciate ligament, besides acting as a mechanical stabilizer, has a sensory function contributing to knee proprioception (Johansson *et al.*, 1991). Deficiency of the anterior cruciate leads to decreased proprioception and, as a result, delayed muscular contractile responses to injury forces (Corrigan *et al.*, 1992). Unstable knees are therefore predisposed to further injuries and progressive deterioration. Meniscal tear is a common secondary effect and it develops in 50% of anterior cruciate deficient knees within 5 years of injury. Articular cartilage lesions increase to about 70% within 10 years. The development of degenerative arthritis ensues in 20–30 years and is correlated with the state of the menisci (McDaniel & Dameron, 1980). The amount of perceived disability depends on the needs of the individual, so that a high-level athlete would perceive more disability than a recreational sportsman with an equal injury. The completeness of the anterior cruciate tear and the presence of additional ligament injury also contribute to the degree of disability. The ability of the individual to compensate functionally for the injury is another factor which is unpredictable.

Posterior cruciate ligament injuries are usually caused by trauma to the tibia with the knee flexed as in dashboard injuries. They are commonly associated with an avulsion fracture of the tibial attachment. Isolated lesions do not usually cause functional disability (Leffers, 1992).

Rehabilitation of knee sprain

Accurate diagnosis of the specific injuries incurred in a knee sprain is vital for proper management. Careful history-taking and clinical examination are essential. Indicators of a significant injury include a history of audible popping or tearing, inability to bear weight immediately after the accident, swelling and haemarthrosis. In the case of anterior cruciate deficiency, a positive pivot shift test indicates rotational instability and correlates highly with functional disability (Leffers, 1992). Examination can be difficult in the acute stage because of pain, muscle spasm and haemarthrosis. Aspiration of the latter and injection of a local anaesthetic can facilitate examination. To test for anterior instability, the Lachman test, applied with the knee slightly flexed, is easier to perform than the anterior drawer test in the acute stage. An examination under anaesthesia may be necessary for accurate assessment. X-rays are useful to exclude associated bony injuries. The advent of magnetic resonance imaging (MRI) as a highly sensitive non-invasive investigation has made it much easier to confirm the diagnosis.

Menisci, cruciate and collateral ligaments are clearly seen on MRI (Munk *et al.*, 1989; Spiers *et al.*, 1993). Arthroscopy is best avoided in the acute stage because of the risk of complications. Leakage of the irrigating fluid through capsular tears can increase swelling and interfere with the process of rehabilitation.

Knee sprain in general is treated initially with rest, ice, compression and elevation to limit local swelling. This is followed by range of movement and progressive muscle strengthening exercises. The latter start with isometric and proceed to isokinetic exercises carried out within the limits of pain tolerance. Wasting is most prominent in the quadriceps muscle which needs most attention. In anterior cruciate injury, the hamstrings are additionally important in view of their restraining effect on anterior tibial translation. The strength of other lower limb muscles should be maintained. In addition to strength, rehabilitation should also aim to regain endurance and agility as these are more relevant to the athlete's performance. Hinged braces that limit valgus and varus stress are used during the initial treatment of more severe collateral ligament injuries. Several types of brace are available to provide stability in anterior cruciate deficiency (Fig. 2). These can be used as an alternative to, or following surgery, but their effect is small and they should not be a substitute for muscle training. Surgery, usually arthroscopic, is needed to deal with associated meniscal tears and for anterior cruciate augmentation or reconstruction. Less common indications for surgery include repair of complete lateral collateral ligament tears and avulsion fractures as bone-to-bone healing is usually excellent.

In anterior cruciate deficiency, the choice between surgical and conservative treatment deserves further consideration. It was hoped that surgery would restore athletic function and prevent the development of degenerative changes. The knee, however, is never returned completely to normal and it is not yet proved that surgery prevents joint degeneration. On the other hand, the success rate of surgery is only 70% to 90%, joint stiffness can be a problem postoperatively and there is the potential for complications such as infection, patellar pain and reflex sympathetic dystrophy. It has been shown that more than one-third of patients improve with conservative treatment in the form of physiotherapy, activity modification and the use of knee braces (Noyes *et al.*, 1983). For those reasons, it is best to have a trial of conservative therapy before deciding upon surgery. Activity modification may not, however, be acceptable to the high-level athlete for whom the decision for surgery will inevitably come earlier.

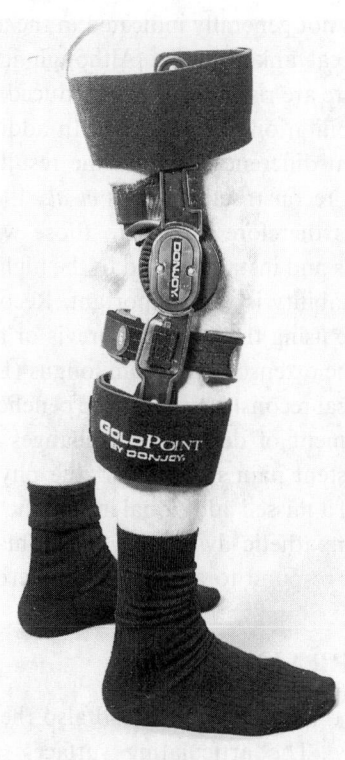

Fig. 2. The Donjoy knee brace is often used as a part of conservative treatment of anterior cruciate tears. The centre of the brace should be situated above the top of the patella and posterior to the midline.

Counselling is vital for the success of postoperative rehabilitation. The full programme of rehabilitation should be adequately explained to ensure patient compliance. Consideration should be given to the time needed out of work. The trend in postoperative rehabilitation is for early exercises and weight-bearing (Stanish & Lai, 1993). Immobilization encourages joint stiffness. Tension increases the tensile strength of ligaments. On the other hand, too much tension may disrupt the newly constructed tendon. Guarded stress is therefore required. It is important to preserve full extension since a flexion deformity can be very disabling. Progressive weight-bearing and isometric exercise starts immediately following surgery. This is followed by active range of movement exercises and, after 4 weeks, progressive resistance exercises for at least a year. Exercises specific for the athlete's sport should be started at about 16 weeks from surgery.

Bibliography

BROOKS, S.C., POTTER, B.T. & RAINEY, J.B. (1981). Treatment for partial tears of the lateral ligament of the ankle: a prospective trial. *Br. Med. J.*, **282**, 606–7.

BYRN, C., OLSSON, I., FALKHEDEN, L. *et al.* (1993). Subcutaneous sterile water injections for chronic neck and shoulder pain following whiplash injuries. *Lancet*, **341**, 449–52.

CAILLIET, R. (1991). *Neck and Arm Pain*, 3rd edn., pp. 81–123. Philadelphia: F.A. Davis.

CARROLL, P.G. (1992). Acute neck strain – the value of judicious early mobilisation. *Aust. Fam. Physician*, **21**, 275–6.

CASS, J.R. & MORREY, B.F. (1984). Ankle instability: current concepts, diagnosis, and treatment. *Mayo Clin. Proc.*, **59**, 165–70.

CASS, J.R., MORRAY, B.F., KATOH, Y. *et al.* (1985). Ankle instability: comparison of primary and delayed construction after long-term follow-up study. *Clin. Orthop.*, **198**, 110–17.

CORRIGAN, J.P., CASHMAN, W.F. & BRADY, M.P. (1992). Proprioception in the cruciate deficient knee. *J. Bone Joint Surg.*, **74B**, 247–50.

COX, J.S. (1985). Surgical and non-surgical treatment of acute ankle sprains. *Clin. Orthop.*, **198**, 118–26.

CROWE, H. (1928). Injuries to the cervical spine. Paper presented at the annual meeting of the Western Orthopaedic Association, San Francisco.

DAVIS, S.J., TERESI, L.M., BRADLEY, W.G. *et al.* (1991). Cervical spine hyperextention injuries: MR findings. *Radiology*, **180**, 245–51.

DEANS, G.T., MAGILLARD, J.N., KERR, M. *et al.* (1987). Neck sprain – a major cause of disability following car accidents. *Injury*, **18**, 10–12.

DIAS, L.S. (1979). The lateral ankle sprain: an experimental study. *J. Trauma*, **19**, 266–9.

EVANS, R.W. (1992). Some observations on whiplash injuries. *Neurol. Clin.*, **10**, 975–97.

FREEMAN, M.A.R. (1965). Treatment of ruptures of the lateral ligament of the ankle. *J. Bone Joint Surg.*, **47B**, 661.

FREEMAN, M.A.R., DEAN, M.R.E., & HANHAM, I.E.F. (1965). The etiology and prevention of functional instability of the foot. *J. Bone Joint Surg.*, **47B**, 678–85.

GARGAN, M.F. & BANNISTER, G.C. (1995). Injuries of the cervical spine. In *Medicolegal Reporting in Orthopaedic Trauma*, 2nd edn. ed. M. Foy & P. Fagg. Edinburgh: Churchill Livingstone.

GATCHEL, R.J., MAYER, T.G., HAZARD, R.G. *et al.* (1992). Editorial: functional restoration. Pitfalls in evaluating efficacy. *Spine*, **17**, 988–95.

HARRINGTON, K.D. (1979). Degenerative arthritis of the ankle secondary to long-standing lateral ligament instability. *J. Bone Joint Surg.*, **61A**, 354–61.

HIRSCH, S.A., HIRSCH, P.J., HIRAMOTO, H. *et al.* (1988). Whiplash syndrome, fact or fiction? *Orthop. Clin. North Am.*, **19**, 791–5.

JOHANSSON, H., SJOLANDER, P. & SOJKA, P. (1991). A sensory role for the cruciate ligaments. *Clin. Orthop.*, **268**, 161–78.

LASSITER, T.E., MALONE, T.R. & GARRETT, W.E. (1989). Injury to the lateral ligaments of the ankle. *Orthop. Clin. North Am.*, **20**, 629–40.

LEFFERS, D. (1992). Dislocations and soft tissue injuries of the knee. In *Skeletal Trauma*, Vol. 2, ed. B.D. Browner, J.B. Jupiter, A.M. Levine & P.G. Trafton, pp. 1715–43. Philadelphia: W.B. Saunders.

LIVINGSTON, M. (1992). Whiplash injury: misconceptions and remedies. *Aust. Fam. Physician*, **21**, 1642–3, 1646–7.

MacNAB, I. (1964). Acceleration injuries of the cervical spine. *J. Bone Joint Surg.*, **46A**, 1797–9.

MacNAMARA, R.M., O'BRIEN, M.C. & DAVIDHEISER, S. (1988). Post-traumatic neck pain: a prospective and follow-up study. *Ann. Emerg. Med.*, **17**, 906.

McDANIEL, W.J., & DAMERON, T.B. (1980). Untreated ruptures of the anterior cruciate ligament. *J. Bone Joint Surg.*, **62A**, 696–704.

MOLLER-LARSEN, F., WETHELUND, J.O., JURIK, A.G. *et al.* (1988). *Comparison of three different treatments for ruptured lateral ankle ligaments. Acta Orthop. Scand.*, **59**, 564–66.

MUNK, P.L., HELMS, C.A., GENANT, H.K. *et al.* (1989). Magnetic resonance imaging of the knee: current status, new directions. *Skeletal Radiol.*, **18**, 569–77.

NOYES, F.R., MATTHEWS, D.S., MOOAR, P.A. *et al.* (1983). The symptomatic anterior cruciate-deficient knee. Part II: The results of rehabilitation, activity modification and counselling on functional disability. *J. Bone Joint Surg.*, **65A**, 163–74.

PORTER, K.M. (1989). Neck sprains after car accidents. A common cause of long term disability. *Br. Med. J.*, **298**, 973–4.

RADANOV, B.P., DI STEFANO, G., SCHNIDRIG, A. *et al.* (1991). Role of psychosocial stress in recovery from common whiplash. *Lancet*, **338**, 712–15.

RADANOV, B.P., STURZENEGGER, M., DE STEFANO, G. *et al.* (1994). Relationship between early somatic, radiological, cognitive and psychological findings and outcome during a one-year follow-up in 117 patients suffering from common whiplash. *Br. J. Rheumatol.*, **33**, 442–8.

RUTHERFORD, W.H., GREENFIELD, A.A., HAYES, H.R.M *et al.* (1985). *The Medical Effects of Seat-belt Legislation in the United Kingdom*. London: HMSO.

SPIERS, A.S., MEAGHER, T., OSTLERE, S.J. *et al.* (1993). Can MRI of the knee affect arthroscopic practice? A prospective study of 58 patients. *J. Bone. Joint Surg.*, **75B**, 49–52.

STANISH, W.D. & LAI, A. (1993). New concepts of rehabilitation following anterior cruciate reconstruction. *Clin. Sports Med.*, **12**, 25–58.

ZWIPP, H. & SCHIENVNIK, B. (1992). Primary orthotic treatment of ruptured ankle ligaments: a recommended procedure. *Prosthet. Orthot. Int.*, **16**, 49–56.

42 Physiotherapy: the contribution

H.R. TRUNDLE

Trauma Service, John Radcliffe Hospital, Oxford, UK

Chapter plan

Introduction
Physiotherapy in the A&E department
Physiotherapy within the fracture clinic
Conclusion

INTRODUCTION

Physiotherapy currently plays an important role in the management of minor trauma where prompt appropriate treatment reduces recovery time and minimizes the risk of recurrent symptoms. This chapter examines the role of the physiotherapist within the accident and emergency (A&E) department and the fracture clinic and details the initial management of the injuries that most commonly require physiotherapy.

PHYSIOTHERAPY IN THE A&E DEPARTMENT

Injuries described as minor often occur in large numbers. Ankle ligament sprains alone, for example, account for 3–5% of all A&E attendances. Inappropriate initial management results in extended treatment time in the physiotherapy department, delayed return to work or recreational activity for the patient, and increased risk of reinjury. Delayed or incomplete recovery therefore carries resource implications for both hospital departments and the individual patient.

The function of the therapist

The primary role is the initial management of minor injury, assessment of the individual's needs for further physiotherapy, and ensuring that referral occurs promptly where necessary.

Advising patients on suitable self-maintenance exercise programmes and detailing the management over the first 48 h after injury helps to avoid possible later complications and in some instances obviates the need for further treatment. A review of referrals from A&E over an 8-month period in Oxford showed that 24% of patients only required one assessment and advice session. Discussing length of time to recovery, reassurance that movement as advised may be painful, but is not harmful, and issuing written information to reinforce advice given in the A&E department are all essential in giving patients confidence in self-management of their rehabilitation.

Assessment of mobility after injury in the elderly is important. Patients who fall and sustain either bruising of the lower limb or fractures of the upper limb are often admitted for mobilization or social reasons. Some of these admissions could be avoided by issuing suitable mobility aids and liaising with the domiciliary services requesting urgent home assessment to identify those at risk.

Many physiotherapy departments have waiting lists. The A&E physiotherapist is in an ideal position to discuss with local centres the urgency of follow-up and the likely number of treatments required. This communication helps to avoid the development of chronic problems following acute lesions while the patient waits for treatment.

The A&E physiotherapist also liaises with the rest of the A&E staff giving input on the initial treatment of minor injuries and soft tissue disorders and correct use of walking aids, braces and taping. A&E staff can consult the in-house physiotherapist about the likely benefits and outcomes of treatment for particular conditions. This will result in appropriate referrals when the A&E

physiotherapist is not available and will also teach junior medical staff the correct treatment of these common minor injuries.

A&E physiotherapists operate review clinics where patients return the following day for further assessment and treatment. Many injuries needing physiotherapy attention occur outside the normal 8 a.m. to 5 p.m. period. If evaluation of these attendances reveals an identifiable busy period occurring regularly then this should be staffed. Weekends should also be considered as A&E physiotherapy ideally should be a 7-day service.

The A&E physiotherapist requires an extensive knowledge of the anatomy, pathology and management of injury and therefore must be an experienced senior clinician. There must be access to a treatment area equipped with an examination plinth (ideally an hydraulic one) strapping and taping materials, knee braces, wrist splints, tubular bandage, an ice machine, walking aids and a telephone.

Individual units need to note how many people are referred from A&E and set aside time to treat them. Physiotherapy is a scarce resource and small A&E departments may not need to have a full-time physiotherapist. Fracture clinics and A&E departments may be able to share the same post.

The place of a sports injury clinic within the A&E unit is often discussed. The majority of injuries to sportsmen are in no way different from those occurring within the population as a whole. The majority of patients suffering injury in sport could be dealt with adequately if the accident services were good enough to cope with the load imposed upon them. Early accurate diagnosis leading to prompt logical treatment is the ideal; delay in supplying this ideal exacerbates the injury and prolongs disability (Williams, 1979). Physiotherapists should aim to offer the same opportunities for advice and treatment to all comers, but would expect commitment on the part of sportsmen to fulfil their share of the responsibility for treatment.

A review of 79 physiotherapy departments in the UK showed that only 12 have a physiotherapist within the A&E unit (unpublished material). Some hospitals have begun an evaluation of the effectiveness of this service. The majority of physiotherapists questioned (90%) believe that an A&E post is an obvious logical extension of their present role. The main functions, as perceived by those responding, are to offer assessment and advice and to begin the definitive treatment of injuries referred.

Many A&E units without a permanent physiotherapist are able to obtain physiotherapy assessment within 1–2 days of injury (85% in the UK survey). However, this relies on physiotherapists seeing A&E patients in addition to the appointment-based service and is disruptive of work in the out-patient department.

Soft tissue injuries requiring physiotherapy

The national review of A&E referrals to physiotherapy shows that the soft tissue injuries discussed below occur frequently. The basic principles of initial management (i.e. rest, ice, elevation, compression, controlled early movement) apply to all soft tissue injuries and are discussed in detail with reference to ankle ligament injury.

Ankle ligament injury

Ankle sprain or lateral ligament injury is common. The majority of these injuries present in the 15–25-year age group and occur in school or recreational sport. The injury may involve time off work as well as attendance for physiotherapy.

There is debate about the detailed management of these injuries, but general agreement that conservative therapy gives at least as good results as surgery for the torn lateral ligament complex (Zwipp *et al.*, 1991). It is not practical in economic terms, nor has it been proved necessary, for all patients with ankle sprains to attend regularly for physiotherapy if the initial treatment is correct.

Treatment of minor sprains presenting with minimal swelling and slight tenderness over the anterior talofibular ligament and mild pain on walking is directed at relief of symptoms and prevention of reinjury by advising cold application, strengthening and balance exercises and avoiding immediate return to sport.

Immediate attention is required for moderate injury with marked swelling, tenderness and difficulty in walking or severe injury with sufficient pain to prevent weight-bearing.

The initial aim of treatment is to limit bleeding and swelling and prevent further injury. The generally accepted approach to immediate management of most minor soft tissue injuries is followed.

Cooling

Cooling the injured limb reduces blood flow, oedema, pain and muscle spasm. This is best achieved either with a cold mains water foot bath, or the application of crushed ice in a wet towel for 20 min. Chemical or gel ice packs are not superior to ice or iced water and are both more expensive and difficult to apply.

Ice is applied as soon as possible after injury, then at 4-hourly intervals over the next 48 h until bleeding and swelling have stabilized. Information on how to continue ice application at home is given to the patient.

TECHNIQUES

Application of ice packs

- Applying an ice pack as soon as possible after an injury helps to reduce the pain and swelling and therefore makes movement easier.
- If you are applying ice packs to ankles, knees, feet, hands, wrists, or elbows, it is important to elevate the area as this will further reduce any swelling.

Using crushed ice

- Use ice cubes from the freezer.
- Place the cubes in a wet towel and crush them.
- Apply the ice pack to the affected area moulding it in place.
- Wrap another towel around the pack to keep it secure.
- Remove after 20 min and repeat every 4 h until the swelling subsides.

Using frozen peas

- Wrap a bag of frozen peas in a wet dish cloth or towel and apply directly, moulding the pack around the swollen area.
- A dry towel wrapped around this will keep the pack in place.
- Remove after 20 min and repeat every 4 h as above.

Compression

Compression further minimizes bleeding and oedema and is a vital part of early management as extensive soft tissue swelling contributes to prolonged joint stiffness and disability. Compression is achieved with strapping, bandaging, pneumatic splints or elasticized ankle supports applied with the ankle in a neutral plantigrade position to facilitate weight-bearing.

Strapping begins with the application of a horseshoe pad of felt around the lateral malleolus to compress the hollows beneath the bone. Zinc oxide stirrup straps over this pad support the ankle in a neutral plantigrade position and continue up over the peroneal muscle group to facilitate proprioceptive reflexes and encourage

dynamic ankle support. Elastoplast bandage is then applied from toes to midcalf with the foot held in dorsiflexion to achieve overall compression. This gives sufficient support to allow some degree of weight-bearing in even the most severely injured ankle.

Strapping is time-consuming to apply; however, tubular bandages alone have not proved helpful and may even have a detrimental effect for those patients who are unable to weight-bear, as they tend to hold the foot in plantiflexion (Muwanga *et al.*, 1986).

Plaster casts should not be used. They do not allow compression of the injured tissues and, even if they allow the patient to take weight on the ankle, their application results in more days off work and longer attendances at physiotherapy and follow-up clinics (Brooks *et al.*, 1981).

Elevation

Patients are advised to elevate the leg for 24 h above the level of the waist whenever they are not exercising as instructed. This includes sleeping with the foot raised on pillows or with a support (e.g. a suitcase) placed under the mattress.

Rest

The advice to rest is often given without guidelines on how to achieve it, or for how long. The injuried tissues must be rested until swelling and bleeding subside. This is achieved by strapping and provision of crutches or a walking stick where walking is difficult, as well as 24–48 h of elevation.

The aim of definitive physiotherapy is to obtain a normal range of movement, muscle power and proprioception or muscle coordination. The first session aims to restore normal gait patterns with sufficient passive or active dorsiflexion to allow the patient to stand with the foot flat, using walking aids if necessary. Reassurance is needed since many patients are fearful of causing more damage by moving the foot or taking weight through the ankle. Explaining the nature of the injury and the course of healing over the ensuing weeks is useful to gain the patient's cooperation with treatment.

Many patients can be given a home exercise programme that allows self-management. This includes active and passive dorsiflexion and plantarflexion, resisted peroneal exercises and balance work to restore muscle coordination. Weak peroneal muscles and slow reflex response to postural sway are factors in chronic instability and recurrent injury. It is essential these potential problems are addressed and emphasized by the home programme. These patients are invited to make a review appointment 2–3 weeks later if recovery is not satisfactory.

TECHNIQUES

Ankle exercises

- Elevate the leg, making sure the foot is above the level of the waist.
- Applying an ice pack as soon as possible after injury helps to reduce pain and swelling.
- Leave the ice pack on for 20 min and repeat four times a day.
- An elastic bandage will help to support the ankle and control swelling.
- Gentle ankle movements done within the limits of pain must be practised frequently to prevent stiffness and stimulate healing.
- You will not damage the ankle further if you attempt to walk on it. Always try to walk normally by putting the heel down first.
- Gradually increase your activity as pain and swelling subside.
- Do not return to sport until you are fully fit.
- The following exercises will help regain strength and movement.

Exercise 1
- Keep your knee straight.
- Pull your foot upwards as far as possible, then use a belt or towel to apply a slight stretch.
- Then point your foot downwards and use the belt to give resistance.

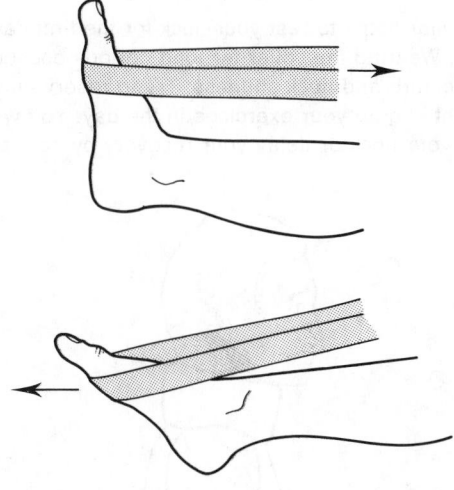

Exercise 2
- Point your foot down away from you, turning the sole inwards. This will gently stretch the injured ligament.
- When you can walk without pain, practice exercises 3–5.

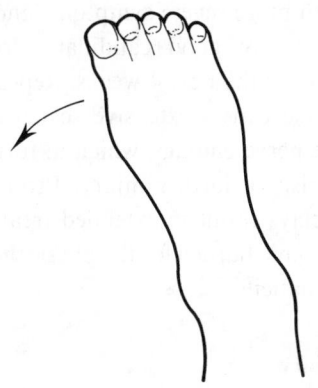

Exercise 3
- Stand on both feet.
- Bend your knees so they move forwards over your feet. Try not to stick your bottom out.
- Hold this position for 10 sec.
- Do this with just your injured leg as you improve.

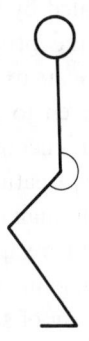

Exercise 4
- Stand on your injured leg and raise yourself onto tiptoes.
- Hold this position for 5 sec then lower slowly.
- Repeat until your calf muscle tires.

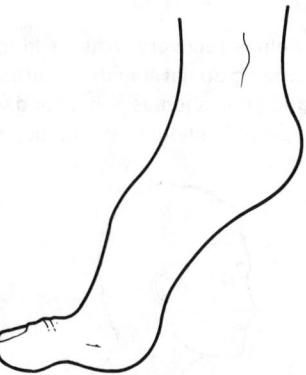

Exercise 5
- Standing on the injured leg alone improves and strengthens the muscles needed for balance. If these muscles are strong you are less likely to injure the ankle again.
- Practice standing whilst brushing your teeth, washing up, etc. until you can manage 3 min without putting the other foot down.

Patients with more severe symptoms and a history of recurrent injury are good candidates for supervised rehabilitation over the next 4 weeks. Repeated injury to the joint capsule causes extensive scarring and loss of proprioceptive nerve endings, which in turn exposes the ankle to the risk of further injury. Prompt referral is essential as delays result in extended treatment and an increased economic burden for the physiotherapy department and the patient.

Acute neck injury

Whiplash injury or acute neck spain is common and occurs in an estimated 20% of all vehicle accidents (MacNab, 1977). Reviews of patients indicate that between 45% and 66% still have symptoms after 2 years (MacNab, 1977; Norris & Watt, 1983). Verbal advice reinforced by written instruction on posture correction, use of collar and analgesia, and performance of mobilization exercises demonstrated by the physiotherapist has been shown to reduce the proportion of those with persistent symptoms at 2 years to 23% (McKinney, 1989).

Written instructions given to patients at the time of injury aid memory and encourage patients to take responsiblity for their own treatment. This enables them to become self-sufficient in managing episodes of minor discomfort and prevents the recurrence or persistence of the cycle of muscle spasm, pain and poor posture, which leads to adaptive shortening of soft tissues.

TECHNIQUES

Neck exercises (after McKinney, 1989)

Posture

- Bad posture delays recovery. When sitting, standing, reading, and driving do not slouch forwards with your chin sticking out and your shoulders hunched. Straighten your back, relax your shoulders and tuck your chin in.

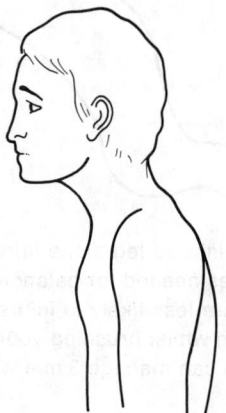

Exercise
- Straighten your back, stretch your shoulders downwards and draw your head backwards on your neck.
- Look straight ahead, not down at your feet.
- Do this ten times an hour.

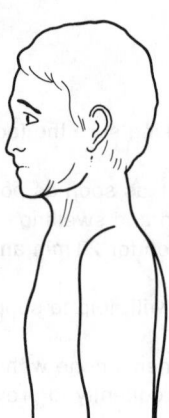

Moving your neck

- These exercises will be painful initially but will not harm your neck. Try and repeat these movements at least ten times an hour. Each day stretch the neck a little further.

Exercises
- Straighten up and look ahead.
- Try to touch your ear down to your shoulder.
- Repeat with the other side.
- Now straighten up again, then look round over each shoulder in turn.
- Finally, straighten up again, look upwards pointing your chin to the ceiling, then downwards putting your chin on your chest.

Soft collar

- The collar helps to rest your neck for the first day after injury. Wearing the collar for long periods encourages bad posture and neck stiffness. Try to reserve it for use at night and do your exercises in the day. You will not harm your neck or delay your recovery by not using the collar.

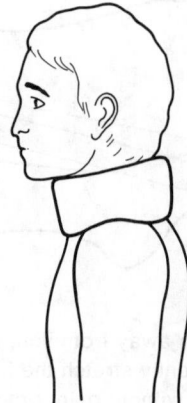

Sleeping

- Do not use too many pillows in bed. Feather or polyester pillows are better than foam as they can be moulded to the shape of your neck. Support your neck either with the collar which you may wear back-to-front, or use a rolled-up hand towel inside the bottom edge of the pillow case. Try not to sleep on your face.

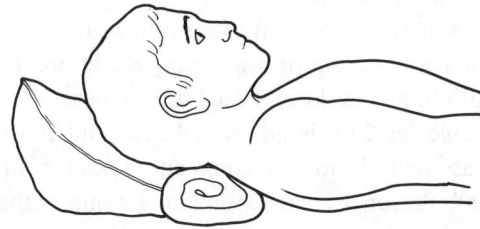

Relieving discomfort

- The pain in your neck will gradually settle as the movement returns. Applying gentle heat often helps. Try a hot water bottle, a heated towel, a heat lamp or a warming liniment. Take any pain-killing tablets that you have been prescribed regularly.

These patients should be reviewed by the A&E physiotherapist after 5 days and those who have not made satisfactory progress may be referred for physiotherapy. It is estimated that as few as 10% of those seen initially will require long-term treatment if managed in this way. It is important this treatment is received immediately. Poor results were shown where the initial management consisted of immobilization in a collar for 10–14 days (Hasheri, 1986).

Knee injury

Injuries to the knee joint, and the medial collateral ligament in particular, are the third most commonly referred injury seen by physiotherapists.

Stable isolated medial collateral ligament sprains are treated symptomatically. Regular application of ice minimizes swelling. Compression is achieved with a double tubular bandage or wool and crepe for 24 h. Reducing the swelling is important as effusion contributes to reflex inhibition of the quadriceps resulting in rapid atrophy, which in turn leads to patellofemoral malalignment and further atrophy through disuse and discomfort (Kannus & Jarvinen, 1990). Muscle wasting is not just a consequence but often a causal factor of poor recovery after knee injury and any measures to prevent it will assist rehabilitation. Immediate static (isometric) quadriceps exercises are encouraged to combat muscle atrophy

which begins within the first 24 h after injury. Active knee flexion and extension within the limits of pain encourages orientation of collagen fibres along the lines of tension stress resulting in strong well-organized scar tissue (Evans, 1980).

TECHNIQUES

Knee exercises

- After injuring your knee the muscles rapidly become weak. These exercises will help your leg to become strong again quickly. Do each exercise at least 20 times. Repeat three times a day, increasing the movement as pain allows. If your knee is swollen you may use an ice pack before starting.

Exercise 1
- Sit with your legs straight out and back supported.
- Tighten your thigh muscles by pushing the back of your knee downwards.
- Hold for 5 sec.

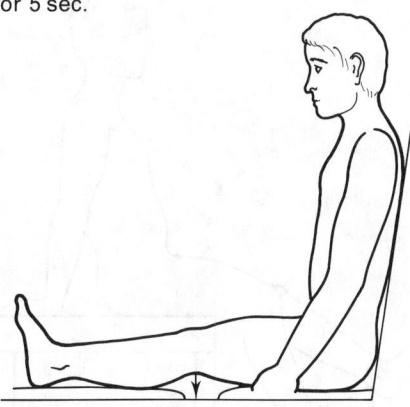

Exercise 2
- Sit as above.
- Roll two towels around a tin to give firm support under your knee.
- Tighten your thigh muscles, lift your foot and straighten your knee. Do not lift your whole leg off the support.
- Hold for 10 sec then lower slowly.

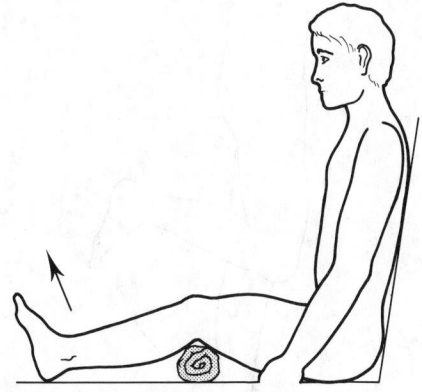

Exercise 3
- Sit as above.

- Place your foot on a tea tray and slide the tray up and down, trying to get as much bend in the knee as possible.

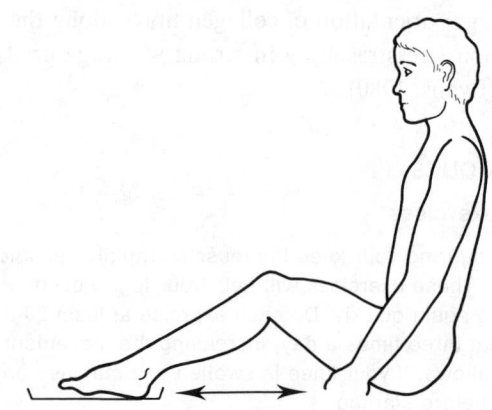

Exercise 4
- Sit on a firm table or kitchen worktop.
- Cross your good leg under the injured one at the ankle.
- Allow gravity to bend the leg towards the floor.

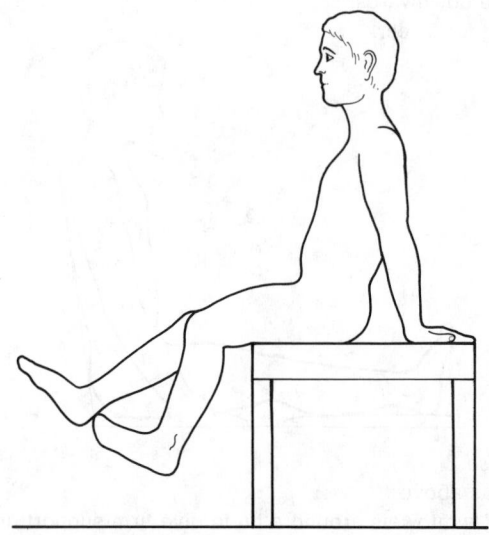

Exercise 5
- Stand on your good leg.
- Bend your other knee up behind you as far as you can, then lower slowly.

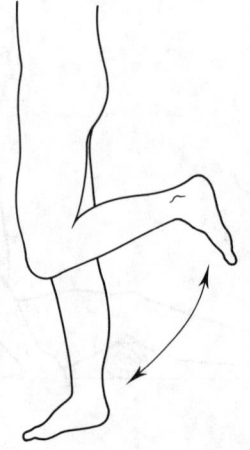

Quadriceps contusions

A direct blow to the anterior, medial or lateral thigh over the muscle bellies of the quadriceps femoris results in pain, swelling and decreased range of knee flexion. The degree of severity has been classified with the loss of flexion: mild has flexion greater than 90°, moderate 45–90° and severe less than 45°.

Those suffering mild contusions follow the basic principles of cooling, compression and elevation. Resting with both hip and knee flexed to as near 90° as is comfortable for 24 h is advised. Active and passive or gravity-assisted flexion is commenced and continued until 120° flexion is reached, again staying within the limits of pain.

Gentle stretches continue until movement is full range. Resistance to active contraction can then begin and sport may gradually be resumed.

Moderate or severe contusion requires formal physiotherapy. The usual first aid management is followed and crutches may be necessary if the patient has difficulty in walking. Early referral is important as myositis ossificans is associated with a treatment delay of 3 or more days and with loss of knee flexion (Ryan *et al.*, 1991).

PHYSIOTHERAPY WITHIN THE FRACTURE CLINIC

Most hospitals have some physiotherapy input to the fracture clinic, even if not on a full-time basis. Smaller hospitals holding clinics only 2 or 3 days a week often have access to an on-call physiotherapist based in the out-patient department. This arrangement is usually reported as being unsatisfactory as it interrupts the out-patient caseload. Ideally, the physiotherapist should be present during the whole time the clinic is running, allowing efficient referral of recent fractures that benefit from prompt physiotherapy input. This also allows detailed advice to be given to those patients emerging from immobilizing casts.

Fractures requiring physiotherapy

Certain fractures are frequently encountered. The physiotherapy approach is detailed below.

Fractures of the humeral neck

The majority of these injuries occur in the over-65 age group. Some 50–80% of these are defined as undisplaced, or minimally displaced, with less than 1 cm of separation between the fracture fragments and less than 45° of angulation (Neer, 1970). These injuries are stable, held by the periosteum, rotator cuff and splinted by the long head of biceps.

Studies of conservative treatment of this group of patients show that there is a significant relationship between early mobilization and the length of time required to achieve a good functional outcome (Clifford, 1980; Livesley *et al.*, 1992). Poor results stem from wearing a sling too long before commencing exercise. Formation of adhesions resulting from tendon, joint capsule and bursal damage obliterates the normal capsular recesses and a painful shoulder results, even after the fracture has healed.

Movement of the distal humerus in relation to the humeral head is palpated while the patient performs gentle pendular exercises to ensure the bone moves as a single unit. Gross movement between the two fragments indicates instability and non-union or malunion may be a consequence of early motion.

Axillary nerve lesions are easy to overlook. Sensory loss is not always present and a deltoid contraction should be looked for and palpated. The inferior subluxation of the humeral head caused either by muscular inhibition of the rotator cuff and deltoid or by nerve damage is painful. A weak deltoid contraction is ineffective in abducting the arm as the effort is spent in reducing the head subluxation. Reduction of the humerus using a supportive triangular sling for the first week, changing to a collar and cuff support if needed, will aid pain relief.

An early attempt to regain abduction must be made to obtain a good result (Maitland, 1986; Young & Wallace, 1985). Appropriate analgesia is given and the arm supported with a sling or collar and cuff. The patient is advised on personal hygiene, washing, dressing and mobility if a walking aid is normally used. Gentle pendular exercises are demonstrated and written instructions supplied.

TECHNIQUES

Shoulder exercises

- After injury your shoulder pain may restrict the use of the arm. It may also be necessary to rest your arm in a sling for a short period. However, it is most important that your shoulder is not allowed to stiffen.
- The following exercises assist return of normal shoulder movement as quickly as possible. Do each exercise ten times and repeat them four times a day.

Exercise 1
- Stand beside a firm support (use a table or the kitchen sink).
- Lean on the uninjured arm, bending forward from the hips as far as possible.
- Let the injured arm hang loosely away from the body.
- Swing the arm gently, like a pendulum, in three directions:

  – Moving backwards and forward as far as possible.
  – Out to the side then back across your body.
  – Circular movements, clockwise, then anticlockwise.

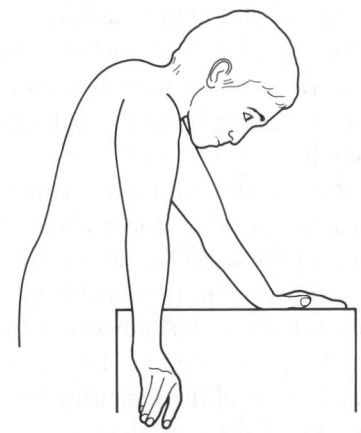

Exercise 2
- Lie down, or, if this is difficult, sit on a firm chair.
- Clasp both hands together, straighten your elbows and raise your arms above your head or as high as you can.
- Use the uninjured arm to support the weight of the other.

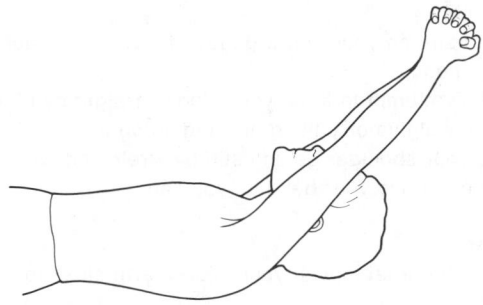

Other exercises
- Make sure that your elbow, wrist and hand all bend and straigthen fully. These all become stiff when your arm is not being used normally. Lifting heavy objects should not be attempted initially.
- Gradually increase the weight you lift. You should be able to do light chores such as washing-up and dusting.
- When getting dressed, remember it is much easier to put the injured arm into sleeves first.

Patients are then referred to the physiotherapy department where further treatment is undertaken as necessary.

Adjustment of the exercise programme at the 3-week stage includes muscle-strengthening exercises as the fracture heals.

Fractures of the radial head

Fractures of the radial head are more common in women and one study reports the average age as 36.5 years (Holdsworth *et al.*, 1987). Joint stiffness is not well tolerated in this age group.

A loss of more than 10° of extension results in discomfort when carrying objects, such as shopping bags, with the elbow extended. Early active movement aids recovery of extension and when combined with aspiration of the elbow joint and the instillation of local anaesthetic is not severely painful. This treatment should be considered for those stable radial head fractures with no or minimal displacement where the fracture involves less than one-third of the articular surface (Jupiter, 1992). Active exercises are demonstrated and patients are given simple written instructions and advised to apply ice over the biceps and anterior elbow joint to reduce flexor muscle spasm. Review of these patients by the fracture clinic physiotherapist at 1 week allows further advice and treatment if necessary.

TECHNIQUES

Elbow exercises

- These exercises should be performed slowly and smoothly.
- Try to stretch your elbow gently at the end of each movement.
- NEVER attempt to force your elbow straight by lifting heavy weights or pulling or hanging on it.
- Stop your shoulder getting stiff by stretching your arm as high above your head as you can.

Exercise 1
- Sit beside a table with your injured arm close to it.

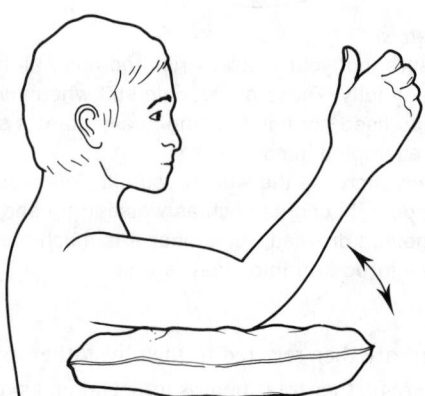

- Support your upper arm on a pillow or cushion so it is in a horizontal position.
- Bend your elbow as much as possible aiming to touch your fingers to your shoulder.
- Then straighten out your elbow as much as possible with the palm of your hand facing upwards.

Exercise 2
- Repeat the exercise above but this time with the palm of your hand facing downwards.

Exercise 3
- Sit beside a table as above.
- Bend your injured elbow to a right-angle.
- Twist your forearm so your palm faces first towards you, then away from you.

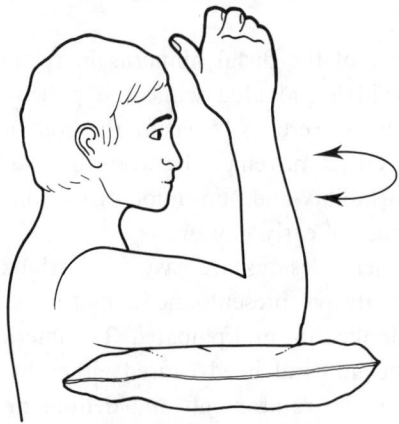

- Repeat all of these exercises ten times each hour.
- If you have been given a sling then try to wear this for short periods only. Take it off when you are sitting or lying down, straighten the elbow and rest the arm on a pillow.
- Use your arm to assist with washing, dressing, eating and other gentle everyday activities.

Removal of limb casts

The physiotherapist working within the fracture clinic also assesses those patients who have had plasters applied or removed. Plaster room staff should alert their patients to problems of plaster tightness or loosening. Plaster suppliers provide instruction sheets that cover maintenance exercises whilst in plaster. These must include active movements for those joints not immobilized, in particular abduction and external rotation of the shoulder for those in forearm casts must not be neglected. Exercises for finger and thumb flexion are especially important following application of external fixation.

When casts are removed the physiotherapist assesses range of motion, muscle strength and the presence of pain or discomfort. Written instructions are given and exercises demonstrated. Exercise sheets may describe general foot and ankle or wrist and hand activities with verbal reinforcement of specific objectives. Advising the patient to 'go away and use it normally' does not help an individual to obtain maximum benefit from treatment.

Many patients have unrealistic expectations of limb function following plaster removal and often need re-assuring that discomfort will decrease and joint stiffness will improve with use. Marked limitation of movement or function indicates the need for formal referral for physiotherapy. The progress of those with reasonable movement and function is reviewed by the physio-therapist on their next attendance at clinic. Patients may be invited to contact the clinic physiotherapist if progress is slow or further problems arise.

The presence of a clinic physiotherapist prevents both unnecessary referrals to the physiotherapy department and the omission of correct advice and treatment within the clinic.

CONCLUSION

The value of input from an experienced physiotherapist within the A&E department and fracture clinic setting has been discussed. In the absence of physiotherapy the same approaches to treatment must be undertaken by the A&E staff but this is not always easy to achieve. Evaluation of the therapist's role in individual units is important to determine the level of input required.

Bibliography

BROOKS, S.C., POTTER, B.T. & RAINEY, J.B. (1981). Treatment for partial tears of the lateral ligament of the ankle; a prospective trial. *Br. Med. J.*, **282**, 606–7.

CLIFFORD, P. (1980). Fractures of the neck of humerus: a review of late results. *Injury*, **12**(2), 91–5.

EVANS, P. (1980). The healing process at cellular level: a review. *Physiotherapy*, **66**(8), 256–9.

HASHERI, K. (1986). Early mobilisation of acute whiplash injuries. *Br. Med. J.*, **292**, 1079.

HOLDSWORTH, B.J., CLEMENT, D.A. & ROTH-WELL, P.N.R. (1987). Fractures of the radial head – the benefit of aspiration: a prospective controlled trial. *Injury*, **18**, 44–7.

JUPITER, J.B. (1992). Trauma to the adult elbow. In *Skeletal Trauma*, ed. B.D. Browner. Philadelphia: W.B. Saunders.

KANNUS, P. & JARVINEN, M. (1990). Non-operative treatment of acute knee injuries. *Sports Med.*, **9**(4), 244–60.

LIVESLEY, P.J., MUGGLESTON, A. & WHITTON, J (1992). Electrotherapy and the management of minimally displaced fracture of the neck of the humerus. *Injury*, **23**(5), 323–7.

MacNAB, I. (1977). The whiplash syndrome. *Orthop. Clin. North Am.*, **2**, 389–403.

MAITLAND, G.D. (1986). Fractures of the humerus. In *Peripheral Manipulation*, pp. 119–20. London: Butterworths.

McKINNEY, L.A. (1989). Early mobilisation and outcome in acute sprains of the neck. *Br. Med. J.*, **299**, 1005–6.

MUWANGA, C.L., QUINTON, D.N., SLOAN, J.P. et al. (1986). A new treatment of lateral ligament injuries of the ankle joint. *Injury*, **17**, 380.

NEER, C. (1970). Displaced proximal humeral fractures. Part 1: Classification and evaluation. *J. Bone Joint Surg.*, **52A**, 1077.

NORRIS, S.H. & WATT, I. (1983). The prognosis of neck injuries resulting from rear end collisions. *J. Bone Joint Surg.*, **65B**, 608–11.

RYAN, J.B., WHEELER, J.H., HOPKINSON, W.J. et al. (1991). Quadriceps contusion. *Am. J. Sports Med.*, **19**(3), 299–303.

WILLIAMS, J. (1979). Injury in sport. Newbury: Bayer UK.

YOUNG, T.B. & WALLACE, W.A. (1985). Conservative treatment of fractures and fracture dislocations of the upper end of the humerus. *J. Bone Joint Surg.*, **67B**, 373.

ZWIPP, H., HOFFMAN, R., THERMANN, H. et al. (1991). Rupture of the ankle ligaments. *Int. Orthop.*, **15**, 245–9.

43 Envenomation

A.F.T. BROWN

Department of Emergency Medicine, Royal Brisbane Hospital, Queensland, Australia

Chapter plan

Hymenoptera envenomation
Snakebite
Arachnid envenomation
Marine envenomation

HYMENOPTERA ENVENOMATION

The insect order Hymenoptera includes bees, wasps, hornets, yellow jackets and ants. The females of the species inject venom by means of a sting, which is barbed and breaks off in honeybees but is unbarbed in wasps and hornets allowing repeated stings (Lok & Chen, 1987).

Stings are common, although fatalities are rare, averaging one fatal bee sting per 5 million population per year. However, in the USA this represents more deaths from anaphylaxis to bee sting than to all other venomous creatures put together (Sutherland, 1983b).

Hymenoptera species are ubiquitous. Those of medical interest include:

EUROPE
European honeybee (*Apis mellifera*)
Africanized honeybee (*Apis mellifera scutellata*)
European wasp (*Vespula germanica*)
Paper-nest wasp (*Polistes annularis*)
European hornet (*Vespa crabro*)

USA
European and Africanized honeybee
Paper-nest wasp
White-faced hornet (*Dolichovespula maculata*)
Yellow jacket (*Vespula pensylvanica*)
Fire ant (*Solenopsis* sp.)

AUSTRALIA
European honeybee
European wasp
Paper-nest wasp
Bulldog ant (*Myrmecia pyriformis*)
Jack-jumper ant (*Myrmecia pilosula*)

Pathophysiology

Local reactions may be inflammatory, or allergic with immediate, generalized or delayed hypersensitivity.

Multiple stings result in a direct toxic action of the venom itself, rather than an allergic reaction. Fifty or more wasp stings may prove fatal. Survival has occurred after over 1000 honeybee stings (Schmidt, 1991).

Honeybee venom includes non-allergenic amines such as acetylcholine, histamine and catecholamines, as well as melittin and apamin polypeptides and major allergens such as phospholipase A_2, hyaluronidase and acid phosphatase.

Clinical presentation

Normal local reactions to the sting include pain, irritation, redness and swelling lasting up to a few hours. Painful vesicles or pustulation may occur, particularly following fire ant stings.

Multiple stings may cause headache, vomiting, diarrhoea, hypotension, fits and coma.

Allergic reactions include extensive local swelling and pain that may persist for several days. This does not necessarily predict systemic anaphylaxis which occurs in 5–10% only (Golden, 1987).

Systemic allergic reactions may appear in minutes and include generalized urticaria, erythema, pruritus, upper airway oedema, stridor, wheeze and dysphagia.

Cardiovascular collapse with hypotension and coma are seen in anaphylactic shock. Non-steroidal anti-inflammatory drugs appear to increase sensitivity to bee stings, while beta-blockers increase the severity and duration of anaphylaxis (Herriott, 1989) and also interfere with treatment with beta-agonists.

Delayed hypersensitivity reactions such as a serum sickness–like illness are rare, but may occur usually within 1 week of envenomation, producing fever, arthralgia, myalgia, lymphadenopathy, headache, glomerulonephritis and vasculitis.

Management

Severe reactions including anaphylaxis require urgent treatment with advanced life support measures in a resuscitation area.

Oxygen, adrenaline, immediate venous access and rapid volume replacement form the mainstay of treatment (see also Chapter 8). Most deaths result from airway obstruction; therefore early tracheal intubation may be life-saving.

Local wound reactions require cleansing of the puncture site and, for honeybee stings, removal of the sting using the back of a knife or piece of card gently scraped over the skin. Ice is applied and the limb elevated. Tetanus prophylaxis is given according to the patient's immune status. Oral antihistamine such as chlorpheniramine 4 mg 6-hourly may decrease local pruritus and swelling.

All patients with systemic anaphylaxis must be admitted, preferably to an intensive care area as in 20%, life-threatening manifestations may recur up to 12 h after treatment of the initial episode. In addition, all multiply stung patients are admitted as rhabdomyolysis and acute renal failure may develop. Serum sickness is treated with a course of oral steroids.

Prevention

Avoid places known to be frequented by bees, wasps, etc.; wear shoes outside, avoid brightly coloured clothes and perfumes. Use a straw to drink from a can. Those with a serious known bee or wasp sting allergy should carry an adrenaline injection kit at all times, on the advice of an allergist or immunologist.

SNAKEBITE

There are 3000 species of snake worldwide, of which only 10% are venomous. In Europe, all venomous snakes are vipers and, although estimates vary, up to 20 deaths may occur annually. In Britain, about 100 people per year are bitten by snakes but only 14 deaths were recorded in the 100 years prior to 1976 (Reid, 1976).

In the USA there are four broad types of venomous snake: three crotalids (the rattlesnakes, copperhead and cottonmouth snakes) and one elapid (the coral snake). Every state except Alaska, Maine and Hawaii has at least one dangerous species. Up to 8000 people per year are bitten, usually between April and October, producing nine to 15 fatalities annually.

In Australia, all venomous snakes are elapids and despite the fact that the ten most venomous snakes in the world are Australian, only one or two fatalities are recorded per year from around 3000 snakebites.

Examples of species of medical interest include:

EUROPE
Vipers
    European adder (*Vipera berus*) – the only venomous snake in the UK
    Asp viper (*Vipera aspis*)
    Latastes viper (*Vipera latasti*)
    Meadow viper (*Vipera ursinii*)
    Sand viper (*Vipera ammodytes*)
Moccasin
    Pallas' viper (*Agkistrodon halys*)

USA
Crotalidae
Rattlesnakes
    Eastern diamondback (*Crotalus adamanteus*)
    Western diamondback (*Crotalus atrox*)
    Timber (*Crotalus horridus*)
    Western (*Crotalus viridis*)
    Sidewinder (*Crotalus cerastes*)
    Mojave (*Crotalus scutulatas*)
    Pigmy (*Sistrurus miliarius*)
    Massasauga (*Sistrurus catenatus*)
Moccasins
    Cottonmouth (*Agkistrodon piscivorous*)
    Copperhead (*Agkistrodon contortrix*)

Elapidae
Coral snakes
    Arizona/Sonoran (*Micruroides euryxanthus*)
    Eastern (*Micrurus fulvius*)

AUSTRALIA

Elapidae

Tiger snakes

    Common (*Notechis scutatus*)

    Western (*Notechis ater occidentalis*)

Brown snakes

    Common (*Pseudonaja textilis*)

    Gwardar (*Pseudonaja nuchalis*)

    Dugite (*Pseudonaja affinis*)

Taipan

    Oxyuranus scutellatus

    Fierce/small scaled (*Oxyuranus microlepidotus*)

Death adder

    Common (*Acanthophis antarcticus*)

    Desert (*Acanthophis pyrrhus*)

Black snakes

    Red-bellied black (*Pseudechis porphyriacus*)

    King brown/Mulga (*Pseudechis australis*)

Copperhead

    Australian copperhead (*Austrelaps superbus*)

Rough scaled snake

    Tropidechis carinatus

Viper envenomation

All European venomous snakes are vipers, with the greatest number and most venomous species found in the Mediterranean region. The only naturally occurring variety found in Britain is the adder or northern viper (*Vipera berus*). The following text refers to envenomation by this species.

Clinical features

Less than 50% of bites by the adder are followed by envenomation. If envenomation does occur, the bite is followed by immediate pain and swelling within minutes, although occasionally these local features are absent despite severe envenomation. Local tender lymphadenopathy is seen. Oedema may increase to a maximum over 2–3 days.

Systemic features include vomiting, abdominal pain, diarrhoea, tachycardia and hypotension. Collapse and coma, or drowsiness with ptosis may occur, but generalized bleeding is rare (Persson & Irestedt, 1981). Nonspecific ECG (electrocardiogram) changes and a neutrophil leucocytosis may be seen. Oliguric renal failure, pulmonary oedema and acute anaphylaxis have occurred on rare occasions.

Management

First aid

The patient is reassured and kept warm. Constrictive clothes are removed and the bitten limb is immobilized in a functional position below the level of the heart. A firm bandage may be applied to restrict venous return, without obstructing the arterial supply. Arterial tourniquets, incision, suction and ice are no longer recommended.

A&E department

The patient is managed in a resuscitation area with cardiac monitoring. Large-bore venous access is gained and blood sent for full blood count, coagulation profile, urea and electrolytes, and creatine kinase. An ECG is performed.

Hypotension is treated initially with oxygen and fluids, and tetanus prophylaxis is given according to the patient's immune status. Frequent observations including limb girth measurements are made.

Use of antivenom

Zagreb antivenom is indicated for persistent or recurrent hypotension, polymorphonuclear leucocytosis greater than 20 000 per mm^3, ECG abnormalities or extensive limb swelling within 4 h of the bite. Two ampoules of Zagreb antivenom are diluted to 50 ml in saline, given intravenously over 30 min to adults or children, and repeated after 1–2 h if there is no clinical improvement. Adrenaline and full resuscitation facilities must be immediately available to treat possible hypersensitivity.

Less severe poisoning with moderate pain and swelling and mild gastrointestinal disturbance requires symptomatic treatment only.

Further management

Every patient with suspected snakebite must be admitted for a period of observation of at least 12 h.

Advice on management and the use of antivenom is available at all times from: New Cross Poisons Unit (tel: 0171 635 9191) or other local Poisons Information Services (see Chapter 11). Information on the supply and use of antivenom for certain other foreign snakes and spiders is also held at New Cross.

Crotalid snake envenomation

Crotalid snakes have a temperature- (prey)-sensitive pit below the eye, hence their common name of pit vipers.

In the USA these include the rattlesnakes, pigmy and massasauga, copperhead and cottonmouth.

Pathophysiology

Venom is injected through a pair of fangs which are rotated from their resting position folded against the roof of the mouth. The venom is a complex mixture of proteins with enzymatic activity including esterase, hyaluronidase, phospholipase and protease, although the lethal fraction may be certain low molecular weight peptides with specific receptor sites.

The venom causes local tissue necrosis with systemic vascular damage, haemolysis, coagulation defects and relatively minor neuromuscular dysfunction (except for the Mojave that has few local effects but significant delayed neuromuscular blockade).

Clinical presentation

Bites by non-venomous snakes are much more common than bites by venomous snakes in the USA. Also, up to 30% of venomous snake bites are 'dry' with no injection of venom and no systemic poisoning. However, as species recognition is difficult, even for experts, every case of snakebite must be treated as an emergency.

Symptoms and signs

Fear and panic are a common reaction to both non-venomous and venomous snake bite and may cause emotional lability, nausea, vomiting, sweating, faintness and tachycardia.

Cardinal signs of envenomation are fang puncture marks with pain out of proportion to the local trauma, and swelling and erythema usually within minutes. If pain is absent at 1 h and oedema and erythema by 4 h, envenomation is highly unlikely.

Systemic features include hypotension and shock in severe envenomation, leading to convulsions, coma and respiratory failure. Other more common signs are perioral paraesthesiae extending peripherally, nausea, vomiting and muscular fasciculation. Intravascular clotting may lead to haematemesis or haematuria.

Envenomation may be graded clinically into four categories, although patients may deteriorate from one grade to another as envenomation progresses (see Table 1).

Table 1. *Classification of severity of envenomation following crotalid bite*

1. Dry bite
   - Mild puncture wound pain only; minimal or no oedema
   - No systemic symptoms or signs
   - Normal laboratory investigation

2. Minimal
   - Localized pain, oedema and erythema
   - No systemic symptoms
   - Normal laboratory investigation

3. Moderate
   - Progressive pain, oedema, erythema and bruising
   - Variable systemic symptoms with stable vital signs
   - Mild laboratory abnormalities

4. Severe
   - Severe pain, massive oedema and ecchymosis
   - Coma, fits, respiratory depression, clinical coagulopathy
   - Unstable vital signs
   - Marked laboratory abnormalities

Investigations

Blood should be sent for a full blood count including platelets as anaemia and thrombocytopenia occur. A coagulation profile including prothrombin time, partial thromboplastin time and fibrinogen level will reveal coagulopathy; serum is sent for electrolytes, urea, creatinine and creatine kinase. Urine is tested for sugar, protein, blood and myoglobin.

A chest X-ray may show pulmonary oedema, and arterial blood gases and an ECG are indicated in severe poisoning.

Management

First aid treatment

The patient is rested, kept warm and reassured. Any restrictive rings or clothing are removed. The injured limb is immobilized in a functional position below the level of the heart. The use of a tourniquet, ice, incision and suction is controversial and is not recommended, particularly when performed by lay people (Gold & Barish, 1992). The patient should be transported immediately to the nearest medical facility.

A&E department

The patient should be managed in a resuscitation area. Rapid venous access is gained using large-bore cannulae. Blood is sent for laboratory studies and shock is treated with a crystalloid infusion. The degree of envenomation is then graded clinically (see Table 1) and antivenin given for any bites showing evidence of envenomation.

In addition, tetanus prophylaxis is given according to the patient's immune status and systemic antibiotics covering Gram-negative organisms are administered for all bites other than trivial scratches (which may still have caused envenomation and require antivenin).

Use of antivenin

Wyeth equine polyvalent *Crotalidae* antivenin remains the mainstay of treatment for snakesbite envenomation. Most therapeutic failures result from inadequate or delayed dosage.

If a definite decision to use antivenin is made, an intradermal skin test should be performed immediately (see antivenin brochure). If positive, the patient may still be given antivenin in an intensive care setting following pretreatment with diphenhydramine, adrenaline and corticosteroids.

Each vial of antivenin is diluted to 10 ml with the supplied diluent, then diluted a further two- to five-fold in crystalloid solution. Three to five vials are given intravenously for minimal envenomation, 8–10 vials for moderate envenomation and 15–20 vials for severe envenomation. A syringe of adrenaline must be ready to treat any signs of anaphylaxis. These amounts are merely a guide, as absolute dosage of antivenin depends on the snake, patient, clinical severity and progression of signs. Children should receive similar or higher doses than adults, although care must be taken with the total amount of fluid used in the dilutions (Gold & Barish, 1990).

Further management

Every patient with suspected snakebite must be observed for a minimum of 6–8 h. Any patient with evidence of envenomation must be admitted to an intensive care or high-dependency area. Mild serum sickness may occur in up to 70% of all patients given antivenin, although only 5% will require oral steroids for fever, rash, arthralgia and tender lymphadenopathy (Corrigan *et al.*, 1978).

Elapid snake envenomation

Elapid snakes have relatively short fangs set in a fixed erect position. In the USA these include the coral snakes, and in Australia all the important venomous species such as the tiger, brown, black, taipan, death adder, copperhead and rough scaled snakes.

Pathophysiology

Australian elapid venoms are the most toxic in the world. The venom is a mixture of active components including neurotoxins, myotoxins, haemotoxins and others (postulated) with direct toxic effects on the nervous system, heart, kidney and histamine release.

Neurotoxins produce a non-depolarizing block at the neuromuscular junction by both a presynaptic action that is slow and progressive, and a postsynaptic action that is rapid and reversed by antivenom. Myotoxins lead to breakdown of skeletal muscle with myoglobinuria and renal failure; haemotoxins include both coagulants and anticoagulants leading to defibrination and coagulopathy.

Clinical presesentation

The majority of bites by elapids are 'dry' with envenomation only occurring in 10–30% cases. Also, unlike crotalid bites, local effects are usually minimal or absent.

Symptoms and signs

Most bites cause little pain and may even go unnoticed, although continued bleeding from the bitten area or marked local swelling (usually following a mulga bite) may be seen. Skin marks from the fangs range from tiny punctures or fine scratches to no apparent injury, yet serious envenomation can still ensue. Local tender lymphadenopathy is common although neither sensitive nor specific for systemic envenomation.

Systemic envenomation may cause sudden collapse, convulsions and occasionally rapid death. This usually follows a common brown snake bite but the exact mechanism is unclear. Headache, nausea, vomiting, abdominal pain and transient hypotension are common. Neurotoxic effects usually affect the cranial nerves first with ptosis, diplopia and dysphagia. Drowsiness progressing to coma and generalized weakness progressing to respiratory failure are seen in severe envenomations. Coagulopathy may be asymptomatic or cause bite site or venepuncture oozing, haematemesis, melaena and haematuria. Rhabdomyolysis causes myoglobinuria.

Investigations

Blood should be sent for full blood count, coagulation profile, urea, electrolytes, creatinine and creatine kinase. Urine is sent for protein, haemoglobin, myoglobin and venom detection.

Venom detection

A skin swab taken from the bite site should be sent for venom detection. The Venom Detection Kit (Commonwealth Serum Laboratories Ltd.) is a micro-ELISA (enzyme-linked immunosorbent assay) designed to distinguish between the five venom groups for which a monovalent antivenom is available. A skin swab or urine sample is used and a result is available within 30 min. Blood has proved far less reliable (Hurrell & Chandler, 1982).

Management

First aid

The 'pressure-immobilization technique' developed in Australia in 1979 is recommended for all elapid bites (and for sea snake bites, funnel web spider bite, severe box jellyfish sting, blue-ringed octopus and cone shell envenomation). A broad, firm bandage is applied around the bite site and up the limb as tight as one would bandage a sprained ankle. A splint is then applied to keep the limb immobile, and transport is brought to the patient. The principle involved is to impede the spread of venom through local lymphatics and capillaries, with the advantage that the bandage is comfortable and may be left on many hours (Sutherland et al., 1979).

Incision, excision, suction and arterial tourniquets are not recommended. The bite site should not be washed so that more reliable skin swabs can be obtained for use with the Venom Detection Kit.

A&E department

The patient is managed in a resuscitation area with cardiac and pulse oximetry monitoring. Large-bore venous access is gained and blood is sent to the laboratory. A pressure-immobilization bandage is applied if not already in place, and a skin swab and urine sample are sent for venom detection.

Use of antivenom

Antivenom is available for the Eastern coral snake in the USA. There is either monovalent equine antivenom for the tiger, brown, taipan, death adder and black snake in Australia, or a polyvalent equine antivenom which covers all five (Commonwealth Serum Laboratories Ltd.).

Indications for antivenom are definite clinical or laboratory evidence of envenomation. The mere suspicion of a venomous bite or a positive skin venom swab alone are not indications for its use. The choice and amount of antivenom depends on clinical circumstances and geographical location (see Figure 1).

Pretreatment is recommended with promethazine 25 mg IV, then hydrocortisone 200 mg IV. Adrenaline 0.3 mg (or 0.01 mg kg^{-1} for a child) is given subcutaneously.

The antivenom is diluted ten-fold and given slowly at 1 ml min^{-1} for 5 min, then the remainder over 30 min in the absence of an allergic reaction. If an acute reaction occurs, the antivenom infusion is stopped and further treatment with adrenaline, fluids and oxygen is given until it resolves, when the antivenom is restarted.

Tetanus prophylaxis is given according to the patient's immune status. All patients who receive polyvalent antivenom or multiple doses of monovalent antivenom should be given a 5-day course of oral steroids to reduce the incidence of delayed serum sickness (Sutherland, 1992).

Further management

Every patient with suspected snakebite must be admitted for a period of observation, even if asymptomatic with minimal or no visible skin abrasion. Repeated clinical and laboratory assessment, particularly for coagulopathy, should be made for at least 12 h after removal of any first aid measures. Suspected envenomation should be treated in an intensive care or high-dependency area. Repeated doses of antivenom may be required (Tibbals, 1992) and, similar to the use of crotalid antivenin, about 10% of patients will develop significant serum sickness following polyvalent antivenom and require steroids (Sutherland, 1983a).

ARACHNID ENVENOMATION

Arachnids as a group include spiders, ticks and scorpions. Thousands of species are known but, although many are capable of envenomation, only a small minority are potentially serious.

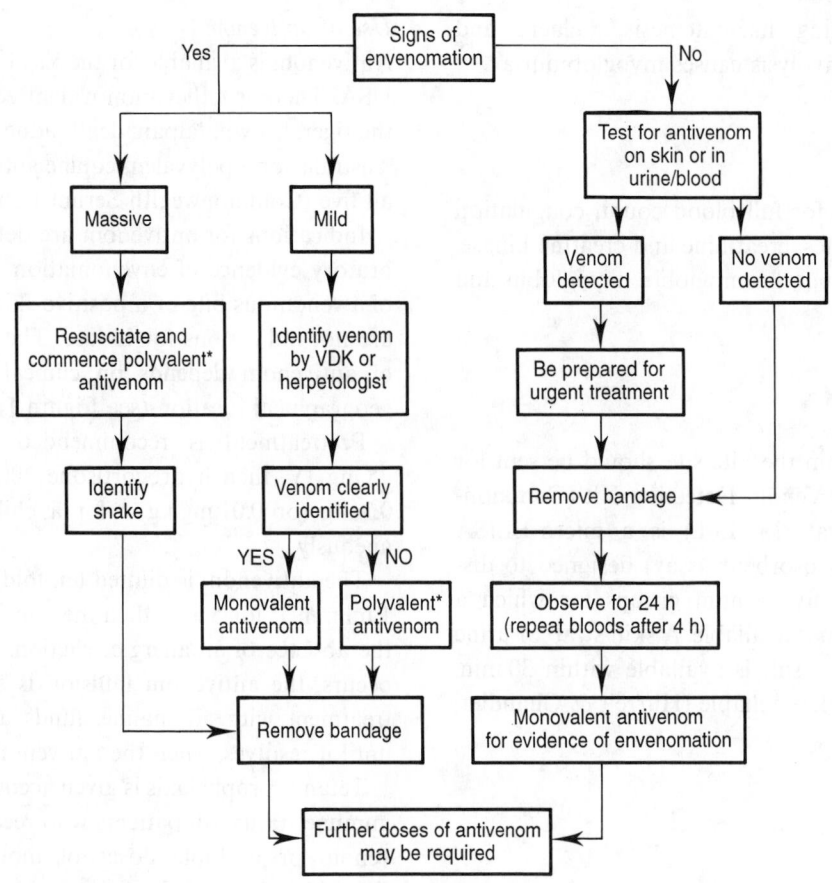

* Victoria: use tiger snake plus brown snake antivenom (not polyvalent)
Tasmania: use tiger snake antivenom (not polyvalent)

Fig. 1. Management of Australian elapid snakebite. VDK, venom detection kit (Commonwealth Serum Laboratories Ltd.). (Adapted and reproduced, with permission, from Myers, C.T. & Dunjey, S.J. (1992). *Emerg. Med.*, **4**, 50–1)

Examples of particular medical interest include:

EUROPE
Spiders
   Latrodectus sp.
Ticks
   Tick paralysis (*Haemaphysalis puncata*)
                  (*Ixodes ricinus*)
   Lyme disease (*Ixodes dammini* as vector for *Borrelia burgdorferi*)

USA
Spiders
   Black widow (*Latrodectus mactans*)
   Brown recluse (*Loxosceles reclusa*)
Ticks
   Tick paralysis (*Amblyomma americanum*)
   Lyme disease
   Rocky Mountain spotted fever (*Dermacentor* sp. as vector for *Rickettsia rickettsiae*)
   Tularemia (*Dermacentor* sp. as vector for *Francisella tularensis*)

Scorpions
   Centruroides sp.

AUSTRALIA
Spiders
   Red back (*Latrodectus mactans hasselti*)
   Sydney funnelweb (*Atrax robustus*)
   White tailed (*Lampona cylindrata*)
Ticks
   Tick paralysis (*Ixodes holocyclus*)
   Lyme disease

Latrodectism

Latrodectus species are common in the USA (black widow), Australia (red back), New Zealand (katipo) and Eastern Europe. Only the female is dangerous; although not naturally aggressive, she will bite if trapped in shoes or clothing.

Pathophysiology

The venom contains alpha-latrotoxin which causes depletion of acetylcholine at motor nerve endings and provokes the release of catecholamines at adrenergic nerve endings.

Clinical features

Although the initial bite may go unnoticed, local pain, erythema and sweating soon occur, followed by painful regional lymphadenopathy. Remote pain in the abdomen or a hitherto unaffected limb, nausea, vomiting and malaise may occur. Generalized sweating, paraesthesiae, mild pyrexia, headache and hypertension all occur in decreasing order of frequency (Brown, 1989).

Bizarre presentations include tingling teeth, tetanic spasms, haemoptysis, trismus, priapism and periorbital oedema (Sutherland & Trinca, 1978). Latrodectism should be considered in the intractable crying baby and may mimic peritonitis and testicular torsion.

Management

First aid consists solely of the local application of cold packs or wrapped, crushed ice. Any local pressure or tourniquet merely increases the pain.

A&E department management depends on the severity of findings. In the USA, symptomatic treatment including diazepam 5–10 mg IV, methocarbamol 15 mg kg^{-1} IV and 10% calcium gluconate (up to 10 ml IV) for muscle cramps, together with oral or parenteral analgesia is favoured. Antivenom derived from horse serum is reserved for severe cases involving marked hypertension for age, protracted pain, pregnancy with symptoms of envenomation, and patients at the extremes of age (Allen, 1992). One 15-ml vial diluted to 50 ml is given intravenously over 15 min.

In Australia, an equine antivenom has been available since 1956 and is recommended for definite or distressing evidence of envenomation. It is given intramuscularly usually within 24 h of the bite, following pretreatment with antihistamine and adrenaline when the patient has a known allergy to equine protein or has received antivenom before. Multiple doses of antivenom may be required. Tetanus prophylaxis is given according to the patient's immune status.

No fatalities have been reported in Australia since 1955, although in North America the black widow is the leading cause of death from spider bites (Kobernick, 1984).

Loxoscelism

Various *Loxosceles* species are known including the violin spider, Arizona brown spider, fiddleback, brown recluse and necrotizing spider.

Pathophysiology

Loxosceles venom contains proteases, esterase, hyaluronidase, collagenase and sphingomyelinase D which cause local and systemic reactions including haemolysis, intravascular coagulation and activation of complement. Skin necrosis is caused by the activation of clotting mechanisms, with aggregation of leucocytes and platelets forming a haemostatic plug in venules and arterioles (Gendron, 1990).

Clinical features

The bite typically causes only minor stinging or burning that begins to itch, swell and may become tender and purpuric over a few hours.

Systemic effects develop over 24–48 h and include fever, chills, malaise, myalgia, arthralgia and a scarlatiniform rash.

Skin necrosis with ulceration can develop from hours to weeks following a bite and is referred to as 'necrotizing arachnidism'. The most severe lesions occur in fatty areas over the abdomen, thigh and buttocks.

Laboratory investigations may show anaemia, leucocytosis, thrombocytopenia and evidence of haemolysis with disseminated intravascular coagulation in severe systemic arachnidism.

Differential diagnosis of necrotizing arachnidism

This includes other causes of skin necrosis such as vasculitis, drug reactions, foreign bodies, artefact, infections and infarction. Necrotizing arachnidism may be caused by species other than *Loxosceles reclusa*, including the orbweaver (*Argiope*), sac spider (*Chiracanthium*), wolf spider (*Lycosa*), jumping spider (*Phidippus*) and Northwestern brown spider (*Tegenaria agrestis*). In Australia, the white tailed spider (*Lampona cylindrata*), black window spider (*Badumna insignis*) and the cupboard spider (*Steatoda* sp.) are all implicated.

Management

Local immobilization and elevation is often all that is required. An oral analgesic or oral antihistamine may be given to reduce pruritus together with tetanus prophylaxis according to the patient's immune status.

Systemic arachnidism requires aggressive, supportive care as fatalities have been reported, particularly in children. Methylprednisolone 1–2 mg kg^{-1} IV 6-hourly may protect against haemolysis.

Various treatments have been advocated for the skin necrosis, ranging from delayed surgical debridement, high-voltage DC, steroids and antibiotics, to dapsone, a polymorphonuclear leucocyte inhibitor (providing the patient has a negative glucose-6-phosphate dehydrogenase screen). The use of hyperbaric oxygen has been reported (Svendsen, 1986) although it is still considered experimental.

Funnel web spider

There are 35 species of funnel web spider grouped into two genera, *Atrax* and *Hadronyche*, distributed throughout South Eastern Australia. The Sydney funnel web spider *Atrax robustus* is confined to a 160 km radius of Sydney, with the male being responsible for severe envenomations.

Pathophysiology

The venom of the Sydney funnel web includes GABA (gamma-aminobutyric acid), a spermine–indole acetic acid complex, hyaluronidase and atraxotoxin. The latter is responsible for the potentially lethal effects by releasing acetylcholine at the motor end-plates, and acetylcholine, adrenaline and noradrenaline throughout the autonomic nervous system.

Clinical features

Envenomation follows less than one in five bites. Severe pain at the bite site is followed by localized muscle fasciculation, generalized fasciculations, nausea, vomiting, abdominal pain, sweating, salivation, lacrimation and piloerection. Initial hypertension and tachycardia give way to hypotension and circulatory collapse. Pulmonary oedema, confusion and coma may occur.

Management

First aid is by the pressure-immobilization technique. If the patient presents with symptoms or systemic signs of envenomation or develops symptoms within 4 h of the removal of first aid, antivenom is indicated. Two vials of antivenom (Commonwealth Serum Laboratories Ltd.) are given slowly intravenously following pretreatment with parenteral antihistamine and hydrocortisone. Otherwise, patients who remain asymptomatic 4 h after the removal of first aid measures may be safely discharged.

Thirteen deaths of humans have occurred since 1927 but since the introduction of the antivenom in 1980 there have been no further fatalities. In addition, the antivenom has proved successful in envenomation by funnel web species other than *Atrax robustus* (Dieckmann *et al.*, 1989).

Tick paralysis

This is a progressive paralysis due to a neurotoxin released from the salivary glands of several species of tick, and has been reported worldwide.

Usually the presence of the tick is unknown to the patient who presents with a vague prodrome of malaise, irritability and paraesthesiae. This is followed within 24 h by progressive motor neuropathy with localized paralysis leading to patchy, generalized, flaccid weakness and decreased tendon reflexes. Rarely, acute allergic reactions to tick bites have been recorded with occasional severe anaphylaxis.

Symptoms occur after 5–7 days of the tick feeding and usually resolve after its removal. This is best performed using the point of a pair of scissors slid under the head which is gently levered out without crushing. Human fatalities have been recorded from bulbar and respiratory failure; in Australia, therefore, patients with significant envenomation are given one to two ampoules of antitoxin intravenously following pretreatment with antihistamine and adrenaline.

MARINE ENVENOMATION

Three-quarters of the world's surface is water. Hazards from marine life include trauma such as shark attack, envenomation from vertebrates and invertebrates and toxic fish ingestion.

Marine trauma

Sharks

Thirty-two of the 300 species of shark are implicated in approximately 100 annual shark attacks worldwide. Seven deaths from shark attacks have been recorded in the USA since 1926 and approximately 186 in Australia since records began in 1788. The commonest species involved include the great white, blue, mako, bull and grey reef sharks (Brown & Shepherd, 1992).

Patient management is based on the standard trauma approach of airway and ventilatory support, haemorrhage control and treatment of circulatory shock. Wounds are prone to contamination with aerobes and anaerobes and require debridement, exploration and delayed primary closure. Antibiotics, such as imipenem 1 g IV 6-hourly, and tetanus prophylaxis are required.

Other fish

The great barracuda in tropical seas, moray eel in tropical, subtropical and temperate waters and the giant grouper in tropical and temperate seas have all caused severe injury. Paradoxically, despite its name, the killer whale (*Orcinus orca*) has never been documented to attack a human, hunting sea lions instead.

Vertebrate marine envenomation

Over 200 species of fish envenomate by spines located on the gill covers, or dorsal, pelvic and anal fins. In addition, envenomation may follow the bite of a sea snake that produces a myotoxic and neurotoxic venom.

Examples of medical interest include:

EUROPE
Stingray
Catfish
Scorpionfish (*Scorpaena* sp.)
Weever fish

USA
Stingray
Catfish
Scorpionfish
Weever fish
Lionfish (*Pterois volitans* – imported)

AUSTRALIA
Stingray
Catfish
Stonefish (*Synanceia verrucosa/trachynis*)
Bullrout (*Notesthes robusta*)
Lionfish
Sea snake (*Hydrophiidae* sp.)

Stingray

Stingrays are the most commonly encountered venomous fish with over 2000 cases per year in the USA. They are peaceful, reclusive, bottom feeders that are inadvertently stepped on by unsuspecting swimmers leading to injury by lashing of their tail causing local lacerations and envenomation.

The venom released by the tail barb is unstable and heat-labile, and includes several toxic compounds producing varying degrees of cardiovascular and neurological disturbance.

Following the sting, local pain is immediate and severe, radiating centrally and sometimes causing disorientation. Systemic symptoms occur within an hour and include nausea, vomiting, weakness and muscle cramps. Hypotension, cardiac arrhythmias and death have occurred.

Treatment involves immediate wound irrigation followed by immersion in hot (but not scalding) water at 45–50°C. Local anaesthetic infiltration or a regional block may be required. Wound exploration to remove the barb fragments under sterile conditions is then indicated, with tetanus prophylaxis and antibiotics such as trimethoprim-sulphamethoxazole (Septrin) two tablets twice a day for 1 week.

Catfish, scorpionfish, weever fish, lion fish, stonefish and bullrout

All these fish have poisonous spines or fins, the most lethal being the stonefish which inhabits Indo-Pacific waters. The extent of envenomation depends upon the species, number and location of stings, amount of venom injected and the size and health of the victim.

Intense, throbbing pain is usually immediate and severe, with local erythema, bruising and oedema. Systemic symptoms include nausea, vomiting, abdominal cramps and weakness. Stonefish envenomation may rapidly lead to respiratory difficulty, hypotension and cardiovascular collapse requiring immediate cardiopulmonary resuscitation.

First aid is by immersion in hot water at 40–50°C which produces symptomatic relief by denaturing the heat-labile toxin. Local anaesthetic or a regional block may be needed, even systemic analgesia. Antivenom is available for stonefish envenomation in Australia and the Indo-Pacific region (Commonwealth Serum Laboratories Ltd.) and is recommended for all but the most mild cases. The dose is one ampoule intramuscularly containing

2000 units in 2 ml for every two skin puncture wounds (Sutherland and Trinca, 1981).

Wound debridement and antibiotic cover such as trimethoprim-sulphamethoxazole (Septrin) are indicated for deep or necrotic wounds. Radiographs should be obtained to rule out retained foreign bodies. Tetanus prophylaxis is given according to the patient's immune status.

Sea snakes

Sea snakes are found in the warmer waters of the Western Pacific and Indian Ocean, but not in the Atlantic Ocean or Caribbean. All 52 species are venomous, the most dangerous being the beaked sea snake *Enhydrina schistosa*. They are an occupational hazard for fishermen when they are entangled in the nets, and for divers.

The highly potent venom is neurotoxic, acting at both pre- and postsynaptic terminals, and myotoxic, containing phospholipase A; it also includes other haemotoxins, cardiotoxins and vasoactive compounds capable of causing acute anaphylaxis.

The initial bite is often painless and may only resemble a scratch (similar to an elapid snakebite). Envenomation is characterized by myalgia within 60 min. Aches, pains, stiffness and weakness occur in the arms, thigh, trunk or neck muscles. Rhabdomyolysis with hyperkalaemia and myoglobinuria becomes evident within 6 h. Vomiting, ptosis, diplopia and mydriasis are all sinister signs.

Management is similar to Australian elapid envenomation and includes the pressure–immobilization first aid technique. Antivenom is only indicated for definite clinical evidence of envenomation, as most bites are 'dry' with no venom introduced. It is available from the Commonwealth Serum Laboratories Ltd. and is given intravenously after pretreatment, as for terrestrial snakes. In an emergency, tiger snake antivenom or even polyvalent (Australia/Papua New Guinea) antivenom may be used. Tetanus prophylaxis is given according to the patient's immune status.

All suspected cases must be admitted, however bizarre or trivial their initial symptoms, until serious poisoning can be excluded.

Invertebrate marine envenomation

Over 100 species of coelenterates are dangerous to man and include the classes Scyphozoa (true jelly fish and sea wasps), Hydrozoa (Portuguese Man-of-War, fire coral) and Anthozoa (sea anemones, true coral). Other venomous invertebrates include Echinodermata (sea urchins, starfish, sea cucumbers) and the molluscs, responsible for cone shell stings, blue-ringed octopus bites and toxic pelecypod ingestion (e.g. clams, oysters, scallops).

Examples of medical interest include:

EUROPE
True jelly fish
 Little mauve stinger (*Pelagia noctiluca*)
Portuguese Man-of-War (*Physalia physalis*)
Sea anemones, true coral
Sea urchins, star fish, sea cucumbers

USA
True jelly fish
 Little mauve stinger
 Sea nettle (*Chrysaora quinquecirrha*)
 Moon jellyfish (*Aurelia aurita*)
Portuguese Man-of-War, fire coral
Sea anemones, true coral
Sea urchins, star fish, sea cucumbers

AUSTRALIA
True jelly fish
 Little mauve stinger
 Box jellyfish or sea wasp (*Chironex fleckeri*)
 Irukandji (*Carukia barnesi*)
Portuguese Man-of-War, fire coral
Sea anemones, true coral
Sea urchins, star fish, sea cucumbers
Cone shells (*Conus* sp.)
Blue-ringed octopus (*Hapalochlaena maculosa*)

Portuguese Man-of-War

This ubiquitous hydrozoan may have a floating sail up to 30 cm across with tentacles up to 30 m long containing millions of nematocysts. Broken-off tentacles washed onto a beach may remain potentially venomous for weeks.

Stings range from mild burning pain, to erythema, blistering, oedema and severe pain with respiratory, cardiac and neurological involvement. Delayed manifestations including cutaneous reactions and renal failure are seen.

First aid includes rinsing with sea water (not fresh water), gentle tentacle removal using forceps and gloves, and the application of cold packs for skin pain. Vinegar, once popular, is no longer recommended as it may cause further nematocyst discharge and does nothing for the existing pain (Exton et al., 1989). Further supportive medical care is given according to symptoms.

Box jellyfish (sea wasp)

Chironex fleckeri, the box jellyfish, is found in the tropical waters of South-East Asia and Northern Australia over the summer months (November to April), often in the shallows. It is the most lethal coelenterate with over 60 deaths recorded in Australia (Lumley et al., 1988) compared with only two recent fatalities due to the Portuguese Man-of-War in the USA.

The venom has neuromuscular and vasopermeable toxic effects causing severe local pain. The tentacles produce a characteristic banded or ladder 'frosted' pattern on the skin. Cardiorespiratory failure may proceed rapidly, particularly in children, necessitating cardiopulmonary resuscitation.

First aid involves immediate dousing with vinegar for at least 30 sec to inactivate remaining nematocysts, removal of adherent tentacles and application of a compression bandage to any major sting (e.g. one covering an area over 50% of a limb or causing impaired consciousness). Urgent transport to hospital is followed by the administration of at least one ampoule of antivenom intravenously (Commonwealth Serum Laboratories Ltd.). Intravenous verapamil for resistant cardiac instability is recommended by some authors (Fenner et al., 1989).

Irukandji syndrome

This is due to the sting of the jellyfish Carukia barnesi found in Northern Australia. Mild initial pain is followed in 20–30 min by severe backache, then waves of cramping chest, muscle and abdominal pain. Headache, sweating, restlessness, dyspnoea, pulmonary oedema and cardiac failure thought to be due to catecholamine release have been reported. The symptoms resulting from this sting may be confused with decompression sickness in scuba divers.

First aid treatment includes vinegar to prevent further discharge of nematocysts. Hospital treatment is supportive but intravenous narcotics may be required for the pain and adrenergic blockade may be needed to control the excessive catecholamine release (Fenner et al., 1986). No deaths have occurred.

Blue-ringed octopus

This tiny octopus, weighing just 10–150 g, is found in Australia inhabiting rock pools and hiding in empty shells. It produces brilliant, irridescent blue rings over its body when provoked.

The venom includes tetrodotoxin which blocks peripheral nerve sodium conduction. After a painless bite, local burning occurs within 10 min followed by pruritus and oedema. Systemic envenomation with paraesthesiae, diplopia, ataxia, nausea and vomiting may progress to generalized weakness with respiratory failure. Two patients have died since 1950.

The pressure-immobilization first aid technique is used. Respiratory failure may require tracheal intubation until the toxin wears off. Mentation is normal in the absence of hypoxia. There is no antivenom.

Cone shells

Eighteen of the 400 beautiful species of cone shells are toxic, the most dangerous being Conus geographus which has been responsible for about 20 deaths worldwide.

A modified radula harpoons its prey releasing neurotoxic conotoxins. Immediate stinging, burning and numbness progress to muscular paralysis and coma.

First aid consists of the pressure-immobilization technique. Other treatment is supportive and includes tetanus prophylaxis. There is no antivenom.

Toxic fish ingestion

The risk from eating seafood is low although illness can occur from allergic, infectious or toxic causes. Toxic fish ingestion includes ciguatera poisoning, scombroid poisoning and paralytic shellfish poisoning.

Ciguatera poisoning

Ciguatera is the most common non-bacterial food poisoning seen in the USA, predominantly in Hawaii and Florida, but it is also endemic in the South Pacific and Australia.

Reef feeders contaminated by toxic dinoflagellates such as Gambierdiscus toxicus are eaten by larger fish which are consumed in turn by humans. The more frequently implicated larger fish in the USA are barracuda, jack, snapper and grouper, and spanish mackerel and barracuda in Australia.

The heat-stable toxin causes a triad of diarrhoea, vomiting and myalgia within 6–24 h of ingestion. Bizarre neurological features include typical hot/cold sensation reversal, paraesthesiae, fatigue and ataxia. Bradycardia, hypotension and respiratory failure have caused death (Bagnis & Legrand, 1987).

Treatment is supportive. Emesis, charcoal, fluids, atropine and inotropes are accepted. Pralidoxime, calcium gluconate, amitriptyline, nifedipine, tocainide and intravenous mannitol all have their proponents, but remain experimental.

Gastrointestinal symptoms are self-limiting although troublesome neurological symptoms may persist for months, especially following recurrent poisoning.

Scombroid poisoning

This pseudoallergic syndrome follows ingestion of improperly preserved or refrigerated fish, usually of the families Scomberesocidae and Scombroidea, such as tuna, mackerel, wahoo, bonito and skipjack. Cases have occurred worldwide.

Toxicity is due to ingestion of histamine and saurine produced by bacterial proliferation on spoiled fish. Flushing, a red rash, headache, nausea, vomiting, diarrhoea and sweating occur within minutes of ingestion. Tachycardia, hypotension and wheeze are seen in severe cases.

Treatment is supportive, including emesis, charcoal and antihistamines. Moderate poisoning should receive parenteral H1-blockers such as diphenhydramine 50 mg, and H2-blockers such as cimetidine 300 mg. Severe cases require aggressive airway control, adrenaline and intravenous fluids in addition (Smart, 1992). No recent deaths have occurred.

Paralytic shellfish poisoning

Shellfish may transmit hepatitis A, typhoid, cholera, *Vibrio vulnificus*, *Vibrio parahaemolyticus*, *Salmonella*, *Shigella* and *Escherichia coli*. When contaminated with dinoflagellates (which may or may not be related to 'red tides'), they produce neuromuscular toxins such as saxitoxin and gonyautoxin, leading to paralytic shellfish poisoning.

Symptoms rapidly follow ingestion of clams, oysters, mussels or scallops and include paraesthesiae, numbness, headache progressing to dysphagia, weakness, ataxia and rarely respiratory failure.

Treatment is supportive, including emesis and charcoal, but may require intensive care with cardiorespiratory support.

Bibliography

ALLEN, C. (1992). Arachnid envenomations. *Emerg. Med. Clin. North Am.*, **10**(2), 269–98.

BAGNIS, R. & LEGRAND, A. (1987). Clinical features on 12,890 cases of ciguatera (fish poisoning) in French Polynesia. In *Progress in Venom and Toxin Research*, ed. P. Gopalakrishnakone & C.K. Tan, pp. 372–84. Kent Ridge, Singapore: National University of Singapore.

BROWN, A.F.T. (1989). Delayed diagnosis of red back spider envenomation: a timely reminder. *Med. J. Aust.*, **151**, 705–6.

BROWN, C.K. & SHEPHERD, S.M. (1992). Marine trauma, envenomations and intoxications. *Emerg. Med. Clin. North Am.*, **10**(2), 385–407.

CORRIGAN, P., RUSSELL, F.E. & WAINSCHEL, J. (1978). In *Toxins: Animal, Plant and Microbial*, ed. P. Rosenberg, p. 457. Oxford: Pergamon Press.

DIECKMANN, J., PREBBLE, J., McDONAGH, A. *et al.* (1989). Efficacy of funnel web spider antivenom in human envenomation by *Hadronyche species*. *Med. J. Aust.*, **151**, 706–7.

EXTON, D.R., FENNER, P.J. & WILLIAMSON, J.A. (1989). Cold packs: effective topical analgesia in the treatment of painful stings by *Physalia* and other jellyfish. *Med. J. Aust.*, **151**, 625–6.

FENNER, P.J., WILLIAMSON, J.A., CALLANAN, V. *et al.* (1986). Further understanding of, and a new treatment for, 'Irukandji' (*Carukia barnesi*) stings. *Med. J. Aust.*, **145**, 569–74.

FENNER, P.J., WILLIAMSON, J.A. & BLENKIN, J.A. (1989). Successful use of *Chironex* antivenom by members of the Queensland Ambulance Transport Brigade. *Med. J. Aust.*, **151**, 708–10.

GENDRON, B.P. (1990). *Loxosceles reclusa* Envenomation. *Am. J. Emerg. Med.*, **8**, 51–4.

GOLD, B.S. & BARISH, R.A. (1990). Venomous snakebites. *Md. Med. J.*, **9**, 833–42.

GOLD, B.S. & BARISH, R.A. (1992). Venomous snakebites: current concepts in diagnosis, treatment and management. *Emerg. Med. Clin. North Am.*, **10**(2), 249–67.

GOLDEN, D.B.K. (1987). Diagnosis and prevalence of stinging insect allergy. *Clin. Rev. Allergy*, **5**, 119–36.

HERRIOTT, R. (1989). Hymenoptera stings and beta blockers. *Lancet*, **ii**, 1159.

HURRELL, J.G.R. & CHANDLER, H.W. (1982). Capillary enzyme immunoassay field kits for the detection of snake venom in clinical specimens: a review of two years use. *Med. J. Aust.*, **2**, 236–7.

KOBERNICK, M. (1984). Black widow spider bite. *Am. Fam. Physician*, **29**, 241–5.

LOK, C.K. & CHEN, J.H.Y. (1987). Hymenopteran stings in Singapore: incidence and deaths in the last 20 years (1966–86). In *Progress in Venom and Toxin Research*, ed. P. Gopalakrishnakone & C.K. Tan. pp. 542–55. Kent Ridge, Singapore: National University of Singapore.

LUMLEY, J., WILLIAMSON, J.A. FENNER, P.J. *et al.* (1988). Fatal envenomation by *Chironex fleckeri*, the

North Australian box jellyfish: the continuing search for lethal mechanisms. *Med. J. Aust.*, **148**, 527–34.

PERSSON, H. & IRESTEDT, B. (1981). A study of 136 cases of adder bite treated in Swedish hospitals during one year. *Acta Med. Scand.*, **210**, 433–9.

REID, H.A. (1976). Adder bites in Britain. *Br. Med. J.*, **2**, 153–6.

SCHMIDT, J.O. (1991). Allergy to venomous insects. In *The Hive and the Honeybee*, ed. J. Graham. pp. 1–90. Hamilton, IL: Dadant & Son.

SMART, D.R. (1992). Scombroid poisoning. A report of seven cases involving the Western Australian salmon, *Arripis truttaceus*. *Med. J. Aust.*, **157**, 748–51.

SUTHERLAND, S.K. (1983a). Treatment of snake bite in Australia. In *Australian Animal Toxins*, ed. S.K. Sutherland. pp. 185–221. Melbourne: Oxford University Press.

SUTHERLAND, S.K. (1983b). Venomous arthopods of medical importance. In *Australian Animal Toxins*, ed. S.K. Sutherland. pp. 320–4. Melbourne: Oxford University Press.

SUTHERLAND, S.K. (1992). Antivenom use in Australia. Premedication, adverse reactions and the use of venom detection kits. *Med. J. Aust.*, **157**, 734–9.

SUTHERLAND, S.K. & TRINCA, J.C. (1978). Survey of 2144 cases of red back spider bites: Australia and New Zealand, 1963–1976. *Med. J. Aust.*, **2**, 620–3.

SUTHERLAND, S.K. & TRINCA, J.C. (1981). Review of the usage of various antivenoms in Queensland. In *Animal Toxins and Man*, ed. J. Pearn. pp. 125–8. Brisbane: Queensland Health Department.

SUTHERLAND, S.K., COULTER, A.R. & HARRIS, R.D. (1979). The rationalization of first-aid measures for elapid snakebite. *Lancet*, **i**, 183–6.

SVENDSEN, F.J. (1986). The treatment of clinically diagnosed brown recluse spider bites with hyperbaric oxygen: a clinical observation. *J. Arkansas Med. Soc.*, **85**, 199–204.

TIBBALS, J. (1992). Diagnosis and treatment of confirmed and suspected snakebite. Implications from an analysis of 46 paediatric cases. *Med. J. Aust.*, **156**, 270–4.

PART III MEDICAL, SURGICAL AND OBSTETRIC EMERGENCIES

44 Adult respiratory emergencies

K. JONES[a] and F. MORRIS[b]

[a] Chest and Heart Unit, Bury General Hospital, Bury, UK
[b] Accident and Emergency Department, Northern General Hospital, Sheffield, UK

Chapter plan

Introduction
Respiratory infections
Inflammatory conditions of the respiratory system
Acute respiratory failure
Toxic lung injury
Mechanical disorders of the respiratory tract
Pulmonary embolism
Adult respiratory distress syndrome
Pulmonary function tests in respiratory emergencies

INTRODUCTION

Respiratory disease places a huge burden on the public health and economy of the UK. It is the commonest reason for consulting a general practitioner and is second only to diseases of the circulation as the commonest cause of death. In 1985, 102 449 deaths were attributed to respiratory disease in England and Wales. This was 17% of the total number of deaths from all causes (Department of Clinical Epidemiology, National Heart and Lung Institute, 1988). From 1979 to 1985, the number of hospital deaths and discharges due to respiratory disease was about 10% of the total for all causes. In 1985 the average number of hospital beds used daily for all respiratory disease was 16 127, or 11% of the total available (Department of Clinical Epidemiology, National Heart and Lung Institute, 1988). Needless to say, against this background, respiratory disease is an important component of emergency medicine. The commonest respiratory diseases presenting as medical emergencies are chronic obstructive pulmonary disease, pneumonia and asthma. All are amenable to therapy.

The incidence of chronic bronchitis and emphysema in the UK is declining, but infective exacerbations lead-ing to respiratory failure and death are a significant part of the workload of any hospital. Accurate figures are difficult to obtain but chronic obstructive pulmonary disease (which includes chronic bronchitis, emphysema, bronchiectasis and chronic asthma) may have a prevalence as high as 3.6% in 45–64-year-old men and 9.3% in men older than that (Royal College of General Practitioners, 1986). Pneumonia accounts for about 60 000 deaths per year which is ten times the number of all other infectious causes of death combined (Macfarlane, 1987). Asthma remains the only potentially treatable disease in the developed world which is increasing in both incidence and severity. It accounts for 2000 deaths per year in England and Wales alone (Burney, 1986).

In this chapter the clinical features, diagnosis and management of respiratory disease presenting as a medical emergency are discussed.

RESPIRATORY INFECTIONS

Acute tracheobronchitis in previously healthy people

This is a common condition which is usually due to a virus infection, although *Mycoplasma pneumoniae* and *Chlamydia psittaci* can cause acute bronchitis in young adults. A dry tickly cough and retrosternal soreness are often associated with upper respiratory tract symptoms. Occasionally, mucoid sputum is produced. If bacterial infection supervenes the sputum may become mucopurulent. The patient is not ill, is rarely pyrexial and the chest radiograph is normal (Seaton et al., 1989).

Treatment should be symptomatic only. Antibiotics are reserved for patients who are pyrexial due to bacterial superinfection when amoxycillin or erythromycin should

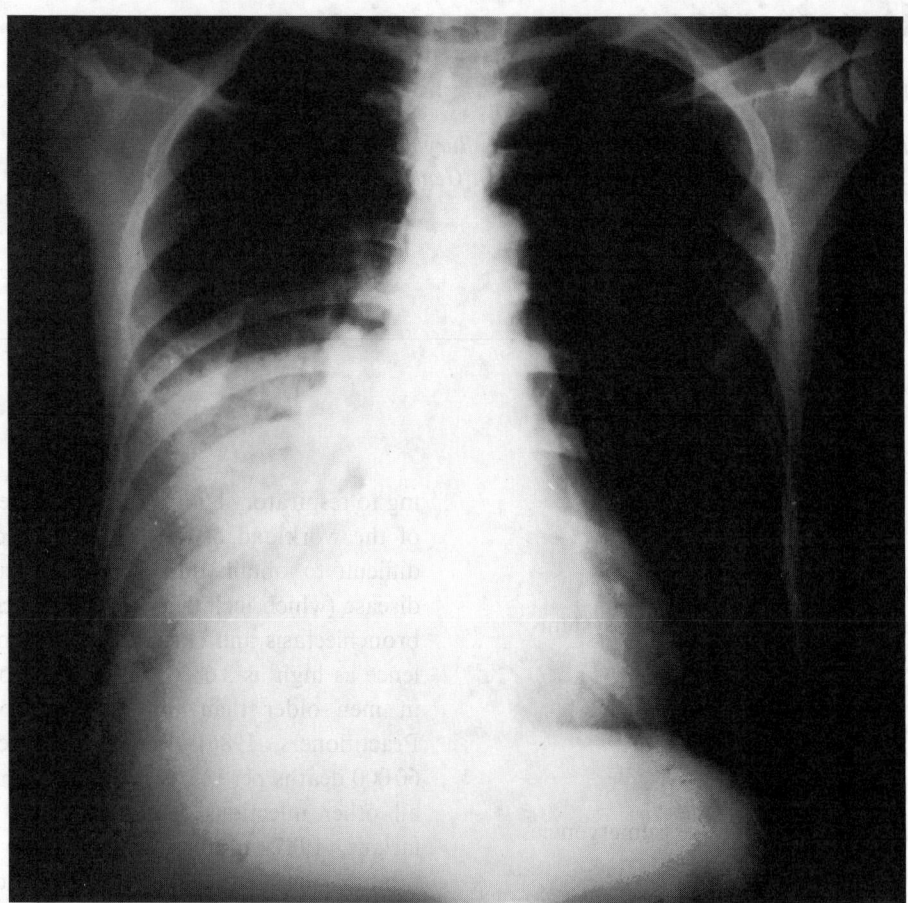

Fig. 1. Chest radiograph showing right lower lobe pneumonia.

be prescribed. It should be remembered that viral bronchitis can precipitate acute asthma in susceptible patients.

Acute bronchitis in patients with chronic lung disease

Patients with chronic bronchitis and emphysema tend to have chronic cough and sputum production. Infective exacerbations are often due to virus infections. *Haemophilus influenzae* and *Streptococcus pneumoniae* are by far the most important bacterial pathogens (Hosker *et al.*, 1994).

Clinical features depend mainly on the severity of the underlying lung disease. Symptoms include cough, increase in amount and purulence of sputum, breathlessness and fever. There may be basal crackles and widespread wheezes on chest auscultation. The chest radiograph may show features consistent with underlying chronic lung disease, but no pneumonia or heart failure. In patients with severe lung disease, acute bronchitis can precipitate respiratory failure.

The management of patients with respiratory failure caused by an acute exacerbation of chronic lung disease is dealt with in the section on respiratory failure. If clinical examination suggests that a patient is severely ill or may be in respiratory failure, arterial blood gas estimation should be carried out immediately. For the uncomplicated case, antibiotic therapy is all that is required. Microscopical examination and culture of sputum rarely alter management and should not be done routinely. Amoxycillin is the drug of choice, except in areas where there is a high incidence of resistant *Haemophilus influenzae*, in which case co-amoxiclav or cefaclor should be given. Prescribing will be influenced by local microbiological advice. Erythromycin and trimethoprim can be used in patients with penicillin sensitivity.

Pneumonia

Pneumonia is defined as a respiratory infection associated with chest radiographic shadowing (Fig. 1). Pneumonia should not be diagnosed if the chest radiograph is normal except when pulmonary infection with *Pneumocystis carinii* is suspected (see below). Sometimes a mistaken diagnosis of pneumonia is made when long-

Table 1. *Differential diagnosis of pneumonia*

- Pulmonary infarction
- Pulmonary oedema
  - Cardiac
  - Non-cardiac (ARDS)
- Eosinophilic pneumonia
  - Bronchopulmonary aspergillosis
- Pulmonary vasculitis
  - Churg–Strauss syndrome
  - Systemic lupus erythematosus
  - Wegener's granulomatosis
  - Polyarteritis nodosa
- Allergic alveolitis
- Alveolar cell carcinoma
- Subphrenic abscess
- Pancreatitis

ARDS, adult respiratory distress syndrome.

standing radiographic shadowing is misinterpreted as new during an intercurrent infection. It is important to review any of the patient's previous radiographs if available. The differential diagnosis of pneumonia is given in Table 1.

Community-acquired pneumonia

Guidelines on the management of community-acquired pneumonia have recently been published by the British Thoracic Society (1993). The important pathogens causing community-acquired pneumonia and their relative frequencies are shown in Table 2. *Streptococcus pneumoniae* remains the single most important organism. *Mycoplasma pneumoniae* is endemic but epidemics tend to occur every 4 years – the last one in 1990. *Haemophilus influenzae* is commoner in patients with coexisting chronic lung disease. Legionnaire's disease may be associated with recent stay in a hotel or hospital and there may be a history of similar symptoms in family or workmates. Infection with *Chlamydia psittaci* and *Coxiella burnetii* may follow contact with birds or farm animals. Staphylococcal pneumonia is commoner during influenza epidemics. Cavitating pneumonia may be caused by staphylococcal, Gram-negative or tuberculous infection.

It is important in all cases of pneumonia to objectively assess and record its severity. Features which are associated with a poor prognosis are listed in Table 3.

Table 2. *Relative frequencies of the common pathogens responsible for community-acquired pneumonia (British Thoracic Society, 1993)*

Organism	%
Bacteria	80–90
Streptococcus pneumoniae	60–75
Mycoplasma pneumoniae	5–18
Haemophilus influenzae	4–5
Legionella	2–5
Chlamydia psittaci	2–3
Staphylococcus aureus	1–5
Gram-negative bacilli	<1
Anaerobes	<1
Rickettsia	
Coxiella burnetii	1
Viruses	10–20
Influenza	8
Others	2–8

Table 3. *Factors associated with increased mortality in pneumonia (British Thoracic Society, 1993)*

- Age >60 years
- Underlying disease
- Confusion
- Respiratory rate >30 min^{-1}
- Diastolic blood pressure <60 mmHg
- Atrial fibrillation
- Multilobar involvement
- PO_2 <8.0 kPa
- White cell count <4000 × 10^9 l^{-1}
- White cell count >20 000 × 10^9 l^{-1}
- Serum urea >7 mmol l^{-1}
- Hypoalbuminaemia
- Bacteraemia

Particularly poor prognostic features of pneumonia

When two or more of the following are present the patient should be managed on an intensive care unit:

- Respiratory rate >30 min^{-1}
- Diastolic blood pressure <60 mmHg
- Serum urea >7 mmol l^{-1}

All patients with pneumonia should have a chest radiograph, haemoglobin estimation, white cell count, and urea and electrolyte measurements. Urine should be analysed for glucose, and blood glucose estimated if positive. Sputum, blood and pleural fluid (if present) should be cultured. It is important, however, especially in the severely ill, that initiation of antibiotic therapy should not be delayed while exhaustive investigations are done. As soon as the diagnosis is made appropriate antibiotics should be given.

Management includes regular measurement of pulse, blood pressure, temperature and respiratory rate. Oxygen should be administered to maintain arterial PO_2 above 8 kPa or oxygen saturation above 92% on pulse oximetry. If necessary, intravenous fluids should be given to correct dehydration or hypotension and renal failure managed appropriately. Analgesics may be required for pleuritic chest pain. Physiotherapy is not helpful in the treatment of pneumonia unless the patient also has coexistent chronic sputum production.

Antibiotics should be given as soon as possible and should not wait until the patient is in a hospital ward or until the next official drug round. Therapy must cover *Streptococcus pneumoniae* and erythromycin should be added if legionella, mycoplasma, coxiella or chlamydial infection is suspected. Antibiotics active against *Staphylococcus aureus* should be considered during influenza epidemics. Choice of antibiotics, dosage and route of administration depend on the severity of the illness and likely organisms plus local microbiological advice. In uncomplicated pneumonia, oral therapy with amoxycillin and/or erythromycin should suffice. In severe pneumonia of unknown aetiology, amoxycillin, flucloxacillin and erythromycin should be given intravenously. Alternatively, intravenous cefuroxime plus erythromycin could be used. Sulphonamides, tetracyclines and oral cephalosporins should not be used in the treatment of pneumonia.

Community-acquired pneumonia in the elderly

The classical symptoms and signs of pneumonia may not be apparent in the elderly who may present with confusion or general deterioration in their health. A chest radiograph should be done in all elderly patients in whom a diagnosis is unclear. Although, *Streptococcus pneumoniae* remains the commonest pathogen, Gram-negative pneumonias are commoner than in the younger population (Verghese & Berk, 1983).

Nosocomial pneumonia

Pneumonia developing in a hospitalized or recently discharged patient has a different spectrum of responsible pathogens. Gram-negative bacteria, anaerobes and *Staphylococcus aureus* are far more common and antibiotic therapy should be tailored accordingly (Macfarlane, 1991). A combination of a third-generation cephalosporin and an aminoglycoside is appropriate. If pseudomonas infection is likely or neutropenia exists, then an antipseudomonal penicillin should be used instead of the cephalosporin.

Aspiration pneumonia

Aspiration of stomach contents or oropharyngeal secretions is associated with impaired conciousness or dysphagia. The acid of stomach contents can lead to chemical pneumonia, pulmonary oedema and acute respiratory failure. Aspiration of particulate matter can lead to bronchial obstruction and Gram-negative and anaerobic bacteria can cause necrotizing pneumonia, lung abscess (Figure 2) and empyema. Community-acquired aspiration pneumonia should be treated with benzylpenicillin or clindamycin. The addition of metronidazole can also be considered. For hospital-acquired aspiration pneumonia, an aminoglycoside or third-generation cephalosporin is needed to cover Gram-negative organisms (Lorber & Swenson, 1974).

Tuberculosis

The incidence of new cases of tuberculosis in Britain has ceased to fall in recent years and with the increase in the number of people with HIV infection, may start to rise (Watson, 1993). A high index of suspicion of tuberculosis should be maintained for all patients with pneumonia (Fig. 3), especially those who are immunosuppressed, diabetic, alcoholic or belonging to ethnic minorities. A history of BCG immunization should be enquired after and sputum sent specifically for mycobacterial staining and culture.

Pneumonia in the immunosuppressed

People with HIV disease are at more risk of developing community-acquired pneumonia than the normal population and, if the chest radiograph shows unilateral shadowing, they should be treated in the conventional manner discussed previously. They can also develop

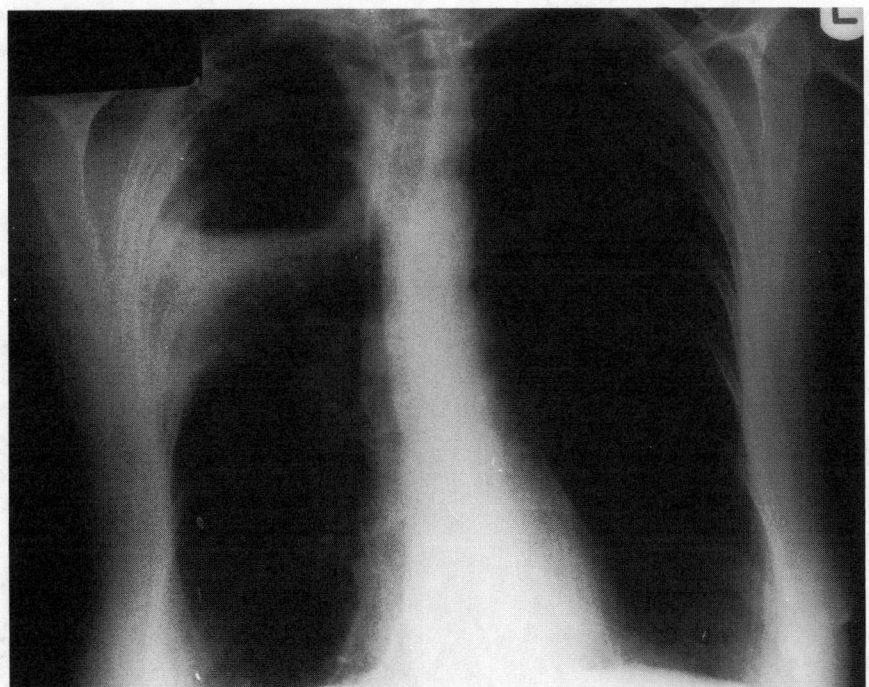

Fig. 2. Chest radiograph showing a lung abscess in the right upper lobe.

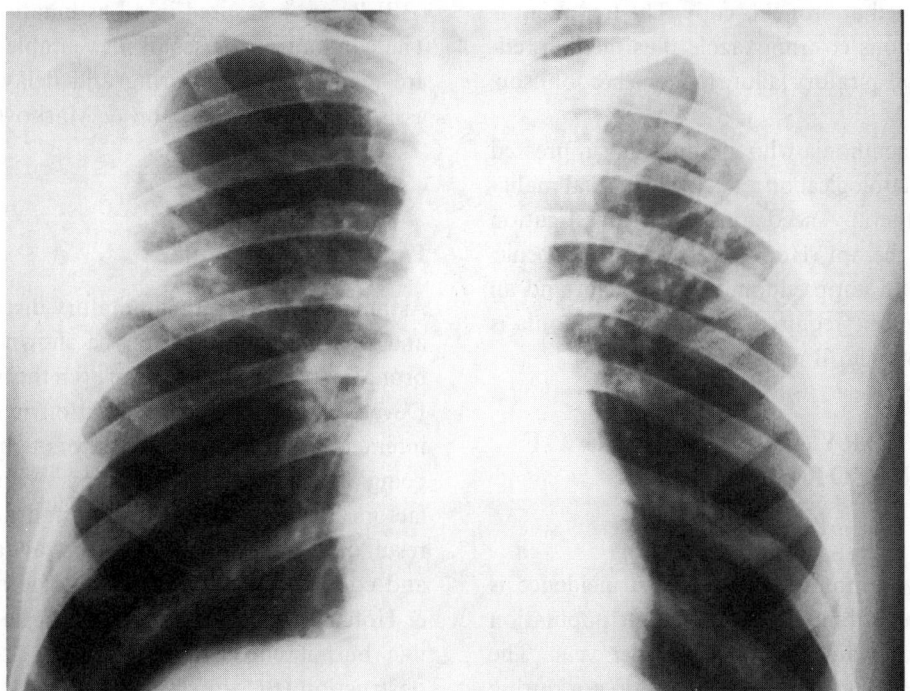

Fig. 3. Chest radiograph showing bilateral upper lobe shadowing due to tuberculosis.

opportunistic infections, the commonest being *Pneumocystis carinii* pneumonia. This usually presents with cough, fever, breathlessness, hypoxaemia and bilateral radiographic shadowing (Fig. 4). However, the chest radiograph can sometimes appear remarkably normal and pneumocystis pneumonia should be considered in any HIV-positive patient or in a patient with risk behaviour associated with HIV disease. The diagnosis is confirmed by cytological examination of sputum (which can be induced by inhaling nebulized hypertonic saline)

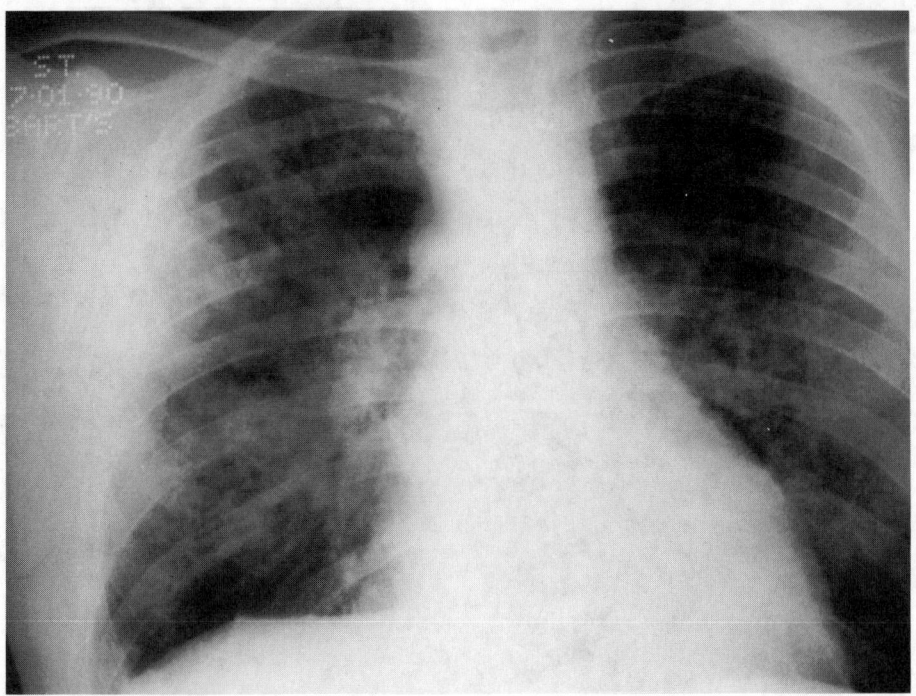

Fig. 4. Chest radiograph showing pneumocystis pneumonia.

or washings obtained at bronchoscopy. The treatment is high-dose intravenous co-trimoxazole plus methylprednisolone if there is respiratory failure (Mitchell & Johnson, 1990).

Patients with pneumonia who are immunosuppressed as a result of haematological or reticuloendothelial malignancy or chemotherapy need aggressive investigation and antimicrobial therapy (Hopkin, 1990). If neutropenic, a combination of an antipseudomonal penicillin and an aminoglycoside will be required. If fungal pneumonia is suspected, amphotericin B may be necessary.

INFLAMMATORY CONDITIONS OF THE RESPIRATORY SYSTEM

Asthma

Asthma is a very common disease whose incidence is increasing. It affects about 2% of the adult population and causes approximately 2000 deaths per year. The majority of asthmatics who die have seen a doctor during their final illness and preventable factors have subsequently been identified in 82% of asthma deaths (British Thoracic Association, 1982). The severity of asthma attacks is often underestimated by the patient, their relatives and doctors alike. This is largely due to a failure to make accurate objective measurements of the patient's condition. It is essential that peak expiratory flow rates

(PEFR) are measured in all asthmatics with symptoms. The commonest causes of preventable death in hospital are inadequate monitoring and delay in institution of assisted ventilation (Eason & Markowe, 1987).

Pathogenesis

Asthma is a chronic inflammatory disease of the airways and this inflammation can be shown to be present in bronchial biopsy specimens of even the mildest asthmatics. Development of the inflammation is dependent on an interaction between genetic factors – the most important being the inheritance of atopy – and environmental factors both specific (allergens) and non-specific. As a result of the inflammation, the airways are hyper-reactive and constrict easily to a wide range of stimuli (Barnes & Holgate, 1990). Airway constriction is usually reversible but, if chronic, may lead to irreversible airway obstruction (Brown et al. 1984).

Pathological changes in the airways of asthmatics include inflammatory cell infiltration, oedema, smooth muscle hypertrophy, shedding of the epithelium and mucus plugging. The mucus produced by asthmatics tends to be thick and tenacious and in postmortem studies has been shown to cause widespread small airway occlusion.

Diagnosis

Asthma is diagnosed when air flow obstruction is documented to be reversible either spontaneously or with treatment. The diagnosis of acute asthma is usually straightforward in the accident and emergency (A&E) department when the patient is young. They are aware of the condition and have presented because of their inability to achieve symptom relief with their usual medication. In older patients, however, it may be difficult to be sure whether the symptoms of breathlessness and wheeze are due to late-onset asthma or infective exacerbations of chronic irreversible airways disease. Patients in whom there is doubt, particularly those who have never smoked or give a good history of previous reversibility to their symptoms, should be treated as for asthma.

Occasionally, patients presenting with wheeze and breathlessness are found to have pulmonary oedema or, on occasion, multiple small pulmomary emboli. These may trap the unwary but the correct diagnosis is usually provided by the history, examination, chest radiograph, ECG and blood gases.

Management of acute asthma

Updated national guidelines on the management of asthma have recently been published (British Thoracic Society *et al.*, 1993). An accompanying chart for use in A&E departments is shown in Fig. 5.

All patients with asthma who present to the A&E department need careful assessment throughout their stay. The random administration of nebulized bronchodilators without such assessment is not condoned but all patients should receive high inspired concentrations of oxygen from the outset. The aim of initial assessment is to identify patients with life-threatening features who are likely to deteriorate and die without aggressive measures. PEFR measurement (before bronchodilator treatment) is essential and patients with acute severe or life-threatening asthma will also need arterial blood gas analysis.

Features of life-threatening asthma

- Exhaustion, confusion or coma
- Bradycardia or hypotension
- A silent chest, cyanosis or feeble respiratory effort
- PEFR < 33% of predicted normal or best
- A normal or high arterial $PaCO_2$ in a breathless asthmatic
- PaO_2 < 8.0 kPa irrespective of treatment with oxygen
- A low arterial pH

From British Thoracic Society *et al.* (1993).

Table 4. *Immediate treatment of life-threatening asthma* (British Thoracic Society *et al.*, 1993)

1. Oxygen	Use highest concentration possible; carbon dioxide retention is not aggravated by oxygen therapy in asthma
2. Bronchodilators	Nebulized salbutamol (5 mg) or terbutaline (10 mg) plus nebulized ipratropium (0.5 mg) Intravenous salbutamol or terbutaline (250 µg over 10 min) Consider intravenous bolus of aminophylline (250 mg over 20 min); do not give to patients already taking oral theophyllines
3. Systemic steroids	Intravenous hydrocortisone 200 mg
4. Exclude pneumothorax	Examination plus chest radiography
5. Consider assisted ventilation	

Life threatening asthma

Patients with life-threatening features should be managed in the resuscitation room and help from a senior anaesthetist must be requested immediately. The initial treatment is outlined in Table 4. Many of these patients will need immediate ventilation, particularly those who present with cyanosis, bradycardia or altered consciousness. Patients not requiring immediate ventilation will need observation on intensive care/high dependency unit with extremely close monitoring. Intravenous adrenaline is not generally required in the treatment of life-threatening asthma but bronchospasm is one of the features of anaphylaxis and adrenaline should be considered for any patient in whom this diagnosis is suspected (see Chapter 8).

Acute severe asthma

Patients without life-threatening features can usually give a brief but essential history. With the patient on a high inspired concentration of oxygen and whilst awaiting the nebulizer, the following aspects of the history should be obtained:

- The frequency and severity of previous attacks – e.g. number of acute attacks per year, number of hospital admissions and particularly whether assisted ventilation has been necessary previously.

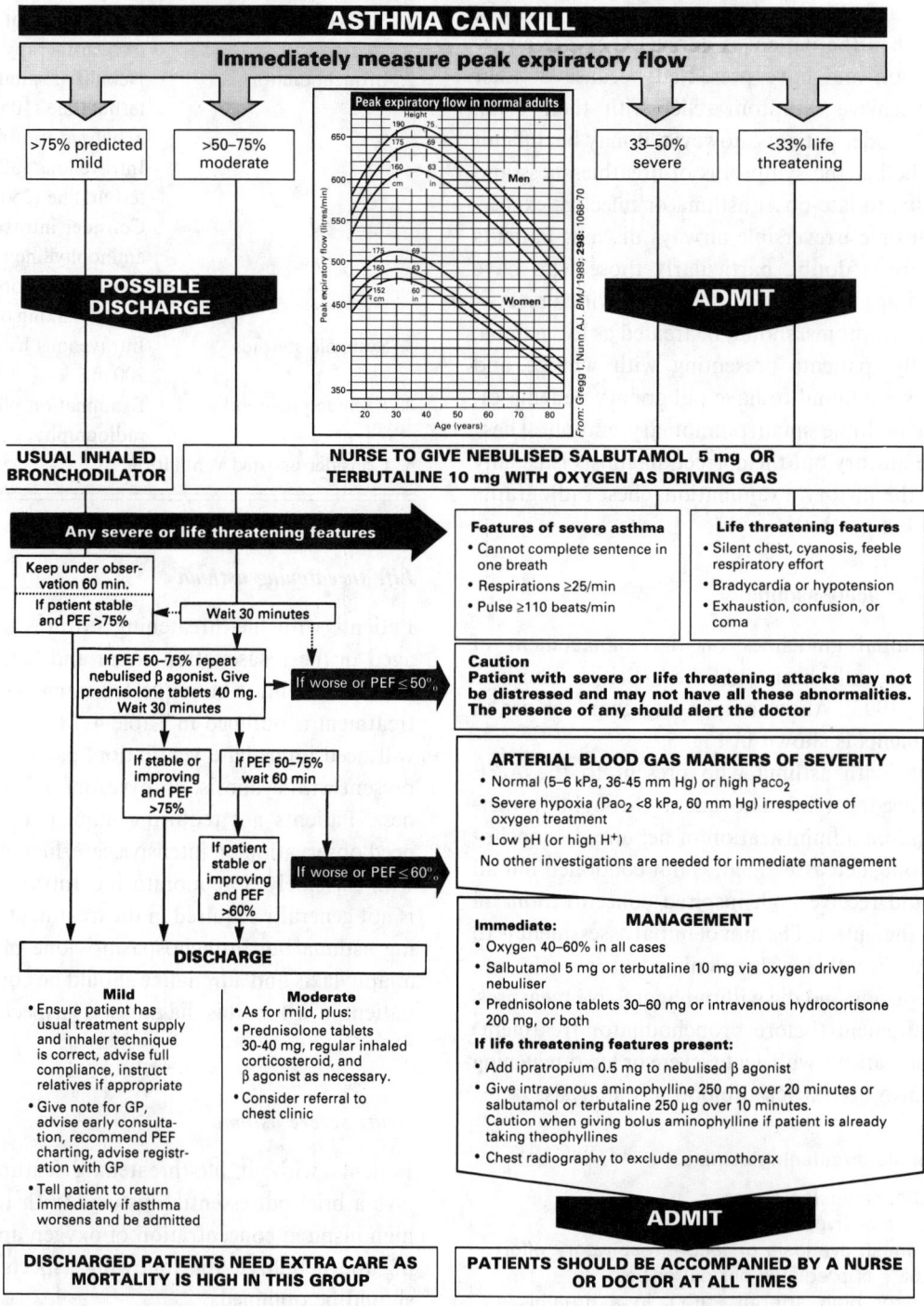

Fig. 5. Algorithm for management of asthma in accident and emergency departments. (Reproduced, with permission, from British Thoracic Society *et al.* (1993). *Thorax*, **48**, S1–S24.)

- Usual maintenance therapy and whether this is taken regularly. It is important to know whether the patient takes theophylline preparations at home, has a home nebulizer or takes inhaled and/or oral steroids regularly.
- What precipitated this attack, what normally precipitates attacks and how quickly can they deteriorate.
- How bad this attack is compared to previous attacks – is this the worse they have ever felt.

The clinical assessment should be designed specifically to exclude a pneumothorax and to report the presence of features leading to a diagnosis of acute severe asthma.

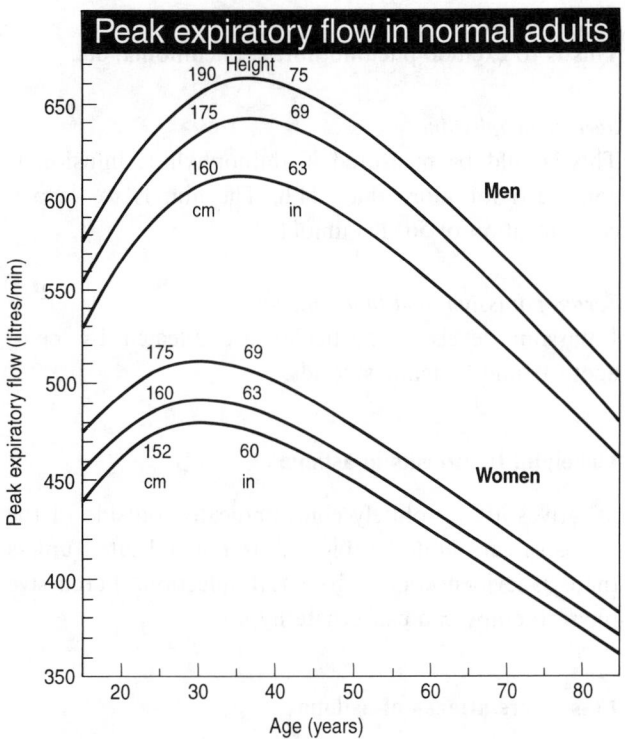

Fig. 6. Peak expiratory flow rates in normal adults. (Reproduced, with permission, from Gregg, I. & Nunn, A.J. (1989). *BMJ*, **298**, 1068–70.)

Features of acute severe asthma

- Unable to complete sentences in 1 breath
- Respiratory rate >25 breaths min^{-1}
- Heart rate >110 beats min^{-1}
- PEFR <50% of predicted normal or best previously obtained
- PEFR <200 litres min^{-1} (if not sure of predicted values)

From British Thoracic Society *et al.* (1993).

The presence of any of these features means the patient requires admission to hospital irrespective of their response to treatment.

Initial treatment should include:

1. High inspired concentrations of oxygen. Retention of carbon dioxide is not aggravated by treatment of oxygen in patients with acute severe asthma so masks delivering 24% or 28% oxygen are inappropriate.
2. Nebulized beta-agonists (e.g. salbutamol 5 mg or terbutaline 10 mg). They must be nebulized with oxygen. Consider the addition of ipratropium (0.5 mg) in patients not responding to initial therapy.
3. Oral prednisolone 40–60 mg. Reserve intravenous hydrocortisone for patients with life-threatening asthma or for those unable to absorb tablets because of vomiting, etc.
4. Consider intravenous infusion of salbutamol (5 µg min^{-1}, range 3–20 µg min^{-1}) or terbutaline (1.5–5.0 µg min^{-1}) in patients who are not responding
5. Consider aminophylline infusion (0.5–0.9 mg kg^{-1} h^{-1}) in patients who are not responding. A loading dose is only required in life-threatening asthma if the patient has not been taking oral theophyllines.

Monitoring of response to asthma treatment

Peak expiratory flow rate

Measurements of PEFR are most easily interpreted when expressed as a percentage of the predicted normal value (Fig. 6) or of the previous best obtainable value on optimal treatment. In patients in whom neither of these is known, decisions have to be taken on the absolute value recorded (see 'features of acute severe asthma', above) remembering that older people, women and shorter people have a lower normal range. PEFR recordings should be obtained before starting treatment and at 15–30-min intervals during nebulizer treatment.

Heart rate

This will fall as the patient improves.

Arterial blood gas tensions

These should always be measured in patients with acute severe asthma. See section on life-threatening asthma (above) for values which suggest a very severe or life-threatening attack.

Chest radiograph
This is to exclude pneumothorax, pneumonia, etc.

Serum theophylline
This should be measured if aminophylline infusion is continued for more than 24 h. The aim is to keep a concentration of $56–111 \,\mu mol\, l^{-1}$.

Serum potassium and blood glucose
Potassium levels in particular are affected by beta-agonists and systemic steroids.

Unhelpful treatments in asthma

Sedatives are absolutely contraindicated outside of the intensive care unit. Antibiotics are not indicated unless there is evidence of a bacterial infection. Percussive physiotherapy can exacerbate hypoxia.

Less severe attacks of asthma

Patients who present to the A&E department without any of the features of acute severe asthma usually respond to treatment with oxygen, nebulized beta-agonists and oral prednisolone. Many of these patients will be able to be discharged home (Figure 5) but it must be remembered that their attendance indicates some failure in their regular symptom control and this will need to be addressed. It is also important to remember that initial response to a nebulized beta-agonist can be short-lived and patients need an adequate period of observation to ensure that improvement is sustained. Asthma tends to deteriorate at night so be especially careful about discharging patients home late in the evening or in the early hours of the morning.

The following points should be assured before discharge:

1. On initial assessment the patient had none of the features of acute severe asthma (see earlier).
2. Response to treatment has been good and PEFR is $> 75\%$ of predicted or previous best.
3. All patients have a short course of oral prednisolone (40 mg of prednisolone for 7 days) and have been observed to have adequate technique to continue inhaled steroids and bronchodilators.
4. Patients should see their general practitioner within 36 h with a letter detailing treatment, PEFR, etc., so that the general practitioner can alter treatment accordingly, arrange for stopping oral steroids as indi-

cated and organize referral to the chest clinic if appropriate.

It is important to stress that if there are any doubts about the safety of discharging an asthmatic from the A&E department, the admitting medical team should see the patient.

Chronic obstructive pulmonary disease

Pathology

The major pathologies accounting for chronic obstructive pulmonary disease are chronic bronchitis, emphysema, bronchiectasis and chronic asthma. Chronic bronchitis has a clinical definition of productive cough lasting over 3 months in 2 consecutive years (Medical Research Council, 1965). Emphysema is defined pathologically as the presence of permanent enlargement of the air spaces distal to the terminal bronchioles, accompanied by destruction of their walls without obvious fibrosis (Snider *et al.*, 1985). The two conditions have similar causes (especially cigarette smoking) and always coexist. Despite popular belief, the classical clinical descriptions of 'pink puffer' and 'blue bloater' do not conform to distinct pathological changes and are opposite ends of a spectrum of clinical manifestations of the combined diseases (Jamal *et al.*, 1990).

We feel a more useful term for management purposes is chronic air flow limitation. This is defined as persistent symptoms (e.g. cough and breathlessness) combined with an obstructive pattern of spirometric values, i.e. $FEV_1/FVC < 0.75$ (see section on respiratory investigations). The important feature clinically is to decide if this air flow limitation has any degree of reversibility or not. It is this factor which will influence treatment. The presence of reversibility can be suggested by the history or proven by response to bronchodilator treatment. No patient should be designated as having irreversible chronic air flow limitation without having a trial of steroids. This usually takes the form of prednisolone 40 mg daily for 2 weeks (Webb *et al.*, 1981). If a 15% or greater improvement in FEV_1 (provided this is at least 0.2 litres) is shown, these patients should be treated as having asthma (Nisar *et al.*, 1990). If not, they are designated as having irreversible chronic air flow limitation and long-term steroid therapy is avoided.

Clinical presentation

Patients with chronic air flow limitation frequently present to hospital with acute exacerbations of cough and breathlessness. They may have cyanosis, wheeze, purulent sputum, peripheral oedema and signs of carbon dioxide retention. There are no specific radiographic changes but they will have a low PEFR and obstructive spirometry. The cause of deteriorating symptoms is most frequently due to a respiratory infection which has added to their airways obstruction. However, other causes of deterioration should always be considered and actively excluded. These include:

1. *Asthma.* Occasionally patients who have been labelled as having irreversible airways disease have late onset asthma or a combination of the two. Asthma is more likely if the patient has never smoked, gives a history of variability of symptoms or was 'chesty' as a child.
2. *Pneumonia.* This may be detected clinically or seen as new shadowing on the chest radiograph.
3. *Pneumothorax.* Initial assessment of patients presenting with signs of chronic air flow limitation should always attempt to exclude this diagnosis. Pneumothoraces are difficult to detect clinically and a chest radiograph is mandatory. Remember that a pneumothorax must be differentiated from an emphysematous bulla.
4. *Pulmonary oedema.* Coexisting left heart failure may be very difficult to exclude clinically as basal crackles are also a feature of chronic obstructive pulmonary disease. A chest radiograph is the investigation of choice but again the radiographic appearances of pulmonary oedema can be considerably distorted by the presence of severe lung disease.
5. *Pulmonary embolism.* Sudden onset of shortness of breath and pleuritic chest pain should always raise the possibility of pulmonary embolism. Further evidence from the clinical history, electrocardiogram (ECG), chest radiograph and arterial blood gases should be sought. The diagnosis is extremely difficult to make and even the results of ventilation/perfusion scanning can be impossible to interpret in patients with chronic air flow limitation.

Management of acute exacerbation of chronic air flow limitation

1. Strong verbal reassurance.
2. 24% oxygen by face mask or nasal speculae at 2 litres min^{-1}.
3. Nebulized salbutamol (5 mg) or terbutaline (10 mg) plus ipratropium (0.5 mg).

4. Order the following urgent investigations:
   a. *Chest radiograph* to exclude the conditions listed above. Specific therapy will be necessary depending on the findings (e.g. diuretics for pulmonary oedema or chest drain for pneumothorax).
   b. *Arterial blood gases.* The degree of hypoxia, hypercapnia and acidosis needs to be documented early. Whether or not controlled oxygen therapy is required will depend on the results (see section on respiratory failure below).
   c. *Electrocardiogram* (ECG). Evidence of ischaemia or changes suggestive of pulmonary embolism should be sought.

Additional therapy

In the absence of any obvious precipitating cause for this deterioration, additional therapy consists of:

1. Controlled oxygen administration if the patient is hypoxic, hypercapnoeic and acidotic (see section on respiratory failure, below).
2. Nebulized beta-agonist and ipratropium 4–6 hourly.
3. Antibiotics orally or intravenously depending on the severity of the illness (see section on respiratory infections, above).
4. Oral prednisolone 40 mg or intravenous hydrocortisone 200 mg if any possibility that steroid reversibility is present. The risks of failing to treat an attack of asthma properly are far more important than the risks of a short course of inappropriate steroid therapy.
5. Intravenous fluids if dehydrated.
6. The use of aminophylline is controversial. It can be dangerous in the presence of hypoxia and should only be used on the advice of senior medical staff. It is best given as an infusion (0.5–0.9 mg kg^{-1} h^{-1}).
7. Diuretics for associated peripheral oedema are probably overused. Fluid retention in chronic air flow limitation is usually due to the effects of hypoxia on renal function rather than true right heart failure (Richens & Howard, 1982). The proper treatment is the careful correction of hypoxia. Diuretics can worsen matters by depleting the circulating intravascular volume.
8. Physiotherapy to aid sputum expectoration by forced expiratory techniques and encouragement of coughing.
9. Respiratory stimulants and assisted ventilation. (This is covered more fully in the section on respiratory failure, below.) The decision to institute these

measures is based on more than just the blood gas levels. It depends on many factors including the patient's previous quality of life and whether reversible causes of respiratory failure exist. Experienced medical advice should be sought.

ACUTE RESPIRATORY FAILURE

Definition

Respiratory failure occurs when the lungs are unable to maintain normal gas exchange at rest. It is arbitrarily defined as a partial pressure of arterial oxygen (PaO_2) of below 8.0 kPa (60 mmHg) or a partial pressure of arterial carbon dioxide ($PaCO_2$) above 6.7 kPa (50 mmHg). Hypoxaemic respiratory failure (type 1) is said to occur when the PaO_2 is less than 8.0 kPa but the $PaCO_2$ is normal or low. The mechanism of this pattern is predominantly ventilation/perfusion mismatching and occurs in conditions such as asthma, pulmonary embolism, pneumonia and pulmonary oedema. In ventilatory respiratory failure (type 2) there is alveolar hypoventilation which leads to hypercapnia as well as hypoxia. Causes of this include respiratory centre depression with sedative drugs (e.g. opiates), acute brain insults (such as head injury, cerebral haemorrhage, etc.), deranged chest wall mechanics (e.g. flail chest) and neuromuscular diseases (e.g. acute infective polyneuritis). In patients with chronic obstructive pulmonary disease, respiratory failure is a combination of both hypoxaemic and ventilatory mechanisms (Gribbin, 1993).

Clinical Signs

Respiratory failure can occur in the context of any major illness. Its signs can be subtle and there is no substitute for performing arterial blood gas analysis. Both hypoxia and hypercapnia can cause sweating, confusion and agitation. Central cyanosis is the cardinal sign of hypoxaemia but can be difficult to detect even when looking at the tongue in a good light. Hypercapnia gives vasodilation with warm sweaty hands, dilated veins, bounding pulse and even retinal vein engorgement and papilloedema. It can also give central nervous system signs of tremor, flap, drowsiness and coma.

Management

Tissue oxygen delivery depends on the haemoglobin concentration, its saturation with oxygen and the cardiac output. Due to the shape of the oxygen dissociation curve, there is little change in the oxygen saturation of haemoglobin until the PaO_2 falls below 8 kPa. After this level, small falls in PaO_2 can cause a significant decrease in oxygen saturation. When the PaO_2 falls below 6 kPa, it can be life-threatening. To improve oxygen delivery to the tissues, measures must be taken to correct anaemia, improve cardiac output and increase alveolar oxygen concentrations. The aim is to raise the PaO_2 above 8 kPa or oxygen saturation of haemoglobin above 90%.

Oxygen therapy

Respiratory failure is treated by attention to the underlying cause and oxygen therapy. The easiest way to increase inspired oxygen concentrations above the 21% in atmospheric air is by use of oxygen face masks or nasal cannulae (Table 5). In principle, the concentration of oxygen that the patient eventually inspires is a function of the type of delivery system, the flow rate of oxygen going to the mask and the breathing pattern of the patient (Leach & Bateman, 1993). Low-flow masks such as MC masks or Hudson masks can give inspired oxygen concentrations up to 60% and are used for patients with type 1 respiratory failure. In type 2 failure, where it is more important to deliver low concentrations of inspired oxygen accurately, high-flow masks (e.g. Ventimask) are preferred. Nasal cannulae give highly variable concentrations of oxygen but have the advantage of comfort.

In patients with type 1 respiratory failure, there is no lack of respiratory drive and hypoxaemia can be corrected without fear of hypercapnia and worsening respiratory acidosis. Once type 1 respiratory failure has

Table 5. *Flow rates and approximate inspired oxygen concentrations for some of the more common oxygen delivery devices*

Device	Flow rate (litres min^{-1})	Inspired oxygen (%)
Nasal cannulae	1–2	24
Nasal cannulae	2–4	28
24% Ventimask	2	24
28% Ventimask	4	28
35% Ventimask	8	35
40% Ventimask	10	40
60% Ventimask	15	60
MC mask	6–10	60
Hudson mask	6–10	60

been proven by arterial blood gases, the patient should be given a high concentration of inspired oxygen to keep the PaO_2 above 8 kPa. Alternatively, if carbon dioxide retention can be excluded confidently on clinical grounds, oxygen therapy can be guided by pulse oximetry with the aim to keep oxygen saturation above 92%. The highest inspired concentration of oxygen possible by conventional face mask is 60%. If this fails to correct hypoxia then assisted ventilation must be considered and anaesthetic advice obtained.

In acute type 2 respiratory failure, oxygen therapy alone will not correct the hypercapnia and treatment of the underlying cause is essential (e.g. naloxone for opiate intoxication). If this cannot be done immediately, then assisted ventilation will be necessary and anaesthetic advice must be requested.

Patients with chronic obstructive pulmonary disease and respiratory failure represent a particularly difficult management problem. Some of these patients have lost the normal increased ventilatory response to hypercapnia and rely on hypoxia alone as a stimulus to breathing. Therefore, even when well, they have hypoxia and hypercapnia but renal retention of bicarbonate prevents acidosis. When decompensation occurs during an infective exacerbation, they become increasingly hypoxic, hypercapnic and acidotic. The level of acidosis is the best guide to the severity of their condition with the mortality much increased if the pH falls below 7.26 (Jeffrey *et al.*, 1992).

In such patients, high inspired oxygen concentrations will reduce respiratory drive, exacerbate hypoventilation and increase respiratory acidosis. The aim, therefore, is to give the lowest concentration of oxygen that will correct hypoxia without worsening acidosis. Initially these patients should be given 24% oxygen and the blood gases repeated after 30 min. The inspired oxygen concentration should be slowly increased to reach a level of PaO_2 above 6.6 kPa (50 mmHg) without a fall in pH below 7.26. If this cannot be achieved by controlled oxygen therapy, respiratory stimulants or assisted ventilation should be considered (see Figure 7). As mentioned in the section on chronic obstructive pulmonary disease, these decisions require experienced medical advice.

TOXIC LUNG INJURY

Introduction

Chemical injury to the lung can arise in three major ways:

- Aspiration of stomach contents.

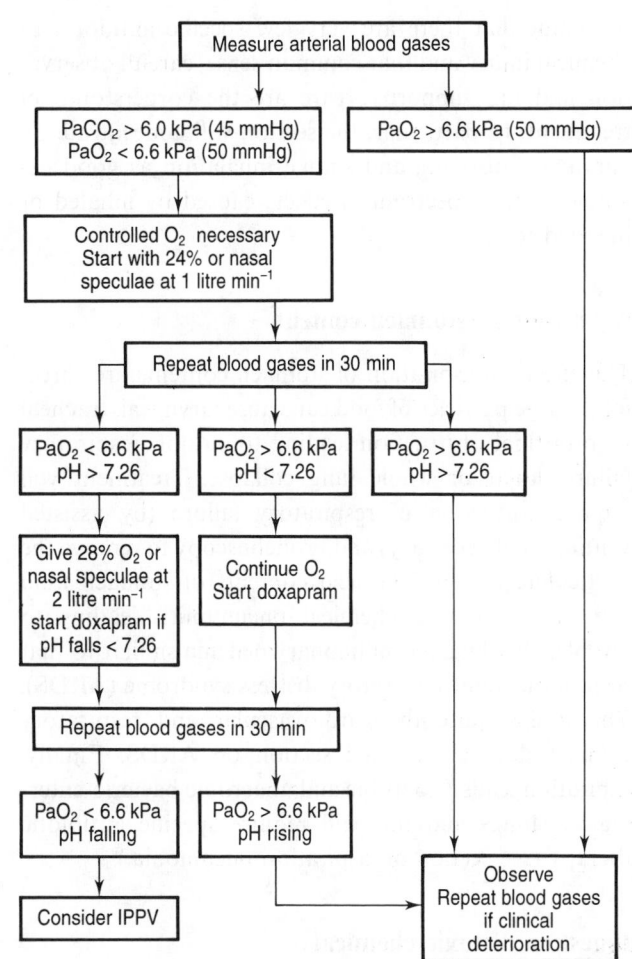

Fig. 7. Algorithm for the management of respiratory failure in chronic air flow limitation.

- Ingestion of toxic chemicals.
- Inhalation of toxic agents.

There may be isolated lung injury or the pulmonary effects may be part of a range of more widespread poisoning involving other organ systems. There is a limited spectrum of response that the lung can manifest to injury (e.g. cough, bronchospasm, pulmonary oedema) and this may be very similar to that seen with other more common conditions such as pneumonia, asthma, vasculitis and cardiac failure. It is very important, therefore, to be aware of the possibility and enquire specifically about environmental exposure to toxic gases and ingested chemicals – including drugs and medicines. It sometimes helps actually to ask the patient if there might be something they have come into contact with at work or home that they think might explain their symptoms.

The following section is not a comprehensive list of every agent that can cause lung damage. Rather, it makes the point that there are very few specific antidotes to chemical injury and that common sense, careful observation and full supportive care are the cornerstones of treatment. In particular, the section will concentrate on paraquat poisoning and smoke inhalation as good examples of the spectrum of effects caused by inhaled or ingested toxins.

Aspiration of stomach contents

The effects of aspiration of stomach contents are three-fold. Large particles of food can cause laryngeal, tracheal or bronchial obstruction leading to stridor, respiratory failure, lobar or whole lung collapse. Treatment will require correction of respiratory failure (by assisted ventilation if necessary) and bronchoscopy to remove the particulate matter. The acid contents of stomach fluid can cause a severe chemical pneumonitis leading to alveolar flooding and pulmonary oedema similar to that seen in the adult respiratory distress syndrome (ARDS). This will require the cardiovascular and respiratory support described in the section on ARDS. Finally, aspiration leads to aerobic and anaerobic bacteria entering the lungs and this will require specific antibiotic therapy (see section on aspiration pneumonia.).

Ingestion of toxic chemicals

Chemicals that can injure the lung may be drugs, toxic products of metabolism, contaminated foodstuffs or substances ingested accidentally or deliberately at work or in the home.

Paraquat

The weedkiller paraquat has been responsible for deaths in humans, usually after oral ingestion. It can rarely be absorbed through the skin or by inhalation. It causes ulceration of the upper gastrointestinal tract and with large doses leads to death in a few hours from pulmonary oedema, metabolic acidosis and multiple organ failure. Smaller doses cause liver damage, acute renal tubular necrosis and progressive pulmonary fibrosis. The onset of pulmonary symptoms may be delayed for some days following ingestion but, once present, death is eventually inevitable from irreversible respiratory failure (Higenbottam et al., 1979). Prognosis after paraquat ingestion depends on the dose absorbed and can be predicted by plotting plasma paraquat concentration against time

Table 6. *Examples of drug-induced pulmonary disease*

Cough	Angiotensin-converting enzyme inhibitors
Bronchospasm	Beta-blockers
	Aspirin
	Non-steroidal anti-inflammatory drugs
Pulmonary oedema	Salicylates
	Thiazides
Pulmonary fibrosis	Cytotoxic drugs
	Amiodarone
Eosinophilic pneumonia	Sulphonamides
	Penicillins
	Sulphasalazine

from ingestion (Proudfoot et al., 1979). Therapy has not been shown to alter outcome but, if the patient presents early enough after exposure, treatment should be aimed at removing paraquat from the gastrointestinal tract (emesis) or preventing absorption (Fuller's earth).

Drugs

Therapeutic agents, even in prescribed dosages, are capable of inducing pulmonary disease as a result of either theoretically predictable actions based on their pharmacology or idiosyncratic reactions. The injury can be extensive and some common examples are shown in Table 6. More comprehensive information can be found elsewhere (Brewis, 1982).

Inhalation of toxic agents

The effect that inhaled toxic agents have on the lung depends on their potency, the dose inhaled, their solubility and particle size. The greater the solubility, the more proximal are the major effects. Particles of 10 μm diameter are deposited in the nose and throat, those of 1–10 μm in the airways and of 0.5–5 μm in the alveoli. The immediate effects of toxic inhalation are fairly predictable with cough followed by an acute inflammatory response. This will comprise tracheobronchitis, bronchiolitis, alveolitis, pulmonary oedema and ARDS depending on site of deposition and severity. If the patient can be kept alive with supportive therapy during the acute illness, there is usually complete recovery without chronic sequelae. Severe secondary infection is a common complication.

Smoke inhalation

Significant inhalation injury is a common cause of death in patients with extensive burns although patients with isolated smoke inhalation usually survive. Smoke inhalation causes two major problems: systemic poisoning and respiratory tract injury.

Systemic poisoning

Noxious substances in smoke are absorbed and act as cellular poisons. The most ubiquitous of these is carbon monoxide, although hydrogen cyanide, hydrogen sulphide and carbon dioxide are also commonly present. Carbon monoxide causes direct cellular damage by competing for haemoproteins such as myoglobin and cytochromes. It also leads to tissue hypoxia by forming carboxyhaemoglobin and shifting the oxygen dissociation curve to the left. Carboxyhaemoglobin levels should always be estimated in patients with suspected smoke inhalation. High levels indicate significant inhalation although normal levels (especially if taken some hours after exposure) do not exclude significant tissue toxicity (Clark & Beeley, 1989).

Inhalation injury to the respiratory tract

Direct thermal damage accounts for a limited percentage of respiratory problems and is usually confined to the upper airways because of the efficient heat-exchanging properties of the nose, pharynx and larynx. However, hot gases may cause damage to the lower airways and lung parenchyma. Irritants contained in the smoke give rise to much of the airway damage, either by direct chemical effects or by injury to the normal protective mechanisms such as mucociliary clearance. Certain irritants (e.g. sulphur dioxide) can cause bronchospasm.

Clinical diagnosis of smoke inhalation

Smoke inhalation can be assumed if more than two of the following risk factors are present:

1. A history of exposure to smoke in a confined space.
2. A history of altered consciousness or confusion at any time since exposure.
3. Symptoms of mucous membrane irritation (watery eyes, sore throat) or respiratory irritation (cough, breathlessness, tight chest, wheeze, etc.).
4. Perioral burns.
5. Signs of respiratory involvement such as tachypnoea, stridor, wheeze.
6. Hoarseness or loss of voice.
7. The production of carbonaceous sputum or soot deposits in the mouth (Clark et al., 1986).

Management of smoke inhalation

Immediate management consists of high inspired oxygen by face mask, nebulized beta-agonist for wheeze and measurement of arterial blood gases and carboxyhaemoglobin levels. An anaesthetist should be informed and admission arranged to a high dependency area or intensive care unit. A chest radiograph can be performed once stabilized as there are no early changes associated with smoke inhalation. It is useful as a baseline investigation and for demonstrating pre-existing disease. Intubation and ventilation with 100% oxygen is necessary for any patient with altered consciousness or coma. Elective intubation should be considered in all patients with the potential for upper airway obstruction (e.g. intraoral burns or pharyngeal oedema) before stridor and respiratory failure develop. Intubation and assisted ventilation are mandatory for patients who cannot tolerate the face mask or maintain a clear airway.

Fibreoptic bronchoscopy is used increasingly frequently to assess the upper and lower airway for evidence of respiratory tract damage. Frank ulceration and bleeding, carbon particles and chemical burn coagulum would all be direct evidence of significant smoke inhalation (Clark & Beeley, 1989).

Carbon monoxide poisoning

Carbon monoxide poisoning should always be considered when there has been exposure to smoke. In other circumstances, however, it can be easily overlooked. Carbon monoxide is produced by car exhausts and poorly ventilated heating systems and inhaled from paint stripper (via the liver).

Symptoms of poisoning are often non-specific and include weakness, nausea, vomiting, headache, lethargy and dyspnoea. Clinical signs are equally unhelpful and are usually attributed to another cause. These include altered consciousness, coma, confusion, hyper-reflexia and cardiac arrhythmias. The so-called typical 'cherry-red' skin colour is rarely seen except in fatalities.

If recognized or suspected, the carboxyhaemoglobin level should be estimated. Levels below 5% are normal. Levels as high as 9% may be found in normal smokers. In the presence of carbon monoxide, PaO_2 levels may be falsely high. This is because a conventional blood gas analyser calculates the PaO_2 on the assumption that only normal haemoglobin is present. The same is true of pulse oximeters.

Treatment consists of giving as high an inspired oxygen concentration as possible via a tight-fitting face mask with rebreathing facility, or assisted ventilation if the patient is unconscious or unable to control the airway. An inspired oxygen concentration of 100% should be continued until carboxyhaemoglobin levels have fallen to less than 5%. Hyperbaric oxygen treatment should be considered if:

- The conscious patient has a carboxyhaemoglobin level greater than 40% at any time following exposure.
- The patient has any neurological symptoms or signs (apart from headache only).
- The patient is pregnant.
- The patient has cardiac ischaemia or arrhythmias (Drugs and Therapeutics Bulletin, 1988).

If contemplating hyperbaric therapy, you should contact the Diving Diseases Research Centre, Fort Bovisand, Plymouth (telephone 01752 261910). They will inform you of your nearest facility.

MECHANICAL DISORDERS OF THE RESPIRATORY TRACT

Massive haemoptysis

Any haemoptysis should be considered massive when it is large enough to endanger life (Jones & Davies, 1990). The mechanism of death is asphyxiation due to inhaled blood rather than hypovolaemia, so the actual volume of blood is not as important as the rate at which bleeding occurs and the state of underlying respiratory function. Massive haemoptysis is a rare event and likely to be due to non-malignant disease (Table 7). The important aspects of acute management are to protect the airway, administer oxygen and encourage the expectoration of inhaled blood. If necessary, the patient should be placed in the head down position lying on the side from which the bleeding is emanating (if that is known). Cough suppressants and sedatives should be avoided and patients should be encouraged to clear their airways with coughing. Blood should be transfused as necessary. Obvious causes of bleeding (e.g. clotting abnormalities) should be remedied. As acute infection can precipitate haemoptysis, all patients should be given broad-spectrum antibiotics intravenously. Patients with depressed conciousness or in imminent danger of asphyxiation should be intubated, ventilated and given adequate suction.

Table 7. *Causes of massive haemoptysis*

- Tuberculosis
- Bronchiectasis
- Lung abscess
- Pneumonia
- Bronchitis
- Aspergilloma

- Bronchial carcinoma
- Endobronchial metastatic malignancy
- Bronchial adenoma

- Mitral stenosis
- Left ventricular failure
- Pulmonary arteriovenous malformations

Once the patient is stabilized, the site and cause of bleeding should be investigated. A chest radiograph may identify the source of haemorrhage but beware of false localizing shadows due to inhaled blood. Most cases of massive haemoptysis will subside within 4 days with supportive treatment alone, and emergency transfer of an unstable patient to a cardiothoracic unit should be avoided. A thoracic physician or surgeon should be involved with the patient's management at an early stage as bronchoscopy may be required to help identify the site and source of bleeding. If bleeding is torrential, the insertion of a double lumen endotracheal tube may isolate the affected lung and protect the healthy side. Bronchial artery embolization should be considered for persistent life-threatening haemoptysis. Emergency surgery should be reserved for those patients with adequate lung function in whom the site of haemorrhage has been identified and who continue to suffer massive haemoptysis despite all other measures (Jones & Davies, 1990).

Massive pleural effusion

Large collections of fluid or blood in the pleural cavity can cause respiratory distress, especially if they accumulate rapidly or the patient has underlying lung disease (Fig. 8). The most common cause is primary or secondary malignancy of the pleura, but spontaneous haemothorax or haemothorax following trauma (which may be relatively minor) can do the same. Pleural aspiration will be required for both diagnostic and therapeutic reasons. If the cause of the effusion is not proven, then pleural aspiration and biopsy must be combined. Pleural fluid is examined macroscopically for the presence of pus,

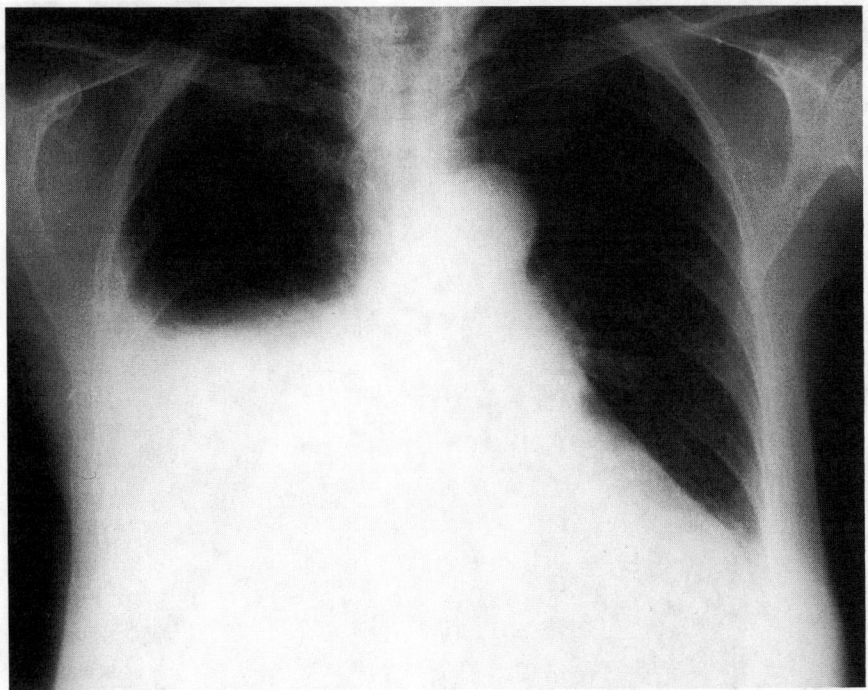

Fig. 8. Chest radiograph showing a right-sided pleural effusion.

blood or chyle and sent for biochemical (e.g. protein, glucose, amylase), microbiological (including mycobacterial) and cytological analysis.

If removal of the pleural fluid is necessary for palliation of respiratory symptoms, a chest drain should be inserted and attached to underwater seal drainage. Always insert a large-bore tube to prevent blockage with fibrin or blood. In traumatic haemothorax the chest drain also gauges the need for surgery by measuring the rate of haemorrhage.

The rate at which pleural fluid should be removed has always been the subject of great debate because of the belief that too rapid removal can cause pulmonary oedema in the underlying lung as it re-expands. Our practice is to allow free drainage of fluid but if the patient complains of chest pain, increasing breathlessness or cough the tube should be clamped and a chest radiograph carried out to exclude any complications such as pneumothorax, poor positioning of the drain or pulmonary oedema. Once the patient has recovered, the rate of fluid drainage can be more gradual and titrated according to symptoms.

Pneumothorax

In health, the visceral and parietal pleura surrounding the lung are in close apposition. If air enters the pleural space either from rupture of alveoli or external chest injury, the normally negative pressure between the two layers of pleura is lost, causing the lung to collapse. The size of the leak determines the degree of collapse. If the leak closes spontaneously, the pneumothorax will cease to enlarge and becomes a closed pneumothorax. If air moves freely into and out of the pleural space with respiration, it is an open pneumothorax. In some patients the defect acts as a valve so that air enters the pleural space with inspiration but cannot escape. This produces a tension pneumothorax with mediastinal shift, compression of the opposite lung, respiratory failure and shock. This can be fatal without prompt treatment.

Primary spontaneous pneumothorax typically occurs in young males and is probably caused by rupture of congenital subpleural blebs or cysts in otherwise healthy lungs. Secondary spontaneous pneumothoraces occur in patients with lung diseases that predispose to pneumothorax, the most common being asthma, chronic bronchitis and emphysema, cystic fibrosis and diffuse pulmonary fibrosis. Causes of non-spontaneous pneumothorax include chest trauma, positive pressure ventilation and interventions such as pleural biopsy.

The clinical features of a pneumothorax will depend on its cause, size and the underlying state of respiratory function. The classical symptoms are pleuritic chest pain and breathlessness. If the pneumothorax is small there

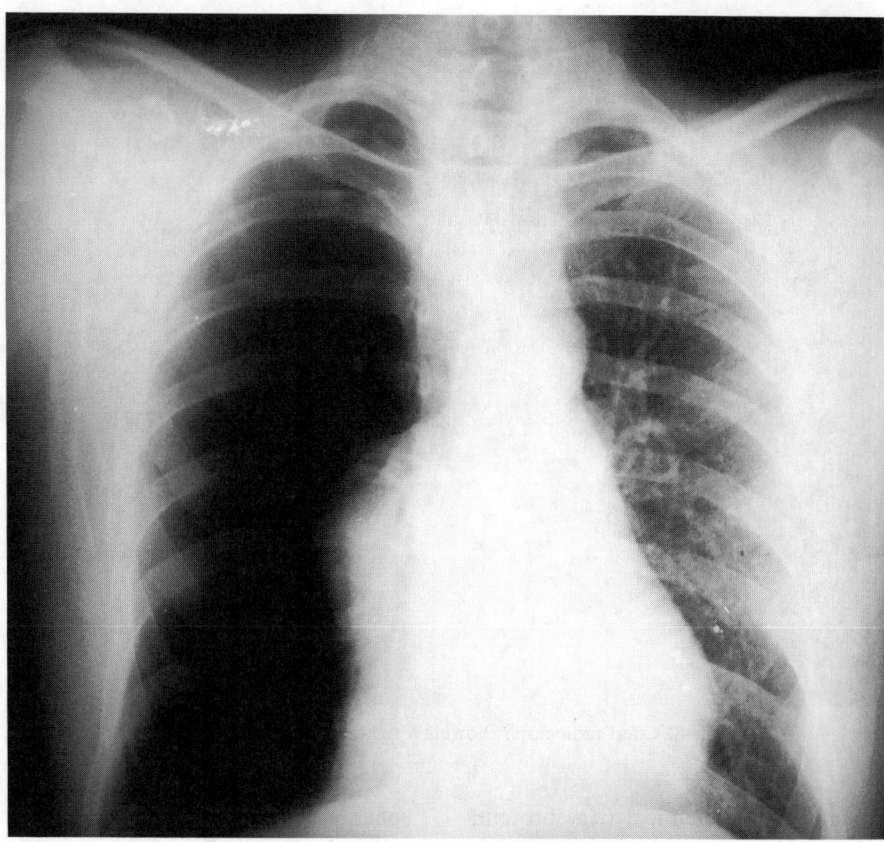

Fig. 9. Chest radiograph showing a right-sided tension pneumothorax.

may be no signs, but decreased chest wall movement and reduced air entry are the commonest manifestations. Increased resonance to percussion is rarely demonstrable. In tension pneumothorax, mediastinal shift produces severe respiratory distress, tachycardia and hypotension (Figure 9).

The diagnosis of a pneumothorax should be confirmed by an erect posteroanterior chest radiograph taken in inspiration. Expiratory films should not be requested routinely. Careful scrutiny for a free lung edge is necessary if small pneumothoraces are not to be missed. In patients with chronic lung disease a large bulla can mimic a pneumothorax radiographically and, if there is doubt, a specialist opinion and comparison with previous films should be obtained before insertion of a chest drain.

A tension pneumothorax is a medical emergency and a wide bore cannula should be inserted immediately into the second intercostal space in the midclavicular line on the affected side. An intercostal tube attached to underwater seal drainage should be inserted as soon as possible after that.

Many pneumothoraces require no drainage and some can be managed with simple aspiration (Miller & Harvey,

1993). The recommended treatment depends on the size of the pneumothorax, the symptoms of the patient and the presence of underlying chronic lung disease (see Fig. 10). Compared with primary spontaneous pneumothoraces, secondary pneumothoraces are more likely to cause breathlessness, less likely to be drained successfully and more likely to need specialist referral.

In a patient without lung disease who has a small or moderately sized pneumothorax without breathlessness, no drainage is required and the pneumothorax can be left to resolve spontaneously with time. The patient can be followed up in the chest clinic after 24 h observation in hospital. If the collapse is complete, or the patient is significantly breathless, aspiration of the pneumothorax should be attempted before resorting to intercostal tube drainage.

TECHNIQUES

Simple aspiration of a pneumothorax

Indications
- Simple aspiration should be attempted on all patients with a spontaneous pneumothorax who are being

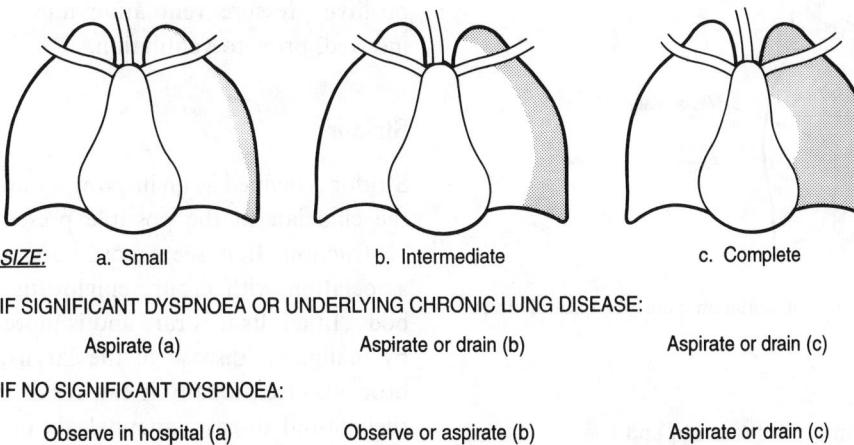

SIZE: a. Small   b. Intermediate   c. Complete

IF SIGNIFICANT DYSPNOEA OR UNDERLYING CHRONIC LUNG DISEASE:

Aspirate (a)   Aspirate or drain (b)   Aspirate or drain (c)

IF NO SIGNIFICANT DYSPNOEA:

Observe in hospital (a)   Observe or aspirate (b)   Aspirate or drain (c)

Fig. 10. Guidelines for the treatment of pneumothorax. Treatment depends on the degree of collapse, the patient's symptoms and the presence of underlying chronic lung disease. The treatment guidelines illustrated are adapted from the recommendations of the British Thoracic Society.

considered for formal drainage, provided emergency relief of breathlessness is not required.

- It is not indicated for tension pneumothorax or traumatic pneumothorax, both of which will require intercostal tube drainage.
- The two broad patient groups who should have simple aspiration are:
  - Patients with no previous history of lung disease who have a complete collapse or significant dyspnoea.
  - Patients with known chronic lung disease who have a moderate or greater degree of collapse or who have significant breathlessness with a smaller collapse.

In both groups the presence of pneumothorax must be proven by chest radiograph.

Practical technique

- This can be carried out without any sedation.
- Local anaesthetic is infiltrated down to the pleura in the mid clavicular line, second intercostal space on the side of the pneumothorax.
- Using a cannula (16G or larger), the pleural space is entered and the needle withdrawn.
- A three-way tap is connected to the cannula and a 50 ml syringe is used to withdraw air from the pleural space and void it to the atmosphere.
- Aspiration should be discontinued if resistance is felt, the patient coughs excessively or more than 2500 ml are withdrawn.
- Technical reasons for failure include inadvertent withdrawal of the cannula from the pleural space or blockage due to kinking.

Following aspiration, a repeat chest radiograph is carried out. If the pneumothorax has resolved or is much smaller, the technique has been successful and no further intervention is required. The patient needs 24 h observation in hospital. If the aspiration has failed, then it is presumed that the pulmonary leak which caused the

pneumothorax is continuing and intercostal tube drainage will be necessary.

Insertion of an intercostal drain

Indications

Intercostal drains are inserted for the following reasons:

- Drainage of a large pleural effusion to relieve breathlessness.
- Drainage of a traumatic haemothorax to relieve symptoms, measure continuing blood loss, prevent empyema and prevent fibrothorax.
- Drainage of a traumatic pneumothorax.
- Drainage of a pneumothorax for any patient requiring assisted ventilation.
- Emergency drainage of a tension pneumothorax.
- Drainage of a spontaneous pneumothorax when simple aspiration has failed.

Practical technique

Throughout the procedure the patient should be reassured and kept informed of progress. Sedation may be required if the patient is very anxious. The side of insertion should be double-checked prior to proceeding by examining the chest radiograph carefully. The best site for insertion is the 'triangle of safety' (Fig. 11). The patient should be positioned comfortably at 30° in the supine position with the arm away from the chest wall, resting behind the head. The site of insertion should be palpated and clearly marked. The drain and attachments must be checked by assembly and dismantling. All connections must fit tightly and the underwater seal drainage bottle containing sterile water must be ready.

Using sterile technique and gloves, local anaesthetic should be generously infiltrated down to the pleural space especially around the periosteum on the upper surface of the lower rib (the neurovascular bundle lies on the lower rib surface). The skin and subcutaneous tissues should be

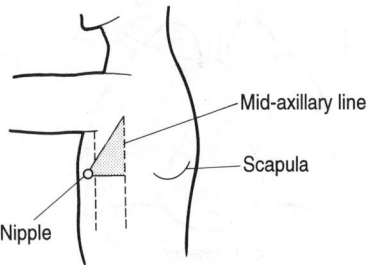

Fig. 11. Diagram of anatomy of optimum point for pleural drain insertion.

incised to ensure a tight fit for the drain and two horizontal sutures put across the incision. These sutures will be used to close the wound when the drain is withdrawn (purse-string sutures are unnecessary). Using forceps, blunt dissection down and through the parietal pleura should make a wide track through the chest wall. After digital examination of the track and confirmation that the pleural space is open the drain should then slide in easily with the assistance of forceps. No force or trocar is required.

Large chest drains should be used for effusions and pneumothoraces to prevent blockage or kinking requiring replacement. For pneumothoraces the drain should be directed towards the lung apex and for pleural effusions directed towards the lung base. The drain must be tightly secured by separate stitches to the skin and the use of plaster dressings. No weight must be attached to the drain and kinking must be avoided.

A properly positioned chest drain will always swing with respiration. If the water level in the distal portion of the drain does not rise on inspiration, the drain is not working and needs to be unblocked or repositioned. A chest radiograph will be required to assess its position. If a drain is bubbling it means that the leak which caused the pneumothorax is continuing and therefore it must not be removed.

In patients with chronic lung disease, if the pneumothorax is small and not causing significant breathlessness, overnight observation is all that is required. If it is no bigger on a chest radiograph the next day, the patient can be followed-up in clinic. When there is moderate or complete collapse of the lung and severe breathlessness, intercostal tube drainage should be carried out immediately. In patients with a moderate or completely collapsed lung who are less breathless, aspiration of air from the pleural space can be attempted prior to intercostal tube drainage (Miller & Harvey, 1993).

Traumatic pneumothoraces more frequently develop tension than spontaneous pneumothoraces and all should be drained. Patients with a pneumothorax who require positive pressure ventilation must have a chest drain inserted, prior to ventilation.

Stridor

Stridor is defined as an inspiratory noise and should alert the clinician to the possible presence of large airway obstruction. It is seen more commonly in children in association with croup, epiglottitis or inhaled foreign body. In adults it is rare and is more likely to be caused by malignant disease of the larynx, trachea or major bronchi. Occasionally it can result from cricoarytenoid rheumatoid disease, anaphylaxis or an inhaled foreign body. Stridor produced by obstruction of the large airways is one of the causes of breathlessness with a normal chest radiograph. Investigation of stridor requires laryngoscopy and/or bronchoscopy. Emergency palliation of stridor caused by malignant disease may be achieved with oral dexamethasone and inhalation of helium/oxygen mixtures while treatment with radiotherapy, chemotherapy, laser ablation or endobronchial stenting is considered.

PULMONARY EMBOLISM

Pulmonary emboli usually occur in patients who are in hospital already, where it constitutes the most common preventable cause of death. Many of these patients are seriously ill or have undergone major surgery – particularly orthopaedic surgery to the pelvis, hips or knees. Pulmonary embolism is also seen in previously well, ambulant patients and it is this group who present to the A&E department.

Pathogenesis

Pulmonary emboli usually originate from clots in the deep veins of the leg. The factors that predispose to the development of venous thrombosis are venostasis, hypercoagulability and vascular damage. The clots begin as small deposits of platelets, fibrin and red blood cells which tend to adhere to the valve cusps of the veins. As these thrombi enlarge, they occlude the lumen of the the vein producing further venostasis which allows the clot to propagate distally and proximally.

When confined to the deep veins of the calf below the knee, the risk of pulmonary embolus is small. However, calf thrombi will propagate to involve the large veins of the thigh and pelvis in approximately 20% of cases. Venous thrombi in the proximal vessels are particularly liable to produce pulmonary emboli (Moser & LeMoine, 1981). Hence patients who undergo major joint surgery are especially susceptible to pulmonary embolism. Only part of the deep vein thrombus embolizes to the lung. Up to 70% of patients with angiographically proven pulmonary embolism have detectable venous thrombosis on investigation (Hull *et al.*, 1985).

It is important to remember that clinical signs for the diagnosis of venous thromboses are notoriously unreliable (Salzman, 1986). The symptoms and signs of a pulmonary embolism will depend on the size of the embolus and the pre-existing cardiorespiratory status of the patient (Benatar *et al.*, 1986).

Clinical features

Patients presenting to the A&E department may be said to have had either an acute non-massive or an acute massive pulmonary embolism depending on the symptoms and signs. Acute non-massive pulmonary embolism is the term used to refer to those patients who present with pulmonary embolism but who are not haemo-dynamically compromised. Patients without pre-existing cardiopulmonary disease require acute occlusion of 50–60% of the pulmonary vascular bed before shock is evident. Significantly smaller emboli can produce shock in patients with poor cardiorespiratory function. The importance of detecting patients with acute non-massive pulmonary embolism is to prevent the subsequent and perhaps fatal development of an acute massive embolism.

Acute non-massive pulmonary embolism

The cardinal feature of a pulmonary embolism is the sudden onset of dyspnoea. This symptom may occur in isolation and be transient. When dyspnoea is associated with pleuritic chest pain (usually lateral and basal) and haemoptysis, pulmonary infarction is likely. This triad of 'classical' symptoms is uncommon and occurs in less than 20% of patients with proven embolism (Wenger *et al.*, 1972). Haemoptysis when it occurs is usually frank and not associated with infected sputum. Patients may complain of pain and swelling in a leg.

On examination, the patient often looks anxious, has a raised respiratory rate and a pleural rub or localized wheeze. A sinus tachycardia is usually present but in a minority of patients there is atrial fibrillation. The jugular venous pressure may be raised and there may be a pulmonary flow murmur caused by partial obstruction of the pulmonary outflow tract. Patients may have

signs of a deep venous thrombosis in one or other leg and a mild pyrexia develops within hours of the event.

None of these symptoms is specific to pulmonary embolism and for each individual symptom or collection of symptoms, alternative diagnoses exist (see below). Pulmonary infection such as viral pleurisy or bacterial pneumonia involving the pleura most commonly give rise to diagnostic difficulty. Pleural inflammation from any cause is exacerbated by breathing and patients tend to alter their respiratory pattern, taking shorter shallower breaths giving rise to a sensation of dyspnoea.

Investigations

Investigations are necessary to look for confirmatory evidence and to exclude alternative diagnoses:

- Pneumothorax.
- Pneumonia.
- Pleurisy.
- Pericarditis.
- Musculoskeletal pain.

Chest radiograph

The chest radiograph is often thought to be normal 24 h after the event. The relevance of subtle abnormalities may only be appreciated retrospectively. The chest radiograph is most useful for excluding pneumothorax or pneumonia. Findings which may suggest pulmonary embolism include a small pleural effusion or linear atelectasis with loss of volume and elevated hemidiaphragm. Radiologically it can be impossible to distinguish between pneumonic consolidation and a pulmonary infarct.

Electrocardiogram

The ECG may be normal in the presence of pulmonary embolism. The commonest abnormalities found are a sinus tachycardia, atrial fibrillation or non-specific T wave changes in the anterior chest leads. Right axis deviation and the oft-quoted S_1, Q_3, T_3 is uncommon and not specific for pulmonary embolism.

Arterial blood gases

Arterial blood gases may be normal in a patient who has suffered a small pulmonary embolism. In a patient without previous cardiopulmonary disease a PaO_2 of less

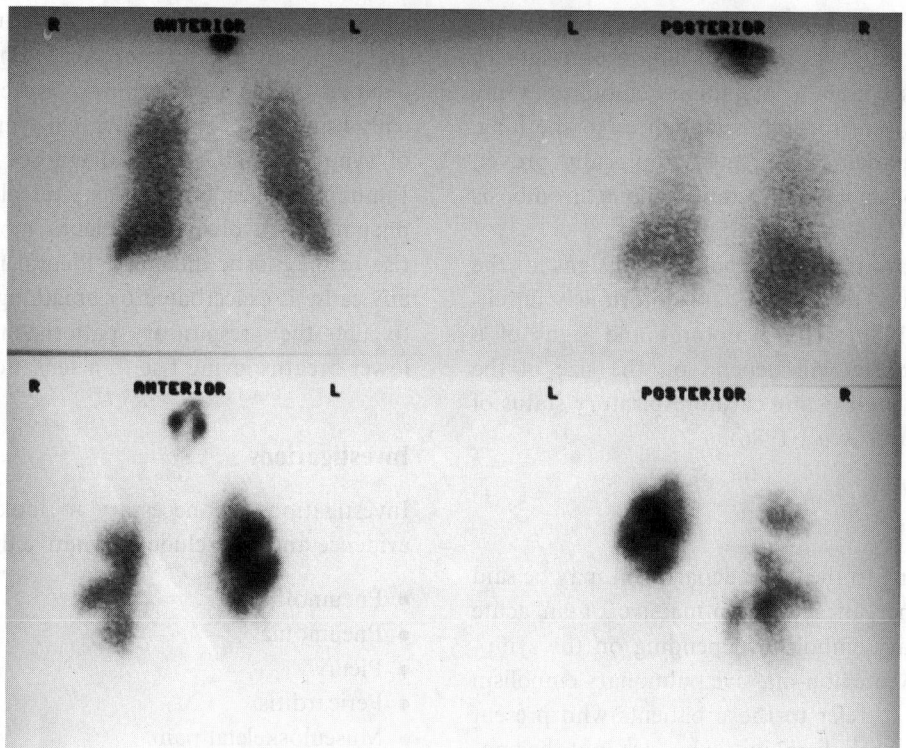

Fig. 12. Radionucleotide scans of ventilation (top) and perfusion (bottom) showing multiple perfusion defects typical of pulmonary emboli.

than 12 kPa should be taken as reduced and compatible with a pulmonary embolism. Patients who have sustained a massive pulmonary embolism will have significant hypoxaemia.

It is therefore possible to have suffered a pulmonary embolism without any abnormality in ECG, chest radiograph or arterial blood gases (Benatar *et al.*, 1986). For this reason it is important that patients with a suggestive history, particularly if there are associated risk factors, should be admitted for further investigation. While awaiting investigations patients should be anticoagulated with intravenous heparin.

Further investigation

Ventilation perfusion scanning (radionuclide lung scanning) is the investigation of choice in making the diagnosis of pulmonary embolism. In patients with a normal chest radiograph, a perfusion scan is usually all that is necessary. A normal perfusion scan excludes a clinically important pulmonary embolism. Other conditions such as pneumonia, chronic air flow limitation and pleural effusion can also give rise to abnormal perfusion scans. With the addition of ventilation scanning, it is possible to demonstrate an area which is abnormally perfused but

normally ventilated (i.e. ventilation/perfusion mismatch). Such a defect suggests a high probability of pulmonary embolism (Fig. 12).

In practice, the interpretation of ventilation/perfusion scans can be very difficult especially in the presence of an abnormal chest radiograph or pre-existing pulmonary disease. The scans are usually reported either as normal, or as indicating a high probability of pulmonary embolism, or intermediate. Patients who have an intermediate scan represent a diagnostic dilemma. A pulmonary angiogram is the gold-standard investigation (Fig. 13) but is not available in many hospitals. An alternative approach is to image the deep veins of the legs (Morrell & Seed, 1992). This is done by venography or ultrasonography. If either proves positive, then pulmonary embolism is more likely and the patient should be treated as such (Dalen, 1993).

Acute massive pulmonary embolism

A massive pulmonary embolism can be fatal despite prompt diagnosis and treatment. It is not uncommon for patients to be admitted from the community having sustained a cardiac arrest who ultimately are shown to have died from a massive pulmonary embolism. Patients

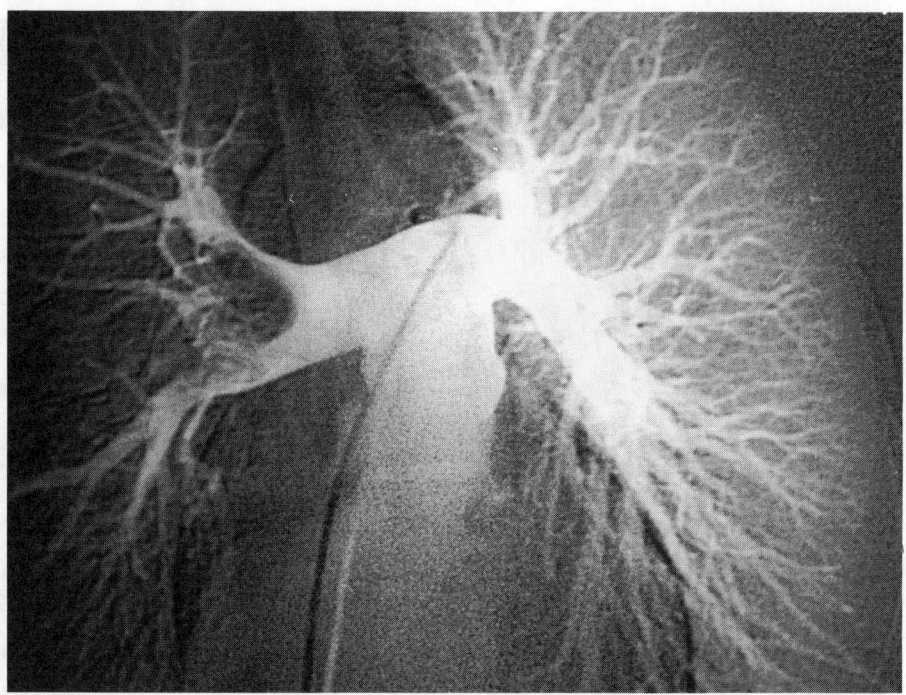

Fig. 13. Pulmonary angiogram showing a filling defect at the bifurcation of the right main pulmonary artery due to an acute pulmonary embolism.

surviving to arrive in hospital need aggressive management but diagnosis can be difficult and misdiagnosis is common. The acute occlusion of a large volume of the pulmonary vascular bed leads to a low cardiac output, hypoxaemia and shock. In patients with pre-existing cardiac disease this can cause ischaemic chest pain due to hypoperfusion of the coronary arteries. It is not surprising, therefore, that many patients with massive pulmonary embolism are diagnosed as having had an acute myocardial infarction.

Clinical examination usually reveals a severely breathless patient who is tachypnoeic, tachycardic, hypotensive and with poor peripheral perfusion. Unlike patients with pulmonary oedema, these patients often prefer to lie flat. Signs of acute right heart failure may be present and should suggest pulmonary embolism if right ventricular infarction can be excluded. The patient will be hypoxaemic. The ECG may not be helpful but should allow the exclusion of a myocardial infarction. The chest radiograph is frequently normal but again allows pulmonary oedema secondary to left ventricular failure to be excluded.

Diagnosis and treatment

Massive pulmonary embolism should be suspected in any patient who presents with dyspnoea, hypoxia and hypotension, especially if there are signs of right heart failure or if there have been risk factors for venous thrombosis or pulmonary embolism. An ECG and chest radiograph are mandatory to exclude cardiac disease. High inspired oxygen is needed to correct hypoxaemia and inotropic support to correct severe hypotension. Diuretics and venodilators are contraindicated as these patients need a high venous pressure to maintain pulmonary perfusion. A heparin infusion should be started as soon as the diagnosis is suspected and further investigations are considered.

If the patient is capable of cooperation, a ventilation/perfusion scan should be performed. However, many patients are too sick to comply and pulmonary angiography is preferable. Once the diagnosis is confirmed, thrombolytic therapy is given either peripherally or perfused directly into the pulmonary artery. The standard contraindications apply to the use of agents such as streptokinase as the bleeding complications associated with their use may be problematical. Many hospitals do not have easy access to radio-isotope scanning or pulmonary angiography. If the clinical suspicion for massive pulmonary embolism is high and the patient is critically ill, there seems little alternative to giving empirical thrombolytic therapy. There have been recent reports of clot fragmentation using a pulmonary artery flotation catheter through which the thrombolytic agent can be

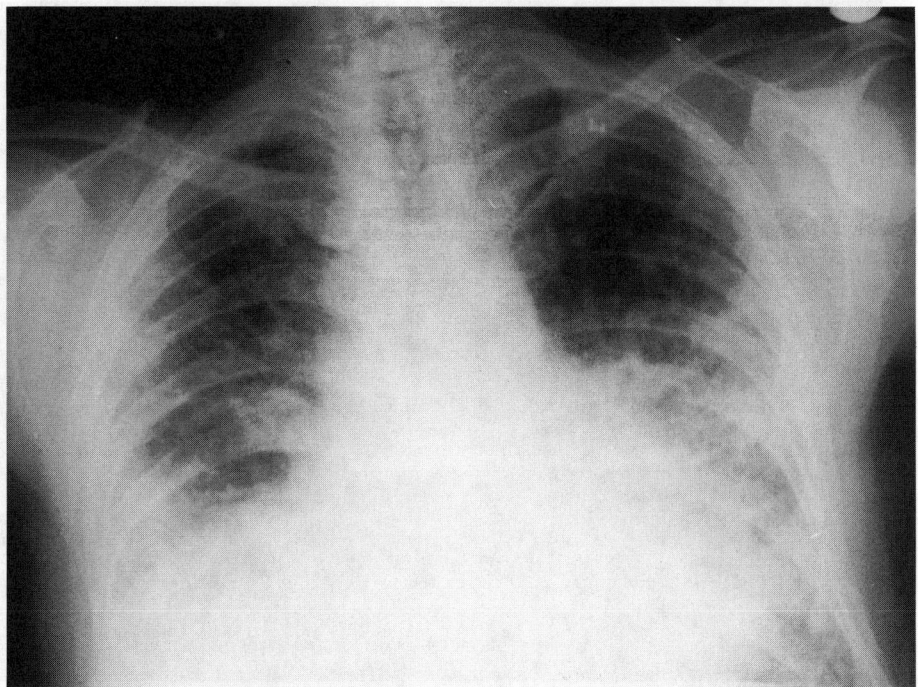

Fig. 14. Pulmonary oedema due to adult respiratory distress syndrome.

given (Brady *et al.*, 1991). For patients not responding to medical treatment, who can be transferred to a cardiothoracic surgical unit, surgery can be life-saving.

ADULT RESPIRATORY DISTRESS SYNDROME

The adult respiratory distress syndrome (ARDS) is a term that has come to describe severe respiratory insufficiency due to permeability pulmonary oedema. It was first described in 1967 as a clinical syndrome consisting of severe dyspnoea, tachypnoea, hypoxia, reduced lung compliance and diffuse alveolar infiltration on the chest radiograph (Ashbaugh *et al.*, 1967). It usually follows 12–72 h after a severe injury or insult (Table 8) which may or may not initially involve the lungs (Fowler *et al.*, 1983). Pathologically, the most striking feature is damage to the components of the alveolar capillary membrane. It is presumed that the initial insult, either directly or by activating cellular, vasoactive and cytotoxic mediators, disrupts the alveolar capillary membrane allowing leakage of blood constituents into the alveoli causing pulmonary oedema and respiratory distress (Murray *et al.*, 1988). Although ARDS probably represents the severe end of a continuum of acute lung injury, there is no specific marker to warn of its development (Jones, 1990). No specific treatment exists and the overall mortality

Table 8. *Some causes of adult respiratory distress syndrome*

- Aspiration of gastric contents
- Severe infective pneumonia
- Drug overdose
- Disseminated intravascular coagulation
- Septicaemia
- Fat embolism
- Hypertension of pregnancy
- Inhalation of toxic fumes
- Multiple blood transfusions
- Near-drowning
- Pancreatitis
- Paraquat poisoning
- Radiation injury
- Pulmonary contusion
- Multiple trauma
- Severe burns
- Cerebral oedema
- Intracranial haemorrhage
- Anaphylaxis
- Diabetic ketoacidosis
- Uraemia

remains around 60% despite all the technology of modern intensive care.

The diagnosis of ARDS is usually made when, in the context of a severe illness, a patient develops respiratory distress and type 1 respiratory failure over a few hours with the later development of pulmonary oedema on the chest radiograph (Fig. 14). Left ventricular failure is excluded by history, examination, ECG and echocardiogram. Insertion of a Swan–Ganz catheter and measurement of pulmonary capillary wedge pressure is not usually necessary for diagnosis, but in severely ill patients can aid management. Hypoproteinaemia is excluded by plasma albumin estimation.

ARDS is not a condition that will present often in an A&E department, but it should be considered as a cause of respiratory failure. If the diagnosis is thought likely, then high inspired oxygen should be given and the intensive care unit staff involved at an early stage. Treatment of patients with ARDS is supportive. Most patients die from associated multiple organ failure and sepsis, rather than respiratory failure. The underlying cause of ARDS should be identified and treated. Any sepsis should be managed aggressively with antibiotics and surgical drainage if indicated. Hypoxia must be corrected with oxygen and/or assisted ventilation. Careful attention must be given to fluid balance, circulatory support and renal function (Macnaughton & Evans, 1992).

PULMONARY FUNCTION TESTS IN RESPIRATORY EMERGENCIES

Arterial blood gases

These are discussed in Chapter 7.

Peak expiratory flow rate

Peak expiratory flow rate (PEFR) is easily measured with cheap and readily available equipment. The meters are accurate at low flow rates but tend to over-read in the middle range and under-read at high flows (Miller & Ouanjer, 1994). There is considerable variability between meters so for serial measurements it is important that the same meter is used. It is also important that the patient's technique is observed during measurement and that the best of three successive manoeuvres is recorded.

A single PEFR value is important in deciding management in a patient with acute severe asthma. Serial PEFR measurements are essential in monitoring treatment response in asthma and assessing reversibility in chronic air flow limitation. However, PEFR values can be low in conditions other than asthma and chronic air flow limitation such as heart failure and tracheal obstruction.

PEFR is more effort-dependent than spirometry and can also fall with diseases causing respiratory muscle weakness such as acute infective polyneuritis. A low PEFR is not, therefore, particularly helpful in making the diagnosis of the cause of a patient's breathlessness.

Spirometry

Spirometry is the best investigation for deciding if a patient's breathlessness is due to air flow obstruction. During spirometry, the patient empties their lungs as quickly and as completely as possible following a full inspiration. Forced expiratory volume in 1 sec (FEV_1) and forced vital capacity (FVC) are recorded. In normal lungs (FEV_1/FVC) × 100 is usually over 75%.

Patients with restrictive lung disease (e.g. heart failure, respiratory muscle weakness, fibrosing alveolitis, etc.) have small lungs and therefore FEV_1 and FVC are reduced proportionally and (FEV_1/FVC) × 100 remains over 75%. In patients with air flow obstruction, FEV_1 and FVC are both reduced but FEV_1 is reduced relatively more so that (FEV_1/FVC) × 100 falls below 75%.

One must beware of one relatively common pitfall in interpreting spirometric values. Patients who are very breathless due to air flow obstruction can sometimes not sustain the forced expiration to fully empty their lungs so that the FVC recorded is spuriously low. Because of this, the FEV_1/FVC ratio may appear normal. It is important to watch the patient doing the test. In the vast majority of cases, an FEV_1 below 1 litre will be due to obstructive airways disease, (chronic bronchitis and emphysema or asthma).

Pulse oximetry

Pulse oximetry is the most convenient non-invasive method of continuously measuring arterial oxygen saturation. In patients with type 1 respiratory failure it can be used to monitor oxygen therapy without the need for repeated arterial blood gas analysis. Oxygen should be administered to keep the oxygen saturation above 95%. Its measurements are not as accurate in the presence of poor peripheral cardiac output, excessive patient movement or nail varnish. It will seriously over-read oxygen saturation in the presence of carbon monoxide poisoning and must never be used as a guide to therapy in this situation. One must also remember that because of the shape of the oxygen dissociation curve, oxygen saturation gives no indication of the underlying PaO_2, which can fall to below 8 kPa before oxygen saturation is affected.

The major pitfall with its use is that it gives no indication of the adequacy of alveolar ventilation in patients who are receiving supplemental oxygen. In patients who hypoventilate while breathing air, $PaCO_2$ will rise and eventually PaO_2 and oxygen saturation will fall. If the patient is receiving extra oxygen, then the saturation will remain normal despite dangerous levels of hypercapnia and ensuing respiratory acidosis (Hutton & Clutton-Brock, 1993). Because of this, pulse oximetry cannot be used in the management of patients in type 2 respiratory failure due to chronic airways disease where monitoring of the $PaCO_2$ and pH using arterial blood gas analysis is mandatory (see section on respiratory failure).

Bibliography

ASHBAUGH, D.G., BIGELOW, D.B., PETTY, T.L. et al. (1967). Acute respiratory distress in adults. *Lancet*, ii, 319–23.

BARNES, P.J. & HOLGATE, S.T. (1990). Asthma: pathogenesis and hyperreactivity. In: *Respiratory Medicine*, ed. R.A.L. Brewis, G.J. Gibson & D.M. Geddes, pp. 558–603. London: Baillière Tindall.

BENATAR, S.R., IMMELMAN, E.J. & JEFFERY, P. (1986). Pulmonary embolism. *Br. J. Dis. Chest*, 80, 313–34.

BRADY, A.J.B., CRAKE, T. & OAKLEY, C.M. (1991). Percutaneous catheter fragmentation and distal dispersion of proximal pulmonary embolus. *Lancet*, 338, 1186–9.

BREWIS, R.A.L. (1982). Respiratory disorders. In *Textbook of Adverse Drug Reactions*, ed. D.M. Davies, pp. 154–87. Oxford: Oxford University Press.

BRITISH THORACIC ASSOCIATION (1982). Deaths from asthma in two regions of England. *Br. Med. J.*, 285, 1251–5.

BRITISH THORACIC SOCIETY (1993). Guidelines for the management of community-acquired pneumonia in adults admitted to hospital. *Br. J. Hosp. Med.*, 49, 346–50.

BRITISH THORACIC SOCIETY, BRITISH PAEDIATRIC ASSOCIATION, RESEARCH UNIT OF ROYAL COLLEGE OF PHYSICIANS OF LONDON, KING'S FUND CENTRE, NATIONAL ASTHMA CAMPAIGN, ROYAL COLLEGE OF GENERAL PRACTITIONERS, GENERAL PRACTITIONERS IN ASTHMA GROUP, BRITISH ASSOCIATION OF ACCIDENT AND EMERGENCY MEDICINE AND BRITISH PAEDIATRIC RESPIRATORY GROUP (1993). Guidelines on the management of asthma. *Thorax*, 48, S1–S24.

BROWN, P.J., GREVILLE, H.W. & FINUCANE, K.E. (1984). Asthma and irreversible airflow obstruction. *Thorax*, 39, 131–6.

BURNEY, P.J.G. (1986). Asthma mortality in England and Wales: evidence for a further increase 1974–84. *Lancet*, ii, 323–6.

CLARK, C.J., REID, W.H., GILMOUR, W.H. et al. (1986). Mortality probability in victims of fire trauma: revised equation to include inhalation injury. *Br. Med. J.*, 292, 1303–5.

CLARK, R.J. & BEELEY, J.M. (1989). Smoke inhalation. *Br. J. Hosp. Med.*, 41, 252–9.

DALEN, J.E. (1993). When can treatment be withheld in patients with suspected pulmonary embolism? *Arch. Intern. Med.*, 153, 1415–18.

DEPARTMENT OF CLINICAL EPIDEMIOLOGY, NATIONAL HEART & LUNG INSTITUTE, London (1988). Respiratory disease in England and Wales. *Thorax*, 43, 949–54.

DRUGS & THERAPEUTICS BULLETIN (1988). Treatment of carbon monoxide poisoning. *Drugs Ther. Bull.*, 26, 77–9.

EASON, J. & MARKOWE, H.L.J. (1987). Controlled investigation of deaths from asthma in hospitals in the North East Thames region. *Br. Med. J.*, 294, 1255–8.

FOWLER, A.A., HAMMAN, R.F., GOOD, J.T. et al. (1983). Adult respiratory distress syndrome: risk with common predispositions. *Ann. Intern. Med.*, 98, 593–7.

GRIBBIN, H.R. (1993). Management of respiratory failure. *Br. J. Hosp. Med.*, 49, 461–77.

HIGENBOTTAM, T., CROME, P., PARKINSON, C. et al. (1979). Further clinical observations on the pulmonary effects of paraquat ingestion. *Thorax*, 34, 161–5.

HOPKIN, J.M. (1990). Respiratory disease in the immunocompromised host: non-AIDS. In *Respiratory Medicine*, ed. R.A.L. Brewis, G.J. Gibson & D.M. Geddes, pp. 961–73. London: Baillière Tindall.

HOSKER, H., COOKE, N.J. & HAWKEY, P. (1994). Antibiotics in chronic obstructive pulmonary disease. *Br. Med. J.*, 308, 871–2.

HULL, R.D., HIRSCH, J., CARTER, C.J. et al. (1985). Diagnostic efficiency of impedance plethysmography for clinically suspected deep vein thrombosis. *Ann. Intern. Med.*, 102, 21–8.

HUTTON, P. & CLUTTON-BROCK, T. (1993). The benefits and pitfalls of pulse oximetry. *Br. Med. J.*, 307, 457–8.

JAMAL, K., FLEETHAM, J.A. & THURLBECK, W.M. (1990). Cor pulmonale: correlation with central airway lesions, peripheral airway lesions, emphysema and control of breathing. *Am. Rev. Respir. Dis.*, 141, 1172–7.

JEFFREY, A.A., WARREN, P.M. & FLENLEY, D.C. (1992). Acute hypercapnic respiratory failure in patients with chronic obstructive lung disease: risk factors and use of guidelines for management. *Thorax*, 47, 34–40.

JONES, D.K. (1990). Markers for impending adult respiratory distress syndrome. *Respir. Med.*, 84, 89–91.

JONES, D.K. & DAVIES, R.J.D. (1990). Massive haemoptysis. *Br. Med. J.*, **300**, 889–90.

LEACH, R.M. & BATEMAN, N.T. (1993). Acute oxygen therapy. *Br. J. Hosp. Med.*, **49**, 637–44.

LORBER, B. & SWENSON, R.M. (1974). Bacteriology of aspiration pneumonia: a prospective study of community and hospital acquired cases. *Ann. Intern. Med.*, **81**, 329–31.

MACFARLANE, J. (1987). Community-acquired pneumonia. *Br. J. Dis. Chest*, **81**, 116–27.

MACFARLANE, J.T. (1991). Pneumonia. *Med. Int.*, **90**, 3732–9.

MACNAUGHTON, P.D. & EVANS, T.W. (1992). Management of adult respiratory distress syndrome. *Lancet*, **339**, 469–72.

MEDICAL RESEARCH COUNCIL (1965). Definition and classification of chronic bronchitis for clinical and epidemiological purposes. *Lancet*, **i**, 775–9.

MILLER, A.C. & HARVEY, J.E. on behalf of Standards of Care Committee, British Thoracic Society (1993). Guidelines for the management of spontaneous pneumothorax. *Br. Med. J.*, **307**, 114–16.

MILLER, M.R. & OUANJER, P.H. (1994). Peak flow meters: a problem of scale. *Br. Med. J.*, **308**, 548–9.

MITCHELL, D.M. & JOHNSON, M.A. (1990). Treatment of lung disease in patients with the acquired immune deficiency syndrome. *Thorax*, **45**, 219–24.

MORRELL, N.W. & SEED, W.A. (1992). Diagnosing pulmonary embolism. *Br. Med. J.*, **304**, 1126–7.

MOSER, K. & LEMOINE, J.R. (1981). Is embolic risk conditioned by location of deep venous thrombosis? *Ann. Intern. Med.*, **94**, 439–44.

MURRAY, J.F., MATTHAY, M.A., LUCE, J.M. *et al.* (1988). An expanded definition of the adult respiratory distress syndrome. *Am. Rev. Respir. Dis.*, **138**, 720–3.

NISAR, M., WALSHAW, M., EARIS, J.E. *et al.* (1990).

Assessment of reversibility of airway obstruction in patients with chronic obstructive airways disease. *Thorax*, **45**, 190–4.

PROUDFOOT, A.T., STEWART, M.S., LEVITT, T. *et al.* (1979). Paraquat poisoning: significance of plasma paraquat levels. *Lancet*, **ii**, 330–2.

RICHENS, J.M. & HOWARD, P. (1982). Oedema in cor pulmonale. *Clin. Sci.*, **62**, 255–9.

ROYAL COLLEGE OF GENERAL PRACTITIONERS, OFFICE OF POPULATION CENSUSES AND SURVEYS, and DEPARTMENT OF HEALTH AND SOCIAL SECURITY (1986). *Morbidity Statistics from General Practice 1981–2. Third National Study.* London: HMSO.

SALZMAN, E.W. (1986). Venous thrombosis made easy. *N. Engl. J. Med.*, **314**, 847–8.

SEATON, A., SEATON, D. & LEITCH, A.G. (1989). Acute infections of the upper respiratory tract, trachea and bronchi. In *Crofton and Douglas's Respiratory Diseases*, 4th edn., ed. A. Seaton, D. Seaton & A. G. Leitch, pp. 270–84. London: Blackwell Scientific.

SNIDER, G.L., KLEINERMAN, J., THURLBECK, W.M. *et al.* (1985). The definition of emphysema. Report of a National Heart, Lung and Blood Institute, Division of Lung Diseases Workshop. *Am. Rev. Respir. Dis.*, **132**, 182–5.

VERGHESE, A. & BERK, S.L. (1983). Bacterial pneumonia in the elderly. *Medicine*, **62**, 271–85.

WATSON, J.M. (1993). Tuberculosis in Britain today. *Br. Med. J.*, **306**, 221–2.

WEBB, J., CLARK, T.J.H. & CHILVERS, C. (1981). Time course of response to prednisolone in chronic airflow obstruction. *Thorax*, **36**, 18–21.

WENGER, N.K., STEIN, P.D. & WILLIS, P.W. (1972). Massive acute pulmonary embolism. The deceivingly nonspecific manifestations. *J. Am. Med. Assoc.*, **220**, 843–4.

45 Cardiovascular emergencies

R. VINCENT and D.A. CHAMBERLAIN (A: Cardiovascular emergencies (excluding arrhythmias))

T.A. MILLANE and A.J. CAMM (B: Cardiac arrhythmias))

Chapter plan

A: Cardiovascular emergencies (excluding arrhythmias)

Introduction
Chest pain
Angina
Acute myocardial infarction
Cardiac failure
Cardiogenic shock
Pulmonary emboli
Aortic dissection
Pericarditis
Accelerated hypertension

B: Cardiac arrhythmias

General introduction
Bradycardia
Tachycardia
Permanent pacemakers
Drug overdose and cardiac arrhythmia
Arrhythmia in infants and children
Arrhythmia in pregnancy and lactation
The future

A: Cardiovascular emergencies (excluding arrhythmias)

R. VINCENT and D.A. CHAMBERLAIN

Department of Cardiology, Royal Sussex County Hospital, Brighton, UK

INTRODUCTION

Cardiovascular emergencies are among the commonest medical conditions to be seen in an accident and emergency (A&E) department. Their frequency reflects the community burden of cardiovascular disease, which still accounts for the single most common cause of death in the UK.

Total mortality in the UK for coronary artery disease is about 160 000 per year (equivalent to the death of a jumbo jet full of passengers each day); roughly half die before the age of 70 years. For every 10 000 persons up to the age of 75 years, 128 years of life are lost through ischaemic heart disease. A further 115 000 patients per year are discharged from hospital with this diagnosis.

In the mid-1980s the national cost of coronary artery disease was estimated at £500m for treatment and £1800m in lost production. In 1991, coronary heart disease accounted for 2.5% of total National Health Service expenditure (Tunstall-Pedoe, 1991).

Patients in whom a *possibility* of cardiac disease is raised by their presenting symptoms provide an important diagnostic challenge. Although many are shown subsequently to have non-cardiac pathology, most need urgent and careful evaluation. To dismiss important vascular disease as benign may have serious consequences, while to attribute an innocent condition mistakenly to heart disease may also have adverse effects – in unnecessary hospital admissions, in matters of employment and insurance, and perhaps in a lifetime of unwarranted anxiety.

In this chapter we will review the following topics:

- Chest pain.
- Angina.
- Acute myocardial infarction.

Presenting symptoms that may indicate cardiac disease but which may also have a non-cardiac cause

- Chest pain
- Palpitation
- Breathlessness
- Wheeze
- Cough
- Peripheral oedema
- Presyncope
- Syncope
- Transient cerebral ischaemic attack
- Stroke
- Peripheral arterial occlusion
- Unaccustomed fatigue

- Cardiac failure.
- Cardiogenic shock.
- Other cardiovascular emergencies
  - Aortic dissection
  - Pulmonary embolism.
  - Pericarditis.
  - Accelerated hypertension.

CHEST PAIN

Although chest pain invariably raises the suspicion of ischaemic heart disease, the range of possible causes is wide:

- Unstable angina.
- Acute myocardial infarction.
- Pericarditis.
- Aortic dissection.
- Pleurisy.
- Pulmonary embolism.
- Pneumothorax.
- Oesophagitis.
- Oesophageal rupture.
- Mediastinitis.
- Costochondral tenderness.
- Nerve entrapment.
- Herpes zoster.
- Other chest wall pain (inflammatory, malignant, traumatic).
- Gallbladder disease.
- Peptic ulcer.
- Hyperventilation.

- Medical 'Munchausen's' syndrome.
- Unknown.

The most valuable tool in the diagnosis of chest pain at rest is the *history*. Make a careful note of the *speed of onset of symptoms*. Pain due to unstable angina and acute myocardial infarction builds up over a few minutes; pain from the chest wall and from acute aortic dissection is 'sudden' – a term ideally used to mean 'instantaneous'. Momentary pains are invariably skeletal, and those lasting persistently for many hours or days have a non-cardiac cause. If the patient uses the word 'sharp' be sure to determine whether he means knife-like or merely severe.

The *character* of the pain is a strong pointer to its cause. Pain worse on inspiration points to pericarditis, pleurisy or pneumothorax, although it also can occur from skeletal causes. 'Squeezing', 'crushing', 'like a weight', or 'a pressure' are frequent descriptions of ischaemic cardiac pain, especially when these sensations apply to the precordium. With milder symptoms patients may be reluctant to use the term 'pain' and even deny it; rather, they may be aware of an intensely disagreeable and frightening substernal discomfort. The patient with ischaemic cardiac pain will usually want to sit up and keep still, and associated breathlessness is common. Do not necessarily be deflected from a diagnosis of ischaemic heart disease if the patient refers to a 'burning' or to a sensation of 'acute indigestion', or by an assertion that it is relieved by burping. Many patients in cardiac care units began their journey there with the conviction that their symptoms were dyspeptic. Beware, too, of the widespread tendency to minimize the severity or significance of chest symptoms.

The *position* of the pain is important. Well-localized, laterally placed symptoms are rarely cardiac, but there are occasional exceptions. Ischaemic pain, although typically retrosternal, is sometimes felt in a single, surprisingly small area, often in the left anterior chest. The radiation of cardiac pain into the arm, neck, jaw and epigastrium is well known, but in a few cases true cardiac pain is felt in only one of these areas with no associated symptoms in the chest. Also, such radiation is not specific for pain of cardiac origin. Radiation of ischaemic pain to the back is much less common and should always raise the suspicion of aortic, oesophageal or gallbladder disease.

A similarity between presenting symptoms and those known previously to be associated with specific pathology can be helpful, but may not always be reliable. The pain of unstable angina or acute myocardial infarction may differ from previous ischaemic symptoms, particularly

Table 1. *Physical signs that can be helpful in the differential diagnosis of chest pain*

Most of these signs need interpretation on the basis of history and/or special investigations.

Signs	Comment
Lipid deposits, arcus senilis, premature earlobe crease	Hints at increased risk of ischaemic heart disease
Herpetic rash	Pain may be out of proportion to skin changes
Hyperaesthetic area at site of pain	Nerve root irritation or early herpes
Diminished breath sounds	May indicate pneumothorax, or effusion, or haemothorax from rupture of aortic aneurysm into the pleural cavity
Obvious chest trauma	
Costochondral tenderness	Commonest tender points in costochondritis are the fourth and fifth left costochondral junctions. Beware a more serious coexisting pathology of cardiac or pulmonary origin
Paravertebral muscle spasm/tenderness	Underlying degenerative spine disease is the commonest cause
High jugular venous pressure	Commonly seen in acute inferior myocardial infarction with right ventricular dysfunction; also with major pulmonary embolism, acute aortic dissection (from pericardial tamponade or superior vena cava obstruction), and ruptured sinus of Valsalva
Dyskinetic left ventricular impulse	Previous or new anterior myocardial infarction
Third or fourth heart sound	Indicative of ventricular dysfunction – a non-specific pointer to acute or long-standing heart disease. Is right-sided in massive acute pulmonary embolism. (A fourth heart sound is a remarkably subtle sign only rarely elicited correctly)
Pericardial rub	Pericarditis – but defining the cause (infarct, viral, malignant, autoimmune) will depend on further tests
Early diastolic murmur	Can be associated with a distorted aortic valve ring due to aortic dissection or a ruptured sinus of Valsalva
Pleural rub	Pleurisy – cause to be further defined
Right hypochondrial or epigastric tenderness	Usually reflects abdominal pathology but may also be due to hepatic congestion from heart failure
Observation of sputum	Blood or pus may be a pointer to diagnosis

after coronary surgery or an earlier infarct. A beneficial response to trinitrine is only a weak pointer to the diagnosis of ischaemic heart disease since both skeletal and oesophageal pain may also improve after nitrate therapy.

Finally, the history may reveal more than one source of pain: for example, both angina and skeletal pain, or aortic dissection and an inferior infarct. (The mechanism for this is illustrated in Fig. 16.) In the elderly, a combination of oesophageal reflux, angina and costochondral pain is common.

The *examination* may elicit one or more of the several physical signs that can be helpful in the differential diagnosis of chest pain. These are set out in Table 1.

Often they need interpretation in the light of the history and subsequent investigations. Persistent autonomic imbalance (a pale clammy patient with tachycardia or inappropriate bradycardia) usually indicates an important pathology but may not distinguish a specific underlying cause. In the overall assessment of the patient, hospital or A&E department records of an earlier examination may be helpful.

A patient presenting with chest pain is likely to undergo a number of *special investigations* of which the *electrocardiogram* (ECG) will be foremost. The following practical points are especially applicable to recording a 12-lead ECG in the A&E department:

- Use a diagnostic quality ECG machine, not one configured only for displaying arrhythmias.
- Ensure that the patient is relaxed with arms, back, and head supported.
- Take care that arm leads are the correct way round and that the chest electrodes are positioned correctly. Errors in lead placement are not uncommon and cause a false interpretation of the trace looked at on its own or in comparison with other records.
- Be prepared to record several 12-lead ECGs within a short time when unstable angina or hyperacute infarction is suspected.
- Record a 12-lead ECG as soon as possible in all cases of broad complex tachycardia (see Chapter 45B).

The trace may be diagnostic, or at least clearly abnormal, but we must reiterate that an apparently normal ECG does not exclude acute myocardial infarction (MI) or another serious underlying condition. In particular, the ECG in pulmonary embolism may show no more than sinus tachycardia or mild ischaemic change, a common appearance also in aortic dissection unless there is a coexistent inferior infarct due to ostial occlusion of the right coronary artery.

ECGs in the A&E department are sometimes noted as showing 'no acute changes'. This phrase is best avoided, however; firstly, because it has no agreed definition (although 'acute changes' are probably taken to mean the ST-T displacement of profound myocardial ischaemia or infarction), and secondly because it may bring an unwarranted sense of reassurance. Describe the record, adding a comment of interpretation.

The appearances of the ECG in unstable angina, acute MI and other cardiac emergencies are described in later sections. But note here that:

- Repolarization (the ST-T-U segment) is usually the most sensitive part of the record to changes in myocardial perfusion.
- Earlier records for comparison can be invaluable: make every effort to find them.
- Specialist advice (perhaps by using a FAX machine) should be sought without hestiation where there is diagnostic uncertainty.

A *chest X-ray* is more likely to be of help in the diagnosis of pulmonary rather than cardiovascular disorders causing chest pain. Pneumonia, neoplasm, peripheral pulmonary embolism, pleural effusion or pneumothorax are seen readily, although these may not always be related directly to the presenting pain. In contrast, the oligaemia of a major pulmonary embolism may be difficult to detect and chest X-ray appearances may be near-normal in this condition in spite of the recent occlusion of a large part of the pulmonary artery tree. Occasionally, the chest X-ray is helpful in showing an unsuspected rib fracture, lung or bone metastases, soft tissue calcification, or abnormalities of the shoulder joint.

Radiographic abnormalities of the mediastinum pointing to a cause for the presenting pain include:

- An enlarged cardiac outline (heart failure/pericardial effusion).
- Mediastinal air (ruptured oesophagus).
- A widened ascending aorta (aortic valve disease or dissection).
- An enlarged aortic arch with double outline (aortic dissection).
- A gastric air bubble behind the heart (hiatus hernia with gastro-oesophageal reflux).

Rarely, subdiaphragmatic gas may be demonstrated, indicating a cause of chest pain that is below the diaphragm.

Simple blood tests – haemoglobin, white count, blood urea and electrolytes, random blood sugar, cholesterol and liver function tests – may contribute to the medical profile of the patient with chest pain, but with the exception of a readily available urgent creatine kinase – or other specific markers of myocardial damage (Adams III *et al.*, 1992) – these are rarely of any diagnostic help.

Echocardiography – if available in the A&E department – will quickly demonstrate the presence of pericardial effusion, and in skilled hands it can show the right ventricular overload of massive pulmonary embolism or the abnormalities of proximal aortic dissection. Occasionally, signs of generalized or regional changes in left ventricular wall movement can be helpful to establish a diagnosis.

The assessment of a patient with chest pain may be straightforward; but it may also pose a diagnostic challenge that defies rapid solution. To reiterate, in most cases the *history* will contribute the most useful data to the decision-making process. Admission of all patients in whom a serious cause cannot be excluded entirely is a counsel of perfection, but is often hindered by the pressure on hospital beds. Where doubt exists, a senior medical opinion should be sought before the patient is sent home.

ANGINA

Definitions

Angina pectoris is a term referring to episodic chest pain of a disagreeable quality that was first described by William Heberden in 1772. It is now equated with the syndrome of precordial pain and breathlessness that arises from transient reversible myocardial ischaemia usually precipitated by exercise or emotion. *Decubitus angina* describes angina prompted by lying down (usually at night) and *unstable angina* indicates a progressive pattern of symptoms that may include pain at rest.

Angina in its various forms is one manifestation of *ischaemic heart disease*, a more general term for the presentations of myocardial ischaemia including stable and unstable angina, acute MI, cardiac failure and sudden cardiac death.

Pathology and presentation

Myocardial ischaemia results from an imbalance between its oxygen demand and oxygen supply through the coronary arteries. *Demand* rises with an increase in ventricular wall tension (determined by blood pressure and end-diastolic dimension), heart rate and contractility. *Supply* may be jeopardized by the effects of tight aortic stenosis, obstruction at the coronary ostia, resistance in the epicardial arteries, increased tone in the subsequent resistance vessels, coronary spasm, and perhaps abnormalities of vessel and cellular behaviour beyond (Fig. 1). Myocardial oxygen delivery may also be hindered by

a decrease in red cell deformability that can accompany ischaemic heart disease.

Atheromatous lesions in the epicardial coronary arteries are by far the commonest cause of both silent and symptomatic ischaemic heart disease. Three main pathological mechanisms are involved:

1. Progressive deposition of atheroma.
2. Plaque disruption causing intraplaque haemorrhage and/or intraluminal thrombosis.
3. An abnormal increase in coronary tone or coronary spasm.

In vitro, animal and human investigations are contributing to our present understanding of the biology of the atheromatous plaque – a lesion which is complex and results from endothelial disruption. Mechanisms of endothelial damage, of subsequent platelet interaction, and of the controlling factors for the cellular processes that follow are under intense investigation. The triggers to cell migration, cell proliferation, lipid accumulation and subendothelial fibrosis (Woolf, 1990; Foegh & Virmani, 1993) have yet to be fully understood. A wide range of vasoactive peptides made and released by platelets, and by the endothelial wall, contribute importantly to the regulation of coronary tone in both normal and abnormal coronary arteries. This, too, is a growing area for research (Luscher *et al.*, 1993).

The interplay of the factors described determines the presentation and progress of patients with ischaemic heart disease. Those whose coronary narrowing is due mostly to slowly progressive atheroma are likely to have chronic stable angina with the familiar precipitating factors of exercise and emotion (Hangartner *et al.*, 1986). But most patients will have an additional component of exaggerated coronary tone accounting in part for exacerbations caused by cold weather or a large meal (Lichtlen *et al.*, 1985).

Where a plaque becomes unstable through disruption or fissuring, a sudden increase in coronary narrowing is likely through several mechanisms (Fig. 2): platelet adhesion, fibrin clot formation in the coronary lumen, enlargement of the atheromatous plaque through intraplaque haemorrhage, abnormal vasconstriction at the site of the plaque, and adventitial inflammation (Davies & Thomas, 1985). The clinical result will depend on a number of factors: the degree of swelling of the plaque itself, the rate of formation, location, extent and stability of the intracoronary clot; the degree of pre-existing vessel narrowing; the intensity and duration of coexisting coronary spasm; the presence of collaterals; and the

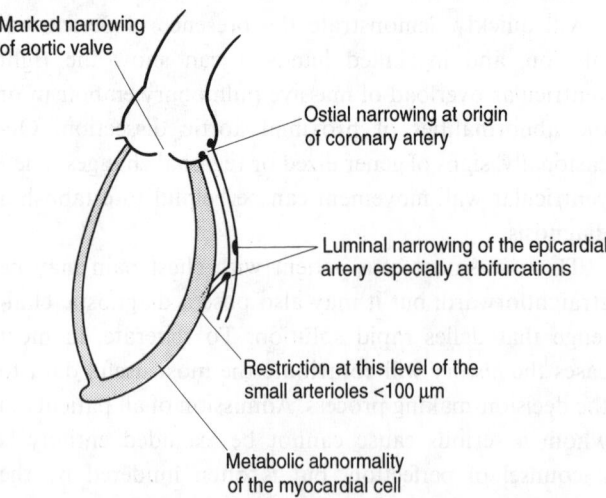

Fig. 1. Sites of restriction to coronary flow that may result in myocardial ischaemia or infarction. Atheromatous obstruction to epicardial coronary arteries is by far the most common mechanism.

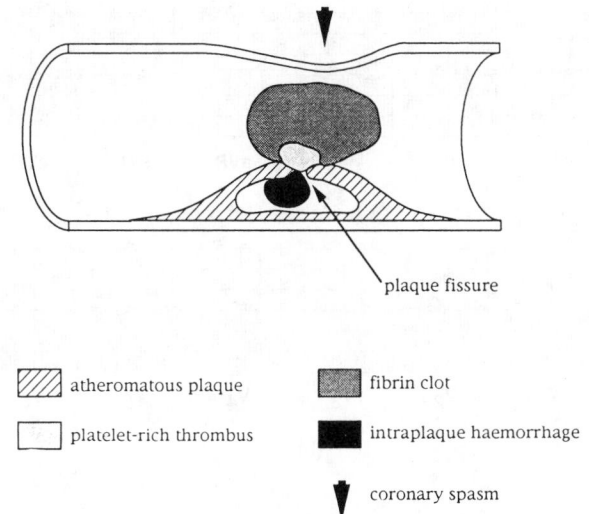

plaque fissure

▨ atheromatous plaque

▨ fibrin clot

☐ platelet-rich thrombus

■ intraplaque haemorrhage

▼ coronary spasm

Fig. 2. The mechanisms of abrupt coronary narrowing through plaque disruption. (Reproduced, with permission, from Skinner & Vincent, 1993.)

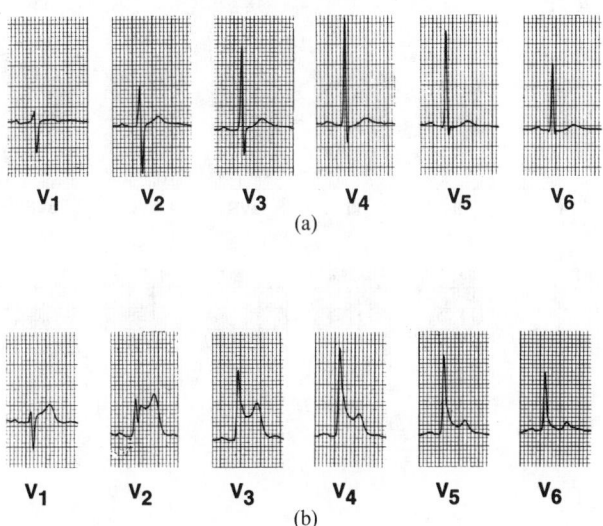

Fig. 3. The electrocardiographic features of Prinzmetal's variant angina. ST segment elevation of characteristic shape (a). As coronary spasm relaxes, both pain and ST abnormalities subside (b).

viability of the cardiac muscle supplied by the artery concerned. It is important to know the common clinical presentations of an unstable coronary lesion since it is this group that demands the most urgent attention and careful management.

Clinical presentations of an unstable coronary lesion

- An abrupt onset of new angina
- A sudden worsening of established angina
- Episodes of pain at rest
- Acute myocardial infarction
- Sudden cardiac death

Endothelial damage may result in a paradoxical vasoconstriction from transmitters that usually cause a relaxation in coronary tone. Where this is superimposed on a proximal atheromatous lesion, rest pain may result; and if symptoms are associated with ST segment elevation on the ECG (Fig. 3) the diagnosis is one of *Prinzmetal's angina* (Prinzmetal *et al.*, 1960). Many patients with this condition (characteristically young male smokers) are at high risk of progression to total coronary occlusion resulting in acute MI.

Occasionally, angina occurs solely on the basis of coronary spasm in the absence of atheromatous obstruction, or because of an unidentified abnormality of flow in small coronary vessels (normal coronary artery or 'NCA' angina) (Hutchison *et al.*, 1989). Sufferers are usually female, middle-aged and present with a fluctuating pattern of symptoms. Pain may be entirely typical, or may be anginal in character and location but occur *after* rather than *with* exertion, lasting longer than usual and being associated with skeletal discomfort and fatigue.

Diagnosis

The *history* is all important. If the character and location of the pain suggests myocardial ischaemia, make a careful note of the timing of symptoms, particularly those features which suggest that a coronary lesion may have become unstable; i.e. the recent development of obtrusive angina in the absence of any previous symptoms, an abrupt deterioration in exercise capacity, or the occurrence of pain at rest.

The *examination* of a patient even with unstable angina may be entirely unrevealing. But note pointers to an increased risk for ischaemic disease (male gender, hypertension, periorbital xanthoma, arcus senilis, ear lobe crease, nicotine-stained fingers, absent peripheral pulses, abnormal retinal vessels). Look carefully for conditions that cause a deterioration in anginal symptoms *without* any worsening of underlying coronary disease: anaemia, thyrotoxicosis, hypothyroidism, aortic stenosis, uncontrolled hypertension, pathological tachycardia (watch especially for new atrial fibrillation (AF)) or cardiac failure.

A wide range of appearances of the ECG is possible in chronic stable angina. Common findings (Fig. 4)

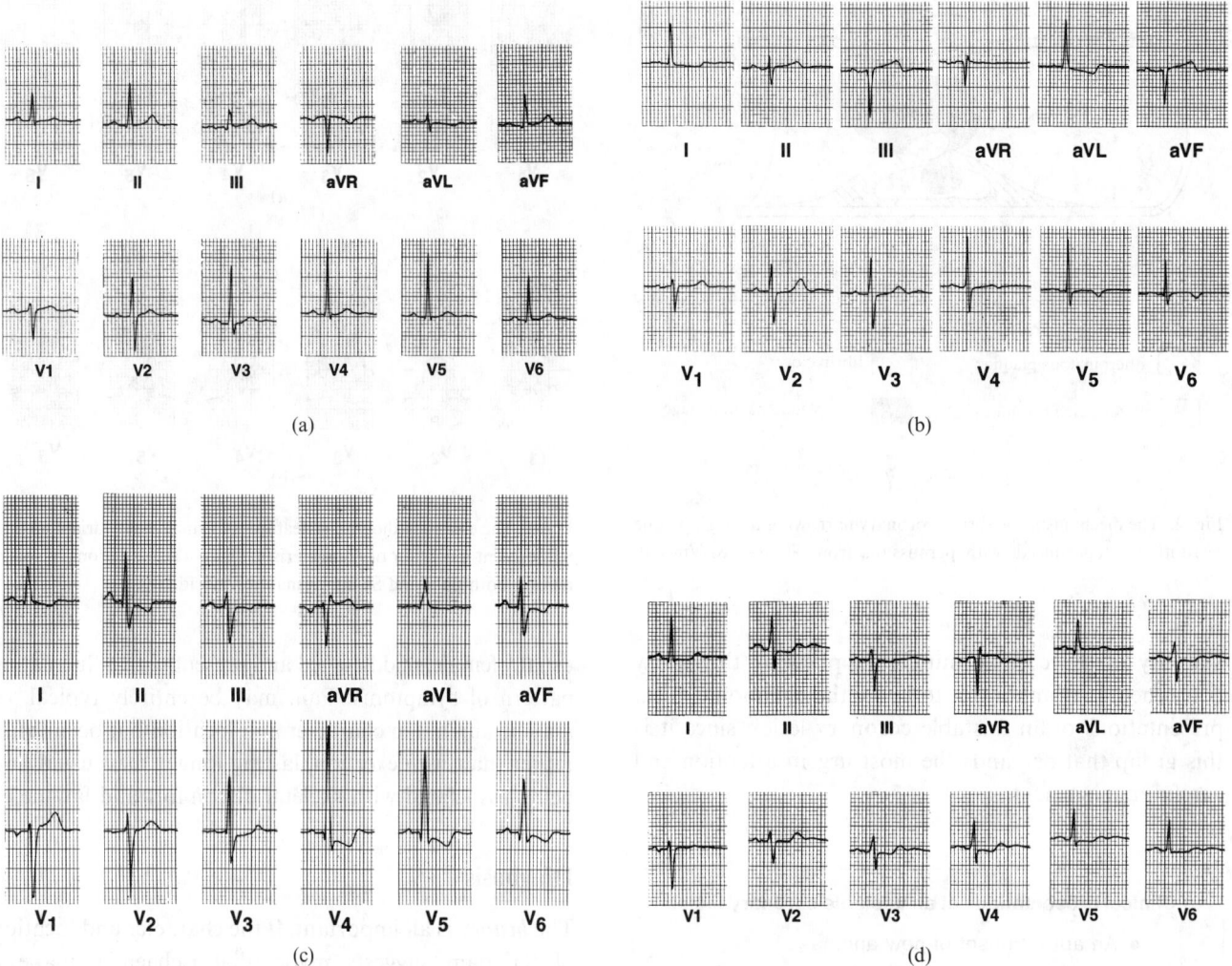

Fig. 4. Common electrocardiographic findings in chronic stable angina: a *normal* trace (a) or ST-T-U changes of varying configuration (b–d).

are that it is normal or that it shows minor ST-T-U wave changes, left ventricular hypertrophy/'strain', or previous MI. In unstable angina the ECG is usually more distinctly abnormal (Fig. 5); ST segment depression and T wave inversion are the most common patterns. Prinzmetal angina is associated with a characteristic form of ST segment elevation (Fig. 3). But to re-emphasize an important point (de Bono & Hopkins, 1993):

A normal electrocardiogram does not exclude a diagnosis of unstable ischaemic heart disease.

Treatment

Chronic stable angina

Patients with chronic stable angina may present to an A&E department for several reasons: slowly worsening symptoms, a single anginal episode of unusual severity, the need for a new supply of their regular medication, or because of a separate condition for which ischaemic heart disease is simply part of their medical background. A discussion of the problem with the patient's usual general practitioner is often valuable and should be attempted whenever possible.

A history of gradually worsening symptoms warrants careful clinical review to discover if:

- Any episodes of rest pain have occurred, or there has been an abrupt change in the pattern of symptoms. (Is the angina becoming unstable?)
- The history, signs, or electrocardiogram suggest recent (possibly silent) MI.
- Uncontrolled hypertension, heart failure or atrial fibrillation has developed
- The patient is anaemic or thyrotoxic.

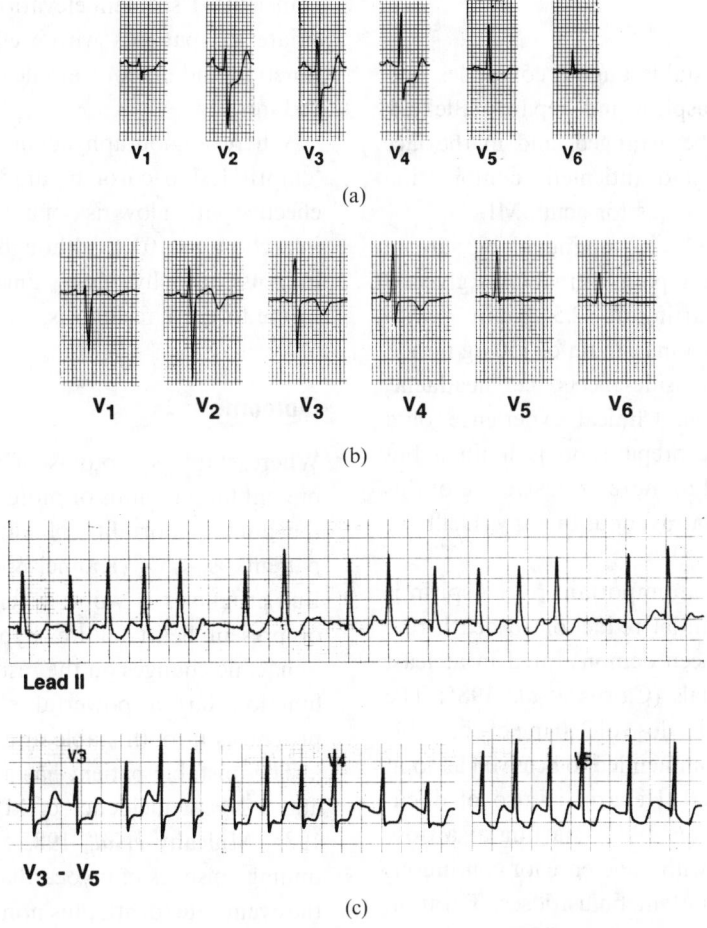

(a)

(b)

(c)

Fig. 5. The electrocardiogram in unstable angina. ST-T abnormalities are usually – though not necessarily – more marked than when symptoms are stable. (a) shows marked ST segment depression; (b) steep T wave inversion; (c) ST segment depression associated with rapid atrial fibrillation.

In the face of any of these conditions, discussion with the on-call medical or cardiology team is appropriate to agree on the best strategy for care, i.e. urgent admission or early out-patient review with additional investigations and treatment before attendance.

Where angina is becoming increasingly obtrusive in the absence of the conditions mentioned, it is often sufficient to arrange rapid referral to the appropriate out-patient clinic and to consider increasing existing antianginal medication (but beware side-effects!). Even at this stage advice on regular aspirin therapy, diet, smoking, alcohol and lifestyle can usefully be reiterated.

An isolated episode of angina that the patient finds more severe or prolonged than usual can pose a perplexing problem of management. This is an occasional pattern in stable patients, particularly in the face of an unusually strong stimulus; it may occur with a transient tachyarrhythmia, or if the patient's usual medication has been omitted. It may *not* harbour any immediate threat of either recurrence or infarction. Alternatively, it may herald instability in an atheromatous plaque that could culminate in complete coronary occlusion.

For a patient who is still in pain the strategy is straight-forward: to admit and treat as unstable angina. For a patient whose 20- or 30-minute episode of pain has already passed off (usually with the help of sublingual or buccal nitrate), careful evaluation of the context of the symptoms is mandatory. On many occasions admission will still be warranted, but discharge home after a few hours' observation may sometimes be considered, particularly where there was a clear precipitating factor, where age is advanced, where the ECG is stable or near-normal, or where there is a previous history of occasional similar episodes without adverse sequelae. The decision for discharge, however, should be made at registrar level or above.

Unstable angina

The early treatment of unstable angina comprises oral and intravenous nitrates, aspirin and heparin (Bleifeld, 1990). Admission should be arranged, and in the face of continuing pain, an opioid/antiemetic combination should be given intravenously as for acute MI.

Nitrates are given initially as sublingual or aerosol nitroglycerin. For continuing pain, intravenous glyceryl trinitrate is appropriate starting at 12.5 μg min^{-1} with increments every 10 min to a maximum of 150 μg min^{-1} in the absence of limiting side-effects, i.e. headache, tachycardia or hypotension. Clinical experience of a slow-release buccal nitrate preparation is limited, but encouraging, and may lead to more extensive use of this agent as a replacement for intravenous therapy (Dellborg et al., 1991).

Antiplatelet agents have an important role. Aspirin is of proven benefit: a substantial reduction in death rate and in non-fatal MI has been demonstrated in at least three large randomized trials (Cairns et al., 1985; The RISC Group, 1990). An initial dose of 300 mg of chewable or dispersible aspirin is recommended to be given as soon as any nausea has subsided. Heparin is also of documented value (Theroux et al., 1990), starting at a dose of 40 000 units per day and with preference for continuous infusion rather than intermittent bolus doses. Titration of the subsequent dose against the APTT (activated partial thromboplastin time) is now recommended (Neri Serneri et al., 1990). Other antithrombotic agents including the leech-related hirudin and its analogues may eventually prove to be a superior agent to heparin both in efficacy and because they can be used without laboratory control. Thrombolytic therapy appears to confer no benefit to patients with unstable angina.

The management of a patient with unstable angina after admission is likely to include continuing intravenous nitrate (changed to regular oral therapy as symptoms subside), beta-blockers and calcium antagonists. With this regimen, up to 80% of patients can be expected to settle within the first 48 h (Von Dohlen et al., 1989). Such patients are mobilized as if they have had an uncomplicated MI, and are considered carefully in the postacute phase for further investigation of their underlying coronary disease by appropriate investigations including exercise electrocardiography, radionucleide scanning and coronary angiography.

Most patients whose pain is resistant to increasing medical therapy in hospital warrant early angiography. This is mandatory without delay for any patient showing transient ST segment elevation and is particularly appropriate for patients with well-preserved left ventricular function and no contraindications to interventional procedures.

Where angiography demonstrates a single proximal 'culprit' lesion, coronary angioplasty can be dramatically effective with a low risk of mortality (<1%) or subsequent infarction (<10%); although – as might be expected from its pathophysiology – unstable lesions are particularly prone to early restenosis.

Outcome

Where stable symptoms of angina pectoris have been present for 3 months or more, the outlook is encouraging; the annual mortality of an unselected group of such patients is <5% (Kannel & Feinleib, 1972; Fry, 1976). But prognosis is worse when there is evidence of past or present heart failure, hypertension, previous MI or ischaemic changes on the resting ECG. Poor myocardial function has a powerful effect in worsening overall prognosis in both stable and unstable patients.

The unstable patient has a 1-year mortality of 8–15% and a 1-year incidence of MI of 10–14% (Cairns et al., 1985; Mulcahy et al., 1985). For those who have continuing episodes of myocardial ischaemia after admission, the event rate (death plus non-fatal MI) is 14–20% within the first 3 months, the majority of events occurring early (Gazes et al., 1973; Gottlieb et al., 1986). In contrast, stable angina is a poor predictor of subsequent MI; many patients with heart attack have neither prior obstructing coronary disease nor a history of effort-related symptoms.

ACUTE MYOCARDIAL INFARCTION

Definition and natural history

Myocardial infarction (MI) refers to the death of heart muscle resulting from a rapid and complete interruption of its blood supply. In its most common presentation, an abrupt thrombotic occlusion of a coronary artery at the site of existing atheroma leads to a circumscribed area of necrosis of the ventricular myocardium. The associated clinical syndrome of chest pain, autonomic overactivity, arrhythmias, progressive ECG changes, and raised 'cardiac' enzymes in the peripheral blood define the classic case.

In practice there is considerable variation in both the pathology and the presentation of this syndrome. In the coronary artery, intraluminal thrombosis secondary to plaque fissuring is usual, but it is often accompanied – or sometimes replaced – by other mechanisms causing coronary narrowing. The coronary lesion is dynamic. It may fluctuate in severity over several hours rather than produce sudden complete occlusion. 'Warning' pains before the onset of major symptoms are therefore not uncommon and in over one-third of patients the infarction process itself also follows a 'stuttering' course. As a result of coronary occlusion myocardial necrosis may be minimal (<10%) or extensive (>50%), discrete or patchy, partial or full-thickness, but its haemodynamic effect and adverse influence on late outcome are proportional to the amount of muscle involved.

The pain of an infarct gives no guide to its severity or to its long-term effect. In the community, silent (painless) infarction is common. Population surveys have shown that up to 30% of subjects with definite ECG evidence of previous myocardial infarction give no history of chest pain at any time (Kannel & Abbott, 1984; Shaper et al., 1984b). In contrast to those who have survived an unnoticed episode of cardiac damage, many patients die suddenly following acute coronary occlusion where myocardial necrosis might not have had time to develop before cardiac standstill or where the extent of muscle loss at postmortem examination appears minimal (one important cause of 'sudden cardiac death') (Davies, 1992).

The variable presentation of acute ischaemic syndromes has hindered the acquisition of true figures for incidence (number of new cases per year), prevalence (number of cases present in the community at any one time), and mortality of acute MI. Nevertheless, studies from Oxford, Edinburgh and London, and a UK General Practice survey point to an incidence of MI of about 12 per 1000 men aged 45–64 years (Armstrong et al., 1972; Kinlen, 1973; Colling et al., 1976; Royal College of General Practitioners, 1979). The condition is more common in Scotland and Northern England than in the South and under the age of 65 years predominates in males. The prevalence of MI in middle-aged men – judged from two British surveys – is of the order of 8% (Reid et al., 1974; Shaper et al., 1984a). The overall mortality rate of MI at 28 days is estimated to be 35–40%. But note that approximately 60% of deaths occur within the first hour after the onset of major symptoms (Armstrong et al., 1972).

Pathology

Following coronary occlusion by a variable combination of intraluminal clot, intraplaque haemorrhage and cor-

onary spasm (Fig. 2), the ventricular muscle supplied by the occluded vessel rapidly becomes abnormal (Poole-Wilson, 1990). Within minutes, myocardial relaxation and then contraction become impaired, giving a stiffened, akinetic muscle segment. If it is undamaged by previous ischaemic disease, the remaining cardiac muscle often compensates by hyperactive contraction to maintain an appropriate cardiac output and ejection fraction. If it fails, left ventricular end-diastolic (filling) pressure rises – a pressure rise that is transmitted back successively to the left atrium, pulmonary veins and lung capillaries.

The segment of functional abnormality of the myocardium at the onset of the attack is often larger than the ultimate size of the infarct: a variable amount of myocardium is 'stunned', but is capable of later recovery. Two important implications follow. Firstly, some patients show an improvement in cardiovascular function in the first few days after presentation. In these, early treatment for clinical heart failure may be reduced before hospital discharge and may not always be necessary long term. Secondly, a major therapeutic task is to ensure that as many potentially recoverable ('jeopardized') myocardial cells survive rather than become necrotic.

Profound myocardial ischaemia causes the disruption of intracellular membranes and abnormal ionic movement, particularly of calcium (Steenbergen et al., 1987). Calcium overload is typical of necrosing myocardial cells. Concentrations of extracellular potassium, hydrogen ions and catecholamines also change rapidly and in a patchy distribution (Webb et al., 1983). This unstable ionic milieu increases electrical excitability and encourages the fragmentation of local electrical pathways predisposing to ventricular arrhythmias. Cellular swelling, a result of ischaemic damage to cell membranes, impedes capillary flow making progression to necrosis more likely.

The death of myocardial tissue is associated with infiltration by neutrophils and macrophages, a process especially evident in late reperfusion (Poole-Wilson, 1990). They both exert a damaging effect on heart muscle that is enhanced by their production of 'free radicals' – short-lived highly reactive oxygen groupings capable of powerfully destructive effects (McCord, 1985; Opie, 1989; Young et al., 1993).

The autonomic nervous system

Profound autonomic imbalance is characteristic of the patient with acute MI. High sympathetic tone and high

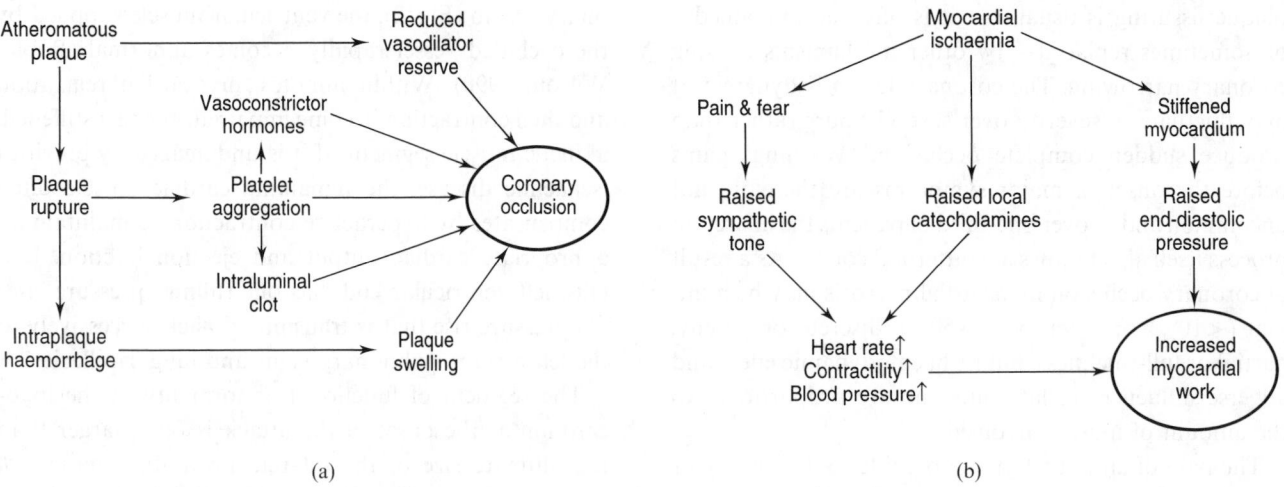

(a)   (b)

Fig. 6. Local and autonomic factors in an evolving myocardial infarction which contribute to continuing or worsening ischaemia: (a) in relation to the coronary artery (supply); (b) in relation to the myocardium (demand).

levels of both local and systemic catecholamines increase myocardial excitability and cause further patchy electrical change – a substrate for malignant arrhythmias. High catecholamine concentrations also propel potassium into skeletal muscle, reducing circulating plasma levels. A concomitant increase in vagal tone further encourages the emergence of ventricular ectopic beats and if dominant may aggravate a pathological bradycardia or block. Autonomic effects – no less than the coronary and myocardial lesions – are unstable and dynamic early in the course of an acute infarct (Fig. 6).

Diagnosis

A *history* of persistent (>20 min) severe pain of myocardial ischaemia at rest gives the strongest initial pointer. Rarely does the pain last for more than a few hours. Many patients, after one or two 'warning' symptoms in the preceding few days, have a single episode of major pain – although even in these obtaining an accurate time of onset can be difficult. Less commonly, a stuttering pattern of symptoms is observed with no one clearly dominant episode. A sensation of breathlessness is common even without overt left ventricular failure. Conversely, patients in severe left ventricular failure may have surprisingly little pain. Others with a painless presentation of acute infarction include the elderly, diabetics and those with very early onset ventricular fibrillation (VF).

Nausea, and occasionally vomiting, are common particularly in the face of high vagal tone. Fear and a sense of impending doom are reported frequently.

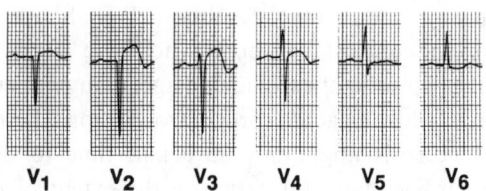

Fig. 7. The characteristic changes of the electrocardiogram in acute myocardial infarction: convex-upwards ST elevation and early formation of Q waves.

Physical signs usually comprise those of autonomic imbalance – abnormalities of heart rate, rhythm and blood pressure – together with evidence of ventricular dysfunction. A third or fourth heart sound and anterior dyskinesia (systolic bulging to the left of the sternum) are common with anterior infarction while a high jugular venous pressure is often associated with an inferior infarct, particularly if this also involves the right ventricle.

The ECG in acute myocardial infarction is abnormal in 90% of cases. The classic appearance of ST segment elevation (Fig. 7) is easily recognized. But with a growing emphasis on early care, the more subtle patterns of a 'hyperacute' infarct are becoming familiar (Schweitzer, 1990). A broad, tall T wave, indistinguishable from the rising ST segment, is characteristic and may progress within minutes to more definite ST segment elevation (Fig. 8).

Hyperacute patterns may pose a diagnostic challenge especially as they can closely resemble a physiological high ST take-off or acute pericarditis. Interpretation is helped by noting the clinical context, and whether the

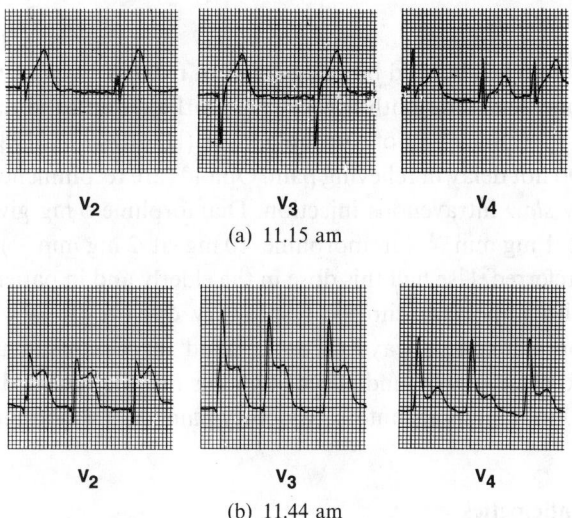

(a) 11.15 am

(b) 11.44 am

Fig. 8. The changes of *hyperacute* myocardial infarction. A broad, tall T wave merges with a just-elevated ST segment (a). Progression to more marked ST elevation is common (b). (The patient is in atrial fibrillation.)

ECG changes are widespread or confined to a lead group representing one of the common infarct locations (Table 2). Associated or 'reciprocal' ST segment depression (Fig. 9) supports the diagnosis of infarction and may be particularly helpful in leads I and aVL when the identity of ST segment elevation in the inferior leads (II, III, aVF) is uncertain.

Although ST segment elevation is the characteristic finding, a variety of studies show that this change occurs in only 18–80% of patients with a discharge diagnosis of MI (Short, 1970; Rude *et al.*, 1983; Adams *et al.*, 1993). Other appearances include modest ST segment depression in V_1 and V_2 (suggesting a true posterior infarct), profound ST segment depression elsewhere, steep T wave inversion, or – rarely – an apparently normal trace.

Left bundle branch block so changes the initial QRS vector and subsequent ST-T pattern that it is said to

---

The diagnosis of myocardial infarction in the presence of left bundle branch block (these signs are highly specific if insensitive)

- Q waves in at least two of the leads I, aVL, V_5 or V_6
- R wave regression from V_1 to V_4
- Notching of the upstroke of the R wave in at least two of the leads V_3–V_5
- Primary ST-T changes in two or more adjacent leads, e.g. T waves pointing in the same direction as the QRS complex or marked ST segment elevation (especially limb leads)

Table 2. *Location of myocardial infarction according to electro-cardiographic appearances*

An infarct may not be confined to one or even two zones. Locating a *second* infarct may not be at all easy.

Location	Abnormal leads
Anteroseptal	V_2–V_4
Anterolateral	V_4–V_6
Lateral	I, aVL
Inferior	II, III, aVF
True posterior	Tall R and ST depression in V_1 and V_2
Indeterminate	Left bundle branch block, previous infarct, Wolff–Parkinson–White syndrome, widespread ST depression only

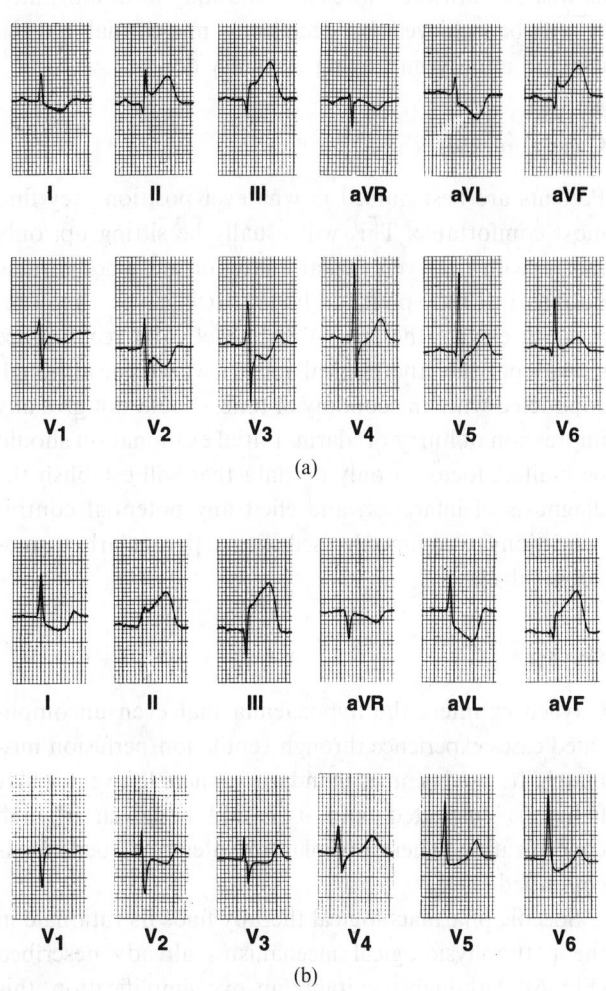

Fig. 9. Myocardial infarction with both ST segment elevation and associated or 'reciprocal' ST segment depression.

preclude the ECG diagnosis of acute MI. But specific abnormalities are accurate diagnostic pointers (Hands *et al.*, 1988) and, in the face of a persuasive clinical presentation, left bundle branch block of any form should be taken as adequate evidence of an infarct. Right bundle branch block does not obscure the development of Q waves, but has ST-T wave changes of its own in the right chest leads. ST segment elevation is always abnormal, however, as is T wave inversion when it *progresses in severity from right to left*.

Management

Aims

The aims of managing acute MI are to relieve pain and distress, to prevent early death from arrhythmias, and to preserve as much myocardium as possible. Myocardial salvage will improve the functional result of the attack as well as both the short-term and long-term mortality. It will be achieved by decreasing myocardial oxygen demand and by improving coronary flow.

General measures

Patients are best nursed in whatever position they find most comfortable. This will usually be sitting up; only rarely (with right ventricular infarction and poor cardiac output) will they prefer to lie flat. It is never a requirement to elevate the legs. A feeling of calm reassurance should pervade the clinical interview, which, although conducted with an economy of time, should not give any impression of hurry or alarm. Initial examination should be limited, focusing only on data that will establish the diagnosis of infarction and elicit any potential contraindications to commonly used agents, particularly thrombolytic drugs.

Oxygen

Oxygen counters the hypoxaemia that even uncomplicated cases experience through ventilation/perfusion mismatch. Its use becomes mandatory where left ventricular failure is suspected, and it should be given in high concentration where alveolar or interstitial oedema is confirmed.

Specific pharmacological therapy finds its rationale in the pathophysiological mechanisms already described (Fig. 6). Although inevitably an oversimplification, this profides a useful framework for selecting the range of drugs currently recommended for routine treatment.

Analgesia

Pain relief, beyond bringing comfort, reduces sympathetic tone, lessening both myocardial workload and the pro-arrhythmic effect of catecholamines (Herlitz *et al.*, 1989). Do not delay in relieving pain. Opioids are recommended by *slow* intravenous injection. Diamorphine 5 mg given at 1 mg min^{-1} (or morphine 10 mg at 2 mg min^{-1}) is preferred. Use half this dose in the elderly and in patients with important chronic respiratory disease. (It is wise for naloxone always to be at hand in case of an unexpectedly profound effect.) Opioids may be repeated at 10-min intervals until satisfactory pain relief is obtained.

Antiemetics

The combination of high vagal tone and the emetic effect of opioid therapy promotes unwelcome and potentially dangerous nausea and vomiting. An antiemetic should therefore be given with the analgesic agent. Cyclizine 25–50 mg is convenient as it can be used to dissolve the opioid for a single combined injection. Metoclopramide 10–20 mg IV is an alternative and should be used where the vasoconstrictor effects of cyclizine must be avoided – in severe left ventricular failure or cardiogenic shock (Tan *et al.*, 1988).

Nitrates

Nitrate therapy mimics the endogenous substance nitric oxide that is released by endothelial tissue and exerts a powerful vasodilatory effect on vascular smooth muscle. Three vascular territories where nitrates are of potential help in acute MI are the coronary arteries themselves, especially at or adjacent to sites of recent plaque disruption, peripheral arterioles and venous capacitance vessels.

Coronary vasodilatation by nitrates improves myocardial blood supply and, because this effect is restricted to the larger vessels, does not cause an unwanted 'steal' effect. Nitrates also favour the perfusion of subendocardial tissue by a second mechanism: by reducing venous return, mechanical pressure on subendocardial cells during diastole is lowered; the pressure gradient between these cells and the blood in the epicardial coronary arteries is enhanced which improves trans-myocardial blood flow. A reduction in venous return also lowers wall tension, a major determinant of myocardial oxygen requirement.

Peripheral arteriolar dilatation reduces myocardial workload but if excessive may lower blood pressure

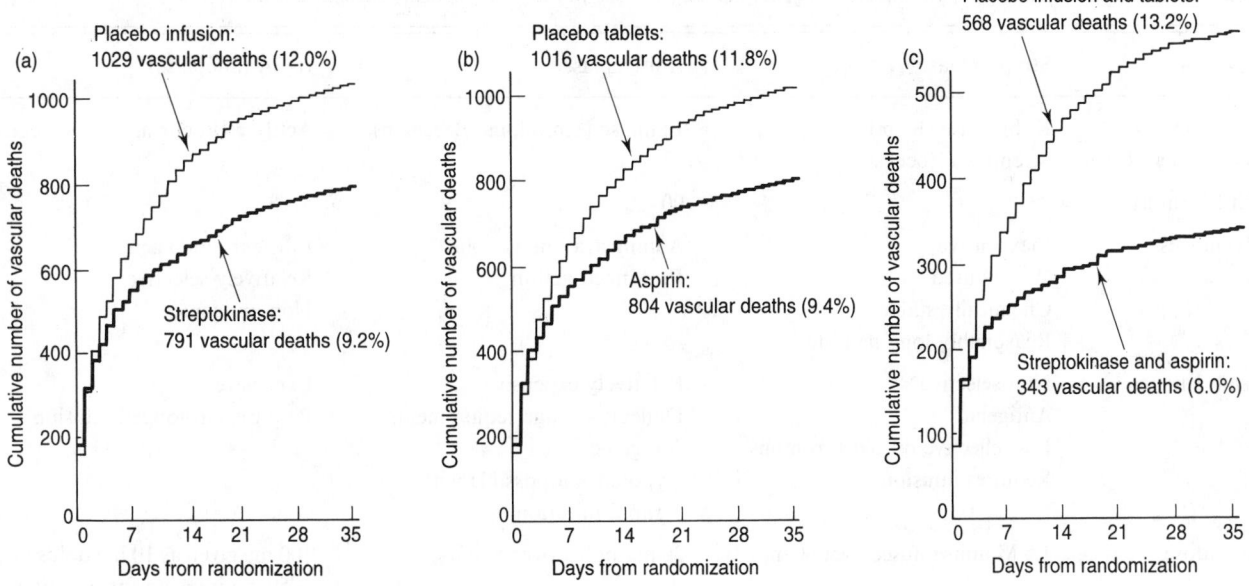

Fig. 10. The salutary effects of streptokinase, aspirin and both on mortality from acute myocardial infarction. (Reproduced, with permission, from the ISIS-2 Collaborative Group, 1988.)

sufficiently to affect cardiac, cerebral and renal perfusion adversely. In practice this effect – and unwanted reflex tachycardia from nitrate therapy – can be avoided by a careful titration of dose.

The evidence for a beneficial effect of nitrate therapy for *all* cases of acute MI was at first encouraging, if rather patchy and incomplete: a meta-analysis by Yusef *et al.* (1988) of a variety of nitrate trials indicated that these agents might confer an improvement in mortality of up to 21%. But the results of ISIS-4, a recent extensive controlled trial of nitrates (and several other agents) in over 40 000 patients, showed no overall benefit from oral nitrates given *routinely* (ISIS-4, 1995).

Nitrates should not be abandoned, however, in the light of these results. Oral glyceryl trinitrate spray or tablets should be encouraged as an immediate therapy unless the patient is profoundly hypotensive. Intravenous nitrate (62.5–250 µg min^{-1}) should be *considered* for patients with continuing ischaemic pain or who have left ventricular failure. It has an almost immediate effect and can be titrated against the patient's response. The half-life of intravenous glyceryl trinitrate (3 min) is shorter than the half-life of the commonly used alternative agent, isosorbide dinitrate (8 min), allowing its action to be withdrawn rapidly if excessive vasodilatation occurs. Hypotension may limit the use of either agent, and special caution is required in inferior infarction (Ferguson *et al.*, 1989).

Aspirin

The value of aspirin in acute myocardial infarction might be predicted from its antiplatelet and anti-inflammatory effects, yet its precise mechanism of action is poorly understood. Its impressive benefit in improving survival from myocardial infarction was shown most dramatically in the large multicentre trial, ISIS-2 (Fig. 10). Not only did it result in a 25% reduction in mortality when used alone, but this advantage could be added to the salutary effects of thrombolysis with streptokinase (ISIS-2, 1988).

In practice, aspirin now forms part of the early management of all patients with suspected acute MI. Its time of administration within the first 24 h may not be critical, but there seems no good reason to delay therapy once the diagnosis is suspected. The recommended dose is 150–300 mg taken once. A common recommendation is that a chewable aspirin tablet be taken to speed absorption (particularly after opioid therapy), although it seems wise to defer aspirin administration in those who are troubled by nausea or vomiting in the early phase of their illness. Its use is contraindicated in those allergic to salicylates, and it should be used with caution with patients with active peptic ulcer.

Thrombolytic therapy

After nearly three decades of obscurity following the first use of streptokinase for acute MI in 1958, thrombolytic agents are now counted as central to the treatment of

Table 3. *Comparative features of thrombolytic agents licensed for use in the UK for acute myocardial infarction*

	Streptokinase	Anistreplase	rt-PA (alteplase)
Tradename (manufacturer)	Kabikinase (Kabi) Streptase (Hoechst)	Eminase (Smithkline Beecham)	Actilyse (Boehringer-Ingelheim)
Half-life (min)	23	90	5
Advantages	Inexpensive Widely-used Chemically stable Reasonably long half-life	Administration as bolus Prolonged action	Efficient lytic agent Relatively selective Non-antigenic
Disadvantages	Non-selective Antigenic Less effective on old thrombus Requires infusion	Relatively expensive Difficult storage requirements Antigenic Hypotension possible with rapid injection	Expensive Requires prolonged infusion
Usual dose	1.5 M units infused over 60 min	30 mg bolus over 5 min	100 mg given as 10 mg bolus then 50 mg infusion for first hour, 40 mg infusion for next 2 h

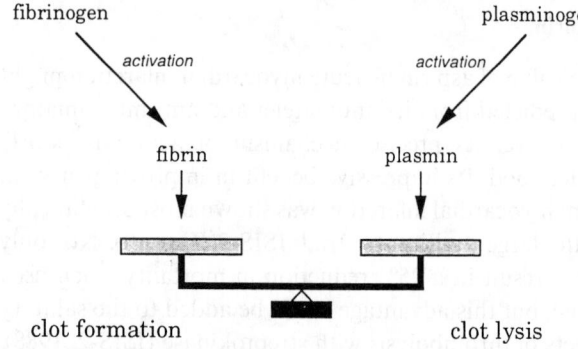

Fig. 11. Activation of the plasminogen system by pharmacological therapy accelerates clot lysis. (Reproduced, with permission, from Skinner & Vincent, 1993.)

this condition. Their beneficial effects on outcome have been documented in over 60 000 patients worldwide (Fibrinolytic Therapy Trialists (FTT) Collaborative Group, 1994). Overall short- and long-term mortality is improved an average of 25%, and there are strong pointers to a favourable effect on infarct size, left ventricular function, and subsequent quality of life.

Mechanism of action

Spontaneous lysis of an intracoronary thrombosis is a natural phenomenon. Physiological thrombolysis leads to reopening of the vessel responsible for infarct in up to 30% of cases within 12 h and in over 50% by 48 h. Pharmacological thrombolytic agents, by activating plas-

minogen (Fig. 11), accelerate this process. More vessels are opened, and recanalization occurs earlier. Within 40 min of the drug being given, up to 80% of arteries are opened by intracoronary agents and up to 70% by intravenous agents.

Activation of clot-bound plasminogen provides the essential mechanism for therapeutic coronary thrombolysis. But even when agents are designed to be 'clot-specific', a systemic effect also occurs. Activation of circulating plasminogen causes degradation of fibrinogen (fibrinogenolysis) leading to a systemic lytic state in which blood clotting throughout the body is impaired. The systemic effect, although slightly increasing the risk of unwanted bleeding, may favour myocardial recovery. But the value of thrombolytic agents in acute MI probably depends on a number of factors in addition to simple recanalization of the culprit vessel, particularly when therapy is given late in the attack (Chamberlain, 1989):

- Clot lysis at the site of intracoronary occlusion.
- Systemic lytic state preventing clot extension.
- Decreased plasma viscosity leading to improved flow in collateral epicardial arteries.
- Improved capillary flow by lysis of microthrombi.
- Modification of platelet activity.
- Cytoprotective effect.
- Vasodilation.
- Improved ventricular remodelling from an open artery.

Available agents

Three thrombolytic agents are licensed in the UK for use in acute myocardial infarction: streptokinase, anistreplase and recombinant tissue plasminogen activator (rt-PA, alteplase). Table 3 shows some comparative features.

Streptokinase – derived from *Streptococcus pyogenes* – is the oldest thrombolytic agent. A complex of streptokinase with plasminogen acts as an activator for further plasminogen molecules. It is non-selective in its action and, being a foreign protein, induces antibodies that *may* cause allergy and/or a diminished therapeutic response for up to 5 years.

Anistreplase was designed as a streptokinase-based thrombolytic agent with a long half-life. An additional advantage lies in its ability to be given as a single bolus injection – of particular benefit in prehospital use.

Tissue plasminogen activator (t-PA) occurs naturally, being made in tiny quantities by many tissues. It has a much stronger affinity for clot-bound plasminogen than for circulating plasminogen. The commercially available product manufactured using recombinant gene technology (hence rt-PA) holds close similarity to the endogenous protein and thus enjoys a very low level of antigenicity. The main disadvantages of rt-PA are its expense and its short half-life.

Other thrombolytic agents potentially suitable for use in acute myocardial infarction include urokinase and prourokinase. These also are non-antigenic, but otherwise seem to resemble streptokinase in time-course and efficacy. At present they are available in the UK only on a named-patient basis.

Thrombolysis in practice

Patient selection for thrombolytic therapy rests on identifying those with early, but definite, evolving MI who are free from major contraindications. Inclusion criteria will vary from unit to unit, but will usually reflect the nature and duration of symptoms, the context of the presentation and the appearance of the ECG.

Typical cardiac pain lasting more than 20 min and not relieved by nitrates is a common prerequisite for thrombolysis, although a patient with somewhat questionable symptoms may also qualify providing the ECG is characteristic. A time window of up to 12 h from the onset of major symptoms is now considered appropriate for thrombolytic therapy, although in some patients symptom onset is difficult to time. The fundamental principle remains:

Thrombolytic therapy should be given as soon as possible after the onset of the attack.

Table 4. *Suggested indications for thrombolytic therapy*

But always take local advice!

Definite
- Typical cardiac pain for more than 20 min
- Onset of major symptoms within 12 h
- Characteristic ECG changes: ST segment elevation
  - 2 mm or more in two adjacent precordial leads, V_2–V_6
  - 1 mm or more in two limb leads representing the same left ventricular wall
- Either gender
- Any age
- No contraindications

Probable
- Characteristic symptoms and *marked* ECG abnormalities (including left bundle branch block) but without ST elevation
- Characteristic ECG but symptoms continuous for >12 h

The need for a characteristic ECG to establish the diagnosis and to qualify patients for thrombolysis remains contentious. Many but not all large trials showing the value of thrombolytic agents have required ST segment elevation. This change (in the appropriate clinical context) also appears both to be specific for the diagnosis and to define those who will receive greatest benefit. Infarct patients with left bundle branch block also fall into a 'high gain' category. In contrast, patients with a normal ECG or with ST segment depression alone have a less favourable response.

Most clinicians currently accept that ST segment elevation, whilst not a unique qualifier for thrombolytic therapy, does define an optimal population for its useful effect. Table 4 summarizes suggested indications for thrombolysis, but local policies may differ and should always be followed.

The *exclusion criteria* for thrombolysis are based on identifying those of increased risk of haemorrhagic complications. Apart from suspected aortic dissection and active bleeding, contraindications are not absolute and most need assessment in the light of diagnostic certainty and the potential benefit of thrombolysis. Weighing the risk/benefit ratio in patients with probable MI but a relative contraindication to thrombolysis should be a task shared with the duty consultant. Other side-effects need be borne in mind when making this decision, but are usually minor (Table 5).

The *choice of thrombolytic agent* in the UK for patients with their first infarct is straightforward. The results of ISIS-3, a 41 000 patient multicentre trial comparing streptokinase, antistreplase and rt-PA, showed an identical outcome for each drug (ISIS-3, 1992). Since it is

Table 5. *Common adverse effects of thrombolytic therapy with an indication of approximate incidence*

Adverse effect	Approximate incidence (%)
Any stroke	1.5
Haemorrhagic stroke	<0.5
Minor bleeding	10.0[a]
Rash	3.0
Severe bleeding	<2.0
Anaphylaxis	<2.0[b]

[a] This figure depends heavily on the definition of minor bleeding.

[b] rt-PA gives substantially fewer allergic reactions.

considerably cheaper than the other agents, streptokinase has become the drug of choice in most UK hospitals.

But this position may not be totally secure. Firstly, a further large trial, GUSTO, has recently shown that rt-PA with early heparin resulted in a mortality of 6.3% as opposed to the 7.3% death rate given by streptokinase (The GUSTO Investigators, 1993). Clinicians are now considering how best to interpret this improvement in clinical practice, particularly as the cost of each extra life saved will be in excess of £10 000. Secondly, the use of streptokinase is resulting in an increasing level of patients with streptokinase antibodies that may hinder the second use of this drug, especially as the antibodies may remain effective in the circulation for over 4 years. Treatment of second and subsequent infarcts may therefore require an

---

Contraindications to thrombolytic therapy

Suspected aortic dissection
Active bleeding
Recent surgery or major trauma
Recent head injury or cerebro-
    vascular accident, even with
    complete recovery
Prolonged cardiopulmonary
    resuscitation
Systolic blood pressure >180 mmHg
Previous allergic reaction
    (streptokinase, anistreplase)
Use of anticoagulants/known
    bleeding diathesis
Active peptic ulcer
Abdominal aneurysm
History of cerebrovascular
    accident with residual
    disability
Possible pregnancy
Proliferative or haemorrhagic
    diabetic retinopathy

---

increasing use of non-antigenic thrombolytic agents – rt-PA and urokinase.

The most important practical aspect of therapy is:

Identify suitable patients for therapy without delay.

Arrangements for the rapid triage of suspected cases must be practicable and reduce time to therapy. The identification of patients with an *unequivocal diagnosis* and *no contraindications* allows a FAST TRACK to therapy – thrombolysis being given in less than 15 min of arrival in the A&E department. Patients with a doubtful diagnosis or ECG or with a relative contra-indication need more careful – though not delayed – consideration and are allocated to a SLOW TRACK category.

The operation of a fast-track system requires motivation, cooperation between specialities, training, and frequent audit. It incurs no additional expense yet produces a measurable improvement in care (MacCullum *et al.*, 1990; Pell *et al.*, 1992).

The use of thrombolytics *before* hospital admission is uncommon though recent Guidelines from the British Heart Foundation (Weston *et al.*, 1994) suggest that this issue should be considered in localities where in-hospital administration may lead to a delay from 'call-to-needle' time in excess of 90 min. In Northern Ireland and in a number of other European countries that operate mobile coronary care units, the use of prehospital thrombolysis may be more practical.

Heparin

Pathological coagulation at three separate sites threatens any patient with MI: within the coronary artery (extending the 'culprit' lesion); adherent to the endocardial surface of the infarct ('mural thrombosis', which carries an important risk of arterial embolism) and the pelvic and lower-limb veins (bringing the risk of potentially fatal pulmonary embolism). A noticeable inflammatory reaction to the MI (fever, high white cell count, raised erythrocyte sedimentation rate, pericarditis) increases circulating fibrinogen levels and intensifies these threats.

Heparin is of undoubted value for prophylaxis against venous thrombosis and seems also to protect against mural thrombus. A beneficial effect on the coronary lesion itself has been difficult to demonstrate. Heparin is used in two distinct settings: after thrombolysis, or in patients for whom thrombolysis has been judged inappropriate. Where thrombolytic therapy has been given, heparin may add little benefit to its early systemic anticoagulant effect and may increase the risk of bleeding complications. Some practitioners now omit heparin altogether in thrombolysed patients while others introduce it late and in low dose (12 500 units subcutaneously starting after 24 h). The exception is following the use of t-PA, when the immediate use of full-dose intravenous heparin is still recommended.

In the absence of thrombolysis, early intravenous heparin is recommended to avoid arterial and pulmonary emboli. A suitable dose is 10 000 units over the first 6 h with subsequent doses being determined by regular haematological monitoring. A reduction in dose is wise in the face of active peptic ulcer, subclavian puncture, temporary pacing, advanced age, pericarditis and haemorrhagic complications. Control with coagulation monitoring is strongly recommended (Chamberlain, 1989; The GUSTO Investigators, 1993).

Antiarrhythmic therapy

Since in early observations of natural history, ventricular arrhythmias accounted for the majority of deaths from acute MI, routine prophylactic antiarrhythmic therapy seemed a logical solution; from the 1970s it was adopted widely. More recently, three important observations have extinguished this enthusiasm. Firstly, even in closely monitored cardiac care units transient ventricular arrhythmias are easily missed. Secondly, the predictive value of 'warning' arrhythmias is disappointingly poor; many patients suffer VF that is unheralded. Thirdly, the routine use of lignocaine – the most benign antiarrhythmic agent – whilst reducing the incidence of VF, may worsen overall mortality.

We now recommend that lignocaine is prescribed for attacks of sustained ventricular tachycardia or as prophylaxis after the successful termination of VF. The suggested schedule is a 100 mg IV bolus followed in 5 min by a further 100 mg, or alternatively four 50 mg boluses given at 5-min intervals. Drug administration should be *slow* to avoid the possibility of inducing convulsions.

Although prophylactic antiarrhythmic therapy has lost favour, reducing the risk of VF by pain relief, by avoiding undue bradycardia, by improving the myocardial oxygen demand/supply ratio, and by the correction of hypoxaemia is encouraged.

A fuller discussion of the treatment of important arrhythmias appears in Chapter 45B.

Beta-blockers

Beta-blockers oppose the effect of sympathetic tone. They lower arterial blood pressure, contractility and heart rate, and thus reduce myocardial oxygen requirement.

Their beneficial effects in acute MI include a reduction in ST segment elevation, cardiac pain, late ischaemia, recurrent MI and death. In the ISIS-1 trial in patients receiving intravenous then oral atenolol mortality was reduced by 21% (ISIS-1 Collaborative Group, 1988). Subsequent analysis has shown that this benefit may have been due to a reduced incidence of myocardial rupture within the first 24 h of admission.

But beta-blockers are not without adverse effects and a reduction in myocardial contractility may precipitate or worsen cardiac failure. They should be used with caution. Intravenous beta-blockade is rarely a feature of the immediate management of MI but should be considered early after admission to the cardiac care unit, particularly in the face of persistent pain, tachycardia or ST segment elevation.

Treatment of complications

Tables 6 and 7 list the possible complications of acute MI. Some will emerge only after the patient has been transferred to the cardiac care unit or ward; others – highlighted in this section – need more immediate care in the A&E department.

A detailed discussion of the diagnosis and treatment of common *arrhythmias* appears in Chapter 45B. Suffice it here to mention some features of the arrhythmias that complicate early acute MI.

Sinus tachycardia is common, usually resulting from enhanced sympathetic tone. Relief of pain and anxiety is the first objective, then to consider whether the patient is in cardiac failure and to treat as necessary. A few patients, particularly those with a 'stuttering' anterior infarction, exhibit a persistent sinus tachycardia with no other signs. Beta-blocking agents are recommended.

Atrial extrasystoles are benign, needing no therapy, but if their rate is high or increasing, AF may follow, and digitalization may be considered.

The treatment of *atrial fibrillation* depends on the ventricular rate and haemodynamic effect. For rates less than 100 min^{-1} a 'watch-and-wait' policy is reasonable. For rates of 100–130 with good clinical condition intravenous digoxin can be used at a dose of 500 µg in 100 ml of 5% dextrose over 30 min with a second, similar dose given over 1 h. An alternative if the haemodynamic state is satisfactory is the use of a beta-blocker, particularly if important ventricular arrhythmias coexist. AF with rates over 130 min^{-1} – or slower if the haemodynamic state is poor – is an indication for DC cardioversion (DCV)

Table 6. *Arrhythmias complicating acute myocardial infarction*

Tachyarrhythmias	Bradyarrhythmias and conduction abnormalities
Sinus tachycardia	Sinus bradycardia
Atrial extrasystoles	Sinoatrial block
Atrial flutter	First degree atrioventricular block
Atrial fibrillation	
Accelerated junctional rhythm	Wenckebach atrioventricular block
Ventricular extrasystoles	2:1 atrioventricular block
Ventricular tachycardia	Mobitz II type AV block
Ventricular fibrillation	Bundle branch block
	Complete heart block
	Asystole with P waves
	Asystole without P waves

Table 7. *Non-arrhythmic complications of acute myocardial infarction*

- Left ventricular failure
- Cardiogenic shock
- Pericarditis, early and late
- Deep venous thrombosis
- Pulmonary embolism
- Mural thrombosis
- Arterial embolism
- Recurrent ischaemia
- Reinfarction or infarct extension
- Ventricular septal defect
- Papillary muscle dysfunction
- Papillary muscle rupture
- Subacute and acute rupture of the free ventricular wall
- Renal failure
- Gastrointestinal haemorrhage

usually followed by maintenance antiarrhythmic therapy. An *accelerated junctional rhythm* is unusual and rarely disadvantageous. If the haemodynamic state is poor (particularly where atrial and ventricular activity occur simultaneously) it may be appropriate simply to speed atrial rate by atropine or (rarely) by atrial pacing.

As noted on page 883, enthusiasm for treating *ventricular arrhythmias* with suppressant drugs has waned. Routine measures for the infarct patient are helpful in themselves; consider also the use of atropine for an inappropriate sinus bradycardia (which predisposes to ventricular arrhythmias), potassium replacement therapy (where serum potassium $<3.5 \text{ mmol l}^{-1}$), and intravenous magnesium (10 ml of a 50% solution diluted in 100 ml of 5% dextrose given over 60 min) (Smith *et al.*, 1986).

Intravenous lignocaine is appropriate as a first-line treatment for recurrent or paroxysmal ventricular arrhythmias when general measures have failed. Second-line measures need careful consideration. The more powerful antiarrhythmic drugs, disopyramide, flecainide, procainamide, amiodarone are likely to be more effective, but at the price of myocardial depression and at a risk of proarrhythmic effect. Electrical treatments, including atrial and ventricular overdrive pacing, may be a better option.

A moderate *sinus bradycardia* can be beneficial in reducing myocardial oxygen demand; but if the rate is less than 40 min^{-1} or if it is associated with a poor haemodynamic state, intravenous atropine is advisable beginning with a dose of 250 µg IV.

First degree atrioventricular (AV) block and *Wenckebach second degree AV block*, commonly associated with inferior MI, are usually benign. Treatment is often unnecessary, but should be considered if the heart rate is less than 40 min^{-1}, if the haemodynamic condition is unsatisfactory, if ventricular arrhythmias prompted by a low heart rate are themselves in need of treatment, if pauses of greater than 3 sec occur, or if the QRS is wide.

Mobitz II type AV block (an abrupt failure of AV conduction without preceding lengthening of the PR interval) or alternating bundle branch block requires specialist consideration of the need for pacing. Pacing is also indicated for patients whose progress is complicated by complete heart block, unless the infarct is inferior in location, the QRS complexes are narrow and occur atgreater than 40 min^{-1} with no unexpected pauses, and any coexistent ventricular ectopic activity does not require suppression.

Only a small number of *non-arrhythmic complications* of MI (Table 7) require attention in the A&E department.

Acute left ventricular failure and *cardiogenic shock* are important mechanical complications whose management is described on pages 888 and 889. Early *pericarditis* is seen occasionally when a patient's presentation to the A&E department has been delayed. Characteristic features are pain worse on inspiration, pericardial rub, fever and a tendency to atrial arrhythmias. The treatment of choice is indomethacin 25–50 mg which may be repeated after 3–4 h; but the drug should be used only while control of troublesome symptoms is essential since it also exerts adverse effects on fluid balance and coronary tone.

While the *thrombotic complications* of MI (deep venous thrombosis, pulmonary embolism, mural thrombosis and arterial embolism) will not be seen on initial presentation, their occurrence should be prevented from the outset. Thrombolytic therapy will provide immediate protection in patients able to receive it, but in others heparin should be commenced (p. 882) in the absence of contraindications.

Recurrent myocardial ischaemia is best treated by introducing or increasing nitrate therapy and by the use of beta-blockers for recurrent symptoms. The addition of calcium channel blocking agents may be necessary, and a small proportion of patients warrant urgent investigation with coronary angiography.

Severe mechanical complications of acute myocardial infarction will be seen occasionally. The presence of an *infarct-related ventricular septal defect* is indicated in a patient in very poor haemodynamic condition by a high jugular venous pressure, a loud truly pansystolic murmur maximum to the left of the sternum and a palpable systolic thrill. With *papillary muscle dysfunction* the systolic murmur often has a more crescendo character, is less than full length, and has no associated thrill. Pulmonary congestion is inevitable and may be severe. The less common but more serious condition of *papillary muscle rupture* is characterized by catastrophic pulmonary oedema, a marked reduction in cardiac output, and a loud mitral systolic murmur.

The most severe mechanical disorder of myocardial infarction – *rupture of the free ventricular wall* – causes cardiac arrest in electromechanical dissociation. Blood in the pericardial space prevents any effective cardiac contraction. The circulation fails while, initially, co-ordinated electrical activity remains; profound brady-cardia, VF and asystole supervene before long in the absence of coronary blood flow. In a few cases this condition is preceded by *subacute rupture* (Pollack *et al.*, 1993).

Further care in hospital

Most patients treated in hospital for acute MI warrant a period of observation in a specialized cardiac care unit before being transferred to the general ward. Exceptions can be made on the basis of time from onset of symptoms and clinical stability, but we do not recommend a cardiac care unit admission policy based solely on age.

A cardiac care unit offers continuous ECG monitoring during the patient's early, unstable phase. It also provides more comprehensive monitoring and special facilities for intracardiac pressure recording and pacing for those with serious complications. More generally, the unit provides a focus for knowledge, expertise, and perhaps research in the management of acute coronary syndromes and important arrhythmias, and in some it is the point of hospital admission for patients with suspected MI rather than the A&E department.

The objectives of hospital care are to confirm the diagnosis through serial ECGs and estimation of cardiac enzymes, to maximize myocardial recovery, to detect and manage complications, to plan long-term treatment on the basis of future risk, and to begin the process of education and rehabilitation of both patients and relatives. Routine treatment of the uncomplicated patient is likely to be simple, perhaps no more than aspirin 75 mg daily. Subcutaneous heparin may be continued until the patient is mobile, especially where thrombolytic therapy has not been used, but policies for the use of heparin vary from unit to unit. Additional treatment will be necessary for specific complications, the commonest being heart failure, recurrent cardiac pain and pericarditis.

An important challenge in the management of each patient is to know how best to prevent the adverse long-term sequelae of myocardial infarction: expansion of the infarct zone, heart failure, angina, fatal and non-fatal reinfarction and sudden cardiac death. Aspirin, beta-blockers, calcium channel blockers, anticoagulants, lipid-lowering agents, ACE (angiotensin-converting en-zyme) inhibitors and coronary bypass grafting are of undoubted benefit. But:

- The beneficial action of these therapies is not shared equally by all patient groups.
- Each treatment has potential adverse effects.
- For some patients the risk of further cardiac events *without* additional intervention is so low that secondary prevention (except perhaps for aspirin) is unnecessary.

Risk stratification is therefore an important component of contemporary cardiac care (Arnold *et al.*, 1993). The patient with none of the features that categorize patients at increased risk has a 1-year mortality in the order of less than 1%. The detailed choice of agents for secondary prevention where this is thought advisable is beyond the scope of this book, but is outlined in several recent texts (Julian & Braunwald, 1994).

Rehabilitation

For most patients and their relatives acute MI is a frightening experience with long-term psychological and social effects even in the face of apparently full 'medical' recovery. Anxiety, depression and fatigue disproportion-ate to cardiovascular status are common and may limit work opportunities as well as social enjoyment.

Cardiac rehabilitation programmes have been devel-oped to address this important aspect of recovery, but are still missing from many hospitals in the UK. Pro-

Features that define a patient at increased risk of subsequent adverse events following acute MI

- Definite cardiac enlargement
- Interstitial or alveolar oedema at any time
- Ejection fraction <40%
- Recurrent ischaemiac cardiac pain after first 24 h
- Serious ventricular arrhythmias (warranting treatment) after the first 24 h
- Previous history of angina requiring treatment
- Previous history of hypertension requiring treatment
- Complex ventricular arrhythmias on 3-h predischarge ambulatory tape
- Ventricular late potentials on signal-averaged electrocardiogram*
  Adverse exercise test within the first 4 weeks
- Plasma fibrinogen >8.5 g l^{-1} at any time
- Presence of diabetes
- Reduced heart rate variability

* Ventricular late potentials are tiny electrical deflections (<10 μV) that can be recorded at the end of the QRS complex using specialized equipment. They indicate a vulnerability to late arrhythmias.

grammes usually include supervised exercise, relaxation, dietary and other lifestyle advice, discussion and counselling both with and without partners.

Staff often make themselves available to answer queries and concerns outside time-tabled classes, acting as an informal but invaluable helpline while the family readjusts to a new, normal life. Commonly, patients join 4–6 weeks after discharge from hospital and attend for several occasions per week for between 4 and 12 weeks.

The benefit of rehabilitation classes is attested by all connected with their operation, but prospective scientific evaluation of rehabilitation has not been rigorous. Retrospective analyses indicate that they have a salutary effect on mood, effort capacity, employment potential, modifiable risk factors and overall as well as cardiovascular mortality (Chua & Lipkin, 1993). They also appear to be cost-effective (Oldridge et al., 1993). Rehabilitation groups should be encouraged, and there seems a role also for well-organized 'self-help groups' where patients can continue to meet after completion of a formal rehabilitation programme.

A summary of management

The management of acute MI now has many facets. Therapy is best tailored to individual presentation, global medical context and subsequent risk stratification. A

therapeutic flow chart that covers the most common steps and decisions from admission to discharge is shown in Fig. 12.

CARDIAC FAILURE

Definition and pathophysiology

'Cardiac failure' does not have a simple definition. Several forms of circulatory impairment are encompassed by the term, although each is characterized by symptoms and signs resulting directly from *ventricular dysfunction*. The main manifestations include poor tissue perfusion – with impaired function if severe – and tissue congestion, the site of which is determined by the type of heart failure present.

Heart failure can be categorized in several ways, according to the detailed functional abnormality of the myocardium, the side of the heart chiefly involved, or the time course of the illness. Systolic and diastolic function of the ventricles can be affected independently according to the underlying aetiology. Systolic failure is the dominant mechanism in dilated hearts; diastolic failure which prevents adequate cardiac filling (especially with tachycardia) is seen especially in patients with small hearts and exertional breathlessness or angina. A mixed picture is common.

A simple physiological diagram of the circulation (Fig. 13) helps our understanding of the pathophysiology of the presentation and management of heart failure. For normal cardiac output the left heart must be filled adequately and must respond to an increase in incoming blood with greater contraction (the Starling relationship; Fig. 14). With left ventricular dysfunction cardiac output is suppressed and rises less than normal in response to an increased load. Where the ventricle is also poorly compliant (diastolic dysfunction) even a small volume of additional blood will cause a rapid rise in filling pressure, a pressure rise that is transmitted sequentially to the left atrium, pulmonary veins and lung capillaries. It is the lungs that fall victim when left ventricular function is depressed, but right ventricular function is normal. Pulmonary venous congestion, alveolar or interstitial oedema stiffens the lungs and causes frightening breathlessness.

In isolated right ventricular dysfunction cardiac output is again reduced but the (normal) left heart is *underfilled*. The lungs are spared; right ventricular overload appears as an elevated jugular venous pressure with subsequent hepatic congestion and, commonly, peripheral oedema. When *both* ventricles fail (the usual pattern of congestive cardiac failure), a mixed picture results, although pul-

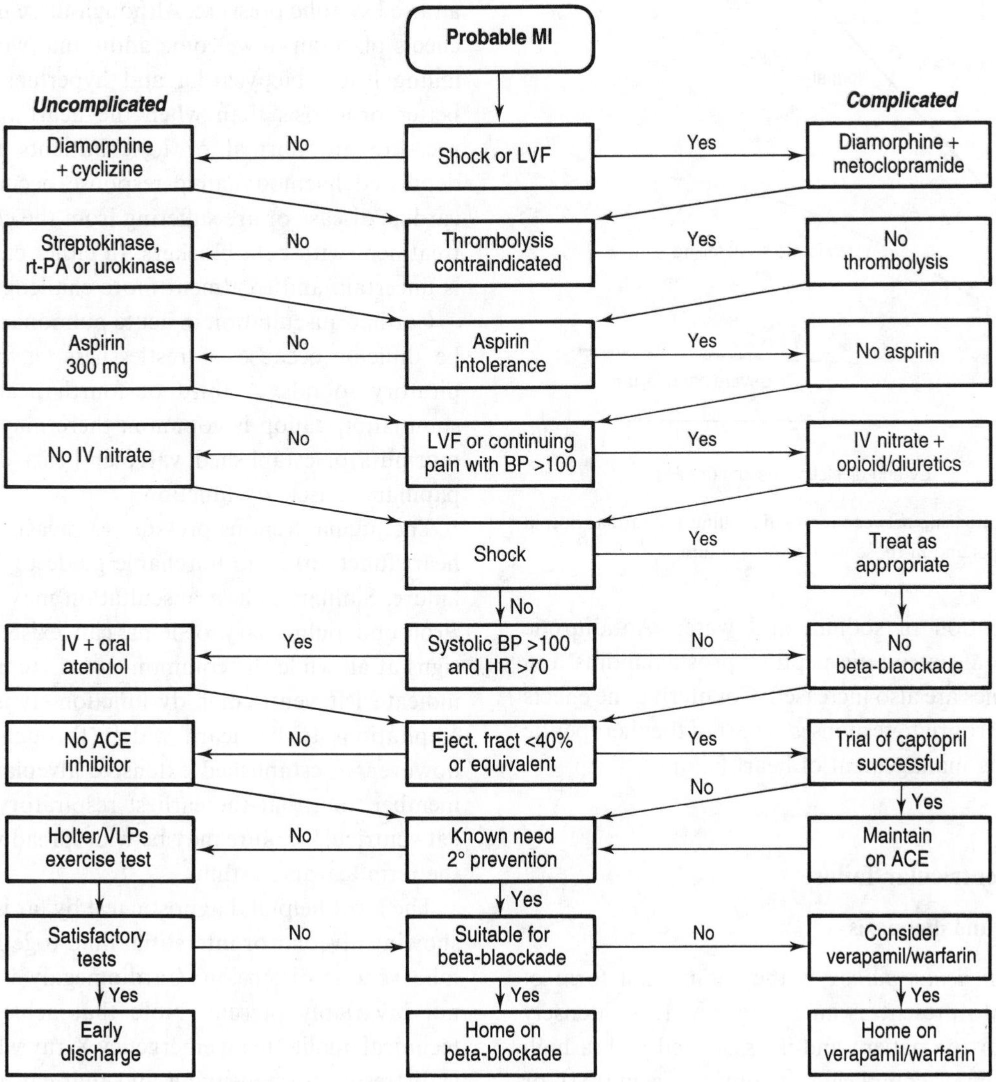

Probable MI
Uncomplicated
Complicated
Diamorphine + cyclizine
No
Shock or LVF
Yes
Diamorphine + metoclopramide
Streptokinase, rt-PA or urokinase
No
Thrombolysis contraindicated
Yes
No thrombolysis
Aspirin 300 mg
No
Aspirin intolerance
Yes
No aspirin
No IV nitrate
No
LVF or continuing pain with BP >100
Yes
IV nitrate + opioid/diuretics
Shock
Yes
Treat as appropriate
No
IV + oral atenolol
Yes
Systolic BP >100 and HR >70
No
No beta-blaockade
No ACE inhibitor
No
Eject. fract <40% or equivalent
Yes
Trial of captopril successful
No
Yes
Holter/VLPs exercise test
No
Known need 2° prevention
Maintain on ACE
Yes
Satisfactory tests
No
Suitable for beta-blaockade
No
Consider verapamil/warfarin
Yes
Yes
Yes
Early discharge
Home on beta-blockade
Home on verapamil/warfarin

Fig. 12. Flowchart of the common treatment steps and decisions in the management of acute myocardial infarction.

Right atrium
Right ventricle
LUNGS
Left atrium
Left ventricle
Body

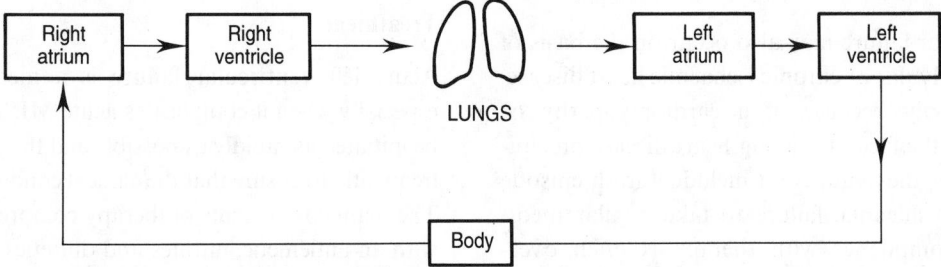

Fig. 13. A block diagram of the circulation showing the interdependence of the two sides of the heart. This is of prime importance in the understanding of heart failure.

monary congestion will be limited as right ventricular dysfunction advances.

Syndromes of heart failure are complicated by the effect of *compensatory mechanisms*, teliologically designed to counter the effects of hypovolaemia. A substantial adrenergic response – marked in acute left ventricular failure – increases heart rate and peripheral resistance adding to cardiac workload and decreasing tissue perfusion. Reduced renal perfusion results in activation of the renin–angiotensin system to cause vasoconstriction

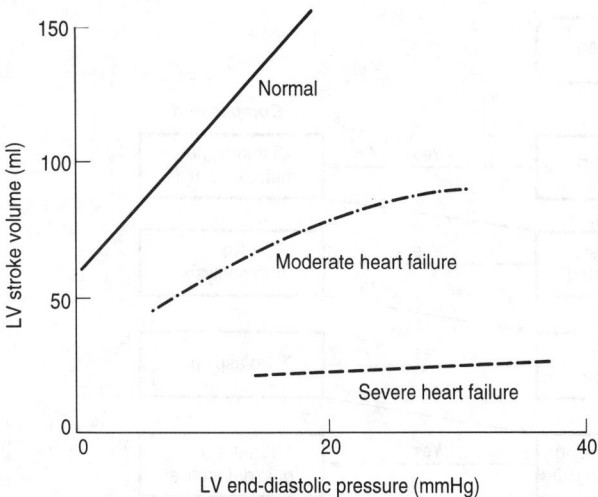

Fig. 14. The relationship between ventricular filling and cardiac output in normal patients and in those with cardiac failure.

and the retention of sodium and water. Antidiuretic hormone, atrial natriuretic peptide, prostaglandins and other hormones are also increased. Countering the effects of these inappropriate responses is part of the therapeutic strategy in the management of heart failure.

Acute left ventricular failure

Presentation and diagnosis

Acute left ventricular failure is the commonest form of heart failure to present as an emergency. It is intensely frightening for the patient and is associated with a high mortality. It may complicate an obvious acute MI or result from a silent (painless) infarct of which the patient is otherwise unaware. In either case diabetes is a predisposing factor.

Left ventricular failure may also occur on the basis of hypertensive, valvular or chronic ischaemic heart disease, or less commonly because of a cardiomyopathy or myocarditis. In the face of existing heart disease precipitating factors for the acute event include a fresh episode of myocardial ischaemia, failure to take regular medication (poor compliance with therapy is often overlooked), a new arrhythmia (commonly AF or VT (ventricular tachycardia)), thyrotoxicosis, or anaemia.

The diagnosis is suggested by the history and by the patient's appearance of distress, severe breathlessness at rest and orthopnoea. Occasionally patients look surprisingly well but most shows signs of the compensatory high sympathetic tone: pallor, sweating, a 'wild-eyed' appearance, peripheral vasoconstriction, tachycardia and

a raised systolic pressure. Although these haemodynamic effects place an unwelcome additional workload on the failing heart, tachycardia and hypertension indicate a better prognosis than when the heart rate and blood pressure are normal or low. Patients in whom this depressed haemodynamic response occurs have severe cardiac disease or are suffering from the effects of earlier treatment with beta-blockers. In either case the outlook is uncertain and treatment more challenging.

Cardiac auscultation in acute pulmonary oedema may be difficult because of restlessness or overriding respiratory sounds. A third or fourth heart sound or a summation gallop is common; there may be additional murmurs of established valvular heart disease or new papillary muscle dysfunction.

The jugular venous pressure (a measurement of right heart function) is an unreliable guide to *left* ventricular failure. Similarly, chest auscultation may be misleading. Profound pulmonary oedema can exist with no chest signs at all while the common 'basal crepitations' rarely indicate left ventricular dysfunction. It is common for crepitations to be heard widely throughout the chest, however, in established extensive alveolar oedema. Remember, too, that the earliest respiratory sign in acute left ventricular failure may be widespread wheezes; hence the term 'cardiac asthma'.

The most helpful diagnostic test by far is a chest X-ray showing alveolar or interstitial fluid together with upper lobe venous distension. Cardiomegaly is often though not invariably present. Note that achieving adequate technical quality in an emergency X-ray when the patient is distressed is challenging and that cardiac size will be exaggerated in an anteroposterior projection.

Treatment

Acute left ventricular failure is a medical emergency, especially when it complicates acute MI. Treatment should be initiated as rapidly as possible and the patient reassessed frequently to ensure that the clinical condition is improving. The main components of therapy comprise oxygen, opioid with an antiemetic, nitrates and diuretics – all drugs being given intravenously (except oxygen!). In severe or refractory cases cardiac glycosides and other inotropes may be required. The need to treat any underlying aggravating factors – anaemia, thyrotoxicosis, the nutritional deficiencies of alcoholism – should also be borne in mind.

In acute left ventricular failure oxygen diffusion is considerably impaired. Alveolar fluid and a marked ventilation perfusion mismatch cause early arterial hypoxia in the face of a normal or reduced level of the more soluble carbon dioxide. In the short term, patients require as high a concentration of *inspired oxygen* as possible, although some may reject the presence of a mask or even nasal spectacles. At this point careful nursing supervision is mandatory! An estimate of arterial blood gases is helpful to confirm that the objectives of therapy are being achieved.

Opioids used with *antiemetics*, as described for acute MI, will relieve some of the severe distress of the internal drowning suffered by the patient in acute left ventricular failure. Unless the patient is close to complete exhaustion, and if the drug is injected at the recommended slow speed, central respiratory depression should not arise. Nevertheless, naloxone should always be readily at hand. By an indirect reduction of sympathetic tone opioids may reduce heart rate and systolic blood pressure with a favourable effect on cardiac workload. This alone may halt or reverse the downward spiral of progressive ventricular failure. Cyclizine should be avoided.

The early introduction of *nitrate therapy* – particularly by the intravenous route – has turned the tide of mortality from acute left ventricular failure. Beneficial effects on venous capacitance vessels (preload) and arterial resistance vessels (afterload) are noticeable almost immediately and favour early recovery. Although nitrates can cause a reflex tachycardia, their judicious use is likely to cause a *reduction* in heart rate where sympathetic tone is high. Use glyceryl trinitrate at $100\,\mu g\,min^{-1}$ for 5–30 min depending on haemodynamic response; then reduce to $50\,\mu g\,min^{-1}$.

Patients whose presenting systolic pressure is 100 mmHg or below need very careful assessment. Nitrates may not be precluded in such patients since any decrease in blood pressure from peripheral arterial vasodilatation may be countered by an improved cardiac output. Starting doses, however, should be modest ($12.5\,\mu g\,min^{-1}$) and titrated against response while other antifailure treatment is introduced.

Diuretic therapy is routine, commonly given as frusemide 40–80 mg or bumetanide 1–2 mg by slow intravenous injection. A beneficial effect often precedes any noticeable diuresis, perhaps by an effect on capacitance vessels. Catheterization may be necessary in the elderly male or severely unwell patient.

Cardiac glycosides have a beneficial action in acute left ventricular failure. Digitalization is best achieved by intravenous administration: digoxin 500 µg in 100 ml of 5% dextrose over 30 min, repeated over 1 h.

Management

The management of acute left ventricular failure with a low systolic blood pressure (<100 mmHg) (cardiogenic shock), especially as a complication of acute MI, is challenging. Specialist help should be sought as soon as possible since such patients often require intracardiac pressure monitoring and the use of several vasoactive infusions including inotropes and dopamine to protect renal function.

Congestive cardiac failure

Patients with congestive cardiac failure present to the A&E department for several reasons: worsening breathlessness or peripheral oedema from increased fluid retention; fatigue because of poor cerebral or skeletal muscle perfusion; nausea and vomiting following progressive renal failure and/or the side-effects of treatment; syncope or presyncope due to intermittent arrhythmias or to iatrogenic or spontaneous hypotension; and abdominal pain from hepatic congestion.

Unless the patient is distressed with breathlessness, profound hypotension (BP <80 mmHg), or a malignant arrhythmia, simple admission without additional treatment is wise. Adjustments to the complex regimens of cardiac glycosides, diuretics, vasodilators, ACE inhibitors and antianginal agents with which many such patients are treated (Davies, 1992; Dargie & McMurray, 1994) are best left to the medical team responsible for the patient's continuing care.

An urgent chest X-ray, ECG, blood urea and electrolyte estimations are valuable while the patient is awaiting an in-patient bed. Intravenous diuretics are appropriate if breathlessness is marked but may not be wise without careful assessment in patients whose failure is predominantly right-sided (i.e. those with poor cardiac output, high jugular venous pressure and relatively clear lung fields). Intravenous potassium and magnesium may be warranted in the face of hypokalaemia, especially if ventricular arrhythmias are threatening.

CARDIOGENIC SHOCK

Shock of any cause is best considered as a profound circulatory disturbance in which tissue perfusion throughout the body is severely impaired (Table 8). Hypotension (systolic BP <90 mmHg) is a central feature but on its own may not define the syndrome (healthy young women often have a blood pressure at this level).

Table 8. *Effect of the severe reduction in blood flow seen in most cases of circulatory shock*

Site of poor perfusion	Effect
Brain	Restlessness; cerebral irritation; drowsiness
Kidney	Urine flow <25 ml h^{-1}; rising urea, creatinine and potassium
Heart	Ischaemic impairment of myocardial contractility
Skin	Pale, cold peripheries (effect enhanced by increased sympathetic tone)
Muscle	Flaccid muscle tone, weakness
Lung	Alveolar capillary leak ('shock lung')
Gut	Gastric and intestinal stasis; very poor absorption

Three main pathological mechanisms cause circulatory shock: loss of effective circulating volume, profound myocardial depression, and circulatory obstruction by a massive pulmonary embolism. Volume depletion may result from loss of fluid externally (gastrointestinal haemorrhage, burns, diarrhoea), internally (ruptured aortic aneurysm), or into the extracellular space (anaphylaxis, septicaemia). The profound venodilatation seen in allergic and toxic reactions causes pooling and a diminished venous return to the heart contributing to the shocked state.

Cardiogenic shock indicates a primary failure of the heart to provide an adequate circulation. The commonest form results from severe left ventricular dysfunction as a result of acute MI. Extensive damage (or, rarely, reversible 'stunning') of the left ventricle results in poor cardiac output and high filling pressures leading to pulmonary oedema. The condition is self-perpetuating since poor coronary flow further jeopardizes ventricular function, high end-diastolic pressures impede transmyocardial perfusion, and pulmonary congestion diminishes arterial oxygenation. The compensatory mechanisms described on p. 888 also add to cardiac embarrassment. There is therefore the need to act urgently to overt a progressively downward spiral. The therapeutic approach for this condition is the following:

- *General*. Patient is placed in the most comfortable position. Venous cannulae are inserted as centrally as possible. Check urea, electrolytes, blood gases.

- Ensure adequate pain relief by careful use of opioids with antiemetics (not cyclizine).
- Correct arrhythmias:
  - DC shock if necessary to avoid further myocardial depression by antiarrhythmic drugs.
  - Consider digoxin for AF.
- Raise PaO$_2$ to >80 mmHg (>10 kPa).
- Use intravenous cardiac glycosides unless ventricular arrhythmias are causing major problems.
- Establish central line for drug delivery and intracardiac pressure monitoring to titrate the response to cardioactive drugs.
- Use inotropic agents:
  - Dobutamine 250–750 µg min^{-1} (higher doses if beta-blockers have been given recently).
  - Dopamine up to 200 µg min^{-1} for its renal effect (higher doses cause harmful vasoconstriction).
  - Enoximone, useful if excessive tachycardia limits use of catecholamines.

Left ventricular function may be impeded by a severe mechanical complication of acute MI. Recovery is usually possible only if this can be corrected, but the hazards are high and recovery from these conditions very unlikely.

Less common forms of cardiogenic shock include the following:

- *Dominant right ventricular infarction*. This condition is characterized by a very high jugular venous pressure and poor cardiac output, but without pulmonary congestion. Differentiation from pulmonary embolism and pericardial tamponade depends on the history and the electrocardiogram. Right ventricular infarction is almost always associated with inferior lateral or true posterior infarction and may be evident in leads V$_{3R}$ and V$_{4R}$. If necessary, an urgent echocardiogram can be used to exclude pericardial effusion.

Two practical points in management. Firstly, such patients *need* a high right-sided filling pressure; diuretics will worsen the haemodynamic state. Secondly, a small amount of fluid loading may be helpful, but the response may be brittle especially as the left ventricle is likely to be impaired as well. Even 200 ml of additional intravenous fluid can precipitate pulmonary oedema.

- *A syncopal response*. Occasionally, poor cardiac output after MI is associated with *low* filling pressures in both ventricles. This may happen after conventional treatment for the usual form of left ventricular failure or after inferior infarction with venodilatation due to high vagal tone whether or not thrombolytic therapy has been used. In the face of a bradycardia *atropine* and time are worthwhile. A short-lived infusion of fluid may be tried (initially 5% dextrose so that it readily diffuses from the vascular space) but these patients, too, are brittle. Where the condition persists, intra-cardiac pressure monitoring is mandatory.

- *Pericardial tamponade.* Shock with a very high non-pulsatile jugular venous pressure and cardiomegaly on chest X-ray characterizes this condition. Pulmonary congestion is usually minimal or absent. The diagnosis is confirmed by echocardiography and treatment is by cautious removal of the pericardial fluid on a monitored unit.

PULMONARY EMBOLI

A physiological function of the pulmonary capillary bed is to filter the circulation of minute clots that are a daily occurrence in health. Pathological obstruction of the pulmonary vessels, however, occurs in one of four types: slowly progressive occlusion of small vessels; occlusion of one or more medium-sized vessels resulting in pulmonary infarction; single or multiple episodes of occlusive emboli to large (lobar and lobular) arteries; massive emboli to the main pulmonary artery or its immediate right or left branches. Each type has a specific clinical presentation and therapeutic approach.

Multiple small pulmonary emboli

Progressive breathlessness in a young or middle-aged woman is the hallmark of this condition. A history of multiple pregnancies or use of the contraceptive pill is common, although not invariable. Characteristically, breathlessness (often with cyanosis) is considerably in excess of clinical or radiographic signs in the lungs. Evidence of right heart overload is more common: tachycardia, a high jugular venous pressure, left parasternal heave, right ventricular gallop and ECG evidence of long-standing right ventricular pressure overload.

This condition needs to be considered in any differential diagnosis of breathlessness, but the clinical context and the long-standing nature of the problem make its presentation more common in a routine out-patient department than in an A&E department.

Segmental emboli with pulmonary infarction

Emboli that block segmental vessels are those that result in areas of peripheral pulmonary infarction. The effects are more visible: pleuritic pain, haemoptysis, a pleural rub, radiological changes of streaky peripheral lung shadowing and a blunted costophrenic angle due to minor blood loss into the pleural space. But even several such emboli will pose little additional resistance to total pulmonary blood flow. The right heart has therefore no additional challenge and both clinical and ECG evidence of right ventricular overload are absent in this condition.

Major pulmonary emboli

Obstruction of the larger branches of the pulmonary tree may be remarkably silent. A sudden episode of breathlessness, transient deterioration of exercise capacity, a brief rise in the heart rate or fall in blood pressure may be the only evidence of occlusion of an important pulmonary artery. Pulmonary infarction (with its attendant signs) rarely occurs, but the event may be repeated in a different artery giving diminution of pulmonary reserve. Not uncommonly a sequence of such events precedes a massive pulmonary embolism. After several emboli into lobar or lobular arteries, total pulmonary vascular resistance may rise and evidence of right ventricular overload emerges. By then the patient will also be cyanosed.

Massive emboli

Emboli to the major pulmonary arteries cause a profound syncopal event with marked tachypnoea, acute right ventricular overload and intense distension of the jugular veins. The conscious patient may complain of precordial discomfort (pulmonary arterial distension and/or right ventricular angina). In severe cases death may be immediate with no response to cardiopulmonary resuscitation or may occur within 1 h. The contribution of 'reflex' or hormonally induced general pulmonary arterial constriction in these patients remains conjectural.

Diagnosis and treatment

The most important factors to prevent death from pulmonary emboli are *adequate prophylaxis* and a *high level of suspicion* of the condition. Over 70% of cases of pulmonary emboli have peripheral venous thrombosis and medical personnel should maintain constant vigilance to protect those at increased risk by prophylactic heparinization.

The signs of pulmonary infarction are usually sufficiently clear to reach a diagnosis although differentiation from pneumonia may be difficult. In these cases a very

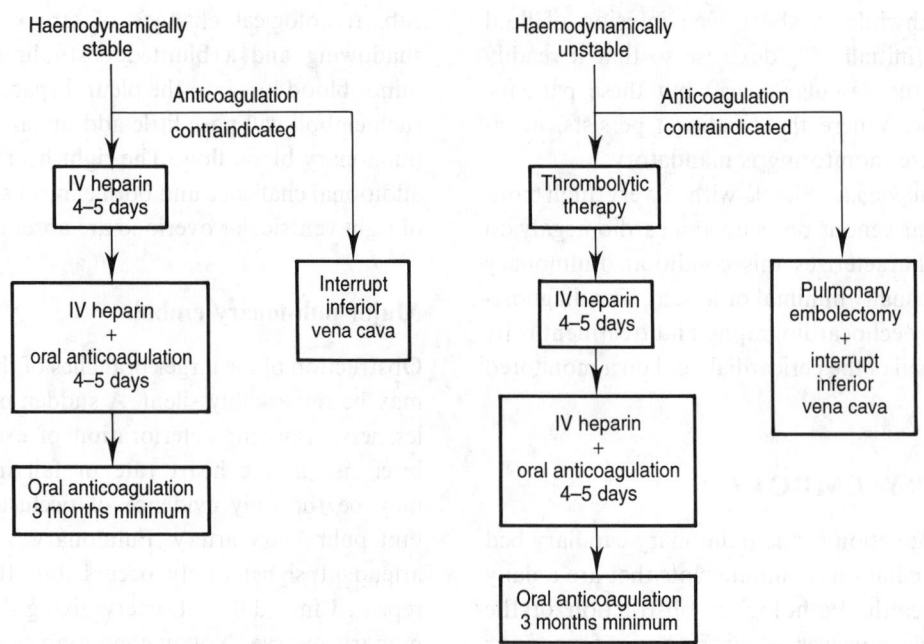

Fig. 15. Suggested treatment protocol for the management of pulmonary embolism. (Reproduced, with permission, from Skinner & Vincent, 1993.)

high fever and normal *blood gases* make pulmonary emboli unlikely. A lung scan – to show areas of ventilation perfusion mismatch – may be helpful, but on occasion the diagnosis may be difficult and treatment with heparin as well as antibiotics may be advisable as a practical course of action in the face of uncertainty.

Unexplained breathlessness with a normal chest X-ray – particularly where a predisposition exists to venous thrombosis – provides a low threshold for undertaking a ventilation/perfusion scan. Where the patient remains symptomatic and non-invasive tests are unclear, consideration should be given to pulmonary arteriography.

The diagnosis of pulmonary embolism is a shocked patient with high venous pressure frequently depends on the demonstration of a normal chest X-ray and the absence of either pericardial tamponade or MI. A persuasive sign is marked cyanosis and profound tachypnoea even when the chest X-ray is unremarkable. The ECG *may* show evidence of acute right ventricular overload, particularly as right bundle branch block, right axis deviation or a prolonged PR interval. The classic $S_1Q_3T_3$ pattern turns out to be both uncommon and non-specific.

The mainstay of therapy for pulmonary embolic disease is anticoagulation with heparin – an agent that can always be given while the diagnosis is being established (Hall & Haworth, 1989); 40 000 units in 24 h by continuous infusion is appropriate initially, with subsequent dosing determined by coagulation monitoring. Massive

pulmonary emboli with loss of cardiac output calls for the standard techniques of cardiopulmonary resuscitation which themselves may disperse a central clot sufficiently to restore the pulmonary circulation and maintain life. Thrombolytic therapy is reserved for patients with severe haemodynamic impairment and can be given in a form now accepted for the treatment of many patients with acute MI. Fig. 15 provides a summary of treatment for the patient presenting with pulmonary embolus.

AORTIC DISSECTION

Pathology

Acute dissection of the thoracic aorta occurs in about 10 per million population per year and accounts for around 5% of cases of sudden death. It is a condition with a high mortality: 90% within 3 months if untreated, 15–20% with combined medical and surgical therapy.

The primary lesion is an intimal tear, most commonly 2–3 cm from the aortic valve about the right coronary sinus. Arterial hypertension is the commonest aetiological factor occurring in 70–90% of cases. In younger patients (<40 years) other predisposing conditions include congenital aortic valve disease, pregnancy and coarctation. (Atheroma plays a surprisingly small part in this condition.) Patients with Marfan's syndrome are at special risk from dissection, especially when weakness of the media has already lead to an aortic root aneurysm.

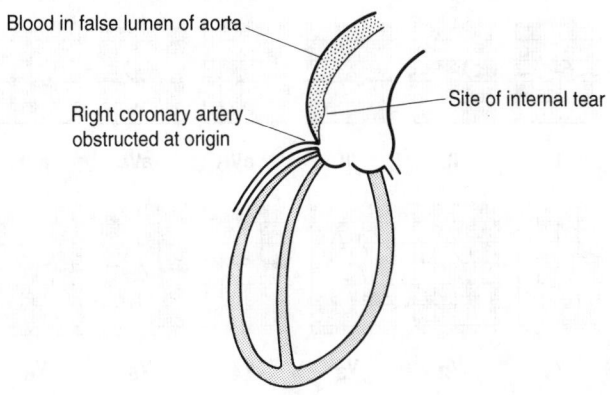

Fig. 16. Dissection of the ascending aorta can occlude the origin of the right coronary artery giving rise to an inferior myocardial infarct complicating the presentation.

The dissecting process usually involves the ascending aorta (type A) with a variable extension into the arch and descending thoracic aorta. Dissection involving the descending aorta only (type B) is less common (20%).

Dissection of the aortic media can result in a number of complications, some fatal. Occlusion of the right coronary artery may cause a simultaneous inferior MI with its own symptoms and signs (Fig. 16). Dissection into branch vessels of the aortic arch may compromise the arterial supply to the arms or cerebral blood flow, with temporary or permanent neurological signs.

Disruption of the aortic valve causes aortic regurgitation and may herald subsequent (fatal) rupture into the pericardium. Rupture may also occur into the left pleural or retroperitoneal space. Distortion of the aortic arch by the additional false lumen may compress the superior vena cava giving a clinically elevated jugular venous pressure.

In some cases, distortion of the aortic arch seems also to alter the control of blood pressure, promoting stubborn hypertension in a condition where this is least desirable. True re-entry of the dissection occurs in 10–20% of cases.

Diagnosis

Severe instantaneous chest pain often radiating to the back in a male hypertensive patient over 50 years of age is strongly suggestive of aortic dissection. Absent peripheral pulses, a raised venous pressure, aortic regurgitation and unilateral neurological signs give supporting evidence from associated complications.

The ECG is usually helpful in excluding an acute MI in the presence of severe chest pain. But an inferior infarct may have resulted from disruption of a right coronary artery confounding the diagnosis. Repolar-

ization (ST-T-U) changes of longstanding hypertension are more common.

The chest X-ray may show widening of the aortic arch, but there are two obscuring factors: firstly, uncomplicated hypertension especially in the elderly often leads to generalized widening of the aorta; secondly, mediastinal widening is reported in only 50–60% of cases of aortic dissection. A double shadow – due to the false and true lumens – is a helpful, but difficult, sign. Enlargement of the cardiac outline is non-specific while a pleural effusion is suggestive, but may be due to a serosanguinous exudate rather than rupture of the aneurysm into the pleural space.

Standard echocardiography may show the abnormal area of the aorta if this extends proximally to the aortic valve; transoesophageal echo provides a much clearer visualization of the aortic pathology and is becoming the initial investigation of choice. In a number of confirmation of the diagnosis requires a thoracic computed tomography (CT) scan with and without contrast enhancement.

Urgent management

After antiemetics and pain relief, a careful reduction in blood pressure and urgent referral to the admitting medical firm are the main requirements. Intravenous opioids with an antiemetic are most appropriate for analgesia, and intravenous antihypertensive therapy will almost certainly be needed. Although intravenous sodium nitroprusside is popular and gives readily adjustable blood pressure control in a sometimes brittle condition, therapy that includes beta-blockade will usefully reduce the rate of rise of systolic pressure as well as its absolute level. Surgery is considered after stabilization of the acute phase. Aortic repair, with or without aortic valve replacement, is common in type A dissections but surgery in type B lesions is reserved for patients in whom the dissection appears progressive or threatens rupture (Miller *et al.*, 1979).

PERICARDITIS

Pathology

Pericardial inflammation may lead to several distinct syndromes:

- Acute pericarditis.
- Recurrent pericarditis.
- Chronic pericarditis.
- Pericardial tamponade.

Table 9. *Causes of acute pericarditis*

Idiopathic	('Benign')
Viral	Coxsackie virus
	Echovirus
	Epstein–Barr virus
Bacterial	Pneumococcus
	Meningococcus
	Haemophilus
	Gonococcus
Ischaemic	Acute myocardial infarction
Immunological	Dressler's syndrome
	– Late after myocardial infarction
	– After cardiac surgery
	Connective tissue disorders
	(SLE, rheumatoid)
Uraemic	
Traumatic	
Malignant	
Postirradiation	

SLE, systemic lupus erythematosus.

● Constrictive pericarditis.

The most common to present in an A&E department is acute pericarditis of either idiopathic or viral origin. Other causes (Table 9) are less common, although an occasional patient will be seen whose recent full-thickness MI presents with a pericardial rather than ischaemic pain.

Diagnosis

Precordial pain worse on inspiration or movement is a key symptom. It may be severe enough to mimic MI. There may be an associated continuous dull ache and occasionally superficial tenderness over the site of maximum discomfort. Radiation of the pain is uncommon, but it may affect the neck or shoulders. Sitting forward is said to be the preferred position. Respiratory excursion limited by pain gives the patient and the doctor an impression of associated breathlessness.

The presence of a pericardial rub is diagnostic and should be heard as a 'scratchy' sound in both systole and diastole. Its intensity may vary with respiration and position. It may be localized to a small area and is best heard with the diaphragm.

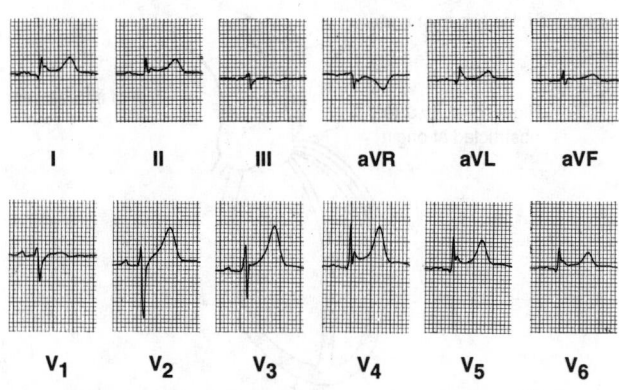

Fig. 17. The typical ECG changes of acute pericarditis.

The ECG may show widespread concave upward ST segment elevation (Fig. 17), although differentiation from a physiological 'high ST take-off' can be difficult, and the change is not central to the diagnosis. Occasionally shallow T wave inversion develops – evidence for involvement of the subpericardial myocardium in the inflammatory process (myopericarditis).

Treatment

Analgesia with indomethacin is appropriate, although rarely small doses of opioid are required for adequate relief. Reassurance is often necessary as the patient will commonly attribute a more serious prognosis to the incident than is necessary. The patient with acute MI needs therapy appropriate to that condition; but even with 'benign' vital pericarditis, admission should be considered for pain relief, and to ensure that the course remains benign – free from arrhythmias and cardiac dilatation.

ACCELERATED HYPERTENSION

Accelerated ('malignant') hypertension is an uncommon but serious condition producing the most severe arterial complications seen with a raised blood pressure. Figures for incidence are difficult to obtain but in Scottish populations suggest a rate of 4–5% of patients presenting to a hypertension clinic at hospital.

An accelerated phase may complicate established hypertension of any aetiology or may be the initial presentation of the hypertensive patient. It is characterized by marked elevation in blood pressure (usually in excess of 200/120) with retinal haemorrhages and exudates. Papilloedema is common but is no longer mandatory to define the malignant phase. Evidence for other target organ damage is likely: cardiomegaly, ECG changes, proteinuria and abnormal renal function.

In untreated patients, death occurs within months as a result of the vascular effects of either an extremely high or rapidly rising arterial pressure. Thrombotic occlusion or increased vascular permeability through overdistension of vessels leads to a mixture of ischaemia and over-perfusion in susceptible areas. The most vulnerable organs are the kidney, brain and retina, but the heart, pancreas and gut may also be involved. Where cerebro-vascular autoregulation is overwhelmed by the raised arterial pressure, hypertensive encephalopathy (head-ache, confusion, coma, fits) may occur.

Hypertensive encephalopathy is a medical emergency requiring immediate care; parenteral therapy is advised. Sodium nitroprusside can be titrated closely against the fall in pressure it produces, but needs very careful monitoring. Labetolol gives an effective and more grad-ual reduction in blood pressure and may be safer. In the absence of encephalopathy admission for investigation and oral therapy for the accelerated phase may be safer than the potentially precipitous fall in blood pressure produced by intravenous agents. With appro-priate medication patients presenting with this condition now have a median survival of 18 years.

Bibliography

ADAMS, III. J.E., BODOR, G.S., DAVILA-ROMAIN, V.G. *et al.* (1992). Cardiac troponin T. A marker with high specificity for cardiac injury. *Circulation*, **88**, 101–6.

ADAMS, J., TRENT, R. & RAWLES, J. (for the GREAT Group). (1993). Earliest electrocardiographic evidence for myocardial infarction: implications for thrombolytic treatment. *Br. Med. J.*, **307**, 409–13.

ARMSTRONG, A., DUNCAN, B. & OLIVER, M.F. (1972). Natural history of acute coronary heart attacks. A community study. *Br. Heart J.*, **34**, 67–80.

ARNOLD, A.E.R., SIMOONS, M.C., DETRY, J.-M.R. *et al.* (1993). Prediction of mortality following hospital discharge after thrombolysis for acute myocardial infarction: is there a need for coronary angiography? *Eur. Heart J.*, **14**, 640–8.

BLEIFELD, W. (1990). Unstable angina: pathophysiology and drug therapy. *Eur. J. Clin. Pharmacol.*, **38** (Suppl. 1), 573–6.

CAIRNS, J.A., GENT, M., SINGER, J. *et al.* (1985). Aspirin, sulfinpyrazone, or both in unstable angina – results of a Canadian multicentre trial. *N. Eng. J. Med.*, **313**, 1369–75.

CHAMBERLAIN, D.A. (1989). Unanswered questions in thrombolysis. In: A symposium on the clinical profile of eminase (APSAC). *Am. J. Cardiol.*, **63** (Suppl. A), 34A–40A.

CHUA, T.P. & LIPKIN, D.P. (1993). Cardiac rehabilitation. *Br. Med. J.*, **306**, 731–2.

COLLING, A., DELLIPIANI, A.W., DONALDSON, R.J. *et al.* (1976). Teeside coronary survey: an epidemiological study of acute attacks of myocardial infarction. *Br. Med. J.*, **2**, 1169–72.

DAVIES, M.J. (1992). Anatomic features in victims of sudden coronary death. *Circulation*, **85** (Suppl. I), I-19–I-24.

DAVIES, M.J. & THOMAS, A.C. (1985). Plaque fissuring – the cause of acute myocardial infarction, sudden ischaemic death, and crescendo angina. *Br. Heart J.*, **53**, 363–73.

DAVIES, M.K. (1992). Modern management of heart failure. *Br. J. Hosp. Med.*, **47**, 16–24.

DARGIE, H.J. & McMURRAY, J.J.V. (1994). Diagnosis and management of heart failure. *Br. Med. J.*, **308**, 321–8.

DE BONO, D.P. & HOPKINS, A. (1993). The investigation and management of stable angina. (Report of a working party of the joint audit committee of the British Cardiac Society and the Royal College of Physicians of London.) *J. R. Coll. Physicians Lond.*, **27**, 267–73.

DELLBORG, M., GUSTAFFON, G. & SWEDBERG, K. (1991). Buccal versus intravenous nitroglycerin in unstable angina pectoris. *Eur. J. Clin. Pharmacol.*, **41**, 5–9.

FERGUSON, J.J., DIVER, D.J., BOLDT, M. *et al.* (1989). Significance of nitroglycerin-induced hypotension with inferior wall acute myocardial infarction. *Am. J. Cardiol.*, **64**, 311–14.

FIBRINOLYTIC THERAPY TRIALISTS (FTT) COLLABORATIVE GROUP (1994). Indications for fibrinolytic therapy in suspected acute myocardial infarction: collaborative overview of early mortality and major morbidity results from all randomised trials of more than 1000 patients. *Lancet*, **343**, 311–22.

FOEGH, M.L. & VIRMANI, R. (1993). Molecular biology of intimal proliferation. *Curr. Opin. Cardiol.*, **8**, 938–50.

FRY, J. (1976). The natural history of angina in a general practice. *J. R. Coll. Pract.*, **26**, 643–8.

GAZES, P.C., MOBLEY, JR., E.M., FARIS, JR., H.M. *et al.* (1973). Preinfarction (unstable) angina – a prospective study – ten year follow-up. *Circulation*, **48**, 331–7.

GOTTLIEB, S.O., WEISFELDT, M.L., OUYANG, P. *et al.* (1986). Silent ischaemia as a marker for early unfavourable outcomes in patients with unstable angina. *N. Eng. J. Med.*, **311**, 1144–7.

HALL, R.J.C. & HAWORTH, S.G. (1989). Disorders of the pulmonary circulation. In: *Diseases of the Heart*, ed. D.G. Julian, A.J. Camm, K.M. Fox, R.J.C. Hall & P.A. Poole-Wilson. pp. 1293–328. London: Baillière Tindall.

HANDS, M.E., COOK, E.F., STONE, P.H. *et al.* (1988). Electrocardiographic diagnosis of myocardial infarction in the presence of complete left bundle branch block. *Am. Heart J.*, **116**, 23–31.

HANGARTNER, J.R.W., CHARLESTON, A.J., DAVIES, M.J. et al. (1986). Morphological characteristics of clinically significant coronary artery stenosis in stable angina. Br. Heart J., **56**, 501–8.

HERLITZ, J., HJALMARSON, A. & WAAGSTEIN, F. (1989). Treatment of pain in acute myocardial infarction. Br. Heart J., **61**, 9–13.

HUTCHISON, S.J., POOLE-WILSON, P.A. & HENDERSON, A.H. (1989). Angina with normal coronary arteries. Q. J. Med., **268**, 677–88.

ISIS-1 (FIRST INTERNATIONAL STUDY OF INFARCT SURVIVAL) COLLABORATIVE GROUP (1988). Mechanisms for the early mortality reduction produced by betablockade started early in acute myocardial infarction. Lancet, **i**, 921–3.

ISIS-2 (SECOND INTERNATIONAL STUDY OF INFARCT SURVIVAL) COLLABORATIVE GROUP (1988). Randomised trial of intravenous streptokinase, oral aspirin, both or neither among, 17,187 cases of suspected acute myocardial infarctions: ISIS-2. Lancet, **ii**, 349–60.

ISIS-3 (THIRD INTERNATIONAL STUDY OF INFARCT SURVIVAL) COLLABORATIVE GROUP (1992). A randomised comparison of streptokinase vs tissue plasminogen activator vs anistreplase and of aspirin plus heparin vs aspirin alone among 41,299 cases of suspected acute myocardial infarction. Lancet, **339**, 753–70.

ISIS-4 (FOURTH INTERNATIONAL STUDY OF INFARCT SURVIVAL) COLLABORATIVE GROUP (1995). A randomised factorial trial assessing early oral captopril, oral mononitrate, and intravenous magnesium sulphate is 58,050 patients with suspected acute myocardial infarction. Lancet, **345**, 669–85.

JULIAN, D.G. & BRAUNWALD, E. (1994). Management of Acute Myocardial Infarction. London: W.B. Saunders.

KANNEL, W.B. & ABBOTT, R.D. (1984). Incidence and prognosis of recognised myocardial infarction: an update on the Framingham Study. N. Engl. J. Med., **311**, 1114–17.

KANNEL, W.B. & FEINLEIB, M. (1972). Natural history of angina in the Framingham Study. Prognosis and survival. Am. J. Cardiol., **29**, 154–62.

KINLEN, L.J. (1973). Incidence and presentation of myocardial infarction in an English community. Br. Heart J., **35**, 616–22.

LICHTLEN, P.R., RAFFLENBENL, W. & FREUDENBERG, H. (1985). Pathoanatomy and function of coronary obstructions leading to unstable angina pectoris – anatomical and angiographic studies. In Unstable Angina, ed. P.G. Hugenholtz & B.S. Goldman. pp. 81–94. Stuggart: Schattauer.

LUSCHER, T.F., EPINONSA, E., DUBEY, R.K. et al. (1993). Vascular biology of human coronary artery and bypass graft disease. Curr. Opin. Cardiol., **8**, 963–74.

MacCULLUM, A.G., STAFFORD, P.J., JONES, C.

et al. (1990). Reduction in hospital time to thrombolytic therapy by audit of policy guidelines. Eur. Heart J., **11**, 48–52.

McCORD, J.M. (1985). Oxygen free radicals in post ischaemic tissue injury. N. Eng. J. Med., **32**, 159–63.

MILLER, D.C., STINSON, E.B., OYER, P.E. et al. (1979). The operative treatment of aortic dissections: experience with 125 patients over a sixteen year period. J. Thorac. Cardiovasc. Surg., **78**, 365–82.

MULCAHY, R., AL AWADHI, A.H., DE BUITLER, M. et al. (1985). Natural history and prognosis of unstable angina. Am. Heart J., **109**, 753–8.

NERI SERNERI, G.G., GENSINI, G.F., POGGESI, L. et al. (1990). Effect of heparin, aspirin, or alteplase in reduction of myocardial ischaemia in refractory unstable angina. Lancet, **335**, 615–18.

OLDRIDGE, N., FURLONG, W., FEENY, D. et al. (1993). Economic evaluation of cardiac rehabilitation soon after acute myocardial infarction. Am. J. Cardiol., **72**, 154–61.

OPIE, L.H. (1989). Reperfusion injury and its pharmacological modification. Circulation, **80**, 1049–62.

PELL, A.C.H., MILLER, H.C., ROBERTSON, C.E. et al. (1992). Effect of 'fast track' admission for acute myocardial infarction on delay to thrombolysis. Br. Med. J., **304**, 87–7.

POLLACK, H., DIEZ, W., SPIEL, R. et al. (1993). Early diagnosis of subacute free wall rupture complicating acute myocardial infarction. Eur. Heart J., **14**, 306–15.

POOLE-WILSON, P.A. (1990). The myocardium in ischaemic heart disease. In Atherosclerosis in Ischaemic Heart Disease: Myocardial Consequences, ed. P.A. Poole-Wilson & D.J. Sheridan. pp. 3.1–3.56. London: Science Press.

PRINZMETAL, M., EKMEKCI, A., KENNAMER, R. et al. (1960). Variant form of angina pectoris. J. Am. Med. Assoc., **174**, 1794–800.

REID, D.D., HAMILTON, P.J.S., KEEN, H. et al. (1974). Cardiorespiratory disease and diabetes among middle-aged male civil servants. Lancet, **i**, 469–73.

ROYAL COLLEGE OF GENERAL PRACTITIONERS (1979). Morbidity Statistics from General Practice 1971–72. Second National Study. London, HMSO.

RUDE, R.E., POOLE, W.K., MULLER, J.E. et al. (1983). Electrocardiographic and clinical criteria for recognition of acute myocardial infarction based on analysis of 3697 patients. Am. J. Cardiol, **52**, 936–42.

SCHWEITZER, P. (1990). The electrocardiographic diagnosis of myocardial infarction in the thrombolytic era. Am. Heart J., **119**, 642–54.

SHAPER, A.G., COOK, D.G., WALKER, M. et al. (1984a). Prevalence of ischaemic heart disease in middle-aged British men. Br. Heart J., **51**, 595–605.

SHAPER, A.G., COOK, D.G., WALKER, M. et al. (1984b). Recall of diagnosis by men with ischaemic heart disease. Br. Heart J., **51**, 606–11.

SHORT, D. (1970). The earliest electrocardiographic evidence of myocardial infarction. *Br. Heart J.*, **32**, 6–15.

SKINNER, D.V. & VINCENT, R. (1993). *Cardiopulmonary Resuscitation* (Oxford Handbooks in Emergency Medicine). Oxford: Oxford University Press.

SMITH, L.F., HEAGERTY, A.M., BING, R.F. *et al.* (1986). Intravenous infusion of magnesium sulphate after acute myocardial infarction: effects on arrhythmias and mortality. *Int. J. Cardiol.*, **12**, 175–80.

STEENBERGEN, C., MURPHY, E., LEVY, L. *et al.* (1987). Elevation in cytosolic free calcium concentrationearly in myocardial ischaemia in perfused rat heart. *Circ. Res.*, **60**, 700–7.

TAN, L.B., BRYANT, S. & MURRAY, R.G. *et al.* (1988). Detrimental haemodynamic effects of cyclizine in heart failure. *Lancet*, **i**, 560–1.

THE GUSTO INVESTIGATORS (1993). An international randomized trial comparing four thrombolytic strategies for acute myocardial infarction. *N. Engl. J. Med.*, **329**, 673–82.

THE RISC GROUP (1990). Risk of myocardial infarction and death during treatment with low-dose aspirin and intravenous heparin in men with unstable coronary artery disease. *Lancet*, **336**, 827–30.

THEROUX, P., OUINET, H., McCANS, S. *et al.* (1990). Aspirin, heparin, or both to treat acute unstable angina. *J. Engl. J. Med.*, **319**, 1105–11.

TUNSTALL-PEDOE, H. (1991). The Health of the Nation: responses: coronary heart disease. *Br. Med. J.*, **303**, 701–4.

VON DOHLEN, T.W., ROGERS, W.B. & FRANK, M.J. (1989). Pathophysiology and management of unstable angina. *Clin. Cardiol.*, **12**, 363–9.

WEBB, S.C., RICKARDS, A.F. & POOLE-WILSON, P.A. (1983). Coronary sinus potassium concentration recorded during coronary angioplasty. *Br. Heart J.*, **50**, 146–8.

WESTON, C.F.M., PENNY, W.J. & JULIAN, D.G. (1994). Guidelines for the early management of patients with myocardial infarction. *Br. Med. J.*, **308**, 767–71.

WOOLF, N. (1990). Atherosclerosis and its genesis. In *Atherosclerosis in Ischaemic Heart Disease: The Mechanisms*, ed. M.J. Davies & N. Woolf. pp. 1.1–1.63. London: Science Press.

YOUNG, I.S., PURVIS, J.A., LIGHTBODY, J.H. *et al.* (1993). Lipid peroxidation and antioxidant status following thrombolytic therapy for acute myocardial infarction. *Eur. Heart J.*, **14**, 1027–33.

YUSUF, S., COLLINS, R., MacMAHON, S. *et al.* (1988). Effect of intravenous nitrates on mortality in acute myocardial infarction: an overview of the randomised trials. *Lancet*, **i**, 1088–92.

B: Cardiac arrhythmias

T.A. MILLANE and A.J. CAMM

Department of Cardiological Sciences, St George's Hospital Medical School, London, UK

GENERAL INTRODUCTION

The purpose of the following discussion is to provide a practical guide to the diagnosis and management of the more common cardiac arrhythmias encountered in an accident and emergency (A&E) department. The text does not encompass the long-term management of cardiac arrhythmia, but some guidance towards immediate follow-up procedure is given. A basic understanding of cardiac conduction is assumed, together with the electrocardiographic features of normal sinus rhythm.

The chapter is extensively subdivided for rapid reference purposes. Both of the first two sections begin with a description of the therapeutic manoeuvres involved in the treatment of the arrhythmia in question, followed by an illustrated discussion of each individual arrhythmia. A troubleshooting approach to problems with permanent pacemakers and implantable cardioverter defibrillators is included in a further section. Treatment of cardiac arrhythmia secondary to drug overdose is followed by a brief description of paediatric cardiac arrhythmia which is complemented by a discussion on the treatment of arrhythmia in pregnancy and lactation.

The common arrhythmias

Arrhythmias are considered as 'bradycardia' or 'tachycardia' with the tachycardias subdivided into 'broad complex tachycardia' and 'narrow complex tachycardia'. The clinical features of each arrhythmia are described, and the electrocardiographic features discussed and illustrated. The common associations of the arrhythmia are listed, and a management protocol suggested. A series of flowcharts are presented to help with interpretation and management of the more complex problems.

Electrocardiography in the A&E department

Most departments have a dedicated ECG (electrocardiographic) machine, and all staff should become conversant with its use. Ideally, the 12-lead ECG should be produced in an 'at a glance' presentation, and include a longer

Table 1. *Sinus rhythm – normal intervals*

	sec
PR interval	0.12–0.20
QRS width	0.06–0.10
QTc interval[a]	0.39–0.44

[a] See section on long QT syndromes.

section or 'rhythm strip' (usually recorded in standard lead II), to aid in the description of the cardiac rhythm. Attention to technique in placing the electrodes will largely avoid the problems of a poor-quality signal. An unstable baseline secondary to fine muscle tremor is difficult to overcome, but an ECG recorded from a warm, comfortable, reassured patient will usually be free of this artefact.

Wherever possible, a 12-lead ECG should be recorded in all patients with suspected cardiac arrhythmia, since a single lead viewed from a single channel monitor may give misleading information. A 12-lead ECG recorded during ventricular tachycardia (VT) can be of enormous help in subsequent decision-making regarding long-term treatment, particularly if the arrhythmia is recurrent.

A 3-lead ECG should be recorded during any anti-arrhythmic manoeuvre, since the mode of termination of an arrhythmia may give vital clues as to its origin and specific type; this is particularly true of the supra-ventricular tachycardias.

Table 1 details normal intervals during sinus rhythm. The ECG is usually recorded at 25 mm sec^{-1}; each 'little square' of ECG paper (0.1 mm) thus represents 0.04 sec (40 msec). For example, the normal PR interval is 0.12–0.20 sec; this is equal to three to five 'little squares' at 25 mm sec^{-1}.

BRADYCARDIA

In general, patients with symptomatic bradycardia will complain of light-headedness or 'dizziness' (particularly on exertion), and may report exertional dyspnoea. If the arrhythmia is intermittent, presyncope or syncope (Stokes–Adams attack) may occur. A normal ECG recorded in the A&E department does not exclude intermittent bradycardia as a cause of collapse – a pathology common in the elderly.

TECHNIQUES

Therapeutic manoeuvres in the management of bradycardia

Drugs

Atropine and isoprenaline are the mainstay of bradycardia pharmacology. Details of dosage, side-effects and interactions are given in Table 2. In the notes on each particular bradyarrhythmia, specific pharmacological approaches are discussed.

External cardiac pacing

It is possible to maintain cardiac rhythm by applying external pacing electrodes fitted to a specialized pacing system with ECG monitoring; a considerably higher voltage is required to achieve ventricular capture than with transvenous pacing and its use is generally limited by the discomfort of associated skeletal muscle contraction. However, it is easy to use and quick to apply; in a difficult situation it is often very useful.

NB: Some pacing generators are oriented to 'current' rather than to 'voltage'; for practical purposes the terms are interchangeable.

Indications
1. Bradycardia unresponsive to atropine with haemo-dynamic compromise.
2. As a bridge, whilst awaiting transvenous pacing.
3. For overdrive pacing (see section on overdrive pacing).

Equipment required
1. External pacing generator.
2. Large specialized electrodes.
3. Defibrillation facilities.
4. Continuous ECG monitoring.

Patient preparation
1. Explanation of technique (if possible).
2. Clean, dry skin areas for electrode placement.
3. Ensure that the patient is electrically isolated and that the patient area is dry (this includes wet sheets, etc.).

Procedure
1. Apply specialized pacing electrodes as per manufacturer's directions (usually anterior left chest over the heart, and posterior left chest opposite anterior electrode).
2. Connect external ECG to pacing generator and ensure adequate signal; the pace generator will sense the patient's own rhythm from the external ECG. If the patient has an underlying rhythm, see instruction 3. If the situation is haemodynamically very serious or if there is no underlying rhythm, see instruction 6.
3. Set pacing generator to 2–3 V output (or lowest current setting) at the required rate (usually 70–90 beats min^{-1}) in 'demand' mode if the patient has some intrinsic rhythm. If no underlying rhythm, see 6 below.

Table 2. *Antiarrhythmic drugs used in the A&E department*

Drug	Initial dose	Maintenance infusion	Indication	Side-effects	Contraindications	Drug interactions
Adenosine	3–18 mg rapid IV bolus	Repeat as necessary	a. Narrow complex tachycardia b. In diagnosis of broad complex tachycardia	Transient flushing Dyspnoea	Asthma	Aminophylline Dipyridamole (see text)
Verapamil	5–15 mg IVI over 2–5 min	Half-life IV 3–4 h	Regular narrow complex tachycardia	Hypotension (reversible with 2.5 mmol calcium)	a. Beta-blockers b. LV dysfunction c. AF and WPW	Beta-blockers
Digoxin	0.5 mg IVI over 30 min (or oral)	See text	a. AF b. Rate control for atrial flutter	No immediate side-effects	Caution with hypokalaemia	Potentiated by amiodarone
Flecainide	2 mg kg^{-1} IVI 20–30 min (max. 150 mg)	Half-life IV 4–6 h	a. Atrial flutter b. Narrow complex tachycardia (third line)	Hypotension	a. LV dysfunction b. IHD	
Amiodarone	300 mg IVI 30 min	1.2 g IVI over 24 h	a. Resistant AF or atrial flutter (especially if LV dysfunction) b. VT	Hypotension if given too quickly	Thyroid disorders (relative contraindication)	Potentiates digoxin and warfarin
Lignocaine	50–100 mg rapid IV bolus	4 mg min^{-1} for 1 h 2 mg min^{-1} for 2 h 1 mg min^{-1} thereafter	VT	Hypotension Cerebral irritability		
Magnesium	4–12 mmol IV bolus 2–5 min	2.5 mmol h^{-1} IVI	a. VT b. Digoxin toxicity	Transient flushing with IV bolus	Caution with IVI if creatinine greater than 300 µmol l^{-1}	
Procainamide	500 mg IVI 30 min	2–6 mg min^{-1} IVI	VT	Conduction defects Hypotension	Caution in LV dysfunction	
Disopyramide	2 mg kg^{-1} IVI 5–10 min (max. 150 mg)	20–30 mg h IVI	a. VT b. AF	Conduction defects Hypotension Anticholinergic	Prostatism LV dysfunction	
Atropine	0.4–0.6 mg IV stat	Repeat as necessary	Bradycardia	VT (if too large a dose used)	Brady-tachy syndrome	
Isoprenaline	No bolus	0.5–10 µg min^{-1}	Bradycardia	VT Hypotension		Anaesthetic agents

IHD, ischaemic heart disease; IVI, intravenous infusion; WPW, Wolff–Parkinson–White syndrome. Other abbreviations, see text.

4. Connect the pacing electrodes. The pace generator should only activate if the intrinsic rate is less than that set. Check the ECG signal if there are problems with failure to detect the underlying rhythm.

5. Paced ventricular beats should be seen. If ventricular capture does not occur, increase the voltage (current) as necessary, limited by patient tolerance. Should there still be no capture despite maximum output, check connections and electrode contact, and consider resiting the electrodes. Meantime, start preparations for an alternative pacing approach.

6. If there is no underlying rhythm and/or there is haemodynamic collapse, set pacing generator to 70 beats min^{-1} in 'fixed' mode at 2–3 V output (or minimum current). Paced ventricular beats should be seen. If ventricular capture does not occur, increase the voltage (current) as necessary, limited by patient tolerance. Should there still be no capture despite maximum output, check connections and electrode contact, and consider resiting the electrodes. Meantime, start preparations for alternative pacing approach.

7. Alter rate for best haemodynamic effect.

Aftercare
This procedure is very temporary, and the patient should be monitored closely. An alternative pacing approach should be instituted as soon as possible.

Complications
Muscle twitch can be very distressing; use an intravenous benzodiazepine as a sedation agent if the use of the external pacer is unavoidable.

Transvenous ventricular pacing

This is best performed with radiographic screening, but flotation pacing wires are available which utilize the inflated balloon technology of Swan–Ganz pulmonary artery catheters. Whilst flotation wires are useful in an emergency situation, it is often difficult to site these wires in a position of electrical and mechanical stability. If possible, radiographic screening should be used in order to shorten procedure time and to maximize benefit to the patient. It is not unreasonable to site a flotation wire in the A&E department and, if necessary, later screen that same wire into a more stable position.

Indications
1. Bradycardia unresponsive to atropine.
2. History of syncope associated with proven conduction disorder.
3. Complete heart block.

Equipment
1. Aseptic technique.
2. Venous sheath 5–7F depending on pacing wire to be used (use sheath with 'side arm' and valve to minimize blood leakage from the puncture wound after the procedure, and to allow concurrent central venous access for drugs, etc.

3.
   a. Bipolar flotation pacing wire with balloon (radiographic screening not required).
      or
   b. Temporary bipolar electrode (radiographic screening required). (Utilize a sterile plastic cover for the flotation pacing wire if further manipulation is anticipated.)
4. Radiographic screening (unless using flotation wire).
5. Pacing box.
6. An assistant familiar with the pacing box is a great advantage.
7. A defibrillator.
8. Continuous ECG monitoring.

Patient preparation
1. Explanation of technique (if possible).
2. Position as for central venous cannulation.
3. Radiation protection if of child-bearing age.
4. If the ventricle is electrically irritable or there is any question of digoxin toxicity, consider prophylactic lignocaine 50 mg IV.

Procedure
1. Under aseptic conditins (whenever possible) establish central venous access and site venous sheath. In an emergency, use the route of cannulation with which you are most familiar. Otherwise, if the patient is right-handed, use a right-sided vein for the temporary wire, and the left side in a left-handed person. (A permanent pacemaker will be placed on the opposite side to the patient's dominant hand, so, if possible, avoid this site.) NB: If using a flotation wire, the procedure is easier from the jugular or subclavian approach than from the femoral vein.

   In the following steps, if manipulation of the wire causes significant ventricular ectopy or VT, stop and administer lignocaine 50–100 mg IV.

2.
   a. *Flotation wire*. Insert the flotation wire into the introducer sheath and advance 10–15 cm. Inflate the balloon and continue to advance the flotation wire up to a depth of 30–40 cm. Some transient ventricular ectopic activity is a good sign since this may indicate the tricuspid valve has been crossed. The balloon is best deflated at the end of the procedure, but, if the wire is unstable (as suggested by a varying threshold or intermittent failure to capture), consider leaving the balloon inflated.
   b. *With radiographic screening*. Check that all personnel and other patients are adequately protected. Screen the pacing wire into the right ventricular apex (see Fig. 1a and b).
3. If patient has an underlying rhythm see instruction 4. If the situation is haemodynamically very serious or if there is no underlying rhythm, see instruction 8.
4. Set pacing box to 2–3 V output at a low rate (30 beats min^{-1} or lower if possible) in 'demand' mode and connect the pacing electrodes (ideally the proximal limb

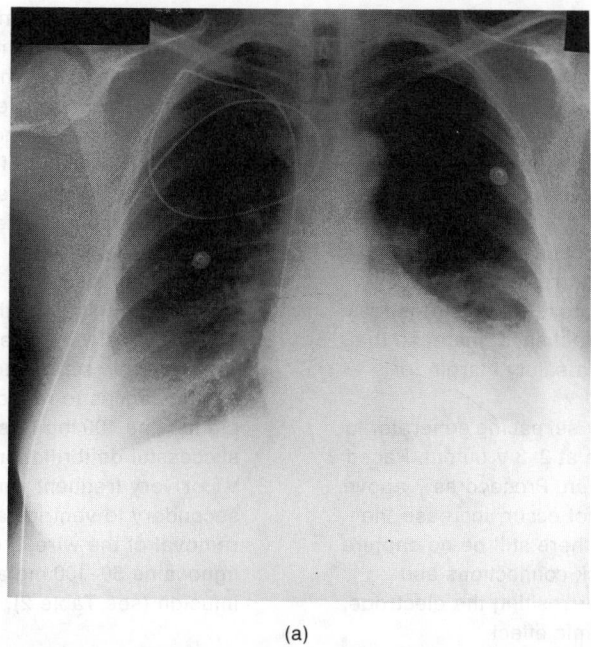

(a)

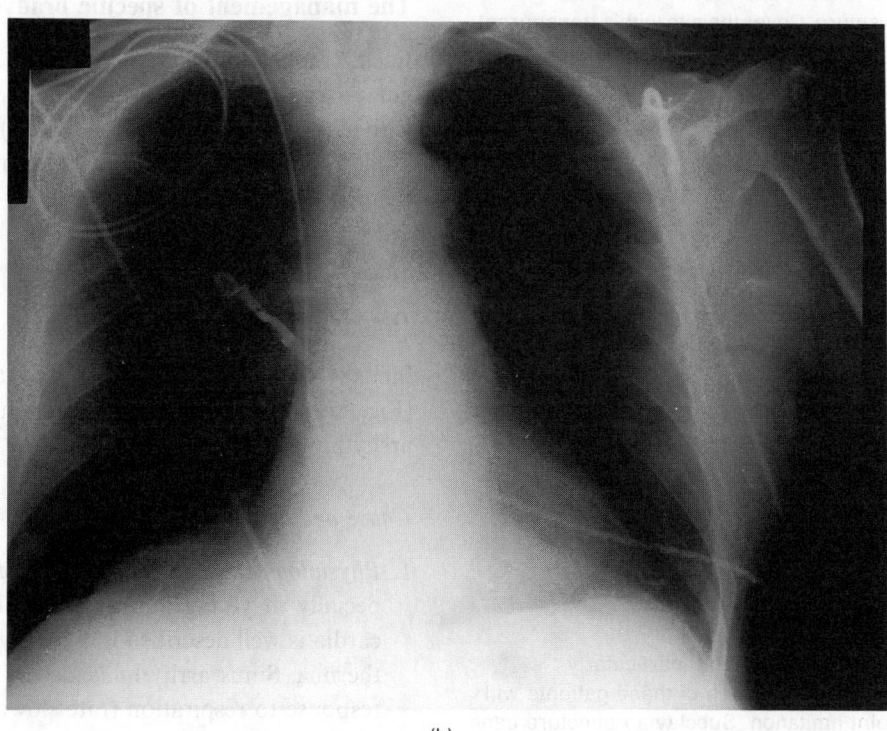

(b)

Fig. 1. (a) Chest radiograph indicating the correct positioning of a temporary ventricular pacing wire. (b) Chest radiograph. The temporary pacing wire is placed insufficiently deeply into the right ventricular cavity. There is an inadequate 'loop' of wire in the right atrium; this can lead to an increased risk of wire displacement.

should be positive (red) electrode). The pace generator should now detect (sense) the patient's own ventricular beat. (If the patient's own rhythm is very disorganized, or if speed is required, set the box to 70–90 beats min^{-1} and skip to instruction 6.)

5. If sensing is absent, turn the pacing box off and adjust the position of the wire. If a satisfactory position cannot be obtained, consider radiographic screening if using a flotation wire. A stiffer wire is sometimes helpful. If the situation deteriorates, see intruction 8 below.

Once sensing is established increase the pacing rate to 70 beats min^{-1} (or a rate greater than the patient's intrinsic rate).

6. Paced ventricular beats should be seen. If ventricular capture does not occur, increase the voltage by 1 V increments as necessary. Should there still be no capture despite 4–5 V output, check connections and consider resiting the wire.

7. Reduce the output of the pace generator until the level at which further reduction would result in loss of capture. The ideal minimum output (threshold) is less than 1 V. Once threshold is established, increase the output by at least 1 V to allow a safety margin for electrode movement.

8. If there is no underlying rhythm, set pacing generator to 70 beats min^{-1} in 'fixed' mode at 2–3 V output. Paced ventricular beats should be seen. Proceed as 7 above.

   If ventricular capture does not occur, increase the voltage as necessary. Should there still be no capture despite maximum output, check connections and electrode contact, and consider resiting the electrode.

9. Alter rate for best haemodynamic effect.

10. Fix the introducer sheath and the wire separately with non-dissolvable suture. Cover the site with a transparent adhesive dressing. Then loop the externalized pacing wire at least twice and fix over the first dressing with a second transparent dressing.

11. Perform a chest X-ray to exclude a pneumothorax and to establish position of the pacing wire.

Aftercare

1. The chest X-ray should be reviewed; this is the responsibility of the operator.
2. Patient movement should be limited, e.g. patient transfer should be passive.
3. Some operators advocate 48 h broad-spectrum antibiotics. This is an empirical practice.
4. The patient should be monitored by staff familiar with transvenous pacing. The wire threshold should be checked after transfer from the A&E department (daily thereafter) and the voltage safety margin adjusted accordingly.

Complications

1. As for central venous cannulation – particularly pneumothorax. A large proportion of these patients will be elderly with joint limitation. Subclavian puncture can be very difficult. If a pneumothorax would be disastrous, consider the femoral or brachial approach.
2. Tamponade (may occur late). Modern pacing wires are relatively flexible and 'soft', so this is rarely a problem. Beware the stiffer wires in patients with enlarged atria, and in patients with dilated cardiomyopathy (the right ventricle can be very thin-walled). If tamponade is suspected, gently remove the wire (if rhythm allows) and observe the patient; such an event is often self-limiting in this circumstance. If there is associated haemodynamic collapse, assess the central venous

pressure (via the pacing sheath) and perform pericardiocentesis if indicated (see Chapter 23).

3. Pleuritic chest pain. This may occur if the wire has perforated the ventricle. Obtain a chest X-ray and consider removal of the wire.

4. Hiccups or twitching of the thoracic wall. This is a result of concurrent diaphragmatic pacing and is usually overcome by reducing the output voltage. The pacing wire should be resited if the problem persists. Hiccups can also be a feature of perforation.

5. VF may be induced either by pacing in fixed mode, or occasionally as a result of wire manipulation. Radiographic screening is very helpful in these circumstances to reduce wire manipulation time. Lignocaine 100 mg IV should be administered after successful defibrillation.

6. VT or very frequent ventricular ectopy may be induced secondary to ventricular irritation by the wire. If removal of the wire is clinically undesirable, administer lignocaine 50–100 mg and consider a lignocaine infusion (see Table 2).

The management of specific bradycardias

Each bradyarrhythmia is described and illustrated. A guide is given as to its cause and association, together with a brief description of its mode(s) of presentation. A suggested management plan is given, with reference to the procedures described above.

Sinus bradycardia

Description

Sinus rhythm with a rate less than 60 beats min^{-1} (Fig. 2a). This may be intermittent and manifest as sinus arrhythmia (Fig. 2b).

Cause and associations

1. *Physiological.* A resting bradycardia is common, especially in young adults and athletes. Sinus bradycardia is well described in hypothyroidism and hypothermia. Sinus arrhythmia occurs as a physiological response to respiration (rate slowing on expiration).
2. *Pharmacological.* Beta-blocker therapy and some calcium antagonists.
3. *Pathological.* In association with sick sinus syndrome (see below).

Symptoms

Sinus bradycardia is usually asymptomatic but may be associated with dyspnoea on exertion. Dizziness, palpitations and syncope occur with sick sinus syndrome.

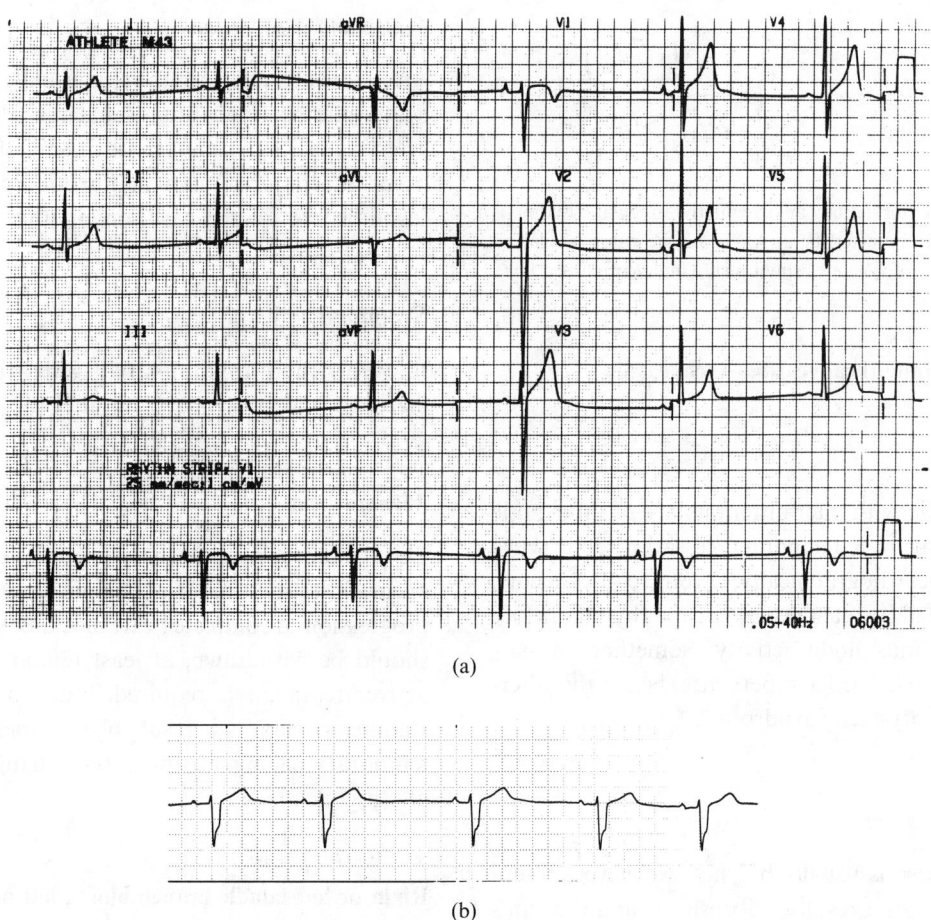

(a)

(b)

Fig. 2. (a) Sinus bradycardia in an athlete's heart (note also the typical high take-off of the ST segments in the anterior chest leads). (b) Sinus arrhythmia.

Management

Specific treatment is not usually required, but atropine may be used short-term whilst attention is directed to the underlying cause. If sinus bradycardia is thought to be drug-induced, consider reducing such therapy (but beware of sudden cessation or beta-blocker therapy in patients with myocardial ischaemia).

Atrial fibrillation with a slow ventricular response

Description

Irregularly, irregular ventricular rhythm with fibrillation waves, often only evidenced by an unstable baseline (Fig. 3). Distinguish AF with complete heart block (CHB) in which the ventricular rate is *regular*.

Cause and associations

Slow AF is usually related to digoxin therapy, but may arise *de novo*, particularly in the elderly.

Symptoms

Often asymptomatic, but may present with dizziness or syncope if the ventricular rate is very slow.

Management

Digoxin should be stopped in the first instance, but the ventricular rate often remains slow, necessitating permanent pacemaker insertion long-term. Emergency temporary pacing is sometimes required.

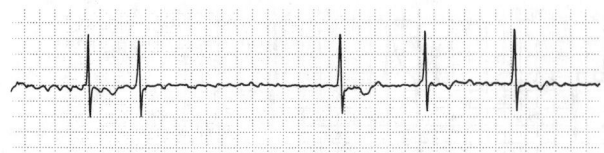

Fig. 3. 'Slow' atrial fibrillation: an irregularly irregular rhythm is seen with a baseline characteristic of AF (a 2.8-sec pause is evident, which, with a history of syncope, would justify intervention; see text).

Sick sinus syndrome (bradycardia–tachycardia syndrome)

Description

Sinus bradycardia with intermittent failure of sinus node function resulting in a temporary cessation of P wave activity. Electrocardiographically, a long pause occurs, usually interrupted by a temporary escape rhythm, before resumption of sinus node activity. Sometimes a paroxysmal atrial tachycardia supervenes, hence the alternative name 'brady-tachy syndrome'.

Cause and associations

Sinus node disease is usually but not exclusively found in the elderly and is a result of fibrosis around the sinus node often associated with more widespread conduction disease.

Management

Any contributory drug medication should be stopped (e.g. beta-blockers, digoxin, etc.) and the patient observed. Should syncope associated with sinus arrest be witnessed, a temporary pacing wire should be sited. Otherwise, a more leisurely decision regarding physiological permanent pacing may be made, in the light of 24 h Holter monitoring and exercise testing. In the event of haemodynamic instability and/or significant delay to the placement of a transvenous electrode, consider external cardiac pacing (if available), atropine (0.4–0.6 mg IV) or an isoprenaline infusion (see Table 2).

Idioventricular rhythm

Description

Narrow complex bradycardia, rate 40–60 beats min^{-1}. P waves are not visible.

Cause and associations

An idioventricular rhythm is usually associated with acute inferior myocardial ischaemia (the right coronary artery supplies the sinus node in 85% of patients). It may occur in conjunction with fibrotic conduction disease secondary to dilated cardiomyopathy.

Symptoms

Idioventricular rhythm rarely gives rise to symptoms; dizziness and presyncope occur if the rate is very slow.

Management

ECG monitoring is essential if idioventricular rhythm occurs in the setting of ischaemia since there is a risk of progression to complete heart block. Beta-blocker therapy should be withdrawn, at least temporarily. Usually no active treatment is required, but if haemodynamic instability occurs as a result of the bradycardia consider temporary pacing; atropine (0.4–0.6 mg IV) is occasionally useful.

Right or left bundle branch block, left anterior hemiblock

Bundle branch block is asymptomatic, and no action is necessary. However, monitoring is advisable if the bundle branch block is a new event. Should it occur or progress in the setting of acute ischaemia (particularly anterior myocardial infarction (MI)), there is a risk of CHB and subsequent circulatory collapse. In this situation, prophylactic siting of a transvenous pacing wire is generally considered judicious (Fig. 4).

First degree heart block

Description

A P wave precedes *each* QRS complex, but the PR interval is prolonged (Fig. 4).

Cause and associations

Idiopathic fibrosis, chronic ischaemic heart disease, acute myocardial ischaemia (particularly inferior MI) and aortic valve disease (local fibrosis and scarring, aortic root abscess) are among the commoner causes of first degree heart block.

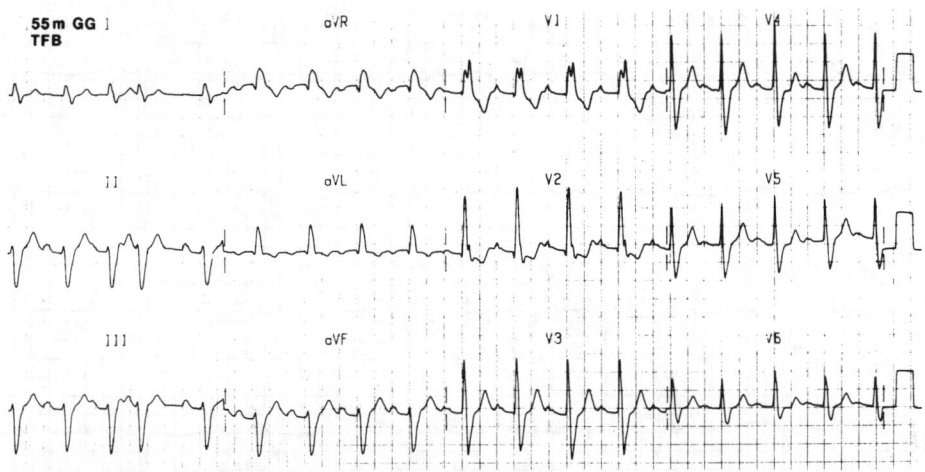

Fig. 4. First degree heart block. There is a P wave associated with each complex but the PR interval is greater than 0.2 sec. (Right bundle branch block and left anterior hemiblock are also apparent in this electrocardiogram.)

Symptoms

None.

Management

No treatment is required, unless associated with acute ischaemia, in which case careful monitoring for progression of the conduction disorder is mandatory. However, if first degree heart block is a feature of aortic valve endocarditis, there is a high risk of sudden complete heart block and temporary pacing is mandatory.

Second degree heart block: Mobitz type 1 (Wenkebach)

Description

A P wave precedes each QRS with the occasional 'missed QRS'. The PR interval is seen to gradually lengthen with successive beats as a result of increasing conduction time in the AV (atrioventricular) node. This continues until the P wave occurs before the previous atrial impulse has reached the ventricle, resulting in a 'missed' or 'dropped' QRS. The subsequent PR interval is once again normal, and the cycle repeats itself (Fig. 5).

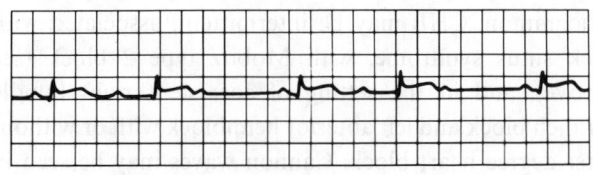

Fig. 5. Wenkebach (second degree heart block: Mobitz type 1).

Cause and association

Wenkebach is commonly associated with a high vagal tone (e.g. during sleep); in this instance the arrhythmia is benign. In the absence of high vagal tone, progression to CHB is recognized. Wenkebach is also associated with inferior MI.

Symptoms

These are usually limited to occasional complaints of a missed beat, or thumping heart.

Management

Wenkebach is nearly always a benign condition and no treatment is required. ECG monitoring is recommended if the arrhythmia occurs in the setting of acute infarction.

Second degree heart block: Mobitz type 2

Description

Regular intermittent failure of conduction of P waves without antecedent increase in the PR interval, usually two P waves for each QRS (Fig. 6).

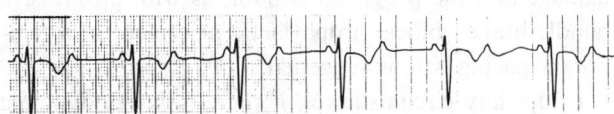

Fig. 6. Second degree heart block (Mobitz type 2). There two P waves for each QRS complex (the second P wave is occurring just after the T wave).

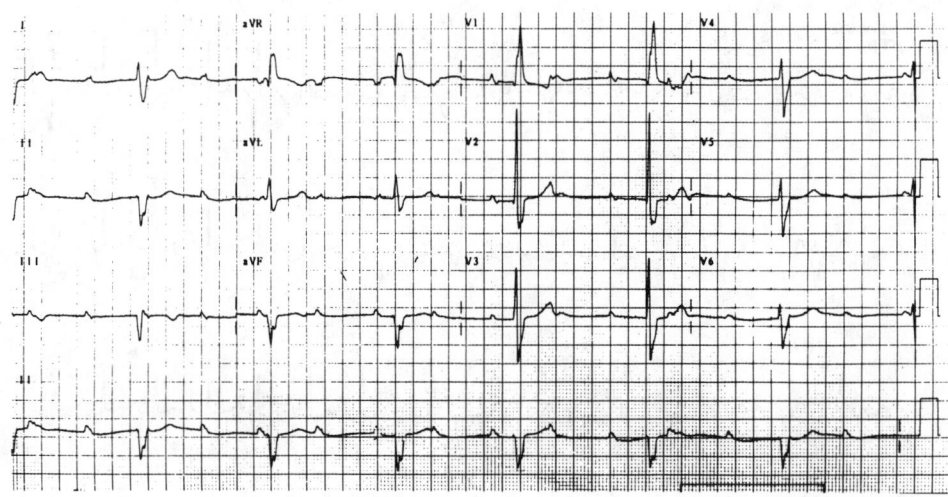

Fig. 7. Complete heart block. There is no relationship between the number or frequency of P waves and QRS complexes (sometimes called AV dissociation).

Cause and associations

Acute and chronic ischaemia; fibrosis.

Symptoms

If the ventricular rate is very slow, then dizziness and syncope can result, particularly on exertion. There is a significant association with sick sinus syndrome (see above); there may be intermittent CHB, resulting in syncope. Associated with acute ischaemia, there is a risk of progression to CHB.

Management

A history of presyncope or syncope in the setting of Mobitz type 2 block should result in further investigation with Holter ECG monitoring and is a strong indication for permanent pacing. However, if associated with recent acute inferior MI, the arrhythmia will resolve spontaneously in approximately 65% of cases and careful haemodynamic and electrocardiographic monitoring are all that is required. If associated with anterior infarction, however, this is suggestive of extensive myocardial damage and the prognosis is poor; as with progressive bundle branch block, prophylactic placement of a temporary pacing wire is suggested.

Under any circumstances, if there is haemodynamic compromise, atropine (0.4–0.6 mg), external pacing (if available), or cautious use of isoprenaline may be helpful pending temporary pacing.

Complete heart block (third degree heart block)

Description

P wave and QRS activity are dissociated with a slow ventricular rate (20–50 beats min^{-1}). This may occur in the setting of AF, in which case, typical fibrillation waves are seen, but with a *regular* ventricular response. QRS complexes may be narrow or wide (Fig. 7).

Cause and associations

The commonest cause of CHB is fibrosis, but it can occur with acute MI, particularly acute inferior MI (in which case it is often transient). Occasionally, CHB can be congenital (associated with maternal systemic lupus erythematosus), or develop as a consequence of dystrophia myotonica. Hypothyroidism and hypothermia may also be complicated by CHB.

Symptoms

CHB may be asymptomatic, or patients may complain of gradually 'slowing up'. Classical Stokes–Adams attacks (i.e. sudden syncope occurring without warning, with rapid recovery) may occur and head injury is not uncommon. CHB may be intermittent, associated with sick sinus syndrome, with Mobitz type 2 block (see above), and in the setting of coexistent right bundle branch block and left anterior hemiblock with or without first degree heart block. Cannon waves may be seen in the neck veins.

Management

In the absence of acute ischaemia:

1. If asymptomatic, and with a narrow complex ventricular response, timely referral for permanent pacing is all that is required.
2. A history of syncope, and/or a broad complex ventricular response, suggesting a high risk of complete conduction failure, are strong indications for temporary ventricular pacing pending implantation of a permanent system.

As with Mobitz type 2 block, CHB in the setting of acute ischaemia may resolve spontaneously, and temporary pacing is only required if there is circulatory embarrassment, or if CHB is associated with acute anterior MI.

Under any circumstances, if there is haemodynamic compromise, atropine (0.4–0.6 mg), external pacing (if available), or cautious use of isoprenaline may be helpful pending temporary pacing.

Electromechanical dissociation

Description

Organized electrical activity with no evidence of cardiac output.

Cause and associations

Electromechanical dissociation (EMD) may be primary or secondary. Primary EMD is due to severe myocardial ischaemia with cessation of effective cardiac output. EMD is considered to be secondary when the underlying cause of loss of cardiac output is extramyocardial (e.g. hypovolaemia, cardiac tamponade, tension pneumothorax, hypoxaemia, acidosis or pulmonary embolus).

Symptoms

Circulatory collapse is universal, with rapid degeneration of the observed electrical rhythm into VF or asystole.

Management

Cardiopulmonary resuscitation (CPR) should be started (see Chapter 3). Adrenaline 1:10 000 (5–10 ml repeated as necessary) should be administered intravenously or via the endotracheal tube (double the dose); consider bicarbonate (50 ml of 8.4% sodium bicarbonate). Strenuous attempts to identify and treat causes of secondary EMD are indicated. Successful resuscitation is unfortunately rare (less than 10% in most series; Charlap et al., 1989).

Agonal rhythm

Description

Wide complex bradycardia, often irregular, with poor cardiac output.

Cause and associations

Ischaemia and acidosis are the usual associated features of this condition. However, hyperkalaemia is a specific and remediable cause recognized by 'sine wave' ventricular complexes, which have progressed from rapidly widening QRS complexes. Hyperkalaemia in this situation is usually a result of renal impairment, either parenchymal renal disease or of prerenal origin (eg. end-stage cardiac failure).

Symptoms

Circulatory collapse is usually established, except in those patients with hyperkalaemia in whom collapse is imminent.

Management (see Fig. 8)

Adrenaline 1:10 000 (5–10 ml repeated as necessary) and atropine (0.6–1.0 mg repeated as necessary) may be helpful. Temporary pacing is often attempted but is rarely effective, unless underlying pathology is rapidly corrected. If hyperkalaemia is suspected, consider calcium chloride (5 mmol) or calcium gluconate (2.5 mmol = 10 ml of 10% solution) and/or dextrose and insulin (50 ml of 50% dextrose with 10 units of soluble insulin stat IV).

Asystole

Description

Complete absence of electrical activity. (NB: Exclude lead displacement and consider 'fine' VF.)

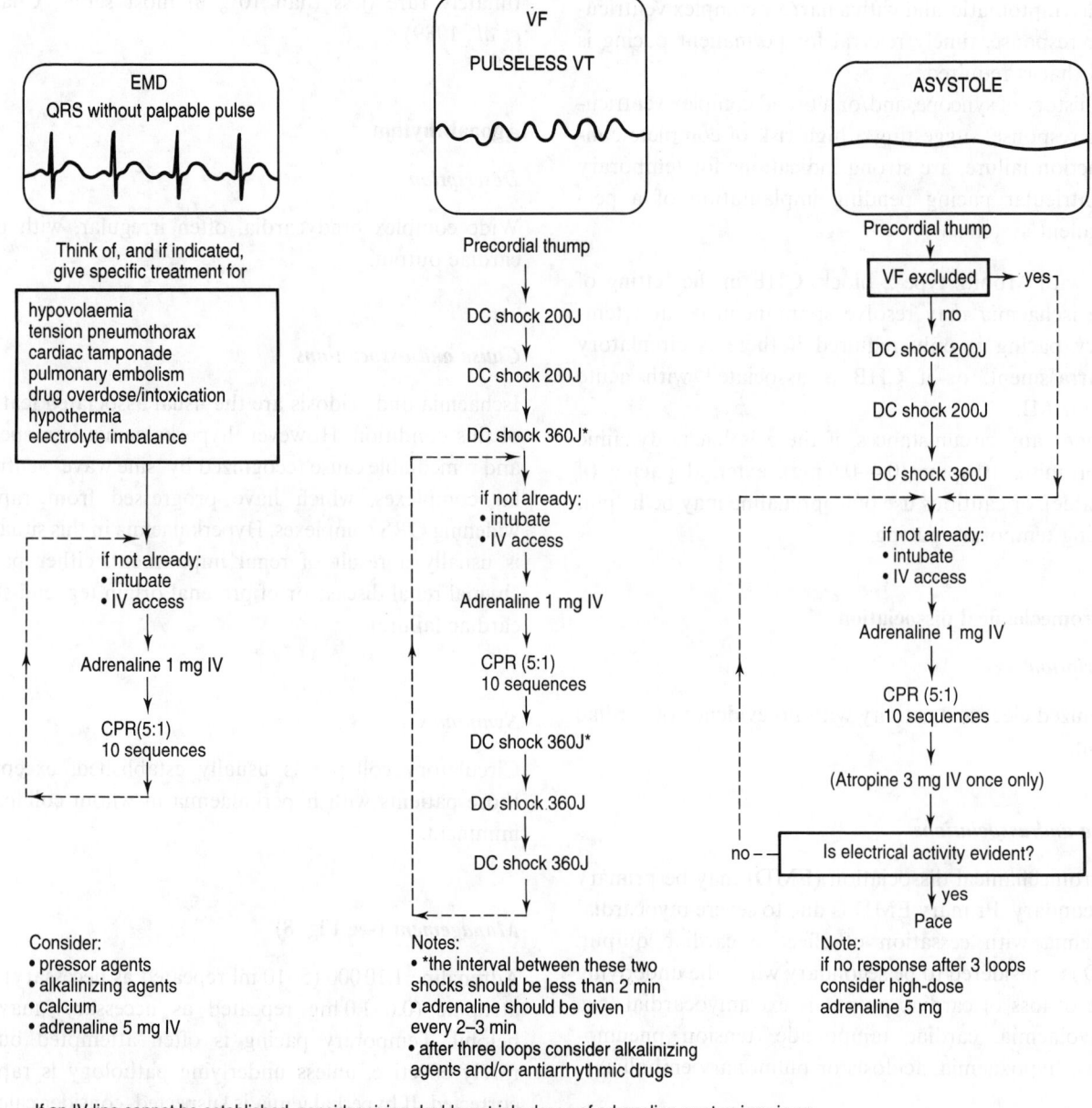

Fig. .8. Guidelines of the European Resuscitation Council (1992). EMD, electromechanical dissociation; CPR, cardiopulmonary resuscitation; VF, ventricular fibrillation; VT, ventricular tachycardia.

Cause and associations

Asystole is usually an end-stage event but may be mimicked by ventricular standstill (P wave activity without QRS complexes) or by very fine VF. Asystole can occur as a result of hyperkalaemia, acidosis, digoxin toxicity or pacemaker failure.

Symptoms

Circulatory collapse.

Management (see Fig. 8)

In the absence of evidence to the contrary, assume that there is very fine VF and administer DC shock (200–400 J). Start CPR and administer adrenaline (1:10 000, 10 ml) repeated as necessary and atropine (3 mg). Temporary pacing (external or transvenous) is occasionally useful and is mandatory in the case of ventricular standstill. Consider bicarbonate (50 ml of 8.4% sodium bicarbonate) if circulatory arrest is prolonged. Treat the underlying cause, if possible.

TACHYCARDIA

There are a wide variety of tachyarrhythmias which, at first sight, may appear bewildering to even the most experienced observer. However, immediate diagnosis and management may be conveniently considered by the division of such tachycardias into 'broad complex tachycardia' (QRS duration more than 120 msec) and 'narrow complex tachycardia' (QRS <120 msec).

A practical guide to the management of broad and narrow complex tachyarrhythmias is given in Figs 8–10. Fig. 8 is a modified version of the European Resuscitation Council recommendations and incorporates the management of VF (covered in more detail in Chapter 3). Fig. 9 outlines the procedure to be followed in broad complex tachycardia; further information about the management of VT is given below. Fig. 10 refers to the management of narrow complex tachycardia, and should be used in conjunction with the notes given below.

General points

1. Whatever the tachycardia, if there is haemodynamic compromise, direct current cardioversion (DCV) is the treatment of choice.
2. Nearly all tachycardias are exacerbated by high sympathetic tone (pain, hypoxia, acidosis) and by electrolyte imbalance (particularly hypokalaemia and hypomagnesaemia). Strenuous attempts to correct and/or avoid such features are advised.
3. Obtain a 12-lead ECG whenever possible before treatment (unless there is haemodynamic instability, in which case DCV is the correct treatment whatever the cause of the arrhythmia), and run a 3-lead ECG during any therapeutic intervention. If this is not possible, use a single rhythm strip to monitor lead II or lead V_2 (P waves are generally at their most visible in these leads).
4. A broad complex tachycardia should be considered to be of ventricular origin until proven otherwise.
5. Intravenous verapamil is absolutely contraindicated if the patient is concurrently receiving oral beta-blocker therapy (asystole is reported).
6. Nothing should be assumed – act on the information to hand. For example, the presenting tachycardia may be different from that seen previously.
7. All antiarrhythmic drugs have the potential to be proarrhythmic.

Drugs used in the diagnosis and management of tachycardia

A full list of drugs, doses, indications and side-effects is given in Table 2. Again, the use of each drug is considered in further detail during discussion of individual arrhythmias. Adenosine is relatively new to the field of tachycardia, but its short half-life and therapeutic efficacy will ensure a large increase in its use (Linker, 1992); this drug is therefore considered in more detail below.

Use of adenosine

Adenosine is a naturally occuring purine nucleoside that is capable of causing rapidly reversible AV nodal block. It is approved for the termination of narrow complex tachycardia in both the USA and the UK. It is additionally licensed as a diagnostic agent in broad complex tachycardia in the UK.

Adenosine has a very short half-life (less than 2 sec); any unwanted side-effects are of very short duration and increasing doses can be administered in rapid succession.

Indications

For the termination or further investigation of regular narrow complex tachycardia, and as a diagnostic agent

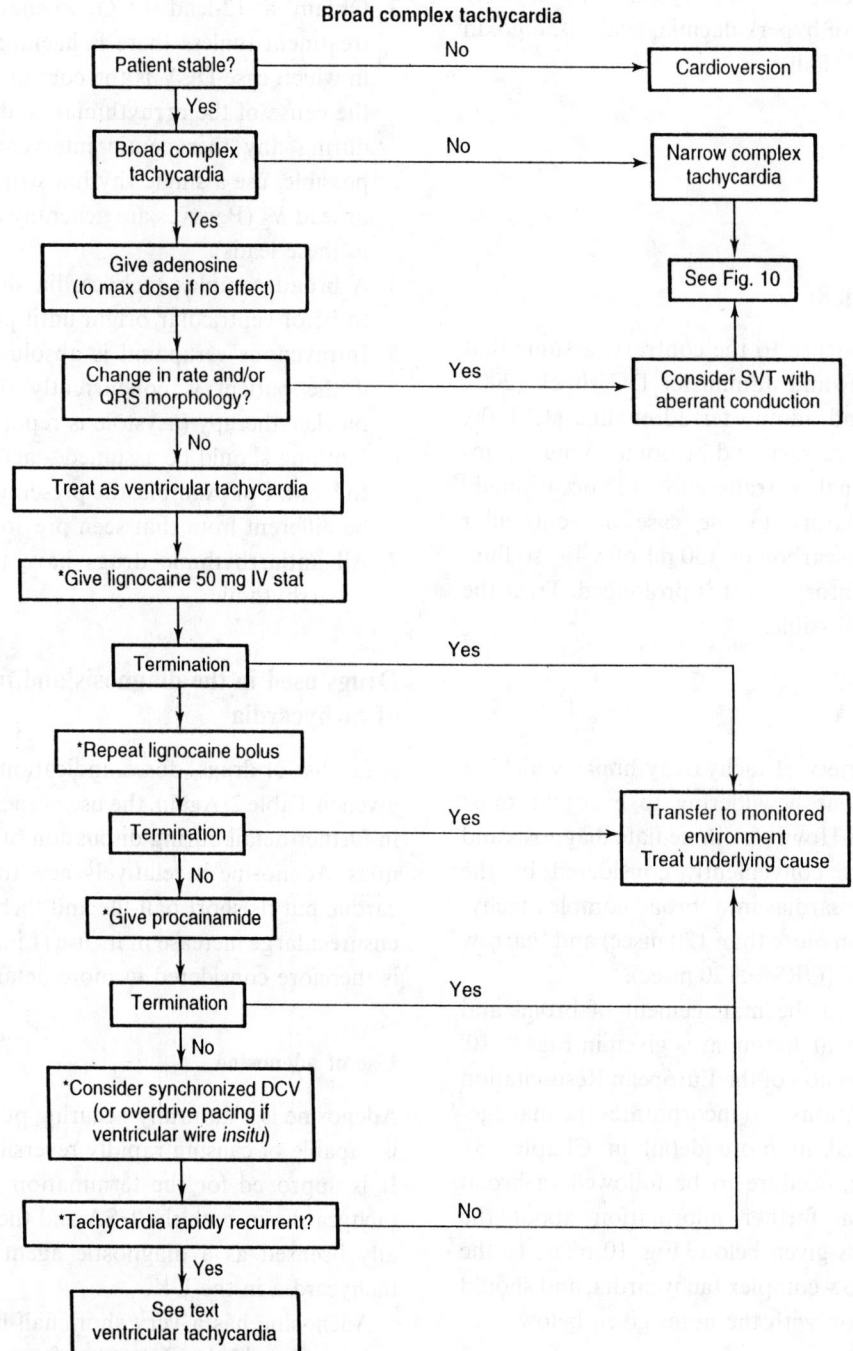

Broad complex tachycardia

* if heamodynamic instability develops, proceed to immediate cardioversion

Fig. 9. Management of broad complex tachycardia. SVT, supraventricular tachycardia; DCV, direct current cardioversion.

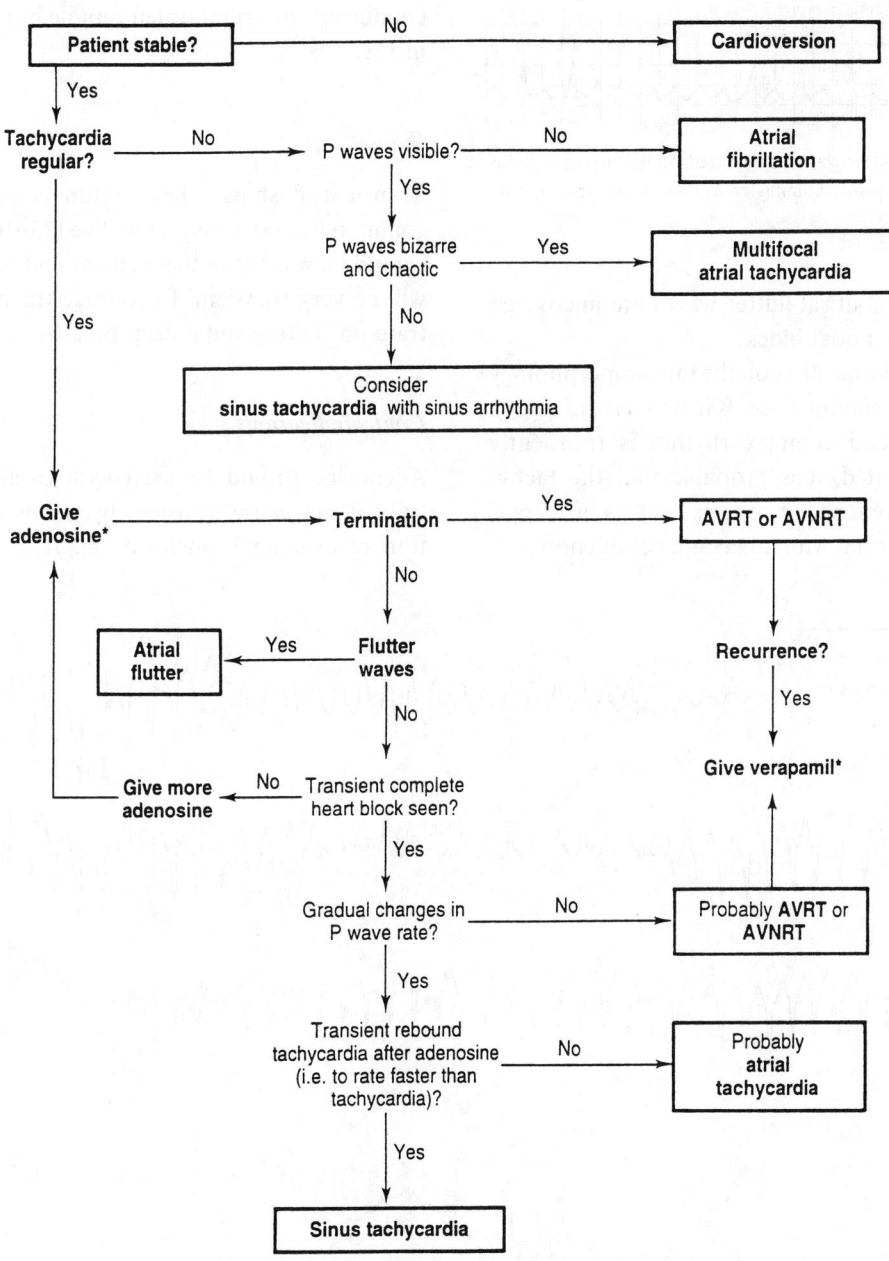

* please see text for dose and contraindications

Fig. 10. Management of narrow complex tachycardia.

in broad complex tachycardia (in the diagnosis of supraventricular tachycardia with aberrant conduction). There is no role for adenosine in AF (Garratt *et al.*, 1992).

Method

Adenosine should be given rapidly into a large peripheral vein, followed immediately by a saline flush (Camm & Garratt, 1991). A low dose is administered initially, with repeated boluses of increasing dose at 1–2 min intervals until AV nodal blockade is seen. The starting dose is 3 mg in adults increasing to 6 mg and then 12 mg. If there is still no effect, higher doses up to 18 mg may be used ($0.05 \, \text{mg} \, \text{kg}^{-1}$ in children increased by $0.05 \, \text{mg} \, \text{kg}^{-1}$ increments to a total dose of $0.25 \, \text{mg} \, \text{kg}^{-1}$). AV nodal blockade may be recognized by a gradual or abrupt prolongation of the PR interval with transient complete heart block. The use of adenosine in the differential diagnosis of narrow complex tachycardia is seen in

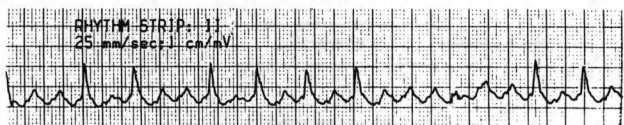

Fig. 11. Typical atrial flutter waves: uncovered transiently by a bolus dose of intravenous adenosine administered 5 sec before this rhythm strip was recorded.

Fig. 11, where typical atrial flutter waves are uncovered during transient AV nodal block.

Adenosine will have no effect on the rate or morphology of VT, even at maximum dose (Griffith *et al.*, 1988). If the observed broad complex rhythm is transiently modified or terminated, it is probable that the tachycardia is not of ventricular origin, but is a supraventricular tachycardia with aberrant conduction (i.e.

conducted with right or left bundle branch block) as seen in Fig. 12a.

Side-effects

Transient flushing, chest tightness and dyspnoea are common but extremely short-lived (5–10 sec). The patient should be warned of these effects and reassured that they will be very transient. Encourage the patient to concentrate on 'taking some deep breaths'.

Contraindications

Adenosine should be used with caution in asthmatics since it can cause transient bronchospasm or exacerbation of existing bronchospasm. If in doubt in narrow

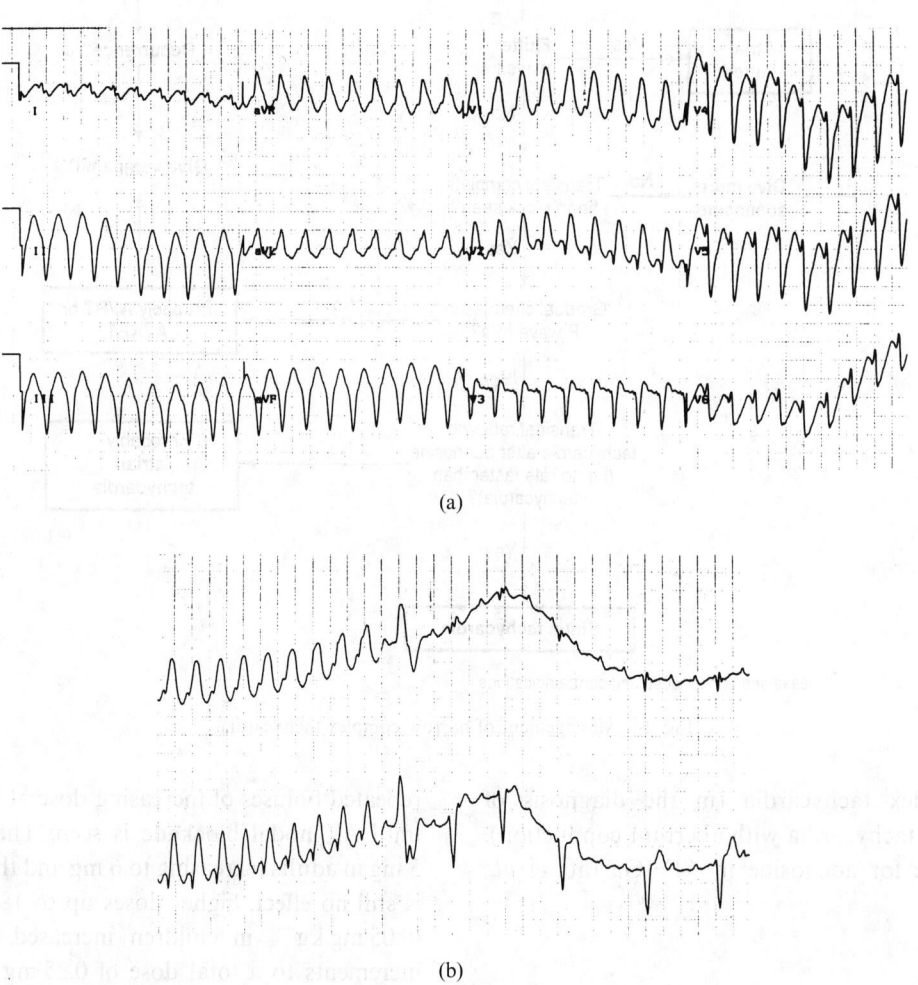

(a)

(b)

Fig. 12. (a) Broad complex tachycardia. Assumed to be ventricular tachycardia, but the P wave activity is very regular, there are no fusion beats and QRS complex morphology is very uniform (cf. Fig. 13a). As per protocol, adenosine was administered (b). (b) Administration of adenosine confirms the clinical impression of atrial flutter with 1:1 (aberrant) conduction. The patient was taking flecainide which slows the rate of atrial flutter facilitating 1:1 conduction. Synchronized DCV resulted in sinus rhythm.

complex tachycardia use verapamil instead. (NB: Never use verapamil for a broad complex tachycardia.)

Drug interactions

Aminophylline is an adenosine antagonist and thus the effect of adenosine is muted. Dipyridamole accentuates and prolongs the effects of adenosine, and adenosine should be used with caution in this circumstance; verapamil may be a safer alternative.

Cautions

Adenosine will also slow sinus node rate to a variable degree, and thus the observation of rate slowing during adenosine administration does not itself suggest a diagnosis of pathological tachycardia. The same rate change will be noted in sinus tachycardia; in this circumstance a reflex tachycardia follows any bolus of adenosine, before the rate settles to pre-adenosine level (see sinus tachycardia).

Efficacy as compared with verapamil for narrow complex tachycardia

There is very little to choose between the two during direct comparison (Garratt et al., 1989). However, adenosine may be given in conjunction with beta-blockers (verapamil is contraindicated). Adenosine is simple and safe, and its short half-life makes it a safer drug to use in inexperienced hands.

TECHNIQUES

Non-pharmacological techniques used in the diagnosis and management of tachycardia

Vagal manoeuvres

These techniques are designed to increase refractoriness of the AV node with vagal efferent stimulation; i.e. to transiently increase vagal tone at the AV node so making the node more sluggish in its ability to conduct an impulse from atria to ventricle. By this technique, any narrow complex tachycardia (often called supraventricular tachycardia) that incorporates the AV node will be modified by this action and many will actually terminate as a direct consequence of a vagal manoeuvre (Mehta et al., 1988).

Indication
1. The assessment and management of narrow complex tachycardia.

Equipment
1. Sphygmomanometer cuff.
2. Ice cold water.
3. Towel.

Patient preparation
1. Explain each procedure carefully.
2. The patient should be monitored if possible, although this is not mandatory.

Methods
1. *Valsalva manoeuvre*. The patient (in a sitting or lying position) is asked to take a deep breath and then to 'bear down' whilst holding the breath for as long as possible. Helpful associations are 'as if you have been constipated for a month' or (for ladies) 'like labour or childbirth'. Should there be a problem, ask the patient to blow into a sphygmomanometer (via the connection normally reserved for the cuff) and maintain the pressure for as long as they can. The Valsalva reflex is by far the most successful of all vagal manoeuvres (approximately 50% of patients, particularly if they are young).
2. *Carotid sinus massage (CSM)*. With the patient supine and the head slightly extended, listen for a carotid bruit on both sides. Presence of a bruit is a contraindication to carotid sinus massage on that side. The most superior point of the artery on either side is identified, and firm pressure applied in a small circular motion. CSM is generally more effective on the right side (15%) than on the left (5%). Simultaneous bilateral CSM is dangerous and should never be performed (asystole reported).
3. *Diving reflex*. Classically the face is submerged in cold water. However, a more practical alternative employs a towel soaked in ice-cold water and applied over the face. This is successful in about 15% of cases.
4. *Intravenous adenosine* (see above). This is conveniently considered as 'very effective carotid sinus massage in a vial' and is successful in over 90% of cases.

Direct current cardioversion

This procedure is the mainstay of treatment for any haemodynamically unstable patient with a tachyarrhythmia (Clark & Cotter, 1991).

Indications
1. Haemodynamic instability and tachyarrhythmia (narrow complex or wide complex).
2. Tachycardia unresponsive to other measures, particularly VT.
3. AF associated with Wolff–Parkinson–White syndrome.
4. VF.

Equipment
1. Defibrillator with a facility for R wave synchronization (not for VF).

2. Electrode patches or jelly (patches are preferable – lower incidence of electrical short-circuiting and burns).
3. Facilities for emergency pacing (external or transvenous).
4. Continuous ECG monitoring.
5. Anaesthetic expertise and suitable sedation (unless an emergency, see below).
6. Facility for immediate CPR.
7. Suction facilities.
8. Dry environment.

Patient preparation

1. If the procedure is to be performed electively, informed consent should be sought and the patient fasted and prepared as for general anaesthesia.
2. Risks of cardioversion include:
   a. Small risk of therapy being ineffective.
   b. Superficial burns to paddle areas.
   c. Some chest discomfort for a day or two.

Procedure
DCV for VF

1. Assume that any cardiac arrest is due to VF (unless there is good evidence otherwise), and defibrillate.
2. It is not essential to have an ECG diagnosis, although it is helpful.
3. ECG monitoring should be instituted as soon as possible, but not so as to delay initial cardioversion.
4. Follow the sequence given in Fig. 8, but check for a pulse between shocks.

Emergency synchronized DCV (i.e. excluding VF)

1. Lie the patient flat if possible. Clear and maintain the airway and supply high-flow oxygen by mask. Remove any nitrate patches (explosion may occur).
2. If cardiac output is minimal, commence CPR.
3. Summon the cardiac arrest team.
4. Establish venous access.
5. See instruction 7 below.

Elective DCV (synchronous, by definition)

1. Check serum potassium and replete prior to the procedure if necessary. Ideally serum potassium should be greater than 4 mmol l^{-1}.
2. Obtain a quality 12-lead ECG.
3. Establish peripheral venous access.
4. Preoxygenate and anaesthetize the patient according to prevailing practice. Propofol is increasingly used as the agent of choice in this situation.
5. Transfer ECG monitoring to defibrillator (either directly or via an accessory lead from the original monitor). Ensure good ECG signal.
6. Synchronize the ECG signal with the defibrillator generator (usually performed by pressing the 'sync' button on the defibrillator). Most models will indicate R wave sensing (synchronization) with high-intensity bars overlying the R wave on the monitor screen, audibly by

bleeping each time an R wave is sensed, or by flashing of the 'sync' button with each R wave sensed. In this mode, the defibrillator will only discharge at the time of R wave sensing, thus avoiding the delivery of a shock on the T wave and precipitation of VF. If the R wave amplitude is variable – poor contact, AF, electrical alternans – there may be intermittent loss of R wave sensing; this is not a problem providing at least some R waves are correctly sensed.

   NB: This is useless in VF since there are no R waves to be sensed. (Inadvertent activation of the synchronization facility is a cause of apparent equipment failure during attempted resuscitation from VF.)

7. Meantime apply electrode patches/jelly to chest wall. The current must pass along the long axis of the heart and the paddle position may have to be altered in cases of anatomical abnormality (severe scoliosis, pectus excavatum, right pneumonectomy). Classically one paddle should be over the base of the heart with the second paddle over the apex of the heart.
8. Charge the defibrillator to the required energy 50–400 J in adults, 2–4 J kg^{-1} in children), starting with a low current unless the arrhythmia is known to be resistant. Caution should be taken in cardioversion in the presence of digoxin (start at 5–10 J; see section on drug overdose).
9. When the defibrillator has charged and the paddles are in position (marked 'apex' or 'sternum'), the operator should check once again that synchronization is adequate, ensure that no other person is in contact with the patient, and indicate to all that the defibrillator is about to be activated.
10. Activate the defibrillator from the paddles or the machine.
    MAINTAIN ELECTRICAL CONTACT. The defibrillator may not fire immediately since it will await a sensed R wave; this may take several seconds. Once fired, remove the paddles, continue oxygenation and review the rhythm.
11. If sinus rhythm has not been restored and there is haemodynamic collapse, continue cardiac massage while the machine is charged up to a higher energy for another attempt. Otherwise, allow a minute or two to elapse before administering a second shock. Further shocks should be administered as necessary.

    NB:
    a. If AF proves refractory, atropinization (0.6 mg IV) is sometimes helpful just prior to a cardioversion attempt.
    b. Front-to-back cardioversion may be tried if maximum energy sternum–apex cardioversion is not successful (not recommended for VT). The patient is turned onto the right side and the paddles placed directly over the heart anteriorly (sternal paddle) and posteriorly (apical paddle).
12. If cardioversion has not been successful despite all these manoeuvres, the attempt should be abandoned,

pending the administration of specific antiarrhythmic agents or pacing techniques.

13. At some stage, if there was no time to administer a formal anaesthetic, give a benzodiazepine for its amnesic effects (diazepam 5–10 mg is the most cardiostable).

14. If sinus rhythm has returned or the attempt has been abandoned, check vital signs and place the patient in the recovery position (unless CPR is in progress).

Aftercare (should sinus rhythm be restored)
1. ECG monitoring in a specialized area is recommended.
2. Serum potassium should be maintained above 4.0 mmol l^{-1}.
3. General postanaesthetic measures.
4. Record a 12-lead ECG in sinus rhythm.

Complications
1. Precipitation of a more serious arrhythmia (particularly in association with hypokalaemia).
2. Bradycardia following successful cardioversion, particularly if associated with acute ischaemia. Atropine is relatively contraindicated in this circumstance, since there would be a risk of precipitating tachycardia. Small doses may be used cautiously (0.4–0.6 mg). Transvenous pacing is probably preferable and may have the added advantage of suppressing recurrent VT.
3. Cardioversion in the presence of digoxin should proceed with care. If the serum digoxin levels are known to be therapeutic, no extra hazard would be expected, providing that hypokalaemia does not coexist. If the digoxin levels are not known, particularly if there is other evidence of toxicity, cardioversion should only be performed if absolutely necessary. There is a risk of serious resistant ventricular arrhythmia or bradycardia. Lignocaine 50 mg and magnesium sulphate 4–8 mmol should be administered intravenously and a prophylactic pacing wire inserted prior to a cardioversion attempt. Shock energy should be very low (5–10 J).

Overdrive ventricular pacing

This procedure is particularly useful for patients with relatively slow VT, especially if the arrhythmia is frequently recurrent. Overdrive pacing is best performed as soon as the tachycardia is noted, since the longer VT persists the more resistant it is to treatment (ischaemia, local acidosis, etc.). It is important to be aware that the tachycardia may merely be accelerated rather than terminated; in some circumstances haemodynamic instability or even VF results, requiring emergency cardioversion. In general, overdrive pacing is best performed by personnel familiar with the technique.

There are early favourable reports of external pacing systems being used for overdrive ventricular pacing; the methodology is much as described below (Grubb et al., 1992). A small dose of benzodiazepine is usually administered as a sedative.

Indication
1. Haemodynamically stable monomorphic VT.

Equipment
1. Ventricular pacing wire in situ (see section on transvenous pacing).
2. Pacing generator with facility for rapid pacing. The commonest such generator is known as a 'times three box'. This is a standard pacing box capable of pacing to rates of 30–150 beats min^{-1}, which is modified to include a knob or key which will instantly produce paced rates of three times that set; for example, a paced rate of 70 can be instantaneously rendered a rate of 210 by activating the 'times three' facility.
3. Defibrillator and resuscitation facility (MANDATORY; see below).

Patient preparation
1. The patient should be warned that there is a moderate risk of the tachycardia getting worse rather than better with this technique.

Procedure
1. Ensure defibrillation facilities are close to hand and that the patient is monitored and well oxygenated.
2. Connect the 'times three box' which should be in 'demand' mode (i.e. sensing the tachycardia) to the pacing wire.
3. The aim is to pace in 'times three mode' at a rate 10–30 beats min^{-1} faster than the tachycardia. Set the pacing rate at a third of this rate: for example, for a VT rate of 170, aim to pace at 180–200 (i.e. set box at 180/3 = 60); for a VT rate of 180, aim to pace at 190–210 (set box to 210/3 = 70).
4. Once all is ready, activate the 'times three mode'; the ventricular complex will change shape as the paced beats start in a few seconds. Allow 5–10 paced beats and then turn the whole pacing box off. Sinus rhythm may be restored; note its rate.
   a. If the tachycardia continues, repeat step 4, this time pacing for 10–20 beats. If the tachycardia fails to respond at all, consider overdrive pacing at a higher rate, first with 5–10 beats and then with 10–20 beats, as before. The rate can be increased as necessary providing the overdrive rate is not greater than 210 (see c).
   b. If the tachycardia recurs after a pause or a period of bradycardia or bizarre rhythm, repeat step 4 but, rather than turning the pacing box off, turn off the 'times three' facility thus immediately pacing the ventricle at the end of the tachycardia at the set rate, which can then be adjusted to suppress any tendency towards bradycardia-facilitated VT; the optimal rate is usually 90–100 beats min^{-1}.
   c. If the tachycardia accelerates, but the rhythm is below 200 and the patient is stable, further attempts at overdrive pacing may be considered. Overdrive pacing at rates above 210 are associated with a high risk of degeneration into VF. In these circumstances, elective cardioversion is advisable.

d. Step 4 onwards may be repeated after the administration of an antiarrhythmic agent. Magnesium sulphate 4–8 mmol is particularly useful since it increases tachycardia cycle length thus reducing the rate; magnesium also appears to increase the chance of successful overdrive pacing (although this is as yet largely anecdotal). Lignocaine or procainamide might also be useful.

5. If there is the expertise available, more sophisticated pacing ramps including the insertion of ventricular ectopic beats are often helpful, but additional equipment and trained personnel are necessary.

Aftercare
1. Keep potassium greater than 4.5 mmol^{-1}.
2. See section on VT.
3. See section on ventricular pacing.

Complications
1. Acceleration of VT as discussed.
2. VF.

Broad complex tachycardia

All broad complex tachycardia should be considered to be of ventricular origin unless proven otherwise.

The majority of broad complex tachycardias seen in an A&E department will be of ventricular origin. However, a smaller number will be due to a supraventricular tachycardia conducted with bundle branch block. A broad complex tachycardia is defined as that where the width of the QRS complex is greater than 0.12 sec (3 mm at 25 mm sec^{-1} paper speed). The immediate management of such tachycardias is described in Fig. 9.

There have been many strategies suggested for the accurate differentiation of these aberrantly conducted rhythms from VT. Few are 100% sensitive or specific (Griffith *et al.*, 1991). The introduction of adenosine has revolutionized this field (Griffith *et al.*, 1988), since a maximum dose intravenous bolus of adenosine will have no effect on the morphology or rate of VT, but will markedly affect any tachycardia with a pathway involving AV node (i.e. all aberrantly conducted supraventricular tachycardias).

Therefore the advice for treatment of sustained broad complex tachycardia is:

1. Get a 12-lead ECG if at all possible.
2. If there is haemodynamic instability, consider DCV.
3. In a stable patient, give a trial of adenosine (see p. 909). If no effect on ventricular rate at the maximum tolerated dose, consider the arrhythmia as VT. If the tachycardia changes or is terminated, this is highly likely to be an aberrantly conducted supraventricular tachycardia; on the whole, higher doses of adenosine are necessary to terminate broad complex supraventricular tachycardia than to terminate classical supraventricular tachycardia.

Fig. 9 depicts a typical management plan, applicable to all broad complex tachyarrhythmias. Further details are given below; as before, each arrhythmia is discussed in detail.

Sustained ventricular tachycardia

Description

Broad complex regular tachycardia, unaffected by an intravenous bolus of adenosine. In contrast to supraventricular tachycardia, the rate of VT may be quite slow (90–120 beats min^{-1}), particularly if the patient is receiving antiarrhythmic medication. Other pointers toward a diagnosis of VT are (see also Fig. 13):

1. The occurrence of independent P wave activity (AV dissociation).
2. Fusion beat – a QRS complex of morphology different from the rest of the tachycardia, resulting from fusion of the QRS from a normally conducted sinus beat with a QRS of ventricular origin. (Supraventricular tachycardia, in contrast, is of entirely regular morphology.)
3. The horizontal axis of the heart may be very bizarre (e.g. all the complexes in V1 to V6 are predominantly negative).

Cause and associations

Usually secondary to ischaemic heart disease, acute MI, or dilated cardiomyopathy, but it can occur with any disease associated with myocardial fibrosis (amyloidosis, sarcoidosis, etc.). In younger patients, right ventricular dysplasia may give rise to a troublesome right ventricular arrhythmia which is increasingly recognized. VT is also recognized to occur in patients with no evidence of heart disease (so-called 'normal heart VT') (Gill *et al.*, 1990).

Symptoms

Palpitations, light-headedness, cannon waves. Angina and/or evidence of ischaemia may occur in association with ischaemic heart disease.

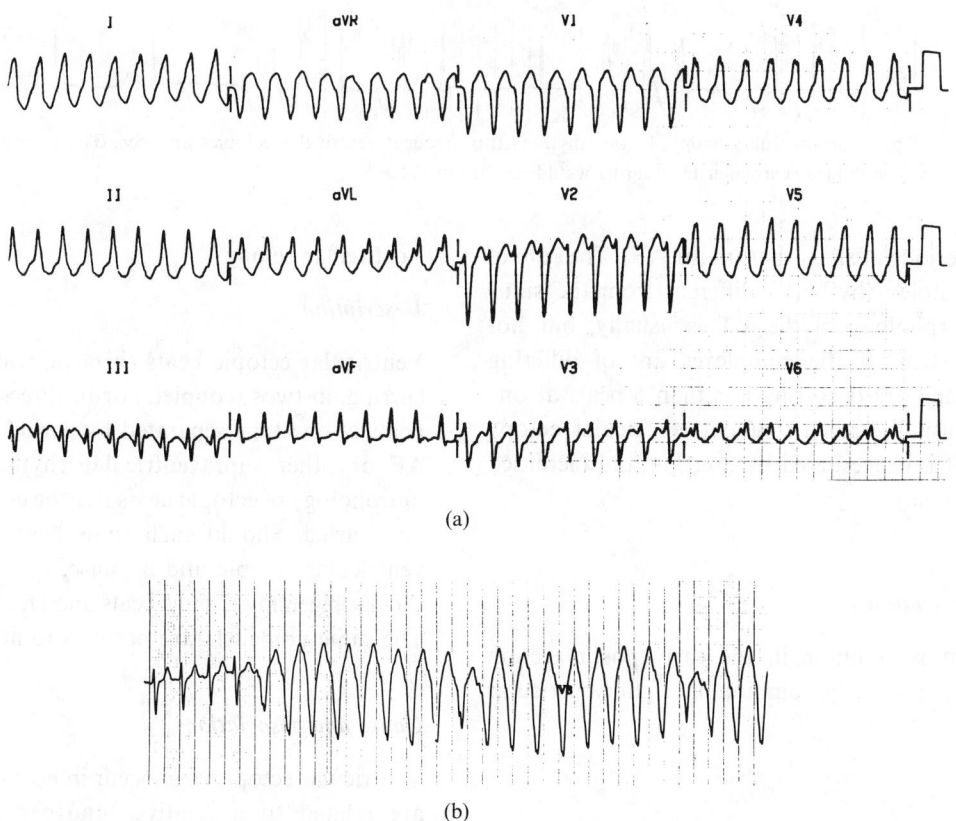

Fig. 13. (a) Ventricular tachycardia: wide complex regular tachycardia. The complexes are irregularly deformed by independent P wave activity, most clearly shown in the penultimate beat of the aVL recording. Adenosine had no appreciable effect on this rhythm. (b) Rhythm strip demonstrating the onset of a broad complex tachycardia. There is evidence of independent P wave activity and fusion beats, suggesting that this rhythm is ventricular tachycardia.

Management

Having excluded aberrantly conducted supraventricular tachycardia with adenosine as described above (see Fig. 9), lignocaine (50–100 mg IV stat) remains the treatment of choice – a role partly justified by a high awareness and large experience of its use, despite the superior efficacy of flecainide and disopyramide (Griffith *et al.*, 1990). The main advantage of lignocaine over the other agents (particularly flecainide) is a much smaller negatively inotropic effect, and lignocaine is particularly indicated in patients with poor LV function. Procainamide is an underused agent with a higher efficacy than lignocaine; it has some negative inotropic effects, which are unfortunately shared by its active metabolite, such that a hypotensive effect may be prolonged. Intravenous magnesium can be a helpful adjunctive agent (4–8 mmol stat); magnesium will tend to modify the tachyardia rather than terminate it, but is associated with an increased success rate for subsequent overdrive pacing (Iseri, 1989).

If these measures are ineffective, consider overdrive pacing or elective synchronized DCV. The longer the period of VT, the more difficult the arrhythmia is to terminate, particularly in association with ischaemic heart disease.

If, despite termination, the arrhythmia is persistently recurrent and the underlying sinus rhythm is slow (less than 85 min^{-1}), consider ventricular pacing at 100 beats min^{-1} (if LV dysfunction is severe, atrial transport may be critical, in which case, ventricular pacing alone will be poorly tolerated; consider referral for temporary sequential atrial–ventricular pacing). Attention to the control of underlying ischaemia is mandatory; this may require coronary vasodilators and/or inotropes.

Frequently repetitive ventricular tachycardia

Description

Short, frequent runs of non-sustained (less than 10 beats) or sustained (more than 10 beats) broad complex tachy-

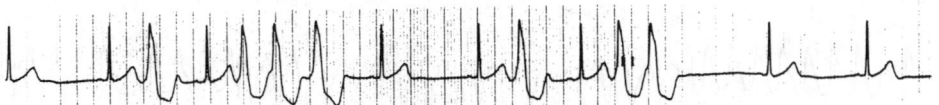

Fig. 14. Frequently repetitive ventricular ectopy. In this rhythm strip, frequent ventricular ectopics are seen. The morphology of the ectopics is identical; a history of sustained ventricular tachycardia would not be unusual.

cardia with periods of sinus rhythm (or AF). The rate of the broad complex rhythm is different from the sinus rate. The morphology of the VT is usually, but not always, consistent. If the complexes are of differing morphology and are occurring less than 5 beats at one time, this is usually called frequent ventricular ectopy (see below). It is exacerbated by exertion and increased sympathetic tone.

Cause and associations

As for VT. It is common in the early postinfarction period; it is particularly common in right ventricular dysplasia.

Symptoms

Often symptomatic, but palpitations are common. It is rarely a haemodynamic problem.

Management

Non-sustained VT occurring in the setting of acute ischaemia has a moderate risk of degenerating into sustained VT or even VF. The arrhythmia is usually very sensitive to lignocaine administered as a 50 mg IV bolus followed by an infusion (Table 2). A magnesium infusion may also be helpful. Should such an arrhythmia occur in a young patient with no history of ischaemic heart disease, this may represent a right ventricular VT or perhaps 'normal heart' VT – an increasingly recognized entity. These forms of VT are usually responsive to lignocaine, and magnesium is particularly useful in VT of right ventricular origin.

NB: Right ventricular VT can be sensitive to calcium antagonists; such patients with VT may therefore be receiving oral medication with calcium antagonists.

Verapamil should never be administered to any patient with VT unless under the supervision of a cardiologist.

Ventricular ectopy

Description

Ventricular ectopic beats (bizarre, wide complexes) occurring, in twos (couplets) or in threes (triplets) up to 5 beats at one time separated by periods of sinus rhythm, AF or other supraventricular rhythm (Fig. 14). The morphology of ectopic beats may be consistent or bizarre and varied. Should each sinus beat be followed by a ventricular ectopic and a pause, this is known as ventricular bigeminy; 2 sinus beats and an ectopic is trigeminy. The same nomenclature pertains to atrial ectopy.

Cause and associations

Ventricular ectopics can occur in normal individuals and are related to a relative bradycardia. Such ectopics disappear on exercise and are generally considered to be benign. Frequent ectopy at rest which is exacerbated by exercise is usually pathological and requires further investigation; it is commonly associated with ischaemia. Ectopy is common in the first 24 h following acute MI, and close monitoring is advised.

Symptoms

Missed beats, thumps in the heart, difficulty sleeping on the left side are frequent complaints. Since the majority of people with ectopy have the benign variety associated with relative bradycardia, symptoms often occur at rest, particularly whilst waiting to go to sleep, when the patient is often more aware of the heart beat. Occurring on exercise, there may be associated short runs of non-sustained VT which may give rise to palpitations and/or transient syncope.

Management

For the majority of patients with benign ectopy, simple reassurance is all that is necessary. For those very symptomatic patients, a beta-blocker may be of benefit in suppression of the ectopic focus.

Patients with increased ectopy on exertion, or who

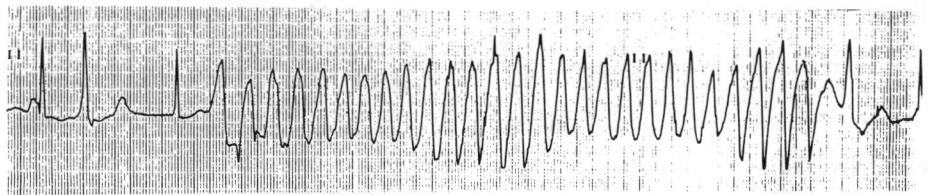

Fig. 15. Self-limiting torsades de pointes. Note the twisting morphology of the ventricular tachycardia and its characteristic initiation at the end of a T wave.

have a history of ischaemic heart disease, should be referred for an exercise test and a 24-h Holter tape (a 24-h recording of a two- or three-channel ECG).

Torsades de pointes

Description

Regular or irregular, fast, wide complex tachycardia with changing focus, reflected in complexes with rapidly changing shape and size, apparently twisting around the isoelectric line (hence the name; see Fig. 15). The arrhythmia may be self-terminating and recurrent and/or degenerate rapidly into VF.

Cause and associations

A complication of long QT syndrome (see below), either congenital or drug-induced. It is occasionally secondary to ischaemia, and may be related to the proarrhythmic effects of concurrent antiarrhythmic therapy.

Symptoms

Usually associated with syncope or presyncope. Torsades de pointes is a cause of unexplained VF.

Management

The arrhythmia is very sensitive to magnesium and will usually stop during the initial bolus dose, which should be followed by an infusion (Tzivoni *et al.*, 1988). If the arrhythmia has persisted for any length of time, there will be haemodynamic collapse and DCV will be required. It is often difficult to sense the R wave of the torsades because of the rapidly changing axis; non-synchronized shock is therefore recommended in this circumstance.

Attention to the underlying cause is mandatory since this arrhythmia is very difficult to control. It will be exacerbated by bradycardia, and high-rate pacing 100–110 min^{-1} is often required to suppress it. Torsades is

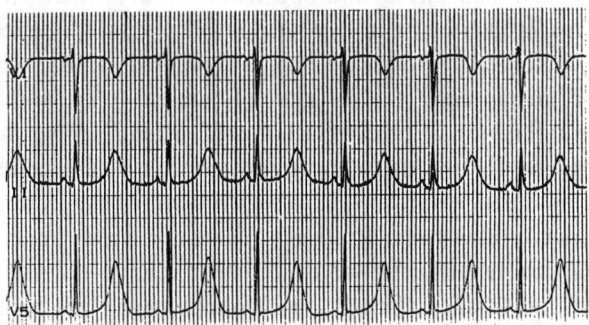

Fig. 16. A 3-lead ECG demonstrating a long QT interval (QT = 520 msec; QTc = 0.58). In this particular case the abnormality was associated with amiodarone therapy, and torsades de pointes resulted. Amiodarone levels were within the therapeutic range.

exacerbated by high sympathetic tone (including exercise), so sedation and/or beta-blockade (plus or minus pacing) are often useful (e.g. propranolol 1–2 mg IV over 2–5 min). Hypokalaemia and/or hypomagnesaemia are frequently associated and should be rigorously treated; this may require central venous cannulation to facilitate high-dose potassium supplementation.

Long QT syndrome

The upper limit of the QT interval is difficult to define, since the QT interval is dependent on heart rate. Several formulae have been proposed for the standardization of the QT interval, but that suggested by Bazett has gained widespread acceptance; i.e. corrected QT (QTc) = QT interval divided by square root of R-R interval. The upper limit of normal is 0.39 sec for men and 0.44 sec for women. Prolongation of the QT interval is usually acquired and is due to antiarrhythmic drug usage (amiodarone, sotalol, quinidine) or poisoning with tricyclic antidepressants (Fig. 16). Torsades de pointes is strongly associated with this abnormality and may be very difficult to control (see above). There are some families with congenital long QT syndrome (rare) in whom a family history of syncope or even sudden death in childhood is not uncommon.

Ventricular fibrillation

See Fig. 8. This arrhythmia is discussed in Chapter 3.

Narrow complex tachycardia (supraventricular tachycardia)

Many of these arrhythmias are paroxysmal, and by their very nature may stop spontaneously. Many are responsive to vagal manoeuvres and/or a reduction in sympathetic tone. They often occur in young people with no evidence of structural heart disease who have suffered palpitations for many years; the patient will present only if the arrhythmia has been unusually persistent, failing to respond to 'the usual measures', or if it is unusually symptomatic. Many will have been prescribed medication which is often taken erratically. There is often an underlying cause for an unusually persistent attack – excessive caffeine intake, anxiety, an alcoholic binge. Patients presenting with an intermittent regular narrow complex tachycardia should be referred for specialist advice (usually as an out-patient) after treatment of the acute arrhythmia since there are now excellent techniques (e.g. radiofrequency transcatheter ablation) whereby many of these patients may be cured of their arrhythmia without recourse to surgery.

NB: The nomenclature of narrow complex tachycardia is rather confusing. The term 'supraventricular tachycardia' is used loosely to describe any narrow complex tachycardia. Strictly speaking, supraventricular tachycardia is a term that applies only to those arrhythmias that incorporate the atrium in the tachycardia circuit; i.e. atrial tachycardias, AF and atrial flutter, and AV re-entrant tachycardia (accessory pathway tachycardia) of which Wolff–Parkinson–White syndrome is a variety. In contrast, AV nodal re-entrant tachycardia is a *junctional* tachycardia which involves an 'accessory pathway' within the AV node itself (i.e. the atrium is not involved in the tachycardia); this is not really a supraventricular tachycardia. However, for the purpose of this discussion, 'supraventricular tachycardia') will be used in the general sense to describe narrow complex tachycardia. (For completeness, there is an exceedingly rare form of VT which arises in the Purkinje system between the AV node and the His bundle; such a tachycardia will therefore be narrow complex. Its rarity limits a discussion of its treatment to electrophysiological texts.)

Fig. 10 can be used to determine the likely cause of any narrow complex tachycardia. Using the notes following, a suitable management programme can then be devised. Alternatively, these notes may be used as a direct source of information.

Sinus tachycardia

Description

An acceleration of normal sinus rhythm. The rate may vary with respiration and is gradually slowed by a reduction in sympathetic tone (e.g. sleep, sedation). The rate may vary by as much as 10 beats min^{-1} in a few minutes; this degree of variability during a regular tachycardia is very unlikely to occur in any other situation. Conversely, a regular tachycardia that varies not at all is unlikely to be a sinus tachycardia.

Cause and associations

High sympathetic tone (e.g. anxiety, pain), exertion, reflex tachycardia (hypovolaemia, vasodilators, etc.), excessive use of beta-agonists (e.g. salbutamol), fever, pregnancy, anaemia, thyrotoxicosis.

Symptoms

Patients may complain of palpitations, sweating, light-headedness and other features of a hyperadrenergic state.

Management

Treatment should be directed to the underlying cause.

Atrial fibrillation

Description

There is an absence of discrete P wave activity which is replaced by a chaotic atrial rhythm (Fig. 17). The narrow complex ventricular rate is irregularly irregular and may at times be very rapid. Wide variation in the ventricular rate occurs at the faster rates, which may reach 200 min^{-1}. AF may be paroxysmal.

Cause and associations

Recent onset AF (particularly in younger people) is typically rather fast and symptomatic. Causes include thyrotoxicosis, mitral valve disease, ischaemic heart disease, any form of cardiomyopathy, idiopathic AF, pneumonia, pericardial effusion, malignant infiltration of the pericardium. Electrolyte imbalance, particularly

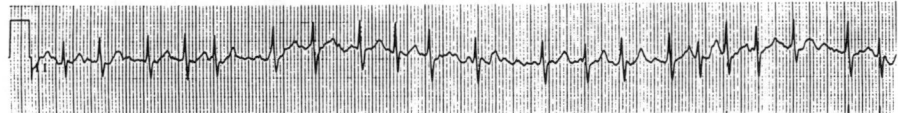

Fig. 17. 'Rapid' atrial fibrillation. The ventricular rate is 130–180 beats min^{-1}.

hypokalaemia, and alcohol poisoning are common precipitants.

The control of longstanding AF may deteriorate in conjunction with any of the above events (particularly pneumonia), and may be related to poor drug compliance. Paradoxically, digoxin toxicity may manifest as rapid AF.

Symptoms

Irregular rapid palpitations (may be paroxysmal), breathlessness, 'thumping heart' (due to variation in stroke volume), light-headedness. Angina may occur in the setting of ischaemic heart disease.

Management

The aim of treatment is two-fold:

1. To control the ventricular rate by slowing AV node conduction.
2. To effect medical cardioversion to sinus rhythm (if possible).

High sympathetic tone will hasten AVN conduction, and associated features such as pain, hypoxia, hypovolaemia, etc. should be remedied. Hypokalaemia and/or hypomagnesaemia should be corrected.

Synchronized DCV remains the treatment of choice if there is severe haemodynamic compromise. This is associated with a 1–2% risk of embolus from left atrial thrombus in patients who have not been on long-term anticoagulant therapy, and synchronized DCV should not be undertaken lightly; embolus is particularly associated with AF of short duration (less than 1 week). Synchronized DCV is rarely required, however, since this arrhythmia is relatively well tolerated.

If the AF is of recent origin (less than 24 h), intravenous disopyramide 2 mg kg^{-1} over 2–5 min (maximum 150 mg) is often effective; if there is no evidence of ischaemic heart disease, intravenous flecainide 2 mg kg^{-1} over 20–30 min (maximum 150 mg) is probably associated with a higher success rate (although conversion to sinus rhythm may take 2 h or more). Both these agents have significant negative inotropic effects which may be undesirable in patients with poor LV function. In these patients, initial control of ventricular rate with digoxin (0.5 mg IV over 30 min or orally, followed by 0.25 mg orally (or IV) at 6 h) will control the rate in the majority of patients (Fig. 18). Consideration should be given to anticoagulation with intravenous or high-dose subcutaneous heparin (if contraindicated, consider aspirin).

Patients with longstanding AF should be digitized as above, since it is unlikely that sinus rhythm will be restored. Should the patient be already taking digoxin, establish the serum level of digoxin (if possible) and supplement the dose if subtherapeutic. In the absence of a facility for digoxin analysis, or should there be rapid AF despite therapeutic levels of digoxin, consider adding verapamil (10–15 mg IV over 2–5 min; 40–80 mg t.d.s. orally) unless there is evidence of significant left ventricular dysfunction, since verapamil is a negative inotrope. In this circumstance, consider intravenous amiodarone 300 mg over 30 min followed by 1.2 g over 24 h. (NB: Intravenous amiodarone should be administered through a central venous catheter since it is extremely irritant to peripheral veins.)

Digoxin modifies ventricular repolarization, resulting in ST changes on the surface ECG (Fig. 18); these should not be confused with those changes secondary to ischaemia.

Atrial flutter

Description

Regular ventricular response with rate occurring in integral divisions of 300 min^{-1}, i.e. 150, 100, 75 min^{-1} (Fig. 19). Atrial flutter waves may be visible (see Fig. 11). May be interrupted by periods of AF.

Cause and associations

Atrial flutter is a troublesome arrhythmia. It is associated with any cause of atrial distension and with extra-atrial irritation (tumours, pericardial effusion).

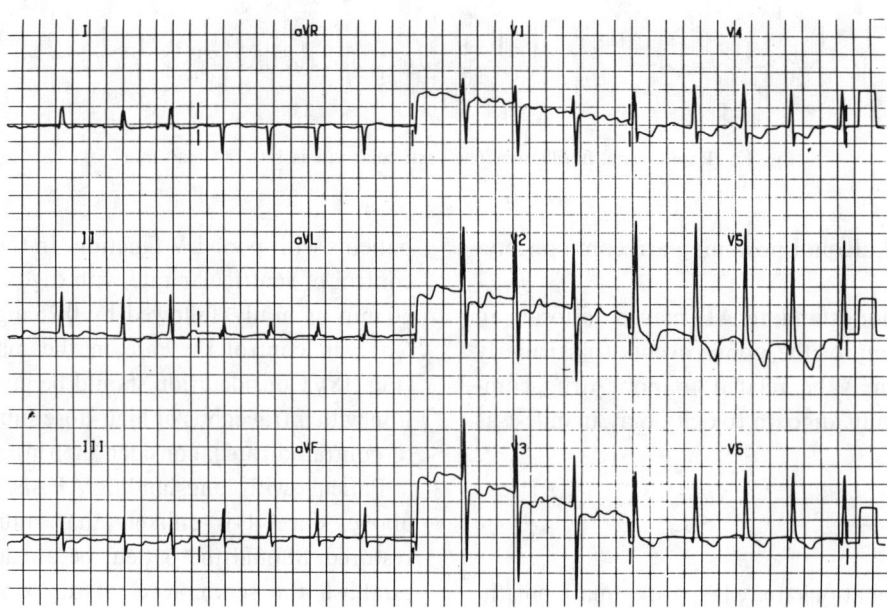

Fig. 18. A 12-lead electrocardiogram illustrating controlled atrial fibrillation, with digoxin-induced repolarization abnormalities (this does not imply digoxin toxicity).

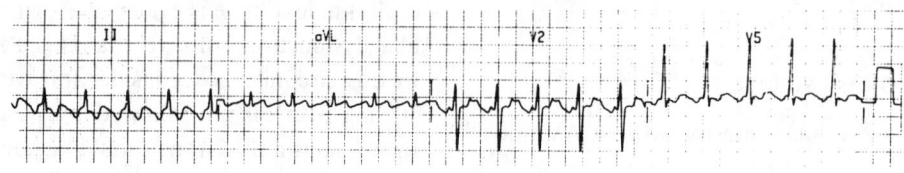

Fig. 19. Atrial flutter with 2:1 block: typical 'saw-tooth' morphology is seen in lead II. The diagnosis might be missed if lead V_5 were the single strip recorded.

Symptoms

Commonly asymptomatic, but patients may complain of palpitations.

Management

The diagnosis can be confirmed by transiently increasing AV conduction time by increasing vagal tone (using the vagal manoeuvre(s) described above). Should these prove unhelpful, a diagnostic dose of adenosine may be used; high-grade AV block is induced and flutter waves are clearly seen (Figs 11 and 12).

Once the diagnosis is confirmed, control of ventricular rate and/or resumption of sinus rhythm are therapeutic objectives as for AF.

Synchronized DCV is probably the treatment of choice, particularly if there is haemodynamic compromise; there is little or no risk of embolism in this circumstance. Other therapeutic options include intravenous flecainide or intravenous disopyramide (see under AF). Intravenous verapamil will control ventricular rate, but is rarely associated with medical cardioversion. Digoxin will also control the ventricular rate, but usually results in conversion to AF.

Atrial tachycardia

Description

This is a rare arrhythmia in which P wave activity is evident, but P wave morphology is often bizarre (but consistent) reflecting an ectopic focus. There is little or no respiratory variation in the P wave rate and physiological reduction of sympathetic tone or vagal manoeuvres is rarely effective. Adenosine results in a gradual slowing of the ectopic focus before complete AV block supervenes. This is identical to its effect in sinus rhythm; the clue lies in the morphology of the P waves.

Cause and association

Atrial tachycardia can occur at any age and may be idiopathic. In young people, this arrhythmia may be long-standing.

Symptoms

It is often asymptomatic, but, if paroxysmal, may give rise to palpitations.

Management

Atrial tachycardia is rarely an acute haemodynamic problem. Atrial tachycardia is very difficult to treat, but beta-blockade is sometimes useful. Cardioversion may be used, but the arrhythmia often recurs.

Multifocal atrial tachycardia

Description

Rare. There is an irregularly ventricular response, but discrete P waves are visible, often with bizarre and varying morphology.

Cause and associations

This usually results from severe electrolyte disturbance, particularly hypokalaemia and/or hypomagnesaemia. It is strongly associated with alcohol abuse. It is also associated with chronic pulmonary disease, usually in conjunction with hypokalaemia, and is a feature of digoxin toxicity.

Symptoms

Palpitations.

Management

Adenosine will have a varying effect on the various atrial foci, but overall the atrial and ventricular rate will slow, facilitating identification of the abnormal P waves; typical flutter waves are not seen.

An intravenous bolus of 4–8 mmol of magnesium sulphate is often successful in restoring sinus rhythm regardless of aetiology. An infusion of magnesium may be necessary (see Table 2) whilst other electrolyte imbalances are resolved. Serum potassium should be checked as soon as possible and any deficit corrected. Treatment

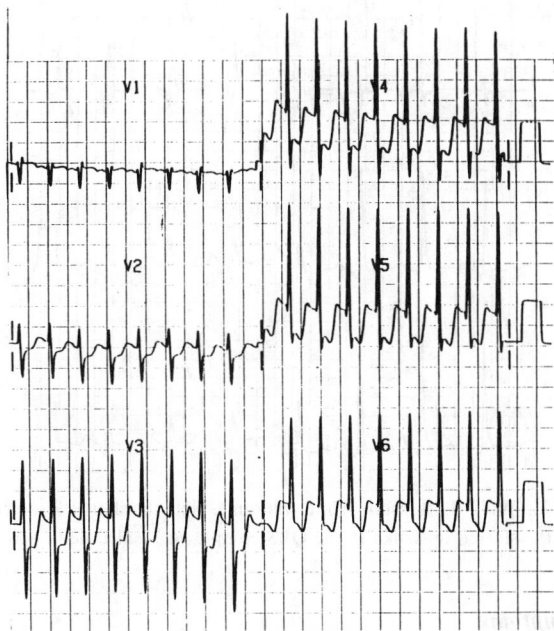

Fig. 20. Narrow complex tachycardia. This arrhythmia would almost certainly terminate with adenosine. Note the profound ST changes; these are rarely indicative of ischaemia, and may persist for some hours after resumption of normal sinus rhythm.

with antiarrhythmic agents is rarely required, and may be detrimental in association with electrolyte disturbance.

AV re-entrant tachycardia and AV nodal re-entrant tachycardia

Description

Narrow complex regular tachycardia (Fig. 20). If P waves are visible, consider AV re-entrant tachycardia. Wolff–Parkinson–White syndrome is a specialized form of AV re-entrant tachycardia in which the presence of the accessory pathway can be detected from the 12-lead ECG in sinus rhythm. Wolff–Parkinson–White syndrome is characterized by a short PR interval and a slurred QRS upstroke, known as a delta wave (Fig. 21).

Cause and associations

These arrhythmias are relatively common and are typically paroxysmal. Very few give rise to troublesome symptoms, and still fewer are persistent enough to precipitate presentation in the A&E department. Wolff–Parkinson–White syndrome may be asymptomatic; a small minority of patients with Wolff–Parkinson–White syndrome will have Epstein's anomaly.

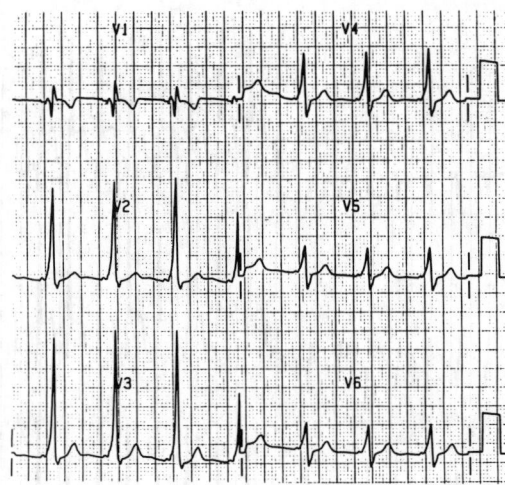

Fig. 21. Wolff–Parkinson–White syndrome. Note the short PR interval and the slurred upstroke to the QRS complex (so-called delta wave).

Symptoms

Fast, regular palpitations possibly associated with dyspnoea and light-headedness. Patients may complain of 'neck pulsations' as a consequence of synchronous contraction of atria and ventricles thus producing cannon waves. The tachycardia may have been transiently responsive to vagal manoeuvres. A previous history of palpitations is common.

Treatment

As with all tachyarrhythmias, cardioversion is the treatment of choice if there is haemodynamic instability. Otherwise, vagal manoeuvres are occasionally successful and should be instituted; these are unlikely to help in a very anxious patient. Adenosine in increasing bolus doses of 4–20 mg will often terminate these arrhythmias, but may be ineffective if the patient is very anxious. If adenosine is ineffective or the tachycardia is rapidly recurrent, consider verapamil 5–15 mg IV over 2–5 min (beware concurrent beta-blocker therapy). Flecainide may be used as a third-line agent (2 mg kg^{-1} over 10–30 min, maximum 150 mg).

Atrial fibrillation associated with an accessory pathway

Accessory pathways rarely give rise to life-threatening arrhythmias or to haemodynamic compromise. The exception to this rule occurs when AF coexists with Wolff–Parkinson–White syndrome. Under normal circumstances, the ventricular rate in AF is controlled by physiological slow conduction in the AV node and rates

in excess of 180–200 min^{-1} are rare. However, in Wolff–Parkinson–White syndrome the accessory pathway may be capable of extremely fast conduction and hence of generating a very fast ventricular response, even VF. Since the impulses are conducted down the accessory pathway the resulting QRS has a very long slurred delta wave, resulting in a wide complex, irregularly irregular tachycardia (Fig. 22). Occasional impulses may conduct down the AV node as well, resulting in a shorter delta wave, and a narrower complex. Treatment is immediate cardioversion.

Description

Wide complex, irregular tachycardia with some narrow beats.

Cause and association

As for AV re-entrant tachycardia.

Symptoms

Palpitations with imminent haemodynamic collapse or hypotension are common.

Management

There is a high risk of degeneration into VF in this circumstance. Immediate cardioversion is required. (Synchrony may not be possible; it is not mandatory in this situation.) Once recovered, intravenous flecainide will prevent recurrence; timely referral to a specialist centre is advised. This is a life-threatening condition.
ADENOSIDE IS CONTRAINDICATED.

PERMANENT PACEMAKERS

The majority of pacemakers are single chamber ventricular lead systems placed in elderly patients for conduction disorders – usually CHB. Single chamber atrial systems will usually present to an A&E department as an incidental finding, and rarely give rise to emergency problems. Dual chamber pacemakers are much more sophisticated and thus are more liable to malfunction; this is rarely of a serious nature, since malfunctions are mostly related to programming problems, and can therefore be referred in good time to the relevant specialist. However, if there are problems with the ventricular lead, they will behave as would a single chamber ventricular system and can be considered as such.

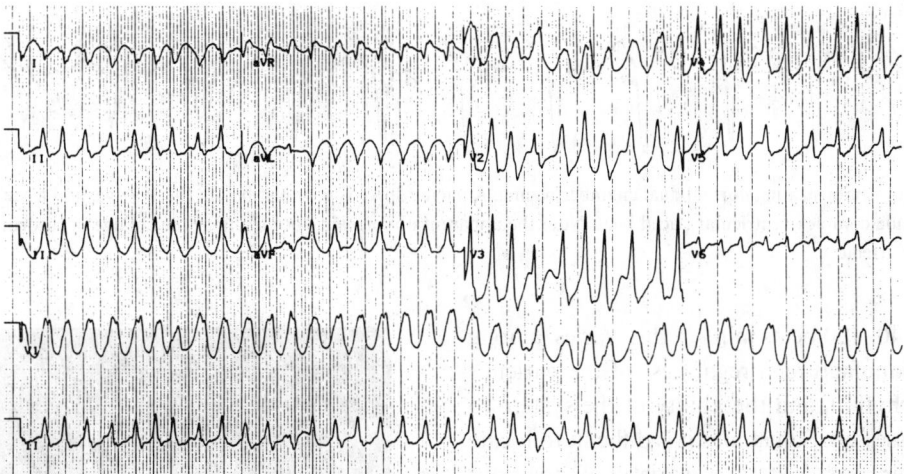

Fig. 22. Atrial fibrillation in the presence of an accessory pathway. The rhythm is irregularly irregular; there are some narrow complexes (conducted normally via the atrioventricular node) and some slurred broad complexes (conducted via the accessory pathway; note the delta wave).

Modern pacemakers rarely fail secondary to unheralded generator malfunction. The problem is usually traced to the pacing lead (e.g. lead displacement, or fracture) or electrical problems with threshold.

All patients should carry a card detailing the type and specification of their pacemaker. Very few pacemakers are affected by environmental electromagnetic radiation; microwaves and metal detectors (such as are found at airports) are not associated with pacemaker dysfunction.

Single chamber cardiac pacemakers

The vast majority of such single chamber pacemakers are sited for AV conduction defects and are thus ventricular pacing systems. This is the commonest form of pacemaker. AV nodal conduction disease is common in the elderly, so it follows that most pacemakers are fitted to older patients, many of whom have several other medical problems. There is a tendency in this circumstance for the patient and relatives to ascribe problems to 'the pacemaker', making life difficult for everyone.

Symptoms

The patient may present with dizzy spells or blackouts, or may complain of missed beats or palpitations. There are many causes of presyncope in the elderly, and in this situation few are due to pacemaker malfunction.

General guide to possible permanent pacemaker malfunction

1. *Examine the patient.* Is there evidence of trauma or infection around the generator box? Are there obvious loose wires? (rare). Is the pacemaker box still in electrical contact with the patient? Many pacemakers are 'unipolar', i.e. the pacing box itself forms part of the pacemaker circuit. Should the pacing box lose contact with the skin surface, the pacemaker will fail to function. This situation occurs when the box erodes out of its subcuticular pocket and hangs free from the patient; in this circumstance thinly wrap the box in a *wet* gauze swab and tape to the chest wall.

2. *The ECG.* Is the patient in their own rhythm, or are paced beats evident? If the patient's own heart rate is higher than that set for the pacemaker, all beats will be sensed and no paced beats will be seen. Paced beats may be distinguished by a sharp upstroke or downstroke (pacing spike) followed by a wide complex ventricular beat. Dissociated P waves may be visible.

   Is there a paced beat after each pacing spike or is there intermittent failure to capture? Do paced beats occur immediately after a native beat suggesting a failure to sense the intrinsic rhythm? Does a change in posture cause loss of sensing? A normal rhythm strip of AV sequential pacing is depicted in Fig. 23. Placing a magnet over the pacemaker box will cause the system to revert to a fixed 'test mode'. In 'test mode' the pacemaker will deliver a pacing signal at

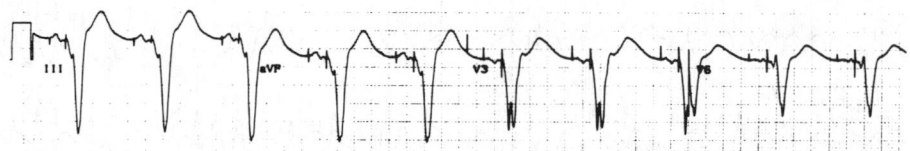

Fig. 23. A 4-lead strip demonstrating normal dual chamber pacing. A pacing spike is seen just before the P wave, and a 'delayed' ventricular pacing spike precedes the wide complex ventricular paced beat. Note the apparent abnormality occurring at the change of recording leads (aVF to V_3 and V_3 to V_6). These are artefacts.

the set rate (40–100 beats min^{-1}; this varies among pacemaker manufacturers) regardless of the patient's own rate or rhythm, and the ability of the system to pace can be assessed. Sometimes it is difficult to locate the pacemaker box, so try a variety of positions of the magnet before assuming a failure to pace. Removal of the magnet will result in reversion of the pacemaker to programmed mode; i.e. as it was before the magnet was placed.

If the patient's own rate is less than 60 min^{-1} and there are no paced beats seen, there is probably (but not necessarily) a problem and close monitoring is required. If the patient has a very slow rhythm, and/or long pauses are seen on the monitor, assume pacemaker failure and consider a temporary pacing wire.

3. On a *penetrated* chest X-ray it should be possible to follow the pacing wire from the generator to the right ventricle. Sometimes a break in the wire may be seen (Fig. 24), or displacement from the ventricular apex may be evident (Fig. 25).

4. *In general*, if pacemaker malfunction is suspected, monitor until a specific check of the pacemaker can be performed. If there is any suggestion of syncope or long pauses, and there is good evidence of malfunction, consider a temporary wire. Otherwise, watch and wait, and request a pacemaker check as soon as is practical.

Dual chamber pacemakers

As suggested above, major problems will occur in these systems if there is a problem with the ventricular wire; such a circumstance should be managed as described above for single chamber systems. Atrial wire problems, in contrast, are rarely an emergency and can be dealt with accordingly.

Pacemaker tachycardia (Dual chamber only)

In a small number of patients the AV node has the capacity to conduct retrogradely, and thus under some

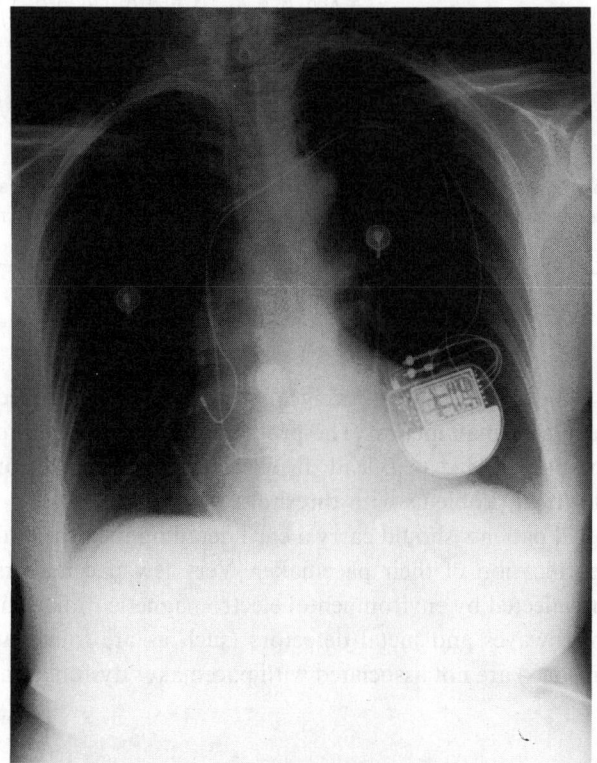

Fig. 24. A dual chamber pacemaker. Note the correct positioning of the atrial J lead and the kink in the ventricular wire as it traverses the tricuspid valve. If the wires are followed from the pacing generator, a clear break in one wire is clearly visible in the midclavicular line.

circumstances ventricular impulses are conducted back up to the atria. The atrial wire then senses the retrogradely conducted beat as a bona fide atrial signal, and the pacemaker system paces the ventricle; the circuit then repeats, producing a pacemaker-induced tachycardia. Most systems are programmed to avoid such pacemaker tachycardia, but it may occur nonetheless. Application of a magnet will cause the pacemaker to revert to a fixed mode thus breaking the loop and terminating the tachycardia; removal of the magnet will allow normal pacemaker function to resume. The patient should then be referred to a pacing centre for assessment.

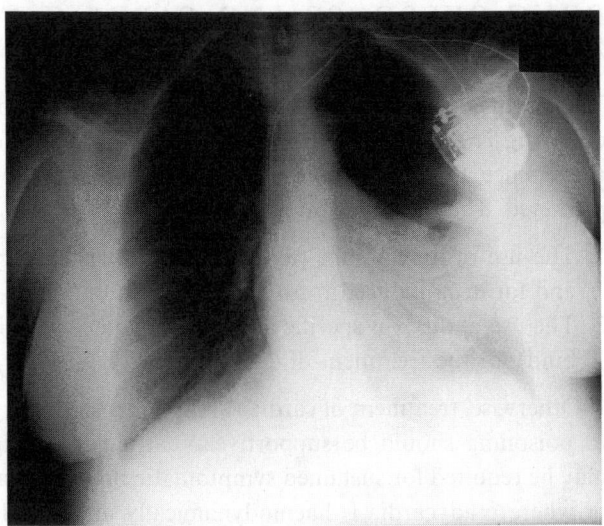

Fig. 25. A dual chamber pacemaker. The ventricular wire is displaced and lies coiled in the right atrium abutting the tricuspid valve. Significant ventricular ectopy can result. The atrial wire appears satisfactory.

DC cardioversion and pacemakers

DCV may be performed quite safely in patients with pacemakers. It is advisable not to position the paddles directly over the generator box, but otherwise cardioversion should proceed normally. Pacemakers are designed to withstand up to 200 DC shocks.

NB: Should diathermy be planned, a similar protocol should be adopted. There is rarely any problem unless the diathermy is applied in close proximity to the generator. If this is absolutely necessary, apply a magnet over the pacemaker converting it to 'set mode' for the duration of the procedure. Removal of the magnet at the end of the procedure will result in reversion to normal pacemaker function.

It is generally advisable to arrange a formal check of pacemaker function after cardioversion or use of diathermy.

Antitachycardia pacemakers

Some patients will arrive in the A&E department with a narrow complex or broad complex tachycardia, clutching a magnet. They will inform you that the magnet should be placed over the generator box and they will be cured! Fewer of these sytems are now placed, as a result of the huge increase in the use of internal cardioverter defibrillators (see below).

These patients have an arrhythmia that is highly sensitive to overdrive pacing and will have a pacemaker fitted that has a preprogrammed 'routine' of overdrive modes that have been specifically designed for that patient. The 'routine' is activated by holding a magnet over the generator, which sets off the first mode. The pacemaker will then sense the rhythm and if tachycardia persists a second mode (of usually three) will activate. Should the rhythm settle, the pacemaker will deactivate and can only be reactivated by removing the magnet and resiting it. Overdrive pacing will stop if the magnet is removed. Overdrive pacing of any description may result in acceleration of the tachycardia or even VF (see overdrive pacing). It is for this reason that the patient has been instructed to report to hospital. Full resuscitation facilities should be available.

Management

If the patient is haemodynamically unstable, defibrillate in the standard manner. Otherwise, perform a 12-lead ECG and attach a cardiac monitor. With full defibrillation and resuscitation facilities to hand, place the magnet over the generator box. If none of the therapies is effective, it may be worth a second attempt with the magnet in a slightly different position. Remove the magnet, wait a minute or two and replace it over the generator. If these methods fail, switch to standard management of the relevant arrhythmia. Synchronized DCV should be used if there is any doubt as to haemodynamic stability.

NB: Many of these antitachycardia pacemakers act concurrently as standard pacing systems.

Internal cardioverter defibrillator

The fastest growing technology in pacing is that of the internal cardioverter defibrillators (ICDs). These devices combine standard pacing systems, antitachycardia pacing and internal defibrillation facilities; they are fitted to the survivors of out-of-hospital cardiac arrest (excluding those with a remediable cause, e.g. acute MI) and/or patients with VT that is poorly controlled by drug therapy. These devices are relatively complicated and there are many different models. Whatever the problem with the device or the patient, DCV (if indicated) is an acceptable mode of treatment and will not damage the device.

Patients with ICDs are usually very knowledgeable about their condition and carry a card documenting the specifications of the device. There is usually an emergency telephone number that the patient will call if a problem is perceived. However, if the device should suddenly start to activate frequently in defibrillation mode, not only will the patient be alarmed, but will also be relatively uncomfortable. The energy of the lowest shock may be only 8 J, but the most commonly used shock energy can approach 35 J, which is not much less than the 50 J used for elective cardioversion (usually performed under general anaesthesia!).

Frequent device activation can be appropriate or inappropriate (which is usually due to misinterpretation by the device of rapid AF as VT or VF). Either way, the application of a magnet over the generator will deactivate its defibrillation mode and the patient can be observed, monitored and/or sedated as necessary, whilst arrangements are made to transfer the patient to a specialist centre. (NB: The generator of older ICD models was rather large and will be found in the abdominal wall in a pouch within the rectus sheath.)

Some devices reactivate automatically when the magnet is removed, others remain deactivated. It is usual practice to tape the magnet firmly in place, ensuring continued deactivation (each patient should carry a card as to the exact characteristics of their device).

If frequent episodes of VT or VF or both occur, suggesting that frequent activation of the device was probably *appropriate*, treat the patient as per the standard protocol and contact the specialist centre; correction of electrolyte disturbances is mandatory (aim for potassium 5.0–5.5 mmol l^{-1}).

NB: Non-sustained VT is very common in these circumstances and, if the patient is asymptomatic, specific therapy is not necessary. Symptomatic bouts may respond to lignocaine and/or magnesium. Sedation to reduce sympathetic tone is also useful. If the arrhythmia proves resistant to these therapies, consider urgent transfer to a specialist centre.

If the device appears to be functioning *inappropriately*, leave the deactivating magnet *in situ*, monitor the patient for genuine problems and transfer when practical. The commonest reason for inappropriate activation is the detection of rapid AF, since the discrimination by the device of AF from VF is still subject to error. Treatment of AF in the standard manner should proceed. However, the patient should be assessed by the specialist centre before discharge, since the drugs used to control AF may interfere with optimal device function. Rarer problems include lead fracture and electrical 'noise' interfering with tachycardia detection; such technical problems require specialist intervention.

DRUG OVERDOSE AND CARDIAC ARRHYTHMIA

The treatment of the arrhythmic effects of toxic levels of one drug is rarely helped by the addition of a second drug, since the interaction of the two can rarely be predicted. The two exceptions to this rule are:

1. The use of magnesium sulphate for digoxin toxicity and for drug-induced torsades de pointes.
2. The use of digoxin specific antibody fragments (Digibind) for the treatment of digoxin toxicity.

Otherwise, treatment of cardiac arrhythmia secondary to poisoning should be supportive. Ventricular pacing may be required for sustained symptomatic bradycardia, or where bradycardia is haemodynamically undesirable (associated trauma, etc.). Sustained VT is very uncommon in drug overdose, with the exception of torsades de pointes associated with tricyclic antidepressant overdose. Correction of electrolyte abnormalities (particularly magnesium and/or potassium in alcoholics and diabetics) is often the only required intervention.

ARRHYTHMIA IN INFANTS AND CHILDREN

The involvement of a paediatrician in the emergency room is strongly recommended. Cardioversion remains the treatment of choice for haemodynamically unstable tachyarrhythmias. The dose energy is 1–4 J kg^{-1}.

Bradycardia

Bradycardia is uncommon, and is usually a feature of severe systemic disease (hypoxia, acidosis, raised intracranial pressure), or it may occur after cardiac surgery. It is rarely an acute event. CHB may be an exception. This is rare in the absence of congenital heart disease, but CHB as an isolated abnormality may be congenital (maternal systemic lupus erythematosus, etc.). Congenital CHB may not need treatment; specialist advice should be sought.

Specific therapies include atropine (dose 15 µg kg^{-1}), isoprenaline (0.02–0.2 µg kg^{-1} min^{-1}) and adrenaline (0.15–0.6 µg kg^{-1} min^{-1}).

Narrow complex tachycardia (supraventricular tachycardia)

This is by far the commonest arrhythmia to occur in children, and can occur as an isolated abnormality at any age. Haemodynamic collapse is rare in the absence of pre-existing heart failure. It is almost always responsive to vagal manoeuvres (the diving reflex is the most useful) and/or adenosine (0.05 mg kg^{-1} increasing in 0.05 mg bolus to total dose of 0.25 mg kg^{-1}). Verapamil should not be used in infants less than 1 year old.

Supraventricular tachycardia is a common problem in children with biventricular failure; a vicious cycle ensues and future digoxin prophylaxis is commonly suggested. If the child is very unwell, synchronized DCV with specialist anaesthetic and paediatric input is advised.

Broad complex tachycardia

This is rare in non-surgical patients, but may be a presenting feature of myocardial tumour, toxic agents (including drugs), congenital long QT syndrome or arrhythmogenic right ventricular dysplasia. Cardioversion is advised as an emergency measure, but specific therapies similar to those recommended for adults may be necessary.

ARRHYTHMIA IN PREGNANCY AND LACTATION

Serious arrhythmia is rare in pregnancy, but should cardioversion be necessary this may safely be performed without risk to the fetus.

Paroxysmal narrow complex tachycardia is the most common problem, as suggested by the age group in question. The mother often prefers to present for treatment if and when necessary, rather than to take prophylactic medication continuously during her pregnancy. Adenosine is safe in pregnancy, mainly because of its extremely short half-life, and can be freely used to terminate such tachycardias. Transient fetal bradycardia does occur, and the interval between incremental doses should probably be increased to allow for stabilization of the fetal heart rate.

Should prophylactic medication for narrow complex tachycardia be necessary, propranolol, oxprenolol and atenolol are considered reasonable choices, and are secreted only in small amounts in breast milk. Maternal beta-blocker usage is associated with bradycardia and hypoglycaemia in the neonate; these effects are short-lived, but a period of close observation of the neonate during the first day of life is mandatory. (NB: The newer short-acting intravenous beta-blocker, esmolol, is *not* free of these neonatal effects.)

Other specific arrhythmias should be treated as de-

Table 3. *Drugs in pregnancy and lactation*

Drug	Crosses placenta?	Present in breast milk?
Adenosine	Yes (but short half-life)	No
Verapamil	No	Yes
Digoxin	Small amounts	Small amounts
Flecainide	No data	?Yes
Amiodarone	No data	Yes
Disopyramide[a]	Yes	Yes
Magnesium	No data	No data
Procainamide	Yes	Yes
Atropine	No data	No data
Isoprenaline	No data	No data

[a] Can precipitate labour.

scribed in the earlier sections, modified as far as possible by the information given in Table 3. In difficult cases, the welfare of the mother is generally considered to override that of the fetus.

THE FUTURE

It is envisaged that there will be the development of an ECG and Arrhythmia Help-line, with FAX facilities for the transmission of ECGs. Many of the major arrhythmia centres already run an informal service, through the on-call cardiology staff.

With the advent of adenosine, the diagnostic dilemmas caused by broad complex tachycardias are largely a thing of the past. A heightened awareness of the need for a 12-lead ECG before considering intervention and a widespread use of adenosine should render cardiac arrhythmia in the emergency room a less stressful circumstance for patients and staff alike.

Bibliography

CAMM, A. & GARRATT, C. (1991). Adenosine and supraventricular tachycardia. *N. Engl. J. Med.*, **325**, 1621–9.

CHARLAP, S., KAHLAM, S., LICHSTEIN, E. *et al.* (1989). Electromechanical dissociation: diagnosis, pathophysiology, and management. *Am . Heart J.*, **118**, 355–60.

CLARK, A. & COTTER, L. (1991). DC cardioversion. *Br. J. Hosp. Med.*, **46**, 114–15.

GARRATT, C., MALCOLM, A. & CAMM, A.J. (1992). Adenosine and cardiac arrhythmias. *Br. Med. J.*, **305**, 3–4.

GARRATT, G., LINKER, N., GRIFFITH, M. *et al.* (1989). Comparison of adenosine and verapamil for termination of paroxysmal junctional tachycardia. *Am. J. Cardiol.*, **64**, 1310–16.

GILL, J., MEHTA, D., POLONIECKI, J. *et al.* (1990). Effect of flecainide, sotalol and verapamil upon ventricular tachycardia in patients with clinically normal hearts. *PACE*, **13**, 522.

GRIFFITH, M., DE BELDER, M., LINKER, N. *et al.* (1991). Multivariate analysis to simplify the differential diagnosis of broad complex tachycardia. *Br. Heart J.*, **66**, 166–74.

GRIFFITH, M., LINKER, N., GARRATT, C. *et al.* (1990). Relative efficacy and safety of intravenous drugs for the termination of sustained ventricular tachycardia. *Lancet*, **336**, 670–3.

GRIFFITH, M., LINKER, N., WARD, D. *et al.* (1988). Adenosine and the diagnosis of broad complex tachycardia. *Lancet*, 672.

GRUBB, B., TEMESY-ARMOS, P., HANN, H. *et al.* (1992). The use of external, non-invasive pacing for the termination of ventricular tachycardia in the emergency department setting. *Ann. Emerg. Med.*, **21**, 174–6.

ISERI, L.T. (1989). Role of magnesium in cardiac tachy-arrhythmias. In *Magnesium in Health and Disease*, ed. Y. Itokawa & J. Durlach, pp. 219–22. Paris: John Libbey & Co.

LINKER, N. (1992). Adenosine – a must for every casualty department. *Br. J. Hosp. Med.*, **47**, 565–6.

MEHTA, D., WAFA, S., WARD, D. *et al.* (1988). Relative efficacy of various physical manoeuvres in the termination of junctional tachycardia. *Lancet*, 8596.

TZIVONI, D., BANAI, S. SCHUGER, C. *et al.* (1988). Treatment of torsade de pointes with magnesium sulphate. *Circulation*, **77**, 392–7.

Further reading

DAVIES, M., WARD, D., CAMM, A. *et al.* (1989). Disorders of rhythm and conduction. In: *Diseases of the Heart*, ed. D. Julian. pp. 486–584. London: Baillière Tindall.

ZIPES, D. & JALIFFE, J. (1990). *Cardiac Electrophysiology. From Cell to Bedside*. New York: W.B. Saunders.

46 Vascular emergencies

D.C. MITCHELL[a] and R.F.M. WOOD[b]

[a] Department of Vascular Surgery, Southmead Hospital, Bristol, UK
[b] Department of Surgery, Northern General Hospital, Sheffield, UK

Chapter plan

Vascular emergencies due to trauma
Vascular emergencies not involving trauma
Venous problems

VASCULAR EMERGENCIES DUE TO TRAUMA

Introduction

Vascular injury presents major problems to clinicians looking after traumatized patients as immediate treatment may be required in order to save life. This applies particularly to penetrating injuries which damage the heart or major vessels.

More sinister, but equally threatening, are blunt injuries to major vessels, when life-threatening haemorrhage may be concealed. Intimal tears can lead to thrombosis of arteries with devastating consequences (e.g. bowel or limb infarction) if the injury is not rapidly detected and treated.

The essential first steps in the management of vascular trauma are to avoid delay in diagnosis and to intervene early. This prevents the problems associated with massive transfusion or prolonged tissue ischaemia. Diagnosis hinges on careful history-taking and detailed clinical examination with particular attention to the pulses in the area supplied by the arteries under suspicion.

Although sophisticated angiographic studies may occasionally be required, this is rarely the case. Most life- and limb-saving procedures can be accomplished with the assistance of portable fluoroscopic screening in the operating theatre to confirm clinical findings. The absence of major angiographic facilities should not be a reason for delay in initiating essential treatment.

Neck

The most common vascular problems in the neck are trauma to the carotid artery or jugular vein, between the clavicle and the angle of the jaw, as a result of stab wound injury or laceration from accidents involving broken glass. The likely site of injury can usually be judged fairly accurately from the position of the external puncture wound. Adequate local pressure will usually control the bleeding while the patient is resuscitated and assessed for the presence of other injuries. Preoperative clinical assessment should include a detailed neurological examination, bearing in mind that signs may be less reliable in the haemodynamically unstable patient. Attempts to use haemostats to achieve local control of haemorrhage should be avoided. This may exacerbate the vascular damage and compromise subsequent repair. In addition, there is a significant risk of causing damage to vital nerves.

Management

Patients presenting with haemorrhage from the neck should never have their wounds explored under local anaesthetic. General anaesthesia with intubation and ventilation is essential. Surgically the first priority is to obtain control of the internal jugular vein and the common carotid artery in the root of the neck, if need be by excision of part of the clavicle or median sternotomy (Pearce & Whitehill, 1988). As dissection proceeds in a cranial direction the site of the bleeding should become

931

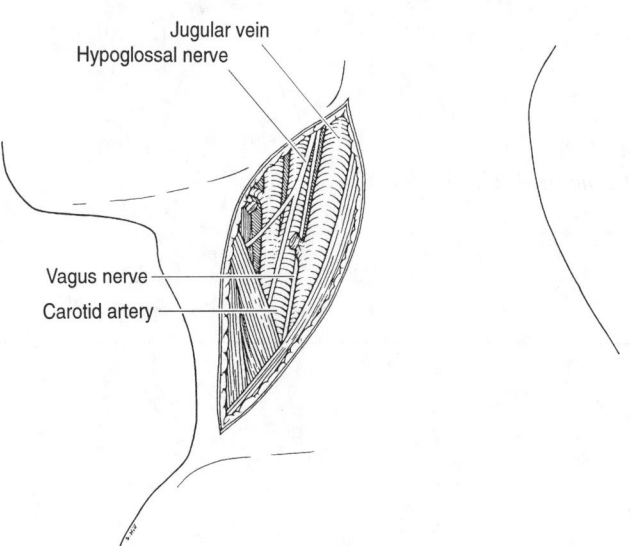

Fig. 1. Line diagram showing the relationship of the carotid vessels to the hypoglossal nerve and the vagus nerve.

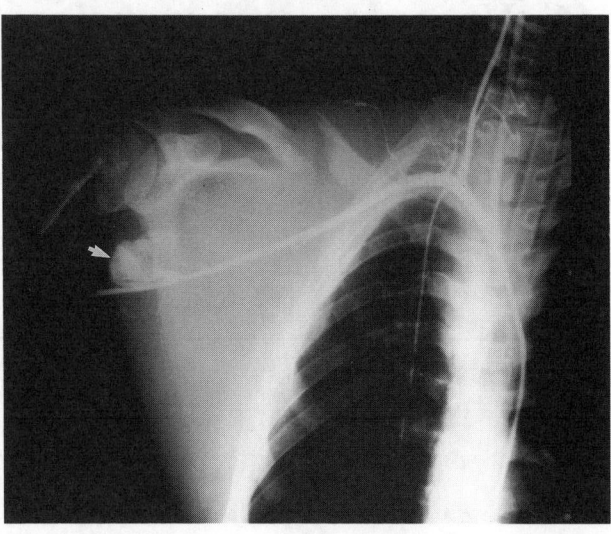

Fig. 2. Angiogram of expanding haematoma of axilla, with a tear in the axillary artery and a false aneurysm (arrowed).

apparent and more precisely directed pressure can be used to maintain control. It should also become clear whether both the artery and vein are involved. The dissection is then taken above the level of the bleeding which may involve separate mobilization of the internal and external carotid arteries. In mobilizing the internal carotid artery it is important to identify and preserve the hypoglossal nerve which runs across in front of the vessel (Fig. 1). Once adequate mobilization has been achieved, traction on vascular slings placed around the vessels should allow the damaged area to be inspected. A decision can then be made whether repair can be effected by direct suture of the vessel. In most cases there will have been trauma to the wall leaving a defect with an irregular edge. In this situation the vessel should be reconstituted with a vein patch of saphenous vein harvested from the thigh. Heparin, $60\,\mathrm{IU}\,\mathrm{kg}^{-1}$, should be given intravenously before applying vascular clamps to the vessels. The clamps should only be applied when the vein has been harvested and the repair is ready to proceed.

If extensive repair is required with prolonged clamping of the common carotid artery, consideration should be given to inserting a shunt to maintain the cerebral circulation.

In patients with total arterial occlusions discovered at surgery, ligation may be the safest option, especially if the patient had no evidence of neurological deficit prior to surgery. In those with neurological defects, restoration of flow by extracranial thrombectomy and arterial repair may offer a better chance of recovery. At the present time opinions are divided as to which is the best course to follow (Pearce & Whitehill, 1988).

Upper limb

The subclavian and axillary arteries

The subclavian and axillary arteries can be injured in high-speed road traffic accidents and this should be suspected if there is a fracture around the shoulder or of the first rib. The case illustrated (Fig. 2) is typical, presenting with an expanding haematoma of the anterior chest wall extending into the axilla. The pulse at the elbow was absent although the arm was viable and there was a strong Doppler signal over the brachial artery. More serious are traction injuries to the axillary vessels and the brachial plexus, which typically occur in motorcyclists. The question of early or delayed repair of the nerve injury remains controversial but prompt vascular repair is certainly indicated (McCready, 1988). Evacuation of haematomas around nerve trunks may improve neurological outcome in a few cases. The longitudinal pull on the vessel usually results in intimal rupture although the adventitia often remains intact. Excision of the damaged section with insertion of an interposition graft of saphenous vein is usually required. The axillary vein is only damaged in the most serious cases. Repair can usually be effected by direct suture although vein patching may be required.

Anterior dislocation of the shoulder can be associated with damage to the axillary artery. Pulses in the arm should always be checked after successful reduction of

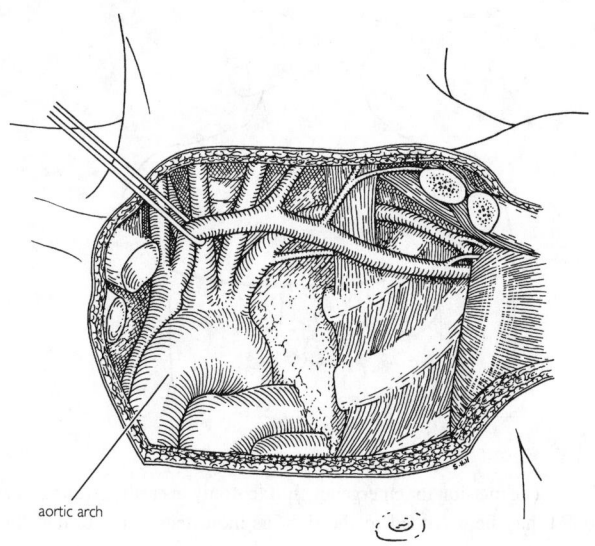

Fig. 3. Line drawing showing exposure of vessels in the root of the neck following division of the clavicle and manubrium. The sling is retracting the innominate vein.

the dislocation. Disruption of the vessel rarely occurs but injury to the vessel wall with the late development of aneurysm or arteriovenous fistula have been described.

Access to the arteries at the root of the neck involves a supra- or infraclavicular approach, with a median sternotomy for proximal subclavian artery injuries (Fig. 3).

The brachial artery

The brachial artery can be damaged in humeral fractures where it winds around the midshaft of the bone. However, this is a relatively rare injury. More common is entrapment of the artery in supracondylar fracture in children with the risk that a missed injury may result in Volkman's ischaemic contracture. Careful checking of the radial pulse following reduction of the fracture is essential. If the pulse is difficult to feel a Doppler pressure should be measured at the wrist. The flow signal at the wrist is first detected with a Doppler probe. A paediatric sphygmomanometer cuff is then placed around the arm and inflated. The pressure at which the flow signal becomes inaudible is noted and compared to a reading obtained in the uninjured arm. If there is a greater than 20 mmHg reduction in the systolic pressure distal to the fracture site then exploration of the vessel should be considered. If the vessel is explored it should always be opened and checked for intimal damage. It is unwise to entertain a diagnosis of vascular spasm (Barros D'Sa, 1992).

In modern medical practice the most common cause

of brachial artery injury is arterial cannulation for coronary angiography or angioplasty. Problems occur with inexperienced staff or when the procedure has been prolonged and several catheter changes have occurred. Presentation is with a cold, pulseless hand. The development of paraesthesia is an indication for urgent exploration. At operation it is not uncommon to find that the back wall of the vessel has been penetrated at some point in the procedure. Local dissection is also not unusual. Repair with a generous vein patch will usually give a good result, even if there is only a relatively narrow strip of the arterial wall remaining in continuity. Interposition vein grafts can be used if the damage is extensive but orientation can be difficult and kinking of the graft as it runs across the elbow joint is a risk.

On-table arteriography should be routinely employed to check the distal circulation at the end of reconstruction and evidence of occlusion is an indication for thrombectomy. In the unusual instance of being unable to retrieve all the clot, local instillation of thrombolytic agents (100 000 U of streptokinase or 5 mg of recombinant tissue plasminogen activator – rt-PA) may clear the distal arterial tree. The use of systemic thrombolytic agents is clearly contraindicated in patients with multiple trauma, or in individuals who have undergone surgery within the last 14 days.

Radial and ulnar artery damage

Isolated damage to the radial artery does not require repair and the vessel can be safely ligated. The blood supply to the hand will be maintained by the ulnar artery via the palmar arch, but patency of the ulnar artery should be checked. Trauma sufficient to divide both the ulnar and radial arteries is usually accompanied by extensive tendon and nerve damage. Such cases require urgent referral to a specialist hand centre with facilities for microsurgical repair of the vessels.

Thoracic (see also Chapter 23)

Aorta

Deep stab wounds causing haemorrhage from the aorta are usually fatal. However, with improvements in prehospital transportation, some of these patients may reach hospital alive. This is one of the few indications for an immediate thoracotomy to arrest life-threatening haemorrhage.

In the era before dished steering wheels and seat belts,

traumatic rupture of the aortic arch was a recognized complication of head-on collisions. The central boss of the steering wheel pushed the ribcage back sufficiently to allow the arterial trauma to occur. The adventitia frequently remained intact and cases were diagnosed on the basis of a marked widening of the mediastinal shadow on chest X-ray. This injury is now rarely seen. If it does occur the intimal rupture is usually at the junction of the relatively mobile aortic arch with the descending aorta which is fixed in position by the intercostal arteries. Thoracotomy and Dacron grafting of the arterial defect are required.

Heart

Injuries to the heart are either penetrating, from knife wound or gunshot, or blunt as seen following high-speed motor vehicle accidents. Both types of injury are being seen with increasing frequency in Britain and the USA, probably because of a real increase in their occurrence coupled with improved prehospital care and transportation (Ivatury & Rohman, 1989).

Penetrating injuries

This should be suspected in any individual with an injury over the cardiac outline, mediastinum or the epigastrium. Pericardial lacerations often seal themselves, and the resulting haemorrhage from the heart fills the pericardial cavity, giving rise to cardiac tamponade. The classic signs of distended neck veins, faint heart sounds and low blood pressure may only be evident in a minority of patients as may the sign of pulsus paradoxus (Ivatury & Rohman, 1989). The key to diagnosis is a high index of suspicion.

In the unstable patient, airway control and rapid infusion with central venous cannulation may improve matters temporarily. In the more severely compromised patient, pericardiocentesis may aid diagnosis and alleviate tamponade to allow time to prepare for thoracotomy, but this procedure carries a significant false negative and false positive rate and findings should be treated with caution.

More severely compromised patients who are moribund or appear to be 'dead on arrival' (but who had signs of life on the way to hospital) should undergo immediate thoracotomy through the 5th intercostal space in the resuscitation room (Fig. 4). Pericardiotomy, avoiding injuring the phrenic nerve, will release blood with improvement in the circulation. Digital control of the cardiac wound can be used whilst adequate exposure is

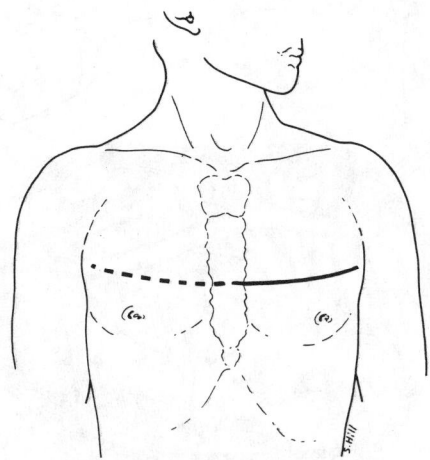

Fig. 4. The incision for emergency thoracotomy in cardiac trauma. The wound may be extended to the right as indicated by the dotted line.

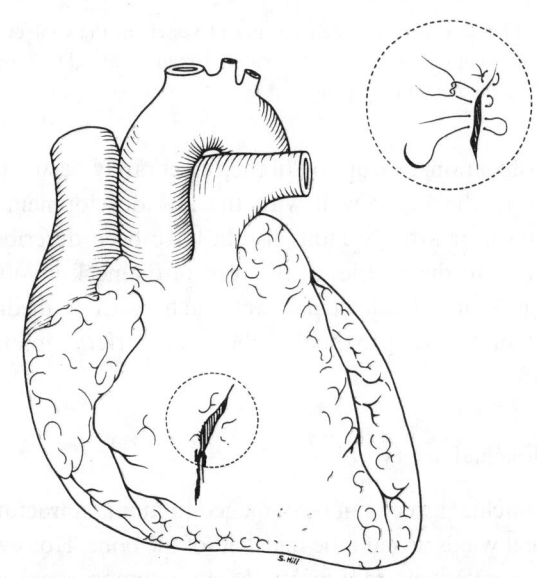

Fig. 5. Line diagram of penetrating cardiac stab wound and insert showing the technique of placing horizontal mattress sutures.

obtained. In about 75% of cases the injury will be in the right or left ventricle; coronary artery injury is the exception rather than the rule. Horizontal mattress sutures should be used to avoid oversewing coronary arteries (Fig. 5). Sutures should ideally be placed over small Teflon pledgets to provide a buttress, but strips of pericardium will suffice in their absence. Using such techniques, survival rates of between 30% and 50% are reported from major centres in the USA. Although the presence of a cardiac surgeon is ideal, cardiopulmonary bypass is rarely required and its absence should not delay thoracotomy in the severely compromised patient.

When the diagnosis is uncertain in an unstable patient, or when laparotomy is required, a subxiphoid approach allows a window to be cut in the pericardium. This may be used to check for the presence of suspected tamponade, before proceeding to thoracotomy.

Gunshot injuries are more likely to be associated with severe haemorrhage due to renting of the pericardium and cardiac chambers. As a result they carry a poorer prognosis than knife wounds. Suture of the cardiac wounds may form an essential part of the initial resuscitation in survivors, using the techniques outlined above.

Blunt injuries

Compression of the heart in road accidents when the ribcage impacts against the steering wheel or safety belt may lead to cardiac contusion or rupture. Management hinges on immediate surgery for the moribund and supportive therapy for those with contusions. The latter diagnosis should be confirmed with serial ECGs (electrocardiograms) and cardiac enzyme estimation.

Following recovery from the immediate injury, all patients with cardiac trauma should be followed up. They should be monitored with echocardiography and ECGs for the presence of unsuspected septal or valvular injury.

Abdominal trauma (see also Chapter 24)

Major bleeding from trauma to the aorta or vena cava is perhaps the most challenging of all surgical emergencies. In the shocked patient with a grossly distended abdomen following stabbing or gunshot injury, urgent laparotomy is clearly required. As with ruptured abdominal aortic aneurysms, a catastrophic fall in blood pressure may occur on induction of anaesthesia. Therefore the patient should be anaesthetized on the operating theatre table with the surgical team scrubbed and prepared. At least 10 units of compatible blood should be available. A long midline incision is made and clot evacuated to allow a rough assessment of the major source of haemorrhage. As far as possible bleeding should be controlled by packs. If the infrarenal aorta is clearly the site of injury, proximal control should be achieved by mobilizing and clamping below the level of the renal arteries. If the area of damage is close to, or above, the renal arteries it may not be possible to control the haemorrhage at this level. In this situation, control should be obtained by cross-clamping at the level of the diaphragm, either abdominally by dividing the lesser omentum and the diaphragm if necessary, or through a 7th intercostal space thoracotomy. This latter approach

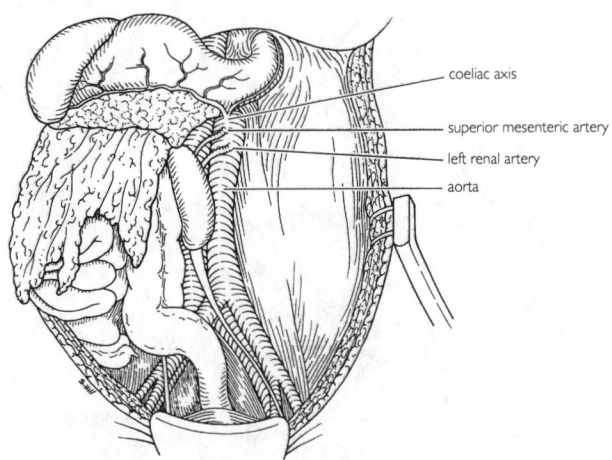

coeliac axis
superior mesenteric artery
left renal artery
aorta

Fig. 6. Line diagram showing the exposure of the abdominal aorta achieved by mobilization of the contents of the left side of the abdomen.

allows cross-clamping of the aorta in the chest. Suction should then be able to cope with the outflow from the traumatized area. The defect is defined by mobilization of all structures lying to the left of the abdominal aorta (Fig. 6) and more precise abdominal control of the aorta achieved. If the aortic defect is readily visualized, passing balloon catheters proximally and distally may be the best way of controlling the problem until adequate mobilization is achieved. It may be possible to suture the defect directly but, if this is likely to lead to narrowing of the aorta, a Dacron or PTFE patch should be inserted.

Major venous bleeding is often more difficult to control than arterial haemorrhage. Blood wells up into the wound and defining the origin can be difficult. In this situation packing is undoubtedly the best option until experienced vascular help is available. It may be necessary to mobilize the duodenum and the iliac vessels in the pelvis to obtain adequate proximal and distal control (Fig. 7). Alternatively, if a large defect is present as for the aorta, balloon catheters may provide the best means of controlling the haemorrhage. Vein patching of the caval defect may be required and if a substantial portion of the wall has been lost it may be necessary to suture two opened segments of saphenous vein together to produce a 'panel' graft of sufficient size to cope with the defect.

Mesenteric vessel injury

Distal vessel injury adjacent to the bowel is best dealt with by ligation and excision of bowel as required. The injured proximal artery should be ligated and a vein bypass implanted between the superor mesenteric artery

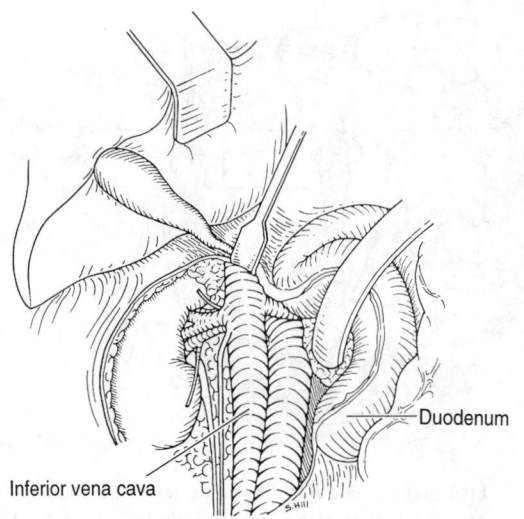

Fig. 7. Line diagram showing the approach to the abdominal infra-hepatic vena cava, with the duodenum and right colon being retracted to the left.

and the aorta at a convenient position. Timely intervention will revascularize bowel, but if there is doubt about bowel viability, a second look laparotomy 24 h later is indicated (Linblad & Hakansson, 1987).

Renal artery (see also Chapter 25)

Direct penetrating injury may devascularize the kidney and blunt injury may lead to intimal tearing and thrombosis. In either case, if there is not an immediate indication for exploration, a patient with haematuria should ideally have an intravenous urogram in the emergency room. This will indicate the presence of functioning renal tissue on the side of injury and the presence or absence of a contralateral kidney.

The absence of function on one side is an indication for renal arteriography. Arterial injuries can be repaired, but are often best left if the patient is stable as exploration may convert a contained haematoma into a frank haemorrhage leading to an avoidable nephrectomy (Carroll et al., 1990). Carefull follow-up and monitoring of renal function and blood pressure, with repeat angiography, is an essential part of the long-term care of these patients.

Pelvic fractures (see also Chapter 31)

These injuries constitute a major threat to life as patients often suffer massive blood loss, especially if the injury is an open one. The priorities are to stabilize the bony injury which may in itself arrest the bleeding. In 'open-book' fracture-dislocations, the application of an external fixation device may be used to reduce and stabilize the fracture. With more extensive fractures it may not be possible to stabilize the fragments in this way and some other form of bracing may be required. The use of pneumatic compression devices such as the MAST garment may help (Mucha & Welch, 1988), although its use remains controversial (Mattox et al., 1986).

Patients with pelvic fractures may have other injuries requiring laparotomy and in such cases the pelvic haematoma should be left undisturbed. If the patient is unstable, pelvic packing may arrest haemorrhage. Failing this, arterial embolization has been used successfully to treat continuing haemorrhage in a few cases (Margolies et al., 1972; Van Urk et al., 1978).

Direct exploration of the internal iliac vessels is a last resort and may provoke new haemorrhage. Vessel ligation may be unsuccessful because of the rich collateral supply around the hip and buttock. In such cases, survival may be bought at the price of extensive amputation.

Lower limb

Assessment of lower limb arterial supply

Careful palpation of lower limb pulses is a vital part of assessing the adequacy of the arterial circulation in patients with potential arterial injury. However, in elderly patients and shocked individuals, pulses may be difficult to feel. Clinical assessment should *always* be augmented by examination with a hand-held Doppler. It is not sufficient to simply detect an audible Doppler signal and examination should include the measurement of the ankle:brachial index (ABPI). The index should normally be 1.0 or greater. A values of 0.9 or lower should raise suspicion of proximal arterial injury. Arteriography should be considered and, if there is clear evidence that the arterial supply is compromised, it may be prudent to undertake the procedure in the operating theatre to avoid additional delay in restoring flow (see below).

Frequent re-assessment using Doppler is helpful in cases with equivocal findings. It is an essential part of post-operative care in patients where arterial reconstruction has been performed. A deterioration in the Doppler signal quality or ABPI is an indication for further arteriography or exploration.

Common femoral artery

The traditional injury to the common femoral artery occurs in butchers boning large joints of meat: the knife slips and lacerates the vessels in the groin. The vessels can also be damaged in crush injuries. The diagnosis is usually readily apparent and angiography to define the lesion is unnecessary. Proximal control of the artery may prove difficult and there may be a temptation to divide the inguinal ligament. However, it is better to achieve control of the external iliac artery above the level of the inguinal ligament. A separate curved incision is made in the iliac fossa deepened through the external oblique aponeurosis and the internal oblique muscle. The transversalis fascia is divided and the peritoneum is reflected from the floor of the iliac fossa allowing access to the external iliac artery and vein. The profunda femoris and superficial femoral artery can then be identified and controlled distal to the common femoral artery. A vein patch is usually required to reconstitute the femoral artery. PTFE patches are best avoided in this situation because of the risk of infection and secondary haemorrhage.

The superficial femoral artery

Fractures of the shaft of the femur, particularly if they are comminuted, can cause damage to the superficial femoral artery. The incidence of arterial trauma is greatest when there has been extensive local trauma (e.g. with blast injuries or high-speed road traffic accidents). The combination of an open wound with an unstable fracture and ischaemia is a complex situation calling for a coordinated approach by vascular and orthopaedic teams. The immediate priority is to revascularize the limb and this is best achieved by performing on-table angiography and exploring the vessels at the site of occlusion.

The femoral vessels should be exposed in the groin and the common femoral artery mobilized. An 18 gauge butterfly cannula is inserted into the superficial femoral artery and the in-flow temporarily occluded by placing an arterial clamp on the common femoral artery. With an X-ray plate placed under the limb at the presumed level of arterial injury 20 ml of suitable contrast material is injected through the cannula. If a mobile screening unit is available the procedure can be carried out using smaller volumes of contrast material and, by moving the screening unit down the limb during the injection, it will be possible to image the run-off vessels below the knee.

Ideally the revascularization should take place before orthopaedic manoeuvres to stabilize the fracture. In very unstable fractures there is a risk that the arterial repair may be compromised during efforts to achieve reduction. If this is felt to be a possible problem, consideration should be given to inserting arterial and venous shunts while the bony injury is dealt with (Barros D'Sa, 1992). Lengths of silastic dialysis tubing can be used with the Teflon vessel tip placed in the common femoral vessels proximally and the popliteal vessels distal to the site of injury. With the use of external fixators, which can be applied fairly rapidly, the need for temporary shunting has receded. Definitive orthopaedic repair can then be delayed until soft tissue healing is well advanced.

When on-table films are assessed there is usually a clearly delineated site of arterial occlusion. Arterial spasm should never be accepted as the diagnosis of an attenuated appearance of the artery. In virtually every case there will be an intimal dissection and the vessel will subsequently thrombose if it is not repaired surgically. Longitudinal arteriotomies and vein patches may be adequate for minor defects, but extensive open wounds of the thigh involving the superficial femoral vessels require grafting. In these cases, the saphenous venous system may be the only route of venous drainage of the limb and vein should be harvested from an uninjured site such as the contralateral limb or arm if this is possible. Grafts should be inserted into clean undamaged tissue where possible and may need to be tunnelled extra-anatomically (e.g. through the obturator foramen) to avoid dirty and devascularized tissues. If this is not possible, then a covering of healthy muscle should be placed over the graft at the end of the procedure.

It is vitally important to check that the arterial run-off is adequate. If the patient is hypotensive and shut down peripherally, pulses may be impalpable despite an adequate arterial repair. Therefore, in trauma cases, on-table angiography on completion of the revascularization procedure is mandatory.

Popliteal artery

This artery is most commonly injured in fracture-dislocation of the knee (Fig. 8) resulting from high-speed motor vehicle accidents, although gun and blast injuries are seen with increasing frequency (Barros D'Sa, 1992; Perry, 1991). The arterial injury is often a contusion with intimal dissection (Fig. 9) and localized thrombosis.

Angiography preoperatively, or on-table should be used to define the level of injury. Exploration of the

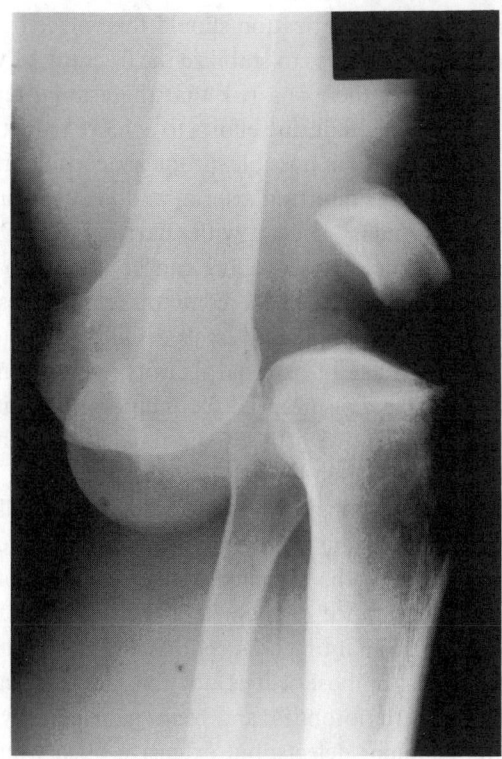

Fig. 8. Dislocation of the knee.

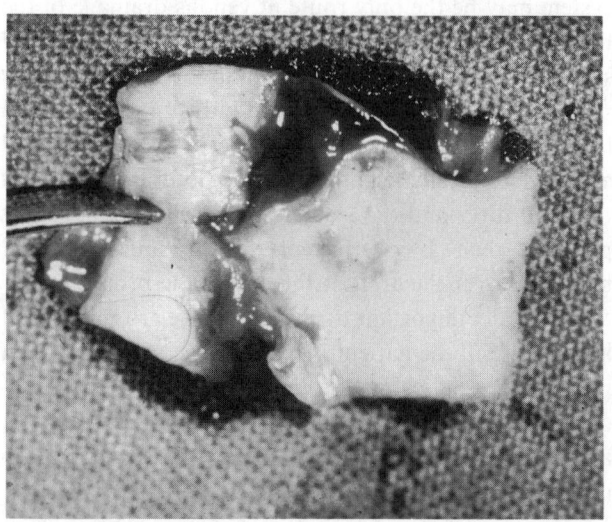

Fig. 9. Resected specimen of popliteal artery from the case in Fig. 8 showing an intimal tear. The artery was thrombosed at exploration.

artery with local vein patching or a short vein graft placed across the damaged artery will usually restore blood flow to the leg. Grafts should be tunnelled along the route of the popliteal artery to avoid compromising the blood supply in any subsequent orthopaedic repair. The arterial run-off should be checked angiographically if foot pulses are not immediately palpable.

Fixation of the fracture by traction or external fixators is essential to stabilize the knee and protect the arterial repair.

Tibial arteries

Injury to all three tibial arteries is rare and may not be compatible with limb salvage. In such conditions amputation may be the safest course in preference to prolonged attempts at revascularization, especially in the severely injured patient with multiple trauma. The decision to amputate should only be taken with the involvement of an experienced vascular surgeon.

Embolization may occur after proximal injury or arterial revascularization and is most easily detected by angiography. As most trauma victims have relatively normal vessels before injury, the absence of arteries on angiography must be attributed to embolism or thrombosis. A timely embolectomy, performed under fluoroscopic control, will often result in restoration of arterial patency. The use of thrombolytic agents in the severely injured patient is fraught with danger and is contraindicated.

Fasciotomy

In both the upper and lower limbs vascular injury will result in muscle ischaemia causing oedema and swelling after revascularization. The division of the deep fascia and skin overlying the muscle compartments reduces the tension in the tissues and improves the circulation. Fasciotomies should always be considered if revascularization cannot be achieved within 4 h of injury. Both skin and fascia should be left open, with antiseptic dressings. Delayed suture of the skin, or split skin grafting can be undertaken when healing is well established.

Open wounds

Any injured vessels or grafts should be covered at least with viable muscle at the end of the procedure, but these attempts should not compromise healing. Contaminated wounds following road accidents or blast injuries should be adequately debrided and left open. Tetanus immunization must be confirmed, and adequate doses of intravenous antibiotics active against clostridia and anaerobes are needed.

Primary closure of dirty wounds may result in the growth of anaerobic organisms, threatening survival of both limb and patient. With exposed graft material, frequent dressings and inspection of the wound will rapidly reveal where an adequately vascularized muscle flap may be found to cover the exposed vessels. Once the wound is clean, early skin grafting will assist in obtaining cover.

Reperfusion injury and the role of amputation

There is a significant risk of muscle infarction if total arterial ischaemia lasts for more than 6 h. Similarly, crush injuries cause both vascular occlusion and muscle necrosis. Reperfusion of infarcted tissues may lead to the massive release of metabolites and myoglobin, which become trapped in the kidneys leading to renal failure. This may prove to be a fatal insult in the multiply injured patient. Where there is evidence of prolonged ischaemia or extensive tissue necrosis in the limb, revascularization may be inappropriate and the patient's future well-being best served by amputation. Such decisions are not made easily and may require the advice of experienced surgeons. It should be remembered that young fit trauma victims have excellent potential for rehabilitation and may achieve near normal mobility on a well-fitting modern prosthesis.

VASCULAR EMERGENCIES NOT INVOLVING TRAUMA

Transient cerebral ischaemia (see also Chapter 53)

The majority of strokes occur as the result of embolism, with a minority being due to haemorrhage (Thomas & Eastcott, 1992). About 20% of patients if questioned when recovering from a stroke will admit to having experienced transient symptoms in the period prior to the stroke. These 'transient ischaemic attacks' (TIA's) are characterized by neurological signs and symptoms which usually completely resolve within a few hours, but always within 24 h. If the neurological deficit persists for a longer period of time it is termed a 'stroke'. In most cases there will be evidence of cerebral infarction on brain imaging.

In a typical TIA the patient experiences numbness and weakness of a limb or a transient hemiparesis. If the blood supply to the dominant hemisphere is involved there may also be speech disturbance. Patients can also experience 'amaurosis fugax' – a temporary blindness usually described as the sensation of a curtain coming down over the visual field. This is due to interruption of flow in the ophthalmic artery caused by cholesterol debris from an ulcerating atheromatous plaque at the carotid bifurcation. In the acute situation cholesterol crystals can sometimes be visualized within the retinal vessels on examination of the fundi.

Management

Patients will frequently be referred to an accident and emergency (A&E) department after having had a TIA. It is important to check that there is *no* residual neurological deficit. If the patient has a carotid bruit the diagnosis can be made with confidence on the basis of the history and clinical findings. Admission is not required but an early neurological/vascular surgical opinion is required. Unless there are any contraindications, the patient should be started on aspirin (150 mg per day) and arrangements made, via the general practitioner, for a carotid duplex Doppler scan prior to specialist assessment. Angiography or magnetic resonance angiography may also be required (Fig. 10). Patients with a stenosis

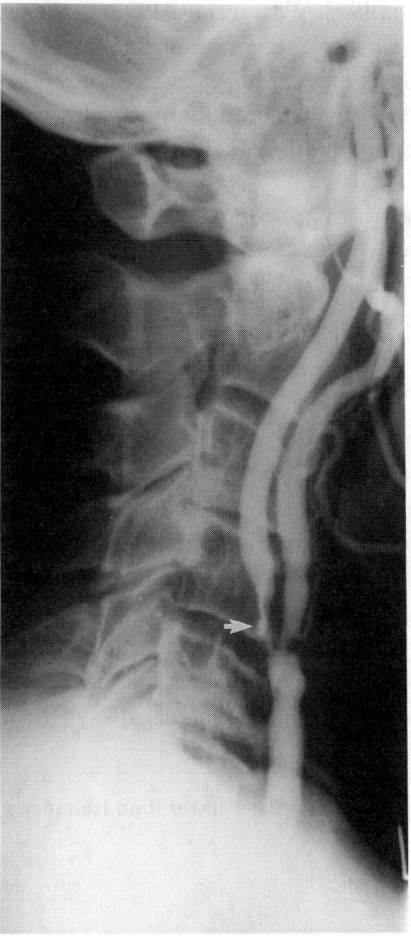

Fig. 10. Carotid angiogram showing tight stenosis of the left internal (arrow) and external carotid artery origins.

of greater than 70% should ideally have a carotid endarterectomy within a week of presentation (European Carotid Surgery Trialists' Collaborative Group, 1991; NASCET Collaborators, 1991). Patients who do not have an obvious carotid source should also undergo echocardiography to seek a possible cardiac source of emboli, in addition to a CT (computed tomography) or MR (magnetic resonance) scan of the brain to exclude other intracerebral pathology.

Crescendo transient ischaemic attacks

Patients may sometimes present with repeated TIAs occurring every few hours, but with full recovery after each episode. Such patients are at increased risk of developing a stroke. They often have a critical stenosis in the internal carotid artery and impending occlusion.

In the past it was held that these patients, although known to be at increased risk of completed stroke, did badly with carotid endarterectomy. Recent reports (Greenhalgh et al., 1993; Wilson et al., 1993) challenge this view and suggest that this group of patients may do better with an emergency carotid endarterectomy. These patients require emergency referral for a neurological and vascular surgical opinion.

The acutely ischaemic lower limb

Acute lower limb ischaemia presents with the five 'Ps' beloved of medical students. The cause of the problem is either embolus or thrombosis-in-situ, the occlusion develops at the site of an established atheromatous narrowing in the vessel. Differentiating between these two causes is vitally important to achieve the best chance of saving the limb. Arterial emboli were once extremely common but have now become a relative rarity. This results from the reduced incidence of rheumatic heart disease and the increased use of maintenance anticoagulant therapy in patients with cardiac arrhythmias.

Unfortunately many doctors still have the impression that an acutely ischaemic limb is always the result of an

---

The five Ps of the acute lower limb ischaemia

- Painful
- Paraesthetic
- Pale
- Pulseless
- Perishing cold

---

embolus. An ill-considered attempt at embolectomy in a patient with thrombosis-in-situ will amost always result in amputation unless the true nature of the problem is recognized at the time and specialist help is available to revascularize the limb. There are a number of features which can be helpful in making the differential diagnosis (Table 1). The Doppler ankle:brachial index should be measured in all patients presenting with lower limb ischaemia.

Management

Embolus

The patient with clear-cut features of an arterial embolus should be transferred to the operating theatre for an embolectomy without delay. As in the management of arterial trauma, the totally ischaemic limb may not recover if revascularization is not effected within 6 h. The femoral vessels in the groin are explored and the thrombus is removed using a Fogarty embolectomy catheter. On-table angiography at the end of the procedure is important to ensure that the distal circulation has been adequately cleared. If full revascularization of the tibial arteries has not been achieved the outcome may be improved by the local infusion of a single dose of streptokinase, 100 000 U in 100 ml of saline, over 30 min. Alternatively, rt-PA may be used in a dose of 5 mg. Repeat X-ray screening should be used to confirm that perfusion of the distal arterial circuit has been improved. Traditionally, embolectomy procedures have been carried out with sedation and local anaesthesia rather than general anaesthesia in the belief that less stress was caused to a patient where the embolus followed a recent myocardial infarct. However, it now seems likely that the stress is just as great with local anaesthesia and the procedure can usually be carried out more quickly and with a better exposure of the femoral vessels under general anaesthesia.

Thrombosis-in-situ

If thrombosis-in-situ is suspected, an angiogram is required. The treatment options are either thrombolytic therapy or reconstructive surgery. The angiogram catheter is left in situ for the delivery of thrombolytic drugs. If the patient has a good femoral pulse on the side of the lesion it may be advantageous for the radiologist to consider an antegrade puncture of the vessel. However, if there is doubt about the arterial in-flow, the arteriogram should be obtained by using a retrograde Seldinger

Table 1. *Clinical features of acute arterial thrombosis and embolism*

Thrombosis-in-situ	Embolus
Often there is a history of ischaemic symptoms – in particular intermittent claudication	No history of ischaemic symptoms
	History of recent myocardial infarction
The patient is in sinus rhythm	The patient may have an irregular pulse (typically atrial fibrillation
Examination of the limb reveals chronic ischaemic changes – muscle wasting, hair loss, nail thickening, ulceration	The limb shows no signs of chronic ischaemia and the pulses on the other side are normal (this does not apply to the patient with a saddle embolus)
There may be signs and symptoms of generalized arterial disease	

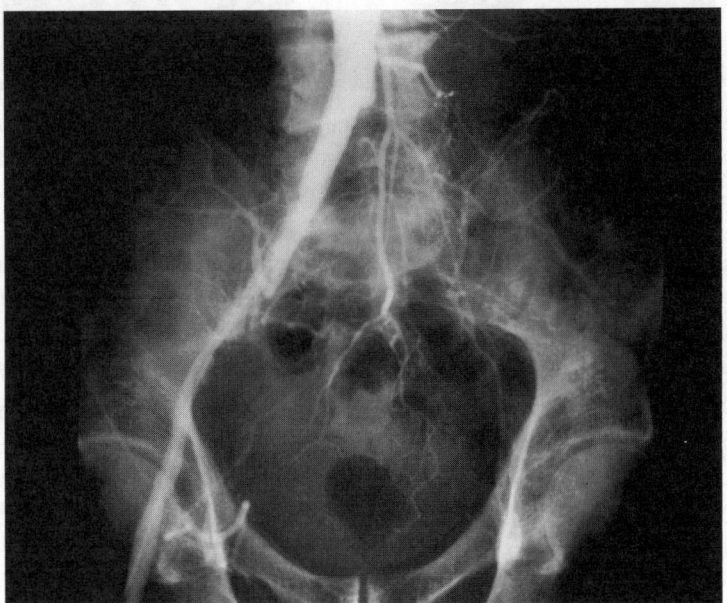

Fig. 11. Arteriogram showing acute occlusion of the left common, internal and external iliac arteries (Mr J.J. Earnshaw's case).

puncture of the contralateral common femoral artery (Fig. 11). This approach retains the possibility of passing the catheter over the bifurcation of the aorta and into the common iliac artery on the side of the occluded artery. The management of these cases requires the combined skills of the interventional radiologist and the vascular surgeon.

Once the site of the block has been identified the possibility of using thrombolytic therapy can be considered. If there are features to suggest that irreversible changes are imminent – severe pain, total loss of movement and staining of the skin – only urgent surgical revascularization has any chance of saving the limb and thrombolytic therapy should not be attempted. If the leg is not in this critical state thrombolysis may be the preferred option. The angiography catheter is left *in situ* or exchanged for a special catheter with multiple side holes at the distal end. The catheter is advanced into the thrombus and either streptokinase at a dose of 5000 units h^{-1}, or rt-PA at 0.5 mg h^{-1}, is infused with heparin, 500 units h^{-1} by syringe pump (Earnshaw, 1991; Berridge *et al.*, 1989). The patient must be closely monitored, on a ward with experienced staff, for improvement in perfusion or haemorrhagic side-effects. If thrombolytic therapy is to be effective there should be evidence of lysis within a few hours. A further X-ray should be obtained at this time (Fig. 12). This may be performed in the radiology department or on the ward using a

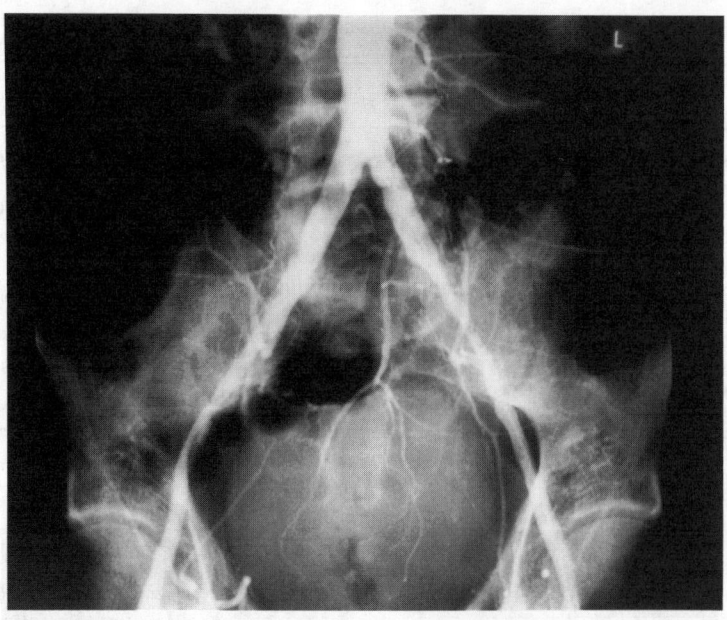

Fig. 12. Arteriogram of the same patient as Fig. 2 following successful thrombolysis. Note the long stenosis of the external iliac artery that was probably the site of initial thrombosis.

portable X-ray machine and injecting contrast material down the catheter. If some lysis has been achieved it may be possible to advance the catheter into the thrombus and deliver a further bolus of thrombolytic therapy. The case should be constantly reviewed over the first 24 h from the start of treatment. In successful cases, the thrombus should be fully lysed by that time and it may then be possible to carry out balloon angioplasty of the underlying atheromatous lesion. If significant thrombus remains and the limb is still ischaemic at 36–48 h, reconstructive surgery will be required. The duration of thrombolysis and decisions regarding the optimal timing of surgery need to be taken by experienced radiologists and vascular surgeons.

Upper limb ischaemia

Significant arterial disease of the axillary and brachial arteries is extremely rare. Acute ischaemia of the upper limb is therefore almost always the result of embolism or trauma.

The typical symptoms of an upper limb embolus are pain and coldness of the hand and forearm. The situation usually improves and by the time the patient is assessed in hospital the pain may have largely subsided. Movement is preserved and the hand, while cooler than on the contralateral side, appears viable. Previously the advice given in these circumstances was to start the patient on systemic heparin but not to pursue more active measures. However, while the arm requires relatively little blood supply to remain viable, muscle function is liable to be compromised unless normal arterial supply is restored. Arteriography may be used to demonstrate the level of occlusion (Fig. 13), but this can now be assessed non-invasively using modern duplex Doppler equipment. If the occlusion is distal to the axillary artery the brachial artery should be explored at the elbow under local anaesthesia and an embolectomy performed using a 2F Fogarty catheter. Propagation of thrombus into the radial and ulnar arteries may have occurred and if adequate clearance cannot be obtained by embolectomy a bolus of streptokinase or rt-PA in the same doses as given above for the lower limb may be infused distally to improve recanalization. Unless the brachial artery is of particularly good calibre, a small vein patch should be inserted at the site of the arteriotomy.

Patients with a cervical rib may occasionally present with an acute ischaemic upper limb (Fig. 14). This occurs when thrombosis supervenes in the dilated segment of the subclavian artery distal to the narrowing created as the vessel arches over the rib. In these cases there will usually be a long history of vascular and neurological symptoms affecting the limb. Appropriate plain X-rays taken in the A&E department should show the cervical rib and the patient can then be urgently referred for specialist treatment.

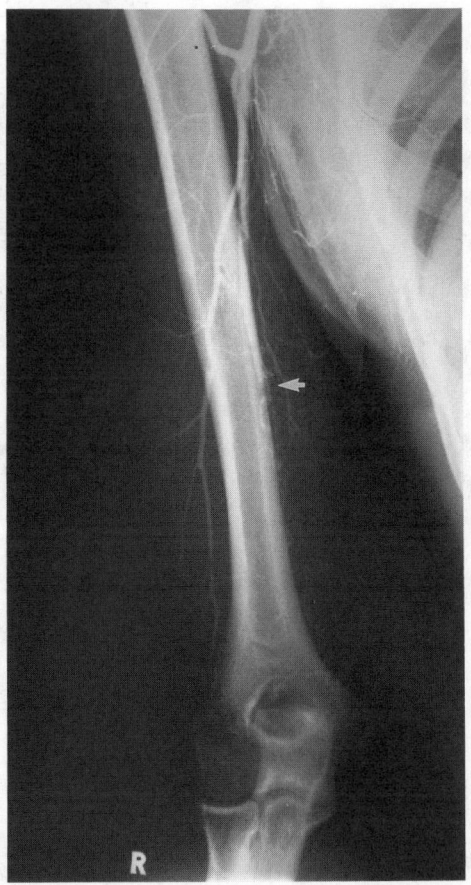

Fig. 13. Arteriogram showing embolus occluding the right brachial artery (arrow).

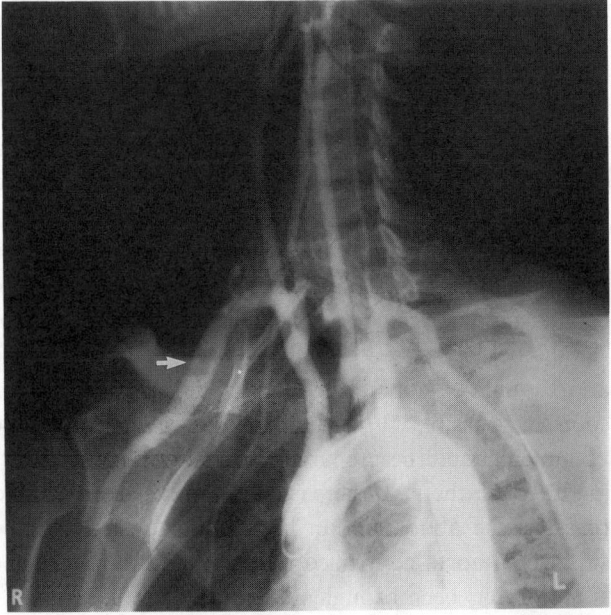

Fig. 14. Arteriogram of patient with cervical rib and acutely ischaemic upper limb. Note poststenotic dilatation and filling defect within artery (arrow).

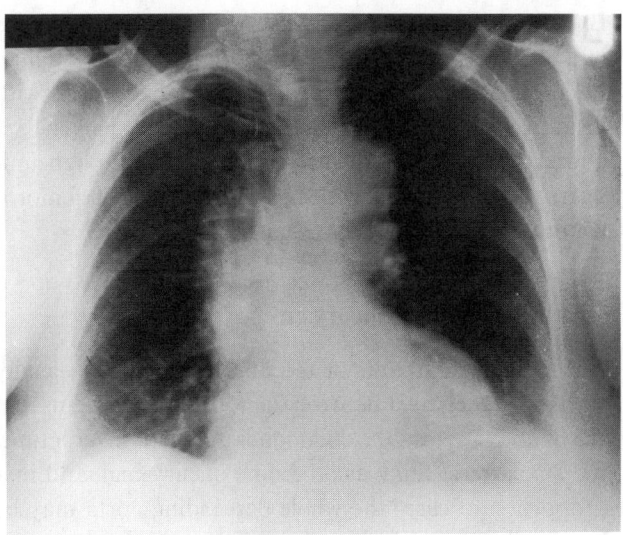

Fig. 15. Chest X-ray showing widened aortic arch due to dissection.

Acute presentation of aneurysmal disease

Dissecting aneurysms of the aorta

The dissection usually originates in the ascending aorta just distal to the aortic valve and the ostia of the coronary arteries. The dissection then tracks around the aortic arch and down the descending thoracic aorta. The patient presents with severe pain in the chest and the upper back. Rupture of the media is caused by excess blood pressure and the patients are usually found to have a systolic pressure close to 200 mmHg. The dissection of the ascending aorta can produce a diastolic murmur and a pericardial friction rub. Blood pressure in the right arm will be reduced if there is dissection around the innominate artery and lower limb pulses may be unequal. Widening of the aortic arch on chest X-ray is a characteristic feature (Fig. 15).

Initial management is to control the hypertension with an intravenous infusion of beta-blockers and nitroprusside. If the patient's condition stabilizes, transfer to a cardiothoracic unit is indicated. Patients require long-term antihypertensive therapy and may need surgical replacement of the aortic arch, either electively at about 4 weeks or as an emergency if cardiac function is compromised by dissection involving the aortic valve, coronary ostia or rupture into the pericardium (Eastcott et al., 1992). If the dissection extends to the abdominal aorta there may be further problems. Dissection around the renal and superior mesenteric artery origins occurs relatively infrequently. However, if these vessels are occluded there is little chance of the patient surviving.

Extension of the dissection into the iliac vessels results in a femoral pulse with a characteristic tapping quality. In complex dissections extending to the iliac vessels with distal ischaemia, aortic bifurcation grafting may be required to restore lower limb blood flow, although unilateral limb ischaemia may be best treated with femoro-femoral crossover grafting.

Abdominal aortic aneurysms

Aneurysmal dilatation of the abdominal aorta usually starts in the segment between the renal artery origins and the bifurcation into the common iliac arteries. With time, the iliac arteries may also become aneurysmal, and in a proportion of cases the whole descending aorta may be involved. These 'thoracoabdominal aneurysms' occur more commonly in patients with familial dilating disease (e.g. Marfan's syndrome). In these patients, aneurysms occur at multiple sites, particularly in the femoral and popliteal arteries. These cases represent a major challenge for elective repair and should they rupture the patient is unlikely to survive.

Although small aneurysms can still rupture, the aortic diameter has normally reached 6 cm before this becomes a significant risk. Anteriorly the lumen of the aneurysm is filled with layered thrombus. However, the posterior wall frequently has little thrombotic covering and as it disintegrates the aneurysm erodes the bodies of the lumbar vertebrae. When the wall gives way, blood may leak retroperitoneally giving rise to severe back pain. Patients who present acutely at this point have the best chance of survival. They may only have leaked a few hundred millilitres of blood and are haemodynamically stable. The pulsatile aneurysmal sac should be readily palpable. If there is uncertainty about the diagnosis, a plain abdominal X-ray (Fig. 16) and particularly an ultrasound or CT scan should be obtained urgently. In most cases it will be possible to stabilize the patient and obtain fully cross-matched blood before proceeding directly to repair.

Anterior rupture of the aneurysm into the peritoneum or massive retroperitoneal haemorrhage constitute a major surgical emergency. Diagnosis is seldom difficult. There is often a history of back pain for 24–48 h prior to sudden collapse of the patient. On admission to the A&E department the patient will be hypotensive and tachycardic with abdominal distension and tenderness. Resuscitation should be commenced immediately; oxygenation of the patient is essential but ideally intubation and ventilation should be delayed until the patient has

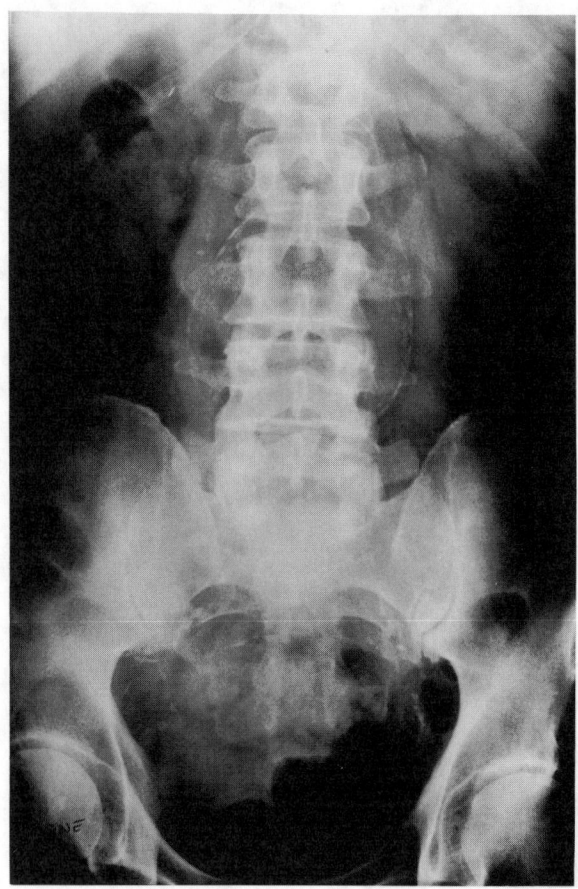

Fig. 16. Plain abdominal X-ray showing calcification in the wall of an abdominal aortic aneurysm.

reached the operating theatre. Vasodilatation associated with the induction of anaesthesia can cause a sudden collapse in blood pressure and result in cardiac arrest.

Although many patients are significantly hypotensive on admission, the situation will have stabilized with a blood pressure of around 90 mmHg. Clotting of blood from the rupture will have produced a temporary tamponade of the defect in the aortic wall. Aggressive efforts to raise the blood pressure in these individuals may be counter-productive and reactivate the bleeding. The patient should be transferred directly to the operating theatre and 10 units of compatible blood should be obtained as soon as possible. For the reasons given above the abdomen should be prepared and drapped before starting the anaesthetic. If there is a sudden collapse in blood pressure the abdomen can be opened rapidly and the suprarenal aorta controlled by direct pressure until the situation has been brought under control.

The preferred operation is to replace the aneurysm with a straight tube graft; bifurcated grafts are only required when the iliac arteries are also aneurysmal (Fig. 17).

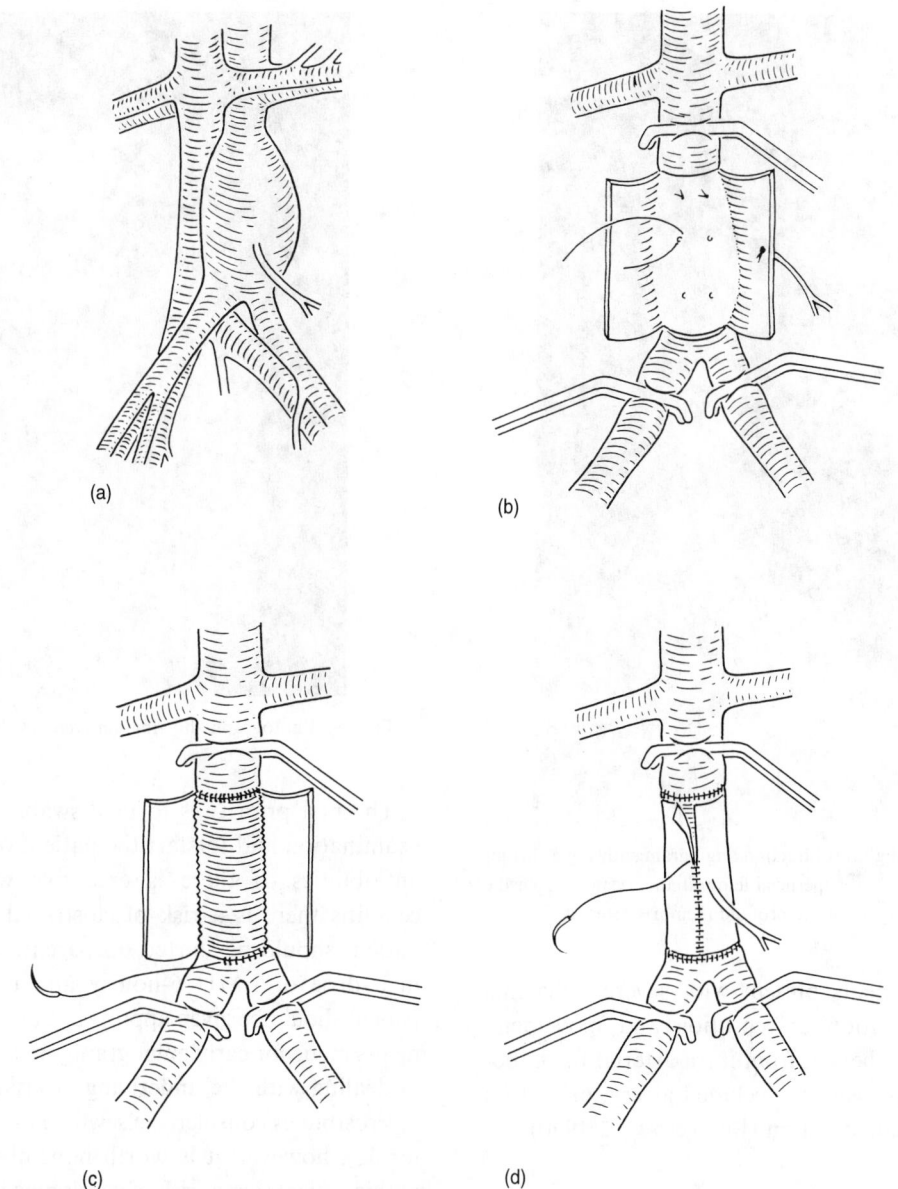

Fig. 17. Line drawing showing the essential steps in grafting an abdominal aortic aneurysm: (a) identify aneurysm; (b) clamps applied above and below aneurysm, sac opened and lumbar vessels oversewn; (c) inlay grafting within sac; (d) sac being closed over graft.

Femoral and popliteal aneurysms

Femoral aneurysms are readily diagnosed and very obvious to the patient. They can thrombose but rarely present as an emergency (Fig. 18). Popliteal aneurysms are potentially a much more serious problem and not infrequently present as an emergency with an acutely ischaemic limb. Rupture is excessively rare but thrombosis relatively common. As in the aorta the lumen of the aneurysm is lined with layered thrombus. In most cases the distal tibial arteries are affected by the thrombotic process and angiography often reveals that there is only a single patent run-off vessel. When the aneurysm thromboses completely, the geniculate collaterals around the knee also become occluded and there is therefore no blood supply to the calf and foot. Unless dealt with rapidly, irreversible ischaemic changes soon supervene. The thrombosed popliteal aneurysm constitutes a vascular surgical emergency and, as in trauma cases, unless flow can be restored within 6 h there is a significant risk that amputation will be required. Without restoration of arterial flow the calf muscles will become infarcted and the leg will have to be amputated above the knee. If revascularization is possible, a fasciotomy is advisable to prevent foot drop and other neurological problems.

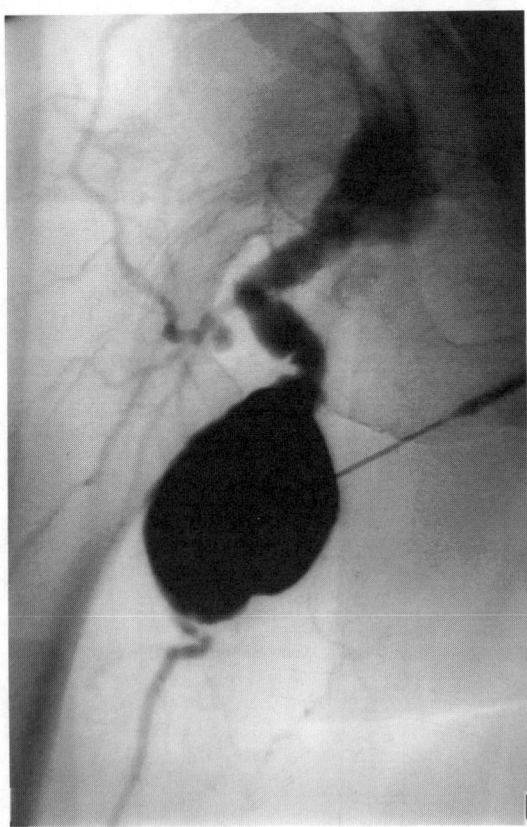

Fig. 18. Intra-arterial digital subtraction angiogram showing a thrombosed common femoral and superficial femoral aneurysm. The needle has punctured an aneurysm of the profunda femoris artery.

Occasionally patients present with severe ischaemia with some preservation of sensation and movement. These patients may benefit from intra-arterial thrombolytic therapy to re-open the occluded artery, prior to a more definitive reconstruction (Bowyer *et al.*, 1990).

The ischaemic foot

Patients with rest pain and distal ischaemia often present as an emergency. The initial appearance of the limb may be worrying but it is important to establish when the patient first had symptoms and how long any ulceration or gangrene has been present. While urgent referral to a vascular surgical clinic is required it is not always essential to admit the patient. The factors which should prompt admission are:

1. A recent deterioration in symptoms and the development of persistent pain.
2. Purplish discoloration of the toes with swelling of the forefoot.
3. Ulceration or gangrene associated with swelling and cellulitis (Fig. 19).

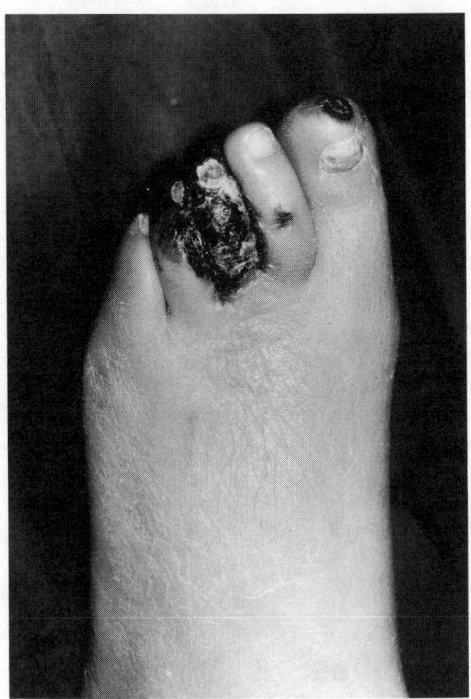

Fig. 19. Photograph showing gangrene of the medial four toes.

The first priority is to take swabs for bacteriological examination and to start the patient on broad-spectrum antiobiotics. If there is extensive wet gangrene and cellulitis there is a risk of clostridial infection and the patient should be started on parenteral benzylpenicillin in a dose of 1 MU 6-hourly and metronidazole. The patient should be given appropriate analgesia and arrangements made for early angiography to assess the possibility of dealing with the underlying arterial lesion.

Frostbite is considered elsewhere in this volume (Chapter 38); however, it is worth remembering that arteriopathic patients are at risk of developing ischaemic problems with their feet in severe winter weather. The classic case is the vagrant sleeping rough on the streets, but elderly patients with a borderline lower limb arterial supply can provoke problems by undertaking tasks like clearing snow from drives and paths while their feet are inadequately protected.

The diabetic foot (see also Chapter 57)

Foot problems in the diabetic are mainly the result of tissue damage secondary to neuropathy. The characteristic problem of the neuropathic foot is the mal perforans ulcer. This is a painless ulcer of the sole of the foot (Fig. 20). Neuropathy affecting the innervation of the small muscles of the foot alters the equilibrium between the

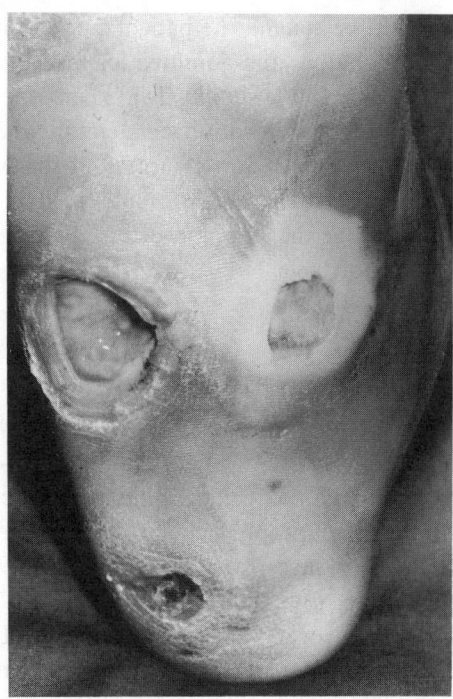

Fig. 20. Extensive neuropathic ulceration on the sole of a diabetic foot.

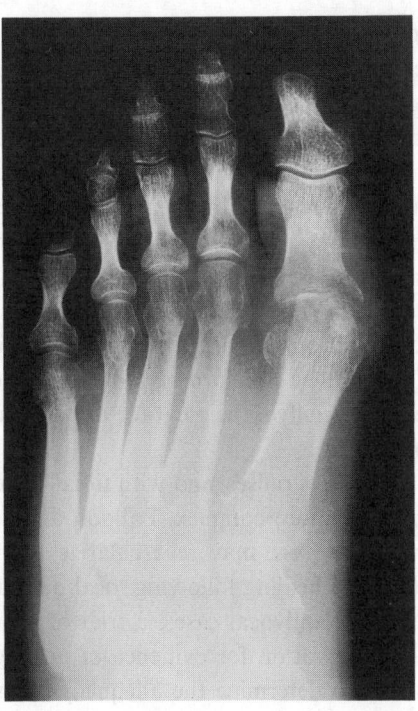

Fig. 21. Osteomyelitis of the first metatarsal in a diabetic with an infected ulcer on the sole of the foot. Note the destruction of the metatarsal head and loss of joint space.

flexor and extensor muscle groups. This results in a change in weight distribution during walking with excess load transmitted to the metatarsal heads. The response is hyperkeratosis and callus formation. Glycosylation of keratin produces a callus that is more rigid than normal and shear forces cause cavitation to develop beneath it. A break in the callus will allow the entry of bacteria and subsequent ulceration. Infection can track back along the tendon sheaths to cause a plantar abscess. Patients with significant neuropathy also develop clawing of the toes with the risk of ulceration over the dorsum of the interphalangeal joints. Pressure from adjacent toes or toenails may produce ulcers on the side of the toes and toe tip breakdown can occur through rubbing on the shoe.

The neuropathic foot with ulceration presents a long-term management problem for the diabetologist, requiring specialist surgical and chiropody input. Patients may from time to time present in the A&E department with a flare-up of infection and spreading cellulitis. The first step is to take swabs for aerobic and anaerobic culture and to start the patient on broad-spectrum antibiotics. Surgery may be required to lay open and drain deep-seated infection in the sole of the foot. Preventing weight bearing through damaged tissue until healing is complete is a very important aspect of management of these ulcers.

A more commom problem in the A&E department is the ischaemic foot in the elderly diabetic. Often the patient presents with one or more ischaemic toes, or an area of necrotic skin in the forefoot or around the heel. There is often surrounding cellulitis and there may be evidence of pus – so called 'wet gangrene'. There is usually an associated neuropathy so the patient feels little pain despite the severity of the physical signs.

A careful history may reveal the initial trauma that led to necrosis and infection, often a new pair of shoes that are too small and pinch the toes. Examination will confirm the absence of pulses, but the ABPI on hand-held Doppler may be more than 1. The surgeon should not reassured, as there is often arterial calcification in diabetic patients and the arteries are incompressible giving a falsely optimistic impression of the ABPI. In the absence of pulses, it is safer to disregard the ABPI if it does not fit with the clinical findings and proceed to arteriography. The picture is often one of severe tibial arterial disease with surprisingly normal looking proximal limb arteries.

If pulses are present in the foot and the arteries are compressible, then it may be safe to perform a local digital amputation of the necrotic tissue and to drain any pus. However, infection tends to track back into the foot via the tendon sheaths. X-ray will often reveal evidence of osteomyelitis affecting the metatarsal head (Fig. 21) and extending periosteal thickening along the shaft of the bone. If exploration reveals pus tracking in the web space, a ray incision or amputation may be required and it is important to obtain consent for this beforehand if there are signs of spreading sepsis in the forefoot. The minimum amount of tissue should be excised and all viable tissue preserved consistent with obtaining adequate drainage of pus. This sometimes leads to unorthodox looking amputations of part of the foot, but it is surprising how useful even a deformed looking foot can be to the patient, especially if the great toe and first metatarsal can be preserved.

In the absence of pulses, and with tibial vessel disease, the situation is more complex. Balloon angioplasty, or distal arterial bypass, may revascularize the foot adequately to allow healing following local debridement or amputation. In equivocal cases, a trial of local surgery with close observation for evidence of healing may be the only way to determine the adequacy of the arterial blood supply. Where revascularization is not possible or fails, then an early below-knee amputation may give better long-term mobility than repeated unsuccessful attempts at local foot surgery.

Infective complications of vascular reconstruction

Graft infection is a potential disaster for the patient with peripheral vascular disease. There is usually no alternative but to remove the graft and achieving revascularization through uninfected tissue planes is a major challenge to the vascular surgeon. The patient who returns to the A&E department with an infected wound after arterial reconstruction does not necessarily have infection of the graft. However, it is prudent to admit the patient, take swabs and start broad-spectrum systemic antibiotics. Discharge of serous fluid from the groin is not uncommon following exploration of the femoral vessels. This is caused by division of lymphatics at the time of surgery. The problem will settle with time and re-exploration of the groin is seldom indicated. More worrying is the patient who presents with secondary haemorrhage from the groin or the site of distal anastomosis in the limb. If this occurs at any time following discharge from hospital it is highly likely to be due to infection of the graft. As these patients may develop catastrophic haemorrhage without warning, they should be admitted as an emergency under the care of a vascular surgeon. Problems are commoner in patients who have had multiple vascular procedures requiring re-exploration of the groin. Special-

ist help should be sought, the patient started on broad-spectrum antibiotics and admitted for investigation.

Aortoduodenal fistula should always be borne in mind in the patient presenting with haematemesis where there is a history of previous aortic surgery. If the patient is fortunate enough to have a warning bleed it may be possible to salvage the situation before there is massive and fatal haemorrhage.

VENOUS PROBLEMS

Deep venous thrombosis

Venous thrombosis is a major cause of in-hospital morbidity although the incidence has reduced considerably with the use of prophylactic heparin and graduated compression stockings (Kakkar & Stringer, 1990). Although there are specific surgical factors which increase the incidence of deep venous thrombosis (DVT), a number of established risk factors apply to patients in hospital and those presenting from the community. These include obesity, malignancy, pregnancy, the oral contraceptive pill, and most potently a past history of DVT. There are a range of situations in which patients may present as an emergency with a DVT:

1. Elderly or at-risk patients following a prolonged period sitting immobile on a plane or bus journey.
2. During late pregnancy from pressure of the gravid uterus on the iliac veins.
3. Spontaneously in women on oral contraceptives.
4. Patients with previously unsuspected malignancy.

The typical presentation is with pain and swelling of the calf. There may be dilatation of the superficial veins and ankle oedema. In patients in late pregnancy, thrombosis affects the iliac veins and in this situation the whole limb will be swollen. Duplex Doppler scanning has revolutionized the diagnosis of DVT (Mitchell et al., 1991). Although the technique has some limitations in the detection of minor calf DVT, an experienced operator will easily identify thrombus in the popliteal and femoral veins (Fig. 22). The procedure is totally non-invasive and has now replaced venography as the investigation of choice.

Patients with calf DVT require treatment with heparin followed by oral anticoagulation for 3 months. In those with more extensive thrombosis involving the popliteal, femoral and iliac veins, longer term anti-coagulation is indicated and should by coupled with follow-up investigation using ultrasound, venography or MR venography

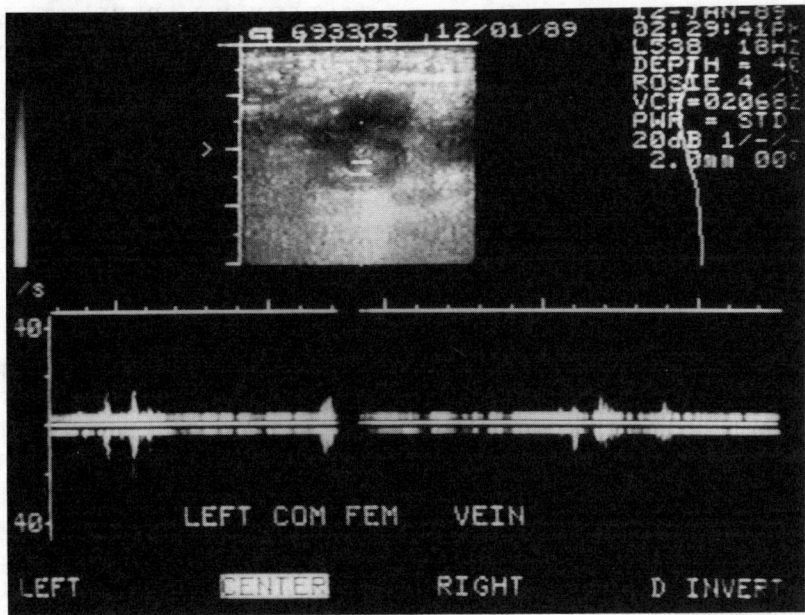

Fig. 22. Duplex scan of femoral deep venous thrombosis. Note absence of normal phasic respiratory flow pattern in Doppler signal.

of pelvin veins to ensure clearance of the thrombus. Compression hosiery may improve swelling and discomfort in these patients.

Massive DVT, the so-called massive blue or white leg constitutes a more complex problem, as the viability of the limb may be threatened. If it complicates pregnancy, then extensive anticoagulation may be contraindicated. In such cases, if limb viability is threatened, consideration should be given to formal thrombectomy, although the results of such surgery are anecdotal. Postoperative anticoagulation will be required as for ilio-femoral DVT.

In non-pregnant patients, thrombolysis may be an option to consider in addition to anticoagulation. It is probably wise to place a temporary inferior vena caval filter prior to lysis to prevent pulmonary embolus. It should be borne in mind that such massive DVT may be the outward manifestation of undetected malignancy, especially in the retro-peritoneum, and these patients should undergo investigation including CT scanning to exclude an obvious tumour. Long-term anticoagulation should be considered in these patients and they should be provided with compression hosiery to prevent subsequent leg ulceration.

Thrombophlebitis

As the name implies this condition is due to thrombosis and an associated inflammatory reaction in the superficial veins. It occurs spontaneously in patients with varicose veins. Full resolution with fibrosis of the thrombosed veins may take 6 weeks to 2 months. The process will be prolonged where the veins were grossly dilated. Treatment is with analgesics. More sinister is the migratory type of superficial thrombophlebitis which may be associated with underlying inflammatory or malignant conditions.

Bleed from varicose veins

In patients with chronic changes from venous hypertension there is a high risk of haemorrhage from the dilated thin-walled veins which commonly surround the area of lipodermatosclerosis at the ankle. Haemorrhage can be profuse and if first aid measures have been inadequate the patient may be hypotensive and in need of resuscitation on admission. Surgical exploration is seldom required. The bleeding will always stop with elevation of the leg. A non-adherent gauze dressing should be applied followed by firm bandaging. Admission and elevation for 24 h is usually effective in achieving control of the problem. The patient should subsequently be referred for surgery to the incompetent veins to prevent recurrent bleeding.

Complications from treatment of varicose veins

The increase in out-patient injection sclerotherapy and day surgery treatment for varicose veins has produced extra problems for the staff of A&E departments. Patients may occasionally develop an allergic reaction to injection sclerotherapy and present with swelling and itching of the affected limb. More commonly the compression has been ineffective and there is extensive tender thrombophlebitis extending well beyond the site of the injection. If there is evidence to suggest an allergic reaction, antihistamines are often helpful. Appropriate non-steroidal analgesics should be prescribed and the patient advised to rest in bed at home with the limb elevated. If the sclerosant has been inadvertently injected into the subcutaneous tissues there is a risk of skin breakdown. There will be redness and blistering of the skin at the injection site. A non-adherent dressing should be applied and the patient should be seen within 48 h at the clinic where the initial treatment was carried out.

Avulsion through small stab incisions is the treatment of choice for calf varicosities. If large-calibre veins have been avulsed there is a risk of bleeding if the patient is up and about at home following discharge from a day surgery unit. Re-exploration is seldom required as elevation and compression – as for patients bleeding from ruptured varicose veins – will rapidly control the problem.

Acknowledgements

We would like to thank Mr J.J. Earnshaw for permission to reproduce Figs. 2 and 3. We would also like to thank Dr J.E. Dacie for permission to reproduce Figs. 4 and 5. The photographs were produced by the Department of Medical Illustration at St. Bartholomew's Hospital and Miss Sandy Hill drew the line diagrams.

Bibliography

Vascular emergencies due to trauma

BARROS D'SA, A.A.B (1992). Arterial injuries. In *Arterial Surgery*, 3rd edn, ed. H.H.G. Eastcott. Edinburgh: Churchill Livingstone.

CARROLL, P.R., McANINCH, J.W., KLOSTERMAN, P. et al. (1990). Renovascular trauma, risk assessment, surgical management and outcome. *J. Trauma*, **30**, 547–52.

IVATURY, R.R. & ROHMAN, M. (1989). The injured heart. *Surg. Clin. North Am.*, **69**, 93–110.

LINBLAD, B. & HAKANSSON, H. (1987). The rationale for second look operation in mesenteric vessel occlusion with uncertain viability at primary surgery. *Acta Chir. Scand.*, **153**, 53–4.

MARGOLIES, M.N., RING, E.J., WALTMAN, A.L. et al. (1972). Arteriography in the management of hemorrhage from pelvic fractures. *N. Engl. J. Med.*, **287**, 317–21.

MATTOX, K.L., PEPE, P.E., BOCKELL, W.H. et al. (1986). Prospective randomized evaluation of the 'MAST' garment in hemorrhagic shock. *J. Trauma*, **26**, 779–84.

McCREADY, R.A. (1988). Upper extremity vascular injuries. *Surg. Clin. North Am.*, **68**, 725–40.

MUCHA, P. & WELCH, T.J. (1988). Hemorrhage in major pelvic fractures. *Surg. Clin. North Am.*, **68**, 757–73.

PEARCE, W.H. & WHITEHILL, T.A. (1988). Carotid and vertebral arterial injuries. *Surg. Clin. North Am.*, **68**, 705–23.

PERRY, P.M. (1991). The popliteal artery – sinister harbinger of pathology. In *Vascular Surgery: Current Questions*, eds. A.A.B. Barros D'Sa, P.R.F. Bell, S.G. Darke & P.L. Harris. pp. 165–76. Oxford: Butterworth-Heinemann.

VAN URK, H., PERLBERGER, R.R. & MULLER, H. (1978). Selective arterial embolization for control of pelvic haemorrhage. *Surgery*, **83**, 133–7.

Vascular emergencies not involving trauma

BERRIDGE, D.C., GREGSON, R.H.S., HOPKINSON, B.R. et al. (1989). Intra-arterial thrombolysis using recombinant tissue plasminogen activator (t-PA): the optical agent at the optimal dose? *Eur. J. Vasc. Surg.*, **3**, 327–32.

BOWYER, R.C., CAWTHORN, S.J., WALKER, W.J. et al. (1990). Conservative management of asymptomatic popliteal aneurysm. *Br. J. Surg.*, **77**, 1132–5.

EARNSHAW, J.J. (1991). Thrombolytic therapy in the management of acute limb ischaemia. *Br. J. Surg.*, **78**, 261–9.

EASTCOTT, H.H.G., HOLLIER, L.H., CRAWFORD, E.S. et al. (1992). Aneurysms. In *Arterial Surgery*, 3rd edn, ed H.H.G Eastcott. Edinburgh: Churchill Livingstone.

EUROPEAN CAROTID SURGERY TRIALISTS' COLLABORATIVE GROUP: MRC EUROPEAN SURGERY TRIAL (1991). Interim results for symptomatic patients with severe (70–99%) or mild (0–29%) carotid stenosis. *Lancet*, **337**, 1235–43.

GREENHALGH, R.M., CUMING, R., PERKIN, D.G., et al. (1993). Urgent carotid surgery for high risk patients. *Eur. J. Vascl. Surg.*, **7** (Suppl. A), 25–32.

KAKKAR, V.V. & STRINGER, M.D. (1990). Prophylaxis of venous thromboembolism. *World J. Surg.*, **14**, 670–8.

MITCHELL, D.C., GRASTY, M., STEBBINGS, W.S.L. et al. Comparison of duplex ultrasound and venography in the diagnosis of deep venous thrombosis. *Br. J. Surg.*, **78**, 611–13.

NASCET Collaborators (1991). Beneficial effect of carotid endarterectomy in symptomatic patients with high-grade stenosis. *N. Engl. J. Med.*, **325**, 445–53.

THOMAS, D.J. & EASTCOTT, H.H.G. (1992). Carotid-vertebral insufficiency. In *Arterial Surgery*, 3rd edn, ed. H.H.G. Eastcott. Edinburgh: Churchill Livingstone.

WILSON, S.E., MAYBERG, M.R., YATSU, F. et al. (1993). Crescendo transient ischemic attacks: a surgical imperative. *J. Vasc. Surg.*, **17**, 249–56.

47 The acute abdomen

B. D. GEORGE[a] and R. CAMPBELL[b]

[a] Department of General Surgery, John Radcliffe Hospital, Oxford, UK
[b] Department of General Surgery, South Tyrone Hospital, Dungannon, Northern Ireland

Chapter plan

Introduction
Pathology
History
Examination
Basic investigations
Preliminary management decisions
Conditions managed without admission to hospital
The need for immediate surgery
Surgery after prompt resuscitation
Admission for further assessment
Medical causes of the acute abdomen
Special problems in the acute abdomen

INTRODUCTION

The term acute abdomen is used to describe patients with clinical features that suggest the presence of significant intra-abdominal pathology of recent onset.

Optimum management presents a challenge to the clinicians involved. Although abdominal pain is usually the dominant symptom, in some circumstances (particularly the elderly, the obese and those on steroids), serious intra-abdominal pathology may be relatively silent. Some causes of the acute abdomen require prompt surgical intervention (e.g. perforated viscus), others require conservative management (e.g. pancreatitis) and others are due to nearby non-abdominal pathology (e.g. basal pneumonia or inferior myocardial infarction) or 'medical' conditions (e.g. diabetic ketoacidosis or porphyria). The major aim of management is to distinguish those cases that require timely surgical intervention from those that do not require surgery and those that require specific medical care.

Table 1. *Pathology of the acute abdomen*

Category	Type	Examples
Inflammation	Localized	Acute appendicitis
		Acute cholecystitis
		Acute diverticulitis
	Generalized	Perforated duodenal ulcer
Obstruction	Simple	Small bowel obstruction due to carcinoma of caecum
	Complicated	Strangulated femoral hernia
	Pseudo	Large bowel pseudo-obstruction
		Post-operative ileus
Haemorrhage	Intraperitoneal	Ruptured ectopic
	Retroperitoneal	Ruptured aortic aneurysm
	Gastrointestinal	Bleeding duodenal ulcer

PATHOLOGY

The pathology of the acute abdomen may be considered in three main categories (Table 1):

- Inflammation.
- Obstruction.
- Haemorrhage.

Features of one or more of these categories may be present simultaneously. For example a patient with acute appendicitis may have features of inflammation localized to the right lower abdomen, but with no features of obstruction or haemorrhage. A patient with a strangulated femoral hernia, however, may have inflammation localized to the site of the hernia and also intestinal obstruction. The clinical presentation depends on the type or types of intra-abdominal pathology.

HISTORY

For the majority of patients presenting with an acute abdomen, the traditional history–examination–investigation approach is employed. In extreme cases, such as a ruptured abdominal aortic aneurysm, the ABC approach (see Chapter 5) may be more appropriate.

The most common presenting symptom of the acute abdomen is abdominal pain. Time spent eliciting the details of this pain is likely to be well spent.

Main site of pain

The site of abdominal pain depends on whether the visceral or parietal peritoneum is stimulated. Most intra-abdominal structures are covered at least partially by visceral peritoneum, the innervation of which depends on its embryological origin. Foregut derivatives include the stomach, the duodenum as far as the ampulla of Vater, the liver, gallbladder and spleen. From the mid-second part of the duodenum to a point two-thirds of the way along the transverse colon, the gut is derived from the midgut. The remainder of the large bowel is derived from the hindgut. Visceral peritoneal sensation travels with the autonomic nerve fibres and tends to produce poorly localized pain. Generally, pain from the foregut is referred to the epigastrium, from the midgut to the periumbilical region and from the hindgut to the suprapubic area.

The parietal peritoneum is supplied by the somatic nervous system. The diaphragmatic peritoneum is supplied by the phrenic nerve (C4). The remainder of the parietal peritoneum is supplied segmentally by intercostal and lumbar nerves. (In parts of the pelvis the obturator nerve is the chief source of supply). Irritation of parietal peritoneum produces pain which is precisely localized to the site of irritation. The site of abdominal pain associated with acute appendicitis provides a good example: in the early phases of appendicitis only the visceral peritoneum is inflamed. As the appendix is embryologically part of the midgut this results in a poorly localized periumbilical pain. As the disease process progresses the nearby parietal peritoneum becomes inflamed and the pain *moves* to the right iliac fossa.

Radiation of pain

Abdominal pain may radiate to other sites in addition to the main site, a feature which may give a clue to the site of origin. Irritation of the undersurface of the diaphagm (for example, due to a subphrenic abscess) may be referred to an area of skin over the shoulder tip. This is because the brain interprets pain 'in the phrenic nerve' as coming from the area of skin with the same segmental innervation (C4). Pain of renal origin is usually felt in the loin, but may radiate into the groin and testis, due to the similar nerve supply of structures which have a common embryological origin. Pain due to inflammation of retroperitoneal structures often radiates to the back (e.g. posterior duodenal ulcer, pancreatitis or an abdominal aortic aneurysm). Referral of pain may also occur due to pressure on a sensory nerve. Pressure on the obturator nerve due to tumour, or rarely an obturator hernia, results in pain radiating down the medial side of the thigh to the knee in the cutaneous distribution of the obturator nerve.

Occasionally the site of the radiating pain may overshadow the main pain, leading to diagnostic confusion. Retroperitoneal rupture of an abdominal aortic aneurysm may present with back pain only, an important consideration if the proposed management is bed rest and non-steroidal anti-inflammatory drugs.

Intensity–time course of pain

The mode of onset of abdominal pain, either instantaneous or gradual, and its subsequent behaviour (e.g. continuous, colicky or progressing) may give important clues to its cause. These features can be represented in an intensity–time graph (Fig. 1). Pain of instantaneous onset must be considered to be due to rupture of an intra-abdominal viscus with release of its contents into the peritoneal cavity (or more rarely an acute vascular accident). This may occur with rupture of a simple ovarian cyst, but more serious pathology, such as a ruptured ectopic pregnancy or a perforated peptic ulcer, must be considered. The pain of pancreatitis typically starts gradually and reaches a crescendo. Pain that waxes and wanes is usually termed colicky pain. Fluctuating severe pain that never entirely subsides is characteristic of ureteric colic. Intermittent spasms of pain that ease off completely between episodes is more typical of acute small bowel obstruction.

Aggravating and relieving factors

- Abdominal pain that is aggravated by movement is suggestive of parietal peritoneal inflammation. Hence, pain that is worse when the patient moves or coughs,

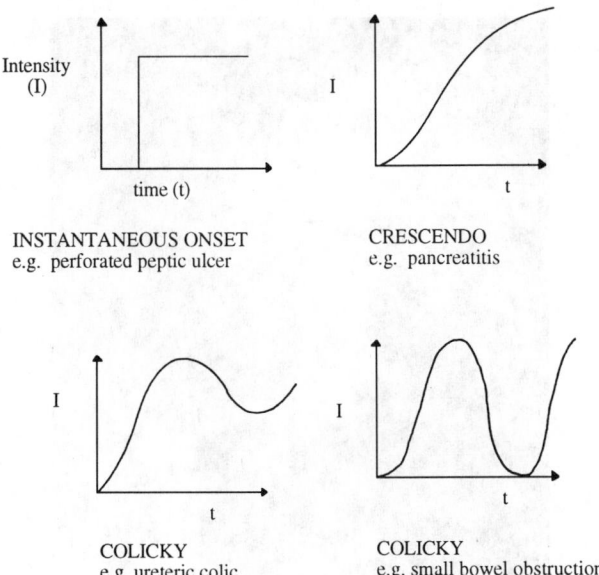

INSTANTANEOUS ONSET
e.g. perforated peptic ulcer

CRESCENDO
e.g. pancreatitis

COLICKY
e.g. ureteric colic

COLICKY
e.g. small bowel obstruction

Fig. 1. Intensity–time course of abdominal pain.

or pain that is worse when a car or trolley travels over bumps, is suggestive of intra-abdominal inflammation.

- Pain that is relieved by leaning forward or lying prone is suggestive of retroperitoneal inflammation (e.g. pancreatitis).
- Patients with renal colic typically move around trying to find a comfortable position but are unable to do so.
- Pain of peptic ulcer disease may be relieved by a trial of antacid medication.
- Pain that is unrelieved by conventional analgesia is characteristic of ischaemic bowel, particularly if the pain appears to be out of proportion to the physical signs.

Past history of similar pain

A previous history of similar pain may give a clue to the diagnosis. Cyclical monthly pain points to a gynaecological cause such as endometriosis. Recurrent right iliac fossa pain associated with diarrhoea and weight loss points to Crohn's disease rather than appendicitis.

Vomiting

Vomiting may occur simply as a response to the abdominal pain, but may also have a cause directly related to the gastrointestinal tract. Vomiting is unusual in a perforated viscus, but is very common in acute cholecystitis. Appendicitis is commonly associated with vomiting,

but the vomiting almost always follows the pain. Conversely, if the vomiting precedes the abdominal pain, a 'surgical' cause is unlikely. Vomiting is almost inevitable in acute small bowel obstruction and may provide temporary relief of the colicky pain. Clear fluid suggests an obstructed pylorus, bilious vomiting suggests obstruction distal to the ampulla of Vater and faeculent vomiting suggests more distal obstruction.

Remainder of history

It is not the remit of this chapter to describe how to take the remainder of a clinical history. Suffice to say that the art of history-taking in the acute abdomen is a combination of attention to detail and comprehensiveness. Time spent eliciting the details of the abdominal pain is likely to be rewarded. Failure to enquire about the family history (e.g. porphyria, sickle cell anaemia), drug history (e.g. warfarin) or past medical history (e.g. Crohn's disease) may have unfortunate consequences.

EXAMINATION

The multitude of causes of the acute abdomen, both abdominal and non-abdominal, dictate that the whole patient is examined rather than the abdomen alone:

- Examination starts with an overall 'end of the bed' impression of the patient.
- Vital signs (pulse, blood pressure, respiratory rate and temperature) are recorded.
- A brief examination of the hands and head/neck region is required, looking for general features such as anaemia, cyanosis, jaundice, pigmentation, dehydration/fluid overload or stigmata of liver disease.
- For most patients with an acute abdomen the examination then concentrates on the abdominal system.
- It is important, however, to include an examination of the cardiovascular, respiratory and neurological systems, particularly in cases where there is not a clear abdominal cause for the patient's symptoms.

Examination of the abdomen

The patient should be lying flat with a single pillow behind the head for comfort and appropriately exposed to permit examination of the whole abdomen. Traditional surgical teaching was that no analgesia should be given until the patient has been assessed by the surgeon responsible for continuing care (Silen, 1979). This approach is no longer generally supported (Editorial, 1979). If the

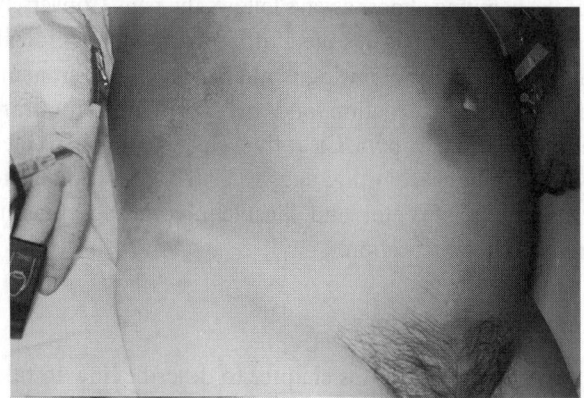

Fig. 2. Periumbilical and loin discoloration in a patient with severe acute pancreatitis. (Courtesy of Oxford Medical Illustration.)

patient is distressed by pain then an appropriately titrated dose of analgesia should be given. Examination proceeds along the lines of inspection, palpation, percussion and auscultation.

Inspection

The skin, the shape of the abdomen and movement of the abdominal wall should be considered.

Skin

Any areas of skin discoloration should be noted. Discoloration in the loins and periumbilically is indicative of severe retroperitoneal inflammation, usually fulminant pancreatitis (Fig. 2). Mild jaundice is sometimes more readily diagnosed in non-sun-exposed abdominal skin than in the sclera, particularly in the artificial light of most hospitals. Areas of redness suggest adjacent inflammation. All scars should be noted.

Contour

The presence of generalized abdominal distension should be considered. If doubt exists, the patient is usually a reliable witness of whether or not his/her abdomen is 'bloated'. Distension may be due to fat, fluid, flatus, faeces or fetus. A scaphoid abdomen suggests malnutrition or dehydration. Non-generalized or asymmetrical swellings should be noted. Most irreducible herniae are visible, although rare herniae such as a lumbar hernia will only be seen if the loins and back are also inspected (Fig. 3). Redness of the skin at the site of a painful irreducible hernia suggests strangulation.

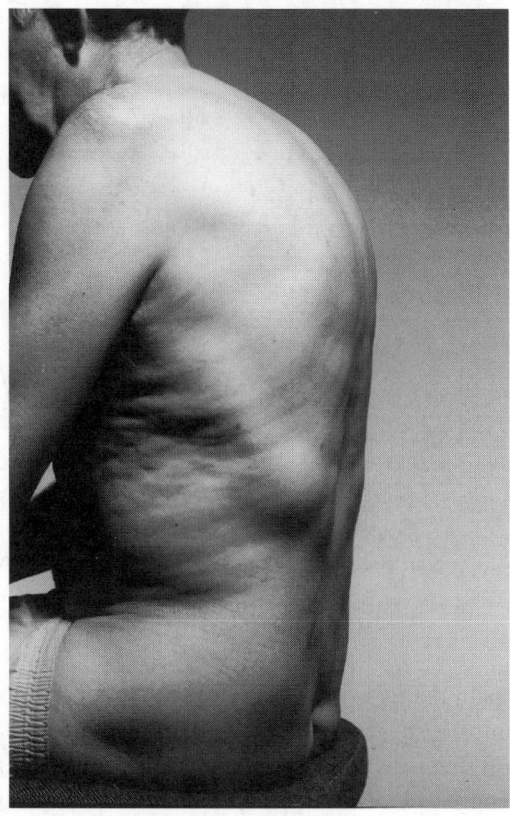

Fig. 3. Irreducible lumbar hernia, illustrating the need to examine the loins and back of patients with the acute abdomen. (Courtesy of Oxford Medical Illustration.)

Movement

Under normal circumstances the abdominal wall moves gently with respiration. Absence of movement occurs in acute peritonitis. Prominent aortic pulsation may be visible in thin normal individuals. An abdominal aortic aneurysm may be visible as a prominent pulsation, usually just to the left of the midline, even in overweight patients. Visible peristalsis is occasionally seen in thin patients with acute small bowel obstruction.

Palpation

Great care is required in palpating the acute abdomen. The examination commences with very light palpation in the quadrant of the abdomen thought least likely to evoke any tenderness. The patient's face is watched for any grimace indicative of tenderness. In children or anxious adults it is helpful to commence palpation using the patient's own hand or even asking the patient to 'press lightly on his/her own abdomen'. Once a degree of confidence has been achieved, the examining doctor asks if he/she 'may gently do the same'. Palpation in the presence of inflammation of the parietal peritoneum causes a reflex increase in tone in the overlying muscles. This is detected as guarding of the muscles concerned. A common problem is distinguishing such involuntary guarding from voluntary guarding. Voluntary guarding is more likely to occur in a patient who is frightened, especially if initial attempts at palpation have produced abdominal pain. Asking the patient to give a deep sigh may help in achieving relaxation of the abdominal muscles. If doubt persists repeated abdominal examinations are useful in distinguishing voluntary from involuntary guarding. In extreme cases of guarding, particularly in the presence of generalized peritonitis, palpation reveals a 'board-like' rigidity of the abdominal wall. Voluntary guarding, especially in very muscular individuals, may be mistaken for a rigid abdomen. Again, repeated examination and interpretation of the finding in the context of the remainder of the history and examination are useful in clarifying the situation.

All four quadrants of the abdomen are palpated lightly for evidence of tenderness, guarding or rigidity. The examination proceeds, pain permitting, with deeper palpation in all quadrants to assess for deeper tenderness or abdominal masses. Specific organs are palpated for (and percussed) in the conventional fashion. Tenderness over the gallbladder should be assessed in all cases of upper abdominal or right-sided pain. The flat of the examining hand is placed gently over the region of the gallbladder and the patient is asked to take a deep breath in. A catch of breath at the zenith of inspiration, known as a positive Murphy's sign, occurs as the inflamed gallbladder moves down with inspiration to touch the examining hand.

Percussion

An important aim of examination of the acute abdomen is to detect parietal peritoneal inflammation. Sudden movement of the inflamed parietal peritoneum results in pain. Deep palpation followed by a sudden release of the examining hand achieves such sudden movement. If pain occurs, rebound tenderness is said to be present. However, the test may be so painful that the patient's confidence is lost, making continued examination difficult. A more subtle method of producing sudden movement of the parietal peritoeum is by gentle percussion. Eliciting pain during percussion is known as percussion tenderness and like rebound tenderness is suggestive of parietal peritoneal inflammation. Percussion is also useful to determine if

distension is resonant or dull and to assist in the assessment of specific organs (e.g. liver and bladder).

Auscultation

The presence or absence of bowel sounds should be recorded in all cases of the acute abdomen. If present, the character, in particular whether obstructive or not, should be recorded. In the absence of bowel sounds, heart and breath sounds may be heard. Easily audible heart or breath sounds, in the absence of bowel sounds, are suggestive of peritonitis.

Examination of the groins, external genitalia and rectal examination

If these are omitted the abdominal examination cannot be considered complete. A strangulated femoral hernia cannot be diagnosed if the groin is not examined. Torsion of the testis may occasionally present with abdominal pain. The diagnosis will be obvious if the scrotum is examined but extremely difficult if it is not. Likewise, tenderness on rectal examination may be the only physical sign of an inflamed appendix lying in the pelvis. In women, a vaginal examination is required if lower abdominal pathology is suspected.

BASIC INVESTIGATIONS

The need for investigations varies from patient to patient. A fit young man with features of appendicitis requires minimal investigation (perhaps urinalysis and full blood count at the most). An elderly patient who is unwell with generalized abdominal pain and no major clue as to the cause requires more extensive investigation.

Urine testing

Urine testing is an essential part of the assessment of the acute abdomen. Simple dipstick testing allows detection of protein, blood or glucose which may give a clue to the diagnosis. If the clinical features point to liver or biliary disease, tests for bilirubin/urobilinogen are indicated. All women of child-bearing potential should have the urinary βhCG (chorionic gonadotrophin) assessed to exclude early pregnancy.

In patients with suspected urinary tract infection, microscopy and culture may provide confirmation. Culture results, however, are not available for at least 24 h. Reagent strips that detect nitrites and leucocyte esterases

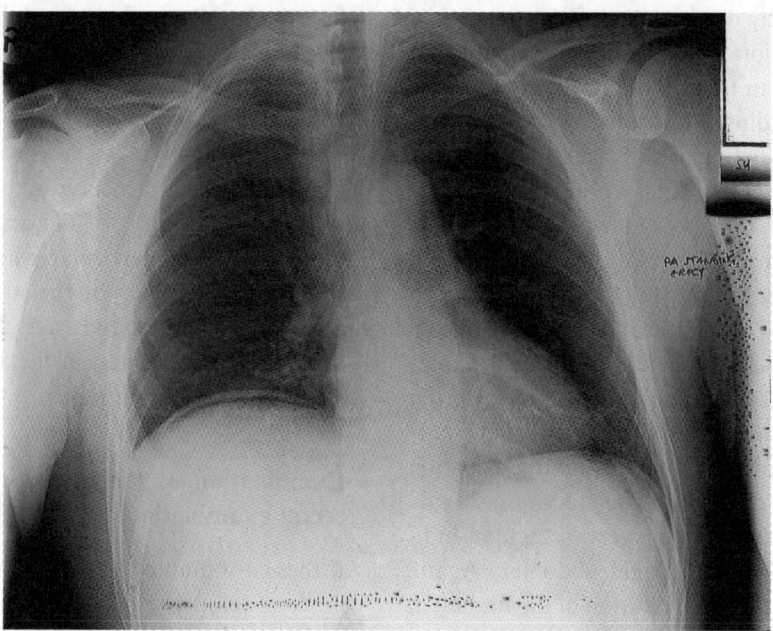

Fig. 4. Erect chest X-ray showing free gas below the diaphragm.

are available which provide useful information immediately (Ravichandran *et al.*, 1994). The nitrite test depends on the ability of bacteria to convert dietary nitrates into nitrites, although false negatives occur in at least 10% of cases. Tests for leucocyte esterase, an enzyme in neutrophil granulocytes, detect the presence of white cells in the urine. However, white cells may be found in conditions other than urinary tract infection, including acute appendicitis.

Full blood count and urea/electrolytes

These are indicated for the majority of patients with an acute abdomen. A leucocytosis provides evidence of inflammation. A raised urea may indicate dehydration, acute gastrointestinal haemorrhage or pre-existing renal impairment.

Amylase

Serum amylase should be checked in all cases of acute abdomen where pancreatitis is considered a possible diagnosis, however remote. Discharging a patient home or undertaking an unnecessary laparotomy in a patient with pancreatitis are major management errors.

Radiology (Figs 4–6)

- An erect chest X-ray is indicated if there is a suspicion of a perforated viscus (sudden onset of pain or features of generalized peritonitis), if the patient has pre-existing cardiopulmonary disease, or if there is a possibility that the presenting abdominal symptoms may be due to pathology in the chest.
- A plain supine abdominal X-ray is indicated if there are features of intestinal obstruction in the history or examination.
- An erect abdominal X-ray rarely provides evidence of obstruction that is not apparent from the supine film.

Electrocardiogram

Myocardial infarction or angina may present with upper abdominal pain. If this is considered a possibility an ECG is mandatory.

PRELIMINARY MANAGEMENT DECISIONS

Once the history, examination and basic investigations have been completed, two issues must be addressed: the diagnosis (or differential diagnosis) and the treatment (or management plan). Ideally, a diagnosis is made first so that specific treatment may be given. However, in many patients with an acute abdomen this is not possible. In other words, treatment may take priority over diagnosis. In a grossly hypovolaemic patient, resuscitation takes priority over making a diagnosis. If the patient is relatively stable more time may be spent making a diagnosis. A critical role of the doctor making the initial assessment

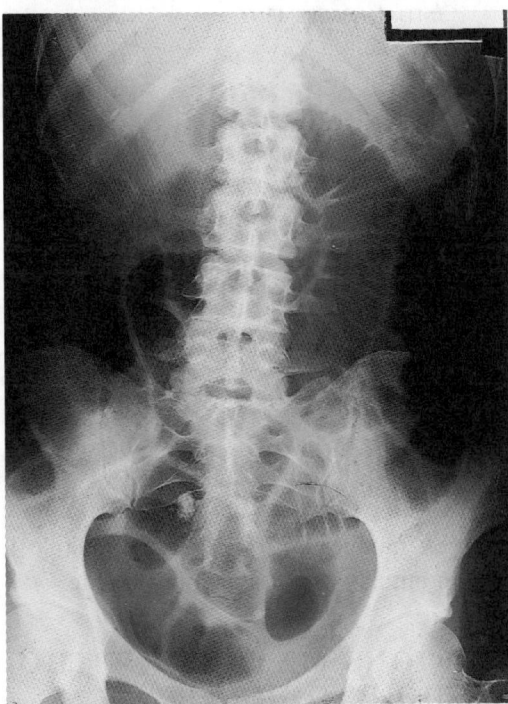

Fig. 5. Abdominal X-ray showing dilated loops of small bowel consistent with small bowel obstruction.

of patients with acute abdominal problems is to determine the degree of urgency for further management.

The diagnosis

In many cases the clinical features and basic investigations will have provided either a definite diagnosis (e.g. strangulated femoral hernia or pancreatitis) or sufficient information (e.g. free gas under the diaphragm; Fig. 4) to make further management clear. In the remainder of patients it may only be possible to make a provisional diagnosis or to categorize the type of diagnosis. It is helpful to attempt to define the type of pathology (Table 1) responsible for the patient's symptoms and to identify the organ or system involved.

Inflammation

Features of localized parietal peritoneal inflammation include:

- Constant pain, exacerbated by movement.
- Tachycardia.
- Pyrexia.
- Localized abdominal guarding or percussion tenderness.
- A leucocytosis.

The site of pain gives a clue to the organ involved. In generalized peritonitis the clinical features will be similar,

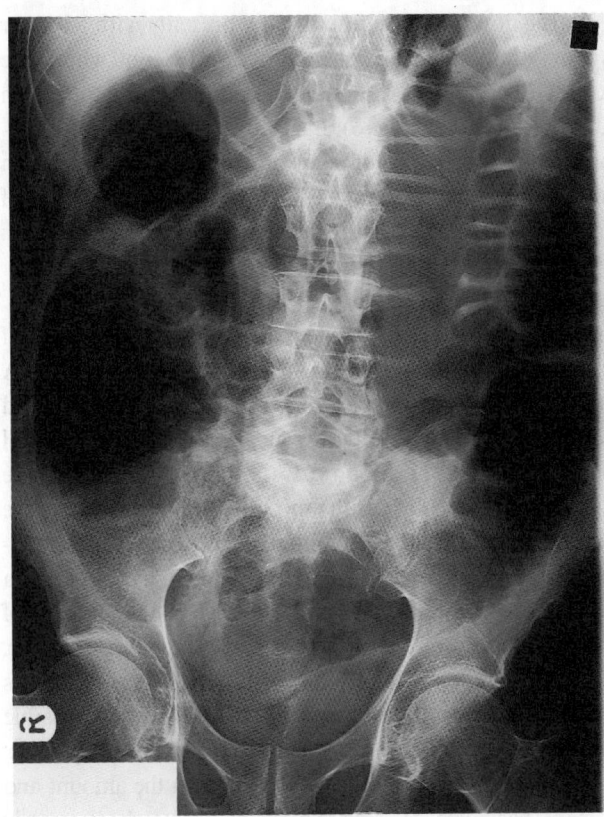

Fig. 6. Abdominal X-ray showing dilated large bowel consistent with large bowel obstruction.

although the pain is generalized, bowel sounds are absent and the patient is more unwell.

Obstruction

Features of uncomplicated small bowel obstruction include:

- Colicky pain.
- Vomiting.
- Distension.
- Absolute constipation.
- Dehydration.
- Obstructive bowel sounds.
- Dilated loops of small bowel on the abdominal X-ray (Fig. 5).

The presence of previous scars or an irreducible hernia may give a clue to the cause.

Small bowel obstruction complicated by intestinal ischaemia is suggested by:

- The pain becoming constant.
- Pyrexia.
- Rising pulse rate.
- Localized abdominal guarding or percussion tenderness.
- Redness or tenderness over an irreducible hernia.
- A leucocytosis.

Large bowel obstruction usually presents with a longer history than small bowel obstruction (except when due to a volvulus) and is usually apparent from the plain abdominal X-ray (Fig. 6). Large bowel obstruction complicated by symptoms or signs of peritoneal inflammation in the right iliac fossa suggests impending perforation of the caecum, which requires urgent surgical intervention.

Haemorrhage

Intraperitoneal haemorrhage may produce features of inflammation due to blood in the peritoneal cavity. A small amount of intraperitoneal blood from a ruptured ectopic pregnancy produces a sudden onset of abdominal pain. Tracking of blood to the undersurface of the diaphragm typically results in pain being referred to the shoulder tip. If a large volume of blood is lost intraperitoneally then the clinical features of hypovolaemia will be present and probably overshadow the features of inflammation. Retroperitoneal haemorrhage (for example, due to a leaking abdominal aortic aneurysm) produces abdominal pain radiating to the back, and possible bruising in the loins or extending into the groins or scrotum. The features of hypovolaemia will depend on the amount and rate of haemorrhage. Gastrointestinal haemorrhage usually presents with haematemesis or melaena and features of hypovolaemia, rather than as an 'acute abdomen'.

Computer-assisted diagnosis

Computer-assisted diagnostic programs have been developed to calculate the probability of various diagnoses given certain clinical features. Clinical information is collected on a structured data sheet and entered into the program. Numerous studies have shown improved diagnostic rates when computer-assisted diagnosis programs are introduced into clinical practice (Gunn, 1976; De Dombal et al., 1974; Wilson et al., 1977). Negative and delayed laparotomy rates are reduced. In the accident and emergency (A&E) environment, the number of patients safely sent home increases. Whether such improvements are soley due to the use of a computer is unlikely. A structured proforma improves the thoroughness of clinical assessment; increased interest in the subject, the degree of peer/superior review and educational feedback all tend to improve clinical performance. Despite this, the catalytic role of computer-assisted diagnosis programs is hard to dispute.

The management

The management of the patient depends on the general state of the patient and on the diagnosis or potential

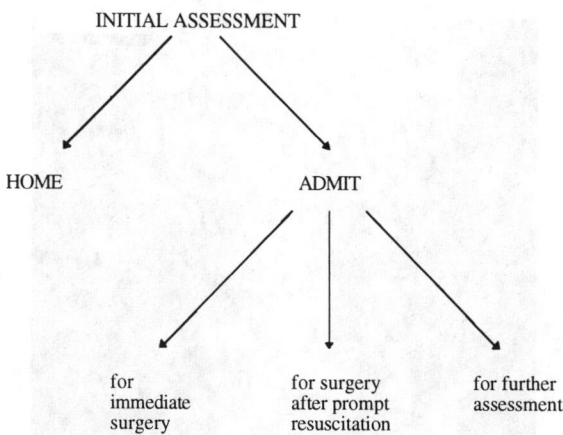

Fig. 7. Management options in the acute abdomen.

diagnoses. A number of options are available to the doctor who initially assesses the patient (Fig. 7).

CONDITIONS MANAGED WITHOUT ADMISSION TO HOSPITAL

Many patients with acute abdominal symptoms do not require admission to hospital.

Broadly, patients may be sent home if:

1. **A diagnosis is made confidently of a condition which may be managed without hospital admission.**

or

2. **There are no features of significant intra-abdominal pathology, or non-abdominal pathology responsible for the acute symptoms, and the overall condition of the patient is satisfactory.**

Further investigations, such as abdominal ultrasound or CT (computed tomography), may be helpful in making the decision about the need for acute admission to hospital. Typical conditions which may be managed without admission are:

- Uncomplicated dyspepsia.
- Uncomplicated gallbladder disease.
- Uncomplicated constipation.
- Uncomplicated renal colic.
- Acute non-specific abdominal pain (ANSAP).

Uncomplicated dyspepsia

An exacerbation of dyspeptic symptoms due to peptic ulcer disease or oesophagitis may result in a patient presenting with features of an acute abdomen. A previous history of similar, albeit less severe, dyspeptic pain and an association with meals support the diagnosis. The presence of retrosternal pain, heartburn, acid regurgitation or symptoms that are worse when bending over suggest reflux oesophagitis. Provided that there are no features of peritoneal inflammation, then it is reasonable to consider not admitting the patient to hospital. Relief of symptoms with a trial of antacid provides supportive evidence of the diagnosis. If the pain was of instantaneous onset, then a perforated peptic ulcer must be excluded. Free gas on a erect chest X-ray is only seen in about 80% of perforated peptic ulcers. If suspicion persists then admission and urgent assessment is required. Consideration should also be given to seemingly dyspeptic symptoms being due to angina or myocardial infarction. An ECG may be helpful, but if doubt exists a medical opinion should be sought. If the patient is sent home with a diagnosis of uncomplicated dyspepsia, then early review by the general practitioner should be organized and the need for an upper gastrointestinal endoscopy considered.

Uncomplicated gallbladder disease

Acute upper abdominal pain, particularly if right upper quadrant, radiating to the shoulder, and associated with vomiting, is typical of gallbladder disease. If the diagnosis is suspected then an ultrasound obtained in the A&E department can give rapid confirmation. It is important to remember that the finding of gallstones does not prove that the patient's symptoms are due to gallstones. Myocardial infarction may present with clinical features which could be confused with biliary colic, especially if incidental gallstones are found on ultrasound. As with dyspeptic symptoms, an ECG may be helpful. Assuming that the clinical picture points to gallbladder pathology, then any features of acute inflammation (acute cholecystitis) or jaundice (in association with acute pain) are indications for hospital admission. If such features are absent and the patient's pain resolves spontaneously or is easily controlled with simple analgesics, then the patient may reasonably be discharged. Follow-up arrangements should be made for early review by the general practitioner and a subsequent out-patient surgical appointment to consider cholecystectomy.

Uncomplicated constipation

Constipation seems to be an increasingly frequent cause of acute abdominal pain. Patients usually present with crampy mid- or lower abdominal pain, the sigmoid is easily palpable and the rectum full of faeces. There is usually no constitutional upset and no other gastro-intestinal symptoms. A recent history of constipating analgesia use supports the diagnosis. Plain abdominal X-ray shows characteristic loading of the colon. Immediate treatment in the A&E department with suppositories or an enema may achieve prompt relief of symptoms. The vast majority of such patients do not require acute admission to hospital. However, constipation of recent onset for no obvious cause, particularly in the elderly, warrants early out-patient follow-up and imaging of the colon. Occasionally it is not possible to make the diagnosis of uncomplicated constipation confidently enough to discharge the patient. If the patient is systemically unwell, if there are signs of parietal peritoneal inflammation, or if there are dilated loops of small bowel on the abdominal X-ray, then other diagnoses such as acute diverticulitis should be considered. It is clearly safer to admit such patients for a period of observation.

Uncomplicated renal colic

Renal, or more properly ureteric, colic is classically an extremely severe, waxing and waning pain felt between the loin and the groin. Occasionally the pain radiates more anteriorly or down into the testis. It is usually described as the most severe pain that the patient has ever experienced and, in contrast to the pain of peritonitis, patients roll around seeking relief. Typically there is microscopic haematuria and a plain abdominal X-ray will show a radio-opaque calculus in about 90% of cases. An immediate intravenous urogram (or ultrasound examination) should provide a definite diagnosis. If the diagnosis is confirmed, there is no gross obstruction to the pelvic-alyceal system, the patient is apyrexial and systemically well, and the pain is well controlled, it is reasonable to manage the patient as an out-patient. The patient should be given a supply of an appropriate analgesic (e.g. diclofenac) and arrangements made for urological out-patient follow-up. Any patient over 50 years of age presenting with their first episode of left renal colic should be considered to have an abdominal aortic aneurysm until proven otherwise.

Acute non-specific abdominal pain (ANSAP)

A significant number of patients have abdominal pain that does not have any specific features of inflammation, obstruction or haemorrhage and insufficient localization to implicate a single organ or system. The pain which is usually self-limiting has been described by the acronym

ANSAP. It is reasonable to consider non-admission in such patients provided the general condition and vital signs are satisfactory, there are no features to suggest non-abdominal pathology responsible for the pain and basic investigations are normal. However, a substantial number of patients labelled as ANSAP do require admission, principally for observation (see below).

THE NEED FOR IMMEDIATE SURGERY

Immediate surgery for non-traumatic acute abdominal problems is rarely required. Uncontrollable haemorrhage which may be intra-abdominal (e.g. ruptured ectopic pregnancy; see Chapter 59), retroperitoneal (e.g. ruptured abdominal aortic aneurysm), or gastrointestinal (e.g. bleeding duodenal ulcer), represents the only indication for emergency laparotomy.

Abdominal aortic aneurysm

Rupture of an abdominal aortic aneurysm presents with sudden onset of severe central abdominal and back pain. Often the patient will have experienced dull backache for several hours or days due to expansion of the aneurysm prior to rupture. On examination the patient will have features of hypovolaemia, the extent of which depends on the amount of blood lost. Abdominal examination will demonstrate a pulsatile central abdominal mass, usually slightly to the left of the midline. If the posterior peritoneum is breached, the patient exanguinates rapidly. Survival after rupture depends on an intact posterior peritoneum, tamponade by the retroperitoneal tissues and emergency surgery. The diagnosis is normally made on clinical grounds alone. A vascular surgeon and anaesthetist should be called immediately, blood taken for cross-matching and the patient transferred directly to theatre.

In a small number of cases with rupture of an abdominal aortic aneurysm, the amount of blood lost initially is small, such that signs of hypovolaemia are absent. The condition may be misdiagnosed as pancreatitis, ureteric colic (especially left) or back pain. In such circumstances an urgent ultrasound or CT scan will make the diagnosis, after which the patient should be transferred to theatre. There is no place for delaying surgery with a ruptured abdominal aortic aneurysm, just because the patient seems stable. The well-tamponaded leak may decompensate at any moment with disastrous results. The operative mortality from ruptured abdominal aortic

aneurysm is high. As the patient is being transferred to theatre, it is essential that one member of the surgical team spends a few minutes explaining the situation and the prognosis to close relatives.

SURGERY AFTER PROMPT RESUSCITATION

The vast majority of inflammatory and obstructive conditions responsible for the acute abdomen do not require immediate surgery. For those in which surgery is considered to be the mainstay of treatment, a period of preoperative resuscitation is usually required:

- Acute appendicitis.
- Perforated peptic ulcer.
- Perforated colon.
- Strangulated hernia.
- Small bowel obstruction with possible ischaemic bowel.
- Large bowel obstruction with possible ischaemia or imminent perforation.

The dangers of inappropriately hasty surgery, particularly by junior surgeons without senior consultation, were highlighted by the CEPOD (Buck et al., 1987) report. Once the patient has been adequately resuscitated it is important not to delay surgery unduly. The optimum timing of surgery is a balance of the benefits of resuscitation weighed against the progression of the disease process (Fig. 8), although opinions vary about the appropriateness of certain operations after midnight (McKee et al., 1991).

Acute appendicitis

In many patients the diagnosis of acute appendicitis may be made confidently on clinical grounds (with a few selected basic investigations). Typically pain starts centrally (midgut visceral) and moves to the right iliac fossa (local parietal). The pain is made worse by moving and coughing and is accompanied by nausea, vomiting and anorexia. The patient is flushed (serotonin levels have been found to be elevated in early appendicitis), tachycardic and has signs of parietal peritoneal inflammation in the right iliac fossa. In otherwise fit patients minimal preoperative preparation is required. Intravenous fluids should be started as the patient is likely to be dehydrated and a broad-spectrum antibiotic (e.g. cefuroxime and metronidazole) commenced. Operation should be undertaken as soon as reasonably possible. Excessive delay increases the risk of perforation, particularly in very young or elderly patients (Koepsell et al., 1981). Perforation

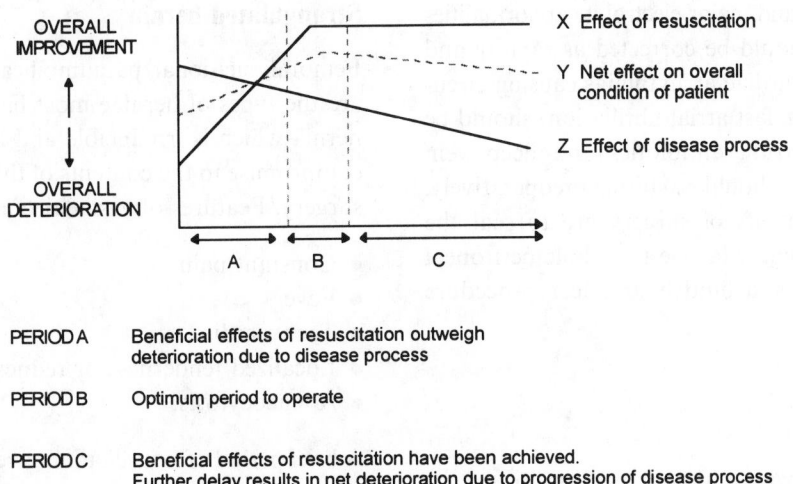

PERIOD A   Beneficial effects of resuscitation outweigh
            deterioration due to disease process

PERIOD B   Optimum period to operate

PERIOD C   Beneficial effects of resuscitation have been achieved.
            Further delay results in net deterioration due to progression of disease process

Fig. 8. Optimum timing of surgery: a balanced assessment.

of the appendix increases the risk of a postoperative wound infection (three-fold), intra-abdominal abscess formation (fifteen-fold) and mortality (fifty-fold) (Lewis *et al.*, 1975; Editorial, 1987). If the diagnosis is less clear-cut, then a period of observation and possible further investigation is necessary (see below).

Perforated peptic ulcer

Perforation of a peptic ulcer usually presents with sudden (instantaneous) onset of severe epigastric pain which rapidly becomes generalized. Retching may occur at the onset of pain, but vomiting is rare. There may be a past history of dyspepsia or a known ulcer (duodenal ulcers are ten times more likely to perforate than gastric ulcers), but perforation without any preceding history is well recognized. The patient lies still, with shallow respirations. The abdomen is tender with guarding or rigidity and absent bowel sounds. An erect chest X-ray shows free gas in the majority of cases (Fig. 4). In some cases this full-blown picture does not develop. Fluid from a perforated ulcer may leak down the right paracolic gutter producing a clinical picture resembling appendicitis. If doubt about the diagnosis exists then a contrast study or CT scan may be helpful.

Recent studies have suggested that some patients with a perforated peptic ulcer, mainly those who are otherwise fit, may be managed non-operatively with intravenous fluids, antibiotics, nasogastric suction and regular examinations to ensure that there is no deterioration (Crofts *et al.*, 1989). The majority of patients, however, are managed surgically. The timing of surgery is critical. It is thought that, initially, peritonitis is chemical, but that

Table 2. *Preparation for urgent laparotomy*

1. Tubes
   - Intravenous cannula
   - Nasogastric tube
   - Urinary catheter
   - ? Central line

2. Correct major abnormalities
   - Hypoxia
   - Cardiac failure/arrhythmias
   - Dehydration
   - Electrolyte imbalance

3. Anticipate problems
   - Bleeding
     —Cross-match blood
     —? Platelets
     —? Fresh frozen plasma
   - Infection
     —Broad-spectrum antibiotics
   - DVT/PE
     —Subcutaneous low-dose heparin
     —TED stockings

4. Consent
   - Possibility of stoma

DVT, deep venous thrombosis, PE, pulmonary embolism, TED, thromboembolic deterrent.

bacterial peritonitis supervenes within about 6 h after the perforation. Preoperative resuscitation (Table 2) therefore needs to be prompt. This should be done in conjunction with the anaesthetist responsible for giving the anaesthetic. A nasogastric tube should be passed to empty the stomach. Dehydration and major electrolyte abnormalities (e.g. hypokalaemia) should be corrected as rapidly and as safely as possible. Cardiac arrhythmias causing circulatory compromise (e.g. fast atrial fibrillation) should be corrected. Broad-spectrum antibiotics and deep vein thrombosis prophylaxis should be started preoperatively. The essential requirements of surgery are to seal the perforation and thoroughly lavage the whole peritoneal cavity. The need for a definitive antiulcer procedure depends on:

- The type of ulcer.
- Its chronicity.
- Previous treatment with antiulcer medication.
- Risk factors such as steroids or non-steroidal anti-inflammatory drugs.
- The degree of contamination at the time of surgery.
- The general condition of the patient.

Individual patients need to be treated on their merits, although the trend in recent years has been towards minimal emergency surgery (seal and lavage), with reliance on aggressive antiulcer therapy postoperatively.

Perforated colon

Colonic perforations occur mainly in the sigmoid in association with diverticular disease, or more rarely profound constipation (stercoral perforation), tumours or instrumentation. Rupture of a diverticular pericolic abscess results in purulent peritonitis. Free perforation of the colon at the site of a diverticulum results in faecal peritonitis. Caecal perforation occasionally occurs secondary to closed loop colonic obstruction or to perforation of a solitary diverticulum. The clinical features are those of generalized peritonitis, with usually a large amount of free gas apparent on the erect chest X-ray. Patients with faecal peritonitis are likely to have features of septicaemia and frequently develop multisystem failure. This is reflected in a mortality of about 50% (Tudor et al., 1994). Preoperative resuscitation (Table 2) is critical to the optimum care of patients with colonic perforations and is likely to be best achieved in an intensive care unit, provided that this does not introduce excessive delays. The majority of patients with colonic perforations will require at least a temporary stoma. Ideally the patient should be seen preoperatively by a stomatherapy nurse and stoma sites marked.

Strangulated hernia

Femoral, incisional, paraumbilical and recurrent inguinal are the types of herniae most liable to strangulate. Any hernia which is irreducible and has features of vascular compromise to the contents of the hernia requires urgent surgery. Features of vascular compromise include:

- Constant pain.
- Fever.
- Tachycardia.
- Localized tenderness or redness over the hernia.
- A leucocytosis.

A brief period of resuscitation is required but the presence of possible strangulation means that the general condition of the patient may deteriorate (i.e. line Z in Fig. 8 is going down steeply). Clearly a balanced judgement needs to be made about the optimum timing of surgery, but this is likely to be within a few hours of presentation. An irreducible hernia may produce small bowel obstruction but without strangulation. Surgical intervention is clearly required, but more time may be spent preoperatively correcting dehydration, electrolyte imbalances, etc., than if features of strangulation are present.

Small bowel obstruction with possible ischaemic bowel

The immediate management of all cases of small bowel obstruction is to correct dehydration and electrolyte abnormalities with intravenous fluids and to decompress the stomach with a nasogastric tube.

Small bowel obstruction may occur by a variety of mechanisms (volvulus, incarceration, intussusception and 'simple' obstruction), which are associated with different risks of intestinal ischaemia. Twisting or volvulus most commonly occurs around an adhesion or tumour. Twisting of the mesentery results in rapid impairment of the blood supply to the bowel with subsequent infarction. A substantial proportion of the small bowel may be affected. Small bowel ischaemia is heralded by constant severe pain, increasing tachycardia, fever, abdominal tenderness with guarding or percussion tenderness, the site of which corresponds to a particularly dilated loop of small bowel on abdominal X-ray. In established cases, especially with extensive ischaemia, an increasing metabolic acidosis occurs. If these features are present, surgery should be undertaken at the earliest opportunity following rapid resuscitation (line Z in Fig. 8). Incarceration is usually due to a loop of bowel being trapped within a hernia.

The urgency of surgery depends on the presence of features of strangulation (see above).

Intussusception is rare in adults, but when it does occur it is usually associated with an intramural or mucosal lesion. Bowel infarction is rare in adults.

Simple obstruction occurs due to progressive narrowing of the bowel lumen from tumour (e.g. carcinoma of the caecum obstructing the terminal ileum) or stricture (e.g. radiation, Crohn's disease or previous ischaemia) and is rarely associated with compromise to the blood supply of the small bowel.

Large bowel obstruction with possible ischaemia or imminent perforation

Large bowel obstruction is most commonly due to a stenosing carcinoma on the left side of the colon or to a stricture related to diverticular disease. The diagnosis is usually suspected from the plain abdominal X-ray (Fig. 6). If the ileocaecal valve is incompetent, secondary small bowel obstruction occurs. Such patients should be resuscitated gradually and plans made for surgery, ideally on an elective list within 1–2 days. It is essential to confirm mechanical large bowel obstruction with a contrast enema preoperatively as pseudo-obstruction may give rise to similar clinical features.

If the ileocaecal valve is competent, then a closed-loop obstruction arises and the caecum progressively distends, with a risk of perforation. In the absence of tenderness over the caecum, surgery should be undertaken within 12–24 h, leaving ample time for preoperative preparation. If the caecum is excessively distended on abdominal X-ray (10 cm or more), or there are signs of caecal tenderness, then perforation is imminent and surgery should be undertaken sooner.

Large bowel obstruction may also occur due to volvulus of the colon, usually sigmoid. Sigmoid volvulus presents with acute colicky abdominal pain, gross distension and usually constipation. These features in an elderly patient or a patient with a chronic psychiatric or neurological disorder should raise the possibility of a sigmoid volvulus. On examination the patient may show features of dehydration and there will be marked generalized tympanitic distension. Provided that there are no features to suggest ischaemia, the initial treatment is to decompress the volvulus peranally. This may usually be achieved with a rigid sigmoidoscope and flatus tube or a colonoscope. If there are features of ischaemia, the patient requires surgical intervention after prompt resuscitation.

ADMISSION FOR FURTHER ASSESSMENT

Patients may be admitted to hospital with no immediate plans for surgical intervention for a variety of reasons. Many will be admitted with the expectation that the abdominal symptoms and signs will resolve with time. Others will have a putative diagnosis, most commonly possible appendicitis, which will be supported or rejected by continued observation and further investigations. Others will be admitted with a probable diagnosis: for example, acute diverticulitis which would be expected to be managed non-surgically in the majority of cases. Admission is required to confirm the diagnosis, treat the condition and observe closely for resolution or the development of complications that may require intervention. Others will have a definite diagnosis already made, such as acute pancreatitis or uncomplicated small bowel obstruction, initially for non-surgical management, with the possibility of surgery if complications supervene. Finally, some patients with an acute abdomen who clearly unwell but no obvious cause or category of diagnosis is apparent. Urgent investigation and consideration of medical causes of the acute abdomen are required.

Repeated observation

Many patients with acute non-specific abdominal pain are admitted for observation, primarily because the diagnosis cannot be made confidently enough at the initial assessment to send the patient home safely. Regular measurement of vital signs and abdominal assessment will rapidly show if the patient is getting better or deteriorating. Very few patients sit on the fence indefinitely. Provided the abdominal symptoms and signs settle, the patient may be discharged home. At least one-third of acute surgical admissions are in this category of ANSAP (De Dombal, 1991). Prospective evaluation of patients categorized as having ANSAP has shown no abnormalities in viral studies or psychological profiles compared to controls (Raheja et al., 1990). Subsequent follow-up of such patients, however, has shown that many will have repeated episodes of pain. In the 20–50-year age group, peptic ulcer or biliary pathology is likely to be responsible. In the older age group, malignant or vascular disease is more likely (McAdam et al., 1978). Thus if the 'diagnosis' of ANSAP is made, the patient should be told that, if further episodes occur, investigation will be required.

Arrangements for follow-up by the general practitioner or as an out-patient should be made accordingly.

Possible appendicitis

The diagnosis of appendicitis is relatively easy to make in young adult men, but at the extremes of age, in women of child-bearing age and pregnant women, it is more difficult. Early surgery risks a high 'normal' appendicectomy rate, whereas prolonged observation of true appendicitis risks perforation and its associated higher morbidity and mortality (Lewis et al., 1975; Editorial, 1987). For most patients with possible appendicitis a brief period of observation will demonstrate if the physical signs (particularly pulse rate, temperature, abdominal tenderness and analgesia requirement) are increasing or resolving. In borderline cases further investigations, particularly ultrasound and laparoscopy, may be useful.

If the appendix is seen on ultrasound, particularly if there is a faecolith in the lumen or adjacent fluid, it is likely to be inflamed. Sensitivity rates of 75–89% and specificity from 86–100% are reported, although early, retrocaecal and perforated appendices are more difficult to diagnose by ultrasound (Hoffmann & Rasmussen, 1989). Ultrasound has the advantage of being able to diagnose other disorders, especially gynaecological, which may be responsible for the patients symptoms.

If diagnostic doubt persists after a period of observation and ultrasound examination, then laparoscopy should be considered. At laparoscopy the diagnosis of appendicitis is made if an inflamed appendix is seen or there are signs of inflammation in the right iliac fossa with no other pathology to account for it (Spirtos et al., 1987). Appendicitis is excluded if another cause for the patient's symptoms is seen or if an unequivocally normal appendix is seen. If doubt exists it is safer to remove the appendix. Although laparoscopy may be used to reduce the negative appendicectomy rate, it is still an invasive procedure requiring general anaesthesia, with a significant complication rate. Its use in cases of suspected appendicitis should not be allowed to lower the threshold for surgical intervention.

Other investigations such as CT scanning (Balthazar et al., 1986) or peritoneal fluid aspiration for cytological examination (Stewart et al., 1986) may occasionally be helpful but are not used routinely.

Probable acute cholecystitis

Acute cholecystitis is characterized by right upper abdominal pain, often radiating around to the back and to the right shoulder, with associated vomiting. On examination, the patient is pyrexial and has signs of tenderness and guarding in the upper right quadrant or a positive Murphy's sign. The diagnosis may be confirmed by ultrasound with the demonstration of gallstones and features of acute inflammation in most cases. If the diagnosis is not supported by ultrasound other diagnoses should be considered:

- Acute peptic ulcer disease.
- Acute pancreatitis.
- Acute appendicitis (high retrocaecal).
- Right pyelonephritis.
- Acute hepatitis.
- Chlamydial perihepatitis (Fitz–Hugh–Curtis syndrome).
- Right heart failure (with hepatic congestion).
- Right lower lobe pneumonia.
- Acute myocardial infarction.

Initial treatment of acute cholecystitis includes analgesia, intravenous fluids and antibiotics (e.g. cefuroxime). Most patients will settle with this regimen but, if the condition deteriorates, for example if an empyema of the gallbladder develops, urgent intervention (either drainage or cholecystectomy) is required. For uncomplicated acute cholecystitis there is controversy over the optimum timing of cholecystectomy. Traditional teaching was that the acute episode should be allowed to settle with conservative treatment and an elective cholecystectomy arranged 6–8 weeks later. In the 1980's several trials resulted in a shift towards cholecystectomy during the initial acute admission (Addison & Finan, 1988). With the advent of laparoscopic cholecystectomy (LC) the pendulum swung back towards a policy of initial conservative management with an elective LC a few months later, because of initial concerns about the safety of LC for an acutely inflamed gallbladder. With increasing laparoscopic experience more units are recommending LC during the acute phase of cholecystitis (Kum et al., 1994), although the conversion rate to open surgery is probably higher.

Probable acute diverticulitis

This presents as pain mainly in the left iliac fossa, often with an alteration in bowel habit and some urinary symptoms. On examination the patient is pyrexial with signs of parietal peritoneal inflammation in the left iliac fossa. The main aims of management are to confirm the diagnosis, treat the condition, monitor for complications and to exclude carcinoma of the colon. Initial treatment is with intravenous fluids and broad-spectrum antibiotics (such as cefuroxime and metronidazole). Progression of clinical features to generalized peritonitis or evidence of free gas on X-ray represent indications for laparotomy after appropriate resuscitation.

In patients with signs localized to the left iliac fossa, an attempt should be made to confirm the diagnosis. Colonoscopy or contrast enema is best avoided in the acute phase because of the risk of perforation. CT scanning is probably the investigation of choice as it usually allows both the diagnosis to be made and complications such as a paracolic abscess to be detected (Nanda & Amini. 1995). Once the acute episode has settled the colon should be imaged by either barium or colonoscopy to rule out an underlying neoplasm.

Uncomplicated small bowel obstruction

Most cases of small bowel obstruction, not due to herniae, and without features of possible ischaemic bowel, are admitted for non-surgical treatment in the first instance. Adhesions represent the commonest cause of small bowel obstruction in Western hospitals. The diagnosis of adhesional obstruction is supported if the patient has had previous abdominal surgery, especially if major, or if there was an episode of small bowel obstruction in the early period after the surgery, if the patient has known adhesions, or if there have been repeated previous episodes with conservative treatment over a long period of time which have resolved. Most episodes of adhesional small bowel obstruction settle with careful non-surgical management, but recurrent attacks eventually become an indication for laparotomy. Water-soluble contrast radiology (Joyce et al., 1992) may be helpful in distinguishing those patients who are likely to settle with conservative management from those who require a laparotomy.

Acute pancreatitis

This typically presents with upper abdominal pain which gradually increases in severity in a crescendo fashion, often radiating to the back. Nausea and vomiting are common. Abdominal examination may reveal upper abdominal tenderness and distension. Periumbilical or flank discoloration are occasionally seen in severe pancreatitis (Fig. 2). Severe pancreatitis is accompanied by shock and multisystem failure. Pancreatitis should be considered in all cases of undiagnosed abdominal pain and the serum amylase checked. Serum amylase levels

Table 3. *Glasgow prognostic scoring system for acute pancreatitis*

• White blood count	$> 15\,000$ per mm^3
• Glucose	> 10 mmol l^{-1}
• Urea	> 16 mmol l^{-1}
• pO$_2$	< 8 kPa
• Albumin	< 32 g l^{-1}
• Calcium	< 2.0 mmol l^{-1}
• Lactate dehydrogenase	> 600 IU l^{-1}
• Aspartate aminotransferase/ alanine aminotransferase	> 200 units l^{-1}

rise within 2–12 h of the onset of symptoms and gradually return to normal over 3–5 days. Levels over 1000 IU l^{-1} (normal range less than 300 IU l^{-1}) are strongly suggestive of acute pancreatitis, although a number of other acute abdominal conditions may be associated with modest hyperamylasaemia (e.g. perforated duodenal ulcer and mesenteric ischaemia). The level of amylase has no prognostic significance in acute pancreatitis although several other factors do. Prognostic factors in the Glasgow scoring system are shown in Table 3. If two or less factors are present the pancreatitis may be considered mild/moderate (mortality $< 2\%$). If three or more factors are present the pancreatitis is severe, with a mortality risk of at least 10%. The initial treatment is with oxygen, intravenous fluids, nasogastric aspiration and analgesia. Antibiotics are of no proven benefit in uncomplicated pancreatitis. Vital signs, oxygenation and urine output should be monitored. Any deterioration in cardiovascular, respiratory or renal function requires careful supportive therapy, usually in an intensive care unit. Progression of abdominal signs or the development of major system failure requires imaging of the pancreas by contrast-enhanced CT, looking mainly for pancreatic necrosis. Evidence of pancreatic necrosis and infection (judged by clinical features or fine-needle aspiraion of necrotic pancreas under radiological guidance) is best treated by surgical debridement. In this situation broad-spectrum antibiotic treatment with imipenem has been shown to be helpful (Pederzoli et al., 1993). For patients with acute pancreatitis secondary to gallstones, the outcome may be favourably influenced by early ERCP (endoscopic retrograde cholangiopancreatography) (Fan et al., 1993). Attempts to 'rest the pancreas' with somatostatin analogues or with H2-receptor blockers have not been shown to be beneficial. The treatment remains purely supportive for the majority of patients.

MEDICAL CAUSES OF THE ACUTE ABDOMEN

Pathology immediately adjacent to the abdomen, particularly in the lower chest, may present with abdominal symptoms. Lower lobe pneumonia, *Legionella* pneumonia and myocardial infarction are the most commonly encountered medical conditions which may cause confusion with an acute abdomen. A high index of suspicion, thorough clinical assessment and basic investigations (especially chest X-ray and ECG) should pick up most cases. A number of miscellaneous other medical conditions which cause confusion are worthy of mention.

Diabetes mellitus

Diabetic ketoacidosis (DKA) is frequently associated with abdominal pain and tenderness. The patient is usually ill, dehydrated and may become drowsy or comatose. The diagnosis of DKA is usually not difficult:

- Glycosuria.
- Ketonuria.
- Hyperglycaemia.
- A metabolic acidosis.

The surgical concern is usually whether the abdominal pain is secondary to the DKA or whether the DKA has been precipitated by an intra-abdominal problem such as appendicitis. The dilemma is usually resolved by frequent repeated examinations, possibly assisted by ultrasound or CT scanning. If the abdominal symptoms and signs persist or progress despite improvement in the metabolic disturbance, then intra-abdominal pathology should be suspected.

Acute adrenal insufficiency

Addison's disease may present with acute abdominal pain and hypotension, usually with a prior history of lethargy and weight loss. The diagnosis should be suspected by the findings of hyperpigmentation (in the palmar creases and buccal mucosa), hypotension and characteristic biochemistry (low sodium, high potassium and urea). In modern practice, acute adrenal crisis is most frequently encountered in patients who have been on long-term steroids which have been abruptly stopped. The acute presentation may be precipitated by a relatively minor illness or infection.

Acute intermittent porphyria

An acute attack of porphyria may cause colicky abdominal pain and vomiting although signs of parietal peritoneal inflammation are absent. The attack may be precipitated by barbiturate ingestion and is usually suspected only if there is a family history of porphyria. The diagnosis is supported by demonstrating porphyrins in the urine. Classically, freshly passed urine looks normal but becomes red on standing or following the addition of Ehrlich's aldehyde reagent.

Sickle cell anaemia

Abdominal pain is common during sickle crises and is most commonly due to splenic infarcts. Associated bone and joint pain suggest that it is part of a generalized sickle crisis. As with DKA, the surgical concern is that the crisis has been precipitated by intra-abdominal pathology. Gallstones are especially common in patients with sickle cell anaemia, making cholecystitis an important consideration. Frequent examinations and scanning (ultrasound or CT) are required in equivocal cases.

Haemophilia

Abdominal pain in haemophiliacs is most commonly due to retroperitoneal haemorrhage, although this may mimic appendicitis. Contrast CT scanning is likely to be helpful in distinguishing haemorrhage from primary intraabdominal pathology.

Drugs

Digoxin toxicity may produce acute abdominal pain, normally with marked anorexia and nausea. Toxicity may be precipitated by hypokalaemia, usually due to concomitant diuretic therapy. If suspected, the blood digoxin level should be measured and hypokalaemia corrected.

Intra-abdominal bleeding due to warfarin (either at therapeutic levels or in excess) may present as an acute abdomen. Clotting studies should be performed on any patient presenting with abdominal symptoms who takes regular warfarin. Excess anticoagulation related to long-term warfarin therapy most commonly occurs following commencement of a new drug which potentiates its action (e.g. broad-spectrum antibiotics, omeprazole and several non-steroidal anti-inflammatory drugs).

SPECIAL PROBLEMS IN THE ACUTE ABDOMEN

Children

The principles of management of the acute abdomen in children are essentially the same as in adults, although the spectrum of diseases encountered is slightly different. Appendicitis and ANSAP account for the majority of acute abdominal symptoms. Constipation and urinary tract infections are quite common. The important diagnosis not to miss is intussusception. This should be considered, especially in children under 30 months of age. Provided that the child does not have features of peritonitis, an air enema should be undertaken which may be both diagnostic and therapeutic.

Intussusception in children should be considered if:

- Pain occurs in severe intermittent spasms.
- There is blood in the stools.
- A mass is palpable abdominally.
- Bowel sounds are abnormal.
- Abdominal X-ray shows dilated loops of small bowel.

The elderly

Acute abdominal problems in the elderly have a high mortality (Faruqi *et al.*, 1991) for several reasons. Vascular and malignant disease is more likely to be responsible for abdominal symptoms than in younger age groups. Acute inflammatory conditions such as appendicitis tend to present at a late stage in their natural history, often with perforation. Physical signs in the early stages of inflammatory conditions may be minimal or masked by other diseases such as dementia or drugs such as steroids. Comorbidity is high, the elderly being particularly susceptible to cardiovascular and respiratory complications, sepsis and deep vein thrombosis/pulmonary embolism (Hobler & Howlett, 1985).

Human immunodeficiency virus infection (Lowy & Barie, 1994)

The broad indications for surgical intervention in a patient with HIV infection presenting with an acute abdomen are no different from those in other patients. However, the decision to operate must take account of the types of pathology likely to be encountered and the high morbidity and mortality in this group of patients.

Cytomegalovirus (CMV) infection is very common in patients with AIDS and may produce an enterocolitis clinically similar to inflammatory bowel disease. Endoscopic biopsies, ideally from the caecum, show typical inclusion bodies. Surgical intervention is required for fulminant toxic colitis or perforation although the mortality is high.

Abdominal involvement of Kaposi's sarcoma or non-Hodgkin's lymphoma in AIDS patients may result in perforation, obstruction or haemorrhage. Unfortunately, this usually represents end-stage disease and surgery should only be considered when medical treatment has failed and there is the prospect of survival with a reasonable quality of life.

Cholecystitis and cholangitis are well recognized in patients with HIV, usually due to opportunistic infections such as *Cryptosporidium* or CMV. Ultrasound examination shows an inflamed thickened gallbladder, usually without any stones. Percutaneous drainage of the gallbladder is probably preferable to cholecystectomy, which also has a high morbidity in this group of patients.

A nihilistic approach to abdominal problems, however, must be tempered with consideration of conditions such as appendicitis, particularly in patients with HIV but no other manifestations of AIDS.

Bibliography

ADDISON, N.V. & FINAN, P.J. (1988). Urgent and early cholecystectomy for acute gall bladder disease. *Br. J. Surg.*, **75**, 141–3.

BALTHAZAR, E.J., MEGIBOW, A.J., HULNICK, D. *et al.*, (1986). CT of appendicitis. *Am. J. Roentgenol.*, **147**, 705–10.

BUCK, N., DEVLIN, H.B. & LUNN, J.N. (1987). *The report of a Confidential Enquiry into Perioperative Deaths.* Nuffield Provincial Hospitals Trust/Kings Fund.

CROFTS. T.J., PARK, K.G.M., STEELE, R.J.C. *et al.* (1989). A randomised trail of non-operative treatment of perforated peptic ulcer. *N. Engl. J. Med.*, **320**, 970–3.

De DOMBAL, F.T. (1991). *Diagnosis of Acute Abdominal Pain*, 2nd ed. p. 20. Edinburgh: Churchill Livingstone.

De DOMBAL, F.T., LEAPER, D.J., HORROCKS, J.C. *et al.* (1974). Human and computer-aided diagnosis of abdominal pain: further report with emphasis on performance of clinicians. *Br. Med. J.*, **1**, 376–80.

EDITORIAL (1979). Analgesia and the acute abdomen. *Br. Med. J.*, 2, 1093.

EDITORIAL (1987). A sound approach to the diagnosis of acute appendicitis. *Lancet*, i, 198–200.

FAN, S.T., LAI, E.C.S., MOK, F.P.T. *et al.* (1993). Early treatment of acute biliary pancreatitis by endoscopic papillotomy. *N. Engl. J. Med.*, **328**, 228–32.

FARUQI, R., GALLAND, R.B. & WILLIAMS, J.M. (1991). An audit of surgical emergencies in the very old. *Ann. R. Coll. Surg. Eng.*, **73**, 285–8.

GUNN, A.A. (1976). The diagnosis of acute abdominal pain with computer analysis. *J. R. Coll. Surg. Edinb.*, **21**, 170–2.

HOBLER, K,E. & HOWLETT, P.A. (1985). Surgery in the very elderly. *Q. R. B.*, **11**, 339–41.

HOFFMAN, J. & RASMUSSEN, O.O. (1989). Aids in the diagnosis of acute appendicitis. *Br. J. Surg.*, **76**, 774–9.

JOYCE, W.P., DELANEY, P.V., GOREY, T.F. *et al.* (1992). The value of water-soluble contrast radiology in the management of acute small bowel obstruction. *Ann. R. Coll. Surg. Engl.*, **74**, 422–5.

KOEPSELL, T,D., INUI, T.S. & FAREWELL, V.T. (1981). Factors affecting perforation in acute appendicitis. *Surg. Gynecol. Obstet.*, **153**, 508.

KUM, C.K., GOH, P.M.Y., ISAAC, J.R. *et al.* (1994). Laparoscopic cholecystectomy for acute cholecystitis. *Br. J. Surg.*, **81**, 1651–4.

LEWIS, F.R., HOLCROFT, J.W., BOEY, J. *et al.* (1975). Appendicitis: a critical review of diagnosis and treatment in 1000 cases. *Arch. Surg.*, **110**, 677–84.

LOWY, A.M. & BARIE, P.S. (1994). Laparotomy in patients infected with human immunodeficiency virus: indications and outcome. *Br. J. Surg.*, **81**, 942–5.

McADAM, W.A.F., WILSON, D.H., MATHARU, S.S. *et al.* (1978). Once a bellyacher always a bellyacher. *Br. J. Surg.*, **65**, 818.

McKEE, M., GINZLER, M., PRIEST, P. *et al.* (1991). Which general surgical operations must be done at night? *Ann. R. Coll. Surg. Engl.*, **73**, 295–302.

NANDA, R. & AMINI, J. (1995). Images in clinical medicine. Diverticulitis. *N. Engl. J. Med.*, **333**, 498.

PEDERZOLI, P., BASSI, C., VESENTINI, S. *et al.* (1993). A randomised multicenter clinical trial of antibiotic prophylaxis of septic complications in acute necrotising pancreatitis with imipenem. *Surg. Gynecol. Obstet.*, **176**, 480–3.

RAHEJA, S.K., McDONALD, P.J. & TAYLOR, I. (1990). Non-specific abdominal pain— an expensive mystery. *J. R. Soc. Med.*, **83**, 10–11.

RAVICHANDRAN, D., DALTREY, I., UGLOW, M. *et al.* (1994). Urine testing for acute lower abdominal pain in adults. *Br. J. Surg.*, **81**, 1460–1.

SILEN, W. (1979). Cope's Early Diagnosis of the Acute Abdomen, 15th edn. p. 5. New York: Oxford University Press.

SPIRTOS, N.M., EISENKOP, S.M., SPIRTOS, T.W. *et al.* (1987). Laparoscopy: a diagnostic aid in cases of suspected appendicitis. *Am. J. Obstet. Gynecol.*, **156**, 90–4.

STEWART, R.J., PURDIE, G.L., GUPTA, R.K. *et al.* (1986). Fine catheter aspiration cytology of peritoneal cavity improves decision making about difficult cases of the surgical acute abdomen. *Lancet.* **ii**, 1414–15.

TUDOR, R.G., FARMAKIS, N. & KEIGHLEY, M.R.B. (1994). National audit of complicated diverticular disease: analysis of index cases. *Br. J. Surg.*, **81**, 730–2.

WILSON, D.H., WILSON, P.D., WALMSLEY, R.G. *et al.* (1977). Diagnosis of acute abdominal pain in the accident and emergency department. *Br. J. Surg.*, **64**, 250–4.

48 Urogenital Diseases

C.A. CARNE and N. BULLOCK

Departments of Genitourinary Medicine and Urology, Addenbrooke's NHS Trust, Cambridge, UK

Chapter plan

Urinary tract infection
Urethritis
Prostatitis
Epididymitis, orchitis and epididymo-orchitis
Genital ulceration
Cystic scrotal swellings
Solid scrotal swellings
Acute retention of urine
Haematuria

URINARY TRACT INFECTION

Differences between age groups

The symptoms and frequency of presentation of urinary tract infections vary with age. In small children symptoms are often non-specific: generalized abdominal pain, vomiting, fever, or failure to thrive. In the elderly, urinary tract infection is often asymptomatic. However, the elderly often have urinary symptoms such as urgency, nocturia and frequency whether or not they have infected urine (Brocklehurst *et al.*, 1968). Urinary tract infection is more widespread in old age than at any other time of life and although still more common in women than in men this difference is less marked than in earlier years (Propper, 1989). The classical features of lower and upper urinary tract infections tend to be seen between childhood and old age and are described below.

Predisposing factors

Children (see also Chapter 60)

Approximately 40% of children who present with a first urinary infection will have some abnormality of the urinary tract (Bullock *et al.*, 1989). Those with reflux or obstruction can suffer a rapid deterioration in renal function.

Adults

Women are more prone to urinary tract infections because of the shortness of the female urethra and its ready contamination by faecal organisms. Sexual intercourse has the effect of massaging bacteria into the urethra and may result in 'honeymoon cystitis'. Instrumentation (e.g. catheterization) is an important predisposing factor to infection. Bladder problems which may predispose to infection are:

- Incomplete emptying (e.g. from prostatic hypertrophy).
- Diverticula.
- Stones.
- Tumours.
- Neuropathic bladder.

Higher in the urinary tract vesicoureteric reflux, ureteric stones, megaureter and obstruction to the ureter are important. Systemic disease such as diabetes mellitus and immunosuppression from whatever cause also predispose to urinary infection.

Upper and lower urinary tract infection

Cystitis

Cystitis commonly causes frequency of micturition, nocturia, dysuria and sometimes symptomatic haematuria. The urine is often foul-smelling. The commonest infecting organism is *Escherichia coli*. Symptoms of frequency and dysuria in the female may also arise in the presence of sterile urine. This is often referred to as the urethral syndrome. In such cases it is prudent to exclude the diagnosis of *Chlamydia urethritis*. Urethritis in the male and prostatitis are described below.

Acute pyelonephritis

This is characterized by loin pain and fever with or without rigors. The patient may also be vomiting and this can lead to dehydration. Symptoms referable to the lower urinary tract are not usually prominent. On examination, fever, tachycardia and marked tenderness in one or both renal angles are found. Rarely a perirenal abscess may form leading to loss of the waist on that side and spasm of the spinal muscles causing scoliosis. In diabetes mellitus, pyelonephritis can precipitate coma which may be the presenting condition. Urinary tract infections are also an important cause of Gram-negative septicaemia.

Emergency diagnosis

A midstream specimen of urine (MSU) should be obtained. In cases of cystitis and pyelonephritis, urinary dipsticks will show protein, blood, leucocytes and nitrites. Urine microscopy will show leucocytes, red blood cells and bacteria. Urine culture must be sent to confirm the diagnosis.

Further investigations for urinary tract infection

- Further investigations should be done if the patient is:
    - Significantly unwell
    - Pregnant
    - Very young
    - Elderly
    - Is known to have a urinary tract abnormality
- Investigations comprise:
    - A full blood count
    - Urea and electrolytes
    - Blood sugar
    - Blood culture
- Hospital admission should be strongly considered in such cases

---

Early treatment

Patients with mild symptoms should be sent home with a course of oral antibiotics after an MSU has been obtained. Acute pyelonephritis may require parenteral treatment if the patient is markedly unwell and/or

vomiting. In such cases ampicillin, a cephalosporin or an aminoglycoside may be used. Effective oral agents include:

- Sulphonamides.
- Tetracyclines.
- Ampicillin.
- Amoxycillin.
- Cinoxacin.
- Cephalosporins.
- Co-trimoxazole.
- Trimethoprim.
- Nitrofurantoin.

Pyelonephritis requires a 7–14-day or longer course of therapy (Andriole, 1988). *Escherichia coli*, the commonest infecting organism, is now often resistant to ampicillin. In cystitis a shorter course of treatment such as 5–7 days will suffice.

Follow-up plan

Patients who are not admitted to hospital should be given a letter to their general practitioner requesting a repeat MSU a few days after completion of antibiotics. Young women with a first episode of cystitis do not require any additional investigation. All other patients should be further investigated with a plain abdominal X-ray and ultrasound of the urinary tract, and the advice of a urologist sought.

URETHRITIS

Causes

The causes of urethritis may be subdivided into gonorrhoea and non-gonococcal urethritis (NGU); 40–50% of cases of NGU are caused by *Chlamydia trachomatis* and approximately 10% by *Ureaplasma urealyticum*. Other causes such as *Trichomonas vaginalis* are very uncommon. It many cases no cause is found and this is referred to as non-specific urethritis. Nowadays in Britain and most of the developed world, NGU is much more common than gonorrhoea.

Clinical features

NGU commonly causes dysuria, urethral discharge and a slight increase in urinary frequency but no nocturia. The discharge may or may not be apparent on examination. If the patient 'milks' his penis this may produce discharge at the meatus when none is initially apparent. The discharge in NGU appears watery, mucoid or mucopurulent. The discharge in gonorrhoea is the most prominent symptom and is commonly thick and purulent, sometimes copious, and usually yellow or yellow-green in colour. It is not, however, always possible to distinguish gonorrhoea from NGU on the appearance of the discharge, even for the specialist. Other symptoms of gonorrhoea such as dysuria and slight frequency tend to be less prominent. In the small minority of cases both gonorrhoea and NGU may be asymptomatic.

Both NGU and gonorrhoea can give rise to complications. The commonest local complication is epididymitis (see later). In about 2% of cases NGU causes Reiter's Syndrome (or sexually acquired reactive arthritis) resulting in arthritis and conjunctivitis or iritis. In less than 1% of cases gonorrhoea may give rise to disseminated infection resulting in fever, a purpuric or vesiculopapular rash, and arthralgia or arthritis.

Diagnosis

A urethral swab should be taken for microbiological investigation prior to the patient passing urine and prior to starting antibiotics. If the local genitourinary medicine clinic is open, immediate referral for investigation is appropriate. If not, a fine cotton swab may be used to take a urethral swab. Unless a specific culture medium for gonorrhoea is available a bacterial transport medium should be used. In uncomplicated urethritis it is not essential to send a swab for *Chlamydia* as this result will not affect the management of the patient. Unless a discharge is readily apparent on examination, the patient should hold his urine for at least 3 h before a swab is taken. After taking the swab the patient should perform a two-glass urine test. To do this the patient should pass the first 20–50 ml of urine into a specimen glass or pot, and the next 50 ml or so into a second glass or pot. In gonorrhoea or NGU, threads of pus will be present in the first but not the second container. In prostatitis or cystitis there will be debris in both containers. If the urine appears turbid, acetic acid should be added to clear the undissolved phosphates so that threads can be observed if present. Urinary dipsticks should be used. If these show haematuria or significant proteinuria, cystitis is more likely. In this situation and when the two-glass urine test suggests prostatitis or cystitis, the second specimen of urine should be sent as an MSU to microbiology.

Treatment and follow-up

In most cases of gonorrhoea the treatment of choice is ampicillin 2 g orally plus probenecid 1 g orally. Where probenecid is unavailable ampicillin 3 g orally may be used. Various areas of the world such as South-East Asia and parts of Africa have a high incidence of penicillin-resistant strains of gonorrhoea. If the patient is thought to be at risk of having such a strain or is allergic to penicillin, the preferred treatment is ciprofloxacin 250 mg orally stat. Whichever initial treatment is used it is wise to prescribe oxytetracycline 250 mg q.d.s. for 1 week as prophylaxis against the development of NGU. In all cases an early appointment at the local genitourinary medicine clinic should be made so that screening for other sexually transmitted diseases and contact tracing can be performed.

In cases of NGU, a 1–2-week course of a tetracycline (e.g. oxytetracyline 250 mg q.d.s.) is required, or erythromycin 500 mg b.d. for 2 weeks. Similarly, such cases should be referred to a genitourinary medicine clinic. Patients should be advised to hold their urine for at least 3 h prior to attendance at the clinic.

PROSTATITIS

Acute prostatitis

Causes

Acute prostatitis is caused by bacteria such as *Escherichia coli*, *Klebsiella*, *Pseudomonas* and *Proteus*.

Clinical features

It causes fever, rigors, frequency of micturition, dysuria and urgency. Pain may be felt in the suprapubic and groin areas. Palpation of the prostate gland reveals it to be tender, irregular and hard. If untreated a prostatic abscess may develop causing intense pain.

Diagnosis

Microscopy and culture of a MSU will reveal infection with one of the bacteria listed above.

Treatment

A suitable antibiotic which penetrates into the prostatic fluid is required (e.g. trimethoprim 480 mg b.d. for

4 weeks). Urine culture and sensitivity testing may indicate a need to change antibiotics.

Follow-up

Acute prostatitis should be investigated by a urologist. Long-term suppressive antibiotic therapy may be required.

Chronic bacterial prostatitis

Causes

This is usually caused by Gram-negative bacteria, sometimes by Gram-positive ones.

Clinical features

It is manifested as relapsing urinary tract infection with the same pathogen.

Diagnosis

A MSU may reveal the causative bacteria (see also section on diagnosis of chronic abacterial prostatitis).

Treatment

The same considerations apply as for acute prostatitis.

Follow-up

This should be by a urologist.

Chronic abacterial prostatitis

This is easily the most common form of prostatitis.

Causes

The cause is unknown. Conflicting evidence exists over whether *Chlamydia trachomatis* plays a role in the aetiology.

Clinical features

'Prostatic' pain may be felt in the perineum, the suprapubic area, the groins, the testicles, the penis and the inner thighs. There may also be frequency, dysuria, urgency and painful ejaculation. In some cases only one symptom is experienced. The course of the condition may be punctuated by relapses and remissions.

Diagnosis

There are no ideal criteria for diagnosing chronic abacterial prostatitis. The best to date (Meares & Stamey, 1968) involves collecting the initial urine, then a MSU, performing prostatic massage to yield prostatic fluid which is collected, followed by a final urine specimen. All four specimens are sent for quantitative bacterial culture. Bacterial prostatitis is diagnosed when the bacterial counts in the third and fourth specimens are more than ten times those in the first and second specimens. The distinction between chronic abacterial prostatitis and normality is somewhat blurred, but the commonest criterion used is the leucocyte count in expressed prostatic secretions (Simmons & Thin, 1983). Diagnosis of chronic abacterial prostatitis, given the vagueness of the symptoms and the lack of an ideal diagnostic method, is the province of the specialist.

Treatment

Treatment should not be given in the A&E department. Such patients should be referred for a specialist opinion and appropriate investigation.

EPIDIDYMITIS, ORCHITIS AND EPIDIDYMO-ORCHITIS

Epididymitis

Causes of epididymitis

- Below 35 years of age, epididymitis is most commonly caused by a sexually transmitted agent:
  - *Chlamydia trachomatis* more often than *Neisseria gonorrhoeae*
- Over the age of 35 years, epididymitis is more likely to arise as a complication of a urinary tract infection with:
  - *Escherichia coli*
  - *Klebsiella*
  - *Pseudomonas*
  - *Proteus*

Diagnosis

Under the age of 25 years, torsion of the testis must be strongly considered in the differential diagnosis. In such cases the testis lies horizontally and is held high in the scrotum. Careful examination is required to distinguish epididymitis from orchitis and epididymo-orchitis. In cases of epididymitis arising as a complication of urethritis, a urethral discharge may or may not be evident. If there is felt to be a possibility of sexually transmitted epididymitis, such cases should be investigated as for urethritis with a MSU to cover the possibility of a urinary tract infection. In other cases a MSU alone will suffice.

Treatment

The antibiotic of choice is indicated by the likely causative agent and subsequent culture and sensitivity results (see under treatment in sections on urethritis and acute prostatitis). Treatment needs to be continued for 4–6 weeks together with scrotal support and rest.

Follow-up

Urethritis-associated cases should be seen at the earliest opportunity in the genitourinary medicine clinic. Cases associated with urinary tract infections need to be investigated by a urologist.

Epididymo-orchitis and orchitis

Causes

These occur secondary to generalized infections such as mumps. Uncommon causes include syphilis, tuberculosis, leprosy and brucellosis.

Clinical features

In most cases pain is an important symptom. However, this is minimal with tuberculosis and absent in syphilis. In most cases the inflammation involves the epididymis as well as the testis; in a minority of cases only the testis is involved.

Diagnosis

Careful scrotal examination is required. In such cases, if there is doubt, a specialist opinion should be sought. Ultrasound examination may often be useful, and is much superior to clinical examination in excluding a diagnosis of malignant disease.

Treatment

This involves treatment of the underlying condition (where possible), analgesia (where appropriate) and rest.

GENITAL ULCERATION

Causes

By far the commonest cause of painful genital ulceration in developed countries is genital herpes. Sometimes in women *Candida* causes minor superficial ulceration accompanied by the more usual symptoms of vulval itching and vaginal discharge. Primary syphilis which characteristically causes a single painless ulcer is now rare in the UK.

Clinical features

Genital herpes commonly causes a characteristic evolution of signs. Vesicles first, followed by ulceration, followed by scabs. The vesicular stage is brief and often missed by the patient. The ulceration may take the form of discrete superficial ulcers about 1–3 mm in diameter with a ring of erythema, or may form a larger confluent area of ulceration. In the first attack the ulceration is often widespread in the genital area and the pain and tenderness are intense. Local tender lymphadenopathy is often present. Patients with true primary genital herpes (i.e. no pre-existing herpes antibodies) usually feel generally unwell with flu-like symptoms and fever. Meningitis may also occur. Hospitalization was required for clinically overt herpes meningitis in 6.4% of women and 1.6% of men with primary genital herpes from herpes simplex virus type 2 (Corey, 1983). In a smaller proportion of cases radiculomyelitis can produce retention of urine. In such cases it is necessary to place a suprapubic urinary catheter. Catheterization per urethram is contraindicated because a herpes urethritis will cause the urethral mucosa to be shed on moving the catheter.

Diagnosis

The diagnosis must be made on clinical grounds so that treatment can be started immediately. Confirmation is provided by viral culture. Prior to starting treatment the ulcerated area should be swabbed with a cotton swab predipped in viral culture medium and the broken-off end of the swab replaced in the culture medium. This should be sent to the laboratory the same day. Culture then takes 5 days.

Treatment

All cases of primary genital herpes presenting within 6 days of onset should be treated with acyclovir tablets

200 mg, 5 per day for 5 days. Oral analgesia may also be needed.

Follow-up

All such patients should be seen at the earliest opportunity in a genitourinary medicine clinic for screening for other sexually transmitted diseases, counselling about herpes, and contact tracing.

CYSTIC SCROTAL SWELLINGS

Hydrocele in adults

Diagnosis

Hydroceles are usually idiopathic in origin but may be secondary to other intrascrotal disease (e.g. trauma, torsion, infection or tumour). Acute presentation is rare but discomfort may lead to the need for emergency assessment. The testis is surrounded by fluid and, especially when the hydrocele is tense, may be impalpable. Diagnosis is primarily clinical, but scrotal ultrasound can be used to confirm the diagnosis and ensure that the underlying testis and epididymis are normal.

Treatment

Emergency treatment is rarely necessary but aspiration of the straw-coloured fluid through a large-bore intravenous cannula produces temporary relief of symptoms. A scrotal support is used after aspiration to ease discomfort. Recurrence of the hydrocele is almost inevitable after simple aspiration but can be prevented by instillation of a sclerosing agent; 500 mg of tetracycline in 10 ml of saline after aspiration produces sclerosis of the hydrocele sac but may cause initial discomfort requiring simple analgesia. Definitive treatment is surgical and involves plication, excision or eversion of the hydrocele sac.

A hydrocele secondary to testicular or epididymal infection which has become secondarily infected (pyocele) is an indication for urgent surgical referral and drainage. Delay in treatment can result in infarction of the testis and epididymis due to infection-induced thrombosis of the spermatic cord.

Hydrocele in children

Diagnosis

Hydroceles in children are usually congenital and may present in neonates as well as in older children. Congenital hydrocele presents as a blue-tinged swelling surrounding the testis which enlarges when the child stands, cries or strains. It usually results from a patent processus vaginalis which communicates with the peritoneal cavity, and a bulge may be found in the groin above the hydrocele where the peritoneal sac contains intraperitoneal fluid.

Treatment

Treatment is not possible or advisable in the A&E department and the patient should be referred for a surgical opinion. Surgical cure of the congenital hydrocele is accomplished by ligation of the patent processus vaginalis in the groin and drainage of the distal hydrocele fluid.

Epididymal cyst

Diagnosis

Epididymal cysts arise from cystic degeneration of the vasa efferentia of the testis and always arise above the testis. Diagnosis is usually clinical with a swelling which transilluminates brilliantly identified separately from the testis. Ultrasound can be used to confirm the nature of the swelling and its relationship to the testis and epididymis.

Treatment

Aspiration of painful epididymal cysts using a large-bore intravenous cannula provides temporary relief of symptoms but, like hydroceles, epididymal cysts tend to reaccumulate within a few weeks of aspiration. Recurrence can be prevented by instillation of tetracycline solution (see above) but definitive treatment requires surgical referral and excision of the cyst.

Haematocele

Blood in the tunica vaginalis may arise following aspiration of an hydrocele or epididymal cyst but is most commonly seen after scrotal trauma.

SOLID SCROTAL SWELLINGS

Tumours of the testis

Clinical features

Testicular tumours usually present with pain, rapid swelling and signs of inflammation. A significant proportion of patients with a testicular tumour have an associated secondary hydrocele. Rarer presentations include gynaecomastia, haematospermia and symptoms of metastatic disease. In 20% of patients, trauma to the testis may be the first time that the attention of the patient has been drawn to a testicular swelling.

Diagnosis

Diagnosis is best accomplished using ultrasound which shows gross disruption of normal testicular architecture and an intratesticular mass. Measurement of serum alpha-fetoprotein and beta-human chorionic gonadotrophin may also help in diagnosis, as well as providing a baseline for future follow-up. Further investigations are directed towards staging the tumour (e.g. abdominal CT scanning) and are not the province of the A&E clinician although it may be possible to identify enlarged para-aortic lymph nodes by palpation or ultrasound in the A&E department.

Treatment

Treatment is primarily the responsibility of the oncologist. Urgent surgical referral is necessary for inguinal orchidectomy which provides a histological diagnosis and, in a proportion of patients, may effect a cure. Patients with metastatic disease or unfavourable histology are treated with radiotherapy or combination chemotherapy.

Tuberculosis of the testis and epididymis

Diagnosis

The commonest manifestation of genital tuberculosis is chronic, relapsing epididymitis, often accompanied by scrotal sinus formation, haematuria and frequency of micturition due to bladder or prostatic involvement. The epididymis, vas deferens and prostate usually feel nodular or irregular and pus may be expressed from chronic sinuses in the scrotal skin. Diagnosis is by culture of acid-fast bacilli from expressed pus or from early-morning urine collections. A chest X-ray shows signs of pulmonary tuberculosis in 60% of patients. Measurement of haemoglobin, erythrocyte sedimentation rate, urea and plasma electrolytes provide a useful baseline for the subsequent treatment of any tuberculous process.

Treatment

Treatment is with antituberculous chemotherapy, although some patients may require orchidectomy because scrotal infection is notoriously slow to resolve, even with appropriate treatment. Referral to a surgeon or urologist is appropriate in most instances because the treatment of urinary tuberculosis can result in rapid fibrosis of the bladder and ureters which must be monitored carefully during treatment.

Syphilis of the testis

Syphilitic gumma of the testis is now very rare. It presents as a painless swelling of the testis in a patient who usually displays the other manifestations of chronic syphilitic infection. Treatment of the testicular swelling is not usually indicated.

Varicocele

A varicocele is a cluster of varicosities formed by dilatation of the veins of the pampiniform plexus. Acute presentation is rare although some patients may experience acute testicular discomfort, especially after scrotal trauma when a haematoma of the scrotum may result.

Diagnosis

Diagnosis is primarily clinical with a 'bag of worms' visible and palpable above the testis, showing a positive cough impulse. The testis below a varicocele is often smaller than the contralateral testis because the shunting of warm blood via the varicocele impairs spermatogenic function in the testis and causes loss of testicular volume. Varicoceles almost invariably occur on the left side and may occasionally be associated with occlusion of the left testicular veins by a left renal tumour. Routine stick testing of the urine is therefore useful, especially in older patients in whom the varicocele has appeared rapidly.

Treatment

Treatment is by surgical ligation of the abnormal veins or by embolization of the testicular vein. This requires referral to a surgeon or urologist.

ACUTE RETENTION OF URINE

Causes

Acute, painful retention of urine is the mode of presentation in approximately 40% of patients with prostatic enlargement (benign or malignant) and the majority of patients with acute retention will fall into this category; 45% of such male patients deny any antecedent symptoms of bladder outflow obstruction and appear to have suddenly developed acute retention. Urethral strictures, phimosis, balanitis xerotica obliterans, haematuria with clots and neurological disorders may also result in acute retention of urine. Retention of urine is rare in women but may be caused by atrophic urethritis and may be seen during childbirth or the later stages of pregnancy. In children, retention of urine is very rare and is usually due to a tight phimosis caused by balanitis xerotica obliterans. Retention of urine may also be precipitated by an intake of certain drugs (e.g. anticholinergic agents, adrenergic agonists, alcohol).

Clinical features

Typically, the patient is unable to pass urine and has an acutely tender bladder palpable above the symphysis pubis. Plain abdominal X-ray should be performed to exclude urinary calculi and ultrasound can confirm the diagnosis although it is not usually indicated. Rectal examination determines the degree of prostatic enlargement and allows an assessment of whether the prostate feels malignant. Vaginal examination in women should be performed to exclude extrinsic pelvic lesions compressing the outlet of the bladder. Measurement of haemoglobin, urea, electrolytes and creatinine is useful as a baseline before any surgical intervention.

Treatment

Urethral catheterization is the treatment of choice in the initial situation. A small (14 or 16 FG) urethral catheter should be passed into the bladder under aseptic conditions and the retained urine allowed to drain freely. Slow decompression of the bladder by periodic clamping of the catheter fulfils no useful purpose, even in patients whose acute retention has resulted from longstanding chronic retention.

If catheterization of the urethra proves impossible, specialist urological help should be sought. The urethra can often be negotiated with the help of urethral sounds and catheter introducers but it is often simplest to insert a suprapubic catheter. Standard suprapubic catheter sets are available employing a small-calibre trocar cannula which is inserted through the lower abdominal midline directly into the bladder, following infiltration of the skin and abdominal wall with local anaesthetic. Occasionally,

a tight foreskin prevents access to the urethra for catheterization; a dorsal slit of the foreskin performed under local anaesthetic may be performed but suprapubic catheterization is probably the preferred option.

Once the retention has been relieved, the patient should be referred for immediate urological assessment and treatment.

HAEMATURIA

The presence of blood in the urine should always be regarded with suspicion, even if the bleeding is only microscopic (i.e. detected on routine stick testing of the urine).

Causes

The commonest cause of haematuria is urinary infection and cystitis. Other causes are shown in Table 1. The trend towards individual fitness had also resulted in increasing numbers of long-distance runners presenting with haematuria after marathon events ('jogger's haematuria').

Clinical features

Lower urinary tract symptoms (e.g. frequency, urgency, strangury and dysuria) suggest cystitis as the cause of the haematuria, but the absence of pain and the lack of disturbance of micturition are typical of bleeding due to a transitional cell carcinoma of the bladder. Penile pain with bleeding at the end of micturition and occasional sudden interruption of the urinary stream are typical of a bladder calculus. Patients with a source of bleeding in the upper tracts may have loin pain or fever and may pass worm-like clots in the urine which have been fashioned by passage down the ureter. It is important to obtain an accurate history regarding drug consumption and bleeding disorders, some of which may be inherited.

Diagnosis

Clinical assessment must include a full assessment of the abdomen (with rectal examination) for enlarged kidneys or bladder. Enlargement of the liver and spleen may be associated with haemopoietic or clotting disorders. A detailed assessment of the general health of the patient is also essential to exclude problems such as endocarditis, arrhythmias or myocardial infarction which have resulted in renal emboli. Pelvic examination is essential in women

Table 1. *Causes of haematuria*

Infection/inflammation	Cystitis
	Glomerulonephritis
	Pyelonephritis
	Parasitic infection
	(e.g. schistosomiasis)
Calculi	Ureteric/bladder stones
Tumours	Urothelial malignancy
	Prostatic carcinoma
	Renal tumours
Congenital disorders	Hydronephrosis
	Renal cystic disease
Haemorrhagic disorders	Leukaemia
	Haemophilia
	Sickle cell disease
	Platelet abnormalities
Vascular	Renal vein occlusion
	Renal artery occlusion
Drugs	Anticoagulants
	Cyclophosphamide
	Aspirin
Other agents which colour the urine	Beetroot
	Rifampicin
	Pyridium
	Haemoglobin
	Myoglobin

and the external genitalia should be examined carefully in both sexes.

Measurements of haemoglobin, urea, creatinine and electrolytes are useful in the assessment of patients with haematuria. Microscopic haematuria found on stick testing of the urine should be confirmed by the finding of red blood cells in the urine on microscopy. Phase-contrast microscopy of the urine may be able to differentiate between the larger red blood cells which have originated in the upper urinary tracts from the more normal, smaller red blood cells shed by lesions in the lower urinary tract. Additional haematological investigation, specifically clotting, may be performed if clinically indicated. A MSU should be sent for bacterial culture and sensitivity whilst dipstick testing of the urine may show leucocytes, red blood cells and bacteria.

The mainstay of investigation is imaging of the urinary tract. Intravenous urography is the investigation most likely to be available and should be performed in all patients; those with an allergy to iodine or contrast media should be referred for a plain abdominal X-ray and ultrasound of the urinary tract. Most patients with haematuria will subsequently require cystoscopy and should be referred for an urgent urological opinion.

Clot retention due to haematuria

Some patients with profuse haematuria and the passage of clots are unable to pass urine and develop 'clot retention'. This is especially likely in elderly men bleeding from prostatic hypertrophy or a bladder carcinoma.

In the patient is unable to pass urine spontaneously and is in extreme discomfort, a urethral catheter should be inserted. To wash clots out of the bladder requires insertion of a large (22FG) three-way irrigating catheter which can subsequently be connected to continuous irrigation to maintain clear urine. Manual washout of the clots from the bladder, using a 50 ml catheter syringe and isotonic saline, should be considered in all patients with clot retention.

Bibliography

ANDRIOLE, V.T. (1988). Urinary tract infections and pyelonephritis. In *Cecil Textbook of Medicine*, ed. Wyngaarden, J.B. and Smith, L.H. pp. 628–32. Philadelphia: W.B. Saunders.

BROCKLEHURST, J.C., DILLANE, J.B., GRIFFITHS, L. *et al.* (1968). The prevalence and symptomatology of urinary infection in an aged population. *Gerontol. Clin.*, **10**, 242–53.

BULLOCK, N., SIBLEY, G. & WHITAKER, R. (1989). *Essential Urology*. p. 132. Edinburgh: Churchill Livingstone.

COREY, L. (1983). Clinical course of genital herpes simplex virus infections in men and women. *Ann. Intern. Med.*, **48**, 973.

MEARES, E.M. & STAMEY, T.A. (1968). Bacteriologic localization patterns in bacterial prostatitis and urethritis. *Invest. Urol.*, **5**, 492–518.

PROPPER, D.J. (1989). Urinary tract infection in old age. In *Urinary Tract Infection*, ed. G.R.D. Catto. pp. 87–112. Dordrecht: Kluwer.

SIMMONS, P.D. & THIN, R.N. (1983). A method for recognising non-bacterial prostatitis: preliminary observations. *Br. J. Vener. Dis.*, **59**, 306–10.

49 Haematological emergencies, blood products and blood transfusion

H.-A. DOUGHTY and M.F. MURPHY

Department of Haematology, St Bartholomew's Hospital, London, UK

Chapter plan

Introduction
Anaemia
Sickle cell disease
Disorders of white cells and host defence
Disorders of haemostasis
Blood transfusion
Major incident procedure

INTRODUCTION

Haematological emergencies are seen daily in accident and emergency (A&E) departments. Most of these emergencies are not related to primary haematological disorders but occur secondary to trauma and other illnesses. In an A&E department, urgent haematology investigations are requested on approximately 10% of the new attenders.

This chapter aims to provide a broad functional outline of the pathophysiology of the blood, together with a practical approach to the investigation and management of patients presenting with haematological problems. Certain conditions have been covered in more detail because they are more commonly encountered in clinical practice. The penultimate section of the chapter covers practical aspects of blood transfusion within the A&E department.

ANAEMIA

Anaemia is defined as a reduction in the concentration of circulating haemoglobin (Hb). The level of Hb depends not only on the absolute amount of Hb but also on the plasma volume. The normal range for Hb and red cell indices vary according to age, sex, pregnancy and population studied. The normal range for adults in the UK is shown in Table 1. An individual may be 'relatively' anaemic despite a normal red cell volume because of an increase in plasma volume. The relationship between red cell volume, plasma volume and Hb concentration is shown in Fig. 1. It should be noted that anaemia does not initially occur after acute blood loss. Following resuscitation with clear fluids, the plasma volume is re-expanded and the Hb falls.

Pathophysiology

The function of red cells is to carry oxygen between the lungs and the tissues. A single red cell contains approximately 640 million Hb molecules. Each molecule of normal adult Hb (Hb A) consists of four globin chains – two alpha chains and two beta chains – together with one iron-containing haem group. Each Hb molecule can combine with four molecules of oxygen. During the loading and unloading of oxygen the globin chains move on one another permitting entry of the metabolite 2,3-diphosphoglycerate (2,3-DPG). 2,3-DPG reduces the oxygen affinity of haemoglobin giving rise to the sigmoid form of the oxygen-dissociation curve.

Red cells are formed in the marrow by erythropoiesis, regulated by the hormone erythropoietin. The mechanism of red cell formation and breakdown is shown in Fig. 2.

The mature red cell is a biconcave disc, 7.5 μm in diameter. The shape provides a large surface area for gas exchange, carriage of oxygen from the lungs to the tissues and the return of carbon dioxide from the tissues to the lungs. The red cell membrane must be extremely flexible to traverse the microcirculation whilst retaining this discoid form. The metabolic pathways of the red cell (i.e. hexose monophosphate and glycolytic pathways) protect

Table 1. *Normal adult values for peripheral blood*

	Male	Female
Haemoglobin, Hb (g dl^{-1})	13–17.5	11.5–15.5
Haematocrit, PCV (l l^{-1})	0.42–0.53	0.36–0.45
Red cell count, RCC ($\times 10^{12}$ l^{-1})	4.5–6.3	3.9–5.4
Mean cell volume, MCV (fl)	80–96	
Mean cell haemoglobin, MCH (pg)	27–33	
Mean cell haemoglobin concentration, MCHC (9 g dl^{-1})	32–35	
White cell count, WCC ($\times 10^9$ l^{-1})	4.0–11.0	
Platelets ($\times 10^9$ l^{-1})	150–400	
Reticulocytes (%)	0.2–2	
Absolute reticulocyte count ($\times 10^9$ l^{-1})	25–75	

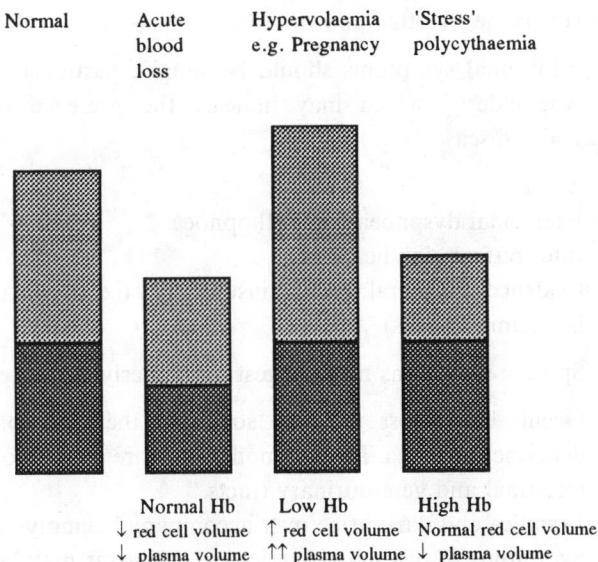

Normal	Acute blood loss	Hypervolaemia e.g. Pregnancy	'Stress' polycythaemia

Normal Hb	Low Hb	High Hb
↓ red cell volume	↑ red cell volume	Normal red cell volume
↓ plasma volume	↑↑ plasma volume	↓ plasma volume

Fig. 1. The relationship between the red cell volume ▓, plasma volume ▒ and Hb concentration in different circumstances.

the membrane proteins from oxidative damage and provide ATP (adenosine triphosphate) to drive the cation pumps which continually pump Na$^+$ out of, and K$^+$ into, the cells. Red cells become increasingly non-viable as the enzymes are not replaced. The mean lifespan of red cells is 120 days. They are removed by the macrophages of the reticuloendothelial system in the marrow, liver and spleen (Fig. 2). Red cell breakdown is increased if either the red cells or their milieu are abnormal.

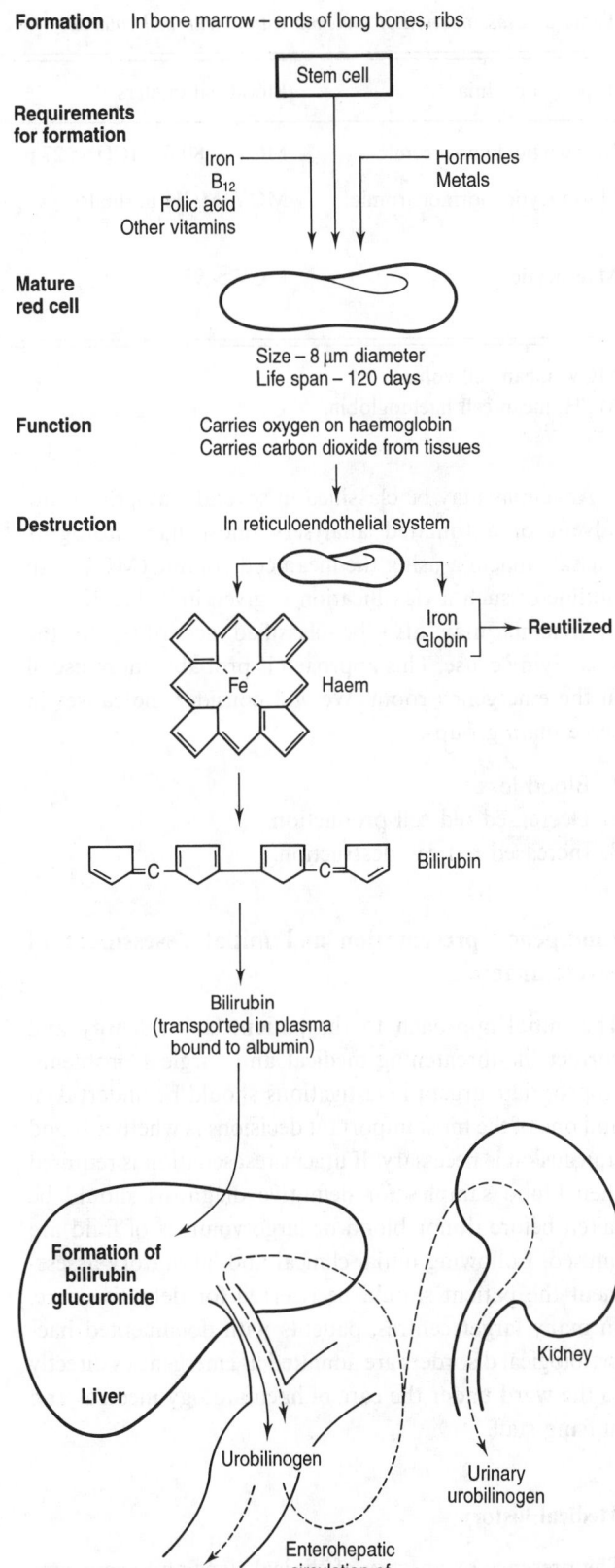

Fig. 2. Red cell formation, haemoglobin breakdown and bilirubin metabolism.

Table 2. *Classification of anaemia using mean cell volume*

Type of anaemia	Blood parameters	Examples
Microcytic, hypochromic	MCV < 80 fl, MCH < 27 pg	Iron deficiency, thalassaemia
Normocytic, normochromic	MCV, MCH normal	Acute blood loss, haemolysis, secondary anaemia, marrow failure
Macrocytic	MCV > 95 fl	Megaloblastic anaemia (vitamin B_{12}/folate deficiency), macrocytosis (alcohol, liver disease)

MCV, mean cell volume.
MCH, mean cell haemoglobin.

Anaemias may be classified in several ways. Since the advent of automated analysers, most haematologists classify anaemia using the mean cell volume (MCV). An outline of such a classification is given in Table 2.

Anaemia may also be classified according to the underlying cause. This approach is probably more useful in the emergency room. We will consider the causes in three main groups:

1. Blood loss.
2. Decreased red cell production.
3. Increased red cell destruction.

Emergency presentation and initial assessment of severe anaemia

The initial approach to the patient is to identify and correct life-threatening medical and surgical problems. Appropriate urgent investigations should be undertaken and one of the most important decisions is whether blood transfusion is necessary. If urgent resuscitation is required then blood samples for definitive diagnosis should be taken before donor blood or large volumes of fluid are infused. Following initial clinical and laboratory assessment the patient should be referred for definitive care. In many larger centres, patients with documented haematological disorders are admitted as emergencies directly to the ward under the care of haematology medical and nursing staff.

Medical history

The presence or absence of clinical signs and symptoms of anaemia depends on the speed of its onset, the severity, the age of the patient, coexisting medical problems and the oxygen-dissociation curve.

The general symptoms of anaemia are similar regardless of the underlying cause. The following symptoms may be elicited:

- Fatigue and faintness.
- Shortness of breath particularly on exercise.
- Palpitations and tachycardia.
- Headaches, vertigo and tinnitus.

Additional symptoms should be sought, particularly in the elderly, which may indicate the presence of vascular disease:

- Angina.
- Exertional dyspnoea and orthopnoea.
- Intermittent claudication.
- Evidence of cerebral vascular insufficiency (i.e. transient ischaemic attacks).

Specific symptoms may suggest the underlying cause:

- Occult blood loss must be sought if there is iron deficiency anaemia. The commonest sites are the gastro-intestinal and genitourinary tracts.
- Jaundice and dark urine may accompany haemolysis.
- Symptoms of other haematological problems may be present, such as easy bruising or bleeding and recurrent infection.
- Glossitis and sensory changes are symptoms of megaloblastic anaemia due to vitamin B_{12} deficiency.

Dietary history

This is important in the assessment of anaemia. Many people have a diet poor in iron and life-long vegans may develop vitamin B_{12} deficiency. Alcoholics, the homeless and the elderly are at high risk of folate deficiency. Acute nutritional deficiencies may occur in pregnancy because of the increased demand for iron and folic acid.

Past medical history

Gastric surgery may result in iron and vitamin B_{12} deficiency. Residence abroad may be associated with tropical sprue, hookworms and malaria.

Family history and ethnic origin

Haemoglobinopathies and enzymopathies are associated with particular ethnic groups. A family history must be taken if the anaemia might be inherited.

Drug history

Identify those patients taking anticoagulants, steroids and aspirin. In G6PD (glucose-6-phosphate dehydrogenase) deficiency, acute haemolysis follows the ingestion of a wide number of drugs. Any exposure to toxins should be noted.

Physical examination

This should cover the following:
- Is the patient unwell? Note the temperature, pulse and blood pressure.
- Skin: pallor (anaemia), jaundice (haemolysis), bruising/petechiae (coagulopathy/thrombocytopenia).
- Mouth: angular stomatitis (iron deficiency), glossitis (megaloblastic anaemia), palatal petechiae (infectious mononucleosis), telangiectasia (iron deficiency), gum hypertrophy (some acute leukaemias).
- Fundi: optic atrophy (vitamin B_{12} deficiency), retinal haemorrhage (severe anaemia of any cause).
- Lymphadenopathy (infection, lymphoid malignancy).
- Nails: koilonychia (iron deficiency), splinter haemorrhages (infective endocarditis).
- Cardiorespiratory system: evidence of cardiac failure in severe anaemia.
- Abdomen: organomegaly (leukaemia, lymphomas, some haemolytic anaemias), abdominal masses, haemorrhoids, rectal mass (iron deficiency).
- Lower limbs: ulceration (haemoglobinopathies and some haemolytic anaemias).
- Nervous system: peripheral sensory neuropathy or combined posterior and lateral column loss (severe vitamin B_{12} deficiency).

Investigation

The following samples should be taken:

1. EDTA (ethylenediaminetetra-acetic acid) 3–5 ml for full blood count (FBC), blood film and reticulocyte count.
2. Serum/EDTA 5–10 ml for blood group, antibody screen and cross-matching.

Full blood count

The FBC will give the level of Hb, MCV and the white cell and platelet counts. In many larger A&E departments, an automated FBC counter is located in the department (see section on blood transfusion). The information is then immediately available to diagnose the presence and severity of anaemia. The type of anaemia may be obvious from the clinical history, level of Hb and MCV but may require further investigation (e.g. examination of blood film and bone marrow by a haematologist). The FBC will distinguish anaemia from pancytopenia, where the white cell and platelet counts are also reduced.

Reticulocyte count

After an acute major haemorrhage the reticulocyte count rises within 2–3 days, reaching a maximum in 6–10 days. The reticulocyte count remains raised until the Hb is normal, providing that iron and folate stores are adequate. A raised reticulocyte count is also usually seen in patients with haemolytic anaemias. If the reticulocyte count is not raised in patients with anaemia this suggests there may be impaired marrow function.

Blood films

These should be examined in all cases of anaemia. The film appearance provides information that cannot be obtained from automated counters and may provide the diagnosis. Examples are the presence of spherocytes in autoimmune haemolytic anaemia, sickle cells in sickle cell disease and the presence of malarial parasites.

Further investigation

If transfusion is required, all other diagnostic blood samples should be taken before blood transfusion is commenced. Many clinicians will take these samples during the initial assessment and cannula insertion to avoid repeated venepuncture. The request for further investigation should follow a provisional diagnosis.

Examples are:

- Microcytic anaemia: serum iron and TIBC (total iron-binding capacity) (10 ml clotted sample), Hb electrophoresis, Hb A_2, Hb F (10 ml, EDTA or heparin).
- Macrocytic anaemia: serum and red cell folate (5 ml EDTA and 5 ml clotted), serum vitamin B_{12} (10–20 ml clotted sample).
- Temporal arteritis, myeloma: ESR (erythrocyte sedimentation rate) (Westergren tube).
- Haemolysis: direct antiglobulin test (FBC/transfusion EDTA sample). Seek advice from a haematologist before taking further samples for other tests in complex cases of haemolytic anaemia.

Samples for clotting screen, blood cultures, urea and electrolytes, liver function tests and immunoglobulins should be taken as indicated.

Blood loss

Acute blood loss from the circulation may not be evident clinically. Massive blood loss may follow pelvic and femoral fractures and trauma involving internal organs. The initial clinical picture is that of hypovolaemic shock. The management of the acute blood loss is covered at the end of the chapter.

Decreased red cell production

A list of causes is shown in Table 3.

Iron deficiency

This common anaemia results predominantly from a diet poor in iron and/or chronic blood loss from the gastrointestinal and genitourinary tracts. It may present suddenly following further bleeding or once cardiac symptoms supervene. The underlying cause of the iron deficiency anaemia must be determined. Treatment should be with oral iron replacement. Transfusion should be given if the anaemia is severe, when blood loss continues or coexisting pathology dictates rapid red cell replacement.

Megaloblastic anaemia

These anaemias are characterized by a macrocytosis, hypersegmented neutrophils and megaloblastic erythropoiesis. In severe cases there may be thrombocytopenia and leucopenia. The mortality associated with severe

Table 3. *Causes of anaemia due to decreased red cell production*

- Inadequate supply of nutrients essential for erythropoiesis, such as:
  - Iron deficiency
  - Vitamin B_{12} deficiency
  - Folic acid deficiency
  - Protein-calorie malnutrition

- Depression of erythropoietic activity, such as:
  - Anaemia associated with chronic disorders, e.g. infection, connective tissue disorders inflammation, disseminated malignancy
  - Anaemia associated with renal failure
  - Aplastic anaemia

- Anaemia due to replacement of normal bone marrow by:
  - Leukaemia
  - Lymphoma
  - Myeloproliferative disorders
  - Myeloma
  - Myelodysplastic disorders

- Genetic defects of haemoglobin, e.g. thalassaemia

megaloblastic anaemia is high, up to 14% if the packed cell volume is less than 25% at initial presentation.

The underlying cause of folate or vitamin B_{12} deficiency must be determined. Folate deficiency is often due to a poor dietary intake alone or in combination with malabsorption or increased folate utilization (e.g. pregnancy or haemolysis). The most frequent cause of vitamin B_{12} deficiency is malabsorption of vitamin B_{12} due to pernicious anaemia. If vitamin B_{12} or folate deficiency is suspected, blood samples must be taken before treatment is given. Often treatment is not required urgently and specific replacement therapy can follow the laboratory diagnosis. Folic acid given in vitamin B_{12} deficiency may precipitate a neurological crisis; large doses of folic acid alone should not be used to treat patients with megaloblastic anaemia unless the vitamin B_{12} level is known to be normal.

Patients presenting with severe anaemia should start combined therapy (vitamin B_{12} 1 mg IM daily for 1 week, folate 5 mg PO daily) after taking blood and bone marrow for diagnosis. Treatment may also be required for heart failure and infection. Profound anaemia presenting with heart failure may require cautious transfusion of red cell concentrates with diuretic cover. In extreme cases an exchange transfusion may be life-saving.

Increased red cell destruction

Haemolytic anaemias result from a shortened red cell lifespan. They are characterized by a variable degree of anaemia, reticulocytosis and hyperbilirubinaemia. A general classification of haemolytic anaemia is outlined as follows:

- Congenital
  - Membrane disorders (e.g. hereditary spherocytosis).
  - Haemoglobin disorders (e.g. sickle cell disease, thalassaemia).
  - Enzyme deficiencies (e.g. G6PD deficiency).
- Acquired
  - Immune: autoimmune, alloimmune (e.g. haemolytic transfusion reactions, haemolytic disease of the newborn), drug-induced haemolysis.
  - Non-immune: malaria, sepsis, burns, mechanical heart valves.

Glucose-6-phosphate dehydrogenase deficiency

G6PD deficiency is widespread in the populations of Africa, the Mediterranean, the Middle East and South-East Asia. It is inherited as an X-linked condition and therefore affects males. The clinical severity is variable, tending to be more severe and even fatal in the Mediterranean variants. Acute haemolysis follows exposure to a variety of drugs, infections and after exposure to the broad bean, *Vicia faba*. Typically haemolysis begins 1–3 days after exposure with rapid onset of anaemia and jaundice. In severe cases the patient describes backache, abdominal pain and dark urine. The blood film shows characteristic 'bite' and 'blister' cells. Management starts by removing the offending drug. In severe cases transfusion may be required. All A&E departments should have a list of drugs which may precipitate a crisis (Table 4).

Autoimmune haemolytic anaemia

Autoimmune haemolytic anaemia (AIHA) is broadly divided into 'warm' and 'cold' types. The aetiology may be idiopathic or secondary to other conditions (Table 5). The clinical course may be acute or chronic. In warm-type AIHA the IgG autoantibody is active at normal body temperature. Haemolysis is typically extravascular, occurring in the spleen. The peripheral blood film may show spherocytosis. Potentially offending drugs should be stopped and treatment started (e.g. prednisolone 60–80 mg PO daily or hydrocortisone 100 mg IV, 4-

Table 4. *Drugs causing haemolysis in glucose-6-phosphate dehydrogenase deficiency*

Analgesics
  Acetylsalicylic acid (aspirin)
  Acetanilide
Antimalarials
  Primaquine
  Pyrimethamine
  Quinine
  Chloroquine
Antibacterials
  Most sulphonamides
  Dapsone
  Choramphenicol
Miscellaneous drugs
  Vitamin K
  Probenecid
  Nalidixic acid
  Quinidine
  Dimercaprol
  Phenylhydrazine
  Para-aminosalicylic acid

Table 5. *Classification of autoimmune haemolytic anaemia*

Warm type (IgG ± complement)	Cold type
• Primary (idiopathic) • Secondary – Other autoimmune diseases e.g. SLE – Lymphoproliferative conditions e.g. CLL, lymphoma – Drugs e.g. methyldopa	• CHAD (IgM + complement) – Acute postinfectious e.g. *Mycoplasma* – Chronic Primary (idiopathic) Lymphoma • Paroxysmal cold haemoglobinuria (IgG + complement) – Postinfectious e.g. measles, syphilis – Idiopathic

SLE, systemic lupus erythematosus; CLL, chronic lymphatic leukaemia; CHAD, acute cold haemagglutinin disease.

hourly). Identification of compatible blood for transfusion may be difficult because cross-matching cannot be easily interpreted due to the presence of autoantibodies; often it is necessary to use blood which is 'as compatible as the patient's own red cells'. However, blood transfusion may be life-saving and such cases should be discussed with a haematologist.

In cold-type AIHA, IgM antibodies with an extended thermal range (above 30°C) may cause clinical problems in cold weather. Agglutination of red cells in the periphery of the body leads to Raynaud's phenomenon and complement activation can result in intravascular haemolysis. Acute cold haemagglutinin disease (CHAD) following *Mycoplasma* pneumonia mainly occurs in the winter. Although this is a self-limiting condition, the haemolysis may be severe. The treatment is to raise the peripheral body temperature. If blood transfusion is indicated, the blood should first be warmed using a standardized blood warming system.

Non-immune haemolytic anaemia

The causes of non-immune haemolysis are listed in Table 6. Non-immune haemolysis is often intravascular and the Hb released into the circulation rapidly saturates the plasma haptoglobins and the excess is filtered by the kidneys. The laboratory features of intravascular haemolysis are haemoglobinaemia, haemoglobinuria, haemosiderinuria and methaemalbuminaemia.

Malaria (see also Chapter 63)

Malaria produces a variety of haematological problems (Phillips, 1988). Acute malaria produces minimal anaemia often accompanied by thrombocytopenia. The most severe disease is associated with *Plasmodium falciparum*. Acute malaria in the non-immune individual may be a medical emergency. The greatest danger remains late

Table 6. *Causes of acquired non-immune haemolytic anaemia*

Acquired membrane defects
    Paroxysmal nocturnal haemoglobinuria (PNH)
Mechanical
    Microangiopathic haemolytic anaemia (MAHA)
    Valve prosthesis
    March haemoglobinuria
Secondary to systemic disease
    Renal and liver failure
Micellaneous
    Infections including malaria
    Drugs and chemicals causing direct toxic damage to red cells
    Hypersplenism
    Burns

diagnosis. All patients who develop fever within 12 months of returning from an endemic zone must have malaria excluded. Blood should be taken for a FBC and reticulocyte count. The blood film will require careful examination for the presence of malarial parasites. If malarial parasites are identified, a screen for G6PD deficiency must be considered in anticipation of using chloroquine or primaquine. Treatment should be discussed with a microbiologist.

SICKLE CELL DISEASE

The term 'sickle cell disease' (SCD) includes all the genetic conditions in which 'sickle' problems may occur. This includes not only HbS/S in which there is a double dose of an abnormal beta-globin gene but also the compound conditions in which Hb S is inherited together with other beta-globin gene disorders such as Hb C (Hb S/C) and beta thalassaemia (Hb S/βthal). SCD is a common inherited haemoglobinopathy seen predominantly in people of Afro-Caribbean descent. The disease is characterized by a partially compensated haemolytic state. In many affected individuals this steady-state is punctuated by crises. The clinical course cannot be predicted from the phenotype (i.e. not all patients with SCD will require repeated emergency medical attention).

Pathophysiology

Hereditary Hb abnormalities may be divided into two main groups:

1. Synthesis of abnormal Hb (e.g. Hb S, C).
2. The reduced synthesis of normal globin chains (i.e. thalassaemia).

Hb S is due to an amino acid substitution in the beta-globin chain. Valine replaces glutamic acid in position 6. Hb S is relatively insoluble and forms crystals when exposed to low oxygen tension. The crystalline Hb deforms the erythrocytes and increases their rigidity. The red cells lose their ability to pass through the microcirculation, causing infarction of tissues and organs.

Clinical features

The clinical manifestations of SCD in early childhood include dactylitis, cerebrovascular accidents and pneumococcal infection. After the first decade of life, painful musculoskeletal crises are the predominant clinical problem. These recurrent attacks of pain are due to bone infarction. The immediate management problem is to treat the painful crisis. The long-term problem due to repeated infarction is bone destruction. Avascular necrosis of the femoral and humeral heads may cause significant morbidity from the second decade onwards. Osteomyelitis caused by *Salmonella* is more common in SCD, compounding the orthopaedic problems. Pigment gallstones may become symptomatic in adolescence and folate deficiency may occur if dietary folate intake is poor. Repeated renal infarction may cause haematuria and failure of urine concentration.

Most adult patients with SCD have a good understanding of their disease. Some may carry a haemoglobinopathy card giving the precise diagnosis, steady-state Hb and reticulocyte count, and the name and address of the haematologist with whom the patient is registered. However, some patients present with life-threatening crises before the diagnosis has been made. The first crises may occur at any age but are most frequent in the first two decades of life. When caring for an individual with SCD it is important to bear in mind that the patient may require repeated visits to hospital, often via the A&E department, and that the family may have other affected members, some of whom may have already died from SCD. It is particularly important that the patient is treated with consideration and that the family's fears are not lightly dismissed.

Many adult patients with SCD coming to A&E require admission. Most attend for one of three reasons:

1. Painful crisis.
2. Life-threatening crisis.
3. Priapism.

The painful crisis

When a patient who is *known* to have SCD presents with a painful crisis similar to previous crises, analgesia should be given as soon as possible before taking a full history.

Medical history

The following are important points to elucidate from the history in all forms of sickle crisis:

- Has the patient got a haemoglobinopathy card? The card will give important administrative and clinical details.
- Has the patient had any symptoms suggesting an infection? Appropriate investigations and treatment can be initiated. Viral infections, particularly *parvovirus*, may precipitate an aplastic crisis.
- Has the patient done anything which may have caused dehydration (e.g. prolonged travel, unaccustomed exercise, excessive alcohol intake)? For many teenagers, parties and raves may combine all three causes.
- Has the patient experienced shortness of breath? Dyspnoea may suggest profound anaemia, chest infection, chest syndrome or pulmonary embolus.
- Has the patient experienced a sudden weakness, sensory disturbance or a fit? CNS (central nervous system) complications require specific emergency and long-term management.
- Does the patient comply with treatment recommendations (e.g. prophylactic antibiotics)? Pneumococcal infection is a common cause of death in children over the age of 3 months and in adults. The risk can be considerably reduced by taking regular prophylactic penicillin, in addition to receiving a pneumovax infection.
- Has the patient undergone a transfusion within the last fortnight? A red cell transfusion may cause a delayed haemolytic reaction, particularly in people who have been previously transfused.

Physical examination

Important points are:

- Has the patient got a temperature? Fever does not necessarily imply infection as a sickle crisis alone often produces a rise in temperature.
- Is there evidence of a focus of infection? Appropriate investigations (e.g. chest X-ray, blood and urine culture) should be initiated.
- Is the patient dehydrated? Is there any reason why they should not drink? Moderate dehydration can be corrected by drinking or fluids given by nasogastric tube. Venous access may be very difficult and precious in these patients.
- Is there organomegaly? Ask the patient or the relatives whether the liver or spleen is larger than usual. Organ sequestration is a life-threatening situation, particularly in young children.
- Are there signs of pulmonary consolidation or tachypnoea? Consider the chest syndrome (see section on life-threatening complications, below), pulmonary embolus or infection.

Investigations

The following should be initiated in all patients:

Full blood count and film

The Hb should be compared with previous results if known. A raised WBC (white cell count) often accompanies a sickle crisis and does not necessarily indicate infection. Circulating nucleated red cells are commonly present during sickle crisis and will be counted by most automated systems as leucocytes.

Reticulocyte count

Most individuals with SCD have a raised count (5–20%). A low or normal reticulocyte count may be an indication of an aplastic crisis.

Serum for blood group, antibody screen and compatibility testing

Many of these patients have red cell antibodies, and the blood transfusion laboratory will require advanced notice if they are to provide compatible blood.

Blood, urine and swabs for culture and sensitivity as indicated

The request should mention any antibiotics already being taken by the patient.

Other investigations

If a chest infection or the chest syndrome is considered then blood gases and a chest X-ray should be checked. If the girdle syndrome is suspected (see section on life-threatening complications), abdominal X-ray films and the serum amylase should be taken on admission and monitored. Urea and electrolytes may be useful if renal impairment or dehydration is suspected. Young children often have poor renal concentrating power with urinary potassium loss. If intravenous fluids are required, appropriate potassium replacement should be given by this route. When interpreting liver function tests, the clinician should take into account that the bilirubin is often elevated due to chronic haemolysis and that the alkaline phosphatase may be raised during adolescence due to rapid bone growth.

Treatment

The main principles of treatment in the A&E department are identification and treatment of life-threatening complications, warmth, rehydration and analgesia. A flow-chart showing the A&E management of SCD is shown in Fig. 3.

Analgesia

The pain of bone infarction may be mild, requiring only simple analgesia. Alternatively, it may be so severe that parenteral opiates are required. Most patients attend after home remedies have failed. Adequate analgesia should be achieved as soon as possible to break the cycle of pain. If no analgesia has been tried, mild pain may respond to paracetamol (1 g stat) together with a non-steroidal anti-inflammatory drug such as naproxen. If no improvement is seen, diamorphine is the opiate of choice for most people. It is more soluble than morphine and has fewer side-effects than pethidine. The dose of diamorphine is 0.1 mg kg^{-1} (5 mg for a 50-kg adult) given either subcutaneously or intravenously over 3–5 min. Intravenous doses should be repeated at 10-min intervals until improvement occurs. If given subcutaneously, reassess at 20-min intervals. Respiratory depression is uncommon if further increments are reduced to 0.05 mg kg^{-1}. Ideally the patient should not be transferred from the A&E department until adequate analgesia has been achieved. Excellent control can be continued using a patient-controlled analgesia system. These are preprogrammed syringe drivers to provide both background analgesia and boluses on demand.

Opiate addiction may become a problem for some patients. The problem appears to be more marked in those patients frequently receiving analgesia with a rapid action and short half-life, such as dextromoramide and pethidine. As a general rule, patients receiving opiate analgesia should be admitted to hospital. If opiates are required for several days they should be discontinued by reducing dosage to achieve a 24-h opiate-free period before discharge.

Life-threatening complications

Rapid action can be life-saving. Important types of life-threatening crises and their management are discussed below. The two commonest crises are acute splenic sequestration and pneumococcal septicaemia.

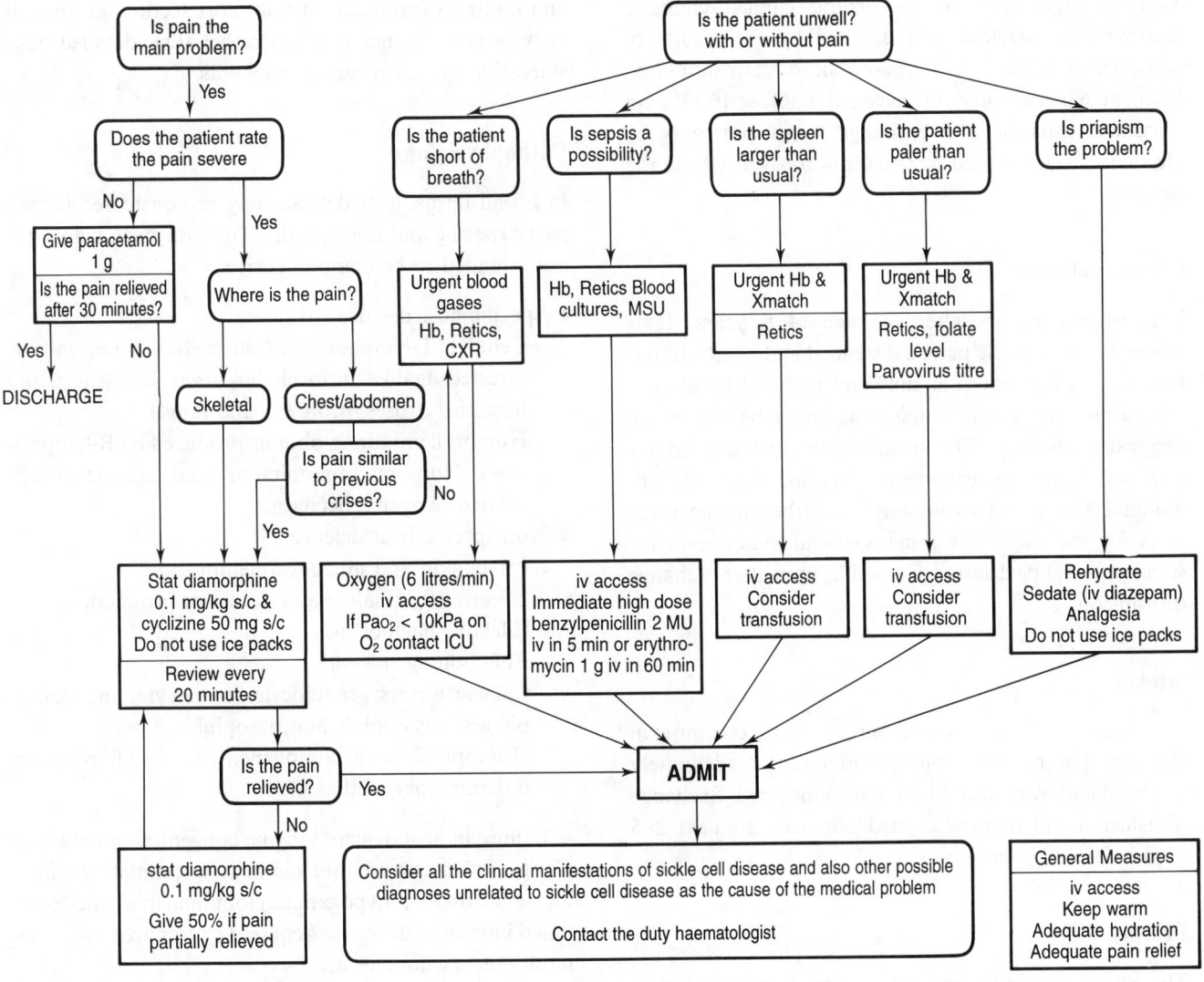

Fig. 3. Management of sickle cell disease in the A&E department. (Courtesy of Dr A.D. Stephens.)

Acute splenic sequestration

This is common in young children and is associated with high mortality. The spleen rapidly enlarges due to sequestered sickled red cells. The Hb falls rapidly. The precipitating cause is often a pneumococcal infection. Treatment is with emergency blood transfusion, intravenous fluids and antibiotics.

Pneumococcal infection

This may cause septicaemia, pneumonia or splenic sequestration. If suspected, antibiotic treatment should be initiated in the A&E department after blood cultures have been taken. The treatment of choice is benzylpenicillin (adult dose: 2 mega units given intravenously

over 5 min) or erythromycin (adult dose: 1 g diluted in 200 ml of 0.9% saline given intravenously over 1 h).

Parvovirus infection

This may be associated with a potentially fatal red cell aplasia in which the reticulocyte count and the Hb drop rapidly. The treatment is emergency blood transfusion.

Chest syndrome

Signs and symptoms include chest pain, pulmonary consolidation which is commonly bilateral, tachycardia and tachypnoea. The syndrome is often associated with infection in young people and infarction in adults. Chest

X-ray changes tend to lag behind clinical changes; treatment is therefore best directed by the results of blood gases. If $PaO_2 < 10\,kPa$ on air, oxygen should be given at 6 litres min^{-1} by mask; if $PaO_2 < 10\,kPa$ on oxygen, ventilation and exchange transfusion may be life-saving. Care should be taken not to overhydrate the patient.

Girdle syndrome

This usually occurs after the age of 8 years. It is associated with girdle pain, a distended abdomen without rebound, absent bowel sounds and bilateral basal consolidation. The precipitating cause may be any acute surgical pathology. The management includes hourly abdominal girth measurements, baseline chest and abdominal X-rays and serum amylase. Other management is as for the chest syndrome. General anaesthesia for surgery should be deferred, if possible, until after exchange transfusion.

Strokes

These can occur at any age but are most common in children. The patient should be maintained adequately hydrated and warm during transfer to the ward. Exchange transfusion will then be carried out over the next 2–3 days before angiography.

Priapism

The patient should be reassured, warmed and rehydrated. The duration of priapism should be determined: many patients are hesitant about presenting for medical attention with this distressing symptom. Surgical drainage will need to be considered if this period is 24 h or more. Initial management is with sedation and analgesia, using a benzodiazepine combined with an opiate. The route will be dictated by the degree of urgency. An exchange transfusion should be undertaken if there is no improvement after 4 h of sedation. After 24 h, deep general anaesthesia should be tried before proceeding to surgical drainage. Ice packs are contraindicated in the management of priapism due to sickle cell disease.

DISORDERS OF WHITE CELLS AND HOST DEFENCE

The body has a complex and well-integrated host defence system for dealing with injury, invasion by organisms and foreign substances. In this short section, an overall view of host defence is taken rather than detailed consideration of its various components.

Pathophysiology

In broad terms, host defence may be considered in two parts: specific and non-specific. The lists given below are not intended to be comprehensive.

- Specific host defence
  - Cellular: T-lymphocytes. Cell-mediated immunity is directed against intracellular organisms (e.g. many bacteria, viruses, protozoa and fungi).
  - Humoral: immunoglobulins produced by B-lymphocytes. Humoral immunity protects against encapsulated pyogenic bacteria.
- Non-specific host defence
  - Intact skin and mucuous membranes.
  - Effective tear, saliva and mucuous production.
  - Effective haemostasis.
  - Functioning spleen.
  - Cellular factors: granulocytes, monocytes and macrophages, eosinophils and basophils.
  - Humoral factors: complement, kinins, fibronectin, inflammatory mediators.

Failure in host defence may be congenital or acquired. Congenital causes are rare and include qualitative granulocyte disorders, hypogammaglobulinaemia and combined immunodeficiency. Acquired causes are more commonly seen; examples are:

- Chronic liver disease.
- Marrow failure.
- Steroids.
- Postsplenectomy.
- Malignancy.
- Immunosuppressive therapy.
- Diabetes.
- Malnutrition.
- Uraemia.
- Shock.
- AIDS (acquired immunodeficiency syndrome).

Presentation

When confronted with a patient with infection, it is important to determine if host factors are present which may cause an increased risk of infection. The clinician should also determine whether host factors are present which may mask clinical signs and limit the response to treatment. In these respects the following should be considered:

- Pre-existing medical conditions as listed above.
- Nutritional state.
- Current state of host defence including haemostasis.
- Current medical and surgical problems.
- State of circulation and adequacy of resuscitation.
- Possible portals of infection (e.g. intravenous cannulae, endotracheal intubation and wounds).
- Nature of invading organisms.

Immunocompromised and elderly patients may present atypically (e.g. without fever). The first sign in these patients may be septic shock within hours of a short period of non-specific illness.

Steroid therapy

Patients on regular steroid therapy should carry a steroid warning card. The dose of steroids will need to be increased during the period of illness. In A&E it should be established that steroids have not been suddenly discontinued. If they have, hydrocortisone (100 mg IV) should be given immediately to prevent shock.

Patients on chemotherapy or immunosuppressive therapy

Individuals undergoing immunosuppressive therapy or chemotherapy may become neutropenic and present in septic shock, most commonly due to Gram-negative organisms from the gut. Staphylococcal infections should be considered if a tunnelled central line (Hickman line) is present. All cases should be discussed with the specialist units concerned. Intravenous antibiotics may need to be started before transfer between hospitals.

Leukaemia

Leukaemias are characterized by the accumulation of abnormal white cells in the bone marrow. The abnormal cells cause bone marrow failure with varying degrees of anaemia, neutropenia and thrombocytopenia. Anaemia may present as fatigue and dyspnoea, neutropenia with mouth ulcers or infections and thrombocytopenia with bruising or bleeding. Organs may be infiltrated (e.g. liver, spleen, lymph nodes, meninges, brain, skin, testes). An accompanying electrolyte imbalance may precipitate a medical emergency. These include:

- Hyponatraemia due to the secretion of inappropriate antidiuretic hormone (SIADH).
- Hypernatraemia due to diabetes insipidus.
- Hypokalaemia due to renal failure.
- Hypercalcaemia due to osteolysis.
- Hyperuricaemia due to lysis of leukaemic cells.

Hyperviscosity syndrome

The causes of this syndrome include a very high white count, polycythaemia, myeloma and Waldenström's macroglobinaemia. The clinical features are fatigue, visual disturbances, headache, confusion and exacerbation of symptoms related to ischaemic heart disease. The clinical sequelae include convulsions, fundal haemorrhage, visual loss, thrombosis, platelet and leucocyte dysfunction and renal failure. Suspected cases must be quickly referred to a haematologist. The treatment is directed at treating the underlying cause. Urgent treatment may involve leucopheresis in leukaemia, venesection in polycythaemia and plasma exchange in myeloma and Waldenström's macroglobulinaemia.

Multiple myeloma

Myelomatosis is a malignant disorder of plasma cells. It is characterized by lytic bone lesions and a monoclonal serum paraprotein. Although relatively rare, the disorder may present with one of the following medical emergencies:

- Uraemia.
- Acute hypercalcaemia.
- Compression paraplegia.
- Painful bony lesions or pathological fractures.
- Severe anaemia.
- Infection related to immunosuppression.
- Hyperviscosity syndrome (see above).

Early treatment such as rehydration, fracture stabilization and analgesia should be initiated prior to referral to an oncologist/haematologist.

The spleen

The spleen is the largest lymphoid organ in the body and is situated in the left hypochondrium. Its functions are:

- Sequestration and phagocytosis of old or abnormal red cells.

- Immunological functions, IgM and tuftsin production.
- Extramedullary haemopoiesis during haematological stress.
- Pooling of red cells and platelets.

Splenomegaly

Splenomegaly may be found in a number of conditions including infective, inflammatory and haematological. Massive enlargement is seen in chronic myeloid leukaemia, myelofibrosis, chronic malaria and kala-azar. Splenomegaly may cause anaemia by shortening red cell lifespan and sequestering red cells. The other complications are hypersplenism causing splenic infarction and splenic rupture following minimal trauma.

Splenectomy

Splenectomy may be performed for trauma, haematological diseases and hypersplenism. Patients are then prone to bacterial infections especially *Pneumococcus* and *Haemophilus*. All patients undergoing splenectomy should receive prophylaxis against pneumococcal infections with the polyvalent antipneumococcal vaccine at least 2 weeks prior to surgery. Phenoxymethylpenicillin 250 mg twice daily should be started after surgery and continued indefinitely (British Committee for Standards in Haematology, 1996). Haematological features post-splenectomy include thrombocytosis, a mild lymphocytosis and monocytosis, a raised MCV and characteristic red cell morphology such as poikilocytosis and Howell–Jolly bodies.

DISORDERS OF HAEMOSTASIS

Haemostasis has two main functions; these are to confine blood to the circulation and to stop bleeding at the site of vessel injury. The process involves a complex interaction between blood vessels, platelets and coagulation factors (Fig. 4). The pathophysiology of haemostasis will be considered under three main headings: vascular disorders, platelet disorders and coagulation disorders.

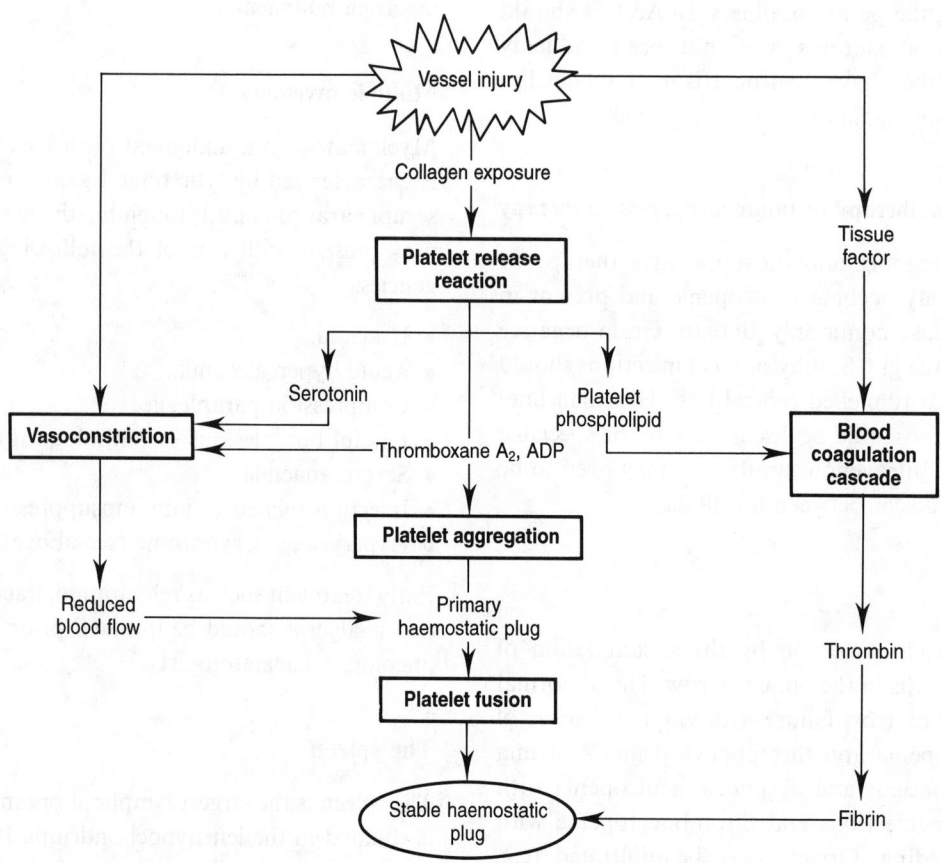

Fig. 4. Reactions involved in haemostasis. (Reproduced, with permission, from A.V. Hoffbrand & J.E. Pettit (1993). *Essential Haematology*. Oxford: Blackwell Scientific.)

Vascular disorders

Vascular endothelial cells comprise a major component of primary haemostasis and serve a variety of functions:

- The supply of nutrients to subendothelial structures.
- Presenting a non-thrombogenic surface for circulating blood.
- Synthesis of prostacyclin, factor VIII:VWF (von Willebrand factor), tissue plasminogen activator (t-PA), antithrombin III and thrombomodulin.

The vascular disorders are a heterogeneous group of conditions. The underlying abnormality is either in the vessels or in the perivascular connective tissues. The defects may be congenital or acquired and in most cases the bleeding is not severe. Bleeding into the skin causes petechiae and ecchymoses and in some disorders there is mucuous membrane bleeding.

Hereditary haemorrhagic telangiectasia

This is an uncommon disorder inherited as an autosomal dominant trait. Telangiectasia are anastomosing thin-walled dilated capillaries and venules. They can be distinguished from petechiae by their blanching on pressure. The telangiectasia appear in childhood and become more numerous with age. They are most commonly found on the face, lips, inside the nose and mouth. Bleeding from these lesions in the gut and nose may give rise to chronic iron deficiency.

Acquired vascular defects are more commonly seen, but in general they rarely cause severe bleeding. Examples are listed in Table 7.

Platelet disorders

Platelets play an essential role in haemostasis. Their main role is the formation of mechanical plugs following vessel injury. Central to this function are:

- Adhesion to the damaged vessel.
- Release of ADP (adenosine diphosphate), serotonin and other factors from their granules.
- Aggregation.
- Fusion.
- Procoagulant properties.

Platelets are produced in the bone marrow by the fragmentation of megakaryocyte cytoplasm. Once released, the normal platelet lifespan is approximately 7–10 days.

Table 7. *Acquired vascular disorders*

Simple easy bruising
Senile purpura
Vascular (non-thrombocytopenic) purpuras
   Infections
   Drugs
   Uraemia
Cushing's disease and steroid administration
Scurvy
Dysproteinaemias, cryoglobulinaemia, macroglobinaemia, multiple myeloma
Henoch–Schölein syndrome (anaphylactoid purpura)
Miscellaneous disorders
   Systemic disorders, e.g. collagen disease, amyloidosis, allergy
   Orthostatic purpuras
   Mechanical purpura
   Fat embolism

Both quantitative and qualitative platelet disorders may result in abnormal bleeding. The bleeding is characterized by spontaneous skin purpura and mucosal haemorrhage and prolonged bleeding after trauma. Thrombocytopenia is a quantitative disorder, and may be classified in four functional groups as shown in Table 8.

Table 8. *Causes of thrombocytopenia*

- Failure of platelet production
  - Selective megakaryocyte depression due to drugs, e.g. cotrimoxazole, tolbutamide, thiazide diuretics, or viral infection
  - Part of general bone marrow failure, e.g. aplastic anaemia, leukaemia, marrow infiltration, megaloblastic anaemia, myelodysplasia
- Increased destruction of platelets
  - Autoimmune thrombocytopenic purpura: acute and chronic
  - Secondary immune thrombocytopenia associated with infection
  - SLE and lymphoproliferative disease
  - Drug-induced immune thrombocytopenia, e.g. quinine, quinidine
  - Disseminated intravascular coagulation (DIC)
  - Malaria
- Increased sequestration of platelets
  - Hypersplenism
- Loss of platelets
  - Massive blood transfusion
  - Extracorporeal circulation

SLE, systemic lupus erythematosus.

Disorders of platelet function should be suspected in patients who clinically demonstrate signs of primary haemostatic failure despite a normal platelet count. A number of hereditary disorders exist (e.g. Bernard–Soulier syndrome and Glanzmann's thrombasthenia) but these are rare. Acquired platelet defects occur much more frequently and may be seen in the following conditions:

- Uraemia.
- Liver disease.
- Hypergammaglobulinaemia.
- Myeloproliferative disorders.
- Antiplatelet drugs (e.g. aspirin).

Aspirin induces a functional platelet disorder which lasts 4–7 days following a single dose. Although it rarely causes purpura it will exacerbate bleeding from other causes.

Coagulation disorders

Blood coagulation involves a cascading biological amplification system culminating in the formation of thrombin (Fig. 5). Patients with a deficiency of a coagulation factor may have a bleeding or thrombotic disorder. The bleeding tends to cause ecchymoses rather than petechiae. If sufficiently severe, these patients may suffer both post-traumatic and spontaneous intramuscular haematomata and haemarthroses. Acquired disorders are more common than inherited deficiencies.

Hereditary defiencies of coagulation factors

The following inherited coagulation disorders are well known but uncommon; haemophilia A (factor VIII deficiency), haemophilia B (factor IX deficiency) and

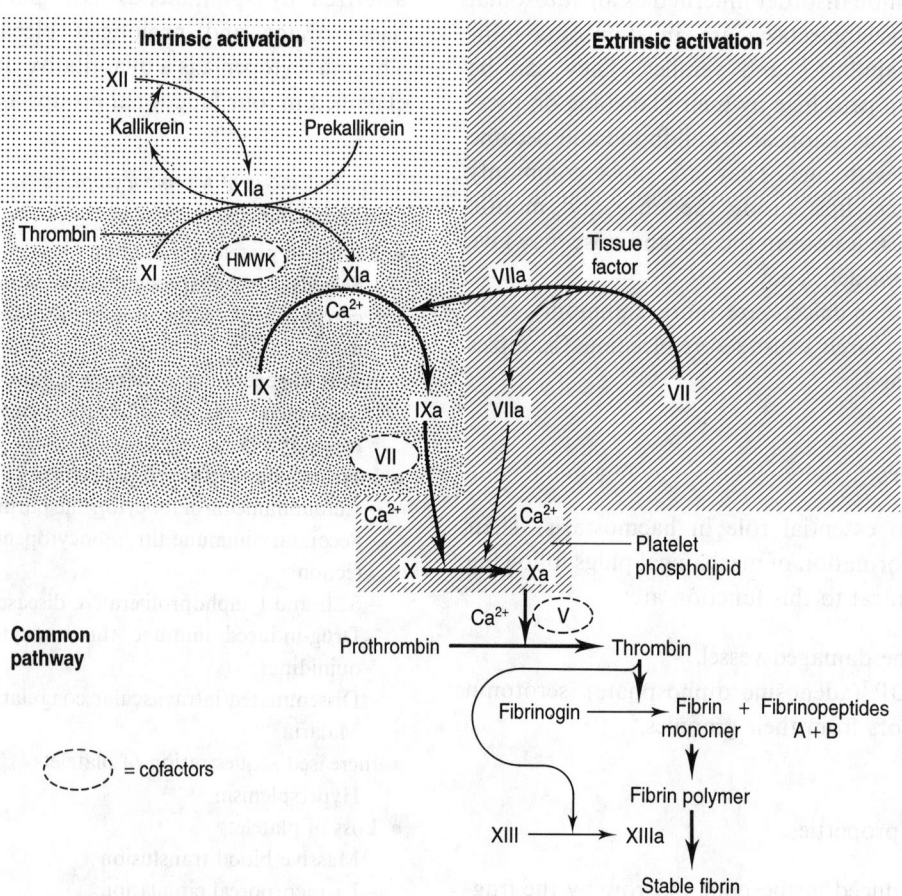

Fig. 5. The pathways of blood coagulation. (Reproduced, with permission from A.V. Hoffbrand & J.E. Pettit (1993). *Essential Haematology*. Oxford: Blackwell Scientific.)

von Willebrand's disease. The other disorders are rare. The clinical severity of the disease correlates with the degree of factor deficiency. Most severely affected children will present as soon as they start to toddle. However, less severely affected individuals may present in later life following trauma or minor operative procedures.

Acquired disorders of coagulation

The commonly seen acquired disorders are discussed below.

Liver disease

This may be complicated by a variety of haemostatic abnormalities which in turn may exacerbate bleeding (e.g. from oesophageal varices):

- Biliary obstruction may lead to vitamin K deficiency resulting in decreased synthesis of factors II, VII, IX and X.
- Hypersplenism may cause thrombocytopenia.
- Platelet function is often abnormal in liver disease.
- Functional abnormalities of fibrinogen may occur.

Vitamin K deficiency

Vitamin K deficiency may occur in children or adults as a result of obstructive jaundice, pancreatic or small bowel disease.

Disseminated intravascular coagulation

In this coagulopathy, widespread deposition of intravascular fibrin leads to the consumption of coagulation factors and platelets (Fig. 6). The spectrum of presentation is wide, ranging from a chronic compensated state to an acute form with widespread bleeding. DIC is associated with a large number of conditions, including:

- Tissue trauma including shock and burns.
- Sepsis.
- Many obstetric complications.
- Haemolysis following a transfusion reaction or drowning.
- Neoplasms or leukaemia.
- Snakebites and other miscellaneous causes.

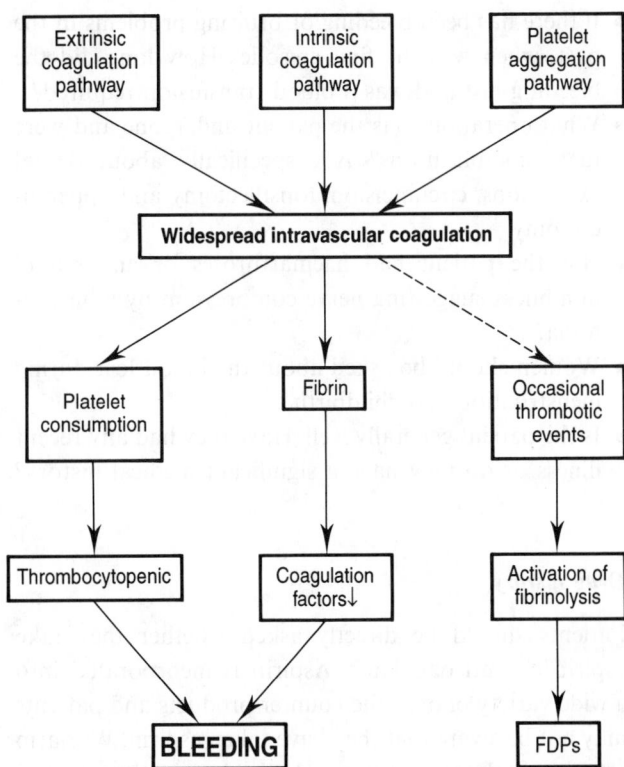

Fig. 6. Disseminated intravascular coagulation. FDPs, fibrin degradation products.

Anticoagulant drugs and fibrinolytics

Overanticoagulation with heparin, oral anticoagulants or thrombolytic therapy may cause bleeding from pre-existing lesions or bruising and bleeding following minimal trauma.

Clinical approach to the patient with bleeding problems

Although the precise diagnosis of a bleeding disorder may depend on laboratory tests, much information may be obtained from the history and physical examination.

The aim should be to determine the following:

- Is there a generalized haemostatic defect?
- Is the defect inherited or acquired?
- Is it a vascular/platelet or a coagulation disorder?

Medical history

The following detailed questions may be relevant:

- Was the bleeding spontaneous or following trauma?

- If there has been bleeding or bruising problems in the past, when was the first episode? How long did the bleeding last and was a blood transfusion required?
- What operations has the patient undergone and were there complications? Ask specifically about dental extractions, circumcision, tonsillectomy and appendicectomy.
- Has the patient had haemarthroses or an area of numbness suggesting nerve compression by a haematoma?
- Women should be asked about the blood lost during menstruation and childbirth.
- Is the patient generally well. Have they had any recent illness or do they have a significant medical history?

Drug history

Patients should be directly asked whether they take aspirin or anticoagulants. Aspirin is incorporated into a wide variety of over-the-counter products and patients may not be aware that they have taken aspirin. Warfarin interacts with many drugs and all other medication and any changes in drugs or dosage should be noted in patients taking warfarin.

Family history

This is helpful in establishing the diagnosis of an inherited disorder. The pattern of inheritance may have great diagnostic relevance.

Physical examination

The physical examination should establish the nature and extent of bleeding. If a bruised patient is unconscious with or without evidence of head injury, a search of the clothing may reveal out-patient appointment and anticoagulation cards. The clinician should determine the urgency with which investigations, emergency treatment and appropriate referrals are to be carried out.

Emergency investigation

The majority of haemostatic problems can be characterized by using simple screening tests. These can be supplemented by further investigations to confirm the diagnosis.

Screening tests

Full blood count and films

A platelet count is required. Examination of the film will exclude a spuriously low count due to platelet clumping. In thrombocytopenia, the presence of large platelets in the blood film suggest that the cause may be peripheral destruction. Diagnostic red cell morphology may be seen in DIC, liver and renal disease and marrow infiltration. The presence of abnormal cells will indicate specific causes such as leukaemia and lymphoma.

Prothrombin time

Prothrombin time (PT) evaluates the extrinsic and common coagulation pathways. Thromboplastin is used to initiate coagulation by reacting with factor VII. The PT is prolonged in patients with acquired or congenital deficiencies of factors II, V, VII, X and fibrinogen. It is used to monitor oral anticoagulation therapy (therapeutic range, INR (international normalized ratio) = 2.0–4.5).

Activated partial thromboplastin time

APTT evaluates the intrinsic and final common pathways. A prolonged APTT is observed if there is a deficiency in factors VIII, IX, XI, XII or 'contact factors'. It is also prolonged in the presence of inhibitors such as the lupus anticoagulant. The APTT is used to monitor heparin therapy (therapeutic range, 1.5–2.5 × control value of APTT).

Thrombin time

Thrombin time (TT) assesses the conversion of fibrinogen to fibrin. The clotting of citrated plasma by thrombin depends on the quantity and quality of fibrinogen and the presence of inhibitors. Fibrin degradation products (FDPs), heparin and paraproteins will inhibit the conversion of fibrinogen to fibrin.

Bleeding time

This is an overall test of primary haemostasis. Although simple and fundamental in haematology, it is rarely appropriate in the A&E room. It is indicated when abnormal bleeding is identified in the presence of a normal platelet count and clotting screen.

Table 9. *The usual laboratory findings in chronic liver disease, disseminated intravascular coagulation and overanticoagulation with warfarin*

	Liver disease	DIC	Overanticoagulation with warfarin
PT (INR)	↑↑	↑	↑↑
APTT	↑	↑	↑
TT	↑	↑	N
Fibrinogen	N/↓	↓	N
FDPs	N	↑	N
Platelet count	N/↓	↓	N

DIC, disseminated intravascular coagulation; PT, prothrombin time; INR, international normalized ratio; APTT, activated partial thromboplastin time; TT, thrombin time; FDPs, fibrin degradation products; N, normal.

Confirmatory tests

Table 9 shows the usual laboratory findings in three common acquired coagulation disorders.

Mixing tests

The approach to a person with a prolonged APTT is to determine whether it is due to a factor deficiency or an inhibitor. A 1:1 mix of normal/patient plasma is retested. Normal plasma will correct the APTT when there is a coagulation factor deficiency but not if an inhibitor is present.

Fibrin degradation products

Excessive fibrinolysis as seen in DIC can be demonstrated by increased FDPs. Local methods and the type of sample required vary; check first with the haematology laboratory.

Fibrinogen

This is best checked on the original citrated sample once the TT has been shown to be prolonged. A plasma level below $0.5 \, g \, l^{-1}$ (normal range $2-4 \, g \, l^{-1}$) may indicate the need for cryoprecipitate therapy.

Bone marrow examination

Decreased production of platelets is characterized by reduced numbers of megakaryocytes, with or without an abnormal infiltrate. Increased megakaryocytes in the presence of thrombocytopenia suggests that the platelets are being prematurely destroyed.

Other tests

Coagulation factor assays and platelet function tests, etc. may be needed to determine the exact diagnosis but are not usually performed as emergency tests.

Early treatment

The nature of most problems should be identified following the history, examination and screening tests. Treatment may not need to be initiated before the final diagnosis is made.

General measures

These include prompt correction of hypovolaemia, sepsis, acidosis and surgical bleeding.

Dextrans impair platelet function and should be avoided as a volume expander in bleeding patients.

Anaemia should be corrected, but the use of large volumes of stored red cell concentrates may exacerbate the haemostatic problem (see section on blood transfusion). Often specific blood component therapy should be started before fully correcting blood loss. Patients with severe haemostatic defects should be moved with great care. Intramuscular injections are contraindicated and venepuncture and arterial puncture sites require sustained moderate pressure after the procedure.

Specific measures

Vitamin K

Factors II, VII, IX and X are vitamin K-dependent. Administration of vitamin K may be indicated in patients with liver and small bowel disease and for reversal of warfarin therapy; 10 mg will start correcting a prolonged PT after 4 h. The full effects are seen 24–48 h later and refractoriness to warfarin therapy may last up to 2 weeks.

Fresh frozen plasma, cryoprecipitate and coagulation factor concentrates

Fresh frozen plasma (FFP) is needed for the replacement of multiple coagulation factor deficiencies, such as DIC

(British Committee for Standards in Haematology, 1992). Cryoprecipitate may be used for fibrinogen replacement (e.g. to treat bleeding after thrombolytic therapy). Single inherited coagulation factor deficiencies are treated using purified single factor concentrates (e.g. factor VIII; see section on blood transfusion).

Specific emergencies and management

Correction of warfarin overanticoagulation

Coumarin anticoagulants interfere with the synthesis of factors II, VII, IX and X. Many drugs and conditions will affect the dose of warfarin required. Changes in either may result in a rapid increase or decrease in the effect of warfarin. Overanticoagulation and bleeds should be managed according to the guidelines outlined in Table 10. Before reversing warfarin therapy the clinician must be clear as to whether effective anticoagulation will be required soon after the event. In view of the risks of infection with blood component therapy, factor II, IX and X concentrates used together with factor VII concentrates are the preferred alternative to FFP if they are available (UK Regional Haemophilia Centre Directors Committee, 1992).

Bleeding following thrombolytic therapy

Agents such as streptokinase and t-PA cause local and generalized fibrinolysis and are used to treat arterial and venous thrombi. Bleeding is unusual when thrombolytic agents are used at the recommended doses with the

Table 10. *Management of overanticoagulation with warfarin* (Recommendations of British Committee for Standards in Haematology, 1991a)

- *Life threatening haemorrhage*
  Immediately give vitamin K 5 mg by slow intravenous injection and either a concentrate of factor II, IX, X with a factor VII concentrate (if these are available) or fresh frozen plasma
- *Less severe haemorrhage, e.g. haematuria or epistaxis*
  Withhold warfarin for 1 or more days and consider giving vitamin K 0.5–2 mg IV
- *INR > 4.5 without haemorrhage*
  Withdraw warfarin for 1 or 2 days and then review
- *Unexpected bleeding at therapeutic levels*
  Investigate possibility of underlying cause such as unsuspected renal or alimentary tract disease

---

INR, international normalized ratio.

contraindications observed. The incidence is approximately 1% in patients being treated for myocardial infarction. The half-lives are short and haemostasis will return to near normal within 2 h of stopping an infusion. If rapid treatment of severe bleeding after thrombolysis is required, the infusion should be stopped and the TT and fibrinogen measured. If the fibrinogen is greater than 0.5 g l^{-1}, correction should be achieved with 2–4 units of FFP. If fibrinogen is less than 0.5 g dl^{-1}, cryoprecipitate or fibrinogen concentrate should be considered for fibrinogen replacement.

Bleeding following heparin therapy

Haemorrhage is more likely to occur with excessive anticoagulation if the APTT is above the therapeutic range than if the dose of heparin is well controlled. The half-life of heparin is approximately 60 min, and so withdrawal of heparin is usually all that is needed to stop bleeding. If rapid correction is required with severe bleeding or with a massive overdose of heparin, intravenous protamine sulphate should be given slowly (1 mg of protamine neutralizes 150 i.u. of heparin but should not exceed 40 mg in one injection).

Disseminated intravascular coagulation

Acute DIC results in a haemorrhagic syndrome which may be very severe. The diagnosis is often suggested by a tendency to generalized bleeding and oozing, especially at venepuncture sites. Treatment must be directed at the underlying cause. If supportive therapy is indicated, FFP (2–4 units) and platelets are given, and the response to treatment is guided by clinical and laboratory responses.

Inherited coagulation disorders

Known haemophiliacs are registered with specialist haemophiliac centres. Patients and their families are trained to deal with bleeding emergencies but may still present to an A&E department. The action which has already been taken should be established and then their haemophilia centre should be contacted for advice.

Thrombophilia

Thrombophilia is a term describing inherited or acquired defects of haemostasis leading to a predisposition to thrombosis. It should be considered in patients with unexpected or recurrent venous or arterial thromboses.

Investigations are usually carried out after anticoagulation has been completed but should be considered before anticoagulants are started. It is important to note that proteins C and S are vitamin K-dependent and are reduced in patients taking warfarin. Basic investigations should include:

- Coagulation screen, including a fibrinogen level.
- Screening for lupus anticoagulant.
- Assays for activated protein C resistance, proteins C and S and antithrombin III.
- Tests of the fibrinolytic pathway.

Local practice varies and these cases are best discussed with a haematologist.

BLOOD TRANSFUSION

Emergency transfusion facilities

Emergency transfusion facilities may be considered in terms of personnel, equipment and materials. Staff are a hospital's greatest asset and good working relationships pay dividends in times of stress. The blood transfusion laboratory should not be abused by overordering blood and blood products and asking for all tests to be performed urgently. Furthermore, time spent on accurate initial assessment of the patient and attention to essential clerical details when requesting blood may save vital time in its provision.

Personnel

Medical laboratory scientific officer

State registered MLSOs have completed a minimum of 3 years' training. The responsibilities they assume are frequently not appreciated by clinicians. Work from different areas of the hospital often arrives simultaneously and must be prioritized. If blood is required urgently, this must be made clear. Although MLSOs are experienced in laboratory aspects of haematology and blood transfusion to varying degrees, they are not able to give clinical guidance (Beal & Isbister, 1985).

Haematologist with special expertise in transfusion medicine

As blood component therapy becomes more complex, haematologists are required to devote more of their time and expertise to providing a specialized consultative service with respect to clinical aspects of blood transfusion. Such staff are also responsible for the hospital blood transfusion laboratory, coordination of the hospital transfusion committee and implementation of major incident procedures.

Equipment

Automated blood count analysers

These are increasingly available in the A&E department alongside blood gas analysers. These machines must be well maintained and used with care if they are to give accurate results. The main haematology laboratory should be responsible for daily maintenance and quality control.

Blood salvage machines

Increasingly, intraoperative blood salvage is practised when surgery causes significant bleeding in the operative field. Salvage should only be performed in the absence of infection and malignancy. Blood is removed by suction, anticoagulated, washed and resuspended prior to re-infusion. Trained staff and equipment are required, but the equipment is now more compact and mobile and, if available, may be considered for use in the emergency room.

Materials

Blood components are red cells, platelet concentrates, FFP and cryoprecipitate; units of each are produced from one donation of blood. Plasma fractions are preparations such as coagulation factor concentrates and albumin produced from pooled donor plasma (McClelland, 1996).

The cells and proteins in the blood express antigens which are controlled by polymorphic genes (i.e. a specific antigen may be present in some individuals but not others; Table 11). A blood transfusion may immunize

Table 11. *Antigens and antibodies in the ABO system*

Phenotype (UK)	Genotype	Antigens	Antibodies	Frequency (%)
O	OO	None	Anti-A and anti-B	44
A	AA or AO	A	Anti-B	45
B	BB or BO	B	Anti-A	8
AB	AB	A and B	None	3

the patient against antigens he or she lacks. All blood components should be ABO-matched and RhD-positive material should not be given to women of child-bearing age. Red cell concentrates provide no functional white cells or platelets but these non-viable cells are still immunogenic and may cause complications. In the absence of blood loss, 1 unit should raise the haemoglobin of an adult by about 1.0 g dl^{-1}.

It is important to note that blood components, unlike plasma fractions, are not virucidally inactivated. They are therefore capable of transmitting any infective agent not detected in routine donor screening.

Whole blood

This is no longer the standard red cell preparation in the UK and is now rarely available in hospital blood banks. It is used only in situations where plasma proteins are also required (e.g. acute blood loss). Coagulation factors with long half-lives will be present in normal amounts but shortlived coagulation factors such as factors V and VIII fall to 10–20% of normal during the first 2 weeks of storage. The volume of 1 unit is approximately 510 ml with a haematocrit of 0.35–0.45 ll^{-1}. Small volume packs (100 ml) may be available in larger centres for paediatric use.

Packed red cells

Plasma (200–250 ml) is removed from a unit of whole blood for further processing. Packed cells are indicated for red cell replacement in acute and chronic anaemia. They should be used together with saline, colloids or plasma when replacing acute blood loss. One unit has a volume of 200 ml with a haematocrit of 0.55–0.75 ll^{-1}.

Red cell concentrates (supplemented)

These are packed cells to which a nutrient solution has been added following removal of nearly all the plasma. The slightly reduced haematocrit (0.50–0.70 ll^{-1}) and lower viscosity allows better flow rates to be achieved than with unsupplemented concentrates.

Fresh frozen plasma

FFP is prepared by freezing the plasma from a unit of blood within 6 h of donation. FFP is used for the replacement of coagulation factors in acquired coagulation factor deficiencies. Packs are stored at −30°C and when thawed contain 200–250 ml. Paediatric units are available in packs of 50 ml. Once thawed, units should be given within 20 min using standard blood giving sets. The dose is 12–15 ml kg^{-1}. Treatment should be monitored using the PT, APTT or TT depending on the coagulation disorder present. Adverse reactions are not uncommon: urticaria is seen in 2–3% and life-threatening anaphylaxis occurs in 1:20 000 patients (British Committee for Standards in Haematology, 1992).

Cryoprecipitate

This is produced by the controlled thawing of FFP; it contains factor VIII:C, von Willebrand factor and fibrinogen. It may be used for fibrinogen replacement therapy following thrombolytic therapy and sometimes in uraemic bleeding. Cryoprecipitate is no longer used to treat patients with haemophilia A or von Willebrand disease because of the greater risk of viral transmission than with treated factor concentrates. The adult dose is 4–6 packs; each unit is from a different donor increasing the risk of viral transmission. Once thawed, each pack containing 10–20 ml plasma can be carefully pooled into one bag and infused through a fresh giving set. To maximize the recovery of cryoprecipitate, saline may be used to flush the bags and giving set. Alternatively the packs can be drawn into 50-ml syringes and slowly injected. As with FFP, adverse reactions do occur; resuscitation staff and equipment should be available.

Platelet concentrates

These are prepared from single red cell donations to give units of approximately 53 × 10^9 platelets in 50–60 ml of plasma. An adult dose is 4–6 packs; each pack can be given over 5 min. Alternatively, platelet concentrates may be prepared by plateletpheresis of a single donor. Platelets are stored at 22°C, unlike blood which is refrigerated at 4°C, and they have a shelf-life of only 5 days. Standard giving sets with 170 μm filters or special platelet giving sets should be used. Not all hospital blood banks store platelet concentrates and there may be a delay while they are delivered from the regional transfusion centre.

Coagulation factor concentrates

These are freeze-dried in vials and made up with saline according to the manufacturer's instructions. Intravenous boluses are given slowly using a syringe and butterfly needle.

Albumin

There are two preparations. Human albumin solution 4.5%, previously called plasma protein fraction (PPF), containing albumin $45\,\mathrm{g\,l^{-1}}$ and sodium $160\,\mathrm{mmol\,l^{-1}}$. It is produced in 50, 100, 250 and 500 ml bottles. Human albumin solution 20%, previously called 'salt-poor albumin', contains albumin $200\,\mathrm{g\,l^{-1}}$ and sodium $130\,\mathrm{mmol\,l^{-1}}$ and is produced in 50 and 100 ml bottles.

Practical aspects of blood transfusion in A&E

In principle, blood transfusion in the A&E department does not differ from transfusion elsewhere. Blood and blood products are not immediately available and their use is associated with acute and chronic complications. The benefits of their use must clearly outweigh any disadvantages.

Fluid choice in resuscitation

The first 20% of blood volume loss can be managed with a plasma substitute. The choice lies between crystalloids, synthetic colloids (dextrans, gelatins and hydroxyethyl starch) and natural colloids (albumin). Crystalloids are thought to be satisfactory for initial replacement but they are rapidly distributed between the intravascular and interstitial spaces. Colloids maintain osmotic pressure better than crystalloids and are less likely to cause pulmonary and peripheral oedema. Albumin solutions are generally not indicated in acute fluid loss and there are no data to suggest that they are more effective than the synthetic colloids which are cheaper. However, their use may be indicated if volume replacement is prolonged and if the serum albumin is less than $20\,\mathrm{g\,l^{-1}}$. Losses of 20–50% of circulating volume require red cell concentrates (up to 3 units) plus a plasma substitute.

Massive transfusion

Massive blood loss presents a serious threat to survival. The anxiety created by the urgent need to replace blood may lead to tension between laboratory staff and those treating the haemorrhage. The definition of massive transfusion is arbitrary, but the term is commonly accepted to mean the replacement of the patient's total blood volume within 24 h (British Committee for Standards in Haematology, 1991b). The aim of transfusion after restoring circulating volume is to maintain a blood composition which achieves adequate oxygen-carrying capacity, haemostasis, oncotic pressure and plasma biochemistry.

The following parameters and target values are used to guide fluid and red cell replacement:

- Systolic blood pressure and pulse.
- Urine output $>30\,\mathrm{ml\,h^{-1}}$.
- Haemoglobin $>10\,\mathrm{g\,dl^{-1}}$.
- Haematocrit $>0.32\,\mathrm{ll^{-1}}$.

Stored blood has no functioning platelets, and dilutional thrombocytopenia should be anticipated after a blood volume replacement of 150%. If there is pre-existing DIC or thrombocytopenia, platelet concentrates will be required much sooner. In order to secure haemostasis the platelet count should be maintained above $50 \times 10^9\,\mathrm{l^{-1}}$.

Coagulation factor depletion is unusual. Stored whole blood contains adequate amounts of all coagulation factors except factors V and VIII. If plasma-reduced blood is used, FFP ($12\,\mathrm{ml\,kg^{-1}}$) may be required after 25% of the blood volume is replaced (Lunsgaard-Hansen, 1992). The critical levels of the plasma haemostatic parameters in injured and massively transfused patients are (British Committee for Standards in Haematology, 1991b):

- Prothrombin time (PT): $1.5 \times$ normal.
- Activated partial thromboplastin time (APPT): $1.5 \times$ normal.
- Fibrinogen: 1.0–$1.5\,\mathrm{g\,l^{-1}}$.

Further complications associated with massive transfusion of stored blood include:

- Hypocalcaemia due to the citrate anticoagulant binding ionized calcium. This is only a significant problem in neonates and if hypothermia is present. Treatment with 10% calcium gluconate should be given if clinical or electrocardiographic (ECG) evidence of hypocalcaemia exists.
- Hyperkalaemia due to the higher potassium content of stored blood. Hyperkalaemia, especially in the presence of hypocalcaemia and hypothermia, may lead to cardiac arrest. In practice it is not common.
- Acidosis due to the excessive lactic acid produced by red cell glycolysis. This is reversed by the improved tissue perfusion following transfusion.
- Hypothermia. If blood stored at 4°C is not prewarmed.

The combination of the above could impair cardiac performance and precipitate cardiac arrest in the shocked patient. Close cardiac and temperature monitoring are essential.

- Oxygen affinity changes. These changes might theoretically be expected to impair tissue oxygenation; however, any effect appears to be transient. There is no objective evidence to support the use of fresh blood for patients with massive blood loss.

Blood ordering

The medical staff in the A&E department are responsible for deciding the degree of urgency when ordering blood. Blood can be provided quickly (see below) but time must be allowed for careful documentation and portering. In the rare situations in which uncross-matched blood is indicated, a sample for later compatibility testing must be taken before transfusion. Full pretransfusion compatibility testing includes:

- Blood grouping.
- Antibody screening.
- Selection of donor blood with the same ABO and RhD group.
- Cross-matching.

Cross-matching may either be a full cross-match or an immediate spin depending on local practice. Categories of compatibility testing and the time taken to prepare them in our own laboratory are as follows:
- O negative, uncrossmatched: 5 min.
- Group-specific, spin-test compatible with no antibody screening: 5–10 min.
- Full compatibility testing: 30 min.

Clinical staff should be familiar with local practice.

Cannulation

The haematocrit of packed red cells is 0.55–0.75 ll^{-1} and to enable adequate rates of transfusion a large cannula (18–14 G) is required. In shock, two large peripheral cannulae or a central line may be necessary. Ideally, cannulae should be positioned in the forearm avoiding joints; if the antecubital fossa is used then the elbow must be well splinted. All cannulae must be well secured. Blood samples must be taken during initial cannulation to expedite tests and cross-match.

Lines and filters

Blood is incompatible with a number of crystalloids. Calcium-containing fluids (e.g. Ringer's lactate) will initiate clotting of the transfused blood. Dextrose 5% (in water) will cause red cell lysis. Blood should be transfused using a new blood giving set primed with 0.9% saline. No drugs should be added to that line. A change of giving set is also indicated when blood of any other ABO group is transfused following the emergency transfusion of group O blood. Blood giving sets have two chambers, the upper one containing a microaggregate filter (170 μm). Additional microaggregate filters (40 μm) are sometimes used in massive transfusion in an attempt to reduce lung injury. However, they are probably ineffective and significantly reduce flow rates. Flow rates may be increased by simultaneously infusing 0.9% saline, raising the blood bag or applying pressure. If blood is given with pressure, care must be taken not to split the bag or cause an air embolus. Blood forced through a 'kinked' or narrow line may be haemolysed. Blood is refrigerated at 4°C and may be safely transfused slowly without warming into a healthy individual. However, large volumes cannot be given safely in shock without warming. With rates above 100 ml min^{-1}, blood should be warmed using a standardized blood warmer (sterile heat-exchange coil) and not on a radiator or in the nearest sink of warm water. Direct excess heat will cause the blood to haemolyse before transfusion.

Infusion rates

All patients must be closely observed for the first 5–10 min. The first 50 ml serves as an *in vivo* compatibility test and should be given slowly before achieving the final flow rate. Standard giving sets allow flow at 15–20 drops ml^{-1}. The infusion should be started within 30 min of removing the blood from refrigeration and completed within 4 h. Blood infusion sets should be changed 12-hourly because bacteria will proliferate in blood kept at room temperature. Blood left out of the refrigerator for more than 30 min should be handed back to hospital blood transfusion laboratory for disposal and not returned to the refrigerator because of the risk of bacterial infection. Insulated blood storage boxes allow blood to be taken out from the laboratory to the scene of accidents and obstetric emergencies.

Transfusion records

Each unit of blood component must be traceable from the donor to the patient (British Committe for Standards in Haematology, 1991c). In the event of immediate or late complications, accurate record-keeping is essential. The laboratory records are kept for not less than 11 years and are the legal responsibility of the haematologist in charge of the hospital blood transfusion laboratory. The patient's record are the responsibility of the medical and nursing staff and must include all laboratory paperwork. The following should be identifiable from the patients notes:

- The donation identification number of blood and blood products.
- The batch number of manufactured products.
- The time of starting and finishing the transfusion.
- Details of blood pressure, pulse rate and temperature recorded at the start and throughout the transfusion. The frequency of observations must be guided by local policy and the condition of the patient.
- Any transfusion reactions and the actions taken.
- The indication for the transfusion and its clinical effectiveness.

Complications and dangers of blood transfusion

As with all forms of therapy, the benefit of transfusion must outweigh the possible risks. Complications may be considered as immediate or delayed. It is the immediate complications which are seen in the A&E department, but staff should be aware of possible later problems.

Acute intravascular haemolysis

The most dangerous complication of blood transfusion is acute intravascular haemolysis due to ABO incompatibility. The underlying cause is nearly always a CLERICAL ERROR. This has been confirmed in a recent survey of UK blood banks (McClelland & Phillips, 1994). It is essential that the patient must be properly identified by staff taking blood for cross-matching and that the blood sample and request form have the same details. For unconscious patients, the details must include the sex and unique A&E or hospital identification number of the patient. If the name and date of birth are unavailable, the patient is recorded as unknown but blood can still be issued.

The frequency of ABO incompatibility is estimated at about 1:34000 units transfused. The mortality is high due to DIC and renal failure. The immediate management is to stop the blood transfusion, continue the infusion with crystalloids and take advice regarding further in-

vestigations. Blood and urine samples will be required to determine the cause of the problem.

Non-haemolytic febrile transfusion reactions

After red cell transfusions, these are caused by white cell antibodies in the recipient reacting with leucocytes in the donor blood. After platelet transfusion, the reactions are often due to cytokines released from leucocytes during storage. These reactions are unpleasant; the signs are flushing, tachycardia, chills and rigors. The transfusion should be stopped and the patient treated with an antipyretic (e.g. aspirin or paracetamol). If further blood transfusion is needed urgently, a new unit of blood and new giving set should be used. The offending unit and a clotted blood sample from the patient should be sent to the laboratory to exclude a haemolytic transfusion reaction. Leucocyte-depleted blood is used for patients with recurrent non-haemolytic transfusion reactions after red cell transfusions.

Urticaria

This complication may be caused by antibodies to plasma proteins but it is often unexplained. It is unpleasant but rarely severe. The transfusion should be slowed or stopped and chlorpheniramine 10–20 mg IV given.

Anaphylaxis due to plasma proteins

This is a rare but life-threatening complication. It is normally associated with IgA deficiency which occurs in 1 in 10 000 of the population. Treat as for other anaphylactic reactions with: adrenaline IM (0.5–1.0 ml of 1:1000), chlorpheniramine IV (10 mg) and hydrocortisone IV (200 mg).

Pulmonary oedema

In the elderly and those with heart disease, the infusion of intravenous fluids may result in pulmonary oedema. This complication should be anticipated and blood transfusion given only when nursing observation is available. Packed red cells should be given either slowly or with diuretic cover. If pulmonary oedema supervenes, it should rapidly respond to an intravenous dose of diuretic (e.g. frusemide 20–40 mg).

Septic shock due to infected blood

This is a very rare complication of blood transfusion. Blood may become contaminated by skin organisms during donation. The organism is commonly *Pseudomonas fluorescens* or other organisms which can survive at low temperatures.

Delayed complications

These include:

- Delayed immune haemolysis due to Rh, Kidd and Kell antigens.
- Post-transfusion purpura.
- Alloimmunization, including the development of anti-D and other antibodies which may cause haemolytic disease of the newborn in subsequent pregnancies.
- Infections such as hepatitis B and C, HIV (human immunodeficiency virus) and malaria.

MAJOR INCIDENT PROCEDURE

All hospitals in the UK should have documented procedures which outline the organization and duties required of staff in the event or a major incident. Different procedures may be required outside normal working hours. All staff should be familiar with the procedures which may affect their own department. The procedure for a haematology department should outline the call-in arrangements for technical and medical staff. The duty haematologist should liaise between the hospital major incident control centre, the regional transfusion centre and the transfusion laboratory. Haematology staff may also act as runners between the laboratory, theatres and the A&E department. The smooth and successful response to a major incident depends on good command, control and communication.

Acknowledgement

We wish to thank Dr Adrian Stephens for allowing us to draw extensively upon the document 'Strategies for the care of patients with sickle cell disease'.

Bibliography

BEAL, R.W. & ISBISTER, J.P. (1985). *Blood Component Therapy in Clinical Practice*. Melbourne: Blackwell Scientific Publications.

BRITISH COMMITTEE FOR STANDARDS IN HAEMATOLOGY (1991a). Oral anticoagulation. In *Standard Haematology Practice*, ed. B.E. Roberts, pp. 73–87. Oxford: Blackwell Scientific Publications.

BRITISH COMMITTEE FOR STANDARDS IN HAEMATOLOGY (1991b). Transfusion for massive blood loss. In *Standard Haematology Practice*, ed. B.E. Roberts, pp. 198–206. Oxford: Blackwell Scientific Publications.

BRITISH COMMITTEE FOR STANDARDS IN HAEMATOLOGY (1991c). Hospital blood bank documentation and procedures. In *Standard Haematology Practice*, ed. B.E. Roberts, pp. 128–38. Oxford: Blackwell Scientific Publications.

BRITISH COMMITTEE FOR STANDARDS IN HAEMATOLOGY (1992). Guidelines for the use of fresh frozen plasma. *Transfus. Med.*, **2**, 57–63.

BRITISH COMMITTEE FOR STANDARDS IN HAEMATOLOGY (1996). Guidlines for the prevention and treatment of infection in patients with an absent or dysfunctional spleen. *Br. Med. J.*, **312**, 430–4.

LUNGSGAARD-HANSEN, P. (1992). Treatment of acute blood loss. *Vox Sang.*, **63**, 241–6.

McLELLAND, D.B.L. & PHILLIPS, P. (1994). Errors in blood transfusion in Britain: Survey of hospital haematology departments. *Br. Med. J.*, **308**, 1205–6.

McCLELLAND, D.B.L. ed. (1996). *Handbook of Transfusion Medicine*. London: HMSO.

PHILLIPS, R.E. (1988). Malaria treatment and prophylaxis. *Prescribers J.*, **28**(3), 72–7.

THE BARTS NHS TRUST (1992). *Strategies for the Care of Patients with Sickle Cell Disease*. London: The Barts NHS Trust.

UK REGIONAL HAEMOPHILIA CENTRE DIRECTORS COMMITTEE (1992). Recommendations on choice of therapeutic products for the treatment of patients with haemophilia A, haemophilia B and von Willebrand's disease. *Blood Coagulat. Fibrinol.*, **3**, 205–14.

Further reading

HOFFBRAND, A.V. & PETTIT, J.E. (1993). *Essential Haematology*. Oxford: Blackwell Scientific Publications.

KUMAR, P. & CLARK, M. (1994). *Clinical Medicine*. London: Bailliere & Tindall.

SKINNER, D., DRISCOLL, P. & EARLAM, R., ed. (1991). *ABC of Major Trauma*. London: British Medical Journal.

50 Acute orthopaedic conditions

H. WARE

Department of Orthopaedic Surgery, St Bartholomew's Hospital, London, UK

Chapter plan

'Whiplash'
Torticollis
Bone infection
Osteochondritis
Slipped upper femoral epiphysis
Irritable hip
Cervical disc disease
Low back pain

'WHIPLASH'

A 'whiplash' (neck sprain) is defined as an extension sprain of the neck after a rear impact injury (MacNab, 1964). However, the neck injury does not always occur in isolation. There may be associated upper or lower backache, often at the thoracolumbar junction. The patient may also complain of headache, either in the occipital area, radiating to the vertex, or a true frontal headache. In considering injuries to the neck after a vehicle accident, a pure whiplash is not that common – the force may be from a side impact and not the rear. Therefore, the prognosis of each type of injury must be considered carefully with respect to the mechanism.

Incidence and pathology

Adhering to the above definition then true whiplash is rare. MacKay (1976) felt it accounted for 8% of all neck injuries after road traffic accidents. However, this was before the introduction of seat belt legislation.

Galasko *et al.* (1993) studied the incidence of neck injuries before and after the introduction of seat belt legislation. Prior to the legislation, 7.7% of road traffic accidents produced soft tissue injuries of the cervical spine. Twelve months after the law had been introduced, this had increased to 20.5%, and several years later it had risen to over 40%.

Galasko also reviewed the type of impact. In over half the cases the injury arose as a result of a force applied directly to the rear of the vehicle. In the other half, the mechanism was almost evenly divided between side and rear impact.

The precise pathology which gives rise to the symptoms has not been clearly defined. Standard radiographic techniques provide no clues, and MRI (magnetic resonance imaging) studies have not conclusively demonstrated a localized lesion, despite the ability of this technique to assess the soft tissues more clearly. Davis (1991), using T2-weighted images, showed separation of the cervical disc from the end-plate, anterior annular tears, occult anterior vertebral end-plate fractures and injuries in the anterior longitudinal ligament – areas which all have an abundant nerve supply. It is likely that the damage is sustained in these areas of the spinal column, causing severe pain, secondary muscle spasm and a rigid neck.

History

The history may vary slightly but there is a common theme. Neck pain is present to a variable degree, along the length of the neck or confined to one part of it. The pain can develop immediately after the impact or several hours later, and it may be associated with radiation to the shoulder blades, and very rarely the upper arm. The patient may also complain of a headache, often in the occipital region.

Rarely, neurological symptoms arise; usually paraesthesia in the arms, occasionally in a dermatomal distribution. Many patients complain of associated low back pain, particularly at the thoracolumbar junction.

Examination

The cervical area must be inspected to assess the posture for loss of cervical lordosis. In my experience this is an unreliable physical sign for which the radiograph will be of greater value. Any superficial injuries are noted, particularly bruising over the forehead which might suggest a more severe injury such as a spinal fracture.

The neck is palpated in the midline assessing for tenderness or malalignment, then either side noting any muscular tenderness or spasm. Tenderness may be present as far laterally as the shoulder girdle.

A neurological examination must be peformed on all patients. In the case of a true 'whiplash' injury this will be normal. Any clinical evidence of a nerve root lesion will require CT (computed tomography) or MRI evaluation to identify a slipped cervical disc or vertebral injury.

Investigation

Anteroposterior and lateral radiographs of the cervical spine may be taken according to clinical need. The lateral view must demonstrate the entire cervical spine. A further lateral view in flexion and extension may be indicated if spinal instability is suspected, but refer such cases to the duty orthopaedic team (see Chapter 22).

A complete cervical series includes an open mouth view to assess the odontoid process and the atlantoaxial area.

Radiography is normal in neck sprains, apart from demonstrating loss of the normal cervical lordosis secondary to muscle spasm.

Treatment

There is no definitive cure for these injuries, except time. A soft cervical collar gives minimal support to the neck, and may be of some value. In normal subjects it allowed 80% of extension and 76% flexion. Indeed many patients find that the collar is both restrictive and uncomfortable. In some cases it even compounds the pain. Systemic or topical anti-inflammatory medication can be prescribed, and physiotherapy can be helpful in the acute phase. However, in the majority of cases recovery is dependent on time (Pennie & Agambar, 1990) and the patient should be told that there is no magic cure and that the pain and spasm may last for several weeks or months.

Prognosis

A significant percentage of these cases are involved in litigation after the road traffic accident. Most of the long-term studies have been based on patients reviewed for medicolegal reports and presumably represent the worst cases.

Parmar & Raymakers (1993) studied victims of pure rear impact injuries and found that the prognosis was worse in patients older than 45 years, when pain develops within 12 h of the injury, and in the presence of cervical spondylosis. All of these prolonged the duration of symptoms; 50% still had significant pain at 8 months, 44% at 1 year and 18% at 3 years.

Gargan & Bannister (1990) noted the presence of pain in the lower back as well as the neck, particularly in the older age group. This study, in common with many others, found no association between duration of symptoms and successful settlement of the legal claim. It is therefore reasonable to say that long-term studies do not incriminate the legal claim as a factor in prolonging symptoms in most cases.

TORTICOLLIS

Torticollis is a rotational deformity of the head on the neck giving the clinical appearance that the head is tilted to one side.

The aetiology is congenital or acquired. The congenital type is caused by fibromatosis within the sternocleidomastoid muscle. In the acquired group, muscle spasm is secondary to pathology elsewhere in the neck.

Congenital torticollis

Coventry & Harris (1959) estimated that the congenital variant was present in 0.4% of all live births. Canale *et al.* (1982) studied 57 cases and concluded that children with established facial asymmetry and limited neck motion usually did badly. The condition usually presents between 1 and 11 months of age when a hard fusiform swelling can be felt in the sternomastoid muscle at the angle of the jaw. The precise aetiology of the 'tumour' is unknown and several theories have been put forward, including intrauterine pressure or obstetric birth trauma.

Congenital torticollis usually regresses within a year of birth and no formal treatment apart from physiotherapy and daily stretching is required. However, a few are resilient to stretching and need surgical correction. This can be performed with a subcutaneous tenotomy, but open surgical release is safer and therefore preferable. As most improve with conservative treatment, surgery can wait until the child is older (about 3 years of age). Facial asymmetry at this stage should resolve following surgery. Rarely there may be a congenital anomaly of the cervical spine such as Klippel–Feil syndrome or atlantoaxial fusion. A thorough radiological as well as clinical assessment is therefore required.

Acquired torticollis

Acquired torticollis can result from several causes, including acute disc prolapse, inflamed neck glands, spinal infection, cervical tumours, and neuritis of the spinal accessory nerve.

Atlantoaxial subluxation can be seen in older children who have often had a history of upper respiratory tract infection within the preceding 1 or 2 weeks. Watson Jones (1932) suggested that this arose as a result of hyperaemic decalcification that developed in the body of the atlas. This in turn loosened the attachment of the transverse ligament of the dens, destabilizing this area. As the torticollis becomes established, the head leans to the affected side and the face to the opposite side.

The first priority is to make the diagnosis. Radiographs must include an open mouth view of the cervical spine to accurately assess the relationship of the atlas to the axis, and a CT scan may be needed to evaluate this further. Treatment consists of Halter traction, and in rare cases (usually when the diagnosis is made late) localized spinal fusion is necessary.

BONE INFECTION

Aetiology

Infection in bone and joints can arise insidiously with no relevant history of trauma or systemic infection. However, one must beware of the immunocompromised individual and those patients with implants. Sepsis can develop from a haematogenous source, direct inoculation, or local spread from an adjacent infection.

Infection can develop with bacteria, viruses or fungi, but the commonest organism is *Staphylococcus aureus*. In a study reviewing the organisms causing osteomyelitis in an English health district over a 10-year period, 44% of all infections were caused by this organism (Cooper & Cawley, 1986). Craigen *et al.* (1992) reported that the commonest organism in children under 13 years in a Glasgow health district was also *Staphylococcus*

aureus, although the incidence was decreasing dramatically. Anaerobes account for under 1% of all infections in otherwise healthy individuals (Clarke & Allum, 1988).

Gonococcal arthritis should be considered. It can present with severe pain, is commoner in females, and there may be an associated history of rash or vaginal discharge. A positive joint aspirate is present in 25% and a positive blood culture in 20% of cases.

Delay in diagnosis is greater with increasing age, pre-existing disease and in deep-seated joints such as the hip.

Diagnosis in young children and the elderly can be difficult and although septic arthritis is rarer in very elderly people, the mortality is higher (Vincent & Amirault, 1990).

Chronic multifocal osteomyelitis

This rare condition of unknown aetiology was first described by Giedion *et al.* in 1972. It can present with lethargy, pain and tenderness in the metaphyses of long bones. The lesions have a tendency to relapse and the condition can last several years, but it is very rare for an organism to be cultured. Histology may vary from relatively normal biopsies to those with features typical of osteomyelitis, with plasma cell, lymphocyte and macrophage infiltration (Carr *et al.*, 1993). Treatment is conservative; non-steroidal anti-inflammatory drugs are prescribed if the pain warrants it but antibiotics have little value.

Pathology of osteomyelitis

The infecting organism settles in the metaphysis of the bone. Pus then develops within the medulla and tracks through Volkmann's canals to the subperiosteal bone from where it may spread to the soft tissues and form a peripheral abscess. Infection is confined by the growth disc to the medullary canal, except in the very young. If the joint capsule extends beyond the growth plate then the pus can track subperiosteally into the joint itself. This is the case in the proximal femur (hip joint), distal femur (knee) and proximal and distal humerus (shoulder and elbow). Under 2 years of age, there is a common vascular supply for the metaphysis and epiphysis which crosses the epiphysial plate, so joint infection can also develop through this route. Once the infection reaches the joint, leucocytic enzymes are released and pus forms within the joint. The articular cartilage is at risk of destruction from the enzymes and from increased pressure within the joint as the volume of pus increases. If the joint is not decompressed and the pus washed out by irrigation, the articular cartilage will be completely destroyed and then fibrosis will occur, ankylosing the joint.

When the bone is surrounded by subperiosteal infection, necrosis can occur primarily, or secondarily by local thrombosis. With time, a separate necrotic segment may be seen – the sequestrum. The periosteum is active in its response to the infection by producing new bone. In time this may form a substantive layer – the involucrum. With the formation of a sequestrum and an involucrum the disease has become chronic.

A Brodie's abscess is a localized form of chronic osteomyelitis. This is often seen in the metaphysis of a long bone and there may be no significant history of infection.

Brucellosis should be considered as a cause of the osteomyelitis in farmers and other professionals dealing with livestock. Indeed, bone and joint infection occurs in 10% of cases with vertebral and disc involvement in 27% (Ganado & Craig, 1958). Congenital syphilis can also cause bone infection, presenting with osteomyelitis or periostitis in the first 6 months of life. Patients with sickle cell disease are reputed to be at risk of infection with *Salmonella*.

In sheep workers, *Echinococcus granulosis* infestation is another disease that is occupationally related. The primary host is the dog but it intermittently infests cows, sheep and man.

Tuberculosis must be considered in the differential diagnosis of all bone and joint infections, especially as the disease is reappearing. The radiographic features may resemble those of a staphylococcal infection, but in a chronic case there may be significant osteoporosis each side of the joint.

Presentation

Septic arthritis

The specific features will depend on the joint involved. Severe pain is common in the acutely infected joint, and in the lower limb the patient is unable to bear any weight at all on the joint. Local examination in a superficial joint reveals heat and tenderness, and the overlying skin may be reddened (but not as red as in cellulitis). In deeper joints nothing abnormal may be seen, but the joint is tender; it lies in a position of flexion and all movements are exceptionally painful.

Osteomyelitis

The presenting features vary, depending on the stage of the disease, the age of the patient, and associated pathology. The patient may be systemically unwell with a fever and lethargy. In the acute phase the pain may be intense and the features of acute infection are evident. In the chronic case, the pain is normally less intense.

Investigations

The patient's temperature must be taken.

Radiographs may be normal in the first 10–14 days, although at this stage soft tissue swelling may be seen. By 3–4 months, 90% of cases have positive radiographic findings (Wheat, 1985). Later features include bone lysis and periosteal new bone formation. A sequestrum may be visible. In chronic cases, a Brodie's abscess cavity may be seen in the metaphysis of long bones. Tomography may be of value, particularly in searching for a sequestrum. In the spinal column, CT scanning can help to assess the degree of bone involvement and define the extent of any abscesses.

A full blood count and ESR (erythrocyte sedimentation rate) or C-reactive protein are useful markers both for diagnosis and for following the course of the infection. A bone scan can be useful in confirming the diagnosis, especially in the first few days when radiographs are normal.

Any discharge should be sent for microbiological analysis and blood cultures taken. All specimens should be tested for aerobic and anaerobic organisms, in addition to tuberculosis.

Differential diagnosis

For septic arthritis, this includes all other causes of joint inflammation, such as rheumatoid arthritis or other arthropathies. In the case of bone infection, sickle cell crisis should be considered, and neoplasms must always be considered in the differential radiographic diagnosis.

Treatment

Acute osteomyelitis

The patient must be referred to the orthopaedic department. Antibiotics are given, initially intravenously then orally. The type of antibiotic will depend on the organism if any are seen on the Gram stain or culture.

It is reasonable to commence therapy with a penicillin-based antibiotic targeting staphylococci. The affected area is rested and elevated. If an abscess has formed, this should be drained under a general anaesthetic, and the bone can be drilled to release any intramedullary pus.

Chronic osteomyelitis

There is no urgency to refer unless the patient is systemically unwell. In most cases oral antibiotics will suffice and, as the commonest organism is a *Staphylococcus aureus*, a penicillin-based antibiotic is appropriate. If the limb is very swollen it may be reasonable to admit the patient for elevation. Surgical drainage is of value if an abscess has developed, or to remove a sequestrum. Other techniques being developed in an attempt to eradicate the infection include bone resection and transport using external fixators.

Septic arthritis

This is an orthopaedic emergency. The patient must be admitted, the joint aspirated and the fluid sent for urgent microscopy, culture and crystal analysis. It may be necessary to lavage the joint under general anaesthaesia, so the patient should be fasted. Antibiotic therapy will depend on the microbiological analysis.

The duration of systemic antibiotic therapy is debatable. Most clinicians are guided by an improvement in the patient's pain, an increase in passive movement, and a falling ESR.

OSTEOCHONDRITIS

This includes a group of conditions which are quite different in appearance and outlook. Three types can be considered:

- Crushing.
- Splitting (osteochondritis dissecans).
- Traction.

A number of eponyms are attached to them (Table 1).

Crushing

This occurs during periods of rapid growth. The precise cause is unknown and theories relating to poor vascular supply, repetitive trauma, infection and congenital anomalies have all been suggested.

Table 1. *Eponyms of osteochondritis*

Eponym	Bone
Perthes	Femoral head
Kienböck	Lunate
Scheuermann	Spine
Köhler	Navicular
Sever	Calcaneum
Osgood–Schlatter	Tibial tuberosity
Preisser	Scaphoid
Panner	Capitulum
Freiberg	Metatarsal
Larsen–Johansson	Lower pole of the patella

Perthes' osteochondritis

Boys outnumber girls 4:1, and the age of presentation is typically between 3 and 10 years. Only 10% are bilateral. The precise cause is unknown, but the final pathway is probably a transient synovitis and an effusion within the hip joint which tamponades the blood supply to the epiphysis, particularly the lateral epiphysial arteries.

The child presents with pain in the hip or limping. The clinical examination reveals limited rotation (usually internal) and limited abduction in flexion. Although the time course may last 4 years, the pain does not persist for that period of time.

The radiographic features depend on the point in the natural history of the condition at which the child presents, as well as the severity of the disease. Either a small part of the head or all of it may be involved. Three radiological phases have been described. The first reflects the initial avascular phase. The area appears porotic, then an opacity develops in the epiphysis over 1 year. Next is the stage of fragmentation when the head breaks up. After another year, repair occurs and normal bone reappears. During this period, the head may remodel completely, flatten or be seen to extrude laterally.

Treatment of Perthes' disease has evolved and the child's hip is now monitored with serial radiographs, in order to identify lateral extrusion. In all other cases, treatment is conservative and symptomatic, involving an initial period of bed rest for the acutely painful hip and then mobilization. If the head is extruding, a femoral osteotomy is indicated.

Köhler's osteochondritis

This presents between 4 and 5 years of age. It is commoner in boys. Radiographs reveal increased density, delayed development, or sometimes fragmentation. Treatment is conservative and there are no long-term complications.

Scheuermann's disease

This is reported to occur in 0.4–8% of the population with equal sex incidence. The aetiology is unknown. The definition is anterior wedging of 5° or more in at least three adjacent vertebrae. It typically presents around puberty with a thoracic or thoracolumbar kyphosis. The natural history is benign, but occasionally a severe kyphosis may develop requiring surgery.

Splitting

A section of bone and cartilage split off from the main segment. Convex surfaces are usually affected, particularly the lateral part of the medial femoral condyle, anteromedial part of the talus, superomedial part of the femoral head, and the humeral capitellum.

Osteochondritis dissecans

Males are more commonly affected. If the segment has completely separated, removal either arthroscopically or via an arthrotomy will be necessary. In some cases, if diagnosed early enough (particularly in the knee), it can be reattached. If the lesion has not separated, the joint can be rested (sometimes in traction) and the situation monitored.

The main fear is of osteoarthritis, particularly in weight-bearing joints. Linden (1977) concluded after an average follow-up of 33 years, that osteochondritis dissecans in the knee did not lead to osteoarthritis, but Twyman et al. (1991) felt that there was an increased risk of osteoarthritis in knees followed-up for a similar timescale. However, this appears to be less likely if the classical site is involved as it is not a weight-bearing area (Linden, 1977).

Capitellum

Early radiographic changes consist of patchy rarefaction of the convexity of the capitellum. Eventually a single punched-out cavity may appear. The head of the radius may also become irregular. Later, loose bodies may be visible, and the capitellum will appear flattened.

Traction

This affects sites near epiphyses where tendons are attached.

Osgood–Schlatter osteochondritis

In the tibial tubercle a single or occasionally double ossific centre (the apophysis) develops, fusing with the main epiphysis around 16 years of age. The segment can be completely separated from the main epiphysis, or more commonly partially avulsed, which affects its blood supply.

A history of trauma is rarely elicited. Symptoms may be vague and include aching in the joint or more specific symptoms of mechanical dysfunction. Local pain, tenderness and difficulty kneeling may be described. Treatment is conservative in all cases. Plaster-of-Paris immobilization should be avoided.

SLIPPED UPPER FEMORAL EPIPHYSIS

This is more frequent in boys than girls (3:2). Girls tend to present with the condition earlier, even under 10 years of age. Bilateral involvement occurs in about 20% of cases.

An endocrine link has been postulated. Harris (1950) found that sex hormones increased the resistance to slipping, whereas growth hormone decreased it, in rabbits.

The classification is:

- Acute.
- Chronic.
- Acute-on-chronic.

An acute slip usually presents with sudden onset of symptoms of less than 3 weeks' duration, whereas a chronic slip has a more gradual onset without sudden deterioration. In practice, this may not always be easy to define, and a more precise definition depends on the radiographic appearance. In the chronic slip there are radiographic signs of remodelling and new bone formation at the epiphysial–metaphyseal junction. These features are absent in the acute case. In the acute-on-chronic slip, the radiographic features are of a chronic slip but the patient presents with severe and acute symptoms suggesting that the slip has suddenly deteriorated (Ward *et al.*, 1992).

Slipped upper femoral epiphysis may present with limping of sudden onset, pain in the groin, or pain in the knee. Examination reveals external rotation of the limb. The hip may appear irritable on movement (see below).

Two radiographs must be taken: an anteroposterior and a frog lateral view. Perkins sign – a very useful guide – is a line drawn along the superior border of the femoral neck. In a slip, the line does not cut across the femoral head and the sign is said to be positive.

Treatment

In an acute slip, the epiphysis should be fixed to prevent further slippage. If the slip is substantial, it is not acceptable to forcefully reduce it as the risk of avascular necrosis is high. However, as the patient is positioned on the reduction table in the operating theatre, the slip may well reduce. If the slip is substantial the pins should be left *in situ* until the epiphysis fuses and some form of osteotomy can be performed at a later date. Chronic slips must be stabilized if osseous fusion has not taken place. Once fusion has occurred, a femoral osteotomy can be undertaken to improve the range of motion in the joint.

Complications of slipped upper femoral epiphysis include chondrolysis and avascular necrosis.

IRRITABLE HIP

The aetiology of this condition is unknown. However, it is important to exclude bacterial infection, congenital dislocation of the hip, Perthes' disease or slipped upper femoral epiphysis.

The symptoms of irritable hip are pain and limping, normally in the absence of a fever. The pain may be felt in the groin or the knee, and abduction and external rotation are often limited and painful.

All radiographic examinations are normal. An increase in the lateral soft tissue capsule around the hip joint was thought to represent capsular thickening associated with the transient synovitis. However, Brown (1975) showed that this was a positional artefact caused by lateral rotation and abduction of the hip.

Ultrasound is of value and if fluid is present this can be aspirated and sent for analysis. The aspiration itself may improve the symptoms by decompressing the joint (Hill *et al.*, 1990).

The traditional management of this condition is to admit the child – usually under the care of the orthopaedic department – for bed rest and skin traction. As the pain subsides and passive movement improves, the traction is removed and the child is mobilized. This philosophy has been challenged; it leads to a number of unnecessary admissions as the child rarely develops any pathology.

Bickerstaff *et al.* (1990) suggest that ultrasound be used instead of radiography, unless the symptoms have not resolved after several days.

Not all units will have ready access to ultrasonography to assess the hip and, if all other pathology has been excluded, it is not unreasonable to consider the patient's domestic circumstances. If these are satisfactory, the child may be allowed to go home and can be reviewed in the next available orthopaedic clinic. When there is doubt about the home circumstances or the diagnosis, an orthopaedic opinion should be sought concerning admission. A child who reattends A&E with persistent or recurrent symptoms should be admitted.

CERVICAL DISC DISEASE

Herniation of the cervical disc is slightly more common in men and is associated with frequent heavy lifting or diving (Kelsey, 1984).

The pathology is similar to that in lumbar disease: disc prolapses in a central or posterolateral direction. The signs and symptoms depend on the direction of the prolapse and the degree of pressure on adjacent structures. In evaluating the neck, one must be aware that other sites (e.g. the shoulder) may mimic cervical pain. Disturbance of nerve function in the arm may be caused by other pathology such as a carpal or cubital tunnel syndrome.

Treatment is conservative unless there is:

- Increasing neurological deficit.
- Progressive cervical myelopathy.
- Failed conservative therapy.

Radiography is performed to assess the degree of degenerative change in the spine or other bony pathology. However, the definitive investigation is MRI.

LOW BACK PAIN

Low back pain is common and most people suffer from at least one attack in their life. In the UK alone,

16 million days a year are lost because of back pain (Wood & Bradley, 1987).

The A&E doctor has to consider many factors before deciding whether orthopaedic referral is appropriate. Management can be based on site of pain and the presence of any neurological symptoms or signs:

1. Low back pain: NO referred pain in the leg or abdomen.
   – No neurological symptoms or signs.
   – Bladder and bowel function normal.
2. Low back pain: referred pain in lower limb.
   – No neurological symptoms or signs.
   – Bladder and bowel function normal.
3. Low back pain: referred pain in leg.
   – Neurological symptoms and signs.
   – Bladder and bowel function normal.
4. Low back pain:
   – Bladder and/or bowel dysfunction.
5. Low back pain:
   – Abdominal symptoms and/or signs.

Consideration should also be given to weight and appetite loss, especially in the older patient.

The causes of low back pain can then be considered as those that arise from pathology extrinsic to the vertebral column and spinal cord, and those that are intrinsic to the column or spinal cord (Table 2). Radiography is normal in the majority of cases, especially when the clinical assessment suggests no extrinsic pathology to be the cause.

Anatomy and pathology

Anteriorly the spinal canal is bounded by the intervertebral disc, the posterior longitudinal ligament and the vertebral body. Posteriorly lies the ligamentum flavum and laminae, and laterally the pedicles. The spinal nerves traverse an area bounded by the facet joints posteriorly, the pedicles superiorly and inferiorly, and the disc and vertebral body anteriorly.

Spinal cord or nerve root compression may be caused by disc herniation superimposed on an already narrowed spinal canal, bony compression (osteophytes), or ligamentous thickening. Compression may occur centrally or laterally (Getty et al., 1981; Epstein et al., 1972).

The three main constituents of the disc are collagen, proteoglycans and water; 80% of the nucleus pulposus and 78% of the annulus fibrosis is water. With ageing the proteoglycan content decreases dramatically and this is responsible for regulating the water content of the

Table 2. *Intrinsic and extrinsic causes of low back pain*

Extrinsic
● Vascular
  – Aortic aneurysm
  Gastrointestinal
  – Peptic ulcer
  – Pancreatitis
  – Neoplasm
● Urogenital
  – Renal colic
  – Pyelonephritis
  – Hydronephrosis

Intrinsic
● Bone
  – Infection and consider tuberculosis/brucellosis
  – Tumour, secondary deposits, myeloma
  – Inflammatory conditions, ankylosing spondylitis
  – Trauma, fracture pars interarticularis defect
  – Spondylolisthesis
● Disc
  – Prolapse, bulge, sequestration
● Joints
  – Osteoarthritis, rheumatoid arthritis
● Spinal cord
  – Myelitis
  – Polio
  – AIDS

Psychological

disc which falls in both compartments to 70%. Thus, with age, the nucleus changes from a gelatinous structure, well delineated from the annulus, to a fibrous structure with an indistinct boundary. The first evidence of degeneration starts as early as the second decade and, by 40 years, 80% of discs are degenerate in males. The result is loss of disc height, and collapse and bulging of the posterior longitudinal ligament.

The position of the nucleus is not static but changes with posture. It moves anteriorly with extension and posteriorly with flexion. Several authors have suggested that discs do not fail in compression but in axial loading with torsion.

The facet joints are synovial and can develop osteoarthritis in just the same way as other synovial joints. Hypertrophy with osteophyte formation can develop, compressing the nerve root as it passes near the joint. The pressure in the intervertebral disc has been measured in relation to posture (Nachemson & Elfstrom,

1970) with a 40% increase in pressure when sitting as opposed to standing.

In most patients the precise source of pain is unclear. Kuslich *et al.* (1991) recorded pain after stimulating areas of the spine under local anaesthaesia. Pain of spinal origin can mimic pain referred from other structures, and vice versa, making diagnosis difficult. There are numerous pain fibres in the spinal column. The outer half of the annulus fibrosus is innervated, whereas the inner half and the nucleus pulposus are devoid of any sensory supply. The dura mater on the nerve root is sensitive, and there are sensory fibres in the vertebral body, the facet joints, the posterior longitudinal ligament and the anterior longitudinal ligament.

Examination

General and specific examinations must be performed. Abdominal examination is essential and, when indicated, digital examination of the rectum should be performed.

The back is examined for areas of tenderness, asymmetry, muscle spasm and scoliosis. The patient should be reviewed in both the erect and supine position. Straight leg examination should assess the degree of movement, the presence and distribution of pain in the elevated leg, and any crossover pain in the other (supine) leg. When indicated, the patient is turned into the prone position and a femoral stretch test is performed.

A full neurological assessment of the lower limb is required, and if necessary an assessment of anal tone, sensation, and the prostate in males. The urine should be tested with a commercial dipstick.

If all the extrinsic causes have reasonably been excluded and the diagnosis falls into any of the categories except low back pain with neurological signs, especially bladder/bowel dysfunction, there are no grounds for admission or urgent referral. The patient can be discharged home to the care of the general medical practitioner, or to orthopaedic out-patients.

Prolapsed intervertebral disc

This typically affects younger adults. As a general principle, the 20-year-old is more likely to have a prolapse and the 60-year-old spinal stenosis. The former condition is rare in the latter age group and vice versa. The majority of lumbar prolapses occur in the L4/5 region, affecting the L5 nerve root; the L5/S1 interspace is the next most frequent region of occurrence, affecting the S1 nerve root. Typically the prolapse is posterolateral, but occasionally

Table 3. *Symptoms and signs resulting from nerve root compression*

L3/4 disc: L4 nerve root affected

Sensation:	posterolateral thigh, anterior knee, medial calf
Motor:	quadriceps, hip adductors
Reflex:	patella

L4/5 disc: L5 nerve root affected

Sensation:	anterolateral calf, dorsum foot, great toe
Motor:	extensor hallucis longus, gluteus medius, extensor digitorum longus and brevis
Reflex:	None lost

L5/S1 disc: S1 nerve root affected

Sensation:	lateral malleolus, lateral heel, foot, lesser toes
Motor:	peroneus longus and brevis, gastrocnemius, gluteus maximus
Reflex:	ankle

the disc prolapses posteriorly, compressing the cauda equina.

If the nerve root is compressed, the symptoms and signs vary from referred pain in the distribution of the nerve to neuropathy affecting one root level (Table 3). The typical presentation of a central compression is saddle anaesthesia over the sacrum, bilateral ankle areflexia and bladder dysfunction.

The management of patients suspected of a prolapse is primarily conservative, except in cases where there is a suspicion of a cauda equina syndrome. These patients should be admitted for urgent spinal imaging with a view to early surgery. Other cases can be referred to out-patients for further investigation.

Spinal stenosis

In this condition, the spinal canal is narrowed centrally or laterally.

Spinal stenosis may be classified as follows:

- Congenital:
  - Chondrodystrophic.
  - Idiopathic.
- Acquired:
  - Degenerative.
  - Spondylitic.
  - Iatrogenic.
  - Post-traumatic.
- Miscellaneous:
  - Paget's disease, etc.

The commonest cause is osteoarthritis. Degenerative changes develop in the synovial joints of the articular facets. Reduction in the joint space, with loss of cartilage, is accompanied by hypertrophy and osteophyte formation narrowing the exit foramina for the spinal nerves as well as the internal diameter of the vertebral canal. Calcification and hypertrophy of the ligamentum flavum further compromise the width of the canal.

Symptoms vary from low back pain to those of nerve root compression, which may not be isolated to one level as the stenosis may extend over many segments. As in the case of the patient with the prolapsed disc, urgent admission is rarely indicated unless there is evidence of spinal cord or cauda equina compression. The majority of cases are treated conservatively, but surgery is occasionally of value in decompressing the affected level.

Bibliography

BICKERSTAFF, D.R., NEAL, L.M., BOOTH, A.J. *et al.* (1990). Ultrasound examination of the irritable hip. *J. Bone Joint Surg.*, **72B**, 549–53.

BROWN, I. (1975). A study of the 'capsular' shadow in disorders of the hip in children. *J. Bone Joint Surg.*, **57B**, 175–9.

CANALE, S.T., GRIFFIN, D.W. & HUBBARD, C.N. (1982). Congenital muscular torticollis: a long term follow-up. *J. Bone Joint Surg.*, **64A**, 810–16.

CARR, A.J., COLE, W.G., ROBERTON, D.M. *et al.* (1993). Chronic multifocal osteomyelitis. *J. Bone Joint Surg.*, **75B**, 582–91.

CLARKE, H.J. & ALLUM, R. (1988). Anaerobic septic arthritis due to bacteroides. *J. Bone Joint Surg.*, **70B**, 847–8.

COOPER, C. & CAWLEY, M.D. (1986). Bacterial arthritis in an English health district a 10 year review. *Ann. Rheum. Dis.*, **45**, 458–63.

COVENTRY, M.B. & HARRIS, L.E. (1959). Congenital muscular torticollis in infancy: some observations regarding treatment. *J. Bone Joint Surg.*, **41A**, 815–22.

CRAIGEN, M.A.C., WATTERS, J. & HACKETT, J.S. (1992). The changing epidemiology of osteomyelitis in children. *J. Bone Joint Surg.*, **74B**, 541–5.

DAVIS, S.J., TERESI, L.M., BRADLEY, W.G. Jr, ZIEMBA, M.A. & BLOZE, A.E. (1991). Cervical spine hyperextension injuries—MR findings. *Radiology*, **180**, 245–51.

EPSTEIN, J.A., EPSTEIN, B., ROSENTHAL, A.D., CARRAS, R. & LAVINE, A.W.F. (1972). Sciatica caused by nerve root entrapment in the lateral recess: the superior facet syndrome. *J. Neurosurg.*, **36**, 584–9.

GALASKO, C.S.B., MURRAY, P.M., PITCHER, M. *et al.* (1993). Neck sprains after road traffic accidents: a modern epidemic. *Injury*, **24**, 155.

GANADO, W. & CRAIG, A.J. (1958). Brucellosis myelopathy. *J. Bone Joint Surg.*, **40A**, 1380–8.

GARGAN, M.F. & BANNISTER, G.C. (1990). Long term prognosis of soft tissue injuries of the neck. *J. Bone Joint Surg.*, **72B**, 901–3.

GETTY, C.J.M., JOHNSON, J.R., KIRWAN, E.O.G. *et al.* (1981). Partial undercutting facetectomy for bony entrapment of the lumbar nerve root. *J. Bone Joint Surg.*, **63B**, 330–5.

GIEDION, A., HOLTHUSEN, W., MASEL, L.F. *et al.* (1972). Subacute and chronic symmetrical osteomyelitis. *Ann. Radiol.*, **15**, 329–42.

HARRIS, W.R. (1950). Endocrine basis for slipping of the upper femoral epiphysis. *J. Bone Joint Surg.*, **32B**, 5.

HILL, S.A., MacLARNON, J.C. & NAG, D. (1990). Ultrasound guided aspiration for transient synovitis of the hip. *J. Bone Joint Surg.*, **72B**, 852–3.

KELSEY, J.L. (1984). An epidemiological study of acute prolapsed cervical intervertebral disc. *J. Bone Joint Surg.*, **66A**, 907.

KUSLICH, S.D., ULSTROM, C.L. & MICHAEL, C.J. (1991). The tissue origin of low back pain and sciatica. *Orthop. Clin. North Am.*, **22**, 181–8.

LINDEN, B. (1977). Oteochondritis dissecans of the femoral condyles: a long term follow up study. *J. Bone Joint Surg.*, **59A**, 769–76.

MacKAY, G.M. (1970). The nature of collisions. Technical aspects of road safety. **43**, 1.

MacNAB, I. (1964). Acceleration injuries of the cervical spine. *J. Bone Joint Surg.*, **46A**, 1797–9.

NACHEMSON, A.L. & ELFSTROM, G. (1970). Intravital dynamic pressure measurements in lumbar disks: a study of common movements, manoeuvres and exercises. *Scand. J. Rehabil. Med. Suppl.*, **12**, 1–40.

PARMAR, V. & RAYMAKERS, R. (1993). Neck injuries from rear impact road traffic accidents: prognosis in persons seeking compensation. *Injury*, **24**, 75.

PENNIE, B.H. & AGAMBAR, L.J. (1990). Whiplash injuries a trial of early management. *J. Bone Joint Surg.*, **72B**, 277–9.

TWYMAN, R.S., DESAL, K. & AICHROTH, P.M. (1991). Osteochondritis dissecans of the knee. *J. Bone Joint Surg.*, **73B**, 461–4.

VINCENT, G.M. & AMIRAULT, J.D. (1990). Septic arthritis in the elderly. *Clin. Orthop.*, **251**, 241–5.

WARD, W.T., STEFKO, J., WOOD, K.B. *et al.* (1992). Fixation with a single screw for slipped capital femoral epiphysis. *J. Bone Joint Surg.*, **74A**, 799–809.

WATSON JONES, R. (1932). Spontaneous hyperaemic dislocation of the atlas. *Proc. R. Soc. Med.*, **25**, 586–90.

WHEAT, J. (1985). Diagnostic strategies in osteomyelitis. *Am. J. Med.*, **78**, 218–24.

WOOD, P.H.N. & BRADLEY, E.M. (1987). Epidemiology of back pain. In *The Lumbar Spine and Back Pain*, ed. M.I.V. Jayson, pp. 1–15. London: Churchill Livingstone.

Further reading

Apley's System of Orthopaedics. (1993). A.G. Apley & L. Solomon. Butterworth-Heinemann.

Campbells Operative Orthopaedics. (1992). A.H. Crenshaw. Mosby, USA.

Orthopaedics in Infancy and Childhood. G.C. Lloyd-Roberts & J.A. Fixsen. Butterworth–Heinemann.

51 Inflamed joints and soft tissues

C.B. COLAÇO[a] and A. WILSON[b]

[a] *Department of Rheumatology, Central Middlesex Hospital, London, UK*
[b] *Accident and Emergency Department, The Royal London Hospital, London, UK*

Chapter Plan

General overview
Specific syndromes
Crystal arthropathies
Polyarthritis
Soft tissue rheumatism
Summary

GENERAL OVERVIEW

Introduction

Joint pains form a major part of general practice workload. There is an equal incidence of axial and peripheral joint disease (Billings & Mole, 1972). In the absence of obvious trauma, painful peripheral joints frequently present as an acute (24–72 h) or often subacute (3–7 days) problem to accident and emergency (A&E) departments. Musculo-skeletal problems account for 20–35% of A&E attendances (Jankowski & Mandalia, 1993).

Inflammatory and degenerative processes can affect any part of the structure of a diarthrodial joint and adjacent tissue. This includes bone, articular cartilage, capsule and synovium. Periarticular bursae and tendons are also lined by synovium and may undergo the same pathological processes. Overlying skin, subcutaneous tissues and ligaments may be involved as, for instance, in cellulitis.

Characteristically, infection will lead to synovial mem-brane activation, infiltration by polymorphs, release of proteases and membrane proliferation resulting in cartilage erosion. As synovial fluid accumulates and joint pressures increase, further destruction results. This may involve reactive oxygen-free radical species as part of an ischaemia-reperfusion effect (Edmonds *et al.*, 1993). Untreated synovitis leads to bony or fibrous ankylosis, and growth plate asymmetry in juveniles. A single painful joint is the commonest presentation. It can herald oligoarticular disease or detract attention from minor inflammation of other joints. The knee, ankle and toes present more frequently than the wrist, shoulders or hips.

An inflamed joint is painful, red, hot and swollen. It may be exquisitely tender and requires a very gentle initial assessment.

These cardinal signs of inflammation are related to functional deficit and a limited range of motion. Delayed presentation following partial treatment or self-medication will alter these signs. The initial examination must try and distinguish between arthritis (synovial inflammation), periarticular inflammation (bursitis, tenosynovitis) and more superficial cellulitis (Fig. 1). The three conditions may co-exist as in gout or bacterial infection. Adjacent bony tenderness may indicate osteomyelitis and is always an important consideration.

Emergency assessment

Triage evaluation

This initial assessment must record the major presenting joints and the apparent level of pain, and also the patient's general systemic condition, noting any history of trauma, rigor or pyrexia.

History

For further assessment it is necessary to maintain a wide differential diagnostic list (Table 1) so as not to miss helpful features at the outset.

The triage record can quickly be extended to question

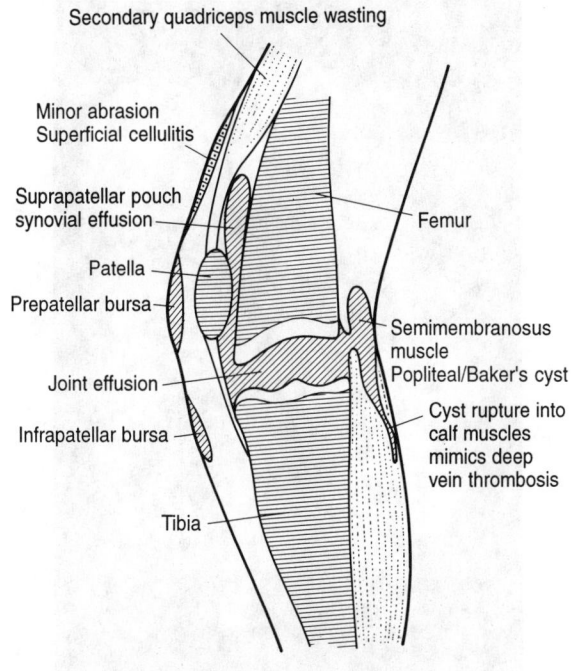

Fig. 1. Signs of an inflamed joint (e.g. knee).

Secondary quadriceps muscle wasting

Minor abrasion
Superficial cellulitis

Suprapatellar pouch
synovial effusion

Femur

Patella

Prepatellar bursa

Semimembranosus
muscle
Popliteal/Baker's cyst

Joint effusion

Infrapatellar bursa

Cyst rupture into
calf muscles
mimics deep
vein thrombosis

Tibia

NB: Also assess anteroposterior and lateral stability

Table 1. *Polyarticular syndromes*

PERIPHERAL SYNOVITIS

- *Inflammatory*
  Rheumatoid disease
  Psoriatic arthritis
  HLA-B27 related
  Ankylosing spondylitis
  Reactive arthritis
  Reiter's disease
  Inflammatory bowel disease
  Psoriatic spondylitis
  SLE vasculitis
  Wegener's granulomatosis
  Sarcoidosis
  Hypertrophic osteoarthropathy
  Infective arthritis
- *Metabolic*
  Hypothyroidism
  Acromegaly
  Gout/pseudogout/hydroxyapatite
  Oxalate/cholesterol/hyperlipidaemia
- *Biochemical*
  Amyloid
  Vitamin C deficiency
  Haemoglobinopathies

ARTHRALGIA

Post-viral
Polymyalgia rheumatica
Myositis
SLE
Fibromyalgia
Vasculitis

SLE, systemic lupus erythematosus.

any minor recent trauma (includes dental and surgical procedures), skin rashes, genital or gastrointestinal infection, diabetes, diuretic or immunosuppressive therapy and previous episodes of arthritis (Table 2).

Further detail identifies risk factors such as alcohol and substance abuse, other causes of immunosuppression and work or recreational overuse injury, which is perhaps more common in joint laxity syndromes. Pain at rest suggests inflammatory conditions. Pain following activity may be mechanical and related to degenerative conditions, and stiffness or 'gelling' after a short period of rest must be questioned for specifically. Children may lose function without expressing obvious pain and in adults, beware of the painless infected neuropathic or chronic Charcot's joint.

Common conditions may be differentiated by direct questioning because the patterns of onset of pain and swelling, or particular joint involvement may be diagnostic. Podagra (gout) of the first metatarsophalangeal joint is often typical. Achilles tendinitis and heel pain characterize Reiter's syndrome if the history of balanitis or urethritis and conjunctivitis is obtained. Arthritis of both ankles may well prove to be part of a reactive spondarthritis, but red lumps (erythema nodosum) on the shins suggests sarcoidosis (Fig. 2). The diagnosis not to miss in A&E is septic arthritis. This is invariably monarticular, but

neisserial disease may have an aseptic flitting polyarthritic phase before localizing to a purulent monarthritis. Despite the typical presenting features of some inflammatory diseases, there is a degree of overlap and non-specificity to be considered when dealing with monarthritis and all possible confirmatory evidence should be obtained. 'Classical' precipitating factors may be irrelevant to the current problem.

Gout, Reiter's syndrome and hip disease in juvenile spondylitis are more common in males, whereas joint laxity, gonococcal septic arthritis and polyarthritis are young female diseases. Postmenopausal diuretic-related gout is now more recognized, and pseudogout is seen in the elderly. Hip disease in the very young may reflect

Table 2. *Emergency (triage) assessment of patient with inflamed joint(s)*

1. One or several joints involved?
2. Level of pain
3. Trauma – history or observed
4. Surgery/dental surgery
5. Systemic illness (fever, sweats, rash)
6. Previous arthritis
7. Diabetes mellitus
8. Diuretics
9. Drug abuse/immunosuppression
10. Genital/gastrointestinal infection

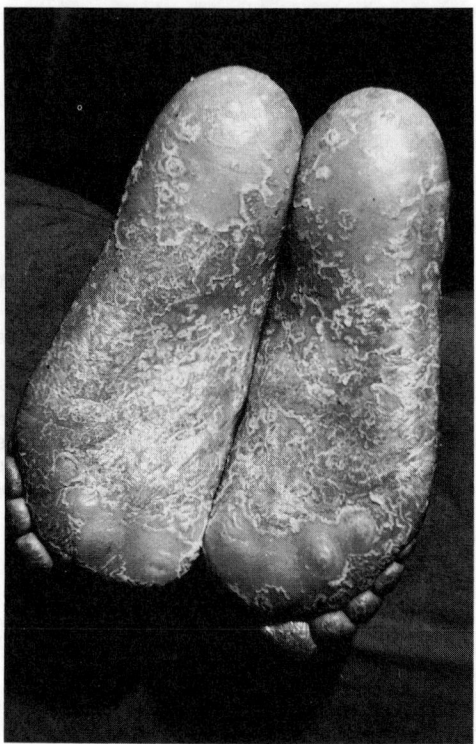

Fig. 3. Psoriasis. Pustular scaly rash on soles of feet and subluxed metatarsophalangeal joints.

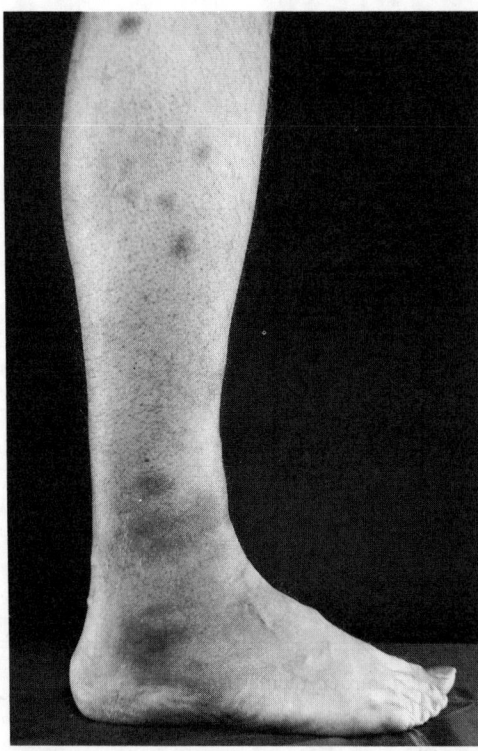

Fig. 2. Sarcoidosis. Note erythema nodosum rash and swelling of the ankle.

congenital dysplasia, but *Haemophilus influenzae* infection to which they are more prone is a surgical emergency. This may now reduce in incidence following introduction in the UK in 1992 of *Haemophilus influenzae* B immunization for children under 2 years of age.

Examination
General

Careful joint and general examination will record important signs, but the mucous membranes and the skin

may define the syndrome by exhibiting features of psoriasis (check hair line, nails, umbilicus and perianal skin), lupus erythematosus (photosensitive), palmoplantar eruptions (Reiter's syndrome, psoriasis; Fig. 3), meningococcal and gonococcal rashes, and the enlarging rash with central clearing which is typical of Lyme disease (borreliosis). The sicca syndrome (dry eyes and mouth) and vasculitis suggest autoimmune disorders, whereas uveitis, conjunctivitis and mouth ulcers might be part of a reactive spondyloarthropathy (see section on polyarthritis). All cardiac lesions are important either as a source or a focus of infection, or target of systemic inflammatory disease (e.g. rheumatic fever or rheumatoid nodules). Chronic pulmonary disease merits careful exclusion of hypertrophic osteoarthropathy by radiology, examining for periosteal reaction (Fig. 4).

Axial joints

Axial stiffness and loss of function may not be noted by the patient. Hip pain and difficulty in climbing stairs in a young male with normal hips might reveal marked lumbar stiffness:

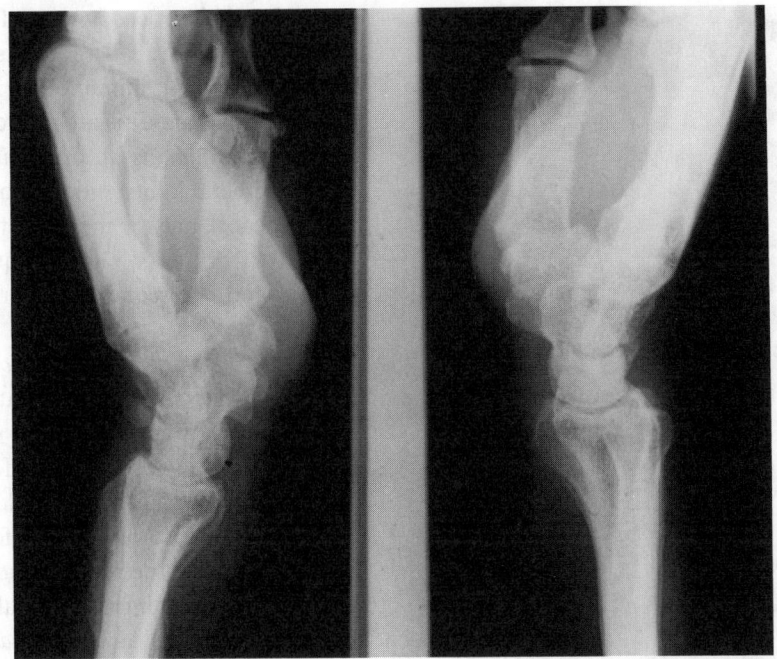

Fig. 4. Hypertrophic pulmonary osteoarthropathy. Note periosteal reaction of distal radius.

- Mark 10 cm posteriorly above the pelvic brim in the midline and 5 cm below with the patient erect.
- Ask the patient to touch his/her toes and measure the segment again.

N.B: Normal Shöber test: 15 cm lumbar segment flexes to 19–23 cm.

Direct compression or forced distraction of the iliac bones by lateral pressure anteriorly causes acute pain localized to the sacroiliac joints in active sacroiliitis. In ankylosing spondylitis or reactive spondarthritis peripheral involvement of knee, ankle and hip disease is common, but dactylitis and second metatarsophalangeal disease is also characteristic. Sternoclavicular, manubriosternal and costovertebral joint involvement leads to reduced chest expansion and a mechanical restrictive lung defect.

Sacroiliac and vertebral infections may be easily missed as a cause of buttock pain and sciatica in drug abusers (Brancos *et al.*, 1991). Sternoclavicular joint involvement may also be infective.

Peripheral joints

Painful peripheral joints must be examined gently to maintain the patient's confidence. Note the extent of skin changes in colour and swelling and look for breaks in the skin. These may be sources of infection, periungually or between digits or on the soles.

In the absence of obvious joint swelling, palpation can confirm an effusion. At the knee, this is felt on ballotting the patella as a 'tap' or by expression of fluid from the medial to the lateral compartment (bulge sign; Fig. 5).

A normal range of motion in the knee is 0°–130°/150°. Evidence of hyperlaxity or loss of passive range is noted. Prepatellar bursae and popliteal cysts (Baker's or semimembranosus) are usually well defined but the latter can rupture into the calf. This causes a tense, hot lower leg mimicking venous thrombosis. Synovial fluid contains proteases and cytokines which cause the myofasciitis in triceps surae.

Every new presentation of a swollen joint must be considered for diagnostic aspiration (see later). A previous diagnosis of gout or a well-defined cause of polyarthritis, which is usual for the patient, may excuse this but the possibility of focal sepsis especially in rheumatoid arthritis and in prosthetic joints must be considered. The causes of a haemarthrosis are:

- Trauma/fractures.
- Tumours.
- Haemophilia/bleeding disorders.
- Anticoagulant therapy.
- Unstable joints (Charcot's).
- Pigmented villonodular synovitis.
- Severe inflammation.
- Haemangioma/arteriovenous fistula.

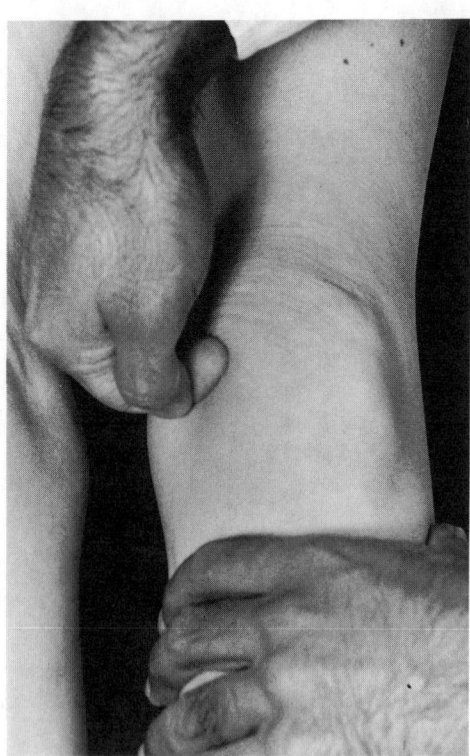

Fig. 5. Knee effusion. Bulge sign. Expression of fluid from medial to lateral compartment of the right knee whilst compressing the suprapatellar pouch.

SPECIFIC SYNDROMES

Infective arthritis

- Staphylococcal/streptococcal.
- Gram-negative.
- Gonococcal.
- Treponemal.
- Mycobacterial.
- Fungal.
- Viral.

Bacterial arthritis

The incidence of non-gonococcal bacterial arthritis is low and has remained stable in the postantibiotic era (Goldenberg & Reed, 1985). Early diagnosis and good management result in a good functional outcome in over 70% of cases (Newman, 1976) but, if the diagnosis is made after a week of symptoms, the results are poor (Goldenberg & Reed, 1985).

Gram-positive infection

Staphylococci and streptococci are the commonest cause of non-gonococcal bacterial infection (Cooper & Cawley, 1986). Staphyloccocus is now often methicillin-resistant (Ang-Fonte *et al.*, 1985). Hosts immunocompromised from HIV (human immunodeficiency virus), drug abuse or rheumatoid arthritis are particularly at risk. *Staphylococcus epidermidis* is an opportunist bacterium that infects prosthetic joints and, like other coagulase-negative staphylococci, may be multiresistant. *Staphylococcus epidermidis* arthritis is a known sequel to urethral catheterization and subsequent bacteraemia (Hutton *et al.*, 1985).

Group A *Streptococcus haemolyticus* arthritis can develop following skin and respiratory infection in normal hosts and has a good outcome when treated promptly. Group B and G streptococcal infections are more serious and are seen in infants or the elderly (Siskind *et al.*, 1975; Lin *et al.*, 1982). Anaerobic infections occur predominantly in hip and knee disease and may be part of a mixed aerobic/anaerobic infection (Hall *et al.*, 1984). *Peptococcus*, *Bacteroides* and *Fusobacterium* are commonly isolated and there are a few reported cases of *Clostridia* and *Listeria*.

Gram-negative infections

Adults develop Gram-negative arthritis because of predisposing debilitating chronic multisystem disease leading to bacteraemia and haematogenous spread. Risk factors include age, sickle cell anaemia, diabetes, other chronic rheumatic disease and prosthetic joints (Fig. 6). Fever may be low-grade but rigors do occur. Involvement of the knee, hip or shoulder is commonest, and usually symptomatic.

Escherichia coli, *Proteus mirabilis*, *Pseudomonas*, *Salmonella* and *Serratia* are the usual agents detected. SLE (systemic lupus erythematosus) victims are especially prone to *Salmonella* (Abramson *et al.*, 1985).

Neonates and infants are prone to hospital-acquired coliform infections commonly related to catheter sepsis and resulting in hip and knee infection (Dan, 1983). The classical description is of an apyrexial neonate with painful hip movements, distal oedema and a hip held flexed in abduction and lateral rotation (Glassberg & Ozonoff, 1978).

Community-acquired disease is usually due to streptococcal or *Haemophilus influenzae* infection. Otherwise normal children between 1 and 24 months who lack specific antibody may develop a septic joint after otitis media or meningitis (Rotbart & Glode, 1985).

Staphylococcus aureus and Gram-negative bacilli cause aggressive and rapid joint destruction. Streptococcal and

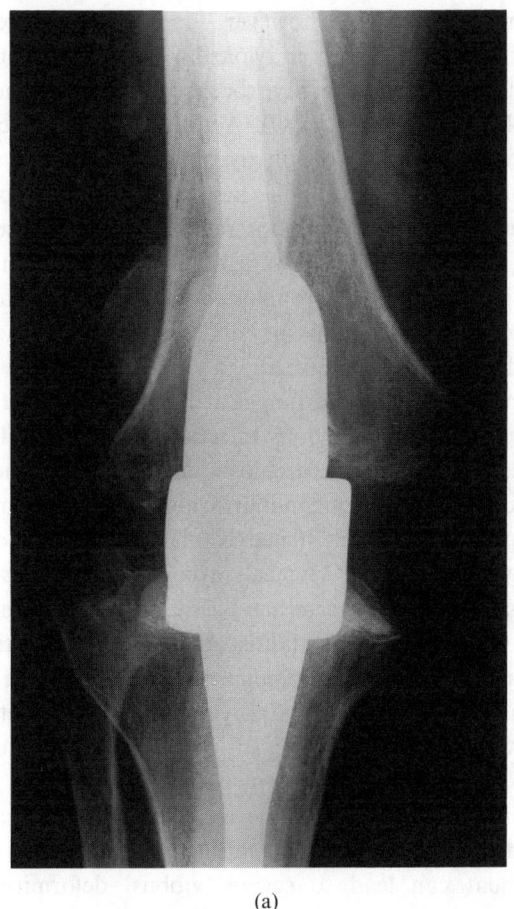

(a)

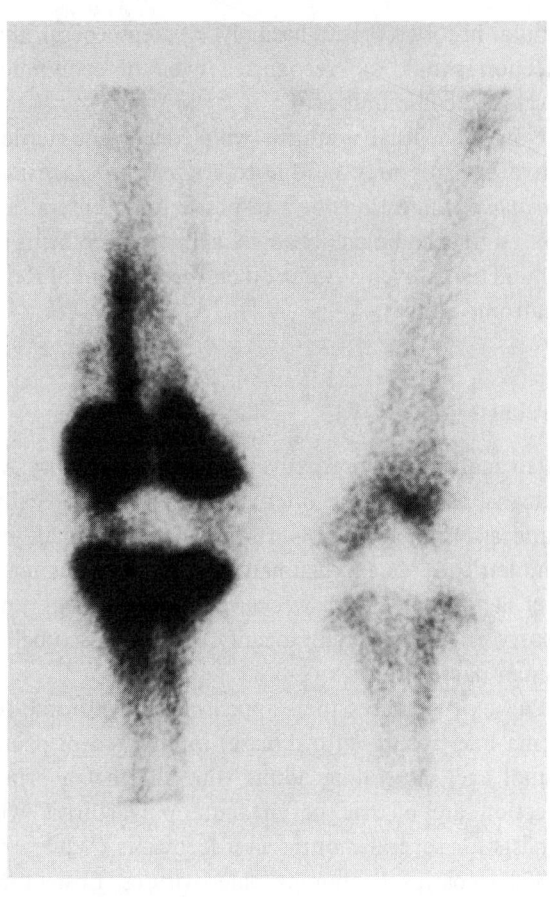

(b)

Fig. 6. Prosthetic joint infection. (a) X-ray; (b) bone scan.

neisserial infections are less damaging and can result in a good functional outcome.

Disseminated gonococcal infective arthritis

This is predominantly a disease of young females (female/male 5:1) with a 3–5-day history of flitting polyarthralgia, often without genitourinary symptoms. Fever, a maculopapular skin rash of the trunk and limbs (distally) with tenosynovitis of wrists, ankles, fingers and toes are typical. The skin lesions may be vesiculopustular, necrotic, or even vasculitic with bullae and erythema nodosum panniculitis. Early blood cultures are usually positive. The non-purulent arthritis and skin rash are related to circulating immune complexes but if left untreated frankly purulent focal arthritis may develop (Holmes *et al.*, 1971). This progression may reflect specific host-strain pathogenetic mechanisms (O'Brien *et al.*, 1983).

Disseminated gonococcal infection must be differentiated from *Neisseria meningitidis* infection in which meningism may be mild but pericarditis is more frequent,

and also from other bacterial arthritides – specifically bacterial endocarditis, in which polyarthralgia and characteristic vascular lesions occur.

Other types of bacterial arthritis

Lyme disease is now clearly defined, but atypical presentations may not show the enlarging rash with central clearing (erythema chronicum migrans) or have any recall of being bitten by the tick *Ixodes damnii*, which carries the spirochaete *Borrelia burgdorferi*. Cerebritis and carditis are serious complications of this disease which is caused by *Borrelia* (Steere *et al.*, 1983). *Borrelia*-specific outer surface protein A DNA has been detected in synovial fluid at the onset of arthritis and is apparently cleared following a complete course of antibiotics. Chronic arthritis may still occur in a proportion of cases in the absence of persisting antigen (Nocton *et al.*, 1994).

Acute rheumatic fever is a rare consideration but may be increasing in incidence. In childhood, flitting arthritis, erythema marginatum and carditis, chorea and nodules with a history of beta-haemolytic streptococcal throat infection should be recognized even in economically developed communities.

Non-gonococcal urethritis with concurrent sterile reactive arthritis may be due to *Chlamydia trachomatis/Ureaplasma* infections or a response to an enteral infection. If the complete triad of arthritis, urethritis and conjunctivitis/uveitis occurs, then the eponym of Reiter's syndrome applies.

Viral arthritis

Often managed conservatively in the community, viral arthritis presents less often to hospitals. Typically it manifests as an acute polyarthritis involving small joints symmetrically as in rheumatoid disease but it usually only lasts from 1 to 2 weeks. Positive serology and a history of exposure may identify the virus as rubella or human parvovirus.

Parvovirus causes the slapped cheek syndrome (erythema infectiosum, fifth disease) in children of primary school age, but young adults who contract a primary infection are at risk of an acute polyarthritis which persists for several months in a few cases (White *et al.*, 1985). Hepatitis B, mumps, enteroviruses, Epstein–Barr virus, herpes virus, varicella zoster or adenovirus can all be related to self-limiting episodes of synovitis, with good functional outcome.

Arthralgia and arthritis occur in rubella and may just precede the onset of the skin rash. Postrubella vaccination arthralgia is also recognized and may be episodic over a few months.

Transient synovitis of the hip in children 5–10 years of age is associated with common upper respiratory viral infections. The child may limp without complaint or pain may be referred to the thigh or knee. Arthritis lasts 1–6 days and specialist attention is required. Aspiration of the hip may be therapeutic in severe cases and to exclude bacterial infection (see later). Late sequelae in less than 1% of cases include osteonecrosis (Legg–Calvé–Perthés disease) or premature osteoarthritis. X-ray may show joint space widening, and ultrasound can confirm an effusion before aspiration is attempted.

Other infections (including HIV)

Acquired immunodeficiency related to HIV infection is a risk factor for septic arthritis and osteomyelitis caused by common and opportunist pathogens. Other rheumatic syndromes, however, such as Reiter's, psoriatic-like disease and spondyloarthropathy with enthesopathy and dactylitis have been described secondary to HIV (Winchester, 1989). Additionally, a few cases of Sjögren's syndrome, polymyositis and vasculitis with characteristic autoantibodies have occurred and demonstrate the disordered immune regulation in this disease. It is imperative to be aware of these associations as occasionally joint disease may be the presenting feature and adequate precautions for handling blood and synovial samples are always required.

Syphilis, leprosy and fungal arthritis are rare. *Mycobacterium tuberculosis* bony infection may be multifocal as part of systemic tuberculosis, or is often diagnosed late following insidious monarthritis when other causes are excluded and insistence is placed upon synovial biopsy and culture. Atypical mycobacteria (*Mycobacterium bovis*, *Mycobacterium kansasii*) can present in small joints or as a dactylitis. Aseptic oligoarthritis of tuberculosis bears the eponym of Poncet's disease but the availability of PCR (polymerase chain reaction) detection of mycobacterial antigen in affected tissue is set to challenge these concepts (Keat, 1993).

Spinal tuberculosis may be mistaken for degenerative spondylosis in the early stages, and late diagnosis and treatment can lead to severe 'gibbus' deformity for which late surgery is usually unhelpful (Fam & Rubenstein, 1993).

CRYSTAL ARTHROPATHIES

Introduction

Crystals form slowly in tissues (particularly damaged joints) when the solute concentration is above saturation point. Monosodium urate (MSU – gout), calcium pyrophosphate dihydrate (CPPD – pseudogout) and hydroxyapatite (HA – calcific periarthritis) are the three crystals most commonly involved in inflammation. The large surface and charge on crystals lead to protein binding, complement, coagulation factor, macrophage and synoviocyte activation, with release of intracellular, and stimulation of extracellular, inflammatory mediators. Urate induces specific polymorphonuclear chemotaxis.

Gout

Clinical

Gout (Latin, *gutta*, 'a drop' of evil humour; Rodnan, 1965) is common, affecting 200–275 persons per 100,000 in Western societies. It results from disordered purine metabolism or excretion. Enzyme defects are rare. Up to 10% of patients with acute gout may have a preceding history of renal urate stones. The first metatarsophalangeal joint is typically involved in up to 75% of cases, but ankles, midtarsal and knee joints also present acutely. The attack is intensely painful with tight shiny overlying tissue which characteristically desquamates as the attack subsides over 3–7 days. Rigors and low-grade fever can occur, meriting exclusion of sepsis at the first presentation.

Asymptomatic hyperuricaemia diagnosed by two fasting urates above the normal laboratory range (0.42 mmol l^{-1}) is not uncommon and is inadequate for the absolute diagnosis of the first gouty attack. Definitive diagnosis can only be made by joint or soft tissue aspirate and demonstration of crystals of MSU. These are negatively birefringent needles seen on polarizing microscopy and are often engulfed by polymorphs.

Risk factors for gout are:

- Hyperuricaemia.
- Age (middle age for men and postmenopausal in females).
- Trauma (often trivial).
- Alcohol (increased urate production and high lactate which reduces renal excretion).
- Perioperative stress.
- Fasting (rise in acetoacetic acid and beta-hydroxy-butyric acids).
- Haematological malignancies.
- Chemotherapeutic drugs, thiazides, frusemide, low dose aspirin.
- Other causes of renal tubular dysfunction.

Intercritical phases of gout are periods of clinical silence despite the occasional persistence of crystals.

Inflamed bunions, psoriatic or Reiter's dactylitis, pseudo-gout, nodal osteoarthritis and septic arthritis in the big toe may be mistaken for gout. Advanced cases without therapy for years develop chronic tophaceous gout. Tophi which occur at sites of pressure and chronic trauma contain chalky material and result from a chronic foreign body reaction to crystals of MSU. They may calcify and show up on radiographs. Other X-ray features are punctate (round or oval) articular or periarticular erosions with sclerotic margins and soft tissue swelling. Signs of chondrocalcinosis or calcific periarthritis should be sought and excluded.

Chronic polyarthritic gout may present subacutely and mimic rheumatoid arthritis. Olecranon bursitis with calcified tophi can be mistaken for nodular rheumatoid disease. Aspiration of bursal fluid and examination for crystals is mandatory to avoid misdiagnosis and inappropriate therapy.

Hyperuricaemia and gout are associated with obesity, excess alcohol intake, hypertension, hypertriglyceridaemia, ischaemic heart disease and renal stones. These need to be considered and managed in conjunction with the gout.

Management

Acute attacks

1. Aspirate the joint and arrange synovianalysis for crystals and microbiological culture.
2. Consider immediate radiology to exclude early bony signs of sepsis.
3. Check blood count and ESR (erythrocyte sedimentation rate), blood urate, urea, electrolytes, liver enzymes. A repeat fasting urate and lipid profile must not be forgotten.
4. Check for causes to be excluded (diet, alcohol, dehydration, drugs). Note that thiazides and frusemide may be weaned and substituted by other classes of antihypertensive agent or by bumetanide which is a loop diuretic with mild uricosuric activity. Stop low-dose aspirin.
5. Prescribe anti-inflammatory and analgesic medication. Potent non-steroidal anti-inflammatory drugs (NSAIDs) are effective: indomethacin 50 mg three times daily, or equivalent doses of flurbiprofen, ketoprofen, diclofenac or naproxen will help within hours. The dose may be weaned off over a week in most acute cases. Contraindications to NSAIDs (heart failure and renal ischaemia in the elderly, active peptic ulcer disease and anticoagulation) may preclude their use and indicate colchicine, reducing from 1 mg three times daily to 0.5 mg three times daily over 7 days. Intravenous colchicine is sometimes required at the onset of therapy. It is an effective inhibitor of chemotaxin release.

Chronic gout

Recurrent renal stones, progressive renal failure, four acute episodes of joint disease in a year, chronic tophaceous gout or polyarticular gout are all indications for long-term hypouricaemic measures. These include:

- Diet with gradual weight reduction.
- Reduction in alcohol intake.

- Stopping diuretics and low-dose aspirin if possible (see above).
- Commencing allopurinol (a xanthine oxidase inhibitor) which is effective and relatively safe, although allergic skin reactions and hepatorenal toxicity are recognized. The dose range is 100–300 mg per day. An initial course of 4–6 weeks of therapy increases risk of acute attacks and NSAID or colchicine should be co-prescribed. A lack of compliance during inactive phases often leads to unnecessary and higher doses being prescribed for persistent hyperuricaemia.
- Uricosuric drugs. These are recommended for under-secretors. Probenecid and tiaprofenic acid and azapropazone are also effective with additional anti-inflammatory activity.
- If other measures are contraindicated, low-dose long-term colchicine can be used.

Calcium pyrophosphate dihydrate crystal deposition disease

Aetiology

There is a familial type in addition to the well-recognized associations with previous trauma and degenerative joint disease, hyperparathyroidism and haemochromatosis. CPPD in cartilage is age-related, and radiological chondrocalcinosis occurs in up to 50% of octogenarians (Ryan & McCarty, 1985). Joint disease is relatively infrequent, so factors governing crystal shedding are important. An association with hypothyroidism has been challenged (Job-Deslandre et al., 1993) and mechanisms for hypomagnesaemia and alkaline phosphatase deficiency being causal have been proposed (McCarty, 1993). The overlap with inflammatory episodes of osteoarthritis can lead to classification difficulty.

Clinical

Pseudogout quite commonly occurs as a monarthritis at the wrist and knees. Polyarthritic disease may be misdiagnosed as rheumatoid because fever, fatigue, morning stiffness, synovitis and a raised ESR can occur. A polymyalgic disease without obvious synovitis is a rare presentation. The diagnosis is made on synovial fluid analysis confirming inflammation and positively birefringent rod-shaped crystals. Occasional extravasation of red cells causes mild haemarthrosis. X-rays must show characteristic calcification in articular cartilage and menisci, e.g. in the knees, hips, symphysis pubis, intervertebral discs (annulus fibrosus) and the triangular ligament in the wrist.

Treatment

Joint aspiration and injection of steroids (crystalline hydrocortisone or prednisolone acetate) is effective (see below). Oral NSAIDs help and occasional use of colchicine (oral/IV) is effective (Bowles et al., 1986).

Hydroxyapatite deposition disease

Calcium hydroxyapatite is the main mineral of bones and teeth. Individual crystals (5–500 nm long) require electron microscopic analysis but clumps of crystals can be detected by alizarin red stain and light microscopy.

HA is the predominant crystal seen in acute calcific periarthritis. This is commonest in the supraspinatus tendon and rotator cuff mechanism of the shoulder. It is seen rarely in the hip. Sudden onset of severe shoulder pain and signs of intense inflammation raise the possibility of sepsis.

Characteristic calcific deposits on X-ray often disperse after resolution of the attack. NSAIDs, aspiration and local steroid injections are effective therapy and recurrence is rare.

Chronic destructive arthritis of the shoulder has been related to HA-mediated chronic synovitis and is known eponymously as 'Milwaukee shoulder' (McCarty, 1993). HA may be detected with other crystals in degenerative osteoarthritic joints and in CPPD disease. Ectopic post-inflammatory soft tissue calcification consists predominantly of HA. Other crystals occasionally detected include cholesterol, injected steroids, prosthetic joint debris and foreign bodies.

TECHNIQUE

Aspiration and injection of joints (and soft tissues)

Objectives
1. Diagnostic aspiration of synovial fluid for laboratory analysis.
2. Therapeutic aspiration of synovial effusion to reduce the pressure and relieve pain.
3. Instillation of corticosteroids and local anaesthetic for treatment of painful inflammatory synovitis and soft tissue lesions.

Indications
- Absolute: in cases of monarthritis of undetermined cause.
- Relative: in acute polyarthritis as part of investigation or management.

Table T1. *Interpretation of results of synovianalysis*

	Inflammatory	Bacterial	Mycobacterial	Viral
Aspirate translucency	Turbid	Purulent	Slightly turbid	Clear/turbid
Cell numbers	$5–25 \times 10^3$	$25–100 \times 10^3$	$10–50 \times 10^3$	$5–25 \times 10^3$
Neutrophils	$>50\%$	$>75\%$	$>50\%$	$<50\%$
Fluid stain	Negative	Gram-positive 50%	AFB positive 30%	Negative
Culture	Negative	90%	80%	Rare

NB: Polarized microscopy for crystal analysis of inflammatory fluids can detect urate, calcium pyrophosphate and other particles. Electron microscopy confirms hydroxyapatite in alizarin red positive samples. AFB, acid-fast bacillus.

Contraindications

- Relative:
  - Anticoagulation and bleeding disorders. Note that there is therapeutic benefit in haemophilic arthropathy under factor VIII cover with cautious aspiration by experienced operators or while the patient is anticoagulated. The use of ice and immobilization for 24 h is advised.
  - Unstable joints.
  - Marked juxta-articular osteoporosis.
  - Intra-articular fracture.
- Absolute:
  - Periarticular sepsis precluding an aseptic joint puncture.
  - Suspected septicaemia/bacteraemia or septic arthritis (i.a. steroid).
  - Prosthetic joint. Consider specialist advice unless the patient is seriously ill with signs of sepsis and the joint is considered to be infected.

Prior investigations/considerations

- Joint X-ray is advisable but is not an absolute requirement. A baseline film for suspected infection is often valuable for comparison later.
- A coagulation screen should be undertaken if indicated by the history.
- Consider carefully any possible risk of HIV or hepatitis B as the arthritis may precede jaundice and an urticarial rash. Take standard precautions and wear gloves especially when handling fluids.
- Operators should be immunized for hepatitis B.

Practical technique

- Strict attention to asepsis is imperative.
- The skin is prepared with iodine or alcohol swabs.
- Disposable needles must be changed after each separate manoeuvre, i.e. after drawing up steroid or anaesthetic and before injection or between joints if more than one is to be injected.
- The use of gloves will assist in the aseptic procedure but is mandatory in high-risk cases to protect the operator.
- Joint aspiration. For large effusions requiring a prolonged procedure, local anaesthetic infiltration of soft tissue is advised. Ethyl chloride spray is effective for quick procedures.
- Examine, palpate and mark the spot for injection. Use a small alcohol swab to clean skin finally and tense the skin prior to injection with a no-touch technique.
- A 21 G needle is adequate for most diagnostic aspirates, but for large effusions or chronic inflammatory joints a 19 G needle will cope with most common debris. If the flow is blocked, gentle reorientation of the needle bevel will free the tip from synovial fronds or loose debris. Positive pressure to flush the tip is rarely required. Fresh syringes to deal with large effusions should be kept available and care must be taken when changing syringes. If the needle lock is accidentally contaminated then the needle should be withdrawn and the procedure recommenced if indicated.
- Joint/soft tissue injection only:
  - Most steroid preparations can be mixed with local anaesthetic if the operator wishes to avoid prior local anaesthesia and a second injection of steroid.
  - Always aspirate prior to injecting to avoid albeit rare intravascular injection.

Postprocedure advice

- Tell the patient that the anaesthetic wears off within 1–2 h.
- A rare inflammatory flare at 12–24 h may occur but settles in a few hours.
- Resting or even splinting the joint for 24 h will maximize steroid uptake into the synovium.
- The effect of the steroid will be noticed between 48 and 72 h.
- Any significant deterioration of the joint at that time or within 7 days must be reported immediately and iatrogenic sepsis must be excluded.

POLYARTHRITIS

Introduction

Acute infective polyarthritis has been discussed earlier. Reiter's disease and reactive arthropathy (grouped as seronegative spondyloarthritis) are the next most common large joint arthritides to present as an emergency. The autoimmune rheumatic diseases such as rheumatoid

Table 3. *Extra-articular emergencies of autoimmune rheumatic diseases*

- Skin: vasculitis
- Renal: glomerular, interstitial or thrombotic causes of failure
- Central nervous system: vascular stroke, cerebritis, sensorimotor neuropathy
- Lung: pleuritis, parenchymal (fibrosis, nodular, embolic)
- Cardiovascular system: peri/myo/endocarditis, renovascular hypertension
- Gastrointestinal tract: peritonitis, pancreatitis, ischaemic crises
- Drug-related: upper gastrointestinal haemorrhage, renal failure, haematological cytopenias (marrow toxicity or peripheral consumption)
- Opportunist infections

arthritis and SLE cannot be dealt with in detail here. They often manifest as subacute or chronic joint disease but can present as emergencies because of a failure of other organ systems as part of the disease process, or because of drug side-effects (Table 3).

Seronegative spondyloarthropathy

The aetiopathology of these syndromes may for the present be grouped under the term 'reactive arthritis'. It implies a casual role for bacterial infections initiating disease in which inflammation may persist or recur in the absence of detectable active infection. Persistence of bacterial antigen within lymphoid tissue at sites remote from inflammation or in synovium is a possible mechanism for recurrence (Highton & Poole, 1993). These disorders share clinical features and have a strong association with the major histocompatibility antigen HLA-B27 (50–90%). Ankylosing spondylitis may be considered the prototype with the strongest association with B27.

Peripheral joint synovitis affects large joints of the lower limbs without the characteristic symmetry of rheumatoid disease. Histology of the synovium is similar to rheumatoid without lymphoid granulomata. Enthesopathy (inflamed ligament or tendon/bone junctions) and periostitis are more characteristic. Axial involvement of large joints (sacroiliac, sternoclavicular, symphysis pubis and intervertebral joints) produces fibrosis followed by ossification. An example of this is the syndesmophyte – a bony outgrowth which develops vertically at the junction of the vetebral plate and the annulus of a disc. This is distinguished from horizontal 'degenerative' osteophytes. Calcaneal spurs associated with plantar fasciitis are another radiological feature.

Sacroiliitis with bony bridging and eventual fusion is usually symmetrical. Unilateral sacroiliitis occurs in psoriatic arthritis but it is important to exclude a tuberculous infection. Juvenile presentation of hip arthropathy in boys over 10 years old is often followed by the insidious development of spondylitis.

Reiter's syndrome defines the triad of arthritis, urethritis/balanitis and conjunctivitis/uveitis. Limited forms do occur.

The clinical assessment to identify axial involvement (see section on examination above) requires measurement of lumbar flexion (Shöber test), lateral flexion of thoracolumbar spine (finger tip to floor), cervical spine (neck) rotation and extension (tragus to wall distance), and chest expansion to assess costovertebral ankylosis.

SOFT TISSUE RHEUMATISM

Introduction

Pain unrelated to acute trauma or systemic disease can affect joint capsules, bursae, tendons and their insertions (enthesopathy), ligaments, muscles and overlying fascia and fibrofatty tissues. The cause may remain obscure though specific functional deficits can help to identify aggravating factors.

Diagnosis is based on the examination. Local tenderness, limited movement and pain reproduced when specific movement is resisted by the examiner confirms the history.

Treatment is often empirical, with rest, supportive splinting occasionally and a programme of re-education. Physiotherapists' use of heat, ice and ultrasound can be effective. Local anaesthetic and hydrocortisone injections can be curative or reduce pain and shorten the period of spontaneous recovery, but there may be a cost in compromised healing and the attendant risk of tendon rupture. Anti-inflammatory medication is restricted to short-term supervised use only. In cases related to chronic overuse, specific attention to ergonomic solutions must be sought in collaboration with 'occupational therapists'. Only in rare instances is referral for surgery required.

Tendon lesions

Traumatic tenosynovitis

This was recognized as an industrial disease in 1947 (Evans, 1988). One form of work-related pain in the extensor mechanism of the forearm just proximal to the tendon sheaths is recognized as peritendinitis crepitans. Features of compartment syndrome have been clearly defined in some cases and, additionally, asymptomatic synovitis at the wrist may occur in the so-called intersection syndrome where extensor pollicis brevis and abductor pollicis longus cross extensor carpi radialis (Grundberg & Reagan, 1985).

Surgical decompression is effective when splinting and local steroids have failed.

The extension of these distinct entities to the all-embracing term 'repetitive strain injury' (RSI) for a variety of upper limb syndromes led to terminological confusion (Fry, 1986) and aetiological debate (Smythe, 1988).

The psychosocial aspects of RSI have led to an epidemic of claims in Australia and its description as an occupational neurosis (Quintner, 1991; Ireland, 1988). Regional pain syndrome is a preferred term (James & Wynn-Parry, 1992) and is increasingly encountered in professional musicians who require particularly sensitive management. Avoidance of the painful task and rest may suffice, but persistence requires coordinated input from therapists, physicians and psychologists. Relaxation, posture, diversional activities and biofeedback are some of the modalities used to achieve specified functional goals and eventual rehabilitation (Brooks, 1993).

De Quervain's disease

This presents with pain at the end of the radius and is recognized in occupations where rapid forearm pronation/supination, or persistent and repeated tension of extensor pollicis brevis or abductor pollicis longus, is required (assembly work, hop-pickers, nappy-pin thumb). The frequency of this condition in postpartum mothers might suggest a causal relationship to transient changes in connective tissue metabolism. In this group the lesion is not recurrent.

Signs of obvious swelling, tenderness and palpable crepitus on moving the related joints may be common to any painful tendon in the hand. Increasing tension by ulnar deviation of the fist while clenching the fully flexed thumb (Finkelstein's test; Finkelstein, 1930) focuses pain at the site of the lesion and distinguishes it from interphalangeal or carpometacarpal disease of the thumb. Mild cases settle with rest, physical measures or topical anti-inflammatory preparations. Prolonged symptoms may respond to local injection of lignocaine and hydrocortisone into the tendon sheath proximal or distal to the swelling. The sheath must be seen to fill without undue pressure during injection. The tendon itself must be spared from iatrogenic insult. Surgical decompression is effective when these measures have failed.

Trigger finger and thumb

These are common. The complaint is of limited extension of a digit which suddenly releases from flexion with a snap or an audible crack. A simple habitual injury may be the cause. Treat these conditions as tenovaginitis (stenosis of tendon sheath) similar to de Quervain's.

Surgical release by incising the sheath to free the thickened portion of tendon is effective in resistant cases. Nodules are not necessarily excised.

Calcific tendinitis

Tendon insertions of flexor carpi ulnaris and radialis (violinists) may become inflamed and occasionally produce calcific tendinitis. Local steroids are effective and surgery is very rarely needed.

Inflammatory tenosynovitis

Painful stiffness of the hands in rheumatoid disease is often caused by palmar tenosynovitis across the metacarpophalangeal joints. Palpable crepitus and nodules facilitate the diagnosis. This condition must be contrasted with the painless nodular fascial contractures of Dupuytren which develop more proximally away from synovium and tendons which do not become tethered. The demonstration of T cell mediated inflammation in this genetically related condition (Baird et al., 1993) may stimulate trials of earlier medical intervention with local steroids as there is a high recurrence after surgical fasciectomy.

Diffuse involvement of all flexor tendons with a limited fist and inability to oppose digits in full extension (positive prayer sign or limited joint mobility) with a waxy oedema of all digits indicates diabetic cheiroarthropathy which may develop independent of diabetic nephropathy (Starkman et al., 1986). Shoulder capsulitis is an associated feature of diabetes and meticulous glucose control is necessary (Isdale, 1993).

Infectious tenosynovitis

Marked swelling of a palmar tendon along the whole digit which is cold and not very painful is the presentation of tuberculous dactylitis. Decompression with biopsy and culture of tissue is essential for diagnosis. Other infections which present in a similar way include gonococcal tenosynovitis and syphilis. *Staphylococcus aureus* tenosynovitis often presents more acutely.

Tennis elbow

This common complaint has a prevalence of 1–3% (Allander, 1974). Spontaneous but gradual onset of symptoms is usual. Pain may be localized to the lateral humeral epicondyle (hence lateral epicondylitis) but referred pain in the hand or up to the shoulder can develop. Spontaneous recovery is most commonly achieved by avoidance of painful manoeuvres related to sport, home improvements or work-related activities. Persistence is associated with tenderness over the epicondyle, the supracondylar ridge or peripherally over the extensor mechanism insertion. The lesion is an enthesopathy and confirmatory signs of pain on resisted supination or dorsiflexion at the wrist, or even resisted extension of the middle finger with the elbow extended, can be elicited. These findings help to distinguish the lesion from other sources of referred elbow pain. Radial nerve compression is a rare cause of persistent symptoms.

If rest and avoidance of strain has failed, management includes physical measures such as local heat/ice, deep friction massage, ultrasound and pressure (epicondylitis clasp), but most frequently a local injection of hydrocortisone and lignocaine is effective (Day *et al.*, 1978). Repeated injections can weaken natural repair so a few resistant cases require surgery which should be as limited a procedure as possible (Calvert *et al.*, 1985).

Golfer's elbow

This is equivalent to medial epicondylitis. Pain is reproduced by pronation of the forearm or wrist flexion against resistance. The principles of management are similar to those of lateral epicondylitis.

Shoulder pain

Minor, often unrecognized, trauma to the rotator cuff muscles is a frequent cause of shoulder pain and limited function. The typical painful arc on active or passive abduction and pain on resisted abduction localizes the lesion to the tendon or tendon sheath of the supraspinatus muscle. The long head of biceps is also easily examined by direct palpation of the tendon in the bicipital groove on the anterior aspect of the shoulder. Secondary inflammation of the subacromial bursa can produce a continuous

nagging pain and if conservative measures of rest or NSAID therapy fail, local injection of lignocaine and hydrocortisone can effect a dramatic cure in the subacute phase. The necessity for local steroids as opposed to simple anaesthetic injections in *acute* rotator cuff lesions has been questioned (Vecchio *et al.*, 1993). Chronic lesions and adhesive capsulitis (often seen in association with insulin-dependent diabetes mellitus) are notoriously slow to respond to injection or physiotherapy. Pain management in these cases can be greatly helped by a judicious bupivacaine and hydrocortisone nerve block to the suprascapular nerve, but this requires an experienced operator to minimize iatrogenic risks such as pneumothorax.

Referred shoulder pain from mediastinal and upper abdominal structures must be considered during clinical assessment.

Bursitis

The common sites of inflamed bursae are:

- Subacromial – shoulder abduction.
- Olecranon – elbow
- Trochanteric – hip flex/abduct, tender.
- Anserine – medial tibial.
- Prepatellar – anterior knee swelling.
- Ischial – tender tuberosity.
- Iliopsoas – hip adduction and internal rotation.
- Achilles – retrocalcaneal, refer to specialist.
- Calcaneal – heel pain, plantar fasciitis.

If infection can be excluded by the history, simple mechanical causes for minor repeated trauma must be sought. Carpet-layers' knee, desk-top olecranon bursitis and sport-related causes are sometimes obvious and are usually managed by rest, temporary support and avoidance of the offending habit. Gout and rheumatoid arthritis are causes of chronic inflammatory bursitis. Beware of greater trochanteric bursitis masquerading as hip osteoarthritis. Stepping out of a low car seat with the hip abducted is an often overlooked cause.

Chronic lesions respond well to local steroid injection. Achilles tendinitis and bursitis should be managed conservatively if at all possible to avoid weakening the tendon with steroids and increasing the risk of rupture.

Infected bursae require aspiration for microbiological analysis (commonly *Staphyloccus aureus*) and appropriate parenteral antibiotics. Resolution is usually prompt and surgery is rarely required.

SUMMARY

Joint pain and swelling is a common emergency presentation. A detailed history and examination can often secure an accurate diagnosis when attention is given to the common patterns of disease presentation covered in this chapter. Local infection or possible systemic infection have to be positively excluded, especially before embarking on steroid injection. Simple exercise, advice and educational measures are often adequate for soft tissue rheumatism. If there is any diagnostic doubt, specialist advice should be sought as the final functional outcome may be compromised by delayed treatment.

Bibliography

ABRAMSON, S., KRAMER, S.B., RADIN, A. et al., (1985). *Salmonella* bacteremia in systemic lupus erythematosus. *Arthritis Rheum.*, **28**, 75–9.

ALLANDER, E. (1974). Prevalence, incidence and remission rates of some common rheumatic diseases and syndromes. *Scand. J. Rheumatol.*, **3**, 145–53.

ANG-FONTE, G.Z., ROZBORIL, M.B. & THOMPSON, G.R. (1985). Changes in non-gonococcal septic arthritis: drug abuse and methicillin resistant *Staphylococcus aureus. Arthritis Rheum.*, **28**, 210–13.

BAIRD, K.S., ALWAN, W.H., CROSSAN, J.F. et al. (1993). T-cell mediated response in Dupuytren's Disease. *Lancet*, **341**, 1622–3.

BILLINGS, R.A. & MOLE, K.F. (1972). Rheumatology in general practice. A survey in World Rheumatism Year. *J. R. Coll. Gen. Pract.*, **27**, 721.

BOWLES, C., HARRINGTON, T., ZINMEISTER, A. et al. (1986). Colchicine prevents recurrent pseudogout: multicenter trial. *Arthritis Rheum.*, **29**, 538.

BRANCOS, M.A., PERIS, P., MIRO, J.M., et al. (1991). Septic arthritis in heroin addicts. *Semin. Arthritis Rheum.*, **21**, 81–7.

BROOKS, P. (1993). Repetitive strain injury. *BMJ*, **307**, 1298.

CALVERT, P.T., MACPHERSON, I.S., ALLUM, R.L. et al. (1985). Simple lateral release in treatment of tennis elbow. *J. R. Soc. Med.*, **78**, 912–15.

COOPER, C. & CAWLEY, M.I. (1986). Bacterial arthritis in an English health district: a 10 year review. *Ann. Rheum. Dis.*, **45**, 458–63.

DAN, M. (1983). Neonatal septic arthritis. *Isr. J. Med. Sci.*, **19**, 967–71.

DAY, B.H., GORINDASAMY, N. & PATNAIK, R., (1978). Corticosteroid injections in the treatment of tennis elbow. *Practitioner*, **220**, 459–62.

EDMONDS, S.E., BLAKE, D.R., MORRIS, C.J. et al. (1993). Imaginative approach to synovitis – the role of hypoxic reperfusion damage in arthritis. *J. Rheum.*, **20** (Suppl. 37), 26–31.

EVANS, G., (1988). Soft tissue rheumatism. ARC proceedings no. 6, 92–9. Arth. Rheum. Council, London

FAM, A.G. & RUBENSTEIN, J. (1993). Another look at spinal tuberculosis. *J. Rheumatol.*, **20**, 1731–40.

FINKELSTEIN, H. (1930). Stenosing tenovaginitis at the radial styloid process. *J. Bone Joint Surg.*, **12**, 509–40.

FRY, H.J. (1986). Overuse syndrome, alias tensosynovitis/tendinitis: the terminological hoax. *J. Plastic Reconstr. Surg.*, **78**, 414–17.

GLASSBERG, G.B. & OZONOFF, M.B. (1978). Arthrographic findings in septic arthritis of the hip in infants. *Radiology*, **128**, 151–5.

GOLDENBERG, D.L. & REED, J.L. (1985). Bacterial arthritis. *N. Engl. J. Med.*, **312**, 764–71.

GRUNDBERG, A.B. & REAGAN, D.S. (1985). Pathologic anatomy of the forearm intersection syndrome. *J. Hand. Surg. [Am.]*, **10**, 229–302.

HALL, B.B., ROSENBLATT, J.E. & FITZGERALD, R.H., Jr., (1984). Anaerobic septic arthritis and osteomyelitis. *Orthop. Clin. North Am.*, **15**, 505–16.

HIGHTON, J. & POOLE, E. (1993). Sexually acquired reactive arthritis: inflammation or sepsis? *Br. J. Rheumatol.*, **32**, 649–50.

HOLMES, K.K., COUNTS, G.W. & BEATY, H.N. (1971). Disseminated gonococcal infection. *Ann. Intern. Med.*, **74**, 979–93.

HUTTON, J.P., HAMORY, B.H., PARISI, J.T. et al. (1985). *S. epidermidis* arthritis following catheter induced bacteremia in a neutropenic patient. *Diagn. Microbiol. Infect. Dis.*, **3**, 119–24.

IRELAND, D.C.R. (1988). Psychological and physical aspects of occupational arm pain. *J. Hand Surg.*, **113**, 5–10.

ISDALE, A.H. (1993). The ABC of the diabetic hand-advanced glycosylation end products, browning and collagen. *Br. J. Rheumatol.*, **32**, 859–61.

JAMES, I.M. & WYNN-PARRY, C.B. (1992). Performing arts medicine. *Br. J. Rheumatol.*, **31**, 795–6.

JANKOWSKI, R.F. & MANDALIA, S. (1993). Comparison of attendance and emergency admission patterns at accident and emergency departments in and out of London. *BMJ*, **306**, 1241–3.

JOB-DESLANDRE, C., MENKES, C.J., GUINOT, M. et al. (1993). Does Hypothroidism increase the prevalence of chondrocalcinosis. *Br. J. Rheumatol.*, **32**, 197–98.

KEATS, A. (1993). TB or not TB?: that is the question. *Br. J. Rheumatol.*, **32**, 769–70.

LIN, A.N., KARASIK, A., SALIT, I.E., et al. (1982). Group G streptococcal arthritis. *J. Rheumatol.*, **9**, 424–7.

McCARTY, D.J. (1993). Calcium pyrophosphate dihydrate crystal deposition disease. *Br. J. Rheumatol.*, **33**, 177–9.

NEWMAN, J.H. (1976). Review of septic arthritis throughout the antibiotic era. *Ann. Rneum. Dis.*, **35**, 198–205.

NOCTON, J.J., DRESSLER, F., RUTLEDGE, B. *et al.* (1994). Detection of *Borrelia burgdorferi* DNA by polymerase chain reaction in synovial fluid from patients with Lyme arthritis. *N. Engl. J. Med.,* **330**, 229–34.

O'BRIEN, J.P., GOLDENBERG, D.L. & RICE, P.A. (1983). Disseminated gonococcal infection: a prospective analysis of 49 patients and a review of pathophysiology and immune mechanisms. *Medicine,* **62**, 395–406.

QUINTNER, J. (1991). The RSI syndrome in historical perspective. *Int. Disabil. Stud.,* **13**, 99–104.

RODNAN, G.P. (1965). Early theories concerning etiology and pathogenesis of the gout. *Arthritis Rheum.,* **8**, 599–609.

ROTBART, H.A. & GLODE, M.P. (1985). *Hemophilus influenzae* type B septic arthritis in children: report of 23 cases. *Pediatrics,* **75**, 254–9.

RYAN, L.M. & McCARTY, D.J. (1985). Calcium pyrophosphate crystal deposition disease: pseudogout, articular chondrocalcinosis. In *Arthritis and Allied Conditions: A Textbook of Rheumatology,* 10th edn, ed. D.J. McCarty, pp. 1515–46. Philadelphia: Lea & Febiger.

SISKIND, B., GALLIGUEZ, P. & WALD, E.R. (1975). Group B hemolytic streptococcal osteomyelitis/purulent arthritis in neonnates. *J. Pediatr.,* **87**, 659.

SMYTHE, H. (1988). The 'repetitive strain injury syndrome' is referred pain from the neck. *J. Rheumatol.,* **15**, 1604–8.

STARKMAN, H.S., GLEASON, R.E., RAND, L.I. *et al.* (1986). Limited joint mobility (LJM) of the hand in patients with diabetes mellitus: relation to chronic complications. *Ann. Rheum. Dis.,* **45**, 130–5.

STEERE, A.C., GRODZICKI, R.L., KORNBLATT, A.N. *et al.* (1983). The spirochaetal aetiology of Lyme disease. *N. Engl. J. Med.,* **308**, 733–40.

VECCHIO, P.C., HAZLEMAN, B.L. & KING, R.H. (1993). A double blind trial comparing subacromial methylprednisolone and lignocaine in acute rotator cuff tendinitis. *Br. J. Rheumatol.,* **32**, 743–5.

WHITE, D.G., WOOLF, A.D., MORTIMER, P.P. *et al.* (1985), Human parvovirus arthropathy. *Lancet,* **i**, 419–21.

WINCHESTER, R. (1989). Immunodeficiency and arthritis. *Curr. Opin. Rheumatol.,* **1**, 199–204.

General reference texts

CASSIDY, J.T. & PETTY, R.E. (1990). *Textbook of Pediatric Rheumatology,* 2nd edn., Edinburgh: Churchill Livingstone.

DIEPPE, P., DOHERTY, M., MACFARLANE, D.G. *et al.* (1985). *Rheumatological Medicine.* Edinburgh: Churchill Livingstone.

ESPINOZA, L., GOLDENBERG, D., ARNETT, F. *et al.* (1988). *Infections in the Rheumatic Diseases.* Orlando: Grune & Stratton Inc.

GATTER, R.A. (1984). *A Practical Handbook of Joint Fluid Analysis.* Phildelphia: Lea & Febiger.

HAZLEMAN, B.L. & SILMAN, A. (1988). Soft tissue rheumatism. *Conference Proceedings* No. 6. Arthritis and Rheumatism Council for Research, London.

KELLEY, W.N., HARRIS, E.D., RUDDY, S. *et al.* (1993). Textbook of Rheumatology, 4th edn. Philadelphia: W.B. Saunders.

52 Dermatological emergencies

H.L. CUGNONI[a] and D.W.S. HARRIS[b]

[a] Accident and Emergency Department, Royal Hospitals Trust, London, UK
[b] Department of Dermatology, The Whittington Hospital NHS Trust, London, UK

Chapter plan

Introduction
Anatomy
Eczema
Psoriasis
Skin infections
Collagen vascular disorders
Systemic disease and the skin
Vascular disorders
Miscellaneous skin disorders
Dermatological tumours
Childhood exanthems and toxic erythema
Infestations
Bullous disorders
Urticaria and angioedema
Drug reactions
Reactive erythema
Ulcers

INTRODUCTION

There is a widely held belief amongst the medical profession that the title of this chapter is, in itself, a contradiction in terms. This potentially dangerous view presumably arises from the knowledge that there are few dermatological conditions that could be considered imminently life-threatening. This perceived lack of potential for death and destruction should not dull the physician's responses in the management of dermatological cases in the accident and emergency (A&E) department. The scarcity of true dermatological emergencies does not render them any less worthy of prompt correct treatment. Naturally, what the patient considers to be an emergency does not necessarily reflect the doctor's view. There are few medical conditions which can cause more anxiety, to the lay person, than a rash. It is a highly visible, often uncomfortable, ill-understood expression of pathology and is hence often perceived as an emergency by the patient. Based on this premise, it should not be surprising that many patients with dermatological complaints present to A&E departments for treatment.

Both life-threatening emergencies and the most common of the less serious conditions encountered by the emergency physician are covered in this chapter.

Acute dermatological emergencies

- Exfoliative dermatitis/erythroderma
- Severe Stevens–Johnson syndrome
- Toxic epidermal necrolysis
- Pemphigus vulgaris
- Pemphigoid in the frail or elderly
- Eczema herpeticum
- Angioneurotic oedema
- Severe cellulitis/erysipelas
- Generalized pustular psoriasis
- Generalized herpes zoster (shingles)

Description of a rash

When confronted by a rash that is completely unrecognizable, it is best to adopt a step-by-step approach. Even if this does not provide the inexperienced doctor with an answer, it may enable the dermatologist to suggest a diagnosis from the description.

Ask the following questions and describe the lesions (see Fig. 1) using the appropriate terms from the glossary in Table 1.

1. When did the rash appear?
2. Where did it start?
3. Has it altered?
4. Have you had it before?

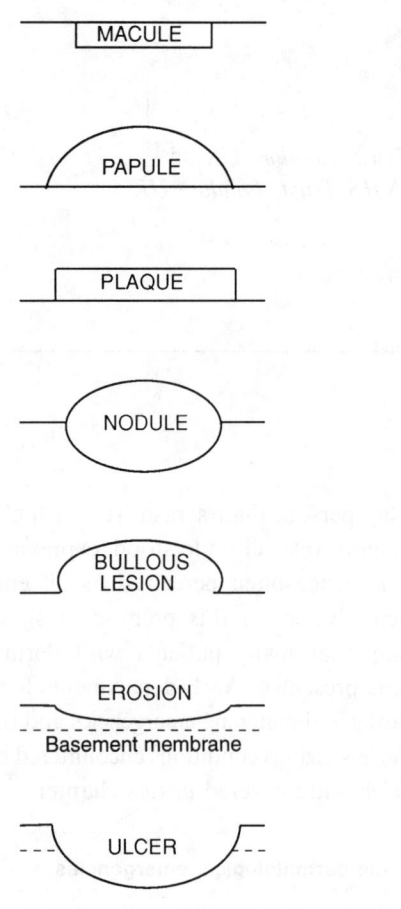

Fig. 1. Diagrams of the more common types of skin lesions.

5. Does it itch/hurt?
6. Does anyone else you know have it?
7. Have you recently started any new medication?
8. Do you feel generally unwell?
9. Are you allergic to anything?
10. Any recent exposure to unusual foods/chemical agents?
11. Any recent foreign travel?
12. Past medical history, including eczema, asthma, hayfever and psoriasis.
13. Drug history.
14. Family history, including eczema, asthma, hayfever and psoriasis.
15. Social history (including occupation).

ANATOMY

The skin consists of two layers – the epidermis and the dermis – which are separated by the basement membrane (Fig. 2). The two layers interdigitate via rete pegs, which are downward projections from the epidermis, and dermal papillae, which are upward projections from the

Table 1. *Glossary of skin lesion types and characteristics*

Lesion	Description
Types	
Macule	A circumscribed, non-raised alteration of skin colour or texture measuring less than 1 cm in diameter
Patch	A macule which measures more than 1 cm
Papule	A solid, raised, superficial lesion less than 1 cm in diameter
Plaque	A superficial, raised, well-circumscribed area of skin measuring more than 2 cm, formed by the coalescence of papules
Nodule	A solid mass within the skin which may be palpated or observed, measuring more than 0.5 cm in diameter
Vesicle	A papule which contains fluid
Pustule	A pus-filled vesicle
Bullous lesion	A vesicle which measures more than 1 cm
Erosion	An area of epidermal loss
Ulcer	An area which has lost the epidermis and at least the upper part of the dermis
Weal	A white raised area of oedema within the skin; it may be any size and is often surrounded by erythema
Telangiectasia	Visible, dilated, small blood vessels
Petechiae	Pin-head-sized macules of blood in the skin
Purpura	A large macule of blood within the skin, which may be raised to form a papule; neither purpura nor petechiae will blanch on pressure
Fissure	A split in the skin
Sinus	A channel to the outer surface of the skin
Characteristics	
Erythematous	Reddened
Hypopigmented	A reduction of melanin pigment
Hyperpigmented	An increase in melanin pigment
Circumscribed	Well-demarcated
Confluent	Individual lesions coalesce to form larger lesions
Crusted	Dried exudate on the surface of the lesion (e.g. blood, pus)
Scaly	Lesions covered with flakes of dry skin which can be very small or large sheets

dermis. The skin performs several functions essential to living:

1. *Temperature control* via vasoconstriction, vasodilatation and evaporation of sweat.
2. *Fluid retention* preventing dehydration and ultimately desiccation.

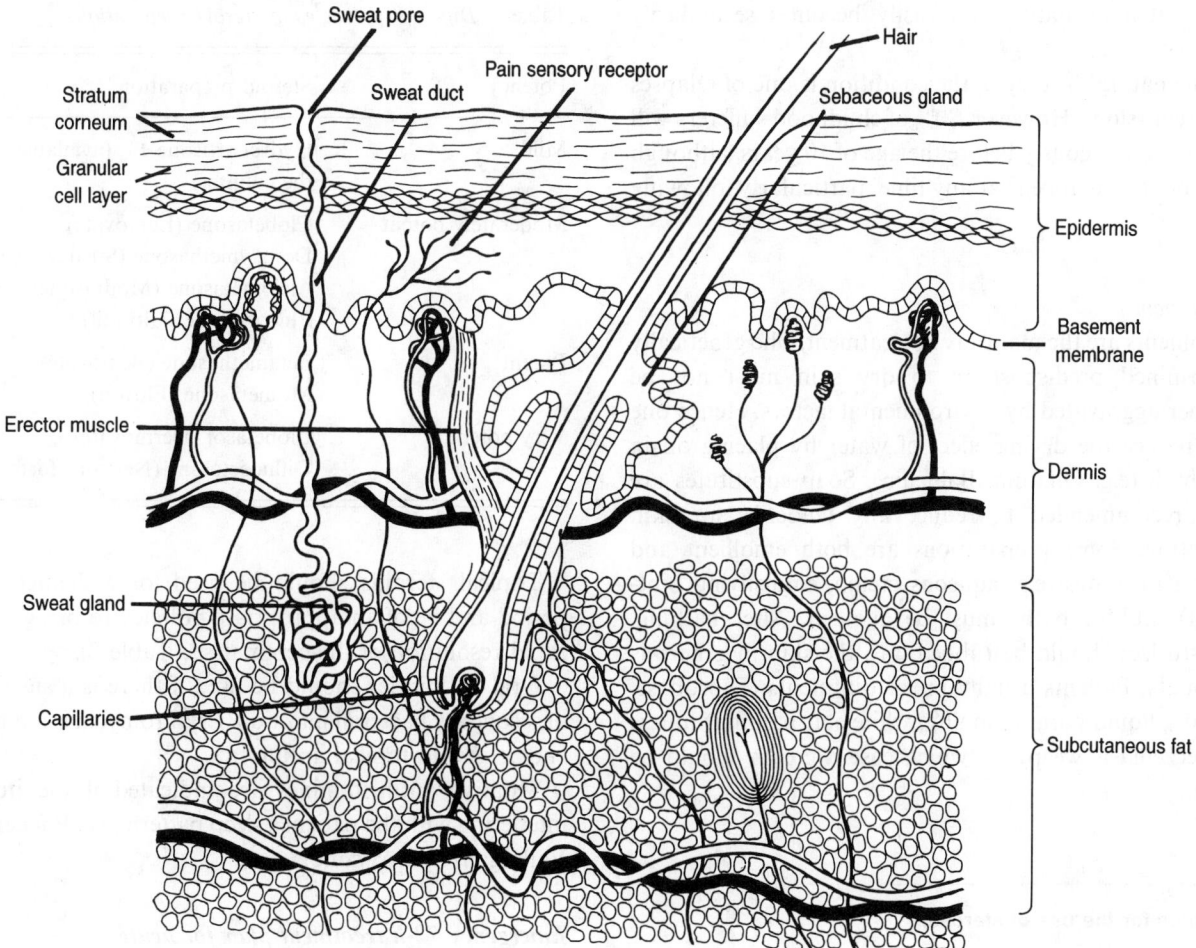

Fig. 2. Cross-section of skin in diagrammatic form.

3. *Protection* from ultraviolet light by melanin.
4. *Barrier to external agents*: the stratum corneum acts as a physical barrier, in addition to which epidermal Langerhans cells are the body's first immunological defence against antigens.
5. *Sensory perception* of pain, temperature and touch is a vital safety mechanism.
6. *Source of vitamin D* via the action of ultraviolet light on dehydrocholesterol.

ECZEMA

There are many forms of this extremely common condition. They fall broadly into two main groups: exogenous and endogenous. Their common histopathological picture is referred to as dermatitis. Eczema is the type of condition that may well prompt a visit to the A&E department as it can be painful (when fissured), infected, unbearably itchy and disfiguring. In almost all cases effective treatment can be initiated in the A&E depart-

ment, but follow-up should be arranged with the general practitioner or a dermatologist if the severity warrants it.

Endogenous eczema

Atopic eczema

This is the commonest form, beginning usually at around 6 months of age. It may, however, present later in childhood or even adulthood. The exact cause is unknown but it is genetically conferred leading to excess formation of IgE antibodies. There is usually a family history of eczema or one of the other atopic conditions (asthma or hayfever). Between 15% and 20% of the population are atopic.

Classically it is a symmetrical erythematous, scaly eruption mainly involving the flexures (e.g. antecubital and popliteal fossae), face, neck, wrists and hands. Rarely it may become generalized. The rash is always extremely itchy and constant excoriation can lead to scarring and ultimately to thickening of the skin (lichenification).

It is often exudative and easily becomes secondarily infected.

The natural history of the condition is one of relapses and remissions. However, 70% of childhood sufferers will remit spontaneously before the age of 10 years, although eczema may reappear at any time, particularly following stress.

Treatment

Emollients are the mainstay of treatment. The genetically determined predisposition to dry skin must not be further aggravated by environmental factors. Hence one can reduce the drying effect of water by placing oil in the bath (e.g. Oilatum, Balneum). Soap substitutes are also recommended to reduce any tendency for skin irritation. Some preparations are both emollient and soap substitutes (e.g. aqueous cream, emulsifying ointment). Bubble baths must be avoided. After bathing, moisturizer should be rubbed into the skin in generous amounts. Patients usually prefer ointments (Diprobase, or 50% liquid paraffin in 50% white soft paraffin) unless the eczema is weepy, in which case a cream should be used.

Rules for the use of steroids

- Topical steroids can cause harm if abused, do not prescribe them lightly
- The strength of steroid is important:
  - Use 1% hydrocortisone on the face or in infants under 1 year old
  - Use a short burst of a higher strength steroid to gain control of the problem and reduce down to a weaker one for longer-term use
  - Never use more than:

    200 g per week – mild
    50 g per week – potent
    30 g per week – very potent

- Lichenified eczema responds best to steroids in an ointment base
- Extensive, persistent eczema may require a 2-week course of potent or very potent steroid application to achieve control; if no improvement can be seen after 72 h oral antibiotics should be considered
- Steroid requirement for twice daily therapy for two weeks:

	4 yr old child	70 kg adult
Trunk (front & back)	40 g	120 g
Both arms & legs	70 g	180 g
Whole body	120 g	340 g

Table 2. *Different potencies of steroid preparations*

Potency	Steroid preparation
Mild	Hydrocortisone 1% (available over the counter)
Moderately potent	Clobetasone (Eumovate)
	Desoxymethasone (Stiedex LP)
	Alclometasone (Modrasone)
	Flucortolone (Ultradil)
Potent	Betamethasone (Betnovate)
	Mometasone (Elocon)
Very potent	Clobetasol (Dermovate)
	Diflucortolone (Nerisone forte)

Topical steroids should be used for a defined time period and be of an appropriate potency to bring about rapid resolution of the eczema (see Table 2).

Oral antibiotics should be used if there is a suspicion of secondary bacterial infection. Erythromycin is a reliable choice. Avoid topical antibiotics.

Sedative antihistamines are indicated if the itch is interfering with the patient's sleep pattern (e.g. Phenergan, Vallergan, hydroxyzine).

Emergency 72-h treatment plan for acute weeping eczema

1. *Dry skin up* with potassium permanganate soaks of a 1 in 10 000 solution. Bathe once or twice daily for 10 min in a 'rose pink' solution. Warn the patient that the solution may stain clothing and nails (temporarily).
2. *Creams* not ointments to be used.
   a. Adult
      - Trunk: Betnovate RD cream b.d.
      - Face: Eumovate cream b.d. (5 days max. then drop to 1% hydrocortisone)
   b. Child (4 yrs)
      - Trunk: Eumovate b.d. or Elocon once daily
      - Face: hydrocortisone 2.5% b.d. (5 days max. then drop to 1% hydrocortisone)
   c. Infant:
      - Trunk: hydrocortisone 2.5% b.d.
      - Face: hydrocortisone 1% b.d.
3. *Antibiotics*: erythromycin q.d.s.
4. *Emollients* only as soap substitutes. Tell the patient to stop placing anything other than the above on the skin to minimize further irritation.

5. *Consider admission* if erythrodermic or in extreme misery.

6. *Remind patient* such therapy is temporary and to book an appointment with their GP to discuss longer term treatment.

Eczema herpeticum

Atopic eczema may become secondarily infected by herpes simplex virus. Clinically a marked systemic upset characterized by fever, headache and tiredness occurs in conjunction with a widespread vesicular eruption. The vesicles turn cloudy and break forming haemorrhagic erosions. The rash is usually localized to the face, neck, upper extremities and back.

Treatment
Systemic treatment with acyclovir should be started immediately. Simple vaseline placed on the skin will keep the lesions moist and hasten healing. The patient remains infectious until all the erosions have dried and may well require admission if unwell.

Seborrhoeic eczema

There are two forms: adult and infantile.

Adult

This eczematous eruption affects the face, in particular the glabella and nasolabial folds, scalp and upper trunk (mainly interscapular and presternal areas). It also affects the intertriginous areas such as the axillae, groins, abdominal skin folds, submammary region, natal cleft and foreskin.

The commonest presentation is mild diffuse scaling of the scalp ('dandruff'). However, thick adherent scales upon a background erythema may occur at this site in more severe disease. On the face, it presents with redness and scaling. On the trunk, the lesions appear similar but may be well-demarcated, discoid or annular. Extensive follicular papules and pustulation can occur (seborrhoeic folliculitis).

In the intertriginous areas, the eczema is moist, red and glazed. It is commonly superinfected with *Candida*.

Infantile

This consists of cradle cap, nappy rash and flexural involvement behind the ears, in the folds of the neck and in the axillae. Occasionally a generalized seborrhoeic rash can occur consisting of confluent ezema emanating from a nappy rash.

Treatment
Topical imidazoles often in combination with hydrocortisone are very effective (Canesten-HC, Daktacort, Nystaform-HC). Cradle cap may be treated with 2% sulphur and 2% salicylic acid in aqueous cream washed out with Polytar shampoo or Capasal.

Pompholyx

A recurrent vesicular or bullous eruption appearing on the palms, sides of the fingers and soles of adults. It is often incapacitating to sufferers as they are unable to use their hands or walk. Secondary infection can occur.

Treatment
Soaking the affected areas in dilute potassium permanganate solution daily for 10–15 min, followed by application of a potent or very potent topical steroid for 7 days improves the condition. Antibiotics may be required.

Varicose eczema

This type of eczema is usually associated with chronic venous stasis of the lower limbs. Complications of treatment are common as patients often become sensitized to local antibiotic preparations or to the preservatives in bandages.

Treatment
Reduction of oedema by elevation and support bandaging should be considered, taking care not to compromise the arterial supply to the limb by injudicious occlusion. Moderately potent topical steroids can be applied to the limb in conjunction with bland applications (e.g. zinc oxide cream, or Ichthopaste bandages).

Discoid eczema

Typified by discrete, coin-shaped, intensely itchy lesion.

Exogenous eczema

This type of eczema is triggered by an external agent. It is further subdivided into allergic contact eczema, where a delayed hypersensitivity reaction is responsible for the cutaneous damage, or non-allergic/irritant eczema where the skin comes into contact with an agent which physically damages the skin by a non-immunologically mediated response.

Allergic contact eczema/dermatitis

Many substances can be responsible for this type of eczema. Some are powerful enough allergens to produce a reaction after a single exposure; others may require years of repeated exposure before the delayed hypersensitivity response is triggered. Once sensitization to an allergen occurs it persists indefinitely and desensitization is seldom possible.

Easily recognizable patterns of contact exist:

- Nickel allergy is the commonest allergy and causes reactions to jewellery (cheap earrings), watch strap buckles, bra fasteners, zips, jean studs and buttons.
- Chromate allergy can occur in building workers who handle cement, as well as from leather products and matches.
- Cosmetic allergy can cause dermatitis of the eyes, lips and cheeks.
- Rubber and elastic allergy may be pertinent in recurrent foot dermatitis, or by fuelling relapses of varicose eczema in a patient who wears support stockings.
- Topical medications may contain neomycin, benzocaine, lanolin or parabens, all of which may be responsible for initiating a contact allergy.
- Adhesive plaster contains colophony which may trigger an eczematous eruption around a wound dressing.

Treatment

Prevention of further exposure is the key element in treatment. Referral to a dermatology department for non-urgent patch testing should be requested. Immediate management is as for an acute eczematous eruption.

Irritant dermatitis

Strong irritants produce an acute eczematous eruption after one or two exposures. This type of eczema is common in industries where acids, detergents, alkalis, solvents and cutting oils are frequently used. The hands, forearms and face are commonly affected. Weaker irritants only induce a response after prolonged or repeated exposure, as in 'housewives' hand dermatitis caused by continual exposure to weak detergents coupled with frequent immersion in water. This leads to dryness of the palms and fissuring, especially at the finger tips.

Treatment

Removal or protection from the harsh environment is achieved either by giving up the offending work (in particular, frequent water immersion) or by wearing protective barriers (e.g. PVC gloves). Copious emollients, in addition to a good hand cream such as Neutrogena should also be prescribed. Active eczematous eruptions should be treated as previously described.

PSORIASIS

This chronic inflammatory disease of the skin affects 2% of the population. It usually presents between the ages of 13 and 40 years but can present at any age above 5 years. It is characterized by well-defined erythematous plaques with adherent silvery scales normally located on extensor surfaces and the scalp. Flexural psoriasis attacks the intertriginous areas. It is prone to exacerbations and remissions. Three specific presentations may require the services of an A&E department.

Erythrodermic psoriasis

This constitutes a dermatological emergency. it follows an irritant trigger such as the effect of tar, dithranol or excessive sun exposure on unstable psoriasis, or drug therapy recently introduced or suddenly withdrawn (e.g. corticosteroids). The skin becomes universally red with no evidence of classical plaques which have been replaced by fine generalized scaling. The skin feels hot and uncomfortable. The patient loses heat rapidly and malaise is accompanied by shivering.

Treatment

The patient should be admitted and a dermatologist contacted. General measures such as bed rest with careful attention to fluid balance and temperature control are essential. Infection if present should be treated. Bland emollients (e.g. zinc and ichthammol cream and emulsifying ointment) should be placed on the skin repeatedly. Dilute topical corticosteroids (Betnovate RD) may be placed on the skin twice a day. The decision to use systemic treatments such as methotrexate should be made by a dermatologist.

Guttate psoriasis

This is usually seen in children or adolescents. It often follows tonsillitis from which a streptococcus can be isolated. The skin is covered in numerous small scaly red macules. The appearance resembles skin that has been 'flicked' with an ink pen. The rash will clear in 6–8 weeks but may herald the onset of plaque psoriais.

Treatment

The skin will respond to weak tar/steroid preparations (e.g. Alphosyl HC). A course of ultraviolet therapy (UVB) will lead to speedier resolution. If a streptococcal sore throat is suspected, appropriate antibiotic therapy should be given.

Pustular psoriasis

This usually affects the palms and soles. These sites become studded with numerous sterile pustules on a background of erythema and scale. There is often a sharp line of demarcation between normal and abnormal skin. The pustules change colour with age from white to brown. Rarely generalized pustulation of the skin can occur with large areas coalescing to form 'lakes' of pus. Successive waves of erythema and pustulation affect the skin, particularly the groins, in association with high fever and severe malaise. Serious metabolic upset and death can occur with this variety of psoriasis.

Treatment

The localized form can be treated with bland emollients to prevent fissuring and a dilute tar/steroid cream (e.g. Alphosyl-HC, Tarcortin) prior to referral back to the general practitioner or to a dermatologist. The generalized form requires immediate admission and assessment of fluid status. Such patients may become profoundly hypo-albuminaemic due to loss of plasma proteins into the tissues. Temperature monitoring with a low-reading thermometer is mandatory, as excessive heat loss occurs. The need for antibiotics should be assessed. Bland emollients can be placed on the skin until a dermatologist has been consulted.

SKIN INFECTIONS

These can be divided into bacterial, viral and fungal.

Bacterial infection

Cellulitis

This infection of the skin and subcutaneous tissues is usually caused by *Streptococcus pyogenes* although rarely a staphylococcus may be responsible. It may affect any part of the body but is commonest on the legs. The affected skin is red, hot and swollen. The erythema is less sharply marginated than in erysipelas. An obvious break in the integument indicating the portal of entry of bacteria may be apparent. Severe episodes can be associated with lymphangitis, lymphadenitis, blistering, necrosis and systemic malaise.

Treatment

Elevation, rest and systemic antibiotics, occasionally needed for up to 6 weeks, are mandatory. Admission for intravenous antibiotics should be considered if the area involved is extensive, the patient's social circumstances are poor or the condition is failing to respond. Regular review should be undertaken.

Erysipelas (St. Anthony's fire)

This is a streptococcal infection which is more superficial than cellulitis and usually involves the face, although it may strike anywhere. The onset is sudden and often heralded by malaise, rigors and a fever. An expanding, red, tender, indurated area with a well-defined margin is characteristic. The patient should be admitted and treated with intravenous penicillin. The condition may recur in the same site. If recurrent, prophylactic penicillin should be considered.

Erysipeloid

This infection, caused by the organism *Erysipelothrix insidiosa*, infects butchers, fishmongers and cooks who accidentally inoculate themselves on the bones of infected animals, birds and fish. It produces a slowly spreading raised reddish-purple area with a well-defined edge. The condition responds rapidly to penicillin.

Erythrasma

This is an infection of the skin, in particular the inter-triginous areas and toe web spaces, caused by *Coryne-bacterium minutissimum*. It causes a macerated white appearance similar to fungal infection as well as slightly scaly pink-brown areas. It responds to topical imidazoles (clotrimazole).

Folliculitis

This is a staphylococcal infection affecting the base of the hair follicle. It presents as tiny pustules on an erythematous base, centred around individual hair follicles. It commonly affects shaved areas and responds to oral flucloxacillin, erythromycin and tetracycline.

Furunculosis (Boils)

A furuncle or boil is an acute pustular infection of a hair follicle with *Staphylococcus aureus*. A tender red nodule enlarges and may later discharge pus before healing with scar formation. Incision and drainage is the correct treatment. Antibiotics will not work.

Carbuncle

This is a deep staphylococcal infection of several adjacent hair follicles. A painful, swollen area of suppuration forms and is associated with marked systemic upset. Deep incision and drainage should be performed if the suppuration is localized. Large axillary abscesses should be drained under general anaesthesia. Diabetes should be excluded.

Paronychia (infection of the nail fold)

This is one of the commonest skin infections to present to the A&E department. Extremely painful collections of pus at the nail fold may extend under the nail. The usual causative organism is *Staphylococcus aureus* and the correct management is drainage. Antibiotics have no place once pus has formed. When draining a paronychia under ring block, always remove enough skin to allow adequate drainage of pus. A linear incision will not suffice – it is better to remove a small ellipse of skin at the point of maximal fluctuance. If there is any suggestion of pus tracking underneath the nail, the overlying portion of the nail should also be removed. The patient should be reviewed in 2–3 days to ensure that the paronychia has resolved.

Impetigo

This is a common bacterial infection with *Staphylococcus aureus*, beta-haemolytic streptococci, or both, affecting any part of the body but particularly the head and neck. Children are at risk. It is highly contagious, spreading rapidly through a family or school class. Autoinoculation is common. Clinically, a thin-walled blister forms leaving a raw, moist area which exudes seropurulent exudate. This exudate dries to form the typical golden crusts.

Management

A swab should be taken to exclude beta-haemolytic streptococcal infection as glomerulonephritis and rheumatic fever may be triggered. Oral penicillin and flucloxacillin should be commenced without delay.

Viral infection

Herpes simplex infection

There are two antigenic types of herpes simplex: HSV-1 and HSV-2. Either can cause a herpes simplex eruption on any part of the body, although the sites of predilection are the lips and the genitalia.

Primary herpes simplex

Most of us are exposed to HSV during childhood. The primary infection may produce a completely subclinical response. However, less commonly, a child who has been exposed may develop an acute gingivostomatitis accompanied by fever, headache, malaise and cervical lymphadenopathy. Painful oral vesicles appear which become ulcerated leading to feeding difficulties. Such children are extremely miserable and fractious. The mucosal surfaces should be cleaned frequently and kept moist with vaseline. Antipyretics should be prescribed. The condition settles within 10 days. If the child is unable to take any liquids at all, admission for parenteral rehydration may be necessary.

A similar picture may be seen in an adult who has had no previous HSV infection. However, the commonest presentation of primary HSV infection in adults is severe vulvovaginitis following exposure to a different form of HSV (usually HSV-2) following sexual contact. Primary infection can also disseminate as in eczema herpeticum and systemic HSV infection (see later).

Recurrent herpes simplex often occurs with or without symptoms (asymptomatic viral shedding can still be infectious). The reasons why some people develop recurrences and some not are as yet unclear, but are in part related to the site of viral infection and the viral type. Following primary infection HSV lies dormant in neural sensory ganglia until it is triggered to migrate along the nerve its cutaneous ending where it produces the typical HSV lesion. Triggers for this process include ultraviolet radiation, fever, menstruation and stress. The typical lesion is of multiple small vesicles clumped together on an erythematous background. These rupture, leaving punched-out erosions which then crust. The eruption resolves within 10–14 days. The whole process may be preceded by an uncomfortable tingling sensation at the affected site in the distribution of the affected nerve (the prodrome). Secondary bacterial infection may cause the vesicles to become pustular prior to crusting.

Treatment

Treatment of the primary attack with oral acyclovir (Zovirax) 200 mg five times a day for 5 days whilst vesicles are forming shortens and reduces the severity of the attack. Commencing treatment after this time has a negligible effect on the length of the attack. Secondary bacterial infection is most likely to be staphylococcal and responds to oral flucloxacillin or erythromycin. Topical acyclovir has been shown to be of no value and oral therapy is to be preferred for recurrences.

Vulvovaginitis and genital herpes (see also Chapter 48)

Any patient presenting to the A&E department with either condition warrants referral to a genitourinary medicine department or similar facility.

Systemic herpes simplex

Very rarely HSV can affect internal organs, specifically the central nervous system, resulting in encephalitis. This may occur at the time of primary infection or during subsequent infections. The immunocompromised are at greatest risk of this potentially fatal complication. If encephalitis is suspected immediate treatment with intravenous acyclovir is indicated.

Eczema herpeticum

See section on eczema.

Herpes zoster infection (shingles)

This is caused by the chicken pox virus (varicella zoster). Individuals who have never had chicken pox can develop it following contact with a patient with shingles. Conversely, shingles cannot be caught from a patient with chicken pox unless both conditions develop simultaneously. Shingles is only seen in people who have had chicken pox. The incidence of shingles is highest in the elderly and the immunocompromised. An attack is due to reactivation of the chicken pox virus which has remained dormant in the dorsal root ganglion since the original infective episode. The virus migrates along the nerve to produce the characteristic dermatomal pattern.

An attack is usually preceded by several days of burning pain or soreness in the affected area, which often leads to confusion over the diagnosis. An erythematous area develops which has multiple clear vesicles (occasionally haemorrhagic) which later turn purulent and cluster together in the distribution of a single dermatome. They do not cross the midline. After 2–4 days the vesicles burst and crust, eventually healing with depressed depigmented scars in 2–3 weeks. The most frequently affected dermatomes are the thoracic or the ophthalmic division of the trigeminal nerve.

Complications

Postherpetic neuralgia is common in the elderly. It is excruciatingly painful and persists for years. Conventional analgesics should be tried first before a trial of carbamazepine. Topical capsaicin cream (Axsain (OTC)) may be beneficial. Referral to a pain clinic may be warranted if the above are unsuccessful.

Corneal ulceration may occur with involvement of the ophthalmic branch of the trigeminal nerve. Patients are at risk of developing conjunctivitis and keratitis. Early ophthalmic assessment must be sought.

Generalized herpes zoster infection, in which the rash may break its dermatomal confines producing prominent necrosis and haemorrhagic lesions, may occur in the immunocompromised. This condition may be fatal. Intravenous acyclovir must be started as early as possible.

Investigations

Where the diagnosis is in doubt blister fluid may be examined under the electron microscope and cultured for the virus.

Treatment

Oral acyclovir (Zovirax) 800 mg 5 times daily for 7 days or Famciclovir (Famvir) 250 mg 3 times daily for 7 days should be given within 48 h of the onset. This may shorten the duration of the eruption. If admitted, patients should be nursed in isolation until crusting occurs as they will be infectious.

Varicella (chicken pox)

See Childhood Exanthems for description. In adults the illness can be much more severe: pneumonitis, secondary infection, purpuric thrombocytopenia, secondary infection and extensive facial scarring may all occur. Treatment should be started once the diagnosis is made.

Treatment

Oral acyclovir (Zovirax) 800 mg 5 times daily for 7 days or Famciclovir (Famvir) 250 mg 3 times daily for 7 days should be given within 48 hours of the onset.

Warts

Warts are a very common viral infection of the skin caused by the human papilloma virus (HPV). There are over 60 HPV subtypes and particular strains cause distinctive clinical entities. They are frequently found on the hands, face and soles of the feet (plantar warts or verrucae). Transmission of the virus occurs by direct contact. The virus is mildly contagious and patients often autoinoculate themselves from hand to foot or from foot to hand. Trauma (e.g. nail-biting) aids successful inoculation of the virus, as does maceration of skin and flat feet. HPV is ubiquitous in the environment, hence there is no reason to prevent children with overt warts from swimming in public baths. Recent evidence confirms the persistence of HPV virus in 'normal' skin from sufferers who have 'cleared' the virus. Successful resolution of HPV depends on the immune response of the individual, especially their cell-mediated immunity. All wart treatments are deliberately irritant in order to precipitate an inflammatory response. If this is marked, upgrading of the host immune response occurs and antibody production against HPV is induced. By 6 months, 30% of warts have cleared spontaneously, 65% by 2 years.

Treatment

Proprietary wart paints should be purchased from the chemist. Preparations containing salicyclic acid (i.e. Salactol, Compound W, Duofilm, Occlusal) should be applied to the wart after firstly softening the skin through bathing and abrasion of the skin with either a pumice stone or emery board. Resolution will only occur after a minimum of 6–12 weeks treatment and only if the patient has persisted religiously with the treatment. The skin surrounding the wart will turn yellow/green and eventually white. Peeling of the area will be prominent. Most patients stop applying paints at this stage as they fear irreparable damage will be caused if they continue to treat. This is precisely the stage to continue treatment. Provoking a healthy reaction will ensure a strong inflammatory response and encourage antibody formation. It is not a chance observation that many patients 'lose' their warts once the lesion becomes painful. Cryotherapy using liquid nitrogen is the next level of treatment. The patient will need to be referred to the dermatology department for this. It would be prudent to warn them that they are unlikely to receive a priority appointment and that the warts may resolve spontaneously in the intervening period.

Molluscum contagiosum

This is a papular epidermal eruption caused by the pox virus. It is commonest in children and the immunocompromised. Atopics are particularly susceptible. The individual lesions are small, shiny, pink or white papules with a central umbilication. Grouped lesions are common, usually on the head, neck or trunk. Autoinoculation is common and it can be spread by direct contact to others (e.g. sexually). Spontaneous resolution eventually occurs, although this process can be hastened by pricking the centre of each lesion with a cocktail stick dipped in phenol or iodine. It is usually a non-scarring condition hence care should be taken not to use a treatment that may cause scarring (e.g. curettage). Untreated lesions clear within 6–9 months, but can occasionally persist for several years.

Orf

This is a pox virus infection of sheep during the lambing season which can spread to humans via direct contact with an infected animal or its carcass. Butchers, farmers and abattoir workers are all at risk. After an incubation period lasting 5–7 days, a solitary red papular lesion on the fingers or hands rapidly becomes haemorrhagic and pustular. It resolves spontaneously 2 months later and does not require any specific treatment. A rare complication is erythema multiforme which can progress to Stevens–Johnson syndrome.

Hand, foot and mouth disease

This condition, due to coxsackie A16 virus infection, is still relatively common in children. It consists of small grey vesicles surrounded by an erythematous rim on the hands and feet in association with buccal apthous ulceration. The condition resolves spontaneously within 2 weeks without treatment.

Erythema infectiosum (fifth disease)

This seasonal spring eruption is caused by parvovirus infection. A 'slapped' cheek erythema in conjunction with a reticulate erythema of the shoulders and upper

Table 3. *Fungal infections of the skin*

Type of fungus	Example of superficial infection	Deep infection
Dermatophytes	Tinea (ringworm) e.g. Tinea capitis Tinea pedis, etc.	Mycetoma (madura foot)
Yeast-like	*Candida* e.g. Intertrigo Balanitis Vulvovaginitis	Paronychia
	Pityrosporum e.g. Pityriasis versicolor	

arms is characteristic. Little systemic malaise is present and the condition spontaneously resolves in 5–7 days with no treatment.

Fungal infections

There are two types of fungus which cause disease in humans: the dermatophytes, of which there are three main genera (*Trichophyton, Microsporum* and *Epidermophyton*), and the yeast-like fungi of which by far the most common is *Candida albicans*. Both types of fungi can cause superficial infections of the skin and mucosal membranes, or deeper infections which may be localized (abscesses or mycetoma) or systemic (see Table 3).

Tinea (ringworm)

Tinea is a superficial infection of the skin by hyphal organisms which invade the stratum corneum of the epidermis and specialized keratinized tissues such as hair or nail. The word 'tinea' is used as a prefix for the body part involved (usually expressed in Latin): e.g. tinea capitis (head), tinea pedis (foot), tinea corporis (body), tinea cruris (groin), and tinea manus (hand).

Some of the dermatophyte fungi involved are pathogenic only to humans (anthrophilic) whilst others can affect both humans and animals (zoophilic). In general, zoophilic fungi cause a more severe inflammation than anthrophilic ones. Contagious ringworm is acquired either through direct contact with an infected animal (e.g. cat or dog) or indirectly following contact with infected keratin debris (e.g. in swimming baths, communal showers), although it is not as virulent as is generally believed.

Tinea capitis

Tinea capitis infection can be caused by either anthrophilic or zoophilic species of dermatophyte. The latter produces a greater inflammatory response than the anthrophilic species. In the UK and Europe, *Microsporum canis* is the commonest pathogen. Transmission occurs following a short contact with an infected person, usually a child. Clinically there is background erythema with patches of scalp hair loss and scaling. Hair tends to break off 1–3 mm above the scalp. A more severe inflammatory response to the dermatophyte leads to the formation of a boggy pustular lesion – kerion. It is important to recognize this before drainage under general anaesthesia is arranged. All boggy masses on the scalps of young children should have a fungal aetiology excluded before surgical intervention is considered. Appropriate antifungal treatment will completely rectify the lesion and hair loss is seldom a permanent problem.

Tinea pedis (athletes' foot)

This is the commonest dermatophyte infection and is most often caused by *Trichophyton rubrum* and *Trichophyton interdigitale*. It is acquired following contact with infected keratin debris on swimming bath or shower room floors. Occlusive footwear encourages relapses. Peeling and maceration between the web spaces of the fourth and fifth toes occurs. Itching and scale formation may progress to the undersurface of the toes. A diffuse dry scaling of the soles occurs with *Trichophyton rubrum*. In persistent infection painful fissuring may occur.

Tinea cruris

This is common and affects men more than women. It starts as an itchy, erythematous bilateral maceration in the crural folds. This may spread down the thighs or extend onto the perineum, in an annular pattern. The edge is raised, red and scaly. It is almost always associated with tinea pedis and is spread from there by hand and towel. Flexural psoriasis may mimic the scaling erythema in the groins and it is important to check for psoriatic lesions elsewhere.

Tinea corporis

The lesions may be multiple and are typically annular, having started as a small, red, often irregular, papule. The edge has a red scaly appearance. The lesions expand slowly leaving a central clearing which helps distinguish them from discoid eczema and the herald patch of pityriasis rosea, both of which are universally red.

Tinea unguium

Fingernail and toenail infection – onychomycosis – is usually associated with tinea pedis. The condition is initially unilateral and affects one or two nails. It can eventually affect all the nails. The dermatophyte usually invades the nail from its distal or lateral margins producing a yellow, crumbly appearance. The nail plate separates from the nail bed – onycholysis – and thickening (subungual hyperkeratosis) then ensues.

Diagnosis of fungal infections

Skin scrapings from the advancing edge of the infection, nail clippings or plucked hair samples should be sent for fungal microscopy and culture. Specimens should be sent in folded black paper.

Treatment

If the infection is not widespread and does not involve hair or nails, topical therapy such as miconazole (Daktarin), clotrimazole (Canesten) or terbinafine (Lamisil) is generally used. These agents should be applied twice a day for 2 weeks.

If the infected area is large, or tinea of the scalp or nails is involved, systemic oral preparations are required.

In adults
- Tinea cruris, corporis, pedis
  Terbinafine (Lamisil) 250 mg daily for 2 weeks
  Itraconazole (Sporanox) 100 mg daily for 2 weeks
  (T. cruris or corporis) or 4 weeks (T. pedis)
- Nail infection
  Terbinafine 250 mg daily for 12 weeks

In children
- Scalp ringworm
  Terbinafine 10 mg kg^{-1} daily for 6 weeks

Candidal infections

Candida albicans is a normal human commensal yeast found in the mouth, gastrointestinal tract and vaginal mucosa. It is less commonly isolated from the skin. Numerous factors predispose an individual to candidal infections: infancy/old age, pregnancy, obesity, high humidity, diabetes, antibiotic therapy, immunosuppres-

sion, iron and zinc deficiency, and chronic immersion in water are all important. The diagnosis can be made on swab culture from an affected area.

Oral candidiasis

This is a common infection of the elderly, denture wearers, infants and the immunosuppressed. Small, white, adherent plaques are seen on the tongue, buccal mucosa, palate and gums. These can be wiped off with a tongue depressor leaving an erythematous base. Sore red areas can be produced under dentures. Oral infection that is refractory to treatment and involvement of the oesophagus and upper respiratory tract should alert one to the possibility of underlying immunosuppression.

Treatment

Treatment is with oral nystatin suspension in infants or amphotericin lozenges (Fungilin) in adults.

Angular cheilitis

Sore red fissuring at the angles of the mouth can accompany signs of oral candidosis. If *Candida* infection is demonstrated it should be treated with topical nystatin or clotrimazole cream. Advice regarding oral hygiene and alteration of dentures may be appropriate in elderly patients. A full blood count and random blood glucose should be checked to exclude iron-deficiency anaemia and diabetes mellitus.

Candidal balanitis and vulvovaginitis

These topics are discussed in Chapter 48.

Candidal intertrigo

This term describes the moist glazed area of erythema and maceration between opposing body folds with occasional satellite papulopustules. These satellite lesions can help distinguish candidal infection from other conditions affecting intertriginous areas. Superinfection is promoted at such sites as the groins, axillae and submammary regions, as well as abdominal folds in the obese. The interdigital folds in hands that are often immersed in water can similarly be affected.

Treatment

This combines cleanliness with thorough drying. Magenta paint can be applied to soggy skin flexures, although this is messy. Antifungal creams with mild topical corticosteroids are often very useful: Daktacort (miconazole with hydrocortisone), Canesten HC (clotrimazole with hydrocortisone) and Nystaform-HC (nystatin and hydrocortisone) are all effective. Topical terbinafine (Lamisil) is a newer effective antifungal.

Chronic paronychia

This occurs in patients who frequently immerse their hands in water, and in patients with severe chilblains. The proximal, and occasionally the lateral nail fold, becomes red and bolstered. The cuticles disappear and pus may appear from the tense swollen nail fold. Eventually the nail plate becomes ridged and discoloured.

Treatment
This involves minimizing exposure of the digits to water and applying topical antifungal therapies. Imidazole as a cream accurately applied to the affected area under clingfilm at night, or a solution applied several times a day for 3 months, may be effective. The only effective treatment for nail plate involvement is oral azoles (e.g. ketoconazole or itraconazole). It should be noted that griseofulvin has no place in the treatment of *Candida* infections.

Pityriasis versicolor

This common condition is caused by overgrowth with the commensal yeast *Pityrosporum orbiculare*. The disease occurs in healthy young adults and is common in the tropics. The pigmentary changes which characterize the infection are thought to follow the inhibition of melanin formation by azaleic acid, produced by yeast enzyme activity.

The rash consists of multiple, superficial, scaly light-brown macules which become hypopigmented after exposure to sunlight. The lesions may coalesce to form patches of varying shapes commonly on the upper trunk, arms and neck. The condition is non-infectious. Affected individuals are asymptomatic and usually present following a beach holiday with a 'ruined' tan.

Treatment
The condition can be treated with shampoo: selenium sulphide (Selsun) lathered onto patches and left to dry for 24 h before being washed off or ketoconazole (Nizoral) once daily for 3 days. Topical antifungal creams (e.g. miconazole) can be applied twice daily for 2 weeks. Oral

antifungal treatments (ketoconazole 400 mg once or 200 mg for 5 days, or itraconazole 200 mg for 7 days) are also effective.

Patients should be told that the skin discolouration takes 3–6 months to fade completely and that its persistence does not indicate the need for further treatment. Relapse is common in patients who live in the tropics.

COLLAGEN VASCULAR DISORDERS

Many of these conditions have cutaneous manifestations. Most sufferers will have chronic problems and will not trouble the A&E department, but occasionally new, unfamiliar cutaneous manifestations will develop prompting an emergency attendance. A brief summary of the dermatological manifestations is given in Table 4 – most can safely be referred to the next rheumatology or dermatology clinic.

Table 4. *Dermatological manifestations of collagen vascular disorders*

Collagen vascular disorder	Dermatological manifestation
Systemic lupus erythematosus	Oropharyngeal ulceration Diffuse scarring alopecia Raynaud's phenomenon Photosensitivity 'Butterfly' malar rash Vasculitis
Discoid lupus erythematosus	Scaling, erythematous plaques, with prominent plugging of follicles in light exposed sites
Dermatomyositis	Facial erythema (heliotrope-pale violet) Periorbital oedema Erythema of dorsa of hands, elbows, knees Erythematous plaques overlying knuckles
Childhood dermatomyositis	Vasculitis with ulceration in axillae and groin
Scleroderma Morphoea	Thickened pale, single, round or oval plaques with smooth shiny surface
Systemic sclerosis	Periorbital furrowing Beaked nose Small mouth with radial furrowing Diffuse hyperpigmentation Raynaud's phenomenon Sclerodactyly Finger pulp infarct, leading to ulcers Calcinosis Telangiectasia

SYSTEMIC DISEASE AND THE SKIN

Many systemic disorders are associated with cutaneous manifestations; some are listed in Table 5. A good history from the patient is the clue to establishing the diagnosis.

Table 5. *Cutaneous manifestations of systemic disorders*

Systemic disorders	Cutaneous manifestation
Diabetes	Neuropathic/ischaemic ulcers
	Necrobiosis lipoidica (see ulcers)
	Xanthomas
	Bullae
	Effects of insulin injection
Hypothyroidism	Dry skin
	'Strawberries and cream' facies
	Coarse hair
	Erythema ab igne
	Pruritus
Hyperthyroidism	Pretibial myxoedema
	Palmar erythema
	Vitiligo
	Pruritus
HIV	Oral candidiasis
	Dry skin
	Itchy folliculitis
	Seborrhoeic dermatitis
	Gingivitis
	Herpes zoster, molluscum contagiosum
	Herpes simplex – severe and atypical forms
	Tinea
	Kaposi's sarcoma
	Oral hairy leucoplakia – ribbed white areas along sides of tongue
Rheumatological	
Gout	Gouty tophi
Rheumatoid arthritis	Rheumatoid nodules
	Vasculitis
	Pyoderma gangrenosum (see Vascular Disorders)
	Palmar erythema
Reiters	Psoriasiform eruption
	Keratoderma blennorrhagica – thickened skin on soles of feet
Vitamin deficiency	
Scurvy	Perifollicular purpura and bruising
	Bleeding gums
Pellagra	Photosensitive dermatitis
Inflammatory bowel disease	Pyoderma gangrenosum
	Erythema nodosum
	Perianal/oral ulcers (Crohn's only)
Hyperlipidaemia	Xanthomas
	– Xanthelasma – on eyelids
	– Tuberous – on knees and elbows
	– Tendinous – on dorsa of hands
	– Eruptive – in crops of small yellow papules
Sarcoidosis	Erythema nodosum
	Papules, nodules, plaques
	Lupus pernio – swollen, purple infiltration of nose and ears
Liver disease	Palmar erythema
	Pruritus
	Spider naevi
	White nails
	Jaundice (bronzed in haemochromatosis)
Malignancy	Dermatomyositis
	Pruritus
	Thrombophlebitis migrans
	Bullous pemphigoid
	Paraneoplastic pemphigus
	Dermatitis herpetiformis
	Erythema multiforme
	Acanthosis nigricans – hyperpigmented thickened skin in axillae and groin

VASCULAR DISORDERS

Vasculitis

Inflammation of the vessel wall brought about by the attachment of circulating immune complexes leading to endothelial cell swelling and fibrinoid change characterizes a vasculitis. The spectrum of physical manifestations (Table 6) which may be caused depends on the size of the blood vessel affected by such a process.

Allergic vasculitis (small vessel)

This may be secondary to antigenic stimuli from bacterial (streptococcal) infections, viral infections, drugs (see section on drug reactions), neoplasia and collagen vascular disorders (e.g. Sjögren's disease, systemic lupus erythematosus and rheumatoid arthritis). The cutaneous lesions are usually purpuric and predominate on the buttocks and lower limbs. The lesions crop, are palpable,

Table 6. *Clinical conditions that might cause vasculitis*

Physical manifestation of vasculitis	Probable cause
Purpuric papules	Allergic vasculitis Henoch–Schönlein purpura
Urticaria	Allergic vasculitis Henoch–Schönlein purpura
Livedo reticularis	Polyarteritis
Nodules	Polyarteritis
Ulcers	Allergic vasculitis Henoch–Schönlein purpura Pyoderma gangrenosum
Haemorrhagic bullae	Pyoderma gangrenosum
Erythema nodosum	Behçet's disease

livid, and can become bullous or frankly necrotic. The lesions may not be limited to the skin as in a systemic allergic vasculitis. This condition may be termed Henoch–Schönlein purpura. Children are more frequently at risk of developing this more widespread vasculitis which causes arthralgia, gastrointestinal bleeding and proliferative glomerulonephritis. The degree of morbidity depends on the severity of the renal involvement.

Treatment
The causal agent must be identified and eliminated. Bed rest is mandatory. Oral non-steroidal anti-inflammatory agents, systemic steroids or even immunosuppressive therapy (for severe renal involvement) are used.

Polyarteritis nodosa (*medium vessel*)

This necrotizing vasculitis affects men more commonly than women. Immune complexes and hepatitis B antigen can precipitate it. The systemic manifestations tend to dominate the clinical picture. The cutaneous manifestations are tender subcutaneous nodules along the line of arteries. The overlying skin may display 'starburst' purpura and often necrosis. Livedo reticularis is prominent. A purely cutaneous form of the condition may exist.

Treatment
Systemic steroids and immunosuppressive drugs are needed, hence patients presenting acutely usually require admission. The purely cutaneous form of polyarteritis nodosa can be controlled with low-dose systemic steroids.

Erythema nodosum

See section on reactive erythema.

Behçet's disease

This condition consists of the clinical triad of recurrent oral ulceration, genital ulceration and uveitis. The disease process may involve the skin in the form of erythema nodosum or pustular lesions. Other systemic manifestations include meningitis, cerebellar disease, cranial nerve palsies, colitis and cardiovascular aneurysms. Eastern Mediterranean races are predisposed to the condition, particularly in early adulthood.

Pyoderma gangrenosum

This is a destructive, non-infective ulceration of the skin which presents as an inflamed nodule or pustule. The nodule breaks down centrally and an ulcer with a characteristic bluish border and undermined edge rapidly enlarges. The pathogenesis is not known but it is included in the spectrum of vasculitides. It is associated with inflammatory bowel disease, rheumatoid arthritis, monoclonal gammopathies and leukaemia. The condition responds to high-dose systemic steroids. It heals with marked scarring.

Purpura

This is a physical sign rather than a disease entity. It is caused by extravasation of red blood cells into the skin. The lesions which are produced by this process are purple, of varying size (small = petechiae, large = ecchymosis) and do not blanch with pressure. The causes broadly fall into three groups:

1. Blood disorders
   a. Thrombocytopenia
      – Idiopathic
      – Secondary to bone marrow infiltration
      – Drugs
   b. Coagulopathies
      – Haemophilia
   The above tend to produce flat ecchymoses.

2. Blood vessel disorders
   a. Congenital
      – Ehlers–Danlos
   b. Increased vascular wall permeability
      – Scurvy
   c. Fragility of vessel wall
      – Senile purpura
      – Steroid therapy
   d. Damage to the vessel wall
      – Vasculitis or emboli
   The above tend to produce palpable purpura.
3. Local causes
   a. Raised venous pressure in association with varicose eczema
   b. Stasis purpura – seen in dependent sites in association with toxic erythema

MISCELLANEOUS SKIN DISORDERS

Pityriasis rosea

The cause of this common skin disorder is unknown. It is thought to be an infective agent, possibly of viral origin.

There is a typical sequence of events starting with the appearance of a 'herald patch'. This is an oval, pink, scaly macule, usually appearing on the trunk and measuring 2–5 cm. It is often mistaken for tinea corporis; however, no central sparing is apparent. It may exist in isolation for 1–2 weeks before other smaller plaques appear. The hallmark of the rash is the presence of a fine collarette of scale within the macule which lifts away with gentle scraping away from, rather than towards, the centre of the lesion. On the back the rash follows the longitudinal lines of the ribs, giving a 'christmas tree' pattern. The rash is usually asymptomatic, although mild itching may be present.

Treatment
As the condition is self-limiting none is required. The patient should be advised that the rash will clear spontaneously within 2–3 weeks. Itching may be soothed with a moderately potent topical steroid (Eumovate). If the diagnosis is in doubt referral to a dermatologist is advisable as secondary syphilis may mimic this condition.

Lichen planus

This is a fairly common dermatological disorder of unknown aetiology. Typical lesions are violaceous or purple, itchy flat-topped papules with fine lace-like patterning on their surface (Wickham's striae). It particularly affects the volar aspects of the wrist and forearm, the ankles and shins. It may, however, occur at any site on the body, particularly the mucous membranes in 50% of patients, where it is typified by white lace-like patterning on the buccal mucosa. Atypically, it can be responsible for annular lesions on the penis, thick plaque-like lesions on the shins and ulcers in the mouth or on the genitals. Certain drugs (e.g. gold, antimalarials and thiazide diuretics) may cause a similar 'lichenoid' eruption.

Treatment
Potent topical steroids are required to relieve symptoms and flatten papules. If painful oral or genital involvement is present then systemic steroids should be used. However, in most cases the condition resolves spontaneously within 18 months.

DERMATOLOGICAL TUMOURS

Benign tumours

Most 'lumps and bumps' are longstanding and do not usually present to A&E. If, however, one is faced with such a problem it is essential to rule out the possibility of malignancy or an instantly rectifiable condition (pyogenic granuloma, abscess). Once this has been done patients can be referred back to their general practitioner for appropriate management.

Pyogenic granuloma

These vascular red nodules often present to A&E departments because of their sudden appearance and their bleeding tendency. They are common benign acquired haemangiomata, often seen in children, which develop at the site of minor trauma.

Treatment
The lesion should be removed by curettage or excision. Histological examination is mandatory to exclude an amelanotic melanoma.

Premalignant skin lesions

These include keratoacanthoma, Bowen's disease (intraepidermal carcinoma) and actinic keratoses.

Keratoacanthoma

This is a rapidly growing tumour which may rarely transform into a squamous cell carcinoma. It appears in sun-exposed sites, usually the face. It starts as a small papule which rapidly enlarges to a 1 cm nodule over a 4–6-week period. The main diagnostic feature is the central keratin core of the lesion. The lesion should be curetted or excised and sent for histological examination.

Bowen's disease (intraepidermal carcinoma)

This is a single, slowly enlarging red scaly plaque with a well-defined border. It is often mistaken for a plaque of psoriasis. Transformation to a squamous cell carcinoma can occur. Referral to a dermatology department for cryotherapy should be requested.

Actinic keratoses

These rough 'sandpaper-like' lesions are commonly found on sun-damaged skin, particularly on the foreheads of bald men and on the dorsa of hands. They can transform into squamous cell carcinoma and are easily treated with cryotherapy or topical 5-fluorouracil cream. They should therefore be referred back to the general practitioner for referral to the dermatology department.

Malignant tumours

Basal cell carcinoma

This is the most common form of skin cancer. It is induced by chronic sun exposure. The incidence is rising, especially in younger age groups, and although they do not metastasize they are a major source of morbidity due to local invasion and tissue destruction. Grossly neglected lesions may invade underlying cartilage and bone.

There are four types: nodular, cystic, morphoeic and superficial. All present as slowly enlarging, glistening, yellow or white lesions which often appear translucent with fine telangiectasia coursing across the surface. The morphoiec type can resemble a scar.

Treatment
Any suspicious lesion should be referred to a dermatology department for biopsy and appropriate treatment planning. Lesions situated on important anatomical areas (e.g. medial and lateral canthi, nose and ears) are especially important to pick up as they can cause extensive tissue destruction with profound cosmetic disability if neglected.

Squamous cell carcinoma

These tumours arise in sun-damaged skin as a result of the oncogenic effects of ultraviolet radiation. They are also commoner in patients who are chronically immuno-suppressed (e.g. following renal transplantation). They arise *de novo* as small keratotic nodules or rapidly growing ulcers. Sites of predilictions are lips, ears, mouth and scalp. Pre-existing lesions such as actinic keratoses, keratoacanthomas or irradiated skin can also undergo malignant transformation. They should be treated urgently in view of their potential to metastasize.

Treatment
Referral to a dermatology department for biopsy and management.

Malignant melanoma

This is an invasive tumour of melanocytes. Its incidence is doubling every 10 years. White, fair-skinned, freckled individuals who burn easily and are of Celtic origin are most at risk of developing a melanoma. In addition, patients with a family history of melanoma and those who have multiple episodic sunburn at an early age are also predisposed to its development. Up to 30% of melanomas arise from pre-existing naevi and patients with atypical moles, incidentally discovered in the course of an examination in the A&E department, should be referred for a dermatology opinion.

There are four types of melanoma:

- Superficial spreading meloma.
- Lentigo maligna melanoma.
- Nodular melanoma.
- Acral melanoma.

Superficial spreading melanoma

This is the most common type. It grows superficially and radially before invading the dermis; hence its early identification. Simple excision with a 0.5 cm margin can prove curative. It is commonly found on backs in men and legs in women. Clinically the lesion is an irregular multicoloured mixture ranging from pink through brown, tan and blue-black. The margins are irregular and show notching or scalloping. A nodule within the lesion signifies dermal invasion with correspondingly poor prognosis.

Lentigo maligna melanoma

This type occurs on the sun-damaged skin of the elderly. An irregularly pigmented macule present for many years develops an invasive nodule within it.

Nodular melanoma

From the start a dark nodule appears without a preceding in situ phase. It is the most aggressive type associated with a poor prognosis. It is commoner in men and usually seen in the middle-aged. It is commoner on the head, neck and trunk. Ulceration and bleeding frequently occur.

An amelanotic melanoma may present as a pyogenic granuloma-like lesion. Any recently noted 'vascular' lesion occurring in a middle-aged person should be viewed with suspicion and referral to a dermatologist urgently requested.

Acral melanoma

This type occurs more frequently in the Japanese and Chinese. It is found mainly on the palmar surfaces and the soles, as well as near to or under the nails. A melanoma involving the nail may be signalled by pigmentation of the proximal nail fold – Hutchinson's sign. A linear streak may also be produced by a melanoma affecting the nail apparatus, although these may commonly be racial in aetiology.

Treatment

Urgent dermatological referral must be sought if a malignant melanoma is suspected and the patient must be strongly counselled to keep the clinic appointment. Many patients find it hard to accept that a small black spot may harbour a lethal condition and they often default. If any surgical biopsy is performed it must be EXCISIONAL, with an initial clearance of at least 0.5 cm. The specimen must be submitted for pathological interpretation. Great care should be taken to ensure that the specimen is not lost. If the lesion is a melanoma then the histopathological depth of invasion, measured from the granular cell layer of the epidermis to the deepest tumour cell (Breslow thickness), provides the only accurate prognostic indicator for the patient. To lose the specimen is, therefore, a disaster.

Differential diagnosis of malignant melanoma

Subungual or periungual haematomas may be confused with a malignant melanoma. A preceding history of trauma will often establish the diagnosis. Talon noir is a pigmented area of petechial haemorrhage within the dermal papillae occurring on the sole or heel of the foot in athletic individuals. Gentle paring of the lesion will dislodge the black dots which come away with the superficial skin squames. Pigmented seborrhoeic 'warts' may resemble melanoma. Their 'stuck on' appearance, similar to squashed chewing gum on the sole of a shoe, often aids the diagnosis. Pigmented basal cell carcinomas can be confused with malignant melanoma.

Suspected malignant change in a pigmented lesion

All medical staff in the A&E department should routinely 'eyeball' patients for malignant melanoma during the course of a clinical examination. This small contribution may help to reduce the inexorable increase in the mortality from this malignancy. If any doubt regarding a pigmented lesion exists do not be afraid to refer to a dermatologist.

A heightened suspicion for melanoma should be provoked if the patient is:

- fair, burns easily and has had numerous episodes of sunburn, with or without blistering, in early childhood
- Has a family history of melanoma
- Has more than 100 moles, many of which are irregularly pigmented and shaped

---

Any change in a pre-existing pigmented lesion must be viewed with suspicion. If more than two of the following criteria, apply to a pigmented lesion, refer to a dermatologist:

A   Asymmetry – benign moles are usually symmetrical, a melanoma is not

B   Border – irregular borders with one area advancing more than the rest of the lesion

C   Colour – benign moles have even colour distribution, usually browns and tans; mixtures of colours and the presence of blue or black are suspicious

D   Diameter larger than 0.5 cm

REMEMBER: Reinforce the use of SPF (sun protection factor) 15 or greater sunscreens, in conjunction with sun avoidance between 11:00 and 15:00 hours, to all patients who present with sunburn or pigmented lesions in the A&E department

CHILDHOOD EXANTHEMS AND TOXIC ERYTHEMA

Childhood exanthems

These conditions, although seen in adulthood in altered forms, are far commoner in children. An adult presenting with any of these conditions will usually give a good history of contact with an affected patient. Vaccination has dramatically reduced the incidence of these illnesses.

Measles

This is primarily a spring eruption. It is infectious for up to 5 days prior to the appearance of the rash until 5 days after the rash has disappeared. After an incubation period of 10 days the exanthem is preceded by a 3–5-day prodrome characterized by a hacking cough, coryza and photophobia. The child is miserable and fractious at this stage. Koplik's spots (white centre with red areolae – 'grains of sand') appear on the soft palate and are pathognomic of the condition. The spots last 12–24 h and occur 2 days prior to the rash appearing. Once the rash manifests itself, an abrupt increase in the child's temperature and concomitant reduction in the severity of symptoms occurs. The eruption is a dark red maculopapular rash which starts behind the ears, spreads to the face and progresses downwards. Upon reaching the feet it gradually fades from the head downwards, taking 7–10 days to disappear. Desquamation may occur, signalling complete resolution.

Rubella (German measles)

This condition is infectious for 7 days before until 7 days after the appearance of the rash. The incubation period is between 14 and 24 days. Children are often asymptomatic although there may be a slight prodrome for 2 days preceding the rash. The eruption starts on the face and spreads rapidly to the trunk. Clinically it consists of discrete maculopapules in large numbers which may become confluent on the face. By the time it is present on the trunk it is absent on the head and neck. It has usually disappeared on day 3. It may be mildly pruritic. Posterior cervical, retroauricular and posterior occipital tender lymphadenopathy can be striking. No treatment is required, but advice *must* be given to accompanying adults regarding exposure to any pregnant women.

Varicella (chicken pox)

An intensely pruritic exanthem which usually occurs in childhood and is caused by the herpes zoster virus. The incubation period is about 14 days. It is infectious for 24 h prior to the appearance of the rash until all the lesions have crusted over – approximately 7 days. Following the prodrome, crops of small red papules appear turning rapidly into clear vesicles on an erythematous base whose contents soon become pustular. Over the next few days the lesions become scabbed, a process that is aided by frantic scratching. New crops of vesicles continue to appear, mainly concentrated on the trunk, face and scalp. Mucous membranes including genitalia and conjunctiva are often involved. The illness can be much more severe in the adult; pneumonitis, secondary infection, purpuric thrombocytopenia, secondary infection and scarring may all occur.

Treatment
This is symptomatic and directed at relieving itching. Oily emollients or oily calamine lotion (rather than plain which is too drying) may be useful. Sedative antihistamines (Phenergan, Vallergan or hydroxyzine) may be helpful.

Scarlet fever (scarlatina)

This is an acute bacterial infection caused by strains of *Streptococcus pyogenes* producing exotoxin. The incubation period is usually 2–5 days. A brief prodrome of 12–48 h is characterized by fever, vomiting, headache and pharyngitis. The tonsils are oedematous and may be covered by exudate. Painful lymphadenopathy is often present. The tongue is heavily coated and its swollen red papillae give the classical 'strawberry' appearance.

The rash appears on the second day and is red and punctate. It first appears on the upper trunk before spreading during the next 24 h. The face is flushed with noticeable perioral pallor. After 7–10 days the rash desquamates, beginning on the face, then the trunk and finally the hands and feet – a process lasting up to 6 weeks. If the streptococcal source of infection is not the pharynx, marked pharyngeal upset may not be evident. Scarlet fever may follow surgical procedures, skin infections or burns.

Treatment
The patient requires admission and intravenous penicillin. The possibility of myocardial or renal damage must always be remembered.

Toxic erythema

In this condition the general impression is of redness. The body is covered by a widespread erythematous, maculopapular rash. The usual cause is infection (viral or bacterial) or a drug, but in many instances the underlying trigger is never positively identified. In such cases the rash may legitimately be termed simply 'toxic erythema'.

Many drugs may be implicated in this type of cutaneous response (e.g. antibiotics such as ampicillin, and sulphonamides, diuretics and oral hypoglycaemics). The commonest bacterial cause is streptococcal infection, but any virus may produce this rash. Occasionally the pattern of the eruption may aid in identifying the virus responsible, as in the 'slapped cheeks' appearance of parvovirus B19 infection – erythema infectiosum or fifth disease.

There are two main types of toxic erythema:

- *Morbilliform.* Red macules starting behind the ears, spreading to the face, trunk and limbs. This is the sort of picture seen in measles and other viral infections. It may also follow drug ingestion when the coryzal features will be absent.
- *Scarlatiniform.* Widespread erythema on the trunk or localized to the palms and soles associated with a burning sensation in the skin. There can be intense engorgement of pharyngeal lymphoid tissue. Desquamation often follows spontaneous resolution. This is often seen in bacterial infection and after drug ingestion.

Management
Routine management for all toxic erythemas should include:

- Throat swabs – bacterial and viral.
- Blood sample for rubella titres if any pregnant women are at risk.

INFESTATIONS

Scabies

This is a common infestation caused by the mite *Sarcoptes scabiei* (Greek = 'flesh cutter'). The female mite burrows into the stratum corneum where she remains for the duration of her life (30 days) and lays her eggs. After 4 days the larvae hatch and moult three times before a fully developed adult mite is formed. Following mating amongst this generation of mites the gravid females burrow into the stratum corneum and lay their eggs, completing the life cycle.

Each time a female mite eats her way into the stratum corneum a 'burrow' is formed. These visible burrows are 0.5–1 cm long, grey-white in colour and often the mite is visible, with the aid of a lens, as a small dark dot at the end of the most recent burrow. Burrows are found on the sides of fingers, in the finger web spaces and on the flexural aspects of the wrists and the extensor surfaces of the elbows. Any site that is frequently handled during intimate contact is prone to infection. In women, lesions are found on the nipples and in men oedematous nodules may be found on the penis and scrotum. In infancy, the soles of the feet and face are affected. In the non-immuno-compromised adult the face is rarely affected.

Transmission
Prolonged contact is required for scabies to spread. Therefore holding hands and sexual contact are the commonest modes of transmission. Clothing and bedding are of NO importance in scabies transmission.

Clinical course
Itching begins slowly and is usually only apparent after 6–8 weeks. The itch is worse when the body is warm and intolerable nocturnal itch is a cardinal symptom. The rash is mainly secondary to traumatic excoriation and does not correspond to the site of the mites.

Complications
Secondary bacterial infection is common. Overzealous use of topical scabetics can induce an irritant dermatitis complicating recovery.

Treatment for scabies

1. Apply thin layer of scabicide to all areas below jaw line
2. Allow to dry. No bath or shower permitted until end of treatment
3. Leave for 24 h
4. If the hands are washed during the treatment period the scabicide should be reapplied
5. Wash off thoroughly. Change into clean clothes and bed linen. It is not necessary to fumigate house or clothing
6. All family members and sexual contacts should be treated simultaneously whether itching or not
7. Residual itching may last up to several weeks. No further scabicide is needed. Crotamiton and 0.25% hydrocortisone cream (Eurax-Hydrocortisone cream) or emollients (e.g. aqueous cream) will suffice

Diagnosis

Direct demonstration of the mite by scraping a burrow and examining the contents under the microscope.

Treatment

This is simple and effective providing the patient is given clear instructions. The two most popular treatments are gamma-benzene hexachloride (Quellada, lindane) or malathion (Derbac-M).

Pediculosis (lice infestation)

Three areas of the body are affected by these blood-sucking wingless insects.

Pediculosis capitis (*head lice*)

The female adult louse lays and cements her eggs (nits) to the base of the hair shafts where they are visible as small white or flesh-coloured specks. They resemble flakes of dandruff, but they cannot be dislodged. The main symptom is itching over the sides and back of the scalp. Secondary bacterial infection leads to matted, malodorous hair and local lymphadenopathy. Spread is by head-to-head contact and sharing of combs.

Treatment

Malathion 0.5% solution is applied to the scalp after washing the hair and is left on for 12 h, then it is washed out. Combing helps to remove the nits and unmatt the hair. One week later the entire process is repeated. All family and schoolmates should be treated.

Pediculosis corporis (*body lice*)

Nowadays this condition is confined to the unhygienic and homeless. Transmission is via infested clothing and bedding as the louse lays its eggs in the seams of the material. The human inhabitant of the clothes is required purely as a source of food. The red macular lesions which result from these bites are extremely itchy and may be associated with excoriation marks and secondary bacterial infection.

Treatment

Treatment consists of washing the patient thoroughly with soap and hot water. Infested underclothing should be laundered at high temperature and outer clothing tumble dried for 15 minutes at high temperature.

Pediculosis pubis (*pubic lice – 'crabs'*)

These lice are passed from person to person by sexual contact. Hairy areas are preferentially affected (pubic, axillae, eyebrows, eyelashes and chest). The scalp is too densely packed for their liking. The lice are visible to the naked eye, as are the brownish eggs which may firmly attach to the hair shafts.

Patients complain of itching and may show signs of secondary bacterial infection.

Treatment

Malathion 0.5% solution should be applied to the pubic, axillary, thigh and perianal hairs. A repeat application should be performed 7 days later. Eyelash infestation should be treated with the aqueous preparation.

Papular urticaria

This is the excessive, allergic response to insect bites. Many insects may be responsible (e.g. fleas, mosquitoes, bed bugs and ticks). The characteristic lesion is an urticarial papule which may become bullous or infected. The lesions, which are usually found on arms and legs, have a tendency to lie in groups or lines.

Unfortunately, scarring may occur and in coloured skins persistent unsightly hyperpigmentation may result.

Treatment

Symptomatic treatment is given with antihistamines for the itch, a weak topical steroid (Eurax-Hydrocortisone ointment) applied twice daily for a week, and insect repellants. Infested animals should be treated with de-fleaing preparations and household furnishings may need to be sprayed every 4 months with permethrin and methoprene (Acclaim Plus).

BULLOUS DISORDERS

In this section only the most common primary disorders will be discussed. The most frequent bullous conditions seen in the A&E department will be those caused by thermal injury following a partial thickness burn. Some of the less common blistering disorders are listed in Table 7.

A knowledge of the location of the blister within the skin will aid in the diagnosis of the condition. As a guide, flaccid and easily disruptible blisters will arise from within the epidermis. In such cases, although patients may give a clear history of blistering, by the time they

Table 7. *Less common blistering disorders*

Congenital	Epidermolysis bullosa	
Acquired	Pemphigus	Disorders in
	Pemphigoid	which bullae
	Dermatitis herpetiformis	are the
	Toxic epidermal necrolysis	predominant
	Epidermolysis bullosa acquisita	feature
	Erythema multiforme (Stevens–Johnson)	
	Eczema (e.g. pompholyx)	
	Lichen planus	
	Vasculitis	
	Urticaria	
Infection	Impetigo	
	Chicken pox	
	Herpes simplex or zoster	
	Smallpox	
	Hand, foot and mouth	
Drug eruptions		

have reached hospital, only excoriations and erosions will remain. Usually, if blisters survive to the A&E department they are subepidermal in location, being tense and non-disruptable.

Intraepidermal

Pemphigus

Pemphigus is a severe, life-threatening autoimmune disease principally affecting middle-aged/elderly people. It is characterized immunologically by the presence of IgG antibodies binding to the intercellular spaces between epidermal cells. This precipitates the dissolution of the intercellular cement and the resultant falling apart (acantholysis) of the keratinocytes. There are four different forms of pemphigus distinguished from each other both histologically (by level of of intraepidermal splitting) and clinically.

Pemphigus vulgaris

Pemphigus vulgaris is the most common type and is characterized by flaccid blisters of the skin and mucous membranes. The bullae rupture easily leaving raw, painful erosions which crust over and frequently become second-arily infected, hindering the diagnosis. The skin adjacent to a blister will often slide over itself causing new lesions to form (Nikolsky's sign).

Investigation

Skin biopsy and immunofluorescence of both perilesional skin and blood are required to establish the correct diagnosis. This will usually show intercellular deposits of IgG and C3. Serum from patients is assayed for the circulating pemphigus antibody which roughly correlates with disease activity and hence can be of some use in drug management.

Treatment

This has to be aggressive from the outset if the disease is to be brought under control and it must involve a dermatologist. Initially, very large doses of systemic steroids, starting at 80 mg per day and doubling daily until the blistering is brought under control, are needed. Once control is achieved, steroid-sparing agents are introduced. It is not surprising that the side-effects of treatment are now the leading cause of death. Prolonged follow-up and treatment is required.

Subepidermal

Pemphigoid

This is a chronic autoimmune blistering disease of the elderly characterized by tense, nondisruptable bullae arising on an erythematous background. The flexures are often affected. The bullae may be extensive and if so fluid balance needs careful monitoring.

Immunologically, IgG and C3 bind along the length of the dermoepidermal junction, giving rise to a linear pattern of immunofluorescence. The binding splits the skin and the entire epidermis becomes the blister roof, accounting for its durability. There are two types of pemphigoid; unlike bullous pemphigoid, the cicatricial type mostly affects the mucous membranes with few bullae in the skin.

There is often an itchy prodromal prebullous eruption, and frequently an annular or urticarial erythema upon which the bullae subsequently arise.

Treatment

This condition is not as life-threatening as pemphigus vulgaris. Control of the eruption is usually achieved with oral prednisolone 40–60 mg per day. The dosage should be tailed off over a relatively short period of time to a low maintenance dose. Like pemphigus, the mortality of this condition is associated with the side-effects of therapy, particularly in the elderly population. The disease is self-limiting, usually lasting 2–4 years.

Dermatitis herpetiformis

This chronic subepidermal vesicular disease is characterized by extremely itchy, grouped vesicles developing over the elbows, knees, shins, buttocks and shoulders. Usually the bullous component is not seen as it has been ruptured by the ferocity of the patient's scratching. Clinical examination reveals only grouped excoriation with added eczematous changes, notably lichenification.

Investigation
Biopsy of a vesicle confirms the subepidermal blister. Direct immunofluorescence of peri-lesional skin shows granular deposition of IgA and C3 in the dermal papillae. A small bowel biopsy should be performed if bowel symptoms are present. (It is associated with coeliac disease.)

Treatment
Gluten-sensitive enteropathy is always present and treatment involves a gluten-free diet in conjunction with oral dapsone or less commonly sulphapyridine. Both drugs cause haematological disorders, notably haemolytic anaemia, leucopenia and thrombocytopenia. Regular blood checks with reticulocyte counts are mandatory. Any suspected undiagnosed case should be referred to the dermatology department.

Pemphigoid (Herpes) gestationis

This can be considered as pemphigoid of pregnancy. It is a very rare pruritic bullous condition occurring at any time from 9 weeks of gestation to 1 week postpartum. It recurs in subsequent pregnancies.

Investigation
Skin biopsy of a bullous lesion shows a subepidermal blister; immunofluorescence confirms the presence in most patients of linear deposits of C3 along the basement membrane. In 25% of cases IgG is also found. The condition usually improves as pregnancy progresses, although flaring postpartum can occur. Usually the disease lasts a matter of weeks, but it can continue for years afterwards.

Treatment
In mild cases, topical steroid can be used with good effect. However, extensive bullous formation requires oral prednisolone. In very severe cases plasmaphoresis is occasionally employed.

Toxic epidermal necrolysis

This constitutes a dermatological emergency and may prove fatal. It is usually a result of drug hypersensitivity or toxicity, occurring 7–10 days following ingestion.

Drugs known to precipitate the condition include sulphonamides, carbamazepine, barbiturates, allopurinol and phenytoin.

Clinical features
It begins as a painful generalized erythema, rapidly progressing to bullous erosion of the epidermis. The skin peels away in sheets resembling a severe scald. Nikolsky's sign is positive and minimal trauma produces extensive skin loss. The mucous membranes are involved and the patients are acutely ill with fever and leucocytosis.

Treatment
This should be carried out in an intensive care unit or burns unit. Management is similar to that of patients with major burns as infection, fluid loss and electrolyte disturbances can all be life-threatening. There is a mortality of around 40%.

URTICARIA AND ANGIOEDEMA
Urticaria (hives)

This is a transient erythematous eruption or oedematous swelling of the dermal and subcutaneous tissues. The lesions occur at any site. They are itchy. Typically a white palpable centre of oedema is surrounded by a halo of erythema. Annular and serpiginous forms occur. Bullae may occasionally be a feature. Individual lesions last a few hours before clearing and leaving normal skin.

Acute urticaria

Most attacks will resolve within hours or days and the cause is not identified. If the allergen is encountered again the urticaria may recur. Several well-recognized triggers should be excluded:

- Plants (nettles).
- Animal fur.
- Foods and food additives (milk, egg whites, shellfish, nuts, strawberries, tartrazine).
- Drugs (aspirin, penicillin).
- Insect bites/stings.

Chronic urticaria

This describes an urticarial eruption which persists for longer than 3 months. The cause is obscure and referral to a dermatology department is advisable.

Treatment

This obviously involves identification and removal of the trigger, if one can be positively identified. No cause can be identified in up to 90% of cases. The main causes are infection (viral and bacterial) and drugs (especially aspirin and penicillins), and should be carefully eliminated. Allergy tests are unhelpful and should not be promised to the patient. They are merely confirmatory and if the patient cannot tell you what is wrong through the clinical history then it is unlikely that the cause will ever be discovered.

Antihistamines (terfenadine 60 mg, b.d., hydroxyzine 10–25 mg q.d.s, cetirizine 10 mg b.d., loratadine 10 mg daily) are the mainstay of treatment. Occasionally, complete blockade of H1–H2-receptors can be beneficial by adding cimetidine 800 mg daily or ranitidine 300 mg daily.

Angioedema

This occurs when swelling of the dermis involves the subcutaneous tissues. The most commonly affected sites are the junctions of skin and mucous membranes (e.g. periorbital, perioral and genital). If the larynx is involved oedema can lead to asphyxiation, hence this complication constitutes an acute medical emergency.

Hereditary angioedema

A family history of sudden attacks of swelling of the face, larynx, gastrointestinal tract and mucous membrane should alert one to the possibility of this rare autosomal dominant condition in which the patient lacks C1 esterase inhibitor. The condition is treatable by replacing the deficient enzyme with reconstituted enzyme or, more inexpensively, fresh frozen plasma. Danazol can also be used.

Treatment

Life-threatening angioedema may be treated with adrenaline 0.5–1 ml of 1:1000 SC or IV, 10 µg kg^{-1} IV in the event of cardiovascular collapse.

A reducing course of oral steroid therapy starting at 30 mg can be used in severe extensive disease but should

not be relied upon as anything other than short-term therapy.

DRUG REACTIONS

The differential diagnosis of any skin eruption should include the possibility of a drug side-effect. Up to one-third of all drug reactions involve the skin. Factors known to provoke drug reactions include polypharmacy (four or more drugs), elderly patients, genetic susceptibility (e.g. acetylator status) and coexisting hepatic and renal disease.

Diagnosis of drug reactions

A careful history and examination are the only tests at the disposal of the diagnostician. The process involves:

- Identification of all drugs including 'over-the-counter' and herbal remedies.
- Time relationships of all the current and recently taken preparations to the onset of the eruption.
- Classification of the morphology of the rash (e.g. eczematous, acneiform, morbilliform).
- Consulting a list of known drug reactions; the pharmacy drug information service can usually provide this knowledge.
- Withdrawal of suspect medication.

Common reaction patterns and their causes

Exanthematous

This is the most frequent cutaneous drug eruption. The majority are symmetrical, erythematous, maculopapular pruritic rashes appearing on the trunk, elbows, back and knees. They usually appear in the first week of therapy but may occur later. The rash resolves within a few days of drug withdrawal. Exfoliation can occur. Drugs involved include sulphonamides, allopurinol, captopril, phenytoin and carbamazepine.

Exfoliative dermatitis

This is a dermatological emergency. The entire skin surface becomes red and scaly. As fluid balance and temperature control become deranged, especially in patients with pre-existing medical conditions, this eruption should be managed in hospital by a dermatologist. Eczematous and exanthematous eruptions can progress to this state 2–4 weeks after drug ingestion. Common drugs known to precipitate this eruption include sulphonamides, gold, para-aminosalicylic acid, carbamazepine, antimalarials, isoniazid and phenytoin. Exfoliative dermatitis in a patient with no previous history of eczema, psoriasis, lichen planus or lymphoma should always raise the possibility of a drug eruption.

Urticaria

Many drugs produce urticaria. Three main reaction mechanisms exist: immediate hypersensitivity (IgE-mediated), histamine-releasing and serum sickness type. All three produce the identical clinical picture of an acutely arising erythematous, itchy eruption consisting of 'geographical map-like' wheals which last less than 24 h and usually disappear within hours of onset. Subcutaneous swelling (angioedema) occurs at junctions between skin and mucous membranes (e.g. around the eyes, lips, tongue and genitals).

Commonly involved drugs

Immediate reaction
- Penicillin.
- Sulphonamides.
- X-ray media.
- Captopril.

Histamine release
- Salicylates.
- Non-steroidal anti-inflammatory drugs (NSAIDs).
- Cimetidine.

Serum sickness
- Penicillin.
- Thiazides.
- Phenytoin.
- Thiouracils.

Allergic vasculitis

Inflammation around small and medium-sized blood vessels can present as a clinical spectrum ranging from urticarial papules, via purpura and livedo, to nodules and necrotic ulceration.

Common incriminants

- Antimicrobials.
- Thiazides.

- Phenytoin.
- Allopurinol.
- Thiouracils.
- NSAIDs.

Fixed drug eruptions

Single or multiple round erythematous or purple plaques occur at exactly the same site each time the drug is taken. The lesion may develop a central bulla. The mucosae, especially the glans penis, may be involved. The lesions arise within hours of taking the drug and subside rapidly leaving an area of postinflammatory hyperpigmentation.

Commonly involved drugs

- Phenolphthalein.
- Barbiturates.
- Tetracyclines.
- Aspirin.
- Quinine.

Bullous eruptions

Pemphigoid and pemphigus-like eruptions can be mimicked by drugs. In addition, blistering resulting from erythema multiforme, fixed drug eruption, photosensitivity and toxic epidermal necrolysis should be considered in the differential diagnosis of drug-induced bullous disease. Bullae may develop in drug-induced coma over pressure points.

Involved drugs

Pemphigoid
- Diclofenac.
- Ibuprofen.
- Frusemide.

Pemphigus
- Penicillamine.
- Captopril.
- Rifampicin.

Photosensitivity

Two types are recognized: phototoxic and photoallergic. Phototoxic reactions are more common than photoallergic reactions. They occur when the drug is activated by ultraviolet light, producing chemical damage to the skin in a light-exposed distribution. Clinically the eruption resembles sunburn. The skin is erythematous and oedematous. Blistering may occur. The light-exposed distribution of the rash is usually obvious, affecting the face, forehead, cheeks and tips of ears, but sparing the periorbital and submental areas. The 'V' of the neck is prominently affected when exposed, as are the dorsa of the hands.

Photoallergic reactions are eczematous in morphology but are identical in distribution to the phototoxic reactions. They may, however, become generalized.

Commonly involved drugs

- Sulphonamide.
- Thiazides.
- Tetracycline.
- Tricyclic antidepressants.
- NSAIDs.

Nalidixic acid can produce a reaction which may persist for up to 2 years postwithdrawal.

REACTIVE ERYTHEMA

Erythema nodosum

This is an acute inflammation of the subcutaneous fat (panniculitis). Tender, raised, red nodules develop singly or in groups on the shins, thighs and extensor surfaces of the upper limbs. There is often associated arthralgia and fever, although not commonly with drug-induced reactions. The lesions resolve after 6–8 weeks.

The main causes are:

1. Idiopathic.
2. Infections
   - Bacterial: Streptococcal, tuberculosis, leprosy, syphilis.
   - Viral: glandular fever.
   - Fungal: blastomycosis, coccidiomycosis, *Mycoplasma*, *Rickettsia*, *Chlamydia*.
3. Drugs
   - Sulphonamides.
   - Oral contraceptive pill.
4. Systemic disease
   - Sarcoidosis
   - Inflammatory bowel disease.
   - Hodgkin's disease.
   - Behçet's disease.

Investigation and management

On presentation to an A&E department it is not unreasonable to arrange full blood count and ASO (antistreptolysin-O) titres and perform a chest X-ray. The patient can then be referred for follow-up. Treatment consists of eliminating the cause, bed rest and NSAIDs.

Erythema multiforme

This is an acute self-limiting inflammatory disorder of the skin and mucous membranes, often in response to an infection (usually herpes simplex) or a drug. Characteristic annular non-scaling plaques appear on the palms and soles extending up the limbs. Individual lesions enlarge leaving a pale central area in which a new lesion may appear, giving rise to the cardinal 'target' lesion. Individual lesions may blister; widespread blistering is an ominous sign which may herald Stevens–Johnson syndrome. This severe variant of erythema multiforme is associated with fever and mucous membrane ulceration. The oral and conjunctival mucosae are usually severely involved. The ulcerative process can extend all the way from the pharynx to the tracheobronchial tree.

The uncomplicated eruption usually resolves in 2–3 weeks, but the Stevens–Johnson variant may persist for longer. The chief complications are those associated with mucous membrane ulceration, in particular conjunctival and corneal ulceration. Urgent advice should be sought from the ophthalmologists to avoid scarring and blindness.

The main causes are:

1. Viral – HSV, hepatitis A and B, orf, *Mycoplasma*.
2. Bacterial – streptococcal, meningococcal.
3. Fungal coccidiomycosis.
4. Parasitic.
5. Drugs – sulphonamides, phenytoin, carbamazepine, mianserin.
6. Pregnancy.
7. Malignancy.
8. Radiotherapy.
9. Idiopathic.

Investigations

Herpes simplex infection should be excluded by viral culture. Other serological tests should be ordered as appropriate. If the condition is prolonged or recurrent, neoplasia should be excluded. In about 50% of cases no cause can be found.

Treatment

Identification and eradication of the cause is the mainstay of treatment. The Stevens–Johnson syndrome requires immediate admission for supportive care. Careful and frequent nursing of the eroded mucous membranes is essential in order to avoid long-term scarring. Systemic steroids should only be used if started within the first 48 h of the eruption and then for only 5–7 days before being tailed off. Prolonged usage is associated with greater morbidity.

Sunburn

This is an extremely common presentation to the A&E department. The length of time taken for an individual to become burnt by ultraviolet B radiation depends upon the skin type. Fair skins are more prone to burning and blistering. Areas of skin exposed to too much UVB become erythematous and painful 2–4 h later. The erythema is maximal after 24 h. Over the next 72–96 h the skin desquamates, eventually healing over with pigmentation.

Treatment

This is symptomatic and includes oily calamine to soothe the damaged skin. Potent topical steroid creams may be used for up to 72 h. Oral salicylates and NSAIDs can be used for analgesia. An important part of the treatment of sunburnt patients should include a strongly delivered warning about the dangers of excessive sunbathing. The epidemiological correlation between frequent episodic sunburn in adolescence and the later development of malignant melanoma should be emphasized. Advice regarding staying out of the sun between the hours of midday and three in the afternoon and the frequent use of an SPF (sun protection factor) 15 or higher sunscreen (ROC SPF A&B, E45 SPF 25, Uvistat 30), as well as covering up, should be given.

Erythroderma/Efoliative dermatitis

See section on drug reactions.

ULCERS

With the exception of traumatic ulcers, most ulcers are not suitable for management in the A&E department because they require long-term follow-up. It is important to establish the underlying cause and refer appropriately.

Causes of skin ulcers:

1. Trauma.
2. Venous hypertension.
3. Infection (streptococcal, staphylococcal, tuberculosis, syphilis).
4. Ischaemia.
5. Vasculitis.
6. Neoplasia (basal cell carcinoma, squamous cell carcinoma, lymphoma).
7. Haematological diseases (sickle cell disease).
8. Necrobiosis lipoidica – well-defined, waxy, yellow lesions on shins, seen in association with diabetes mellitus.
9. Pyoderma gangrenosum (see section on vascular disorders).

Treatment

Keep it simple and give it time to work by not altering management too frequently.

TECHNIQUE

1. Clean: normal saline washes. If very mucky use potassium permanganate 1:10 000 soaks for 15 min for 7 days. Immersion of the affected limb in a bucket containing the 'rose pink' solution is handy.
2. Dress: keep moist with paraffin gauze dressing (Jelonet or Bactigras), or colloid dressing (e.g. Granuflex).
3. Oral antibiotics only if surrounding cellulitis is present.
4. Support stockings (e.g. Medi-UK) of appropriate pressure should be applied only if a Doppler assessment of the arterial function of the lower limb has been carried out to ensure that vascular compromise does not occur.
5. Topical steroid ointment (e.g. Eumovate, Elocon) if pronounced varicose or stasis eczema is present.

Bibliography

BUNNEY, M.H., BENTON, C. & CUBIE, H.A. *Viral Warts. Biology and Treatment*, 2nd edn. Oxford: Oxford University Press.

CERIO, R. & JACKSON, W.F. (1992). *A Colour Atlas of Allergic Skin Disorders*. London: Wolfe.

COHEN, B.A. (1993). *Atlas of Paediatric Dermatology*. London: Wolfe.

DU VIVIER, A. (1993). *Atlas of Clinical Dermatology*, 2nd edn. London: Gower Medical.

GAWKRODGER, D.J. (1992). *Dermatology: An Illustrated Colour Text*. Edinburgh: Churchill Livingstone.

GRAHAM-BROWN, R.A.C. & BURNS, D.A. (1990). Lecture Notes on Dermatology, 6th edn. Oxford: Blackwell Scientific.

MACKIE, R.M. (1989). *Skin Cancer*. London: Martin Dunitz.

PENNEYS, N.S. (1990). *Skin Manifestations of AIDS*. London: Martin Dunitz.

WEISMANN, K., PETERSON, C.S., SONDER-GAARD, J. *et al.* (1988). Skin Signs in AIDS. Copenhagen: Munksgaard.

Textbook of Dermatology, 5th edn. Oxford: Blackwell Scientific.

53 Neurological emergencies

M.K. SHARIEF and P. ANAND

Department of Neurology, London Hospital Medical College and Royal London Hospital, London UK

Chapter plan

Stroke
Seizures
Vertigo
Syncope
Headache
Acute weakness
Meningitis in adults
Viral encephalitis in adults
Cerebral abscess

This chapter deals with neurological emergencies that are commonly encountered by internists or accident and emergency (A&E) physicians. Neurological diseases account for about 20% of admissions to general hospitals in the UK. An increasing proportion of these admissions are emergencies, and the responsibility for their management falls on primary care physicians, A&E clinicians, general physicians, neurologists and neurosurgeons.

STROKE

Stroke is a common worldwide cause of death and disability. It is the third commonest cause of death in most developed countries, and accounts for more than 5% of the UK National Health Service resources. Each year in the UK more than 100 000 people have a first stroke, and almost 25 000 seek medical attention because of transient ischaemic attacks (TIAs).

Stroke and TIAs are defined primarily by their clinical features rather than by laboratory investigations. A TIA is defined as an acute loss of focal cerebral function with symptoms lasting less than 24 h, which after adequate investigations is presumed to be caused by embolic or thrombotic vascular disease. A stroke may be defined in the same way, except that the symptoms last more than 24 h, or lead to death within that time.

The abruptness of the neurological deficit is the main factor that characterizes the disorder as 'vascular'. Embolic strokes usually begin suddenly and the deficit reaches its peak almost at once, whereas in many thrombotic strokes the onset is somewhat slower, over a period of several minutes, hours, or even days, and usually occurs in a stepwise fashion. In cerebral haemorrhage the onset is usually sudden, and the deficit steadily progressive over a period of minutes or hours. The neurological deficit reflects both the location and size of the infarct or ischaemia, and the territory of the artery involved. The consequent neurovascular syndromes enable the physician to locate the lesion, sometimes down to the affected arterial branch (see below), to provide a prognosis, and to initiate appropriate treatment.

Anatomy of brain blood supply

Arterial blood flows to the brain by way of three major vascular trees: the right and left internal carotid arteries, which supply the anterior two-thirds of the corresponding hemisphere, and the vertebrobasilar system, which supplies blood to the brainstem and the posterior parts of both hemispheres. Anastomotic connections between the internal carotid and vertebrobasilar systems occur at the base of the brain surrounding the optic chiasma and pituitary stalk. This ring-like series of vessels, the circle of Willis (Fig. 1), consists of the anterior communicating artery, which unites the two anterior cerebral arteries, and the posterior communicating

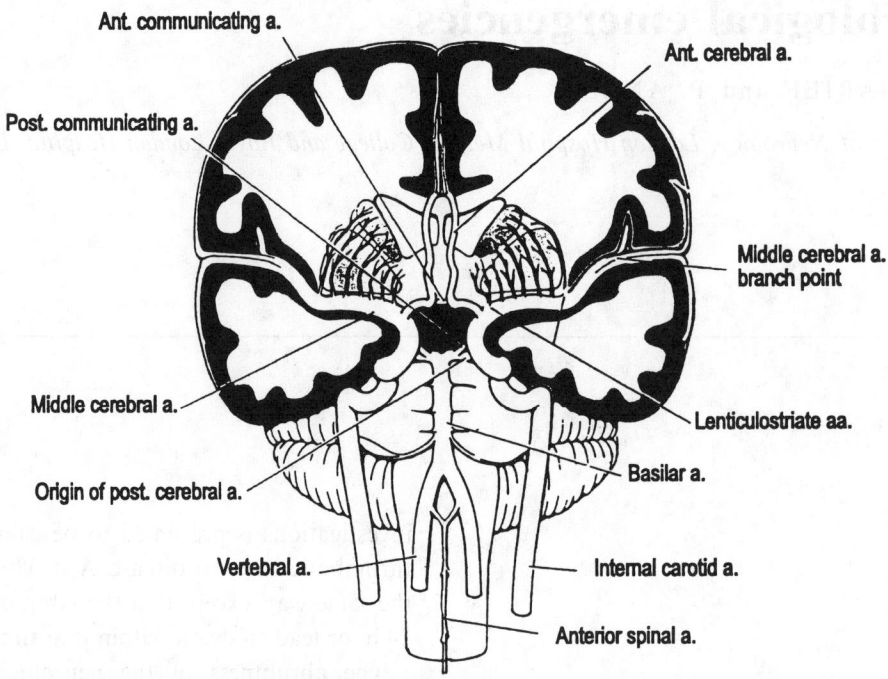

Fig. 1. The cerebral arterial supply showing the major branches of the circle of Willis at the base of the brain.

arteries, which join the internal carotid arteries with the posterior cerebral arteries.

The medial surface of the cerebrum and the superior border of the frontal and parietal lobes are supplied by the anterior cerebral artery. The middle cerebral artery supplies most of the lateral surface of the cerebral hemispheres, including the lateral portions of the frontal lobe, the superior and lateral portions of the temporal lobes, and the deep structure of the frontal and parietal lobes. The entire occipital lobe and the inferior and medial portions of the temporal lobes are supplied by the posterior cerebral artery. Deeper structures of the cerebral hemispheres are supplied by penetrating branches of the larger arteries.

Classification of stroke

In the classification devised by a committee of the National Institute for Neurological Disorders and Stroke in the USA, stroke was subdivided according to pathological mechanism, clinical category, and arterial distribution (Table 1). Cerebral infarction has been further subclassified into four clinical syndromes: total and partial anterior circulation syndromes, posterior circulation syndrome, and lacunar syndrome (Table 1). The clinical features of these syndromes are discussed below.

Although subclassification of stroke serves to identify

Table 1. *Classification of stroke*

NINDS classification

Mechanism: thrombotic, embolic, haemodynamic, haemorrhagic

Clinical: atheroembolic, cardioembolic, lacunar

Arterial side: Internal carotid, middle cerebral, anterior cerebral; vertebral, basilar, posterior cerebral

Syndromic classification

Total anterior circulation syndrome
Partial anterior circulation syndrome
Posterior circulation syndrome
Lacunar syndrome

NINDS, National Institute for Neurological Disorders and Stroke.

the underlying pathophysiological processes and provide a more accurate prognosis, a simple classification is needed to provide a universal applicability in clinical practice. Thus, it is practical from the clinical point of view to preserve the classical division of stroke into thrombotic, embolic and haemorrhagic types. This clinical classification therefore will be adopted throughout this chapter, and the causes, criteria for diagnosis, and management of the three main types of stroke will be considered in subsequent sections.

Table 2. *Causes of stroke*

Thrombotic stroke (due to cerebrovascular disease)
1. Large artery atheroma, with or without ulceration
2. Intracranial artery atherosclerosis, with or without ulceration
3. Small vessel disease
4. Arterial dissection: cystic medial dissection, fibromuscular dysplasia, pseudoxanthoma elasticum, arteritis
5. Inflammatory arterial disease: systemic lupus erythematosus, polyarteritis nodosa, giant cell arteritis, Behçet's, sarcoid
6. Infectious arterial disease: syphilis, mycobacterial, bacterial, fungal
7. Traumatic or postirradiation
8. Venous sinus thrombosis
9. Migraine (?vasospasm)

Embolic stroke
1. Cardiac origin
   −Left atrium: atrial fibrillation, myxoma, aneurysm
   −Mitral valve: infective endocarditis, prolapse, prosthetic valve
   −Left ventricle: mural thrombus, aneurysm, cardiomyopathy
   −Paradoxical embolism with congenital heart disease
2. Non-cardiac origin
   −Ulcerating thrombus of carotid arteries
   −Mural thrombus of aorta and carotid arteries
   −Fat, air, or tumour cells

Haemorrhagic stroke
1. Hypertension
2. Berry aneurysms (and postsubarachnoid haemorrhage vasospasm)
3. Arteriovenous malformations, cavernous angiomas
4. Traumatic haematomas
5. Amyloid angiopathy
6. Bleeding diathesis, warfarin treatment

Aetiology of stroke

The causes of stroke are usually thrombosis (or vascular occlusion), thromboembolism, or haemorrhage (Table 2). Of all causes of cerebrovascular disease, atheroma is by far the most important, and patients often have evidence of peripheral or coronary vascular disease. Atheroma tends to be most marked at branch points in the major vessels and in the carotid syphon. It may cause stenosis or complete occlusion, and a thrombus may form on atheromatous plaques with small fragments breaking off and lodging distally.

In most cases of cerebral embolism, the embolic material consists of a fragment which has broken away from a thrombus within the heart. Less frequently the source is intra-arterial, from an ulcerated atheromatous plaque in the carotid sinus or internal carotid artery. Cerebral embolism due to fat, air or tumour cells is quite rare and seldom enters into the differential diagnosis of stroke. Any region of the brain may be affected, but the upper division of the middle cerebral artery is most frequently involved. The two hemispheres are approximately equally affected.

Haemorrhagic stroke is due to bleeding into brain parenchyma with formation of a focal haematoma, or into the subarachnoid space from a ruptured berry aneurysm or arteriovascular malformation. It accounts for about 10% of all strokes, and most are attributed to chronic or acute arterial hypertension. Aneurysms and vascular malformations are a common cause in young normotensive individuals, whereas amyloid angiopathy accounts for up to a third of haematomas in elderly patients. Occasionally haematomas develop in regions reperfused after brain infarction or after use of anticoagulant or fibrinolytic agents.

Pathophysiology of stroke

Under normal circumstances, the adult human brain is entirely dependent on the oxidation of glucose to generate high-energy phosphate compounds to meet its energy needs. Reversible alteration in cell function due to decreased blood flow and consequent lack of oxygen occurs in ischaemia, and irreversible alteration in infarction. After occlusion and deprivation of cerebral blood flow, a series of events unfold, the ischaemic cascade (Westmoreland *et al.*, 1994), which consists of the following alterations, leading ultimately to neuronal dysfunction and death:

1. Decreased cerebral blood flow and cerebral oxygen and glucose consumption in the centre of the ischaemic area. These functions are less impaired at the periphery of the ischaemic area, the ischaemic penumbra, where blood flow is sufficient to prevent irreversible cell damage.
2. Impairment of local autoregulatory mechanisms, and initiation of anaerobic glycolysis as oxygen and glucose supply decrease. Tissue lactate increases, pH decreases.
3. Failure of mitochondrial function and inefficient ATP generation as substrate depletion continues. This is associated with leakage of K^+ from cells, and intracellular accumulation of Na^+, Cl^-, Ca^{2+} and free fatty acids. The net effect is neuronal depolarization, loss

of the transmembrane potential, and impairment of ATP-dependent neurotransmitter reuptake.

4. Release of excitatory neurotransmitters such as glutamate, which may be neurotoxic via activation of N-methyl-D-aspartate receptors, causing increased permeability to Na^+, cellular swelling and lysis, and massive influx of Ca^{2+} into postsynaptic neurons.

5. Increased intracellular Ca^{2+} activates proteases and phospholipases and generates oxygen free radicals and nitric oxide. This leads to membrane, mitochondrial and microtubular damage and eventual cell destruction.

Clinical presentation

> **The clinical diagnosis of stroke is highly specific provided the following definition is observed:**
>
> A neurological deficit of sudden onset with focal rather than global neurological dysfunction, and with symptoms lasting more than 24 h which are presumed to be of a non-traumatic vascular origin.

Diagnostic errors could arise in patients with intracerebral malignancy, especially if there has been haemorrhage into areas of necrosis. The presence of features that are unusual in uncomplicated stroke, (e.g. papilloedema or unexplained fever) should call into question the clinical diagnosis.

When occlusion of a major cerebral artery occurs, the extent of infarction will depend on the degree of collateral blood supply. The features of ischaemia due to arterial occlusion are defined by its location, severity and duration. The term 'stroke in progression or evolution' is used when deterioration is observed after the initial insult, which can occur for as long as 48 h if the stroke affects the anterior circulation, and sometimes for as long as 96 h in those of the posterior circulation. In a *partial stroke*, only a portion of an arterial territory has been affected. A *completed stroke* occurs if the entire cerebral tissue perfused by an artery is damaged at the onset of the stroke, or if a partial stroke progresses to completion.

The clinical presentation of stroke depends on the nature of the primary pathological abnormality and the vessel or vessels involved. However, a few general principles may be stated here, provided it is recognized that there is no certain means to distinguish clinically between haemorrhage and infarction. In general, the onset of cerebral embolism is abrupt, with the appearance

of neurological deficit in a few seconds or minutes. Cerebral haemorrhage is often accompanied by headache or vomiting at the onset, and loss of consciousness is not uncommon, with neurological deficit progressing over 10–30 min. The condition often presents during waking hours, usually during exertion or other circumstances which raise the blood pressure. Non-embolic cerebral infarction (thrombotic stroke) usually occurs during sleep or soon after rising, with a neurological deficit developing over 30 min or more. Sometimes, the established stroke is preceded by warning symptoms in the form of TIAs (see below).

Cerebral infarction may be caused by occlusion of cerebral veins (phlebothrombosis) or thrombophlebitis of dural sinuses. Bacterial infection of the middle ear and mastoid cells, paranasal sinuses, or skin around the upper lip, nose and eyes may extend to the large dural sinuses causing thrombophlebitis and venous occlusion. Other clinical settings known to favour the occurrence of venous thrombosis include hypercoagulable states, polycythaemia, cyanotic heart disease, the puerperium, antithrombin III, protein S and C deficiency, and Behçet's disease. A stroke due to venous thrombosis is characterized by slow evolution of the clinical syndrome, and a greater epileptogenic and haemorrhagic tendency.

Localization of affected part of brain

The clinical picture resulting from occlusion of any one artery is sufficiently uniform to justify the description of a typical syndrome related to each major artery. The following description applies particularly to infarction and ischaemia due to embolism or thrombosis. The clinical picture of intracerebral haemorrhage is apt to differ because, in its deep extension and associated mass effect, haemorrhage involves the territory of more than one artery. Patients with completed anterior circulation stroke present with the combination of higher mental integrative cerebral dysfunction, homonymous visual field defect, and contralateral motor or sensory deficit of at least two areas of face, arm and leg. Patients with partial anterior circulation stroke present with only two of the three components of the total anterior circulation stroke, with higher cerebral dysfunction alone, or with a restricted motor/sensory deficit (e.g. confined to one limb or to the face). Patients with posterior circulation stroke present with any of the following: ipsilateral cranial nerve palsy with contralateral motor or sensory deficit; bilateral motor or sensory deficit; disorder of conjugate eye movement; cerebellar dysfunction; or isolated homonymous visual field defect.

Middle cerebral artery occlusion

The classic picture of total occlusion is contralateral hemiplegia, affecting the arm and face more than the leg, hemianaesthesia, and homonymous hemianopia. The patient may be stuporous in the beginning and there is aphasia with dominant hemisphere lesions. This artery is the most frequent vessel occluded by emboli from the heart.

Anterior cerebral artery occlusion

Occlusion of this artery results in contralateral hemiparesis and hemisensory loss, in which the leg is often more severely affected than the arm. Urinary incontinence, contralateral grasp reflex and paratonic rigidity may be evident. With occlusion in the dominant hemisphere, there may be non-fluent dysphasia and contralateral motor dyspraxia.

Posterior cerebral artery occlusion

Occlusion of the posterior cerebral artery produces a greater variety of clinical features than occlusion of any other artery. Thus, although homonymous visual field defects predominate, hemiparesis, sensory disturbances and sometimes hemiballismus may also occur. Patients with extensive lesions may deny being blind (Anton's syndrome) and if the angular gyrus is involved, finger agnosia, dyscalculia and right–left disorientation (Gerstmann's syndrome) may occur.

Posterior inferior cerebellar artery occlusion

Also termed lateral medullary infarction or Wallenberg syndrome, occlusion of this artery results in specific neurological signs (Fig. 2). These include ipsilateral facial pain or numbness, severe vertigo and vomiting, dysphagia, ataxia, and contralateral spinothalamic sensory impairment. There is also ipsilateral Horner's syndrome and horizontal nystagmus to the side of the cerebellar lesion. The syndrome could also be caused by occlusion of the vertebral artery. There are additional ischaemic syndromes, which are discussed in detail elsewhere (Adams & Victor, 1993).

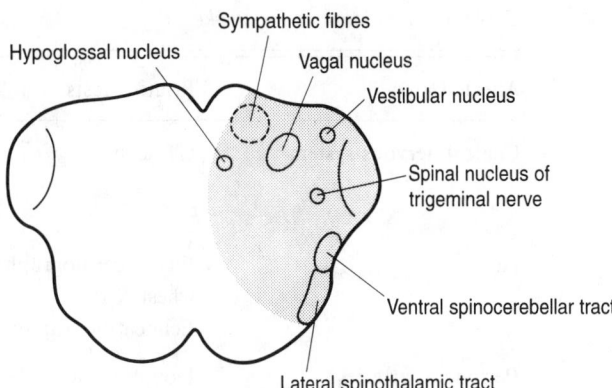

Fig. 2. The lateral medullary syndrome. The grey area shows the extent of infarction, and the structures affected.

Other neurovascular syndromes

Pontine infarction, due to basilar artery thrombosis, is often fatal. The signs are coma, multiple cranial nerve palsies, quadriplegia and cardiorespiratory abnormalities. Medullary infarction, due to vertebral artery occlusion, results in lower cranial nerve palsies and tetraparesis or hemiparesis. Pure cerebellar infarction is rare, and most infarcts involve the brainstem, though cerebellar signs predominate.

Diagnosis and management of stroke

When the patient is admitted, a definitive diagnosis of the nature and location of stroke is necessary. The clinical syndrome is classified as a TIA, a partial stroke, a progressive stroke, or a completed stroke. Investigations are based on the clinical evaluation, and include both essential routine tests and special investigations (Table 3). A CT (computed tomography) scan or MRI (magnetic resonance imaging) of the brain (Fig. 3) should be performed as soon as possible to rule out haemorrhage or an unsuspected space-occupying lesion. Other diagnoses should be considered when the history is atypical or inadequate. These include chronic subdural haematoma, cerebral abscess, or encephalitis, particularly due to herpes simplex. MRI of the brain or intravenous digital subtraction angiography may be required to exclude venous sinus thrombosis. Investigations for TIA are essentially similar to those for stroke. Carotid and vertebral angiography remain the most accurate means of determining the extent and site of atherosclerotic lesions in the extracranial cerebral vessels (Fig. 4). Echocardiogram, ECG (electrocardiogram) and 24-h ECG monitoring are indicated if a cardiac cause of TIA is suspected.

Table 3. *Investigations for stroke*

Affected area	Routine tests	Special tests
Central nervous system	CT scan	Magnetic resonance imaging
		Electroencephalogram
		Lumbar puncture
Heart	Electrocardiography	Catheterization
	Chest X-ray	24-h ECG, Holter monitor
	Echocardiography	Continuous ambulant ECG
Peripheral arteries	Doppler studies	Intra-arterial angiography
		Intravenous digital subtraction angiography
		Magnetic resonance arteriography
		CT angiography
Systemic	Full blood count	Coagulation studies
	ESR	Autoantibody screen
	Blood glucose	Lupus anticoagulant
	Lipid profile	Antithrombin III level
	Liver function tests	Proteins C and S levels
	Syphilis serology	Fibrinogen
		Haemoglobin electrophoresis
		Other tests

ESR, erthyrocyte sedimentation rate.

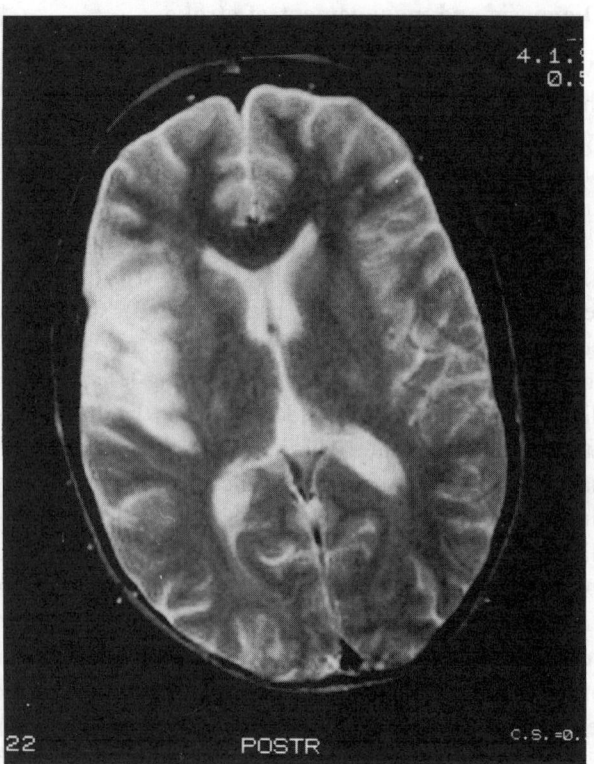

Fig. 3. An ischaemic infarct of the right cerebral hemisphere in the distribution of the middle cerebral artery.

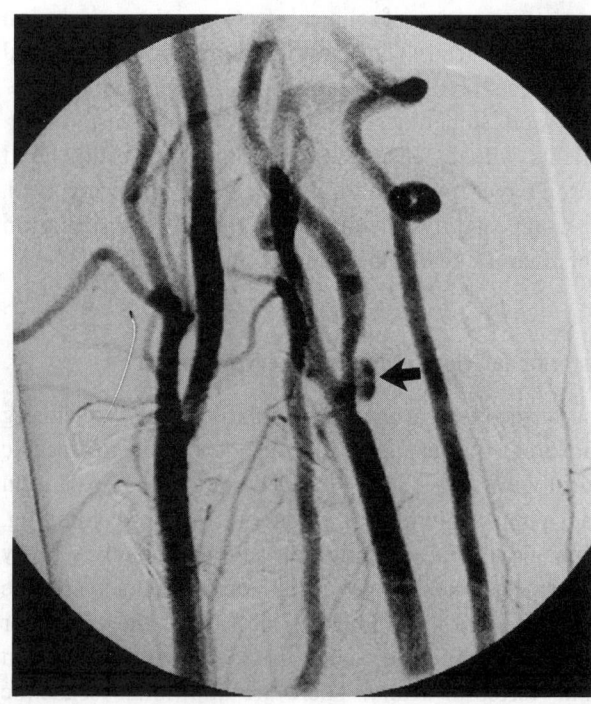

Fig. 4. Conventional angiography showing an ulcerated plaque in the left carotid bifurcation (arrow).

Table 4. *Clinical trials for early medical treatment of acute ischaemic stroke*

Mechanism	Medical treatment
Restore cerebral artery patency	Fibrinolytic agents
	Tissue plasminogen activator
Prevent progressive arterial occlusion	Heparin
	Antiplatelet agents
Improve cerebral haemodynamics	Avoid systemic hypotension
	Cerebral vasodilators/calcium antagonists
Prevent neurotoxicity	Calcium antagonists
	Inhibitors of excitatory amino acids
Reduce cerebral oedema	Corticosteroids
	Glycerol
Improve cerebral oxygen delivery	Haemodilution
	Hyperbaric oxygen

Early treatment

The aim of early treatment for acute stroke is to reverse or limit the degree of brain dysfunction. When the patient is comatose or semiconscious, the usual measures necessary in the management of the unconscious patient are required. The treatment of previously undetected hypertension is preferably deferred until the neurological deficit has stabilized. In severe strokes, if severe oedema of the affected hemisphere is suspected, treatment with dexamethasone may be indicated. However, analysis of trials conducted so far suggests that treatment is unlikely to reduce mortality.

Once an ischaemic stroke has fully developed, no available treatment could restore the damaged cerebral tissue or its function. Effort should, therefore, be directed to preventing the progression of ischaemia and improving cerebral circulation. Table 4 describes some clinical trials that have been conducted in the early treatment of ischaemic stroke. Treatment with hyperbaric oxygen or glycerol are unlikely to be valuable, whereas treatment with calcium antagonists may be useful in certain situations (e.g. in postsubarachnoid haemorrhage vascular spasm) and haemodilution may be used in polycythaemia.

Approach to thrombotic stroke

The treatment of completed stroke aims essentially to prevent further episodes, detect and treat any complications, and ensure that a complete cardiovascular assessment has been made. The role of anticoagulant therapy in cerebral ischaemia has been a source of controversy for many years. A formal overview of several controlled trials of heparin in acute ischaemic strokes suggests uncertain effects on mortality and haemorrhagic transformation of the cerebral infarct. There is, therefore, no place for routine anticoagulation in stroke, except in patients with a cardiac source of emboli, particularly in the presence of arrhythmias. In critical stenosis of the internal carotid artery associated with cerebral vascular insufficiency, anticoagulation and urgent consideration of endarterectomy have been indicated.

An overview of all randomized trials of antiplatelet agents demonstrated that drugs such as aspirin reduce the risk of further vascular events, including recurrent stroke and myocardial infarction, by about 25%. Doses of aspirin as low as 75 mg have been shown to be effective. No other antiplatelet agent is clearly more effective than aspirin. The role of carotid endarterectomy is discussed below.

Treatment of venous sinus thrombosis consists of large doses of antibiotics, if suppuration is suspected, and anticoagulant therapy. In other causes of thrombophlebitis, specific treatment is indicated. For instance, regular venesection can be used in patients with polycythaemia to maintain the haematocrit below 0.42.

Approach to embolic stroke

Management decisions concerning anticoagulant therapy for patients with a cardiac source of brain embolus should balance the benefit of reduction in early recurrent embolism against the risk of potentiating secondary brain haemorrhage. Cardioembolic strokes have a propensity for secondary haemorrhagic transformation, so early

Table 5. *Symptoms of transient ischaemic attacks*

Focal deficit	Carotid artery TIA	Vertebrobasilar TIA
Motor deficit	Contralateral weakness	Bilateral or shifting weakness Ataxia or unsteadiness
Sensory deficit	Contralateral numbness or paraesthesia	Bilateral or shifting numbness
Speech deficit	Dysphasia, dysarthria	Dysarthria
Visual deficit	Amaurosis fugax	

anticoagulation is often hazardous. If intravenous heparin is given, it should be avoided until at least 48 h after stroke. In patients with severe neurological deficit, it is prudent to wait 7–10 days before starting anticoagulation. Low-dose subcutaneous heparin or antiplatelet agents are acceptable alternatives to intravenous heparin. Anticoagulation is not indicated in acute embolic stroke due to infective endocarditis; initiation of antibiotic therapy is associated with a marked reduction in embolism.

Approach to haemorrhagic stroke

Warfarin anticoagulation should be reversed quickly with vitamin K or fresh frozen plasma. Other bleeding diatheses should be treated specifically when possible. Calcium antagonists are used for postsubarachnoid haemorrhage arterial spasm. Surgical evacuation of large cerebral hemisphere haematomas is sometimes undertaken in patients whose condition is deteriorating. Evacuation of cerebellar haematomas with progressive hydrocephalus is essential, in association with ventricular cerebrospinal fluid shunting. Artificial hyperventilation may be needed to reduce raised intracranial pressure. Neurosurgical treatment is also indicated for aneurysms and arteriovenous malformations.

Transient ischaemic attacks

A TIA is an important predictor of the subsequent development of a stroke. If no therapy is instituted, cerebral infarction develops in about 30% of cases. Because the risk of stroke cannot be predicted, all patients with TIAs are considered at risk, and those with recent onset should be evaluated on an urgent basis.

The diagnosis of TIA is made on the basis of the history, and the symptoms should be analysed to ascertain whether the carotid or vertebrobasilar territory is affected (Table 5). Differential diagnosis includes migraine, epilepsy, structural brain lesions, and non-vascular causes such as hypoglycaemia, multiple sclerosis and Ménière's disease.

Management of TIAs includes modification of atherosclerotic risk factors, such as hypertension, diabetes, or hypercholesterolaemia, and the use of antiplatelet agents. At present, aspirin is the best medical therapy in the management of TIA. Recent evidence suggests that, in patients with carotid TIA or minor ischaemic strokes who have carotid stenosis of 70% or more, carotid endarterectomy reduces the risk of subsequent stroke despite surgical morbidity and mortality. Unlike aspirin, carotid endarterectomy only has an effect on the risk of ipsilateral stroke, and is unlikely to prevent myocardial infarction.

SEIZURES

Seizures are amongst the most common neurological disorders. It is important to recognize that a seizure is a symptom of dysfunction of the cerebral grey matter rather than a disease in itself. The normal brain can be driven to a seizure with a variety of acute insults. Such an occurrence is distinguished from epilepsy, a chronic condition in which seizures occur repeatedly. A seizure may be described basically as a condition in which individuals experience paroxysmal changes in behaviour caused by abnormalities in the electrical activity of the brain. Seizures can take many forms, ranging from a sudden loss of consciousness and convulsions to a brief lapse of attention or a change in perception of the environment. The diagnosis of seizures is essentially a clinical one. Paroxysmal cortical electrical activity as seen in seizures may occur intermittently without clinical abnormality, and the incidental finding of such activity on electroencephalography (EEG) does not necessarily imply a diagnosis of epilepsy.

Epidemiology

The annual incidence rates of epileptic seizures in most studies are between 20 and 120 cases per 100 000 with a point prevalence of 4–10 per 1000. Incidence rates vary considerably with age. They are highest in childhood, trough from 15 to 65 years, and rise again in the elderly. The age of onset also depends on the cause of the seizures. In general, seizures with onset before the age of 10 years or after the age of 30 years are best not considered to be manifestations of primary epilepsy, but suggestive of symptomatic seizures.

About 2–5% of a general population have at least one seizure at some time in their lives, and seizures probably recur in more than 50% of these individuals. Around 5–12 per 1000 of the population suffer chronic or active epilepsy, and only about 3% of those require institutional care, usually because of associated mental or neurological handicap. There is good epidemiological evidence that epileptic seizures remit permanently in a majority of cases. In general, remission tends to occur early after the onset of seizures; the longer the seizures continue, the poorer is the prognosis. Similarly, relapses are relatively uncommon after a substantial remission has been achieved. The underlying cause of the seizures is also an important factor for prognosis.

Pathophysiology

Although much is known about the physiological basis of the abnormal discharges accompanying seizures, the cellular mechanisms responsible for epileptogenesis remain conjectural. The anatomical and histological characteristics and functional organization of the cerebral cortex make it particularly susceptible to the development of excessive paroxysmal synchronized activity that is manifested as seizures. The two primary factors that produce seizures are increased excitability of cortical neurones and synchronization of the neuronal population. Mechanisms that may cause these processes include:

- Alteration of intrinsic membrane properties.
- Local changes in neuronal environment.
- Impairment of local inhibitory mechanisms, mainly of the gamma-aminobutyric acid (GABA)-related system.
- Increased recruitment and recurrent excitation of neuronal populations via synaptic input or electrical coupling.

Seizures can become generalized as a result of synchronization between the two hemispheres, recruitment of synchronizing thalamocortical circuits, or involvement of subcortical structures. Repeated activation of a neuronal population may produce a persistent increase in neuronal excitability via long-term potentiation, including long-term changes in cytoarchitecture and genetic expression.

Aetiology

The aetiology of seizures is quite varied and multi-factorial. Almost all cerebral grey matter diseases, many white matter diseases, most metabolic disorders and several systemic diseases may cause epileptic seizures. In most patients, however, no cause can be determined, and are best referred to as cryptogenic. These cases should not be confused with the syndromes of primary generalized epilepsy or the other well-defined epileptic syndromes. From an aetiological viewpoint, factors that have to be considered include heredity, structural cerebral lesions, age and biological changes.

Seizure disorders may be divided into two main categories. The first includes those patients with a strong genetic factor in the causation of their seizures in whom acquired focal or diffuse cerebral disease plays little or no role. These are often termed primary or idiopathic epilepsies. The second category includes those patients in whom seizures are secondary to acquired cerebral or systemic disease. Aetiology also varies considerably with the age at onset of seizures (see Table 6).

The incidence of neonatal seizures varies from 1.5 to 14 per 1000 live births, and they are always symptomatic. Narcotic withdrawal may cause convulsions in babies born to addicted mothers, but irritability is much more common. Epileptic seizures are more common in infancy and childhood than at any other period of life. The epilepsies of childhood are also much more variable in expression and outcome than those of adults as a result of incomplete development of synaptic and intra-hemispheral connections. Seizures in paediatric practice are discussed in more detail in Chapter 60. The spectrum of causes of adult-onset seizures is quite wide and overlaps with that of childhood. Although seizures may result from numerous causes, only some of which are given in Table 6, the remarkable fact remains that, in the majority of cases, no cause is found.

Classification and description of types

Epileptic seizures can be classified in several ways, such as by clinical events, aetiology, pathophysiology, EEG changes, or age. The International League Against Epilepsy (1981) introduced, and later modified, a classi-

Table 6. *Causes of seizures*

Neonatal seizures
Birth asphyxia
Cerebral haemorrhage
Developmental defects
Meningoencephalitis
Hypoglycaemia
Hypocalcaemia
Metabolic disorders
Narcotic withdrawal
Unknown cause

Infantile and childhood seizures
Infantile spasms (West's syndrome)
Lennox–Gastaut syndrome
Specific epileptic syndromes
Early myoclonic epilepsies
Neurodegenerative diseases
Chromosomal disorders
Structural brain abnormalities
Toxic/metabolic causes
Central nervous system infections/trauma
Febrile convulsions
Idiopathic/cryptogenic

Adult-onset seizures
Idiopathic
Cerebral infections
Intracranial tumours
Cerebral trauma
Cerebrovascular diseases
Hypertensive vascular diseases
Systemic diseases
Metabolic disorders
Autoimmune diseases
Neurodegenerative diseases
Progressive myoclonic epilepsies
Specific epileptic syndromes
Deficiency states
Toxic causes
Drug induced
Cryptogenic/pseudoseizures

Table 7. *International classification of seizure type*

I. Partial seizures
  A. Simple partial seizures
    (1) With motor signs
    (2) With somatosensory hallucinations
    (3) With autonomic features
    (4) With psychic symptoms
  B. Complex partial seizures
    (1) Simple partial onset followed by impairment of consciousness
    (2) With impaired consciousness at onset
  C. Partial seizures evolving to secondary generalized seizures
    (1) Simple partial seizures evolving to generalized
    (2) Complex partial seizures evolving to generalized
    (3) Simple partial seizures evolving to complex partial seizures evolving to generalized

II. Generalized seizures
  A. (1) Absence seizures
    (2) Atypical absence
  B. Tonic–clonic seizures
  C. Myoclonic seizures
  D. Clonic seizures
  E. Tonic seizures
  F. Atonic seizures

III. Unclassifiable epileptic seizures

1. *Simple partial seizures* in which there is no alteration of consciousness.
2. *Complex partial seizures* in which consciousness is lost or impaired.
3. *Secondary generalized seizures* in which the epileptic discharge spreads to the entire brain.

The seizure discharge in generalized seizures involves both cerebral hemispheres simultaneously from the onset of the attack, and there is no clinical or EEG evidence of a focal onset. Consciousness is invariably impaired. Generalized seizures are divided into several clinical types.

- *Tonic–clonic seizures* are the typical 'grand mal' attacks. The attack may start with a cry and the patient will fall and stiffen (the tonic phase). This phase is succeeded by the clonic phase, when convulsive movements take place for several minutes. This is followed by a phase of relaxation with deep respiration and atonia.
- *Absence seizures* are the typical 'petit mal' attacks. They take the form of a sudden impairment of

fication of seizure type in which EEG data, pathophysiology and aetiological data are taken into account (Table 7).

Partial seizures start in a small area (focus) of the cerebrum, usually in the temporal or frontal lobes. The features of the seizure reflect the function of the part of the brain involved, and the symptoms produced by the seizure may therefore vary widely. These seizures are divided into three main categories:

Table 8. *Choice of drug for initiation of anticonvulsant therapy for common seizure types in adolescents or adults*

Seizure type	First-line	Second-line
Partial	Carbamazepine	Phenytoin, sodium valproate Vigabatrin, lamotrigine, gabapentin
Tonic–clonic	Sodium valproate Carbamazepine	Phenytoin Lamotrigine
Absence	Sodium valproate	Ethosuximide
Myoclonic	Sodium valproate	Clonazepam
Unclassified	Carbamazepine Sodium valproate	Phenytoin Vigabatrin, lamotrigine

consciousness lasting from a few seconds to a minute or so, during which the patient remains motionless and unresponsive.

- *Myoclonic seizures* are brief jerks of a muscle group or several muscle groups; they may be single or rapidly repetitive.

Diagnosis

The diagnosis of epileptic seizures is essentially clinical, and on occasions no investigation can conclusively confirm or refute this. A clear witnessed account of the attack is therefore necessary. The list of conditions commonly mistaken for epileptic seizures is long and includes syncope, migraine, cardiac arrhythmias, paroxysmal vertigo, hypoglycaemia, panic attacks, pseudo-seizures, abnormal illness behaviour, night terrors and other sleep disorders, and TIAs.

Having established that the patient has seizures, a primary task of the physician is to determine whether a specific aetiology for the patient's seizures can be identified. It is not possible to list the investigations appropriate to all cases, and these should be planned on an individual basis. The range of investigations varies from haematological and biochemical screening to EEG and neuroimaging by either CT scan or MRI. Cerebro-spinal fluid examination is needed in a small number of patients to exclude meningitis or encephalitis.

Treatment of seizures

A single fit in an adult is rarely an indication to start anticonvulsant treatment, except when an underlying structural cause is likely or confirmed. Otherwise, most neurologists would wait until two or three seizures have occurred before starting treatment. Having decided that treatment is necessary, the choice of drug to initiate therapy depends on seizure type. Consideration may be given to efficacy, side-effects, and ease of use.

Treatment should be started using a single drug at low dose, and subsequent titration should be undertaken on an individual basis. For most patients, carbamazepine or sodium valproate represent the drug of choice (Table 8). Phenytoin is as effective as carbamazepine against partial and generalized tonic–clonic seizures, but is now regarded as a second-line therapy because of its potential to produce cosmetic and psychological side-effects, and its complex pharmacokinetics.

Anticonvulsant monotherapy should be the rule in initial treatment and, in the event of treatment failure, anticonvulsant drugs should be exchanged rather than added. Combination therapy should be embarked upon only as a last resort. Treatment of patients with established active epilepsy is more difficult than that of newly diagnosed patients, since the former have a generally poorer prognosis, are more drug-resistant and will often have additional neurological handicap. Specialist assessment is often desirable in these circumstances.

Status epilepticus

Status epilepticus can be defined as a condition in which prolonged or recurrent seizures persist for 30 min or more. There are several forms of status epilepticus, including tonic–clonic status, absence status, complex partial status, and epilepsia partialis continua. Tonic–clonic status epilepticus, unlike other types, is a medical emergency and carries about 5–10% risk of mortality. Immediate control of seizures is therefore necessary.

For patients presenting as an emergency in status

Table 9. *Emergency anticonvulsant drug treatment for adult patients with status epilepticus* (modified from Shorvon, 1994)

Stage	Drug treatment
Prodromal stage	Diazepam 10–20 mg given rectally or IV Midazolam 5–10 mg given rectally, IV or IM Paraldehyde 10–20 ml given rectally or IM *If seizures continue, treat as below*
Early status (0–30 min)	Lorazepam 0.07 mg kg^{-1} given as IV bolus, repeated once after 10–20 min *If seizures continue, treat as below*
Established status (30–60/90 min)	Phenytoin 15–18 mg kg^{-1} IV infusion at a rate of 50 mg min^{-1} *and/or* Phenobarbitone 10 mg kg^{-1} IV bolus at a rate of 100 mg min^{-1} Chlormethiazole 320–800 mg IV infusion at a rate of 40–120 mg min^{-1} *If seizures continue, treat as below*
Refractory status (after 60/90 min)	General anaesthesia, with either thiopentone or propofol, continued for 12–24 h after last clinical or EEG seizure

IV, intravenous; IM, intramuscular.

epilepticus, it is first essential to assess cardiorespiratory function, administer oxygen, set up intravenous lines and institute regular monitoring. Intravenous glucose (50 ml of 50% solution) should be given immediately if hypoglycaemia is suspected, and intravenous thiamine (250 mg) should be administered if there is a history of alcoholism. Emergency investigations to establish aetiology depend on the clinical circumstances. If status epilepticus has followed the withdrawal of a particular anticonvulsant drug, the same drug should be rapidly reintroduced. It is helpful to plan anticonvulsant drug therapy in a series of progressive phases (Table 9). In patients with established epilepsy, status epilepticus is usually preceded by a prodromal phase during which seizures become increasingly frequent or severe. Urgent drug treatment will often prevent the evolution into true status epilepticus. If the patient is at home, treatment should be given before transfer to hospital. Once status epilepticus has developed, treatment should be carried out in hospital under close supervision as outlined in Table 9.

Prognosis and follow-up

The overall prognosis of epilepsy is much better than is often suggested. In the majority of cases, the total number of seizures experienced is small, duration of active epilepsy is short, and once remission is achieved it is usually permanent. About 75% of patients overall will enter permanent remission and 50% will successfully withdraw medication.

The question of complete withdrawal of anticonvulsant therapy from a patient in remission is difficult. Withdrawal of therapy can be considered if a patient has been 3–5 years without a fit, but studies in this area have been contradictory. A long history of active epilepsy, the presence of a structural neurological disease, and partial seizure types are associated with a poorer prognosis for withdrawal of treatment.

VERTIGO

Vertigo refers to an illusory sensation of movement or rotation. Vertigo and dizziness are common complaints, and because the entire physical examination and all diagnostic tests may be normal, the diagnosis depends primarily on the history. A history of episodic symptoms accompanied by double vision, slurred speech or paralysis would suggest transient vestibulobasilar ischaemic episodes; a long history of severe episodes of imbalance followed by severe headaches may be suggestive of basilar artery

Table 10. *Causes of vertigo*

Peripheral causes
Benign paroxysmal positional vertigo
Peripheral vestibulopathy (acute or recurrent)
Ménière's disease
Post-traumatic (cupulolithiasis)

Central (intracranial) causes
Cerebellopontine angle tumours (acoustic neuroma, meningioma, etc.)
Brainstem ischaemia, infarction, or structural lesions
Demyelinating diseases affecting the brainstem
Geniculate herpes zoster (Ramsay Hunt syndrome)
Hereditary cochleovestibular atrophies (Alport's and Refsum's, Gardner's syndrome, etc.)

Systemic causes
Vestibulotoxic drugs (aminoglycosides, antihypertensives, etc.)
Vasculitis (giant cell arteritis, connective tissue diseases)
Endocrine diseases (hypothyroidism, diabetes mellitus)

migraine; episodic positional vertigo following head trauma suggests cupulolithiasis. Ménière's disease is characterized by recurrent attacks of vertigo associated with fluctuating tinnitus and deafness. Benign positional vertigo is characterized by paroxysmal vertigo and nystagmus that occur only with the assumption of certain critical positions of the head, particularly lying down, bending over or tilting the head backward.

Causes of vertigo and dizziness could be broadly divided into peripheral vestibulopathy, central vestibular lesions, and systemic causes (Table 10). The distinction between a peripheral and central lesion causing vertigo can usually be made clinically. Acute episodes with nausea and vomiting, but without other neurological symptoms, are nearly always due to peripheral vestibular disturbance. Peripheral disorders are much more likely to be associated with tinnitus or deafness than central lesions.

The Hallpike test for positional nystagmus is particularly helpful in differentiating between central and peripheral lesions. The patient is seated on the edge of the examination table, having him or her lie down abruptly with the head hanging 45° backward and to one side. The development of nystagmus and vertigo is observed and the test is repeated with the head turned to the opposite side. The response is prompt with relatively severe symptoms in positional vertigo.

Management of vertigo

In a classical peripheral vertigo, no further investigations are necessary. A vestibular sedative, such as cinnarizine, is occasionally required if symptoms are severe or persistent. Vestibular exercises may be helpful, such as gait-training, visual-vestibular exercises, and positioning manoeuvres. Further neuro-otological assessment is indicated in those with recurrent episodes of vertigo or associated cochlear symptoms. CT brain scanning to rule out cerebellopontine angle tumours may be indicated, and is essential in patients with additional sensorineural deafness or facial weakness.

SYNCOPE

Syncope may be defined as an episode of altered consciousness triggered by a reduction of cerebral perfusion. Common causes of syncope include vasovagal attacks (common faints), postural (orthostatic) hypotension, and cough or micturition syncope, particularly in the elderly. Other causes of episodic faintness and syncope are listed in Table 11. Loss of consciousness in these different types of syncope must be ultimately caused by a change in the neural elements in parts of the brain that subserve consciousness, such as the brainstem reticular activating system.

Diagnosis and management

Syncope should be distinguished from other cerebral disturbances causing loss of consciousness, the most frequent of which are akinetic seizures or other forms of epilepsy. Syncope is usually postural, with prodromal symptoms before loss of consciousness, whereas seizures occur regardless of the position of the patient. Loss of consciousness in syncope lasts less than a minute, in contrast to most seizures. Headache, confusion and drowsiness are common after seizures, but not after syncope.

Distinguishing different types of syncope depends on characteristic clinical features and results of investigations, such as ECG, haematocrit, blood glucose and, in patients with extracranial cerebral vessel stenosis, digital subtraction angiography (see above). Similarly, treatment depends on the specific cause of syncope. However, patients seen during the preliminary stages of fainting or after they have lost consciousness should be placed in a position which permits maximal cerebral blood flow (e.g. in the supine position with legs elevated). If the

Table 11. *Causes of syncope*

Mechanism	Causes
Cardiac arrhythmias	Atrioventricular block
	Sinus bradycardia, sinoatrial block
	Carotid sinus syncope
	Tachyarrhythmias
Reduced cardiac output	Left ventricular outflow obstruction
	Pulmonary flow obstruction
	Cardiomyopathy, pericardial effusion
Reduced cardiac venous return	Cough or micturition syncope
	Valsalva manoeuvre
Hypotensive	Hypovolaemia
	Autonomic failure
	Addison's disease
Cerebrovascular disease	Carotid or vertebrobasilar disease
	Large vessel arteritis
Other mechanisms	Anoxia, hypoglycaemia
	Hyperventilation
	Emotional syncope

temperature is subnormal, the body should be covered with a warm blanket. Nothing should be given by mouth until the patient has regained consciousness.

HEADACHE

Headache is by far the commonest single symptom in surveys of neurological out-patients. The vast majority of such patients have no physical signs, and there is a complex interaction of various clinical subtypes of headache with psychiatric symptoms. A number of intracranial and extracranial structures may give rise to headache. It may be due to referred pain from the muscle and joints of the cervical spine, or caused by diseases of sinuses, teeth, ears, eyes and temporomandibular joints. Raised and reduced intracranial pressure, subarachnoid haemorrhage, meningitis and encephalitis usually produce headache. Spasm, dilatation or inflammation of branches of the external carotid artery may lead to headache. A number of metabolic disturbances such as hypoglycaemia and hypercapnia are also associated with headache.

Classification

A definitive classification of headache is hindered by the relatively limited knowledge of its fundamental patho-physiology. Classification based on structural causes is often unsatisfactory since it does not include functional or 'vascular' headaches. The classification presented in Table 12 is an expanded adaptation of the diagnostic criteria published by the Headache Classification Committee of the International Headache Society in 1988.

Pathophysiology

Current knowledge of the pathogenesis of headache is fragmentary and incomplete. Most spontaneous cranial pains can be caused by one of the following mechanisms:

1. Traction or dilatation of intracranial arteries and distension of extracranial arteries.
2. Traction of intracranial veins or their dural sheaths.
3. Compression or inflammation of sensory nerves.
4. Meningeal hyperaemia.
5. Spasm or interstitial inflammation of cranial muscles.

Migraine is generally considered to have a vascular basis, although it has been proposed that the primary event in migraine is neuronal, the vascular changes being secondary.

Table 12. *Classification of headache*

1. Migraine
   A. Migraine with aura
   B. Migraine without aura
2. Tension-type headache
   A. Episodic tension-type headache
   B. Chronic tension-type headache
3. Cluster headache
4. Functional headaches
   A. Post-traumatic headache
   B. Cough and exertional headaches
   C. Coital headache
   D. Drug- or food-induced headache
5. Raised intracranial pressure
6. Vascular headache
   A. Subarachnoid haemorrhage
   B. Arteritis
   C. Acute onset systemic hypertension
7. Inflammatory or infectious headache
   A. Meningitis or encephalitis
   B. Disorders of cranium or cranial structures
   C. Systemic infections

Diagnosis and management

A basic task when assessing a patient with headache is to differentiate specific headache syndromes listed in Table 12 from headaches caused by a structural lesion. The next task is to differentiate migraine from various non-migrainous headaches and from cluster headaches. A few structured questions, followed by examination, will usually serve to eliminate a possible structural cause. An abrupt onset of headache raises the suspicion of a subarachnoid haemorrhage from a berry aneurysm or arteriovenous malformation, or a parenchymal haemorrhage associated with hypertension. Coital headache may have a similar onset and, until the diagnosis is established following repeated episodes, should be regarded as a potential indication of subarachnoid haemorrhage. An evolving headache over hours or days raises the possibility of meningitis or encephalitis. If the evolution is over days or weeks, the question of raised intracranial pressure due to either a tumour or a subdural haematoma should be considered. Intermittent or periodic headache is seen in migraine or cluster headache, whereas longstanding and constant headache is suggestive of tension headache, although raised intracranial pressure may occasionally present in this way.

In the elderly patient and in patients with localized tenderness and changes in the arterial vessels and skin, the subacute onset of headache should raise the question of temporal arteritis. In the majority of patients the erythyrocyte sedimentation rate will be grossly elevated, in which case it is necessary to institute immediate treatment with intravenous corticosteroids followed by high-dose oral steroids before referring the patient for temporal artery biopsy, so as to reduce the risk of involvement of the retinal artery and consequent loss of vision.

Features of headache in patients with raised intracranial pressure usually include a postural relationship, often wakening the patient from sleep, and being made worse by stooping, coughing and bending. In addition, there may be an association with vomiting, altered conscious level and seizures. Examination may show papilloedema or focal neurological signs. Indications for CT brain scan, therefore, include headaches of increasing severity or frequency, papilloedema or lateralizing signs, seizures, persistent vomiting, altered mental state, and headaches exacerbated by coughing or sneezing. Suspicion of subarachnoid haemorrhage or subdural haematoma are other indications for CT scanning. The remainder of this section will discuss headaches that are not associated with structural neurological abnormalities.

Migraine

Migraine affects about 5% of the population and is more common in women. It may start in childhood, adolescence or early adult life, and rarely starts after the age of 35 years. Migrainous headache usually lasts for 6–24 h and may be preceded by a visual aura of flashing moving dots or fortification spectra. Nausea, vomiting, photophobia and phonophobia are common. The headache itself is characterized by its unilateral location, pulsating quality and moderate or severe intensity. It is aggravated by walking upstairs or similar routine physical activity. Rare forms of the condition include:

- Hemiplegic migraine, with transient hemiplegia and dysphasia.
- Basilar migraine, presenting as transient brainstem dysfunction.
- Ophthalmoplegic migraine.

The International Headache Society classifies migraine as either 'migraine without aura' (previously termed common migraine) or 'migraine with aura' (previously termed classical migraine). Migraine without aura is characterized by headache lasting between 4 and 72 h associated with at least one of the following:

- Nausea or vomiting.
- Photophobia.
- Phonophobia.

In addition, at least two of the following features of the headache must apply:

- Unilateral location.
- Pulsating quality.
- Moderate or severe intensity.
- Aggravation by routine physical activity.

In migraine with aura, three of the following must be present: one or more fully reversible aura symptoms indicating focal cortical or brainstem dysfunction; at least one aura symptom developing over four minutes or two or more symptoms occurring in succession; no aura symptoms lasting more than 60 minutes; and headache following the aura with a free interval of less than 60 minutes (it may begin before or simultaneously with the aura).

Treatment of migraine

An acute attack of migraine can be treated with early administration of adequate doses of analgesics, such as aspirin, paracetamol, or dihydrocodeine. Antiemetic agents, such as metoclopramide or domperidone, may be necessary.

Ergotamine is an effective drug in migraine, but is frequently associated with nausea and vomiting and, rarely, peripheral ischaemia. It exerts its action by interacting with 5-HT (serotonin) receptors. Sumatriptan, a selective 5-HT$_1$ receptor agonist, is a potent vaso-constrictor of the cerebral vessels, but is best avoided in cases of coronary artery disease.

Prophylactic treatment of migraine could be achieved by pizotifen, or 5-HT antagonists with a central action, and beta-blockers such as propranolol. Methy-sergide is another effective drug in migraine prophylaxis, but its use is limited by serious side-effects such as retroperitoneal fibrosis. Avoidance of stimuli that may trigger an attack is an important aspect of management.

Tension-type headache

These are by far the commonest type of headache. The pain is usually described as pressing or tightening (non-pulsating), is of bilateral location and mild to moderate intensity, and is not aggravated by physical activity. The headache lasts from minutes to days, or even months, and is not associated with nausea or vomiting, although anorexia may occur. If the average frequency of headache is more than 15 days per month for more than 6 months, the condition is called chronic tension-type headache.

Treatment with analgesics is not usually successful. Explanation, reassurance and instructions in techniques of relaxation may reduce the headache. The use of small doses of amitriptyline has been found to be effective in some cases.

Cluster headache

This is the most easily definable syndrome among patients with headache. It occurs predominantly in young adult men and is characterized by severe constant unilateral orbital, supraorbital or temporal pain lasting for 15 min to 3 h. The pain is associated with conjunctival or nasal injection, lacrimation, rhinorrhoea, ptosis, miosis or eyelid oedema. The frequency of attacks varies from 8 per day to 2–3 per week. The picture of cluster headache is characteristic, but a diagnosis of migraine, trigeminal neuralgia, or sinusitis may have to be entertained.

Treatment of cluster headache

Treatment of cluster headache is more difficult than of migraine, and no analgesic is appropriate for routine use. Pizotifen and methysergide have been used successfully in the prevention of cluster headaches. Oxygen inhalation can also be effective during the acute attack. Lithium therapy is the most effective treatment in the unremittent type of cluster headaches, and treatment with indo-methacin has been advocated in some cases.

Post-traumatic headache

Post-traumatic headache is a chronic persistent headache that follows head injury. It may be associated with dizziness, sleep disturbance and intolerance of alcohol. The headache is intermittent, with episodes lasting from a few hours to several days, and is of very variable severity and character. The relative contribution of organic and psychogenic factors in the aetiology of post-traumatic headache is poorly understood. The headache may respond to a small dose of amitriptyline.

ACUTE WEAKNESS

Guillain–Barré syndrome

Acute inflammatory polyneuropathy, commonly known as Guillain–Barré syndrome (GBS), is an acute demyelinating disorder of peripheral nerves. The majority of cases are preceded by non-specific illness, and some follow specific infections, such as campylobacter, mycoplasma, cytomegalovirus or HIV (human immunodeficiency virus) infection. A similar clinical syndrome may occur in lymphoma, porphyria, abnormalities of potassium metabolism, and exposure to various toxic agents (e.g. organophosphorus or thallium).

The disease typically begins with paraesthesiae in the feet and hands, but rapidly involves the motor system, with ascending weakness and hypo- or areflexia. Autonomic dysfunction is common. Cerebrospinal fluid examination may show markedly elevated total protein, with normal glucose and cell count or slight pleocytosis. About 70% fully recover, 20% develop some motor disability, and 10% die.

Management of Guillain–Barré syndrome

A combination of falling vital capacity and poor bulbar function is an indication for intubation and artificial ventilation. There is no evidence that corticosteroid treatment improves the outcome, but plasma exchange has been shown to reduce the duration of disability by up to 30%. It is only effective when carried out within the first 2 weeks. It is usually carried out for bulbar failure and respiratory muscle involvement. Infusion of high doses of human polyclonal IgG from healthy donors has been shown to ameliorate the disease in some patients. It has been speculated that polyclonal IgG contains anti-idiotype antibodies, which inactivate putative pathogenic antibodies directed to myelin.

Myasthenia gravis

Myasthenia gravis is an autoimmune disease that is caused by antibodies against acetylcholine (nicotinic) receptors at the neuromuscular junction of striated muscle. It is characterized by fatiguable weakness of striated muscle, and there is an association with the presence of thymic hyperplasia or a thymoma. Women are more commonly affected than men. The initial presentation is weakness, which may be sometimes restricted to the external ocular muscles and the eyelids.

However, any muscle may be involved, including bulbar, respiratory, trunk and limb muscles.

The diagnosis is confirmed by improvement of power in a muscle with excessive fatigue after intravenous edrophonium (the 'Tensilon' test). Electromyography shows a decremental response on repetitive stimulation, and acetylcholine receptor antibodies are raised in about 90% of patients.

Management of myasthenia gravis

Initial treatment is with the long-acting anticholinesterase agents pyridostigmine or neostigmine. Thymectomy is likely to benefit patients if undertaken relatively early in the course of the disease, particularly in female patients with thymic hyperplasia. Immunosuppression with prednisolone and azathioprine is indicated in patients with limited response to pyridostigmine, and plasma exchange in patients with severe respiratory and bulbar weakness.

Botulism

Botulism is a rare form of food poisoning, caused by the exotoxin of *Clostridium botulinum*. The primary site of action of botulinus toxin is at the presynaptic ending of the neuromuscular junction, interfering with the release of acetylcholine. Symptoms appear within 12–36 h in the form of nausea and vomiting followed by blurred vision and diplopia. Extraocular muscle palsies, bulbar involvement and progressive muscle weakness may then follow. These symptoms are associated with severe constipation. The diagnosis is confirmed by electrophysiological studies.

Treatment is with trivalent antiserum as soon as the clinical diagnosis is made. Guanidine hydrochloride (50 mg kg^{-1}) may be useful in reversing muscle weakness. Respiratory care and maintenance of fluid and electrolyte balance are required in severe cases.

Other causes of acute weakness

Acute episodes of weakness are known to occur with derangement of potassium metabolism, mainly hypokalaemia. There are at least three hereditary syndromes of recurrent muscle weakness:

- Hypokalaemic periodic paralysis.
- Normo- or hyperkalaemic periodic paralysis.
- Paramyotonia with periodic paralysis.

Periodic paralysis should be clinically distinguished from cataplexy and drop attacks. Taking a detailed family

Table 13. *Cerebrospinal fluid findings in meningitis*

Cause	Pressure	Microscopy	Biochemistry
Bacterial	Elevated	Polymorphs and organisms	Low glucose High protein
Viral	Normal/mild increase	Lymphocytes, but no organisms	Normal glucose Mild increase in protein
Tuberculous	Elevated	Lymphocytes and tuberculosis bacilli on special staining	Low glucose High protein
Malignancy	Elevated	Mixed inflammatory and malignant cells	Low glucose High protein

history, measurement of serum potassium and electrodiagnostic testing are helpful in making the diagnosis.

Weakness associated with hypokalaemia could also be due to excessive use of diuretics and laxatives, barium poisoning, aldosteronism, and abuse of thyroxine.

MENINGITIS IN ADULTS

Inflammation of the leptomeninges and the subarachnoid space may be due to bacterial, viral, spirochaetal, protozoal, or fungal infection. Involvement of the meninges may also occur in malignant infiltration within the subarachnoid space.

Aetiology

Common bacterial causes of meningitis is the UK include *Neisseria meningitis*, *Haemophilus influenzae*, and *Streptococcus pneumoniae*. Tuberculous meningitis is common worldwide, and in patients with immunosuppression, including those with AIDS (acquired immunodeficiency syndrome). Meningitis could also be caused by several viruses, including echo, coxsackie, Epstein–Barr, mumps and herpes viruses. Microorganisms reach the meninges either by direct extension from the nasopharynx, ears, a cranial injury or congenital meningeal defect, or by spread via the bloodstream.

Presentation

Bacterial meningitis may develop rapidly, and clinical features are due to a combination of sepsis, meningism and raised intracranial pressure. Symptoms include acute onset of fever, lethargy, generalized headache, vomiting and photophobia. Clinical signs include neck stiffness,

Kernig's sign (inability to straighten the leg below the knee once the hip is flexed to 90°), drowsiness and, occasionally, papilloedema. The onset may be fulminating in meningococcal meningitis, with rapid onset of coma. Symptoms and signs are usually less severe in viral meningitis.

There are some clinical clues as to the causative organism. Petechial rash or profound shock may occur in meningococcal meningitis. Pneumococcal meningitis may be associated with skull fracture, ear infection or congenital brain abnormalities.

Diagnosis

A lumbar puncture should be performed and rapidly analysed (Table 13) unless there is evidence of increased intracranial pressure (papilloedema, confusion, obtundation) or focal neurological signs. If such complications are present, brain imaging should precede the lumbar puncture. A preponderance of polymorphonuclear leucocytes and low cerebrospinal fluid glucose ($<60\%$ of concomitant blood glucose) strongly suggest bacterial meningitis. Bacteriological studies are required to identify the causative organism and to determine antibiotic sensitivity.

Early management

Specific antibiotic treatment for bacterial meningitis depends upon identification of the organism. In meningococcus and pneumococcus meningitis, treatment is with intravenous benzylpenicillin 1.2–2.4 g 4-hourly, or a cephalosporin, particularly intravenous cefuroxime 3 g 6-hourly. *Haemophilus influenzae* meningitis is treated with chloramphenicol 3–4 g daily. Treatment of presumed bacterial meningitis before microbiological confirmation is usually with penicillin and chloramphenicol. Treatment of viral meningitis is generally symptomatic except for herpes simplex, which is treated with acyclovir, and cytomegalovirus, which is treated with ganciclovir.

VIRAL ENCEPHALITIS IN ADULTS

Viruses can affect the brain by at least two mechanisms: direct invasion of brain cells and autoimmune damage. It has been increasingly recognized that viruses do not only produce acute, sometimes self-limiting, neurological diseases, but also involve the central nervous system in slowly progressive pathological processes extending over months to years. This section, however, will only discuss acute encephalitides caused by conventional viruses.

Presentation

Viral encephalitis usually presents as an acute illness producing maximal neurological deficits within a period of hours to days, from which surviving hosts may make a gradual recovery. The extent of the disorder is conditioned by several factors, such as the nature of the infecting agent and the age and immune status of the host. Some viral encephalitides are sporadic (e.g. herpes simplex virus, HSV), whereas others are predominantly epidemic or geographically restricted (e.g. Japanese B encephalitis).

The clinical features of viral encephalitis arise from focal areas of pathology within the brain (e.g. epileptic seizures, focal weakness, visual changes, or speech disturbances) and general effects of raised intracranial pressure (e.g. headache, impairment of consciousness, or delirium). These features are generally accompanied by signs and symptoms of systemic infection. Many viruses can cause sporadic encephalitis, including HSV, varicella zoster, Epstein–Barr, measles, mumps, rubella, adeno-viruses, and HIV.

HSV encephalitis

HSV encephalitis is one of the commonest forms of sporadic encephalitis. Type I is usually responsible for the large majority of cases. The disease carries a 50–60% mortality if untreated. The disease begins with a prodromal phase of headache, fever, and general malaise lasting for 3–4 days. This is followed by progressive impairment of cortical functions, with the appearance of focal neuro-logical signs and epileptic seizures. Unusual behaviour and hallucinations have been observed. Coma rapidly supervenes in many cases.

Diagnosis of encephalitis

The disease should be differentiated from cerebral abscess, when focal neurological signs are detected, and from bacterial or other forms of infective meningitis when such signs are absent. Brain imaging, such as CT or MRI, is important to exclude structural pathologies. If not contraindicated, cerebrospinal fluid examination should be performed to exclude other infective diseases requiring antimicrobial therapy, and to perform viro-logical analysis. Cerebrospinal fluid pleocytosis, mostly lymphocytes, and raised protein are the usual findings in viral encephalitis. Other body fluids, and a throat swab, should be sent for microbiological analysis. A focal EEG abnormality is seen in 65–80% of patients during the acute phase of HSV encephalitis. In some instances it is feasible to perform a brain biopsy to establish the diagnosis.

Specific treatment of encephalitis

Specific treatment with acyclovir has greatly improved the outlook in HSV encephalitis. Intravenous acyclovir (30 mg kg^{-1} per day) for 10 days reduces the overall mortality to less than 20%, and also reduces the incidence of residual neurological damage. Recent observations indicate that a longer course of the drug (14 days) may be necessary to prevent relapse. In many cases, intra-venous steroids are also given. The efficacy of the drug is greater if given early after the onset of encephalitis. Thus, successful treatment depends on enhanced clinical awareness of the condition, and rapid administration of acyclovir in patients with suspected HSV encephalitis.

CEREBRAL ABSCESS

A cerebral abscess consists of suppurative necrosis of the brain parenchyma. It is most prevalent in patients under the age of 40 years, as a result of congenital heart disease and middle ear and sinus infection, and is encountered twice as often in males as in females. A cerebral abscess starts as an area of cerebritis which then develops into a pus-filled cavity surrounded by a wall of variable thickness and, outside this, cerebral oedema. Some abscesses are single, others multilocular or multiple.

Pathogenesis

Cerebral abscess is usually formed through the contiguous spread of infection from parameningeal foci, such as sinusitis, otitis media, dental abscess or osteomyelitis. Adjacent areas of the brain are often affected; thus ear infection spreads to the temporal lobe or cerebellum, whereas frontal sinus infection spreads to the frontal lobe. A cerebral abscess may also result from the direct introduction of organisms from the outside following penetrating head injury or during neurosurgical procedures. Haematogenous spread from remote sources of infection, such as bronchiectasis or bacterial endocarditis, often spawns multiple abscesses with a predilection for forming at the grey/white matter junction, the functional watershed between cortical and deep penetrating vascular systems. Immunosuppression is an increasingly important predisposing factor for cerebral abscess. In children, more than 50% of cerebral abscesses are associated with congenital heart disease, probably due to hyperviscosity of the blood, chronic hypoxaemia and impaired filtering function of the lungs. In about 15% of patients with cerebral abscess, no obvious primary site of infection or predisposing cause can be identified.

The most common organisms causing cerebral abscess are *Streptococcus* species, many of which are anaerobic or microaerophilic. *Bacteroides*, Enterobacteriaceae and staphylococci are other important groups. In the immunosuppressed host (e.g. patients with AIDS), cerebral abscess is often caused by *Toxoplasma gondii* or *Listeria monocytogenes*.

Clinical presentation

Onset of symptoms is usually subacute with about 80% of cases presenting for diagnosis within 2–3 weeks of initial manifestations. Acute, stroke-like onset has been described. The most common clinical presentation of a cerebral abscess consists of headache and signs of raised intracranial pressure (nausea, vomiting, altered sensorium, and occasional papilloedema). Focal neurological signs, such as hemiparesis, cranial nerve palsies, dysphasia and visual field defects, are common and reflect the location of the abscess. Seizures occur in about 40% of cases. Patients may also present with signs of meningeal irritation, which may be due to spread of the infection to the meninges or rupture of an intracerebral abscess into the subarachnoid space or into a ventricle. Meningeal irritation may be mimicked by herniation of the cerebellar tonsils in the foramen magnum secondary to raised intracranial pressure.

When there is an obvious primary infection, the development of focal neurological signs or features of raised intracranial pressure will be likely to suggest the correct diagnosis. The severity of the general symptoms, however, is usually proportional to the acuteness of the abscess. In acute cases an irregular pyrexia is the rule; in chronic cases the temperature may be intermittently, but not invariably, raised. Systemic symptoms may be absent in the immunosuppressed host.

Early investigations and management

Early recognition requires a keen alertness to the possibility of the diagnosis, and if possible the definition of a source of infection. Lumbar puncture is contraindicated when a cerebral abscess is suspected because of the risk of herniation. CT brain scan is the investigation of choice for both diagnosis and follow-up. The diagnosis must be confirmed by operation, and samples of pus should be sent for aerobic and anaerobic cultures.

The treatment of cerebral abscess is primarily surgical, but a successful outcome depends on early diagnosis and adjuvant antibiotic treatment. Most supratentorial abscesses can be sterilized by aspiration through a burr hole (under CT control) under full antibiotic cover. Frequent aspirations may be needed in the early stages to keep the abscess cavity empty. Cerebellar abscesses should be treated by primary excision under antibiotic cover.

Once the content of an abscess has been aspirated, antibiotic treatment is able to sterilize the remainder of the cavity. Antibiotics alone may sterilize areas of developing cerebritis and very small abscesses. Appropriate therapy depends on the likely primary cause and the site of the abscess. For otogenic abscesses a combination of high-dose intravenous penicillin (20 mega units daily) and gentamicin should be given for 3 weeks. The addition of a second- or third-generation cephalosporin is indicated for treatment of resistant coliforms, or in patients who are allergic to penicillin. Metronidazole should also be given initially until anaerobes have been excluded on culture. For frontal abscess, high-dose penicillin and metronidazole are indicated. Fusidic acid and high-dose flucloxacillin are given for staphylococcal abscesses.

Early management should also be directed towards reducing the effect of raised intracranial pressure and avoiding the risk of seizures. Cerebral oedema may be reduced by intravenous mannitol or supported ventilation to reduce arterial carbon dioxide concentration. Dexamethasone can also be used in conjunction with surgical drainage to reduce brain swelling. Antiepileptic therapy should be started at the time of diagnosis and continued for 3–5 years to reduce the risk of seizures.

Bibliography

ADAMS, R.D. & VICTOR, M. (1993). *Principles of Neurology*, 5th edn. pp. 669–748. New York: McGraw-Hill.

SHORVON, S.D. (1994). *Status Epilepticus in Children and Adults. Pathogenesis and Management.* Cambridge: Cambridge University Press.

WESTMORELAND, B.F., BENARROCH, E.E., DAUBE, J.R., et al. (1994). *Medical Neurosciences. An Approach to Anatomy, Pathology, and Physiology by Systems and Levels*, 3rd edn. pp. 273–306. Boston: Little, Brown & Co.

54 The management of psychiatric emergencies

W.D.A. BRUCE-JONES[a] and P.D. WHITE[b]

[a] *Bath Mental Health Care Trust, Royal United Hospital, Bath, UK*
[b] *Department of Psychological Medicine St Bartholomew's Hospital, London, UK*

Chapter plan

Introduction
Models of liaison
Common clinical presentations and their management
Specific psychiatric disorders and their management in A&E
Side-effects of psychotropic medication
Mental health legislation
Conclusion

INTRODUCTION

In 1959 a royal commission recommended a move from hospital-based care to community care for the mentally ill. Since then the number of beds in England and Wales has decreased from 160 000 to 60 000. With under-developed and underresourced community services, more patients with psychiatric illness are inevitably presenting to accident and emergency (A&E) departments and at least one-fifth of patients attending A&E suffer from a psychiatric disorder (Bell *et al.*, 1990). However, patients presenting with bizarre, uncooperative or aggressive behaviour often provoke anxiety and hostility in A&E staff. Those who deliberately harm themselves directly or by abusing alcohol and other drugs are often treated unsympathetically. These are understandable reactions in a busy A&E department, particularly if there is not a close liaison with the local department of psychiatry. Proper training, support and back-up will allow all staff to be able to cope with and help such patients (Brown *et al.*, 1990).

Those commonly presenting to A&E will include the homeless. One-third of the homeless suffer from psychiatric illnesses, especially schizophrenia and alcohol dependence (Marshall & Reed, 1992). Close links between A&E, psychiatry and social services are vital for their successful treatment and rehabilitation. Other common presentations to A&E include those with substance misuse, panic attacks, suicidal intentions, threatening or violent behaviour, victims of violence and those who deliberately harm themselves.

The assessment and management of psychiatric disorders in A&E should follow three main principles:

1. Make sure the patient and other staff are safe from immediate harm.
2. Take a history, which will often include a corroborative story from others.
3. Perform an appropriate physical and mental state examination.

The essential mental state examination

- Appearance
- Behaviour
- Affect (objective evidence of mood)
- Suicidal intentions
- Thought disorder
- Delusions
- Hallucinations
- Orientation
- Memory
- Insight

The essential information to give a psychiatrist when referring a patient should include:

- The presenting history of the illness.
- The past and family psychiatric history.
- Drug history (including alcohol).
- The mental state examination.

Practical arrangements

Careful consideration must be given to the practical arrangements for the management of patients with psychiatric illness in A&E. A separate interview room should be provided. This should have two doors and be comfortably furnished with two chairs and a desk. Most importantly, the room should have a clearly marked and easily accessible alarm button. Arrangements for liaison with psychiatric staff should be clearly agreed and written into operational policies, preferably with expected response times. Operational policies should also include arrangements for the use of security staff in emergencies.

MODELS OF LIAISON

The move to provide care for the mentally ill in the community has meant that psychiatric services are increasingly based in general hospitals rather than in isolated mental hospitals. As a result, psychiatric staff are increasingly available for active liaison or consultation with A&E departments. Psychiatrists may provide an important service to A&E departments which goes beyond simply responding to emergencies. Individual hospitals should develop services appropriate to their needs to ensure the best possible service to their patients.

Consultation model

The most common liaison model depends on A&E staff requesting help or advice when emergencies arise. This may be provided by junior doctors, by specialist psychiatric nurses or a combination of both. Operational policies should ideally include expected response times as well as cover and referral arrangements. Consultations may comprise assessments in A&E, telephone advice or provision for outpatient follow-up.

Liaison model

Closer liaison may be developed by psychiatric staff attending regular meetings with A&E staff, teaching, supervision, and developing a psychiatric clinic in the A&E department. This can be a particularly useful way of managing patients who are repeat A&E attenders (see below), allowing assessment of patients who would not otherwise attend psychiatric clinics. These arrangements require an extra allocation of resources but encourage closer cooperation and may act as a forum for support and the continuing education of staff from both departments.

COMMON CLINICAL PRESENTATIONS AND THEIR MANAGEMENT

Severe behavioural disturbance

Patients with bizarre, aggressive and violent behaviour present some of the most difficult problems to A&E staff. Doctors and nurses who are accustomed to managing cooperative patients feel deskilled. Considerable distress may be caused to other patients and their relatives. Behavioural problems of this kind are seen increasingly frequently in general hospitals. In part, this is accounted for by the widespread abuse of drugs as well as the present inadequacies of community care of the mentally ill.

History-taking and examination are often difficult in these situations but every attempt should be made to obtain information from anyone accompanying the patient including police or carers. Important information may be obtained from descriptions of the patient's behaviour which may be useful when trying to assess the underlying problem. For example, the patient may have been seen brandishing an empty bottle of alcohol or apparently responding to voices. The main causes of disturbed behaviour encountered in A&E are:

- Drug intoxication (especially alcohol).
- Delirium (acute confusional state).
- Acute psychosis.
- Personality disorder.

Management of the severely disturbed patient

The primary aims of management should include control of dangerous behaviour and establishment of a provisional diagnosis. In many cases there is an urgent need to control behaviour before any further steps can be taken. Three specific strategies may be necessary when dealing with the violent patient:

- Reassurance and explanation.
- Physical restraint.
- Medication.

Reassurance and explanation

The majority of disturbed patients are themselves frightened as well as frightening and feel threatened by those around them. Patients with delirium or a psychosis are unsure of their surroundings and easily misinterpret the actions of others. These patients should not be left alone and staff should always explain the situation and their intentions. This simple strategy of reorientation may be all that is required to calm a patient sufficiently to be interviewed and allow an appropriate examination.

Physical restraint

If the behaviour remains severely disturbed it may be necessary to restrain the patient from harming themself or others. Once this decision has been made staff must act decisively and a restraint team should be formed. This must comprise as many staff as is necessary to control the patient with minimal risk of injury. The team leader, usually the senior nurse, should coordinate the task and designate one member of staff to be responsible for each limb of the patient. Once the patient is immobilized and brought to the ground gently he should be held in the prone position. This will help to protect the airway and allow access for intramuscular medication.

Medication

If it has become necessary to physically restrain the patient it is almost certain that they will require some form of tranquillizing medication (Silverstone & White, 1992). In these circumstances it is usually necessary to administer medication while the patient is restrained and they should not be released until they are visibly calmed. A treatment strategy known as 'rapid tranquillization' has been advocated; this involves the administration of moderate doses of a tranquillizer (neuroleptic or benzodiazepine) at regular, comparatively short, intervals (30–60 min) (Dubin, 1988). It is not recommended that such treatment be carried out in the A&E department unless a diagnosis of psychosis has been made and the appropriate legal steps have been taken (see below). In most situations a single dose of medication should be enough to allow more definitive management to take place. The intramuscular route gives a faster response than the oral route and is practical in the restrained patient. The intravenous route has been advocated by some clinicians but is not generally recommended because of the cardiotoxicity of some agents and respiratory depression by others.

Both neuroleptic drugs and benzodiazepines may be used as tranquillizers. Used in combination they have a synergistic action and it has been shown to reduce the total amount of neuroleptic required to treat psychotic illnesses. There has long been concern that benzodiaze-

pines are not only respiratory depressants but have the potential for disinhibiting and worsening disturbed behaviour. Therefore a simple regimen of an intramuscular butyrophenone (a neuroleptic) may be used in most situations. Haloperidol or droperidol may be used in similar dosage although droperidol has a more pronounced sedative action. The regimen recommended in patients under the age of 60 years who are physically fit is droperidol 5–10 mg. Patients over the age of 60 years should not be given more than 5 mg in the first instance and the dose should be significantly reduced in patients with known cardiac or hepatic disease. Neuroleptics given by the intramuscular route reach peak plasma concentrations after approximately 30 min. It is therefore advisable to observe the patient for up to 1 h before a further dose is administered. In the case of continuing disturbance it may be preferable to administer an adjunctive intramuscular benzodiazepine (lorazepam 2 mg) rather than a further dose of neuroleptic. After the administration of parenteral neuroleptics, pulse and blood pressure should be monitored for hypotension and arrhythmias. Attention should be paid to the possible development of acute dystonia, especially in the young and those who have not previously received neuroleptics (see below). In this case, an intramuscular anticholinergic agent such as procyclidine or orphenadrine should be given without delay.

Once the patient's behaviour has settled it is important to try to clarify the cause of the disturbance. In taking the history particular attention should be paid to:

- Past psychiatric illness and treatment.
- Use of prescription and/or illicit drugs.

Mental state and physical examinations are of particular importance in differentiating between acute psychosis and delirium. It is important to make this distinction as conditions presenting with delirium are medical emergencies in their own right and require urgent investigation and treatment. Some of the features which help to distinguish delirium from other psychoses are:

- Developing or damaged brain.
- Rapid onset.
- Prodromal physical illness (e.g. infection).
- Sleep reversal.
- Fluctuating course – worse at night.
- Impairment of attention.
- Delusions of harm by others.
- Visual illusions or hallucinations.
- Abnormal vital signs.

The presentation and management of delirium are discussed in detail in the next section.

Acute psychosis

Psychoses induced by illicit psychotropic drugs such as ecstasy, amphetamine, lysergic acid, phencyclidine and cocaine are frequently seen in inner city hospitals. It is sometimes difficult to distinguish initially between drug-induced psychosis, mania and schizophrenia. Behaviour is erratic, thinking is disordered and perceptual abnormalities may be reported in all three. A history of illicit drug-taking may be elicited from either the patient or an accompanying friend. Patients with psychoses who present with severe behavioural disturbance will almost invariably require treatment in hospital. It may be necessary to use the mental health legislation which is discussed below.

Personality disorder

The diagnosis and management of patients with personality disorders are much disputed by psychiatrists. Although sometimes difficult in practice, it is very important to set limits on behaviour which cannot be tolerated in hospital. Individual units should develop policies which are agreed and known by all staff and outside agencies, including the police. The label of 'personality disorder' may act as a barrier to proper medical and nursing care. Habitually disturbed behaviour or repeated suicidal threats may understandably result in frustration and hardened staff attitudes. This must not prevent the appropriate assessment and management of individual patients who are more liable to develop coexistent physical and psychiatric disorders. The advice of a psychiatrist is often required to decide appropriate management.

Confusion

The term 'confusion' is often applied to those patients who suffer from significant impairment of their thinking and memory. The two clinical syndromes which may present with 'confusion' are delirium (acute confusional state, toxic psychosis) and dementia. Although these syndromes may develop at any age they are most commonly seen in children (delirium) and the elderly (delirium and dementia). Two specific causes of delirium, delirium tremens and the Wernicke–Korsakoff syndrome, constitute medical emergencies.

Delirium

Lipowski (1990) has written the definitive review of delirium. The syndrome occurs most frequently in those with a developing, damaged, or deteriorating brain. Thus the extremes of age are over-represented and those with a long history of excessive alcohol consumption, a brain damaged by a previous or current cerebrovascular accident or head injury.

The clinical features of delirium were listed in the previous section. Impairment of consciousness is the cardinal feature of delirium. On a continuum ranging from full alertness to coma a mild condition may fluctuate and be characterized by distractibility and a diminished capacity to pay attention. Diminished ability to register and retain new information is characteristic. Disorientation in time and place is the commonest consequence of this and is probably the most useful clinical sign. Registration may be more formally tested by asking the patient to recall a set of digits. Retention and recall of memory may be tested by asking the patient to learn a standard piece of information (most usually a name and address) and recall it after 5 min.

Disturbance of mood is common and may dominate the presentation. Anxiety and perplexity are most common, exacerbated by illusions, hallucinations and delusions of harm. Visual disturbances including misinterpretations (illusions) and true hallucinations are characteristic, and allow provisional differentiation from schizophrenia and mania. Auditory and tactile hallucinations occur less commonly.

Causes of delirium

It is difficult to produce a comprehensive list of causes of delirium as virtually any systemic disturbance may be responsible. Table 1 lists some of the causes of delirium encountered in A&E, the most common being infections and drugs.

Management of delirium

Investigation and treatment should be directed to the underlying cause. As far as possible attempts should be made to avoid worsening the patient's confusion. They should be observed in a quiet, well-lit area. The number of different nurses and doctors dealing with the patient should be kept to a minimum. Reassurance and careful explanation are very important. If the patient is distressed or their behaviour becomes disturbed medication should

Table 1. *Common causes of delirium in A&E*

- Infections
  - Urinary tract
  - Respiratory tract
  - Septicaemia
- Drugs
  - Anticholinergics
  - Dopaminergic
- Drug withdrawal
  - Alcohol
  - Barbiturates
  - Benzodiazepines
- Trauma
  - Head injury
- Epilepsy
  - Postictal states
- Vascular
  - Transient ischaemic attack
  - Cerebrovascular accident
- Metabolic
  - Hypoglycaemia
  - Electrolyte disturbance

be used with caution. Haloperidol (0.5–5 mg) or thioridazine (10–25 mg) may be given with careful attention paid to the effect on the cardiovascular system.

Dementia

Dementia is an acquired global deterioration of intellect, memory and personality. Patients with dementia are seen frequently in A&E with coexisting physical illness or trauma, such as a fractured hip. Because of their cognitive problems these patients are difficult to assess, particularly if a collateral history is not available. A sudden deterioration in the behaviour of a patient with pre-existing dementia may indicate a superadded episode of delirium, commonly resulting from infection. This has been found in 40% of admitted patients with dementia.

Acute anxiety

Clinical features

The physical symptoms of acute anxiety are responsible for many sufferers seeking help in A&E. Panic attacks are associated with a spectrum of disorders, the most common of which are panic disorder and agoraphobia. They are characterized by intense fear accompanied by a sense of impending doom. Physical symptoms include palpitations, chest pain, choking, difficulty in breathing and light-headedness. Attacks may develop spontaneously and are always of rapid onset. Sufferers often fear that they are about to collapse, are suffering a 'heart attack' or are going to die. These 'catastrophic interpretations' of physical symptoms are thought to be partly responsible for the rapid escalation of attacks (Barlow, 1988).

Management of acute anxiety

This depends on the severity of symptoms. Careful reassurance and straightforward explanation of the diagnosis may significantly reduce symptoms and distress. However, if the patient is so distressed that any discussion of underlying problems is impossible, then immediate treatment with an anxiolytic drug is indicated. Oral administration of 10–20 mg of diazepam liquid is likely to ameliorate symptoms within 1–2 h (Pollard & Lewis, 1989). It is unlikely that symptoms will be so severe that parenteral administration is necessary. It should be remembered that individual panic attacks are self-limiting and therefore the use of benzodiazepines usually should be limited to treatment of the acute episode. If overbreathing is pronounced, particularly if it is resulting in paraesthesiae or tetany, rebreathing into a paper bag or breathing 5% carbon dioxide may rapidly improve symptoms. This technique may also demonstrate to the patient the ways in which behaviour (hyperventilation) may exacerbate symptoms. When panic attacks have been triggered by a particular situation, another simple behavioural technique used in A&E may improve the prognosis of sufferers. After careful explanation of the rationale, patients are instructed to return to the situation where the panic attack took place as soon as possible and wait there until their anxiety diminishes (Swinson *et al.*, 1992). In a similar way, exposure techniques may help to limit the development of post-traumatic stress disorder in people who have been exposed to trauma which is outside the normal range of human experience.

Stupor

Clinical features

This is a state in which the patient is apparently fully conscious but makes no spontaneous movements and little response to external stimuli (Joyston-Bechal, 1966). Purposeful eye movements may be the only indication of awareness. The self-neglect accompanying stupor of any duration may result in serious physical morbidity. Pressure sores, malnutrition, dehydration, electrolyte disturbance and orthostatic chest infection are sequelae of prolonged stupor.

Causes of stupor

Organic causes of stupor are comparatively uncommon. They include delirium, a cerebrovascular accident and raised intracranial pressure. The most common causes of stupor are depressive illness and catatonic schizophrenia. 'Psychogenic' stupor occurs but is less common. In the case of schizophrenia and mood disorders the onset of stupor is insidious and a collateral history is likely to reveal prior clear-cut mood disturbance or bizarre behaviour. 'Psychogenic' stupor is a dissociative state, usually related to a major stressful event and the onset is sudden.

Management of stupor

Careful assessment, including neurological examination and appropriate investigations, should identify an organic aetiology as well as any physical complications which may be exacerbating an apparently 'functional' state. These complications may need to be treated before definitive psychiatric management can take place.

Amnesia

The patient with apparent sudden loss of memory is uncommon and may be difficult to assess. As in the case of stupor, the first task of the physician in A&E is to identify organic aetiologies. These include head injury, delirium, postictal states and transient global amnesia. Clinical features of the underlying pathology will, in most cases, distinguish these disorders from psychogenic amnesia. Both anterograde and retrograde amnesia will usually be present in organic states, but information about personal identity will not be lost, except in the severest of cases (Kopelman, 1987).

Psychogenic amnesia is a dissociative disorder in which there is a sudden, temporary alteration in the normally integrated functions of consciousness. Fugue states, in which the patient suddenly travels or wanders away from home, often accompany amnesic episodes. Localized amnesia for a circumscribed period of time is most common and may include important personal information such as an address and telephone number.

Commonly, generalized amnesia will include all information about the individual's life. Paradoxically, common skills including reading and writing are likely to be retained. The underlying mechanisms of psychogenic amnesia are not clear but it is often associated with severe stress such as the breakdown of a personal relationship or legal problems. Dissociative states are found to be frequently complicated by an abnormal premorbid personality and abuse of alcohol. Psychogenic amnesia usually lasts only a few days, resolving as rapidly as it developed. Patients should usually be admitted to hospital to allow a more thorough assessment.

Mutism

There are two groups of patients who do not speak although they appear to be able to. Collateral history and examination will distinguish these patients from those who suffer aphasia as the result of a cerebrovascular accident.

Elective mutism of childhood

It is unlikely that this rare condition, which occurs equally in boys and girls, will be seen in A&E. It usually has an insidious onset and is often associated with other developmental problems (Kolvin & Fundundis, 1981).

Mutism associated with psychiatric illness

This form of mutism is usually associated with the states of stupor described above. It is most often found in psychotic illness, particularly in schizophrenia presenting with bizarre motor phenomena (catatonic schizophrenia). These patients will usually need admission to hospital for further assessment and treatment.

Repeat attending

A&E staff are at times frustrated by a group of patients who present repeatedly with apparently trivial complaints. The pressure of time often does not allow full assessment of underlying problems which frequently fall into two categories.

Chronic psychiatric illness

Many of these patients will not be registered with a general practitioner. They may use A&E not only as a source of primary health care but also as a refuge and a place to socialize. Their mental state should be regularly monitored in order to identify as early as possible any relapse of their condition. In addition it is recommended that A&E staff should liaise regularly with psychiatric staff.

Somatization

The core feature of this common phenomenon is that symptoms are described for which there is no sufficient underlying physical cause (Bass, 1990). It may form part of normal behaviour but is also associated with a wide range of psychiatric disorders. Although the mechanisms of somatization are not known it is often assumed that the symptoms are produced for some form of psychological gain. This assumption must be treated with particular caution when dealing with patients from other than a Western cultural background. In non-Western cultures, somatic concerns are frequently expressions of psychological distress and may be the only indication of serious psychiatric disorder. For example, the patient with 'total body pain' may be suffering a depressive illness or anxiety disorder which is likely to go unrecognized. Particularly problematic are patients with chronic physical illness such as diabetes, epilepsy or ulcerative colitis who appear to exaggerate symptoms or produce symptoms which appear to be unrelated to their primary disorder. This may be related to life problems and relationship difficulties or may indicate the development of a coexistent psychiatric disorder. Although often difficult in practice, both careful physical and psychiatric evaluation of these patients should be carried out as well as close liaison with other medical staff involved.

SPECIFIC PSYCHIATRIC DISORDERS AND THEIR MANAGEMENT IN A&E

Schizophrenia

Patients with schizophrenia may present to A&E for a wide variety of reasons including relapse, physical illness, social problems and the side-effects of drugs. The label of mental illness and the unconventional ways in which these patients can sometimes present should not be a barrier to proper assessment of their individual problems.

Acute schizophrenia

An acute episode of this condition may be the first presentation of the illness or may be the relapse of a chronic disorder. The behaviour of someone presenting to A&E with acute schizophrenia may range from apparent normality to gross disturbance, including bizarre motor phenomena (catatonia). The history is likely to reveal a gradual onset of symptoms and, in the case of relapse of a chronic illness, may be related to non-compliance with maintenance treatment. Where the presenting complaints are clearly of a delusional nature the diagnosis may be relatively easy. The patient who complains that aliens are controlling his thoughts by the use of special computers is clearly likely to be suffering a serious psychiatric illness. On the other hand, the complaints may be of a simple, physical type. The patient complaining of headache may only later reveal that he believes this to be caused by a device implanted in his head by the secret services. A careful mental state examination including direct questions will usually reveal the extent and nature of the patient's abnormal beliefs and perceptions. Management will depend on a careful consideration of the severity of the episode together with the availability of social and professional support. Patients with a first episode of psychotic illness should be admitted to allow for the thorough assessment of what is potentially a lifelong illness.

Chronic schizophrenia

Perhaps the most disabling aspect of the chronic illness is the so-called negative symptoms which led to the disorder being named 'dementia praecox'. The patient loses his drive and motivation and, with this, his capacity to organize his life effectively. His emotional range is blunted and the content and quality of his thoughts and speech are diminished, preferring his own company to that of others. Self-neglect, significant social problems and physical morbidity are commonly associated with this stage of the illness (Kendell, 1988).

Depressive illness

Depression is a cause of significant unrecognized morbidity in medical practice as well as in the community, where the prevalence is at least 5% (Angst, 1992). A&E staff should be particularly aware of its clinical features and the different ways in which depression can present.

Clinical features of depressive illness

A lowering of mood is the cardinal feature of a depressive illness. The patient takes a gloomy view of himself and the world around him. This is often accompanied by a loss of energy and drive. Appetite is diminished and as a result there may be a significant loss of weight. The pattern of sleep may be disturbed throughout the night. Motor behaviour may vary from retardation to agitation. The patient has difficulty in concentrating on everyday tasks and his thoughts are taken up with pessimistic themes. Hopeless thoughts about the future are frequently expressed. Accompanying these, patients may harbour suicidal thoughts which vary from wishing that they were dead to actively planning suicide.

Management of depressive illness in A&E

The most important aspect of the assessment is to judge severity, in particular the risk of suicide. It is mistakenly believed that questioning about suicide will implant the idea in the mind of the patient. This is not the case and it is imperative that all patients with depression are asked sensitively about morbid and suicidal thoughts. Other important information to elicit at this stage should include contact with other professionals (e.g. general practitioner or social worker) as well as family and social support available. The management of all patients with severe depressive illness should be discussed with psychiatric staff or the general practitioner. Admission to hospital should be considered in the following circumstances:

- Active suicidal thinking.
- Delusions and/or hallucinations.
- Severe physical self-neglect.
- Social isolation.

Post-traumatic stress disorder

Post-traumatic stress disorder may develop in any individual who has been exposed to trauma that is outside the range of normal human experiences. Incidents such as sexual and physical assaults, 'natural' disasters and road traffic accidents are common precipitants for the syndrome whose onset is sometimes delayed by several months. It should be remembered that not only victims but also witnesses of a particularly horrific incident may suffer from the disorder. This includes medical and nursing staff, particularly if they attended the scene of the incident. Anxiety, hypervigilance, insomnia, nightmares and flashbacks are the core features of the syndrome. Fear of a repeat of the incident leads to avoidance which may in itself become disabling. For example, the

victim of a road traffic accident may be unable to drive or even travel in a car. 'Flashbacks' or sudden powerful recollections or images of the original incident are intrusive and distressing. Sleep is frequently disturbed and accompanied by vivid nightmares of the incident (Ramsay, 1990).

Post-traumatic stress disorder is more likely to occur in people with a prolonged exposure to the trauma and where the trauma is extraordinary. There is some evidence that early intervention may help to limit the frequency and severity of post-traumatic psychological morbidity. Counselling takes the form of debriefing, encouraging victims to relive the event in detail and facilitating the expression of their feelings. Major incident policies should include provision for coordinating counselling services from the hospital, social services and voluntary agencies (Rosser et al., 1991). Victims should not leave A&E without a short leaflet explaining the symptoms of post-traumatic stress disorder, and how to get help. If a major incident, with an attendant counselling programme, is not declared the patient's general practitioner should be informed.

Management of rape victims by all staff in A&E should pay special attention to the psychological consequences which include the development of post-traumatic stress disorder. Important aspects include careful explanation of the interview, examination and necessary investigations (Martin et al., 1983). The patient should be encouraged to talk through the experience with a close friend or counsellor and be given written information about local rape victim support organizations.

Victims of repeated physical or sexual abuse deserve careful management. They should be referred to a social worker and their case discussed with their general practitioner.

Eating disorders

The two eating disorders anorexia nervosa and bulimia nervosa involve pathological attitudes to food and body shape and weight. Anorexia nervosa is characterized by a morbid fear of fatness and an overestimation of body weight. This results in starvation causing marked weight loss (15–20% below that expected for the individual's age, sex and height) and amenorrhoea. Sufferers use a number of ways of controlling their weight. They will not only diet to extreme but exercise excessively and may abuse laxatives and diuretics. Patients with anorexia may therefore have a number of physical complications. At the most severe stage, collapse may result from cardiac arrhythmia, hypotension, cardiac failure, hypo-thermia or hypoglycaemia. If the body mass ratio (Quetelet Index: weight in kilograms, divided by the height in metres squared) is less than 15, an urgent combined psychiatric and medical opinion is required.

Bulimia nervosa may occur comorbidly with anorexia nervosa, although usually they occur separately. The patient's eating is chaotic. Bulimic episodes of gross overeating are followed by purging and self-induced vomiting. The sufferer's weight is often normal or fluctu-ant and they have fewer physical complications than those with anorexia. Intermittent oedema, lethargy and abdominal pain are frequently encountered but are rarely of serious consequence. Hypokalaemia should be ex-cluded. Regurgitation of acidic gastric contents may lead to severe dental erosions and caries, especially on the dorsal aspects of the upper teeth. Calluses may be present on the dorsum of the first and second fingers, from inducing vomiting (Russell, 1983).

Anorexia nervosa or bulimia nervosa should be con-sidered in women who repeatedly present to A&E with minor gastrointestinal complaints, especially when there is significant weight loss. These patients will often not disclose their underlying problem, particularly when they are abusing laxatives, and may react dramatically to confrontation. Discussion with their general practitioner is often worthwhile. Patients with eating disorders should be referred to the appropriate psychiatric service for out-patient treatment except where physical complica-tions or weight loss are of a severity which warrant medical admission.

Somatoform disorders

These are a heterogeneous group of disorders in which the patient presents with physical symptoms for which there is insufficient explanatory physical pathology. They include conversion and dissociative disorders, previously described as hysterical disorders, as well as hypochondriasis (overvalued self-belief that the patient is suffering from a physical disease) and psychogenic pain. Somatization disorder (Briquet's syndrome) is a cause of repeated A&E attendance. This condition describes a lifetime illness career of multiple and different physical complaints for which there is no physical explanation (Bass, 1990).

The aetiology of these disorders is complex but it has long been recognized that they are frequently associated with both organic and other psychiatric disorders. For this reason, a careful physical and psychiatric assessment is mandatory in these cases. Most patients with a somatoform disorder present to specialists or to their general practitioner. Occasionally a patient with the acute onset of a conversion disorder such as an 'hysteri-cal' hemiplegia may present to A&E. There is evidence that early intervention is important for a good prognosis. Close liaison between physicians and psychiatrists is essential from the outset.

Factitious disorders

These are conditions in which the patient deliberately produces symptoms of physical or psychiatric illnesses. Sufferers have an overwhelming need to assume the sick role and this may be related to unmet dependency needs early in life because of parental neglect or abuse. Patients are often young women who may work in the caring professions, getting the personal approval and warmth they previously lacked. This heterogeneous group of disorders includes some cases of 'brittle' diabetes, feigned unconsciousness, dermatitis artefacta and factitious py-rexia. Patient's with Munchausen's syndrome or 'hospital addiction' repeatedly present with an apparent medical or surgical emergency, such as an acute abdomen (Asher, 1951). The presentation is dramatic, often very realistic and they may even undergo surgery. They frequently attend numerous different hospitals, do not live locally, assume aliases, and have either no general practitioner or a fictitious one. Comparatively little is known about the aetiology of the disorder but it most commonly presents in socially isolated men with disturbed personali-ties. Confrontation usually results in rapid self-discharge. Patients will rarely agree to a psychiatric assessment. A variant of the medical or surgical presentation is the patient who reports psychiatric symptoms, including perceptual disturbances and suicide intent, in order to gain admission to a psychiatric hospital. They may describe complicated life stories, sometimes involving murders and multiple accidents killing close relatives. It is usually impossible to obtain corroborative histories.

More recently, attention has been drawn to women who repeatedly seek medical attention for their children by inducing physical illness in them (see Chapter 61). This is known as 'Munchausen's syndrome by proxy' (Meadow, 1977). It is a complex and potentially very serious disorder and when recognized demands careful but urgent intervention. Admission of the child to a paediatric ward is a necessary first step to allow further assessment of the child and relative.

These disorders are a source of considerable frustration in A&E departments and are all difficult to manage. The most important aspect of management is close liaison with all the agencies involved with the patient. Confrontation in the A&E department should only occur for Munchausen's syndrome. For this disorder, many departments keep a confidential 'frequent attender file' with physical and behavioural descriptions of patients. Information from these files is circulated among different hospitals.

Malingering

Patients may be regarded as malingering when they deliberately produce symptoms for an easily identifiable goal. For example, pethidine addicts may feign the symptoms of renal colic. The reasons for malingering are diverse. In reality there is no clear-cut distinction between these patients and those with factitious disorders. The underlying motivation in both groups is often mixed and poorly understood by patients and their doctors.

SIDE-EFFECTS OF PSYCHOTROPIC MEDICATION

An increasing number of drugs are being used to treat mental illness. Troublesome side-effects are associated with the majority of these and they may be sufficiently severe to result in presentation to A&E. The sometimes bizarre nature of these side-effects may result in their being mistakenly attributed to the mental illness itself (Silverstone & Turner, 1988).

Neuroleptic drugs

Drugs used in the treatment of schizophrenia have a wide range of side-effects. The most common and potentially most distressing are caused by the blockade of central dopamine receptors.

Acute dystonia

This reaction to neuroleptic drugs usually occurs shortly after starting treatment. It may present as an oculogyric crisis, protrusion of the tongue, opisthotonos or torticollis. The patient is usually very distressed and therefore unable to describe the problem. This, together with the bizarre nature of the symptoms, may lead to misdiagnosis. Acute dystonic reactions should be treated promptly with an anticholinergic drug given intramuscularly (e.g. procyclidine 5–10 mg). This dose may need to be repeated after half an hour.

Pseudoparkinson's syndrome

This extrapyramidal syndrome may also develop in the early stages of treatment. It has many features in common with Parkinson's disease, in particular rigidity, akinesia and a 'pill-rolling' tremor. It is caused by dopamine blockade in the basal ganglia and is treated with anticholinergic drugs (e.g. procyclidine or orphenadrine) as well as considering a reduction of the dose of neuroleptic.

Akathisia

The patient experiences an uncomfortable motor restlessness which may result in an inability to sit still, constant movement in the lower limbs and tense muscles. This is a particularly distressing side-effect which may be difficult to treat. The dose of neuroleptic should be reviewed by the psychiatrist or general practitioner and specific treatment given with propranolol or a benzodiazepine.

Neuroleptic malignant syndrome

This underestimated disorder consists of hyerpyrexia and autonomic instability together with severe muscular rigidity. It is thought to arise as an idiosyncratic reaction to antidopaminergic drugs, in the presence of comorbid factors such as infection or dehydration. Mortality rates of 20% have been reported for this medical emergency. Supportive measures such as rehydration and cooling are vital. Admission to the intensive care unit is often needed for muscle paralysis and supported ventilation. Specific treatment with the dopamine agonist bromocriptine and the muscle uncoupling agent dantrolene sodium may be necessary (Sakkas et al., 1991).

Antidepressants

The most commonly prescribed antidepressants form part of the group known as monoamine reuptake inhibitors. The majority of these have a wide range of side-effects, the most frequent of which are related to their anticholinergic action. Dry mouth, tremor and blurred vision are common complaints. Related acute urinary retention and severe constipation may cause the patient to attend A&E. In these circumstances it may be necessary to stop the medication after consultation with a psychiatrist or the general practitioner. A newer class of antidepressants, selective serotonin reuptake inhibitors, is more frequently being prescribed. The most frequent side-effects associated with these drugs are nausea, vomiting and headache.

The tyramine or 'cheese' reaction is a potentially serious consequence of interactions with the monoamine oxidase inhibitor class of antidepressants. Peripheral inhibition of monoamine oxidase prevents the metabolism of tyramine. The interaction with tyramine-rich foods or certain drugs may therefore lead to a dramatic rise in blood pressure presenting as a pounding headache. For mild elevations of blood pressure, treatment with a calcium antagonist may be effective. For more severe reactions, intravenous phentolamine should be used with close monitoring.

Lithium

Lithium preparations are prescribed for the prophylaxis of recurrent mood disorders, particularly bipolar mood disorder (manic-depressive psychosis). Patients taking lithium may experience a wide range of side-effects which include a fine tremor, polyuria and polydipsia, sleepiness, nausea, diarrhoea, and a metallic taste. Lithium toxicity requires urgent intervention. Serum lithium levels of between 1.5 and 2.0 mmol l^{-1} cause diarrhoea and vomiting, a coarse tremor, ataxia, dysarthria and drowsiness. A serum level above 2 mmol l^{-1} causes impairment of consciousness and seizures. Toxicity may be precipitated by dehydration as a result of physical illness (commonly infection) or interaction with other drugs such as diuretics and non-steroidal anti-inflammatory agents. In the earliest stages of toxicity, rehydration, treatment of the precipitating cause, and temporarily stopping lithium may be sufficient. Specific treatment is with saline infusion and osmotic diuretics. In the most severe cases haemodialysis may be necessary.

Anxiolytics

The benzodiazepines are widely prescribed as hypnotics and anxiolytics. In overdosage, a toxic syndrome may develop with features of delirium. Falls and subsequent fractures in the elderly may partially result from overuse of benzodiazepines. There is increasing awareness of a sometimes severe withdrawal syndrome which may develop after abrupt cessation of treatment. Symptoms include irritability, anxiety, insomnia with nightmares and perceptual disturbances, especially skin sensitivity (Ashton 1986).

MENTAL HEALTH LEGISLATION

Patients may sometimes require admission to hospital against their will. In England and Wales the 1983 Mental Health Act provides for the compulsory admission, detention and treatment of patients with mental disorders. This includes mental illness, mental impairment (learning difficulties), and psychopathic disorder (personality disorder) which results in 'abnormally aggressive or seriously irresponsible conduct'. Legislation can only be invoked when the patient is unwilling to be admitted or detained in hospital voluntarily and it is judged that detention is in the interests of the patient's health or safety, or for the protection of others (Bluglass, 1983). It should be remembered that the Mental Health Act is only of relevance when the patient is suffering a mental disorder and may not be used to admit or treat a patient with physical illnesses. The only exception to this is when the mental disorder is the result of a physical illness, most commonly delirium. Intoxication or misuse of drugs or alcohol is not considered to be a mental disorder under the terms of the Mental Health Act. Only a small proportion of mental health legislation is relevant to A&E staff. Table 2 shows the relevant sections of the Mental Health Act (1983) (England and Wales) and their equivalents in the Mental Health (Scotland) Act (1984) and the Mental Health (Northern Ireland) Order (1986).

Section 136: police powers

This section authorizes the police to remove to a place of safety anyone in a public place who is judged to be suffering a mental disorder and is in immediate need of care and control. The order lasts for 72 h and the person must be assessed by an approved social worker and a registered doctor. The designated 'place of safety' varies locally and may often be the A&E department.

Table 2. *Mental health legislation in the UK*

England and Wales (1983)	Scotland (1984)	Northern Ireland (1986)
Section 4	Section 24	Article 4[a]
Section 2	Section 26	
Section 136	Section 118[c]	Article 130[b]

[a] Admission for assessment for 48 h or 7 days if recommendation is by an approved doctor.
[b] 48 h.
[c] 72 h.

Section 4: emergency admission

The powers of admission under Section 4 may be invoked when the situation is considered to be an emergency and fulfilment of the requirements of Sections 2 or 3 would involve unnecessary delay. There is only one recommendation which may be made by any medical practitioner. This should preferably be a doctor with previous knowledge of the patient, but urgent circumstances may require this to be the A&E officer. The application is made by an approved social worker or the nearest relative who should have seen the patient within the last 24 h. This is clearly a difficult and important management decision to take and, where possible, guidance should be sought from the local psychiatrist. As soon as is practical the patient must be reassessed to consider further detention. This is usually under Section 2.

Section 2: admission for assessment and treatment

This allows for compulsory admission for assessment and treatment for up to 28 days. Two medical recommendations are required, one of which should be by a doctor approved under Section 12 of the Act. In hospital practice this usually implies a psychiatrist at senior registrar grade and above. The other recommendation should preferably be made by a doctor with prior knowledge of the patient who does not work in the same unit as the first. This usually means the general practitioner. The application is made by an approved social worker or nearest relative.

Section 3: admission for treatment

The requirements for the recommendations and application are the same as for Section 2. Section 3 allows for admission for treatment of a mental disorder for up to 6 months in the first instance. Section 3 is usually only used when the patient and diagnosis are known and it is less often used in emergency situations.

Section 5(2): detention of a patient already in hospital

This allows a patient who is already admitted to hospital to be detained for up to 72 h. The recommendation is made by the doctor responsible for the patient or their nominated deputy. It is important to remember that a patient attending an A&E department is not legally regarded as being admitted to hospital and, therefore, may not be detained using Section 5(2).

CONCLUSION

A&E staff will increasingly be called upon to assess and provide primary care for patients with psychiatric disorders or emotional distress. Taking a history, with corroboration, a mental state examination, and asking for advice if unsure, will enable the doctor in A&E to be confident of providing professional help to a much neglected group of patients.

Bibliography

ANGST, J. (1992). Epidemiology of depression. *Psychopharmacology*, **106** (Suppl.), 71–4.

ASHER, R. (1951), Munchausen's syndrome. *Lancet*, **i**, 339–41.

ASHTON, H. (1986). Adverse effects of prolonged benzodiazepine use. *Adverse Drug React. Bull.*, **118**, 440–43.

BARLOW, D.H. (1988). *Anxiety and Its Disorders: The Nature and Treatment of Anxiety and Panic*. New York: Guildford Press.

BASS, C.M., ed. (1990). *Somatization: Physical Symptoms and Psychological Illness*. Oxford: Blackwell Scientific.

BELL, G., HINDLEY, N., RAJIYAH, G., *et al.* (1990). Screening for psychiatric morbidity in an accident and emergency department. *Arch. Emerg. Med.*, **7**, 155–62.

BLUGLASS, R. (1983). *A Guide to the Mental Health Act 1983*. London: Churchill Livingstone.

BROWN, T.M., SCOTT, A.I.F. & PULLEN, I.M. (1990). *Handbook of Emergency Psychiatry*. Edinburgh: Churchill Livingstone.

DUBIN, W.R. (1988). Rapid tranquillization: antipsychotics or benzodiazepines? *J. Clin. Psychiatry*, **49** (Suppl. 12), 5–11.

JOYSTON-BECHAL, M.P. (1966). The clinical features and outcome of stupor. *Br. J. Psychiatry*, **112**, 967–81.

KENDELL, R.E. (1988). Schizophrenia. In *Companion to Psychiatric Studies*, R.E. Kendell & A.K. Zealey. ed. pp. 310–34. Edinburgh: Churchill Livingstone.

KOLVIN. I. &. FUNDUNDIS, T. (1981). Elective mute children: psychological development and background factors. *J. Child Psychol. Psychiatry*, **22**, 219.

KOPELMAN, M.D. (1987). Amnesia: organic and psychogenic. *Br. J. Psychiatry*, **150**, 428–42.

LIPOWSKI, Z.J. (1990). *Delirium: Acute Confusional States*. New York: Oxford University Press.

MARSHALL, E.J. & REED, J.L. (1992). Psychiatric morbidity in homeless women. *Br. J. Psychiatry*, **160**, 761–8.

MARTIN, C.A., WARFIELD, M.C. & BRAEN, G.R. (1983). Physician's management of the psychological aspects of rape. *JAMA*, **249**, 501–3.

MEADOW, R. (1977). Munchausen syndrome by proxy: the hinterland of child abuse. *Lancet* **ii**, 343–5.

POLLARD, C.A. & LEWIS, L.M. (1989). Managing panic attacks in emergency patients. *Curr. Pract. Emerg. Med.*, **7**, 547–52.

RAMSAY, R. (1990). Post-traumatic stress disorder; a new clinical entity? *J. Psychosom. Res.*, **34**, 355–65.

ROSSER, R., DEWAR, S. & THOMPSON, J. (1991). Psychological aftermath of the King's Cross fire. *J. R. Soc. Med.*, **84**, 4–8.

RUSSELL, G.F.M. (1983). Anorexia nervosa and bulimia nervosa. In *Handbook of Psychiatry*, Vol. 4, ed. G.F.M. Russell & L. Hersov. *The Neuroses and Personality Disorders.* pp. 285–98. Cambridge: Cambridge University Press.

SAKKAS, P., DAVIS, J.M., JANICAK, P.G. *et al.*

(1991). Drug treatment of the neuroleptic malignant syndrome. *Psychopharmacol. Bull.*, **27**, 381–4.

SILVERSTONE, T. & TURNER, P. (1988). *Drug Treatment in Psychiatry*. London: Routledge.

SILVERSTONE, T. & WHITE, P.D. (1992). Management of the acutely disturbed patient. *Postgrad. Update*, **1**, 842–8.

SWINSON, R.P., SOULIOS, C., COX, B.J. *et al.* (1992). Brief treatment of emergency room patients with panic attacks. *Am. J. Psychiatry*, **129**, 944–6.

55 Deliberate self-harm and substance misuse

C.V.R. BLACKER[a] and B. CHARNAUD[b]

[a] Cornwall Healthcare Trust, Royal Cornwall Hospital, Truro, UK
[b] Trengweath Mental Health Unit, Redruth, UK

Chapter plan

Introduction
Deliberate self-harm
Substance misuse
Appendix

INTRODUCTION

Patients who harm themselves, threaten to harm themselves or have histories of self-harming behaviour commonly present to accident and emergency (A&E) departments. So do those who abuse substances – including alcohol and illicit drugs. A&E departments are also the medical (and social) port of call for large numbers of persons with psychiatric disorders, especially those with chronic psychotic disorders and personality disorders, many of whom are indigenous or not in contact with existing medical and social services. Finally, A&E departments are the port of call for many persons in social crises of one kind or another who are not necessarily mentally ill but are nonetheless seeking help. Not surprisingly, there are large areas of overlap between these populations.

A few studies have attempted to estimate prevalence rates for these populations of patients, but they are conditioned by their geographical setting. For example, in inner-city A&E departments one normally finds proportionally more patients with psychotic disorders and substance abuse disorders because these disorders are more common in urban, city and inner-city areas.

Bell *et al.* (1991) and Salkovskis *et al.* (1990) both report a prevalence rate of 37% for all psychiatric disorders in A&E attenders in city-based hospitals. This rate is high and clearly demonstrates that, for the smooth running of A&E departments, staff benefit from familiarity with the basic management of the commoner forms of mental illness.

In most A&E departments access to psychiatric assistance is via a junior doctor on call; only occasionally are additional staff and resources (such as psychiatric nurses) available and then only usually on a p.r.n. (as required) basis. Few departments as yet have fully established psychiatric liaison services and until they do it is probably more realistic to provide basic guidelines around which can be wrapped the details relevant to the local situation so that each department has its own policies. This is the rationale for the present chapter.

DELIBERATE SELF-HARM

Actual self-harm

Deliberate self-harm is responsible for approximately 100 000 admissions (or 10% of all acute medical admissions) per annum in the UK (Office of Health Economics, 1991). Most of these come through A&E departments and/or admissions units. The majority are admitted to medical wards but around 15% are sent home directly from A&E. There are some signs of a decline in rates of self-harm nationally, but the rate for suicide, especially in young males, is increasing and, after road traffic accidents, is now the second commonest form of death in that age group. Patients who harm themselves are also at risk from other problems such as mental illness, drug and alcohol abuse, violence to self or others, or social crises of one kind or another. This means that it is important that these patients are adequately assessed. Of prime importance in the assessment is the issue of suicide risk, especially when considering whether to allow them to return home. These patients also have a right to be assessed and offered help from the social and psychiatric point of view. This can be done by duty social workers and psychiatrists. A&E medical and nursing staff should

```
NAME = _____

Age = _____ Sex _____ Date = _____

Name of GP = _____

Other individual professionals = _____

Describe the attempt, the method used, how "dangerous" in your
estimation it was, and any other relevant medical information

_____

_____

1.   Why did they do it?_____

2.   Was the act premeditated or impulsive? _____

3.   Did the patient intend to die? _____

4.   Did the patient intend to be discovered? _____

5.   Is there continuing suicidal intent? _____

6.   Has the precipitating crisis resolved? _____

7.   What are the patient's social circumstances and
     potential support? _____

     _____

8.   Are there any young children at home who might be at
     risk? _____

9.   How hopeless are they? _____

10.  How many times have they harmed themselves before? ____

11.  Is there a family history of suicide ? _____

12.  What are the main psychiatric symptoms (if any)? _____

     _____

     _____

13.  Do they currently have a problem with Alcohol or Drug
     Abuse ? _____

14.  Is this, in your opinion, a "high" or "low" risk case?
     (all high risks should be seen by a psychiatrist) _____

     _____

15.  Indicate follow-up:  GP ___   Medical Social Worker ____

     Community Social Services _____

     Psych. outpatient app _____

     Immediate psychiatric opinion _____

     Day Centre/Community Care Team _____

     Other (please specify) _____

     _____
```

(a)

Fig. 1. Deliberate Self Harm Assessment Form (Blacker *et al.*, 1992).

conduct a preliminary enquiry by asking the patient about their social circumstances, the circumstances of the overdose and by making a brief examination of the mental state. This will at least identify the patients who are most at risk and determine the right course of action should the patient suddenly decide to leave.

There are positive advantages in A&E staff involvement in this area:

- A speedier decision regarding the most appropriate form of disposal can be reached.

- Potentially difficult situations can be anticipated (e.g. whether to call in the social worker/police/psychiatrist now or wait until the patient, fed-up with waiting, is already half-way through the door).

- Staff become more adept at spotting the high-risk cases.

- Experience usually begets confidence and a reduction in fear and hostile attitudes (which only lead to mutual antagonism and unnecessary unpleasantness).

For A&E junior doctors their last brush with psychiatry

```
┌─────────────────────────────────────────────────────────────────────┐
│ GUIDELINES FOR ASSESSMENT AND REFERRAL OF DELIBERATE SELF-HARM        │
│                                                                       │
│ 1.  Identify the precipitating cause and assess the degree of suicidal│
│     intent ..                                                         │
│                                                                       │
│        .. was there a clear precipitant?                              │
│        .. was the act premeditated or impulsive?                      │
│        .. what was the patient's state of mind at the time?           │
│        .. did they take steps not to be discovered?                   │
│        .. was anyone expected to appear/return home?                  │
│        .. was the attempt in familiar or unfamiliar surroundings?     │
│        .. did they leave a suicide note?                              │
│        .. how did this attempt come to light?  Did they summon help   │
│           themselves?                                                 │
│        .. is there continuing suicidal intent?                        │
│                                                                       │
│                                                                       │
│ 2.  Mental State Examination                                          │
│                                                                       │
│        .. does the patient have any psychiatric symptoms?             │
│        .. does the patient have a history of psychiatric disorder?    │
│        .. have they harmed themselves before?                         │
│        .. do they have a problem with alcohol/drugs?                  │
│        .. are they expressing hopelessness?                           │
│                                                                       │
│                                                                       │
│ 3.  Other relevant factors                                            │
│                                                                       │
│        .. has anyone in the family taken their life?                  │
│        .. what is their social support system like?                   │
│        .. has the precipitating crisis resolved since admission?      │
│        .. what have they done to help themselves?                     │
│        .. do they have a physical illness?                            │
│        .. if young female, are there children at home who might be at │
│           risk?                                                       │
│                                                                       │
│                                                                       │
│ INDICATIONS FOR PSYCHIATRIC REFERRAL                                  │
│                                                                       │
│ = Clinical Depression present                                         │
│ = Psychosis (delusions/hallucinations/bizarre behaviour etc)          │
│ = Evidence of clear premeditation or continuing suicidal intent       │
│   (the more detailed the plans the more serious the risk)             │
│ = Violent method chosen                                               │
│ = Alcoholics and Drug Addicts                                         │
│ = Older (over 45) and younger (under 16) age                          │
│ = Serious or chronic physical illness present                         │
│ = Those in a major life crisis which has not yet resolved             │
│ = DSH recidivists and those who have harmed themselves recently       │
│ = Any patient who gives you, the nurses or the family cause for concern│
│                                                                       │
│ If possible, always try to speak to a member of the family or other   │
│ close associate and check the details with them.   Always telephone the│
│ GP for further information and advice.  If you decide not to make an   │
│ immediate psychiatric referral consider alternative options e.g. Social│
│ Services, GP, Day Centre, routine Psychiatric Outpatients or Samaritans│
│ Befriending Scheme.  Either way patients should always be advised to   │
│ consult their GP after discharge and to return to casualty for         │
│ psychiatric assessment if things deteriorate.  It can be helpful to give│
│ the patient a relevant contact telephone number to take with them in  │
│ case of a further crisis.                                             │
└─────────────────────────────────────────────────────────────────────┘
```

(b)

Fig. 1. *Continued*

was during their medical student training. In addition, time is in short supply in A&E. For this reason it is not expected that these psychosocial assessments should be as long or as comprehensive as those taught on psychiatric firms in medical school. With these problems in mind the best way to make sure that the essential elements of assessment are covered is to provide junior doctors with written guidelines such as the Deliberate Self-Harm Assessment Form (Fig. 1), which was developed and validated at St. Bartholomew's Hospital (Blacker *et al.*, 1992). This form is now in use in a number of hospitals in the UK. Although designed originally for use by junior physicians on medical wards, it is just as effective in A&E and admissions units. On side 1 of the form (Fig. 1a) are written guidelines specifying the various factors that contribute to the assessment of 'risk'. Side 2 (Fig. 1b) specifies the key questions that should be asked in such an interview. The form is self-explanatory and, providing that the patient is cooperative, or not too drowsy or intoxicated to answer the questions, takes approximately 10 min to complete. Patients are categorized into one of only two groups: 'high-risk' and 'low-risk'. This is deliberate because it reflects the clinical dilemma that underlies all questions to do with deliberate self-harm, i.e. should the patient be allowed home? All such decisions are binary and to write 'medium' in that space introduces an unnecessary complication. In cases of doubt, such patients automatically become high-risk and appropriate action is taken. It is the *nature* of that action that the remainder of the chapter addresses.

The policy of most hospitals in this country is that patients presenting to hospital following an act of deliberate self-harm are admitted for observation, assessment and treatment. This is usually to a medical ward, although some hospitals have overnight-stay or observation wards. In three-quarters of cases admission is usually a fairly straightforward procedure and A&E staff do not need to pursue management far beyond the immediate medical care of the patient. However, in some cases the patient is reluctant to go into hospital or refuses to accept treatment. The decision of what to do next tends to depend solely upon the question of the 'medical lethality' (e.g. paracetamol level) of what the patient took or did. Such assessments are often unreliable because patients may fail to declare other medication they have taken, they may underestimate or deny the number of tablets they took and there are uncertain interactions between medication and alcohol, the effects of which may take time to develop. In addition, the patient may have other supplies at home. The decision whether or not to let the patient go home after presenting with an overdose is therefore difficult and there are good grounds for admitting all patients for observation overnight in the first instance. So, what if the patient refuses? Guidelines such as those in the Appendix and Fig. 2 may well prove useful.

The Mental Health Act (UK)

The disturbed, violent or suicidal patient presents special problems to the A&E department. Not all patients are there voluntarily and some have been brought in by police or relatives and are unwilling to accept examination, assessment or treatment. Such patients are not deemed to have been formally admitted to hospital and thus Sections 5(2) or 5(4) cannot be employed.

If the situation warrants it and emergency treatment is necessary to save life, to prevent a serious incident or a serious deterioration in health, then treatment should be given under 'common law' with the guiding principle that one is seen to be acting in the patient's best interests. Likewise, patients who are at risk medically or psychiatrically and who are unwilling to stay to be assessed should be detained under 'common law' until such time

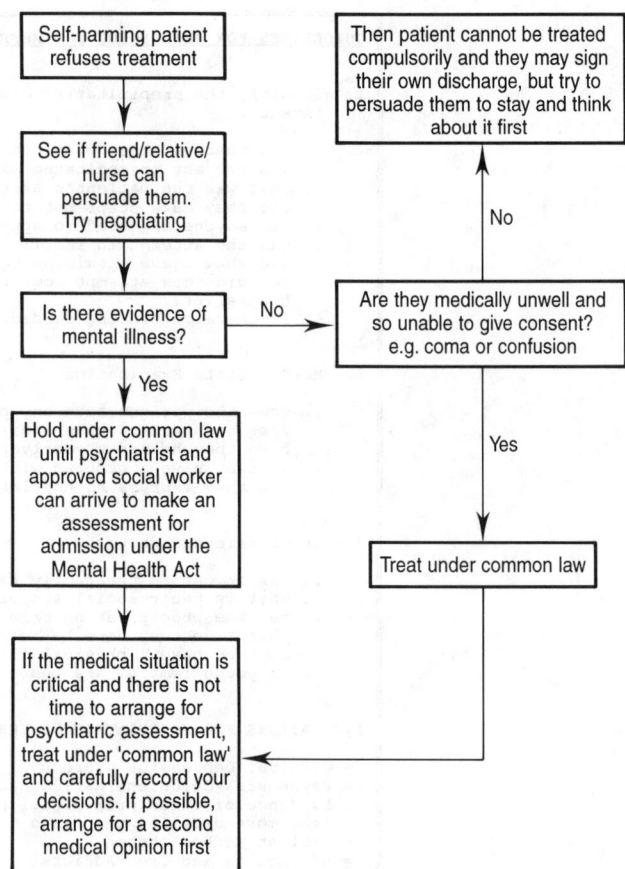

Fig. 2. Guidelines for the management of the deliberate self harm patient who refuses treatment.

as they can be assessed by those with responsibility under the mental Health Act. In extreme circumstances where it is known that the patient has a mental illness and a psychiatrist is not readily available, the use of an emergency section (Section 4 involving a senior doctor plus a social worker) may be appropriate.

In every department there should be a flowchart to assist A&E and junior psychiatric staff with the correct procedures to be followed. There should also be clarification with regards to the powers under Section 136.

In view of the increasing violence towards medical staff, it should also be mandatory for all A&E and psychiatric liaison staff to receive regular training in the use of control and restraint techniques.

Threatened self-harm

Many patients with depression, panic attacks, alcohol dependence, personality disorder and those in social and relationship crises experience suicidal thoughts. A proportion declare them to the doctor or nurse. In some cases the concern is genuine; in others the threat of self-harm has a more manipulative tone. There is no hard-and-fast way to deal with this but the following suggestions may be helpful. Much depends upon the patient and whether they are well known to the department or the psychiatric team.

A typical kind of patient who makes repeated suicide attempts or threats is the person with borderline personality or other kind of personality disorder. These patients are very difficult to handle and A&E staff should not be left to carry the responsibility for deciding what to do. Such patients require a coordinated, planned, multi-departmental, multidisciplinary treatment strategy – copies of which should be held in A&E for future occasions. This will stipulate who should be called, whether there is a risk of violence, and whether the patient should be 'sectioned'. Less well-known patients who make suicide threats are probably best taken at face value and a psychiatric opinion obtained. Patients who are intoxicated are a particularly difficult group to assess: the presence of alcohol is well recognized as facilitating suicide attempts, but equally it makes a reliable mental state examination difficult. In such cases it is probably wise to admit the patient for observation until they are sober and they can be assessed properly. Such patients will need regular observations.

Management of deliberate self-harm

Once equipped with the appropriate skills, instruments and confidence, the management of deliberate self-harm can be rewarding. The purpose of this chapter is to make things less difficult for all concerned by providing a model for the quick and smooth processing of these patients. We recommend supplementing these guidelines with DSH Assessment Forms, flowcharts on noticeboards and regular teaching, debriefing and feedback from the local psychiatric team. Ideally, district general hospitals should have a designated consultant psychiatrist with responsibility for overseeing the deliberate self-harm patients. A&E departments should also have a designated psychiatric team with whom they can liaise on a 'cold' as well as 'hot' basis. Regular review of those patients who are discharged home directly from the A&E department, guidelines and policies from the local psychiatric teams on what to do with known recidivists and operational policies for the management of violence should be in place. The remaining patients who threaten suicide can be assessed using the DSH Assessment Form which, although pertaining to completed overdoses, nonetheless covers most of the points that determine suicide risk.

In all cases it is essential that the A&E officer records his/her opinion, details of the examination and the reasons for the course of action they subsequently follow. This is not only good clinical practice but it has important and protective medicolegal functions as well.

SUBSTANCE MISUSE

Patients who misuse drugs and present to A&E usually fall into one of two categories:

1. Those who present as a result of the unwanted effects of the drug they are taking (including overdoses – accidental or intended).
2. Those requesting further prescriptions for their drug of abuse (including those experiencing withdrawal symptoms).

The unwanted effects of these drugs can be subdivided into psychological/psychiatric and physical sequelae and further subdivided in terms of their short- or long-term effects and the dose (or doses) of drug(s) which have been taken. Generally speaking, the effects of most drugs of abuse are considered desirable by those who take them whereas the symptoms associated with overdose or excessive use are not (see Table 1).

The commonest drugs of abuse in the UK are opioids and amphetamines, but it is important to recognize that the majority of addicts and regular users take multiple drugs simultaneously in order to trade the effects of one drug off against another. Thus, benzodiazepines are used extensively, often in very high doses, to come down from the 'highs' associated with stimulants, or to self-medicate against the insomnia associated with stimulants and opioids. Many addicts who use benzodiazepines in this way do not regard them as part of their habit and therefore fail to acknowledge that they are taking them unless asked. Generally speaking, patients who present requesting further prescriptions overestimate the dose of drug they normally take and a more accurate picture can be gained by enquiring how much they actually spend on their habit.

Many drug users have underlying personality disorders, low self-esteem, and have come from damaging backgrounds where they have been subject to considerable trauma and abuse, and they therefore have a high incidence of deliberate self-harm. Depression (either chronic or acute) is also common in these patients and in those who misuse drugs. Intentional drug overdoses

Table 1. *Effects of illicit drugs*

Effects	Effects in excess	Effects in withdrawal
Amphetamines		
Stimulant	Pyrexia	Lethargy
Increased confidence	Tachycardia	Low mood
Wakefulness/insomnia	Weight loss	Depression following prolonged use
Appetite suppressant	Anorexia	Exhaustion
Sociability	Chronic anxiety	Tension
	Paranoia: abnormal suspiciousness and aggression	Craving
	Hallucinations	
	Amphetamine psychosis, often when in combination with alcohol or benzodiazepines	
Amyl/butyl nitrates ('Poppers' or 'Rush')		
Short-acting stimulant	Overstimulation of the heart	No physiological effect
Euphoria	Vasodilatation and collapse	
Light-headedness	Vomiting	
	Headaches	
	Dermatitis	
	Loss of memory	
	Confusion	
	Unsteady gait	
	Erratic heartbeat	
	Cardiac failure	
Anabolic steroids		
Muscular hypertrophy aggressive	Masculinization	Uncontrolled outbursts on sudden cessation of use
	Liver, kidney and bowel problems	
	Aggression	
Barbiturates		
Sedative	Easy development of tolerance, psychological dependency and physical dependency	Convulsions and coma may lead to death
Tranquillizer		Sweating, anxiety and tremor common
Disinhibitor	High potential for fatal overdose because of narrow therapeutic margin	
Occasional euphoria		
Relaxation and sociability as with alcohol	Use in conjunction with other drugs, particularly alcohol, greatly potentiates effects and risks	
Benzodiazepines		
Sedative	Respiratory depression	Anxiety
Tranquillizer	Loss of consciousness	Insomnia
Disinhibitor	Impaired memory	Perceptual disturbance
Euphoriant	Exaggerated emotional responses, including aggression and irrational behaviour; these are potentiated if the drugs are taken in combination, particularly with alcohol, but also with other sedative drugs	Fits
	Irrational behaviour may mimic a psychotic episode and the individual may become confused and suspicious	

Table 1. *Continued*

Effects	Effects in excess	Effects in withdrawal
Cannabis		
Relaxation	Anxiety	Possible effects similar to mild
Euphoria	Panic	benzodiazepine withdrawal in regular
Mild sedative	Confusion/disorientation	cannabis users
Possible anxiety	Hallucinations	
Confusion	Psychosis	
Dry mouth	Hypotension	
Increased appetite	Nausea	
	Respiratory problems	
Cocaine		
Stimulant	Weight loss	Lethargy
Increased confidence	Anxiety	Low mood
Wakefulness	Paranoia: abnormal suspiciousness and	Depression following prolonged use
Appetite suppressant	aggression	
Excitability	Hallucinations	
Sociability	Irritability	
	Agitation	
	Nausea	
	Tremor	
	Convulsions	
Hallucinogenic amphetamines (Ecstasy)		
Increased confidence	Insomnia	Drowsiness
Euphoria	Weight loss	Muscle aches
Friendliness/empathy	Poor concentration	Headache
Sociability	Moodiness	Underlying depression
Increased energy	Anxiety	
Wakefulness	Depression	
Nausea	Hallucinations	
Hyperthermia	Paranoia	
Dehydration	Hyperthermia leading to collapse	
	Respiratory failure	
	Disseminated intravascular coagulation	
Hallucinogenic mushrooms		
Euphoria	Nausea	Nothing of note
Excitement	Vomiting	
Increased energy	Stomach pain	
Abnormal perception	Anxiety	
Depersonalization	Confusion	
Anxiety	Panic	
	Hallucinations	
	Psychosis	
Solvents and gases		
Similar to drunkenness:	Pseudohallucinations	Psychological craving
dizziness, unreality,	Feeling of hangover	
euphoria, slurred	Acute physiological shock	
speech, double vision,	Heart failure	
nausea and drowsiness	Neurological damage and high psychological	
	dependence may both occur with long-term	
	heavy use	

Table 1. *Continued*

Effects	Effects in excess	Effects in withdrawal
LSD		
Euphoria	Mood changes	Nothing of note
Excitement	Anxiety	
Poor concentration	Confusion	
Mood changes	Panic	
Abnormal perception	Hallucinations	
Depersonalization	Psychosis	
Anxiety		
Wakefulness		
Opioids		
Physical and psychological analgesia, i.e. blocking of pain sensations and reduction of reaction to them	Respiratory failure	Sleep disturbance and restlessness
	Coma	Any combination of hot and cold sweats
	Death	runny nose, stomach cramps, nausea,
	These effects are potentiated by alcohol	vomiting, diarrhoea and muscular pain
Psychological distancing from hunger, pain, fear, anxiety and all other emotions	Tolerance will develop after a few weeks of regular use	which may be severe
		Psychological distress and sleep disturbance may persist for up to 6 months
Rush feeling on injection, i.e. sensation of intense pleasure; this is experienced, but to a lesser degree, with other modes of administration		Craving (a sense of psychological compulsion to seek and use the drug) may persist for much longer

are therefore common in this class of patient and can be fatal. Accidental overdoses also occur as a result of fluctuations in the quality (and potency) of street drugs; this is especially common after theft from pharmacies. They also occur as a result of fluctuations in neuro-pharmacological tolerance following abstinence to certain classes of drug; for this reason it is vital to inform patients that their tolerance to some drugs can reduce drastically if they have not taken them for any length of time.

Patients who abuse drugs are often unpopular in A&E departments for a variety of reasons. However, a significant proportion (especially amongst those requesting further prescriptions or experiencing withdrawal) are genuinely asking for help and, indeed, go on to accept help from local drug rehabilitation services. In such cases A&E staff may be the first contact they have made with these services and it is essential that A&E staff try and keep an open mind, are non-confrontational and provide the patient with details and telephone numbers of local drugs services where they can get the specialist help they need. This group of patients can be helped, as shown by the successful reduction in the incidence of HIV (human

immunodeficiency virus), hepatitis B and other infections as a consequence of needle exchange schemes, as well as the proportion of patients who give up their drug-taking lifestyle. A&E staff therefore have an important role to play in the pathway to recovery from this medical and social problem. To assist with the efficient care and disposal of these patients, A&E departments should regularly invite their local drugs teams to come and teach staff how best to approach these patients, to provide hand-outs for the patients and to put together policies and systems for dealing with particular groups such as known A&E recidivists, psychotic or disturbed patients, those who request new prescriptions and those who are medically ill but refuse treatment.

Psychiatric and behavioural sequelae of drug use

Most of the problems associated with drug misuse encountered in A&E consist of the acute effects of the drugs themselves. These can include various forms of psychosis with paranoid ideation, excitement and over-activity and possibly auditory, visual and tactile hallucinations (especially with the hallucinogens). The patient may respond to these hallucinations, or act out on the fears arising from their paranoid beliefs and so become disturbed or even violent. It is important to obtain a history (perhaps from a third party) of what was taken and when. If there is a history of violence or it seems that the patient may become violent, summon assistance before any violence occurs. The patient can then be encouraged to move to a quieter area where there is less chance of their interfering with other patients.

If it is necessary to sedate the psychotic and/or intoxicated patient in order to examine them or for their own safety or the safety of others, the safest and most effective medication is intramuscular haloperidol 10 mg every 30 min and/or intramuscular lorazepam 1–2 mg every hour (maximum doses: haloperidol 40 mg; lorazepam 6 mg). Very often such intervention proves effective well in advance of any pharmacological effect because the action of taking charge of the situation and giving an injection paradoxically makes the patient feel contained and 'safe'. Pharmacological efficacy from this medication usually reveals itself within 20–30 min, which is why 30-min intervals between injections are necessary to avoid dose accumulation. Whilst waiting for the medication to take effect staff should continue to sit with the patient, reassuring them and allaying whatever anxieties and fears there may be. If, as a result of the medication, the patient becomes sedated they will require regular observation while awaiting transfer to an appropriate ward and will need to be accompanied by adequate staff, including a nurse or doctor, while transfer is taking place.

Medical sedation can be given under common law if it is clearly in the patient's best interests and intended to prevent a serious deterioration in health or harm to themselves or others. A psychiatric opinion should be sought since a proportion of psychoses seen in drug misusers are not merely the effects of intoxication but persist beyond the time that the drug is active. Generally speaking drug-induced psychoses are short-lived and resolve spontaneously when the drug wears off; but, if the patient has a history of multiple such psychoses with heavy chronic drug use, or psychoses occurring outside the context of acute ingestion, or a coincidental history of schizophrenia or bipolar affective disorder, some form of continuing psychiatric treatment will be necessary. This is not always welcome. Patients who simply abuse drugs and repeatedly appear in A&E requesting this or that whilst declining psychiatric (or medical) help are *not* eligible for detention under the Mental Health Act. Drug

misuse and/or intoxication are not grounds for detaining a patient under the Act. However, patients who develop psychotic or other serious psychiatric symptoms consequent upon their drug use (e.g. depression or psychosis) and who refuse help may well be eligible. If in doubt obtain an opinion from a psychiatrist and approved social worker.

Certain behavioural and psychological states arising from acute drug intoxication can be treated pharmacologically. The atropinic psychosis of *Datura* can be treated by giving intravenous physostigmine. Opioid intoxication can be treated by naloxone 0.4–2 mg IV every 3–5 min until the patient improves. (Further their intramuscular injections are often required over the following couple of hours because of short half-lives.) The use of flumazenil in benzodiazepine overdose is more hazardous. Flumazenil is not licensed for this indication and there are several reports of patients with mixed benzodiazepine and tricyclic overdoses who have developed seizures after flumazenil. However, this drug may be useful if there are signs of respiratory depression. Finally, the behavioural excitement seen with psychostimulants can be treated by giving oral or intramuscular lorazepam 1–2 mg and/or haloperidol 10–15 mg, repeated an hour later if necessary.

Various psychiatric and behavioural states can also arise as a consequence of drug withdrawal. This often occurs when users have moved from one area to another without organizing their prescription to follow them. The various symptoms of withdrawal from each class of drug are listed in Table 1, but the only one that is of acute medical concern is barbiturate (and benzodiazepine) withdrawal in which there is a substantial risk of seizures. Fortunately, barbiturate misuse is now relatively uncommon.

A&E departments often lack guidelines on when it is appropriate to refer drug-abusing patients to specialist drug teams. It is important to establish locally agreed criteria for referral but patients who are simply intoxicated by virtue of their drug use and not displaying psychiatric symptoms need to be managed medically (i.e. in the context of the physical risk imposed by their intoxication). For patients who abuse drugs and are displaying prominent psychiatric symptoms referral to local psychiatric teams or the on-call psychiatrist is probably the best way to proceed. However, it is often difficult to make a mental state assessment on someone who is intoxicated; in such cases it is probably wise to let them sober up first (the same applies to alcohol). Referral to specialist drug teams should be restricted to those who are requesting help with their addiction or who are placing themselves physically and psychiatrically at risk because of their habit.

APPENDIX

What to do if a patient presents to A&E/admissions with a suspected overdose and refuses investigation and treatment

1. If the patient agrees to wait a few minutes then use that time to find out all you can about their present circumstances, the circumstances of the overdose (using the specially prepared DSH Assessment Form) and their past medical and psychiatric history. Start with the ambulance men, and any police, friends and relatives who may have accompanied the patient to hospital. Find out if the patient has any previous history of deliberate self-harm (medical notes) or a known psychiatric history. Speak to any psychiatric units who may know the patient and be able to give further information and advice.

   If possible, speak to the patient's general practitioner. On the basis of this information you will then be in a stronger position to know what to do next.

2. See if friends or relatives who have accompanied the patient to hospital can persuade the patient to accept treatment. If none are available find out whether the patient will give permission to contact family or friends at home and then arrange for them to come in. Alternatively, try seeing whether one of the nurses will be able to persuade the patient to accept help. Most DSH patients are angry, frightened or upset and will accept treatment once they have gained trust in the staff; nurses may be better able to do this than doctors.

3. If (1) and (2) fail then you have to make two decisions:
   a. Is the patient at significant medical risk and has the overdose impaired the patient's judgement (e.g. confusion and intoxication)? If so, then one can and should go ahead and treat the patient under common law, especially if their physical health is deteriorating. Severely physically or mentally ill patients can also be restrained from leaving under common law so long as it is clear that such an action is in the patient's best interests and so long as that patient is subsequently assessed by a psychiatrist and approved social worker at the earliest possible convenience.

   b. Is there any evidence to suggest the presence of mental illness? (The taking of an overdose does not automatically indicate mental illness.) If it is suspected, then the patient will need to be seen by the duty psychiatrist and held under common law until such time as this opinion can be obtained. Assessment for the purposes of admission under the Mental Health Act requires a psychiatrist, an approved social worker, and another doctor – preferably the patient's general practitioner. Incidentally, the Mental Health Act does not empower doctors to administer compulsory physical treatment for physical illness even in patients with mental illness; in such cases waiting for implementation of the Mental Health Act may merely introduce an unnecessary delay to medical treatment.

Common law requires further explanation. Whereas it confers certain rights to patients empowering them to make decisions concerning the acceptance or refusal of treatment (even those which would endanger life), it is also true that under common law a doctor can be found negligent of a 'failure of duty to care' by letting a patient go or by not instituting appropriate treatment. Thus, if the patient has mental illness and/or impaired judgement as a result of a medical condition, and if urgent treatment to prevent serious deterioration of health or to save life is required, then one can, and should, physically detain the patient and administer whatever treatment is necessary. However, such a decision needs to be regularly reviewed and discussed with the patient, senior medical and psychiatric staff and the patient's next of kin.

If the patient is not mentally ill and their judgement is not impaired by the overdose, yet persists in the wish not to have medical treatment, then a compulsory imposition of such treatment could be deemed an assault and the doctor is thus exposing himself to a possible legal action. However, a decision to let a patient leave hospital and/or to continue to decline treatment is not one that can be taken lightly and it is strongly recommended that these patients receive careful assessment from senior psychiatric and medical personnel before such a decision is reached or before letting them go. All reasons for any decisions subsequently taken should be fully recorded in the notes. Fortunately this sort of scenario is fairly uncommon in clinical practice and most patients do eventually agree to have treatment.

Bibliography

BELL, G., REINSTEIN, D.Z., RAJIYAH, G. *et al.* (1991). Psychiatric screening of admissions to an accident and emergency ward. *Br. J. Psychiatry*, **158**, 554–7.

BLACKER, C.V.R., SILVERSTONE, T. & JENKINS, R. (1992). A deliberate self-harm assessment form for use by junior medical staff. *Psychiatric Bulletin*, **16**, 262–3.

OFFICE OF HEALTH ECONOMICS (1991). *Suicide and Deliberate Self-harm.* London: Office of Health Economics.

SALKOVSKIS, P.M., STORER, D., ATHA, C. *et al.* (1990). Psychiatric morbidity in an accident and emergency department. Characteristics of patients at presentation and one month follow-up. *Br J. Psychiatry*, **156**, 483–7.

56 Endocrine emergencies

R. SHEAVES and J. WASS

Department of Endocrinology, St Bartholomew's Hospital, London, UK

Chapter plan

Thyroid emergencies
Disorders of calcium metabolism
Adrenocortical insufficiency
Acute pituitary emergencies
Hypertensive crisis and suspected phaeochromocytoma

THYROID EMERGENCIES

Thyroid crisis

Definition

Thyroid crisis represents a life-threatening exacerbation of the manifestations of thyrotoxicosis. This leads to a decompensation and critical failure of a number of organ systems. The abrupt deterioration is usually related to a precipitating factor such as acute infection or surgery and the cardinal features of thyroid crisis require prompt recognition since the condition is associated with a very significant mortality (Waldstein *et al.*, 1960).

Clinical history

The attending physician may be asked to assess a patient whose condition has deteriorated to a degree that obtaining a clear history is difficult. However, a careful history of thyrotoxicosis should be sought and the typical complaints of weight loss, weakness, breathlessness, irritability and heat intolerance may be elucidated. Rarely, however, apathetic thyrotoxicosis may present in crisis with extreme weakness, exhaustion and apathy. A past history or family history of thyroid disorder is important, the latter because autoimmune thyroid disease may run in families. The acute precipitating factor for the crisis may be identifiable and includes thyroid surgery or general surgery on a thyrotoxic patient, infection and the recent administration of iodine either as contrast dyes or radioiodine therapy (Blum *et al.*, 1976).

Prior to the availability of adequate pharmacological control of thyrotoxicosis, thyroid crisis was often seen in the immediate postoperative period following thyroidectomy. With improved preparation of patients for surgery this complication is now rarely seen although it still may occur in a poorly prepared patient or one undergoing general surgery in whom thyrotoxicosis is undiagnosed. Nowadays infection probably represents the most common precipitating factor (Nelson & Becker, 1969).

Clinical examination

A patient in thyroid crisis may demonstrate features of a multisystem decompensation, and the combination of tremor, a high fever, warm peripheries, tachycardia, bounding pulse and signs of shock makes the distinction from septicaemia extremely difficult. It is therefore necessary to examine specifically for signs of thyroid disease and in particular look for a goitre. Commonly the patient appears agitated or delirious and, on a systems review, typical features include tachyarrhythmias, congestive cardiac failure, respiratory distress and congestive hepatomegaly. The associated vomiting and diarrhoea may precipitate a state of severe dehydration, hypotension and prerenal failure. The most characteristic feature of thyroid crisis is pyrexia which may rise to above 40°C. Specific thyroid signs include a bilateral tremor of the hands, a goitre and signs of thyroid eye disease. The patient may also have a profound proximal myopathy.

Staff in the accident and emergency (A&E) department may be alerted to a diagnosis of thyroid crisis if a patient presents with a high fever, has a hyperdynamic circulation and has cardiac failure. It is important that the appropriate laboratory investigations are organized although treatment should be initiated immediately.

Laboratory investigations

Routine haematology, biochemistry and an infection screen should be requested although it should be remembered that a leucocytosis is well recognized in thyrotoxicosis, even in the absence of infection. Hypercalcaemia associated with a raised alkaline phosphatase is relatively common in severe thyrotoxicosis although it rarely requires independent emergency treatment.

Thyroid function tests, total or free T4 (thyroxine), T3 (tri-iodothyronine) TSH (thyroid-stimulating hormone) and thyroid antibodies will be required to confirm the diagnosis although treatment should not be delayed awaiting the results. The levels of thyroid hormones will be above the normal range but the values are not grossly elevated and are usually within the order of otherwise uncomplicated thyrotoxicosis.

Treatment

The patient is best managed in an intensive care unit where close attention can be paid to the cardiorespiratory status and fluid balance. The treatment can thus be divided into general supportive therapy and specific thyrotoxic treatment.

General supportive therapy

Monitoring of cardiovascular status is necessary for the delicate adjustment of fluid balance in the presence of potential cardiac failure. Standard antiarrhythmic drugs can be used including digoxin for atrial fibrillation after correction of hypokalaemia. If anticoagulation is indicated because of atrial fibrillation then it must be remembered that the thyrotoxic patient is very sensitive to warfarin. It is usually sufficient to treat the hyperpyrexia with external cooling although inhibition of central thermoregulation can also be obtained with chlorpromazine (50–100 mg IM) which should in addition be standard treatment for the agitation. Appropriate nutritional support with vitamin supplements should be considered early in the management since these patients are often undernourished and grossly hypermetabolic. There is no general indication for antibiotics unless the diagnosis of infection is supported.

Specific therapy for thyrotoxicosis

The drug treatment for thyroid crisis can be divided into the following categories which also serve as useful reminders of the various stages of thyroid hormone synthesis, secretion, metabolism and mode of action susceptible to pharmacological intervention.

Inhibition of thyroid hormone synthesis

Propylthiouracil (PTU) is the drug of choice, being preferred to carbimazole or methimazole since not only is new hormone synthesis inhibited but there is also an inhibitory effect on the peripheral conversion of T4 to T3. The recommended dose of PTU is 200 mg 6-hourly orally or via a nasogastric tube.

Inhibition of thyroid hormone release

The effects of iodides in blocking thyroid hormone secretion are immediate. They should be administered about 1 h after the first dose of PTU since iodination will enrich the hormone stores within the thyroid gland and thereby generate the possibility of massive hormone release and subsequent exacerbation of thyrotoxicosis. If, however, the iodides are administered in conjunction with PTU then decreases in serum thyroid levels are seen within a few days.

Traditional preparations include potassium iodide (60 mg orally three times daily), Lugol's iodine (use 10 drops of a solution containing 130 mg of iodine ml^{-1} diluted in milk or water twice daily), potassium iodide saturated solution (8 drops 6-hourly orally or 1 g IV twice daily) and sodium iodide 1 g (10 ml of 10% solution) IV.

Recently the radiographic contrast dyes containing iodine have been used in place of traditional iodide preparations. The cholecystographic contrast agent ipodate is metabolized to yield large amounts of iodide capable of inhibiting thyroid hormone secretion and also the peripheral conversion of T4 to T3. Some authors have recommended that iodides be replaced by these contrast agents and suggest that ipodate (oragrafin) is administered in a 3 g oral daily dose (Burger & Philippe, 1992).

In the occasional patient who may be allergic to iodine, lithium carbonate may be used to block thyroid release. Care should be taken with lithium (300 mg 6-hourly) to avoid toxic symptoms and the dose must be adjusted to maintain serum lithium levels of approximately 1 mmol l^{-1}.

Inhibition of peripheral thyroid hormone conversion

The use of propranolol to block the beta-adrenergic effects of thyroid hormones also inhibits T4 to T3 conversion (Hellman *et al.*, 1977). Despite the temptation to choose a more cardioselective beta-blocker in thyrotoxicosis, propranolol maintains a role in for this reason.

Corticosteroids are used in the treatment of thyroid crisis although many would say that a beneficial role is still unproven. However, since the conversion of T4 to T3 is reduced by glucocorticoids, their routine use in thyroid crisis can be justified. High doses of prednisolone (60 mg daily) can be used in the initial stages of management and are also effective in reducing the hyperthyroid state in amiodarone-induced thyrotoxicosis (Wimpfheimer *et al.*, 1982).

Inhibition of peripheral thyroid hormone action

Beta-adrenergic blockade with propranolol (80 mg orally 8-hourly) causes rapid reduction of heart rate and cardiac work. Intravenous therapy with 2 mg bolus doses can be given whilst awaiting the effects of the orally administered drugs. Beta-blockers would be contraindicated in patients with moderate or severe cardiac failure although they can be used with caution in patients with minor degrees of cardiac failure precipitated by their thyrotoxicosis. A further contraindication is bronchospasm and selective beta$_1$-blocking agents can be prescribed although the risk of bronchospasm still exists with high doses. In this situation guanethidine (30–40 mg orally 6-hourly) can be given, although this should not be used in the presence of cardiovascular collapse.

Summary and conclusions

Thyroid crisis is rare but clinical suspicion should be high in a patient with a past history of thyroid disease who develops a decompensated state characterized by fever, tachycardia, cardiac failure, atrial fibrillation and agitation. Immediate treatment is mandatory even before confirmation of thyrotoxicosis from the laboratory. The patient should be managed in an intensive care setting and specific therapy is directed at the inhibition of thyroid hormone synthesis, release and peripheral conversion. The effects of the thyroid hormones on the cardiovascular system and central nervous system (CNS) can be treated with propranolol and chlorpromazine respectively. A specific therapeutic plan is set out below.

1. *Propranolol* 2 mg IV over 5 min. Continue 80 mg orally 8-hourly.

2. *Chlorpromazine* 50 mg IM.
3. *Propylthiouracil* 200 mg orally 6-hourly.
4. *Iodide*: 1 g (10 ml of 10%) of sodium iodide IV followed by potassium iodide 60 mg orally q.d.s. This should be started 1 h *after* the first dose of propylthiouracil.
5. *Prednisolone* 60 mg orally daily.

Graves' ophthalmopathy

Definition

Graves' ophthalmopathy is a chronic infiltrative disorder of the orbits which, although it is most often associated with hyperthyroidism, may also occur in the absence of thyroid disease. Although patients with Graves' ophthalmopathy often complain of gritty eyes, diplopia or temporary visual blurring it is very important to identify the ocular emergencies such as corneal ulceration, congestive ophthalmopathy and optic neuropathy. Early recognition of these complications and immediate treatment is critical for the preservation of sight.

Symptoms

The proptosis associated with Graves' ophthalmopathy results in failure of lid closure and therefore protection of the cornea and this increases the likelihood of exposure keratitis. The sensation of gritty eyes is common and can be treated with artificial tears. However, the development of severe conjunctival pain associated with erythema indicates corneal ulceration and is an indication for urgent referral to an ophthalmologist.

The deposition of mucopolysaccharides and development of lymphocytic infiltrates and orbital oedema displaces the globe anteriorly and is sometimes associated with a deeper pain behind the eyes. If there is visual blurring it is very important to examine the eyes carefully for the typical features of congestive ophthalmopathy and optic neuropathy. Momentary visual blurring is associated with fluid on the surface of the cornea and is cleared on blinking. This is because the displaced orbit results in less efficient lacrimal drainage. Visual blurring may also be due to minor degrees of extraocular muscle imbalance and the resulting diplopia is abolished on closing one eye. Persistent visual blurring, especially associated with gradual deterioration in visual acuity, may indicate an optic neuropathy and requires urgent treatment.

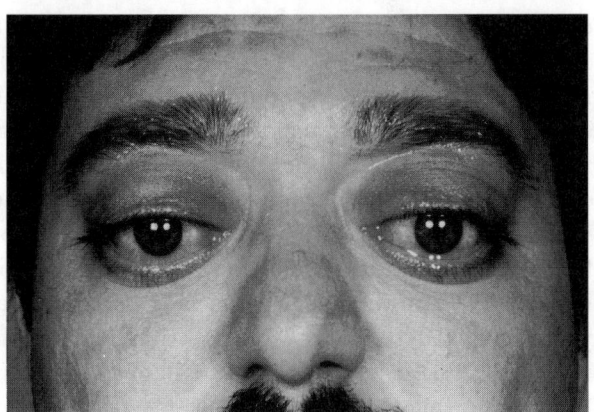

Fig. 1. A patient with thyroid eye disease demonstrating bilateral proptosis and chemosis

Clinical signs

Careful observation will detect even mild proptosis but it is useful also to document the disease with a Hertel exophthalmometer. Lid retraction will be obvious by identifying the sclera between the upper lid and the limbus of the cornea with the patient looking straight forward. The eyelids themselves may be swollen and this is common when the globe has been displaced anteriorly within the limited size of the orbit. However, if either the lid or inferior margin of the orbit is oedematous, this may indicate significant venous congestion or conjunctival oedema (Fig. 1) which are signs of potentially dangerous congestive ophthalmopathy.

Visual actuity should be formally tested and the causes of deterioration should be considered. Optic neuropathy is usually associated with a gradual deterioration rather than the abrupt loss of vision seen with an ischaemic event or optic neuritis. The visual fields should be tested by confrontation to a red pin and by formal Goldman perimetry. Graves' ophthalmopathy produces a variety of defects, the most frequent being a combination of a central scotoma and an inferior arcuate field loss. The pupils should be examined for the presence of an afferent pupillary defect; this is performed by shining a torch alternately between the two eyes and identifying dilatation rather than constriction to light in the affected eye. It indicates an abnormal afferent neural pathway such as would be produced by an optic neuropathy. The suspicions may be confirmed on fundoscopy by finding disc pallor, papilloedema or venous congestion.

Limitation of both upward gaze and convergence are common abnormalities of eye movements in Graves' ophthalmopathy. These abnormalities may produce diplopia or may progress to cause a permanent strabismus

with suppression of the visual image of one eye and subsequent loss of the diplopia.

Investigations and differential diagnosis

The differential diagnosis of proptosis is wide and includes infiltration of the orbits with tumours, granulomas and cysts. The condition may also be caused by pituitary tumours, brain tumours and vascular anomalies such as retrobulbar haemorrhage and cavernous sinus thrombosis. Consideration of this differential diagnosis is particularly important when there is unilateral proptosis or when the patient does not have associated thyroid disease. In these cases a CT (computed tomography) scan of the orbits is helpful and may also show the typical radiological appearances associated with optic neuropathy.

Treatment

Graves' opthalmopathy may improve on antithyroid medication and this should be started without delay if the patient is thyrotoxic. More radical thyroid ablation has been performed in the past although there did not appear to be any significant improvement in the ophthalmopathy in patients treated with thyroidectomy, radioiodine or antithyroid drugs (Barbosa et al., 1972). There have also been reports of a deterioration in eye disease following radioiodine ablation and many centres now avoid this treatment for thyrotoxicosis in patients with severe eye signs. The emergency treatment of severe eye complications such as optic neuropathy and venous congestion comprise the use of corticosteroids, orbital radiotherapy and surgery.

Urgent medical and ophthalmological advice must be sought.

Summary and conclusions

Many patients present for the first time in the A&E department with typical symptoms and signs of thyrotoxicosis. In these uncomplicated cases, biochemical tests to confirm the thyroid status can be organized together with a follow-up appointment in the endocrine clinic. Only those patients with significant complications such as arrhythmias, cardiac failure or extreme agitation would normally require admission. Graves' ophthalmopathy is a frequently discovered finding, and, unless a threat to sight can be demonstrated, this too can be assessed in the out-patient clinic.

Patients may frequently complain of gritty eyes and blurred vision, but it is the sudden development of severe eye pain or the detection of a deterioration in visual acuity which alerts the physician to some of the more serious complications. Specific signs of corneal ulceration, congestive ophthalmopathy or optic neuropathy necessitate prompt referral to an ophthalmologist.

Myxoedema coma

Hypothyroidism presents with a great diversity of symptoms and signs and some patients are severely affected. It is important, however, to identify patients with severe hypothyroidism from those suffering from the rare decompensation state known as myxoedema coma. Myxoedema coma can be characterized by clinical features of hypothyroidism accompanied by changes in mentation ranging from confusion to coma and associated with hypothermia (see Chapter 38). There is often an identifiable precipitating factor such as infection, cerebrovascular accident or the administration of chlorpromazine and the diagnosis can be further suspected by finding raised plasma levels of intracellular enzymes such as creatine phosphokinase.

Patients presenting to the A&E department with unexplained coma or confusion should be suspected of being hypothyroid if there is associated hypothermia (see Chapter 38). Further clues may be gained from a detailed history from a relative and from the clinical examination.

History

Typical features of hypothroidism include lethargy, cold intolerance, weight gain, hoarse voice and acroparaesthesiae. A precipitating cause for the deterioration such as an infection or recent drug treatment (beta-blockers, narcotics, vasodilators or sedatives) may precede the change in mental state. Significant past medical history includes previous thyroid disease, antithyroid medication and also specific drugs such as lithium and amiodarone which are known to precipitate hypothyroidism. A family history of thyroid or other organ specific autoimmune disease is also important.

Clinical signs

Some of the general features include pale, dry skin with subcutaneous swellings around the eyes. Periorbital oedema and macroglossia are also typical but loss of the lateral third of the eyebrows is not a specific sign. The neck should be examined for a thyroidectomy scar or a goitre and a sparsity of body or secondary sexual hair may indicate associated hypopituitarism. Other general features include hypothermia and delayed relaxation of the tendon reflexes. In the comatose patient hypoventilation may be severe enough to cause hypoxia and hypercapnia requiring ventilatory support. In this type of patient a respiratory infection may well be the precipitating factor. Cardiovascular signs include a bradycardia, hypotension and soft heart sounds. Although cardiac output is reduced severe cardiac failure is unusual. Cardiomegaly may be seen on the chest X-ray and may be associated with a pericardial effusion which seems to accumulate slowly and rarely causes cardiac tamponade. There is hypofunction of the intestine, resulting in paralytic ileus and decreased motility of the bladder with urinary retention. Neuropsychiatric signs are typical and seizures and cerebellar signs have been well described. A range of psychiatric features, including depression, paranoia and hallucinations, may be present.

Laboratory investigations

Routine investigations may reveal a normocytic or megaloblastic anaemia and hyponatraemia due to water overload and inappropriate secretion of antidiuretic hormone (ADH). Raised cardiac enzymes (creatine phosphokinase, lactate dehydrogenase, aspartate transaminase) help to confirm the diagnosis and may either be confused with an acute myocardial infarct or reflect a cardiac event in a susceptible patient. The raised enzymes in myxoedema coma remain high for several days unlike the acute changes seen after a myocardial infarct. An ECG (electrocardiogram) is helpful in the differential diagnosis and typical changes of hypothyroidism include small voltages and a prolonged QT interval.

Thyroid function tests should be urgently requested together with a serum cortisol. Most commonly the tests reveal a primary thyroid disorder (low T4, high TSH) but they occasionally show secondary pituitary or tertiary hypothalamic hypothyroidism (low T4, low TSH) with a possibility of adrenal insufficiency.

Treatment

A patient with myxoedema coma requires accurate monitoring of cardiac and pulmonary status preferably on an intensive care unit. Ventilatory support may be necessary in a patient exhibiting hypoventilation and respiratory acidosis. The treatment of hyponatraemia is fluid restriction (500 ml in 24 h) but, if sodium depletion is severe and accompanied by seizures, an infusion of hypertonic saline (50–100 ml of 5% sodium chloride) should be administered under carefully monitored conditions. Similarly, hypertonic glucose (50 ml of 50% dextrose) may be required to treat hypoglycaemia and this should be administered cautiously. The hypothermia should be monitored using a rectal temperature probe and treated by slow rewarming to avoid a sudden decrease in peripheral vascular resistance precipitating vascular collapse.

Glucocorticoids (hydrocortisone 100 mg IM 6-hourly) should be given before laboratory confirmation of the serum cortisol and continued until the cortisol result is available. The patient may be suffering from relative adrenal insufficiency resulting from the hypothyroid state or directly from pituitary disease. In the intensive care setting it should be remembered that hypothyroid patients are particularly sensitive to CNS depressants and digoxin, and relatively resistant to anticoagulation.

Specific thyroid treatment

In uncomplicated severe hypothyroidism, treatment with low-dose thyroxine in gradual increments limits the cardiac complications such as arrhythmias and myocardial infarction caused by an imbalance in myocardial oxygen supply and demand. However, in myxoedema coma, the immediate mortality is so high (Lindberger, 1975) that treatment with high-dose thyroid replacement has been justified. The rarity of this clinical situation has limited the therapeutic trials necessary to define a consistent approach to treatment so there is controversy surrounding the use of either thyroxine (T4)or liothyronine, (T3) the dose and the route of administration. The aim, however, is to balance the risk of high mortality of the untreated condition against the risks of inducing cardiac complications.

Advocates of T4 would suggest that the smooth onset of action limits the risks of side-effects. The response, however, is slow and those physicians recommending T3 argue that the rapid onset is beneficial despite large, fluctuating T3 levels and their cardiac risks (Chernow *et al.*, 1983). It has been argued that a large intravenous bolus of T4 should replace the depleted thyroid hormone pool and that adequate levels of T4 would be available for peripheral conversion. However, the conversion of T4 to T3 in sick patients is reduced (Wartofsky & Burman, 1982) and this therefore provides a reasonable argument for adding a small supplement of T3 to the T4 therapy. In addition, there does not seem to be agreement on whether oral replacement or intravenous therapy confer specific advantages. Theoretically, if the documented disorders of gut motility are common, this is likely to interfere with the absorption of oral drugs.

Finally the recommended dose of thyroid replacement varies widely and this again reflects the rarity of this condition and a sparsity of clinical trials with thyroid hormone replacement. The various regimens used lack scientific justification. Large boluses of T4 and smaller supplements of T3 are recommended by some (Wartofsky 1991) but we advocate a gradual approach to limit cardiac complications, starting with a small dose of T3 (2.5 µg initially increasing to 2.5 µg 8-hourly).

Summary and conclusions

Myxoedema coma represents a decompensated hypothyroid state. There is a high mortality and intensive therapy is required both for supportive management and the monitoring of cardiac complications induced by thyroid replacement therapy. In severe hypothyroidism without decompensation, gentle T3 replacement is recommended (2.5 µg initially followed by 2.5 µg 8-hourly orally) whereas in myxoedema coma the replacement regimen is controversial. We would advise using the same approach but intravenous therapy will be required until the patient is conscious and able to take oral therapy in gradual increasing doses. When T3 replacement reaches 20 µg twice daily the patient can be switched to maintenance T4.

DISORDERS OF CALCIUM METABOLISM

Introduction

The total serum calcium concentration is normally maintained within a narrow range (2.20–2.67 mmol l^{-1}) allowing for the regulation of the many calcium-dependent processes. Since a large proportion of the total calcium measured is bound to serum proteins it is customary to adjust this according to the serum albumin and so calculate a corrected value. A reasonable correction factor is to add 0.02 mmol to the calcium level per gram of albumin higher or lower than 40 g l^{-1}.

The control of calcium metabolism is complex and involves the influences of vitamin D and parathyroid hormone on calcium absorption from the intestine, the regulation of calcium metabolism in bone and the renal

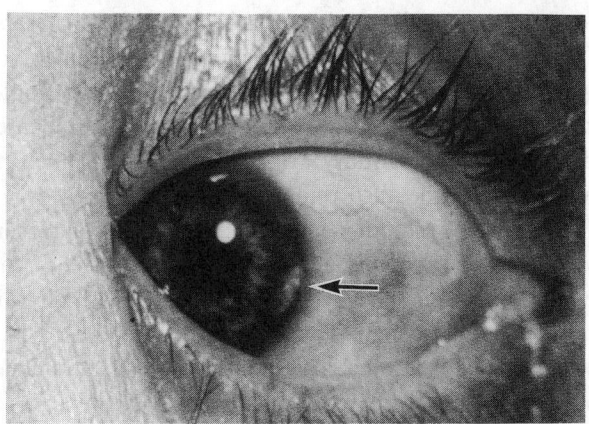

Fig. 2. Demonstration of corneal calcification

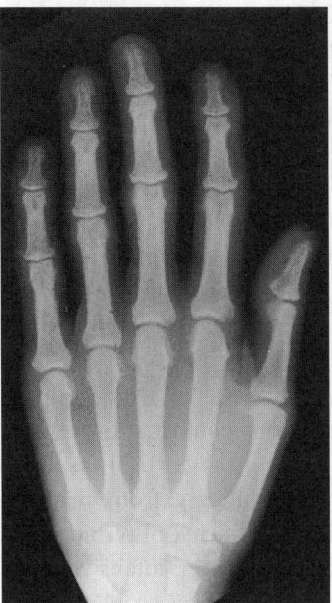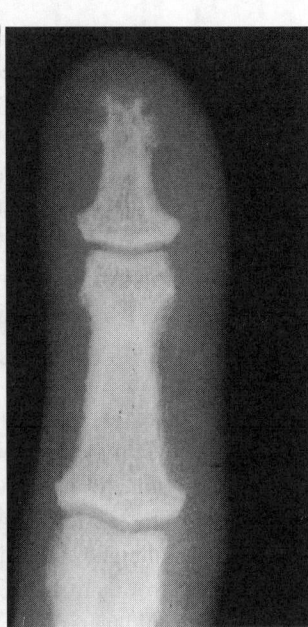

Fig. 3. X-ray of a hand from patient with primary hyperparathyroidism demonstrating subperiosteal bone resorption (a) and demineralization of the phalangeal tuft (b)

excretion of calcium. Symptoms resulting from a disorder of calcium metabolism must be recognized in the A&E department since the conditions represent reversible medical emergencies.

Hypercalcaemia

Symptoms and signs

The symptoms of hypercalcaemia may be non-specific gastrointestinal complaints but they may also present as an acute emergency with mental changes, including drowsiness, confusion, mania, psychosis and ultimately coma. In this case a relative may provide the history of recent tiredness and general weakness associated with anorexia, nausea, vomiting and constipation. Pruritus is also typical and there may be a good description of polydipsia and polyuria in the preceding months. The latter reflects impaired renal concentrating ability as calcium interferes with the action of ADH on the distal tubules which can result in significant dehydration. Long-standing hypercalcaemia can produce nephrocalcinosis and renal calculi, visible on plain abdominal X-rays. Calcification of the conjunctiva may also be seen on careful inspection of the corneoscleral junction (Fig. 2).

An understanding and search for the causes of hypercalcaemia is necessary so that associated disorders can be identified and treated appropriately.

Causes of hypercalcaemia

The most frequent cause for hypercalcaemia detected in the out-patient clinic is primary hyperparathyroidism. Excess parathyroid hormone results most commonly

from a parthyroid adenoma but is also associated with hyperplasia of the parathyroid glands and, more rarely, parathyroid carcinoma. Hyperparathyroidism results in a typical X-ray appearance of the hand (Fig. 3).

The principal cause of hypercalcaemia in hospitalized patients is malignancy (Fisken et al., 1980). There does not appear to be a correlation between the level of hypercalcaemia and the presence of bone metastases and this prompted the proposal that the hypercalcaemia was in part due to a humoral factor. The identification of a parathyroid hormone related protein, sharing the parathyroid hormone receptor and demonstrating similar physiological actions to parathyroid hormone, has advanced our understanding of malignancy-related hypercalcaemia (Broadus et al., 1988).

A number of less common causes of hypercalcaemia (see Table 1) have also been identified. Granulomatous diseases such as sarcoidosis and tuberculosis are associated with unregulated production of 1,25-dihydroxyvitamin D (Bell, 1985). A variety of medications precipitate hypercalcaemia and drugs such as thiazide diuretics may worsen the condition when coincidental hyperparathyroidism already underlies a high bone turnover state. The cause of lithium-related hypercalcaemia is unclear although restoration to normal calcium levels quickly follows cessation of the medication. The recognition of familial hypocalcuric hypercalcaemia is important since the condition is asymptomatic and is not

Table 1. *Causes of hypercalcaemia*

Primary hyperparathyroidism
Malignancy, including myeloma
Granulomatous diseases
– Sarcoidosis
– Tuberculosis
Medication
– Vitamin D
– Thiazide diuretics
– Lithium
Rare causes
– Familial hypocalciuric hypercalcaemia
– Thyrotoxicosis
– Immobilization
– Vitamin A intoxication
– Milk-alkali syndrome
– Renal failure with tertiary hyperparathyroidism
– Adrenal failure

associated with other endocrine abnormalities. Patients with this condition should not be referred for parathyroid surgery. The biochemistry of these patients, however, may be similar to those with primary hyperparathyroidism with raised levels of parathyroid hormone (Marx *et al.*, 1981) and the condition can be confirmed by screening family members.

Treatment of hypercalcaemia

One of the initial stages in the management of hypercalcaemia is to identify the underlying disorder. This is particularly important since beneficial effects of glucocorticoids have been shown in vitamin D intoxication and granulomatous diseases such as sarcoidosis and haematological malignancy but not with primary hyperparathyroidism or solid cancers (Percival *et al.*, 1984; Sandler *et al.*, 1984). A recommended steroid regimen would be 100 mg of hydrocortisone IM every 6 h or 60 mg of prednisolone per day orally.

In the emergency situation the patient is often severely dehydrated in addition to suffering the life-threatening complications of hypercalcaemia. Management is therefore aimed at correcting dehydration and introducing drug therapy to inhibit bone resorption.

Correcting dehydration

Isotonic saline should be infused at a rate based on the level of dehydration and the tolerance of the cardio-vascular system to volume expansion. It is important to maintain the plasma osmolality within the normal range ($280–290$ mOsm kg^{-1}). Loop diuretics have been used together with rehydration since their impairment of calcium resorption from the ascending limb of Henle may encourage quicker normalization of the serum calcium. However, it has also been argued that such a small percentage of the resorbed calcium occurs in the ascending limb of Henle that a role for loop diuretics in this situation is of dubious efficacy (Rizzoli & Bonjour, 1992).

Biphosphonates as inhibitors of bone resorption

Biphosphonates inhibit resorption of bone by binding to hydroxyapatite and inhibiting the dissolution of the crystals. Their high affinity and long half-life in bone makes them ideal drugs in the management of hypercalcaemia (Davis & Heath, 1989). Most derivatives are poorly absorbed from the intestine and are therefore administered intravenously. The effects, however, are relatively slow in onset taking 2–3 days to decrease the serum calcium level and approximately 1 week to achieve the nadir (Bilezikian, 1992). The biphosphonates currently available include etidronate given as 7.5 mg kg^{-1} IV over 4 h, pamidronate given as a single 90 mg IV infusion over 24 h, and clodronate given as a single 600 mg IV infusion over 4 h.

Alternative hypercalcaemic medication

For a more rapid hypocalcaemia some authors recommend using calcitonin although others doubt its effectiveness in maintaining the initial hypocalcaemic effect (Hosking & Gilson, 1984). When life-threatening complications seem imminent the osteoclast RNA synthesis inhibitor, mithramycin, has been used to produce significant falls in serum calcium within 12 h (25 µg kg^{-1} IV with 1 litre of normal saline over 4 h). Its main limitation is marrow, renal and hepatic toxicity. It can, however, be a useful drug in the early stages of acute management (Bilezikian, 1992) although the effect is short-lived.

Hypocalcaemia

Symptoms and signs

General symptoms include fatigue, irritability and anxiety. More specific clues to hypocalcaemia relate to the neuro-muscular irritability seen when the serum calcium falls below 2.0 mmol l^{-1}. Thus patients may give a history of circumoral and peripheral paraesthesia and carpopedal spasm. The spasm is rarely dangerous but its alarming nature often precipitates hyperventilation and the subsequent alkalosis worsens the condition. Occasionally hypocalcaemia can precipitate laryngeal spasm and it is also a well-established cause of seizures. Hypocalcaemia may in less common circumstances be a chronic condition and it is then associated with different clinical signs. These includes the presence of cataract, choreoathetosis resulting from calcification in the basal ganglia, and mental retardation (Friedman *et al.*, 1987).

The typical facial twitch following tapping of the facial nerves is Chvostek's sign. Trousseau's sign may be demonstrated by observing paraesthesia and carpal spasm following the inflation of a blood pressure cuff above the systolic pressure for 3 min. Characteristically there is adduction of the thumb followed by flexion of the metacarpophalangeal joints, extension of the interphalangeal joints and flexion of the wrist.

Hypocalcaemia may contribute to the development of cardiac failure. Calcium has a positive inotropic effect on the myocardium and, besides congestive cardiac failure, it can be associated with conduction defects. There are delays in ventricular repolarization and a lengthening of the QT interval on the ECG.

Causes of hypocalaemia (Table 2)

The inadvertent removal of the parathyroid glands during thyroidectomy results in postoperative hypocalcaemia requiring frequent monitoring and calcium replacement. Similarly, the removal of a parathyroid adenoma is likely to render the patient hypocalcaemic because the remaining glands are suppressed. In both these situations it is also advisable to monitor the serum magnesium since deficiency contributes to the symptoms directly and also indirectly by impairing parathyroid hormone secretion and action (Rude & Singer, 1981)

Disorders of vitamin D metabolism result in hypocalcaemia; clues to this may include malabsorption, hepatic disease or renal failure. Anticonvulsant drugs are known to induce hepatic microsomal mixed oxidase activity and this may lead to accelerated breakdown of some of the vitamin D metabolites.

In the absence of disorders of parathyroid hormone or vitamin D metabolism the most likely cause for symptomatic hypocalcaemia is sudden sequestration of plasma calcium. This occurs in pancreatitis with the intra-abdominal saponification of fat and also with sudden phosphate excess resulting in calcium phosphate

Table 2. *Causes of hypocalcaemia*

Hypoparathyroidism
- Surgery involving parathyroid glands
- Autoimmune
- Infiltration (metastatic, granulomatous, amyloid)
- Associated magnesium deficiency
- Pseudohypoparathyroidism
- Congenital aplasia of parathyroid glands

Abnormal vitamin D metabolism
- Dietary deficiency
- Malabsorption
- Liver disease
- Renal disease
- Drugs (anticonvulsants)

Calcium sequestration
- Pancreatitis
- Rhabdomyolysis
- Blood transfusion
- Burns

deposition in the tissues. Muscle trauma and rhabdomyolysis are common causes, in addition to cytotoxic therapy and malignant hyperthermia. Rapid blood transfusion with citrated blood, severe burns and situations which accelerate bone formation have all been said to cause hypocalcaemia.

Treatment of hypocalcaemia

Hypocalcaemia is associated with cardiac arrhythmias and continuous monitoring is needed, especially since intravenous calcium replacement may precipitate a life-threatening arrhythmia if given too rapidly. The recommended replacement dose is 10 ml of 10% calcium gluconate IV over 10 min. This can then be followed by 40 ml of 10% calcium gluconate in 1 litre of normal saline over 8 h. The infusion rate can be adjusted according to the serum calcium. When the patient is stable, longer term maintenance of the serum calcium can be achieved with oral calcium supplements (1–2 g of elemental calcium per day) and vitamin D supplements (1–4 μg of One-alpha (alfacalcidol) per day) if deficiency is proven. Measurement of plasma magnesium is also important in the hypocalcaemic patient and if necessary 1–5 mmol of magnesium sulphate can be given intravenously over 15 min.

Summary and conclusions

Hypercalcaemic patients presenting to the A&E department may also be severely dehydrated. The mainstay of treatment at this stage is to provide adequate rehydration and consider the relevance of glucocorticoid therapy. Rapid reduction in the serum calcium can be achieved with mithramycin, but biphosphonates should be regarded as first choice agents in general since they are virtually free from side-effects.

Patients found to be suffering from hypocalcaemia also require prompt medical attention. This may be given in the form of intravenous calcium gluconate with continuous cardiac monitoring to detect the development of cardiac arrhythmias.

ADRENOCORTICAL INSUFFICIENCY

Introduction

This is the most important endocrine emergency since missing the diagnosis can be fatal. The clinical features of acute adrenocortical insufficiency are dramatic but often non-specific and the precipitating cause may also feature in the differential diagnosis of shock. It is therefore important to maintain a strong index of suspicion of adrenocortical failure in any shocked patient in the A&E department. This is especially true for patients with a history of pituitary or adrenal disease, or those previously treated with glucocorticoids and whose pituitary–adrenal axis may be impaired (Schlaghecke et al., 1992). The diagnosis is further suggested if the patient gives the typical clinical history of Addison's disease and is found to be pigmented. This represents primary adrenal failure with excess pituitary secretion of ACTH (adrenocorticotropin). Routine laboratory abnormalities may be the first clue to adrenocortical failure. A resumé of the various causes of adrenal insufficiency provides the basis for further management (Burke, 1985).

Causes of adrenal insufficiency

It is convenient to consider adrenal failure as resulting from either primary adrenal causes or secondary hypothalamic–pituitary disease. Within both of these groups the condition can present acutely and the patient becomes dramatically unwell. Alternatively, there may be a more insidious development of symptoms with a final acute stress precipitating a rapid deterioration (Table 3).

Acute primary adrenocortical failure is rare but is well described in meningococcal septicaemia, classically known

Table 3. *Causes of adrenocortical insufficiency*

Acute primary adrenocortical failure
– Adrenal haemorrhage (anticoagulation, septicaemia)
– Acute on chronic adrenocortical failure
– Drugs (mitotane, ketoconazole)
Chronic primary adrenocortical failure (Addison's disease)
– Autoimmune adrenalitis
– Tuberculosis
– Metastatic infiltration
– Granulomatous infiltration (e.g. sarcoid)
– Amyloid
– Fungal infiltration (cryptococcus, histoplasmosis)
– AIDS
– Haemochromatosis
– Congenital adrenal hyperplasia
Acute secondary adrenocortical failure
– Pituitary apoplexy
– Sheehan's syndrome
– Withdrawal of glucocorticoid administration
Chronic secondary adrenocortical failure (hypopituitarism)
– Hypothalamic tumours and infiltrations
– Pituitary tumours and infiltrations
– Pituitary vascular anomalies
– Pituitary surgery and radiotherapy
– Empty sella syndrome
– Isolated CRH or ACTH deficiency

CRH, corticotropin releasing hormone.

as Waterhouse–Friderichsen syndrome. It is also seen with other septicaemic crises (Migeon et al., 1967). Acute adrenal failure may also be precipitated by haemorrhage associated with the use of anticoagulants and other drugs such as mitotane and ketoconazole for the treatment of Cushing's syndrome. Ketoconazole, when used as an antifungal, may also cause adrenal failure (Khosla et al., 1989). These forms of adrenal failure are not associated with pigmentation and can be missed.

Chronic primary adrenal failure, Addison's disease, is caused by a variety of pathological conditions, most commonly autoimmune adrenalitis and tuberculosis. Other significant causes include metastatic infiltration and, although fungal infiltration of the adrenal glands is extremely rare, it is much more likely in immunosuppressed patients such as those with AIDS (acquired immunodeficiency syndrome) (Membreno et al., 1987).

An unpredictable cause of acute secondary adrenocortical failure is previous glucocorticoid therapy (Schlaghecke et al., 1992). Glucocorticoid tablets, creams and inhalers are all relevant since cessation of treatment can result in either temporary or permanent pituitary adrenal suppression. Acute secondary adrenal insufficiency can result from two other clinical situations. First, pituitary apoplexy from sudden haemorrhage into a pituitary tumour may, in addition to adrenal failure, cause a severe headache and visual deterioration. Prompt recognition is necessary to treat the adrenal failure and to refer to the neurosurgical department for consideration of emergency trans-sphenoidal surgery. Secondly, Sheehan's syndrome, due to ischaemic necrosis of the pituitary in the postpartum period, may result in a variable degree of hypopituitarism often first recognized by absent lactation.

Clinical features

Symptoms common to both primary and secondary insufficiency include general weakness, weight loss, anorexia, nausea, vomiting and diarrhoea. These gastro-intestinal symptoms may also be associated with abdominal pain and it would not be uncommon to find that patients have been previously investigated for gastro-intestinal disease before adrenal failure is suspected (Burke, 1985). Other significant symptoms include my-algia, arthralgia, depression, confusion and dizziness relating to postural hypotension although the systolic blood pressure may be maintained until late into the course of the disease.

The clinical signs of acute adrenal crisis are shock (tachycardia and hypotension in a patient with peripheral shutdown). The presence of pigmentation, especially in the palmar creases, knuckles, elbows, buccal mucosa and gums, supports the diagnosis of Addison's disease (Fig. 4). The absence of pigmentation but features of

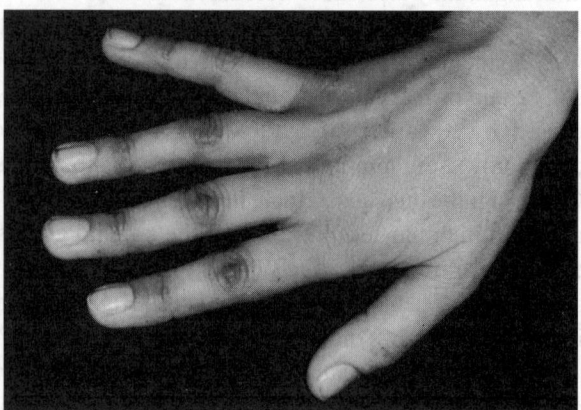

Fig. 4. Marked pigmentation on the hand of a patient with Addison's disease

hypogonadism (sparse axillary and pubic hair with small testes) or hypothyroidism favours a diagnosis of hypopituitarism. The patient in this case may demonstrate typical features of fine wrinkled skin associated with hypopituitarism. Whatever the cause of the adrenal crisis the treatment is essentially the same although interpretation of the laboratory investigations is slightly different. This is because with primary adrenal failure there is loss of both glucocorticoid and mineralocorticoid hormones whereas with secondary adrenal failure the renin–angiotensin system, which is not ACTH-dependent, continues to control aldosterone output.

Laboratory investigations

It is worthwhile following an organized list of routine investigations since once the confirmatory endocrine tests have been performed the patient should be treated with hydrocortisone without delay. Confirmation of the diagnosis is then made later when the results are available. A list of recommended investigations is presented in Table 4.

Routine haematology may reveal a normocytic anaemia and a moderate eosinophilia which is common in Addison's disease. Typical biochemical features of Addison's disease include hyponatraemia, hypoglycaemia, hyperkalaemia and a raised plasma urea. In secondary adrenal failure the hyponatraemia and hypoglycaemia again feature but a normal serum potassium

Table 4. *Investigations for acute adrenal insufficiency*

Haematology
– Full blood count and ESR
Biochemistry
– Electrolytes
– (urea and creatinine, calcium, glucose)
Immunology
– Autoantibody screen, including adrenal antibodies
Endocrine
– Cortisol, ACTH, aldosterone
– Basal pituitary function including LH, FSH, oestradiol, testosterone, T4, TSH, prolactin and growth hormone
Radiology
– Chest X-ray
– Abdominal X-ray
– Skull X-ray – if pituitary disease suspected
– CT scan of the adrenals – if Addison's disease suspected

ESR, erythrocyte sedimentation rate; FSH, follicle stimulating hormone.

reflects the functioning renin–angiotensin–aldosterone system. Blood should be taken for basal cortisol and aldosterone and, if facilities are available for cold spinning and immediate freezing of the sample, a plasma ACTH is useful since it will be raised in Addison's disease and low in pituitary disease (Besser et al., 1971).

Routine radiology includes a chest X-ray which may identify the small heart of Addison's disease or demonstrate signs of tuberculosis. A plain abdominal film may reveal adrenal calcification making tuberculosis a much more likely diagnosis (Vita et al., 1985). An abdominal CT scan can be arranged at a later date to assess the size of the adrenals. Autoimmune adrenalitis causes small glands with lymphocytic infiltration, whereas enlarged glands are seen with infiltrative processes and adrenal haemorrhage.

Treatment

Initial management is emergency glucocorticoid replacement and correction of hypovolaemia, electrolyte disorders and hypoglycaemia using an infusion of 0.9% sodium chloride and 5% dextrose. The speed of the infusion depends upon the degree of hypovolaemia but may require careful monitoring in the intensive care unit. The simplest steroid replacement regimen is 100 mg of hydrocortisone IV followed by 100 mg IM every 6 h. The definitive test for primary adrenal insufficiency is a Synacthen test and this can be incorporated into the treatment programme. A basal blood test is taken for cortisol before giving steroid replacement in the form of dexamethasone (2 mg IV) which does not interfere with the cortisol measurement. Then Synacthen 250 μg IV is given and blood taken at 30 min and 60 min for cortisol. If the cortisol rises by more than 190 nmol l^{-1} to greater than 550 nmol l^{-1} then Addison's disease is excluded. Following the last blood test, hydrocortisone replacement therapy can be started on a regular basis with 100 mg IM every 6 h. Separate mineralocorticoid replacement is not needed until later because of the high mineralocorticoid activity of hydrocortisone at high dosage.

After stabilization, maintenance therapy can be considered in the form of oral hydrocortisone, 20 mg on awakening and 10 mg in the evening. The dose can be adjusted later. Fludrocortisone replacement (50–300 μg daily) may be needed, depending on postural symptoms, plasma electrolytes and renin activity. During the later stages of the patient's management the results of all the initial screening tests will become available and confirm

the diagnosis. A reversible form of biochemical hypothyroidism is common in Addison's disease and does not necessarily indicate coincidental autoimmune thyroid disease.

Conclusions

Acute adrenal insufficiency should be considered in any patient presenting with shock. Clues to the diagnosis can be gained from the typical symptomatology of chronic adrenal failure and excess pigmentation. A history of pituitary disease or of previous glucocorticoid administration is relevant to a diagnosis of secondary adrenal insufficiency. Further support for the diagnosis is obtained by findings of hyponatraemia, hyperkalaemia and hypoglycaemia. Routine blood tests to confirm the diagnosis of adrenal failure should be taken before steroid administration and hydrocortisone therapy are commenced without delay.

ACUTE PITUITARY EMERGENCIES

Introduction

Expanding lesions within the pituitary fossa result in local compression of the optic pathways and surrounding structures. Although most pituitary tumours grow slowly and produce gradual visual deterioration, others develop rapidly and require immediate investigation and treatment to prevent permanent visual loss. Pituitary apoplexy (in which there is sudden pituitary haemorrhage and infarction) may also result in a rapidly expanding mass and compression of the optic pathways. Emergency surgery may save life and prevent blindness.

The development of hypopituitarism in association with pituitary tumours and other lesions (Table 5) may be insidious and reasonably well tolerated. However, under certain conditions such as acute stress or pituitary apoplexy, the loss of an appropriate pituitary–adrenal response results in cardiovascular collapse. Although an acute deficiency of the majority of the pituitary hormones is well tolerated, absence of glucocorticoids is not and requires urgent replacement therapy. Similarly, impaired control of vasopressin release from the posterior pituitary results in diabetes insipidus and abnormalities of fluid balance control. Both of these situations should be considered in the A&E department if a pituitary gland disorder is suspected.

Table 5. *Pituitary tumours*

Secretory pituitary adenomas
– Prolactinoma
– Growth hormone secreting tumours
– ACTH-secreting tumours
– TSH-oma
– LH/FSH-oma
Non-functioning pituitary adenomas
Craniopharyngioma
Primary CNS neoplasms
– Meningioma
– Glioma
– Chordoma
Secondary metastatic deposits
Infiltrative diseases
– Infective
– Granulomatous
– Immune lymphocytic hypophysitis
Vascular lesions

Pituitary tumours and visual complications

Unless the patient arrives in the A&E department with a previous diagnosis of a pituitary tumour, it is unlikely that a definitive diagnosis will be made in time to guide therapy. However, it is worthwhile considering the differential diagnosis of pituitary lesions (see Table 5) since prolactinomas, which are relatively common, respond well to bromocriptine therapy without the need to refer for urgent surgery. This situation is especially relevant during pregnancy when tumour expansion occurs in approximately 20% of patients with macroadenomas (Grossman & Besser, 1985).

Clinical features

Expanding pituitary lesions cause pressure on the dura and this results in headache which is characteristically bitemporal and retro-orbital. Superior extension of the lesion may involve the optic pathways and cause visual deterioration. It is imperative in these patients to accurately record the visual acuity and to document the visual fields by confrontation with a red pin. Although a bitemporal hemianopia is more commonly associated with chiasmal compression from pituitary lesions, other field defects including subtle superior temporal defects are also well described. An afferent pupillary defect may be demonstrated as evidence of optic nerve compression, and disc pallor and papilloedema may be viewed on fundoscopy. Any acute threats to visual integrity should be regarded as an indication for emergency treatment since permanent visual loss may result from delayed management (Gaillard, 1992).

Lateral extensions of the pituitary tumour into the cavernous sinus may involve the third, fourth or sixth cranial nerves and cause diplopia. The patient may readily describe double vision but eye movements should be tested systematically to detect subtle abnormalities.

Diagnosis and treatment

Routine haematological, biochemical and radiological investigations may reveal no abnormalities. A skull X-ray, however, provides simple radiological confirmation of a pituitary tumour if an abnormal pituitary fossa is found (Fig. 5). If vision is compromised, urgent referral to an endocrine and neurosurgical centre is indicated. Basal pituitary function tests should be performed and a rapid prolactin result is useful if available. A macroprolactinoma can be immediately treated with bromocriptine which not only reduces the hyperprolactinaemia but also causes significant tumour shrinkage (Molitch et al., 1985). Rapid responses can be achieved with a 50 mg intramuscular depot injection of bromocriptine and improvement of visual fields may be seen within hours of treatment (Grossman & Besser, 1985).

A reduction in serum prolactin may be seen following bromocriptine in the presence of pituitary tumours other than prolactinomas. However, in these cases the tumours do not diminish in size (Grossman et al., 1985) and the risk to vision remains. These situations may need urgent surgery to decompress the lesion. Medical therapy with octreotide may also be appropriate in acromegaly (Lamberts, 1988). However, although approximately 50% of patients may show tumour shrinkage, the effects are much less dramatic than with bromocriptine (Anderson et al., 1992). Trans-sphenoidal surgery is therefore the treatment of choice for these situations and all patients require hydrocortisone cover in the perioperative period.

Pituitary apoplexy

This rare clinical syndrome is characterized by haemorrhagic infarction of the pituitary gland and is associated with sudden onset of headache, visual impairment, ophthalmoplegia, meningism and altered consciousness. The situation most commonly occurs in the presence of a pituitary adenoma (for review see Cardoso & Peterson, 1984) although it has also been described following the

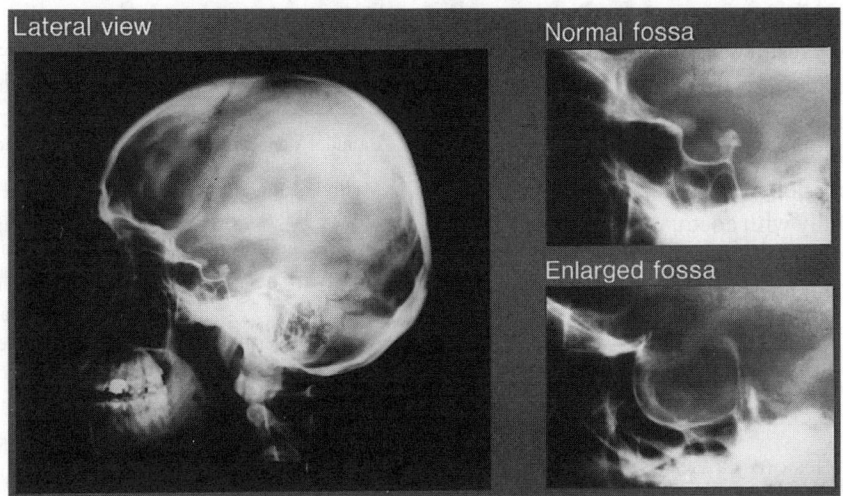

Fig. 5. Plain X-rays showing a lateral view of the skull with coned views demonstrating a normal pituitary fossa and an enlarged fossa of a patient with a pituitary tumour

use of anticoagulants, after head injury and also following dynamic pituitary function tests using TRH (thyrotrophin releasing hormone) and LHRH (luteinizing hormone releasing hormone).

The clinical features are difficult to differentiate from other sudden-onset CNS catastrophes such as subarachnoid haemorrhage. An urgent CT scan is mandatory to provide anatomical confirmation. The patient should be immediately referred to a neurosurgical unit where emergency surgery may be life-saving and prevent permanent visual loss and hypopituitarism (Arafah *et al.*, 1990). Multiple hormone deficiencies are common in the long term but diabetes insipidus is rare. The most important part of endocrine management is to anticipate acute adrenal insufficiency and provide glucocorticoid replacement therapy (hydrocortisone 100 mg IV stat followed by 100 mg IM 6-hourly).

Hypopituitarism and diabetes insipidus

Chronic hypopituitarism may be incomplete and well tolerated until an acute stress supervenes. The management of acute adrenal insufficiency is a priority (see above). It would be exceptional for a patient to also require thyroid replacement but if myxoedema coma is suspected then the management protocol described previously can be followed. It must be remembered that thyroid hormone replacement will aggravate adrenal insufficiency which should be corrected before giving thyroid hormone therapy.

Cranial diabetes insipidus results from impaired secretion of vasopressin from the neurohypophysis and is characterized by polyuria and thirst. An understanding of the basic mechanisms of water balance is essential so that diabetes insipidus can be promptly diagnosed. Water balance is achieved by feedback mechanisms involving thirst and control of water intake, and by the pituitary secretion of vasopressin and its antidiuretic action on the kidney. As a result plasma osmolality is maintained within a narrow range (280–290 mOsm kg^{-1}) and small changes influence vasopressin secretion.

Cranial diabetes insipidus may be associated with the many causes of hypopituitarism but may also result from head injuries, pituitary apoplexy and post partum necrosis. The diagnosis may be suspected after documentation of polyuria (e.g. urine >200 ml min^{-1}) with confirmation provided by finding a high plasma osmolality (>295 mOsm kg^{-1}) and an inappropriately low urine osmolality. The decision to treat depends very much on the clinical situation. Complete diabetes insipidus results in the passage of many litres of urine per day and inadequate fluid replacement may quickly result in hypernatraemia, hypovolaemia and cardiovascular collapse. The effect of acute hypernatraemia is to cause brain dehydration by intracellular fluid shift and this results in the neurological signs of lethargy, confusion and coma. The treatment of choice for diabetes insipidus is desmopressin (1 µg of DDAVP subcutaneously), which is a long-acting vasopressin analogue with minimal pressor activity but potent antidiuretic activity.

Situations in which care must be taken with adjustment of fluid balance include those patients in whom the hypernatraemia has developed chronically (Snyder *et al.*, 1987). These patients would have few symptoms of acute hypernatraemia, but rapid restoration of the serum sodium to normal may result in cerebral oedema, seizures and death. In addition, there are clinical situations such as head trauma in which the patient is deliberately managed with a high plasma osmolality to limit cerebral oedema. Provided the polyuria of diabetes insipidus can be managed successfully with adequate fluid replacement it may be relevant to withdraw desmopressin therapy and adjust the fluid balance according to clinical requirements.

Conclusions

Expanding pituitary lesions cause visual symptoms by compressive effects on the optic pathways. Rapid visual deterioration requires urgent assessment and treatment in order to prevent permanent visual failure. When the problems are caused by an enlarging macroprolactinoma, treatment with bromocriptine has been shown to result in rapid tumour shrinkage and improvement in visual fields. It is likely that urgent surgery will be required to relieve the visual failure caused by other pituitary tumours. Hypopituitarism in its acute form is life-threatening and it is most relevant to treat impending adrenal insufficiency. Diabetes insipidus may also be a feature but this is easily managed with desmopressin.

HYPERTENSIVE CRISIS AND SUSPECTED PHAEOCHROMOCYTOMA

It is not uncommon for patients with a hypertensive crisis to be assessed in the A&E department. This may be defined as a severely elevated blood pressure (e.g. diastolic >120 mmHg) and may be considered a hypertensive emergency if there is associated cardiac, renal or CNS deterioration. There are many causes for both hypertension and a hypertensive crisis. However, clinical suspicion of a phaeochromocytoma is critical since pharmacological mismanagement can have disastrous effects and contribute to the high mortality of this condition. An understanding of the typical symptoms and associated physical signs increases the likelihood that phaeochromocytoma will be included in the list of differential diagnoses.

Incidence

Phaeochromocytoma represents a rare cause of hypertension (<1%) but a significant number are unsuspected clinically and are diagnosed at autopsy (St John Lutton *et al.*, 1981). The 10% rule is a useful reminder of some

Table 6. *Familial syndromes associated with phaeochromocytoma*

Syndrome	Characteristics
Familial phaeochromocytoma	No typical features
Multiple endocrine neoplasia	
Type IIa	Phaeochromocytoma
	Medullary carcinoma of thyroid
Type IIb	Phaeochromocytoma
	Medullary carcinoma of thyroid
	Multiple mucosal neuromas
	Marfanoid habitus
	Medullated corneal nerve fibre
Neurofibromatosis	Phaeochromocytoma
	Neurofibromata
	Café au lait pigmentation
	Axillary freckling
Von Lippel–Lindau	Phaeochromocytoma
	Retinal angiomas
	Cerebellar haemangioblastomas

of the features of phaeochromocytoma: 10% are diagnosed in childhood, 10% are extra-adrenal, 10% are bilateral, 10% are malignant and 10% are associated with a familial syndrome. Knowledge of the familial syndromes and the characteristic physical signs is helpful (Table 6).

Presentation

Hypertension is invariantly present (90% of cases) and this may be sustained or paroxysmal. Additional features include paroxysms of headache, sweating, palpitations, anxiety, chest pain and abdominal pain (Ross & Griffith, 1989). The paroxysm may be precipitated by a variety of factors including exercise, positional change and abdominal palpation. Medical intervention including some pharmacological agents, CT contrast dyes, anaesthesia and surgery are also known to precipitate paroxysms and should not be considered until the patient has been adequately treated.

Clinical signs

During a paroxysm the patient may appear pale and anxious with cold clammy extremities. Despite the hypertension there may be a postural drop in blood pressure associated with blood volume contraction and impaired sympathetic reflex control. Signs of chronic hypertension such as hypertensive retinopathy, cardiomyopathy and renal failure may be present. An adrenal phaeochromocytoma is rarely palpable. Signs of a familial syndrome should be actively sought; these include neurofibromatosis, mucosal neuromas, retinal angiomas and cerebellar signs of Von Hippel–Lindau disease. In addition, the neck should be palpated since an associated medullary carcinoma of the thyroid suggests multiple endocrine neoplasia type II (Thakker, 1993).

Routine investigations

A full blood count may show an increased haematocrit and this reflects the volume contraction caused by constant alpha-adrenergic stimulation. Impaired glucose tolerance is also associated with adrenergic stimulation and adds further to the clinical suspicion of a phaeochromocytoma. Hypercalcaemia has also been recognized and may be related to the secretion of parathyroid hormone related protein from the tumour which is also known to secrete a number of neuroendocrine tumour markers. Confirmation that the patient has a phaeochromocytoma is obtained by measuring plasma catecholamines and collecting 24-h urine samples in acid for catecholamine estimations (Sheps et al., 1990). Localization of the tumour can be investigated later using CT or MRI (magnetic resonance imaging) and with MIBG (^{131}I-labelled meta-iodobenzylguanidine) scanning. The latter technique detects the uptake of MIBG into chromaffin cells.

Management of a hypertensive crisis

A hypertensive crisis without any of the features of a phaeochromocytoma can be treated with oral nifedipine. The aim is to achieve a gradual reduction in blood pressure reducing the diastolic by approximately 25%. However, a hypertensive emergency is by definition associated wth cardiac, renal or CNS deterioration. The aim is to admit the patient for cardiac and blood pressure monitoring and to produce a prompt but gradual decrease in blood pressure to approximately 25% of the diastolic over a few hours. This blood pressure is maintained for several days and gradually reduced to normotensive levels over a few weeks. Too rapid a reduction in blood pressure may cause end-organ ischaemia or infarction with permanent CNS or cardiac deficit.

Many pharmacological agents are available for blood pressure control but sodium nitroprusside is recommended for the patient in whom the cause of the hypertension is unknown (Calhoun & Oparil, 1990). An intravenous infusion of this short-acting agent provides an easily adjustable regimen. Labetolol has also been widely used although it should not be used if a phaeochromocytoma is suspected because the drug has weaker alpha-blockade than beta-action and may therefore be associated with a pressor crisis (Sever et al., 1980).

Hypertensive control and phaeochromocytoma

In the case of a hypertensive emergency the short acting alpha-adrenergic blocker phentolamine (1–5 mg boluses IV) is the drug of choice. The longer-acting alpha-blocker, phenoxybenzamine (10 mg orally four times daily or 40 mg in 500 ml of 5% dextrose IV over 2 h), can then be used to stabilize the blood pressure. A beta-blocker such as propranolol (80 mg 8-hourly) is indicated for tachycardia and arrhythmias but should only be started after alpha-blockade to avoid paradoxical hypertensive crisis.

Summary

Labile or hypertensive crises represent a common problem in A&E departments. The attending physician should always be aware of the possibility of an underlying phaeochromocytoma and take a careful history and a detailed clinical examination. If phaeochromocytoma is suspected then it is important to follow certain pharmacological guidelines and avoid drugs known to precipitate a pressor crisis. Thus the patient should receive adequate alpha-blockade before a beta-blocker is introduced.

Bibliography

ANDERSON, S.W.J., CHARLESWORTH, M., BESSER, G.M. et al. (1992). Effects of preoperative treatment with the somatostatin analogue octreotide on pituitary tumour size in acromagelic patients. J. Endrocrinol., **132** (Suppl.), 260.

ARAFAH, B.M., HARRINGTON, J.F., MADHOUN, Z.T. et al. (1990). Improvement of pituitary function after surgical decompression for pituitary tumour apoplexy. J. Clin. Endocrinol Metab., **71**, 323–8.

BARBOSA, J., WONG, E. & DOE, R.P. (1972). Ophthalmopathy of Graves disease. Outcome after treatment with radioactive iodine, surgery or antithyroid drugs. Arch. Intern. Med., **130**, 111.

BELL, N.H. (1985). Vitamin D – endocrine system. J. Clin. Invest., **76**, 1–6.

BESSER, G.M., CULLEN, D.R., IRVINE, W.J. et al. (1971). Immunoreactive corticotrophin levels in adrenocorticol insufficiency. Br. Med. J., **374**, 374–6.

BILEZIKIAN, J.P. (1992). Management of acute hyper-calcaemia. *N. Engl. J. Med.*, **326**, 1196–203.

BLUM, M., KRANJAC, T., PARK, C.M. *et al.* (1976). Thyroid storm after cardiac angiography with iodinated contrast medium. *JAMA*, **235**, 2324.

BROADUS, A.E., MANGIN, M., INSOGNA, K.L. *et al.* (1988). Humoral hypercalcaemia of cancer: identification of a novel parathyroid hormone-like peptide. *N. Engl. J. Med.*, **319**, 556–63.

BURGER, A.G. & PHILIPPE, J. (1992). Thyroid emergencies. In *Endrocrine Emergencies. Baillière's Clinical Endocrinology and Metabolism*, Vol. 6(1), ed. A.G. Burger & J. Philippe. pp. 77–93. London: Baillière Tindall.

BURKE, C.W. (1985). Adrenocortical insufficiency. *Clin. Endocrinol. Metab.*, **14**, 947–76.

CALHOUN, D.A. & OPARIL, S. (1990). Treatment of hypertensive crisis. *N. Engl. J. Med.*, **323**, 1177–83.

CARDOSO, E.R. & PETERSON, E.W. (1984). Pituitary apoplexy: a review. *J. Neurosurg.*, **14**, 363–73.

CHERNOW, B., BURMAN, K.D., JOHNSON, D.L. *et al.* (1983). T_3 may be a better agent than T_4 in the critically ill hypothryoid patient: evaluation of transport across the blood–brain barrier in a primate model. *Crit. Care Med.*, **11**, 99–104.

DAVIS, J.R.A. & HEATH, D.A. (1989). Comparison of different dose regimes of aminohydroxypropylidene-1,1-diphosphonate (APD) in hypercaelcaemia of malignancy. *Br. J. Clin. Pharmacol.*, **28**, 269–74.

FISKEN, R.A., HEATH, D.A. & BOLD, A.M. (1980). Hypercalcaemia – a hospital survey. *Q. J. Med.*, **49**, 405–18.

FRIEDMAN, J.H., CHIUCCHINI, M.A.J.I. & TUCCI, J.R. (1987). Idiopathic hypoparathyroidism with extensive brain calcification and persistent neurologic dysfunction. *Neurology*, **37**, 307–9.

GAILLARD, R.C. (1992). Pituitary gland emergencies. In *Endocrine Emergencies. Baillière's Clinical Endocrunology and Metabolism*, Vol. 6 (1), ed. A.G. Burger & J. Philippe. pp.57–75. London: Baillière Tindall.

GROSSMAN, A. & BESSER, G.M. (1985). Regular review: prolactinomes. *Br. Med. J.*, **290**, 182–4.

GROSSMAN, A., ROSS, R., CHARLESWORTH, M. *et al.* (1985). The effect of dopamine agonist therapy on large functionless pituitary tumours. *Clin. Endocrinol.*, **22**, 679–86.

HELLMAN, R., KELLY, K.L. & MASON, W.D. (1977). Propranolol for thyroid storm. *N. Engl. J. Med.*, **297**, 671.

HOSKING, D.J. & GILSON, D. (1984). Comparison of the renal and skeletal actions of calcitonin in the treatment of severe hypercalcaemia of malignancy. *Q. J. Med.*, **211**, 359–69.

KHOSLA, S., WOLFSON, J.S., DEMERJIAN, Z. *et al.* (1989). Adrenal crisis in the setting of high-dose ketoconazole therapy. *Arch. Intern. Med.*, **149**, 40–4.

LAMBERTS, S.W.J. (1988). The role of somatostatin in the regulation of anterior pituitary hormone secretion and the use of its analogs in the treatment of human pituitary tumours. *Endocr. Rev.*, **9**, 417–36.

LINDBERGER, K. (1975). Myxoedema coma. *Acta Med. Scand.*, **198**, 87–90.

MARX, S.J., ATTIE, M.F., LEVINE, M.A. *et al.* (1981). The hypocalciuric or benign variant of familial hypercalcaemia. Clinical and biochemical features in 15 kindreds. *Medicine*, **60**, 397–412.

MEMBRENO, L., IRONY, I., DERE, W. *et al.* (1987). Adrenocortical function in acquired immuno deficiency syndrome. *J. Clin. Endocrinol. Metab.*, **65**, 487.

MIGEON, C.J., KENNY, F.M., HUNG, W. *et al.* (1967). Study of adrenal function in children with meningitis. *Pediatrics*, **40**, 163–83.

MOLITCH, M., ELTON, R.L., BLACKWELL, R.E. *et al.* (1985). Bromocriptine as primary therapy for prolactin-secreting macroadenomas: results of a prospective multicenter study. *J. Clin. Endocrinol. Metab.*, **60**, 698–705.

NELSON, N.C. & BECKER, W.F. (1969). Thyroid crisis: diagnosis and treatment. *Ann. Surg.*, **170**, 263.

PERCIVAL, R.C., YATES, A.J.P., GRAY, R.E.S. *et al.* (1984). Role of glucocorticoids in the management of malignant hypercalcaemia. *BMJ*, **289**, 287.

RIZZOLI, R. & BONJOUR, J.-P. (1992). Management of disorders of calcium homeostasis. In *Endrocrine Emergencies. Baillière's Clinical Endocrinology and Metabolism*, Vol. (6) 1, ed. A.G. Burger & J. Philippe. pp. 129–42. London: Baillière Tindall.

ROSS, E.J. & GRIFFITH, D.N.W. (1989). The clinical presentation of phaeochromocytoma. *Q. J. Med.*, **266**, 485–96.

RUDE, R.K. & SINGER, F.R. (1981). Magnesium deficiency and excess. *Annu. Rev. Med.*, **32**, 245–59.

SANDLER, L.M., WINEARLS, C.G., FRAHER, L.J. *et al.* (1984). Studies of the hypercalcaemia of sarcoidosis: effect of steroids and exogenous vitamin D3 on circulating concentration of 1,25-dihydroxy vitamin D3. *Q. J. Med.*, **53**, 165–80.

SCHLAGHECKE, R., KORNELY, E., SANTER, R. *et al.* (1992). The effect of long term glucocorticoid therapy on pituitary–adrenal responses to exogenous corticotrophin-releasing hormone. *N. Engl. J. Med.*, **326**, 226–30.

SEVER, P.S., ROBERTS, J.C. & SNALL, M.E. (1980). Pheochromocytoma. *Clin. Endocrinol. Metab.*, **9**(3), 543–68.

SHEPS, S.G., JIANG, N.S., KLEE, G.G. *et al.* (1990). Recent developments in the diagnosis and treatment of pheochromocytoma. *Mayo Clin. Proc.*, **65**, 88–95.

SNYDER, N.A., FERGAL, D.W. & ARIEFF, A.I. (1987). Hypernatraemia in elderly patients. *Ann. Intern. Med.*, **107**, 656–64.

ST JOHN LUTTON, M.G., SHEPS, S.G. & LIE, J.T. (1981). Prevalence of clinically unsuspected pheochromocytoma: review of 50 year autopsy series. *Mayo Clin. Proc.*, **56**, 354–60.

THAKKER, R.V. (1993). The molecular genetics of the multiple endocrine neoplasia syndromes. *Clin. Endocrinol.*, **38**, 1–14.

VITA, J.A., SILVEBERG, S.J., GOLAND, R.S. *et al.* (1985). Clinical clues to the cause of Addison's disease. *Am. J. Med.*, **78**, 461–66.

WALDSTEIN, S.S., SLODKI, S.J., KAGONIEC, G.I. *et al.* (1960). A clinical study of thyroid storm. *Ann. Intern. Med.*, **52**, 626.

WARTOFSKY, L. (1991). Myxoedema coma. In *Werner's The Thyroid. A Fundamental Clinical Text*. 6th Edition. ed. L.E. Braverman. & R.D. Utiger. pp. 1084–91. Philadelphia: J.B. Lippincott Co.

WARTOFSKY, L. & BURMAN, K.D. (1982). Alterations in thyroid function in patients with systemic illness: the 'Euthyroid Sick Syndrome'. *Endocr. Rev.*, **3**, 164–217.

WIMPFHEIMER, C., STAUBLI, M., SCHADELM, J. *et al.* (1982). Prednisolone in amidarone-induced thyrotoxicosis. *BrMJ*, **284**, 1835–36.

57 Diabetic emergencies

J. ANDERSON and E. GALE

Department of Diabetes and Metabolism, St Bartholomew's Hospital, London, UK

Chapter plan

Pathophysiology
Clinical and laboratory diagnosis
Classification of diabetes
Diabetic emergencies
Conditions presenting to A&E departments in which
  diabetes may play a significant part
Prevention

PATHOPHYSIOLOGY

Diabetes mellitus is a state of chronic hyperglycaemia resulting from absolute or relative deficiency of insulin in the circulation. Insulin has a vital action in the metabolism of many carbohydrates (Ferrannini & DeFronzo, 1992), lipids (Kissebah, 1992) and proteins (DeFronzo & Ferrannini, 1992), and is of pivotal importance in the maintenance of steady blood concentrations of glucose and other metabolites (Walker & Alberti, 1992). The actions of insulin are balanced by those of counter-regulatory hormones including glucagon, adrenaline, noradrenaline, cortisol and growth hormone. Homeostasis is maintained by a dynamic balance between these opposing forces.

Although insulin is important in several areas of metabolism, its effect on blood glucose captures the attention of most clinicians. This is because glucose is easy to measure and because the effects of insulin on lipids, ketones and protein are less easy to quantitate. It is, however, important to remember that insulin has metabolic actions other than those on blood glucose, and that these contribute to the acute and chronic disorders produced by diabetes.

Glucose is poorly absorbed from the stomach but enters the circulation rapidly from the small intestine. Anything which delays gastric emptying reduces the bioavailability of glucose taken by mouth. Glucose passes to the liver via the portal venous system, as does insulin secreted by the β-cells of the pancreas. It is taken up by liver cells under the influence of insulin and either used as a fuel, converted into lipids and other substances, or stored as glycogen. Some glucose and insulin move on into the systemic circulation where glucose acts as the major aerobic metabolic fuel and insulin modulates glucose entry into target tissues.

Glucose entering the circulation postprandially is stored in muscle cells as glycogen or taken up into fat cells and metabolized into lipid. Once food is digested, no more glucose enters the circulation from the gut but the circulating blood glucose concentration remains regulated within narrow limits. This is achieved by reduced insulin secretion and a rise in counter-regulatory hormones. This combination stimulates release of glucose from the liver by glycogen breakdown (glycogenolysis) or synthesis of glucose from amino acids, glycerol or lactate (gluconeogenesis).

The kidneys actively reabsorb glucose from the glomerular filtrate. Glycosuria occurs when the concentration of glucose in the glomerula filtrate rises sufficiently to overcome the renal threshold for reabsorption. The renal threshold for glucose varies, and a few individuals have asymptomatic glycosuria despite normal blood glucose levels. This also occurs in pregnancy as the renal threshold for glucose falls. Conversely, the renal threshold may be elevated in the elderly. Asymptomatic hyperglycaemia is one consequence of this since the threshold for osmotic diuresis is elevated, and urine tests for glucose may give false reassurance, or at least a misleading impression of glycaemic control.

CLINICAL AND LABORATORY DIAGNOSIS

Diabetes is usually easy to diagnose, with characteristic symptoms such as thirst, polyuria, nocturia, weight loss, pruritus vulvae or balanitis and blurred vision. When symptoms are present, a single fasting plasma glucose of $8 \, \text{nmol} \, l^{-1}$ or more, or a random plasma glucose concentration of $12 \, \text{nmol} \, l^{-1}$ or more, will clinch the diagnosis. Almost all patients are diagnosed in this way and the glucose tolerance test should be reserved for the minority with borderline hyperglycaemia and few or no symptoms. Transient hyperglycaemia may develop in the course of many acute illnesses, and the label of diabetes should not be bestowed until it is apparent that hyperglycaemia persists when the acute stress has passed.

The World Health Organization criteria (WHO Study Group, 1985) by which diabetes is diagnosed using a standard 75 g glucose tolerance test are set out in Table 1. Many regard the criteria for diagnosis of diabetes or impaired glucose tolerance as arbitrary. This is not the case. The levels of hyperglycaemia defining diabetes were chosen because epidemiological studies have shown that microvascular complications rarely develop until these have been exceeded. They have important practical relevance.

An intermediate category of *impaired glucose tolerance* has also been designated by the WHO. This is based on the oral glucose tolerance test, and indeed can only be diagnosed by this means (Yudkin *et al.*, 1990). People in this category are relatively immune from microvascular disease but the risk of arterial disease due to atherosclerosis is as high as in frank diabetes. Impaired glucose tolerance is therefore an important cardiovascular risk factor. One-third of individuals with impaired glucose tolerance will progress to frank diabetes within 5 years. The risk of progression increases with a sedentary lifestyle and obesity. Patients should be advised to keep as slim and as fit as possible. Steps should be taken to correct other cardiovascular risk factors such as smoking. The blood glucose concentration should be measured at least once a year to detect any worsening in glucose tolerance.

Many patients are screened for diabetes in accident and emergency (A & E) departments. Urine tests are painless and simple, but have poor sensitivity and specificity in detecting diabetes for the reasons set out above. Blood tests are more useful, but it is important not to rely on fingerprick tests performed by untrained staff. Alarmingly few nurses have been trained to use a glucose meter correctly.

CLASSIFICATION OF DIABETES

Secondary diabetes

Whenever diabetes is diagnosed, the possibility that this might be secondary to another disorder should be considered. All of the following secondary causes of diabetes are rare. Their importance is that the treatment of the patient is often different from the treatment of primary diabetes alone.

- Pancreatic:
  - Haemochromatosis.
  - Chronic pancreatitis.
  - Cancer of the pancreas.
  - Cystic fibrosis.
- Hormonal:
  - Thyrotoxicosis.
  - Acromegaly.
  - Cushing's syndrome.
  - Phaeochromocytoma.
  - Glucagonoma.
- Drug-induced:
  - Steroids.
  - Antihypertensive drugs (e.g. thiazides).
  - Others.

Table 1. *The glucose tolerance test*
- 75 g of glucose (or 375 ml of Lucozade)
- Only a fasting and a 120-min sample are needed (results are for venous plasma)

	Not diabetic	Impaired glucose tolerance	Diabetes mellitus
Fasting	$< 7.8 \, \text{mmol} \, l^{-1}$	$< 7.8 \, \text{mmol} \, l^{-1}$	$> 7.8 \, \text{mmol} \, l^{-1}$
2 hr after 75 g of glucose	$< 7.8 \, \text{mmol} \, l^{-1}$	$7.8–11.0 \, \text{mmol} \, l^{-1}$	$11.1 \, \text{mmol} \, l^{-1}$ or more

Notes
- There is no such thing as mild diabetes. All patients who meet the criteria for diabetes are liable to disabling long-term complications.
- When glucose is measured in whole venous blood, subtract $1.1 \, \text{mmol} \, l^{-1}$ from the above values.

- Neurological syndromes:
  - –Friedreich's ataxia.
  - –Myotonic dystrophy.

Weight loss is characteristic of undiagnosed diabetes, but thyrotoxicosis should be suspected when this is marked, whether or not the thyroid is enlarged. Other features such as excessive sweating, tremor, agitation, palpitations, tachycardia, a goitre, lid-lag, Graves ophthalmopathy, muscular weakness and hyper-reflexia (see Chapter 56) may be present.

Cushing's syndrome, acromegaly and phaeochromocytoma are much rarer causes of secondary diabetes but are important since they are treatable and considerable morbidity can result if they remain undetected. The features of Cushing's syndrome (truncal obesity, hypertension, hirsutism, backache and depression) are common in the general population, but clinical suspicion should be aroused by vertebral crush fractures, purple abdominal striae or a proximal myopathy. The best way to exclude Cushing's syndrome is with a low-dose dexamethasone suppression test (see Chapter 56). Acromegaly is suggested by facial appearance, or more specific features including excessive sweating, greasy skin, and enlargement of the hands and feet (or of hat size) after the age of 21 years (see Chapter 56 for the biochemical diagnostic criteria). Phaeochromocytoma may be suspected from a history of hypertension, particularly if intermittent, associated with palpitations, flushing and headache (a surprisingly unusual feature of essential hypertension). Diagnosis is by 24-h urinary catecholamine measurement (see chapter 56).

Cancer of the pancreas should be suspected in any middle-aged person who has recent-onset diabetes associated with abdominal pain, unexplained jaundice or marked weight loss. An ultrasound scan of the pancreas is the initial diagnostic test. Sadly, there is no evidence that early detection affects prognosis.

Non-insulin-dependent diabetes mellitus (NIDDM) is associated with hypertension in 30% of patients of European extraction and 50% of Afro-Caribbeans. Many new patients present with this combination and are on treatment with thiazide diuretics which may have precipitated the onset of diabetes. Patients on steroids should be actively screened for diabetes.

Non-insulin-dependent diabetes

Most people with diabetes presenting over the age of 40 years do not need insulin treatment, at least initially. Such patients are classified as having non-insulin-dependent diabetes (NIDDM). Although the presenta-

tion is often less dramatic than with insulin-dependent diabetes (IDDM), these patients are also at risk of microvascular disease. The risk of myocardial infarction and stroke is two to three times higher than in similarly aged non-diabetic people (Pranzram, 1987), while the risk of peripheral vascular disease is greatly increased. The morbidity and mortality from diabetic retinopathy, cataract, neuropathy, foot disease and renal failure are also considerable.

Between 1.5% and 3% of the white population, and a higher proportion in Afro-Caribbean and Asian ethnic groups, suffer from diabetes (Odugbesan et al., 1989; Mather & Keen, 1985). Studies of identical and non-identical twins with diabetes have revealed that the tendency to develop NIDDM is strongly inherited (Lo et al., 1991). The age at which the disease is manifest is influenced by body weight, diet and level of physical activity. If one member of an identical twin pair develops NIDDM the other twin will almost always develop the disease provided that he/she lives long enough.

Because its onset is often insidious, NIDDM is often discovered in patients attending A & E departments with unrelated problems.

Insulin-dependent diabetes

Patients with insulin-dependent diabetes (IDDM) have sustained pancreatic beta-cell damage resulting in severe insulin deficiency and are therefore prone to ketosis. The risk of developing IDDM is HLA-linked, and autoimmune processes play an important role in its pathogenesis (Bingley & Gale, 1991). Most newly diagnosed patients have circulating autoantibodies directed against antigens present in islet cells. Environmental factor(s) are assumed to trigger autoimmunity in genetically susceptible individuals, but their nature remains uncertain. Although about two-thirds of patients with IDDM present before the age of 30 years, it can develop at any age. Age is therefore a poor criterion for insulin treatment, and the decision should be based on the clinical condition of the patient together with such pointers as short duration or severe symptoms, moderate or heavy ketonuria, major weight loss, coexistence of other autoimmune disease or a first-degree family history of IDDM.

DIABETIC EMERGENCIES
Ketoacidosis

Diabetic ketoacidosis is still a significant cause of death in IDDM patients under the age of 45 years and many of these deaths are potentially avoidable (Tunbridge, 1981). Reasons for death have included late presentation, self-neglect, poor clinical management, or coexistence of another severe disease process. The overall mortality ranges from 5% to 10% in published series, with worse prognosis in children under 10 years and in the elderly.

The hallmarks of diabetic ketoacidosis are (Marshall & Alberti, 1986):

- Hyperglycaemia.
- The presence of ketones in the blood (and urine).
- A metabolic acidosis.
- Dehydration.
- Electrolyte imbalances.

Ketoacidosis is differentiated from the hyperosmolar non-ketotic state and from lactic acidosis by the presence of ketones.

Pathophysiology of ketoacidosis

The combination of insulin deficiency and excess production of stress hormones (glucagon, catecholamines, growth hormone and cortisol) promotes accelerated hepatic glucose production via glycogen breakdown and unrestrained gluconeogenesis. This glucose is unavailable to cells in the absence of insulin, and is flushed through the kidneys causing an osmotic diuresis with loss of water, sodium, potassium, phosphate and other electrolytes.

The same hormonal changes result in rapid lipolysis and release of triglycerides and non-esterified fatty acids from fat cells. Circulating triglycerides may render the plasma lipaemic, and electrolyte measurement may show pseudohyponatraemia for the same reason. The fatty acids are broken down in liver cells and (under conditions of insulin deficiency and stress hormone excess) are metabolized to ketones in hepatic mitochondria. Ketone bodies in excess produce acidosis, leading to hyperventilation, prostration, nausea and (sometimes) abdominal pain.

In early ketoacidosis the rise in plasma glucose is partly compensated by the loss of glucose in the urine, but this compensatory mechanism is later overwhelmed by the rate of hepatic gluconeogenesis. Glycosuria may have one beneficial side-effect since the diuresis that results preserves renal function in the presence of hypoperfusion. The fluid lost is initially replaced by drinking, but eventually nausea makes this impossible, while vomiting compounds the problem. The patient has entered a vicious spiral which – untreated – would inevitably result in death.

Causes of ketoacidosis

About 25% of patients with ketoacidosis have previously undiagnosed diabetes. Another 25% are diabetic patients who have omitted or reduced their dose of insulin themselves, or been advised to by a doctor. This has usually been done because patients are unable to eat because of nausea or vomiting and are afraid of hypoglycaemia if they take their normal dose of insulin. Another 25% have an intercurrent illness such as an infection or a heart attack which has precipitated ketoacidosis. In the final quarter, no clear cause can be found.

The insulin dose should NEVER be reduced because of nausea or vomiting.

Instead the patient should check the blood glucose frequently, should take a normal or increased insulin dose as appropriate, and should balance this with sugary drinks or other easily absorbed forms of rapidly digestible carbohydrate. If oral fluid cannot be retained, hospital admission and intravenous fluids are necessary.

Presenting features of ketoacidosis

Patients present with the symptoms of uncontrolled diabetes and signs of dehydration and acidosis. The symptoms typically develop over hours or even days. In elderly patients, confusion and urinary incontinence may also be present. Dehydration (dry mouth, sunken eyes, postural hypotension) is almost universal. Ketones have a distinctive smell. Acidosis causes warm dry skin, hyperventilation, vomiting and – occasionally – abdominal pain which has been known to trap the unwary surgeon into laparotomy. Most patients in ketoacidosis, even those severely ill, are conscious. Stupor is unusual and coma is now extremely rare. The symptoms of the precipitating illness (e.g. urinary tract infection, pneumonia, or heart attack) may contribute to the clinical features, but chest infection is easy to overlook on clinical examination of a hyperventilating patient.

The differential diagnosis should present little difficulty provided a history is available. The possibility of overdose, stroke or subarachnoid haemorrhage should be considered in unconscious patients (even if ketoacidosis is also present). Some textbooks provide a detailed list of features which distinguish hypoglycaemic coma from diabetic ketoacidosis, but these resemble each other so little that one might be forgiven for wondering if the authors had ever encountered either condition!

Patient management

Immediate management

Classic ketoacidosis can be diagnosed at a glance, or by inhaling as you enter the examination cubicle. Confirmation proceeds through three stages. The first is to establish that the patient has diabetes from the history or by fingerprick blood testing. The second is to establish that ketosis is present. This can be shown by moderate or heavy ketonuria (traces of ketones appear in many other conditions), or by testing the plasma with a ketone stick after centrifugation. A potential pitfall is that standard bedside tests do not detect the ketone beta-hydroxybutyrate which may rarely be the dominant anion. For this reason, and as good practice, it is useful to establish that an anion gap acidosis is present by calculating the anion gap from the plasma electrolyte concentrations (one reason why chloride measurement should always be requested if not routinely reported by your laboratory). Finally, acidosis is confirmed by measurement of blood gases. Measurement of venous pH is sufficient in those who are clinically well. Arterial blood gas measurement contributes little to management unless the illness is complicated by respiratory problems.

These investigations can be set on track within minutes of admission, and should not delay treatment which should begin as soon as the diagnosis has been made. The need for rapid treatment often falls foul of the perceived competing need for 'a full history, examination and special investigations' (as in the classic scenario of the patient who spends an hour in X-ray with his drip turned off before going up to the ward).

Blood should be sent to the laboratory as a matter of urgency, intravenous access should be established and simple fluid therapy started. After that a brief history and examination are needed to answer three principal questions:

1. What is the precipitating cause?
2. How badly dehydrated is the patient?
3. Is there coincident cardiac or renal disease which will complicate therapy?

Subsequent management

Treatment can be subdivided into three phases (see Technique section) During the first phase of treatment, there is an enormous excess of glucose in the blood and a deficiency inside cells. Insulin allows glucose to enter cells. The plasma concentration of glucose falls and potassium, water and phosphate are also driven into the cells. This flux of potassium into cells is initially rapid and can endanger the patient from hypokalaemia unless an adequate supply of potassium is provided. Since it is impossible to estimate the size of the potassium deficit within cells in any given patient, regular monitoring of electrolyte concentrations during the initial phases of treatment, and adjustment of the rate of potassium infusion, is mandatory. Even a patient with complete anuria will have a large potassium flux into cells when insulin treatment is started and will require potassium intravenously in the first hour or two of treatment. It is clearly vital to measure urine output from the beginning of treatment and to rapidly stop potassium supplementation once it is clear that urine output is inadequate.

We have found that the main risk of providing guidelines is that they tend to be followed mindlessly regardless of the situation. The fluid and electrolyte replacement regimen proposed assumes that the patient is severely dehydrated and that the patient is not elderly and does not have cardiac or renal insufficiency. Treatment should always depend on individual clinical evaluation plus careful monitoring of the response to treatment. Renal failure and hypokalaemic death can occur due to under-replacement of fluids or electrolytes. Cerebral and pulmonary oedema can occur following overenthusiastic application of a standard recipe in inappropriate circumstances.

TECHNIQUE

Management of diabetic ketoacidosis
(a didactic scheme for modification in the light of each patient's particular circumstances)

Phase I

1. *Confirm diagnosis*
   - Capillary blood glucose test
   - Measure urine or plasma ketones
2. *Take blood*
   - Glucose, sodium, potassium,
   - Urea, bicarbonate
   - Full blood count
   - Blood cultures
   - Cardiac enzymes
   - Venous/arterial gases
3. *Intravenous fluids*
   - Normal saline +20 mmol KCl 1 litre in 30 min; then 1 h; then 2 h; then 4 h

4. *History and examination*
   a. Precipitating cause
      - ?Stopping insulin
      - ?Chest or urine infection
      - ?Heart attack
   b. How severe is dehydration?
      - Blood pressure
      - Capillary filling
      - Temperature of extremities
      - Peripheral cyanosis
      - Poor tissue turgor
   c. Underlying diseases
      - Pre-existing heart/renal disease
5. *Insulin*
   - 6 units h^{-1} IV
6. *Further investigations*
   - Chest X-ray
   - ECG
   - Midstream urine
7. *Other measures*
   - Nasogastric tube – gastric dilation
   - Coma – position patient
   - Catheterize if poor urine output
   - Oxygen if shocked
   - Blood/plasma expander for persistent hypotension
   - Heparin if severely dehydrated
   - Consider central venous pressure line
   - Consider bicarbonate (pH < 7.0)
8. *Reassess*
   - Hourly – capillary blood glucose test
   - 2-hourly – clinically assess volume status
   - 2-hourly – sodium, potassium
   - Blood gases

Phase II (blood glucose < 12 mmol l^{-1})

1. *Change fluids to:*
   - 1 litre 5% dextrose +20 mmol KCl 6-hourly
2. *Change fixed insulin dose to:*
   - Variable-dose regimen (example)

Blood glucose concentration (mmol l^{-1})	Insulin infusion rate (units h^{-1})
0–3.5	0
3.6–6.0	1
6.1–9.0	2
9.1–12.0	3
12.1–16.0	4
16.1–20.0	5
20.1–	6

Phase III

When
- Acidosis has resolved
- Able to eat and drink

1. *Stop all intravenous therapy*
2. *Start regular premeal subcutaneous insulin*
   - Four times daily dose regimen
   - 24 h total dose of insulin is equal to the last 24-h insulin consumption
3. *Search for precipitating cause*

What sort of fluid replacement?

There is some debate as to whether plasma expanders should be used instead of simple crystalloid solutions in the early phase of treatment. Our view is that most patients with ketoacidosis have relatively normal capillary permeability and are deficient in water and electrolytes but not in plasma proteins, and that water and electrolytes should therefore be given. Hypotension will usually correct itself rapidly once adequate quantities of crystalloid solution are given to the patient. We use plasma expanders only when there is evidence that a patient is failing to perfuse his/her brain and kidneys at presentation, and that this situation is failing to respond to treatment with crystalloid solutions.

When to use bicarbonate?

Another controversy surrounds use of sodium bicarbonate to correct severe acidosis – a controversy which, incidentally, antedates the introduction of insulin! The hazards of bicarbonate are:

- Increased anaerobic glycolysis.
- Hypokalaemia.
- Slightly impaired oxygen delivery to the tissues.
- A paradoxical fall in the pH of cerebrospinal fluid.

The potential benefit is in reversing consequences of severe acidosis such as vasoconstriction, reduced cardiac output, insulin resistance and impaired enzyme function. The issue has never been tested in a clinical trial and probably never will be. We give bicarbonate if the pH is less than 7.0, particularly if the patient is slow to respond to other treatment.

It is vital that 8.4% bicarbonate solution (readily available for use during cardiac arrest) should not be used. The osmotic strength of 8.4% bicarbonate is just over six times that of normal plasma and this would therefore produce a sudden and enormous osmotic load in a patient who is already badly dehydrated, with resultant damage to capillary beds and possible induction of thrombosis.

The solution of choice is 1.26% sodium bicarbonate solution, which is iso-osmolar with normal plasma. A 500-ml bag of 1.26% bicarbonate solution provides a useful unit dose of approximately 75 mmol of bicarbonate. Bicarbonate can be given as multiples of this, with repeated measurement of blood gases, until the pH has risen above 7.0.

Further aspects of treatment

Ketoacidosis causes ileus, gastroparesis and a superficial gastritis. The stomach fills with watery 'coffee grounds' fluid. A nasogastric tube should be inserted in moderately or severely ill patients to avoid vomiting and aspiration. Measurement of the central venous pressure, or of the left atrial pressure, may prove necessary in a patient with severe cardiac or renal disease. In the majority of patients with ketoacidosis, the kidneys are functioning adequately and fluid therapy can be administered in the light of clinical assessment with regular observation of the jugular venous pressure and blood pressure. The general rule seems to be that clinicians rely less on invasive investigation as they become more experienced in the management of ketoacidosis. The ECG (electrocardiogram) is a very poor guide to the presence of either hypo- or hyperkalaemia, and reliance should be placed on regular laboratory measurement.

A small quantity of insulin in an infusion set will adsorb onto the plastic tubing. This interesting pharmacological observation is of no clinical relevance. The common practice of adding protein to infusion solutions to prevent insulin adsorption has little point. The main danger of giving insulin by infusion is that the infusion will for some reason be stopped or disconnected. Insulin infusion pumps should *only* be used in high-dependency wards, and insulin should be given by hourly intramuscular injection if the patient is unlikely to receive close supervision.

Common problems in the assessment and treatment of patients with ketoacidosis

Ketoacidosis may come on particularly rapidly during pregnancy, in patients using subcutaneous insulin infusion devices which stop or become disconnected, and in some adolescent patients. Hospital admission is potentially avoidable in most of the remainder.

Infection and ketoacidosis

There are many pitfalls in diagnosis of infection in a patient with ketoacidosis. A marked neutrophil leucocytosis appears, even in the absence of infection, and the temperature is typically normal or subnormal even when infection is present. Blood and urine cultures and a chest X-ray should be taken on all patients but it is unnecessary to give broad-spectrum antibiotics to every patient with ketoacidosis. Hidden sepsis (e.g. a perinephric abscess) will manifest in a few patients and failure to respond to treatment may be the clue to this. 'Blind' antibiotic treatment should be reserved for patients whose life is in clear danger, or who do not respond swiftly to standard therapy.

Other biochemical changes

A number of abnormalities appear during ketoacidosis. Hypertriglyceridaemia can cause a mild pancreatitis and elevation of the serum amylase concentration. Underperfusion of muscle beds and acidosis cause damage to skeletal muscle with a resulting increase in cardiac enzymes. Liver enzymes also often show transient abnormalities. Some methods of measuring serum creatinine will give artificially high readings because of interference by ketone bodies.

Complications

Cerebral oedema is uncommon, but can be fatal. It is a particular hazard in small children. Its cause is uncertain and probably multifactorial, but some cases may result from failure to tailor 'standard regimens' of fluid replacement to the particular clinical circumstances. Use of hyperosmolar bicarbonate solutions or excessive hypotonic fluids can exacerbate the problem.

Arteriovenous thrombosis can occur in older patients as a result of dehydration, and low-grade disseminated intravascular coagulation can also complicate ketoacidosis.

Hypothermia is an occasional complication in the elderly and is surprisingly easy to overlook. Failure to recognize this will almost inevitably mean that the patient will drown in intravenous fluid.

Prevention

Most instances of ketoacidosis could be prevented. The admission provides a useful opportunity to re-educate the patient on how to cope when an intercurrent illness interferes with diabetes.

TECHNIQUE

Management of intercurrent illness in an insulin-treated patient with diabetes.

- Blood sugar rises with infections and there is a risk of diabetic ketoacidosis

Mild or moderate illness

- Monitor blood glucose 3–6-hourly
- Increase the dose of insulin in 10% increments should persistent hyperglycaemia occur

Vomiting

- Take usual insulin dose
- Measure blood glucose every 2 h
- Measure urine for ketones
- Take an additional 4 units of soluble insulin, repeated 2-hourly, if the blood glucose remains over 15 mmol l^{-1}.
- Maintain normal energy intake by drinking carbohydrate-containing fluids
- There are 10 g carbohydrate in:
  - Lucozade 50 ml (eggcupful)
  - Fruit juice 100 ml (wineglassful)
  - Milk 200 ml (one-third of a pint or full glass)

One in four patients admitted in diabetic ketoacidosis has stopped, or been advised to stop, their insulin!

NEVER stop insulin

There are a small number of children and young adults who have repeated admission to hospital with ketoacidosis. Some patients are genuinely ketosis-prone but many others have psychological and social problems which need exploration.

Hyperosmolar non-ketotic hyperglycaemia

More than 50% of patients presenting with this condition have previously undiagnosed diabetes (Marshall & Alberti, 1988). It often affects the elderly, but can occur at any age. Residual insulin secretion probably determines whether a patient will present in ketoacidosis or in a hyperosmolar non-ketotic state. Those developing the latter usually have sufficient insulin to inhibit unrestrained ketogenesis, whilst those developing keto-acidosis have very little. This is why ketoacidosis

is considered the hallmark of IDDM. Those with true ketoacidosis almost always need long-term insulin therapy, those with the non-ketotic state often do not. Hospital discharge summaries often fail to make this valuable distinction, mislabelling an admission with a hyperosmolar state as ketoacidosis just because a modest quantity of ketones was present in the urine.

The mortality rate in patients with hyperosmolar non-ketotic hyperglycaemia is much greater than for ketoacidosis, partly because the patients are older. Quoted rates range from 14% to 60%.

The clinical features are identical to those for keto-acidosis except that the duration of symptoms is longer and features attributable to acidosis (nausea, vomiting and abdominal pain) are usually absent.

Treatment of hyperosmolar non-ketotic hyperglycaemia

Treatment is similar to that of diabetic ketoacidosis (see previous section) but some differences exist. There is a therapeutic 'trade-off' between the conflicting needs of the cardiovascular system and the kidneys for a swift repletion of circulating volume. Aggressive fluid therapy may cause rapid osmotic shifts which can precipitate cerebral oedema, neuronal damage and even intra-cerebral haemorrhage. There are no large randomized trials to guide the clinician. We almost always rely on isotonic (0.9%) saline for fluid replacement and avoid hypotonic fluids for fear of precipitating cerebral oedema or worse. Normal (0.9%) saline is usually more dilute than the patient's own plasma. Fluid administration should be tailored to the individual but as a guide we suggest giving approximately one-third to one-half of the estimated fluid deficit in the first 12 h, approxi-mately two-thirds of the deficit over the next 12 h, with repletion of the remainder of the deficit in the 12 h following that.

Normal saline (0.9% sodium chloride solution) has a sodium concentration of 150 nmol l^{-1}. When patients are rehydrated with it their serum sodium concentration, which may start off above 155 or 160 mmol l^{-1}, will rise further with time. This is due to water leaving the vascular compartment to correct the intense dehydration within cells. This increase in serum sodium concentration is to be expected and should be regarded as a consequence of improving the intracellular environment rather than a hazard. The urge to abandon 0.9% sodium chloride and to give half normal saline when faced with this predictable rise in plasma sodium concentration should be resisted unless there are compelling circumstances.

Skilled fluid replacement is the mainstay of management of hyperosmolar non-ketotic hyperglycaemia and insulin should be regarded as an adjunct to this. Since some patients are very sensitive to insulin we start insulin infusion at half the rate normally used in ketoacidosis (i.e. 3 units h^{-1}), and monitor carefully for the first 2–3 h. If the plasma glucose concentration fails to fall satisfactorily, the insulin infusion rate can be increased to 6 units h^{-1}, although this rarely proves necessary. The aim should be to return the plasma glucose concentration to normal within a period of 6–10 h and to avoid a more rapid change.

Patients with hyperosmolar non-ketotic hyperglycaemia have a thrombotic tendency, and most clinicians anticoagulate with heparin as early as possible unless strong contraindications exist.

Diabetic lactic acidosis

Lactic acidosis is a rare complication of uncontrolled diabetes (Park & Arieff, 1983), although relatively common when use of the biguanide phenformin was widespread. Lactate and pyruvate are both produced by glycolysis. In the presence of adequate oxygenation and adequate functioning of the mitochondria, both are further metabolized by aerobic metabolism and concentrations within cells and in the blood remain constant. If oxygenation or mitochondrial function are impaired, lactate will accumulate when glycolysis outstrips the rate at which its products can be metabolized. When lactic acidosis occurs in diabetes there is often an underlying condition promoting lactate overproduction (e.g. biguanide therapy) or producing poor tissue oxygenation (e.g. cardiogenic, septic or other causes of shock, carbon monoxide or cyanide poisoning, methaemoglobinaemia, liver failure, alcohol poisoning, inherited glycolytic enzyme deficiencies).

In lactic acidosis, ketonuria and ketonaemia are absent. In other respects, patients present in a similar manner to ketoacidosis and may have symptoms and signs of a precipitating illness. The anion gap (which is the sum of serum sodium and potassium minus the sum of serum chloride and bicarbonate), normally 15–20 mmol l^{-1}, is enlarged. The diagnosis is confirmed by finding excess lactic acid in plasma.

Treatment of lactic acidosis in diabetes is the same as that for ketoacidosis except that identification and treatment of any underlying condition which has predisposed to poor tissue oxygenation is vital. Mortality is

very high, mainly because of such underlying conditions. High concentrations of oxygen should be given.

As with ketoacidosis, there is a debate as to whether bicarbonate should be used to treat cases in which acidosis is severe. We would suggest avoiding bicarbonate unless the pH is less than 7.0. For more severe acidosis it is important to avoid full correction with bicarbonate. We suggest correcting the pH to approximately 7.1 by a method similar to that outlined for ketoacidosis.

Hypoglycaemia

Episodes of hypoglycaemia are almost inevitable when people with diabetes are treated adequately with insulin (Cryer et al., 1989). Hypoglycaemia is less frequent, but more often fatal, in patients treated with sulphonylureas (Ferner & Alberti, 1989). From the biochemical point of view, hypoglycaemia is present when blood glucose falls below 2–2.5 mmol l^{-1}, measured by a reliable method (not a reflectance meter). Associated symptoms may vary considerably, from none at all to coma. Many diabetic patients experiencing hypoglycaemia outside hospital have a normal or even elevated blood glucose by the time they reach the A & E department because of treatment or spontaneous recovery.

The symptoms of hypoglycaemia arise from three sources:

- Adrenergic symptoms result from activation of the autonomic nervous system and the adrenal medulla (e.g. sweating, palpitations, tremor).
- Neuroglycopenic symptoms are caused by lack of glucose supply to brain cells (e.g. light-headedness, blurred/double vision, clumsiness, excitation, paranoia, aggression, confusion, disorientation, automatism, fits, abnormal neurological signs, coma).
- General malaise (e.g. depression, headache) also accompanies hypoglycaemia.

The concentration of blood glucose at which symptoms occur varies from one individual to another and also with time in any individual. Patients who habitually over-control their diabetes may appear asymptomatic at relatively low blood glucose concentrations. Others who are habitually exposed to hyperglycaemia may experience hypoglycaemic symptoms at higher than usual blood glucose concentrations. As a general rule, autonomic symptoms appear as the blood glucose falls below 3 mmol l^{-1} and neurological symptoms and signs appear when the concentration falls below 2 mmol l^{-1}.

Some patients feel shaky, unwell and sweaty when their

blood glucose concentration falls rapidly from hyperglycaemic values to the normal range. Anxiety reactions and hyperventilation can also produce many of the symptoms of hypoglycaemia.

Hypoglycaemia should be treated as soon as it is suspected, but it is important to take blood for laboratory confirmation of the diagnosis. This may have vital clinical or even medicolegal importance.

Unusual presentations of hypoglycaemia

Fits

Severe hypoglycaemia can cause fits. However, idiopathic epilepsy is no more common in patients with diabetes than it is in the general population. A fit in any diabetic patient should be regarded as due to hypoglycaemia until proved otherwise. EEG (electroencephalogram) abnormalities appear in the postictal period and the test should be delayed for a week. Referral to a diabetologist is usually more appropriate than to a neurologist.

Hemiplegia

Severe hypoglycaemia may present with hemiplegia associated with classical upper motor neurone signs. Very often this is present when patients awake, as a result of nocturnal hypoglycaemia. It usually responds to treatment with glucose within a short period of time. One confusing factor is that the blood glucose concentration may be normal by the time the patient has sought medical advice. In more elderly patients, hypoglycaemic hemiplegia may be very difficult to differentiate from a transient ischaemic attack.

Pseudodementia

Sulphonylurea drugs, and occasionally insulin, can accumulate in elderly patients, particularly as renal function declines. Such patients may gradually enter hypoglycaemia over a period of days and weeks, rather than hours. With such a gradual onset, many of the acute symptoms and signs of hypoglycaemia are absent and patients can present with progressively failing mental function which can be mistaken for dementia.

Hypothermia

Hypoglycaemia impairs thermoregulation and inhibits shivering in a cold environment. It should be excluded in any patient presenting with hypothermia. Patients with moderate hypothermia due to hypoglycaemia begin to shiver within seconds of glucose administration.

Nocturnal hypoglycaemia

At night many of the early warning symptoms and signs of hypoglycaemia pass unnoticed. Excessive sweating at night, or headaches and mental dullness or malaise on waking, may provide a clue. Relatives and friends of the patient may be alerted by irregular breathing, excessive sweating or thrashing movements whilst the patient is asleep.

Tablet-treated patients

Severe hypoglycaemia is of greatest concern when it occurs in a patient on tablet treatment, and it is often mismanaged. All sulphonylurea drugs (e.g. chlorpropamide and glibenclamide) and their active metabolites persist in the body for some hours. These drugs 'prime' the beta-cell to respond to rising blood glucose levels, and their hypoglycaemic effect often lasts more than a day. A patient with sulphonylurea-induced hypoglycaemia can thus be treated and discharged only to rebound into hypoglycaemia (Ferner & Alberti, 1989). Elderly people are particularly at risk. Avoidable brain damage may result. Admission to hospital, intravenous infusion of 5% or 10% dextrose with the infusion rate titrated against regular blood glucose testing, and careful in-patient supervision is required. Tolbutamide is safer for elderly patients since it has a much shorter elimination half-life.

Insulin-induced hypoglycaemia

As a general rule about one-third of young insulin-treated diabetic patients will have a hypoglycaemic coma at some stage during their lives. Approximately one in ten of all insulin-treated patients will have a hypoglycaemic coma in any given year and approximately three out of every 100 patients will suffer recurrent hypoglycaemia. Unfortunately, attempts to improve glycaemic control in diabetic patients (and therefore hopefully to reduce the risk of long-term complicatons) by using multiple daily injections or continuous subcutaneous infusion of insulin appear to increase the risk of severe hypoglycaemia (Diabetes Control and Complications Trial Research Group, 1993). Single episodes of hypoglycaemia are unlikely to have long-term sequelae. Since hypoglycaemia is so common, its rarer complications (which include permanent disability) are still encountered from time to time. The adverse sequelae of hypoglycaemia are well reviewed elsewhere (Frier, 1992).

Since insulin has a relatively short half-life, hypoglycaemia occurring in an insulin-treated patient is often easy to treat. Hospital admission is required infrequently, and patients can usually be discharged from the A&E department once the precipitating cause has been identified and corrected. The most common factors are:

- Exertion (the effects of which may be delayed several hours).
- A delayed meal.
- Alcohol.
- Erratic absorption from the injection site (due, for example, to lipohypertrophy).

After a decade of IDDM, at least a third of patients lose some or all of the 'early warning' autonomic symptoms of hypoglycaemia and are forced to rely on symptoms of neuroglycopenia. Since neuroglycopenia itself impairs judgement, patients may fail to perceive or even deny changes in their behaviour or appearance which are obvious to an experienced observer. Loss of awareness of hypoglycaemia is associated with a reduced counter-regulatory hormone response, which further predisposes the patient to severe hypoglycaemia. Loss of awareness of hypoglycaemia is sometimes transient, and a single severe hypoglycaemic attack can result in an impaired counter-regulatory response which persists over several days. This is one reason why hypoglycaemic attacks tend to come in runs. Patients should be advised to monitor their control with extra care after an episode of severe hypoglycaemia to guard against a cascade of repeat attacks.

There has been considerable publicity in the lay press suggesting that, compared to animal insulins, human insulin is associated with a loss of the warning signs of hypoglycaemia. This has been extensively investigated and two double-blind placebo-controlled trials have revealed no clear difference between the effects of human and animal insulin on hypoglycaemic reactions (Gale, 1989). It is likely that problems have been caused by the different pharmacokinetics of human and animal insulins (human insulin is absorbed more swiftly), and also because a loss of awareness of hypoglycaemia occurs with time irrespective of the type of insulin used. Patients who are concerned about this issue, however, should be offered the choice of treatment with animal insulins if, after discussion, they would still like to change.

Treatment of hypoglycaemia

Intravenous 50% dextrose solution frequently scleroses veins and is often used unnecessarily. Many patients arriving at an A&E department with hypoglycaemia have an altered level of consciousness but are not unconscious and can guard their airway. Surprisingly small amounts of orally administered glucose solution given by a sympathetic attendant can wake patients sufficiently to allow them to eat their way out of hypoglycaemia. Fat delays gastric emptying, thus glucose should not be given in milk.

If a patient is truly unconscious, 25 ml of 50% dextrose should be given intravenously over 60 s (a surprisingly long period once the needle is in the vein), followed after 3 min by a further 25 ml of 50% dextrose if an adequate response has not occurred. All injections of 50% dextrose should be followed by a 10 or 20 ml flush of normal saline in an attempt to preserve the vein. It is a tragedy if injudicious use of 50% dextrose results in the loss of all available peripheral veins in a patient who is prone to repeated attacks of hypoglycaemia.

Injection of 1 mg of glucagon intramuscularly is an alternative treatment of severe hypoglycaemia in an unconscious patient. It has the advantages that it can be used when venous access proves problematic (e.g. in an aggressive patient) and that it can be injected into the thigh by a patient's relatives or friends if medical help is unavailable. Glucagon mobilizes glucose from hepatic glycogen stores, and will not work in a fasted patient or if an earlier dose has been given. It should always be followed by oral carbohydrate when the patient wakes, to replenish glycogen stores.

Glucose gels can also be useful. The gel is supplied in a squeezable plastic dispenser and can be absorbed directly from the buccal mucosa. Gels are effective if squirted into the cheek pouch even when the teeth are tightly clenched, and can terminate an acute attack whilst further medical help is being sought. The main disadvantage is that they tend to be very messy as consciousness returns.

On recovery from hypoglycaemia the patient should be given a carbohydrate-rich meal as a precaution against recurrent hypoglycaemia. The cause of the attack should be sought and advice given on prevention. Do not assume the episode was accidental – deliberate insulin overdose is probably more common than most people realize. Patients typically underestimate a lethal dose of insulin but might not make the same mistake twice.

Coma unresponsive to treatment

If a patient has not responded to glucagon within 5–10 min, intravenous glucose should be given. Further intravenous bolus doses of glucose in excess of 50 ml of 50% dextrose should not be given since severe hyperglycaemia and an intense osmotic imbalance across the blood/brain barrier may result. This can cause cerebral oedema. Such patients should be admitted and put onto a slow infusion of 10% dextrose, adjusted to give blood glucose concentrations in the range of 10–15 mmol l^{-1}. Mannitol or dexamethasone are sometimes given in prolonged coma to protect against cerebral oedema but there is no evidence of benefit. Prolonged coma despite treatment should prompt consideration of other potential causes such as intracerebral haemorrhage, drug overdose, hypothermia, alcohol intoxication, meningitis or overwhelming sepsis. At this stage you may bitterly regret failing to put some blood into a fluoride tube before treatment was given. The prognosis after severe prolonged hypoglycaemia seems to be inversely proportional to the duration of coma. The worst outcome is not death but survival with severe cortical brain damage.

Recurrent hypoglycaemia

Overaggressive or poor management by doctors, and fecklessness or manipulation by patients, account for the vast majority of cases of recurrent hypoglycaemia in insulin-treated patients. There is no clearly documented case of an insulinoma occurring in a patient with IDDM.

Deliberate insulin overdose

Hypoglycaemia after insulin overdose is surprisingly variable in its presentation. Coma may be severe and prolonged, but some patients walk into the A&E department after massive overdoses. In one such case, the injection site was resected by a surgeon, but heroic measures such as this are unnecessary. Intravenous glucose is given through a peripheral vein followed swiftly by the insertion of a central venous cannula. It is always possible to give dextrose in sufficient quantity to control the hypoglycaemic effect of an insulin overdose since the body does not have an infinite capacity to dispose of glucose. An infusion of 20% dextrose is titrated against repeated bedside measurement of blood glucose by a competent member of staff. Large amounts of dextrose are sometimes needed.

The newly diagnosed diabetic patient

Hospital is an unsuitable place for the vast majority of newly diagnosed people with diabetes (Gale & Tattersall, 1990). Non-specialist teams are much more likely to admit such patients and keep them in longer – often on wards where the nurses and doctors have little practical experience in diabetes management. The patient is surrounded by sick and dying people with other medical conditions and the quality of information available from busy clinical teams is limited. We admit newly diagnosed patients only for ketoacidosis, social reasons or other illness.

Management of the newly diagnosed diabetic patient in the A&E department will depend upon local arrangements. The threshold for admission will depend upon the availability of out-patient care. Education and management should usually be initiated by a specialist diabetic physician with a team including diabetes nurse specialists, diabetes dietitians and chiropodists.

The plasma glucose concentration is often immaterial in deciding whether admission is necessary. The key issues are whether the patient is unwell, has particularly severe symptoms, a very swift onset of symptoms, or moderate ketonuria. If these are absent, as they usually are, out-patient management is appropriate (Chase et al., 1992). Some patients will need to be seen the next day, while those with mild symptoms should be seen within a maximum of 2 weeks. The route of urgent referral should be clearly established between the A&E department and the physicians and paediatricians routinely involved in the management of diabetic patients.

Intercurrent illness in diabetic patients

Infections, trauma, myocardial infarction, surgery and other common illnesses produce a complex series of hormonal and metabolic changes. These result in reduced insulin secretion and overproduction of counter-regulatory hormones, causing glucose levels to rise in patients with diabetes. Anorexia, vomiting and erratic foood intake may compound the problem.

Management of patients with intercurrent illness should not aim for near normoglycaemia; mild hyperglycaemia will be less of a risk to a sick patient than an episode of hypoglycaemia. It is particularly important to avoid hypoglycaemia in patients who have had myocardial infarcts (when arrhythmias could be induced), impaired consciousness, or require anaesthesia (since such patients will not be in a position to detect or correct the hypoglycaemia).

Non-insulin-dependent patients

NIDDM patients have limited insulin reserves, and mild to moderate stress will produce a deterioration in control. Careful monitoring may be all that is needed until the underlying illness has resolved, but a temporary increase in tablets may be required if the illness is likely to persist more than a few days.

Admission for treatment with insulin and intravenous fluids is needed for more severe intercurrent illness, for illnesses that interrupt regular food intake, and for patients who are already poorly controlled.

Insulin-treated patients

Insulin should never be reduced or stopped in ill insulin-dependent patients who are vomiting or who have gone off their food. This is a common error of management and can result in ketoacidosis.

Patients should be advised to monitor their blood glucose regularly during mild or moderate intercurrent illness and to increase the dose of insulin in 10% increments should hyperglycaemia develop. Patients who are reasonably well, but off their food, should be advised to consume regular carbohydrate-rich drinks (such as fruit juice) to ensure an adequate intake of glucose against which the insulin dose can be balanced.

More severely ill insulin-treated patients, and less ill patients unable to maintain an adequate carbohydrate intake, will require admission and treatment with insulin and intravenous glucose. These are two ways of doing this. The first is to use two separate infusions (often running into the same intravenous cannula): one containing glucose at a rate of 100 ml h^{-1} of 10% dextrose solution (or 200 ml h^{-1} of 5% dextrose) and the other containing insulin delivered via a syringe pump (usually 100 ml of soluble insulin in 100 ml of 0.9% saline infused at 2–4 units h^{-1}). The rate of insulin infusion is adjusted according to the results of regular (1–2-hourly) capillary blood glucose test results.

An alternative, which we prefer, is the glucose–potassium–insulin (GKI) system (Husband *et al.*, 1986). A bag of 500 ml of 10% dextrose containing 10 mmol of potassium chloride and 15 units of soluble insulin is infused over 5 h, preferably via an infusion pump. The great advantage of this system is that, even if the drip runs too slowly, or too fast, insulin and glucose continue to be given to the patient in the correct proportion. The risk of hyper- or hypoglycaemia is thus reduced. The blood glucose concentration should be measured 2-hourly with the aim of keeping it between 6 and 11 mmol l^{-1}. If it dips below 6 mmol l^{-1}, a similar infusion solution containing only 10 units of insulin per bag should be substituted. If it rises above 11 mmol l^{-1}, the current infusion bag should be taken down and a replacement bag containing 20 units of insulin substituted. Further adjustments of the insulin dose per bag (carried out in 5-unit increments) are rarely needed.

Ill patients requiring GKI infusion often need other fluids intravenously, and we strongly recommend the establishment of a second intravenous line for all 'other fluids'. This helps all grades of staff understand that treatment for the diabetes needs to be carried on without interruption, regardless of the need for other forms of intravenous therapy.

Childbirth and caesarean section

It is very important to maintain strict glycaemic control during labour because hyperglycaemia in the mother will cause an increased production of insulin by the fetus which would then be at risk of neonatal hypoglycaemia. Diabetic patients in labour, and all those undergoing caesarean section, will be starved and catabolic. There is clearly a need for a continuous supply of glucose and insulin. The mother's insulin requirements are usually very high towards the end of pregnancy and swiftly decline following delivery of the fetus and placenta. For this reason, separate control over the administration of insulin and dextrose is required and a GKI infusion as described above is less satisfactory.

We recommend giving 500 ml of 10% dextrose containing 10 mmol of potassium chloride 5-hourly, and, through a separate infusion line, 100 units of soluble insulin in 100 ml of 0.9% saline infused at a rate equal to the mother's rate of insulin consumption during the latter weeks of pregnancy. (This value is obtained by adding up the total dose of insulin taken in 24 h and dividing by 24.) The mother's capillary blood glucose concentration should be tested 2-hourly and the insulin infusion rate adjusted accordingly with the aim of keeping the blood glucose concentration between 6 and 9 mmol l^{-1}. After delivery of the fetus and placenta, women who were diabetic before conception should have their insulin infusion rate reduced to their prepregnancy insulin requirement. Women who developed gestational diabetes can safely have the insulin infusion stopped after delivery. Profound hypoglycaemia may develop if insulin is not reduced following delivery and maternal death or disability have occurred as a result.

CONDITIONS PRESENTING TO A&E DEPARTMENTS IN WHICH DIABETES MAY PLAY A SIGNIFICANT PART

Eye problems

Both IDDM and NIDDM patients are at risk of developing diabetic retinopathy (Kohner, 1989). After 15 years of diabetes, approximately 96% of IDDM patients have background retinopathy. The majority will be asymptomatic. After 20–25 years of diabetes, 40% will have proliferative retinopathy – the major threat to vision (Kohner, 1991). In people of working age, diabetes is the commonest cause of registrable blindness in the UK, and any new eye symptom in a diabetic patient warrants investigation.

Proliferative retinopathy usually has no effect on vision until the disease is well advanced. At this stage, retinal ischaemia has stimulated the growth of new blood vessels into ischaemic areas. These vessels are very fragile and easily bleed. Leakage of blood may be localized, or may fill the vitreous humour causing blindness in the affected eye. Diagnosis is usually easy. With a large vitreous haemorrhage, the red reflex will be lost and it will be impossible to see the retina. With a smaller haemorrhage, the area of the bleed should be easily visible and the rest of the retina typically shows signs of advanced diabetic eye disease.

Proliferative retinopathy requires urgent referral to an ophthalmologist. Patients with small haemorrhages from new vessels require urgent laser photocoagulation to induce regression of the new vessels and hopefully prevent further haemorrhage. Patients with larger vitreous haemorrhages can be offered vitrectomy once the condition of the eye has stabilized. Diabetic maculopathy is much harder to diagnose. It may produce a swift reduction in visual acuity with minimal signs in the optic fundus. If haemorrhages or exudates are visible around the macula, the diagnosis is made relatively easily. However, the only lesion may be macular oedema. This is exceedingly difficult to diagnose with an ophthalmoscope. Therefore, any diabetic patient suffering an unexplained loss of visual acuity should be referred for an ophthalmic opinion. Photocoagulation treatment of clinically significant macular oedema reduces the risk of blindness by over 50% (British Multicentre Study Group, 1983).

Glaucoma is no less common in diabetics than in the normal population and it can also produce a loss of visual acuity with normal retinal appearances. This is another reason for obtaining an ophthalmic opinion in any diabetic patient presenting with an acute reduction in visual acuity.

Conjuctivitis is a common problem in patients with poorly controlled diabetes. Recognition should not only prompt treatment with antibiotic eye-drops or ointment but it should also lead to referral to a diabetic clinic in the hope of preventing or detecting other complications.

Skin problems

About 30% of diabetic patients will suffer skin disorders at some stage in the course of their disease, and a number of conditions may be seen in the A&E department.

Lipodystrophy

This can occur in any diabetic patient who ignores advice to rotate injection sites and repeatedly injects insulin into a localized area (Boyd et al., 1982). In such an area, the fatty tissue may hypertrophy (resembling a fibrotic lipoma) or atrophy. Apart from the cosmetic problems that such lesions cause, the absorption of insulin from these areas is erratic and can be responsible for both hyper-and hypoglycaemia. Examination of the injection sites of any patient presenting with poor diabetic control is mandatory since it might reveal the cause of the poor control.

Skin abscesses

Skin abscesses occur spontaneously in patients with poor diabetic control but rarely with moderately deranged glycaemic control. Many patients with abscesses and poor control are not receiving adequate supervision and present to the A&E department. If the opportunity for referral is missed, further complications are likely.

Abscesses at injection sites

These are exceedingly uncommon and usually indicate a major problem in insulin administration. They most commonly result from bacterial contamination and growth within an insulin vial. All insulin contains preservatives but bacterial growth can become established if these are degraded or if repeated contamination occurs. The abscesses usually resolve spontaneously following adjustment of the insulin administration technique and provision of fresh insulin. Many patients with diabetes are advised to reuse their syringes until the needle becomes blunt. This practice does not predispose to abscess formation and should not be discouraged (Anonymous, 1983).

Rarer skin problems

Insulin allergy occurs but is usually a reaction to the preservative or protamine used to stabilize the insulin within the vial. The key diagnostic feature is the temporal relationship to the administration of insulin.

The glucagonoma syndrome is undoubtedly the rarest cause of a rash in a diabetic patient but it is of some importance since recognition of the rash permits surgical removal of the tumour (Anderson & Bloom, 1986). Erythematous patches may erupt at any site which goes on to develop blistering, secondary infection, and then heal within a week or two. Similar patches then erupt elsewhere. The rash is well named 'necrolytic migratory erythema'.

Neurological problems

A symmetrical, predominantly sensory, peripheral neuropathy is a common complication of diabetes (Thomas et al., 1982). This type of neuropathy is usually seen in the A&E department when ulceration of the foot has supervened.

An acutely painful neuropathy (Ward, 1989) may also occur in patients with diabetes. In this condition the pain is distressing and occurs typically in the legs. The symptoms are associated with muscle weakness and wasting, and very often with generalized weight loss. Unusually, the knee and ankle reflexes are preserved in patients with this variant of diabetic neuropathy and there is often very little sensory deficit. This acute neuropathy normally occurs in patients with poor diabetic control. Improving control usually produces a gradual recovery over a period of many months.

Diabetic amyotrophy presents with a relatively sudden onset of severe pain in one thigh accompanied by marked muscle wasting (Garland, 1955). The condition is usually unilateral. Tendon reflexes are reduced but there are rarely any sensory signs. The cause of this myopathy is unknown, but it is usually associated with a period of poor diabetic control. Most patients recover over a period of weeks or months after control is improved. The differential diagnosis includes other causes of pain and unilateral muscle wasting in the legs. It is particularly important to exclude spinal tumours or an acute disc protrusion.

Diabetes predisposes to the development of acute mononeuropathies assumed to be caused by sudden occlusion of intraneural blood vessels. Acute third and sixth cranial nerve palsies are relatively common in diabetic patients. Diabetes underlies approximately 20% of all isolated ocular nerve palsies. The main feature which differentiates a diabetic mononeuropathy from other causes (including intracerebral tumours and aneurysms) is the very sudden onset in an otherwise well, pain-free and asymptomatic diabetic patient. When the third cranial nerve is affected by diabetic mononeuropathy the pupil responses are usually spared. Spontaneous resolution normally occurs.

Nerves in diabetic patients are at risk of entrapment neuropathies. Carpal tunnel syndrome is the most frequent. Diabetic cheirarthropathy which results in stiffening and thickening of the tendons, particularly in the hand and wrists, may be a precipitating factor (Rosenbloom et al., 1981).

The diabetic foot

Many diabetics with foot problems have a combination of peripheral neuropathy and arterial disease, but one disease process usually predominates (Jones et al., 1986).

The neuropathic foot is often warm and dry (deranged neural control of sweating) and the pulses are bounding because of arteriovenous shunting. The toes tend to become retracted onto the dorsum of the foot, exposing the metatarsal heads. The loss of sensation then predisposes to ulceration over the metatarsal heads, or other points of abnormal pressure. In severe disease, loss of sensory feedback can result in a Charcot joint.

Ischaemic feet are usually cool, with reduced or absent pulses, and ulceration may result from localized pressure necrosis or thrombotic obliteration of small or large arteries.

Ulceration

Ulceration is the most common emergency presentation of diabetic foot disease. Treatment is usually more effective if the patient's care is managed from the start by a multidisciplinary team, including a physician, surgeon, nurse, chiropodist and shoe fitter.

Neuropathic ulcers

These are treated by swabbing the ulcer for infecting organisms and immediate oral antibiotic therapy. We use flucloxacillin 500 mg 6-hourly and metronidazole 400 mg 8-hourly (adding amoxycillin 500 mg 8-hourly if spreading cellulitis is present). Antibiotic therapy is adjusted according to the results of swab cultures. Patients with localized infection can be treated as out-patients, but spreading cellulitis is an indication for admission, bed rest and intravenous antibiotic therapy.

Abnormal pressure on the plantar surface of the foot must be avoided to encourage healing. This can be achieved by bed rest, the use of special insoles in extra-depth shoes, and the use of casts made of plaster or lightweight plastic materials.

In Charcot's disease of the foot, an episode of minor trauma such as tripping produces a warm, red, swollen and sometimes painful foot (Sinha et al., 1972). X-rays are usually normal in the first instance but, as days go by, radiological evidence of fractures, bone lysis and callous formation develops. Because the process is largely painless, the patient continues to walk on the affected foot and anatomical disorganization eventually results. This leads to severe deformity. Early diagnosis is achieved by recognizing the typical history and performing a bone scan which will show markedly increased uptake in the affected foot, even if plain X-ray films are normal.

The patient should be treated by immobilization (often with a plaster cast and crutches) until all swelling, warmth and redness have resolved. Gradual mobilization is then undertaken using moulded insoles in special extra-depth custom-fitted shoes.

Ischaemic ulcers

Ischaemic ulcers are often painful and usually result from excessive pressure on an underperfused area of the foot, particularly the heel. They may develop on the ends of toes as a result of arterial occlusion and gangrene.

Treatment consists of prompt antibiotic therapy, as for neuropathic ulcers. Chiropody will be needed to debride the ulcer whilst avoiding damage to surrounding viable tissues. Deep, widely fitting shoes should be worn to protect the foot.

An ulcer that is not clearly responding to medical treatment within a month requires further investigation and management. Angiography should be considered with a view to angioplasty or reconstructive surgery. Amputation may be required. Sympathectomy is generally of little use in patients with diabetes.

Education about diabetic foot disease and its prevention by regular inspection of the feet and chiropody are of vital importance in preventing diabetic foot disease in at-risk patients (Edmonds et al., 1986).

PREVENTION

Fifty per cent of diabetics undergo no formal review of their diabetic management. Identifying such patients when they present to A & E departments with coincidental illness can provide an unrepeatable opportunity to refer the patient to a diabetic clinic for education and screening for treatable diabetic complications.

Bibliography

ANDERSON, J.V. & BLOOM, S.R. (1986). Neuro-endocrine tumours of the gut: long term therapy with the somatostatin analogue SMS 201-995. Scand. J. Gastroenterol., 21 (Suppl. 119), 115–28.

ANONYMOUS (1983). Re-use of disposable plastic insulin syringes. Lancet, i, 570.

BINGLEY, P.J. & GALE, E.A.M. (1991). Lessons from family studies. Baillière's Clin. Endocrinol. Metab., 52, 261–83.

BOYD, S.G., INNES, S.M. & CAMPBELL, I.W. (1982). Skin manefestations of diabetes mellitus. Practitioner, 226, 253–64.

BRITISH MULTICENTRE STUDY GROUP (1983). Photocoagulation for diabetic maculopathy: a randomised controlled clinical trial using the xenon arc. Diabetes, 32, 1010–16.

CHASE, H.P., CREWS, K.R., GARG, S. et al. (1992). Outpatient management vs inhospital management of children with new-onset diabetes. Clin. Pediatr., 31, 450–6.

CRYER, P.E., BINDER, C., BOLLI, G.B. et al. (1989). Hypoglycaemia in IDDM. Diabetes, 38, 1139–99.

DeFRONZO, R.A. & FERRANNINI, E. (1992). Insulin actions in vivo: protein metabolism. In International Textbook of Diabetes, Vol. 1, ed. K.G.M.M. Alberti, R.A. DeFronzo, H. Keen & P. Zimmet. pp. 467–512. Chichester: Wiley.

DIABETES CONTROL AND COMPLICATIONS TRIAL RESEARCH GROUP. (1993) The effect of intensive treatment of diabetes on the development and progression of long-term complications in insulin-dependent diabetes mellitus. N. Engl. J. Med., 329, 977–86.

EDMONDS, M.E., BLUNDELL, M.P., MORRIS, M.E. et al. (1986). Improved survival of the diabetic foot: the role of a specialised foot clinic. Q. J. Med., 4, 475–9.

FERNER, R.E. & ALBERTI, K.G.M.M. (1989). Sulphonylureas in the treatment of non-insulin dependent diabetes. *Q. J. Med.*, **73**, 987–95.

FERRANNINI, E. & DeFRONZO, R.A. (1992). Insulin actions *in vivo*: glucose metabolism. In *International Textbook of Diabetes*, Vol. 1, ed. K.G.M.M. Alberti, R.A. DeFronzo, H. Keen & P. Zimmet. pp. 409–38. Chichester: Wiley.

FRIER, B.M. (1992). Hypoglycaemia – how much harm. *Hosp. Update*, 876–84.

GALE, E.A.M. (1989). Hypoglycaemia and human insulin. *Lancet*, **ii**, 1264–6.

GALE, E. & TATTERSALL, R. (1990). Starting treatment in the new patient with insulin dependent diabetes. In *Diabetes Clinical Management*, ed. R.B. Tattersall & E.A.M. Gale. pp. 17–25. Edinburgh: Churchill Livingstone.

GARLAND, H. (1955). Diabetic amyotrophy. *Br. Med. J.*, **2**, 1287–90.

HUSBAND, D.J., THAI, A.C. & ALBERTI, K.G.M.M. (1986). Management of diabetes during surgery with glucose–insulin–potassium infusion. *Diabetic Med.*, **3**, 69–74.

JONES, E.W., PEACOCK, I., McLAIM, S. *et al.* (1986). A clinicopathological study of diabetic foot ulcers. *Diabetic Med.*, **4**, 475–9

KISSEBAH, A.H. (1992). Insulin actions *in vivo*: insulin and lipoprotein metabolism. In *International Textbook of Diabetes*, Vol. 1, ed. K.G.M.M. Alberti, R.A. DeFronzo, H. Keen & P. Zimmet, pp. 439–58. Chichester: Wiley.

KOHNER, E.M. (1989). Diabetic retinopathy. *Br. Med. Bull.*, **45**, 148–73.

KOHNER, E.M. (1991). The natural history of diabetic retinopathy. *Eye*, **5**, 222–5.

LO, S.S., TUN, R.Y.M., HAWA, M. *et al.* (1991). Studies of diabetic twins. *Diabetes Metab. Rev.*, **7**, 223–38.

MARSHALL, S.M. & ALBERTI, K.G.M.M. (1986). Diabetic ketoacidosis. In *The Diabetes Annual 3*, ed. K.G.M.M. Alberti & L.P. Krall. pp. 498–526. Amsterdam: Elsevier.

MARSHALL, S.M. & ALBERTI, K.G.M.M. (1988). *Hyperosmolar non-ketotic coma. The Diabetes Annual 4*, ed.

K.G.M.M. Alberti & L.P. Krall. pp. 235–47. Amsterdam: Elsevier.

MATHER, H.M. & KEEN, H. (1985). The Southall diabetes survey: prevalence of known diabetes in Asians and Europeans. *Br. Med. J.*, **291**, 1081–4.

ODUGBESAN, O., ROWE, B., FLETCHER, J. *et al.* (1989). Diabetes in the U.K. West Indian community: the Wolverhampton survey. *Diabetic Med.*, **6**, 48–52.

PARK, R. & ARIEFF, A.I. (1983). Lactic acidosis: current concepts. *Clin. Endocrinol. Metab.*, **12**, 339–58.

PRANZRAM, G. (1987). Mortality and survival in type 2 (non-insulin-dependent) diabetes mellitus. *Diabetologia*, **30**, 123–31.

ROSENBLOOM, A.L., SILVERSTEIN, J.H., KUBILIS, P.S. *et al.* (1981). Limited joint mobility in childhood diabetes. *N. Engl. J. Med.*, **305**, 191–4.

SINHA, S., MUNICHOODAPPA, C.S. & KOZAK, G.P. (1972). Neuroarthropathy (Charcot joints) in diabetes mellitus. *Medicine*, **51**, 191–210.

THOMAS, P.K., WARD, J.D. & WATKINS, P.J. (1982). Diabetic neuropathy. In *Complications of Diabetes*, 2nd edn, ed. H. Keen & J. Jarrett. pp. 109–36. London: Edward Arnold.

TUNBRIDGE, W.M.G. (1981). Factors contributing to deaths of diabetics under 50 years of age. *Lancet*, **i**, 569–72.

WALKER, M. & ALBERTI, K.G.M.M. (1992). Insulin actions *in vivo*: its role in the regulation of ketone body metabolism. In *International Textbook of Diabetes*, Vol. 1, ed. K.G.M.M. Alberti, R.A. DeFronzo, H. Keen & P. Zimmet. pp. 4459–66 Chichester: Wiley.

WARD, J.D. (1989). Diabetic neuropathy. *Br. Med. Bull.*, **45**, 111–26.

WHO STUDY GROUP (1985). Diabetes mellitus. *WHO Tech. Rep. Ser.*, **727**.

YUDKIN, J.S., ALBERTI, K.G.M.M., McLARTY, D.G. *et al.* (1990). Impaired glucose tolerance. *Br. Med. J.*, **301**, 397–402.

58 Obstetric emergencies

P. NASH[a] and J. PRICE[b]

[a]Accident and Emergency Department, Neath General Hospital, Neath, UK
[b]Obstetrics and Gynaecology Department, Hillingdon Hospital, Uxbridge, UK

Chapter plan

Introduction
Physiology of pregnancy
Vaginal bleeding related to pregnancy
Preterm labour
Non-obstetric causes of abdominal pain
Pre-eclampsia and eclampsia
Medical emergencies in pregnancy
Puerperal depression

INTRODUCTION

The majority of women approaching the 20th week of pregnancy have booked at an antenatal clinic and therefore have direct access to maternity services if they require emergency treatment. However, on occasion, women do present to the accident and emergency (A&E) department in the 2nd or 3rd trimesters of pregnancy for various reasons. They may have medical problems which they perceive as being unrelated to pregnancy, they may be away from home or they may have denied pregnancy until labour ensued. Some hospitals have an A&E department but no obstetric unit on site. It is therefore important that the emergency physician has an understanding of the physiology of pregnancy, is aware of the common emergency complications of pregnancy and has knowledge of how pregnancy affects the presentation and management of common medical and surgical emergencies, so that he can manage the patient whilst waiting for obstetric help to arrive.

PHYSIOLOGY OF PREGNANCY

During the 1st trimester the uterus enlarges so that by the 12th week it rises above the symphysis pubis and becomes palpable in the abdomen. Thereafter the fundal height is a guide to gestational age.

Respiration

As pregnancy advances the shape of the chest alters, with flaring of the lower ribs and elevation of the diaphragm by up to 4 cm. The respiratory rate in pregnancy is unchanged but tidal volume increases by 40% and residual volume falls by 25%. This causes 'physiological hyperventilation' of pregnancy which results in a Pco_2 of 4.0 kPa (30 mmHg). The finding of an apparently normal Pco_2 of 5.3 kPa in pregnancy reflects both maternal and fetal acidosis.

Circulation

During pregnancy the cardiac output increases by 1.0–1.5 litres min^{-1}, although in the supine position the pressure of the uterus on the great vessels (aortocaval compression) may decrease cardiac output by 30–40%. The cardiac output is distributed differently in pregnancy, with peripheral vasodilatation and increased blood flow to the uterus and kidneys. Resting pulse increases by 15–20 beats min^{-1} in the 3rd trimester and both systolic and diastolic blood pressure fall by 15 mmHg in the 2nd trimester, returning to normal by term. Blood volume increases by 50% by 34 weeks of gestation. Oedema occurs in 50% of pregnancies because of increase in total body water. Early or midsystolic functional murmurs develop by the 12th week of pregnancy in many women but disappear soon after delivery.

Gastrointestinal tract

During pregnancy there is reduced motility of the intestinal tract. Constipation and cholestasis are common. Heartburn results from a rise in intragastric pressure without a concomitant increase in tone of the gastro-oesophageal sphincter. Stretching of the peritoneum and abdominal musculature by the gravid uterus diminishes rebound tenderness and guarding as signs of intra-abdominal pathology.

Urinary tract

The glomerular filtration rate and renal plasma blood flow increase during pregnancy causing falls in blood urea and creatinine. Urinary frequency and nocturia are common. The renal calyces, pelvices and ureters are dilated. Tubular function changes during pregnancy and can result in protein loss of up to 300 mg per 24 h and glycosuria in the absence of raised blood sugar.

Endocrine system

The maternal endocrine system is modified during pregnancy by the addition of the fetoplacental unit which produces human chorionic gonadotropin, human placental lactogen and other hormones which affect the mother's endocrine organs. Raised progesterone levels may produce tiredness and dyspnoea and contribute to changes in maternal psyche.

During pregnancy the mass of the pituitary gland increases by up to 50% because of an increase in prolactin-secreting cells. Haemorrhagic shock can cause necrosis of the anterior pituitary resulting in pituitary insufficiency.

The serum level of insulin rises during the second half of pregnancy although there is relative insulin resistance. As a result the upper limit of normal blood sugar in a glucose tolerance test increases from 7.5 mmol l^{-1} in the 2nd trimester to 9.6 mmol l^{-1} in the 3rd trimester.

Musculoskeletal system

Ligamentous laxity results in widening of the symphysis pubis by up to 8 mm and relaxation of the sacroiliac joints.

Blood composition

Dilutional anaemia occurs because of a smaller increase in red cell mass than circulatory volume. The white cell count is increased because of a raised neutrophil count. Although lymphocyte numbers remain constant their function is suppressed, rendering the pregnant woman more susceptible to viral infections and malaria. Serum fibrinogen and clotting factors are increased and pro-thrombin time and partial thromboplastin time may

be shortened. Platelet counts decrease slightly and the erythrocyte sedimentation rate is raised to up to 100 mm h^{-1}.

VAGINAL BLEEDING RELATED TO PREGNANCY

Vaginal bleeding is a common symptom in pregnancy. Bleeding in early pregnancy and ectopic pregnancy are discussed in Chapter 59. Women who present to an A&E department with vaginal bleeding after 20 weeks of gestation should not have an internal examination, unless performed by a senior obstetrician with facilities for urgent surgical intervention, for fear or precipitating massive haemorrhage from a placenta praevia.

Antepartum haemorrhage

Antepartum haemorrhage is defined as bleeding from the genital tract after the 28th week of pregnancy. The widespread use of ultrasound in the 2nd trimester has enabled the early diagnosis of asymptomatic placenta praevia, a common cause of antepartum haemorrhage. Nowadays babies born before 28 weeks are often viable, rendering the lower limit of gestation in antepartum haemorrhage open to debate.

Antepartum haemorrhage occurs in approximately 3% of single pregnancies (Paintin, 1962). Causes include placental abruption, placenta praevia, vasa praevia and unexplained haemorrhage. Bleeding also occurs from other specific causes unrelated to the placenta (e.g. polyps, carcinoma of the cervix or vulval varices).

Placental abruption

Placental abruption occurs when a normally sited placenta separates from the myometrium because of haemorrhage. Bleeding may be localized behind the placenta (concealed haemorrhage) or may track between the membranes and decidua and pass through the cervix (revealed haemorrhage). Placental abruption may be complicated by disseminated intravascular coagulation and amniotic fluid embolus (Chamberlain, 1991a).

The incidence of placental abruption is unrelated to age and parity but is increased in smokers (Naeye, 1980). Raised blood pressure and proteinuria are more common at the time of an abruption but it is unclear whether this is a causative effect of pre-eclampsia or a result of placental separation (Paintin, 1962; Hibbard & Hibbard, 1963). Placental abruption may follow abdominal trauma, including external cephalic version. Maternal mortality following placental abruption is uncommon, accounting for only four deaths in the UK between 1985 and 1987 (Department of Health, 1991). However fetal mortality is more common, ranging from 20% to 35% (Lowe & Cunningham, 1990).

In placental abruption the patient presents with pain over the uterus, usually accompanied by vaginal bleeding with clots. If the placenta is posteriorly sited, low back pain may be the only symptom. If separation is extensive there will be signs of shock. Abdominal examination reveals a woody, hard, tender uterus. Preterm labour may have commenced. Fetal parts may be difficult to palpate and there may be no audible fetal heart beat.

Initial management of placental abruption includes prompt resuscitation from maternal shock with monitoring of central venous pressure and attention to clotting disorders. Early involvement of a senior obstetrician, anaesthetist and haematologist is mandatory. Guidelines or the management of massive obstetric haemorrhage are detailed in the Report on Confidential Enquiries into Maternal Deaths in the United Kingdom 1985–1987 (Department of Health, 1991) and summarized here:

- Summon help from obstetricians, anaesthetists, midwives and nurses.
- Alert the haematologists and blood transfusion service.
- Take blood for group, cross-match (minimum 6 units) and coagulation studies.
- Establish two 14-gauge peripheral intravenous lines and give warmed, preferably grouped, blood via compression cuffs. (Remember O negative can be lifesaving.)
- Monitor pulse, blood pressure, central venous pressure, urinary output, ECG (electrocardiogram) and blood gases.
- Do not give fresh frozen plasma or platelet concentrates until major haemorrhage has been stopped or until 5 units of blood have been given rapidly.
- Consider early transfer to an intensive care unit and/or obstetric intervention.

If the fetus is mature and alive, emergency caesarean section should be performed. If the fetus is dead, artificial rupture of the membranes usually leads to a rapid labour. After a mild abruption, with an immature fetus, the obstetrician may allow the pregnancy to continue, but the woman will need to remain in hospital with antenatal monitoring. On occasion it may be necessary to transfer the woman to a regional centre with neonatal intensive care facilities prior to delivery of an immature fetus.

Placenta praevia

Placenta praevia occurs when the placenta is wholly or partially inserted into the lower uterine segment. The routine use of ultrasound screening has assisted in the diagnosis of asymptomatic placenta praevia. A low-lying placenta occurs in up to 28% of patients in the 2nd trimester but, as pregnancy progresses and the uterus grows, the placental site migrates upwards so that by term only 3% are praevia. Placenta praevia is more common with advancing maternal age, parity and in women who smoke (Paintin, 1962; Naeye, 1980). It is also more common following caesarean section and uterine instrumentation (Rose, 1986). There were no maternal deaths from placenta praevia in the UK between 1985 and 1987. Perinatal mortality is lower than with placental abruption, occurring in 4–12% of cases in recent studies (Lavery, 1990).

Placenta praevia usually presents with painless vaginal bleeding in the 3rd trimester. The bleeding is usually unprovoked but may follow coitus. It can be torrential, especially after 34 weeks' gestation or when ill-advised vaginal examination is performed. The degree of maternal shock is proportional to the degree of haemorrhage. Abdominal examination may reveal breech presentation or a transverse lie because the placenta acts as a pelvic tumour. The fetal heart is unaffected. The diagnosis can be confirmed with ultrasound scan.

Following resuscitation, the aim of treatment is to maintain the pregnancy until the fetus is mature enough to be delivered. Caesarean section by an experienced obstetrician is indicated unless there is a minor degree of praevia with the presenting part below the placenta.

Vasa praevia

Vasa praevia is a rare cause of antepartum haemorrhage. Bleeding occurs at the time of membrane rupture from fetal blood vessels crossing the internal cervical os. The fetus becomes bradycardic and prompt diagnosis is essential as caesarean section must be performed before it exsanguinates. Fetal haemoglobin in the vagina suggests vasa praevia.

Postpartum haemorrhage

Postpartum haemorrhage accounted for 60% of maternal deaths from haemorrhage in the UK between 1985 and 1987 (Department of Health, 1991). Primary postpartum haemorrhage is defined as blood loss from the genital tract in excess of 500 ml in the first 24 h after delivery (Zahn & Yeomans, 1990). Secondary postpartum haemorrhage occurs when there is excessive bleeding from the genital tract after the first 24 h until 6 weeks after delivery.

Primary postpartum haemorrhage

Although primary postpartum haemorrhage is most frequently encountered in the labour ward, occasionally the A&E doctor may have to treat this problem when a woman has concealed her pregnancy and presented in labour or immediately after delivery.

As with all potentially life-threatening haemorrhage, the woman should be resuscitated with intravenous fluids through two 14-gauge cannulae using O negative blood if necessary prior to cross-match. Because uterine atony is a common cause of postpartum haemorrhage, contraction of the uterus should be stimulated by mechanical compression and the use of oxytocics (e.g. Syntocinon, 10 units IV or as an infusion).

The vulva and vagina must be inspected for tears, which should be repaired. Any arterial bleeding points should be ligated. The patient requires admission to the obstetric unit and may need exploration under anaesthetic proceeding to removal of retained placental fragments or ligation of internal iliac arteries. On occasion hysterectomy is the only means by which haemorrhage can be controlled.

Secondary postpartum haemorrhage

Secondary postpartum haemorrhage is more often seen in the A&E department. The patient may present with profuse vaginal bleeding or a change in the lochia, most commonly in the 2nd week postpartum. To assess the significance of vaginal bleeding in the puerperium it is important to understand changes in normal lochia. The median duration of red lochia is 4 days, with brown-pink lochia lasting for 22 days. Yellow-white discharge persists for an average of 33 days (Oppenheimer et al., 1986).

Secondary postpartum haemorrhage most commonly results from retained products of conception and/or infection. Dehiscence of a caesarean section scar, rupture of a vulval haematoma and, rarely, development of choriocarcinoma are other causes. The management priorities are to resuscitate the patient, give ergometrine, screen for infection and start broad-spectrum antibiotics; then organize for the woman to be admitted. Clearly early

involvement of an obstetrician in the patient's management is important.

PRETERM LABOUR

Preterm labour is defined as the occurrence of regular contractions producing cervical change (dilatation or effacement) prior to 37 completed weeks of pregnancy.

Causes of preterm labour include:

- Antepartum haemorrhage.
- Cervical incompetence.
- Premature rupture of the membranes.
- Overdistension of the uterus (e.g. with twin pregnancy or polyhydramnios).
- Maternal illness or infection, especially urinary tract infection.

The patient with preterm labour presents most commonly with uterine contractions accompanied by abdominal, suprapubic or back pain (Wilkins & Creasy, 1990). She may describe the characteristic gush of fluid from ruptured membranes or vaginal bleeding from abruption or placenta praevia. The presence of vaginal loss precludes digital vaginal examination for fear of introducing infection through ruptured membranes or causing profuse bleeding with antepartum haemorrhage. The diagnosis of preterm labour in patients without vaginal loss is confirmed by finding greater than 2 cm cervical dilatation and 80% effacement on vaginal examination. The presence of regular contractions is confirmed by cardiotocography, which is also used to assess fetal heart rate for signs of distress.

Having made the diagnosis of preterm labour the obstetrician must decide whether the patient is a candidate for tocolytic therapy to abolish contractions, based on the following criteria:

- Healthy fetus.
- Firm diagnosis of preterm labour.
- Cervical dilatation <4 cm.
- Gestation <34 weeks and >18–20 weeks.
- No significant vaginal bleeding.
- No contraindication to prolongation of pregnancy.
- No contraindication to individual drugs.

Tocolytic drugs include beta-adrenergic stimulants (e.g. ritodrine, terbutaline), magnesium sulphate, calcium channel blockers and prostaglandin synthetase inhibitors (e.g. indomethacin) (Caritis et al., 1988). Because patients with preterm labour are at high risk of preterm delivery, corticosteroids may be used to reduce the incidence of neonatal respiratory distress. After bacteriological screening, antibiotics may be required for maternal infection.

Once preterm labour has advanced to the stage where delivery is imminent, the obstetrician must decide whether vaginal or surgical delivery is appropriate. Clearly there is a need for paediatricians to take over the care of the premature infant, and transfer to a unit with neonatal intensive care facilities may be required prior to delivery for infants of 24–28 weeks' gestation.

NON-OBSTETRIC CAUSES OF ABDOMINAL PAIN

Abdominal pain in pregnancy can result from obstetric causes (e.g. the onset of labour or placental abruption), but the pregnant woman is also likely to experience pain caused by other intra-abdominal pathology. The relative frequency with which gastrointestinal surgery is performed for various non-obstetric causes of abdominal pain is shown in Table 1.

Diagnosis of abdominal pain in pregnancy can be difficult because of the displacement of abdominal organs by the enlarging uterus and diminution in guarding and rebound tenderness by stretching of the peritoneum and abdominal wall musculature. Alders' sign helps to differentiate uterine from non-uterine abdominal pain (Alders, 1951). With the patient lying supine the point of maximal abdominal tenderness is palpated. With the fingers still in contact with the abdominal wall the patient is asked to turn onto the opposite side. If abdominal

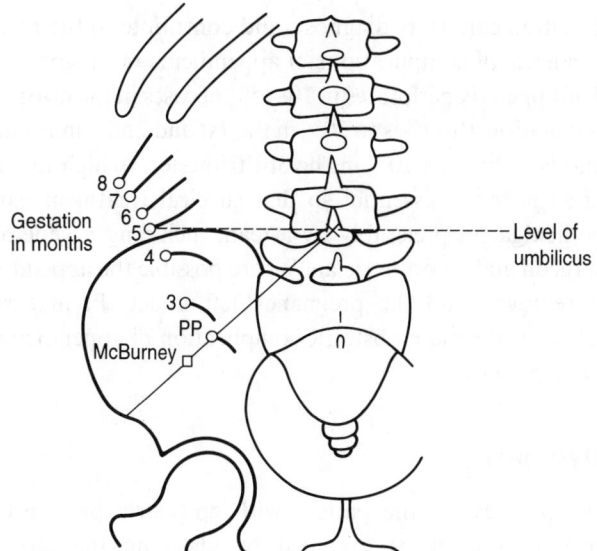

Fig. 1. Changes in position of the appendix during pregnancy. PP, prepregnancy. (Reproduced, with permission, from Baer, J.L., Reis, R.A. & Arens, R.A. (1932). *J. Am. Med. Assoc.*, **98**, 1359–64. Copyright 1932, American Medical Association.)

tenderness has diminished or disappeared (shifting tenderness) the cause of pain is uterine. If, however, the pain is unchanged the lesion is likely to be extrauterine.

Appendicitis

The incidence of appendicitis in pregnancy is approximately 1 case per 1000 deliveries, an incidence similar to that in non-pregnant women (Weingold, 1983). The position of the appendix after the 3rd month of pregnancy rises above McBurney's point and its base rotates horizontally (Fig. 1). The appendix reaches the level of the umbilicus at 5 months and approaches the right costal margin at 8 months' gestation (Baer *et al.*, 1932).

Abdominal pain is the commonest symptom of appendicitis in pregnancy. Initially there is epigastric or central abdominal pain which localizes to the site of the displaced appendix as the parietal peritoneum becomes inflamed. Anorexia, nausea and vomiting are common symptoms that may easily be overlooked because of their high prevalence in normal pregnancy. Abdominal tenderness is present in 90% of cases but rebound tenderness and guarding are less common, occurring in only 58% and 33% of cases, respectively (Weingold, 1983). Absence of fever occurs in almost half of the cases and an elevated white blood cell count may be physiological.

The relative absence of localized signs of peritoneal

Table 1. *Gastrointestinal surgery in pregnancy*

Surgical condition	Percentage of operations
Appendicitis	63.5
Abdominal exploration (including trauma)	12.5
Biliary tract problems	11.0
Intestinal obstruction	3.7
Anorectal disease	2.5
Tumours	2.5
Peptic ulcer	1.5
Pancreatitis	1.2
Inflammatory bowel disease	1.2
Miscellaneous	0.4

irritation can delay diagnosis and contribute to the high incidence of complications of appendicitis in pregnancy. The appendix perforates in 10–15% of cases in the normal population: this rises to 30% in the 1st and 2nd trimesters and is as high as 70% in the 3rd trimester. A high index of suspicion is essential so that surgical treatment can be instigated, preferably by a team including a general surgeon and an obstetrician. Where possible the appendix is removed and the pregnancy left intact. Premature labour is the main obstetric complication of appendicitis in pregnancy.

Dyspepsia

When assessing the patient with epigastric pain, pre-eclampsia must be excluded by checking the blood pressure and the urine for protein. Heartburn is a common symptom in normal pregnancy, caused by the increase in intragastric pressure without concomitant rise in oesophagogastric sphincter tone. The patient experiences epigastric burning pain and acid regurgitation into the mouth, exacerbated by specific foods, heavy meals and lying flat. Symptoms are usually improved by avoiding these precipitating factors and taking antacids.

The incidence of peptic ulcer in pregnancy is lower than in the normal community because of the protective effect of oestrogen and histaminase in pregnancy (Becker-Anderson & Husfeldt, 1971). Most women with peptic ulcers have a history that predates their pregnancy and will have noticed improvement of their symptoms with pregnancy. Women rarely present with complications of peptic ulcer disease. Perforation is characterized by epigastric pain, a rigid silent abdomen and clinical shock, and can be confirmed by finding free air on an erect chest X-ray. Following resuscitation prompt laparotomy is indicated.

Cholecystitis

Cholecystitis is relatively common because pregnancy encourages the formation of gallstones as a result of stasis in the biliary tract and increased secretion of lithogenic bile (Simon, 1983). Half of the patients with gallstones have a history that antedates pregnancy. The symptoms of gallbladder disease in pregnancy are the same as in the non-pregnant patient, namely right hypochondrial pain radiating to the shoulder or loin with nausea and vomiting. In early pregnancy a positive Murphy's sign assists diagnosis. In the second half of pregnancy diagnosis may be more difficult because superior displacement of

the appendix makes appendicitis more likely. Ultrasound is useful in confirming the presence of gallstones. Most cases settle with conservative management including bed rest, intravenous fluids, nasogastric suction and antibiotics. Cholecystectomy should be delayed until the 2nd trimester whenever possible, and reserved for treatment of cases that fail to settle with conservative management or are associated with cholangitis, pancreatitis or empyema of the gallbladder.

Intestinal obstruction

Intestinal obstruction is an unusual finding in pregnancy but the incidence is similar to that in the general population. Over 60% of cases are caused by adhesions which usually result from a previous appendicectomy or gynaecological surgery. Volvulus and intussusception are next most common, with hernias and carcinomas seldom the cause (Davis & Bohon, 1983). The incidence of obstruction in pregnancy is triphasic, occurring at 4–5 months when the uterus becomes intra-abdominal and exerts traction on adhesions, at 8–9 months when the head engages, and during delivery and the puerperium when the rapidly changing size of the uterus alters the relations of adhesions to adjacent bowel. The classical symptoms of intestinal obstruction are abdominal pain, vomiting and constipation. The last two are common symptoms in normal pregnancy. Clinical examination of the abdomen is hampered by the enlarged uterus, but Alders' sign and abnormal bowel sounds on auscultation assist diagnosis. Plain abdominal X-rays are also useful. Adequate fluid resuscitation followed by early laparotomy for intestinal obstruction is advocated to give optimal outcome for mother and child. Caesarean section may be required to gain access to the surgical field. Maternal mortality from intestinal obstruction is approximately 10–20%. Fetal death or premature labour occurs in over 30% of cases in the 3rd trimester.

Pyelonephritis

Asymptomatic bacteriuria occurs in 2–8% of pregnancies, usually before the 12th week. Between 20% and 40% of women with asymptomatic bacteriuria go on to develop pyelonephritis if they remain untreated (Phillips & Kwart, 1983). Screening for bacteriuria is therefore an important part of routine antenatal screening.

Symptoms of pyelonephritis include loin pain, spikes of fever and preterm labour. Urine microscopy shows white blood cells and bacteria. Treatment should be commenced with intravenous antibiotics and fluids before the result of culture is available, and continued until the patient is afebrile. This should be followed by a full course of oral antibiotics. Repeat urine culture should be analysed after stopping treatment and every 4 weeks thereafter throughout pregnancy. If bacteriuria persists, further investigation of the urinary tract is indicated to diagnose underlying structural abnormalities of the kidneys, ureters or bladder.

Uterine fibroids

Uterine fibroids are found in up to 5% of pregnancies. They are often asymptomatic and are detected by routine ultrasound screening in the 2nd trimester. Fibroids enlarge and soften during pregnancy and at times of maximal growth, usually in the 2nd trimester, may outstrip their blood supply, resulting in red degeneration (Amias, 1989). The patient complains of acute abdominal pain and vomiting and may develop a low-grade fever. There is exquisite localized tenderness over the fibroid. Diagnosis can be confirmed with an ultrasound scan. The patient is managed with bed rest, sedation and analgesia. The application of ice packs to the abdomen helps to resolve the condition. Surgery is indicated for cases which fail to settle with conservative management, where the diagnosis is in doubt (to exclude appendicitis or torsion of an ovarian cyst) or when a pedunculated fibroid has undergone torsion and secondary degeneration.

Ovarian cyst

The unexpected presentation of an ovarian cyst with abdominal pain in pregnancy is relatively rare because most are detected on routine clinical and ultrasound antenatal screening. Between 10% and 20% of pregnant patients with ovarian cysts require laparotomy for complications including torsion, rupture and haemorrhage. Torsion of an ovarian cyst is more common on the right and presents with a slow onset of intermittent, severe abdominal pain usually between the 8th and 12th weeks of pregnancy (McGowan, 1983). Nausea and vomiting occur in one-third of patients. Examination reveals a tense, tender, lower abdominal or pelvic mass. Urgent surgery is indicated as, if the torsion is unrelieved, haemorrhage and necrosis will lead to secondary rupture of the cyst, suggested by signs of increasing shock and spreading peritonitis. The differential diagnosis of torsion of an ovarian cyst in early pregnancy includes ectopic pregnancy, fibroids and appendicitis.

PRE-ECLAMPSIA AND ECLAMPSIA

Hypertensive disorders of pregnancy are a major cause of maternal death, accounting for almost 20% of maternal mortality in the UK. Undue delay in making or implementing critical clinical decisions and inappropriate delegation of clinical responsibility have been shown to be the main defects in hospital obstetric management of these patients (Department of Health, 1991).

Early recognition of pre-eclampsia and appropriate referral are essential skills for all doctors who treat pregnant women.

Pre-eclampsia

Pre-eclampsia can be defined as pregnancy-induced hypertension, usually associated with proteinuria. Patients with a blood pressure or greater than 140/90 mmHg are considered hypertensive, but those with a high systolic pressure (e.g. 160/80 mmHg) or an increase in diastolic pressure from a low baseline (e.g. from 65 to 85 mmHg) may also be classified as hypertensive. The presence of oedema is common in pregnant women with and without pre-eclampsia, rendering this an unhelpful sign in diagnosis.

Those at high risk of pre-eclampsia are primigravid patients, especially those aged over 35 years. Other risk factors include a family or previous history of pre-eclampsia, chronic hypertension or renal disease, and migraine. Those who are underweight and of short stature are also more prone to pre-eclampsia (Redman, 1989).

The majority of patients with pre-eclampsia are asymptomatic and routine screening for raised blood pressure and proteinuria is therefore important. Pre-eclampsia can be classified into three grades, each of increasing severity (Table 2). Those with isolated elevation of blood pressure should be referred to the next antenatal clinic for assessment, including doppler measurements of placental blood flow, and in the interim should rest in bed at home.

The combination of proteinuria and hypertension warrants obstetric admission that day. In hospital, bed rest can be enforced, doppler studies performed and fetal monitoring undertaken using the cardiotocogram. A rise in plasma urate levels and a fall in platelet count reflect deteriorating disease. Antihypertensives have been shown to protect the mother's circulation reducing the risk of a stroke, maintaining the pregnancy and allowing the fetus to become more mature.

Table 2. *Progression of pre-eclampsia*

	Stage 1	Stage 2	Stage 3
Hypertension	+	+	+
Proteinuria	−	+	+
Symptoms	−	−	+
Eclampsia	−	−	−
Duration	2–12 weeks	2–3 weeks	2–72 h
Time of admission	Elective	Today	Flying squad
Anticonvulsants	No	No	Yes
Delivery	After 38 weeks	After 34–36 weeks	After stabilization

The onset of symptoms heralds stage 3 pre-eclampsia which is an obstetric emergency necessitating urgent intervention to prevent the onset of fits.

Clinical features of stage 3 pre-eclampsia

- Headache
- Visual disturbance
- Epigastric pain
- Facial itching
- Rapidly increasing blood pressure
- Increasing proteinuria
- Hyper-reflexia

Frontal headaches are common and often associated with visual disturbance such as jagged, angular flashes at the periphery of the visual field and visual loss. These symptoms are caused by cerebral oedema. Stretching of the peritoneum over an oedematous liver causes epigastric pain. The patient may complain of facial itching. Examination reveals brisk tendon reflexes with clonus (Chamberlain, 1991b). Failure to test urine and check blood pressure in a pregnant woman with any of these clinical features may have fatal results. The blood pressure will be greatly elevated above previous readings and there will be a quantitative increase in proteinuria.

Early involvement of a senior obstetrician in the management of the symptomatic pre-eclamptic is mandatory but treatment should not be delayed while waiting for obstetric help to arrive. Intravenous diazepam should be given to prevent fits and reduce blood pressure.

Hydralazine is the favoured antihypertensive which can be given either as an intravenous bolus or as a continuous infusion. Once stage 3 pre-eclampsia has been reached urgent delivery of the fetus, regardless of gestational maturity, is advocated to reduce the risk of eclampsia and maternal death.

Eclampsia

The onset of eclampsia is characterized by convulsions in a woman with pregnancy-induced hypertension. Usually fits develop in labour or the puerperium of women with hypertension and proteinuria. Eclamptic women are at risk of disseminated intravascular coagulation, renal failure and adult respiratory distress syndrome.

When a woman has an eclamptic fit the priorities are to maintain the airway, stop the convulsions, control the blood pressure and expedite delivery of the fetus:

- The woman should be nursed on her side in the recovery position and the airway should be kept clear.
- Intravenous diazepam should be given immediately to stop the fits.
- Anticonvulsant therapy should then be commenced with a phenytoin infusion. Magnesium sulphate is an alternative anticonvulsant which is widely used in the USA.
- Intravenous hydralazine should be used to control blood pressure.
- If the woman is in labour or about to have labour induced, epidural anaesthetic is useful in reducing blood pressure and the tendency to fit.

The ultimate treatment of eclampsia is delivery of the infant. The decision as to the best mode of delivery (i.e. induction or caesarean section) should be made by a senior obstetrician.

MEDICAL EMERGENCIES IN PREGNANCY

Asthma

Pregnancy does not have a consistent effect on the severity of pre-existing asthma. Some women notice improvement in their symptoms, others deteriorate and the majority remain unchanged. In general, therapeutic regimens which were effective prior to pregnancy will continue to be so; therefore inhaled steroids, bronchodilators and oral theophyllines should not be interrupted during pregnancy. Cough preparations containing iodine must not be used as they cause fetal goitre. The use of a home peak flow meter will help in assessing the degree of asthma control.

During pregnancy, maternal oxygen consumption increases by 25% and the fetus tolerates hypoxia poorly. In an acute asthmatic attack hypoxia poses a greater threat to the fetus than the side-effects of drugs used to treat the attack; therefore treatment of the attack is the same as in the non-pregnant patient. Rapid correction of hypoxia is essential and treatment includes the use of high-concentration oxygen, nebulized beta-agonists such as salbutamol, and parenteral steroids. Early mechanical ventilation may be required.

Epilepsy

The frequency of seizures increases in almost half of epileptic women when they become pregnant (Montouris *et al.*, 1979). This is caused by a fall in the plasma levels of anticonvulsants during pregnancy despite maintenance of prepregnancy dosage. Known epileptics should have their anticonvulsant levels monitored on a monthly basis so that drug levels can be kept in the therapeutic range. The risk of teratogenicity to the fetus from anticonvulsant drugs has to be balanced against the damage caused by uncontrolled convulsions. The ideal is to establish a maintenance regimen using the least number of drugs with the fewest side-effects whilst providing optimal seizure control.

If a pregnant woman presents to the A&E department with a fit, the management priorities are the same as for the non-pregnant patient:

- The airway must be cleared, supplemental oxygen given and the patient protected from self-injury.
- Intravenous diazepam is the best drug for control of fits in the emergency situation (Chamberlain, 1991c).
- Blood should be taken for anticonvulsant levels as subtherapeutic concentrations are almost always the cause of seizures in known epileptics.
- Eclampsia must be excluded by assessment of blood pressure and urinalysis for proteinuria.

Deep vein thrombosis

Deep vein thrombosis (DVT) occurs in up to 3 per 1000 pregnancies and, if left untreated, pulmonary emboli will complicate 15–24% of cases (Chatelain & Quirk, 1990). DVT is more common in pregnant than in non-pregnant women because of increased concentrations of clotting factors and fibrinogen, production of fibrinolysis inhibitors from the placenta and venous stasis.

The clinical features of DVT are the same as in the non-pregnant patient:

- Pain.
- Swelling.
- Tenderness.
- A positive Homan's sign.
- Change in limb colour.

Doppler ultrasound is a non-invasive test which is useful in diagnosis of venous thrombosis above the knee. The technique has a 30% false positive rate and is unhelpful in the diagnosis of calf thrombosis.

The most accurate test for DVT is venography. Because this investigation is associated with a significant radiation dose to the fetus, it is contraindicated in the 1st trimester (Department of Health, 1991). Later in pregnancy venography should be performed to confirm the diagnosis prior to starting treatment because of the risks of prolonged anticoagulation. Isotope scanning with labelled fibrinogen is contraindicated in pregnancy because this test involves injection of a radioisotope.

Anticoagulation in pregnancy is restricted to the use of heparin because warfarin crosses the placenta and is associated with fetal abnormalities. Chatelain advocates intravenous anticoagulation with heparin for the first 7–10 days to prolong the activated partial thromboplastin time to 1.5–2 times the control. Thereafter, treatment is changed to subcutaneous heparin, 5000 units twice daily, throughout pregnancy and for the first 3–6 weeks postpartum. Warfarin can be started after delivery if the woman is not breastfeeding.

Obstetric septic shock

Septic shock during pregnancy often has a subtle presentation, and a high index of suspicion is required so that life-threatening infections are promptly diagnosed and treated. During pregnancy it is caused by urinary tract infection, septic abortion and prolonged rupture of the membranes (greater than 48 h). In the puerperium retained products of conception (often presenting as secondary postpartum haemorrhage) and endometritis following caesarean section are common causes (Pearlman & Faro, 1990).

Recognition of early signs of sepsis – namely, clinical evidence of infection together with fever or hypothermia, tachypnoea, tachycardia and signs of renal, cerebral or respiratory disturbance – facilitates early therapeutic intervention. If left untreated, hypotension, adult respiratory distress syndrome, disseminated intravascular coagulation and renal failure ensue.

Treatment of septic shock requires adequate oxygenation, fluid replacement with haemodynamic monitoring and administration of broad-spectrum intravenous anti-biotics once blood cultures and bacteriological samples have been taken. The patient should then be transferred to the intensive care unit if urgent surgical removal of infected tissue is not required.

Cardiopulmonary resuscitation

The priorities in cardiopulmonary resuscitation of the pregnant patient are the same as for the non-pregnant patient – namely airway, breathing and circulation – ABC (see Chapter 3). However, modifications need to be made to take account of the physiological changes of pregnancy. In the supine position the weight of the gravid uterus causes aortocaval compression reducing venous return to the heart and rendering conventional cardio-pulmonary resuscitation ineffective. To reduce aortocaval compression whilst still delivering a suitable force during chest compression, the patient should be inclined 30° to the left. This patient position can be maintained using a Cardiff wedge (Rees & Willis, 1988). Alternatively the uterus can be manually displaced to the left. If the patient does not respond after 5 min of cardiopulmonary resuscitation in the appropriate position, immediate caesarean section should be performed. Delivery of the infant improves maternal circulation and increases venous return, giving the mother the best chance of survival (Oates et al., 1988).

PUERPERAL DEPRESSION

Adjustment to the demands of parenthood puts consider-able strain on the psyche. On or about the 3rd day following the delivery of the infant it is common for the mother to experience 'baby blues' characterized by tearfulness, feelings of inadequacy and an inability to cope. She may also experience anorexia and nausea. Her symptoms are caused by the demands of the neonate, fatigue from the delivery and lack of sleep, and the hormonal changes following the birth. Usually such symptoms are self-limiting and resolve within a few days, but approximately 5% of women will seek medical help because of the severity of their symptoms. The majority of cases of puerperal depression are best treated with counselling and reassurance rather than sedatives or psychotropic drugs.

On occasion the mother will develop symptoms of psychotic illness (e.g. schizophrenia or mania). Such patients should be referred for psychiatric assessment.

Bibliography

ALDERS, N. (1951). A sign for differentiating uterine from extrauterine complications of pregnancy and puerperium. *Br. Med. J.*, **2**, 1194–5.

AMIAS, A.G. (1989). Abdominal pain in pregnancy. In *Obstetrics*, ed. A Turnbull & G. Chamberlain, pp. 605–21. Edinburgh: Churchill Livingstone.

BAER, J.L., REIS, R.A. & ARENS, R.A. (1932). Appendicitis in pregnancy with changes in position and axis of the normal appendix in pregnancy. *J. Am. Med. Assoc.*, **98**, 1359–64.

BECKER-ANDERSON, H. & HUSFELDT, V. (1971). Peptic ulcer in pregnancy. *Acta Obstet. Gynecol. Scand.*, **50**, 391–5.

CARITIS, S.N., DARBY, M.J. & CHAN, L. (1988). Pharmocologic treatment of preterm labour. *Clin. Obstet. Gynecol.*, **31**, 635–51.

CHAMBERLAIN, G. (1991a). Antepartum haemorrhage. A.B.C. of antenatal care. *Br. Med. J.*, **302**, 1526–30.

CHAMBERLAIN, G. (1991b). Raised blood pressure in pregnancy. A.B.C. of antenatal care. *Br. Med. J.*, **302**, 1454–8.

CHAMBERLAIN, G. (1991c). Medical problems in preg-nancy. A.B.C. of antenatal care. *Br. Med. J.*, **302**, 1262–6.

CHATELAIN, S.M. & QUIRK, J.G. (1990). Amniotic and thromboembolism. *Clin. Obstet. Gynecol.*, **33**, 473–81.

DAVIS, M.R. & BOHON, C.J. (1983). Intestinal obstruc-tion in pregnancy. *Clin. Obstet. Gynecol.*, **26**, 832–41.

DEPARTMENT OF HEALTH, WELSH OFFICE, SCOTTISH HOME AND HEALTH DEPART-MENT, DEPARTMENT OF HEALTH AND SOCIAL SERVICES, NORTHERN IRELAND (1991). Report on Confidential Enquiries into Maternal Deaths in the United Kingdom, 1985–1987. London: HMSO.

HIBBARD, B.M. & HIBBARD, E.D. (1963). Aetiological factors in abruptio placentae. *Br. Med. J.*, **2**, 1430–6.

LAVERY, J.P. (1990). Placenta praevia. *Clin. Obstet. Gynecol.*, **33**, 414–21.

LOWE, T.W. & CUNNINGHAM, F.G. (1990). Placen-tal abruption. *Clin. Obstet. Gynecol.*, **33**, 406–13.

McGOWAN, L. (1983). Surgical diseases of the ovary in pregnancy. *Clin. Obstet. Gynecol.*, **26**, 843–51.

MONTOURIS, G.D., FENICHEL, G.M. & McLAIN, L.W. (1979). The pregnant epileptic. *Arch. Neurol.*, **36**, 601–3.

NAEYE, R. (1980). Abruptio placentae and placenta praevia: frequency, perinatal mortality and cigarette smoking. *Obstet. Gynecol.*, **55**, 701–4.

OATES, S., WILLIAMS, G.L. & REES, G.A.D. (1988). Cardiopulmonary resuscitation in late pregnancy. *Br. Med. J.*, **297**, 404–5.

OPPENHEIMER, L.W., SHERRIFF, E.A., GOODMAN, J.D.S. et al. (1986). The duration of lochia. *Br. J. Obstet. Gynaecol.*, **93**, 754–7.

PAINTIN, D. (1962). The epidemiology of antepartum haemorrhage. *J. Obstet. Gynaecol. Br. Commonw.*, **69**, 614–24.

PEARLMAN, M. & FARO, S. (1990). Obstetric septic shock: a pathophysiologic basis for management. *Clin. Obstet. Gynecol.*, **33**, 482–92.

PHILLIPS, M.H. & KWART, A.M. (1983). Urinary tract disease in pregnancy. *Clin. Obstet. Gynecol.*, **26**, 890–901.

REDMAN, C.W.G. (1989). Hypertension in pregnancy. In *Obstetrics*. ed. A. Turnbull & G. Chamberlain, pp. 515–41. Edinburgh: Churchill Livingstone.

REES, G.A.D. & WILLIS, B.A. (1988). Resuscitation in late pregnancy. *Anaesthesia*, **43**, 347–9.

ROSE, G. (1986). Aetiological factors in placenta praevia – a case controlled study. *Br. J. Obstet. Gynaecol.*, **93**, 589–93.

SIMON, J.A. (1983). Biliary tract disease and related surgical disorders during pregnancy. *Clin. Obstet. Gynecol.*, **26**, 810–21.

WEINGOLD, A.B. (1983). Appendicitis in pregnancy. *Clin. Obstet. Gynecol.*, **26**, 801–9.

WILKINS, I. & CREASY, R.K. (1990). Preterm labour. *Clin. Obstet. Gynecol.*, **33**, 502–13.

ZAHN, C.M. & YEOMANS, E.R. (1990). Postpartum haemorrhage, placenta accreta, uterine inversion and puerperal haematomas. *Clin. Obstet. Gynecol.*, **33**, 422–31.

59 Gynaecological emergencies

C. GILLING-SMITH, L. REGAN and R. TOUQUET

Department of Obstetrics and Gynaecology, St Mary's Hospital, London, UK

Chapter plan

Introduction
Assessment of the gynaecological patient
Gynaecological conditions
Pregnancy ⩾20 weeks/puerperium
Appendix: Advice on miscarriage

INTRODUCTION

We have set out in this chapter our recommended management guidelines for gynaecological problems presenting to accident and emergency (A&E) departments. In order to ensure swift referral and treatment, particularly in the case of potentially life-threatening conditions such as ectopic pregnancy, it is important to avoid unnecessary duplication of certain procedures (e.g. pelvic examinations, taking swabs, arranging ultrasound). Therefore A&E and gynaecological staff must make time to discuss which team is primarily responsible for each stage of management. It is perfectly acceptable for A&E doctors to carry out most of the procedures discussed below, including performing pelvic examinations, provided they receive sufficient training to interpret their findings correctly and act appropriately (note exceptions in section on pelvic examinations).

Ultimately the extent to which A&E doctors take responsibility will be determined by the geographical situation of the gynaecological unit, and the degree of training/supervision given to them. A telephone discussion with the on-call gynaecologist will help prevent many potential problems.

A&E departments must have available:

- An examination room with a door, and angled headlight for performing speculum examinations.
- A gynaecological tray with essential equipment (Table 1 and Fig. 1).

Table 1. *Recommended contents of the gynaecological tray*

- Gloves
- Speculum – Cusco's medium ×3, small ×1, large ×1
  – Sims ×1
- Sponge forceps
- Gauze swabs, cotton-wool swabs
- Bacterial swabs – high vaginal swabs
- Histology specimen pots (×2):
  1. containing formalin saline to fix tissue;
  2. dry and sterile for cytogenetics
- Sanitary towels
- KY jelly, Hibitane obstetric jelly
- Ultrasound jelly
- Portable Doppler sonicaid

- On-site ultrasound scanning facilities and portable Doppler sonicaid.
- 24-h access to blood grouping and Rh (rhesus) typing.

Finally, when patients are discharged home directly from the A&E department, we advocate the use of simple explanatory leaflets and careful follow-up, either by their family doctor or by the hospital specialist. Every patient should have a discharge letter for their general practitioner.

We shall first describe general principles of gynaecological examination and investigation before describing in more detail management of specific problems.

ASSESSMENT OF THE GYNAECOLOGICAL PATIENT

History

More than 50% of women presenting with lower abdominal pain will have an eventual gynaecological

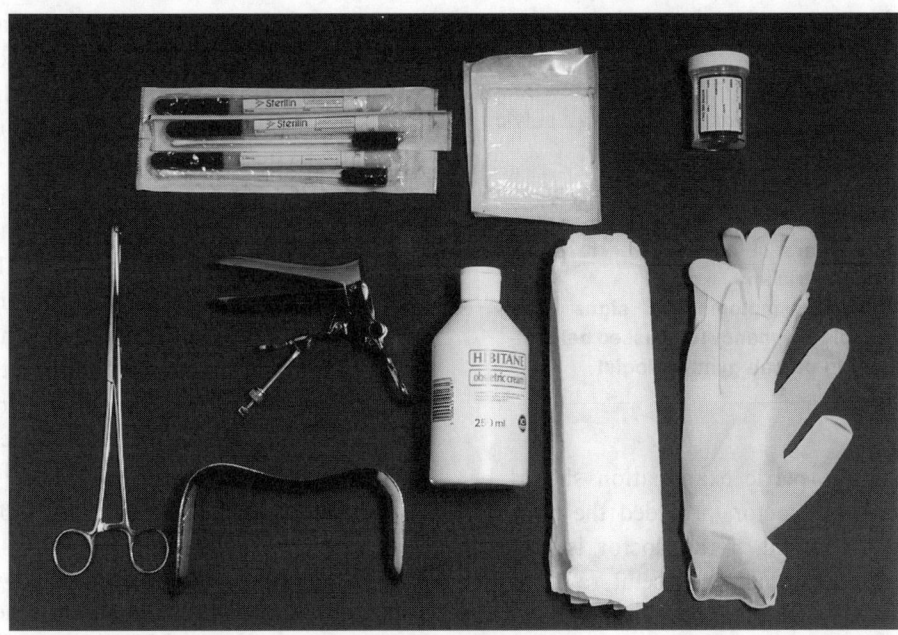

Fig. 1. Contents of the gynaecological tray. From left to right: sponge forceps, bacterial swabs, Cusco's speculum (top), Sims speculum (bottom), gauze swabs, chlorhexidine obstetric cream, sanitary towels, histology specimen pot and gloves.

diagnosis (Gilling-Smith *et al.*, 1995). The points which should generally be noted are outlined in Table 2. In addition, all women of child-bearing age presenting with abdominal pain, vaginal bleeding or fainting should have a urinary (human beta-chorionic gonadotropin, βhCG) pregnancy test performed on arrival.

General examination

Examination must take place in a room with a door for privacy. General physical signs such as temperature, pulse and blood pressure must be measured and note must be taken of any scars during the routine abdominal examination. Subumbilical (laparoscopy), Pfannenstiel and midline scars are all suggestive of previous gynaecological surgery – information which may not be volunteered by the patient during the history-taking. If an abdominal mass is felt, its relationship to the pelvic brim should be noted along with its size, mobility, consistency and presence of tenderness. Percussion can be useful in distinguishing between free fluid and a large ovarian cyst.

At this stage the doctor should be able to make an informed judgement as to whether a pelvic examination is warranted. As discussed below, in certain cases it may be more appropriate to refer the patient immediately to the on-call specialist.

Table 2. *Specific points to note in the gynaecological history*

Menstrual history	Date of last menstrual period
	Length of cycle
	History of cycle irregularity
Obstetric history	Number of viable pregnancies
	Previous ectopic pregnancies
	Previous miscarriages
Contraception used	Current and recent
Presenting complaint	Nature and duration
	Relation to cycle
	Associated symptoms – vaginal discharge, dysmenorrhoea and dyspareunia
	Previous attendance with the same complaint
	Results of any investigations and treatment given
Past gynaecological, medical, surgical and psychiatric history	Previous attendance/treatment for same problem
Drug history	Hormone replacement therapy
	Injectable progestagens
Social history	Marital status, sexual partners
	Smoking, drinking
	Recent travel

Pelvic examination

The A&E doctor should *not* perform a pelvic examination in the following situations:

- Woman with a pregnancy ⩾ 20 weeks – refer to on-call obstetrician
- Patient under 16 years of age – refer to on-call gynaecologist/paediatrician
- Patient with clinical symptoms and signs *highly suggestive* of ectopic pregnancy (discussed below) – refer immediately to on-call gynaecologist

In other circumstances pelvic examination should be performed by the A&E doctor, provided the patient's consent has been given and, if the doctor is male, a chaperone is present. It is always useful to have an assistant present to help with handling instruments and swabs, adjusting the overhead light and comforting the patient.

The bladder should be empty. The patient is placed in the dorsal position with feet together and knees flexed and apart. The perineum and vulva are first inspected and the labia separated. One hand should be placed on the patient's lower abdomen and either one or two gloved and lubricated fingers of the other hand should be inserted into the vagina and the cervix identified.

The following points should be noted:

- *State of the internal cervical os – open or closed.* The internal os is 'open' if it admits a finger tip or contains products of conception. Confusion can arise in the case of a multiparous patient where the external os is often patulous (gaping). Nevertheless the internal os should be closed.
- *Presence of cervical excitation.* This is intense pain experienced on moving the cervix and is suggestive of peritoneal irritation.
- *Size, shape, position and mobility of the uterus.* This is best assessed by pushing the uterus gently up from the vagina against the fingers of the abdominal hand which, initially, is kept still. The position of the cervix is usually the best guide as to whether the uterus is anteverted, retroverted or axial. Judging size is a matter of clinical experience but as a rough rule of thumb a non-gravid uterus is just palpable bimanually and about the size of an egg. By 8 weeks' gestation the uterus is usually the size of an orange and by 12 weeks the size of a grapegruit. Thereafter it starts to rise out of the pelvis and should be palpable abdominally.

The aim of the speculum examination is to visualize the vaginal walls and then the cervix. A Cusco's bivalve speculum of the appropriate size (the examiner should be guided by his findings at bimanual examination) is usually the instrument of first choice, although in women with a degree of vaginal prolapse or uterovaginal descent a Sims speculum should be used. In this case the patient is placed in the left lateral position. The speculum should be warmed first under a hot tap, lubricated and inserted slowly and gently into the vagina to avoid causing any pain. It is only by paying attention to these details that any information is to be gleaned from the procedure. Bleeding from the vaginal walls, the appearance of the cervical os and the presence and character of any discharge should be noted and swabs taken from the vaginal walls and cervical os where appropriate. Sponge forceps should be used to remove visible products of conception. If products are distending the cervical os they prevent the uterus from contracting and can provoke cervical shock. Any tissues removed should be sent for histological analysis.

Investigations

Doppler sonicaid

This simple piece of equipment should be available in every A&E department and its use understood by all A&E doctors (Fig. 2). The fetal heart should be audible

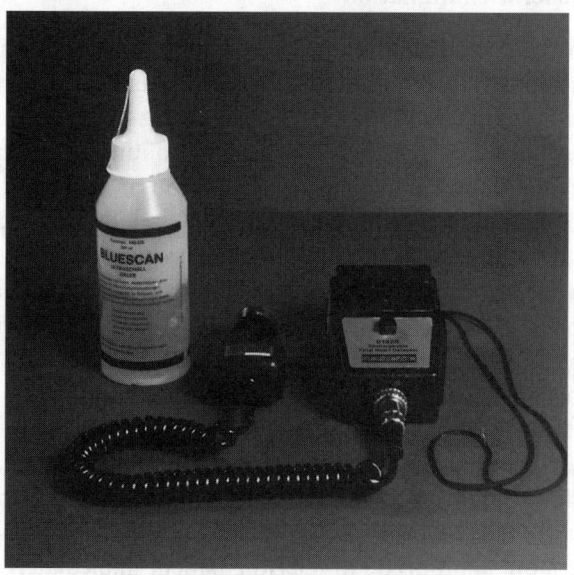

Fig. 2. Doppler sonicaid.

from 12 weeks. The pregnant patient will be very reassured by hearing the fetal heart amplified by the sonicaid.

Ultrasound

In recent years, pelvic ultrasound scanning has become a vital diagnostic tool in the assessment of women with lower abdominal pain and/or vaginal bleeding. It is a simple non-invasive test which should be immediately available to all A&E departments between the hours of 9 a.m. and 5 p.m.

Pelvic ultrasound can be performed by two routes:

1. Transabdominal (TA).
2. Transvaginal (TV).

The TA route requires the patient to have a distended bladder which provides an 'acoustic window' by displacing small bowel out of the pelvis. In practice, the patient needs to drink about one litre of fluid and wait until the bladder is adequately distended. This can cause considerable delay (prior pelvic examination requires an empty bladder), be uncomfortable for the patient and if the fluid cannot be taken by mouth (general anaesthesia a possibility or patient is vomiting) it necessitates the insertion of a urinary catheter or an intravenous infusion to fill the bladder. In hospitals with the necessary equipment and expertise the TV route is undoubtedly the method of choice (Goswany, 1992). A distended bladder is not required (important in an emergency situation) and image resolution is significantly improved (particularly noticeable in obese women) as the probe is much closer to the pelvic organs. Heavy vaginal bleeding should not interfere with the procedure and the only contraindication is if the patient is virgo intacta. In general women find the TV route more acceptable than the TA route.

Ultrasound plays a key role in the investigation of women with abnormal vaginal bleeding or lower abdominal pain. This is rarely a problem during normal working hours when A&E departments should have ready access to ultrasound facilities. Out of hours, particularly at weekends, it may be more prudent to refer and admit the patient, although in certain cases (discussed below) advice to return the following day for an ultrasound examination may be justified. When a portable sector scanner is available in A&E, this dilemma is resolved and, by reducing the number of unnecessary admissions, it is invariably cost-effective. Most registrars in gynaecology receive sufficient training in ultrasound interpretation to be able to diagnose an intrauterine pregnancy, the presence or absence of a beating fetal heart, or any large pelvic adnexal masses – critical findings which will determine subsequent management. With the wider availability of high-resolution ultrasound equipment this training could be extended to A&E doctors in well-organized A&E departments, especially those without gynaecological services on site.

Urinary pregnancy testing

The rapid measurement of urinary βhCG to detect pregnancy is now routine practice. The monoclonal antibody enzyme-linked immunoassay technique provides a rapid and sensitive test with a colour end-point and can easily be performed by nursing or medical staff in A&E. A review of a number of such tests in the management of patients with suspected ectopic pregnancies has shown a 100% sensitivity and specificity along with a 100% predictive value for normal and abnormal results (McCready et al., 1978).

The Clearview test (Unipath, Bedford) and the rapid Absorbent Matrix Pad are both simple 5-min qualitative tests and will detect βhCG levels as low as 50 IU per litre, levels which are reached approximately 10 days post-conception in a normal pregnancy (in other words before the woman even knows she is pregnant). A recent evaluation of the Clearview test for the assessment of gynaecological emergencies in A&E indicated a 100% sensitivity and negative predictive value. The additional cost of the test was clearly offset by a reduction in the number of unnecessary admissions where the test was negative (Kingdom et al., 1991).

Urinalysis

Reagent strips (Nephur-test sticks) are a simple but useful investigation in women presenting with lower abdominal pain with or without urinary symptoms. These detect not only blood, glucose and protein but also leucocytes and nitrates which are indicative of urinary tract infection (Wilkie et al., 1992). In all cases a midstream urine (MSU) must be sent for culture.

Microscopic haematuria should not be assumed to be caused by infection. Further urine testing (when there is no menstrual bleeding) must be arranged, preferably by the general practitioner, to exclude neoplastic lesions of the urinary tract.

Haematological indices

Haemoglobin should always be checked in patients presenting with menorrhagia. Anaemia may also be present in a patient with an undiagnosed ectopic pregnancy where symptoms have been present for more than 48 h. The white cell count and erythrocyte sedimentation rate (ESR) may be raised in pelvic inflammatory disease (PID).

Blood cultures should be taken in any patient with a clinical diagnosis of septic abortion, toxic-shock syndrome or puerperal sepsis prior to starting any antibiotic therapy.

Rh testing

The risk of maternal immunization following miscarriage ranges from 2% to 9% at 8 to 12 weeks respectively (Huggon & Watson, 1993; National Blood Transfusion Service Immunoglobulin Working Party, 1991). The risk of sensitization through transplacental bleeding is almost twice as high in threatened abortion. It is for this reason that A&E departments should have 24-h access to Rh testing so that prophylactic anti-D immunoglobulin (250 IU IM) can be given to all Rh negative patients discharged home with a diagnosis of threatened abortion within 72 h of the first bleed.

Swabs

As a general rule, the taking of high vaginal swabs in A&E should be limited to cases of suspected vulvovaginal thrush (candidiasis). All other conditions should be referred to the genitourinary clinic (or on-call gynaecologist) for detailed screening, definitive diagnosis, treatment and follow-up with contact tracing (see section on vaginal discharge).

Human immunodeficiency virus

A&E departments *should not take blood samples for HIV testing* unless they can provide a pre- and post-test counselling service (Bor *et al.*, 1991).

All A&E departments must have a reliable system for checking pathology results and informing general practitioners of abnormal results.

GYNAECOLOGICAL CONDITIONS

Vaginal bleeding in early pregnancy (≤ 20 weeks)

Vaginal bleeding is the commonest complication of early pregnancy with a reported incidence of 16–25% (Anonymous, 1980; Niswander & Gordon, 1973). The bleeding is frightening to the woman and consequently this is one of the most frequent gynaecological emergencies presenting to A&E. In one teaching hospital where the gynaecology department is located on a different site, early pregnancy bleeding represents 0.7% of the total A&E workload (Gilling-Smith *et al.*, 1988). Overall management of this problem remains poor, both in general practice (Everett *et al.*, 1987) and A&E (Gilling-Smith *et al.*, 1994).

A rapid assessment should be made through careful history-taking, pelvic examination, βhCG urinalysis and demonstration of fetal viability by ultrasound or Doppler sonicaid. In this way, delay in the diagnosis of various life-threatening complications of early bleeding can be prevented. These include rupture of an ectopic pregnancy, septicaemia and disseminated intravascular coagulation secondary to a missed abortion, shock from excessive vaginal haemorrhage and, in the long term, the risk of Rh isoimmunization in Rh negative patients. This approach significantly reduces the rate of unnecessary admission, referral to the on-call gynaecologist and re-attendance to the department with further episodes of bleeding (Gilling-Smith *et al.*, 1988).

Table 3 summarizes the causes, diagnosis and management of early pregnancy bleeding.

Miscarriage

Although synonymous, the term miscarriage is preferable to spontaneous abortion because many patients believe that an 'abortion' describes the voluntary termination of a pregnancy. The vast majority of miscarriages occur before 12 weeks' gestation. Aetiological factors may include chromosomal abnormalities of the embryo, structural abnormalities of the genital tract, infection, endocrine and immunological abnormalities. In many cases detailed investigations fail to identify an obvious cause. Second trimester miscarriage is usually associated with heavier bleeding and simple resuscitative measures in A&E (intravenous line, etc.) may be required.

There are several types of miscarriage.

Table 3. *Differential diagnosis and management of early pregnancy bleeding*

Symptoms	Pelvic examination	Ultrasound	Diagnosis	Management
Bleeding + Pain +/−	Cervix closed No adnexal tenderness	IU pregnancy FH present	Threatened miscarriage	• Anti-D if Rh − ve • Discharge home • Advice sheet
Bleeding + + (clots) Pain + +	Cervix open +/− lower abdominal tenderness	IU pregnancy FH absent	Inevitable miscarriage	• IV line • +/− Syntocinon • FBC/G&S • Admit for ERPC
Bleeding + Pain +/−	Cervix closed No adnexal tenderness	IU gestational sac FH absent	Missed abortion	• FBC/G&S • Admit for ERPC
Bleeding + Pain + + (L or RIF) Shoulder tip pain Fainting	Cervical excitation + + Cervix closed Adnexal tenderness +/− mass	No IU pregnancy +/− adnexal mass/ectopic +/− free fluid	Ectopic pregnancy	• Avoid pelvic exam if this is suspected • IV line • Cross-match at least 2 units of blood • Refer
Bleeding + + (clots) Pain +	Cervix open POC + +	Mass in uterine cavity 'Snowstorm appearance'	Hydatidiform mole or incomplete miscarriage	• Send POC for histology • FBC/G&S • Admit for ERPC and follow-up

L, left; RIF, right iliac fossa; IU, intrauterine; FH, fetal heart; POC, products of conception; ERPC, evacuation of retained products of conception; FBC, full blood count; G&S, group and save; Rh, rhesus; IV, intravenous.

(a) Threatened miscarriage

This refers to vaginal bleeding in association with a viable intrauterine pregnancy.

Clinical presentation There is a small amount of vaginal bleeding with little or no abdominal pain.

Pelvic examination The uterus is enlarged corresponding to gestational size and the cervical os closed. There is usually little or no pelvic tenderness.

Diagnosis In all women presenting with early pregnancy bleeding, fetal viability should be verified using pelvic ultrasound. The Royal College of Radiologists and the Royal College of Obstetricians and Gynaecologists have recently produced guidelines to assist in this (Guidance on Ultrasound Procedures in Early Pregnancy, 1995). The single most important diagnostic sign is the presence of a pulsating fetal heart (Hertz, 1984). If present, the chances of the pregnancy continuing successfully are greater than 95%. Using real-time ultrasound, an intrauterine gestation sac is detectable from 5 weeks and a pulsating fetal heart from 6 (TV) or 7 (TA) weeks of amenorrhoea. If no intrauterine pregnancy is demonstrable and an adnexal mass is present, the probability of an ectopic pregnancy is of the order of 95% (Robinson & De Crespigny, 1983). From 12 weeks, the fetal heart should be audible using a portable Doppler ultrasound machine (sonicaid) (Robinson, 1972; Romero et al., 1984). If not easily audible at this gestation, the presence or absence of a fetal heart beat should be verified promptly by ultrasound.

If there is doubt about the presence of a fetal heart in a 6–7-week fetus or confusion about the menstrual dating, arrangements should be made to repeat the scan one week later. During this interval the gestation sac would be expected to have doubled in size and the fetal heart to be visible in a viable pregnancy. The repeat scan should be arranged either by the ultrasound department or by the on-call gynaecologist following referral.

Referral Whether findings need to be discussed with the on-call gynaecologist are largely dictated by the clinical and mental state of the woman as well as her home circumstances.

Treatment The patient should be reassured and discharged home with an advice sheet (see Appendix). If she is Rh negative, 250 IU (50 µg) of anti-D should be given intramuscularly. She should be advised to book for antenatal care and, if already attending, details of ultrasound results and any treatment given (anti-D, etc.) should be written on her antenatal notes or shared care card.

Complications If there are further episodes of bleeding the woman should be advised to see her general practitioner or obstetrician.

(b) Incomplete miscarriage

The fetus is dead and miscarriage inevitable. The cervix has started to open and the membranes have often ruptured. Products of conception (POC) and blood clots may be passed through the cervix but some decidua and products are retained which defines the miscarriage as incomplete.

Clinical presentation Bleeding is often profuse with clots, and severe abdominal cramping pains may accompany uterine contractions. If POC are in the cervical os there may be signs of cervical shock (faintness, rapid pulse, low blood pressure).

Pelvic examination The uterus is enlarged, often tender and the cervical os open. On speculum examination, POC may be seen in the os and should be carefully removed with sterile sponge forceps and sent for histopathological examination. The purpose of this is to:

- Reduce the risk of cervical shock.
- Reduce uterine bleeding by allowing the uterus to contract.
- Allow histological confirmation of diagnosis of pregnancy.
- Exclude hydatidiform mole.

If chromosomal analysis is also required (e.g. recurrent miscarriage), the POC must be sent promptly to the cytogenetics department in a dry container.

Diagnosis Clinical findings alone are often sufficient to make the diagnosis, particularly if POC are visible. However, many patients find it difficult to accept the diagnosis of a lost pregnancy without ultrasound evidence that the fetal heart is absent. Ultrasound is also helpful in determining whether there are retained POC within the uterine cavity. An empty cavity is evidence that the patient does not need surgical evacuation of retained products of conception provided the possibility of ectopic pregnancy has been excluded (histological confirmation that POC have been passed and/or serum βhCG measurements).

Referral This must be to the on-call gynaecologist for admission. If transfer to another hospital is required, basic resuscitation should be carried out before transfer (see below).

Treatment Admission and surgical evacuation of the uterus is required. If the bleeding is profuse and/or clinical signs of shock are present, an intravenous line should be sited, blood volume replaced with either saline or colloid and oxytocics (Syntocinon 10 units IV or IM) administered. Blood should always be taken first for haemoglobin estimation and grouping.

(c) Complete miscarriage

The contents of the uterus have been completely expelled and the cervical os is usually closed. This type of miscarriage is common in very early pregnancies (<5 weeks) complicated by bleeding.

Clinical presentation Symptoms will depend on the gestation. The patient will give a history of heavy bleeding associated with cramping lower abdominal pain and the passage of fetal tissue.

Pelvic examination The uterus will be of near normal size (non-pregnant) and the cervix is usually firm and closed.

Diagnosis This is based on the clinical findings and ultrasound demonstration of an empty uterus and thin endometrium. Failure to recognize that the uterus contains fetal products may result in long-term sequelae. If the diagnosis is in any doubt, the ultrasound scan should be repeated by a qualified ultrasonographer.

Referral   If the diagnosis is conclusive the patient should be discharged and the general practitioner notified. Counselling and follow-up by the general practitioner is advisable.

(d) Missed abortion

The embryo has died and been partly absorbed but the uterus has not expelled the decidua and gestation sac.

Clinical presentation   The woman may complain of a dull weight in her pelvis and a brown, watery vaginal discharge.

Pelvic examination   Uterine size is less than expected for dates but the cervix is closed.

Diagnosis   The ultrasound scan demonstrates an intra-uterine gestation sac containing a fetal pole but no heart pulsation is visible. Absence of a fetal heart should always be confirmed by a repeat scan.

Occasionally a large gestation sac (>2.5 cm) is seen without a feltal pole. This is known as a blighted ovum and is managed in the same way as a missed abortion.

Referral   To the on-call gynaecologist.

Treatment   Admission for evacuation of uterus.

(e) Septic abortion

Septic abortion is nowadays rare, but the potential severity of the infection demands prompt diagnosis and treatment. It follows the ascent of organisms, usually *Escherichia coli*, *Bacteroides* and *Streptococcus faecalis*, from the vagina into the uterus and colonization of any retained POC. This situation may arise after an incomplete miscarriage or an induced abortion (termination of pregnancy) when the uterus has been incompletely evacuated.

Clinical presentation   Along with pain and vaginal bleeding, the woman presents with fever, signs of endotoxic shock and occasionally disseminated intra-vascular coagulation.

Referral   Resuscitative measures for the treatment of shock should be initiated in A&E, specimens including blood culture sent to the laboratory and the patient referred immediately to the on-call gynaecologist.

Treatment   Intensive antibacterial treatment followed by surgical evacuation of retained POC 12–24 h after starting therapy to reduce the risk of bacteraemia secondary to uterine instrumentation.

(f) Recurrent miscarriage

This is diagnosed when a woman has had three or more consecutive miscarriages. Any woman presenting to A&E with early pregnancy bleeding and a history of two or more miscarriages must be discussed with the on-call gynaecologist. If the miscarriage is inevitable, it is essential that any products of conception are sent for chromosomal analysis (place in a dry sterile container, *not* formalin) and proper follow-up arranged. These women require detailed investigation for any under-lying genetic, anatomical, endocrine or immunological abnormality which may be present Clifford *et al.*, 1994).

Miscarriage advice sheet

Much has been written on the high incidence of long-term psychological sequelae after miscarriage. Providing the patient with a definitive diagnosis and giving her both verbal and written advice should minimize these sequelae. In a recent study of 42 patients reviewed 6 weeks after a first trimester miscarriage, only 40% were able to recall any of the detailed verbal information about miscarriage given to them in hospital (Hamilton, 1989). This is also the case with threatened miscarriage emphasizing the need for written information which the patient can absorb more readily at home (see Appendix).

Hydatidiform mole

This is a benign tumour of trophoblastic tissue. In the UK it affects about 1 in 1500 pregnancies but in some parts of the world (e.g. Asia) the incidence is as high as 1 in 200 pregnancies. The aetiology is unclear although the male genetic contribution is an important factor. There are basically two types of mole: a partial mole where fetal tissue is present and a classical mole in which it is not.

Clinical presentation Classically, the woman presents at about 12 weeks with vaginal bleeding often accompanied by severe nausea (hyperemesis gravidarum).

Pelvic examination The uterus is larger than expected for dates and on speculum examination grape-like trophoblastic tissue may be seen in the cervix and vagina. This should always be removed and sent for histology.

Diagnosis The ultrasound shows the uterine cavity to be filled with a mass. The appearance is often described as 'snow storm'. No fetal pole or fetal heart is present. Differentiation from retained products of conception is difficult and definitive diagnosis is based on histological examination of the tissue removed at surgical evacuation of the uterus.

Referral Haemorrhage can be severe so an intravenous line should be sited in the A&E department, the patient grouped and cross-matched and referred to the on-call gynaecologist.

Treatment This involves evacuation of the uterus, usually in conjunction with an intravenous infusion of oxytocin to reduce blood loss, and careful follow-up; 10% of women with hydatidiform mole will subsequently develop choriocarcinoma and need chemotherapy which is only undertaken in specialized centres.

Ectopic pregnancy

An ectopic pregnancy is a gestation in which the fertilized ovum implants outside the uterine cavity.

Ectopic pregnancy is the most important gynaecological condition seen in A&E as the natural history of acute rupture of an ectopic is fatal haemorrhage.

Ectopic pregnancy is also the most common gynaecological cause of medicolegal complaints since the clinical presentation is variable and diagnosis easy to miss (Touquet *et al.*, 1994). It unfortunately remains a major cause of mortality in the first trimester of pregnancy, accounting for 8% of all direct maternal deaths in the most recent Confidential Enquiry into Maternal Deaths in England and Wales (DHSS, 1994). As in previous years, this report reinforced the point that '*any woman*

presenting with unexplained abdominal pain with or without vaginal bleeding should not be allowed home until every means available has been used to exclude an ectopic pregnancy'. Early diagnosis substantially reduces the woman's morbidity and mortality and increases her chances of bearing children in the future.

Incidence In the last 20 years, almost certainly because of an increase in the aetiological factors listed below, the incidence of ectopic pregnancy has almost doubled and is now 1 in every 100 clinically recognized pregnancies Coste *et al.*, 1994).

Aetiology The main aetiological factors are fallopian tube narrowing and/or decreased motility of the cilia which normally brush the fertilized ovum into the uterine cavity. Predisposing factors in the patient's history which should alert suspicion include:

- Previous ectopic pregnancy (10%).
- Pelvic inflammatory disease (25–30%).
- Contraception: intrauterine contraceptive device or progestagen-only pill.
- Tubal surgery (including sterilization) or infertility treatment (e.g. *in vitro* fertilization).

Age Most ectopics occur in women between the ages of 20 and 29 years. A quarter are nulliparous.

Site The majority (95%) implant in the fallopian tube and tend to present between 5 and 7 weeks. Rarer sites include the ovary (1%), the cervix (1%) and the abdominal cavity (1%) and these present later (>10 weeks). More severe haemorrhage is likely at later gestations. It is extremely rare to find a coexisting intrauterine pregnancy (heterotopic gestation).

Clinical presentation The cardinal symptom is amenorrhoea with lower abdominal pain which is usually unilateral. Abnormal vaginal bleeding is present in 85% of cases. These symptoms may have been present for more than 1 week (Clancy & Illingworth, 1989). The patient may then be anaemic. Symptoms suggestive of tubal rupture include fainting and shoulder tip pain caused by subdiaphragmatic irritation.

Examination General physical signs and internal bleeding may be present. There may be reflex bowel distension caused by blood in the peritoneal cavity and guarding with rebound tenderness. If the history and examination suggest an ectopic pregnancy pelvic examination should not be undertaken. An intravenous line should be sited and the patient referred immediately to the on-call gynaecologist. Where the likelihood of ectopic pregnancy is low and pelvic examination is undertaken (preferably with an intravenous line *in situ*), characteristic findings are cervical excitation and adnexal tenderness.

Diagnosis This is one of the most difficult diagnoses to make in gynaecological practice (Tindall, 1987). The aim is to make a diagnosis before tubal rupture occurs. This will prevent severe haemorrhage/death, maximize the chances of conserving the affected tube and prevent the long-term sequelae of tubal damage. Although cervical excitation and adnexal tenderness may be present, a mass is rarely palpable.

Ultrasound examination has an increasing role to play in the differential diagnosis of lower abdominal pain where ectopic pregnancy is suspected (DeCrespigny, 1988; Stabile *et al.*, 1988). It carries no risk of rupture of the ectopic and in most cases yields more information than bimanual examination. Diagnosis is easy if an ectopic gestation sac or complex adnexal mass can be visualized. However, even when TV scanning is used, an extrauterine fetus can only be demonstrated in 9% of cases. In most cases the ultrasound diagnosis of ectopic pregnancy depends upon the absence of an intrauterine gestation sac in the presence of a thickened endometrium together with a positive βhCG test (Bradley *et al.*, 1983). The presence of free fluid in the pelvis should also arouse some concern as this may indicate the ectopic has already ruptured.

Difficulty arises if the patient presents before any intrauterine structures can be visualized by ultrasound. In experienced hands, TV ultrasound can detect an intrauterine pregnancy within 5 days of a missed period and a beating fetal heart within 10 days (i.e. 1 week earlier than by the TA route) and hence this is the preferred method of scanning when ectopic pregnancy is suspected (Goswany, 1992). A positive pregnancy test in the presence of an empty uterus may reflect a complete miscarriage, since a pregnancy test may remain positive for up to 2 weeks after fetal death. If there is any doubt, prompt referral is required. Diagnosis is then by laparoscopy or, in selected low-risk cases, serial measure-

ments of serum βhCG together with repeated ultrasound scans (Shephard *et al.*, 1990). A serial rise in the βhCG titre with no evidence of an intrauterine sac is highly suggestive of ectopic pregnancy. Conversely, a falling titre suggests that the pregnancy is non-viable whether it is sited in the fallopian tube or in the uterus.

Serial scanning and repeated βhCG estimations should not be A&E-based investigations.

Referral

The woman must be referred as soon as clinical suspicion is raised. An intravenous line should be sited and blood sent for group and cross-match. Blood volume should be restored where necessary with colloid solutions until whole blood is available.

Treatment Subsequent management will be determined by the location and gestation of the pregnancy and whether it has ruptured. Traditionally laparotomy followed by salpingostomy or salpingectomy was used. The use of minimally invasive laparoscopic techniques in cases not complicated by tubal rupture may allow the affected tube to be conserved. The gestation sac can be milked out of the tube, removed piecemeal via a small tubal incision or injected with hypertonic solutions under direct vision or ultrasound guidance (Grainger & Seifer, 1995).

Abnormal vaginal bleeding – pregnancy test negative

Menstrual disorders are a common source of gynaecological referral to hospital. In inner cities these patients frequently present to A&E rather than to their general practitioner or gynaecologist. In the A&E department, careful history-taking and examination must aim to exclude acute pathology requiring immediate referral (e.g. severe anaemia). The majority of cases will prove suitable for referral to gynaecology out-patients or preferably back to the general practitioner who holds all the patient's records. Our experience is that many of these patients make multiple presentations to various A&E departments and may already be attending another hospital. In order to avoid conflicting advice, the A&E doctor must ensure that communication is made with the general practitioner.

Table 4. *Pathological causes of menorrhagia*

Cause	Comment
IUCD *in situ*	Maximum loss begins in the second cycle; 50% of women experience double their previous loss
Infection	Chronic PID
Benign neoplasms	Fibroids, oestrogen-producing cysts of the ovary
Malignant neoplasms	Carcinoma of the endometrium, cervix
Metabolic disorders	Hypothyroidism
Congenital abnormalities of the uterus	
Blood dyscrasia and coagulation disorders	

IUCD, intrauterine contraceptive device; PID, pelvic inflammatory disease.

Menorrhagia

Normal menstrual loss is between 30 and 50 ml (mean 35 ml). Blood loss greater than 80 ml per cycle is considered excessive and will lead to iron-deficiency anaemia. In practice only 40% of women complaining of excess loss lose more than 80 ml blood per month (Fraser *et al.*, 1984).

Objective clinical assessment of the blood loss is difficult. When taking the history, useful questions to ask are how often sanitary pads/tampons need to be changed on the days when the flow is heavy, whether flooding occurs at night and the degree of disruption caused to everyday life. A woman who is unable to go shopping for fear of staining her clothes has an unacceptable menstrual blood loss and needs medical help.

Pathological causes of menorrhagia are numerous and are listed in Table 4. The most common are fibroids and endometrial hyperplasia associated with anovulation. Fibroids are found in up to 20% of women after the age of 35 years. Enlarged ovaries with multiple peripheral cysts (polycystic ovaries) are also a common finding in women of reproductive age, with a much higher incidence in women with menstrual cycle disturbance (Franks, 1989).

Clinical presentation Endometriosis, chronic PID and intrauterine contraceptive devices (IUCD) are the most likely causes if the bleeding is associated with pain. Endometrial hyperplasia and carcinoma are associated with a long history of anovulatory cycles.

Pelvic examination This can determine if there is any irregular uterine enlargement (fibroid) or adnexal mass (ovarian tumour or hydrosalpinx). Speculum examination should identify any abnormality of the cervix.

Referral The patient should be referred for proper out-patient evaluation by the gynaecologist as ultrasound, dilatation and curettage, hysteroscopy and possibly laparoscopy will be required for a definitive diagnosis. Fibroids are diagnosed on ultrasound as masses arising from the uterus. Endometrial thickening (hyperplasia) is also seen on ultrasound and may well be associated with polycystic ovaries.

Treatment It is helpful to check the patient's haemoglobin as treatment for iron deficiency anaemia should always be started in A & E.

If there is no obvious underlying cause, treatment with a progestagen (e.g. norethisterone 5 mg t.d.s. for 15 days in every cycle, usually days 10–25) or a prostaglandin synthetase inhibitor (non-steroidal anti-inflammatory drug; e.g. mefenamic acid 500 mg q.d.s.) during menstruation may reduce the loss until the patient is seen in clinic.

If the excess blood loss is thought to be secondary to an IUCD, the woman should be advised to return to her family planning clinic or general practitioner for removal and advice on alternative contraception.

Dysfunctional uterine bleeding

In 50% of cases there is no underlying organic disease and excessive bleeding is referred to as dysfunctional uterine bleeding. This is a diagnosis of exclusion following appropriate investigations in out-patients.

Dysfunctional uterine bleeding is often due to endocrine imbalances associated with either ovulatory or anovulatory cycles.

(a) Anovulatory cycles

These tend to occur close to the menarche and menopause and in women with polycystic ovaries throughout their reproductive life. Excessive menstrual loss is generally due to lack of progesterone, which is secreted by the corpus luteum in the second half of ovulatory cycles. As a result the endometrium remains in its proliferative phase and becomes increasingly thick.

Clinical presentation   Typically a prolonged cycle which ends in heavy and persistent vaginal bleeding.

Referral   The problem may be discussed with the on-call gynaecologist and then treated. Follow-up should be undertaken by the general practitioner or in gynaecology out-patients.

Treatment   Progesterone (e.g. norethisterone 5 mg t.d.s.) in the second half of the cycle (days 10–25) will usually diminish the loss considerably.

(b) Ovulatory cycles

The excess loss is thought to result from abnormal levels of prostaglandins in the uterus (Rees, 1989).

Clinical presentation   The excess loss is often accompanied by lower abdominal discomfort, dysmenorrhoea and dyspareunia and it affects women in the 35–45-year age group.

Referral   The woman should be referred to gynaecology out-patients or back to her general practitioner for further assessment.

Treatment   Progesterone treatment is unlikely to be any help but prostaglandin synthetase inhibitors such as mefanamic acid 500 mg q.d.s. during menstruation may reduce the loss.

Amenorrhoea or oligomenorrhoea

The normal menstrual cycle is defined as occurring every 21–35 days. Abnormalities of cycle length are unlikely to present to A&E in the absence of other symptoms. Once pregnancy has been excluded the patient should be referred to her general practitioner for proper evaluation and subsequent gynaecological referral if required.

Bleeding from the cervix, vagina or vulva

Abnormal bleeding from these sites may be due to trauma, neoplastic lesions or infection.

Trauma and forensic causes are discussed in Chapter 58.

If rape or abuse is suspected, gynaecological assessment should be undertaken by the police doctor.

Clinical presentation   Abnormal bleeding from a neoplastic lesion is usually intermittent – often after intercourse (postcoital bleeding) or intermenstrually. Pain is not usually a feature unless the tumour has metastasized. The woman should be asked if she has had routine (3-yearly) cervical smear tests and the date and result of her last test.

Pelvic examination   An attempt should be made to locate the site of the bleeding and identify any lesion present by speculum examination. The inguinal nodes may be enlarged if there is a vulval tumour.

Referral   If a neoplasm is suspected the patient should be referred promptly to the next gynaecological clinic.

Secondary haemorrhage following pelvic surgery

Secondary haemorrhage may occur from the vaginal vault following vaginal or abdominal hysterectomy or from the cervix following cone biopsy and local ablative therapy. Bleeding typically occurs about 10 days after surgery due to secondary infection.

Pelvic examination   Careful speculum examination may locate the site of bleeding.

Referral   The patient should be referred promptly to the on-call gynaecologist.

Treatment   The A&E doctor should site an intravenous line and start replacing lost blood volume. If there is no on-site gynaeocologist and the bleeding is profuse, the vagina should be packed with a large gauze swab to staunch the haemorrhage before transferring the patient.

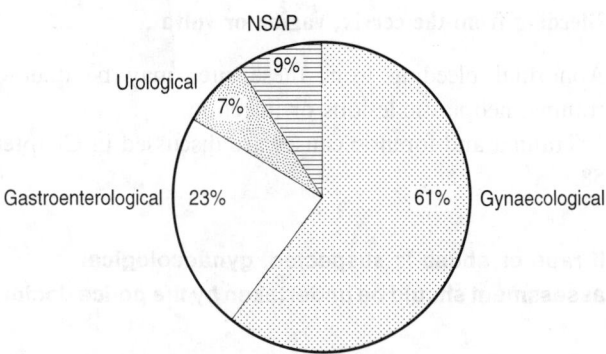

Fig. 3. Causes of acute lower abdominal pain in 322 women presenting to the A&E department at St Mary's Hospital, London, over a 6-month period according to A&E doctor's diagnosis. Percentages refer to the total number of women seen. NSAP, non-specific abdominal pain. (Reproduced from Gilling-Smith et al., 1995.)

Lower abdominal pain

A recent study revealed that acute lower abdominal pain in women represented 1.5% of the total A&E workload (Gilling-Smith et al., 1995). Furthermore, 61% of these women were found to have pain of gynaecological origin as shown in Fig. 3. Previous studies have highlighted the difficulty in diagnosing the cause of acute lower abdominal pain in the A&E department (Gatzen et al., 1991). A&E doctors need to be particularly aware of gynaecological causes of abdominal pain.

Table 5 shows the causes of lower abdominal pain. Early pregnancy bleeding was one of the commonest causes. Ectopic pregnancy and accidents to ovarian tumours caused the greatest diagnostic dilemma, reinforcing the need for a sensitive urinary pregnancy test and, where an adnexal mass is suspected, pelvic ultrasound.

Lower abdominal pain in women of reproductive age should be attributed to an ectopic pregnancy until proven otherwise. These patients should not be discharged home until a sensitive pregnancy test has been reported negative.

Having excluded an ectopic pregnancy, other gynaecological causes of lower abdominal pain associated with a negative pregnancy test need to be considered.

Pelvic inflammatory disease (PID)

PID is an inflammation of the upper genital tract (endometrium, salpinges) secondary to the spread of microorganisms from the lower genital tract (vagina and

Table 5. *Common causes of lower abdominal pain in 322 women presenting to an A&E department* (Gilling-Smith et al., 1995)

Gynaecological
- Miscarriage – threatened and incomplete (34%)
- Dysmenorrhoea (12%)
- Pelvic inflammatory disease (9%)
- Accident to an ovarian or uterine tumour (4%)
- Ectopic pregnancy (1%)
- Retained products of conception (1%)

Gastroenterological
- Constipation (10%)
- Gastroenteritis (8%)
- Appendicitis (3%)
- Irritable bowel sydrome (1%)

Urological
- Urinary tract infection (7%)

Non-specific abdominal pain (9%)

endocervix). It is a broad term which encompasses endometritis, salpingitis, oophoritis, tubo-ovarian abscess and pelvic peritonitis. Unfortunately, the condition is often missed or inadequately managed. It is particularly important not to label a woman with pelvic pain as having PID until a firm diagnosis has been made (Pearce, 1990).

Incidence Age-specific incidence rates show a marked increase in PID up to the early 1980s (the greatest increases occurring in women under 25 years), followed by a fall together with a tendency towards milder disease (Westrom, 1980, 1988).

Aetiology Acute infections are caused by two major groups of organisms:

- Sexually transmitted agents: *Neisseria gonorrhoeae, Chlamydia trachomatis, Mycoplasma hominis.*
- Endogenous lower genital tract organisms: group B streptococci, *Escherichia coli, bacteroides.*

Sexually transmitted infections tend to occur in young, sexually active women, whereas infection with endogenous flora is more prevalent in slightly older women, those who have had previous PID or are using an IUCD. Chlamydial PID is now the most common sexually transmitted disease in industrialized countries, responsible for 50% of PID cases in Europe (Smith et al., 1991).

Pathogenesis The cervix provides a natural barrier to pelvic infection. Any event which breaches this barrier (e.g. miscarriage, termination of pregnancy, childbirth or the presence of an IUCD) will increase the risk of infection.

Clinical presentation Acute infections vary from asymptomatic to life-threatening. Symptoms include:

- Bilateral lower abdominal pain.
- Vaginal discharge.
- Irregular vaginal bleeding.
- Dysuria.
- Dyspareunia.
- Rectal discomfort.
- Lower back pain.
- Fever.

General examination This reveals pyrexia and bilateral lower abdominal tenderness with rebound and guarding in severe cases.

Pelvic examination Cervical excitation and bilateral pelvic tenderness are characteristic and occasionally an adnexal swelling is palpable.

Differential diagnosis Other causes of acute pain (accident to an ovarian cyst, appendicitis) and chronic lower abdominal pain (endometriosis, pelvic congestion) must be considered.

Diagnosis Clinical findings alone are usually unreliable and laboratory tests such as an elevated white cell count, ESR and C-reactive protein are non-specific. If an adnexal mass is palpable it may be possible to demonstrate a tubo-ovarian mass on ultrasound. Bilateral masses are highly suggestive of infection. Definitive diagnosis requires laparoscopy to exclude other causes of acute pain. Mild to moderate symptoms are usually treated empirically with antibiotics although failure to respond is generally an indication for diagnostic laparoscopy.

Referral Acute severe systemic infection (with fever, etc.) should be referred to the gynaecologist for admission and intravenous therapy. Mild or moderate infection can be referred to the genitourinary medicine clinic. All sexual partners will need to be traced and screened for sexually transmitted infection.

Treatment Treatment should only be started after appropriate swabs have been taken. This is not usually possible in the A&E department unless the on-call genitourinary doctor can be called. Inadequate treatment can lead to chronic PID (see below). Treatment should only be started in A&E in those patients who cannot attend a genitourinary clinic within 48 h (Friday night presentations, imminent travel). In these cases a letter must be given to the patient to ensure that she is followed-up. The patient also needs to be advised that her male partner should attend the genitourinary clinic as he may also require treatment.

When symptoms are mild, combination therapy is started (e.g. ciprofloxacin 500 mg stat followed by doxycycline 100 mg b.d. and metronidazole 400 mg b.d. for 14 days). More severe infection with systemic symptoms demands admission for treatment with an intravenous combination of the above drugs. If an IUCD is present, it should be removed at the earliest opportunity and sent for culture if symptoms fail to settle with treatment.

Complications Most women with acute PID recover completely. A minority will develop complications, particularly if diagnosis and treatment has been delayed. Short-term sequelae include perihepatitis (Fitz-Hugh–Curtis syndrome) and pelvic abscess. Long-term sequelae include:

- The risk of further PID increasing six- to ten-fold.
- The risk of ectopic pregnancy increasing seven- to ten-fold.
- Tubal infertility – 10% risk.
- Chronic lower abdominal pain – 15%.

Accident to an ovarian or uterine tumour

Ovarian cysts up to 3 cm in size are a normal feature of the female pelvis during reproductive years. The prevalence of polycystic ovaries (enlarged ovaries with multiple peripheral cysts) is high in women of reproductive age (Polson *et al.*, 1988), and they are unlikely to be the cause of pain unless associated with pelvic congestion (Adams *et al.*, 1990). Fibroids are rarely a cause of pain unless they undergo degeneration.

Ovarian tumours usually only cause lower abdominal

pain when very large (pressure symptoms on bladder or bowel) or undergo the following complications:

- *Torsion.* Acute spasmodic lower abdominal pain may be accompanied by signs of shock, abdominal guarding and a palpable pelvic mass. Alternatively, the signs may be mild in relation to the severity of the pain.
- *Rupture.* Signs and symptoms vary according to the contents of the cyst. Dermoid and endometriotic cysts contain very irritant substances.
- *Haemorrhage into or from a cyst.* Signs and symptoms vary according to the extent of blood loss. Blood in the peritoneal cavity does not necessarily excite a peritoneal reaction. On the other hand, exquisite tenderness may be elicited in the pouch of Douglas on vaginal and rectal examination.
- *Infection.* This is a rare complication of ovarian tumours.
- *Degeneration.* Acute red degeneration of a uterine fibroid can cause intense pain and is most commonly seen during pregnancy.

Diagnosis   The non-specific history and examination findings often preclude a definitive diagnosis. If the patient is stable, emergency pelvic ultrasound should be arranged. If the patient shows signs of shock, immediate resuscitation and referral to the on-call gynaecologist should take precedence.

Ultrasound is a very sensitive means of detecting ovarian cysts, as pressure over the cyst will indicate whether or not the cyst is the cause of pain. Features suggestive of painful complications (torsion, haemorrhage or infection) include internal echoes, irregular wall thickening and fluid in the pouch of Douglas. Fibroid degeneration can be detected with ultrasound.

Dysmenorrhoea

This is a term used to describe lower abdominal pain accompanying menstruation (Roberts, 1984).

Clinical presentation   Cramping lower abdominal pain is often associated with pain in the thighs and lower back.

Primary (spasmodic) dysmenorrhoea

This is usually related to the first ovulatory cycles of adolescence. It is usually limited to the first few days of menstruation.

Treatment   This is best achieved in A&E with prostaglandin synthetase inhibitors (i.e. mefenamic acid 500 mg 4-hourly). Recurrent episodes should be referred back to the general practitioner for further investigation. In the long term, suppression of ovulation with the oral contraceptive pill may be required. In the majority of cases the condition resolves with time.

Secondary dysmenorrhoea

The pain is secondary to underlying organic or psychosexual disease and warrants an out-patient referral for thorough gynaecological investigation via the general practitioner. In the majority of cases treatment with mild analgesics is appropriate; symptoms may sometimes be sufficiently severe to warrant referral to the duty gynaecologist.

(a) Endometriosis

This is caused by implantation of endometrial tissue outside the uterine cavity which causes pain during menses. The pain characteristically starts several days before the onset of menstruation and is often relieved once the bleeding starts.

(b) Chronic pelvic inflammatory disease

This is a delayed complication of acute PID and frequently follows inadequate treatment. The patient has non-specific symptoms which may include secondary dysmenorrhoea, dyspareunia, intermittent purulent vaginal discharge and irregular, heavy menstrual bleeding. On examination the uterus may be fixed and retroverted and tender adnexal masses palpable. Tubo-ovarian masses are often visualized on pelvic ultrasound.

(c) Pelvic congestion (pelvic pain syndrome)

Some patients presenting with chronic pelvic pain have dilated pelvic varicosities (Beard *et al.*, 1984) and the cause of their pain has been attributed to pelvic congestion. The diagnosis is usually made following laparoscopic exclusion of other gynaecological and non-gynaecological causes of pain.

The following features in the patient's history are suggestive of pelvic pain syndrome:

- Dull pain in one or other iliac fossa or vague lower abdominal discomfort. The pain is often relieved by lying flat.

- Dysmenorrhoea, deep dyspareunia, postcoital ache, nervous tension, fatigue, insomnia, premenstrual breast pain and irregular menses.
- Unhappy social, marital and sexual history.

Referral These women should be referred to the gynaecological clinic by the general practitioner, whose more detailed knowledge of the patient will help to avoid repetition and conflicting advice in the management of this difficult problem.

Treatment Medroxyprogesterone acetate 50 mg daily for 6 months has been shown to be effective in selected patients (Farquar *et al.*, 1989).

Urological problems (see also urinalysis)

Acute retention of urine

Although uncommon in women, several well-recognized gynaecological conditions may compress the urethra or cause sufficient pain to cause acute retention. These include:

- Painful vulval lesion (herpetic ulcer).
- Irreducible vaginal prolapse.
- Pelvic tumour (fibroid or ovarian cyst).
- Pelvic haematocoele (secondary haemorrhage following pelvic surgery).
- Haematocolpos (imperforate hymen or vaginal septum).
- Incarceration of a retroverted pregnant uterus (often cited, rarely seen).

Treatment The patient should be catheterized in A&E and referred to the on-call gynaecologist for definitive management. The catheter stream urine must be checked for blood, protein and sugar.

Urinary tract infection

This should always be considered in a woman who presents with lower abdominal pain and generalized malaise, whether urinary symptoms are present or not.

The urine should be checked with a Nephur-test stick (leucocyte esterase and nitrate test) and sent for culture and sensitivity prior to starting any antibiotic treatment. More than one plus of protein in the urine demands that the patient is examined to exclude oedema and hyper-tension, and that creatinine and electrolyte levels are measured to exclude underlying renal disease.

Treatment If a urinary tract infection is suspected on clinical grounds, antibiotic treatment should be started in A&E. Amoxycillin and cephalexin are suitable in pregnancy but tetracyclines must be avoided as these are teratogenic. The general practitioner must be informed of all test results and advised to arrange a post-treatment MSU to confirm that the infection has been eradicated.

Hyperstimulation syndrome

This life-threatening syndrome has emerged in the last decade as a rare but well-recognized iatrogenic complication of ovulation induction (drug treatment of infertile women to stimulate the ovaries to release eggs). Excess stimulation results in massive ovarian enlargement, multiple cyst formation and in more severe cases ascites, pleural effusions and electrolyte disturbances (Schenker & Weinstein, 1989). Since a large percentage of infertility treatment is carried out in private units with no out-of-hours on-call service, these patients may present to A&E departments and doctors must be aware of the diagnosis in any patient with a recent history of infertility treatment. The syndrome is more likely to be severe if the patient has polycystic ovaries (MacDougall *et al.*, 1992) or is pregnant.

Clinical presentation The patient presents with abdominal pain and distension and, in severe cases, respiratory symptoms.

Examination Abdominal tenderness, distension, ascites and signs of pleural effusion.

Diagnosis Pelvic ultrasound will reveal massive ovarian enlargment and cyst formation (severity is usually related to the number and size of the ovarian follicles). Ascites may also be evident. An elevated haematocrit and electrolyte disturbances are further indications of the severity of the syndrome.

Referral Immediate referral must be made to the on-call gynaecologist who will arrange treatment and liaise with the infertility unit in cases for whom transfer is appropriate.

Treatment This consists of intravenous fluid replacement and correction of electrolyte disturbance.

Non-gynaecological causes of lower abdominal pain

An acutely *inflamed appendix* can be visualized on ultrasound as a tubular structure which remains distended when adjacent small bowel loops are compressed by the transducer. A chronically inflamed appendix with an appendix mass may be harder to identify because of adherent gas-filled loops of bowel that cannot be compressed away from the appendix.

Other causes of acute lower abdominal pain in women of reproductive age which can be diagnosed ultrasonically include mesenteric lymphadenopathy, colonic masses (diverticulitis, tumours), cholecystitis and renal abnormalities.

Non-specific abdominal pain is defined as abdominal pain lasting a maximum of 7 days for which no cause can be found (Gray & Collin, 1987) (Table 5).

Infections/vaginal discharge (Table 6)

A wide range of acute infections can affect the genital tract. In the vast majority of cases the patient should be referred to the genitourinary clinic, or the on-call gynaecologist if the symptoms warrant urgent treatment. These cases should be referred to specialists who can ensure that the correct investigations and treatment are organized, and that contact tracing, counselling and follow-up are arranged. Incomplete treatment must be avoided because of the risk of the patient developing chronic PID.

In children, vaginal discharge may be caused by foreign bodies, threadworms (refer to the gynaecologist) or trauma (see Chapter 58).

If there is any suspicion of sexual abuse the A & E doctor should only inspect the perineum (no digital examination), and refer immediately to a *senior paediatrician*.

Symptoms and signs vary with the organisms involved and the site of infection. With the exception of candidiasis, treatment should only be given in A & E in exceptional cases (patient travelling and unable to attend genitourinary clinic; see section on treatment of PID). Patients must be advised to attend a genitourinary clinic in the near future and be given a letter for follow-up.

Vulvovaginal candidiasis (thrush)

Epidemiology In over 85% of cases the causative organism is the yeast *Candida albicans*. Asymptomatic genital tract candidiasis is present in up to 50% of women of child-bearing age. The organism flourishes where the vaginal pH is less than 4.5; hence the incidence is higher in pregnant women and those taking oral contraceptives. The incidence is also increased amongst diabetics, patients on antibiotics or immunosuppressant drugs and women in tropical climates.

Clinical presentation Vulval pruritus is the commonest symptom accompanied by an odourless, white, cheese-like discharge. There is erythema of the vulva and vagina. Discharge varies from minimal to copious with vaginal plaque formation causing the patient much distress.

Referral This is the only cause of vaginal discharge which should be treated by an A & E doctor. Referral to the genitourinary clinic or gynaecologist is appropriate if symptoms recur or are resistant to conventional therapy.

Diagnosis A high vaginal swab should be taken in A & E to confirm the clinical diagnosis. This is the only type of swab which should be taken routinely in A & E. Diabetes should be excluded by a glucostick blood or urine test.

Treatment Topical therapy with an antifungal (e.g. clotrimazole intravaginal pessary 500 mg stat with 1% clotrimazole cream to the vulva). If the patient is unable to use a topical preparaton, an oral preparation (fluconazole 150 mg stat) may be given provided that the patient is not pregnant. It is not usually necessary to treat asymptomatic male sexual partners.

Bacterial vaginosis

Epidemiology This is the commonest cause of vaginal discharge worldwide. The precise aetiology remains unclear but is related to a marked decrease in vaginal lactobacilli, associated with an overgrowth of other vaginal commensals such as *Gardnerella vaginalis*, mycoplasmas and other anaerobic bacteria. There is increasing evidence of an association between bacterial vaginosis

Table 6. *Causes and treatment of genital tract infections*

Infection	Organism	Treatment
Candidiasis	Candida Albicans	Clotrimazole pessary and cream
Bacterial vaginosis	*Gardnerella vaginalis* *Mycoplasma* Other anaerobic bacteria	Metronidazole (in 1st trimester of pregnancy low dose metronidazole or clindamycin vaginal cream)
Trichomonas vaginalis infection	Protozoon	Metronidazole (in 1st trimester of pregnancy clotrimazole pessaries or low dose metronidazole)
Streptococcal vulvovaginitis	Group B streptococcus	Penicillin or erythromycin
Staphylococcal toxins	Toxins from organisms in vaginal foreign body (e.g. tampon)	Removal of foreign body
Pelvic inflammatory disease	*Neisseria gonorrhoeae* *Chlamydia trachomatis* *Mycoplamsa hominis* Group B streptococci *Escherichia coli* Bacteroides	Ciprofloxacin, doxycycline and metronidazole
Herpes simplex	Herpes simplex virus	Acyclovir
Vulval warts	Human papilloma virus	Analgesia and salt water bathing
Infection of Bartholin's or Skene's glands	*Neisseria gonorrhoeae* *Chlamydia trachomatis* Gram-negative bacteria Anaerobes	Ciprofloxacin, erythromycin and metronidazole If abscess formation, surgical marsupialization of gland
Puerperal sepsis	All known pathogens	Ciprofloxacin, doxycycline and metronidazole

and ascending genital tract infection, premature labour and chorioamnionitis.

Clinical presentation The vaginal discharge is characteristically offensive and if profuse may be associated with vulval irritation.

Referral Swabs should be taken before treatment. There is no evidence that asymptomatic male sexual partners require treatment.

Diagnosis This is based on the presence of at least three of the following four criteria:

- Characteristic white homogeneous discharge.
- Vaginal fluid pH > 4.5.
- Release of an amine odour when 10% potassium hydroxide is added to vaginal fluid.
- Presence of 'clue cells' (vaginal epithelial cells covered with secondary organisms) on microscopic examination of vaginal secretions.

Treatment Metronidazole 400 mg b.d. is given for 5 days. High dose metronidazole is not recommended in the first trimester of pregnancy. Metronidazole 200 mg t.d.s. or clindamycin vaginal cream may be used.

Trichomonas vaginalis infection

Epidemiology The incidence of this protozoon is decreasing.

Clinical presentation There is vaginal discharge, often non-offensive, vulval and vaginal soreness and occasionally dysuria. Erythema of the vulva and vagina often spreads to include the cervix. The discharge is typically copious, yellow/green and frothy.

Referral   Refer to the genitourinary clinic for follow-up and contact tracing as male sexual partners need to receive treatment.

Diagnosis   This is based on the microscopic detection of trichomonads in a 'wet-mount' of vaginal fluid.

Treatment   Metronidazole 2 mg should be given as a single oral dose. Infection during the first trimester of pregnancy should be treated with clotrimazole pessaries or metronidazole 200 mg t.d.s. for 1 week.

Streptococcal vulvovaginitis

Epidemiology   This is caused by colonization of the vulva and vagina with group B streptococci. Although usually asymptomatic, the organisms may occasionally cause acute vulvovaginitis.

Clinical presentation   Vulval or vaginal soreness, with or without discharge and dysuria. On examination, patchy erythema of the vagina may extend to the vulva. Discharge is often minimal.

Referral   Refer to the genitourinary clinic.

Diagnosis   This is usually based on clinical findings, where vulvovaginitis is evident in the absence of candida or *trichomonas vaginalis* infection, but it can be confirmed by culture of group B streptococci from a high vaginal swab.

Treatment   The organisms are usually sensitive to penicillin and erythromycin.

Staphylococcal toxins

Epidemiology   Staphylococcal toxins produced by organisms in tampons and other vaginal foreign bodies are a rare cause of vaginal ulceration and toxic shock syndrome.

Clinical presentation   This is characterized by a variable rash followed by desquamation with or without fever, hypotension and multisystem involvement. Inflammation of the mouth, conjunctiva and vagina can sometimes be accompanied by hepatic, haematological and central nervous system involvement.

Referral   The patient will need to be admitted under the medical or gynaecological team.

Diagnosis   The finding of a foreign body or retained tampon in the vagina should raise suspicion. Vaginal swabs and blood cultures should confirm the diagnosis.

Treatment   A penicillinase-resistant antibiotic will be required. Since the symptoms are toxin-mediated, general supportive measures (often in the intensive therapy unit) are usually necessary.

Pelvic inflammatory disease

This is not a common cause of vaginal discharge and is discussed in detail in the section on lower abdominal pain.

Herpes simplex virus infection

Epidemiology   Genital herpes simplex virus (HSV) can be isolated in up to 5% of asymptomatic patients. Seroprevalence data indicate that exposure to HSV is even higher than this (Daling *et al.*, 1987). The virus is shed from genital ulcers of infected individuals and is transmitted by direct inoculation on to a susceptible mucosal surface (cervix or oropharynx) or damaged skin of a contact.

Clinical presentation   A typical attack is characterized by the appearance of multiple painful genital ulcers on the vulva, less commonly on the vaginal walls or cervix, accompanied by tender enlargement of inguinal lymph nodes. Primary attacks have an incubation period of 2–14 days and are frequently accompanied by systemic symptoms such as fever and headache. Primary genital herpes is accompanied by herpetic cervicitis in 90% of cases.

Differential diagnosis   This includes:

- Primary syphilis (chancre is usually painless).
- Chancroid and lymphogranuloma venereum (seek relevant travel history).
- Non-infectious ulceration, e.g. Behçet's disease, inflammatory bowel disease.
- Vulval trauma.

Referral The patient should be directed to the genito-urinary clinic or obstetrician/gynaecologist if the woman is pregnant.

Diagnosis Swabs taken from vesicle fluid or directly from an ulcer must be placed immediately in viral transport medium. HSV can only be detected in early lesions so a negative result does not exclude the diagnosis.

Treatment To relieve pain and shorten the duration of symptoms, treatment is recommended for all moderate and severe primary attacks of HSV. This is best achieved by a combination of analgesia, saline bathing and acyclovir 200 mg, five times daily for 5 days. Antibiotics (e.g. co-trimoxazole) and antifungals are occasionally required for secondary infection.

Complications These include secondary infection with bacteria or fungi, aseptic meningitis and in rare cases cutaneous and visceral spread due to disseminated infection. Patients presenting with any of these complications must be referred immediately for admission under the gynaecological team. Women presenting with HSV infection in pregnancy should be discussed with the obstetrician. In early pregnancy, a primary attack of HSV may be teratogenic and in late pregnancy vaginal delivery in the presence of open genital sores is best avoided to minimize the risk of neonatal herpetic septicaemia.

Vulval warts

Epidemiology Human papilloma virus (HPV) is a common cause of clinical and subclinical infection in differentiating squamous epithelium of the genital tract.

Clinical presentation The warts have a characteristic flat topped appearance. Occasionally patients may present with acute symptoms due to excoriation, bleeding or secondary infection.

Differential diagnosis

- Molluscum contagiosum (common).
- Skin tags (common).
- Malignant and premalignant vulval lesions (increasingly common).
- Condylomata lata of secondary syphilis (rare).

Referral The patient should attend the genitourinary clinic.

Diagnosis This is based on clinical examination since the virus does not grow in tissue culture. In doubtful cases excision biopsy and histological examination is necessary.

Treatment Analgesia and salt water bathing are all that is required. The genitourinary clinic will provide definitive treatment and follow-up. HPV is a recognized risk factor for cervical cancer and follow-up with regular cervical smear testing is needed.

Infection of Bartholin's glands

Epidemiology These are paired glands located at 5 and 7 o'clock in the labia majora. Causative organisms include *Neisseria gonorrhoeae*, *Chlamydia trachomatis*, Gram-negative bacilli and anaerobes.

Clinical presentation The patient typically presents with acute pain and unilateral swelling in the posterior part of the vulva. The tender swelling can be easily palpated and sometimes purulent material can be expressed from the duct.

Referral The on-call gynaecologist will arrange definitive (surgical) treatment.

Treatment If the gland is non-fluctuant, a course of antibiotics can be administered (ciprofloxacin 500 mg followed by erythromycin 500 mg b.d. for 10 days and metronidazole 400 mg b.d. for 7 days). Urethral and endocervical swabs for *Chlamydia trachomatis* and *Neisseria gonorrhoeae* should be taken before starting this treatment so the patient is best referred to the on-call gynaecologist or genitourinary clinic. If abscess formation has occurred, the patient needs formal marsupialization of the gland to prevent a recurrence. No form of vaginal or vulval surgery should be carried out by A&E doctors as the area is very vascular and sensitive. Poor surgical technique may produce introital narrowing and dyspareunia.

Infection of Skene's glands

These glands lie adjacent to the female urethra. Investigation and treatment of the infection is essentially the same as for Bartholin's glands.

Puerperal sepsis

Severe infection of the endometrium following birth is nowadays rare, but may follow prolonged rupture of the membranes, instrumental delivery and retained POC. Almost all known pathogenic organisms can be responsible. This once fatal disease may not be considered by the inexperienced doctor, to whom the woman may present out of hours.

Clinical presentation

The woman characteristically presents within 6 weeks of delivery with offensive heavy lochia, lower abdominal pain and generalized malaise.

Diagnosis Ultrasound will demonstrate any retained POC.

Referral All women presenting within 6 weeks of delivery should be discussed with the on-call obstetric team.

Treatment Appropriate pathology specimens should be taken including high vaginal swab and blood cultures. Broad-spectrum antibiotic treatment (as for treatment of PID) can then be started by the duty obstetric team.

Postcoital contraception

Each year 170 000 abortions are carried out in England and Wales. Many of these could be avoided with emergency (postcoital) hormonal contraception (Anonymous, 1993). Whenever possible the woman should be advised to attend her local family planning clinic. Treatment is effective within 72 h of unprotected intercourse.

Clinical assessment Details of the patient's current method of contraception will dictate whether postcoital contraception is needed. It is important to note the last menstrual period, normal cycle length, calculated day of ovulation and number of hours since unprotected intercourse. If there is any uncertainty, pregnancy should be excluded by urinary βhCG testing. A pelvic examination is only necessary if pathology is suspected or a cervical smear required.

Table 7. *Indications for providing postcoital contraception*

Indication	Comment
Unprotected intercourse	May not have volition to attend family planning clinic
Condom rupture/misuse[a]	
Diaphragm/cap misuse[a]	Incorrectly inserted, torn or removed too early
IUCD expulsion	
Missed progestogen-only pills	If intercourse has taken place from the time of the missed pills to 48 h after recommencing the pills
Missed combined (oestrogen/progestogen) pills	If missed pills lengthen the pill-free interval to 9 or more days *or* if more than 3 pills are missed at any time in the cycle
Sexual assault	Rape discussed in Chapter 58
Recent use of teratogenic drugs	

[a]May be too embarrassed to relate problem to reception staff.

The indications for postcoital contraception are shown in Table 7.

Two basic methods are available and choice depends on the delay since unprotected intercourse.

(a) *If unprotected intercourse has taken place within the last 72 h – Yuzpe method*

This involves a high-dose oestrogen/progestogen preparation which is suitable for prescription by the A & E doctor. Two doses of 100 μg of ethinyl oestradiol combined with 500 μg of levonorgestrel given 12 h apart results in withdrawal bleeding within 21 days in 98% of women (Yuzpe *et al.*, 1982). Implantation of the fertilized ovum is prevented by blocking oestrogen and progesterone receptors which makes the endometrium hostile to implantation.

The standard preparation available consists of four tablets of ethinyloestradiol 50 μg plus 250 μg norgestrel (Schering PC4). Two tablets are taken immediately and two 12 h later. They should be stocked in the A & E department. The patient must be warned that there is still a risk of pregnancy if she has further unprotected intercourse before her next period.

If the woman is already pregnant, breastfeeding or has a past history of thrombosis, the combined preparation should not be given.

Patients taking liver enzyme inducing drugs (e.g. Rifampicin) should take three tablets immediately with a further three 12 h later.

Unfortunately the high-dose oestrogen causes nausea in up to 50% of women and vomiting in 24%. If the patient vomits within 3 h of taking the tablets she must return to the department either to take two further tablets with an antiemetic or discuss the alternative of inserting an IUCD. An oral antiemetic such as metoclopramide may be routinely prescribed with the preparation.

(b) If unprotected intercouse has taken place more than 72 h but less than 5 days before presentation – insertion of IUCD

Insertion of a copper-based IUCD (which prevents implantation) should only be performed by the on-call gynaecologist for the patient who cannot attend a family planning clinic within 5 days of unprotected intercourse, or when the combined oestrogen/progestogen method is contraindicated e.g. past history of thombosis. This is not a suitable treatment for the A&E doctor to perform.

Follow-up The woman should be told to expect a menstrual bleed within the following 3 weeks and must be advised to attend her general practitioner or family planning clinic as soon as possible. Details of post-treatment bleeding will then be discussed, pregnancy excluded and definitive contraception advised. A&E departments should provide details of local family planning clinics.

PREGNANCY ≥ 20 WEEKS/PUERPERIUM

Patients more than 20 weeks pregnant attending A&E with any condition which may affect the pregnancy should be discussed with the on-call obstetrician. The condition and treatment given must be recorded in the the obstetric notes (if hand-held) or cooperation card. The same applies to women in the puerperium (up to 6 weeks postpartum).

Road Traffic Accident injury or abdominal trauma in pregnancy

Rh negative pregnant women are at risk of Rh immunisation if they are involved in a road traffic accident (seatbelt injury) or receive a direct blow to the abdomen. Immunisation due to anti-D not being given may result in claims for medical negligence. Rh testing should therefore be performed in the A&E department on all such cases. Where the woman in Rh negative, anti-D immunoglobulin should be administered with 72 h of the injury, at a dose of 250 IU IM if the gestation is ≤ 20 weeks and 500 IU IM if greater than 20 weeks. In the latter case Kleihauer testing is advisable and should be discussed with the on-call gynaecologist.

ACKNOWLEDGEMENTS

We would like to thank Dr E. Claydon, Consultant in Genito-Urinary Medicine, St Mary's Hospital and Dr M. Crofton, Consultant Radiologist, St Mary's Hospital, for their contributions.

APPENDIX: Advice on Miscarriage

1. *Why does the doctor keep talking about abortions?* The medical term for a miscarriage is a 'spontaneous abortion'. This is quite different from an induced abortion, but it can sound the same, so we try to remember to say 'miscarriage' instead.
2. *Is all bleeding a miscarriage?* No – most women that bleed during pregnancy are experiencing what is called a 'threatened' abortion. Only some women with a 'threatened' go on to lose their baby.
3. *How common is it?* Very common. Altogether at least one-fifth of pregnancies end in miscarriage, sometimes before the woman even knows she is pregnant.
4. *What are the chances for my baby?* More than three out of four women who have a threatened miscarriage will go on to give birth as normal.
5. *Why does it happen?* Unfortunately we don't know in most cases, although in many instances there is evidence to show that the baby was not developing 'properly'.
6. *Could I have prevented this happening?* It is difficult to accept the fact that usually nothing could have been done to prevent a miscarriage happening. It is very important to remember that miscarriages are no one's fault.

7. *Does that mean if the bleeding stops my baby will be handicapped?* Definitely not! While it is true that most miscarriages happen when the embryo is abnormal, those that continue have no more risk of producing an abnormal baby than anyone else.

8. *How does the doctor know whether it is a miscarriage?* The doctor will question and examine you. There are four things that are important:

> How much bleeding?
> Is there any pain?
> Has the neck of your womb opened up?
> Is the baby all right?

The doctor will assess these things. If you are less than 3 months pregnant, an ultrasound scan may be arranged to look at the baby and make sure it is alive and well. If you are more than 3 months pregnant then a special stethoscope may also be used to make sure that the baby's heart is beating well.

9. *Aren't all these 'internals' dangerous?* No, although you may worry about an internal examination making the bleeding worse, if done by the doctor or midwife they will not affect your baby's chances. Although it can be embarrassing to be examined, it is important. If you would very much prefer not to have an internal examination you do have the right to refuse it and request an ultrasound examination instead, but this may mean that some serious problems are not detected.

10. *Will I have to come into hospital?* Not necessarily. Every woman is different, but on the whole, if you and your baby are all right and you are not bleeding too much, there is no need for you to come into hospital.

11. *Why don't I need to come in?* Since there is no evidence that bed rest, whether at home or in hospital, is effective in preventing miscarriage, just do what feels right for you. Do be aware that while bleeding often stops if you lie down, it may well start again if you get up, even to go to the toilet. Don't feel guilty about this.

12. *What do I do at home?* Do what feels right for you, but it may be wise to avoid strenuous or tiring work or exercise. If the bleeding continues for more than a week, your GP may want to give you another check-up (bleeding for a long time isn't necessarily anything to worry about).

13. *What about sex?* You should avoid intercourse while the bleeding or pain continues. Some women find that sex starts the bleeding again and they have to avoid intercourse for quite a long while.

14. *What should I do if the bleeding gets heavier?* If it gets heavy or you pass blood clots or you get abdominal pain, you should call your GP in to check up on you and decide whether you need to come into hospital.

15. *What about future pregnancies?* There is no reason why you shouldn't go on to have more children. Most women who have a miscarriage go on to have trouble-free pregnancies in the future. You can get pregnant again as soon as you feel ready.

16. *Remember*:

> Threatened miscarriages are very common.
> Most women go on to have healthy babies.
> If you do miscarry, it probably will not affect your chances of a normal pregnancy next time, especially if this is the first time this has happened to you.

17. *What follow-up treatment is available?* You should see someone for follow-up after a miscarriage. Make an appointment with your GP to discuss the miscarriage with her/him, and also to ask questions about the future.

Further information and support for patients who have experienced miscarriage may be obtained through national miscarriage associations. For the UK this is located c/o Clayton Hospital, Northgate, Wakefield, West Yorkshire WF1 3JS. Tel: 01924 200799.

Bibliography

ADAMS, J., REGINALD, P.W., FRANKS, S. *et al.*, (1990). Uterine size and endometrial thickness and the significance of cystic ovaries in women with pelvic pain due to congestion. *Br. J. Obstet. Gynaecol.*, **97**, 583–7.

ANONYMOUS (1980). Vaginal bleeding in early pregnancy (Editorial). *Br. Med. J.*, **281**, 470.

ANONYMOUS (1993). Hormonal emergency contraception. *Drug Ther. Bull.*, **31**(7), 27–8.

BEARD, R.W., HIGHMAN, J.H., PEARCE, S. *et al.* (1984). Diagnosis of pelvic varicosities in women with chronic pelvic pain. *Lancet*, **ii**, 946–9.

BOR, R., MULLER, R. & JOHNSON, M. (1991). A testing time for doctors: counselling patients before an HIV test. *Br. Med. J.*, **303**, 905–7.

BRADLEY, W.G., FISKE, C.E. & FILLY, R.A. (1983). The double sac sign of early intrauterine pregnancy: use in the exclusion of ectopic pregnancy. *Radiology*, **143**, 223–6.

CLANCY, M.J. & ILLINGWORTH, R.N. (1989). The

diagnosis of ectopic pregnancy in an accident department. *Arch. Emerg. Med.*, **6**, 205–10.

CLIFFORD, K., RAI, R., WATSON, H. & REGAN, L. (1994). An informative protocol for the investigation of recurrent miscarriage: preliminary experience of 500 consecutive cases. *Hum. Reprod.*, **9**, 1328–32.

COSTE, J., JOB-SPIRA, N., AUBLET-CUVELIER, B., *et al.* (1994). Incidence of ectopic pregnancy. First results of a population-based register in France. *Hum. Reprod.*, **9**, 742–5.

DALING, J.R., WEISS, N.S., HISLOP, G. *et al.* (1987). Sexual practices, sexually transmitted diseases and the incidence of anal cancer. *N. Engl. J. Med.*, **317**, 973–7.

DeCRESPIGNY, L. Ch. (1988). Demonstration of ectopic pregnancy by transvaginal ultrasound. *Br. J. Obstet. Gynaecol.*, **95**, 1253–6.

DHSS (1994). *Report on Confidential Enquiries into Maternal Deaths in the United Kingdom 1988–90*. London: HMSO, **6**, 66–7.

EVERETT, C., ASHURST, H. & CHALMERS, I. (1987). Reported management of threatened miscarriage by general practitioners in Wessex. *Br. Med. J.*, **295**, 583–6.

FARQUAR, C.M., ROGERS, V., FRANKS, S. *et al.* (1989). A randomized controlled trial of medoxyprogesterone acetate and psychotherapy for the treatment of pelvic congestion. *Br. J. Obstet. Gynaecol.*, **96**, 1153–62.

FRANKS, S. (1989). Polycystic ovary syndrome: a changing perspective. *Clin. Endocrinol.*, **31**, 87–120.

FRASER, I.S., McCARRON, G. & MARKHAM, R. (1984). A preliminary study of factors influencing perception of menstrual blood loss volume. *Am. J. Obstet. Gynecol.*, **149**, 788–93.

GATZEN, C., PATERSON-BROWN, S., TOUQUET, R. *et al.* (1991). Management of acute lower abdominal pain: decision making in the A&E department. *J. R. Coll. Surg. Edinb.*, **36**, 121–3.

GILLING-SMITH, C., ZELIN, J., TOUQUET, R. *et al.* (1988). Management of early pregnancy bleeding in the accident and emergency department. *Arch. Emerg. Med.*, **5**, 133–8.

GILLING-SMITH, C., TOOZS-HOBSON, P., POTTS, D.J. *et al.* (1994). Management of bleeding in early pregnancy in accident and emergency departments. *Br. Med. J.*, **309**, 574–5.

GILLING-SMITH, C., PANAY, N., WADSWORTH, J., BEARD, R.W. & TOUQUET, R. (1995). Management of women presenting to the Accident and Emergency department with lower abdominal pain. *Ann. R. Coll. Surg. Engl.*, **77**, 193–7.

GOSWANY, R.K. (1992). Transvaginal ultrasonography. *Br. Med. J.*, **304**, 331–2.

GRAINGER, D.A. & SEIFER, D.B. (1995). Laparoscopic management of ectopic pregnancy. *Curr. Opin. Obstet. Gynaecol.*, **7**, 277–282.

GRAY, D.W.R. & COLLIN, J. (1987). Non-specific abdominal pain as a cause of acute admission to hospital. *Br. J. Surg.*, **74**, 239–42.

HAMILTON, S.M. (1989). Should follow-up be provided after miscarriage ? *Br. J. Obstet. Gynaecol.*, **96**: 743–4.

HERTZ, J.B. (1984). Diagnostic procedures in threatened abortion. *Obstet. Gynecol.*, **64**, 223–9.

HUGGON, A.M. & WATSON, D.P. (1993). Use of anti-D in an accident and emergency department. *Arch. Emerg. Med.*, **10**, 306–9.

KINGDOM, J.C.P., KELLY, T., MACLEAN, A.B. *et al.* (1991). Rapid one step urine test for human chorionic gonadotrophin in evaluating suspected complications of early pregnancy. *Br. Med. J.*, **302**, 1308–11.

MacDOUGALL, M.J., TAN, S.L. & JACOBS, H.S. (1992). *In-vitro* fertilisation and the ovarian hyperstimulation syndrome. *Hum. Reprod.*, **7**, 597–600.

McCREADY, J., BRAUNSTEIN, G.D., HELM, D. *et al.* (1978). Modification of the chorionic beta-subunit radio-immunoassay for determination of urinary choriogonadotrophin. *Clin. Chem.*, **24**, 1958–61.

NATIONAL BLOOD TRANSFUSION SERVICE IMMUNOGLOBULIN WORKING PARTY (1991). Recommendations for the use of anti-D immunoglobulin. *Prescribers J.*, **31**, 137–45.

NISWANDER, K. & GORDON, M. (1973). *The Collaborative Perinatal Study: The Women and their Pregnancies*. Philadelphia: W.B. Saunders.

PEARCE, J.M. (1990). Pelvic inflammatory disease. *Br. Med. J.*, **300**, 1090–1.

POLSON, D.W., ADAMS, J., WADSWORTH, J. *et al.* (1988). Polycystic ovaries – a common finding in normal women. *Lancet*, **i**, 870–2.

REES, M.C.P. (1989). Heavy, painful periods. *Baillière's Clin. Obstet. Gynaecol.*, **3**(2), 341–56.

ROBERTS, D.W.T. (1984). Dysmenorrhoea. In: *Contemporary Gynaecology*, ed. G.V.P. Chamberlain. p. 1. London: Butterworths.

ROBINSON, H.P. (1972). Detection of fetal heart movement in the first trimester of pregnancy using pulsed ultrasound. *Br. Med. J.*, **4**, 466–8.

ROBINSON, H.P. & DeCRESPIGNY, L. (1983). Ectopic pregnancy. *Clin. Obstet. Gynaecol.*, **10**, 407–21.

ROMERO, R., JEANTY, P. & HOBBINS, J.C. (1984). Diagnostic ultrasound in the first trimester of pregnancy. *Clin. Obstet. Gynaecol.*, **27**, 286–313.

ROYAL COLLEGE OF RADIOLOGISTS AND ROYAL COLLEGE OF OBSTETRICIANS AND GYNAECOLOGISTS (1995). Guidance on ultrasound procedures in early pregnancy. London.

SCHENKER, J.G. & WEINSTEIN, D. (1989). Ovarian hyperstimulation syndrome: a current survey. *Fertil. Steril.*, **30**, 255–62.

SHEPHARD, R. W., PATTON, P.E., NOVY, M.J. *et al.* (1990). Serial β-hCG measurements in the early detection of ectopic pregnancy. *Obstet. Gynecol.,* **75**, 417–20.

SMITH, J.R., MURDOCH, J., CARRINGTON, D. *et al.* (1991). Prevalence of *Chlamydia trachomatis* in women having cervical smear tests. *Br. Med. J.,* **302**, 82–4.

STABILE, I., CAMPBELL, S. & GRUDZINSKAS, J.G. (1988). Can ultrasound reliably diagnose ectopic pregnancy? *Br. J. Obstet. Gynaecol.,* **95**, 1247–52.

TINDALL, V.R. (1987). In: *Jeffcoate's Principles of Gynaecology*, 5th edn. p. 212. London: Butterworths.

TOUQUET, R., FOTHERGILL, J. & HARRIS, N.H. (1994). In: *Medical Negligence*, ed. M.J. Powers & N.H. Harris, 2nd edn. p. 631. London: Butterworths.

WESTROM, L. (1980). Incidence, prevalence and trends of acute pelvic inflammatory disease and its consequences in industrialised countries. *Am. J. Obstet. Gynecol.,* **138**, 880–92.

WESTROM, L. (1988). Disease incidence in women treated in hospital for acute salpingitis in Sweden. *Genitourin. Med.,* **64**, 59–63.

WILKIE, M.E., ALMOND, M.K. & MARSH, F.P. (1992). Diagnosis and management of urinary tract infection in adults. *Br. Med. J.,* **305**, 1137–41.

YUZPE, A.A., PERCIVAL SMITH, R. & RADEMAKER, A.W. (1982). A multicentre clinical investigation employing ethinylestradiol combined with dl-norgestrel as a postcoital contraceptive agent. *Fertil. Steril.,* **37**, 508–13.

60 Paediatric emergencies

E.M. MOLYNEUX

Accident and Emergency Department, Royal Liverpool Children's Hospital NHS Trust, Liverpool, UK

Chapter plan

Fever
Respiratory emergencies
Ear infections
Gastroenteritis
Urinary tract infections
Meningitis
Convulsions
Coma
Cardiac emergencies
Sudden infant death syndrome

FEVER

Assessment

Fever is a common symptom in childhood illness. The height of the temperature is often out of proportion to the severity of the disease. It is important to record body temperature accurately. In a baby less than 6 months of age a rectal temperature is reliable (normal range 36.7–37.9°C). In this age group the oral temperature is difficult to measure, and axillary temperature readings (normal range 35.6–37.2°C) may be 0.5–3°C below core temperature (Morley *et al.*, 1992). A fever can of itself cause headaches, nausea, myalgia and sweating. A rapid rise in body temperature can cause rigors and convulsions. Delirium is common with body temperatures greater than 39°C.

Management

Fever can be reduced with oral or rectal paracetamol (15 mg kg^{-1}), oral fluids and, if necessary, by tepid sponging and fanning. Serious causes of fever must be excluded by history and careful examination. In particular, meningitis, bacteraemia, pneumonia, urinary tract infection and ear infection must be specifically looked for and excluded. In an older child who is not toxic a thorough clinical examination with urine microscopy and culture may be sufficient. In younger children in whom the signs and symptoms of serious infection are less specific it is important to consider additional investigations. All infants under 3 months of age who are febrile and in whom a benign cause of fever, such as upper respiratory tract infection, cannot be clinically confirmed need to have a full blood count, urine microscopy and culture, blood culture and chest X-ray. A lumbar puncture should be done if the child appears unwell. These investigations are usually necessary even when there is a focus of infection such as otitis media because there is the strong likelihood of systemic spread of the disease. Broad-spectrum antibiotics should be prescribed.

If a child is between 3 months and 1 year of age and has a temperature greater than 39°C and no focus of infection is clinically evident, a urine sample should be sent for microscopy and culture and a full blood count done. If the child is delirious or there is a leucocytosis ($>15\,000$ cells μl^{-1}), the child should be admitted for observation and a blood culture considered. If the child is unwell, toxic or has had a febrile convulsion, the full range of tests for sepsis must be carried out including a lumbar puncture.

Any child who is toxic with or without a purpuric rash, cellulitis or other focal infection with peripheral circulatory shutdown and hypotension needs urgent circulatory support and intravenous broad-spectrum antibiotics.

RESPIRATORY EMERGENCIES

Emergency respiratory problems are common in children. It is important that the clinician should rapidly assess not only the cause of the condition but also the *degree of respiratory effort and/or difficulty*, because understanding these will contribute to appropriate management decisions. Respiratory effort and the potential for respiratory failure are best assessed by looking at:

- The work of breathing.
- The effectiveness of breathing.
- The effects of respiratory inadequacy on other organs.

The work of breathing

In chest disease there is an increase in the work of breathing which leads to tachypnoea at rest. This can only be judged if normal respiratory rates at different ages are known (Table 1). However, there are other

Table 1. *Normal respiratory rates in children*

Age (years)	Normal resting respiratory rate (breaths min^{-1})
<1	30–40
2–5	20–30
5–12	15–20
>12	12–16

causes of a rapid respiratory rate such as fever, anxiety, exercise or metabolic acidosis. If a child is exhausted the respiratory rate and effort will decrease; this is a dangerous preterminal sign.

Suprasternal, intercostal and subcostal recession become evident as the work of breathing increases. This is particularly obvious in infants as they have compliant chest walls. In a child over 5 years old it is a sign of severe respiratory difficulty. In older children sternomastoid muscles are used to assist ventilation causing 'tracheal tug'. In infants this leads to the head nodding with each respiratory effort; at the same time the ala nasi flare with each inspiration.

Noisy breathing indicates respiratory difficulty. *Stridor* is a sign of upper airway obstruction; it is more obvious in inspiration than in expiration. *Wheezing* indicates lower airway narrowing and is more pronounced in expiration. The severity of obstruction cannot be judged by the loudness of the noise.

Infants in severe respiratory distress *grunt* with each breath. The sound is made by exhaling against a partially closed glottis. This has the effect of generating a positive end-expiratory pressure and minimizing airway collapse at the end of expiration.

Increased work of breathing, manifested as increased respiratory rate, recession and noise, will not be present if the respiratory drive is inadequate. These signs may therefore not be present in patients with raised intracranial pressure, some poisonings and encephalopathy.

The work of breathing may suddenly fail if the child becomes exhausted. This is a dangerous development which may rapidly lead to respiratory failure.

Effectiveness of breathing

The depth of breathing is assessed by auscultation and looking for chest expansion (or, in infants, abdominal excursion). In exhaustion the chest may be silent despite severe respiratory distress. Pulse oximetry will help evaluate saturation of arterial oxygen.

The effect of respiratory inadequacy on other organs

Hypoxia causes tachycardia in children but anxiety, fever and pain will also contribute to this sign. The heart rate varies with age (Table 2).

Table 2. *Normal heart rate in children*

Age (years)	Normal resting heart rate (beats min^{-1})
<1	110–160
2–5	95–140
5–12	80–120
>12	60–100

Prolonged or severe hypoxia causes bradycardia; this is a dangerous preterminal sign. Hypoxia causes peripheral vasoconstriction leading to skin pallor and cooling which in turn lead to peripheral cyanosis. Hypoxia and/or hypocapnia cause mental confusion and agitation. As this progresses the child becomes increasingly drowsy and then unconscious. Early signs of confusion are important to note. Parents may say that their child is 'not himself'. It is essential to look for signs of decreasing alertness, lack of eye contact or a sluggish response to pain or voice. Generalized hypotonia accompanies profound hypoxia.

Upper airway obstruction

Upper airway obstruction may range in severity from very mild to life threatening. The causes are many (Table 3) and it is important to differentiate between them in order to decide appropriate management. *Croup* is the most common cause of acute inflammatory obstruction in childhood. Fortunately it usually takes a benign course. By contrast, *epiglottitis* is a severe rapidly progressive infection that nearly always requires management by intubation and assisted ventilation.

Table 3. *Causes of acute upper airway obstruction*

Cause	Example
Infection	Viral croup (acute laryngotracheobronchitis)
	Epiglottitis
	Bacterial tracheitis
	Tonsillitis, infectious mononucleosis
	Retropharyngeal abscess
	Diphtheria
Trauma	Foreign body inhalation
	Inhalation burns from heat or chemicals
	External neck trauma
Others	Angioneurotic oedema
	Spasmodic croup
	Tumours
Congenital	Choanal atresia
Newborn	Facial/skeletal anomaly (e.g. Pierre Robin syndrome)
	Treacher Collins syndrome
	Laryngomalacia, vocal cord paralysis, laryngeal web, subglottic stenosis
	Vascular ring
	Macroglossia, oropharyngeal tumour, ectopic thyroid

Croup

Croup is a clinical syndrome characterized by a barking cough, inspiratory stridor, hoarseness and a variable degree of respiratory distress. There are several disorders which cause this syndrome. The most common is *viral laryngotracheobronchitis* (90% of all cases of croup). Three-quarters of these cases are caused by parainfluenza

viruses; adenovirus and respiratory syncitial virus can cause the same clinical picture (McKenzie, 1992). Viral croup presents between the ages of 3 months and 5 years, the highest incidence being in the second year of life. Typically there are 1 or 2 days of coryza and mild fever ($<38°C$) followed by the onset of a barking cough, hoarseness and inspiratory stridor. The cough and stridor are often worse at night. Most children do not become severely ill, and recover after two to five days. Many will develop stridor only if they are upset or when hyperventilating. In some, however, the disease becomes severe. Stridor may then be present on both inspiration and expiration, and signs of upper airway obstruction become evident: nasal flaring, suprasternal, intercostal and infracostal recession, increasing restlessness, pallor and eventually cyanosis and altered consciousness.

Some children have recurrent episodes of croup with or without preceding coryza and fever. The onset is sudden, often at night and the episode is usually short-lived (3–6 h). The majority of these children, who are usually aged 1–3 years, are atopic and suffer from asthma, eczema or hay fever. There may be a family predisposition to croup. Although these episodes of spasmodic croup are sometimes severe, they are usually self-limiting and occur with diminishing intensity on 2–3 successive nights. This form of croup often responds to nebulized salbutamol.

Bacterial tracheitis is a rare but life-threatening form of croup. The tracheal mucosa is infected by *Staphylococcus aureus*, beta-haemolytic streptococci, *Haemophilus influenzae* B and, more rarely, *Branhamella catarrhalis*. These organisms cause extensive mucosal necrosis, oedema and the production of copious purulent secretions. The child, usually under 3 years of age, looks ill and toxic and has a high temperature and signs of progressive upper airway obstruction. Hoarseness and a croupy cough lead on to worsening inspiratory stridor. Sudden occlusion of the trachea by secretions or slough may result in death.

Bacterial tracheitis can be distinguished from epiglottitis by the absence, in tracheitis, of drooling and the presence of a cough. Suctioning secretions gives temporary relief but most patients will need tracheal intubation or a tracheostomy to maintain an adequate airway. All will need treatment with intravenous antibiotics.

Assessment of croup

The degree of hypoxia does not correlate well with physical signs but respiratory rate and sternal recession are helpful. A rise in respiratory rate may be the first sign of impending trouble. The arterial oxygen saturation (SaO$_2$) should be measured by pulse oximetry.

Treatment

Mild croup (no stridor at rest)
This needs no active treatment. The parents and child will benefit from gentle reassurance and the child can be supervised by the parents at home.

Moderate croup (can be placated, interested in surroundings)
These children are often miserable and frightened. They need to be comforted and carefully observed in hospital. Crying makes them worse and increases their oxygen requirements, so they should be disturbed as little as good observation allows. Steam is seldom of benefit and clouds the child from view. They are often best on their mother's lap where they feel secure.

Severe croup (apathetic, restless, marked retractions)
These children need humidified oxygen, preferably by face mask. Nebulized adrenaline (1–5 ml of 1:1000) given through the face mask will often produce improvement lasting 30–60 min; repeated doses have diminishing effects. These children need close observation in a paediatric intensive care unit, where continuous electrocardiographic (ECG) monitoring and measurements of arterial oxygen saturation are possible. About 3% of all children admitted to hospital with croup will require intubation and assisted ventilation (McKenzie, 1992).

Should systemic steroids be used in the treatment of croup? In patients who require intubation, steroids reduce the required duration of intubation and lessen the likelihood that reintubation will be necessary (Karys et al., 1989). Recently, nebulized steroids have been used in moderate croup with more sustained benefit than placebo (Husby et al., 1993). The decision to ventilate should be based on signs of increasing respiratory rate, increasing tachycardia, recession, the appearance of cyanosis, exhaustion and confusion. Intubation is difficult and, except in dire circumstances, should only be attempted by an experienced paediatric anaesthetist.

Epiglottitis

Epiglottitis is a life-threatening infection of the supraglottic tissues. Although it shares some features with croup it is a distinct entity and must be differentiated from croup as it is managed differently. If treatment is incorrect it may rapidly progress to acute tracheal obstruction and death. Intense swelling of the epiglottis and aryepiglottic folds is caused by infection with *Haemophilus influenzae*. Young children aged between 2 and 7 years are most commonly affected but 25–30% are less than 2 years of age and 5–10% are infants.

The onset is often acute with high fever ($>38.5°C$), a soft inspiratory stridor and rapidly increasing respiratory difficulty over a few hours. In contrast to children with croup these children do not cough (coughing is too painful). Infants may present with poor feeding, fever and stridor. They drool saliva and appear toxic, with poor peripheral skin perfusion and pallor. A child with epiglottitis tends to take up a particular position and remain quiet and immobile. An infant may lie with his neck hyperextended, but older children prefer to sit forward with the mouth open and chin jutted forward. The child refuses to drink and will not swallow saliva. Any disturbance such as trying to lie the child flat, look in their throat or attempt venepuncture will cause distress and may precipitate laryngeal obstruction and death.

Do's and don'ts in epiglottitis	
Do	**Don't**
Be gentle	Lie flat
Supervise the child	Look in throat
Give oxygen by face mask	Venepuncture
Call anaesthetist	
Admit to intensive therapy unit	

The diagnosis is made on the history and appearance of the child (Table 4). Lateral neck X-rays are unneces-

Table 4. *Differences between croup and epiglottitis*

	Croup	Epiglottitis
Onset	2–3 days	Over hours
Prodroma	Coryza	No
Cough	Barking	Absent
Ability to drink	Yes	No
Drooling saliva	No	Yes
Appearance	Unwell	Toxic
Fever	<38.5°C	>38.5°C
Stridor	Harsh	Soft
Voice	Hoarse	Muffled
Severity	Variable	Severe

sary and by disturbing the child may add to the danger of sudden laryngeal obstruction. Once the diagnosis is suspected the child must not be left unsupervised. They should be allowed to stay in the position they prefer (often on their mother's knee). Any examination must be gentle and cautious and no painful procedures should be undertaken. If 100% humidified oxygen is tolerated this should be applied by face mask. It is less disturbing if the mother holds the mask close to, but not applied to, the child's face. An experienced anaesthetist must be called and the intensive care unit informed. The child should go straight from the resuscitation room in the accident and emergency (A&E) department to theatre or intensive care where elective tracheal intubation can be performed by an experienced paediatric anaesthetist. Provision must be made for an emergency tracheostomy should it prove necessary. Tracheal intubation can be very difficult, as supraglottic oedema distorts the anatomy of the larynx. A narrower tube than usual will be needed and a gum bougie may be needed to help pass the tube through the larynx. When the larynx is so distorted that no airway can be seen, it helps if an assistant compresses the chest and a bubble of air passes up through the trachea to reveal the opening into the airway.

If a child comes into an A&E department *in extremis*, and if tracheal intubation fails, a needle cricothyroidotomy can be performed. This will relieve asphyxia for about 15–20 min while arrangements are made for a tracheostomy to be performed in theatre. Once the airway is established venous access must be secured. Blood samples should be taken for full blood count and culture and intravenous antibiotics should be commenced. Cefuroxime, 30 mg kg^{-1} 8 hourly, or chloramphenicol 25 mg kg^{-1} 6 hourly are appropriate.

Most children can be extubated within 36 h and fully recover within 5 or 6 days.

Differential diagnosis: other causes of upper airway obstruction

Croup and epiglottitis account for over 98% of cases of acute upper airway obstruction but several other conditions need to be considered.

A *retropharyngeal abscess*, although uncommon, may present with signs of upper airway obstruction. There is often a history of recent throat infections accompanied by 2 or 3 days of fever. The child has been unwell with increasing difficulty in swallowing and stridor. The treatment is surgical drainage and intravenous antibiotics.

Angioneurotic oedema of the face and mouth can develop over a few minutes as part of an anaphylactic reaction. Allergies to food, especially nuts, drug reactions and insect stings are common causes of this. The treatment is 100% oxygen by face mask, intravenous adrenaline, hydrocortisone and an antihistamine; intubation may be required. If the oedema is less severe and not life-threatening it sometimes responds to nebulized adrenaline by face mask, and oral steroids.

Marked tonsillar swelling, as in *infectious mononucleosis* or occasionally in *acute tonsillitis*, can compromise the upper airway. *Diphtheria* is a rare infection seen in children who are not immunized against the disease, particularly if they have recently been abroad.

Toddlers are at risk of *inhaling a foreign body*. Coins, watch batteries, pieces of food and small toy parts are common offending items. Of the objects which cause obstruction 6–7% lodge in or above the larynx; most slip through the larynx and lodge in the bronchial tree where they cause a persistent cough of very acute onset and unilateral wheezing.

If the presence of a foreign body is highly likely, but the child is not in immediate danger, no attempt should be made to remove or visualize the object. Disturbing the child may dislodge the item, only for it to be relodged in a more difficult and obstructive position. If the obstruction is life-threatening, attempts to remove the foreign body must be made by chest compression and back blows in an infant and the Heimlich manoeuvre in older children (see Chapter 4). Blind finger sweeps should *not* be made in a child's mouth as the foreign body may be pushed further into the trachea and lodge below the glottis where the trachea is most narrow. It is better to look for a foreign body by direct vision using a tongue depressor and torch or laryngoscope. If a foreign body is seen and is accessible it should be removed with Magill forceps. In a less urgent situation, where the foreign body has slipped into the bronchial tree, inspiratory and expiratory chest X-rays may show mediastinal shift on expiration due to gas trapping distal to the bronchial foreign body. The foreign body should be removed through a bronchoscope under general anaesthesia as soon as possible. There is always a risk that coughing or changes of posture may cause the object to move into a more severely obstructive position within the bronchial tree.

Lower airway obstruction

Lower airway obstruction is characterized by cough, wheeze and a prolonged expiratory phase. In older children *asthma* is the most common cause; in infants the most likely causes are *bronchiolitis, asthma* and *pneumonia*. Foreign body inhalation, upper airway obstruction, bronchial obstruction by intra- or extra-luminal masses and pulmonary oedema need to be considered.

Bronchiolitis

Bronchiolitis is the most common serious respiratory infection in childhood. It occurs in young children under the age of 18 months; 90% of children are 1–9 months of age, with a peak incidence around 6 months. Epidemics of bronchiolitis occur in winter or early spring. Respiratory syncytial virus is the cause in 75% of cases; other causative agents include parainfluenza B, adenovirus and mycoplasma. Adenovirus infection can lead to residual lung disease as bronchiolitis proliferans may develop. Bronchiolitis is due to inflammatory obstruction of small airways in which mucosal oedema, secretions and cellular debris block these channels. Young infants with small airways are particularly prone to obstruction, as resistance to air flow is inversely proportional to the fourth power of the radius of the airway. A minor degree of oedema may therefore lead to a major increase in airway resistance. As resistance is greater in expiration than in inspiration, air trapping develops beyond the obstruction and the lungs become overinflated.

Clinical findings

Typically, other members of the family have minor upper respiratory tract infections. The baby develops a dry cough and runny nose. Over 2–3 days there is increasing breathlessness. Feeding becomes increasingly difficult and tiring. A wheeze may be present and in infants there may be recurrent periods of apnoea. Bronchiolitis may remain a mild illness; but premature babies and children with chronic underlying disease (cystic fibrosis, broncho-pulmonary dysplasia, cardiac disorders) are at particular risk of developing severe respiratory difficulties. A low-grade fever may be present, and on auscultation some wheeze and characteristic end-inspiratory, early-expiratory fine crackles are heard. A chest X-ray shows air trapping, thickening of bronchial walls, scattered areas of interstitial pneumonia and atelectasis. The liver and spleen are often palpable because they have been pressed down into the abdomen by the distended lungs. Characteristic findings are:

- Tachypnoea.
- Recession.
- Sharp dry cough.
- End-inspiratory fine crackles.
- High-pitched wheeze.
- Tachycardia.
- Pallor or cyanosis.
- Recurrent apnoea or irregular breathing pattern.

Management

Mild bronchiolitis, in which the baby is alert and feeding, can be treated at home. Parents should be told to seek medical attention if the baby has any increased difficulty in feeding, pallor, tachypnoea or tachycardia. The baby should be reviewed the following day by a doctor. A child with moderate or severe bronchiolitis, with difficulty in feeding, restlessness, marked recession or hypoxia (as measured by pulse oximetry or suggested by clinical signs such as pallor, cyanosis, tachypnoea or irregular breathing) must be admitted and given supportive treatment. These children need close clinical observation with continuous or frequent ECG monitoring and pulse oximetry. Antibiotics are not warranted unless a chest X-ray shows evidence of pneumonia. The baby should be given 100% humidified oxygen in a head box. Nasal and upper airway secretions may need removal by suction. Fluids can be given by nasogastric tube or intravenously. If there is evidence of increasing hypoxaemia and respiratory fatigue, or in the presence of recurrent apnoeic attacks, elective intubation and assisted ventilation are necessary.

Steroids and bronchodilators have not been shown to help. Nebulized ribovarin, an antiviral agent, is reserved for the use of children with pre-existing disease which makes them prone to severe infections. About 2% of infants admitted to hospital with bronchiolitis will require ventilation because of hypoxia, increasing hypercapnia or exhaustion and apnoea. Most children make a full recovery from bronchiolitis within 2 weeks.

Asthma

Acute exacerbations of asthma account for 10–20% of medical admissions of children in the UK (Couriel, 1993). Over the last 15–20 years there has been a great increase in the number of children with asthma and, despite improved understanding of the disease, more informed treatment schedules and better delivery apparatus for medication to children, there are still 40–50 deaths each year (Couriel, 1993).

Clinical findings

Asthma is characterized by cough, wheeze and breathlessness. In the preschool child symptoms are most commonly precipitated by viral upper respiratory tract infection. In older children exercise may induce an attack. Some episodes are triggered by excitement or emotional upset. Allergy may induce asthma; the house mite, grass pollens, moulds and contact with animals have all been implicated.

Physical irritation of the airway by smoke, chemicals or a sudden drop in temperature can trigger an attack.

Assessment of severity

The diagnosis of asthma is not usually in doubt except in infants, in whom it may be difficult to differentiate pneumonia or bronchiolitis, but severity is not easily ascertained in a child. Wheeze and respiratory rate are poor indicators of severity, but the use of accessory muscles, chest recession and pulsus paradoxus are fairly reliable measures. In the history it is important to include the duration of symptoms, what treatment has already been tried and what the previous pattern of attacks has been. A clinical assessment score is helpful in assessing severity (Table 5).

The peak expiratory flow rate (PEFR) is an objective measure of airway obstruction and should be used both in diagnosis and in the monitoring of treatment. PEFR is unreliable in children under 4 or 5 years of age and in the very dyspnoeic child. It varies with the height of the

Table 5. *Clinical asthma score* (Heaf, 1992)

	Score		
	0	1	2
Cyanosis	None	In air	In 40% O_2
Inspiratory sounds	Normal	Wheeze	Decreased/Absent
Expiratory sounds	Normal	Wheeze	Decreased/Absent
Accessory muscles	None	Moderate	Marked
Alertness	Normal	Agitated	Reduced

Score >5 = severe asthma.
Score >7 = respiratory failure.

Consider requesting a chest X-ray (once the child is stable) if:

1. No previous history of wheezing.
2. Any possibility of inhaled foreign body.
3. Irregular breath sounds or deviated trachea.

Table 6. *Predicted values of peak expiratory flow rate (PEFR) in children*

Height (cm)	Peak flow (litres min^{-1})
110	150
120	200
130	250
140	300
150	350
160	400
170	450

child (Table 6) and should be recorded as a percentage of normal after two or more readings have been taken, not as a single reading.

Arterial oxygen saturation (SaO_2) measured by pulse oximetry is helpful in assessing severity and outcome. It should not be the sole measure of hypoxaemia and should be interpreted in the light of clinical signs and symptoms (Bishop & Nolan, 1991).

A chest X-ray is seldom helpful. It should be done in first asthma attacks, if there is pain in the chest, or if the presence of a foreign body is being considered. Pain in the chest should suggest the possibility of a pneumothorax. Many children complain of abdominal pain which is muscular in origin and due to respiratory effort.

The British Thoracic Society has issued guidelines (1993) for assessment and management of severe asthma in childhood.

British Thoracic Society Guidelines for severe asthma in children

Features of severe asthma
- Too wheezy or breathless to talk or to feed
- PEFR <50% predicted normal or best
- Heart rate >140 beats min^{-1}
- Respiratory rate >50 breaths min^{-1}.

Features of life-threatening asthma
- PEFR <33% predicted or best
- Silent chest, cyanosis, poor respiratory effort
- Fatigue, exhaustion
- Agitation, reduced level of consciousness

Patients with life-threatening attacks may not have all these signs and may not appear distressed. Any one sign indicates the presence of a severe attack.

Arterial blood gas estimates are not necessary for initial management but in severe or refractory attacks may be useful in deciding further treatment.

Table 7. *Drugs in the treatment of acute asthma*

Oxygen	100% high-flow
Nebulized beta-agonist	Salbutamol 2.5–5 mg 0.5–4 hourly
	Terbutaline 5–10 mg 0.5–4 hourly
Prednisolone	1–2 mg kg^{-1} day^{-1} for 3 days or hydrocortisone 100 mg IV 6 hourly
Aminophylline	[a]Loading dose 5 mg kg^{-1} IV over 20 min
	Maintenance infusion 1 mg kg^{-1} h^{-1}
Intravenous salbutamol	Loading dose 4–6 µg kg^{-1} over 10 min
	Continuous infusion 0.5–1.0 µg kg^{-1} min^{-1}
Nebulized ipratropium	125–250 µg 6 hourly

[a] Omit if child is already on oral theophylline therapy.

Treatment

Oxygen, nebulized beta-agonists and steroids are the basis of treatment in acute asthma (Table 7). All children with acute asthma should be given nebulized beta$_2$-bronchodilator (salbutamol or terbutaline) driven by 100% oxygen at a high flow of 4–6 litres min^{-1}. Improvement should be judged by pre- and postnebulizer PEFR readings and clinical score. The postnebulizer reading should be taken 15 min after finishing the treatment and the child should be watched for a further 45 min. If there is no relapse in symptoms the child may be sent home with a short course of oral steroids. Ensure that the child has their usual treatment supply and uses correct inhaler technique. Parents must be asked to return at once if they are worried or symptoms reappear or worsen.

Moderate or severe cases need admission. Immediate treatment consists of 100% oxygen by face mask and nebulized beta-agonist. Prednisolone 1–2 mg kg^{-1} body weight (maximum 40 mg) should be given by mouth. The beta-agonist can be repeated every 1–2 h until there is improvement. If there is no improvement or the attack is life-threatening give 100% oxygen and a nebulized beta-agonist and commence an intravenous infusion of aminophylline 5 mg kg^{-1} to run through in 20 min, followed by a maintenance dose of 1 mg kg^{-1} h^{-1}. The loading dose of aminophylline should be omitted if the child is already on oral theophylline. Intravenous hydrocortisone 100 mg 6 hourly can replace the oral steroids if the child is vomiting. Ipratropium (250 µg, or 125 µg in the very young child) may be added to the nebulized beta-agonist. Assess the response to treatment. If the SaO$_2$ remains or falls below 92% consider a chest X-ray to exclude a pneumothorax. If there is improvement continue treatment with oxygen, steroids and nebulized beta-agonist. If the child is not improving after 15–30 min

continue oxygen and steroids and give nebulized beta-agonist up to half hourly and repeat ipratropium 6 hourly. If the child is still not improving continue treatment with maintenance aminophylline infusion but monitor the blood levels and consult a paediatric chest physician.

> **Monitor progress and treatment of severe asthma in children by:**
> * Peak expiratory flow, 15–30 min after starting treatment (<33% = severe)
> * Pulse oximetry, to maintain SaO$_2$ at >92%
> * PaO$_2$ (<8 kPa = severe hypoxia)
> * PaCO$_2$ (5–6 kPa) or higher levels denote severity)

Fig. 1 shows a management protocol for children with severe asthma.

Exhaustion, confusion, a deteriorating peak expiratory flow, hypoxia or rising hypercapnia require urgent admission to a paediatric intensive care unit where mechanical ventilation may be necessary.

Pneumonia

Pneumonia is caused by many pathogens in children, but at certain ages children are more commonly affected by particular agents. Children with underlying lung disease such as cystic fibrosis, bronchiectasis, tracheo-oesophageal fistula or with congenital abnormalities such as cleft palate are prone to infection. Also, viral chest infections temporarily disrupt the epithelium of the lung respiratory passages and predispose to secondary bacterial infection. Newborn infants may be infected by pathogens from the parturient tract and develop pneumonia due to

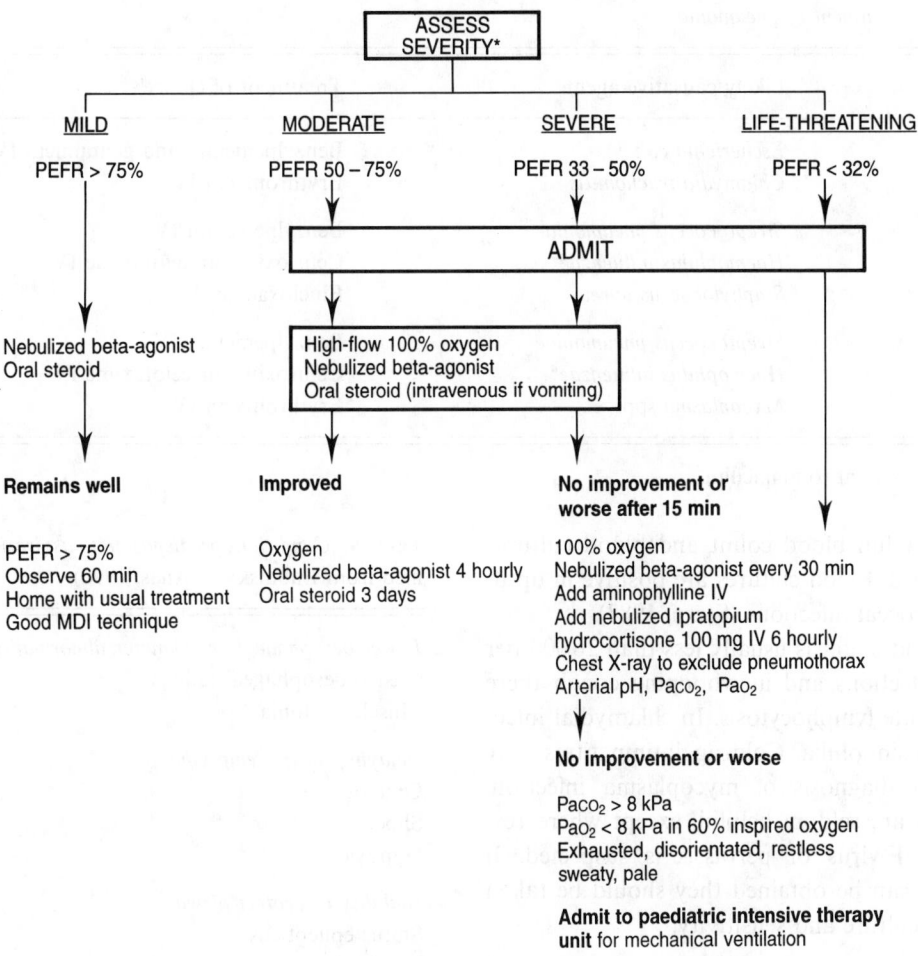

Fig. 1. Management protocol for children with severe asthma. MDI, metered-dose inhaler. (Modified from British Thoracic Society, 1993.)

Escherichia coli, beta-haemolytic streptococcus or, increasingly, *Chlamydia trachomatis*. Infants develop pneumonia most commonly from viruses such as respiratory syncytial virus or adenovirus, but *Haemophilus influenzae* and pneumococcus and occasionally *Staphylococcus aureus* may cause a primary infection or, more typically, a secondary bacterial chest infection. In the older child pneumonia is less likely to be viral in origin and pneumococcus or mycoplasma are often the cause of illness.

Clinical findings

In older children the signs of pneumonia are not difficult to elicit. The child is febrile and there is a dry cough, which may become productive over 2 or 3 days. There are signs of consolidation in one or more areas of the lungs with reduced air entry, bronchial breathing and added breath sounds. The child is tachypnoeic and (in lower lobe pneumonia) may complain of abdominal or low chest pain. In infants, the signs of a chest infection are less explicit. The baby may have a low-grade or no fever. Respiratory rate is raised and feeding difficulties may be apparent. There may be chest retractions or signs of respiratory failure. There may be recurrent episodes of apnoea. However, listening to the chest may demonstrate little that is abnormal. For this reason a chest X-ray should be done in infants suspected of pneumonia. The X-ray changes are often considerable and varied. In viral infections, the chest X-ray will show patchy gas trapping, hyperinflation, bronchial tree thickening and atelectasis. In bacterial infections, there are patches of consolidation, lobar in pneumococcal pneumonia but widespread and patchy in most other types of pneumonia. Staphylococcal infections can lead to multiple

Table 8. *Antibiotic treatment of pneumonia*

Age of child	Likely causative agent	Treatment of choice
<4 weeks	*Escherichia coli*	Benzylpenicillin and gentamicin IV or cefotaxime IV
	Chlamydia trachomitis	Erythromycin IV
0.5–2 years	*Streptococcus pneumoniae*	Benzylpenicillin IV
	Haemophilus influenzae[a]	Cefuroxime or cefotaxime IV
	Staphylococcus aureus	Flucloxacillin IV
2–12 years	*Streptococcus pneumoniae*	Benzylpenicillin IV
	Haemophilus influenzae[a]	Cefuroxime or cefotaxime IV
	Mycoplasma spp.	Erythromycin IV

[a]15% of cases are resistant to ampicillin.

lung abscesses. A full blood count and blood cultures should be obtained. Blood cultures are positive in up to 30% of pneumococcal infections (Stern, 1983).

The white blood count is usually less than 20 000 per mm^3 in viral infections and in whooping cough there may be an absolute lymphocytosis. In chlamydial infections, there is eosinophilia. Cold agglutinin titres may help establish a diagnosis of mycoplasma infection. Postnasal swabs are seldom helpful, except where respiratory syncytial virus or pertussis is suspected. If sputum samples can be obtained they should be taken for microscopy, culture and sensitivity.

Treatment

Treatment should be started on clinical suspicion of pneumonia and targeted at the most likely pathogens, given the age of the child and history of the illness. If the child is not severely ill and is well hydrated and not vomiting, oral medication can be prescribed. In more sick patients, intravenous therapy and supportive treatment should be given in hospital. Monitoring should include pulse oximetry, respiratory rate and checking for signs of respiratory effort. Appropriate therapy for pneumonia is shown in Table 8.

Recovery from most types of pneumonia is quick and complete within 2 weeks; however, mycoplasma pneumonia can lead to a prolonged illness over several weeks and staphylococcal infections can be prolonged and require antibiotic therapy for 4–6 weeks.

Aspiration pneumonia

Table 9 illustrates some conditions that predispose to aspiration pneumonia. It is usually gastric contents that

Table 9. *Conditions predisposing to aspiration pneumonia* (modified from Lubinsky & Anas, 1990)

Lower oesophageal or sphincter abnormalities
Gastro-oesophageal reflux
Muscle dystonia

Delaying gastric emptying
Opioids
Shock
Hypoxic

Inability to protect airway
Status epilepticus
Head injury
Alcohol intoxication
Opioids
Cardiopulmonary resuscitation
Uncoordinated swallowing
Unconscious

Anatomical problems
Cleft palate
Vocal cord paralysis
Epiglottitis
Tracheo-oesophageal fistula
Nasogastric feeding

are aspirated. After a brief latent period (usually less than 1 h), fever, tachypnoea and cough develop. Apnoea and shock can also occur. Examination of the chest reveals diffuse scattered crackles and wheezing. The patients may be cyanotic. A chest X-ray shows extensive bilateral patchy infiltrates. Prevention is of the utmost importance. However, should aspiration occur, the airways should immediately be suctioned and oxygen administered. In severe cases mechanical ventilation will be required. Many of these patients develop secondary bacterial infections of the chest (Lubinsky & Anas, 1990).

Pertussis

Pertussis is caused by *Bordetella pertussis*. There are three distinct phases in the progress of the illness. The *coryzal stage* lasts 1–3 weeks, in which the child has signs of an upper respiratory infection. In the second or *paroxysmal stage* (2–8 weeks) the child has bouts of coughing which may be associated with vomiting. In older children a fit of coughing ends in a characteristic sharp intake of air which sounds like a whoop. These bouts of coughing are worse at night and when the child is out in the cold air.

Infants do not whoop but have bouts of coughing. In severe cases the cough leads to recurrent episodes of cyanosis and apnoea. In some children feeding can be a real problem and loss of weight and dehydration ensue. The third or *convalescent stage* is of variable duration; the coughing bouts are less frequent and gradually abate. The diagnosis is a clinical one, although early in the illness an absolute lymphocytosis may be present and *Bordetella pertussis* may be found in a postnasal aspirate. A chest X-ray is not helpful unless a secondary infection has occurred. The child is infectious in the first stage and for a few days into the paroxysmal stage of the disease.

Management

Early in the illness, while the child is still infectious, erythromycin 30 mg kg^{-1} per day for 7 days will reduce the infectivity of the child, but not alter the course of the illness. This is important for a child in a family with a small baby, as young infants may have marked respiratory difficulty with pertussis. Parents and the child need reassurance. If the child is vomiting it is often better to let them eat immediately after a bout of coughing and vomiting. Separating drinks from solids seems to reduce vomiting. If there is a history of apnoea, cyanosis or respiratory distress, the child must be admitted for close observation and further treatment as appropriate.

EAR INFECTIONS

Acute otitis media

Bacterial otitis media is usually secondary to a viral upper respiratory tract infection. It is especially common in children under 4 years of age, with most infections occurring in infants (Glover, 1990). *Streptococcus pneumoniae* and *Haemophilus influenzae* (usually non-capsulated) are the most common causative agents but *Branhamella catarrhalis* and beta-haemolytic streptococci are also found. In newborns, Gram-negative *Escherichia coli* or *Staphylococcus aureus* may be the cause. *Mycoplasma pneumoniae* may give rise to infection at any age.

Clinical findings

In an infant the signs of otitis media are non-specific. There may be a history of fever, diarrhoea, poor feeding and vomiting. Older children complain of earache which may be severe. Head banging and pulling the ears are not diagnostic signs and may imply referred otalgia from erupting teeth or even distressing abdominal pain (Glover, 1990).

All children warrant a thorough examination to exclude other causes for the generalized symptoms. In suppurative otitis media the eardrums are dull red and bulging; but eardrums can appear red or injected with fever, crying and viral upper respiratory tract infections. Some viral infections may lead to an opaque immobile drum behind which bubbles may be seen. In mycoplasma and some viral infections the eardrum may have haemorrhagic blisters on it (myringitis bullosa haemorrhagica). This can be exquisitely painful.

In suppurative otitis media, if the drum ruptures the pain is reduced and the ear discharges pus.

Complications

If the pain does not settle with treatment, or if pus continues to discharge or increases in quantity, the child may have developed mastoiditis. Classical signs (oedema and tenderness over the mastoid process with downward displacement of the pinna caused by a subperiosteal abscess) may not be present in partially treated cases. Other complications, which are rare, are due to infection spreading beyond the middle ear cleft into petrous temple bone; these include facial palsy, lateral sinus thrombophlebitis and suppurative labyrynthitis. Spread within the cranial cavity can lead to meningitis or abscess formation (Ludman, 1988).

Management

Adequate analgesia and antipyretic treatment must be given. In bacterial infections a course of oral ampicillin, co-trimoxazole or cefaclor should be prescribed for 5 days. If a mycoplasma infection is suspected, erythromycin is the antibiotic of choice. If pus is discharging from the ear, take a swab for microscopy, culture and sensitivity and clean the canal by dry mopping. Antibiotic treatment should be guided by the culture findings if there is no clinical improvement. Nasal decongestants do not help (Ludman, 1988). If complications have developed the child should be admitted: take blood samples for a full blood count and culture, commence intravenous antibiotic therapy and arrange for the child to be evaluated by an ear, nose and throat (ENT) surgeon. Recurrent otitis media needs an ENT referral as tonsillectomy and adenoidectomy may be required. Recurrence also predisposes to persistent middle ear effusions and grommets may be necessary.

Acute otitis externa

Acute otitis externa may be generalized or confined to a furuncle. A generalized infection causes diffuse inflammation of the lining of the external auditory canal and usually follows local trauma (e.g. attempts to clean the ear), frequent swimming or the presence of a foreign body. Debris in the auditory canal promotes infection. There is often a mixed growth of bacteria with a predominance of pseudomonas or *Proteus mirabilis*. Pain in the ear is worsened by chewing, yawning or pulling on the pinna. Tender lymph nodes may be palpable in front of or behind the ear. Fever develops if the infection spreads in front of the ear as a cellulitis.

A *furuncle* is a localized infection within the external auditory canal. It is exquisitely painful and is usually caused by a staphylococcal infection.

Differential diagnosis

Impetigo can affect the auditory canal but has usually spread over the pinna and on to surrounding skin. Herpes simplex infections or herpes zoster (Ramsay Hunt syndrome) can give rise to ear pain and vesicle formation.

Management

Swabs are seldom useful in directing treatment as there is a mixed growth on culture. Treatment consists of adequate systemic analgesia and careful cleaning of the ear. Cleaning can be done with a cotton bud, the tip of which has been pulled out to make it wispy. Daily cleaning may be required for the first few days. A few drops of antibiotic/steroid solution (e.g. Sofracort) should be instilled in the ear every 2–4 h when the child is awake. If there is a lot of swelling of the auditory canal a ribbon gauze wick soaked in the drops may be helpful. However, this is not easy to accomplish in a small wriggling child and it is better to leave it to an experienced ENT surgeon. Systemic antibiotics are not necessary unless there is spreading cellulitis, when an antistaphylococcal agent such as flucloxacillin should be prescribed. The furuncle will usually discharge naturally. Incision is seldom necessary and could predispose to perichondritis.

Infection around a pierced ear lobe causes oedema and the stud can become imbedded in the tissues. It may be possible to pinch the oedematous tissue between two fingers, expose the stud and lift it out with forceps. If this is not possible it should be removed under local anaesthesia through a small incision at the back of the ear lobe where the scar will not be visible. Antibiotics are seldom necessary.

GASTROENTERITIS

Acute diarrhoea and vomiting are common symptoms in children. Infective gastroenteritis is the most usual cause, but other conditions, some potentially serious, must be excluded:

- Gastroenteritis – viral, bacterial, parasitic.
- Appendicitis.
- Poisoning.
- Extraintestinal disease – urinary tract infection.
- Respiratory infection, otitis media.
- Antibiotics.
- Intussusception.
- 'Overflow' diarrhoea.
- Toddler diarrhoea.
- Malabsorption.
- Milk allergy.
- Inflammatory bowel disease.
- Disaccharide intolerance.
- Cystic fibrosis.
- Haemolytic-uraemic syndrome.
- Staphylococcal toxic shock syndrome.

Gastroenteritis, usually a mild disease, may be severe. It causes 4 000 000 deaths worldwide annually in children less than 5 years of age. Most of these deaths occur in the developing world (World Health Organization, 1990). The complications (dehydration and electrolyte loss) tend to be more severe in children than in adults.

Viruses cause about 80% of all childhood gastrointestinal infections. *Rotaviruses* account for 30–60% of all episodes of gastroenteritis. Rotavirus infections are most common in infants in the winter months. The typical illness is a 7–8-day episode of vomiting and the passing of watery and foul-smelling stools which are occasionally bloodstained. Rotavirus can be seen on microscopy of the stool sample. *Norwalk virus* causes diarrhoea and vomiting which may be severe. The illness is commonly brief (2–3 days) and may be associated with myalgia. *Calicivirus, adenovirus* and many other viruses cause gastroenteritis.

Common *bacterial* causes of gastroenteritis are pathogenic *Escherichia coli*, shigellae, salmonellae, campylobacter, *Clostridium difficile* and *Yersinia enterocolitica*. The protozoon *Giardia lamblia* and cryptosporidium also cause gastroenteritis in children. In mild cases of gastroenteritis, testing stool samples is unrewarding. Over 50% will give negative results. Stool samples should be sent for analysis from patients with bloody diarrhoea or prolonged diarrhoea, even if the child is well, and samples should be taken from all children with severe gastroenteritis. Stool samples should be sent for microscopy, bacterial culture and sensitivity and viral assay. In prolonged diarrhoea a further stool sample should be analysed for reducing sugars; a result of >1% implies sugar intolerance.

The younger the child, the more likelihood of severe effects of gastroenteritis. The clinical signs are those of fluid and electrolyte loss.

History

Note how long the child has been ill. Has diarrhoea been accompanied by fever and other systemic symptoms? Is the child drinking and active, or listless and refusing to drink? Is the child passing urine (have there been wet nappies in the past few hours)? How frequent is the diarrhoea and are the stools bloodstained, watery or foul-smelling? Bloodstained stools are seen in shigella infections and also in viral gastroenteritis and in the haemolytic-uraemic syndrome.

Examination

Take careful note of any possible extraintestinal cause for the symptoms. Assess the degree of dehydration, indicated by loss of skin turgor, dry mouth, sunken fontanelle, sunken eyes and deep, rapid (acidotic) breathing. The child should be weighed; if a recent weight is

Table 10. *Degrees of dehydration*

Signs/symptoms	Mild (<5%)	Moderate (5–10%)	Severe (>10%)
Dry mouth	Slight	Present	Present+
Skin turgor	Normal	Reduced	Reduced+
Eyes	Normal	Sunken	Sunken+
Fontanelle	Normal	Normal	Sunken
Tachypnoea	Normal	Increased	Increased+
Tachycardia	Normal	Increased	Increased+
Oliguria	None	Present	Nil passed
Acidotic	No	Slight	Usually present
Conscious state	Normal	Drowsy	May be comatose
Skin perfusion	Normal	Normal	Poor

known this should also be noted. Dehydration is assessed as mild (less than 5%), moderate (5–10%) or severe (greater than 10%). Table 10 shows how to assess the degree of dehydration by signs and symptoms.

Clinical assessment of degree of dehydration

Dehydration is not detectable clinically below 5%, which is equivalent to a fluid deficit of 50 ml kg^{-1}. Dehydration may be isotonic, hyponatraemic or hypernatraemic. If isotonic dehydration is present there has been equal loss of water and electrolytes. In hypotonic dehydration, more electrolytes than water have been lost; in hypernatraemic dehydration, the predominant loss has been of water. Hypernatraemic dehydration should be suspected in a child with a 'doughy' feel to the skin, and in a patient with neurological signs such as convulsions, neck stiffness and marked irritability (usually in the absence of circulatory collapse). Normal water and electrolyte requirements need to be known before fluid loss and replacement can be assessed. These requirements are shown in Table 11.

Table 11. *Normal water and electrolyte requirements in children*

Body weight	Fluid requirement (ml kg^{-1}) per day	per hour	Sodium (mmol kg^{-1} per day)	Potassium (mmol kg^{-1} per day)
First 10 kg	100	4	2–4	1.5–2.5
Second 10 kg	50	2	1–2	0.5–1.5
Subsequent kg	20	1	0.5–1	0.2–0.7

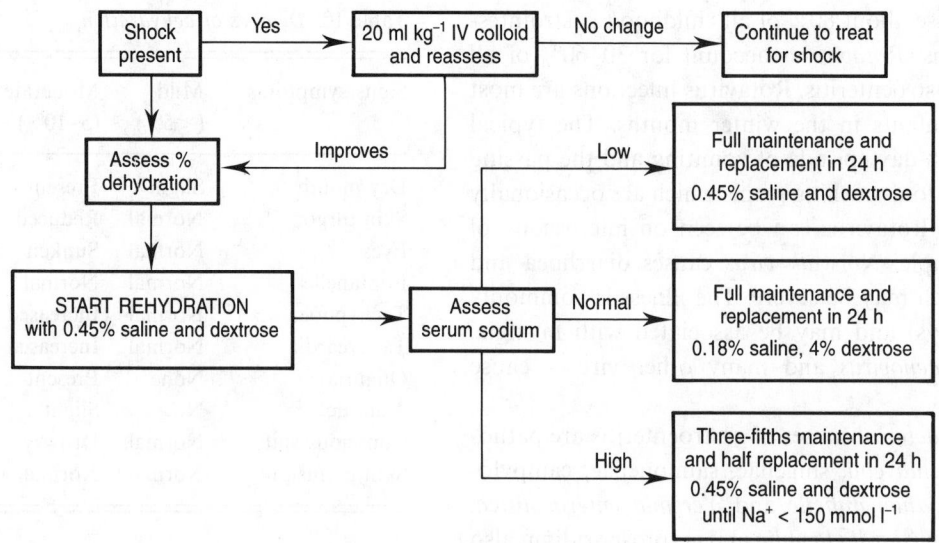

Fig. 2. Initial rehydration therapy in children with gastroenteritis. (Courtesy of Advanced Paediatric Life Support (UK); Advanced Life Support Group.)

Management

Treatment consists of replacing fluid and electrolytes. In most cases increasing oral fluids will suffice. The use of ORS (oral rehydration salts) should be encouraged (Table 12).

Oral fluids should be given little and often. Breastfeeding should be continued. Recent studies have shown no disadvantage to continuing other feeds (Hafferejee, 1993) but in most cases where nutrition is not an acute problem it often helps to stop all other fluids and solids and gradually reintroduce them after 12–24 h. Milk should be reintroduced at quarter strength and, if tolerated, rapidly increased to full strength. The child who is moderately or severely dehydrated needs to be admitted to hospital. Intravenous access must be secured and blood samples sent for full blood count, urea and electrolytes, and blood culture. Intravenous fluid and electrolyte replacement must be calculated. If the child is in shock, plasma or colloid should be administered at $20 \, \text{ml kg}^{-1}$ and the child reassessed. If the situation is stable, fluids should be replaced as:

- Replacement fluid.
- Maintenance fluid.
- Continuing losses.

Replacement fluids are calculated by the formula: Percentage dehydration × weight × 10. Thus a 10 kg infant who is 7.5% dehydrated requires the replacement of 750 ml. In all types of dehydration the deficit is mainly extracellular fluid loss and should be replaced as 0.9%

Table 12. *Electrolyte content of reconstituted oral rehydration salts (mmol l^{-1})*

	Sodium	Potassium	Chloride	Bicarb-onate	Glucose
Glucolyte	35	20	37	18	200
Rehidrat	50	20	50	20	91
Dioralyte	60	20	60	0	90
WHO solution	90	20	80	0	111

sodium chloride solution. Maintenance fluids are best replaced as 0.18% sodium chloride in 4% dextrose. However, in practice, 0.45% sodium chloride with 2.5% dextrose can be used for the first 24 h. Once urine is passed, 20 mmol of potassium should be added to every 500 ml of infusion fluid to replace potassium losses. In isotonic or hypotonic dehydration maintenance and replacement fluids are replaced over 24 h. In hypernatraemic dehydration it is dangerous to reduce the serum sodium level too quickly; thus replacement fluid should be given over 48 h and maintenance calculated for the first 24 h as three-fifths of the normal requirement (Fig. 2). Acidosis will usually improve with correction of dehydration and electrolyte loss. If the child is profoundly acidotic (pH less than 7.1) despite fluid replacement, sodium bicarbonate should be given as $1 \, \text{mmol} \, l^{-1}$.

The use of drugs in gastroenteritis

Antibiotics should only be used for invasive dysentery (co-trimoxazole) or for cholera. Erythromycin is sometimes used in prolonged or severe cases of campylobacter gastroenteritis. Antiparasitic drugs are used for amoebiasis (metronidazole 10 mg kg^{-1} t.d.s. for 10 days) and giardiasis (metronidazole 5 mg kg^{-1} t.d.s for 5 days).

"Antidiarrhoeal drugs and antiemetic drugs should never be used. There is no evidence that kaolin and pectin reduce the duration or severity of diarrhoeal illness; they do not reduce fluid or electrolyte losses and may interfere with efficacy of antibiotics where these are indicated." (World Health Organization, 1990)

URINARY TRACT INFECTIONS

The urinary tract is a common site for bacterial infections in childhood. Between 1% and 2% of all girls, 5% of school girls and nearly 1% of boys will acquire at least one urinary tract infection. Below the age of 6 months, boys and girls are equally affected.

An infection results from colonization and then invasion of the urinary tract by normal bowel commensal bacteria. *Escherichia coli* causes more than 90% of infections; *Proteus mirabilis, Enterococcus faecalis, Klebsiella aeruginosa* and pseudomonas infections are usually associated with urinary outflow obstruction or previous urinary surgery. Most bacteria gain access up the urethra but, in infants, infections are commonly bloodborne. In 90% of reinfections 'new' organisms are found, suggesting a host susceptibility to infection and not bacterial resistance (Smellie & Normand, 1992).

The urinary tract is kept free of infection by flushing and voiding. Urine stasis predisposes to infection (Table 13). Poor fluid intake or local genital irritation (e.g. with bubblebath salts or threadworms) can lower defences against urinary tract infection.

An infection is defined as a bacteriuria of 10 cfu (colony-forming units) ml^{-1} in a midstream specimen of urine, or bag specimen, and any growth from a properly taken suprapubic tap or catheter specimen. Urinary tract infections (UTIs) are accompanied by pyuria (>50 white cells ml^{-1}) and microscopic or macroscopic haematuria.

Diagnosis

Clinical features

UTIs are difficult to diagnose in children. Urinary tract infections present differently in differing age groups. In *neonates* there may be excessive weight loss, prolonged jaundice, diarrhoea and vomiting, lethargy with or without fever.

Under 2 years of age, failure to thrive, poor feeding and so-called 'teething' are common presenting symptoms.

In *older children* dysuria, frequency, abdominal pain and urinary incontinence are more typical features of urinary tract infection. Thirty per cent of daytime enuretics and 2% of nocturnal enuretics aged 5 years have urinary tract infections on investigation (Hellström *et al.*, 1991). A thorough physical examination should include measuring the blood pressure, checking carefully for the presence of a palpable bladder, descending colon and kidneys. Any sick child may have a urinary tract infection and this important diagnosis needs to be excluded by investigation.

The differential diagnosis depends on the age group, but in older girls threadworms, vulvovaginitis, local chafing from wet pants and adherent labia with urinary dribbling must be considered. In any child, sexual abuse must be excluded.

Diagnosis

It is difficult to obtain a reliable specimen of urine.

In older children, a clean catch urine specimen can be collected. In younger children, bag collections are used. To lessen the likelihood of contamination and mixed growth culture (results that make interpretation difficult), it is important to:

- Clean the perineum with water and not with an antiseptic, which can cause irritation.
- Leave the urinary bag on for as little time as possible.

Table 13. *Causes of urinary statis*

- Mechanical outflow obstruction
  - — Stones
  - – Ureterocoele
  - – Urethral folds/valves
  - – Constipation
- Functional outflow obstruction
  - – Neuropathic e.g. spina bifida, cerebral palsy
  - – Inadequate bladder emptying
  - – Bladder instability
  - – Detrusor/sphincter dyssynergia
- Vesicouretic reflux

- If possible, the child should be up and about so that urine drops into the bottom of the bag and does not splash back on to the periurethral skin.
- Empty the bag into the sterile collection bottle by cutting a corner off the bottom of the bag and not by tipping the urine back through the opening.

A 'negative' bag specimen is an important finding. A pure growth on culture suggests a urinary tract infection; mixed growth results require repeating. A suprapubic aspiration specimen is the most reliable method of collection in infants. The procedure should be carried out only by a person experienced in the technique. A bag specimen should be collected first; a paediatrician may then decide to take a suprapubic aspirate. A catheter specimen taken by inserting a fine feeding tube (F5) into the bladder through the urethra should be avoided if possible because this procedure may *cause* an infection. It is *not* a technique of choice in an accident and emergency (A&E) department. In both suprapubic aspiration samples and catheter samples any bacteria seen or grown indicate the presence of infection.

Urine samples should be examined by microscopy and plated for culture and sensitivity as soon as possible. If delay is envisaged, the urine can be stored in a refrigerator at 4°C for up to 12 h before investigations are undertaken. Treatment should be started if microscopy of the unspun urine shows organisms or if there are more than 100 white blood cells per high-power field. Dipstick tests are available for the quick assessment of urine specimens. The dipstick nitrite test can demonstrate the presence of pathogenic bacteria on the basis of their property of converting nitrate to nitrite. False negative results will be found with enterococcal infections which do not split nitrate or when there has been insufficient incubation time in the bladder (i.e. if the child has frequency). The leucocyte esterase test indicates the presence of more than 10 leucocytes per mm^3. The presence of leucocytes alone is not a reliable indicator of infection. The nitrite and esterase tests combined have a good sensitivity and specificity for urinary infection. Proteinuria is a non-specific finding, being present in any febrile illness and many renal diseases. Haematuria has many causes other than infection of the urinary tract.

Haematuria

The most common cause of haematuria is a urinary tract infection but other causes must be excluded, especially in the presence of frank haematuria (Table 14).

Table 14. *Causes of haematuria*

Cause	Example
Infection	Bacteria
	Viral (especially adenovirus)
	Schistosomiasis
	Tuberculosis
Trauma	
Glomerular disease	
Stones	Urolithiasis
	Idiopathic hypercalciuria
Anatomical abnormalities	Pelviureteric junction obstruction
Tumours	Nephroblastoma
Exercise-induced	
Factitious	Münchausen by Proxy
Vascular	Renal vein thrombosis (especially in infants)
	Infarction
Haematological	Sickle cell disease
	Coagulopathies
Drugs	

UTIs are usually benign, but there is a risk of renal damage. It is difficult to be sure that a UTI in a child has only affected the lower renal tract. Smellie & Normand (1992) advise that, in any sick child with bacteriuria, renal involvement should be assumed when planning immediate treatment. Further investigations of the renal tract must be carried out to demonstrate underlying disorders such as vesicoureteric reflux or outflow obstruction that increase the risk of renal damage. UTI with vesicoureteric reflux is strongly associated with renal scarring and is the main cause of renal insufficiency and hypertension in childhood.

Management schemes (Table 15) have been suggested to help the clinician to minimize the number of expensive and invasive investigations necessary to identify disorders that may lead to renal damage (White, 1987; Rickwood *et al.*, 1992). These investigations, most of which are organized by the paediatrician, may be summarized briefly as follows:

- In all children, another urine sample should be examined after completing antibiotic treatment to ensure that the infection has cleared.
- All children should have an ultrasound scan of the

Table 15. *Suggested scheme for imaging of urinary tract infections* (adapted from Smellie & Normand, 1992)

This scheme is not exhaustive. Investigations will depend on availability. Rickwood *et al.* (1992) substitute radioisotope examinations for intravenous urography.

Age (years)	USS	AXR	DMSA scan	MCU	IVU
<1	+	+	+	+	+[a]
1–2	+	+	+	+	
2–7	+	+	+	+[b]	+[b]
>7	+	+			+[c]

USS, ultrasound renal tract – demonstrates obstruction. AXR, plain abdominal X-ray – demonstrates radio-opaque stones and special defects. DMSA, ^{99m}Tc dimercaptosuccinic acid scan – demonstrates renal function and scarring. MCU, micturating cystourethrography – demonstrates bladder structure and VUR. IVU, intravenous urography – comprehensive overview of renal tract.
[a] Needed if DMSA or urine abnormal.
[b] If recurrent UTIs, family history of vesicoureteric reflux or abnormal DMSA scan.
[c] If recurrent UTIs.

renal tract to exclude obstruction. A plain abdominal X-ray will identify most urinary calculi (90% of stones are radio-opaque).

- The younger the child the more extensive are the imaging investigations needed to exclude renal pathology. In older children further investigations will be necessary if the initial investigations are abnormal or clinical features such as fever and vomiting or repeated infections suggest upper renal tract disease.
- *There is a tendency for UTIs to recur*: 50% of urinary tract infections will recur within 1 year and 75% will recur within 2 years (Smellie & Normand, 1992).

Treatment

Neonates and infants will need intravenous antibiotics suitable for bacterial septicaemia (e.g. penicillin and gentamicin).

In older children, trimethoprim is the first antibiotic of choice but cephalosporins, nitrofurantoin and nalidixic acid are suitable alternatives. Nalidixic acid should not be prescribed in children under the age of 1 year as there is an increased likelihood of benign intracranial hypertension. Only children who are not well enough for home treatment should be admitted to hospital since there is a risk of nosocomial infection with drug-resistant

Table 16. *Antibiotics for treating urinary tract infections*

Age	Therapy (mg kg^{-1} day^{-1})	Prophylaxis (mg kg^{-1} day^{-1})
Neonates 5–7-day course	Benzylpenicillin IV 45–60 Gentamicin IV 3–6	
'Sick' children 5–7-day course	Cefuroxime IV 100–200 Cefotaxime IV 100–200	
'Well' children 3-day course	Trimethoprim PO 8 Nitrofurantoin PO 3 Nalidixic acid PO 25–50 Cefaclor PO 20 Cefadroxil PO 25	Trimethoprim 2 Nitrofurantoin 1 Nalidixic acid 12

Amoxycillin is widely used in the community for non-urinary tract infections and gut bacteria may be resistant to it.
IV, intravenous; PO, per os.

organisms in the hospital environment. Treatment is urgent as delay in starting treatment is associated with an increase in renal scarring. Table 16 suggests appropriate antibiotic treatment in UTIs.

Improvement should occur within 48 h of the start of chemotherapy, by which time microscopy, culture and sensitivity of the urine specimen should be available to help target treatment. Repeat urine sampling during and after treatment will show a resolving pyuria. Urine must be tested again after completion of treatment and referral made to a paediatrician for follow-up and further investigations. Local policy will dictate whether prophylactic antibiotics should be given after the first confirmed UTI by A&E staff or paediatricians. Parents must be advised of the importance of a good fluid intake, the need to get their child to empty the bladder frequently and efficiently and to seek medical advice should the child have any symptoms suggestive of a recurrence of infection. If the presence of threadworms or vulvovaginitis has predisposed to urinary tract infection these should be treated. Bubblebath salts or other irritants should be avoided.

MENINGITIS

Eighty per cent of patients with bacterial meningitis are children, the incidence being greatest in infants. This incidence has not declined in the past 40 years, but the mortality is lower. In 1985–87, the mortality in meningitis in the age group 1 month to one year was 5.4% compared with double that figure 20 years previously (Mellor, 1992). However, in neonates the mortality rate remains

19.8% (De Louvois *et al.*, 1991). The bacteria commonly causing neonatal meningitis are beta-haemolytic streptococcus, *Escherichia coli*, other Gram-negative bacteria and *Listeria monocytogenes*. In infants and children over 3 months of age, *Neisseria meningitidis*, *Streptoccoccus pneumoniae* and *Haemophilus influenzae* are the most common aetiological agents. In infants below 3 months of age, any of these bacteria may be found (Klein *et al.*, 1992). In neonates, meningitis is often a component of the clinical syndrome of septicaemia.

Meningitis is inflammation of the meningeal covering of the central nervous system. This inflammation leads to the appearance of *inflammatory cells* in the cerebrospinal fluid (CSF), *leakage of protein* across damaged capillary cells into the CSF, *loss of autoregulation of cerebral blood flow* with *raised intracranial pressure* and *brain oedema*. These effects may in part be mediated by cytokines released from mononuclear cells in the inflammatory exudate and by the inappropriate release of antidiuretic hormone.

Clinical findings

In *infants and young children* the signs and symptoms of meningitis are non-specific (refusal to feed, irritability, a 'far-away vacant look', high-pitched cry, and convulsions). Vomiting and fever are frequent symptoms. A tense fontanelle may be present but in dehydration this valuable sign may disappear. A bulging fontanelle, neck retraction or stiffness and positive Kernig's sign are features that occur late in bacterial meningitis. Papilloedema, also a late sign, appears in some patients. A petechial rash, though not pathognomonic of the disease, should be assumed to be due to meningococcal septicaemia.

An *older child* with meningitis may complain of headache, nausea, photophobia and neck pain. The child lies still, turns away from light and protects the extended neck from movement. Convulsions occur in 20–30% of children with meningitis (Rudd, 1992), usually in the early stages of the illness. Most convulsions are of short duration.

Raised intracranial pressure is the rule rather than the exception in children with acute bacterial meningitis. It is probably due to generalized cerebral oedema exacerbated in some cases by convulsions. A purulent exudate obstructing the flow of CSF may be an additional mechanism. Raised intracranial pressure is the direct cause of death in 30% of cases of fatal meningitis (Mellor, 1992). Cerebral herniation is found in 5% of children who die of bacterial meningitis. The signs of meningitis are therefore often signs of raised intracranial pressure, such as abnormal posturing, coma, seizures, irregular breathing, bradycardia, hemiparesis, or unequal pupils. The physical examination should be directed towards a full assessment of neurological signs, and also towards the identification of any possible source of infection or any evident cause for raised intracranial pressure.

Differential diagnosis

Acute hydrocephalus, posterior fossa tumours, cerebral abscess and subdural haematoma may present with signs of raised intracranial pressure. Herpes encephalitis and Reye's syndrome may also present a similar clinical picture. Patients with viral meningitis (Coxsackie, ECHO, mumps, polio, varicella) commonly have other physical signs which help in diagnosis, or have a typical history of prodromal illness. In tuberculous meningitis there is usually (not invariably) a history of gradually increasing neurological disability, and there may be a family history of tuberculosis.

Management

Bacterial meningitis is a medical emergency: delay in treatment will increase morbidity and mortality. The diagnosis is confirmed by typical findings in the CSF (raised protein level, lowered glucose concentration, pleocytosis, bacteria and/or bacterial growth on culture). However, a lumbar puncture is contraindicated in many circumstances:

- Convulsion within the preceding 30 min.
- Recent or current prolonged seizure.
- Coma.
- Septic shock or purpuric rash .
- Papilloedema.
- Abnormal posturing.
- Bradycardia.
- Raised blood pressure.
- Irregular or slow breathing.
- Fixed and dilated or unequal pupils.
- Absent doll's eyes reflex.
- Hemiparesis.

Intravenous antibiotic treatment should be started as soon as meningitis is suspected and after blood cultures and throat swabs have been taken. Throat swabs will identify *Haemophilus influenzae* and pneumococcal infections in 90% of patients with disease due to these organisms. In children with meningococcal meningitis the organism can be grown from throat swabs in 50% of cases (Mellor, 1992). A delayed lumbar puncture can be carried out 24–48 h after the start of treatment.

Table 17. *Normal cerebrospinal fluid values in children*

	Neonates	Infants and children
White blood cells (per mm^3)	<9 (60% PMN)	0
Glucose (mmol l^{-1})	>3	>2.5
Protein (mg ml^{-1})	<90	<40

PMN, polymorphonuclear neutrophils.
To correct CSF protein in a traumatic tap, subtract 1–1.5 mg ml^{-1} for every 1000 red blood cells ml^{-1}.

Table 18. *Antibiotic choices for treatment of bacterial meningitis* (Klein, 1992)

Age	Drug	Dose (mg kg^{-1} per day)
1/12–3/12	Ampicillin	200
	+Cefotaxime	200
Older infants and children	1. Cefotaxime or ceftriaxone	200 100
	2. Ampicillin and chloramphenicol	200 75–100

7-day course for *Neisseria meningitidis*.
10-day course for *Streptococcus pneumoniae* or *Haemophilus influenzae*.
15% of *Haemophilus influenzae* infections are resistant to ampicillin.

A CT (computed tomography) scan of the head will help in the differential diagnosis. Acute hydrocephalus, posterior fossa tumours, abscesses and haematomas may be demonstrated. In Reye's syndrome or herpes encephalitis the findings are non-specific. If herpes encephalitis is suspected, intravenous acyclovir (30–50 mg kg^{-1} per day) should be added to the treatment regimen. In many cases a lumbar puncture can be safely performed and the findings can only be interpreted if normal CSF values are known (Table 17).

The choice of antibiotics will depend on the likely causative bacterial pathogen. Table 18 suggests appropriate treatment for different age groups.

Some neonatal meningitis infections may require more prolonged treatment courses. Table 19 gives typical findings in different cerebro-spinal infections.

Dexamethasone (0.15 mg kg^{-1} per dose, 6 hourly for 4 days) has been shown to lessen the likelihood of sensory neural deafness following *Haemophilus influenzae* meningitis. It is most effective if given very early in the disease (Lebel *et al.*, 1988). Its use in other forms of bacterial meningitis is controversial. Care must be taken not to overload the child with fluid as this increases the likelihood of secondary cerebral oedema. Unless hypotension is present intravenous fluids should be kept to a minimum. Hypoglycaemia and convulsions must be treated promptly.

Prophylaxis

The immediate family and anyone who has had prolonged contact with a child with meningococcal meningitis or meningococcal septicaemia should receive a

Table 19. *Typical findings in cerebrospinal infections*

Condition	WBC per mm^3	Cell differential	Protein (mg ml^{-1})	Glucose (mmol l^{-1})
Acute bacterial meningitis[a]	100–>30 000 (N.B. <100 in EARLY disease)	Mostly PMN (Monocytes in *Listeria monocytogenes*)	>100	<2.5
Herpes encephalitis	Normally <500	Mostly lymphocytes (PMN in EARLY disease)	Slight increase or normal	Normal
Cerebral abscess	10–200	PMN or lymphocytes	>100	Normal
TB meningitis	50–500 (sometimes higher)	Lymphocytes (PMN in early disease)	>100	<2.5

[a] Findings are altered by partial treatment with antibiotics.
WBC, white blood cells; PMN, polymorphonuclear neutrophils.

2-day course of rifampicin. Hospital staff only require treatment if they have been in contact with the blood of a patient with meningococcal septicaemia, or who have been coughed over by the infected child. All contacts should have throat and nasal swabs taken before prophylaxis is given.

Prophylactic rifampicin doses for *Neisseria meningitis*:

- Under 1 year   Rifampicin 10 mg kg^{-1} (total daily dose) given 12 hourly for 2 days.
- 1–7 years   20 mg kg^{-1} (total daily dose) give 12 hourly for 2 days.
- 7–14 years   300 mg twice daily for 2 days.
- Adults   600 mg twice daily for 2 days.

In the case of a child with *Haemophilus influenzae* meningitis and household members under 5 years of age, all the family should be treated with a 4-day course of rifampicin (hospital staff and other contacts do not require treatment).

Prophylactic dose requirements for *Haemophilus influenzae*:

- Less than 1 year   10 mg kg^{-1} (total daily dose) given daily for 4 days.
- 1–7 years   20 mg kg^{-1} (total daily dose) given daily for 4 days.
- 7–14 years   300 mg daily for 4 days.
- Adults   600 mg daily for 4 days.

If a neonate is jaundiced, prophylactic treatment should be discussed with a pharmacist or microbiologist. A patient who is also taking oral contraceptives must be informed that rifampicin can interfere with the metabolism of the contraceptive drug: extra precautions should be advised for the remainder of their cycle. Rifampicin can impart a red colour to secretions, stools, urine, and even contact lenses. Patients or parents should be warned about this. Prophylaxis for contacts who are pregnant should be amoxycillin 500 mg t.d.s. for 5 days; rifampicin should not be given. *Haemophilus influenzae* B (HiB) vaccine is now part of the primary vaccination programme for children under the age of 2 years. It is hoped that this will lessen the severity and number of invasive *Haemophilus influenzae* infections in small children.

CONVULSIONS

A convulsion is an abnormal paroxysmal discharge of cerebral neurones.

Status epilepticus

This is a convulsion lasting for more than 30 min or a series of convulsions occurring so frequently that there is no recovery of consciousness between them. Status epilepticus is most commonly tonic/clonic in type. Between 1% and 5% of children with epilepsy, and 5–10% of children with febrile seizures, develop at least one episode of status epilepticus. Infants are particularly susceptible to status epilepticus, and it is in this age group that the incidence of neurological complications is greatest. Status epilepticus causes new neurological sequelae or cognitive problems in 9% of children (Maytal *et al.*, 1989).

Convulsions are less commonly fatal in children than in adults, but the mortality associated with status epilepticus lies in the range 3–20% (Appleton, 1993). Death may result from complications of the convulsion (airway obstruction, aspiration of vomit, overmedication) or from the underlying cause of the convulsion. Injury to the brain during status epilepticus may occur because of:

- The underlying disease, e.g. meningitis.
- Systemic complications of the convulsion, especially hypoxia, hypertension or metabolic acidosis.
- Direct neuronal cell damage from repetitive neuronal discharge.

During a generalized convulsion, cerebral metabolic rate is increased three-fold. The increased energy requirements of the brain are met by increased cerebral perfusion which results from increased sympathetic activity and the systemic release of catecholamines. Initially catecholamines produce peripheral vasoconstriction and increased systemic blood pressure; there is concomitant loss of autoregulation of cerebral blood flow which therefore increases. However, if the convulsions continue, the systemic blood pressure falls and cerebral blood flow decreases. Lactic acid accumulates, the blood/brain barrier breaks down, and cerebral oedema develops, leading to raised intracranial pressure. This in turn causes a further reduction in cerebral blood flow. Calcium enters brain cells, damaging the mitochondria and causing cell death. The sodium–potassium pump fails, causing leakage of potassium from the cells and further cell death. After 20–30 min of continuous convulsions, the brain shows evidence of ischaemia and oedema, and after 1–1.5 h irreversible damage may occur. Treatment is aimed at preventing this downhill spiral of energy/demand mismatch and progressive cell damage.

Common causes of status epilepticus

These depend on the age of the child.

Neonates
- Asphyxia (hypoxic-ischaemic encephalopathy).
- Intra- and periventricular haemorrhage.
- Metabolic dysfunction, e.g. hypoglycaemia, hypocalcaemia, hyponatraemia.
- Infection, e.g. congenital infections, septicaemia, meningitis.
- Cerebral malformations.
- Trauma.

Children
- Febrile convulsions (3 months to 5 years of age).
- Sudden reduction in antiepileptic medication.
- Trauma.
- Epilepsy.
- Infection, e.g. meningitis, septicaemia.
- Encephalopathy, e.g. Reye's syndrome.
- Poisoning.

Febrile convulsions

Febrile convulsions occur in 3% of children aged 3 months to 5 years who have no evidence of acute brain disease or chronic disorder. There is often a strong family history of convulsions. A simple febrile convulsion is generalized, short-lasting (<15 min, usually much shorter), not focal in nature and recovery is rapid and complete. A full neurological examination is normal, and postictal electroencephalography (EEG) done more than 1 week after the convulsion is normal. Thirty per cent of children with a febrile convulsion will have a recurrence, one-third of whom will have a third seizure; 2–5% of children with febrile convulsions will subsequently develop epilepsy. (Wolf, 1979).

All children having their first febrile convulsion need admission to hospital for evaluation and investigation. The parents will be frightened and need to be taught what to do should this happen again. In obtaining the history from parents of a child who is convulsing, particular attention must be paid to the following questions:

- Has the child used any drugs recently or regularly?
- Is the child a known epileptic or diabetic, or suffering from a chronic respiratory or cardiac disorder?
- Is there a precipitating cause such as fever, diarrhoea, vomiting, upper respiratory tract infection or trauma?

- Is there any possibility of poison ingestion?
- Has the child any evidence of a rash?
- Has the child suffered previous convulsions?
- Is there a family history of convulsions?

A brief description of this convulsive episode is then necessary.

Management of the convulsing child in the A&E department

Airway and breathing

An airway must be established and adequate oxygenation and ventilation ensured; 100% oxygen is given. The oropharynx must be sucked out as necessary. Bag and mask ventilation should be used if the child is hypoxic or not ventilating adequately. It may be necessary to proceed to intubation, although this is rare. An anaesthetist should perform this as rapid sequence induction and muscle relaxation will be necessary.

Circulation

Establish intravenous access, take blood samples and carry out an immediate BM stix test. If the blood glucose is below 3 mmol l^{-1}, give intravenous glucose 0.5 g kg^{-1} as a 25% solution. If there is no evidence of shock give minimal isotonic fluid ($2–3 \text{ ml kg}^{-1} \text{ h}^{-1}$ of 0.45% saline and 5% dextrose) to discourage cerebral oedema. Take the core temperature and if it is greater than 39°C give paracetamol 15 mg kg^{-1} rectally and take other antipyretic measures. Measure the blood pressure as soon as feasible.

Anticonvulsant drug therapy (Appleton, 1992b)

Give diazepam $0.3–0.4 \text{ mg kg}^{-1}$ IV slowly at the rate of 1 mg min^{-1}. If venous access is difficult diazepam can be given rectally (0.5 mg kg^{-1}). If there is no response within 10 min, repeat the same dose. If the convulsion is still not controlled, give paraldehyde 0.4 mg kg^{-1} rectally in arachis oil and at the same time give a loading dose of phenytoin (18 mg kg^{-1} IV). This should run in over 20 min. The drip fluid should be normal saline. Omit the loading dose if the child is already on phenytoin therapy but continue with the maintenance dose of 5 mg kg^{-1} in 24 h. When phenytoin is administered, the child must be monitored as phenytoin can cause arrhythmias, bradycardia and hypotension. If the convulsion is still not controlled, further drugs will be necessary and advice should be sought from a paediatric neurologist. Local protocols will dictate the next drug to be used. Pheno-

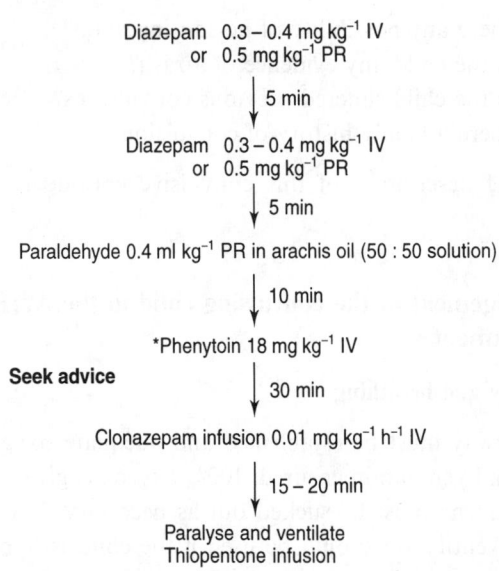

Diazepam   0.3 – 0.4 mg kg⁻¹ IV
or   0.5 mg kg⁻¹ PR

↓ 5 min

Diazepam   0.3 – 0.4 mg kg⁻¹ IV
or   0.5 mg kg⁻¹ PR

↓ 5 min

Paraldehyde 0.4 ml kg⁻¹ PR in arachis oil (50 : 50 solution)

↓ 10 min

Seek advice   *Phenytoin 18 mg kg⁻¹ IV

↓ 30 min

Clonazepam infusion 0.01 mg kg⁻¹ h⁻¹ IV

↓ 15 – 20 min

Paralyse and ventilate
Thiopentone infusion

* Avoid if already on phenytoin therapy and check serum phenytoin level.
Prepare phenytoin infusion as soon as paraldehyde is administered.

Fig. 3. Drug therapy for status epilepticus.

barbitone (loading dose 10–15 mg kg⁻¹ IV; maximum single dose 750 mg) can be used, but this drug will cause respiratory depression, especially in a child who has already received diazepam. The combination of phenobarbitone and diazepam should not be used in an A&E department without an anaesthetist standing by.

Further measures may be to induce barbiturate coma, but this requires a general anaesthetic with intubation, assisted ventilation and EEG monitoring. Paralysing a child will control the abnormal movements but will not suppress the neuronal discharges, and EEG monitoring is essential to monitor effective management of the convulsive episode. Throughout treatment continual reassessment of the metabolic state of the child (blood gases, acid–base levels, blood glucose levels) is necessary. Treatment must be directed not only at the convulsion but also at the underlying cause. The postictal state and anticonvulsant drugs may disguise neck stiffness and pupillary reflexes. In some patients a full search for bacterial sepsis is necessary.

A summary of drug therapy for status epilepticus is provided in Fig. 3.

Diazepam

Dose: 0.25–0.4 mg kg⁻¹ IV bolus given over 30–40 sec.
0.5 mg kg⁻¹ PR (e.g. Stesolid).
100–400 µg kg⁻¹ h⁻¹ by infusion.

This is an effective, quick-acting anticonvulsant, which takes effect within 5–10 min but whose action is short-lasting (about 40 min to 1 h). It has a depressant effect on respiration and this is enhanced by the addition of anticonvulsants such as phenobarbitone. Repeated doses make side-effects more marked. The rectal dose is well absorbed and acts almost as quickly as the intravenous dose.

Lorazepam

Dose: 0.05 mg kg⁻¹ IV bolus given over 30–40 sec.
0.1 mg kg⁻¹ PR.

This drug has a similar rapid action to diazepam but with a more sustained result, usually lasting 6–8 h. It causes little respiratory depression.

Paraldehyde

Dose: 0.4 ml kg⁻¹ PR, made up as a 50:50 solution in arachis oil.

This can cause rectal irritation, but intramuscular paraldehyde causes severe pain and may lead to sterile abscess formation.

Paraldehyde causes little respiratory depression. It should not be used in patients with liver disease or chronic respiratory diseases. Paraldehyde takes 10–15 min to act and its action is sustained for 2–4 h.

Do not leave paraldehyde standing in a plastic syringe for longer than a few minutes.

Phenytoin

Dose: 18 mg kg⁻¹ IV over 20–30 min.
Rate of infusion no greater than 1 mg kg⁻¹ min⁻¹.
Infusion to be made up in 0.9% sodium chloride solution to a maximum concentration of 1 mg in 1 ml.

Measure plasma phenytoin levels 90–120 min after the completion of the infusion. Phenytoin can cause arrhythmias and hypotension; an ECG monitor should therefore be used and the blood pressure should be checked regularly. Phenytoin has little depressant effect on respiration. Do not use parenteral phenytoin if the child is known to have been taking oral phenytoin until the blood level of phenytoin is known to be <2.5 µg ml⁻¹. Phenytoin has a peak action within 1 h but a long half-life that is dose-dependent. Its action is more sustained than that of diazepam; phenytoin is therefore useful in status epilepticus.

Thiopentone sodium

Induction dose: 4–8 mg kg^{-1}.

This is an alkaline solution which will cause irritation if it leaks into subcutaneous tissues. It has no analgesic effect and is a general anaesthetic agent. Repeated doses have a cumulative effect. It is a potent drug with marked cardiorespiratory effects and should be used only by experienced staff who can intubate a child. It is not an effective long-term anticonvulsant and its principal use in status epilepticus is to facilitate ventilation and the subsequent management of cerebral oedema due to the prolonged seizure activity. Other antiepileptic medication must be continued. A baseline EEG should be obtained as soon as possible after the child has been paralysed and ventilated.

Clonazepam

Dose: infusion of 10 µg kg^{-1} h^{-1}.

This anticonvulsant can cause hypersalivation and hypotonia. It has a marked respiratory depressant effect and should be used under specialist supervision, preferably in an intensive therapy unit.

Alternative anticonvulsant infusion regimens

These are available, but should only be tried if there is a recurrence of seizures after initial control of status and despite maximum rates of infusion of either diazepam or clonazepam. In decreasing order of preference these are infusions of chlormethiazole, paraldehyde, lignocaine.

The role of cerebral function analysis monitoring is as yet unclear. Clinical features and standard EEG are the preferred method of assessing seizure activity at present (Appleton, 1993). Additional treatments will depend on the clinical situation.

Investigations

Mandatory investigations for a child with status epilepticus are:

- Blood glucose.
- Plasma calcium and phosphate.
- Plasma magnesium.
- Full blood count.
- Plasma electrolytes.
- Urinalysis.
- Arterial blood gases.

Optional investigations depend on the history and examination and include:

- Toxicology.
- Screening for bacterial infection.
- Blood ammonia.
- Liver function tests.
- Metabolic screening.
- Clotting screen.
- Chest X-ray.
- CT scan.

Lumbar puncture should not be done in children with prolonged seizures or a Glasgow Coma scale score (GCS) of less than 13.

Monitor

Monitoring should include:

- ECG.
- Blood pressure.
- Pulse oximetry.
- Core temperature.
- Urine output.

Medical complications which may be associated infrequently with status epilepticus and which usually follow prolonged convulsions include cardiac arrhythmias, pulmonary oedema, disseminated intravascular coagulation, myoglobinuria and hyperthermia.

Differential diagnosis

Convulsions may be confused with other disorders with altered consciousness or abnormal movements (Appleton, 1992a).

Episodes with altered consciousness
- Syncope.
- Cyanotic breath-holding attacks.
- Pallid breath-holding attacks.
- Rigors and delirium.
- Migraine with an aura or confusion.
- Cardiac arrhythmias (especially supraventricular tachycardia).
- Night terrors.

Episodes without altered consciousness
- Jitteriness (especially in neonates).
- Tics or rhythmic motor habits.
- Rigors.

- Pseudoseizures.
- Cardiac arrhythmias.
- Gastro-oesophageal reflux (Sandifer's syndrome).
- Daydreaming.
- Benign myoclonus of infancy.
- Benign paroxysmal choreoathetosis.
- Benign sleep myoclonus of infancy.

Breath-holding attacks

There are two types of breath-holding attack:

1. *Cyanotic breath-holding attacks.* These are common in children under 5 years of age; they are usually precipitated by minor trauma or an emotional upset and frequently occur as part of a tantrum. The child seems to stop breathing in expiration and rapidly becomes cyanosed and may lose consciousness and fall limply to the ground. Shortly after this the attack ends or may be followed by a few clonic jerks. There is a rapid recovery which is complete. These attacks, although alarming, are harmless and will usually stop within the second year of life. No specific treatment is necessary or effective and careful calm handling of the child during a temper tantrum is the best way of dealing with these attacks.

2. *Pallid breath-holding attacks* (reflex anoxic seizure) occur in a similar way. They are often precipitated by minor trauma. The child suddenly becomes pale and limp and loses consciousness. There may be brief clonic jerking of the limbs and the whole episode is over within 0.5–1 min. The child appears lifeless and very pale during the episode. These episodes are caused by a reflex asystole due to increased vagal responsiveness and they appear to be familial in origin. No treatment is required unless they are very frequent, in which case atropine is effective (Stephenson, 1978).

Syncope or fainting

This is particularly common in young female teenagers and appears to be vasovagal in origin. Fainting attacks are often brought on by emotional upset, experiencing or hearing unpleasant things, or standing still for a long period of time. These girls have often not had breakfast before going to school. They can usually describe the feelings of coldness, sweating and light-headedness with difficulty in focusing their vision prior to losing consciousness. Friends say they went very white before falling very gently to the ground. This collapse is some-times followed by stiffening of the limbs and a few brief clonic jerks. Recovery is usually rapid and complete, but they may complain of nausea and a headache following a faint. A BM stix should be taken at the time that the child is seen and, if low, a sugary drink may make the child feel much better. If faints are frequent and do not respond to simple measures of sitting and eating normally, an ECG should be taken to exclude a cardiac arrhythmia or congenital abnormality such as prolonged QT syndrome.

COMA

The level of consciousness may be altered by disease processes, injury or poisoning. Common terms for different degrees of altered consciousness (*drowsiness, obtundation, stupor, coma*) are imprecise, and coma scores have therefore been developed to produce a semiquantitative measure of altered consciousness. The Glasgow Coma Scale can be used in children over the age of 4 years, and a modified version has been devised for use in younger children (Table 20).

Coma is caused by diffuse interference with brain cell function or metabolism. It is a sign of significant 'brain failure' and requires emergency treatment to prevent or minimize central nervous system (CNS) damage. In children, coma is usually caused by a toxic or metabolic process (95% of cases in temperate countries). Coma may also result from structural damage to the brainstem reticular activating system from compression or direct trauma to the brain.

The most likely causes of coma

- Hypoxic-ischaemic brain injury following respiratory or circulatory failure
- Epileptiform seizures
- Trauma – intracranial haemorrhage or brain swelling
- Infections – meningitis, encephalitis, intracranial abscess, cerebral malaria
- Poisons – especially opioids, tricyclic antidepressants, barbiturates, alcohol and carbon monoxide
- Metabolic – uraemia, hepatic failure, hypoglycaemia, dehydration (especially hyponatraemic), diabetes, Reye's syndrome, hypothermia and hypercapnia
- Vascular lesions – haemorrhage, embolus, arteriovenous malformations, arterial or venous thrombosis
- Hypertension

The management of coma is based on:

- Treating any treatable cause.

Table 20. *The Glasgow Coma Scale and its modified version for children*

Glasgow Coma Scale		Children's Coma Scale	
4–15 years		<4 years	
Eyes		*Eyes*	
Open spontaneously	4	Open spontaneously	4
Open to verbal command	3	React to speech	3
React to pain	2	React to pain	2
No response	1	No response	1
Best motor response		*Best motor response*	
Obeys verbal command	6	Spontaneous or obeys verbal command	6
Localizes pain	5	Localizes pain	5
Flexion withdrawal with pain	4	Withdraws in response to pain	4
Abnormal flexion with pain	3	Abnormal flexion with pain (decorticate posture)	3
Extension with pain	2	Abnormal extension with pain (decerebrate posture)	2
No response	1	No response	1
Best verbal response		*Best verbal response*	
Orientated and talking	5	Smiles, follows, interacts	5
Disorientated and talking	4	Crying, but consolably, inappropriate interaction	4
Inappropriate words	3	Crying, sometimes consolable, moaning	3
Inappropriate sounds	2	Inconsolable, irritable	2
No response	1	No response	1

- Preventing secondary brain damage from raised intracranial pressure (ICP) or from metabolic instability.

In infants with unfused cranial sutures, a gradual increase in intracranial volume can be accommodated by separation of the bones of the vault. However, rapid expansion in young children, or any increase in volume in a child whose cranial sutures are closed, will result in increased ICP. This increase in intracranial volume may be caused by brain swelling, intracranial haemorrhage or blockage of CSF drainage. Initially, the expansion is compensated by a reduction in the volume of venous blood and CSF within the cranium. When this limited compensating mechanism fails, ICP begins to rise. This leads to a fall in cerebral perfusion pressure (CPP), although CPP may be temporarily maintained by increased mean arterial pressure (MAP):

$$CPP = MAP - ICP$$

If cerebral perfusion pressure is reduced, cerebral blood flow is decreased. Normal cerebral blood flow is over 50 ml per 100 g brain tissue per min. If this falls below 20 ml per 100 g brain tissue per min, the brain will suffer from ischaemia. Increasing ICP may push brain tissue against rigid intracranial structures, causing clinical syndromes to develop which are recognizable by the site of localized brain compression.

Central syndrome

The whole brain is pressed down towards the foramen magnum and the cerebellar tonsils herniate through it ('coning'). Clinical signs include neck stiffness, a slowing pulse rate, rising blood pressure and irregular respiration which may lead to apnoea.

Uncal Syndrome

If the intracranial volume increase is mainly in the supratentorial space, the uncus (part of the hippocampal gyrus) is forced through the tentorial opening and pressed against the fixed free edge of the tentorium. If the pressure is unilateral (e.g. from a subdural or extradural haematoma), this leads to third nerve compression and an ipsilateral dilated pupil. Progressive pressure leads to external ocular motor palsies and a hemiplegia may then develop on either or both sides of the body.

History

> **Important points to note when obtaining the clinical history**
> - Any history of *injury* or recent *illness*
> - *Medications* used by the child or anyone else in the family
> - Does the child suffer from a *known chronic problem*, such as renal, cardiac or neurological disease or diabetes?
> - Has there been travel abroad recently?
> - When was the last meal taken?

Coma is of sudden onset in epileptic seizures, vascular accidents and poisoning. A slower onset suggests a metabolic disturbance or an intracranial mass lesion. Accompanying signs and symptoms such as headache, pain, sweating, fever, neck stiffness or a rash may help elicit the cause of coma.

Management of coma in children in the A&E department

Management can be divided into a primary and a secondary phase.

Primary phase

In the primary phase, the airway, breathing and circulation must be assessed and stabilized. Urgent treatable problems such as hypoglycaemia, infection, opioid overdose or raised intracranial pressure are treated.

Airway

The airway must be secured and maintained.

Breathing

High-flow 100% oxygen should be given by face mask. If breathing is shallow and inadequate, if there is no protective cough reflex or gag reflex, the Glasgow Coma Scale is less than 8 or there are signs of impending herniation (abnormal posturing, unequal pupils, fixed dilated pupils, irregular breathing pattern, papilloedema), *intubation* and *ventilatory support* will be needed.

Circulation

Intravenous access must be established. If there is evidence of shock, the blood pressure must be restored with fluids (20 ml of crystalloid or colloid per kg) and the child reassessed. If there is no response and no continuing blood loss from haemorrhage the central venous pressure should be monitored before further fluids are given. In the absence of shock there should be fluid restriction ($2 \, \text{ml} \, \text{kg}^{-1} \, \text{h}^{-1}$). This is to minimize the development of cerebral oedema. If significant hypertension is present, this should be treated. However, hypertension must not be treated aggressively because a fall in blood pressure may impair cerebral or renal perfusion; paediatric advice should be sought urgently before commencing treatment.

Other treatment

When an intravenous line has been established, all necessary blood samples should be taken. Blood glucose concentration should be measured at the bedside and, if hypoglycaemia is present (blood glucose less than 3 $\text{mmol} \, \text{l}^{-1}$), intravenous 25% glucose should be given immediately ($2 \, \text{ml} \, \text{kg}^{-1}$). If the history or clinical signs suggest the possibility of opioid ingestion, an intravenous bolus of naloxone ($10 \, \mu\text{g} \, \text{kg}^{-1}$) should be given. If this is unsuccessful the dose can be increased up to 100 μg kg^{-1} (maximum 2 mg per dose). Naloxone is short-acting; if a long-acting opioid such as methadone has been ingested, an infusion of naloxone will be required. Convulsions must be treated. If the temperature is greater than 39°C, paracetamol 15 mg kg^{-1} should be given rectally. Hypothermia should be treated with an overhead heater and blankets. If the child is stable at this stage, specific conditions may have been identified and treatment should be commenced; for example,

- Intravenous antibiotics for meningitis.
- Intravenous acyclovir for herpes encephalitis.
- Supportive and specific treatment for poisons.
- Management of diabetes.
- Intravenous antibiotics for meningococcal septicaemia.

Unless meningitis can be excluded by the clear identification of another cause for coma, antibiotic therapy should be commenced with intravenous penicillin and cefotaxime.

Monitoring

This should include:

- Pulse rate and rhythm.
- Respiratory rate and pattern.
- Core temperature.

- Pulse oximetry.
- Blood pressure.
- Fluid balance.
- Coma score.

Early investigation should include:

- Glucose.
- Electrolytes and urea.
- Calcium, magnesium, phosphate.
- Full blood count.
- Blood culture.
- Arterial blood gases.
- Chest X-ray.
- Toxicology.

If the situation is stable, a thorough investigation should be undertaken to find the cause of the coma. If, however, the situation remains unstable or is deteriorating, immediate aims are to maintain homeostasis and treat the treatable.

Clinical evidence of raised ICP must be sought. Absolute signs of raised ICP such as papilloedema, a bulging fontanelle and absence of venous pulsation in retinal vessels are late signs. These are often absent in acutely raised ICP. Abnormal decorticate and decerebrate posturing, which are stimulus-sensitive are suggestive of raised ICP. Positive oculocephalic reflexes (a test that should not be carried out in patients with neck injuries), variable pupillary abnormalities and abnormal breathing patterns suggest raised ICP.

Cushing's triad of a slow pulse, raised blood pressure and abnormal breathing pattern are very late signs of raised ICP.

Acutely raised ICP is an emergency and a paediatric neurologist or neurosurgeon should be consulted urgently. The following treatment should be commenced:

- The child's head should not be flexed unnecessarily.
- The head end of the bed should be elevated 30° above horizontal.
- The child should be paralysed, intubated and hyperventilated to keep the PCO_2 at 26–28 mmHg and PO_2 at >90 mmHg.
- Frusemide $1\,\mathrm{mg\,kg^{-1}}$ IV may be given. Mannitol 0.25–$0.5\,\mathrm{g\,kg^{-1}}$ IV should be given only after the child has been catheterized and anuria has been excluded. After giving mannitol, there may be a rebound increase in ICP after 2–3 h.
- Restrict fluids to two-thirds maintenance requirements.

Table 21. *Summary of pupillary changes* (APLS, 1993)

Pupil size and reactivity	Cause
Small reactive pupils	Metabolic disorders Medullary lesions
Pin-point fixed pupils	Metabolic disorders Narcotic/barbiturate/opioids Organophosphate ingestions
Fixed middle-size pupils	Midbrain lesions
Fixed dilated pupils	Hypothermia Severe hypoxia Barbiturates (late signs) During and post seizure Anticholinergic drugs Irreversible brain damage
Unilateral dilated pupil	Rapidly expanding ipsilateral lesion (e.g. subdural haematoma) Tentorial haematoma Third nerve nucleus lesion Epileptic seizures

Secondary phase of assessment and management

At this stage the findings of the first phase should be reassessed and efforts made to localize the site and cause of neurological dysfunction. Neurological examination should include examination of the eyes for deviation, reflex ocular movements, pupil size and reactivity (Table 21) and fundal changes. Fundal changes may demonstrate acute haemorrhage or papilloedema.

Signs of *lateralization* should be looked for in *posture* and *tone*, and in the assessment of deep tendon *reflexes* and plantar responses. The *coma score* should be reassessed regularly.

Specific points to include in the general physical examination are:

- There may be evidence of a rash, haemorrhage, trauma or evidence of neurocutaneous syndrome.
- Scalp – examination may demonstrate concealed trauma.
- Ears and nose – a bloody or clear discharge suggests a basal skull fracture. Otitis media may be the source of spreading infection.
- Neck tenderness, rigidity, or a tilt should be recorded.
- Odour – certain metabolic disorders and poisoning have a distinctive odour.
- Abdomen – the presence of an enlarged liver is suggestive of hepatic failure. A reduced area of percussion dullness over the liver may be found in acute hepatic necrosis.

The conclusions from a full examination may lead to further investigations, including:

- Toxicology screen.
- Liver enzymes.
- Blood ammonia.
- Urinary metabolic screen.
- CT scan.
- Blood smears for parasites.
- Chest X-ray.
- Store serum for further investigations.

Lumbar puncture is contraindicated until after neurological consultation.

Fig. 4 summarizes the management of coma.

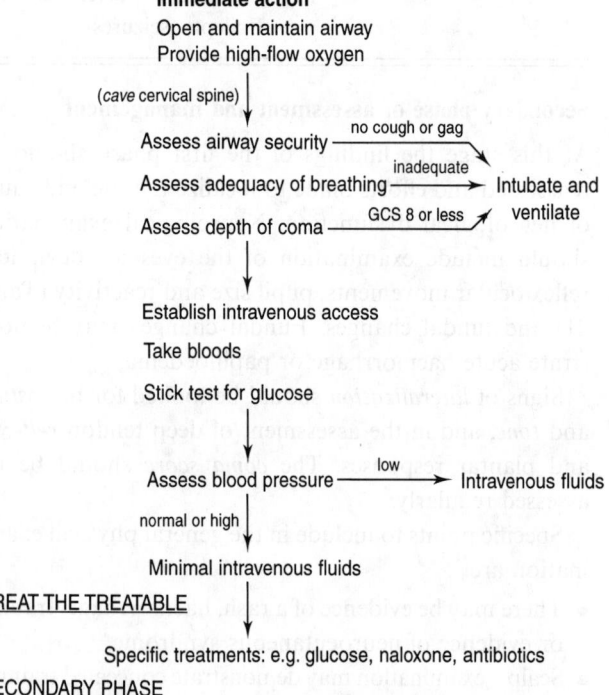

PRIMARY PHASE

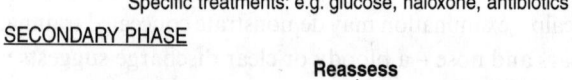

TREAT THE TREATABLE

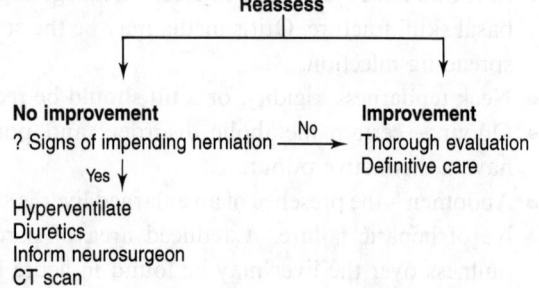

Fig. 4. Algorithm for the management of coma.

Table 22. *Common causes of cardiac failure*

Pump failure	Myocarditis
	Cardiomyopathies
Increased pulmonary blood flow	Ventricular septal defect
	Patent ductus arteriosus
	Atrioventricular septal defect
	Common arterial trunk
Outlet obstruction	Critical aortic stenosis
	Coarctation of the aorta
	Hypoplastic left heart syndrome
Arrhythmias	
Decreased systemic vascular resistance	Sepsis
	Anaphylaxis
	Arteriovenous fistula
Metabolic causes	Hypoxia
	Hypoglycaemia
	Hypocalcaemia
	Hypomagnesaemia
	Acidosis

CARDIAC EMERGENCIES

The clinician must be able to recognize the patient in whom either cardiac failure or shock is imminent. They must deal with life-threatening conditions and call for appropriate specialist help.

Cardiac failure may be due to intrinsic cardiac disease, arrhythmias and mechanical difficulties caused by congenital disorders, or to impaired cardiac function in septicaemia, severe anaemia or metabolic disturbance. Some common causes of cardiac failure are listed in Table 22.

Clinical manifestations

Infants in heart failure are unable to feed, and are sweaty and restless with rapid, grunting respiration. There may be evidence of failure to thrive. Older children complain of tiredness, are anorexic and have abdominal pain. They may have a cough. On examination, the peripheries are mottled and cool, respiration and heart rate are rapid; on auscultation there is often a cardiac gallop rhythm and basal crepitations in the lungs. Hepatomegaly is common in infants.

Urgent investigations include a full blood count, blood culture, electrolytes, chest X-ray and electrocardiographic (ECG) monitoring. If structural lesions are suspected an echocardiogram and urgent cardiac opinion are needed.

Management

General measures include giving 100% oxygen by face mask, and correcting anaemia, electrolyte abnormalities and hypothermia. Hypovolaemia must be corrected and intravenous broad-spectrum antibiotics given if sepsis is suspected. Cardiac arrhythmias (see below) require correct diagnosis and prompt treatment. If the systemic circulation is dependent on a patent ductus arteriosus, this should be kept open by the administration of intravenous prostaglandin E_2. The drugs used most commonly in heart failure are diuretics (frusemide, 1 mg kg^{-1}), digoxin and, in cardiogenic shock, inotropic agents.

Arrhythmias

The emergency recognition and management of arrhythmias depends on the answers to a few simple questions:

- Is the heart rate too fast or too slow?
- Is the rhythm regular or irregular?
- Is the QRS complex broad or narrow?
- Is the child's clinical condition stable or unstable?

A cardiac monitor using lead II or a full 12-lead ECG should be used to make the diagnosis.

Is the rate too fast?

Sinus tachycardia can cause a heart rate of up to about 230 beats min^{-1}. The rate is rapid but varies slightly. P waves are seen and precede each QRS complex, all of which are identical (Fig. 5). This tachycardia is caused by underlying fever, dehydration, pain or anxiety; and treatment should be directed to the underlying cause.

Supraventricular tachycardia (SVT) gives rise to a heart rate of 150–300 min^{-1} (mean 240 min^{-1}). The QRS

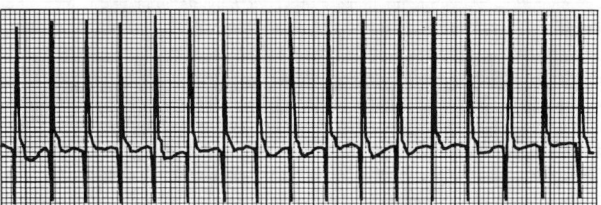

Fig. 6. Supraventricular tachycardia, rhythm strip. (Courtesy of Advanced Paediatric Life Support (UK); Advanced Life Support Group.)

complexes are identical and regular (Fig. 6); each is preceded by a P wave but this may not be identifiable due to the rapid heart rate. This rhythm has a sudden onset and may last from minutes to hours. Some children tolerate it well but infants usually present in heart failure or are irritable and screaming. SVT may degenerate into ventricular fibrillation. SVT is the most common primary cardiac arrhythmia in children. It results from an abnormal conductive mechanism that originates proximal to the bifurcation of the bundle of His but does not have the ECG features of atrial flutter. Commonly there is aberrant retrograde entry of electrical impulses through the atrioventricular node and an accessory pathway such as the bundle of Kent or James. A rapid rhythm is possible in children because the conducting tissues repolarize quickly. When the SVT has been treated and sinus rhythm restored, a Wolff–Parkinson–White phenomenon may be seen in the rhythm strip (this is a short PR interval with a slow delta wave upstroke to the beginning of the QRS complex). In a few children there is a short PR interval without a delta wave (Lown–Ganong–Levine syndrome), but most children have a normal ECG. In a few patients with SVT the QRS complexes are wide, but in an emergency it is safer to assume that all wide QRS complexes are ventricular in origin (Till & Shinbourne, 1991).

In *ventricular tachycardia* (VT) there are runs of three or more ectopic ventricular beats (Fig. 7). It is called sustained if lasting over 30 sec. The rate varies between 120 and 300 beats min^{-1}. The QRS complexes are wide

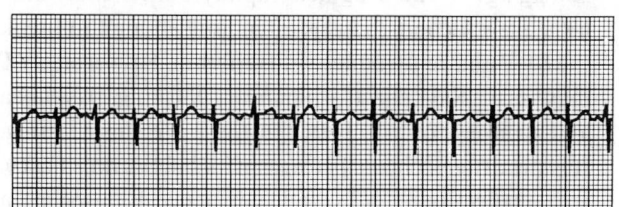

Fig. 5. Sinus tachycardia, rhythm strip. (Courtesy of Paediatric Life Support (UK); Advanced Life Support Group.)

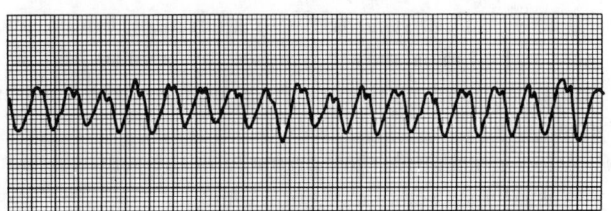

Fig. 7. Ventricular tachycardia rhythm strip. (Courtesy of Advanced Paediatric Life Support (UK); Advanced Life Support Group.)

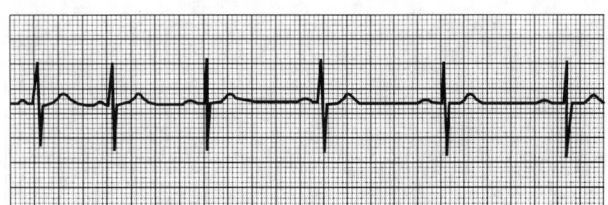

Fig. 8. Bradycardia invoked by pharyngeal stimulation. (Courtesy of Advanced Paediatric Life Support (UK); Advanced Life Support Group.)

and almost regular. However, in children, the complexes are not necessarily grossly widened. A helpful sign is the presence of fusion or capture beats (Till & Shinbourne, 1991). There are no preceding P waves as the QRS complexes arise from within the ventricles. VT is rare in children. It may be caused by myocarditis, cardiomyopathy or cardiac surgery. Systemic causes are poisoning with drugs that prolong the QT interval (e.g. procainamide, quinidine), or with tricyclic antidepressants, or phenothiazines. VT may occur in hypocalcaemia or hypomagnesaemia and in rare congenital conduction disorders such as Romano–Ward and Jervell–Lange–Neilson syndromes in which the QT interval is prolonged. The onset of VT is sudden and there may be rapid deterioration into ventricular fibrillation.

Is the rate too slow?

Bradyarrhythmias are often the final response to hypoxia and acidosis and herald cardiac arrest.

Sinus bradycardia is a slow heart rate which is variable (Fig. 8). The QRS complexes are normal, identical and preceded by P waves. Heart rates below 100 in an awake infant, 80 in an under 5-year-old child and 60 in a child over 5 years of age are abnormal. Fit athletic adolescents often have a slow heart rate. Bradycardia may be caused by raised intracranial pressure, vagal stimulation such as pharyngeal suctioning, acidosis, hypoxia, hypercalcaemia, hypoglycaemia or hypothermia. Digitalis and propranolol poisoning may also cause a bradycardia.

The *sick sinus syndrome* with alternating brady- and tachyarrhythmias may be caused by myocarditis, hypoxia, cardiomyopathies or direct injury to the heart as in surgery.

Idioventricular rhythms originate in the ventricles and are usually slower than 40 beats min^{-1}.

Heart block causes bradycardia. This may be congenital or acquired and may be complete or incomplete.

Are the QRS complexes narrow or wide?

Narrow complexes arise in the atria; broad QRS complexes sometimes arise through aberrant conduction but most commonly arise from within the ventricles. The complexes are wide because ventricular myocardium depolarizes slowly.

Management of arrhythmias

The pulse rate, blood pressure and cardiac rhythm must be monitored continuously. An intravenous or intraosseous line must be established. DC shock must not be delayed to achieve vascular access in a shocked or pulseless child. Treatment depends on the rhythm, rate and complex type and on whether the child is stable or unstable.

Sinus tachycardia

This requires no specific treatment. Management should be directed towards the underlying cause.

Stable supraventricular tachycardia

In the infant who is not in shock, vagal stimulation with continuous cardiac monitoring should be attempted. A diving reflex may be elicited which, by raising vagal tone and slowing atrioventricular conduction, may interrupt the tachycardia. A baby should be held firmly, wrapped in a towel and the whole face immersed for 3–5 sec in cold water. The baby will be temporarily apnoeic (there is no need to occlude the nose or mouth). In an older child ice cubes in a cloth are placed on the nose and mouth, or one-sided carotid body massage is given. An older cooperative child can try a Valsalva manoeuvre and some children with recurrent SVT know that a certain position or action will usually effect a return to sinus rhythm. If these manoeuvres are unsuccessful drugs may be used.

- Intravenous or intraosseous *adenosine* may be given starting with a bolus of 50 µg kg^{-1} and increasing the dose by 50 µg kg^{-1} every 2 min to a maximum of 500 µg kg^{-1}. The drug acts rapidly but its effect only lasts a few seconds. This is often long enough to break the SVT and reintroduce sinus rhythm. However, SVT may recur. Side-effects are nausea, flushing, dyspnoea and tightness of the chest, but these are short-lasting. It is the drug of choice because of its safety and efficacy. It is ineffective in VTs and can hence be used as a diagnostic tool if the origin of a tachycardia is unknown.

- *Verapamil* should not be used in children under 1 year of age. It can cause hypotension and asystole. It should not be used if beta-blockers have been given already. The intravenous dose in 1–5-year-olds is $15 \, \mu g \, kg^{-1}$ IV slowly, and $50 \, \mu g \, kg^{-1}$ in 5–10-year-olds. In 10–15-year-olds, $100 \, \mu g \, kg^{-1}$ is given. As soon as sinus rhythm is restored the administration of the drug should be stopped.
- Intramuscular *digoxin* may be used to control SVT; $10 \, \mu g \, kg^{-1}$ 8-hourly for 24 h is given, then reducing to $4 \, \mu g \, kg^{-1}$ every 12 h (maximum $250 \, \mu g$ per dose). Digoxin must not be used until Wolff–Parkinson–White syndrome is excluded as it may increase conduction through the accessory conduction pathway and precipitate ventricular fibrillation.
- *Propranolol* $10–15 \, \mu g \, kg^{-1}$ can be given by slow intravenous injection. This drug should not be used if verapamil has been prescribed as asystole may occur and pacing be required.
- *Flecainide* is negatively intropic and proarrhythmic. It exerts a profound effect on the retrograde conduction in an accessory connection. It should only be used by those familiar with its use.

Unstable supraventricular tachycardia

If SVT has resulted in a state of clinical shock, cardioversion must be used to attempt to restore sinus rhythm quickly. Apply a synchronized DC shock, $0.5–1 \, J \, kg^{-1}$ body weight, increasing to $2 \, J \, kg^{-1}$ if this is unsuccessful. Recurrent arrhythmias should be treated with the lower electrical charge. Intravenous adenosine may be used as an alternative to electrical cardioversion if vascular access is already established. DC shock should be used without delay if intravenous access is not available.

Fig. 9 shows an algorithm for the management of SVT.

Stable ventricular tachycardia

Stable VT is treated with intravenous lignocaine $0.5–1$ $mg \, kg^{-1}$ as a bolus followed by an infusion of $10–50 \, \mu g$ $kg^{-1} \, min^{-1}$. If this is ineffective, amiodarone $5 \, mg \, kg^{-1}$ over 2 h in 5% dextrose may be successful. Phenytoin $20 \, mg \, kg^{-1}$ as a loading dose in normal saline over 20 min followed by $5 \, mg \, kg^{-1}$ per day is especially useful in tricyclic antidepressant-induced VT.

Unstable ventricular tachycardia

The patient requires non-synchronized shock at $0.5–1.0$ $J \, kg^{-1}$ followed by a bolus and infusion of lignocaine. If

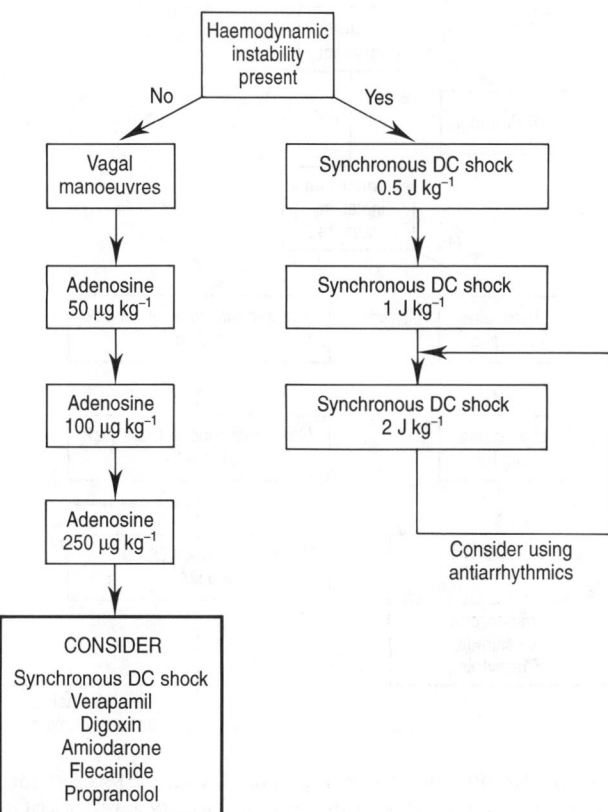

Fig. 9. Algorithm for management of supraventricular tachycardia. (Courtesy of Advanced Paediatric Life Support (UK); Advanced Life Support Group.)

lignocaine is unsuccessful, phenytoin or amiodarone should be used.

Fig. 10 is an algorithm for the management of VT.

Bradycardia in neonates

Bradycardia of less than 60 beats min^{-1} in a newborn usually responds to oxygen, ventilatory support and external cardiac compressions. If these are unsuccessful, adrenaline $10 \, \mu g \, kg^{-1}$ is given. (Atropine is not effective in this age group.)

Bradycardia in an unstable child

Bradycardia is usually caused by underlying hypoxia and acidosis which must be corrected with oxygen and ventilation and volume expansion. If these measures are ineffective a bolus of intravenous adrenaline, $10 \, \mu g \, kg^{-1}$, or an infusion of isoprenaline, $0.02–0.2 \, \mu g \, kg^{-1} \, min^{-1}$, is given. Atropine, $0.02 \, mg$ IV (minimum $0.1 \, mg$, maximum $2.0 \, mg$, per dose) may help. Cardiac pacing should be considered if other measures are unsuccessful.

Fig. 11 is an algorithm for the management of bradycardia.

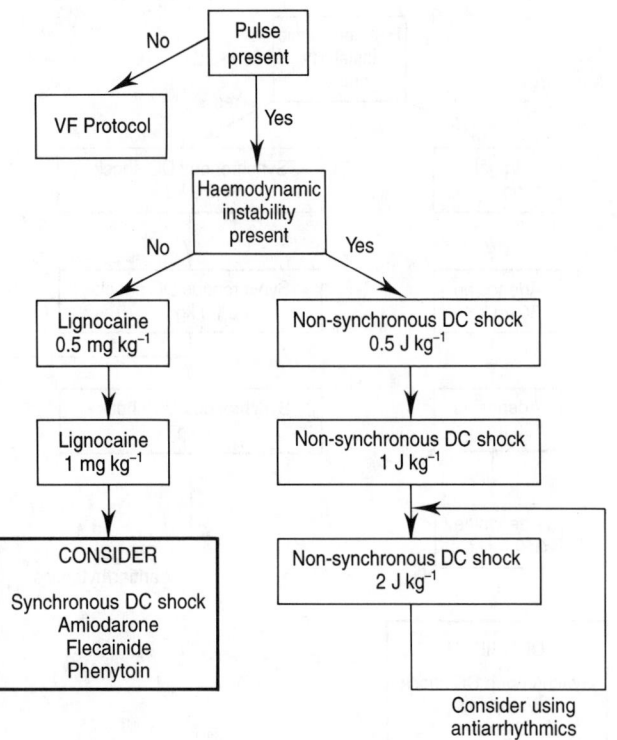

Fig. 10. Algorithm for the management of ventricular tachycardia. (Courtesy of Advanced Paediatric Life Support (UK); Advanced Life Support Group.)

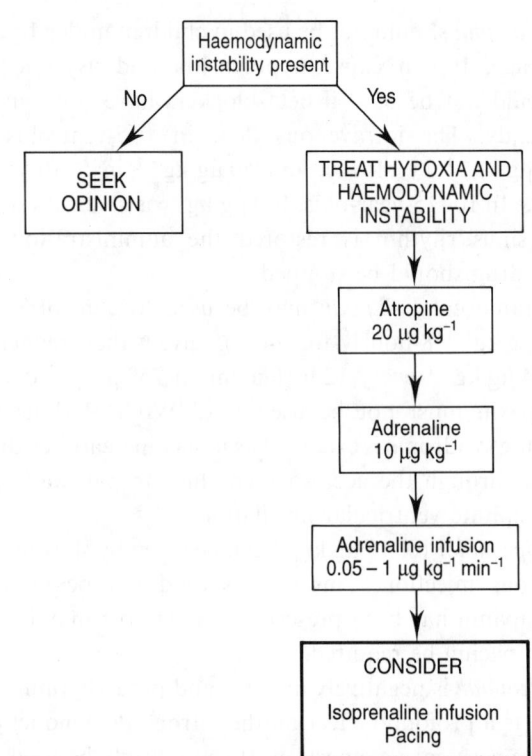

Fig. 11. Algorithm for the management of bradycardia. (Courtesy of Advanced Paediatric Life Support (UK); Advanced Life Support Group.)

Duct-dependent systemic circulation

The ductus arteriosus normally closes within 24 h of birth. However, in some cardiac congenital abnormalities this is delayed. When the patent ductus arteriosus does close the child may present with sudden heart failure and cyanosis. Duct-dependent disorders may be due to inadequate pulmonary blood flow (e.g. tricuspid atresia, severe Fallot's tetralogy and critical pulmonary stenosis), or when there is marked intracardiac mixing of pulmonary and systemic circulations as in transposition of the great vessels, or if there is outlet obstruction as in aortic atresia, coarctation of the aorta or hypoplastic left heart syndrome.

Babies with inadequate pulmonary circulation may present in the first few days of life with breathlessness, cyanosis and shock. When there is a duct-dependent systemic circulation due to outlet obstruction, the baby will have difficulty feeding, become grey, clammy and peripherally shutdown. Femoral pulses will be impalpable or very thready.

Management

These babies need prompt treatment with prostaglandin E_2 infusion $0.5 \, \mu g \, kg^{-1} \, min^{-1}$ to maintain a patent ductus arteriosus. Intubation and assisted ventilation will be necessary on transfer to a neonatal unit. High concentration of oxygen precipitates the closure of the duct. Nevertheless these babies are hypoxic and should be given oxygen and ventilated as the clinical situation and pulse oximetry dictate. Hypothermia must be avoided, and hypoglycaemia and electrolyte imbalance and acidosis corrected.

Cyanotic spells

Children with Fallot's tetralogy may develop acute episodes of cyanosis due to sudden reduction in pulmonary blood flow from right ventricular infundibulum spasm. The child or baby appears pale or cyanosed as deoxygenated blood is diverted through a septal defect or patent ductus arteriosus to the systemic circulation. Attacks may be self-limiting or fatal. Treatment consists of 100% oxygen by face mask and intravenous morphine, $0.2 \, mg \, kg^{-1}$. If this is ineffective propranolol, $0.1 \, mg \, kg^{-1}$ IV is usually successful.

Hypertensive crises

Hypertension is uncommon in children. Blood pressures are not routinely recorded in childhood and a child may present in hypertensive crisis. The causes are numerous:

- Haemolytic uraemic syndrome.
- Glomerulonephritis.
- Renal vascular disease.
- Renal arterial embolism (neonates).
- Chronic renal failure.
- Phaeochromocytoma.
- Lupus erythematosus.
- Essential hypertension.

In children hypertension is often secondary to renal disease.

Clinical findings

Headaches, convulsions and coma occur due to raised intracranial pressure; focal neurological abnormalities are not infrequent. Nausea and vomiting, poor urine output and evidence of congestive cardiac failure are found. Fundoscopic examination will show retinal haemorrhages and papilloedema.

The blood pressure is greater that the 95th percentile for age and sex and it must be checked several times with the correct arm cuff size.

Management

Blood pressure must be reduced very slowly and with extreme caution. Sudden drops in blood pressure are associated with increased mortality and morbidity (Deal et al., 1992). The diastolic blood pressure should be reduced to the upper limit for age and sex over 3 days (120 diastolic if less than 5 years; 130 diastolic if greater than 5 years). Do not treat without consulting a paediatric nephrologist who may request transfer prior to treatment, in which case intravenous access should be established. A nephrologist may request sublingual nifedipine to give temporary relief prior to transfer.

If the child is in coma with raised ICP, urgent ventilation and diuretics will be required and specialist consultation is necessary.

Suitable drugs to reduce the blood pressure are labetalol $1-3 \, mg \, kg^{-1} \, h^{-1}$ IV, or sodium nitroprusside $0.5-8 \, \mu g \, kg^{-1} \, min^{-1}$. The drugs are given by infusion and the rate titrated against the blood pressure (Deal et al., 1992). If the blood pressure falls too rapidly the infusion of the drug is stopped and boluses of normal saline are given until the blood pressure is restored to the level required. The blood pressure needs to be monitored continuously.

A full blood count and differential, urea and electrolytes and creatinine must be checked urgently.

SUDDEN INFANT DEATH SYNDROME

Sudden infant death syndrome (SIDS) is defined as 'the sudden death of an infant or young child which is unexpected by history, and for which a thorough postmortem examination fails to demonstrate an adequate cause'. The diagnosis cannot be made without autopsy. SIDS must not be presumed when a dead baby is brought into an A&E department. Some other unexpected causes of death are overwhelming sepsis, meningitis, myocarditis, intracranial haemorrhage, pertussis and non-accidental injury. SIDS is a diagnosis of exclusion. It is the leading cause of death in postneonatal infants in Britain (Table 23).

The incidence of SIDS in the general population is 2 per 1000 live births and appears to be decreasing. How much this is due to changes in baby care, and how much to developments in postmortem diagnosis and reporting, is difficult to measure (Wigglesworth et al., 1987). There are certain factors that increase the risk of sudden infant death: low birth weight, previous infant death in the family, maternal smoking, maternal drug addiction, and a previous apparent life-threatening event. The babies of young mothers in social classes IV and V are at increased risk. Various studies have suggested that sleeping in the prone position is significantly more common in children who subsequently have a cot death and that the supine sleeping position is less common in such infants (Beal, 1988). Mothers are now advised not to put their babies

Table 23. *Common causes of death by age group* (England & Wales; OPCS, 1991)

In parentheses, percentage of total in each age group.

	Age group		
	4–52 weeks	1–4 years	5–14 years
SIDS	880 (42)	0 (0)	0 (0)
Congenital abnormality	349 (18)	194 (20)	116 (10)
Infection	279 (13)	143 (15)	59 (5)
Trauma	86 (14)	211 (22)	382 (34)
Neoplasm	16 (1)	118 (12)	237 (21)
Other	276 (12)	290 (31)	337 (30)

down to sleep in the prone position (Chief Medical Officer 1991). Department of Health figures show a 55% reduction in SIDS between 1991 and 1992 (The Economist, 1993). Overheating a sleeping child is also associated with sudden infant death (Fleming *et al.*, 1990). Overlying a child in bed is very rare and usually occurs when a parent has been drunk or drugged (Bass *et al.*, 1986). Geographical differences in the incidence of SIDS (e.g. there is a lower incidence in Asian infants than Caucasian infants) may have both a cultural and a genetic basis.

Clinical findings

Sudden infant death is most common between the ages of 2 and 8 months with the peak at 3 or 4 months; in rare cases it has occurred in the second year of life (Brooks, 1990). It is most common in the winter months, in males, and there is often a history of minor upper respiratory tract infection which can be identified at postmortem but has not been implicated as the cause of death. Death usually occurs at night, unobserved, apparently in sleep, and the death is discovered in the early hours of the morning. The baby may have been dead for several hours and appear pale with postmortem lividity. If the death is recent, the baby is warm. In most cases the bedclothes are undisturbed and death appears to have been quiet and quick. In others, the bedclothes are disturbed as in a terminal struggle or convulsion. Sometimes milk and food have regurgitated into the mouth, sometimes there is frothy blood-stained mucus at the nose and lips (Sibert & Davies, 1992).

Management

A baby suspected of sudden infant death must be taken straight to resuscitation and quickly examined for signs of life. If any sign is present, full resuscitative measures must be taken. Unfortunately, in most cases the baby is obviously dead and it is pointless to start token resuscitation attempts. In this situation the baby should be fully examined for evidence of the cause of death (rash, dehydration, bruising). The rectal temperature should be recorded, and the baby's clothes should be carefully kept in a hospital bag as these will be required by the police. Swabs for microscopy, culture and sensitivity should be taken from the nose, throat, ears and rectum. There should be an agreed policy as to which other specimens (blood, skin snips, urine, CSF) should be taken for the attention of the local pathologist. As long as there are

no suspicious circumstances, the baby should then be dressed in clean clothes and put into a baby snug. A photograph should be taken of the baby and kept in the notes. This can be given to the parents at a later date if they have no suitable baby pictures and desire one. The parents and family can hold the baby in the baby snug; the wrapping disguises the lack of body warmth.

All the time the baby is being cared for, the parents should be with an experienced senior nurse or social worker in a quiet room. It helps if the room is near to the resuscitation department and has a small sofa in it where parents can sit close and comfort one another. When the most senior doctor involved in the care of the family has confirmed that the baby cannot be resuscitated, he or she should give the bad news to the parents. It is better if this is done to both parents together. It is important to be gentle and clear; euphemisms for death are unhelpful. Nothing makes bad news any better, but such devastating news should be given as gently and sympathetically as possible. It may help to sit or crouch down beside a mother or father so that news is not delivered standing over them. It is important to use the baby's name and explain how sorry one is but that nothing could have been done to alter the outcome.

The news is not often unexpected. Reactions are as variable as people and any reaction is legitimate. The news may cause numbness, an inability to take it in, or wild anger and loud grief. The parents will need time by themselves, time with a member of staff and, most importantly, time with their baby. Slowly and gently it is important to obtain a clear history of the past few days and hours. When was the baby last seen? Was the baby well? The past history and family history should be thorough. Record the baby's date of birth and address at which the death occurred. History-taking cannot be hurried. Parents should be encouraged to hold their baby and say a proper goodbye. There is often fear of this, but with gentle encouragement most parents are glad to be able to hold their baby. It is a precious memory for them. There are no hard and fast rules to follow. Some parents need to be left alone at this time with a doctor or nurse hovering nearby. They may feel awkward about when to put the baby down; this should be anticipated. Parents should be allowed to take as long as they wish with their baby and when they finally leave the hospital, they should be told they can come back at any time to see the baby. It is helpful if this is preceded by a phone call so that arrangements can be made for the parents to be met and taken to the chapel or similar location.

The parents should be asked if they would like anyone

to be contacted (e.g. a member of the family or a religious leader). They may want the baby baptized. The parents must be told that police and coroner are informed of all sudden deaths and that the police will ask some routine questions. It must be explained that a postmortem is required, that the coroner will arrange this and that it will be done as soon as possible. Parents will want to know the cause of death and it is wise not to guess but to say that the postmortem will give the answer. It is important to stress that the parents could not have prevented the death or altered the outcome and that no-one could have anticipated it.

The doctor should find out what address the family are going back to so that the family practitioner can be informed and can visit. The health visitor should also be told as soon as possible. They can prevent computerized requests for vaccination and baby clinic appointments being sent to the family. The family should have transport home; this should be arranged for them. No bereaved parent should return alone to an empty house.

The checklist below summarizes the necessary actions when a child is brought into hospital having died of an unknown cause.

The baby
- Full and thorough examination.
- Core temperature.
- Swabs – throat, nose, rectum.
- Specimens – blood, etc., as agreed with local pathologist.
- Keep clothes in labelled hospital bag.
- Wrap the baby in clean, warm baby clothes for parents to hold.
- Take photographs of baby and keep in notes.

The parents
- Explain that the child (use name) has died and that nothing they could have done would have prevented it.
- Gently get as full a history as possible.
- Ask if they would like a priest/religious leader present.
- Ask if they want any close relative to be contacted.
- Encourage the parents to see and hold the baby.
- Let them know that a postmortem needs to be carried out.
- Let them know that police are always informed at sudden, unexpected deaths and will need to ask a few simple questions of the carers.
- Ask what address the family will be going to on leaving hospital.

- Arrange transport from hospital to home. If a parent is alone, make sure they are accompanied and not left alone at home.
- Be gentle, unhurried, calm and careful.
- Do not guess at the diagnosis.

Obtain details of:
- Baby's and parents' names.
- Baby's date of birth.
- Address at which death occurred.
- Time of arrival in department.
- Time last seen alive.
- Usual address if different from above.

Inform
- General practitioner of the death and address to which parents will be going from hospital.
- Health visitor.
- Social worker.
- Any relative as requested by the family.
- Coroner – who will need to know the full name and address and date of birth of the child, time of arrival, place of death, brief recent history, any suspicious circumstances. The coroner will inform the police and pathologist.

The result of the postmortem should be told to the parents as soon as possible, usually within 24–48 h. This is usually done by a social worker.

About 6 weeks later, when histology reports are available, an appointment should be offered to the parents to come and discuss the death and postmortem findings with the doctor concerned. It is often useful to have the social worker present who can remind parents of questions they wanted to ask, and can hear what they are told by the doctor. This interview can take place in the hospital; alternatively, it may be necessary to go to the parents' home or meet them in a neutral place, as the hospital may still bring back very painful memories to them.

TECHNIQUES OF VASCULAR ACCESS

Vascular access is essential in most life-threatening situations. Not all resuscitation drugs may be given via the tracheal tube, and fluids can only be infused by venous or intraosseous routes.

Arterial cannulation provides a means of measuring blood pressure and of obtaining blood samples for oxygen levels and acid–base balance.

There are several percutaneous techniques for intravenous, arterial and intraosseous cannulation.

Surgical venous cannulation (a cut-down) may be required. In an emergency the largest vein that can easily be cannulated is used. Peripheral venous access can be attempted on the scalp, arm, hand, leg or foot. The disadvantages are the small size of the veins and the fact that they are often collapsed or 'shut down'.

Central access can be obtained through the femoral, external jugular or internal jugular veins and, in older children, subclavian veins. The femoral vein is preferred as it is easy to cannulate and is well away from cardiopulmonary resuscitation measures. Central venous access through the neck veins is not without danger and can be difficult in children.

Infusion pumps should be used to give intravenous fluids to small children so that large amounts are not infused inadvertently. If infusion pumps are not available, paediatric infusion-giving sets should be used.

Types of cannulae

Butterfly needles
These are useful for peripheral venous access but dislodge easily. They come in sizes 19–27, the most useful sizes being 21 and 23.

Over-the-needle cannulae
These cannulae can be used in peripheral veins or the femoral or external jugular vein. Sizes vary from 24 (for neonates) to 14 (for a large child). The most useful sizes are 22, 18 and 16.

Catheter-introducing sheaths
The Seldinger method (described below) is used to introduce relatively large-bore catheters into small veins. The introducer sheath can be used for giving large volume fluids quickly. The catheter can be used for infusions and for assessing central venous circulation.

Peripheral venous access

The frontal, superficial temporal, posterior auricular, supraorbital and posterior facial veins may be used on the *scalp*. At the *upper and lower extremities*, veins on the dorsum of the hand, at the elbow, on the dorsum of the feet or the saphenous vein can be used for cannulation.

Scalp veins

Equipment
1. Skin cleansing swabs.
2. Butterfly needle sizes 21 and 23 (25 for neonates).
3. 2 ml syringe.
4. Short piece of tubing or bandage to use to obstruct the vein to be cannulated.

Procedure
1. Restrain the child.
2. Shave the appropriate area of the scalp.
3. Clean with antiseptic swabs.
4. An assistant should hold a taut piece of tubing or bandaging perpendicular to the vein to be punctured and proximal to the site of puncture, to distend the vein.
5. Check the patency of a butterfly needle with suitable sterile fluid and leave the needle and tubing full of infusion fluid.
6. Disconnect the syringe and leave the end of the tubing open.
7. Use a butterfly needle or cannula to puncture the skin and enter the vein. Blood will flow back through the tubing. Infuse a small quantity of fluid to see that the cannula is properly placed and then tape into position.

Seldinger technique of cannulation of a vein

This technique allows cannulation of a vein with a relatively large sheath, or the introduction of a long catheter for administration of infusion fluids and assessment of central venous pressure. The technique can be used in an antecubital vein, the jugular or subclavian vein or femoral vein. Femoral vein and external jugular vein are the preferred sites as there are fewer possible complications at these sites.

Equipment
1. Skin cleansing swabs.
2. Syringe with 2 ml of 0.9% normal saline.
3. Seldinger cannulation set, including needle, guideline and cannula (21 gauge needle).
4. Fully prepared infusion set.
5. Adhesive taping.

Procedure (cannulation of femoral vein)
1. The child lies supine with the groin exposed and leg slightly flexed and abducted at the hip. If the child is conscious the leg and body must be restrained to prevent movement.
2. Cleanse the area well and wear gloves if time allows.
3. Attach the syringe to the needle and locate a femoral vein by palpating the femoral artery. The vein lies immediately adjacent to the artery on the medial side.
4. Keep one finger on the artery to mark its position and introduce the needle at a 45° angle pointing towards the patient's head directly over the femoral vein. Keep the syringe in line with the child's leg and introduce the needle with the plunger withdrawn so that blood will flow freely into the syringe when the vein is entered.
5. Remove the syringe and put a finger over the hub of the needle to prevent blood loss. Insert the guidewire down the needle and then remove the needle.
6. Nick the skin near the guidewire with a scalpel to ease the cannula through the skin.
7. Pass the cannula over the guidewire until it is placed in the vein and then remove the guidewire.
8. Attach the infusion set to the cannula. Fix the cannula in place with tape and a suture.

Venous cut-down

If venous access cannot be secured through peripheral or central veins, a cut-down may need to be done. It takes time (about 15 min) and it may be more appropriate to use the intraosseous route for immediate access and the cut-down route for continued fluid and drug therapy.

Sites
The long saphenous vein at the ankle or the brachial vein at the elbow are preferred sites.

Equipment
1. Antiseptic and swabs to clean.
2. 1% lignocaine for local anaesthetic with 2 ml syringe and fine needle (size 25).
3. Cut-down set which includes two curved mosquito forceps, suture material, fine scissors in good condition, scalpel with a fine blade (size 15).
4. Catheter or cannula sizes 14, 16, 18 and 22 as appropriate.

Procedure
1. Immobilize the lower leg and foot.
2. Clean the skin over the lower leg and foot.
3. Scrub hands and wear gloves if there is time, and drape the area.
4. The long saphenous vein courses anterior to the medial malleolus at the ankle. The site for incision is one finger's breadth superior and anterior to the medial malleolus in children and half a finger's breadth superior and anterior to the medial malleolus in infants.
5. Infiltrate the overlying skin with 1% lignocaine and make an incision perpendicular to the course of the vein through the skin.
6. Use the curved haemostat tips pointing downwards and held perpendicular to the incision to separate the subcutaneous tissue and identify the vein.
7. When the vein is identified pass a long loop of suture material under it. Cut the loop so that two strands of suture material now lie under the vein. Tie the lower strand and ligature the distal end of the vein. Keep the ends of the tie long (Fig. 12).
8. Make a small hole in the upper part of the exposed vein with a scalpel blade or fine pointed scissors and feed a cannula or catheter into the vein. Secure this in place with the upper ligature. Do not tie this too tightly and occlude the cannula.
9. Attach a syringe filled with isotonic fluid to the cannula and ensure that fluid flows freely up the vein. If it does not, the tip of the cannula may be up against a venous valve and by shifting it slightly the flow will improve; otherwise, the cannula may be wrongly placed in the adventitia surrounding the vein. If fluid flows freely, tie the distal ligature around the catheter to help immobilize it and close the incision site with interrupted sutures. Fix the catheter or cannula to the skin and cover with a sterile dressing.

Intraosseous infusion

The technique of intraosseous infusion is not new. It was used in the 1940s as a quick method of gaining vascular access when the only alternatives were to use a reusable,

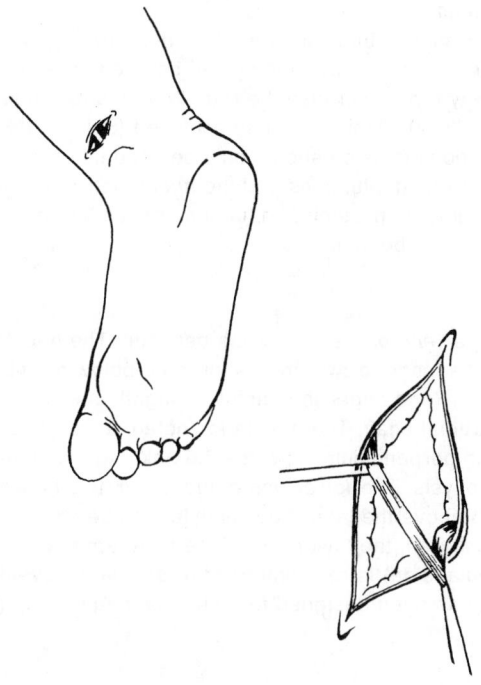

Fig. 12. Cut-down on saphenous vein, at the ankle. (Courtesy of Advanced Paediatric Life Support (UK); Advanced Life Support Group.)

resharpened metal needle or perform a venous cut-down (Tocantins *et al.*, 1941). When plastic venous cannulae were designed, and thus the cannulation of central veins made possible, the technique of intraosseous infusion went out of fashion. However, over the years, it has become clear that central venous lines are not always as easy, safe and reliable as was hoped, especially in small children, and despite all the modern techniques and equipment available there are still times when venous access is very difficult to achieve in a short time. Because vascular access is important to achieve quickly in many life-threatening situations the technique of intraosseous infusion has been revived. Specially designed needles make the technique quick and easy. It is a technique with which everyone dealing with children in life-threatening situations should be familiar and be able to use if other attempts at venous access fail or will take longer than 5 min to carry out.

Uses
Intraosseous infusion is especially useful in infants and toddlers. It can be used for fluid replacement – crystalloids, colloids or blood can be transfused – and all emergency drugs can be given by this route except bretylium. Marrow aspirate samples can be used for group and cross-match, biochemical analysis, culture and sensitivity (Ummenhofer *et al.*, 1992).

Limitations

An intraosseous infusion, if left to run by gravity, will drip at 5–10 ml min^{-1}. A syringe should be used on a three-way tap to increase the rate. With this technique a rate of 35–40 ml min^{-1} can be achieved (Spivey, 1987). Intraosseous infusion should only be used in life-threatening situations and the needle left *in situ* for as short a time as possible, i.e. until a venous line or cut-down can be achieved.

Sites

The *upper end of the tibia* is the best site. The needle should be inserted two fingers' breadth below the tibial tuberosity (one finger in infants) or slightly medially into the flat tibial shaft. The needle is angled at about 10° away from the perpendicular towards the ankle to avoid injuring the epiphysis. The *lower end of the femur*, two fingers' breadth above the lateral epicondyle, can be chosen; in older children, the lower end of the tibia (approached from the medial side) is recommended. A special screw-like needle has been designed for use in this age group (3–6 years).

Complications

The bone may fracture. The needle may pierce the bone through and through; fluid will then infuse into the surrounding soft tissues. If the calf is involved a compartment syndrome can occur. There is a small chance (0.6%) of osteomyelitis at the needle site (Heinild *et al.*, 1947). This chance increases if the needle is left *in situ* for more than 6–8 h. The needle may block. The fluid may not flow freely; there is a theoretical risk of fat embolism which has not given rise to problems in practice.

Equipment

1. Swabs/antiseptic to cleanse the skin.
2. Intraosseous needle size 16 or 18. If not available, size 19 butterfly or angiocath.
3. 10 ml and 20 ml syringes; three-way tap.
4. Infusion-giving set.

Procedure

1. Clean and prepare the skin over the upper tibia with an antiseptic solution.
2. Note the site for the intraosseous infusion which is two fingers' breadth below the tibial plateau and one finger medial to the midline on the flat shaft of the tibia.
3. If the child is conscious infiltrate this area with local anaesthetic down to the periosteum.
4. The intraosseous needle should be directed almost perpendicularly into the bone. A 10° angle caudally helps avoid injury to the tibial epiphyseal plate. The needle is pressed firmly into the bone with a to-and-fro twisting motion. A clunk is heard and the needle 'gives' when the marrow is entered. Attach a three-way tap and 10 ml or 20 ml syringe (depending on the size of the patient). Attempt to aspirate marrow. If successful,

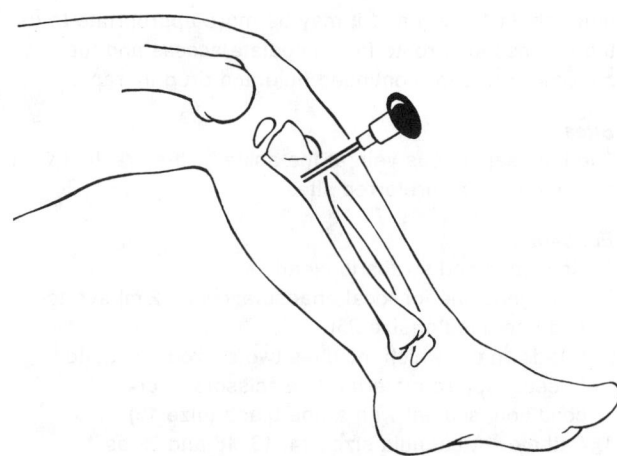

Fig 13. Intraosseous infusion needle in upper tibia. (Courtesy of Advanced Paediatric Life Support (UK); Advanced Life Support Group.)

keep the marrow sample for haematological, biochemical and bacteriological analyses.

5. If the needle is correctly sited it should stand upright without support in the bone (Fig. 13). Marrow may be aspirated through the needle (in about 50% of cases) and fluid will flow freely through the needle.
6. Using the syringe, flush isotonic saline through the needle and watch for free flow of fluid, without extravasation into subcutaneous tissues. If this is successful attach an infusion set to the three-way tap but use the syringe to pump boluses of fluid into a child requiring large fluid volumes. All resuscitative drugs can be given via the intraosseous needle, including anaesthetic drugs, muscle relaxants, glucose, inotropes, blood, antibiotics, etc.
7. Secure the needle in position.
8. Do not leave the needle in situ for longer than necessary. As soon as it is feasible establish an alternative vascular route.

Umbilical vein access

Cannulation of an umbilical vein is rapid and simple and is used during neonatal resuscitation. An umbilical tape should be tied loosely around the base of the cord and after thorough cleaning the cord should be cut with a scalpel, leaving a 1 cm stump distal to the tape. An umbilical vein should be identified within the stump. Three vessels are visible: two are small and contracted – these are arteries; the vein is larger and dilated. A 5F catheter should be prefilled with normal saline solution and inserted 5 cm into the vein. The umbilical tape should then be tightened to secure the catheter and a purse-string suture or adhesive tape can be used to secure its position.

Arterial puncture and cannulation

Blood gas analysis is required in children suffering from serious illness or trauma and cannulation will allow the frequent analysis and the assessment of arterial blood pressure.

Equipment

1. Heparinized syringe.
2. 23 gauge butterfly needle or needle.
3. Cleansing swabs for the skin.
4. Gauze, pad and tapes.

Procedure

1. The preferred sites for arterial puncture are the radial or posterior tibial arteries. Before using the radial artery check that an ulnar artery is present and patent by occluding both arteries at the wrist. Release the pressure on the ulnar artery and the circulation should return to the hand (it will flush pink). If this does not happen do not proceed with a radial puncture on that side.
2. Palpate the radial artery and keep the wrist hyperextended and restrained.
3. Cleanse the area thoroughly.
4. Insert the needle or catheter over the artery at 45° to the skin, directed proximally. When the artery is punctured, blood will be seen to pulsate into the syringe.
5. Collect the required amount of blood, withdraw the needle and compress the puncture site firmly for at least 5 min to prevent the formation of a haematoma.
6. Ensure there are no air bubbles in the blood sample and send it for analysis immediately or place it on ice if any delay is anticipated.

In very small babies a 23 gauge needle can be used to puncture the artery and blood collected from the well of the needle into a heparinized capillary tube.

Summary

Figure 14 shows the suggested sequence of intravenous access in children.

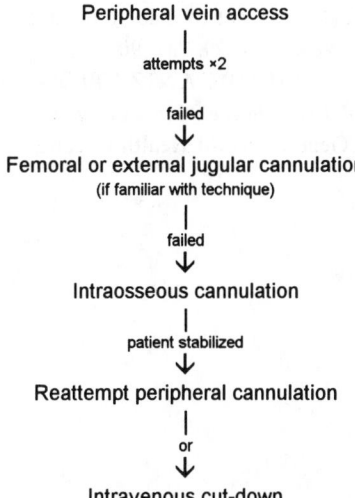

Peripheral vein access
|
attempts ×2
|
failed
↓
Femoral or external jugular cannulation
(if familiar with technique)
|
failed
↓
Intraosseous cannulation
|
patient stabilized
↓
Reattempt peripheral cannulation
|
or
↓
Intravenous cut-down

Fig. 14. Suggested approach to intravenous access in children.

Bibliography

APLS (1993). *Advanced Paediatric Life Support – A Practical Approach*, ed. K. Mackway-Jones, E. Molyneux & B. Phillips. London: BMJ Publications.

APPLETON, R. (1992a). Diagnosis and investigation of epilepsy. In *Epilepsy*, ed. R. Appleton, G. Baker, D. Chadwick & D. Smith. London: Martin Dunitz.

APPLETON, R. (1992b). Anticonvulsant drugs. In *Therapeutic Guidelines*. Royal Liverpool Children's Hospital (NHS) Trust.

APPLETON, R. (1993). Convulsions. In *Advanced Paediatric Life Support – A Practical Approach*, ed. K. Mackway-Jones, E. Molyneux & B. Phillips. London: BMJ Publications.

BASS, M., KRAVATH, R.E. & GLASS, L. (1986). Death scene investigations in sudden infant death syndrome. *N. Engl. J. Med.*, **315**, 100–5.

BEAL, S. (1988). Sleeping positions and sudden infant death syndrome (Letter). *Lancet*, **ii**, 512.

BISHOP, J. & NOLAN, T. (1991). Pulse oximetry in acute asthma. *Arch. Dis. Child.*, **66**, 724–6.

BRITISH THORACIC SOCIETY (1993). Guidelines for acute severe asthma in children. *Thorax*, **48** (Suppl.), S1–S24.

BROOKS, J.G. (1990). Sudden infant death syndrome and acute life threatening events. In *Essentials of Paediatric Intensive Care*, ed. D. Levin & C. Morris, pp. 262–67. St Louis: Quality Medical Publications.

CHIEF MEDICAL OFFICER (1991). Sleeping position of infants and the risk of cot death (sudden infant death). *Letter to All Doctors in England*, PL/CMO(91)16.

COURIEL, J. (1993). Respiratory emergencies. In *Advanced Paediatric Life Support – A Practical Approach*, ed. K. Mackway-Jones, E. Molyneux, B. Phillips. London: BMJ Publications.

DEAL, J.E., BARRATT, T.M. & DILLON, M.J. (1992). Management of hypertensive emergencies. *Arch. Dis. Child.*, **67**, 1089–92.

DE LOUVOIS, J., BLACKBOURNE, J., HURLY, R. *et al.* (1991). Infantile meningitis in England and Wales – a two year study. *Arch. Dis. Child.*, **66**, 603–7.

FLEMING, P.J., GILBERT, R., AZAZ, Y. *et al.* (1990). Interaction between bedding and sleeping position in the sudden infant death syndrome: population based case control study. *Br. Med. J.*, **301**, 85–89.

GLOVER, G.W. (1990). Otitis media. *Prescr. J.*, **30** (5), 218–28.

HAFFEREJEE, I.(1993). Nutritional management during acute infantile diarrhoea. *Postgrad. Doct. Africa*, **15**, 8–10.

HEAF, D.H. (1992). Clinical asthma score. In *Therapeutic Guidelines*. Royal Liverpool Children's Hospital (NHS) Trust.

HEINILD, S., SONDERGAARD, J. & TUDVAD, F. (1947). Bone marrow infusions in childhood: experience from 1,000 infusions. *J. Pediatr.*, **30**, 400–11.

HELLSTRÖM, A., HANSEN, E., HANSON, S. *et al.* (1991). Association between urinary symptoms at seven years old and previous urinary tract infections. *Arch. Dis. Child.*, **66**, 232–4.

HUSBY, S., AGERLOFT, L., MORTENSEN, S. *et al.* (1993). Treatment of croup with nebulised steroid (budesonide): a double blind, placebo-controlled study. *Arch. Dis. Child.*, **68**, 352–5.

KARYS, S.W., OLMSTEAD, E.N. & O'CONNOR, G.T. (1989). Steroid treatment of laryngotracheitis: a meta-analysis of the evidence from randomised trials. *Pediatrics*, **83**, 683–93.

KLEIN, N.J., HEYDERMAN, R.S. & LEVIN, M. (1992). Antibiotic choices for meningitis beyond the neonatal period. *Arch. Dis. Child.*, **67**, 157–9.

LEBEL, M.H., FREIJ, B.J., SYROGIANNOPOULOS, G.A. *et al.* (1988). Dexamethasone therapy for bacterial meningitis: results of two double-blind placebo-controlled studies. *N. Engl. J. Med.*, **319**, 964–71.

LUBINSKY, P. & ANAS, N.G. (1990). Aspiration pneumonia. In *Essentials of Pediatric Intensive Care*, ed. D. Levin, & F.C. Morriss, pp. 693–8. St Louis: Quality Medical Publications.

LUDMAN, H. (1988). Pain in the ear. In *ABC of Ear Nose and Throat*. London: BMJ Publications.

MAYTAL, J., SHINNAR, S., MOSHE, S.L. *et al.* (1989). Low morbidity and mortality of status epilepticus in children. *Pediatrics*, **83**, 323–31.

McKENZIE, S. (1992). Respiratory tract infections. In *Forfar and Arneil's Textbook of Paediatrics*, ed. A.G.M. Campbell & N. McIntosh, pp. 633–44. London: Churchill Livingstone.

MELLOR, D. (1992). The place of computed tomography and lumbar puncture in suspected bacterial meningitis. *Arch. Dis. Child.*, **67**, 1417–20.

MORLEY, C.J., HEWSON, P.H., THORNTON, A.J. *et al.* (1992). Axillary and rectal temperature measurements in infants. *Arch. Dis. Child.*, **67**, 122–5.

RICKWOOD, A.M.K., CARTY, H.M., McKENDRICK, T. *et al.* (1992). Current imaging of childhood urinary infections: prospective study. *Br. Med. J.*, **304**, 663–5.

RUDD, P.T. (1992). Acute bacterial meningitis. In *Forfar and Arneil's Textbook of Paediatrics*, ed. A.G.M. Campbell & N. McIntosh, pp. 1344–8. London: Churchill Livingstone.

SIBERT, J. & DAVIES, P.A. (1992). Suddent infant death syndrome. In *Forfar and Arneil's Textbook of Paediatrics*, ed. A.G.M. Campbell & N. McIntosh, pp. 1793–7. London: Churchill Livingstone.

SMELLIE, J.M. & NORMAND, I.C.S. (1992). Urinary tract infection. In *Forfar and Arneil's Textbook of Paediatrics*, ed. A.G.M. Campbell & N. McIntosh, pp. 1031–48. London: Churchill Livingstone.

SPIVEY, W.H. (1987). Medical progress: intraosseous infusions. *J. Pediatr.*, **111**, 639–42.

STEPHENSON, J.B.P. (1978). Reflex anoxic seizures (while breath holding); non-epileptic vagal attacks. *Arch. Dis. Child.*, **53**, 193–200.

STERN, R. (1983). Bacterial pneumonias. In *Nelson's Textbook of Pediatrics*, ed. R.E. Behrman & V.C. Vaughan, pp. 1046–54. Philadelphia: Saunders.

THE ECONOMIST (1993). Britain in brief. *Economist*, April 3–9, p. 40.

TILL, J.A. & SHINBOURNE, B.A. (1991). Supraventricular tachycardia: diagnosis and current acute management. *Arch. Dis. Child.*, **66**, 647–52.

TOCANTINS, L.M., O'NEILL, J.F. & JONES, H.W. (1941). Infusions of blood and other fluids via the bone marrow. *J. Am. Med. Assoc.*, **117**, 1229–34.

UMMENHOFER, W., FREI, F., URWYLER, A. *et al.* (1992). Emergency laboratory studies in paediatric patients: does bone marrow aspirate give accurate results? PO20 (poster at Silver Jubilee, British Accident and Emergency Medicine). *Arch. Emerg. Med.*, **9**, 93.

WHITE, R.H.R. (1987). Management of urinary tract infection: personal practice. *Arch. Dis. Child.*, **62**, 421–7.

WIGGLESWORTH, J.S., KEELING, J.W., RUSHTON, D.I. *et al.* (1987). Pathological investigations in cases of suddent infant death. *J. Clin. Pathol.*, **40**, 1481–3.

WOLF, S.M. (1979). Controversies in the treatment of febrile convulsions. *Neurology*, **29**, 287–90.

WORLD HEALTH ORGANIZATION (1990). *The Rational Use of Drugs in the Management of Acute Diarrhoea in Children*. Geneva: World Health Organization.

61 Management of non-accidental injury

T.F. BEATTIE

Accident and Emergency Department, Royal Hospital for Sick Children, Edinburgh, UK

Chapter plan

Introduction
Physical abuse
Sexual abuse
Emotional abuse/physical neglect
Munchausen by proxy
Systems in A&E to detect child abuse
Legal system
Conclusion

INTRODUCTION

Dealing with non-accidental injury (or child abuse) is unfortunately one of the more unpleasant tasks in the accident and emergency (A&E) department. Children present in one of two ways. Firstly, they may be referred for investigation by an outside agency which has reason to suspect that the child has been abused. The child will usually have been referred for the opinion of a senior member of the medical staff either in A&E or paediatrics. The use of the A&E department for these purposes is entirely appropriate. It is open 24 h a day with trained nurses available to give comfort and support as necessary. In addition, the facilities exist to treat injuries such as wounds or burns; in rare circumstances resuscitation will be needed.

Secondly, children may present to the A&E department with an apparently benign history, but the features of the history, physical examination or clinical investigation suggest that the child may have been abused. In this situation junior doctors should seek the advice of senior staff at an early stage. It is not appropriate for junior staff in A&E to manage child abuse. They should, however, be able to identify suspicious injuries and refer for immediate senior advice. They should remain involved in such cases as an observer to further their training.

Every A&E department should have a quiet, well-decorated examination room together with an adjacent interview room so that the history, examination and interview can be carried out as discreetly and as privately as possible.

Non-accidental injury takes five forms:

1. Physical abuse.
   – Trauma.
   – Burns/scalds.
2. Sexual abuse.
3. Emotional abuse/neglect.
4. Physical neglect.
   – Failure to thrive.
   – Neglected medical conditions.
   – Unsupervised avoidable accidents.
   – Cold injury.
5. Munchausen by proxy.

Several of these five forms may coexist in one child and in one family (Hobbs & Wynne, 1990). They are not mutually exclusive. The true incidence of each is unknown.

Factors which predispose to child abuse include:

1. Parents who were abused as children.
2. Lack of bonding (e.g. prolonged period in the neonatal unit).
3. Unwanted child/pregnancy.
4. Previous history of abuse.
5. Siblings on the 'at-risk' register.

PHYSICAL ABUSE

Physical abuse entails actual bodily harm to the child. Usually blunt trauma is involved but thermal injury and wounding are included.

Diagnostic features

No single criterion should be used in isolation to make a diagnosis of child abuse. The following are indicators that abuse may have taken place. Used in isolation they will lead to distress for all involved. Used appropriately in conjunction with a full physical examination and with other circumstantial evidence they are good pointers to the diagnosis:

1. Delay in seeking medical help. It should be borne in mind that many parents consult health visitors, district nurses, neighbours in paramedical professions or first aiders. The fact that they have not seen a doctor does not always mean that medical help has been delayed.
2. Poor history from the guardians. Often the history will be vague and change in detail and substance.
3. The history given does not account for the injuries witnessed, or the pattern of injury is different to that expected from the history.
4. There may be failure to thrive or developmental delay. Previous normal development followed by regression may also be significant.
5. The history does not fit with the developmental age of the child, e.g. babies of a few weeks rolling off a settee or young babies turning taps on.

Pattern of injury

Determination of the pattern of injury includes observation of physical signs and X-ray findings.

Belt marks, finger tip imprints, teeth marks and cigarette burns are all indicative of non-accidental injury. In the case of finger tip imprints it is important to look for the pattern of finger and thumb pressure applied on different surfaces (e.g. fingerprints over the scapula with a thumbprint over the pectoral region).

A torn frenulum may be the result of a bottle being forced into a child's mouth. It may also be associated with 'shaken baby' syndrome which is usually associated with other bruising. Many more cases of torn frenulum are associated with a fall or other benign causation.

Retinal haemorrhages are very often associated with the shaken baby syndrome. Children with an altered level of consciousness and retinal haemorrhages should be assumed to have been shaken until proved otherwise. Subdural haemorrhages in the absence of accidental injuries are also indicative of abuse.

Liver and splenic trauma may be associated with punches or kicks, which may also cause mesenteric tears or duodenal perforation.

Blood loss from intra-abdominal bleeding will cause hypovolaemic shock. Babies and infants will readily lose their level of consciousness in this situation. The presence of bruises or abrasions to the head or face may wrongly cause attention to be focused on head injury as a cause of coma. It is important to remember that abdominal injury may coexist with head injury. The shocked child should be fully resuscitated with oxygen (via an endotracheal tube if necessary) and adequate fluid therapy. After examination, injury to intra-abdominal structures can be assessed by ultrasound examination or computed tomography (CT).

Mesenteric tears and intestinal rupture may cause delayed shock with symptoms and signs taking 6–12 h to develop. Again, intensive resuscitation should precede any further assessment.

Hobbs (1984) has indicated that the pattern and site of skull fractures can help to determine whether the injury is accidental or non-accidental. Fractures which involve one skull bone, which are narrow and are not depressed are more likely to have been caused in an accidental fashion. Fractures which cross suture lines, are multiple, wide and growing are more likely to be associated with non-accidental injury (Figs 1–4). Growing fractures occur only in infancy and are characterized by enlargement beyond 0.5 cm to form a cranial defect.

X-ray signs

Certain X-ray findings are highly suggestive of physical abuse. These include rib and skull fractures. Other X-ray features which may indicate child abuse include:

1. Multiple fractures in different stages of healing.
2. Multiple metaphyseal/epiphyseal injuries.
3. A single fracture with multiple bruises.

Thermal injury

Approximately 2% of children who attend A&E departments each year in the UK have sustained thermal injury. This includes scalding, contact with hot surfaces, electrical burns and chemical burns.

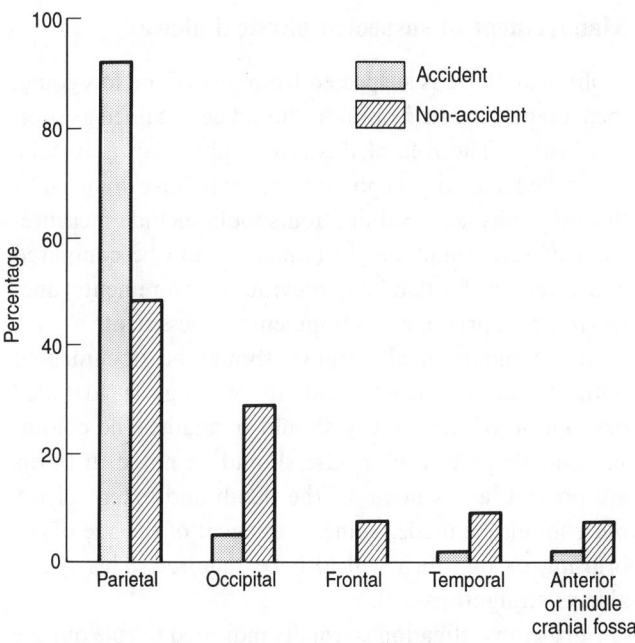

Fig. 1. Site of cranial fracture in accidental and non-accidental injury. (After Hobbs, 1984, with permission.)

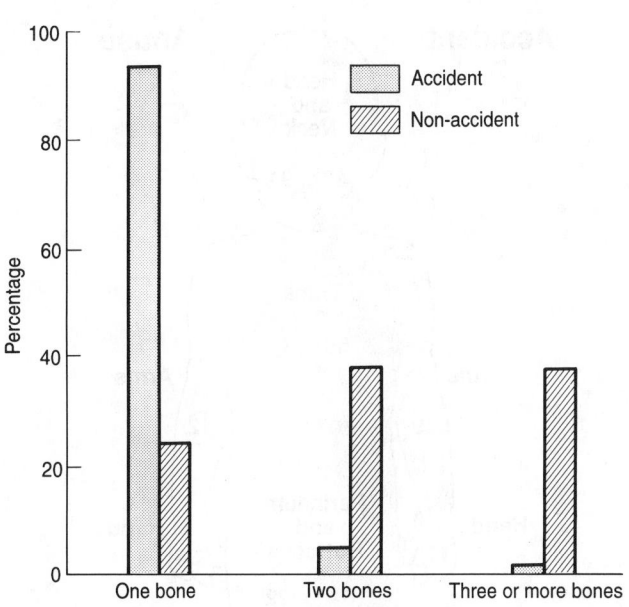

Fig. 3. Number of skull bones involved in accidental and non-accidental injury. (After Hobbs, 1984, with permission.)

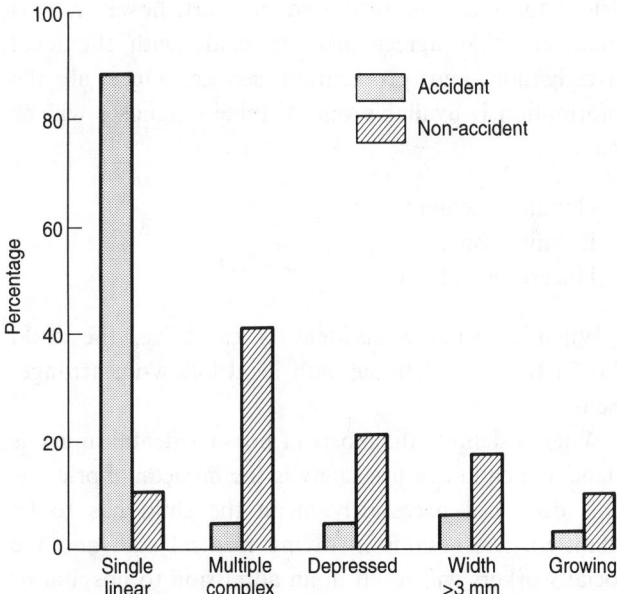

Fig. 2. Types of skull fractures in accidental and non-accidental injury. (After Hobbs, 1984, with permission.)

Fig. 4. Wide and growing fractures.

Scalding is by far the most common. The typical pattern is for a child to reach up and pull hot liquid on itself. The usual areas affected are the head, shoulders and upper chest. Children who have hot liquids accidentally dropped on them by adults usually have the same signs.

Children who touch hot objects normally do so with the palm rather than the dorsum of the hand. Injuries which follow this pattern are usually accidental (Hobbs, 1986). Burns to the dorsum of the hand, the perineum, buttocks and feet should be regarded with much more suspicion (Fig. 5).

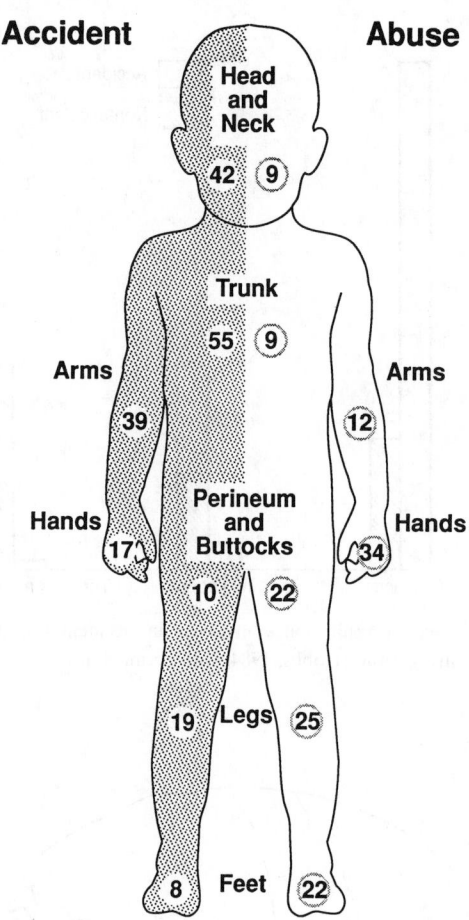

Accident   **Abuse**

Head and Neck 42 9

Trunk 55 9

Arms 39   Arms 12

Hands 17 Perineum and Buttocks 10 22 Hands 34

Legs 19 25

Feet 8 22

Fig. 5. Incidence of burns in particular sites expressed as the percentage in each group (accident and abuse) with burns involving that site. (Reproduced, with permission, from Hobbs, 1986.)

Underlying disease

Before one can confidently proceed with investigation or management of suspected physical abuse it is important to rule out underlying causes. It should be borne in mind that bruising may be present as the result of a bleeding diathesis (e.g. haemophilia, idiopathic thrombocyto-penia). The latter in particular can arise spontaneously.

With regard to fractures, it is important to exclude underlying bone diseases as very rarely these can mimic the signs of non-accidental injury. Bone diseases implicated include osteogenesis imperfecta and Caffey's disease (Hobbs, 1989). If suspected, further radiological, biochemical or haematological investigations will be indicated.

Management of suspected physical abuse

If physical abuse is suspected from any of the foregoing, then a senior medical opinion should be obtained as soon as possible. The role of this senior physician is to take as detailed a history as possible from all those involved. A thorough physical examination should include measurement of height and weight (which should be compared with a centile chart and any previous measurements) and, where appropriate, a developmental assessment.

At examination, all injuries should be documented both diagrammatically and in writing. A detailed description of each injury should be made. The colour, size and shape of each bruise should be noted. If burns are present, an estimate of the depth and extent of the burn should be made. Some assessment of the age of the bruising or the burn will also be required. This is not always straightforward.

Further investigation is usually indicated to rule out the possibility of underlying disorder. Minimum haematological investigations include a full blood count, platelet count and clotting screen. Skeletal surveys may be helpful in younger children and photographs should be taken. Before these can be produced in court, however, it is important that agreements are made with the local investigation and prosecution service. Once all the information is available one of three diagnoses will be made:

1. Genuine accident.
2. Definite abuse.
3. Uncertain/not proven.

When a genuine accident is causative, the child should be allowed home with local follow-up arrangements.

When a definite diagnosis of non-accidental injury is made, the child's future safety is the immediate priority. This does not necessarily mean the child has to be admitted. Discussions involving medical staff and the social workers will result in an admission to hospital or temporary foster care. In certain circumstances the child may be allowed home (e.g. abuse by a relative who is now in police custody and is likely to remain there for some time).

If the cause of the injury is unclear, the child should be allowed home following discussion with the social work department. In this instance, and in the case of genuine non-accidental injury, a case conference will be called. The clinician involved in making the diagnosis should then be present.

SEXUAL ABUSE

Sexual abuse presenting *de novo* to the A&E department is rare. Occasionally children will attend for treatment of an acute injury caused by sexual abuse. In rare circumstances haemorrhage may arise from the genitals or the anus and resuscitation may be required.

Sexual abuse should be suspected in the following circumstances:

1. Prepubertal vaginal bleeding
2. Sexually transmitted disease proven by bacteriology
3. Anal trauma
4. Teenage pregnancy
5. Altered behaviour:
   - Truancy
   - Suicide attempt
   - Increased promiscuity/inappropriate sexuality
6. Suggestive physical signs

Role of the A&E department in managing child sexual abuse

Any junior doctor who suspects a child of being sexually abused should immediately obtain advice from senior medical staff who will be responsible for further management.

Physical examination should ideally be performed by a paediatrician in conjunction with a doctor skilled in forensic examination. Usually this will be a police surgeon. Only in exceptional circumstances should more than one examination be made.

While waiting for forensic examination it is important that the clothing is not disturbed and that the child is not washed, particularly in cases of acute or recent rape. Valuable forensic evidence may otherwise be lost.

Forensic examination (Royal College of Physicians, 1991) *must* record any signs of:

1. Bruising to the external genitalia/anus/perineum.
2. Tears to the external and internal genitalia/anus/perineum.
3. Ruptured hymen.
4. Scar tissue.
5. Torn frenulum (males).
6. Intraoral petechiae or lesions.
7. Any other physical injury (e.g. bruising to thighs or lower spine).

The size of the introitus is measured and evidence of forced intercourse sought. Swabs may be appropriate if the abuse is recent to detect the presence of semen. Bacteriology samples may be sent. Any hairs should be collected and stored separately.

In the case of peripubertal or postpubertal girls consideration should be given to emergency contraception. If abuse has taken place over a long period of time a pregnancy test may be indicated and if positive, abortion may be offered. Consideration should also be given to hepatitis B and HIV (human immunodeficiency virus) testing.

Abuse may not be admitted at the initial presentation, and may take many hours of patient discussion and consultation. Much of the treatment of sexual abuse will take place over a long period of time with extensive counselling. While A&E specialists are closely involved in the initial diagnosis and management of sexual abuse, it is not appropriate for them to be involved in the extensive and long-term counselling aspects. However, A&E medical staff should be able to initiate and follow agreed local guidelines for the management of sexual abuse.

EMOTIONAL ABUSE/PHYSICAL NEGLECT

Emotional abuse and physical neglect commonly co-exist with other forms of abuse. Evidence of failure to thrive and delayed speech or development should be sought in the presence of other signs of abuse (Hammond *et al.*, 1989). Indeed, all children who have suffered physical or sexual abuse should have their development assessed.

If the abuse is proven and the child has spent some time in care, an improvement in developmental milestones may often be detected. This in itself is evidence that the child has suffered either emotional abuse or physical neglect. Similarly, physically or sexually abused children may show improved development and behaviour when out of the harmful environment.

Management of these children requires careful multi-disciplinary assessment involving community paediatricians, social workers, speech therapists and psychologists.

There are many other causes of failure to thrive or developmental delay which must be considered before they are attributed to emotional abuse or physical neglect.

MUNCHAUSEN BY PROXY

This is a rare, but possibly underdiagnosed, syndrome. The child is not ill but suffers repeated hospital admissions for investigation of vague and undetermined clinical signs and symptoms. Various aetiologies include:

1. Repeated smothering of the child, often leading to seizure.
2. Bogus haematuria.
3. Repeated poisonings.

In all of these cases the child has apparently genuine symptoms. A&E departments should be particularly aware of this type of presentation. Any signs or symptoms which do not fit with the normal pattern of disease should be carefully documented.

With regard to suffocation, evidence of petechial bruising to the face and eyes should be sought particularly.

Once diagnosed, priority must be given to child protection. The mother should be offered psychiatric treatment as soon as possible. The social work department should make arrangements for the continued safety of the child and siblings.

SYSTEMS IN A&E TO DETECT CHILD ABUSE

About 1 child in 7 attends an A&E department in Britain every year. A large proportion of these children will have suffered accidents, but a significant minority will have an injury that is non-accidental in nature. Great vigilance is needed to try to identify these children. Various mechanisms should exist in every A&E department to help detect the child who has been abused so that prompt action may be taken. These measures include the following:

1. *Staff education*. Each induction programme for new staff should include a discussion on child abuse and its detection. All medical and nursing staff should be made aware of the local policies for investigation and protection of abused children.
2. *Record linking*. Each attendance of a child at an A&E department should automatically be linked to its previous attendances. Great care should be taken to look for changed names and aliases. The process is enhanced by a computerized record system which can search for different names at the same address automatically. Where manual systems still exist a

search should be made for each child in the records already stored. Wherever possible, new case sheets should be presented to the doctor together with all previous records.
3. *A specific social worker in the A&E department*. Each A&E department that deals with children should have a specific social worker allocated to it. This enables close contact to be maintained, building up camaraderie and fellowship. The social worker should have easy access to community-based colleagues. A regular audit of all children referred for social work assessment should be made and presented at A&E department meetings.
4. *Liaison health visitor*. A liaison health visitor should be appointed to the A&E department. All children presenting under the age of 5 years are referred to the health visitor who can then arrange for follow-up to be carried out in the community. Frequent attenders and problem families can be investigated by this mechanism.
5. *Access to the child abuse register*. Social work departments regularly update the 'at-risk' or child abuse register. An up-to-date copy of this should be available at all times in every A&E department that regularly sees children. Some departments have difficulty obtaining access to it. It is important that all children on the register should be identified as early as possible so that prompt social work contact can be made. Early review of these attendances should be made by the senior doctor in A&E looking for signs of injury incompatible with the history or other signs and symptoms compatible with non-accidental injury.

LEGAL SYSTEM

Every case of suspected child abuse will be investigated by the legal system. This will begin with a police statement and may well be followed up with reports to the court. Evidence will have to be given by all people concerned with the case. It is crucial that accurate, concise notes are made at the time of the examination. These will invariably be produced in court and have to withstand vigorous cross-examination by the defence counsel.

Evidence given must be factual and based on extensive clinical experience. It is obviously more appropriate for senior doctors to do this. Junior doctors should not be intimidated by the defence counsel and if in doubt should seek guidance from the magistrate or judge presiding. Both senior and junior doctors will be asked to give their opinion as to how these injuries have been caused. If either are unable to say, with certainty, how the injuries were caused, they should say so.

CONCLUSION

Child abuse is not a new problem. As society has changed so the threshold for diagnosing child abuse has altered. It is not for the clinician to say that a mother who slaps her child's bare bottom and leaves a hand imprint is right or wrong. The doctor examining the case must be non-judgemental. It is up to society to decide, in the form of court judgements and jury pronouncements, what is and what is not child abuse.

The principal role of the physician in managing child abuse is to provide unbiased, accurate medical evidence and informed opinion as to how the injuries may or may not have been caused. It is crucial that the physician joins with social workers and other agencies in reaching optimal decisions for the future protection of the child.

Bibliography

HAMMOND, J., NOBEL-GOULD, A. & BROOKS, J. (1989). The value of speech/language assessment in the diagnosis of child abuse. *J. Trauma*, **29**, 1258–60.

HOBBS, C.J. (1984). Skull fracture and the diagnosis of abuse. *Arch. Dis. Child.*, **59**, 246–54.

HOBBS, C.J. (1986). When are burns not accidental. *Arch. Dis. Child.*, **61**, 357–61.

HOBBS, C.J. (1989). Fractures. In *ABC of Child Abuse*, ed. Meadows Orr, pp. 8–11. London: British Medical Journal.

HOBBS, C.J. & WYNNE, J.M. (1990). The sexually abused and battered child. *Arch. Dis. Child.*, **65**, 423–7.

ROYAL COLLEGE OF PHYSICIANS OF LONDON WORKING PARTY. (1991). *Physical Signs of Sexual Abuse in Children*, p. 53. London: RCP Publications.

62 Care of the elderly

C. BOWMAN

Department of Gerontology, General Hospital, Weston-super-Mare, UK

Chapter plan

Introduction
Falls and immobility
Confusional states
Iatrogenic disease and therapeutics
Abuse and neglect
Ethnic minorities

INTRODUCTION

The definition of 'the elderly' remains curiously imprecise; for practical purposes, a simplistic age-based categorization will be avoided here, but the patients that are the concern of this chapter are those who do not fit into simple diagnostic boxes and are widely identified as geriatric. The approach used is based on the common presentational patterns of functional impairments rather than organ/system-based diseases.

The Western world's population is 'greying', the aged, particularly the old old (chronologically and physiologically), constituting a large and rapidly increasing group. In the UK, the population over 85 years is projected to increase by 66% between 1989 and 2026 (Central Health Monitoring Unit, 1992). This group presents an increasing burden of chronic and acute health problems with increasing social dependence, isolation and economic deprivation.

A key requirement for health services to respond adequately to the challenges of the aged is for clear practices to ensure that 'treatment success, outcome failure' cases are infrequent, which demands that not only are treatments given correctly but are defensible as the appropriate treatments to give. Many very frail elderly fear morbidity more than mortality and have low expectations of health services. It is incumbent on attendant staff to be aware of these issues. This difficult area is compounded by the diminished mental capacity of those with dementia and allied conditions who cannot make decisions with informed consent. In such circumstances, if a formal advocate exists for the patient, their guidance should be sought. In a similar manner, family, medical attendants or friends may be able to help. Where no patient-related opinion can be obtained regarding decisions, discussion with other preferably more experienced staff should be routine. For more junior medical staff the support of senior experienced nursing staff is invaluable but should be underpinned by ready access to senior medical opinion. In situations such as cardiorespiratory arrest, treatment must be active until its correctness is found wanting or failure is agreed as the outcome.

In the UK, many systems of health care exist in the hospital service for the delivery of medical care to the elderly. Some geriatric services operate an age-related service, others a needs-based policy while increasingly, particularly in smaller district hospitals, an integrated emergency policy exists. The common objective is that emergency presentations in the elderly should be dealt with on the basis of need and not be discriminated against on grounds of age (Royal College of Physicians, 1994). The level of response to life-threatening illness must be appropriate and acknowledge likely benefits in terms of outcomes and be mindful of premorbid health status and life quality. This is demanding of clinical skills and decision-making, and within the accident and emergency (A&E) department the greatest requirement is adequate, competent clinical time and attentive nursing care.

Equipment requirements of the elderly are generally as for other patients. In particular, there must be appropriate seating in waiting areas; this means a range of seat heights, good arm supports and toilet facilities that are not only wheelchair-accessible and well served with grab-rails but are also clearly signposted. Frail aged patients being admitted should be moved to proper ward settings and beds as soon as clinically and logistically possible. Some elderly patients may remain on hard trolley surfaces for several hours whilst diagnosis and management plans are formulated and are at considerable risk of developing pressure sores. Sores will not become apparent until several days after admission but the awareness of tissue viability in the A&E department and its promotion by the use of large-cell pressure-relieving mattresses is essential.

A significant proportion of presentations to an emergency service are subacute and clear arrangements for managing these in terms of communication with primary healthcare teams and referral to hospital services should be practised. Similarly, procedures for the management of patients whose medical status is well understood but in whom the need is primarily personal care and social support depend on good working practices between health and social services. Such arrangements should be the subject of written policy agreements with built-in audit facilities allowing service development by evolution rather than crisis management. Services for the very frail elderly are seldom if ever adequate and tend to be developed through inadequacy, leading to a definition of minimum standards. Awareness of consumer rights and limited resources dictate that referral processes must be clear if only for medicolegal purposes. Prudent practice requires that, when cases discharged from A&E units are dependent on services arranged by telephone negotiation, they are documented clearly and liaison contacts identified. Verbal arrangements should be backed up by written confirmation, ideally faxed and copied to the primary care team.

Elderly patients presenting with typical symptoms and signs of medical conditions are generally best served by being dealt with in the same manner as younger patients; indeed, the health benefits of prompt treatment usually are greater, relatively, in this patient group. Delayed treatment will frequently lead to protracted management courses and impaired outcomes. The history obtained from ill, often confused, patients is limited; many are anxious regarding hospitalization, and the attitude of staff towards the patient is crucial. It is often remarkable how, having confirmed that the patient can hear and communicate, an orientating greeting to the patient reduces an alleged confusional state to one of a stress reaction. A useful opening line is:

'*Good morning Mrs X, my name is Dr. Y. You are at Z hospital. You have been brought here I understand because . . . ; could you tell me what's been happening?*'

If the patient is accompanied by a family member, carer or friend, it is frequently productive and expeditious to ask if they may be present during clerking. Furthermore, as the range of normality becomes increasingly diverse at great age with regard to cognitive function, the unwary may dismiss a slight confusion as of no significance when in fact the patient's usual state is of a much higher level of cognitive competence. Confirmation of the patient's usual status is often a significant factor in decision-making and should be painstakingly sought, this being particularly relevant for the increasingly very frail patients that are referred to A&E units from nursing and residential care settings.

Several factors in the initial assessment of the very elderly should be routine. Firstly, whilst undeniably important, conventional vital signs may be misleadingly normal due to impaired physiology; for example, a pulse rate may be 'normal' because of autonomic denervation in spite of significant heart failure, and fever may often be absent in the presence of infection. A more useful sign is that of respiratory rate, although its accurate measurement is unusual (best done by casual observation whilst taking a relaxed history). Secondly, classical physical signs may be of no relevance whatsoever to the presentation and, whilst always noteworthy, they should not prove a distraction to the active problems!

Assessments both of mental state and of functional performance prove particularly useful in making management decisions; their universal application to aged patients in the A&E department is inappropriate, but they are helpful in cases where doubt exists regarding a patient's competence. It is quite remarkable how a moderately severe cognitive impairment can be hidden by a sophisticated confabulation. The 10-point Abbreviated Mental Test (Royal College of Physicians, 1992) questionnaire is sufficient as a screening process (Table 1). A thorough assessment of daily living skills is not expected of an A&E department, but use of the Barthel Index (Royal College of Physicians, 1992) as an aide-memoire in questioning functional ability (Table 2) will make the likelihood of missing a significant deficit in living skills unlikely and form a useful basis for referral to geriatric and social services.

Enthusiastic diagnosis poses a major risk to the aged, producing problems of inappropriate treatment. Slowness

Table 1. *Abbreviated Mental Test (AMT) score*

1. Age
2. Time (to nearest hour)
3. Address for recall at end of test – this should be repeated by the patient to ensure it has been heard correctly: *42 West Street*
4. Year
5. Name of institution
6. Recognition of two persons (doctor, nurse, etc.)
7. Date of birth (day and month sufficient)
8. Year of First World War
9. Name of present monarch
10. Count backwards from 20 to 1

Scoring: Each correct answer scores 1 mark. A guide to rating cognitive impairment: 0–3, severe impairment; 4–7, moderate impairment; 8–10, normal.

Table 2. *Barthel Activities of Daily Living Index (BAI ADL)*

Function	Score	Description
Bowels	0	Incontinent (or enema-dependent)
	1	Occasional accident (once a week)
	2	Continent
Bladder	0	Incontinent, or catheterized and unable to manage
	1	Occasional accident (max. × 1/24 h)
	2	Continent (for more than 7 days)
Grooming	0	Needs help with personal care: face, hair, teeth, shaving
	1	Independent (implements provided)
Toilet use	0	Dependent
	1	Needs help but can do something alone
	2	Independent
Feeding	0	Unable
	1	Needs help in cutting, spreading butter, etc.
	2	Independent (food within reach)
Transfer	0	Unable – no sitting balance
	1	Major help (physical, one or two people), can sit
	2	Minor help (verbal or physical)
	3	Independent
Mobility	0	Immobile
	1	Wheelchair-independent, including corners, etc.
	2	Walks with help of one aid (verbal or physical)
	3	Independent
Dressing	0	Dependent
	1	Needs help but can do about half unaided
	2	Independent (including buttons, zips, laces, etc.)
Stairs	0	Unable
	1	Needs help (verbal, physical, carrying aid)
	2	Independent up and down
Bathing	0	Dependent
	1	Independent (bath/shower, unsupervised/ unaided)

of movement and tremor may be due to parkinsonism, but opportunistic initiation of therapy is not helpful; firstly, because the patient is diagnostically labelled and, secondly, because subsequent out-patient review will often be frustrating, there being a paucity of typical signs – because of excellent treatment response or misdiagnosis. A more useful approach is a clear description of the signs and further specialist opinion, which should also be fed back to the referring A&E department doctor as part of an educational process. Other diagnoses vulnerable to overzealous management include:

- Dependent oedema (diuretics).
- Epilepsy (anticonvulsants).
- Diabetes (oral hypoglycaemics).
- Hypertension (various).

The converse also applies, particularly in mental illness where, for example, depression may be easily missed. When history-taking, consideration of depressive symptoms by direct questioning should be routine and acted on, most often by advising the patient's usual medical attendant. Where necessary, referral to psychiatric teams should respect local arrangements (and it is important to be aware of these before becoming frustrated through promising actions to patients and their carers that cannot be guaranteed).

Attempted suicide in the elderly must be taken seriously, initial attempts being more serious and likely to succeed than in younger age groups. It is seldom that overdoses are used as attention-seeking gestures in older people, and particular anxiety should be expressed regarding recently bereaved men. Elimination of poisons should be at least as vigorous as in younger groups, and gastric lavage in particular should not be overlooked even if airway protection with an endotracheal tube is necessary.

Hypothermia in the aged may occur through one or more problems such as an insensitivity to cold, impaired thermogenesis, environmental risk and other predisposing illness. The important measurement is core temperature and when this is between 32°C and 34°C the situation is described as moderate hypothermia; below 32°C the hypothermia is rated severe. It is common for ill patients to have cool peripheries, but a cold abdomen necessitates core temperature measurement using a low-reading thermometer rectally. Conscious levels deteriorate with severity of hypothermia, but not predictably so. Common complicating features are cardiac arrhythmias and aspiration of gastric contents from a dilated stomach.

The guiding principle of treatment within the A&E department should be the initiation of management that allows core temperature to rise gradually. Warming of peripheries is potentially dangerous, being complicated by cardiovascular collapse. Severe hypothermia may require more active measurements such as a warming colonic or gastric lavage, or peritoneal dialysis. The exact method used will be dependent on local expertise and the individual case circumstances; these may be beyond the scope of an A&E unit but an awareness of what is possible in a given hospital is useful for the A&E unit.

Many old patients will present with a multiplicity of problems and pathology and are in what is usefully described as 'status geriatricus'. A reliable way of dealing with such cases is the formulation of an active problem list with issues being prioritized. From this, a management plan is developed and logical onward referral. Generally, these cases can prove particularly rewarding for staff to exercise their clinical skills and often to stretch their abilities in a manner that medicine increasingly fails to allow, with the increasing prevalence of guidelines and protocols; a dismissive approach is unacceptable.

FALLS AND IMMOBILITY

Elderly fallers presenting to A&E in whom no trauma requiring specific intervention has occurred offer the prospect of case finding and the potential to avert significant injury and morbidity. Those presenting with a clear history describing an accidental trip in understandable circumstances may be discharged, but unexplained collapses and, particularly, repeated presentations with no action to determine the aetiological circumstances are the mark of a negligent service.

Falls are frequently symptomatic of underlying disease processes and a methodical approach is necessary. There are a number of diagnostic possibilities that should be routinely considered:

- Sensation
  - Visual acuity
  - Proprioception, vitamin B_{12} deficiency, cervical myelopathy
- Locomotor function
  - Arthritis
  - Muscle power
- Nervous system
  - Dementia
  - Cerebrovascular disease
  - Parkinsonism and allied disorders
  - Autonomic dysfunction
  - Epilepsy
  - Vestibular lesions
  - Spinal cord compression
- Cardiovascular/respiratory
  - Heart failure/infarction
  - Arrhythmia
  - Airway disease
  - Autonomic dysfunction
- Other physical illness
  - Infarction/infection
  - Anaemia
- Metabolic
  - Diabetes
  - Thyroid
  - Electrolyte disturbance
  - Dehydration
  - Metabolic bone disease
- Psychiatric/psychological
  - Depression and major psychoses
  - Loss of confidence
- Drug-related
  - Diuretics and other cardiovascular agents
  - Sedatives
- Environmental (examples)
  - Poor clothing, especially footwear
  - Loose rugs

A general history and examination are essential and should routinely include an observation of mobility; indeed, in the absence of a clear diagnosis from the history and obvious trauma, the observation of mobility at the commencement of an examination may concentrate limited clinical time more effectively.

Specific mention must be made of spinal lesions; the combination of weakness leading to falls, a full bladder and a sensory loss below the level of the lesion is easily recognized, but early symptoms can be very vague and only by specifically considering cord compression will the diagnosis be made. The advances of surgical techniques and/or the prompt administration of radiotherapy in cases of malignancy mean that real life quality gains can be easily lost. Particular cases where a high index of suspicion should exist are those with chronic rheumatic conditions and malignancy known to frequently metastasize to bone (particularly prostate, bronchus and breast).

Attention to detail is important; physical examination may reveal significant arthritis affecting hips and knees, but mobility may be compromised because of unmanicured nails, poorly fitting footwear, or even worn-out non-slip end-rubbers of a stick or frame.

Frequently it will be impossible to identify a discrete substantive physical reason for falls, and although generally unremarkable to clinical examination a patient may just not be capable of standing and walking. These patients should be admitted, but a clear pathology may remain elusive with rather nebulous final diagnoses such as minor cerebrovascular disease and loss of confidence. Such patients often respond well to rehabilitative care and must be seen as medically ill rather than as social problems; inappropriate transfer to residential or nursing home care is unacceptable. Finally, it is a regular occurrence for elderly patients to arrive in A&E departments having spent prolonged periods on floor surfaces; in addition to determining the likely reasons why, particular attention should be made to minimizing the risk of pressure sore development.

CONFUSIONAL STATES

The incidence of dementia increases to above 2% in the elderly over 80 years of age; by implication, a majority of the old are not demented and whilst the demented are more frequently involved in accidents the loose usage of the term 'dementia' to confused, previously undiagnosed patients is unacceptable. In the A&E unit, the non-perjorative 'confusional state' should be preferred. Information regarding the patient's normal functional state from accompanying persons familiar with the patient is important and should never be dismissed. In addition to seeking information regarding behavioural changes, particularly useful lines of enquiry are recent life changes, medication, recent head injury, shortness of breath and pain.

Where confusion is longstanding, understood and the presentation is principally related to behavioural problems, the most appropriate transfer from the A&E

unit may be to a psychogeriatric service. It should be recognized that the pressure on these resources is often severe and that what seems to the A&E department to be the most deserving case may not in fact be so; indeed, if the most expeditious route to a psychogeriatric bed becomes a presentation to the A&E department it will surely become the most popular. An agreed policy for such cases should minimize the potential for episodes of frustration and improve the prospects for an equitable service.

There are a number of common investigations that should be considered for an ill, acutely confused elderly patient:

- Infection
  - Urine dipstick, macroscopic and laboratory
  - Blood cultures
  - Sputum
  - Aspiration of synovial fluid
  - Lumbar puncture
  - Chest X-ray
- Infarction
  - ECG cardiac enzymes (creatine kinase – CK-MB)
  - CT (computed tomography) head scan
- Haematological/metabolic
  - Blood count
  - Urea and electrolytes
  - Blood sugar
  - Calcium
  - Thyroid biochemistry

In the frail elderly with diminished physiological reserves, acute illness will often provoke a 'toxic confusional state'. Frequently, familiar history patterns emerge; for example, the constipated, dehydrated patient who after feeling strange (myocardial infarction, stroke, etc.) took to their bed, stops drinking to avoid incontinence, subsequently becoming increasingly confused and then presents with a urea of 40+. Infection, particularly of the urinary tract, is a very frequent cause of confusional states, but minor proteinuria or a macroscopically non-turbid urine is unlikely to be sufficiently infected to be an adequate, sole cause of confusion. Attribution of all of a patient's problems to urinary infection may encourage a dismissive approach and failure to adequately identify other problems. This is of importance, particularly when medical teams are very busy; such a patient may remain inadequately diagnosed once admitted, one confused elderly person of 80 years plus being very similar in characteristics to another from a nursing care observation perspective on a busy mixed ward.

Several other infective episodes warrant special attention in relation to confusional states. The joint swollen with an effusion must be aspirated and urgently examined by Gram stain and subsequent culture; similarly, meningitis will be missed unless a low threshold for lumbar puncture prevails. Bacterial endocarditis similarly needs to be actively considered. Inspection of pressure areas and the examination of leg ulcers hidden underneath extensive bandaging will often be unpleasantly revealing.

Elderly chest signs may be misleading or notable for their absence and a chest film – posteroanterior if possible – should be considered part of the routine examination. The finding of significant heart failure is often a surprise; the classical chest pain symptoms of myocardial infarction are frequently absent in the aged, but a story can be obtained of a short illness followed by several courses of antibiotics to which no improvement occurred with increasing confusion. Similarly, the finding of abdominal masses should not lead to a sudden diagnosis of widespread malignancy until an abdominal X-ray clarifies the extent of constipation, and the prudent will await a bowel clearance before reconsidering the diagnosis.

Finally, the difficult question of the urgent CT head scan – the question is only difficult because of frequent limited access to the investigation. This is unacceptable and if a clear diagnosis and management plan cannot be made, particularly on a previously cognitively intact elderly patient, a scan should be obtained and if the neurological signs are of deterioration this should be urgently dealt with.

IATROGENIC DISEASE AND THERAPEUTICS

Virtually all areas of therapeutics can be implicated in producing iatrogenic disease and when a presentation doesn't make sense it is worth methodically looking through the registered side-effects of medication. Often a pill box containing an assortment of medicaments will be produced; these should be readily identifiable through colour, size and markings using charts that are available from hospital pharmacies. Although the elderly are widely credited with non-compliance, at times they adhere remarkably to prescribed treatments in the presence of adverse reactions. Multiple pathology leads to polypharmacy and it is often difficult to understand the logic of therapeutic regimens, if indeed one exists, when confronted by a patient possessing a wide array of prescribed drugs.

Particular attention should be paid to psychoactive drugs. The problems relating to tricyclic drugs (falls, confusion, postural hypotension, constipation and visual disturbance) are often overlooked, and whilst drug-induced parkinsonism is recognized with major tranquillizer usage it may be missed with combination preparations containing antidepressant and major tranquillizer. Cardiovascular drugs frequently give problems. Digoxin toxicity may cause severe dysrhythmias and digoxin-specific antibody should be readily available within A&E departments. Overdiuresis, electrolyte disturbance and, increasingly, uraemia secondary to ACE (angiotensin converting enzyme) inhibitory prescribed for cardiac failure occur. Postural hypotension complicating treatment for heart failure or the overenthusiastic management of hypertension will only be diagnosed by careful measurement of blood pressure – both supine and standing; while a small drop of 10 mmHg or so in systolic pressure may not be important, a drop of greater than 20 mmHg of systolic pressure and over 10 mmHg of diastolic pressure constitutes orthostatic hypotension. Not uncommonly, pressure drops will be significantly greater, but, as always, caution must be exercised in basing a diagnosis on single measurements.

There is a natural, laudable temptation to stop medication when presentations are apparently due to adverse reactions, but there needs to be clarity on the original prescribing rationale – requiring liaison with the patient's usual doctor. If doubt exists, the correct course is often to advise the patient's doctor and to defer from radically changing the therapy. If potentially long-term medication is initiated in the A&E department, good communication is necessary not only with regard to the need for therapy but also for review, as this will rarely be the responsibility of the A&E unit.

The longstanding maxim of 'go low, go slow' is worth remembering when prescribing for the elderly – particularly considering the range of pharmokinetic possibilities between the thin frail old man and the obese old woman.

It is important to give the patient a clear explanation of treatment expectations, together with a description of likely side-effects. It is good practice for elderly patients being discharged from the A&E department to have their complete drug regimen written legibly so that they and their attendants are reliably informed; it is also useful to identify the purpose of individual drugs in a simple manner (e.g. heart, diabetes, etc.).

Analgesia is frequently dispensed on an 'as required basis', but it must be realized that many elderly persons are stoical and too conservative in analgesic use while others will abuse treatment. It is far more constructive to advise routine analgesia to avoid breakthrough pain. While potent anti-inflammatory drugs are good for inflammation, pain such as that from vertebral crush fractures needs more analgesia and in such circumstances low-dose morphine sulphate in controlled-release formulations may be particularly useful. It is worth remembering that simple regular analgesia such as paracetamol 6-hourly will often be sufficient for minor conditions. Generally, elderly patients make light of pain, and anticipatory management with analgesia often provides a much safer functional capacity. Finally, when patients are given medication in the A&E department, labelling should be particularly clear and so-called child-proof containers avoided as they are in fact more usually impossible to open by many elderly subjects.

ABUSE AND NEGLECT

Abuse towards an elderly person may occur in a variety of guises. Circumstances that may contribute include:

- Increasing dependency.
- Personality or behavioural problems.
- Multiple dependants within the family.
- Financial difficulties.
- Environmental problems.
- History of abuse within the family.
- History of psychiatric/psychological problems within the family.
- Poor communication problems within/between family/ carers.

It can be particularly difficult to diagnose abuse in the case of the very frail, agitated person in whom reasonable handling may on occasion produce significant bruising. Within the A&E department suspicious signs should be clearly documented and when a high level of concern exists photographs should be taken if possible. Accusation of abuse should be avoided as circumstances often require sensitive assessment; but anxieties should be recorded and emotions controlled. Often such patients will be well known to geriatric psychiatric departments as well as to social workers. Physical abuse can be easily hidden and emotional abuse may never be witnessed; above all, if abuse is not considered it will be missed.

Sexual abuse is not uncommon; for example, the elderly man whom following a small stroke has a heightened drive may make abusive demands of a retiring spouse, or, conversely, the severely handicapped women whose catheter is always removed by her spouse to facilitate intercourse. These are not simple matters and require very mature clinical guidance which is beyond the responsibility of the A&E department. Failure to respond to such issues is, however, nothing short of an acceptance of the abuse continuing.

Financial abuse occurs in various guises and often amounts to extortion; the identification of cases and individuals at risk – for example, the forgetful widow who coincidentally is found to be carrying a large amount of money – is important. The appropriate action is referral to a medical social worker who can, for example, advise the individual to appoint a power of attorney or, where the individual is unable to give reasoned agreement, refer their case to the Court of Protection. One of the sadder observations is the situation where a family becomes dependent on the benefits and accommodation of an elderly person for their own viability and yet are unable to meet the care needs; typically these patients will be known to hospital and community teams who should be advised of A&E department attendances.

Legislation in the UK fails to adequately safeguard the elderly from abuse, although in some circumstances Section 47 of the National Assistance Act (1948) may enable a local authority to remove a patient from their home to a place of safety when they pose a danger to themselves or others. Section 135 of the Mental Health Act (1983) allows a mentally ill person who has been ill treated or is unable to look after themselves to be detained for 72 h. Most situations fall outside these legislations and rely on complaint to the police and a subsequent willingness to press charges – a process many victims are unwilling to pursue. In many instances, counselling and revision of care circumstances are required. The purpose of detailing these issues here is to emphasize the difficulties and to encourage A&E department policies of careful documentation and constructive disclosure to those with the power and resources to case manage.

Self-neglect, often to extremes, is occasionally encountered and while frontal cerebral lobe disease and dementia may account for a proportion of such patients many will be remarkably free of identifiable psychopathology. The importance of this is that with sensitive handling by staff an opportunity to intervene helpfully may be created – a patronizing or dissenting attitude may create alienation.

Senile recluses pose a further challenge; they are often notable for their lack of poverty, large amounts of money commonly being found. They are typically independent, quarrelsome people of above average intelligence, who over a long period increasingly shun contact except with perhaps a visiting relative. It is difficult to rationalize this behaviour – perhaps regarding such cases as representing the late stage of a personality disorder is the most helpful! These cases may come to the A&E unit having sustained an injury a considerable time before presentation and, while beyond comprehension, management will not be helped by confrontation. Infestation with lice and scabies should be anticipated and the misguided temptation to treat pruritic eruptions with corticosteroids resisted (scabies may be mistaken for excoriated eczema).

Alcohol abuse in the elderly is often overlooked. The life-long heavy drinker who displays typical stigmata may be identified readily, but others turn to drink in old age for a variety of reasons which may be understood and generate much sympathy. More usefully, referral for psychiatric counselling may be effective in avoiding serious injury.

ETHNIC MINORITIES

Multicultural society poses several challenges with regard to care of the elderly, the most common being the difficulty of communication with those with limited or no English. An interpreter is highly desirable – ideally a family member – and if this is not possible, access to a bilingual volunteer. For hospitals with large ethnic populations in their catchment area this should not pose a problem. Communication may depend on simple communication boards, and where such difficulties occur frequently in A&E departments it is useful for a core of nursing staff to be familiar with their use – many languages scan text differently from English and some orientation may be required. The ability of an attending doctor or nurse to be able to introduce themselves in the patient's language will frequently break communication barriers and allow for a more satisfactory consultation.

Although it may seem mundane, the importance of reception staff making sure of the correct details, in particular the spelling and pronunciation of names, is considerable. Where significant ethnic populations exist, signs in the A&E department should be duplicated in the appropriate language and/or leaflets made available to enable an understanding of the working of the department. Inappropriate use of accident services is to be discouraged and should a department feel misuse is occurring this should be investigated by an audit, followed by liaison with public health departments, health promotion and the family health services authority to develop a plan of appropriate action.

Immunization records may be deficient for many immigrants and tetanus prophylaxis may be overlooked. Finally, the possibility of tuberculosis as an active pathology should not be forgotten, and in areas with a high prevalence of this disease clear arrangements for screening and surveillance should be operational.

Bibliography

CENTRAL HEALTH MONITORING UNIT (1992). *The Health of Elderly People: An Epidemiological Overview.* London: HMSO.
ROYAL COLLEGE OF PHYSICIANS (1992). Standardized assessment scales for elderly people. A report of joint workshops of the Research Unit of the Royal College of Physicians and the British Geriatric Society.
ROYAL COLLEGE OF PHYSICIANS (1994). Ensuring equity and equality of care for elderly people. A report of the Royal College of Physicians of London.

Further reading

BROCKLEHURST, J.C., TALLIS, R. & FILLITT, H.M., ed. (1992). *Textbook of Geriatric Medicine and Gerontology*, 4th edn. Edinburgh: Churchill Livingstone.
SQUIRES, A., ed. (1991). *Multicultural Health Care and Rehabilitation of Older People.* London: Edward Arnold.
TALLIS, R., ed. (1989). *The Clinical Neurology of Old Age.* Chichester: Wiley.

63 The febrile patient

A.D. HARRIES[a] and C. PARRY[b]

[a] Department of Medicine, Queen Elizabeth Central Hospital, Blantyre, Malawi, Central Africa
[b] Wellcome Trust Clinical Research Unit, Centre for Tropical Diseases, Cho Quan Hospital, Ho Chi Minh City, Viet Nam, and
Centre for Tropical Medicine, John Radcliffe Hospital, Oxford, UK

Chapter plan

Introduction
Normal body temperature and thermoregulation
Fever and pathogenesis of fever
Patterns of fever
The emergency assessment of the febrile patient
General management
The acutely febrile patient
Specific febrile problems
The febrile illness shortly after returning from international travel
Appendix: Sources of advice on travel-associated illness

INTRODUCTION

Well before the introduction of the thermometer in the middle of the nineteenth century, fever was recognized as a sign of disease. Although usually the result of infection, fever may also result from non-infectious causes such as drugs, tumours and connective tissue disorders. In this chapter, we review the current understanding of thermoregulation, the pathogenesis of fever and discuss the assessment of febrile patients in the accident and emergency (A&E) department, particularly patients presenting with fever after returning from international travel.

NORMAL BODY TEMPERATURE AND THERMOREGULATION

Body temperature

The normal body temperature measured orally is usually considered to be 37°C although it can vary between 36°C and 37.8°C. The core temperature (the temperature of aortic blood and internal organs) is about 0.25°C higher than oral temperature, and rectal temperature averages about 0.5°C above the core. A rectal temperature of 37.7°C is taken as the norm. Skin temperature is lower and varies with the degree of vasoconstriction and distance from the aorta. Hand skin temperature is about 30°C, while that of the axilla is normally about 36.2°C.

Circadian temperature rhythm

There is a circadian rhythm of body temperature with a low point in the early morning, a peak at 4–6 p.m. and a diurnal variation of 1°C or more. The temperature changes are related to exercise and feeding and are much less marked in people kept in bed or starved. Body temperature also varies with age and sex. Temperatures are lower in the elderly than in the young and young women have greater temperature fluctuations between morning and evening than young men. Two weeks before the start of menstruation many women have peak temperatures of 37.8°C, an effect probably mediated by progesterone.

Thermoregulation

Body temperature is maintained by balancing heat gain and loss (Murphy, 1992). This balance is controlled by the thermoregulatory centre of the anterior hypothalamus which has a preferred temperature or 'set point'. The heat generated from basal tissue metabolism and normal daily activities is usually greater than that necessary to maintain a temperature of 37°C. Thermoregulation is principally directed at controlling heat loss from the skin by regulating skin blood flow and water evaporation. These physiological processes maintain body temperature in the face of moderate climatic changes. Behavioural thermoregulation is more important when severe environmental heat or cold is encountered. Clothing adjustments and alteration of physical activity enable humans to adjust to almost any outside thermal conditions.

FEVER AND PATHOGENESIS OF FEVER

Fever

Fever is a controlled elevation of body temperature above the peak normal range and occurs when the hypothalamic thermostat is reset at a higher level (Dinarello et al., 1988). An oral temperature above 37.8°C is usually considered indicative of fever. When the hypothalamic set point is raised to a higher setting the vasomotor centre stimulates peripheral vasoconstriction, blood is shunted from the periphery and heat loss reduced. This raises body temperature by 2–3°C. Behavioural changes such as curling up in bed and pulling up the covers also occur. If the body temperature does not reach the new set point, shivering (rhythmic bursts of muscle contraction) further increases muscle heat production. When the temperature of the blood bathing the hypothalamus matches the higher setting, the hypothalamus maintains the new temperature just as it does in the normal state (i.e. with diurnal variation). If the hypothalamic set point is regulated downwards, heat loss is mediated by vasodilatation and sweating and behavioural changes such as flinging off bed covers and adopting the extended position.

Hyperthermia (see also Chapter 39)

Hyperthermia is an elevated body temperature in the presence of a normal hypothalamic set point (Dinarello et al., 1988). Hyperthermia occurs when the mechanisms for heat loss have been impaired by drugs or disease, or overwhelmed by environmental or internal (metabolic) heat. Examples of hyperthermia include heat stroke, occurring as a result of sustained vigorous exercise in hot climatic conditions, the increased temperature that may occur in untreated hyperthyroidism and malignant hyperthermia associated with anaesthetic agents. Differentiating fever from hyperthermia can be difficult and the history is often crucial. The skin in hyperthermia is usually very hot, but dry. Anti-inflammatory agents such as aspirin may reduce the temperature in fever but not hyperthermia.

Hyperpyrexia

Hyperpyrexia is an uncommon condition in which the body temperature rises above 41.5°C. Levels of 43°C or higher are usually lethal. Infections are the commonest cause of hyperpyrexia (Speck, 1986), particularly Gram-negative bacteraemia, Legionnaire's disease, bacterial meningitis, viral encephalitis, typhoid fever and malaria. Non-infectious causes include heat stroke, intracerebral haemorrhage, haemorrhagic pancreatitis, malignant hyperthermia and neuroleptic malignant syndrome. A recent addition to this list is recreational abuse of 3,4-methylenedioxymethamphetamine – 'ecstasy' (Henry et al., 1992).

Pathogenesis of fever

Substances that cause fever are called pyrogens. Exogenous pyrogens (viruses, bacteria, bacterial products and toxins) originate outside the body but actually cause fever by inducing the production of endogenous pyrogens (Dinarello et al., 1988). Endogenous pyrogens are cytokines derived from the host cells, principally monocytes and macrophages. Endogenous pyrogens may also be induced by antigen–antibody complexes in the presence of complement, complement components and some lymphocyte products.

Endogenous pyrogens enter the circulation from sites of infection or inflammation and cause fever by acting on structures in the thermoregulatory centre. Several endogenous pyrogens have been indentified and characterized, including interleukins IL-1 alpha and IL-1 beta, tumour necrosis factor, and interferon-alpha (Dinarello & Wolff, 1990). Although pyrogenic cytokines do not appear to cross the blood/brain barrier, cytokine receptors have been detected in several areas of the brain including the hypothalamus and third cerebral ventricle. It is thought that the fenestrated capillary endothelium in the wall of the third ventricle allows neurones (projecting to the hypothalamus) to sample cytokines in the bloodstream. Metabolic changes initiated in the hypothalamic thermoregulatory centre by these cytokines include the synthesis of prostaglandin E2. The ability of drugs such as aspirin to inhibit the synthesis of prostaglandins at the hypothalamic level explains their anti-pyretic effect. Serotonin, noradrenaline and cyclic AMP also interact at the cellular level to alter the hypothalamic set point although the precise mechanisms are unclear. When the hypothalamic set point is raised,

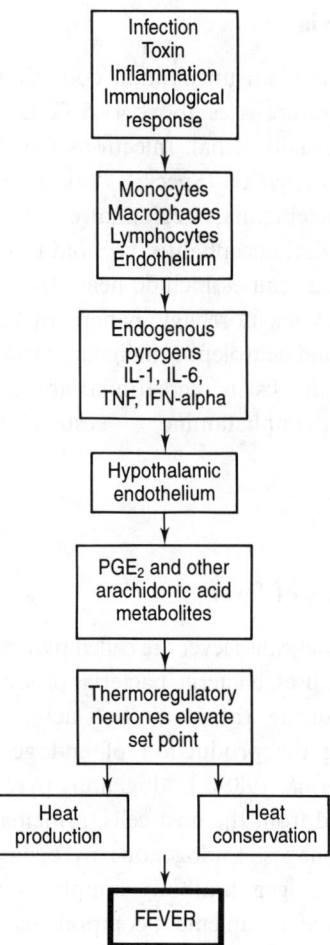

Fig. 1. The pathogenesis of fever. IL, interleukin; TNF, tumour necrosis factor; IFN, interferon; PGE, prostaglandin E.

the mechanisms for raising body temperature are initiated and fever follows (Fig. 1).

Acute phase changes associated with fever and infection

Some of the main acute phase responses are shown in Table 1. These changes result from the fever and also the direct action of invading microorganisms and pyrogenic cytokines. Agents which can block the effects of these cytokines and so reduce some of their deleterious effects in severe infection are being actively sought (Cohen & Glauser, 1991; Hinds, 1992).

PATTERNS OF FEVER

The pattern of fever was once stressed as an important aid to diagnosis. Although fever patterns cannot be

Table 1. *Acute phase changes associated with fever*

Physiological

- Increased metabolic rate, approximately 12% with each 1°C elevation; leads to increased catabolism and body wasting
- Increased sleep, lethargy and poor appetite
- Increased loss of water and electrolytes, water loss approximately 500 ml per m^2 per °C per day
- Increased heart rate, approximately 15 beats min^{-1} per °C increase in temperature
- Increased respiratory rate, which may lead to respiratory alkalosis

Metabolic

- Changes in liver protein synthesis: Increased production of fibrinogen (responsible for increased ESR), haptoglobins; new synthesis of C-reactive protein and amyloid-A association protein
- Reduced levels of serum iron and serum zinc

Haematological

- Increase in polymorphonuclear leucocytes, increase in leucocyte mobility, increased bactericidal activity of leucocytes
- Anaemia due to dyserythropoeisis

ESR, erythrocyte sedimentation rate.

considered pathognomonic for particular infections, they occasionally provide diagnostic clues.

Intermittent fever

Short paroxysms of high fever, accompanied by rigors, are separated by periods when the temperature is normal. Paroxysms may occur daily (quotidian fever), every third day (tertian fever) or every fourth day (quartan fever). The causes of intermittent fever include pyogenic abscesses, bacteraemia, acute pyelonephritis, disseminated tuberculosis, malaria and the intermittent use of antipyretics.

Remittent fever

The pattern is similar to intermittent fever except that the temperature fluctuates less dramatically and does not return to normal. Most fevers are of this type.

Continuous fever

The temperature remains elevated throughout the day with minimal fluctuations (less than 1°C). Miliary tuberculosis and enteric (typhoid) fever are examples.

Table 2. *Factitious fever – diagnostic clues*

1. Failure of the temperature to follow a diurnal variation
2. Rapid defervescence unaccompanied by other signs such as profuse sweating
3. Temperatures of 42°C or greater
4. Normal physical examination
5. Normal laboratory studies
6. Normal oral and rectal temperatures when these measurements are made under careful supervision
7. Patients are often medical or paramedical
8. Urinary temperature should be within 1–1.5°C of a simultaneously taken oral temperature and within 2°C of a simultaneously taken rectal temperature[a]

[a] Murray *et al.* 1977.

Table 3. *Infectious disease in relation to occupation*

Anthrax	Traders/workers in raw animal materials such as hides, wool, hair and bone
Brucellosis	Farmers, butchers, slaughtermen, meat packers, veterinary workers, laboratory personnel
Leptospirosis	Farmers, agricultural workers, sewer workers, abattoir workers, miners, fish workers, veterinary workers
Q fever	Farmers, veterinarians, abattoir workers
Psittacosis	Pet shop owners, zoo workers, veterinary surgeons
Histoplasmosis	Persons who explore bat caves, clean chicken houses, and those involved in demolition work – endemic in USA

Relapsing fever

Periods of fever alternate with periods of normal temperature. During febrile episodes, the fever may follow any of the above patterns. Causes include lymphomas (in Hodgkin's disease this fever is termed Pel–Ebstein fever), brucellosis and the relapsing fevers due to *Borrelia*. In the condition of cyclic neutropenia there is a 14–21-day cycle of fever and low peripheral neutrophil counts, often with concurrent ulceration of mucous membranes.

Fever and pulse rate

For every 1°C the temperature rises above normal the pulse rate rises about 15 beats min^{-1} A slower pulse rate than would be predicted from the temperature chart (relative bradycardia) may be seen in typhoid fever, meningitis and central nervous system (CNS) infections with raised intracranial pressure, hepatitis, Legionnaire's disease, psittacosis and brucellosis as well as hepatitis and cholecystitis. A relative bradycardia may also indicate a factitious fever; other clues to this are in Table 2. Factitious fever should be distinguished from fraudulent fever, in which the fever is authentic but induced by self-inoculation of foreign material by the patient.

Attenuated fever

Fever is sometimes absent even in the presence of severe infection. This is particularly important in seriously ill newborns, the elderly, patients with chronic renal failure and those taking corticosteroids or continuous antipyretics.

THE EMERGENCY ASSESSMENT OF THE FEBRILE PATIENT

History

Occupation

Occupations, such as those in Table 3, may be associated with particular infectious diseases.

Geographical status

Important questions include geographical origins and current residence, travel undertaken in the last year, information concerning immunizations received prior to international travel and details of malaria prophylaxis.

Past medical and surgical history

A history of valvular heart disease, either congenital or acquired, and the presence of medical conditions such as diabetes mellitus, rheumatic disease, chronic renal failure or alcoholism are important. Asplenia, either functional or anatomical (removed following trauma or for haematological conditions), predisposes the patient to infection with encapsulated bacteria, particularly *Streptococcus pneumoniae* and *Salmonella* spp., and malaria.

Family history of fever

Recurrent polyserositis (Familial Mediterranean fever) is an autosomal recessive disorder which occurs among inhabitants of the Near and Middle East. Patients present with fever and abdominal pain, pleurisy, arthritis and skin rashes.

Social history

Many illnesses can be acquired from pets (Elliot *et al.*, 1985). Psittacosis is a potential risk for those who keep pet birds. Campers, swimmers, windsurfers and canoeists exposed to contaminated water are at risk of leptospirosis.

A history of exposure to febrile or ill patients within the recent past or risk habits such as intravenous drug abuse can be important.

Drug history

Drugs are a relatively common cause of fever (Young *et al.*, 1982), usually as a result of an allergic (hypersensitivity) reaction, but sometimes for other reasons. Atropine, for example, and some antidepressants interfere with heat regulatory mechanisms causing hyperthermia rather than true fever. Amphotericin B and bleomycin cause fever by directly stimulating the production of endogenous pyrogenic cytokines. All drugs are capable of causing fever, with the exception of digoxin, chloramphenicol, tetracycline and insulin. Fever usually develops 7–10 days after the drug has been started, although it can start with the first dose. There is often a rash and eosinophilia, although with some drugs fever occurs with no other clinical manifestations (Table 4). When the drug is discontinued the temperature usually returns to normal within 48 h and almost always within 4 days.

Two important types of drug fever are potentially life-threatening. *Malignant hyperthermia* is a genetically determined condition in which the skeletal muscles generate massive heat production in the presence of anaesthetic agents, in particular halothane and suxamethonium (Nelson & Flewellen, 1983). Following anaesthetic induction, muscle contractions develop, the skin becomes extremely hot and the central temperature rises rapidly (see also Chapter 10). The anaesthetic must be stopped, the patient ventilated and cooled. Intravenous dantrolene (which interferes with calcium efflux from the muscle cell and inhibits the contractile process) should be given in a dose of $1–10 \, mg \, kg^{-1}$. A suspicious family history and an abnormal resting creatine phosphokinase level suggests the diagnosis and should lead to avoidance of anaesthesia, particularly with the above-mentioned agents.

The *neuroleptic malignant syndrome* is an idiosyncratic reaction to neuroleptic agents, particularly chlorpromazine, haloperidol and flupenthixol, which results in hyperthermia, muscle rigidity and impaired consciousness (Smego & Durack, 1982). Unlike malignant hyperpyrexia, the condition develops insidiously over 1–3 days and the temperatures are not so high. There is a significant mortality from respiratory infection. Creatine phosphokinase levels are elevated during the illness. The drug should be stopped and dantrolene and bromocriptine have been used with some success. Recovery generally takes several days while the neuroleptic responsible is cleared from the circulation.

Recent hospitalization and hospital procedures

Phlebitis related to intravenous cannulae is a common cause of fever. Patients discharged with indwelling central venous catheters for the administration of home parenteral nutrition, cytotoxic drugs or antimicrobials are at risk of infection, particularly with *Staphylococcus aureus*, *Staphylococcus epidermidis* and *Candida* spp. Wound infections, urinary tract infections, deep venous thrombosis, pulmonary emboli and deep operative infection may complicate early discharge after surgery. Vascular, orthopaedic and cardiac prostheses may become infected.

Blood transfusions may be followed weeks and months later by hepatitis B, hepatitis C, Epstein–Barr and cytomegalovirus infections and, rarely, exotic infections such as malaria and Chagas' disease.

Sexually transmitted disease exposure

The sexual orientation of the patient (homosexual, bisexual or heterosexual) and potential sexual exposures, particularly during travel to areas of the globe highly endemic for human immunodeficiency virus (HIV) such as sub-Saharan Africa and Thailand, may be relevant (Noone *et al.*, 1991). Groups at particular risk for HIV infection are listed in Table 5.

Table 4. *Drugs which produce fever without other manifestations*

Allopurinol	Penicillins
Antihistamines	Phenytoin
Barbiturates	Quinidine
Iodides	Salicylates
Isoniazid	Sulphonamides
Methyldopa	Thiouracils

Adapted from Speck (1986) with permission.

Table 5. *Groups at particular risk of human immunodeficiency virus infection*

- Homosexual or bisexual males, particularly those with numerous partners and who indulge in passive rectal intercourse
- Intravenous drug abusers, including both men and women
- Blood product recipients, particularly haemophiliacs
- Sexual partners of patients with acquired immunodeficiency syndrome (AIDS), AIDS-related complex or at high risk of acquiring HIV infection
- Indigenes from areas of the tropics with a high level of HIV (e.g. areas of sub-Saharan Africa, Thailand, India, Brazil)
- Travellers to high-risk areas of the world, particularly those who have had blood transfusions or sexual contact with local people (especially prostitutes)
- Children (< 4 years of age) whose parents (one or both) either have or are at high risk of HIV infection
- Any promiscuous individual, whether homosexual or heterosexual

The immunocompromised patient

The immunocompromised host is at risk of a wide range of infections depending on the type of immunosuppression (Geddes & Ellis, 1985). Special categories of patient that need to be recognized include intravenous drug users, transplant recipients (kidneys, bone marrow, heart, liver and cornea), patients with the acquired immunodeficiency syndrome (AIDS), patients taking corticosteroids and those with haematological malignancies and neutropenia due to cytotoxic drugs.

The current illness

Febrile illnesses may be acute (< 2 weeks' duration) or chronic (> 2 weeks' duration) and the differential diagnosis differs between the two categories. Most acute fevers are self-limiting and probably viral.

Symptoms common to all febrile patients, such as headache, anorexia, lassitude and sweating, have no diagnostic or localizing value. Symptoms which cannot be attributed to the pyrexia, however, may provide a clue to the anatomical site of disease (Table 6). Symptoms suggesting HIV infection are summarized in Table 7.

Table 6. *Localizing symptoms and signs of infection*

Cough, pleuritic chest pain, rusty sputum
Tachypnoea, localized inspiratory crackles, bronchial breathing
= PNEUMONIA

Severe headache, pain in back of neck, vomiting, photophobia
Neck stiffness, positive Kernig's sign
= MENINGITIS

Diarrhoea with or without blood, abdominal pain, vomiting
= GASTROENTERITIS

Frequency, dysuria and loin pain
Loin tenderness
= ACUTE PYELONEPHRITIS

Severe lower abdominal pain in a sexually active woman
Lower abdominal tenderness and guarding
On vaginal examination, the presence of tenderness on moving the cervix, adnexal tenderness and palpable adnexal swelling
= PELVIC INFLAMMATORY DISEASE

Severe pain in a bone
Soft tissue swelling, erythema, warmth, point tenderness
= OSTEOMYELITIS

Pain and swelling of a joint/joints
Signs of joint inflammation, tenosynovitis
= PYOGENIC ARTHRITIS

Table 7. *Symptoms suggesting human immunodeficiency virus infection*

- Recurrent skin problems (seborrhoeic dermatitis, generalized itchy dermatitis, herpes simplex, dermatophyte infections, herpes zoster, new-onset psoriasis)
- Oral mucosal problems (oral candidiasis, hairy leucoplakia, aphthous ulceration, gingivitis, dental abscesses)
- Generalized lymphadenopathy
- Marked weight loss, chronic diarrhoea, prolonged night sweats, malaise
- Recurrent pneumonia (especially intravenous drug abusers)
- Recurrent sexually transmitted diseases
- Numerous presentations with common childhood illnesses (e.g. otitis media, tonsillitis)

Examination

Important points in the examination of a febrile patient

- General appearance and toxicity of the patient
- Vital signs
- Skin rash or skin lesions*
- Lymphadenopathy
- Mucosal, conjunctival and genital lesions
- Cardiac murmurs
- Hepatosplenomegaly
- Mental or neurological dysfunction
- Dental sepsis
- Rectal/vaginal examination

* Kingston & MacKey, 1986.

A complete and careful physical examination must be carried out. The testicles and epididymis are often neglected and should be examined carefully. Rectal and pelvic examinations should be performed if the diagnosis remains uncertain after completion of the physical examination.

Laboratory evaluation

Investigations should be used to confirm or refute a clinical diagnosis or to help when the apparent cause of the fever is unclear. If the cause is felt to be a non-specific upper respiratory viral infection, a clinical diagnosis is usually sufficient, without further investigation. Useful screening laboratory tests are listed in Table 8. Other investigations depend on the clinical situation.

GENERAL MANAGEMENT

Whether the fever *per se* should be treated is debated. Although *in vitro* and animal studies suggest that some host defence functions (lymphocyte activation, immuno-globulin synthesis) are enhanced by elevated temperatures (Murphy, 1992), the evidence in humans is inconclusive. Furthermore, suppressing the fever may be misleading in patients with fever of unclear aetiology. It also removes a marker which helps to judge the patient's response to treatment when aetiology is known.

Suppression of fever is justified:

1. If the fever makes the patient feel uncomfortable.
2. To avoid potentially harmful secondary effects such as tachycardia in those with heart disease and the

Table 8. *Useful investigations*

Blood tests
- Full blood count with differential white cell count and film
- Erythrocyte sedimentation rate
- Thick and thin blood films in patients with overseas exposure
- Serum biochemical profile, including liver function tests, urea and electrolytes, blood glucose
- Two sets of blood cultures (aerobic and anaerobic). If empirical antibiotics are to be given in the presence of systemic infection, it is advisable to take two or three sets of blood cultures first
- Serum for storage, acute and convalescent antibody titres, antigen detection and acute phase reactants

Other specimens
- Urinalysis, with microscopy and culture when relevant
- Sputum microscopy and culture
- Stool microscopy and culture

Radiology
- Chest radiography

---

elderly, febrile convulsions in children under the age of 5 years and to reduce a hypercatabolic state.
3. To reduce extremely high temperatures above 41.5°C where there is danger of cerebral, cerebellar and other organ damage.

Antipyretics such as aspirin and paracetamol effectively reduce body temperature, particularly if given regularly. Salicylates should be avoided in children under 12 years of age because of the risk of Reye's syndrome (Committee on Safety of Medicines, 1986), and also in patients with a history of peptic ulcer disease. Physical methods such as sponging with tepid water (cold water causes peripheral vasoconstriction) and use of a fan to encourage evaporation are also valuable. In extreme hyperpyrexia the temperature should be reduced quickly to avoid either sudden death or irreversible cerebral or cerebellar damage. The most effective method is to immerse the patient in an ice-water bath until the temperature is below 40°C when the moderate measures discussed above can be adopted.

THE ACUTELY FEBRILE PATIENT

The common causes of acute fever can usually be diagnosed clinically with the aid of simple laboratory tests. Management depends on whether the patient requires hospitalization or can take medication at home. If antimicrobial agents are required the route and dosage will depend on the severity of infection and other factors such as age, weight and renal function. Where possible, microbiology samples should be obtained before antibiotics are started.

The following section contains some general comments relating to common infection syndromes seen in adults. More detail in each area will be found in other chapters. The management of the febrile returning traveller, however, will be addressed in detail.

Upper respiratory tract infections

Acute pharyngitis and tonsillitis is usually viral although 15–20% of cases are due to *Streptococcus pyogenes*. Distinguishing bacterial from viral infection can be difficult, although tender, enlarged cervical lymph nodes and leucocytosis point to a bacterial aetiology. Oral penicillin (erythromycin if penicillin-allergic) should be given if there is doubt about bacterial infection, and continued for 10 days. In severe cases, including peritonsillar abscess (quinsy) which may need drainage, the patient should be admitted and given intravenous benzylpenicillin for 1–2 days, followed by oral therapy. Exudative pharyngitis or tonsillitis occurs in one-half of patients with infectious mononucleosis due to Epstein–Barr virus. Additional clues to this diagnosis are splenomegaly, bilateral enlargement of cervical lymph nodes, thrombocytopenia, atypical mononuclear cells in the peripheral blood film and a positive Monospot test. If given amoxycillin, about 50% of these patients will develop a rash. Acute herpetic pharyngitis should be suspected if pharyngitis is associated with vesicles or ulcers on the lips, buccal mucosa and palate. Treatment involves admission to hospital and administration of acyclovir.

Sinusitis and otitis media may be treated with amoxycillin. Failure to respond may be due to a beta-lactamase-producing strain of *Haemophilus influenzae* or *Moraxella catarrhalis*, when co-trimoxazole or co-amoxyclav (amoxycillin/clavulanic acid) could be used, or *Mycoplasma pneumoniae* which would require erythromycin. Dental infections usually respond to amoxycillin. Unresponsive or severe cases of these infections are best seen by appropriate specialists.

Skin infections

The most common skin infections with fever are caused by *Streptococcus pyogenes* or *Staphylococcus aureus*, and include cellulitis, erysipelas, and subcutaneous abscesses (see also Chapter 52). Flucloxacillin (with or without

benzylpenicillin) is an appropriate empirical antibiotic. Anaerobic soft tissue infections, which should be suspected if the patient is toxic, has soft tissue crepitus and gas on X-ray of the affected limb, are serious conditions warranting hospital admission and intravenous antibiotics which should include an aminoglycoside, benzylpenicillin and metronidazole. Bite wounds, both animal and human, may become infected with a variety of organisms (Goldstein, 1992) (see also Chapter 12). Antibiotic coverage should include an agent with activity against anaerobes and tetanus status should be checked.

Community-acquired pneumonia

The commonest causes are *Streptococcus pneumoniae* and *Mycoplasma pneumoniae*. In mild illness, treatment can be given at home with either amoxycillin or erythromycin (Macfarlane, 1988). Erythromycin is effective against atypical organisms (mycoplasmas, legionella, psittacosis and Q fever), as well as pneumococci, and should be considered particularly during mycoplasma epidemics, which in Britain occur every 3–4 years. Seriously ill patients with community-acquired pneumonia of unknown cause could be treated with a combination of intravenous co-amoxiclav or cefuroxime and erythromycin. In patients with an aspiration pneumonia, when oropharyngeal anaerobes are involved, a regimen including metronidazole, co-amoxiclav (amoxycillin/clavulanic acid) or clindamycin would be appropriate.

Complicated urinary tract infection (see also Chapter 48)

A patient (usually female) with symptoms of urinary tract infection and fever often has an upper urinary tract infection and may need in-patient treatment. Amoxycillin, an oral cephalosporin, trimethoprim or a quinolone could be chosen for out-patient treatment. Older patients, those with vomiting and those who are bacteraemic or toxic need hospitalization and intravenous antibiotics. An aminoglycoside, second- or third-generation cephalosporin or a quinolone in the penicillin-allergic patient would be suitable for community-acquired infections (Wilkie *et al.*, 1992).

Pelvic inflammatory disease (see also Chapter 59)

Patients with systemic disturbance are best admitted under the appropriate specialist as specimens need to be taken from the urethra and cervix and possibly laparoscopically. Antibiotic treatment might include cipro-floxacin (against gonorrhoea), an aminoglycoside or second-generation cephalosporin (against Gram-negative organisms) and metronidazole (against anaerobes), followed by a course of doxycycline or erythromycin to prevent persistence of chlamydia and mycoplasma (Pearce, 1990).

Gastroenteritis

Many patients with gastroenteritis due to *Salmonella*, *Campylobacter*, or *Shigella* have fever associated with gastrointestinal symptoms. Patients needing admission often require no more than oral or intravenous fluids. Toxic patients and those clinically bacteraemic with shock and confusion may need systemic antibiotics. Quinolones, such as ciprofloxacin, are active against most important gut pathogens (Gorbach, 1988). An exception is *Clostridium difficile* induced pseudo-membranous colitis which must be suspected if the patient has taken antibiotics prior to developing diarrhoea. The microbiology laboratory should look for the *Clostridium difficile* toxin. Treatment is with oral metronidazole or oral vancomycin.

Meningitis (see also Chapter 53)

Patients with suspected meningitis must be admitted, and the cerebrospinal fluid examined. The two common causes of pyogenic meningitis in adults, *Streptococcus pneumoniae* and *Neisseria meningitidis*, are treated with high-dose parenteral benzylpenicillin. In a pyogenic meningitis of unknown aetiology, an empirical antibiotic regimen should include a third-generation cephalosporin (eg cefotaxime) and ampicillin may be added (to cover against the unlikely event of *Listeria* infection).

Bacterial infections of bone and joints (see also Chapter 50)

Such patients require hospital admission. Pyogenic arthritis is caused principally by *Staphylococcus aureus*, occasionally *Neisseria gonorrhoeae*, and antibiotics should initially be selected to cover these pathogens. Adults with acute osteomyelitis are likely to have *Staphylococcus aureus* or enteric Gram-negative bacteria. Flucloxacillin and an aminoglycoside or a third-generation cephalosporin would be suitable choices.

Septicaemia

Septicaemia should be clinically suspected if there is fever, tachycardia, tachypnoea, change in mental status and/or evidence of organ failure. Septic shock is present if the systolic blood pressure is less than 90 mmHg, providing there are no other causes of shock such as hypovolaemia, myocardial infarction or pulmonary embolism. Antibiotic treatment should be started without delay to cover the likely pathogen(s). The clinical presentation may provide a clue, such as a purpuric rash in meningococcal infection or pneumonia in pneumococcal infection. If no clues are present, initial blind antibiotic treatment could consist of an aminoglycoside plus a broad-spectrum penicillin such as co-amoxyclav (amoxycillin/clavulanic acid), or a combination of cefotaxime and metroidazole. Common organisms causing bacteraemia include staphylococci, streptococci and Gram-negative bacteria such as *Escherichia coli*. The illness could, however, also be due to an exotoxin. The toxic shock syndrome is an example, caused by a toxin-producing *Staphylococcus aureus*. This may occur in young women using tampons at the time of menstruation, although many cases are not associated with menstruation (Williams, 1990).

In the immunocompromised patient, particularly the neutropenic patient, blind antibiotic treatment needs to cover Gram-negative bacteria of which *Pseudomonas aeruginosa* is particularly important. An aminoglycoside plus anti-pseudomonal beta-lactam antibiotic would be a good initial option (Hughes *et al.*, 1990). Antibiotics active against Gram-positive organisms would be important if there were signs of a central venous line infection.

SPECIFIC FEBRILE PROBLEMS

Fever in intravenous drug abusers.

Infectious complications are common (Levine & Sobel, 1991). Skin infections at the sites of needle injections include cellulitis, superficial and deep abscesses, necrotizing fasciitis, and pyomyositis. *Staphylococcus aureus* is a common organism in these situations, but infection can also occur with beta-haemolytic streptococci, Gram-negative organisms and anaerobes. Co-amoxiclav, with or without an aminoglycoside, is a suitable antibiotic choice. Clindamycin is a good alternative in a patient allergic to penicillins.

Endocarditis with tricuspid valve involvement, usually

caused by *Staphylococcus aureus*, is a well-recognized and common complication of intravenous drug abuse. CNS infections (brain abscess, subdural empyema and meningitis) and pulmonary infections (pneumonia, empyema and lung abscess) must be remembered. Hepatitis is also very common. Drug withdrawal itself may cause fever although infection should always be excluded first.

Shortlived fever with transient bacteraemia is common after injection of contaminated material. Rarely the cause is fungal and signs of endophthalmitis and embolic rash should be looked for.

Acute fever with rash

Several important questions should be considered when evaluating a patient with a fever and rash:

- Is the patient so ill as to require immediate resuscitative procedures?
- Is the rash consistent with meningococcal disease requiring immediate antibiotic therapy?
- If the patient is returning from international travel is isolation required?

Correct diagnosis of the rash requires attention to its characteristics (Table 9), the timing of its development (Table 10; Weber *et al.*, 1990) and its distribution and pattern of progression. Particular attention must be paid to the presence of a coagulopathy, valvular heart disease, travel, sexual history, immunological status and prior use of drugs (especially antibiotics). A Gram stain of exudate from the lesion or from a biopsy lesion may allow a rapid diagnosis.

Several life-threatening infections, such as meningococcaemia, may present with erythematous, maculo-

Table 9. *Fever and rash in the acute febrile patient according to classification of rash*

Petechiae/purpura	Vesicles/bullae	Macules/papules
Bacteraemia	Varicella	Viral exanthem
Vasculitis	Disseminated herpes zoster	Scarlet fever
Enterovirus	Disseminated herpes simplex	Secondary syphilis
Drug reaction	Erythema multiforme	Erythema multiforme
	Drug reaction	Drug reaction

Adapted from Foltzer & Reese (1986) with permission.

Table 10. *Timing of rash in relation to onset of illness*

Early-onset rash: at or up to 3 days after start of illness

a. Diffuse purpuric lesions: bacteraemias, especially Gram-negative organisms

b. Macronodular lesions: bacteraemias or fungaemias; *Candida* should be considered; lesions with blackening suggest *Pseudomonas*

c. Diffuse erythema, especially if desquamation or peeling: scarlet fever, erysipelas (well-defined edge), toxic shock syndrome, Stevens–Johnson syndrome and other drug rashes, Kawasaki disease

Late-onset rash: more than 3 days after onset of illness

a. Erythema gangrenosum and macronodular lesions: *Pseudomonas* and other Gram-negative organisms

b. Macules/papules/vesicles: often immune-mediated: if involves distal portions of extremities, consider gonococcal infection; if in travellers, consider tick typhus (eschar not always present)

papular lesions before evolving into petechiae or purpura, and if there is any doubt parenteral penicillin should be given. Secondary syphilis may present with a rash of highly variable morphology and should be suspected if there is no other obvious diagnosis. Erythema multiforme is typically symmetrical on the trunk and extremities with a predilection for knees, elbows, palms and soles. When mucosal involvement occurs with fever then the term Stevens–Johnson syndrome is used. About half of the cases of erythema multiforme are idiopathic but the disease may be related to drugs (particularly sulphonamides) or infections such as herpes simplex or mycoplasma. Erythema nodosum can be associated with fever and arthralgia and occur with a streptococcal sore throat, sulphonamide exposure, sarcoidosis, tuberculosis and inflammatory bowel disease.

Human immunodeficiency virus

Patients may have fever as part of the virus infection itself or due to other disseminated infections (Shanson, 1990; Table 11). These are best managed by admission to the appropriate local unit.

Chronic febrile illness

A pyrexia of unknown origin is a febrile illness of more than 3 weeks' duration with no diagnosis apparent after

Table 11. *Causes of fever in human immunodeficiency virus infected patients*

Opportunistic pathogens	Conventional pathogens
Mycobacterium avium complex	*Salmonella* spp.
Cytomegalovirus	*Streptococcus pneumoniae*
Cryptococcus neoformans	*Pseudomonas aeruginosa*
Pneumocystis carinii	*Mycobacterium tuberculosis*
Toxoplasma gondii	
Histoplasma capsulatum	

Table 12. *Common causes of pyrexia of unknown origin*

Infections (30–40%)
Common: Tuberculosis, infective endocarditis, intra-abdominal abscesses, perinephric abscess, biliary tract infections, dental abscess, osteomyelitis, cytomegalovirus, Epstein–Barr virus
Uncommon: Q fever, brucellosis, salmonellosis, toxoplasmosis, disseminated mycosis, spirochaetes (relapsing fever, leptospirosis, rat bite fever)

Neoplasms (20–30%)
Lymphoma, leukaemia, renal cell carcinoma, gastrointestinal tumour, metastatic ovarian carcinoma, hepatoma

Connective tissue disease (15–20%)
Systemic lupus erythematosus, vasculitis, polyarteritis nodosa, Still's disease, mixed connective tissue disease

Miscellaneous (15–20%)
Drug fever, multiple pulmonary emboli, inflammatory bowel disease, temporal arteritis, sarcoidosis, factitious fever

Undiagnosed (10%, up to 30% in children)

one week of investigation in hospital. The A&E doctor will not be involved in the work-up of such patients but at least should be familiar with the common causes Table 12 (Larson *et al.*, 1982; Knockaert *et al.*, 1992).

THE FEBRILE ILLNESS SHORTLY AFTER RETURNING FROM INTERNATIONAL TRAVEL

General

With rapid modern travel, infections contracted abroad may still be incubating as the traveller returns home. Those at risk include British travellers (tourists, busi-

Table 13. *Causes of fever in admissions to the Hospital for Tropical Diseases, London*

Common causes	
Malaria	44%
Hepatitis	11%
Typhoid, paratyphoid	5%
Pneumonia	2%
Gastroenteritis	2%
Upper respiratory tract infections	2%
Amoebiasis (liver abscess)	2%
Tuberculosis	2%

Uncommon causes
Typhus
Trypanosomiasis
Schistosomiasis
Human immunodeficiency virus related
Brucellosis
Visceral leishmaniasis

Adapted from Bryceson (1987) with permission.

nessmen, ship and air crews, children visiting expatriate parents during school holidays), immigrants and settled immigrants visiting their country of origin, and foreign visitors. Countries of residence and areas visited must be documented. Although the 6 weeks before the onset of symptoms are especially important, sometimes a period of many years is relevant.

Fever is a common presentation in this group of patients: 51% of admissions to the Hospital for Tropical Diseases in London in 1986 were in response to fever (Bryceson, 1987); the causes are listed in Table 13. Laboratory-confirmed imported infections reported to the Communicable Diseases Unit in Scotland between 1975 and 1987 (Walker & Williams, 1989) are shown in Table 14. Most infections occur among holidaymakers during the summer and autumn. Some imported infections

Table 14. *Imported infections into Scotland 1975–1987*
Total number of laboratory-confirmed cases = 5646.

Salmonellosis	46%
Campylobacter enteritis	14%
Bacillary dysentery	12%
Malaria	8%
Viral hepatitis	4%
Enteric fever	2%

Adapted from Walker & Williams (1989) with permission.

have an importance out of proportion to their incidence, such as falciparum malaria, Legionnaire's disease and the haemorrhagic fevers. Early diagnosis is essential for optimal treatment in these cases and others with public health implications such as typhoid fever. Useful sources of advice for travel-associated illnesses are given in the Appendix.

In the initial assessment of febrile patients returning from abroad, a thick and thin blood film and a full blood count with differential white cell count are invaluable investigations.

Diagnoses from the thick and thin blood films (Fig. 2)

Malaria

General

Thirty million people visit malaria-endemic areas from non-tropical countries every year (Steffen & Behrens, 1992). Fig. 3 shows the worldwide distribution of malaria. Malaria transmission is high in all countries in sub-Saharan Africa, the Indian subcontinent and in Papua

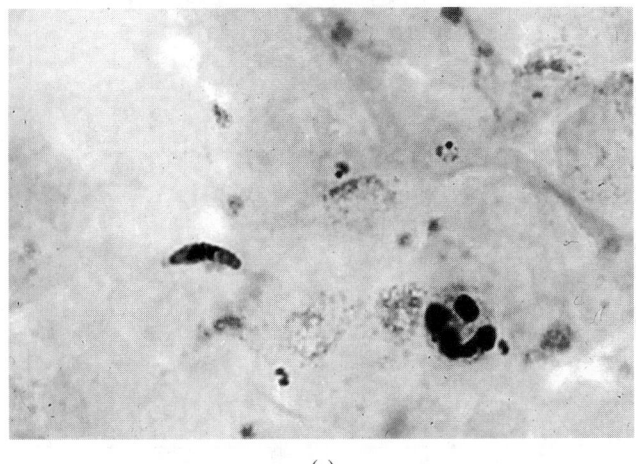

(a)

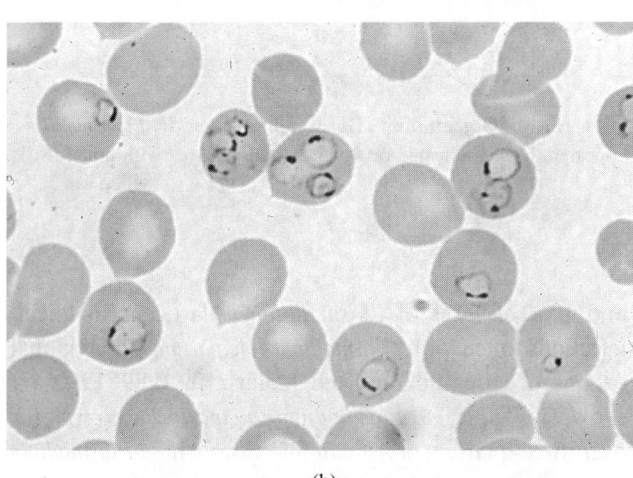

(b)

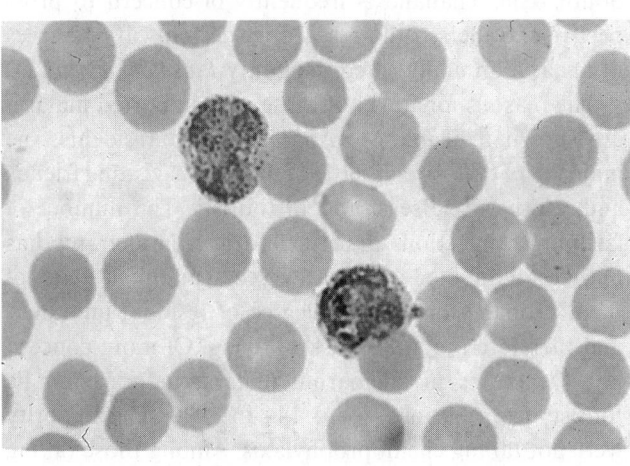

(c)

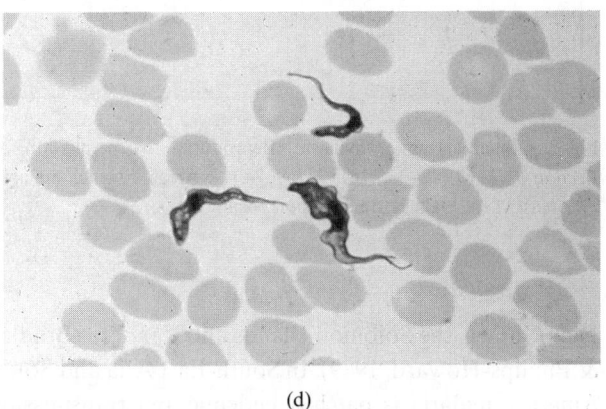

(d)

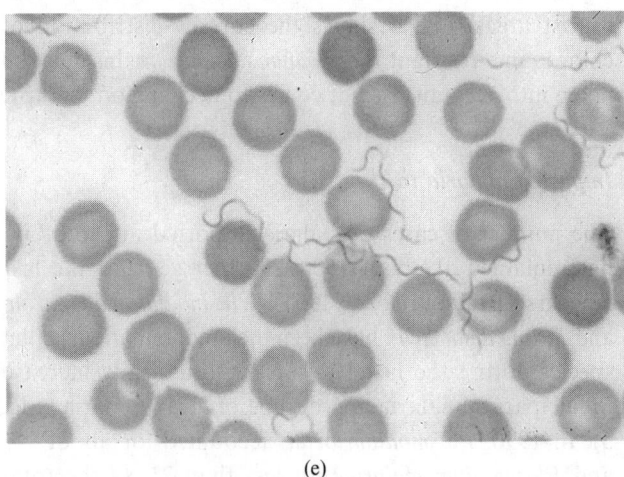

(e)

Fig. 2. Thick and thin blood films: thick blood film of *Plasmodium falciparum* (a), thin blood films of *Plasmodium falciparum* (b), *Plasmodium vivax* (c), *Trypanosoma rhodesiense* (d) and *Borrelia* (e).

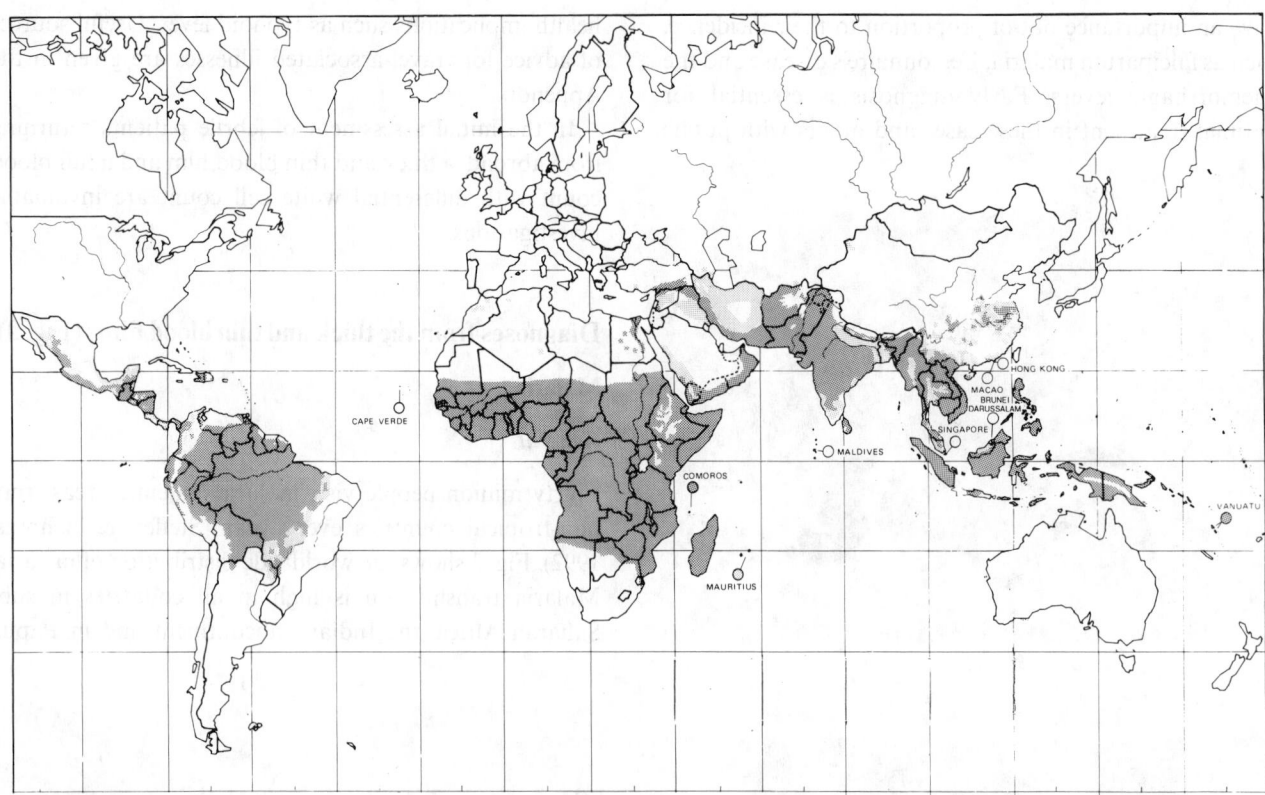

Fig. 3. Global status of malaria. (Reproduced, by permission of the World Health Organization, Geneva, from *Weekly Epidemiological Record*, 1992; **67** (22–23), 161–7, 169–74.) ◯ Areas in which malaria has disappeared, been eradicated or never existed. ◯ Area with limited risk. ◉ Areas where malaria transmission occurs.

New Guinea, the Solomon Islands and Vanuatu (Bradley & Phillips-Howard, 1989). In South-East Asia and South America, malaria is patchily endemic, but transmission either does not occur or is extremely low in the main tourist areas. Fig. 4 shows the current distribution of chloroquine-resistant *Plasmodium falciparum*: this must be taken into account when it comes to deciding on therapy.

Imported malaria to the UK

The number of cases of malaria imported into the UK has remained at about 1500–2500 per year for the last 10 years (Bradley *et al.*, 1991). *Plasmodium falciparum* and *Plasmodium vivax* have been the predominant infecting species during the last 10 years, with a steady increase in falciparum malaria and decline of vivax malaria (Fig. 5). In 1990, *Plasmodium ovale* accounted for about 7% and *Plasmodium malariae* for less than 2% of the total number of malaria infections. The number of mixed species infections has increased in the last 3 years, and in fact a third of all instances of *Plasmodium malariae*

and 10% of cases of *Plasmodium ovale* occur in mixed infections, often with *Plasmodium falciparum*. The regional origins of cases of imported malaria in 1989–1990 are shown in Table 15. *Plasmodium falciparum* accounts for over three-quarters of African infections whilst *Plasmodium vivax* accounts for over 90% of malaria contracted in South Asia. Thailand is frequently of concern to prospective travellers, although it provides only 10–12 cases of malaria annually (predominantly *Plasmodium vivax*).

The reasons for travel of those with imported malaria are shown in Table 16. Among British residents, the majority of cases are in settled immigrants visiting friends and relatives overseas, and in tourists. The number of falciparum infections in settled African immigrants has more than doubled in the last 5 years, although many of them probably have some degree of residual immunity and therefore are at less risk of dying. Of more concern is the increase in falciparum malaria in non-immune tourists from 82 in 1986 to 144 in 1990. The majority were not taking chemoprophylaxis. Among those taking chemoprophylaxis, a significant proportion were non-

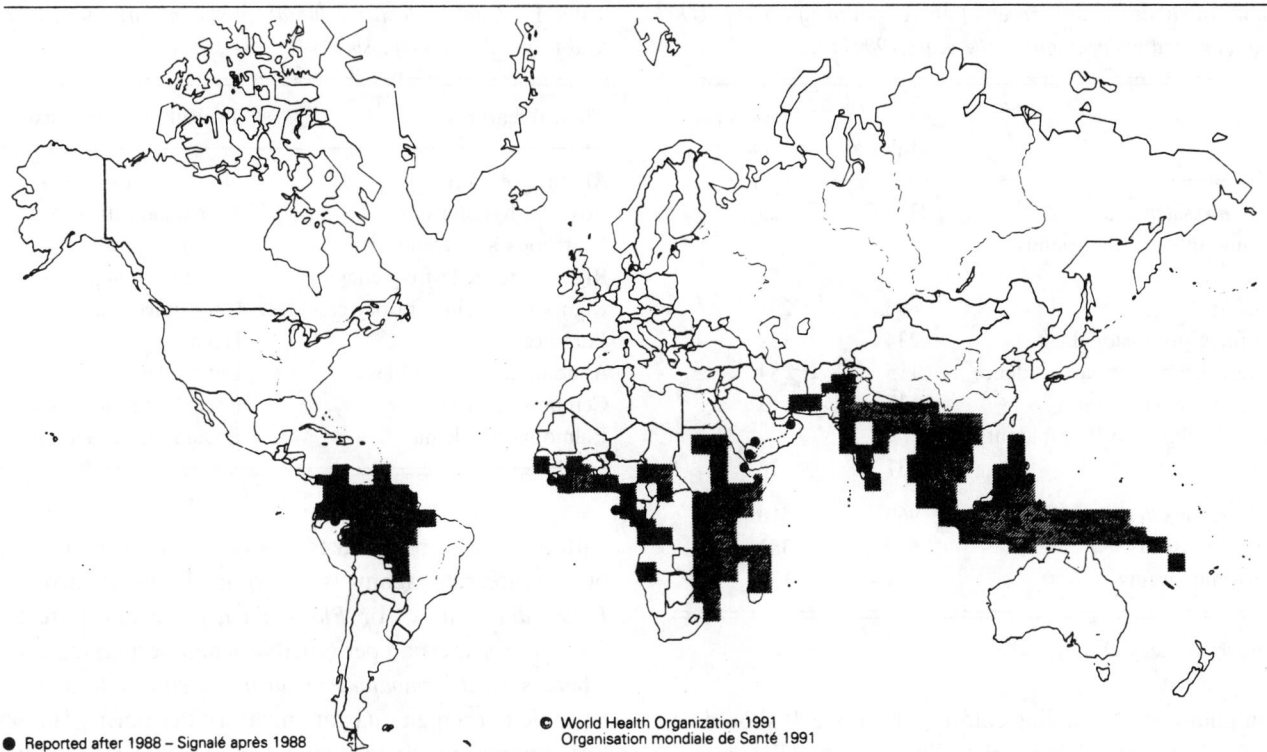

Fig. 4. Areas where chloroquine-resistant falciparum malaria has been reported. (Reproduced, by permission of the World Health Organization, Geneva, from *Weekly Epidemiological Record*, 1991; **66** (22), 162.)

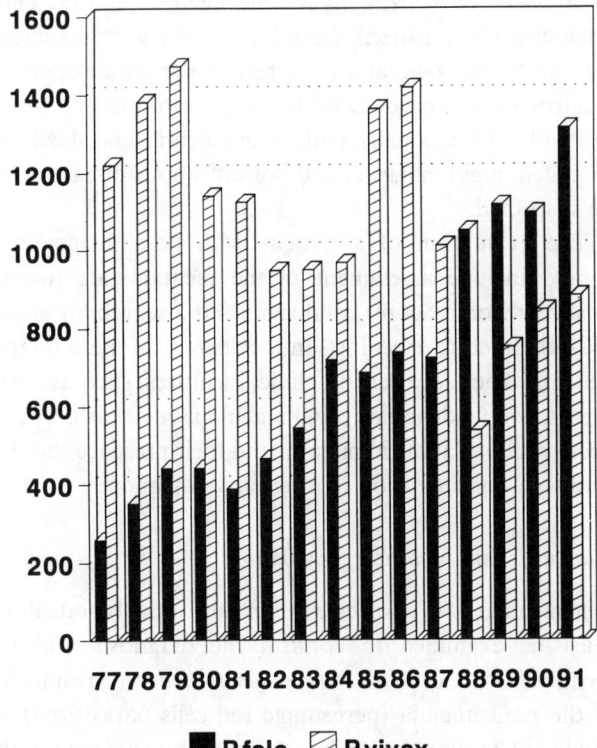

Fig. 5. *Plasmodium falciparum* and *Plasmodium vivax* infections 1977–1991.

Table 15. *Geographical source of malaria imported to the UK during the years 1989–1990*
Cases with mixed infections are excluded from the species-specific data.

	Malaria	Plasmodium falciparum	Plasmodium vivax	Plasmodium ovale
Africa	2275	1845 (81%)	111	218
Middle East	16	6	9	1
South Asia	1244	81	1144 (92%)	1
South-East Asia	63	16	44	2
Asia unstated	18	1	17	–
Latin America	36	4	30	–
Oceania	40	7	31	1
Unstated	391	169	179	27
Total	4083	2129	1565	250

Source: Bradley *et al.*, (1991).

Table 16. *Reasons for travel of those returning to the UK with imported malaria during the years 1989–1990*

	Malaria	*Plasmodium falciparum*
British residents	2373	1229
Immigrants visiting friends/family	1453	654
Tourist	496	291
Business/professional	234	152
Return from overseas residence	115	84
Air/sea crew or military	38	13
Schoolchildren visiting parents abroad	37	26
Overseas residents	969	516
Foreign visitors	620	383
New immigrants	349	133

Source: Bradley *et al.* (1991).

compliant or were taking chloroquine alone. It should be realized, however, that strict adherence to UK recommendations for chemoprophylaxis does not guarantee protection against infection or death. In the last decade, four to 12 people have died of imported falciparum malaria each year. Of the 11 deaths due to falciparum malaria in 1991, four were taking chemoprophylaxis and one of the patients was taking chloroquine and proguanil (Bradley & Warhurst, 1993).

Clinical assessment of a patient with malaria

A patient presenting with fever and who has passed through a malarious area must be regarded as having malaria. Over 85% of patients with falciparum malaria present within 1 month of return to the UK, although some patients may present much later. In contrast only about one-quarter of vivax malaria cases present within 1 month, and 5–10% may present more than 1 year later (Source: PHLS Malaria Reference Laboratory). Relapses in *Plasmodium vivax/Plasmodium ovale* malaria occur for up to 10 years in the absence of radical cure with primaquine. *Plasmodium malariae* malaria does not relapse, but a low-grade, undetected parasitaemia may give rise to intermittent fever (from recrudescence) for 30–40 years.

The common clinical features (fever, anaemia, splenomegaly and jaundice) of the four species of malaria relate to the release of pyrogens and red cell destruction consequent upon red cell schizogony. In non-immunes

Table 17. *Clinical features in falciparum malaria which can lead to pitfalls in diagnosis*

Clinical features	Typical misdiagnosis
Absence of fever	Non-infectious illness
Postural hypotension	Vasovagal attack
Diarrhoea and vomiting	Gastroenteritis
Rigors/backache/frequency	Acute pyelonephritis
Rigors/cough/inspiratory crackles	Chest infection
Jaundice	Hepatitis
Abdominal pain and fever	Enteric fever
Cerebral malaria	Encephalitis/intoxication
Pulmonary oedema	Pneumonia/heart failure

with malaria, it often takes 3–4 days before the rhythm of parasite schizogony is determined. In synchronous *Plasmodium vivax* or *Plasmodium ovale* infection, the fever shows a tertian periodicity (benign tertian malaria), whereas in *Plasmodium malariae* it shows a quartan periodicity (benign quartan malaria). Periodicity is often less apparent in *Plasmodium falciparum* malaria in which the fever is variable and irregular. The spleen is not always palpable in falciparum malaria (Harries, 1989).

Falciparum malaria may cause organ-specific damage as a result of schizogony in the deep capillaries and adherence of parasitized red cells to capillary endothelium leading to microcirculatory arrest. These organ-specific syndromes may produce misleading symptoms and signs (Table 17). Occasionally, patients are afebrile and shocked, so-called 'algid malaria', and non-infectious disease may be suspected.

The evaluation of a patient with possible malaria should include assessment of the mental state (using Glasgow Coma Score), vital signs and a search for signs of spontaneous bleeding and evidence of pulmonary oedema. There are certain clinical features, such as sore throat, lymphadenopathy and maculopapular rash, which occur rarely, if at all, in malaria and their presence should lead to a consideration of alternative diagnoses.

Diagnosis and laboratory evaluation

When malaria is suspected, thick and thin blood films must be examined to confirm the diagnosis and to identify the species. With *Plasmodium falciparum* an estimate of the parasitaemia (percentage red cells parasitized) is needed. The film should be examined by someone with experience so that a low parasitaemia is not missed. Sometimes no parasites are found in peripheral blood

Table 18. *Laboratory abnormalities in falciparum malaria which can lead to pitfalls in diagnosis*

Laboratory abnormality	Typical misdiagnosis
Raised liver transaminases	Hepatitis
Raised prothrombin time	Hepatocellular dysfunction
Raised creatine phosphokinase	Myocardial infarction
CSF: raised protein and lymphocytes	Viral meningitis
Urine: blood/protein/casts	Nephritis
Thromocytopenia	Dengue fever, typhoid, septicaemia

CSF, cerebrospinal fluid.

smears as a result of scanty parasitaemia (partial antimalarial treatment, malaria prophylaxis) or sequestration of parasitized red cells in deep capillaries. If malaria is still suspected it is best to admit the patient and perform repeated blood films. A bone marrow aspirate or blood-stained tissue from intradermal puncture may be of help in difficult cases (Bradley *et al.*, 1987). The presence of schizonts in blood films suggests severe infection.

In a non-immune patient the presence of malaria parasites indicates that malaria is the cause of the illness. In the semi-immune patient (i.e. foreign visitor), parasitaemia may be asymptomatic, and although it should be treated it is worth remembering that the current illness may have an alternative explanation.

Pancytopenia is a common accompaniment of malaria although a leucocytosis may occur in severe infection or intravascular haemolysis. Thrombocytopenia is a valuable pointer to malaria although it may be due to an arbovirus infection or septicaemia. Electrolyte disturbance, hypoglycaemia, impaired renal function, disseminated intravascular coagulation and secondary bacteraemia may be seen. Important investigations include full blood count, urea and electrolytes, blood glucose, blood cultures and clotting screen if there is severe illness or high parasitaemia. In malaria, abnormal investigations occasionally lead to misdiagnosis (Table 18).

Treatment of malaria (Warrell *et al.*, 1990; Gilles, 1991; Molyneux & Fox, 1993)

Plasmodium falciparum

Patients with falciparum malaria in the UK should be admitted to hospital. Non-immune patients or those with any complications should be monitored in a high-dependency or intensive care unit. Local expert advice should be obtained at the outset. Because of the widespread prevalence of chloroquine-resistant strains, all patients should receive quinine either parenterally (quinine dihydrochloride) or orally (quinine sulphate). Parenteral quinine should be given if there is vomiting, severe illness or parasitaemia exceeds 2%. If quinine is unavailable in the pharmacy, then quinidine can be given.

- *Parenteral quinine.* Quinine dihydrochloride given at a dose of 10 mg salt kg^{-1} (up to maximum 700 mg) in 10 ml kg^{-1} (maximum 500 ml) 5% dextrose over 4 h. This is administered 4-hourly (i.e. 4-h infusion followed by 4-h rest) until the patient can swallow or is less severely ill.

  Some authorities recommend a loading dose of quinine, particularly in severe illness or high parasitaemia, PROVIDED the patient has not already received quinine, quinidine or mefloquine in the preceding 24 h. The purpose of the loading dose is to achieve the desired blood concentration of quinine more quickly. The loading dose may be given as quinine dihydrochloride 20 mg salt kg^{-1} (up to maximum 1.4 g) in 10 ml kg^{-1} (maximum 500 ml) 5% dextrose over 4 h *or* quinine dihydrochloride 7 mg salt kg^{-1} (up to a maximum of 490 mg) by infusion pump over 30 min.

- *Parenteral quinidine.* Quinidine gluconate 7.5 mg salt kg^{-1} (up to a maximum of 525 mg) over 4 h, repeated 8-hourly until the patient is able to swallow. A loading dose may be given (see comments above) PROVIDED the patient has not already received quinine, quinidine or mefloquine in the preceding 24 h. The loading dose would be quinidine gluconate 15 mg salt kg^{-1} (up to a maximum of 1.0 g) over 4 h.

- *Oral quinine.* Quinine sulphate (adult 600 mg, child 10 mg kg^{-1}) given 8-hourly usually to complete a course of 7 days' quinine treatment.

- *Completion of quinine treatment.* Fansidar (sulphadoxine 500 mg plus pyrimethamine 25 mg per tablet) will usually be given at the end of treatment. Doses are:

  - Adults: 3 tablets as a single dose.
  - Children > 5 years: 1/2 tablet.
  - Children 5–6 years: 1 tablet.
  - Children 7–9 years: 1½ tablets.
  - Children 10–14 years: 2 tablets.

Fansidar is contraindicated if the patient has a history of sulphonamide sensitivity. Some experienced tropical doctors prefer to administer mefloquine at the end of quinine treatment instead of Fansidar.

Ill patients should also receive broad-spectrum antibiotics after blood cultures have been taken because of the association with Gram-negative septicaemia; parenteral cefuroxime 1.5 g 8-hourly would be an acceptable choice.

Parasite counts should be measured daily until no parasites are detected and a final count is performed at the end of treatment. Hypoglycaemia may be induced by quinine, especially in pregnant women. Patients should have blood glucose measured daily while receiving parenteral quinine and every 6 h in severe illness or during pregnancy. In severe illness or high parasitaemia, daily estimations of urea, electrolytes and haemoglobin are necessary. If patients deteriorate during treatment, hypoglycaemia, concurrent Gram-negative bacteraemia, gastrointestinal bleeding (from disseminated intravascular coagulation), spontaneous rupture of the spleen and resistant parasites should be considered. Chloroquine and quinine do not kill *Plasmodium falciparum* gametocytes, and their presence after a course of treatment is not an indication of failure or an indication for retreatment.

In cerebral malaria, the use of dexamethasone is contraindicated as it prolongs coma and is associated with an increased incidence of complications (Warrell *et al.*, 1982). Quinine can be safely given to the pregnant woman with falciparum malaria. Its main toxic effect is not an oxytocic action but rather its capacity to release insulin and provoke hypoglycaemia (Looareesuwan *et al.*, 1985). Exchange blood transfusion is an option that might be considered in non-immune travellers who are ill with falciparum malaria and whose parasite levels are above 15%, but only after expert specialist advice (Editorial, 1990).

In view of the worrying spread of multiresistant *Plasmodium falciparum* strains, new antimalarial drugs such as Qinghaosu and its derivatives (Hien & White, 1993) and halofantrine are being evaluated. In a recent study (Weinke *et al.*, 1992), halofantrine (3 × 500 mg tablets) taken within a 12 h period followed by 500 mg on day 7 had a 100% efficacy rate in non-immune travellers with falciparum malaria.

Plasmodium vivax, ovale and malariae
These parasites are usually chloroquine-sensitive, although there have been recent reports of chloroquine-resistant *Plasmodium vivax* in New Guinea (Murphy *et al.*, 1993). Chloroquine is given as 25 mg base kg⁻ over 3 days. The time-honoured regimen for adults is:

- Day 1: 600 mg base stat (i.e. 4 tablets chloroquine sulphate)
  300 mg base 6 h later (i.e. 2 tablets)
- Day 2: 300 mg base (i.e. 2 tablets)
- Day 3: 300 mg base (i.e. 2 tablets)
- If further chloroquine is needed in obese people then administer as 300 mg base on day 4/day 5.

If vomiting precludes administration of oral chloroquine, quinine dihydrochloride is given by intravenous infusion until the patient can swallow; a full chloroquine course is then administered. In cases of mixed infections with falciparum malaria, treatment is carried out as for falciparum malaria.

For radical cure of *Plasmodium vivax* and *Plasmodium ovale*, primaquine is given after completing a course of chloroquine EXCEPT in pregnant women and patients deficient in glucose-6-phosphate dehydrogenose. The usual dose is 7.5 mg b.d. for 14 days (for vivax malaria acquired in South-East Asia and Papua New Guinea, primaquine 7.5 mg bd for 21 days is given).

Malaria – species undetermined
Treatment is carried out as for falciparum malaria.

Follow-up
One week after completing quinine and Fansidar or chloroquine, malaria prophylaxis is resumed to complete a total of 4 weeks' prophylaxis after leaving a malaria-endemic area.

Acute infection with *Trypanosoma rhodesiense*

This potentially fatal infection is acquired through the bite of infected tsetse flies which may be found in several of the game parks in Central and Southern Africa. About 2 weeks after an infected bite, a 'chancre' or painful swelling develops, followed within 7–14 days by fever, headache, an erythematous rash and splenomegaly. The diagnosis should be considered in anyone who has visited games parks in Central Africa within the previous month. Patients should be managed in a specialist tropical unit.

Relapsing fever due to infection with *Borrelia* spp.

This is found in most tropical countries and is acquired either through the bites of lice or ticks. The spirochaetes are easily recognized in blood films and the infection responds to tetracycline (1–2 g a day for 7 days). In louse-borne relapsing fever there is often a Herxheimer

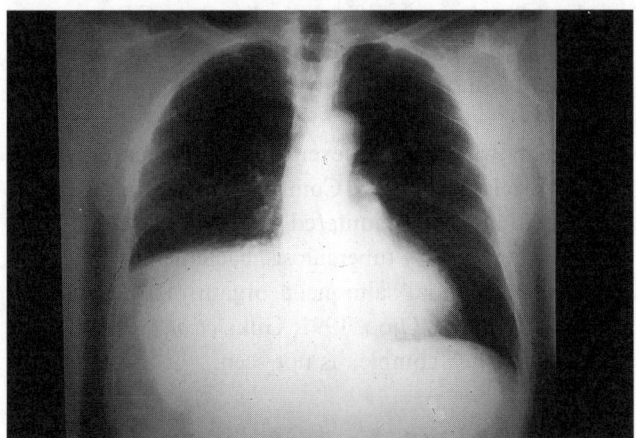

Fig. 6. Chest X-ray showing elevated right hemidiaphragm in amoebic liver abscess.

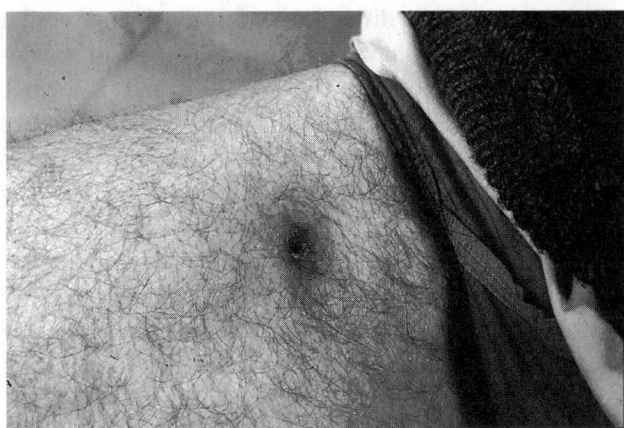

Fig. 7. Eschar in patient with tick typhus.

reaction following antibiotics which may be dramatically alleviated by intravenous meptazinol 300–500 mg.

Diagnoses from the white blood count

Neutrophil leucocytosis

Pyogenic infections and deep sepsis should not be forgotten. There are several specific infections to be considered, including spirochaetal infections such as leptospirosis (suspicious findings are conjunctival suffusion, muscle tenderness, jaundice and urine sediment abnormalities) and relapsing fevers due to *Borrelia* spp.

An amoebic liver abscess can cause both acute and chronic fever and only about half the patients give a preceding history of dysentery. Pain in the right hypochondrium is common with a cough if there is a lung involvement. The liver is enlarged and tender with possible signs at the right lung base. Occasionally patients present just with fever. Anaemia, neutrophil leucocytosis, raised serum alkaline phosphatase and an elevated right hemidiaphragm on chest radiography (Fig. 6) are usual. An ultrasound scan of the liver will demonstrate the abscess although it may be negative early in the illness. The amoebic IFAT (immunofluorescent antibody test) will usually be positive although it can be negative in 5–10% during the first week of symptoms. Treatment with metronidazole 400 mg three times a day for 10 days should be followed by a good intestinal contact amoebicide–diloxanide furoate 500 mg t.d.s. for 10 days. Indications for aspiration of amoebic liver abscesses include marked swelling of the rib cage, marked local tenderness or a very raised hemidiaphragm. The temptation for routine aspiration should be resisted.

Normal white count and differential with a negative blood film

The most important causes of acute fevers in this category are viral, rickettsial and typhoid fever.

Viral fevers often have non-specific features and are rarely diagnosed specifically. Dengue fever, caused by an arbovirus and endemic in South-East Asia and the Caribbean, occasionally presents with a characteristic pattern. There is fever, severe headache, myalgia and sore eyes. The fever settles after 4 days but recurs a few days later in association with a maculopapular rash (double humped fever pattern). Other arbovirus infections (e.g. sandfly fever from the Middle East) can cause a similar illness.

Forms of typhus are endemic the world over. Cases of typhus imported into the UK are usually tick-borne and acquired in East and South Africa following visits to game parks. An eschar appears at the site of bites (Fig. 7) and there is local lymphadenopathy. Fever is accompanied by a generalized maculopapular rash and generalized lymphadenopathy. Ticks may climb up the legs before they feed and eschars may therefore be found on the thighs and buttocks. Serology for rickettsial antibiotics retrospectively confirms the diagnosis. Treatment can be instituted on clinical grounds with either tetracycline 500 mg 6-hourly for 7 days or a single dose of doxycycline 200 mg.

Typhoid fever must be considered in any patient with an indefinite illness continuing for a week or more, especially if the patient is withdrawn and apathetic (Adams, 1987). Headache is the most common symptom and the diagnosis should be questioned if headache is absent. Other symptoms include constipation, diarrhoea (occasionally bloody), abdominal discomfort and cough. The few physical signs include scattered rhonchi in the chest and a slightly distended tender abdomen. About a quarter of patients have an enlarged liver and/or spleno-megaly. Rose spots on the abdomen and a relative bradycardia are helpful signs. Three sets of blood cultures and a stool culture should be taken. The Widal test is often unhelpful. It gives false positive results if there has been previous typhoid vaccination, prior infection with other *Salmonella* spp., and in patients with chronic liver disease. It may also remain negative despite positive cultures. Empirical treatment is advisable because delay leads to an increased risk of complications. Multiresistant strains of *Salmonella typhi* have become increasingly prevalent in the Indian subcontinent, Mexico, South Asia, China and South Africa (Mandal, 1991). A quinolone should now be regarded as the drug of choice in the treament of typhoid fever (Mandal, 1991). With oral ciprofloxacin 500 mg b.d. for 14 days the fever usually resolves in 5 days and the convalescent carriage rate is low. In pregnant women and children, quinolones are contraindicated and a third-generation cephalosporin is an alternative.

Normal or low white blood count

The causes of chronic fever in patients with a normal or low white cell count are similar to those listed in Table 12.

Tropical infections associated with neutropenia include malaria, visceral leishmaniasis, brucellosis and dissemi-nated tuberculosis. A negative malaria IFAT effectively rules out a diagnosis of blood film negative malaria.

Visceral leishmaniasis, a disease caused by the protozoan *Leishmania donovani*, is widely distributed around the Mediterranean basin, the Middle East, tropical Africa, parts of South America and East and South Asia. It is transmitted by the bite of a sandfly and causes fever with marked splenic enlargement and pancytopenia. The diag-nosis is established by a positive Leishmania IFAT and finding the classical amastigotes 'Leishman–Donovan bodies' in bone marrow or splenic aspirate. Therapy with pentavalent antimony drugs should be supervised in a centre with tropical expertise.

The diagnosis of brucellosis should be considered in a patient returning particularly from the Middle East or South and Central America. The diagnosis is established usually by serology and occasionally by isolation of the organism from blood or bone marrow cultures after prolonged incubation. Treatment is with a combination of rifampicin and tetracycline/doxycycline (Acocella *et al.*, 1989).

Disseminated tuberculosis in immigrants or foreign students can be very difficult to diagnose. CT scans and biopsy of lymph nodes, bone marrow or liver for histology, microscopy and culture may be needed to establish the diagnosis.

Patients with chronic fever and leucopenia may have an HIV-related illness. Common HIV-related febrile illnesses that are encountered in Africa are pulmonary and extrapulmonary tuberculosis, bacteraemia (especially with non-typhoidal salmonella organisms) and crypto-coccosis (Gilks & Ojoo, 1991; Gilks *et al.*, 1992). *Myco-bacterium avium* complex is not seen.

Eosinophilia

Causes of fever with eosinophilia are listed in Table 19. In the returning traveller such illness is usually caused

Table 19. *Causes of eosinophilia and systemic illness from the tropics*

	Diagnosis
Infections	
Acute schistosomiasis	Ova of schistosome species in stool
	Positive schistosomal serology
Acute fascioliasis	Positive fasciola serology
	Fasciola eggs in the stool
Trichinellosis	Periorbital oedema
	Elevated creatine phosphokinase
	Positive trichinella serology
Toxocariasis	Children
(visceral larva migrans)	Positive toxocara serology
Strongyloides	Abdominal pain ± diarrhoea
	Positive stool microscopy and serology
Loa Loa	West African travel, transient multiple swellings of arms, hands
	Positive blood film
Gnathostomiasis	Travel in Far East, periorbital and other swellings
Loeffler's syndrome	Short-lived illness
(ascaris, hookworm)	Ova in stools when worms mature
Others	
Neoplasia – lymphoma, carcinoma	
Polyarteritis nodosa	
Drugs	
Hypereosinophilic syndrome	

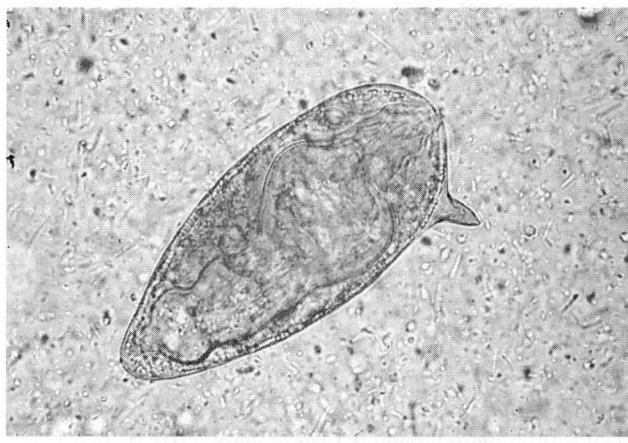

Fig. 8. Ova of *Schistosoma mansoni*.

Table 20. *Distribution of viral haemorrhagic fevers of public health importance*

Lassa fever	West Africa (principally Nigeria, Liberia and Sierra Leone)
Ebola virus	East and Central Africa (Southern Sudan and Zaire)
Marburg virus	East and Central Africa (Kenya and Zimbabwe)
Congo-Crimean haemmorrhagic fever	Wide distribution in Africa Sporadic cases in Southern Africa Endemic in Middle East, Pakistan, Eastern Europe
	Vector: tick Natural host reservoir: small mammals

by the early stages of a helminthic infection. Acute schistosomiasis (Katayama fever) is the commonest cause in trans-Africa travellers. *Schistosoma mansoni* is usually responsible for this acute illness occurring in individuals exposed for the first time to this helminth. After swimming in water infested with cercariae (the infective form of the schistosome helminth), the individual may notice itching for 1–3 days – the 'swimmer's itch'. The cercariae penetrate into skin lymphatics and blood vessels and make their way to the liver where they develop into adult flukes. The mature worms mate in the liver, and migrate to the venous plexus of the intestine where the females lay their eggs. The illness commences at the time of first oviposition (usually about 4–6 weeks after the initial infection) and is probably immune complex mediated. Clinical features include fever, arthralgia, diarrhoea with or without blood, tender hepatomegaly, cough with expiratory wheezes and urticarial skin rashes. The differential diagnosis is wide. The diagnosis is made by finding ova of *Schistosoma mansoni* in the stool (Fig. 8) and a positive schistosomal ELISA (enzyme-linked immunosorbent assay). At the onset of the illness, stool microscopy may be negative and eosinophilia mild, so a high index of suspicion is sometimes required to make the diagnosis (Harries *et al.*, 1987). Treatment requires a combination of praziquantel (to kill the adult flukes) and corticosteroids (to prevent exacerbation of immune complex mediated disease as a result of killing the worms), and is best carried out in hospital.

Is it viral haemorrhagic fever?

The rare possibility of viral haemorrhagic fever (VHF) should be considered, particularly in all patients with fever who have been in Africa south of the Sahara or the Middle East during the 3 weeks before the onset of their symptoms. The arboviruses that are responsible for these illnesses are widely distributed in Africa, Asia, Europe and Oceania, and sporadic cases may occur in travellers who visit these endemic areas (Glover, 1987). Most of the viruses cause no public health concern, but unfortunately four – Lassa fever, Ebola virus, Marburg virus and Congo-Crimean haemorrhagic fever virus – are capable of person-to-person transmission through close contact with infected blood and other body secretions. Health and laboratory personnel are particularly at risk. The distribution of the viruses is shown in Table 20. The illnesses are similar (Glover, 1987). The initial illness is characterized by fever, headache, myalgia, pharyngitis, conjunctival suffusion and maculopapular rash, followed after 5–7 days by rapid deterioration with multiple organ failure and bleeding. Laboratory investigations often show thrombocytopenia and highly elevated serum transaminase levels. The mortality is high, although tribavirin is useful in Lassa fever and possibly Congo-Crimean haemorrhagic fever (Huggins, 1989).

It is impossible to make a definitive diagnosis on clinical grounds as the differential diagnosis is wide:

- Malaria.
- Trypanosomiasis.
- Bacterial septicaemia.
- Tick typhus.
- Viral hepatitis.
- Epstein–Barr virus.
- Streptococcal pharyngitis.

- Leptospirosis.
- Haemorrhagic states due to clotting deficiences.

A high index of suspicion is thus needed. Febrile patients who should be strongly suspected as having VHF are the following:

1. Patients with an unexplained fever who have been in rural areas or large towns where VHF is known to be endemic *within* 3 weeks of becoming ill. Particular risk factors include:
   - Camping in the bush.
   - Sleeping on the ground or staying in a rural farming area
   - Contact with sick animals or their carcasses.
   - Contact with a tick-infested environment or tick bites.
2. Medical and nursing staff from country hospitals in these endemic areas.
3. Laboratory workers who handle viral haemorrhagic viruses, both in the UK and abroad.
4. Febrile contacts of confirmed cases of VHF.

If a patient is suspected of having a viral haemorrhagic fever it is vitally important to seek IMMEDIATE advice from a specialist in infectious or tropical diseases and to inform the local consultant in communicable disease control and the medical microbiologist.

Such patients are managed along nationally accepted guidelines using a high-security laboratory and isolation facilities (Department of Health and Social Security, 1986). No blood specimens or body secretions are sent to the routine laboratory. Although only a few imported cases of VHF have been managed in the UK in the last 20 years, there are many more who have been suspected of having VHF and have required isolation. It is vital to seek expert advice because many of these patients turn out to have falciparum malaria which requires rapid diagnosis and treatment. If delay in the diagnosis is likely, the patient should be treated for falciparum malaria anyway.

Useful sources of advice for patients at risk of a VHF are listed in the Appendix.

ACKNOWLEDGEMENTS

We thank Dr N.J. Beeching and Professor C.A. Hart for helpful comments on the manuscript and Dr G. Wyatt, Mr M. Guy and Mr K. Jones at the Liverpool School of Tropical Medicine for the illustrations.

APPENDIX: Sources of advice on travel-associated illness

Advice is often available from the local medical microbiology or infectious diseases service. The following centres will provide up-to-date medical advice on travel-associated febrile illness:

Hospital for Tropical Diseases, London	0171-387-4411
Liverpool School of Tropical Medicine	0151-708-9393

Infectious diseases units

City Hospital, Aberdeen	01224-681818
East Birmingham Hospital, Birmingham	0121-772-4311
Southmead Hospital, Bristol	0117-950-5050
Addenbrookes Hospital, Cambridge	01223-245151
City Hospital, Edinburgh	0131-447-1001
Ruchill Hospital, Glasgow	0141-946-7120
Seacroft Hospital, Leeds	0113-264-8164
Fazakerley Hospital, Liverpool	0151-525-5980
Groby Road Hospital, Leicester	0116-287-4141
Coppetts Wood Hospital, London	0181-883-9792
Northwick Park Hospital, London	0181-864-3232
St Georges Hospital, London	0181-672-1255
Monsall Hospital, Manchester	0161-205-2393
Newcastle General Hospital, Newcastle	0191-273-8811
City Hospital, Nottingham	0115-969-1169
Churchill Hospital, Oxford	01865-741841
Royal Hallamshire Hospital, Sheffield	0114-276-6222
City General Hospital, Stoke-on-Trent	01782-715444

Bibliography

ACOCELLA, G., BERTRAND, A., BEYTOUT, J. *et al.* (1989). Comparison of three different regimens in the treatment of acute brucellosis: a multicenter multinational study. *J. Antimicrob. Chemother.*, **23**, 433–9.

ADAMS, E.B. (1987). Typhoid and paratyphoid fevers. In *Oxford Textbook of Medicine*, 2nd edn, Vol. 1, ed. D.J. Weatherall, J.G.G. Ledingham & D.A. Warell, pp. 5.218–5.224. Oxford: Oxford University Press.

BRADLEY, D.J. & PHILLIPS-HOWARD, P.A. (1989). Prophylaxis against malaria for travellers from the United Kingdom. *Br. Med. J.* **299,** 1087–9.

BRADLEY, D.J. & WARHURST, D.C. (1993). Malaria imported into the United Kingdom 1991. *Communicable Disease Report*, Vol. 3, Review No. 2 (PHLS).

BRADLEY, D.J., NEWBOLD, C.I. & WARRELL, D.A. (1987). Malaria. In *Oxford Textbook of Medicine*, 2nd edn, Vol. 1, ed. D.J. Weatherall, J.G.G. Ledingham & D.A. Warrell, pp. 5.474–5.502. Oxford: Oxford University Press.

BRADLEY, D.J., WARHURST, D.C., BLAZE M. *et*

al. (1991). Malaria imported into the United Kingdom 1989 and 1990. *Communicable Disease Report*, Vol. 1, Review No. 5 (PHLS).

BRYCESON, A. (1987). Imported fevers. In *Advanced Medicine 23*, ed. R.E. Pounder & P.L. Chiodini, pp. 344–55. London: Baillière Tindall.

COHEN, J. & GLAUSER, M.P. (1991). Septic shock: treatment. *Lancet*, **338**, 736–9.

COMMITTEE ON SAFETY OF MEDICINES (1986). Reye's syndrome and aspirin. *Br. Med. J.*, **292**, 1590.

DEPARTMENT OF HEALTH AND SOCIAL SECURITY (1986). *Memorandum on the Control of Viral Haemorrhagic Fevers*. London: HMSO.

DINARELLO, C.A. & WOLFF, S.M. (1990). Pathogenesis of fever. In *Principles and Practice of Infectious Diseases*, 3rd edn, ed. G.L. Mandell, R. Gordon Douglas & J.E. Bennett, pp. 462–7. New York: Churchill Livingstone.

DINARELLO, C.A., CANNON, J.G. & WOLFF, S.M. (1988). New concepts on the pathogenesis of fever. *Rev. Infect. Dis.*, **10**, 168–89.

EDITORIAL (1990). Exchange transfusion in falciparum malaria. *Lancet*, **335**, 324–5.

ELLIOT, D.L., TOLLE, S.W., GOLDBERG, L. *et al.* (1985). Pet-associated illness. *N. Engl. J. Med.*, **313**, 985–95.

FOLTZER, M.A. & REESE, R.E. (1986). Bacteraemias and sepsis. In *A Practical Approach to Infectious Diseases*, 2nd edn, ed. R.E. Reese & R. Gordon Douglas Jr., pp. 47–74. Boston: Little, Brown.

GEDDES, A.M. & ELLIS, C.J. (1985). Infection in immunocompromised patients. *Q. J. Med.*, **55**, 5–14.

GILKS, C.F. & OJOO, S.A. (1991). A practical approach to the clinical problems of the HIV-infected adult in the tropics. *Trop. Doct.*, **21**, 90–7.

GILKS, C.F., OTIENO, L.S., BRINDLE, R.J. *et al.* (1992). The presentation and outcome of HIV-related disease in Nairobi. *Q. J. Med.*, **82**, 25–32.

GILLES, H.M. (1991). *Management of Severe and Complicated Malaria. A Practical Hand Book*. Geneva: World Health Organization.

GLOVER, S.C. (1987). Imported viral haemorrhagic fevers: what to do and why. In *Advanced Medicine 23*, ed. R.E. Pounder & P.L. Chiodini, pp. 344–55. London: Baillière Tindall.

GOLDSTEIN, E.J.C. (1992). Bite wounds and infection. *Clin. Infect. Dis.*, **14**, 633–40.

GORBACH, S.L. (1988). Bacterial diarrhoea and its treatment. In *Infection Today. A Lancet Review*, pp. 31–42. London.

HARRIES, A.D. (1989). Malaria: the principal cause in Europids for acute medical admission to a general hospital, Malawi. *Ann. Trop. Med. Parasitol.*, **83**, 187–9.

HARRIES, J.R., HARRIES, A.D. & COOK, G.C.

(1987). *100 Clinical Problems in Tropical Medicine*. London: Baillière Tindall.

HENRY, J.A., JEFFREYS, K.J. & DAWLING, S. (1992). Toxicity and deaths from 3,4-methylenedioxymethamphetamine ('ecstasy'). *Lancet*, **340**, 384–7.

HIEN, T.T. & WHITE, N.J. (1993). Qinghaosu. *Lancet*, **341**, 603–8.

HINDS, C.J. (1992). Monoclonal antibodies in sepsis and septic shock. *Br. Med. J.*, **394**, 132–3.

HUGGINS, J.W. (1989). Prospects for treatment of viral haemorrhagic fevers with ribavirin, a broad-spectrum antiviral drug. *Rev. Infect. Dis.*, **11** (Suppl. 4), S750–S761.

HUGHES, W.T., ARMSTRONG, D., BODEY, G.P. *et al.* (1990). Guidelines for the use of antimicrobial agents in neutropenic patients with unexplained fever. *J. Infect. Dis.*, **161**, 381–96.

KINGSTON, M.E. & MACKEY, D. (1986). Skin clues in the diagnosis of life threatening infections. *Rev. Infect. Dis.*, **8**, 1–11.

KNOCKAERT, D.C., VANNESTE, L.J., VANNESTE, S.B. *et al.* (1992). Fever of unknown origin in the 80s: an update of the diagnostic spectrum. *Arch. Intern. Med.*, **152**, 51–5.

LARSON, E.B., FEATHERSTONE, H.J. & PETERSDORF, R.G. (1982). Fever of undetermined origin: diagnosis and follow up of 105 cases, 1970–1980. *Medicine*, **61**, 269–92.

LEVINE, D.P. & SOBEL, J.D. (1991). *Infections in Intravenous Drug Abusers*. New York: Oxford University Press.

LOOAREESUWAN, S., PHILLIPS, R.E., WHITE, N.J. *et al.* (1985). Quinine and severe falciparum malaria in late pregnancy. *Lancet*, **ii**, 4–8.

MACFARLANE, J.T. (1988). Treatment of lower respiratory infections. In *Infection Today. A Lancet Review*. pp. 43–51. London.

MANDAL, B.K. (1991). Modern treatment of typhoid fever. *J. Infect.*, **22**, 1–4.

MOLYNEUX, M.E. & FOX, R. (1993). Diagnosis and treatment of malaria in Britain. *Br. Med. J.*, **306**, 1175–80.

MURPHY, P.A. (1992). Fever. In *Infectious Diseases*, ed. S.L. Gorbach, J.G. Bartlett & N.R. Blacklow, pp. 79–84. Philadelphia: W.B. Saunders.

MURPHY, G.S., BASRI, H., PURNOMO, *et al.* (1993). Vivax malaria resistant to treatment and prophylaxis with chloroqine. *Lancet*, **341**, 96–100.

MURRAY, H.W., TUAZON, C.V., GUERRERO, I.C. *et al.* (1977). Urinary temperature: a clue to early diagnosis of factitious fever. *N. Engl. J. Med.*, **296**, 23–24.

NELSON, T.E & FLEWELLEN, E.H. (1983). The malignant hyperthermia syndrome. *N. Engl. J Med.*, **309**, 416–18.

NOONE, A., GILL, O.N., CLARKE, S.E. *et al.* (1991).

Travel, heterosexual intercourse and HIV-1 infection. *Communicable Disease Report* No. 4, R39–43.

PEARCE, J.M. (1990). Pelvic inflammatory disease. *Br. Med. J.*, **300**, 1090–1.

SHANSON, D.C. (1990). Septicaemia in patients with AIDS. In Parasites and Otyer Infections in AIDS. *Trans. R. Soc. Trop. Med. Hyg.*, **84** (Suppl. 1), 14–16.

SMEGO, R.A. & DURACK, D.T. (1982). The neuroleptic malignant syndrome. *Arch. Intern. Med.*, **142**, 1183–5.

SPECK, E.L. (1986) Fever and fever of unknown etiology. In *A Practical Approach to Infectious Diseases*, 2nd edn, ed R.E. Reese & R. Gordon Douglas. pp. 1–17. Boston: Little, Brown.

STEFFEN, R. & BEHRENS, R.H. (1992). Travellers' malaria. *Parasitol. Today*, **8**, 61–6.

WALKER, E. & WILLIAMS, G. (1989). Infections on return from abroad. In *ABC of Healthy Travel*, pp. 28–33. London: British Medical Journal.

WARRELL, D.A., LOOAREESUWAN, S., WARRELL, M.J. *et al.* (1982). Dexamethasone proves deleterious in cerebral malaria. A double-blind trial in 100 comatose patients. *N. Engl. J. Med.*, **306**, 313–19.

WARRELL, D.A., MOLYNEUX, M.E. & BEALES, P.F. (1990). Severe and Complicated Malaria, 2nd edn. WHO Division of Control of Tropical Diseases. *Trans. R. Soc. Trop. Med. Hyg.*, **84**, (Suppl. 2) 1–65.

WEBER, D.J., GAMMON, W.R. & COHEN, M.S. (1990).The acutely ill patient with fever and rash. In *Principles and Practice of Infectious Diseases*, 3rd edn, ed. G.L. Mandell, R. Gordon Douglas Jr & J.E. Bennett, pp. 479–89. New York: Churchill Livingstone.

WEINKE, T., LOSCHER, T., FLEISCHER, K. *et al.* (1992). The efficacy of halofantrine in the treatment of acute malaria in nonimmune travellers. *Am. J. Trop. Med. Hyg.*, **47**, 1–5.

WILKIE, M.E., ALMOND, M.K. & MARSH, F.P. (1992). Diagnosis and management of urinary tract infection in adults. *Br. Med. J.*, **305**, 1137–41.

WILLIAMS, G.R. (1990). The toxic shock syndrome. *Br. Med. J.*, **300**, 960.

YOUNG, E.J., FAINSTEIN, V. & MUSHER, D.M. (1982). Drug-induced fever: cases seen in the evaluation of unexplained fever in a general hospital population. *Rev. Infect. Dis.*, **4**, 69–77.

Index

A&E department
  appointment of consultants, 3
  appointment of registrars, 3
  audit, 1992 Report, 7
  creation of specialty, 3
  design and equipment, 4–6
  management, 15–19
  staffing and training, 6–9
  trauma teams, 9–10
ABCs
  airway with cervical spine control, 330
  breathing, 330
  circulation, 330
  consciousness, 330–1
  +DE (ATLS system), new approaches to
    resuscitation, 102, 133–4, 423–4
  primary survey in trauma, 692
  see also resuscitation
abdominal assessment and acute abdomen,
  112–13, 951–68
  acute non-specific abdominal pain
    (ANSAP), 959–60, 963–4
    gynaecological conditions, 1160
  admission for further assessment, 963–5
    appendicitis, 964, 1141
    cholecystitis, 964
    diverticulitis, 964
    pancreatitis, 965
    small bowel obstruction, 965
  children, 967
  ectopic pregnancy, 1156–7
  elderly patients, 967
  examination, 953–5
  gynaecological emergencies, 1152–70
  history, 952–3
  immediate surgery, 960
  investigations, 955–6
  non-admission decisions, 958–60
  pathology, 951, 966
  pregnant woman, non-obstetric causes,
    1141–3
  radiology, 956
    acute cholecystitis, 386
    appendicolith and abscess, 385
    bowel rupture, 388
    intraperitoneal air, 384
    IVU criteria, 383
    liver damage, 367
    renal colic, 386
    renal trauma, 388, 389
    small bowel obstruction, 383
    splenic damage, 367
    toxic megacolon, 384
    ultrasonography vs CT scanning, 380,
      383–8
  surgery after prompt resuscitation, 960–3
abdominal thrust, 31–2
abdominal trauma, 558–67, 935–6
  assessment and resuscitation, 560–3
  diagnostic peritoneal lavage, 560–1
  elderly people, 710
  emergencies, 935–6
  paediatrics, 699
  radiology, 562
  surgical intervention, 563–7
  suspicion of intra-abdominal injury, 558
ABO system, antigens and antibodies, 997
abortion
  missed/inevitable, 1153, 1155
  septic, 1155
  threatened
    assessment, 1152–5
    Rh testing, 1152
  unlawful, uterine trauma, 720
abscess
  amoebic, liver, 1245
  diabetes-related conditions, 1133
abuse, 1213–19
  emotional, 1217
  Munchausen by proxy, 1218
  physical, 1214–16
  sexual, 1217
accidents
  by nation, 412
  falls, 417
  International Classification, 418–19
  kinematics and patterns of injury, 413–17
  major incident plan *see* disasters
  prevention, 417–18
  standardized reporting forms, 331
  see also road traffic accidents (RTAs)
acetylcysteine, antidote to paracetamol
  poisoning, 219, 224–6
Achilles tendon
  bursitis, 666
  rupture, 641, 666
  tendonitis, 666
acid–base homeostasis, 140–1
  disorders of, 142–7
  hyperthermia, 793
acidaemia, following cardiac arrest, 70–1
acidosis, defined, 140, 141

acrocyanosis, 784
acromioclavicular subluxation, 603–4, 678
  radiology, 351
actinic keratoses, 1045
activated charcoal, 215
activated partial thromboplastin time
  (APTT), 994
acute abdomen *see* abdominal assessment;
  abdominal assessment and acute
  abdomen
acute intravascular haemolysis, 1001
acyclovir, herpes infections, 1037
Addison's disease, 1111–13
  adrenal insufficiency, acute abdomen,
  966
adenosine
  compared with verapamil, 913
  contraindications, 899, 912–13
    atrial fibrillation, 924
  indications, 899
    tachycardias, 909–11, 923
  interactions, 899
  method of administration and dosage, 899,
    911–12
  paediatrics, 92, 929, 1202
  pregnancy and lactation, 929
  side-effects, 899, 912
adrenal insufficiency, acute abdomen, 966
adrenaline
  anaphylactic shock, 120, 162
    self-injection, 120, 165–6
  asystole, 909
  in cardiac arrest, 69–70
  contraindicated practices, 235, 238
  endobroncheal route, 69, 89
  with local anaesthesia, maximum doses
    and duration of action, 194
  paediatrics, 92
    newborns, 96
  tetracaine, adrenaline and cocaine (TAC),
    239
adrenocortical insufficiency, 1111–13
advanced (cardiac) life support (ACLS), 71–3
  airway management, 333–4
  breathing, 335
  cardiac prehospital care, 302–3, 310–12
  circulation, 335–6
  defined, 314
  early ACLS, 302–3, 310–12
  paediatrics, 84–93
    algorithm, 90

prehospital care of trauma patient, 329–36
training, 345
advanced (trauma) life support (ATLS), 423–4
Aeromonas hydrophila, 246
agonal rhythm, 907
air embolism, scuba diving injuries, 760
airport major disaster plan, 273
airway
  see also airway management techniques
  ABCs, assessment, 329–30, 423
  anatomy, 22–5
    paediatrics, 24
    in pregnancy, 25
  assessment, 25–6, 103–5, 423
  basic/advanced life support, 332–4
  burns, 722–3, 724–6
  cardiovascular response to intubation, 55–6
  cervical spine control, 330
  chemical injuries, 736–7
  Combitube airway, 37
  emergency
    cricothyroidotomy, 48–50, 58, 485–6
      contraindications, 684, 694
      paediatrics, 87–8, 1177
  facial trauma, 441
  foreign bodies, 391–2
  infections, 84
  local anaesthesia, 55
  obstruction
    convulsions, paediatrics, 1193–5
    lower, 1177–8
  paediatrics
    acute, vital signs and equipment, 693
    lower/upper obstruction, 1175–8
    obstruction, convulsions, 1193–5
    structural differences (from adults),
      684–5
  pathophysiology, 26–7
  rewarming method in hypothermia, 774–5
airway management techniques, 29–50
  advanced direct manoeuvres, 34–48
  airway adjuncts, 33–4
  airway obstruction, 25, 27, 83
    clearance, 31–3, 83
  basic manoeuvres, 29–33
  in cardiopulmonary resuscitation, 66–7
  facial trauma, 442–3
  percutaneous approaches
    tracheostomy, 50, 485–6
    transtracheal jet ventilation, 47–8
    see also cricothyroidotomy
  pharmacological adjuncts, 55–8
  toilet and suction, 30–1
  summary, 59
  *see also specific equipment and
    procedures*; tracheal intubation
akithesia, 1087
albumin
  blood products, 999
  and serum calcium, 1107
alcohol poisoning, 217, 222–3
alcuronium, 203
aldosterone, 150
alfentanil 192, *see also* opioids
algorithms
  acute respiratory failure, 851
  advanced life support paediatrics, 90
  asthma, 846
  asystole, 72, 90
    paediatrics, 90
  basic life support paediatrics, 82
  bradycardias, 1203

choking, paediatrics, 83
coma, 1200
dispatch, trauma prehospital care, 328
electromechanical dissociation (EMD), 73
poisoning, management, 208
prehospital triage, 329
sickle cell disease, 987
supraventricular tachycardia, 1203
ventricular fibrillation, 72
alkali burns, 737
alkalosis, defined, 140, 141
allergic contact eczema, 1034
allergic vasculitis (small vessel disease),
  1042–3
  drug reaction, 1053
alpha-agonists, contraindications, severe
  hyperthermia, 794
alteplase, thrombolytic therapy, 879–82
Amanita phalloides poisoning, 209, 211
amaurosis fugax, cerebral ischaemia, 939
ambulance control point (APC), HMIP,
  274–5, 277
ambulance liaison officer, 281
ambulance service
  choice of vehicle, 343
  equipment, 343–4
  helicopters, 287, 343, 347
  and prehospital care, 284–8
  pretransport checklist, 345
  special considerations, 346
  training schools, 286
  transport of patient, 340–7
  see also transport of patient
ameloblastoma, 472
amiodarone, 70
  cardiac arrhythmias, 899
  pregnancy and lactation, 929
amoebic liver abscess, 1245
amphetamines
  illicit use, psychological sequelae, 1096–100
  poisoning, 227
amylase, serum, 956
amyotrophy, diabetic, 1134
anaemia, 978–84
  blood loss, 982
  classification
    autoimmune haemolytic, 983
    haemolytic, 983
    iron deficiency, 982
    megaloblastic, 982
    nonimmune haemolytic, 984
    using mean cell volume, 980
  due to malaria, 984
  emergency presentation, 980
  examination, 981
anaesthetic agents
  causing anaphylaxis, 165
  see also general anaesthesia; intravenous
    regional anaesthesia; local
    anaesthesia
anaesthetic problems, elderly people, 714
analgesic agents and routes, 184–93
  inhalational, 186–9
  oral, 184–6
  parenteral, 189–93
  patient-controlled analgesia, 189–90
  rectal, 186
  sublingual, 186
  topical, 186
anaphylaxis, 159–66
  acute and secondary management, 162–3,
    165–6

anaphylactic shock, 120
anaphylatoxins, C3a and C5a, 160–1
bee and wasp stings, 822–3
blood transfusion, 1001
causes, 164–6
clinical presentation, 161–2
differential diagnosis, 162
epidemiology, 160
immediate generalized reactions, 160
immunization, 253
local anaesthesia, 194–5
paediatrics, 1177
pathogenesis, 160–1
prognosis, 166
second-phase reaction, 161
aneurysmal disease, acute presentation, 943–6
angina pectoris
  ECG, stable/unstable angina, 872, 873
  outcome, 874
  pathology and presentation, 870–1
  Prinzmetal's variant, 871
  treatment, 872–4
    chronic stable, 872–3
    unstable, 874
angioedema, 163, 1052
angioneurotic oedema, 1177
animal bite wounds, 248–50
ankle, functional anatomy, 807–8
ankle injuries, 644–6
  classification, 644
  paediatrics, 631
  sport causes, 665–8
  sprain
    physiotherapy techniques, 813–16
    rehabilitation, 807–9
ANSAP *see* abdominal assessment and
  acute abdomen
antiarrhythmic drugs 70, 899, *see also* named
  drugs
antibiotics
  bacterial meningitis, 1191
  bite wounds, 250
  contraindications in burn patient, 731
  gastroenteritis, 1187
  pneumonia, 1182
  prophylaxis of wound infection, 245–6,
    250, 583
  topical, 245
  urinary tract infections, 970, 1189
  wound irrigation, 242
antibodies, antilipopolysaccharide Abs, 136
anticholinergic agents, antidote, 217
anticoagulants
  poisoning, 217
  pregnancy, 1145
anticonvulsants
  paediatrics, 1193–5
  poisoning, 229
antidepressants
  poisoning, 214, 226
  side-effects, 1087–8
antidiuretic hormone (ADH), release, 149
antidotes, 215, 217–19
  chemical injuries, 738
antiplatelet agents, for angina, 874
antipyretics, contraindications, severe
  hyperthermia, 794
Anton's syndrome, 1061
anxiolytics 1088, *see also* benzodiazepines
aorta
  abdominal aortic aneurysms, 945, 960

dissection, 369, 892–3
  aneurysms, 943–5
  complications, 893
  diagnosis, 893
  urgent management, 893
grafts, 945
injury, urgent management, 935
mediastinal widening, 369
patch, 935
rupture, 371, 380, 552
aphonia, 25
appendicitis, 960–1, 964, 1141, 1164
  appendicolith and abscess, 385
arachnids, envenomation, 827–30
arboviruses, 1247
arm *see* upper limb
arrhythmias *see* cardiac arrhythmias
arterial blood gases
  normal values, 28, 67, 143, 537
  sampling, principles, 142–3
arterial embolus
  air embolism, scuba diving injuries, 760
  clinical features, 941
  management, 940
arterial puncture and cannulation, 1207,
  1210–11
arteriography, indications, 388, 937–8
arthritis
  bacterial, 1018
  differential diagnosis, 1015
  disseminated gonococcal infective, 1019
  infective, 1018–19
  Lyme disease, 1019
  polyarthritis, 1023–4
  septic, 375–6, 1006–7, 1015
  viral, 1020
ascorbic acid, antidote to opioids poisoning,
  218, 227–8
Asian cultural practice in event of death, 403
aspiration, gastric, and lavage, 213–14
aspiration pneumonia, paediatric
  emergencies, 1182–3
aspiration of stomach contents, 852
aspirin, 185, 186
  for angina, 873
  contraindications, severe hyperthermia,
    794
  for myocardial infarction, 879
assault, facial trauma, 440–1
assessment procedures
  airway, 25–6, 103–5
  circulation, 106–7
  fluid loss, 130
  multiply injured patient
    primary, 102–8
    secondary evaluation of body systems,
      108–14
  shock, 125–7
  ventilation, 28, 105–6
asthma, 844–8
  algorithm for management, 846
  British Thoracic Society Guidelines for
    severe asthma, paediatrics, 1179–81
  chronic, 849
  croup, 1175
  less severe attacks, 848
  life-threatening features, 845
  paediatric emergencies, 1178–80
    management protocol, 1181
  in pregnancy, 1144–5
asystole, 907–9
  algorithms, 72, 90

differentiation from ventricular fibrillation,
  317
atheroma, mechanism of coronary
  narrowing, 870
athlete's foot, tinea pedis, 1039
athlete's heart
  bradycardia, 903
ATLS system, ABCDE, 423–4
atracurium besylate, 58, 203
atrial fibrillation
  with accessory pathway, 925
  adenosine, contraindications, 924
  management, 883
  with slow ventricular response, 903–4
atrial flutter, 921–2
atrial natriuretic peptide (ANP), 150
atrioventricular block, following AMI, 884
atropine
  antidote to organophosphates, 218
  arrhythmias, 71
  cardiac arrhythmias, 899
  endobronchial route, 69, 89
  paediatrics, 92
  pregnancy and lactation, 929
  sinus bradycardia, 884
audit, 1992 Report, 7
Augustine guide, 44–5
autoimmune haemolytic anaemia, 983
autonomic nervous system, in AMI, 875–6
AVPU, 424
axillary arteries, trauma, 932
axonal injury, 429

back pain, 1009–12
  cold effects, 785
  prolapsed intervertebral disc, 1011
  spinal stenosis, 1011–12
bacterial infections *see* infections
bacterial meningitis *see* meningitis, bacterial
bag–valve–mask ventilation technique, 52–3,
  66, 67, 88–9
ballistic injuries, 798–804
  abdominal trauma, 563
  incidence, 798
  management, 802–4
  missiles, 799–802
  weapons, 798
barbiturates, illicit use, and psychological
  sequelae, 1096–100
barotrauma, 758
  of ascent, 759–60
  of descent, 759
  pulmonary, 759
basal cell carcinoma, 1045
base excess, defined, 143
basic (cardiac) life support, 65–6
  airway management, 332–3
  ambulance attendant, 344–5
  breathing, 334
  circulation, 335
  paediatrics, 82–4
  prehospital care of trauma patient,
    329–36
basilar artery
  migraine, 1068–9
  thrombosis, 1061
basophil mediators, anaphylaxis, 161
baton rounds, 800–1
Beck's triad, 545
bees and wasps, stings, 160, 822–3
behavioural disturbance, severe, 1079–84
Behçet's disease, 1043

Belgium, cardiac prehospital care, 304, 308
Bell's palsy, 491
'bends', scuba diving injuries, 760
benzodiazepines, 57, 240
  antagonist (flumenazil), 204, 217
  illicit use, and psychological sequelae,
    1096–100
  mode of action, 203
  pharmacological data, 203
  side-effects, 1088
  see also named agents
bereaved relatives, 398–404
Berlin blue, antidote to thallium poisoning,
  219
beta-blockers
  contraindications, anaphylactic shock, 165
  following myocardial infarction, 883
  labetolol, contraindications, 1117
  paediatrics, 1203
  poisoning, 217, 229
bicarbonate system, 142
  see also sodium bicarbonate
bicipital tendonitis, 679
bilirubin metabolism, 979
biphosphonates, 1109
birth *see* neonate; obstetrics
bite wounds, 248–50
bleeding disorders *see* coagulopathies;
  haemophilia
bleeding *see* haemorrhage
blind nasal intubation, 45
blood
  ABO system, 997
  composition, 979
    trauma, pregnancy changes, 704
  haematological indices, 1152
  normal adult values, 979
  pathophysiology, 978–9
  specimen, assessment of poisoning, 211
  transmission of viruses, 246–7
blood giving set, blood transfusion, 1000
blood pressure
  comatose patient, 171
  estimation, 330
  monitoring during ventilation, 54
  paediatrics, 85
blood products, 995–6, 997–9
  albumin, 999
  coagulation factor concentrates, 998
  cryoprecipitate, 995, 998
  fresh frozen plasma (FFP), 995–6, 998
  leucocyte-depleted blood, 1001
  ordering, 1000
  packed red cells, 998
  platelet concentrates, 998
  red cell concentrates, 998
  whole blood, 998
blood salvage machines, 997
blood tests, hyperthermia, 791
blood transfusion, 997–1002
  cannulation, 1000
  complications and dangers, 1001–2
  lines and filters, 1000
  massive, complications, 999–1001
  practical aspects, 999–1002
  pretransfusion compatibility testing, 1000
  rates, 1000
  record-taking, 1000–1
body fluids
  24 h water balance, 150
  water excess and depletion, 150–1
body lice, pediculosis corporis, 1049

body temperature, 1228
  regulation, 766–7
boils, 1036
Bolam test, 18
bone infection, 1005–7
bone injuries, terminology, 350–3
bone marrow, examination, 995
bone pain, osteomyelitis, 587–8, 1005–7
Borrelia spp., 1019, 1244–5
botulism, 1073
Bowen's disease (intraepidermal carcinoma),
  1045
brachial arteries, trauma, 933
  paediatrics, 933
brachial plexus injury, 514
brady-tachy syndrome, 904
bradycardia *see* cardiac arrhythmias
brain
  blood supply, 1057–8
  paediatrics, 686–7
  see also cerebral; intracranial
brain injury *see* head injuries
breast milk, drugs entering, 929
breath–holding attacks, 1196
breathing
  basic/advanced life support, 334–5
    child, 694
  burn patients, 725
  see also ABCs; resuscitation; ventilation
bretylium tosylate, 70
  paediatrics, 92
British Association for Immediate Care
  (BASICS), 274–5, 286–7
Brodie's abscess, 1006
bronchi
  foreign bodies, 443, 495, 1177
  trauma, 554
  see also airway, lower
bronchiectasis, 848
bronchiolitis, paediatric emergencies, 1178
bronchitis
  acute, 839–40
  chronic, 848–50
bronchospasm, anaphylaxis, 163
brucellosis, 1246
buffers, 142–3
  and alkalizing agents, 70–1
  sodium bicarbonate, 148
Bullard laryngoscope, 42–3
bullous disorders, 1049–51
bullous eruptions, drug reaction, 1053
bundle branch block, bradycardia, cardiac
  arrhythmias, 905–6
bupivacaine
  contraindications, 200, 238
  maximum doses and duration of action,
    194, 238
buprenorphine 185, 186, 192, *see also*
  opioids
burns, 721–32
  chemical, 737–8
  classification, 722
  elderly people, 712
  electrical injuries, 742–50
  flash and arc burns, 744
  hypovolaemic shock, 129
  lignocaine gel, 187, 239
  Lund and Browder charts, 729
  management, 724–32
    immediate, 724–30
    subsequent, 730–2
  pathophysiology, 722–4

in pregnancy, 707
surgical intervention, 731

C1 esterase inhibitor
  in angioedema, 163
  deficiency, 162
caesarean section
  diabetes mellitus, 1132
  post mortem delivery, 707
calcaneus
  Bohler's angle, 380, 381
  fractures, 631, 641
calcific tendinitis, 1025
calcium, normal range, 1107
calcium alginate dressings, wound care, 245
calcium gluconate
  IV, 154, 155
  use in hydrofluoric acid poisoning, 218, 737
calcium ions
  balance, 154–5
  EMD, 71, 93
  NMDA receptor, 75
calcium metabolism disorders, 1107–11
  hypercalcaemia, 1108–9
  hypocalcaemia, 1109–11
calcium pyrophosphate dihydrate crystal
  deposition disease, 1022
call–response interval, defined, 314
candidal infections, 478, 1040
  intertrigo, 1040–1
  oral candidiasis, 1040
cannabis, illicit use, and psychological
  sequelae, 1096–100
carbamates, poisoning, antidote, 738
Carbicarb, 148
carbon dioxide
  arterial blood, normal values, 28, 67, 143
  capnography, 67
  detection, tracheal tube, 55
carbon monoxide poisoning, 28–9, 216, 217,
    853
  treatment, 738
carbuncle, 1036
cardiac arrest, paediatric emergencies, 1200–5
cardiac arrest *see* cardiac prehospital care;
    resuscitation
cardiac arrhythmias, 72, 897–929, 1201–4
  brady-tachy syndrome, 904
  bradycardias, 898–909
    agonal rhythm, 907
    algorithm, 1204
    asystole, 907–9
    athlete's heart, 903
    atrial fibrillation with slow ventricular
      response, 903–4
    bundle branch block, 905–6
    drugs used in diagnosis and
      management, 899
    electromechanical dissociation, 907
    general management, 898–902
    heart block, 904–7
    idioventricular rhythm, 904
    right or left bundle branch block, 904–5
    sick sinus syndrome, 904, 1202
    sinus bradycardia, 884, 902–3, 1202
    transvenous ventricular pacing, 900–1
  drug overdose, 928
  electrical injuries, 747
  electrocardiography, 897–8
  European Resuscitation Council
    guidelines, 908
  heart block

first/third degree, 904–7
  Wenckebach second degree AV block,
    884, 905
  hypocalcaemia, 1110
  management, 1202
  neonates, 1203
  pacemakers, 924–8
  paediatrics, 91–2, 928–9, 1201–3
  permanent pacemakers, 924–8
  in pregnancy, 928
  prophylaxis following myocardial
    infarction, 883
  tachycardias, 909–24
    atrial fibrillation, 883, 903–4, 920–1,
      924–5
    atrial flutter, 921–2
    atrial tachycardia, 922–3
    broad complex tachycardias, 910–13,
      916–20
    drugs used in diagnosis and
      management, 899
    frequently repetitive ventricular, 917–18
    lignocaine, 883, 899
    long QT syndrome, 919–20
    multifocal atrial tachycardia, 923
    narrow complex tachycardias, 910–13,
      920–4
    overdrive ventricular pacing, 915–16
    re-entrant AV tachycardia, 923–4
    sinus tachycardia, 883, 920, 1201
    supraventricular tachycardia, 317, 883,
      910–13, 920
    sustained ventricular, 916–17
    torsade de pointes, 919
    treatment principles, 909
    vagal manoeuvres, 913–15
    ventricular ectopy, 918
    ventricular tachycardias, 317, 884,
      910–13, 916–20
cardiac care unit, 885
  rehabilitation, 885–6
cardiac emergencies, paediatrics, 1200–5
cardiac failure, 886–9
  acute left ventricular failure, 888–9
  causes, 1200
  congestive cardiac failure, 889
  definition and pathophysiology, 886–8
  Starling relationship, 886
cardiac pacemakers, 924–8
cardiac prehospital care, 288–323
  chain of survival, 294, 299–300
    early access link, 299–300, 303, 308–9,
      313
    early advanced life support, 302–3,
      310–12, 313
    early CPR, 294–6, 309, 313
    early defibrillation, 296, 301–2, 310, 313
  emergency medical systems, Europe/USA,
    292–6, 299–323
    medical emergency telephone numbers,
      308
    response intervals, 303
    two-tiered approach, 303
  England, 304, 308
  European and USA perspectives, 298–323
  first MCCU (Belfast), 290
  outcomes, model, 292–4
  time to definitive care, statistics, 292
  trauma patient, 329–36
  Utstein Consensus Conference, 296–7, 313
  Utstein glossary of terms, 313–14
  Utstein II recommendations, 296–7, 321–3

Utstein template, 315–19
Utstein time points and time intervals, 319–21
summary and recommendations, 312–13
see also resuscitation
cardiac rupture, 885
cardiac tamponade, 545
cardiac thoracic pump concept, 64
cardioactive drugs, poisoning, 228–9
cardiogenic shock, 889–91
dominant right ventricular infarction, 890
syncopal response, 890
cardiovascular emergencies (excluding arrhythmias), 866–95
acute myocardial infarction, 874–86
angina, 870–4
aortic dissection, 369, 892–4
cardiac failure, 886–9
chest pain, causes, history and investigations, 867–9
drowning injury, 752
malignant (accelerated) hypertension, 894–5
pulmonary embolism, 858–62, 891–2
signs of poisoning, 209
see also paediatrics; resuscitation
cardiovascular system, paediatrics, 686
cardioversion
DC, and pacemaker, 927
internal cardioverter defibrillator (ICD), 927–8
carotid arteries
angiography, 939–40
endarterectomy, indications, 939–40
relationship with nerves, 932
shunt, 932
carotid body tumours, 477–8
carpal injuries, paediatrics, 621
carpal tunnel syndrome, 593
cat bites, 249
cathartics, 214–15
cavernous sinus thrombosis, 463
cellulitis, 1035
cement burns, 737
central syndrome, 169
central venous cannulation
during CPR, 68, 89, 107, 423
paediatrics, 89
pneumothorax following, 116
central venous pressure, monitoring, 127
cerebellar artery occlusion, posterior inferior, 1061
cerebellar herniation (coning), 1197
cerebellar infarction, 1061
cerebellopontine angle, trigeminal neuralgia, 460
cerebral abscess, 1075–7
cerebral air embolism, scuba diving injuries, 760
cerebral artery anatomy, 1057–8
cerebral artery occlusion, 1061
cerebral blood flow (CBF), and head injury, 421
cerebral haemorrhage, 1060
cerebral ischaemia
crescendo ischaemic attacks, 940
TIAs, 939–40
cerebral oedema
causing coma, 169
ketoacidosis, 1126
treatment, 180

cerebral perfusion pressure, 169, 421, 1197
and intracranial pressure, 169
cerebral protection, following cardiac arrest, 74–5
cerebral resuscitation, near drowning, 756
cerebrospinal fluid
nasal leakage, 441–2
normal values, paediatrics, 1191
cerebrospinal infections, paediatrics, 1191
cervical lymphadenopathy, 461, 476–7
cervical rib, upper limb ischaemia, 942
cervical spine, physical examination, 806–7
cervical spine trauma, 359
disc disease, 1009
elderly people, 709–10
neck sprain (whiplash injury), 366, 513, 805–7, 816–17, 1003–4
paediatrics, 626–7, 683–5, 699
retropharyngeal space, 525
policy guidelines, 362
radiology, 359, 362–7, 519–25
adequacy, 520
clay shovellers' fractures, 366, 529
dens fractures, 367
facet joint dislocation, 364, 523–5
five-view series, 521–4
hangman's fracture, 366, 526
hyperflexion sprain, 366
Jefferson fracture, 522, 523
malrotation, 522–3
odontoid peg view, 365, 522
pillar fracture, 367
subluxation, 521
swimmer's view, 520–1
tear-drop fracture, 526
suspected injury
moving patient, 30
tracheal intubation, 45–7
torticollis, 1005
treatment, 528
see also neck injuries
chancre, 1244
charcoal, activated, 215
Charcot's disease, 1135
cheese (tyramine) reaction, 1088
cheilitis, 1040
chemical hazards
CHEMDATA, 733
decontamination, 734
HAZCHEM codes, 733–5
chemical injuries, 733–9
antidotes, 738
respiratory effects, specified substances, 736
to lung, 851–4
chest, paediatric, structural differences (from adults), 685
chest injuries, 533–56
aorta, disruption, 552–3, 933–4
assessment
life-threatening conditions, 538, 550
primary survey, 110–12, 537–49
secondary survey, 549–54
blast injuries, 534
capnography, 549
cardiac contusion, 551–2
cardiac tamponade, 545
chest drain placement, 539–44, 556
chest wall, 535–6
circulation assessment, 544
compression (traumatic asphyxia), 555
elderly people, 710

emergency thoracotomy and sternotomy, 547–8
flail chest, 544
management, 554–5
massive haemothorax, 548
mediastinum, 536
monitoring and reassessment, 548–9
open chest wound, 544
paediatrics, 699
basic life support, compression, 83
pathophysiology, 537
pericardiocentesis, 545–7
primary/secondary/tertiary effects, 533
pulmonary contusion, 550–1
pulse oximetry, 549
rib fractures, 363, 554–5
ruptured diaphragm, 552
ruptured oesophagus, 553
sports injuries, 675
transfer, 555–6
vascular injury, 933–5
see also pneumothorax
chest pain
causes, history and investigations, 867–9
physical signs and differential diagnosis, 868
chest radiology, 363, 368
acute dyspnoea, 371
diaphragm trauma, 369, 370
intraperitoneal air, 384
rib fractures, 363
tension pneumothorax, 371
X-ray, interpretation, 869
chicken pox, 1037, 1047
chilblains, 783–4
child abuse see abuse; non-accidental injury
child see paediatrics
childbirth see neonate; obstetrics
chin lift and jaw thrust, 29–30
chlorhexidine, 241
chloroquine, poisoning, 230
choking
algorithm, 83
in child, 32, 83–4
in infant, 31, 83
unconscious victim, 32–3
cholecystitis
acute, 964
pregnancy, 1142
radiology, 380, 386
chronic obstructive pulmonary disease (COPD), 848–50
oxygen therapy, 850–1
Chvostek test, 155
circadian temperature rhythm, 1228
circulation, block diagram, 887
circulation and volume replacement
assessment, 106–7
microcirculation
nutritive flow improvement, 133
pharmacological manipulation, 133–4
pregnancy changes, 703
trauma
burns, 723–4, 726
paediatrics, 694
pregnancy, 703
circulatory shock, 890
clavicle
fractures, 602–3, 604
osteolysis, 678
Clonazepam, paediatrics, 1195
Clostridium botulinum, 1073

Clostridium tetani, 252
coagulation factors
    concentrates, 998
    depletion, 999
    in stored whole blood, 999
coagulopathies, 443, 992–7
    clinical approach, 993–4
    early treatment, 995–7
    following myocardial infarction, 882
    hereditary, 992
    investigations, emergency, 994–5
dicobalt edetate, antidote to cyanide
        poisoning, 217
cocaine
    illicit use, and psychological sequelae,
        1096–100
    poisoning, 228
    tetracaine, adrenaline and cocaine
        (TAC), 239
cochleovestibular emergencies, 489–90
codeine 185, 186, 192, *see also* opioids
cold erythema, 784
cold haemagglutinin disease (CHAD), 984
cold injury, 776–85
    after-effects, 782–3
    conjunctivitis, 783
    frostbite, 776–81
    non-freezing (NFCI), 781–2
    other effects, 783–5
    trench foot, 781–3
    wind-chill chart, 766
cold urticaria, 784
collagen vascular disease, 1041
Colles' fracture, 351, 373, 614, 711
    radiology, 351
colloids, fluid replacement, 157, 728
colon
    injuries, 565
    irrigation, 215
    ischaemia, 962–3
    obstruction, 963, 1142
    perforation, 962–3
    whole bowel irrigation, 215
coma
    assessment, 172–8
    causes, 1196
    causes and pathophysiology, 167–9
        primary and secondary, 170
    classification of lesions, 167
    defined, 167
    Glasgow Coma Scale, 175, 424–5
        paediatric version, 695, 1197
    head injuries, causing coma, 167–9, 174–8
    investigations, 178
    management, 170–2
        algorithm, 1200
        early, 179–80
    myxoedema coma, 1106–7
    paediatric emergencies, 1196–200
    pupillary changes, 1199
    respiratory assessment, 173
communication
    skills, 9
    staff, 12
    transport of patient, 346
compartment syndromes, acute, 643–4
Congo–Crimean haemorrhagic fever virus,
        1247
coning, cerebellar herniation, 1197
conjunctivitis, 505
    cold injury, 783
consent, patients' rights, 14–15

constipation, acute abdomen, 959
consultants, first appointment, 3
contraception, postcoital contraception, 718
contusions *see* wound care
convulsions, 1064–8
    differential diagosis, 1195–6
    paediatric emergencies, 1192–6
    treatment, 195
cooling methods, management of
        hyperthermia, 793
cornea, retrieval, 407
coronary arteries, mechanism of narrowing,
        871
coronary artery bypass surgery,
        extracorporeal warming, 775
coroner, notification of death, 396, 406
coronoid process fractures, 449
corticosteroids, in hypothermia, 776
costochondritis, 675
cough reflex, 177
counselling, 13
crabs, 1049
cradle cap, 1033
cranial nerves, palsies, diabetes-related, 1134
creatine phosphokinase isoenzyme
        (CPK-MB), 551
cricoid pressure, 38
cricothyroid airway, 333–4
cricothyroidotomy, 48–50, 58, 485–6
    paediatrics, 87–8, 1177
        contraindications, 684, 694
crime, forensic evidence, 396–7
critical incident stress debriefing (CISD), 13
croup, paediatric emergencies, 1175–6
cryoprecipitate, 995, 998
crystal arthropathies, 1020–3
cuboid, fractures, 642
cupulolithiasis, 1069
cutis marmorata, 760
cyanide poisoning, 28–9, 216–19
    antidotes, 217, 738
cyanoacrylate glue, wound closure, 244
cyanosis
    paediatrics, 1204
    persistent central, COPS, 97
cyclizine
    contraindications, 878
    indications, 878
cyclo-oxygenase, inhibition by NSAIDs, 184
cystitis, 969–70
cytokines, proinflammatory, 123–4
    immune responses, 123

dacrocystocele, 456
dacryoadenitis, 504
dactylitis, tuberculous, 1025
dantrolene, use in severe hyperthermia, 794
DC cardioversion, pacemakers, 927
de Quervain's disease, 1025
death certificate, 396
deaths, 395–407
    Asian cultural practices, 403
    checklist, 403
    management of deceased patient, 395–8
    management of relatives, 398–404
    multiple deaths 406, *see also* disasters
    organ donation, 406–7
    staff support, 404–6
debriefing
    deaths, 405
    operational, 12
    psychological, 13–14

decompression sickness, 758, 760
    A&E management, 762–3
    prehospital care, 761–2
    recompression therapy, 762
    terminology, 761
deep venous thrombosis
    as an emergency, 948
    elderly people, 713
    emergency, in pregnancy, 1145
    massive, 949
defibrillation, 67–8
    paediatrics, 91
    see also prehospital cardiac care, chain of
        survival
defibrillators, automated external (AEDs),
        314
dehydration
    degrees of, paediatric emergencies, 1185
    hypovolaemia, 130
dementia, differention from hypoglycaemia,
        1129
Dengue fever, 1245
Denmark, cardiac prehospital care, 304, 308
dental abscess, 460–1, 468
dental caries/decay, 464, 467–9
dental pain, 460, 462
dental radiology, 465, 471
dental trauma, 451–2
dentoalveolar fractures, 451–2
depressive illness, 1085
    puerperium, 1146
dermatitis herpetiformis, 1051
dermatological emergencies, 1029–55
    bullous disorders, 1049–51
    burns, electrical injuries, 746
    childhood exanthems, 1047
    collagen vascular disease, 1041
    diabetes-related conditions, 1133–4
    drug reactions, 1052–4
    eczema, 1031–4
    erythema, 1054
    infections, 1035–41
    infestations, 1048–9
    lesions, 1030
    psoriasis, 1034–5
    skin contamination, chemical injuries, 737
    systemic disease, 1042
    toxic erythema, 1048
    tumours, 1044–5
    ulcers, 1055
    urticaria, 1051–2
    vascular disorders, 1042–4
desferrioxamine
    antidote to iron poisoning, 218, 229–30
    iron poisoning, 230
desmopressin, diabetes insipidus, 1115–16
dextrans
    capillary effects in decompression
        sickness, 762
    contraindications, 995
dextropropoxyphene, 186
dextrose, IV, properties, 157–8
dextrose saline, properties, 157–8
diabetes insipidus, 1115–16
diabetes mellitus
    acute abdomen, 966
    childbirth and caesarean section, 1132
    classification, 1121
        secondary causes, 1121–2
    emergencies, 1122–35
        hyperosmolar non-ketotic
            hyperglycaemia, 1127–8

hypoglycaemia, 1128–31
ketoacidosis, 1122–7
lactic acidosis, 1128
glucose tolerance test (WHO), 1121
glucose–potassium–insulin (GKI)
system, 1132
insulin-treated patients, 1132
intercurrent illness, 1131–5
newly diagnosed, 1131
NIDDM patients, 1132
pathophysiology, 1120–1
related conditions
diabetic foot, 1134–5
eye problems, 1133
neurological problems, 1134
skin conditions, 1133–4
diagnosis, litigation risk management, 17
diamorphine 191, see also opioids
diaphragm trauma, 369–70, 564
rupture, 552
Diazemuls, 195, 204
diazepam
paediatrics, 1194
pharmacological data, 203, 240
dichloroacetate, 148
diclofenac, 185, 186
dicobalt edetate, antidote to cyanide
poisoning, 217
digital nerve block, 195–6, 239
digoxin
acute abdomen, 966
acute left ventricular failure, 889
atrial fibrillation, 883
dosage, 899
indications/contraindications, 899
interactions, 899
paediatrics, 1203
poisoning, 217, 228–9
pregnancy and lactation, 929
side-effects, 889
dimercaprol, antidote to heavy metal
poisoning, 218
diphtheria, 1177
diplopia, 508
disasters
bereaved relatives, 398–404
British Association for Immediate Care
(BASICS), 274–5, 286–7
Control of Industry Major Accident
Hazard (CIMAH) Regulations (1984),
266
hospital major incident plan (HMIP),
257, 272–82
action cards, 273
administrative coordinator, 277
ambulance control point (APC),
274–5, 277
ambulance liaison officer, 281
communications, 277
debriefing, 282, 405
hospital coordination team, 276–7
hospital information centre, 280
incident stand-down, 281–2
medical incident coordinator (MIC),
276
medical incident officer (MIO), 272,
274–5
mobile medical team, 275–6
news media, 281
police, 281
putting into action, 273–7
relatives' reception officer (RRO), 280

training, 282
triage, 277–8
types and causes, 257–72
chemical incidents, 266–7
civil disturbances, 271
fire, 260–5
gas explosions and building collapse,
267–9
mine explosions and collapse, 269
natural disasters, 257–8
nuclear accidents, 271
public health incidents, 272
shooting, 269–70
sports stadia, 270–1
terrorism, 265
transport, 258–60
see also deaths
disopyramide
cardiac arrhythmias, 899
pregnancy and lactation, 929
disorientation, right–left, 1061
disseminated intravascular coagulation,
993–7
screening tests, 994–5
distributive shock, 120
diuretics, treatment of cerebral oedema,
180
diverticulitis, 964
diving injuries, 757–63
emergency telephone numbers, 763
management, 761–3
pathophysiology, 757–61
diving reflex, 1202
hypothermia, 753–4
DMSA, DMPS, antidotes to heavy metals,
217
dobutamine, 890
inotropy, 132
dog bite wounds, 248–50
dopamine, 890
Doppler sonicaid, 1150–1
drawer test, 669
dressings, wound care, 244–5
drowning, near, 751–7
epidemiology, 751
immersion hypothermia, 753
pathophysiology, 752–4
prehospital care, 754
prognosis, 757
salt water vs fresh water, 752–3
'secondary' drowning, 752
see also hypothermia
drug abuse, 1095–100
infections, 1236–7
drug delivery routes, 68–9
endobronchial route, 69, 89
drug overdose, cardiac arrhythmias, 928
drug reactions, 1052–4
acute abdomen, 966
allergic vasculitis, 1053
bullous eruptions, 1053
dermatological emergencies, 1052–4
exanthematous, 1052
exfoliative dermatitis, 1052–3
fixed drug eruptions, 1053
photosensitivity, 1053–4
urticaria, 1053
drug-induced pulmonary disease, 852
drugs
causing malignant hyperthermia, 789–90
illicit
effects (table), 1096–8

psychological and behavioural
sequelae, 1099–100
duct–dependent systemic circulation, 1204
duodenum, injuries, 564
dyscalculia, 1061
dyspepsia, pregnancy, 1142
dyspnoea, acute, radiology, 371
dystonia, side-effects, neuroleptic drugs,
1087

ear, nose and throat emergencies, 481–96
ear
foreign bodies, 487–8
infections, 488–9
scuba diving injuries, 483, 759
trauma, 481–2
ear infections, paediatric emergencies,
1183–4
eating disorders, 1085–6
Ebola virus, 1247
eclampsia and pre-eclampsia, 1143–4
traumatic changes, 704
ecstasy (E, MDMA)
illicit use, and psychological sequelae,
1096–100
poisoning, 227
severe hyperthermia, 794
ectopic pregnancy, 1156–7
incidence, 1156
eczema, 1031–4
EDTA tube, blood, assessment of
poisoning, 211
elbow
dislocations, 610–11
paediatric, 625
exercises, 820–1
fractures, paediatric, 622, 624
golfer's elbow, 1026
pulled, 623
sports injuries, 679
tennis elbow, 1026
see also upper limb
elderly people, 1220–7
abdominal assessment and acute
abdomen, 967
abdominal trauma, 710
abuse and neglect, 1226–7
anaesthetic problems, 714
confusional states, 1224–5
deep venous thrombosis, 713
ethical aspects of resuscitation, 714–15
ethnic minorities, 1227
hypothermia, 712, 1223
iatrogenic disease, 1225–6
intercurrent drugs, 713
metabolism and nutrition, 713–14
pressure sores, 713
trauma, 708–15
burns, 712
cervical spine trauma, 709–10
chest injuries, 710
epidemiology, 708
ethical aspects of resuscitation, 714–15
falls, 1223–4
femur, 655, 656
head and neck injuries, 709
lower limb, 712
and osteoporosis, 710–13
pelvic fractures, 652, 710
specific injury patterns, 709–13
electrical injuries, 742–50
A&E protocol

domestic supply injury, 748–9
    high-voltage burns, 749
cardiac arrhythmias, 747
epidemiology, 742–3
pathophysiology, 743–8
rescuer and propagation distance of
    current, 748
secondary injuries, 745
voltages, 742–3
electricity, characteristics, 742–4
electrocardiography
    12-lead ECG, 897–8
    interpretation of ECG, 868–9
        cardiac arrhythmias, 897–8
    pericarditis, 893
    sinus rhythm, normal intervals, 898
electrolytes see fluids and electrolytes
electromechanical dissociation (EMD)
    algorithm, 73
    paediatrics, 91
embolus see air embolism; thromboembolism
emergencies, civil see disasters
emergency telephone numbers, 308
    diving injuries, 763, 854
emesis, in poisoning, 212–13, 214
EMLA cream, 186
emotional abuse, 1217
emphysema, 848–50
    surgical, 554
encephalitis
    herpes simplex infection, 1075, 1190
    specific treatment, 1075
encephalopathy, hypertensive, 895
endocrine emergencies, 1102–17
    acute pituitary emergencies, 1113–16
    adrenocortical insufficiency, 1111–13
    calcium metabolism disorders, 1107–11
    myxoedema coma, 1106–7
    thyrotoxicosis, 1102–7
    see also diabetic emergencies
endotracheal intubation see tracheal
    intubation
enoximone, 890
Entonox, 188
envenomation, 222, 822–34
    arachnids, 827–30
    bees and wasps, 822–3
    snakes, 823–7
eosinophilia, 1246–7
epididymal cyst, 974
epididymitis, 972–3
epididymo-orchitis, 388, 973
epiglottitis, 462
    paediatric emergencies, 1176–7
epilepsy
    following head injury, 422
    pregnancy, 1145
    seizures, 1064–8
epiphysis, slipped upper, femur, 1008–9
epistaxis see nose bleeds
erysipelas, 1035
erythema
    necrolytic migratory, 1134
    reactive, 1054–5
erythema infectiosum (fifth disease), 1020,
    1038–9
erythema multiforme, 1038, 1054
erythema nodosum, 1054
erythrasma, 1035
ESR
    pelvic inflammatory disease, 1152
    pregnancy, 1138

ethanol
    antidote to ethylene glycol poisoning, 217
    poisoning, 222–3
ethical aspects of resuscitation, elderly
    people, 714–15
ethnic differences, deaths, 403
ethylene glycol poisoning, ethanol as
    antidote, 217
etomidate, 57
Europe
    ambulance provision, 285
    controlled studies of survival of cardiac
        arrest, Europe/USA, 291
    emergency medical systems,
        Europe/USA, 292–6, 299–323
European Resuscitation Council guidelines,
    cardiac arrhythmias, 908
eustachian tube pathology, 467
exanthems, childhood, 1047
expired air ventilation, 50–2, 82–3
external chest compression (ECC), 83
extracellular fluid
    composition, 150
    osmolality, 149
    volume, role of sodium, 150
extremities, assessment, 113–14
eye
    acute diplopia, 508
    acute visual loss, 507–8
        ischaemic optic neuropathy, 508
        optic neuritis, 508
        retinal detachment, 507
        retinal vascular occlusion, 507–8
        vitreous haemorrhage, 507
    diabetes-related conditions, 1133
    emergencies other than trauma, 504–8
    essential medical equipment, 498
    foreign bodies, 499
        intraocular, 502–3
    hyphaema, 500, 698
    inflammatory disorders, 504–7
        anterior uveitis, 506
        conjunctivitis, 505
        corneal ulceration/keratitis, 505–6
        episcleritis, 506–7
        glaucoma, 506
        herpes zoster, 506
        lacrimal gland, 504
        orbital cellulitis, 504–5
        scleritis, 507
    lens opacity and displacement, 501
    orbital complications of acute sinusitis,
        492–3
    pain relief, 737
    proliferative retinopathy, 1133
    pupillary changes in coma, 1199
    trauma, 442, 498–508
        burns, 503–4, 732
        chemical injuries, 503–4, 737–8
        choroidal tears, 501
        corneoscleral lacerations, 502
        globe rupture, 502
        iris and pupil damage, 501
        non-penetrating injury, 500–2
        optic nerve injury, 501
        orbital fracture, 501–2
        retinal breaks and oedema, 501
        superficial, 499
        ultraviolet keratoconjunctivitis, 499
eyelids
    inflammatory disorders, 504
    trauma, 442, 500

Fab antibody, antidote to digoxin
    poisoning, 217
face, skin conditions, 474–5
facial injuries, 439–58
    aetiology, 440–1
    assessment, 109–10, 236–7, 444, 456
    complications, 455
    fractures, 444–53
        Le Fort I, II and III fractures, 452
        summary, 454–5
    management, 442–3
    paediatrics, 698
    radiology, 456
    sutures, 457
    timing of treatment, 443–4
facial nerve
    paralysis, 491
    trauma, 442
facial pain, 459–61
faciomaxillary trauma, 439–59
factitious disorders, 1086–7
factitious fever, 1231
fainting (syncope), 1069–70, 1196
falls, 417
fascioliasis, 1246–7
fasciotomy, indications, 938
fat embolism, 587
febrile illness, 1228–48
    acute, 1234–6
    acute phase responses, 1230
    chronic, 1237–8
    drug history, 1232
    emergency assessment, 1231–4
    fever, defined, 1229
    fever and pathogenesis of fever, 1229–30
    management, 1234
    paediatrics, 1173
        convulsions, 1193
    pathogenesis, 1229–30
    patterns, 1230–1
    pulse rate, 1231
    sources of advice, 1248
    specific illnesses, 1236–8
    telephone numbers in emergencies, 1248
    thermoregulation, normal body
        temperature, 1228–9
    travel-associated illness, 1238–48
femoral arteries
    aneurysms, 945–6
    injury, 937
    tapping pulse, 943
femoral vein, ultrasonography, 372
femur
    avascular necrosis of femoral head,
        712
    fractures and dislocations, 373–80
        birth injuries, 628
        elderly people, 655, 656
        paediatrics, 628, 655–7
    Perthes' osteochondritis, 1007–8
    slipped upper femoral epiphysis, 1008–9
fentanyl 193, 240, see also opioids
fetus
    heart rate, 705
    maternal trauma, 702–7
        assessment, 705–6
fever see febrile illness
fibrin degradation products, 993, 995
fibrinogen, 995
fibroblast growth factor, in wound healing,
    237
fibrocartilage, sports injuries, 662

field assessment and treatment *see* cardiac prehospital care; injuries, prehospital care
fifth disease, 1020, 1038–9
finger agnosia, 1061
Finland, cardiac prehospital care, 305, 308
firearm injuries *see* ballistic injuries
fish
  envenomation, 831–2
  toxins, 834
  trauma, 830–1
flail chest, 544
flecainide
  paediatrics, 1203
  pregnancy and lactation, 929
  properties, 899
fluid, 24 h balance, 150–1
fluid and electrolyte requirements, 140–58
  body fluids, 149
  choice of fluid, 157–8
  maintenance, estimation, 156
  paediatric emergencies, 1185–6
fluid loss
  assessment, 130
    burns, 728
    Muir and Barclay plan, 730
    newborn resuscitation, 97
    paediatrics, 93
    replacement, 157
  see also hypovolaemia
flumenazil
  benzodiazepine antagonist, 204
  in benzodiazepine poisoning, 217, 226–7
folate deficiency, 980, 982
folliculitis, 1035–6
food-induced anaphylaxis, 164
foot *see* lower limb
forearm *see* upper limb
foreign bodies
  bronchi, 495
  chest X-ray, 443
  detection methods, 247–8, 391–3, 443
  ear, 487
  eye, 499, 502–3
  hands, 592–3
  inhalation, 495, 1177
  larynx, 495
  nose, 491
  oesophagus, 494–5
  throat, 493–4
  trachea, 495
  see also choking
forensic evidence, 396–7
Fournier's gangrene, 572
fractures
  open, 581–8
    classification, 582
    debridement of wound, 584
    emergency treatment, 582
    examination, 584–5
    limb salvage/amputation, 586–7
    post operative care, 587–8
    stabilization, 585–6
    wound coverage, 586
  terminology, 350–3
  see also specific regions and named bones
fractures, paediatric, 618–32
  growth plate (Salter–Harris types I–IV) injuries *see* physeal injuries
  hip fractures, 627–8
  lower limb, 628–32
  mnemonic CRITOE, 356

ossification centres, 356, 623
  pattern of injury, 618
  pelvic fractures, 627
  periosteum, 619
  physeal injuries, 353–4, 619–20, 621
  remodelling, 619
  spinal injuries, 626–7
  types of fractures, 618
    greenstick fractures, 621
    shaft fractures, 354
    supracondylar fractures, 354–8
    torus fractures, 621
  upper limb, 620–6
    radial head dislocation, 356, 625
    radial head fractures, 625
France, cardiac prehospital care, 305, 308
fresh frozen plasma (FFP), 995–6, 998
frontal bones, injuries, 453
frostbite, 776–81
  analgesia, 780
  countering infection, 780
  hydration and haemodilution, 780
  see also hypothermia
frusemide, treatment of cerebral oedema, 180
fundal examination, 177
fungal infections
  head and neck, 466
  skin, 1039–41
furuncle, otitis externa, acute, 1184
furunculosis, 1036

gag reflex, 177
Galeazzi fractures, 612
  paediatrics, 621
gallbladder disease, acute abdomen, 959
gases, Dalton's law, 758
gastric aspiration and lavage, 213–14
gastric regurgitation, patients at risk, 38
gastroenteritis
  antibiotics, 1187
  fever, 1236
  paediatric emergencies, 1184–7
gastrointestinal signs
  coma, 173–4
  poisoning, 209
  see also abdominal assessment
gastrointestinal tract
  pregnancy changes, 703
  surgery, 1141
general anaesthesia, 201–4
  agents, 203
  anaphylaxis, 165
  classification, 202
  contraindications, 201
  indications, 201
  induction, 56–7
    on admission, 183
    inhalational induction, 59
    rapid sequence, 58–9
  patient preparation, 202–3
genital herpes, 973–4, 1166–7
genital injuries, 571–2, 578
  sexual assault, 572, 719–20
genital tract infections
  summary, 1165
  see also sexually transmitted diseases
German measles, 1047
Germany, cardiac prehospital care, 306, 308
Gerstmann's syndrome, 1061
giant cell arteritis, 475
giardiasis cryptosporidiosis, 1185
Gibbs–Donnan law, 149

gingival swelling (infections), 461, 463–4, 469–71
  gingivostomatitis, 1036–7
girdle syndrome, sickle cell disease, 988
Glasgow Coma Scale, 174–6, 424
  paediatric version, 695
  paediatrics, 176, 1197
glaucoma, 1133
gloves, integrity, 247
glucagon, antidote to beta-blockers, 217
glucagonoma syndrome, 1134
glucocorticoids, previous therapy, adrenocortical insufficiency, 1111–12
glucose
  levels in hypothermia, 776
  paediatric resuscitation, 93, 96
glucose tolerance test, 1121
glucose-6-phosphate dehydrogenase deficiency, 983
glucose–potassium–insulin (GKI) system, 1132
glue, wound closure, 244
glue sniffing, 207
glyceryl trinitrate *see* nitrates
gnathostomiasis, 1246–7
golfer's elbow, 679
gonococcal arthritis, 1005
gonorrhoea, 970–1
gout, 1015, 1020–2
grafts, organ donation, 406–7
grand mal attacks, 1066
Graves' ophthalmopathy, 1104–6
grey baby syndrome, 1204
guardsman's fracture, 450
Guedel oropharyngeal airway, 33–4, 85
Guillain–Barré syndrome, 1073
gums, 463
gunshot injuries *see* ballistic injuries
gynaecological emergencies, 1148–70
  assessment, 1148–52
    pelvic examination, 1150

haematemesis, signs of poisoning, 209
haematocele, 974
haematocrit, haemorrhagic shock, 132
haematological emergencies, 978–1002
  anaemia, 978–84
  blood transfusion, 997–1002
  haemostasis disorders, 990–7
  major incident procedure, 1002
  sickle cell disease, 984–8
  white cell disorders, 988–90
haematological indices, 1152
haematomas
  haematoma block, 199
  investigations, 428–30
  radiology, 428–30
  subungual, 664
haematuria, 976–7
  causes, 977
    paediatrics, 1188
  clot retention, 977
haemoglobin, 979
haemolytic anaemia, 983
haemophilia, 992
Haemophilus influenzae infection
  hip disease, 1016, 1018
  meningitis, 1074
haemoptysis, massive, 854
haemorrhage
  abdominal trauma, 935–6
  acute abdomen, 958, 966

assessment, 106–7
chest trauma, 933–4
face, 443
following heparin therapy, 996
following thrombolytic therapy, 996
haemorrhagic telangiectasia, 991
massive obstetric, 1139
menorrhagia, 1152, 1158
neck trauma, 931–2
overanticoagulation with warfarin, 996
pituitary apoplexy, 1112, 1114–15
upper limb trauma, 932–3
vaginal bleeding in pregnancy, 1138–40
venous bleeding, 935
haemorrhagic shock
class I–IV, 131
fluid replacement regimens, 131
haematocrit, 132
and hypovolaemia, 129
haemostasis disorders, 990–7
reactions involved, 990
haemothorax
management, 554
massive, 548
hair removal, 240
Hallpike test, positional nystagmus, 1069
hallucinogens, illicit use, and psychological
sequelae, 1096–100
hand, anatomy, 589–91
hand injuries
bites, 248–50, 597
burns, 598
clinical examination, 591
cold injury, 598, 783–4
foreign bodies, 592–3
fractures and dislocations, 594–5
lunate/perilunate dislocation, 594–5
metacarpal fractures, 595
metacarpophalangeal dislocations,
595
paediatrics, 620–1
phalangeal dislocations, 595
scaphoid fracture, 594
thumb metacarpophalangeal injuries,
595
infections, 595–7
cellulitis and lymphangitis, 597
hand, foot and mouth disease, 1038
paronychia, 596
pulp space infection, 596
pyogenic granuloma, 598
tendon sheath infections, 596
local anaesthesia
digital nerve block, 195–6
peripheral nerve blocks, 196–8, 599
ring block, 598–9
mallet finger, 593
mutilation, 594
nerve injury, 593
ring avulsion injuries, 593
soft tissue injuries, 591–4, 1025
splintage, 600
traumatic amputations, 595–6
trigger finger, 1025
wound care, 599
see also wrist
Hartmann's fluid (sodium lactate),
composition, 157
HAZCHEM codes, 733–5
hCG test
acute abdomen, 955, 1151
ectopic pregnancy, 1157

head
surface area and heat loss, 766, 772
see also face; facial
head and neck infections
blood tests, 464
normal flora, 466
pathogens, 466
symptomatology, 459–62
head and neck injuries, 420–37
elderly people, 709
investigations, 425–30
brain contusions, 429
CT scan pathology, classification and
criteria for arranging, 427–8
diffuse axonal injury, 429
haematomas, 428–30
management plan, 430–2
criteria for hospital admission, 432
criteria for referral to neurosurgeon, 434
emergency management, 432–5
neurosurgical unit, 435–7
neurological assessment, 109, 114, 422–5
AVPU system, 424
comatose patient, 167–9, 174–8
responsiveness, 107–8
paediatrics, 200, 686–7, 697
pathophysiology, 420–2
policy guidelines, 360
primary/secondary brain injury, 420–2
radiology, 359
safe transfer, 435
seizures, 434
skull fractures, 360–1, 425–8
treatment at neurosurgical unit, 435–7
head and neck masses, 476–8
headache, 1070–2
cluster, 1072
post–traumatic, 1072
tension–type, 1072
healing see wound care
hearing loss, sudden, 489
heart
blunt injuries, 935
electrical injuries, 746–7
paediatrics, 686
penetrating injuries, 934–5
heart block
first degree, 904–5
second degree AV block, Mobitz, 905–6
third degree, 906–7
Wenckebach second degree AV block,
884, 905
heart rates, normal, paediatrics, 1174–5
heart valves, retrieval, 407
heat production
central mechanisms, 790
peripheral mechanisms, 789–90
heavy metals, antidotes, 217, 218
Heimlich manoeuvre, 31–3
Henderson–Hasselbalch equation 143
Henoch–Schonlein purpura, 1043
heparin
for angina, 874
bleeding following, 996
following myocardial infarction, 882
hepatitis B, blood transmission, 246–7
hereditary angioedema, 163
hereditary haemorrhagic telangiectasia, 991
heroin, poisoning, 227–8
herpes simplex infection, 478–9, 1036–7
eczema herpeticum, 1033
genital herpes, 973–4, 1166–7

HSV encephalitis, 1075, 1190
meningitis, 973
herpes zoster infection, 479, 1037
eye inflammation, 506
hip
fractures and dislocations, 373–80
paediatrics, 627, 653–4
hip pain, paediatrics, 375–6, 379
infection
Haemophilus influenzae, 1016
transient synovitis, 1020
tuberculosis, 379
irritable, 1009
Perthes' osteochondritis, 1007–8
slipped upper femoral epiphysis, 1009
hirudin, leech-related, 874
history-taking
mnemonic, 108
poisoning, 211
wound care, 235–6
HIV infection and AIDS, 479
acute abdomen, 967
bite transmission, 250
blood transmission, 246–7
causes of fever, 1238
deaths, precautions to be taken, 398
groups at particular risk, 1233
post sexual assault, 719
symptoms suggesting, 1233
hives, 1051
homeostasis, normal values, 179
Horner's syndrome, 1061
hospital major incident plan (HMIP),
271–82
summary, 257
see also disasters
host defence, infections, 988–9
human bite wounds, 249–50
human papilloma virus, 1038
humerus
fractures and dislocations, 605–9
distal humerus, 610
management, 606–7
paediatrics, 623, 625
proximal humerus, 605–7
radiographic classification, 606
shaft, 609–10
see also upper limb injuries
Hutchinson's sign, 1046
hydatidiform mole, 1155–6
hydrocele
adults, 974
children, 974
hydrocephalus, acute, 1190
hydrocolloid dressings, wound care, 244–5
hydrofluoric acid poisoning, calcium
gluconate, 218, 737
hydrogen ion homeostasis, 140–1
hydrogen sulphide, antidote, 738
hydrophobia in rabies, 251
hydroxyapatite crystal deposition disease,
1022
hydroxycobalamin, antidote to cyanide
poisoning, 217
hydroxyethyl starch (HES), osmolarity and
oncotic pressure, 158
hymenoptera envenomation, 822–3
hyperbaric chamber, 761–2
hyperbaric oxygen therapy, 29, 761–2,
854
telephone number, 854
hypercalcaemia, 155, 1108–9

hyperglycaemia, hyperosmolar non-ketotic, 1127–8
hyperkalaemia, 154
hypermagnesaemia, 156
hypernatraemia, 152
hyperosmolar non-ketotic hyperglycaemia, 1127–8
hyperpyrexia, 58, 1229
hypertension
  crisis and phaeochromocytoma, 1116–17
  emergencies, 1117
  hypertensive encephalopathy, 895
  malignant (accelerated) hypertension, 894–5
  paediatrics, 1204–5
  in pregnancy (eclampsia), 1143–4
  protective, 171
hyperthermia, 787–95, 1229
  clinical features, 790–3
  clinical presentation, 787–8
  complications, 792–3
  defined, 787
  differential diagnosis, 791
  pathophysiology, 788–90
  treatment, 793–5
hyperviscosity syndrome, 989
hyphaema, 500, 698
hypocalcaemia, 155
hypoglycaemia, 1128–31
  insulin-induced, 1129–30
  nocturnal, 1129
  recurrence, 1131
  tablet-treated patients, 1129
  treatment, 1130
  unusual presentations, 1129–30
hypokalaemia, 153–4
hypokalaemic periodic paralysis, 1073–4
hypomagnesaemia, 156
hyponatraemia, 152–3
hypopituitarism, and diabetes insipidus, 1115–16
hypothermia, 765–85
  chest compression rate, 754
  classification, 767–9
  cold risk in industry, 765
  defined, 767
  diagnosis, 769–70
  diving reflex, 753–4
  heat loss, 766
  and hypoxia, 767
  immersion, 753
  insulation care, 754
  rescue, 770
    death following rescue, 770–1
  resuscitation, 771–6
  rewarming methods, 772–6
  symptoms and signs, 769
  and trauma, elderly people, 712, 1223
  see also cold injury; frostbite
hypovolaemic shock, 119, 122–3, 129–34, 587
  assessment, 106–7
  choice of fluid, 157–8
  classification I–IV, 129
  pathogenesis, 121
  treatment, 133–4, 171
  see also fluid loss
hypoxia
  and hypothermia, 767
  see also coma

ibuprofen, 185, 186
iliac arteries, angiography, 941
immersion hypothermia, 753
immunization
  anaphylaxis, 253
  tetanus, 252, 253
immunocompromised host, 1233
immunoglobulin E, anaphylaxis, 159–66
impetigo, 1036
impingement syndromes, 667
indomethacin, 185, 186
industrial hazards, hypothermia, 765
infant see neonate; paediatrics
infections
  abdominal trauma, 563–4
  bite wounds, 248–50
  burns, 724
  deaths, precautions to be taken, 398
  host defence, 988–9
  jaw, 471–2
  principal sites, 135
  protection of staff, 10
  signs, 1233–6
    gastroenteritis, 1233, 1236
    meningitis, 1233, 1236
    osteomyelitis, 1233–6
    pelvic inflammatory disease, 1233, 1235–6
    pneumonia, 1233, 1235
    pyelonephritis, 1233
    pyogenic arthritis, 1233–6
  skin, 1035–6
  see also fungal infections; septic shock; viral infections; specific organs and infections
infectious mononucleosis, 1177
infiltration anaesthesia, 195, 239
inflammatory responses, in shock, 123–4
inhalational anaesthesia see general anaesthesia
injuries
  chemical injuries, 733–9
  elderly people, 708–15
  fractures and dislocations, 350–68
  Injury Severity Score, 341
  multiply injured patient, 100–17
    assessment, 102–14
    documentation, 116–17
    resuscitation, 114–16
      recommended equipment, 101
  prehospital care, 326–47
    dispatch algorithm, 328
    field assessment, 328–32
    field treatment, 332–6
    interhospital transport, 340–7
    quality management and research, 336–7
    system features, 326–8
    treat vs transport, 332
    triage, 328
  radiation injuries, 739–40
  trauma admission record, 117
  trauma teams, 9–10, 101
  see also accidents
inner ear and temporal bone fractures, 482–3
inotropic agents, 890
  dobutomine, 132, 890
insect venom sensitivity, 160, 822–3
insulin
  administration to insulin-treated patients, 1132
  allergy, 1134

  childbirth and caesarean section, 1132
    cessation, 1133
  glucose–potassium–insulin (GKI) system, 1132
  insulin-induced hypoglycaemia, 1129–30
  and ketoacidosis, 1123, 1127
  overdose, 1131
  pregnancy changes, 1138
  see also diabetes mellitus
interdigital neuroma, 665
internal cardioverter defibrillator (ICD), 927–8
interstitial fluid, composition, 150
intervertebral disc, prolapse, 1011
intestinal radiology see abdominal assessment; colon; small bowel
intracellular fluid, composition, 150
intracranial pressure, 1199–200
  and cerebral perfusion pressure, 169, 421
  elevated
    effects, 421–2
    signs, 179
    treatment, 179–80, 421
  meningitis, 1190
  primary and secondary coma, 170
intraosseous infusion, paediatrics, 1209–10
intraperitoneal air, 384
intraperitoneal haemorrhage, 958
intravenous access, paediatrics, summary, 1211
intravenous (IV) fluids, 158
  prehospital care, 336
  rewarming method in hypothermia, 775
intravenous regional anaesthesia (IVRA), 200–1
intravenous urography (IVU), 383, 573–5
intubation see tracheal intubation
invertebrates
  insects, 822–3
  marine, envenomation, 832–3
iodide, in thyroid emergencies, 1103
iodine compounds, 241
ionizing radiation
  injuries, 739–40
  types, 739
  units, 739
ipecacuanha, as emetic, 212–13, 214
iron, poisoning, 218, 229–30
iron deficiency anaemia, 982
irradiation, injuries, 739–40
irrigation of wounds, 241
isoprenaline
  antidote to beta-blockers, 217
  cardiac arrhythmias, 899
  paediatrics, 928
IUCD, menstrual loss, 1158

jaw infections, 471–2
jaw thrust, 29–30, 82
jaws, see also faciomaxillary trauma; mandible; maxilla
jellyfish, envenomation, 832–3
Jervill–Lange–Neilson syndrome, 1202
jogger's nipple, 675
joint pain, 1014–27
  axial and peripheral joints, 1016–17
  crystal arthropathies, 1020–3
  emergency assessment, 1014–16
  inflammatory disease, 1014–17
  polyarthritis, 1023–4
  soft tissue rheumatism, 1024–6
  specific syndromes, 1018–20

joints
   aspiration and injection of joints, 1022–3
   injuries see specific joints
Jones (metatarsal) fractures, 631, 643

kaolin, contraindications, 1187
keloids, 238
KEMLER scale, chemical hazards, 734
keratoacanthoma, 1045
Kernig's sign, 1074
ketamine, 57, 193
   paediatrics, 240
   side-effects, 240
ketoacidosis, 1122–7
   management, 1124–6
   pathophysiology, 1123
   presentation, 1123
ketorolac, 193
kidneys, injuries see renal trauma
Kleihauer test, 705
knee
   arterial injury, 937–8
   brace, 810
   fractures and dislocations, 635–8, 938
      paediatrics, 628–9
   ligamentous injury, 809
   patellar fracture, 352, 636–7, 672
   physiotherapy techniques, 817–18
   sports injuries, 668–74
   sprain, rehabilitation, 809–10
knee pain, causes, 673
Köhler's osteochondritis, 1008
Kussmaul's sign, 545

labetolol, contraindications, 1117
lacerations see wound care
Lachman's test, 669
lactation
   absent, Sheehan's syndrome, 1112
   drugs in breast milk, 929
lactic acidosis, 146
   diabetes mellitus, 1128
laparotomy, urgent, preparation, 961
large bowel see colon
laryngeal mask airway, 35–6, 67
laryngoscopes, 39–43
   paediatrics, 41
laryngotomy, 485–6
laryngotracheobronchitis, viral, 1175
larynx
   anatomy, 25
   foreign bodies, 495
   injuries, 553
   neonates, 684
   thyromental distance, 26
   trauma, 486–7
Lassa fever, 1247
latex sensitivity, 164–5
law and litigation
   errors in radiology, 349
   mental health, 1088–9, 1094, 1100
   risk management, 16–19
   in diagnosis, 17
laxatives, 214–15
Le Fort I, II and III fractures, facial
   bones, 452
leech-related hirudin, 874
leg see lower limb
legislation see law
Leishmania donovani, 1246
leucocyte-depleted blood, 1001

leukemias, 989
lice infestation, 1049
lichen planus, 1044
life support
   advanced, 71–3
   basic, 65–6, 332–3, 344–5
      paediatrics, 82–4
   paediatrics, 82–93
ligaments, injury, 662
light reflexes, 175–7
light wand, 43
lightning, electrical injuries, 743, 749–50
lignocaine
   cardiac arrhythmias, 899
   endobronchial route, 69, 89
   following myocardial infarction, 883, 884
   indications, 899
   interactions, 899
   lignocaine gel, 187, 239
   maximum doses and duration of action,
      194, 238, 899
      paediatrics, 93
      with/without adrenaline, 194, 238
   side-effects, 899
   skin infiltration technique, 195, 239
   in VT and VF, 70, 883, 884
   see also local anaesthesia
limbs
   assessment, 113–14
   see also lower limb; upper limb
lime burns, 737
lithium
   lithium toxicity, 1088
   side-effects, 1088
   in thyroid emergencies, 1103
litigation see law and litigation
Little's area, 462, 463
liver abscess, amoebic, 1245
liver damage
   injuries, 566
   radiology, 367, 369
liver disease
   bleeding, 993
   investigations, 994–5
loaiasis, 1246–7
local anaesthesia, 193–201
   digital nerve block, 195–6
   drug pharmacology, 194–5
      maximum doses and duration of
      action, 194
   femoral nerve block, 198
   haematoma block, 199
   intravenous regional anaesthesia, 200
   lateral cutaneous nerve of thigh,
      199
   radial nerve block, 197
   skin infiltration technique, 195, 239
   toxicity, 194–5
   ulnar nerve block, 196–7
   wounds, 238–9
   see also topical analgesic agents and routes
lochia, 1140
   abnormal, 1168
long QT syndrome, 919–20
lorazepam, paediatrics, 1194
low back pain see back pain
lower limb
   ankle:brachial index (ABPI), 936
   avascular necrosis of femoral head, 712
   cold injury to feet, 781–4
   diabetic foot, 1134–5
   feet, mid/hindfoot, sports injuries, 664–5

fractures and dislocations, 373–80, 382,
   633–46
   ankle injuries, 644–6
   calcaneus, 631, 641
      Bohler's angle, 380, 381
   elderly people, 712
   femoral shaft, 633–5
   hind/midfoot, 376–80, 641–3
   knee, 635–8
   Lisfranc fracture, 380
   paediatric fractures, 628–32
intravenous regional anaesthesia (IVRA),
   200–1
ischaemia, 940–8
   5Ps, 940
   cause, thrombosis-in-situ vs embolus,
      940
   diabetic foot, 946–8
   ischaemic foot, 946
   management, 940–2
Köhler's osteochondritis, 1008
local anaesthesia, 198–9
pretibial lacerations, 251
sports injuries, 664–5, 668
vascular injury, 936–8
see also specific parts and joints
Ludwig's angina, 459, 462, 468–9, 496
lumbar spine injury, 528
lunate fractures, 373
lung function see pulmonary function
Lyme disease, 1019
lymph node cytology, 465–6
lymphadenopathy, 463, 464
lysergic acid (LSD)
   illicit use, and psychological sequelae,
      1096–100
   poisoning, 228

magnesium
   balance, 155–6
   cardiac arrhythmias, dose and
      indications, 899
   pregnancy and lactation, 929
magnesium salts, in VT, 71
major accidents see disasters
malaria, 1239–44
   anaemia, 984
   cases 1977–1991, 1241
   chloroquine–resistant areas, 1241
   clinical assessment, 1242
   differential diagnosis, 1248
   treatment, 1243–4
malignant hyperpyrexia, 58, 1229
malingering, 1087
mandible
   dislocation, 448–9
   fractures, condylar head, 447–8
   growth failure, 442
   limitation of movement, 442
   temporomandibular joint
      dysfunction syndrome, 474
   fractures, 446–50
mangled extremity severity score (MESS),
   640
mannitol, treatment of cerebral oedema, 180
Marburg virus, 1247
march fracture, 665
marine envenomation, 830–4
mast cells, anaphylaxis, 160
mastoiditis, 489
maxillary trauma, 439–58
McCoy levering laryngoscope, 41–2

MDMA (ecstasy, E), poisoning, 227
measles, 1047
Mecca body-cooling unit, 793
mechanoceptors, 183
median nerve, 590
median nerve block, 196
mediastinal X-ray, interpretation, 869
Medic-Alert foundation, addresses (UK and USA), 165
medical emergency telephone numbers, 308
medical incident coordinator (MIC), 276
medical incident officer (MIO), 274–6
medical negligence, 16–19
medical staff, 6
    training, 8–9
medullary infarction, 1061
megaloblastic anaemia, 982
melanoma, malignant, 1045–6
Mellinghof's sign, 760
meningitis
    adults, 1074–5
    bacterial
        antibiotics, 1191
        Haemophilus influenzae, 1074
        Streptococcus pneumoniae, 1074
    fever, 1236
    intracranial pressure, 1190
    paediatric emergencies, 1189–92
    prophylaxis of contacts, 1191
meningococcal septicaemia,
        Waterhouse–Friderichsen syndrome, 1111
menstrual loss, 1158
    dysmenorrhoea, 1162
    menorrhagia, 1152, 1158
Mental Health Act, 1088–9, 1094, 1100
mental health legislation, 1088–9, 1094
mental state examination, 1078, 1221–2
meperidine (MPC), contraindications, 240
mercurials, poisoning, antidote, 738
mesenteric arteries, involvement in dissecting aneurysms, 943
mesenteric vessel injury, 935–6
metabolic acidosis, 145
    drowning, near, 756
metabolic alkalosis, 147
metabolism
    burns, 724
    and nutrition, elderly people, 713–14
    signs of poisoning, 210–11
metacarpal nerve block *see* digital nerve block
metacarpophalangeal joint injuries, 249–50
metatarsal bones
    fractures, 631, 642–3
        sports injuries, 664–5
    traction apophysitis, 665
methaemaglobin poisoning, 218
methanol, poisoning, 218
methionine, antidote to paracetamol poisoning, 219, 224–6
metoclopramide, indications, 878
mexiletine, 70
midazolam
    paediatrics, 240
    pharmacological data, 203, 204, 240
middle ear
    scuba diving injuries, 759, 760
    trauma, 482
middle ear squeeze, 759
migraine, 1071–2
minor injuries, paediatrics, 691

miscarriage
    advice sheet, 1155, 1169–70
    complete/incomplete, 1154–5
    missed/inevitable, 1153, 1155
    recurrence, 1155
    threatened
        assessment, 1152–5
        Rh testing, 1152
molluscum contagiosum, 1038
Monteggia fractures, 612
    paediatric, 621
morphine, 191
    see also opioids
mortality, paediatric trauma, 680–3
Morton's neuroma, 665
motor responses, 178
mouth, anatomy, 23, 26
mouth opening, difficulty, 442, 464
mouth ulcers, 461, 463, 470
mouth-to-mouth ventilation, 50–2
multiple myeloma, 989
multiply injured patient *see* injuries
mumps, 473
Munchausen by proxy, 1218
muscle injury, 661–2
musculoskeletal burns, electrical injuries, 746
musical distraction, 240
myasthenia gravis, 1073
Mycobacterium tuberculosis infection, 479
mycoplasma infection, 1183
myocardial dysfunction
    primary and secondary, 119–20
    recurrent ischaemia, 885
myocardial infarction, 874–86
    complications
        risk factors, 886
        treatment, 883–5
    diagnosis, 874–7
    epidemiology, 874–5
    management, 878–83
        analgesia, 878
        antiarrhythmic therapy, 883
        antiemetics, 878
        aspirin, 879
        beta-blockers, 883
        fast track therapy, 882
        flowchart, 887
        heparin, 882
        lignocaine, 883
        streptokinase and analogues, 879–82
    pathology, 875
    prophylaxis of cardiac arrhythmias, 883
    rehabilitation, 885–6
myringitis bullosa haemorrhagica, 1183
myxoedema coma, 1106–7

nalbuphine, 192
    see also opioids
naloxone, antidote to opioids poisoning, 218, 227–8
narcotics, babies of dependent mothers, 97
nasal bones, fracture, 444
nasal cavity and nose, anatomy, 22–3
nasal discharge, 463
nasoethmoid complex, fractures, 452–3
nasopharyngeal airway, 33–4, 85–6, 443
naviculares, 642
neck injuries
    assessment, 110, 931
    sprain
        incidence and pathology, 1003

physiotherapy techniques, 816–17
    rehabilitation, 805–7
    treatment and prognosis, 1004
    with/without seat belt, 513
    torticollis, 1004–5
    vascular trauma, management, 931–2
    see also cervical spine
neck masses, 476–8
neck veins, 107
necrotizing fasciitis, 475
needle cricothyroidotomy, 1177
needle placement, tibia, 696
needle thoracostomy, tension pneumothorax, 538–9
needlestick injuries, 246–7
Neisseria meningitis, 1074
neonate
    cardiac arrhythmias, 1203
    larynx, airway problems, 684
    persistent central cyanosis, COPS, 97
    poisoning, 207
    prematurity, 97
    resuscitation, 93–8
        external chest compression, 83
        intubation, 86–7, 95–6
        problems, 97
    see also paediatrics
neurochemicals, damage by, 422
neuroleptic drugs
    neuroleptic malignant syndrome, 789, 1087
    side-effects, 1087
neurological assessment *see* head injuries
neurological problems, diabetes-related, 1134
neurological signs, poisoning, 209–10
neuromuscular blocking drugs, 57–8
neuroprotective drugs, 437
neutrophil leucocytosis, 1245–6
nifedipine, hypertensive crisis, 1116–17
nitrates
    for angina, 874
    for cardiac failure, 889
    illicit use, and psychological sequelae, 1096–100
    for myocardial infarction, 878
nitrogen narcosis, 758
nitrous oxide, 188, 240
    contraindications, 188–9
NMDA receptor, calcium ions, 75
nociceptors, 183–4
non-accidental injury, 1213–19
non-steroidal antiinflammatory agents
    dosage, 185
    inhibition of cyclo-oxygenase, 184
    list and routes of administration, 185
    parenteral route, 193
    topical NSAIDs, 187
Norway, cardiac prehospital care, 306–7, 308
nose
    foreign bodies, 491
    trauma, 483–4
nose bleeds, 463, 491–3
    unilateral recurrent, 462
nursing incident coordinator (NIC), 277
nursing staff, 7–8

Oakley paediatric resuscitation chart, 39
obstetric emergencies, 1138–44
    caesarean section, 707, 1132
    diabetes mellitus, 1132

haemorrhage
   massive, 1139
   postpartum, 1139–40
high risk deliveries, 94
meconium-stained liquor, 97
preterm labour, 1140–1
septic shock, 1145
vasa praevia, 1139
obstructive shock, 120
occupations, infectious disease, 1231
ocular trauma see eye
oculocephalic reflexes, 177
oculovestibular reflexes, 177
oedema, cold effects, 785
oesophageal detector, 55
oesophagus
   foreign bodies, 494–5
   ruptured, 553
oncotic pressure, 149
onychomycosis, 1040
open fractures see fractures, open
ophthalmic see eye
ophthalmopathy, Graves', 1104–6
opioids
   babies of dependent mothers, 97
   for cardiac failure, 889
   illicit use, and psychological sequelae,
      1096–100
   list and routes of administration, 185
   poisoning, 218, 227–8
   prescribing, 190–1
   in sedation, 240
   terminology and classification, 190
   variable responses to, 189
oral analgesic agents and routes, 184–6
oral and maxillofacial diseases, 459–69
oral rehydration salts, 1186
orbit
   foreign bodies, 392–3
   roof, wall and floor injuries, 450–1
orchitis and epididymo-orchitis, 388, 972–3
orf, 1038
organ donation, 406–7
organophosphates, poisoning, 218–19, 221
   antidote, 738
   muscarinic effects, 739
oropharyngeal airway, 33–4, 85
oropharynx, anatomy, 23–4
orthopaedic conditions
   acute, 1003–27
   see also specific areas and conditions
os trigonitis, 666
Osgood–Schlatter osteochondritis, 1008
osmotic pressure, 149
osteoarthropathy, hypertrophic pulmonary, 1017
osteochondritis, 1007–8
   dissecans, 664, 667, 675, 1008
   eponyms, list, 1007
   Perthes', 1007
osteomyelitis, 587–8, 1005–7
   acute, 1006–7
   aetiology, 1005
   chronic, 1007
   chronic multifocal, 1005
   jaws, 471–2
   pathology, 1005–6
   septic arthritis, 1006, 1007
osteoporosis, trauma in elderly people,
   710–13
otitis externa, acute, 1184
otitis media, paediatric emergencies, 1183–4
ovarian cyst, 1143, 1161–2

ovulation induction, hyperstimulation
   syndrome, 1163
oxygen
   antidote to carbon monoxide, 217
   antidote to cyanide poisoning, 217
   arterial blood, normal values, 28, 67, 143
   in hypothermia, 776
   for myocardial infarction, 878
oxygen consumption
   hypoxaemia in shock-associated
      conditions, 124–5, 132
   pulse oximetry, 54, 85
oxygen pathway, causes of blockade, 213
oxygen therapy, 29, 850–1
   flow rates, common delivery devices,
      850–1
   hyperbaric, 29
   new approaches to treatment of shock, 133
   paediatrics, 84–5
   preoxygenation, 34
oxygen-powered resuscitators, 53–4

pacemakers, 924–8
   antitachycardia pacemaker, 927
   DC cardioversion, 927
   internal cardioverter defibrillator (ICD),
      927–8
   malfunction, 925–6
   paced beats, 925
   pacemaker tachycardia, 926
packed red cells, 998
paediatric emergencies, 1173–211
   cardiac emergencies, 1200–5
   coma, 1196–200
   convulsions, 1192–6
   croup, 1175–6
   ear infections, 1183–4
   electrolytes required, 1185–6
   epiglottitis, 1176–7
   fever, 1173
   fluid requirements, 1185–6
   gastroenteritis, 1184–7
   Glasgow Coma Scale, 695, 1197
   meningitis, 1189–92
   non-accidental injury, 1213–19
   pertussis, 1183
   pneumonia, 1180–3
   rehydration therapy, 1186
   respiratory emergencies, 1174–83
   sudden infant death syndrome, 398, 403,
      1205–11
   urinary tract infections, 1187–9
paediatrics
   see also main subject headings
   abuse and non-accidental injury, 1213–19
   acute abdomen, palpation, 954
   airway anatomy and physiology, 24
   anaphylaxis, 1177
   anatomy, 24–5
      structural differences from adults,
      683–5
   arrhythmias, 929
   bradycardia, 928
   brain, 686–7
   cardiovascular system, 93–4, 686
   central nervous system, 94
   cervical spine, 683–5
      trauma, 525
   coma, management, 1196–200
   deaths, 398, 403
   and drug abuse, narcotics in babies of
      dependent mothers, 97

drugs, 207
   adenosine, 92, 929
   adrenaline, 928
   atropine, 92, 928
   bretylium tosylate, 92
   delivery routes, 69
   isoprenaline, 928
   ketamine, 240
   lignocaine, 93
   midazolam, 240
   salicylates, 224
   sedation, 203–4, 239–40
   sodium bicarbonate, 91, 92, 96
   verapamil, 929
exanthems, 1047
fluid loss, 93, 97
foreign bodies, 247–8, 391–3
fractures see fractures, paediatrics
growth and development: effects on
   management of injury, 688
heart, 686
heart rates, normal, paediatrics, 1174–5
hip pain, 375–6, 379
hydrocele, 974
immobilization on backboard, 691
lung functional residual capacity (FLC),
   24
mortality
   by age group, 1205
   SIDS, 1205–6
needle cricothyroidotomy, 87–8, 1177
non-accidental injury, 721–2
osteochondritis, 1007–8
peripheral venous cannulation, 89, 96
poisoning, 206–7
psychosocial development, 687
pulse, in infant, 83
respiratory rates, normal, 1174
respiratory system, 93
resuscitation, 81–99, 695–6
   advanced life support, 84–93
   airway obstruction, 31–3, 82
   algorithms
      for ACLS, 90
      for asystole, 90
      for BCLS, 82
   arrhythmias, 91–2
   basic (cardiac) life support, 82–4
   blood pressure, 85
   central venous cannulation, 89
   choking, 31, 32, 83–4
   cricothyroidotomy, 87–8, 1177
   defibrillation, 91
   see also prehospital cardiac care,
      chain of survival
   electromechanical dissociation (EMD),
      91
   external chest compression, 83
   Oakley paediatric resuscitation chart, 39
   oxygen therapy, 84–5
   tracheal intubation, 41, 86–7, 95–6
resuscitation (newborn), 93–8
   external chest compression, 83
   intubation, 86–7, 95–6
   problems, 97
sickle cell disease, life-threatening
   complications, 986–8
status epilepticus, 1192–3
structural anatomical differences from
   adults, 683–5
sudden infant death syndrome (SIDS),
   398, 403

tachycardias, 928–9
techniques, vascular access, 1207–11
temperature control, 94
trauma, 680–700
    acute, vital signs and equipment, 693
    immobilization on backboard, 691
    incidence and consquences, 680–3
    minor injuries, 691
    primary survey, 692–5
    resuscitation, 695–6
    secondary survey, 696–7
    serious injuries, 692–700
    trauma score (PTS), 689
    triage, trauma team and transport,
        689–91
    see also fractures, paediatrics
urinary tract infections, 969
ventilation techniques, 86–9
ventricular fibrillation, 91
whole bowel irrigation, 215
see also neonate
pain
    acute non-specific abdominal pain
        (ANSAP), 959–60, 963–4
    nature of pain, 183–4
    see also abdominal assessment and acute
        abdomen
pancreas, injuries, 566
pancreatitis, acute, 965
    Glasgow scoring system, 965
pancuronium bromide, 58
pancytopenia, malaria, 1243
papaveretum 192, see also opioids
papilloedema, 177
paracetamol, 185
    poisoning, 219, 224–6
paraldehyde, paediatrics, 1194
paramedics, 285–6
paramyotonia with periodic paralysis,
    1073–4
parapharyngeal abscess, 459, 462
paraquat ingestion, 852
parasitic infestations, skin, 1048–9
parasuicide see poisoning
parenteral analgesic agents and routes,
    189–93
Parkinson's disease, pseudoparkinson's
    syndrome, 1087
paronychia, 1036, 1041
parotid fistula, 442
paroxysmal cold haemoglobinuria, 784–5
parvovirus infection, sickle cell disease, 987
patellar fracture, 352, 636–7, 672
    see also knee
patent ductus arteriosus, 1204
patients' rights, 14–15
peak expiratory flow rate, 847, 863
    normal adults, 847
pectin, contraindications, 1187
pediculosis, 1049
pediculosis pubis, 1049
PEEP, drowning, near, 755
pelvic fractures, 388, 567, 648–53
    elderly people, 652, 710
    MAST garment, 936
    paediatrics, 653
    sports injuries, 675
    vascular injury, 936
pelvic haemorrhage, 388
pelvic inflammatory disease, 1160–1
pelvic stability, examination, 113
pemphigoid, 1050

pemphigus vulgaris, 1050
penicillamine, antidote to heavy metal
    poisoning, 218
penicillin, anaphylaxis, 160
peptic ulcers
    perforation, 961–2
    uncomplicated, 958–9
perforated viscus
    appendix, 960–1
    colon, 962–3
    palpation, 954–5
    ulceration, 961–2
pericardial tamponade
    assessment, 107, 115
    diagnosis, 894
pericarditis, 893–4
    ECG changes, 894
    treatment, 894
periodic paralysis, 1073–4
periodontal disease, 461, 469–71
peripheral vascular disease, 946–50
peripheral venous access, paediatrics, 1208
peripheral venous cannulation
    during CPR, 68, 89
    newborn, 96
    paediatrics, 89
peritoneal dialysis rewarming method in
    hypothermia, 775
peritoneal lavage
    cooling method in hyperthermia, 793
    diagnosis of intra-abdominal injury, 560–1
peritonsillar abscess, 496
pernio, 783–4
peroneal tendon subluxation, 668
pertussis, paediatric emergencies, 1183
pethidine, 185, 186, 191
petit mal attacks, 1066
pH values, 141
phaeochromocytoma, 1116–17
pharynx
    anatomy, 25
    pharyngeal/laryngeal oedema, 47
    pharyngotracheal lumen airway, 36, 67
    sore throat, 461–2, 463, 466–7
    trauma, 487
phencyclidine derivatives, 193
phenobarbitone, poisoning, 229
phenol, burns, 737
phenoxybenzamine, 1117
phenytoin
    indications, severe hyperthermia, 795
    paediatrics, 1194
    poisoning, 229
photosensitivity, drug reaction, 1053
phycomycosis, 466
physeal injuries, paediatrics, 353–4,
    619–20, 621
physiotherapy
    role in A&E department, 812–21
    role in fracture clinic, 818–21
piroxicam, 185, 186
pituitary apoplexy, haemorrhage, 1112,
    1114–15
pituitary emergencies, 1113–16
    hypopituitarism and diabetes insipidus,
        1115–16
    pituitary apoplexy, 1112, 1114–15
    tumours, 1113
pituitary gland, pregnancy changes, 704,
    1138
pityriasis rosea, 1044
pityriasis versicolor, 1041

place of safety order, 1088
placenta praevia, 1139
placental abruption
    presentation, 1138–9
    trauma in pregnancy, 706
plantar fasciitis, 664–5
plants (inc. mushrooms, berries), poisoning,
    221–2, 223
plasma, osmolality, 149
plaster casts, removal, 820–1
platelet concentrates, 998
platelet disorders, 991–2
Platt Report (1962), 3
pleural effusion, massive, 854–5
pneumonias, 840–4
    antibiotics, 1182
    aspiration, 842
        paediatrics, 1182–3
    community-acquired, 841–2, 1235
    and immunosuppression, 842–4
    nosocomial, 842
    paediatric emergencies, 1180–3
    tuberculosis, 842
pneumothorax
    aspiration, 856–8
    closed pneumothorax, 855
    diagnosis, 849, 856
    open pneumothorax, 334, 855
    tension pneumothorax, 107, 371, 538–47,
        855
        following central line insertion, 116
        needle thoracostomy, 538–9
        paediatrics, 699
        scuba diving, 759
        signs, 538
        tube thoracostomy, 540–4
    treatment guide, 857
pneumothorax see chest injuries
poisoning, 206–32
    age and aetiology, 206–7
    antidotes, 215, 217–19, 738
    cardiopulmonary resuscitation, 231
    deaths, precautions to be taken,
        398
    diagnosis and assessment, 207–12
        clinical signs, 209–11
        laboratory investigations, 211
    history-taking, 211
    in infants, 207
    list of agents, 215–31
        antidepressants, 214, 226
        carbon monoxide, 28–9, 216
        cardioactive drugs, 228–9
        chlorinated hydrocarbons, 221
        chloroquine, 230
        corrosives, 220
        cyanide, 28–9, 216–19
        ethanol (ethyl alcohol), 222–3
        ethylene glycol, 221
        gaseous agents, 215–16, 219–20
        heavy metals, 218–19
        hydrocarbons, petroleum distillates
            and oils, 220–1
        insect stings, 222
        iron, 229–30
        liquid agents, 220–1
        methanol (methyl alcohol), 221
        paracetamol, 224–6
        plants (inc. mushrooms, berries), 221–2,
            223
        salicylates, 224
        sedatives and hypnotics, 226–7

smoke, 219–20
substances of abuse, 227–8
theophylline, 230
management, 212–15
algorithm, 208
immediate, 208
preventing ingestion, 212–15
National Poisons Information Service, 231–2
in neonates, 207
pathogenesis and mechanisms, 212
respiratory assessment, 207
police powers, mental health, 1088–9
polyarteritis nodosa (medium vessel), 1043
polyarthritis, joint pain, 1023–4
polyneuropathy, 1073
pompholyx, 1033
pontine infarction, 1061
popliteal artery
aneurysms, 945–6
injury, 937–8
porphyria, acute abdomen, 966
positional nystagmus, Hallpike test, 1069
postcoital contraception, 718, 1168–9
posterior fossa tumours, 1190
postherpetic neuralgia, 1037
posttraumatic stress disorder (PTSD), 11, 1085
potassium iodide, in thyroid emergencies, 1103
potassium ions, balance, 153–4
povidone–iodine, 241
power lines, electrical injury, propagation distance, 748
pralidoxime, antidote to organophosphates, 219
precordial thump, 66
pregnancy
anticoagulants, 1145
appendicitis, 1141
bleeding, differential diagnosis, 1153
cardiac arrhythmias, 928
cholecystitis, 1142
drugs that cross placenta, 929
dyspepsia, 1142
eclampsia and pre-eclampsia, 704, 1143–4
ectopic, 1156–7
fundal height, by gestation time, 703
gastrointestinal surgery, 1141
medical emergencies, 1144–6
asthma, 1144–5
deep vein thrombosis, 1145
epilepsy, 1145
obstetric emergencies, 1138–44
pemphigoid (herpes), 1051
physiology, 1137–8
seat belt wearing, 706
small bowel obstruction, 1142
suspected, hCG testing, 955, 1151, 1157
test, in acute abdomen, 955
test, βhCG, 1151
trauma, 702–7
assessment of fetus, 705–6
assessment of mother, 704–5
blunt trauma, 705–6
burns, 707
penetrating trauma, 706–7
placental abruption, 706
post mortem caesarean section, 707
uterine rupture, 706
vaginal bleeding, 1138–40

prehospital care
and ambulance service, 284–8
see also cardiac prehospital care
pressure sores, elderly people, 713
pretibial lacerations, 251
priapism, 988
prilocaine, maximum doses and duration of action, 194
Prinzmetal's variant angina, ECG, 871
procainamide
cardiac arrhythmias, 70, 899
pregnancy and lactation, 929
Procurator Fiscal, notification of death, 396, 406
professional chairs, 4
promethazine, 240
propionic acid derivatives, list and routes of administration, 185
propofol, 57
contraindications, 203
propranolol
paediatrics, 1203
in thyroid emergencies, 1104
proprioceptive reflexes, 178
proptosis, Graves' ophthalmopathy, 1104–6
propylthiouracil, thyroid emergencies, 1103, 1104
prostatitis, 971–2
prothrombin time (PTT), 994
psoriasis
erythrodermic, 1034
guttate, 1034
pustular, 1035
psychiatric emergencies, 1078–89
depressive illness, 1085
eating disorders, 1085–6
factitious disorders, 1086–7
malingering, 1087
mental state examination, 1078
models of liaison, 1079
post-traumatic stress, 1085
schizophrenia, 1084
somatoform disorders, 1086
psychological debriefing, 13–14
psychotropic medication, side-effects, 1087–8
pubic lice (crabs), pediculosis pubis, 1049
puerperal depression, 1146
pulmonary artery flotation catheter (PAFC), 127–8
pulmonary barotrauma, 759
pulmonary contusion, 550–1
pulmonary disease, drug-induced, 852
pulmonary embolism, 849, 858–62, 891–2
acute massive, 860–1, 891
diagnosis and treatment, 891–2
flowchart, 892
investigations, 859–60
multiple small, 891
pathogenesis, 858–9
radiology, 369–70, 372, 858–9
segmental emboli, 891
treatment protocol, 892
pulmonary function, 537
lung functional residual capacity (FLC), 24
pulmonary function tests
peak expiratory flow rate, 847, 863
pulse oximetry, 54, 85, 549, 863–4
spirometry, 863
pulmonary injury, near drowning, 752
pulmonary manifestations, decompression sickness, 760–1

pulmonary oedema
blood transfusion, 1001–2
electrical injury, 747
pulse, in infant, 83
pulse oximetry, 54, 85, 549, 863–4
pulse rate, in fever, 1231
pupillary changes, coma, 1199
pupillary light reflexes, 175–7
purpura, 1043–4
pyelonephritis, 1233
pregnancy, 1142–3
pyoderma gangrenosum, 1043
pyogenic granuloma, 1044
pyrexia, malignant hyperpyrexia, 58, 1229
pyrexia of unknown origin, causes, 1238
pyrogens, defined, 1229–30

quadriceps, contusions, 818
quality management and research, prehospital trauma care, 336–7
quinine, quinidine, 1243

rabies, 251
radial arteries, trauma, 933
radial nerve block, 197
radiation dose, unshielded gravid uterus, 705
radiation injuries, 739–40
radiography staff, 8
litigation, risk management, 16–19
radioiodine, release to atmosphere, 740
radiology, 349–93
errors in interpretation, 349
selection of modality, 350
unnecessary, 349–50
radius
fractures, 357, 820
radial head dislocation, 356
see also upper limb
Ramsay Hunt syndrome, 479
rape, 716–20
postcoital contraception, 718, 1168–9
rash, description, 1029–30
RAST detection of IgE, 165
Raynaud's syndrome, 783–4
reactive erythema, 1054–5
erythema nodosum, 1054
sunburn, 1054
recovery position, 30–1
contraindications, 332–3
rectal analgesic agents and routes, 186
rectal examination, 112
rectum, injuries, 565
red cells, 979
concentrates, 998
loss, burns, 728
packed, 998
reflexes
assessment, 175–7
proprioceptive reflexes, 178
regional anaesthesia (IVRA), 200–1
regional pain syndrome, 1025
registrars
entry requirements, 3–4
first appointment, 3
rehabilitation, soft tissue injuries, 805–10
rehydration therapy, paediatric emergencies, 1186
Reiter's syndrome, 971
relapsing fever, 1244–5
relatives of deceased, management, 398–404

renal colic
  radiology, 380, 386
  uncomplicated, 959
renal failure
  burns, 724
  radiology, hydronephrosis, 386
renal trauma, 567, 569–70
  diagnosis and assessment, 573–4
  management in A&E department, 578–9
  radiology, 388, 389
  retrieval of kidneys, 407
  vascular injury, 936
reperfusion injury, 939
repetitive strain injury, 1025
reporting forms, standardized, 331
respiration, pregnancy changes, 703
respiratory acidosis, 144–5
respiratory alkalosis, 145
respiratory assessment
  causes of blockade of oxygen pathway, 213
  coma, 173
  poisoning, 207
respiratory emergencies, paediatric
  emergencies, 1174–83
respiratory emergencies, adult, 839–64
  acute respiratory failure, 850–1
  adult respiratory distress syndrome
    (ARDS), 862–3
  infections, 839–44
  inflammatory conditions, 844–50
    asthma, 844–8
    chronic obstructive pulmonary disease,
    848–50
  mechanical disorders, 854–8
  pulmonary embolism, 849, 858–62
  pulmonary function tests, 54, 85, 549,
    863–4
  toxic lung injury, 851–4
respiratory failure
  acute, 850–1
    algorithm for management, 851
respiratory infections, 839–44
respiratory rates, normal, paediatrics, 1174
responsiveness
  determining level, 107–8
  mnemonic, 108
resuscitation
  ABCs + DE (ATLS system), new
    approaches to resuscitation, 102,
    133–4, 330–1, 423–4, 692
  advanced life support, 71–3, 195, 314
    ALC courses, 75
    defined, 314
    paediatrics, 84–93
    prehospital care of trauma patient,
    329–36
    assessment, 114–16
    coma, 172–3
    poisoning, 207–8
  at birth, 93–8
    equipment, 94
  attempted/not attempted, 316
  basic life support, 65–6, 115
    paediatrics, 82–4
    prehospital care of trauma patient,
    329–36
  bystander CPR, 290, 313, 318
  caesarean section, 1146
  cardiac arrest, 62–77
    cardiac/non-cardiac aetiology, 317
    causes, 288–9
    'clocks, four', 320

complications, 66
controlled studies of survival,
Europe/USA, 291
defined, 313
diagnosis, 63
out-of-hospital resuscitation attempts,
320
pathophysiology, 62–3, 289
rhythm and outcome, 290
syndromes of sudden cardiac death, 289
team, 10, 75–6
times vs intervals, 314–15
Utstein style template for reporting
data, 316–19
chest trauma see chest injuries
drowning, near
  A&E management, 755–7
  prehospital care, 754
drugs
  antiarrhythmics, 70
  bicarbonate, 148
  buffers and alkalizing agents, 70–1
  calcium and magnesium salts, 71
  vasopressors, 69–70
equipment, recommended, 101
European Resuscitation Council
  guidelines, cardiac arrhythmias, 908
factors associated with successful
  resuscitation, 289–90
fluid choice, 999–1001
  see also blood products; blood
  transfusion
forward blood flow, 63–4
injured patient, 114–16
neonate, 83, 86–7, 93–8
new approaches see resuscitation, ABCs
Oakley paediatric resuscitation chart, 39
open chest CPR, 73–4
outcome predictions, 76–7
paediatrics, 82–94
in poisoning, 231
post-resuscitation care, 74–5
in pregnancy, 1146
prehospital care, trauma patient, 329–36
resuscitation room, 6
resuscitation techniques, 50–4
return of spontaneous circulation
  (ROSC), 318
times vs intervals, 314–15
see also cardiac prehospital care;
  paediatrics, resuscitation
reticular activating system (RAS), arousal,
  167–8
retinal conditions see eye
retropharyngeal space, paediatrics, cervical
  spine trauma, 525
rewarming methods, 772–6
Reye's syndrome, 1191
Rh testing, 1152, 1169
  seatbelt injury, 1169
rhabdomyolysis, 795
rheumatic fever, acute, 1019–20
rheumatism, 1024–5
rib fractures, 363, 554–5
rickettsial fever, 1245
right–left disorientation, 1061
Ringer's fluid, composition, 157
ringworm, 1039
risk management, 16–19
  Bolam test, 18
road traffic accidents (RTAs), 412–17
  categories of fatalities, 414

facial trauma, 440–1
injury patterns, 415–17
neck sprain, 805–7
  with/without seat belt, 513
paediatric trauma, 680–3
Rh testing, 1169
statistics, by nation, 412–13
see also accidents
rocuronium bromide, 58, 203
Romano–Ward syndrome, 1202
rubella (German measles), 1047
rule of nines, and paediatrics modification,
  727

sacral fractures, 529–30
sacroiliitis, 1024
salbutamol, in anaphylaxis, 163
salicylates
  poisoning, 224
    promoting excretion, 215, 216
saline, osmolarity and oncotic pressure, 158
saline (0.9%), wound irrigation, 241
saline (7.5%), osmolarity and oncotic
  pressure, 158
saline, dextrose, properties, 157
saline (HSD), prehospital care, 336
saline, normal, properties, 157–8
salivary glands
  infections, 472–3
  swellings, 461
  trauma, 442
  tumours, 473–4
Salmonella typhi, 1246
Salter–Harris types I–IV injuries, 354–5
sandfly, 1246
sarcoidosis, 476
scabies, 1048
scalds see burns
scalp injuries, 236, 425
  sutures, 243
scaphoid fractures, 373
scapular fractures 601-2, see also shoulder
scapulothoracic dissociation, 604–5
scarlet fever, 1047
scars
  factors increasing, 242
  hypertrophic, 238
  keloids, 238
  prevention of hyperpigmentation, 243
Scheuermann's disease, 675, 1008
schistosomiasis, 1246–7
schizophrenia, 1084
scorpion bites, 827–30
Scotland, cardiac prehospital care, 307
scrotal pain, 388–90
scrotal swelling
  cystic, 974
  solid, 974–5
scuba diving injuries, 757–63
seat belts, RTA in pregnancy, 706
sedation, 203–4, 239–40
  antagonist (flumenazil), 204
  see also named agents
seizures, 1064–8
  aetiology, 1065
  diagnosis, 1067
  epidemiology, 1065
  head-injured patients, 434
  paediatrics, febrile illness, 1193
  pathophysiology, 1065
  treatment, 1067
self-harm, actual and threatened, 1091–5

senior house officers, 6, 8–9
septic arthritis, 375–6, 1006–7
septic shock, 123–4, 134–7
  pharmacological manipulation, 136
  pregnancy, 1145–6
  principal infections, 135
  transfused blood, 1002
septicaemia, toxic shock, 1236
sexual assault
  child abuse, 1217
  genital trauma, 719–20
  postcoital contraception, 718, 1167–8
  rape, 716–20
  suspected, procedure, 1164
sexually transmitted diseases, 1164–7
  bacterial vaginosis, 1164–5
  candidiasis, 1164
  PID, 1160–1
  and sexual assault, 718–19
  summary, 1165
  Trichomonas vaginalis infection, 1165
  urethritis, 970–1
Sheehan's syndrome, 1112
shellfish, toxins, 834
shin, pretibial lacerations, 251
shingles, 479, 1037
Shöber test, 1017, 1024
shock
  assessment, 125–7
  clinical presentation, 119–25
    cellular and subcellular response, 122
  defined, 118
  management procedures, 126–8
    investigations, 128
    monitoring, 127–8
  new approaches to treatment, ABC+DE,
    133–4
  pathophysiology, 120–5
    cellular and subcellular response, 122
    pathogenesis, 121
    supply-dependent oxygen
      consumption, 124–5
  types, classification, 118
  types and management
    anaphylactic, 120
    cardiogenic, 119–20
    distributive, 120
    hypovolaemic, 122–3, 129–34
    obstructive, 120
    refractory, 125
    septic, 123–4, 134–7
shoulder exercises, 819–21
shoulder girdle
  anatomy and biomechanics, 605
  dislocations, 370–3, 607–9
    management, 608–9
    posterior, 608
    recurrence, 609
    subglenoid, 608
  fractures, 601–4
    elderly people, 711
  sternoclavicular joint, 601–2
  see also humerus
shoulder pain, 1026
  Milwaukee shoulder, 1022
sialadenitis, 472
sialocele, 442
sick sinus syndrome, 904, 1202
sickle cell disease, 984–8
  acute abdomen, 966, 988
  analgesia, 986
  chest syndrome, 987

investigations, 986
  life-threatening complications, 986–8
  management, algorithm, 987
  painful crisis, 985
  parvovirus infection, 987
  priapism, 988
sinus bradycardia, 902–3, 1202
  following AMI, 884
sinus tachycardia, 920, 1201
  following AMI, 883
sinusitis, 462, 467, 492–3
Sjögren's syndrome, 473
skier's thumb, 679
skin, *see also* dermatological emergencies
skin area, rule of nines, and paediatrics
  modification, 727
skin conditions, face, 474–5
skin grafts, pretibial lacerations, 251
skin infiltration anaesthesia, 195, 239
skin manifestations, scuba diving injuries,
  760
skin staples, 243–4
skin surface, head surface area, 766, 772
skin tumours, 475
skull *see* head injuries
slapped cheek syndrome, 1020, 1038–9
small bowel injury, 564
  management of vascular injury, 935–6
small bowel obstruction
  admission, 965
  diagnostic features, 957
  intussusception, 963
  possible ischaemia, 962–3
  pregnancy, 1142
  radiology, 383
smoke inhalation, 853
snakebite, 823–7
sodium bicarbonate, 71, 91, 92
  bicarbonate system, 142
  as buffer, 148
  newborns, 96
  normal values, 143
  paediatrics, 91, 92
sodium calcium edetate, antidote to heavy
  metal poisoning, 218
sodium chloride 7.5%, osmolarity and
  oncotic pressure, 158
sodium ions, balance, 151–3
sodium lactate, composition, 157
sodium nitrite, antidote to cyanide
  poisoning, 217
sodium nitroprusside, 1117
sodium thiosulphate, antidote to cyanide
  poisoning, 217
sodium valproate, poisoning, 229
soft tissue
  injuries, rehabilitation, 805–10
  rheumatism, 1024–6
solvents, illicit use, and psychological
  sequelae, 1096–100
somatoform disorders, 1086
sore throat, 461–2, 463, 466–7
spider bites, 827–30
spinal anatomy and physiology, 1010–11
spinal cord injury
  diagnosis injury, 518–19
  elderly people, 709
  mechanisms, 514
  partial cord injuries, 519
  treatment, 528–9
  without radiographic abnormality
    (SCIWORA), 699

spinal decompression sickness, 760
spinal immobilization, 336, 515
spinal infections, paediatrics, 1192
spinal stenosis, 1011–12
spinal trauma
  casualty positioning and movement,
    515
  diagnosis of spinal cord injury, 518–19
  nerve root compression, 1011
  neurological examination, 518–19
  paediatrics fractures and dislocations,
    627–8, 699
  primary and secondary survey, 517–18
  radiological examination, 519–20
  sacral fractures, 529–30
  spinal columns concept, 510–11
  sports injuries, 675
  stable injuries, 529–30
  suspected injury
    moving patient, 30
    paediatrics, 699
    tracheal intubation, 45–7
  unstable injuries, 510–29
    causation and incidence, 512–13
    classification, 511–12
    clinical anatomy and pathogenesis,
      513–14
    definition, 510–11
  see also cervical spine; spinal cord injury
spirometry, 863
spleen
  injuries, 367, 565–6
  sequestration in sickle cell disease, 987
  splenectomy, 990
  splenomegaly, 990
splint, inflatable, contraindications, 335
spondyloarthropathy, seronegative, 1024
spondylolysis, paediatrics, 627
sports injuries, 659–79
  acute/chronic injuries, treatment, 661–3
  classification, 659
  diagnosis and transplantation, 660–1
  diving, 757–63
  prevention, 661
  sports injury clinics, 660
  wind-chill chart, 766
sprains
  ankle, 813–16
  knee, 809–10
  neck, 366, 513, 805–7, 816–17, 1003–4
  rehabilitation, 805–10
squamous cell carcinoma, 1045
  tongue, 470
stab wounds, abdominal trauma, 563
staff, support of carers following deaths,
  404–6
staffing and training, 6–9
  advanced life support, 345
  bereavement service, 406
  entry requirements for registrars, 3–4
  medical staff, 6, 8–9
  nursing staff, 7–8
  paramedics, 285–6
  performance reviews, 15
  protection of staff, 10–11
  registrar grades, 9
  stress, 11–14
Starling relationship, 888
status epilepticus, 1067–8
  paediatrics, 1192–3
sternoclavicular joint injuries, 601–2
sternum, fractures, 554

steroids, 989
  for eczema, 1032
  in hypothermia, 776
  illicit use, and psychological sequelae,
    1096–100
  spinal cord injury (NASCIS 1 and 2), 529
  treatment of cerebral oedema, 180
Stevens–Johnson syndrome, 1038, 1054
stings, 160, 822–3
  bees and wasps, 822–3
  jellyfish, 832–3
stomach, trauma, 564
Streptococcus pneumoniae, meningitis, 1074
streptokinase, thrombolytic therapy, 879–82
stress, 11–14
  critical incident stress debriefing (CISD),
    13
  debriefing, 12–14
stridor, 25, 858
stroke, 1057–64
  anatomy of brain blood supply, 1057–8
  causes, 1059
  cerebral artery occlusion, 1061
  classification, 1058
  clinical presentation, 1060
  diagnosis and management, 1061
  pathophysiology, 1059–60
  sickle cell disease, 988
  TIAs, 939–40
strongyloidiasis, 1246–7
subclavian arteries, trauma, 932
sublingual analgesic agents and routes, 186
substance misuse, 1095–100
subtentorial lesions, 167–8
sudden infant death syndrome (SIDS),
    398, 403, 1205–11
sufentanil, 192
  intranasal, 240
  see also opioids
suicide
  and deliberate self-harm, 1091–5
    assessment form, 1092
  see also poisoning
sunburn, reactive erythema, 1054
supratentorial lesions, 167–8
supraventricular tachycardia, 1201
  algorithm, 1203
  management, 1202–3
surface area, rule of nines, and paediatrics
    modification, 727
sutures, 242–3
  facial injuries, 457
suxamethonium, 57–8, 203
swallowing difficulty, 461
sweat gland activity, suppression, 789
Sweden, cardiac prehospital care, 307
sympathectomy, after frostbite, 780–1
Synacthen test, 1113
syncope, 1069–70, 1196
synovitis, 1020–3
syphilis
  gumma, 975
  head and neck, 480

tachycardias, 909–24
talus, fractures, 631, 641
tarsal coalition, 667
tarsometatarsal bones, fractures
    (Lisfranc's), 643
teeth
  avulsed, storage, 451
  fracture, 451–2

see also dental
telephone numbers
  emergency, 308
    diving injuries, 763, 854
temperature regulation, 1228–9
temporal arteritis, 475
temporomandibular joint
  dislocation, 448
    joint meniscus, 448–9
  dysfunction syndrome, 474
  fractures, 446–50
  infections, 474
tendonitis, bicipital, 679
tendons, injury, 641, 662, 666, 675
tennis elbow, 679, 1026
tenosynovitis, 667
  de Quervain's disease, 1025
  infectious, 1025–6
  inflammatory, 1025
  traumatic, 1024–5
Terry Thomas sign, 377
testis
  injuries, 389–90
  syphilis, 975
  tuberculosis, 975
  tumours, 974–5
tetanus, 252–3
  prophylaxis, 583
tetracaine, adrenaline and cocaine (TAC),
    239
  contraindications, 239
thalassaemias, 984
thallium poisoning, Berlin blue, 219
theophylline, poisoning, 230
thermoregulation, 1228–9
  central mechanisms, 790
  peripheral mechanisms, 789–90
thigh
  local anaesthesia, 199
  sports injuries, 674–5
thiopentone sodium, 56–7
  paediatrics, 1194–5
thoracotomy, emergency, for injury, 934
thorax
  paediatrics, structural differences (from
    adults), 685
  spinal injury, 526, 528
  vascular injury, 933–5
throat
  foreign bodies, 493–4
  sore throat, 461–2, 463, 466–7
  trauma, 484–5
thrombin time (TT), 994
thrombocytopenia, 991–2
  malaria, 1243
thromboembolism, arterial embolus,
    management, 940
thrombolytic therapy
  adverse effects, 882
  bleeding following, 996
  comparative features of agents, 880
  contraindications, 882, 941
  indications, 71, 881, 941
  myocardial infarction, 879–82
thrombophilia, 996
thrombophlebitis, 949
thrombosis-in-situ, management, 940–2
thyroglossal duct cysts, 477
thyroid emergencies, 1102–7
  Graves' ophthalmopathy, 1104–6
  myxoedema coma, 1106–7
  thyroid crisis, 1102–4

thyrotoxicosis, 1102–4
thyroid swellings, 477
thyromental distance, 26
tibia
  fractures
    amputation role, 640
    open, 639–40
    paediatrics, 629
    stress fractures, 668, 669–70
    tibial plafond, 640
    tibial plateau, 637
    tibial shaft, 638–9
  needle placement, 696
  Osgood–Schlatter osteochondritis, 1008
tibial arteries, injury, 938
tick bites, 827–8, 830
tick–borne infections, 1244–5
time (of cardiac arrest), defined, 314–15
tinea, and ringworm, 1039
tinea unguium, 1040
tissue plasminogen activator, 881
tocolytic drugs, 1140
tongue, squamous cell carcinoma, 470
tonsil suction, 30
tonsillitis, 466–7, 496, 1177
topical analgesic agents and routes, 186–9,
    239
  tetracaine, adrenaline and cocaine
    (TAC), 239
  see also local anaesthesia
torsade de pointes, 71
torticollis, 1004–5
torus fractures, paediatric, 621
toxic epidermal necrolysis, 1051
toxic erythema, 1048
toxic megacolon, 384
toxic shock, septicaemia, 1236
toxocariasis, 1246–7
trachea
  foreign bodies, 495
  obstruction, 1177–8
    paediatrics, 1193–5
  trauma, 486–7, 553–4
  see also airway
tracheal intubation, 38–47, 66
  blind nasal intubation, 45
  confirming correct tracheal tube
    placement, 54–5
  digital blind oral intubation, 43
  emergency airway control, rapid
    sequence, 58–9
  fibreoptic techniques, 45
  indications, 171
  oral intubation
    blind, with Augustine guide, 44–5
    blind, with light wand, 43
    using Bullard laryngoscope, 42–3
    using McCoy levering laryngoscope,
      41–2
  orotracheal intubation using direct
    laryngoscopy, 39–41
  paediatrics, 41, 86–7
    Cole pattern tube, 96
  with pharyngeal/laryngeal oedema, 47
  retrograde tracheal intubation, 45
  suspected cervical spine injury, 45–7
tracheitis
  bacterial, 1175
  laryngotracheobronchitis, viral, 1175
tracheobronchitis, acute, 839
tracheostomy, 50, 485–6
training *see* staffing and training

transcutaneous electrical nerve stimulation, 239
transient ischaemic attacks, 1064
transport of patient
    contraindications, 116
    personnel/escorts, 344
    pretransport checklist, 345
    protocols, 345–6
    referral, 343
    trauma patient, 341–2
    see also ambulance service
transthoracic impedance, 67–8
trauma centres, 287
trauma prehospital care, 328
trauma see accidents; injuries
trauma teams, 9–10, 101
triage, 7, 277–8
    algorithm, 329
    assessment of injury mechanism, 331–2
    trauma prehospital care, 328
trichinellosis, 1246–7
tricyclic antidepressants, poisoning, 214, 226
trigeminal nerve
    spinal nucleus, 460
    trauma, 442
trigeminal neuralgia, 460
trigger finger, 1025
trimeprazine, 240
tromethamine, 148
Trousseau test, 155
trypanosomiasis, 1244
tsetse flies, 1244
tube thoracostomy, tension pneumothorax, 540–4
tuberculosis, 476, 842
    disseminated, 1246
    of hip, 379
    of testis, 975
tympanic rupture, scuba diving injuries, 759
typhoid fever, 1245
typhus, 1245
tyramine (cheese) reaction, 1088

ulcers
    genital, 973–4
    ischaemic, 1135
    mouth, 461, 463, 470
    neuropathic, 1135
    skin, 1055
    see also peptic ulcer
ulna, greenstick fracture, 357
ulnar arteries, trauma, 932
ulnar nerve, 590
ulnar nerve block, 196–7
ultrasound
    ectopic pregnancy, 1157
    pelvic, 1151
ultraviolet radiation, 1055
    keratoconjunctivitis, 499
umbilical vein, access and cannulation, 96–7, 1210
uncal syndrome, 169, 1197
upper limb injuries, 601–16
    forearm
        compartment syndrome, 612–13
        distal radius, 614–15
        elbow involvement, 373, 611–12
        fractures, 611–16
        Galeazzi fracture–dislocation, 375, 612, 613
        management, 613

Monteggia injury, 612, 613
olecranon fracture, 611
radiology, 373
fractures and dislocations, elderly people, 712
intravenous regional anaesthesia (IVRA), 200–1
local anaesthesia, 195–8
paediatric radiology, 354–9
shoulder dislocations, 370–3, 374
sports injuries, 676–9
vascular injuries, 932–3
wrist
    Colles' fracture, 351, 373, 614, 711
    intra-articular fractures, 615–16
    lunate fractures, 373, 377
    scaphoid fractures, 373, 376
    sports injuries, 679
    triquetral fractures, 373, 377
    see also elbow; hand; humerus; shoulder
upper limb ischaemia, 942
upper respiratory tract, infections, 466–7
ureteric injuries, 570, 574–5
urethral injuries, 388, 571–2
    investigations, 568, 576–7
    paediatrics, 699
urethral syndrome, 970
urethritis, 970–1
    non-gonococcal, 970–1
urinary bladder injuries, 388, 390, 567, 570–1
    investigations, 575–6
    paediatrics, 699
urinary tract, pregnancy changes, 703
urinary tract infections, 969–70
    antibiotics, 1189
    complications, 1235
    imaging, paediatrics, 1188–9
    paediatric emergencies, 1187–9
urinary tract injuries
    criteria for transfer, 579
    management, 578–9
    see also specific parts
urine
    acute retention, 975–6
        gynaecological conditions, 1163
    analysis, gynaecological emergencies, 1151
    haematuria, causes, 977
    investigations, 1188
        test, in acute abdomen, 955–6
        test, in urethritis, two-glass test, 971
    output in shock, 127
    specimen, paediatrics, 1187–8
urography (IVU), 385, 573–5
urticaria, 1051–2
    in anaphylaxis, 163
    blood transfusion, 1001
    cold, 784
    drug reaction, 1053
    papular, 1049
USA
    accidents, all causes, 413
    ambulance service, 285
    cardiac arrest, controlled studies of survival, Europe/USA, 291
    cardiac prehospital care, 306, 308
    emergency medical systems, 292–6
        survival outcomes, 295
        types, 293
    road traffic accidents (RTAs), 412–13
uterus
    dysfunctional bleeding, 1158–9

fibroids, in pregnancy, 1143
hydatidiform mole, 1155–6
pelvic examination, 1150
    miscarriage, 1152–5
    trauma, 720
    rupture in pregnancy, 705
    tumours, 1161–2
Utstein Consensus Conference, 296–7, 313–23
    recommendations
        clinical data, 322–3
        out of hospital cardiac arrest, 296–7, 321–3
    Utstein style template for reporting data on cardiac arrest, 315–19, 316
    Utstein time points and time intervals, CPR, 319–21

vaccination, anaphylaxis, 253
vagal blockade, atropine, 71
vaginal bleeding
    abnormal, 1157–8
    in pregnancy, 1138–40
vaginal infections, 1164–9
vaginal trauma, 719–20
vanillylmandelic acid, 477
varicella, 1037–8, 1047
varicocele, 975
varicose veins
    bleeding from, 949
    complications from treatment, 949–50
vascular access, techniques, paediatrics, 1207–11
vascular disorders, 991
vascular emergencies, 931–50
    not involving trauma, 939–48
    reperfusion injury, 939
    traumatic, 567, 931–9
    venous problems, 948–50
vasculitis, 1042
vasodilators, 132
vasopressin deficiency, diabetes insipidus, 1115–16
vasopressors, 69–70
vasospastic attacks, 784
vecuronium, 58, 203
vehicles, chemical hazards, signs, 733–4
vena cava, approach, 936
venous access see central venous cannulation
venous bleeding, major, 935
venous cut–down, paediatrics, 1208–9
ventilation
    expired air, 50–2, 82–3
    external chest compression (ECC), 83
    near drowning, indications, 755
ventilation and ventilation techniques, 27–9, 50–4
    ABCs, 102, 133–4, 330–1, 423–4, 692
    assessment, 28, 105–6
    bag–valve–mask system, 52–3, 66, 67, 334
    basic life support, 65–6
    in cardiopulmonary resuscitation, values, 66
    causes of blockade of oxygen pathway, 213
    expired air ventilation, 50–2, 82–3
    flail chest, 334
    hypoventilation, peripheral causes, 28
    monitoring, 54–5
    oxygen-powered resuscitators, 53–4
    paediatrics, 86–9, 694
        decreased excursion, 694
        newborn resuscitation, 95–8

PEEP in hypovolaemic shock, 132
peripheral control, 27–8
pneumothorax, open, 334
positive pressure ventilation, 52–3, 66, 67, 84–5
protective appliances, 51–2
respiratory control, 27
ventricular failure *see* cardiac failure
ventricular fibrillation, 67
  algorithm, 72
  differentiation from asystole, 317
  paediatrics, 91
  prophylaxis, 883
  treatment, 69–71
ventricular rupture, 885
ventricular septal defect, infarct-related, 885
ventricular tachycardia, 317, 1201–3
  algorithm, paediatrics, 1204
  lignocaine, 883
  see also cardiac arrhythmias
verapamil
  dosage, 899
  indications/contraindications, 899
  interactions, 899
  paediatrics, 1202–3
  pregnancy and lactation, 929
  side-effects, 899
vertebral artery occlusion, 1061
vertigo, 1068–9
  acute, 489–90
violence
  protection of staff, 10–11
  risk management, 16
viral haemorrhagic fever, 1247–8
viral infections
  encephalitis, 1075
  fever, 1245
  gastroenteritis, 1185–7
  laryngotracheobronchitis, 1175
  skin, 1036–9
viruses, blood transmission, 246–7
visceral larva migrans, 1246–7

visceral leishmaniasis, 1246
visceral trauma, 387–8
visual emergencies, pituitary tumours, 1113
vitamin B-12 deficiency, 980, 982
vitamin K
  administration, 995
  deficiency, 993
vomiting, acute abdomen, 953
vulval trauma, 719
vulvovaginal candidiasis, 1164
vulvovaginitis, 1036–7
  Bartholin's glands, infection, 1167
  HPV, 1167
  HSV infection, 1166–7
  staphylococcal, 1166
  streptococcal, 1166
  Trichomonas, 1165–6

warfarin
  acute abdomen, 966
  contraindications in pregnancy, 1145
  overanticoagulation, 996
warts, 1038
wasp venom sensitivity, 160, 822–3
water
  24 h balance, 150
  excess and depletion, 150–1
  see also fluid
water and electrolyte requirements, paediatrics, 1185–6
Waterhouse–Friderichsen syndrome, meningococcal septicaemia, 1111
weakness, acute, 1073–4
weapons, ballistic injuries, 798
Wee oesophageal detector, 55
Wenckebach second degree atrioventricular block, 905
  following AMI, 884
whiplash injury *see* neck sprain
white cells
  blood count, 1245–8
  normal, 1246

disorders, 988–90
WHO, oral rehydration salts, 1186
whole blood, 998
Wolff–Parkinson–White syndrome, 923, 924, 1201
Wolff's law, 661
workload, 7–8
wound care, 235–53
  bacterial contamination, 237
  bite wounds, 248–50
    rabies, 251
  burns, 730
  delayed primary closure, 237
  dressings, 244–5
  examination and classification, 236–7
  foreign bodies, 247–8
  history-taking, 235–6
  management, 238–46
    antibiotics, 242
    cleansing, 241
    closure, 242–4
    contraindicated practices, 235, 238
    debridement, 242
    local anaesthesia, 238–9
    precautions against cross-infection, 246–7
    skin staples, 243–4
    sutures, 242–3
  pretibial lacerations, 251
  puncture wounds, 250
  tetanus, 252–3
  underlying structures, 236
  wound healing, types, 237–8
  see also injuries
wrist *see* hand injuries; upper limb injuries

xerographs, detection of foreign bodies, 248

zinc, wound healing, 245
zygoma, fracture, 444, 447